# FOR REFERENCE

**Do Not Take From This Room**

# HANDBOOK
## *of*
# NUTRITION
## *and*
# FOOD
### *Third Edition*

## Edited by
## CAROLYN D. BERDANIER
## JOHANNA T. DWYER
## DAVID HEBER

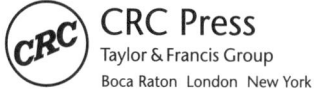

CRC Press
Taylor & Francis Group
Boca Raton   London   New York

CRC Press is an imprint of the
Taylor & Francis Group, an **informa** business

CRC Press
Taylor & Francis Group
6000 Broken Sound Parkway NW, Suite 300
Boca Raton, FL 33487-2742

Printed on acid-free paper
Version Date: 20130531

International Standard Book Number-13: 978-1-4665-0571-1 (Hardback)

---

### Library of Congress Cataloging-in-Publication Data

Handbook of nutrition and food / editors, Carolyn D. Berdanier, Johanna T. Dwyer, David Heber. -- Third edition.
    p. ; cm.
Includes bibliographical references and index.
ISBN 978-1-4665-0571-1 (hardcover : alk. paper)
    I. Berdanier, Carolyn D., editor of compilation. II. Dwyer, Johanna T., editor of compilation. III. Heber, David, editor of compilation.
    [DNLM: 1. Food. 2. Nutritional Physiological Phenomena. 3. Diet Therapy. 4. Diet. 5. Research. QU 145]

QP141
612.3--dc23
                                                            2013019697

---

**Visit the Taylor & Francis Web site at**
**http://www.taylorandfrancis.com**

**and the CRC Press Web site at**
**http://www.crcpress.com**

*This book is dedicated to Elaine Feldman, MD. Elaine coedited the first and second editions of this handbook and was instrumental in organizing the clinical nutrition section. Her broad understanding of the role of nutrition in the management of so many clinical conditions added much to the science of nutrition as it stands today.*

*Thanks, Elaine*

# Appreciation

We would like to express our appreciation to all those who helped us organize this massive undertaking and converting it into a useful manuscript. We are especially grateful to Katie Crane and Susan Bowerman, who organized the assessment and clinical sections. They kept the authors and the editors on task and on time.

We would also like to express our appreciation to Randy Brehm, our editor at Taylor & Francis Group, and Amy Blalock, the book's project coordinator at Taylor & Francis Group, for their encouragement and support.

# Contents

## PART I  Food

## PART II  Nutrition Science

## PART III  Nutrition throughout Life

# Preface

Five years have elapsed since the second edition of this handbook was published. During that time, nutrition scientists have become increasingly reliant on the World Wide Web for access to large databases. As with the second edition, many of the chapters in this edition provide web addresses for the readers to use as they need information about specific topics. There are, as a consequence, fewer large tables of data in this book than in past books. The organization of the handbook follows that of the earlier editions. Part I is devoted to food: its composition, its constituents, its safety, its labeling, and its analysis. In addition, there is a chapter on the laws that regulate food and its production.

Part II focuses on nutrition as a science. Basic terminology, nutritional biochemistry, nutrition and genetics, food intake regulation, and the micronutrients (minerals and vitamins) are included in this part. Although this handbook is oriented toward human nutrition, we have included a chapter on the nutritional needs of a variety of species and a chapter on finding appropriate mouse models for the study of human diseases. These two chapters will be useful to the bench scientist as inquiries are made about the relevance of specific nutrients in specific metabolic processes or in the pathophysiology of disordered nutrition states.

Part III provides information on the nutrient needs of humans throughout their lives. Infants, children, adolescents, adults, older adults, and human nutritional needs under special circumstances are addressed in this part. Nutrient needs for the active adult, the elite athlete, the vegetarian, and for the space traveler are special concerns.

Although we have good information about nutrient needs, the means to discover whether these needs are being met are a special concern. The question of nutrient intake adequacy is addressed in Part IV. Nutrition assessment from a variety of perspectives, nutrition education, and the provision of healthy eating recommendations all contribute to the assessment paradigm.

Finally, Part V addresses all the special clinical conditions in which nutrition plays a part. Many of the authors of the chapters in this part are familiar names in the clinical nutrition world. The part begins with nutritional assessment in the clinical setting and progresses through the many conditions the clinician is likely to see in medical practice.

Many of the authors in this edition have graciously updated the material they prepared for the second edition, but other authors are new, providing their unique perspectives on the large and interesting world of nutrition. We are grateful to these authors for generously sharing their expertise and providing wide coverage of the field of nutrition. We hope that you will find this edition an excellent addition to your professional library.

**Carolyn D. Berdanier**
**Johanna T. Dwyer**
**David Heber**

# Editors

**Carolyn D. Berdanier**, PhD, is professor emerita, nutrition and cell biology, University of Georgia in Athens. She earned her BS from the Pennsylvania State University and her MS and PhD from Rutgers University. She has had a long and productive career in nutrition, beginning with her first position as a nutrition researcher for the USDA at Beltsville, Maryland. She then moved to a faculty position at the College of Medicine, University of Nebraska, and then moved to the University of Georgia. Her research was widely supported by grants from the USDA, NIH, Department of Commerce, and a number of commodity research boards. Her publication record includes 135 research publications in peer-reviewed journals, 20 books either authored or edited, 55 chapters in multiauthored books, 30 invited reviews, and numerous short reviews in *Nutrition Reviews* and papers in the lay nutrition magazine, *Nutrition Today*. She has received numerous awards for her scientific work. She is a member of the American Society of Nutrition Science, Society for Experimental Biology and Medicine, the American Physiology Society, and the American Diabetes Association.

**Johanna T. Dwyer**, DSc, is professor of medicine (nutrition) and community health at the Tufts University Medical School and professor of nutrition at Tufts University Friedman School of Nutrition Science and Policy. She is also a senior scientist at the Jean Mayer/USDA Human Nutrition Research Center on Aging at Tufts University. Her major research interest is in flavonoids, population-based nutrition surveys, and nutrition policy. Dr. Dwyer is the director of the Frances Stern Nutrition Center at Tufts Medical Center. From 2003 to 2011, Dr. Dwyer served part time as senior nutrition scientist, Office of Dietary Supplements, National Institutes of Health. She now serves as a scientific consultant in the same capacity, where she is responsible for several large projects, including studies of dietary supplement motivation and use, development of an analytically substantiated dietary supplement database and other dietary supplement databases, development of research on the assessment of dietary supplement intake, and other topics.

Dr. Dwyer received her DSc and MSc from the Harvard School of Public Health, an MS from the University of Wisconsin, and completed her undergraduate degree with distinction from Cornell University. She is the author or coauthor of more than 250 research articles and 300 review articles published in scientific journals on topics including dietary treatment of end-stage renal disease, the role of dietary flavonoids in health, preventing diet-related disease in children and adolescents, maximizing quality of life and health in the elderly, vegetarian and other lifestyles, and databases for bioactive substances other than nutrients. She also serves as the editor of *Nutrition Today*.

Dr. Dwyer has served on many committees, including the 2000 Dietary Guidelines Committee, served as a member of the Food and Nutrition Board of the National Academy of Sciences, was elected member of the Institute of Medicine, National Academy of Sciences in 1998, and served as councilor of the Institute of Medicine from 2001 to 2003. She received the Conrad V. Elvejhem Award for public service in 2005 from the American Society for Nutrition Sciences, the Alumni Award of Merit from the Harvard School of Public Health in 2004, the W.O. Atwater award in 1996, the Medallion Award of the American Dietetic Association in 2003, and was recently honored with the Dean's Medal from the Tufts University Friedman School of Nutrition Science and Policy. She is a fellow of the American Society of Nutrition, the Society for Nutrition Education, and the American Society of Parenteral and Enteral Nutrition.

**David Heber**, MD, PhD, is professor of medicine and public health, chief of the Division of Clinical Nutrition, and director of the Center for Human Nutrition at UCLA. He received his medical degree from Harvard Medical School and his PhD in physiology from UCLA. Dr. Heber is board certified in internal medicine and endocrinology and metabolism by the American Board of Internal Medicine and as a physician nutrition specialist by the American Board of Physician Nutrition Specialists. He served as a director of the Certification Board for Nutrition Specialists and is a former chair of the Medical Nutrition Council of the American Society for Nutrition. He is a councilor and fellow of The Obesity Society. He has written over 200 peer-reviewed scientific articles, over 60 book chapters, 2 professional texts, and 4 books for the public. His main research interests are obesity treatment and nutrition for cancer prevention and treatment.

# Contributors

**Kelly M. Adams**
Department of Nutrition
University of North Carolina
    at Chapel Hill
Chapel Hill, North Carolina

**Caroline M. Apovian**
Section of Endocrinology, Diabetes,
    and Nutrition and Weight
    Management
Boston Medical Center
Boston University School of
    Medicine
Boston, Massachusetts

**Judith Ashley**
College of Agriculture,
    Biotechnology, and Natural
    Resources
University of Nevada, Reno
Reno, Nevada

**Suzanne Domel Baxter**
Institute for Families in Society
College of Social Work
University of South Carolina
Columbia, South Carolina

**Jimmy D. Bell**
Metabolic and Molecular Imaging
    Group
Medical Research Council Clinical
    Sciences Centre
Imperial College London
London, United Kingdom

**Carolyn D. Berdanier**
Department of Foods and Nutrition
University of Georgia
Athens, Georgia

**Lynnette A. Berdanier**
Department of Biology
Gainesville State College
Gainesville, Georgia

**Odilia I. Bermudez**
School of Medicine
Tufts University
Boston, Massachusetts

**Laura L. Bernet**
Department of Internal Medicine
Kaiser Permanente Santa Clara
    Medical Center
Santa Clara, California

**Jatinder Bhatia**
Division of Neonatology
Department of Pediatrics
Georgia Health Sciences University
Augusta, Georgia

**Jeffrey Blumberg**
Jean Mayer United States
    Department of Agriculture
Human Nutrition Research
    Center on Aging
Tufts University
Boston, Massachusetts

**Susan Bowerman**
Center for Human Nutrition
The University of California,
    Los Angeles
Los Angeles, California

**Lynda M. Brown**
Department of Nutrition
University of North Carolina,
    Greensboro
Greensboro, North Carolina

**Erin Bury**
Friedman School of Nutrition Science
    and Policy
Tufts University
Boston, Massachusetts

**Courtney Byrd-Williams**
Michael & Susan Dell Center for
    Healthy Living
School of Public Health
The University of Texas at Austin
Austin, Texas

**Catherine L. Carpenter**
Center for Human Nutrition
and
Schools of Medicine, Nursing, and
    Public Health
The University of California,
    Los Angeles
Los Angeles, California

**Ricardo Carvajal**
Hyman, Phelps & McNamara P.C.
Washington, District of Columbia

**Ronni Chernoff**
Geriatric Research Education and
    Clinical Center
Central Arkansas Veterans Healthcare
    System
and
Donald W. Reynolds Department
    of Geriatrics
University of Arkansas for Medical
    Sciences
Little Rock, Arkansas

**Wm. Cameron Chumlea**
Department of Pediatrics
and
Department of Community Health
Lifespan Health Research Center
Boonshoft School of Medicine
Wright State University
Dayton, Ohio

**Deborah J. Clegg**
Department of Internal Medicine
Touchstone Diabetes Center
Southwestern Medical Center
The University of Texas at Dallas
Dallas, Texas

**Rikki S. Corniola**
Department of Medical Education
College of Medicine
California Northstate University
Elk Grove, California

**Gary R. Cutter**
Department of Biostatistics
and
Section on Research Methods and
    Clinical Trials
School of Public Health
The University of Alabama
    at Birmingham
Birmingham, Alabama

**Stefan A. Czerwinski**
Division of Epidemiology
Lifespan Health Research Center
Boonshoft School of Medicine
Wright State University
Dayton, Ohio

**Cindy D. Davis**
Office of Dietary Supplements
National Cancer Institute
National Institutes of Health
Bethesda, Maryland

**R. Sue McPherson Day**
Michael & Susan Dell Center for
   Healthy Living
School of Public Health
The University of Texas at Houston
Houston, Texas

**Ellen W. Demerath**
Division of Epidemiology &
   Community Health
School of Public Health
University of Minnesota
Minneapolis, Minnesota

**Michael P. Doyle**
Center for Food Safety
University of Georgia
Griffin, Georgia

**Johanna T. Dwyer**
Jean Mayer United States
   Department of Agriculture
Human Nutrition Research
   Center on Aging
and
School of Medicine
and
Friedman School of Nutrition Science
   and Policy
Tufts University
Boston, Massachusetts

**Robert H. Eckel**
Division of Endocrinology, Metabolism
   and Diabetes
Anschutz Medical Center
University of Colorado
Aurora, Colorado

**William J. Evans**
Muscle Metabolism Discovery Unit
GlaxoSmithKline
Research Triangle Park, North Carolina

and

Geriatrics Program
Duke University
Durham, North Carolina

**Annie Ferland**
Division of Endocrinology,
   Metabolism, and Diabetes
Anschutz Medical Center
University of Colorado
Aurora, Colorado

**Claudia S. Plaisted Fernandez**
Department of Nutrition
University of North Carolina
   at Chapel Hill
Chapel Hill, North Carolina

**Joan G. Fischer**
Department of Foods and Nutrition
University of Georgia
Athens, Georgia

**J.A. Fitzpatrick**
Metabolic and Molecular Imaging
   Group
Medical Research Council Clinical
   Sciences Centre
Imperial College London
London, United Kingdom

**John P. Foreyt**
Department of Pediatrics—Nutrition
United States Department of
   Agriculture
Agricultural Research Service
Children's Nutrition Research Center
and
Department of Medicine
Baylor College of Medicine
Houston, Texas

**Gary D. Foster**
School of Medicine
Temple University
Philadelphia, Pennsylvania

**Gary Frost**
Department of Investigative
   Medicine
Imperial College London
London, United Kingdom

**Constance J. Geiger**
Division of Nutrition
The University of Utah
Salt Lake City, Utah

and

Geiger & Associates, LLC
Fort Bridger, Wyoming

**Jeanne Goldberg**
Friedman School of Nutrition Science
   and Policy
Tufts University
Boston, Massachusetts

**David J. Greenblatt**
Department of Molecular
   Physiology and
   Pharmacology
School of Medicine
and
Tufts Medical Center
Tufts University
Boston, Massachusetts

**Harry L. Greene**
Division of Pediatric Gastroenterology
   and Nutrition
Department of Pediatrics
Vanderbilt University Medical Center
Nashville, Tennessee

**Alyson Haslam**
Department of Foods and
   Nutrition
College of Family and Consumer
   Sciences
University of Georgia
Athens, Georgia

**Daniel Hatfield**
Friedman School of Nutrition Science
   and Policy
Tufts University
Boston, Massachusetts

**David Heber**
David Geffen School of Medicine
Center for Human Nutrition
The University of California,
   Los Angeles
Los Angeles, California

**Deanna M. Hoelscher**
Michael & Susan Dell Center for
   Healthy Living
School of Public Health
The University of Texas at Austin
Austin, Texas

**Sergio Huerta**
Southwestern Medical Center
The University of Texas at Dallas
and
Dallas VA Medical Center
Dallas, Texas

**Katherine H. Ingram**
Department of Health, Physical
    Education and Sport Science
WellStar College of Health and Human
    Services
Kennesaw State University
Kennesaw, Georgia

and

Department of Nutrition Sciences
The University of Alabama
    at Birmingham
Birmingham, Alabama

**Lisa Jahns**
United States Department of
    Agriculture
Agricultural Research Service
Grand Forks Human Nutrition
    Research Center
Grand Forks, North Dakota

**Elizabeth J. Johnson**
Jean Mayer United States
    Department of Agriculture
Human Nutrition Research
    Center on Aging
Tufts University
Boston, Massachusetts

**Mary Ann Johnson**
Department of Foods and Nutrition
College of Family and Consumer
    Sciences
University of Georgia
Athens, Georgia

**Craig A. Johnston**
Department of Pediatrics—Nutrition
United States Department of
    Agriculture
Agricultural Research Service
Children's Nutrition Research Center
and
Department of Medicine
Baylor College of Medicine
Houston, Texas

**Nancy L. Keim**
United States Department of
    Agriculture
Agricultural Research Service
Western Human Nutrition Research
    Center
Davis, California

**Eileen Kennedy**
Friedman School of Nutrition Science
    and Policy
Tufts University
Boston, Massachusetts

**Lalita Khaodhiar**
Section of Endocrinology, Diabetes,
    and Nutrition
Boston Medical Center
Boston University School of
    Medicine
Boston, Massachusetts

**Christina N. Kim**
Department of Medicine—Dermatology
David Giffen School of Medicine
The University of California,
    Los Angeles
Los Angeles, California

**Dong Wook Kim**
Section of Endocrinology, Diabetes,
    and Nutrition
Boston Medical Center
Boston University School of
    Medicine
Boston, Massachusetts

**Jenny Kim**
Department of Medicine—Dermatology
David Giffen School of Medicine
The University of California,
    Los Angeles
Los Angeles, California

**Vickie Kloeris**
Johnson Space Center
National Aeronautics and Space
    Administration
Houston, Texas

**Martin Kohlmeier**
Department of Nutrition
The University of North Carolina
    at Chapel Hill
Chapel Hill, North Carolina

**Kathryn M. Kolasa**
Department of Family Medicine
and
Department of Pediatrics
Brody School of Medicine
East Carolina University
Greenville, North Carolina

**Anup Kollanoor-Johny**
Department of Animal Science
University of Connecticut
Storrs, Connecticut

**Doina Kulick**
School of Medicine
University of Nevada, Reno
Reno, Nevada

**Theodore Kyle**
ConscienHealth
Pittsburgh, Pennsylvania

**Emma M. Laing**
Department of Foods and Nutrition
University of Georgia
Athens, Georgia

**Michael J. LaMonte**
Department of Social and Preventive
    Medicine
School of Public Health and Health
    Professions
University of Buffalo
Buffalo, New York

**Helen W. Lane**
Johnson Space Center
National Aeronautics and Space
    Administration
Houston, Texas

**Donald K. Layman**
Department of Food Science and
    Human Nutrition
University of Illinois at
    Urbana-Champaign
Urbana, Illinois

**Edward H. Leiter**
The Jackson Laboratory
Bar Harbor, Maine

**Leslie Lewinter-Suskind**
Department of Medical Education
California Northstate University
Elk Grove, California

**Hsiao C. Li**
Southwestern Medical Center
The University of Texas at Dallas
Dallas, Texas

**Zhaoping Li**
David Geffen School of Medicine
and
Center for Human Nutrition
The University of California,
    Los Angeles
Los Angeles, California

**Edward H. Livingston**
*Journal of the American Medical
    Association*
Chicago, Illinois

**David Martins**
Charles R. Drew University of
    Medicine and Science
Los Angeles, California

**Margaret A. McDowell**
Division of Nutrition Research
    Coordination
National Institutes of Health
Bethesda, Maryland

**John P. McNamara**
Department of Animal Sciences
President's Teaching Academy
Washington State University
Pullman, Washington

**John A. Milner**
Nutritional Science Research Group
Division of Cancer Prevention
National Cancer Institute
National Institute of Health
Bethesda, Maryland

and

Agricultural Research Service
United States Department of
    Agriculture
Beltsville, Maryland

**Diane C. Mitchell**
Department of Nutritional Sciences
The Pennsylvania State
    University
University Park, Pennsylvania

**Jennette P. Moreno**
Department of Pediatrics
Agricultural Research Service
United States Department of
    Agriculture
Children's Nutrition Research Center
Baylor College of Medicine
Houston, Texas

**Cynthia Mundy**
Division of Neonatology
Department of Pediatrics
Georgia Health Sciences University
Augusta, Georgia

**Krishna K. Murthy**
Department of Virology and
    Immunology
Southwest Foundation for Biomedical
    Research
San Antonio, Texas

**Marian L. Neuhouser**
Division of Public Health Sciences
Fred Hutchinson Cancer Research
    Center
Seattle, Washington

**Forrest H. Nielsen**
United States Department of
    Agriculture
Agricultural Research Service
Grand Forks Human Nutrition
    Research Center
Grand Forks, North Dakota

**Keith Norris**
Charles R. Drew University of
    Medicine and Science
Los Angeles, California

**Melissa Page**
School of Dentistry
Tufts University
Jamaica Plain, Massachusetts

**Carole A. Palmer**
School of Dental Medicine
Tufts University
Boston, Massachusetts

**Thai Pham**
Southwestern Medical Center
The University Texas at Dallas
and
Dallas VA Medical Center
Dallas, Texas

**Suzanne Phelan**
Department of Kinesiology
California Polytechnic State
    University
San Luis Obispo, California

**Rebecca S. Reeves**
School of Public Health
The University of Texas
Fredericksburg, Texas

**Richard S. Rivlin**
Strange Cancer Prevention Center
Scarsdale, New York

**Donato F. Romagnolo**
Department of Nutritional Sciences
and
The University of Arizona Cancer Center
The University of Arizona
Tucson, Arizona

**Christine Rosenbloom**
Georgia State University
Atlanta, Georgia

**Sammy Saab**
Department of Medicine
and
Department of Surgery
The University of California,
    Los Angeles
Los Angeles, California

**Andrew J. Schile**
The Jackson Laboratory—West
Sacramento, California

**Barbara J. Scott**
Department of Pediatrics
School of Medicine
University of Nevada, Reno
Reno, Nevada

**Ornella I. Selmin**
Department of Nutritional Sciences
The University of Arizona
    Cancer Center
The University of Arizona
Tucson, Arizona

**Wenyuan Shi**
Section of Oral Biology
Division of Oral Biology and
    Medicine
School of Dentistry
The University of California,
    Los Angeles
Los Angeles, California

**Gary W. Small**
Department of Psychiatry and
    Biobehavioral Sciences
Longevity Center
and
Division of Geriatric Psychiatry
Semel Institute for Neuroscience and
    Human Behavior
and
David Geffen School of Medicine
The University of California,
    Los Angeles
Los Angeles, California

**Helen Smiciklas-Wright**
Department of Nutritional Sciences
The Pennsylvania State
    University
University Park, Pennsylvania

**Scott M. Smith**
Johnson Space Center
National Aeronautics and Space
    Administration
Houston, Texas

**David L. Suskind**
Division of Pediatric
    Gastroenterology
Department of Pediatrics
School of Medicine
University of Washington
and
Seattle Children's Hospital
Seattle, Washington

**Robert M. Suskind**
Department of Pediatrics and
    International Health
College of Medicine
California Northstate University
Elk Grove, California

**E.L. Thomas**
Metabolic and Molecular Imaging Group
Medical Research Council Clinical
    Sciences Centre
Imperial College London
London, United Kingdom

**Kumar Venkitanarayanan**
University of Georgia
Griffin, Georgia

and

Department of Animal Science
University of Connecticut
Storrs, Connecticut

**Rohini Vishwanathan**
Jean Mayer United States Department
    of Agriculture
Human Nutrition Research
    Center on Aging
Tufts University
Boston, Massachusetts

**David G. Weismiller**
Department of Family Medicine
Brody School of Medicine
East Caroline University
Greenville, North Carolina

**Dara Wheeler**
Department of Nutritional Sciences
The Pennsylvania State
    University
University Park, Pennsylvania

**Michelle L. Wilkinson**
Michael & Susan Dell Center for
    Healthy Living
School of Public Health
The University of Texas at Houston
Houston, Texas

**Sara R. Zwart**
Johnson Space Center
National Aeronautics and Space
    Administration
Universities Space Research
    Association
Houston, Texas

# Part I

*Food*

# 1 Food Composition

*Carolyn D. Berdanier*

## CONTENTS

## INTRODUCTION

The composition of food in terms of its nutrient content has a long history of interest by scientists concerned with the adequacy of man's diet. The energy content of food was explored by Lavoisier in the 1700s. The fat content and the protein content were determined in the late 1800s and early 1900s. As vitamins and minerals were found to be essential, food chemists developed ways of determining how much of each was found in food. Studies of nutrient composition were focused not only on the nutrient content of a given food but also on the methodology available to give the requisite information. New methodology is published in one of many peer-reviewed journals. Among these are the *Journal of Food Composition and Analysis, The Journal of Food Science*, Food Science Biotechnology, and the *Journal of International Network of Food Data Systems*.

The U.S. Department of Agriculture (USDA) is the lead government agency for food composition analysis. Scientists within the Agricultural Research Service, Food Composition Laboratory, have accumulated and organized nutrient composition data as they have become available. Large tables of food composition are available online to the public.[1,2] Food analysts continue to expand the database, adding foods that previously had not been analyzed and included. The composition tables are periodically updated as new methods for analysis are developed and used to provide more accurate nutrient analysis. Other organizations have also contributed to the knowledge base about the nutrient content of food. Table 1.1 provides web addresses to these data sets. There are a number of tables devoted to special interests such as vitamin D, vitamin K, carotenoids, lysine, total sugars, and trans fatty acids. To access these tables, one must first go to the primary USDA website, then click on the SR tables. Tagatose (Table 1.2) is a food additive used to reduce the amount of sugar in food.[3] It has a sweet taste, yet does not have the same energy value as sucrose. Other sugar substitutes are also used in the preparation of reduced-energy foods; however, data on their quantitative occurrence are not as readily available because of the proprietary interests of food producers. Chapter 2 provides information about food additives. Additives are used to improve the quality of the food or to enhance its appearance or to increase its shelf life or to change its flavor or to enhance its safety.

In order to evaluate the nutrient content of the daily diet, one must know how much of each food has been consumed. The tables provide nutrient information in 100 g quantities, whereas food records are in terms of servings. One must know the serving size (weight/volume) and convert it to a 100 g portion. The following conversion factors will be helpful: 1 oz = 28 g, 1 lb = 454 g, 1 mg = 1/1000 g, 1 μg = 1/1000 mg, 1 kJ = 1/4 kcal, 1 kcal = 4.2 kJ, and 1mL of water = 1 g.

Included in Table 1.1 is a web address that provides for the composition of fast-food restaurant items. Some of the fast-food restaurants also have a website for their menu items. The composition of fast-food items is particularly valuable because Americans eat more of their meals away from home than ever before. In addition, the data are from combination foods, that is, the information is for a particular menu item complete with its "fixings." Other entries in this table are for specific country foods, that is, from Nigeria, West Africa, Tanzania, and France. European foods are included in a website that covers several European countries.

A number of organizations, both governmental and nongovernmental, are interested in providing food intake recommendations (listing both kinds and amounts of foods) to promote good health and reduce the risk of disease. Table 1.3 provides websites for these recommendations. Additional information on healthy eating by different age groups are provided in Chapters 17–27. Healthy eating focuses on food choices that promote optimal nutrition. Mainly these recommendations address the food needs of adults. The recommendations for infants, children, adolescents, and the aged are not usually included. Special disease states such as recommendations for children with type 1 diabetes mellitus can be found in the care recommendations for these disease states. Chapters 18, 19, and 21 address some of these recommendations.

There are several concerns about food intake that are separate from food composition, yet food composition can influence food intake. The regulation of food intake by internal and external signals can quantitatively affect what food is consumed and how much. This in turn will influence the nutritional status of the consumer. Food intake regulation is discussed in Chapter 7. The signals that regulate the impulse to eat and to stop eating are integrated ones.[4] Not all of these signals are known. Research

**TABLE 1.1**
**Web Addresses for Information on the Composition of Food**

| Data Set | Web Address |
| --- | --- |
| Primary nutrient data sets (results of USDA composition analysis) | http://www.nal.usda.gov/food composition |
| Selenium | Use USDA web address, then click on this file to open |
| Vitamin D | Use preceding address, then click on these files to open |
| Daidzein, genistein, glycitein, isoflavone content of 128 foods | Use preceding address, then click on this file to open |
| Carotenoid content of 215 foods | Use preceding address, then click on this file to open |
| Choline content | Use preceding address, then click on this file to open |
| Trans fatty acid content of 214 foods | Use preceding address, then click on this file to open |
| Sugar content of 500+ foods | Use preceding address, then click on this file to open |
| Nutritive value of foods (HG-72) data from 1274 foods expressed in common household units | http://www.nal.usda.gov/fnic/foodcomp, Click on nutritive value of foods to open |
| Vitamin K | Use USDA web address, then click on this file |
| Soy foods (beneficial compounds) | Use USDA web address, then click on this file to open |
| Individual amino acids and fatty acids | Use USDA web address, then click on this file to open |
| Nutrient retention factors: calculations of retention of specific micronutrients | Use preceding address, then click on Nutrient Retention Factors, Release 5 (2003) |
| List of key foods (foods that contribute up to 75% of any one nutrient) | Use preceding address, then click on Key Foods to open |
| Nutrition information on restaurant foods (insert name of chain in web address) | www.calorielab.com/restaurant/ (insert restaurant name) |
| McDonald's menu items | www.mcdonalds.com |
| African foods | www.fao.org/infoods/tables/africa-ev.stm |
| Food tables for international use | www.fao.org; see also www.hsph.harvard.edu |
| Nigerian food | www.nutrientdataconf.org/pastconf/ NDBC31/2-3 |
| West African food | www.biodiversityinternational.org |
| World food program | www.wfp.org/fais/nutritionalreporting/food composition-table |
| European foods | www.food-info.net/uk/foodcomp/table.htm; also www.briannac.co.uk/food htm |
| Hemp oil | hempoil.com/nutrition_composition.php |
| Lysine | www.traditionaloven.com/tutorials/l-lysine_ amino_acid.htm |
| French food | www.anses.fr/PNB610.htm |

a  A PDF file can be obtained on the USDA home page. Among the publications available in this way are Agricultural Handbook No. 74, No. 102, and Nos. 8–16. The special interest tables are superseded by SR. A CD-ROM is being prepared for purchase from the government printing office.

**TABLE 1.2**

**Occurrence of D-Tagatose in Foods**

| Food | Result (mg/kg) | Sample Preparation | Apparatus |
|---|---|---|---|
| Sterilized cow's milk | 2–3000 | Extracted with methanol; prepared trimethylsilyl (TMS) derivatives | Gas chromatography (GC), fused-silica capillary column (18 m × 0.22 mm) coated with AT-1000; carrier gas N2; flame ionization detector (FID) |
| Hot cocoa (processed with alkali) prepared with milk | 140 | Extracted with deionized (DI) water | High-performance liquid chromatography (HPLC); used Bio-Rad Aminex® HPX-87C column (300 mm × 7.8 mm) heated to 85°C; mobile phase DI water; flow rate 0.6 mL/min; refractive index (RI) detector |
| Hot cocoa prepared with milk | 190 | Extracted with DI water | HPLC; Bio-Rad Aminex HPX-87C column heated to 85°C; mobile phase DI water; flow rate 0.6 mL/min; RI detector |
| Powdered cow's milk | 800 | Extracted three times with distilled water for 3 h at 60°C; column chromatography to remove organic acids and bases; fractionation by partition chromatography | Paper partition chromatography, descending method on Whatman no.1 paper; used three solvent systems |
| Similac® infant formula | 4 | Extracted with 90% ethanol; prepared TMS derivatives | GC; DB-5 fused-silica capillary column (15 m × 0.53 mm, 1.5 mm film thickness); carrier gas He; FID detector |
| Enfamil® infant formula | 23 | Extracted with 90% aqueous ethanol; prepared TMS derivatives | GC; DB-17 fused-silica capillary column (15 m × 0.53 mm, 1 mm film thickness); carrier gas He; FID detector |
| Parmesan cheese | 10 | Extracted with 80% aqueous methanol; prepared TMS derivatives | GC; DB-5 fused-silica capillary column (30 m, 0.25 mm film thickness); carrier gas He; FID detector |
| Gjetost cheese | 15 | Extracted with 80% aqueous methanol; prepared TMS derivatives | GC; DB-5 fused-silica capillary column (30 m, 0.25 mm film thickness); carrier gas He; FID detector |
| Cheddar cheese | 2 | Extracted with 80% aqueous methanol; prepared TMS derivatives | GC; DB-5 fused-silica capillary column (30 m, 0.25 mm film thickness); carrier gas He; FID detector |
| Roquefort cheese | 20 | Extracted with 80% aqueous methanol; prepared TMS derivatives | GC; DB-5 fused-silica capillary column (30 m, 0.25 mm film thickness); carrier gas He; FID detector |
| Feta cheese | 17 | Extracted with 80% aqueous methanol; prepared TMS derivatives | GC; DB-5 fused-silica capillary column (30 m, 0.25 mm film thickness); carrier gas He; FID detector |
| Ultra high-temperature milk | ~5 | Dried under vacuum; water was added, then volatile derivatives extracted with isooctane | GC; Rescom-type OV1 capillary column (25 m × 0.25 mm, 0.1 or 0.25 mm film thickness); carrier gas H2; FID detector |
| BA Nature® yogurt | 29 | Extracted with DI water; passed through a strong cation exchange column followed by an amine column | HPLC; Bio-Rad Aminex HPX-87C column heated to 85°C; mobile phase DI water; flow rate 0.6 ml/min; RI detector |
| Cephulac®, an orally ingested medication for treatment of portal-systemic encephalopathy | 6500 | DI with Amberlite IR-120 (H) and Duolite A-561 (free base); diluted to 20 mg/ml with a 50:50 mixture of acetonitrile and water | HPLC; Waters Carbohydrate Analysis Column (300 mm × 3.9 mm); mobile phase water: acetonitrile, 77:23 (w/w); flow rate 2 mL/min; RI detector |
| Chronulac®, an orally ingested laxative | 6500 | DI with Amberlite IR-120 (H) and Duolite A-561 (free base); diluted to 20 mg/mL with a 50:50 mixture of acetonitrile and water | HPLC; Waters Carbohydrate Analysis Column (300 mm × 3.9 mm); mobile phase water: acetonitrile, 77:23 (w/w); flow rate 2 mL/min; RI detector |

*Sources:* Lee Zehner, Beltsville, MD, 2000; Lentner, C. et al., *Geigy Scientific Tables*, Vol. 1. CIBA-Geigy, West Caldwell, NJ, 1981.

**TABLE 1.3**

**Websites for Food Intake Recommendations**

| Recommendation | Website |
| --- | --- |
| Daily recommended intake (DRI) | www.nap.edu and http://www.nal.usda.gov/fnic/etext/000105.html |
| Dietary guidelines | www.health.gov/dietary guidelines |
| Food pyramid | www.mypyramid.gov/tipsresources/menus.html |
| Cancer risk reduction | www.cancer.org/docroot/PED/content/PED |
| Food from plants | www.5aday.gov/ |

in this area is particularly active as interest in the prevention of obesity as well as in weight reduction may well involve modifying the urge to eat and the signals to stop eating.

## REFERENCES

1. Lentner, C., *Geigy Scientific Tables*, Vol. 1. CIBA-Geigy, West Caldwell, NJ, pp. 241–266, 1981.
2. USDA. http://www.nal.usda.gov/fnic/foodcomp/data (accessed June 8, 2012).
3. Lee Zehner, Beltsville, MD, 2000. Unpublished data.
4. Harris, RBS and Mattes, RD *Appetite and Food Intake, Behavioral and Physiological Considerations*. CRC Press, Boca Raton, FL, 360pp., 2008.

# 2 Food Constituents

*Carolyn D. Berdanier*

## CONTENTS

Animals, including man, consume food to obtain the nutrients they need. Throughout the world, there are differences in food consumption related to socioeconomic conditions, food supply, and cultural dictates. If a variety of fresh and cooked foods is consumed in sufficient quantities to meet the energy needs of the consumer, then the needs for protein and the micronutrients should be met. Having this in mind, it is surprising to learn that some people are poorly nourished and indeed may develop one or more nutrition-related diseases through either excessive intake or inadequate intake of one or more essential nutrients and/or destruction of essential nutrients during preparation.

The early years of nutrition research focused on diseases related to inadequate vitamin and mineral intake. Nutrient deficiency diseases were identified and described. An important component of this research was the determination of the vitamin and mineral content of a vast array of foods. The composition of these foods has been compiled by the USDA and other organizations (see Chapter 1). The adequacy of one's diet can be determined by assessing the nutrient value of a careful record of the foods consumed. There are a number of computer programs designed to help the individual assess intake adequacy (see Chapter 6). In general terms, one can calculate diet adequacy by calculating the nutrient content of the foods consumed versus the nutrient needs of the consumer. This assumes that the estimate of intake is correct and that the food is prepared with a minimum loss of nutrient content and that there are no interfering substances that hinder nutrient availability and use. There are a number of websites that provide information about healthy eating. These are listed in Table 2.1.

Today, few people prepare all of their food from raw ingredients. Instead they purchase some foods that are partly or fully ready to eat. Food manufacturers have devised products that are tasty, reasonable in cost, and easy to prepare. These so-called convenience foods are a regular component of the shopper's grocery list. In order to provide such convenience, food manufacturers have used a variety of additives that stabilize the food product, extend its shelf life, and improve its quality and flavor. All food additives must be approved by the U.S. Food and Drug Administration (FDA). The FDA publishes a list of approved food additives called the GRAS list. GRAS means "generally recognized as safe." The approval is based on a detailed review of the scientific literature reporting on the clinical and toxicological responses to the additive. Some additives are naturally occurring substances that have

been in general use for long periods of time and are accorded GRAS approval due to that history.

A common additive is a sweetener. Sweeteners can be either naturally occurring compounds with a sweet taste or artificial sweeteners that mimic the sweet taste of natural ingredients.[1–3] Foods with a sweet taste are often consumed and contribute to an excess energy consumption perhaps leading to obesity and other health problems. There is current concern and interest in developing food products that have a lower energy content. Both sugar substitutes and fat substitutes have been developed that are useful in new food product development. Some of the sugar substitutes, the sugar alcohols (maltitol, sorbitol, xylitol, and others), are naturally occurring compounds that have 50% less available energy than sucrose.[3] These compounds are frequently used in foods designed as "sugar-free" foods for people with diabetes. Unfortunately, overconsumption of these sugar alcohols can lead to digestive upset characterized by diarrhea. When consumed in moderation, this characteristic can be avoided. Food manufacturers have developed products in which sugar alcohols are used to provide the bulkiness that sucrose provides but not the sweetness. The sweetness is then provided by inclusion of nonnutritive, high-intensity sugar substitute. A list of sweeteners added to foods is provided in Table 2.2.[1–3] Some of these are not allowed in the United States but may be allowed in other countries.

The sweetness characteristic is but one characteristic that food manufacturers might want to alter. Flavor is another. There are many flavoring agents that are included in the FDA list of approved additives. Other FDA-approved additives alter food characteristics such as texture, color, or shelf life. These characteristics are listed in Table 2.3. Some additives are nutrients added to a specific food to increase its nutritive value. Vitamins, minerals, and amino acids are added to food products to either restore the levels of these nutrients to those levels in the food prior to processing or improve the overall nutritional quality of the food. Enriched flour used in the preparation of bread is an example. Grain used for the preparation of flour loses some of its nutritional value when it is milled. The enrichment of this flour restores the nutrients lost during the milling process. In other foods, vitamins or minerals are added to improve the nutritional quality of the food so as to reduce the incidence of malnutrition in the consumer. Examples include the enrichment of milk with vitamin D to prevent rickets or vitamin D deficiency in the

**TABLE 2.1**

**Websites for Food Intake Recommendations**

| Recommendation | Website |
|---|---|
| Daily recommended intake (DRI) | www.nap.edu and http://www.nal.usda.gov/fnic/etext/000105.html |
| Dietary guidelines | www.health.gov/dietaryguidelines/ |
| Food pyramid | www.mypyramid.gov also myplate.gov www.hc-sc.gc.ca (Canada); www.chose my plate.gov |
| Cancer risk reduction | www.cancer.org/docroot/PED/content/PED |
| Food from plants | www.5aday.gov/ |
| Food guidance | www.hanefesh.com/edu/kosher; www.fnic.nal.usda.gov www.mypyramidtracker.gov; www.who.int/foodsafety/publications/general/en/terrorist www.kitchenfoodguide; www.mealtime.org www.dhcs.ca.gov; www.nefoodguide.cee.cornell.edu |

consumer, the addition of folacin to a number of foods to prevent folacin-related deficiency problems, and the enrichment of certain cereals with iron to prevent iron-deficiency anemia. Amino acids are frequently added to foods having an inadequate amino acid array. This addition improves the quality of the protein in that food. All of these nutrient additions are considered food additives and many are listed in Table 2.4.[4]

A number of food additives and food processing techniques are used to improve the safety of the food. Foods can be contaminated by a wide variety of organisms some of which are listed in Table 2.5.[5,6] Some of these contaminants can produce toxins that if consumed can be lethal. Table 2.6 is a list of mycotoxins and bacterial toxins that can occur in food.[5,6] The reader should also review Chapter 3 for an extensive list of pathogens known to cause food-borne illness.

Some foods such as soy protein, cabbages, and other vegetables contain compounds referred to as antinutrients. Table 2.7 provides a list of antinutrients sometimes found in food.[7] Antinutritives are compounds that interfere with the use of essential nutrients. They are generally divided into three classes: A, B, and C. Type A antinutritives are substances primarily interfering with the digestion of proteins or the absorption and utilization of amino acids. They are also known as antiproteins. Strict vegetarians, for example, are in danger of nutritional inadequacy by this type of antinutritive. The most important type A antinutritives are protease inhibitors and lectins.

Protease inhibitors, occurring in many plant and animal tissues, are proteins that inhibit proteolytic enzymes by binding to the active sites of the enzymes. Proteolytic enzyme inhibitors were first found in avian eggs around the turn of the century. They were later identified as ovomucoid and

ovoinhibitor, both of which inactivate trypsin. Chymotrypsin inhibitors also are found in avian egg whites. Other sources of trypsin and/or chymotrypsin inhibitors are soybeans and other legumes and pulses, vegetables, milk and colostrum, wheat and other cereal grains, guar gum, and white and sweet potatoes. The protease inhibitors of kidney beans, soybeans, and potatoes can additionally inhibit elastase, a pancreatic enzyme acting on elastin, an insoluble protein in meat. Animals given food containing active inhibitors show growth depression. This appears to be due to interference in trypsin and chymotrypsin activities and to excessive stimulation of the secretory exocrine pancreatic cells, which become hypertrophic. Valuable proteins may be lost in the feces in this case. In vitro experiments with human proteolytic enzymes have shown that trypsin inhibitors from bovine colostrum, lima beans, soybeans, kidney beans, and quail ovomucoid were active against human trypsin, whereas trypsin inhibitors originating from bovine and porcine pancreas, potatoes, chicken ovomucoid, and chicken ovoinhibitor were not. The soybean and lima bean trypsin inhibitors are also active against human chymotrypsin. Many protease inhibitors are heat labile, especially with moist heat. Relatively heat-resistant protease inhibitors include the antitryptic factor in milk, the alcohol-precipitable and nondialyzable trypsin inhibitor in alfalfa, the chymotrypsin inhibitor in potato, the kidney bean inhibitor, and the trypsin inhibitor in lima beans.

Lectin is the general term for plant proteins that have highly specific binding sites for carbohydrates. They are widely distributed among various sources, such as soybeans, peanuts, jack beans, mung beans, lima beans, kidney beans, fava beans, vetch, yellow wax beans, hyacinth beans, lentils, peas, potatoes, bananas, mangoes, and wheat germ. Most plant lectins are glycoproteins, except concanavalin A from jack beans, which is carbohydrate-free. The most toxic lectins in food include ricin in castor bean (oral toxic dose in man, 150–200 mg; intravenous toxic dose, 20 mg) and the lectins of kidney bean and hyacinth bean. The mode of action of lectins may be related to their ability to bind to specific cell receptors in a way comparable to that of antibodies. Because they are able to agglutinate red blood cells, they are also known as hemagglutinins. The binding of bean lectin on rat intestinal mucosal cells has been demonstrated in vitro, and it has been suggested that this action is responsible for the oral toxicity of the lectins. Such bindings may disturb the intestines' absorptive capacity for nutrients and other essential compounds. The lectins, being proteins, can easily be inactivated by moist heat. Germination decreases the hemagglutinating activity in varieties of peas and species of beans.

Type B antinutritives are substances interfering with the absorption or metabolic utilization of minerals and are also known as antiminerals. Although they are toxic per se, the amounts present in foods seldom cause acute intoxication under normal food consumption. However, they may harm the organism under suboptimum nutriture. The most important type B antinutritives are phytic acid, oxalates, and glucosinolates.

**TABLE 2.2**
**Sweetening Agents, Sugar Substitutes**

| Name | Sweetness[a] | Classification | Uses |
|---|---|---|---|
| Acesulfame-K (Sunette) | 130 | Nonnutritive; artificial | Tabletop sweetener, chewing gum, dry beverage mixes, puddings. This is actually the potassium salt of the 6-methyl derivative of a group of chemicals called oxathiazinone dioxides; approved by the FDA in 1988. |
| Aspartame | 180 | Nutritive; artificial | In diet sodas; also used in cold cereals, drink mixes, gelatin, puddings, toppings, dairy products, and at the table by the consumer; not used in cooking due to lack of stability when heated. Composed of the two naturally occurring amino acids, aspartic acid and phenylalanine; sweeter than sucrose. |
| Cyclamate | 30 | Nonnutritive; artificial | Tabletop sweetener and in drugs in Canada and 40 other countries. Banned by FDA in 1969. |
| Dulcin (4-ethoxy-phenyl-urea) | 250 | Nonnutritive; artificial | Not approved for food use in the United States; used in some European countries; also called Sucrol and Valzin. |
| Fructose (levulose) | 1.7 | Nutritive; natural | Beverages, baking, canned goods; anywhere invert sugar or honey may be used. |
| Glucose (dextrose) | 0.7 | Nutritive; natural | Primarily in the confection, wine, and canning industries. |
| Glycine | 0.8 | Nutritive; natural | Used to modify taste of some foods. |
| Mannitol | 0.7 | Nutritive; natural | Candies, chewing gums, confections, and baked goods; a sugar alcohol or polyhydric alcohol (polyol); occurs naturally in pineapples, olives, asparagus, and carrots. |
| Monellin | 3000 | Nutritive; natural | None; only a potential low-calorie sweetener. |
| Neohesperidin dihydrochalone (Neo DHC, NDHC) | 1250 | Nonnutritive; artificial | None approved; potential use in chewing gum, mouthwash, and toothpaste. |
| P-4000(5-nitro-2-pro-poxyaniline) | 4100 | Nonnutritive; artificial | None approved in United States. |
| Phyllodulcin | 250 | Nonnutritive; natural | None approved in United States. |
| Saccharin (0 benzosulfimide) | 500 | Nonnutritive; artificial | No longer approved by FDA for use in food. |
| Sorbitol | 0.6 | Nutritive; natural | Chewing gum, dairy products, meat products, icing, toppings, and beverages. |
| SRI Oxime V (perilla sugar) | 450 | Nonnutritive; artificial | None approved by FDA for use in food. |
| Stevioside (Stevia, Truvia) | 300 | Nutritive; natural | FDA approved in 2008; Truvia is a blend of rebiana and erythritol. Rebaudioside A, isolated from the same plant, is chemically similar but sweeter than stevioside. |
| Sucrose (table sugar) | 1.0 | Nutritive; natural | Many beverages and processed foods. |
| Splenda (dextrose/maltodextrin/ sucralose) | 4.0 | Nonnutritive | Used in many beverages and processed foods. Stable to heat. |
| Thaumatins | 1600 | Nutritive; natural | None; from the tropical fruit Thaumatococcus daniellii. |
| Xylitol | 0.8 | Nutritive; natural | Chewing gums and "sugar-free" foods; a sugar alcohol or polyhydric alcohol (polyol). |

*Sources:* http://www.nlm.nih.gov/medlineplus/ency/article/002444htm (accessed October 26, 2011); http://www.fda.gov/Food/FoodIngredientsPackaging/ucm094211.htm (accessed October 26, 2011); Hosoya, N. ed., *Proceedings of International Symposium on Caloric Evaluation of Carbohydrates*, Research Foundation For Sugar Metabolism, Tokyo, Japan, pp. 257, 1990.

[a] Compared to sucrose.

**TABLE 2.3**

**Terms Used to Describe the Functions of Food Additives**

| Term | Function |
|---|---|
| Anticaking agents and free-flow agents | Substances added to finely powdered or crystalline food products to prevent caking |
| Antimicrobial agents | Substances used to preserve food by preventing growth of microorganism and subsequent spoilage; these agents include fungicides, mold and yeast inhibitors, and bacteriocides |
| Antioxidants | Substances used to preserve food by retarding deterioration, rancidity, or discoloration due to oxidation |
| Colors and coloring adjuncts | Substances used to impart or enhance the color or shading of a food, including color stabilizers, color fixatives, color-retention agents |
| Curing and pickling agents | Substances imparting a unique flavor and/or color to a food, usually producing an increase in shelf life stability |
| Dough strengtheners | Substances used to modify starch and gluten, thereby producing a more stable dough |
| Drying agents | Substances with moisture-absorbing capacity used to maintain an environment of low moisture |
| Emulsifiers and emulsifier salts | Substances that modify surface tension of two (or more) immiscible solutions to establish a uniform dispersion of components; called an emulsion |
| Enzymes | Substances used to improve food processing and the quality of the finished food |
| Firming agents | Substances added to precipitate residual pectin, thus strengthening the supporting tissue and preventing its collapse during processing |
| Flavor enhancers | Substances added to supplement, enhance, or modify the original taste and/or aroma of a food without imparting a characteristic taste or aroma of its own |
| Flavoring agents and adjuvants | Substances added to impart or help impart a taste or aroma in food |
| Flour-treating agents | Substances added to milled flour, at the mill, to improve its color and/or baking qualities, including bleaching and maturing agents |
| Formulation aids | Substances used to promote or produce a desired physical state or texture in food, including carriers, binders, fillers, plasticizers, film formers, and tableting aids |
| Fumigants | Volatile substances used for controlling insects or pests |
| Humectants | Hygroscopic substances incorporated in food to promote retention of moisture, including moisture-retention agents and antidusting agents |
| Leavening agents | Substances used to produce or stimulate production of carbon dioxide in baked goods to impart a light texture, including yeast, yeast foods, and calcium salts |
| Lubricants and release agents | Substances added to food contact surfaces to prevent ingredients and finished products from sticking to them |
| Nonnutritive sweeteners | Substances having less than 2% of the caloric value of sucrose per equivalent unit of sweetening capacity |
| Nutrient supplements | Substances that are necessary for the body's nutritional and metabolic processes |
| Nutritive sweeteners | Substances having greater than 2% equivalent unit of sweetening capacity |
| Oxidizing and reducing agents | Substances that chemically oxidize or reduce another food ingredient, thereby producing a more stable product |
| pH control agents | Substances added to change or maintain active acidity or alkalinity, including buffers, acids, alkalis, and neutralizing agents |
| Processing aids | Substances used as manufacturing aids to enhance the appeal or utility of a food or food component, including clarifying agents, clouding agents, catalysts, flocculants, filter aids, and crystallization inhibitors |
| Propellants, aerating agents, and gases | Gases used to supply force to expel a product or used to reduce the amount of oxygen in contact with the food in packaging |
| Sequestrants | Substances that combine with polyvalent metal ions to form a soluble metal complex and to improve the quality and stability of products |
| Solvents and vehicles | Substances used to extract or dissolve another substance |
| Stabilizers and thickeners | Substances used to produce viscous solutions or dispersions, impart body, improve consistency, or stabilize emulsions, including suspending and bodying agents, setting agents, gelling agents, and bulking agents |
| Surface-active agents | Substances used to modify surface properties of liquid food components for a variety of effects, other than emulsifiers but including solubilizing agents, dispersants, detergents, wetting agents, rehydration enhancers, whipping agents, foaming agents, and defoaming agents |
| Surface-finishing agents | Substances used to increase palatability, preserve gloss, and inhibit discoloration of foods, including glazes, polishes, waxes, and protective coatings |
| Synergists | Substances used to act or react with another food ingredient to produce a total effect different or greater than the sum of the effects produced by the individual ingredients |
| Texturizers | Substances that affect the appearance or mouth feel of the food |

*Source:* http://www.fda.gov/Food/FoodIngredientsPackaging/ucm094211.htm (accessed October 26, 2011).

**TABLE 2.4**
**Specific Food Additives and Their Functions**

| Name | Function[a] |
| --- | --- |
| Acacia | Emulsifier, foam agent, gelling agent, stabilizer, suspending agent, thickener, whipping agent |
| Acesulfame potassium | Sweetener |
| Acetaldehyde | Flavoring agent |
| Acetanisole | Flavoring agent |
| Acetic acid | pH control, preservative, flavoring |
| Acetic and fatty acid esters | Emulsifier, foaming agent, whipping agent |
| Acetion acetophenone | Flavoring agent |
| Acetone | Extractant, solubilizer, solvent, vehicle |
| Acetone peroxides | Bleaching agents, dough conditioner, flour treatment agent, maturing agent, oxidizing agent |
| Acetylated distarch adipate | Gelling agent, stabilizer, suspending agent, thickener |
| Acetylated distarch phosphate | Emulsifier, foaming agent, gelling agent, thickener, whipping agent |
| Acetylated monoglycerides | Antisticking agent, coating agent, emulsifier, texturizer, foaming agent, lubricant, solvent |
| Acid-treated starch | Binder, filler, gelling agent, plasticizer, stabilizer, suspending agent, thickener |
| Activated carbon | Decolorizing agent, odor-removing agent, taste-removing agent |
| Adipic acid | Buffer and neutralizing agent |
| Agar | Emulsifier, foaming agent, gelling agent, stabilizer, suspending agent, thickener, whipping agent |
| Ammonium alginate | Stabilizer and thickener, texturizer |
| Alginic acid | Emulsifier, foaming agent, gelling agent, stabilizer, suspending agent, whipping agent |
| Alkaline-treated starch | Binder, filler, gelling agent, plasticizer, stabilizer, suspending agent, thickening agent |
| Allura red Ac | Color |
| Allyl α-ionone | Flavoring agent |
| Allyl cyclohexanepropionate | Flavoring agent |
| Allyl heptanoate | Flavoring agent |
| Allyl hexanoate | Flavoring agent |
| Allyl isothionate | Flavoring agent |
| Allyl isovalerate | Flavoring agent |
| Allyl tiglate | Flavoring agent |
| Almond oil | Flavoring agent |
| α-Amyl cinnamic aldehyde dimethyl, alcohol | Flavoring agent |
| α-Amylase | Enzyme |
| α-Ionone | Flavoring agent |
| α-Methyl cinnamic alcohol, aldehyde | Flavoring agent |
| α-Phellandrene | Flavoring agent |
| α-Pinene | Flavoring agent |
| α-Terpinene | Flavoring |
| Aluminum ammonium sulfate | Color fixative, firming agent |
| Aluminum potassium sulfate | Buffer, firming agent, neutralizing agent |
| Aluminum powder | Color |
| Aluminum silicate | Anticaking agent, drying agent |
| Aluminum sodium sulfate | Buffer, firming agent, neutralizing agent |
| Aluminum sulfate | Firming agent |
| Aluminum ammonium sulfate | Buffer, neutralizing agent |
| Amaranth | Color |
| Ambrette seed oil | Flavoring agent |
| Ammonium adipate | Buffer, neutralizing agent |
| Ammonium alginate | Emulsifier, foam agent |
| Ammonium bicarbonate | Alkali, leavening agent |
| Ammonium carbonate | Buffer, leavening agent |
| Ammonium chloride | Dough conditioner |
| Ammonium dihydrogen phosphate | Buffer, dough conditioner, leavening agent |
| Ammonium hydrogen carbonate | Alkali, leavening agent |
| Ammonium hydroxide | Alkali |
| Ammonium persulfate | Flour treatment agent |

*(continued)*

**TABLE 2.4 (continued)**
**Specific Food Additives and Their Functions**

| Name | Function[a] |
|------|-------------|
| Ammonium phosphate dibasic | Buffer, dough conditioner, leavening agent |
| Ammonium phosphate monobasic | Buffer, dough conditioner, leavening agent |
| Ammonium salts of phosphatidic acid | Emulsifier, foaming agent |
| Ammonium sulfate | Dough conditioner |
| Amyl acetate | Carrier solvent, flavoring agent |
| Amyl cinnamate | Flavoring agent |
| Amyl octanoate | Flavoring agent |
| Amyl propionate | Flavoring agent |
| Amyloglucosidases | Enzyme agent |
| Amyris oil | Flavoring agent |
| Anethole | Flavoring agent |
| Angelica root oil | Flavoring agent |
| Anise oil | Flavoring agent |
| Anisole | Flavoring agent |
| Anisyl acetate, alcohol | Flavoring agent |
| Annatto | Color |
| Anoxomer | Antioxidant |
| Arabinogalactan | Stabilizer and thickener, texturizer |
| Ascorbic acid (vitamin C) | Nutrient, antioxidant, preservative |
| Aspartame | Sweetener; sugar substitute |
| Avian pepsin | Enzyme |
| Azodicarbonamide | Flour-treating agent |
| Azorubine | Color |
| Balsam Peru oil | Flavoring agent |
| Basil oil | Flavoring agent |
| Bay oil | Flavoring agent |
| Beeswax | Coating agent |
| Beet red | Color |
| Benzoic acid | Antimicrobial agent, preservative |
| Benzaldehyde, acetate, alcohol | Flavoring agent |
| Benzoyl peroxide | Flour-treating agent, bleaching agent |
| Bergamot oil | Flavoring agent |
| β-Apo-8′-carotenal | Color |
| β-Carotene | Color, nutrient |
| β-Caryophyllene | Flavoring agent |
| β-Glucanase | Enzyme |
| β-Ionone | Flavoring agent |
| β-Pinene | Flavoring agent |
| Butylated hydroxyanisole (BHA) | Antioxidant, preservative |
| Butylated hydroxytoluene (BHT) | Antioxidant, preservative |
| Biotin | Nutrient |
| Birch tar oil | Flavoring agent |
| Black pepper oil | Flavoring agent |
| Black current extract | Color |
| Bleached starch | Binder, filler, gelling agent, plasticizer, stabilizer, suspending agent |
| Bois de rose oil | Flavoring agent |
| Bone phosphate | Anticaking agent |
| Bornyl acetate | Flavoring |
| Brilliant Black Pn | Color |
| Brilliant Blue FCF | Color |
| Bromelain | Enzyme |
| Brominated vegetable oil | Cloud-producing agent, flavoring adjunct, stabilizer |
| Brown FK, HT | Color |
| Butadiene styrene | Chewing gum component |

**TABLE 2.4 (continued)**
**Specific Food Additives and Their Functions**

| Name | Function[a] |
| --- | --- |
| Butan-1-ol | Solvent |
| Butan-3-one-2yl butyrate | Flavoring agent |
| Butyl acetate, alcohol, butyrate, isobutyrate | Flavoring agent |
| Butyl P-hydroxybenzoate | Antimicrobial agent |
| BHA, hydroxymethylphenol, hydroxytoluene | Antioxidant |
| Butyraldehyde | Flavoring agent |
| Butyric acid | Flavoring agent |
| Caffeine | Flavoring agent |
| Calcium 5′-guanylate | Flavor enhancer, intensifier |
| Calcium 5′-inosinate | Flavor enhancer, intensifier |
| Calcium 5′-ribonucleotides | Flavor enhancer, intensifier |
| Calcium acetate | Anti-mold agent, antirope agent, buffer, neutralizing agent, sequestrant, stabilizer, suspending agent |
| Calcium alginate | Stabilizer and thickener, texturizer |
| Calcium aluminum silicate | Anticaking agent, drying agent |
| Calcium ascorbate | Antioxidant |
| Calcium benzoate | Antimicrobial agent, preservative |
| Calcium bromate | Dough conditioner, maturing agent |
| Calcium carbonate | Alkali, anticaking agent, mineral supplement, dough conditioner, firming agent |
| Calcium chloride | Firming agent, sequestrant |
| Calcium citrate | Buffer, firming agent, sequestrant |
| Calcium ferrocyanide | Anticaking agent, drying agent |
| Calcium DL-L-glutamate | Flavor enhancer, intensifier, salt substitute |
| Calcium dihydrogen phosphate | Buffer, firming agent, leavening agent, neutralizing agent, texture-modifying agent, texturizer |
| Calcium disodium ethylenediamine-tetraacetic acid (EDTA) | Preservative, sequestrant, antioxidant synergist |
| Calcium gluconate | Buffer, firming agent, neutralizer, sequestrant |
| Calcium glycerophosphate | Dietary supplement |
| Calcium hydrogen sulfite | Firming agent, preservative |
| Calcium hydroxide | Buffer, firming agent |
| Calcium iodate | Dough conditioner |
| Calcium lactate | Preservative, dough conditioner, buffer |
| Calcium lactobionate | Firming agent |
| Calcium DL-malate | Buffer, neutralizing agent, seasoning agent |
| Calcium monohydrogen phosphate | Dough conditioner |
| Calcium oxide | Alkali, dough conditioner, dietary supplement |
| Calcium pantothenate | Dietary supplement |
| Calcium peroxide | Bleaching agent, dough conditioner, oxidizing agent |
| Calcium phosphate | Leavening agent, sequestrant, nutrient |
| Calcium polyphosphates | Emulsifier, foaming agent, humectants, moisture-retaining agent, sequestrant, texturizer |
| Calcium propionate | Preservative |
| Calcium pyrophosphate | Buffer, dietary supplement |
| Calcium silicate | Anticaking agent |
| Calcium sorbate | Antimicrobial agent, preservative |
| Calcium stearate | Anticaking agent, binder, drying agent, emulsifier, filler, foaming agent, plasticizer |
| Calcium stearoyl lactylate | Dough conditioner, emulsifier, foaming agent, stabilizer |
| Calcium sulfate | Dietary supplement, dough conditioner, firming agent, sequestrant |
| Camphene | Flavoring agent |
| Cananga oil | Flavoring agent |
| Candelilla wax | Chewing gum base, coating agent, film former, glaze, polish, surface-finishing agent |
| Canthaxanthin | Color |
| Caramel | Color |
| Caraway oil | Flavoring agent |

*(continued)*

**TABLE 2.4 (continued)**
**Specific Food Additives and Their Functions**

| Name | Function[a] |
|---|---|
| Carbohydrase | Enzyme |
| Carob bean gum | Stabilizer and thickener |
| Carrageenan | Emulsifier, stabilizer, and thickener |
| Cellulose | Emulsifier, stabilizer, and thickener |
| Citric acid | Preservative, antioxidant, pH control agent, sequestrant |
| Citrus Red No. 2 | Color |
| Cochineal | Color |
| Corn endosperm oil | Color |
| Cornstarch | Anticaking agent, drying agent, formulation aid, processing aid, surface-finishing agent |
| Corn syrup | Flavoring agent, humectant, nutritive sweetener, preservative |
| D-α-Tocopherol (acetate, succinate) | Antioxidant, nutrient |
| D-Carvone | Flavoring agent |
| D-Dihydrocarvone | Flavoring agent |
| D-Limonene | Flavoring agent |
| Dammar gum | Gelling agent, stabilizer, suspending agent |
| Decanal | Flavoring agent |
| Dehydroacetic acid | Preservative |
| Δ-Decalactone | Flavoring agent |
| Δ-Dodecalactone | Flavoring agent |
| Desoxycholic acid | Emulsifier, foaming agent, whipping agent |
| Dexpanthenol | Dietary supplement |
| Dextrin | Binder, filler, gelling agent, plasticizer, stabilizer, suspending agent, thickener |
| Dextrose (glucose) | Flavoring agent, humectant, nutritive sweetener, synergist |
| Diacetyl | Flavoring agent |
| Diacetyl tartaric acid esters | Emulsifiers, foaming agent |
| Diammonium hydrogen phosphate | Buffer, dough conditioner, leavening agent, neutralizing agent |
| Diatomaceous earth | Filter aid |
| Dibenzyl ether | Flavoring agent |
| Dibutyl sebacate | Flavoring agent |
| Dicalcium pyrophosphate | Buffer |
| Dichloromethane | Extraction solvent |
| Diethyl ether | Extraction solvent |
| Diethyl malonate | Flavoring agent |
| Diethyl pyrocarbonate | Antimicrobial agent, preservative |
| Diethyl sebacate | Flavoring agent |
| Diethyl succinate | Flavoring agent |
| Diethyl tartrate | Carrier solvent, flavoring agent |
| Diglycerides | Emulsifiers |
| Dihydrocarveol | Flavoring agent |
| Dihydrocoumarin | Flavoring agent |
| Dilauryl thiodipropionate | Antioxidant |
| Dill seed oil | Flavoring agent |
| Dimethyl anthranilate | Flavoring agent |
| Dimethyl benzyl carbonyl acetate | Flavoring agent |
| Dimethyl dicaronate | Preservative |
| Dimethylpolysiloxane | Defoaming agent |
| Dioctyl sodium sulfosuccinate | Emulsifier, processing aid, surface-active agent |
| Diphenyl | Fungistatic agent |
| Dipotassium 5′-guanylate | Flavor enhancer, intensifier |
| Dipotassium hydrogen phosphate | Buffer, sequestrant |
| Disodium guanylate | Flavor enhancer |
| Disodium inosinate | Flavor adjuvant |
| Disodium pyrophosphate | Buffer, leavening agent, sequestrant, stabilizer |
| Distarch phosphate | Binder, filler, plasticizer, stabilizer, suspending agent, thickener |

## TABLE 2.4 (continued)
## Specific Food Additives and Their Functions

| Name | Function[a] |
| --- | --- |
| DL-Alanine and other amino acids | Nutrients |
| Dodecyl gallate | Antioxidant |
| Edible gum | Emulsifier, foam agent, gelling agent, stabilizer, suspending agent |
| EDTA | Antioxidant, sequestrant |
| Erythorbic acid | Antioxidant, preservative |
| Ethoxylated mono and diglycerides | Emulsifiers |
| Ethoxyquin | Antioxidant |
| Ethylene dichloride | Solubilizer, solvent |
| Ethylene oxide | Fumigant |
| Ethyoxylated mono- and diglycerides | Dough conditioners |
| Eucalyptol | Flavoring agent |
| Eucalyptus oil | Flavoring agent |
| Eugenyl acetate | Flavoring agent |
| Farnesol | Flavoring agent |
| Fast Green FCF | Color |
| Fast Red E | Color |
| Fatty acid esters | Antispattering agents, emulsifiers, foaming agents |
| Fennel oil | Flavoring agent |
| Ferric ammonium citrate | Anticaking agent, nutrient, drying agent |
| Ferric phosphate | Nutrient |
| Ferric pyrophosphate | Nutrient |
| Ferrous ammonium citrate | Nutrient, anticaking agent, drying agent |
| Ferrous fumarate | Nutrient |
| Ferrous gluconate | Color adjunct, nutrient |
| Ferrous lactate | Color adjunct |
| Ferrous sulfate | Nutrient |
| Ficin | Enzyme |
| Fir needle oil | Flavoring agent |
| Folic acid | Nutrient |
| Food starch | Filler, binder, gelling agent, plasticizer, stabilizer, suspending agent, thickener |
| Formic acid | Flavoring adjunct, preservative |
| Fructose | Sweetener, carrier, disintegrating agent, dispersing agent, tableting aid, formulation aid |
| Fumaric acid | Acidifier, flavoring agent |
| Furfural | Extraction solvent, flavoring agent |
| γ-Butyrolactone | Flavoring agent |
| γ-Heptalactone | Flavoring agent |
| γ-Nonalactone | Flavoring agent |
| γ-Octalactone | Flavoring agent |
| γ-Terpinene | Flavoring agent |
| γ-Undecalactone | Flavoring agent |
| γ-Valerolactone | Flavoring agent |
| Garlic oil | Flavoring agent |
| Gellan gum | Gelling agent, stabilizer, suspending agent, thickener |
| Geraniol | Flavoring agent |
| Geranium oil | Flavoring agent |
| Geranyl benzoate | Flavoring agent |
| Geranyl acetate, acetoacetate, butyrate, formate, phenylacetate, propionate | Flavoring agents |
| Gibberellic acid | Enzyme activator |
| Ginger oil | Flavoring agent |
| Gluconolactone | Acid, acidifier, leavening agent |
| Glucose isomerase | Enzyme |
| Glucose oxidase | Enzyme |

(continued)

**TABLE 2.4 (continued)**
**Specific Food Additives and Their Functions**

| Name | Function[a] |
| --- | --- |
| Glycerine (glycerol) | Humectant |
| Glycerol | Bodying agent, bulking agent, carrier solvent, humectant |
| Glycerol diacetate | Carrier solvent |
| Glycerol esters of rosins | Component of chewing gum |
| Glycine | Nutrient |
| Grape skin extract | Color |
| Grapefruit oil | Flavoring agent |
| Green S | Color |
| Guaiac resin | Antioxidant |
| Guar gum | Stabilizer and thickener, texturizer |
| Gum arabic | Stabilizer and thickener, texturizer |
| Gum ghatti | Stabilizer and thickener, texturizer |
| Gum guaiac | Antioxidant |
| Hemicellulase | Enzyme |
| Heptanol | Flavoring agent |
| Heptane | Extraction solvent |
| Heptyl alcohol | Flavoring agent |
| Heptylparaben | Antimicrobial agent, preservative |
| Hexabe | Extraction solvent |
| Hexanoic acid | Flavoring agent |
| Hexyl-2-butenoate | Flavoring agent |
| Hexyl 2-methylbutyrate | Flavoring agent |
| Hexyl alcohol | Flavoring agent |
| Hexyl isovalerate | Flavoring agent |
| Hops oil | Flavoring agent |
| Hydrochloric acid | Acidifier |
| Hydrogen peroxide | Bleaching agent |
| Hydroxycitronellal | Flavoring agent |
| Hydroxylated lecithin | Cloud-producing agent, emulsifier, foaming agent, whipping agent |
| Hydroxypropyl cellulose | Coating agent, emulsifier, film former, thickener |
| Hydroxypropyl starch | Binder, thickener, emulsifier |
| Hydrolyzed vegetable protein | Flavor enhancer |
| Indigotine | Color |
| Indole | Flavoring agent |
| Inositol | Nutrient |
| Insoluble polyvinylpyrrolidone | Colloidal stabilizer, color stabilizer |
| Invert sugar | Humectant, nutritive sweetener |
| Iron | Nutrient |
| Iron oxide red or yellow | Color |
| Iron ammonium citrate | Anticaking agent |
| Iso-α-methyl ionone | Flavoring agent |
| Isoamyl acetate | Flavoring agent |
| Isoamyl butyrate | Flavoring agent |
| Isoamyl formate | Flavoring agent |
| Isoamyl gallate | Antioxidant |
| Isoamyl hexanoate | Flavoring agent |
| Isoamyl isovalerate | Flavoring agent |
| Isoamyl salicylate | Flavoring agent |
| Isobornyl acetate | Flavoring agent |
| Isobutanol | Extraction solvent |
| Isobutyl acetate | Flavoring agent |
| Isobutyl alcohol | Flavoring agent |
| Isobutyl cinnamate | Flavoring agent |
| Isobutyl-2-butenoate | Flavoring agent |

## TABLE 2.4 (continued)
## Specific Food Additives and Their Functions

| Name | Function[a] |
| --- | --- |
| Isobutylene–isoprene copolymer | Chewing gum component |
| Isobutyraldehyde | Flavoring agent |
| Isobutyric acid | Flavoring agent |
| Isoeugenol | Flavoring agent |
| Isomalt | Sweetening agent |
| Isopropyl acetate | Extraction solvent, flavoring agent |
| Isopropyl alcohol | Solubilizer, solvent, vehicle |
| Isopropyl citrate mixture | Antioxidant, sequestrant |
| Isopropyl myristate | Carrier solvent |
| Isopulegol | Flavoring agent |
| Isoquinoline | Flavoring agent |
| Isovaleric acid | Flavoring agent |
| Juniper berry oil | Flavoring agent |
| Kaolin | Anticaking agent, drying agent |
| Karaya gum | Stabilizer and thickener |
| Kelp(fiber) | Nutrient |
| Lactic acid | Preservative, pH control |
| L-Amino acids | Nutrients |
| L-Menthol | Flavoring agent |
| L-Menthone | Flavoring agent |
| Labdanum oil | Flavoring agent |
| Lactated glycerides | Emulsifiers, foaming agents, stabilizers, suspending agents |
| Lactic acid | Acidifier |
| Lactitol | Sweetener, texture modifier, texturizer |
| Lactylic esters of fatty acids | Emulsifiers, foaming agents, surface-active agents, wetting agent |
| Lanolin | Chewing gum component |
| Laurel leaf oil | Flavoring agent |
| Lauric acid | Defoaming agent, Flavoring agent |
| Lauryl alcohol, aldehyde | Flavoring agent |
| Lavandin oil | Flavoring agent |
| Lavender oil | Flavoring agent |
| Lecithin (phosphatidylcholine) | Emulsifier, surface-active agent |
| Lemon oil | Flavoring agent |
| Lemon grass oil | Flavoring agent |
| Lime oil | Flavoring agent |
| Limestone, ground | Chewing gum component |
| Linaloe wood oil | Flavoring agent |
| Linalyl acetate | Flavoring agent |
| Lipase | Enzyme |
| Lithol rubine | Color |
| Locust bean gum | Emulsifier |
| Lovage oil | Flavoring agent |
| Mace oil | Flavoring agent |
| Magnesium carbonate | Alkali, antibleaching agent, anticaking agent, dispersing agent, drying agent, tableting aid |
| Magnesium chloride | Color-retention agent, firming agent |
| Magnesium DL-L-glutamate | Flavor enhancer, intensifier salt substitute |
| Magnesium lactate | Buffer, dough conditioner, neutralizing agent |
| Magnesium gluconate | Buffer, firming agent, neutralizer |
| Magnesium hydrogen carbonate | Carrier, color-retention agent, disintegrating agent, dispersing agent, formulation aid |
| Magnesium hydrogen phosphate | Nutrient |
| Magnesium hydroxide | Alkali, anticaking agent, color adjunct, drying agent |
| Magnesium hydrogen carbonate | Alkali, anticaking agent, drying agent |
| Magnesium lactate | Buffer, nutrient, dough conditioner, neutralizing agent |

(continued)

**TABLE 2.4 (continued)**
**Specific Food Additives and Their Functions**

| Name | Function[a] |
| --- | --- |
| Magnesium oxide | Alkali, anticaking agent, buffer, drying agent, neutralizing agent |
| Magnesium phosphate | Nutrient |
| Magnesium silicate | Filter aid, anticaking agent, drying agent |
| Magnesium stearate | Anticaking agent, binder, drying agent, emulsifier, filler, foaming agent |
| Magnesium sulfate | Nutrient |
| Malic acid | Acidifier, flavoring agent |
| Malt, malt carbohydrases | Enzyme |
| Maltitol | Humectant, sweetener |
| Maltol | Flavoring agent |
| Mandarin oil | Flavoring agent |
| Manganese chloride, gluconate | Nutrient |
| Mannitol | Anticaking, nutritive sweetener, stabilizer and thickener, texturizer |
| Marjoram oil | Flavoring agent |
| Mentha arvensis oil | Flavoring agent |
| Menthol | Flavoring agent |
| Methanol | Extraction solvent |
| Methylcellulose | Bulking agent |
| Methylparaben | Preservative |
| Mineral oil | Antisticking agent, release agent, sealing agent |
| Modified food starch | Drying agent, formulation aid, processing aid, surface-finishing agent |
| Monoglycerides | Emulsifiers |
| Monosodium glutamate (MSG) | Flavor enhancer |
| Myrcene | Flavoring agent |
| Myristic acid | Defoaming agent |
| Myrrh oil | Flavoring agent |
| Nerol | Flavoring agent |
| Nerolidol | Flavoring agent |
| Niacin | Nutrient |
| Niacinamide | Nutrient |
| Niacinamide ascorbate | Nutrient |
| Nisin | Preservative |
| Nitrogen | Freezing gas |
| Nitrous oxide | Propellant |
| Nonanal | Flavoring agent |
| Nonyl acetate, alcohol | Flavoring agent |
| Nordihydroguaiaretic | Antioxidant |
| Nutmeg oil | Flavoring agent |
| O-Phenylphenol | Preservative |
| Octanal | Flavoring agent |
| Octanoic acid | Defoaming agent |
| Octyl acetate, formate | Flavoring agent |
| Octyl gallate | Antioxidant |
| Oleic acid | Antisticking agent, binder, filler, lubricant, plasticizer |
| Orange GGN | Color |
| Orange oil | Flavoring agent |
| Orris root oil | Flavoring agent |
| Oxidized starch | Binder, filler, gelling agent, plasticizer, thickener |
| Oxystearin | Antifoaming agent |
| Palmitic acid | Defoaming agent |
| Papain | Texturizer, enzyme |
| Paprika | Color, flavoring agent |
| Paraffin wax | Chewing gum component, defoaming agent |
| Parsley herb oil | Flavoring agent |
| Patent Blue V | Color |

**TABLE 2.4 (continued)**
**Specific Food Additives and Their Functions**

| Name | Function[a] |
|---|---|
| Pectin | Stabilizer and thickener, texturizer |
| Pennyroyal oil | Flavoring agent |
| Pentapotassium triphosphate | Texture-modifying agent, texturizer |
| Peppermint oil | Flavoring agent |
| Pepsin | Enzyme |
| Perlite | Filter aid |
| Petroleum jelly | Antifoaming agent, antisticking agent, lubricant, release agent, sealing agent |
| Phosphoric acid | pH control |
| Pimaricin | Fungicidal preservative |
| Pimenta oil | Flavoring agent |
| Piperonal | Flavoring agent |
| Polyethylene glycols | Antisticking agent, binder, carrier solvent, dispersing agent, filler, film former |
| Polyphosphates | Nutrient, flavor improver, sequestrant, pH control |
| Polypropylene glycol | Defoaming agent |
| Polysorbates | Emulsifiers, surface-active agent |
| Potassium alginate | Stabilizer and thickener, texturizer |
| Potassium bromate | Flour-treating agent |
| Potassium iodide | Nutrient |
| Potassium nitrite | Curing and pickling agent |
| Potassium sorbate | Preservative |
| Propionic acid | Preservative |
| Propyl gallate | Antioxidant, preservative |
| Propylene glycol | Emulsifier, humectant, stabilizer and thickener, texturizer |
| Propylparaben | Preservative, fungicide |
| Quillaia extracts | Emulsifiers |
| Quinine hydrochloride | Flavoring agent |
| Quinine sulfate | Flavoring agent |
| Quinoline | Yellow color |
| Red 2G | Color |
| Rennet | Enzyme |
| Rhodinol | Flavoring agent |
| Riboflavin | Nutrient, color |
| Rice bran wax | Chewing gum component |
| Rose oil | Flavoring agent |
| Rosemary oil | Flavoring agent |
| Rue oil | Flavoring agent |
| Saccharin | Nonnutritive sweetener |
| Saffron | Color, flavoring agent |
| Sage oil | Flavoring agent |
| Shellac | Coating agent, film former |
| Silicon dioxide | Anticaking agent |
| Sodium acetate | pH control, preservative |
| Sodium alginate | Stabilizer and thickener, texturizer |
| Sodium aluminum sulfate | Leavening agent |
| Sodium benzoate | Preservative |
| Sodium bicarbonate | Leavening agent, pH control |
| Sodium chloride (salt) | Flavor enhancer, formulation acid, preservation |
| Sodium citrate | pH control, curing and pickling agent, sequestrant |
| Sodium diacetate | Preservative, sequestrant |
| Sodium nitrate (Chile saltpeter) | Curing and pickling agent, preservative |
| Sodium nitrite | Curing and pickling agent, preservative |
| Sodium propionate | Preservative, fungicide, and mold preventative |
| Sorbic acid | Preservative |

*(continued)*

**TABLE 2.4 (continued)**
**Specific Food Additives and Their Functions**

| Name | Function[a] |
|------|-------------|
| Sorbitan monostearate | Emulsifier, stabilizer, and thickener |
| Sorbitol | Humectant, nutritive sweetener, stabilizer and thickener, sequestrant |
| Sucrose | Nutritive sweetener, preservative |
| Tagetes (Aztec marigold) | Color |
| Talc | Anticaking agent, coating agent, film former, dusting powder, texturizer |
| Tangerine oil | Flavoring agent |
| Tannic acid | Clarifying agent |
| Tara gum | Gelling agent, stabilizer, suspending agent, thickener |
| Tarragon oil | Flavoring agent |
| Tartaric acid | pH control |
| Tartrazine | Color |
| TBHQ | Antioxidant |
| Titanium dioxide | Color |
| Tocopherols (vitamin E) | Antioxidant, nutrient |
| Tragacanth gum | Stabilizer and thickener, texturizer |
| Triacetin | Carrier, solvent, humectants, solubilizer |
| Trypsin | Enzyme |
| Turmeric | Color |
| Undecanal | Flavoring agent |
| Undecyl alcohol | Flavoring agent |
| Valeric acid | Flavoring agent |
| Vanilla | Flavoring agent |
| Vanillin | Flavoring agent and adjuvant |
| Vitamins A, D, E, $B_6$, $B_{12}$ | Nutrients |
| Wintergreen oil | Flavoring agent |
| Yellow prussiate of soda | Anticaking agent |

*Source:* Helmenstine, A., *Food Additives*, http://www.chemistry.about.com/od/foodcookingchemistry/a/additives.htm (accessed October 26, 2011).
[a] Function refers to those defined in Table 2.3.

**TABLE 2.5**
**Microbial Contaminants of Fresh Food**

| Foods | Microorganism | Common Contaminants |
|-------|---------------|---------------------|
| Fruits and vegetables | Bacteria | *Erwinia, Pseudomonas, Corynebacterium* |
| | Fungi | *Aspergillus, Botrytis, Geotrichium, Rhizopus, Penicillium, Cladosporium, Alternaria, Phytopora,* various yeasts |
| Fresh meat | Bacteria | *Acinetobacter, Aeromonas, Pseudomonas* |
| Fish, poultry | Bacteria | *Micrococcus, Achromobacter, Flavobacterium, Proteus, Salmonella, Escherichia* |
| | Fungi | *Cladosporium, Mucor, Rhizopus, Penicillium, Geotrichum, Sporotrichum, Candida,* Torula, *Rhodotorula* |
| Milk | Bacteria | *Streptococcus, Leuconostoc, Lactococcus, Lactobacillus, Pseudomonas, Proteus* |
| High-sugar foods | Bacteria | *Clostridium, Bacillus, Flavobacterium* |
| | Fungi | *Saccharomyces,* Torula, *Penicillium* |

*Sources:* Jensen, M. et al., *Microbiology for the Health Sciences*, 4th edn., McGraw Hill, New York, 1997;
Chenault, A.A., *Nutrition and Health*, Holt, Rinehart and Winston, New York, 1984.

## TABLE 2.6
## Mycotoxins/Bacterial Toxins in Foods

**Toxins from Bacteria**

*Staphylococcus aureus*:

α-Exotoxin (lethal, dermonecrotic, hemolytic, leucolytic)

β-Exotoxin (hemolytic)

γ-Exotoxin (hemolytic)

Δ-Exotoxin (dermonecrotic, hemolytic)

Leucocidin (leucolytic)

Exfoliative toxin

Enterotoxin

*Clostridium botulinum* (four strains):

Toxins are lettered as A, B, Ca (1,2,D), Cb, D (C1 and D), E, F, and G. All of the toxins are
proteolytic and produce $NH_3$, $H_2S$, $CO_2$, and volatile amines. The toxins are hemolytic and
neurotoxic

*Escherichia coli* (several serotypes): induces diarrhea, vomiting; produces toxins that are heat labile

*Bacillus cereus* (several types): produces heat-labile enterotoxins that induce vomiting and diarrhea

Mycotoxins are also produced by the following fungi:

*Aspergillus flavis, Claviceps purpurea, Fusarium graminearum, Aspergillus ochraceus,
Aspergillus parasiticus,* and *Penicillium viridicatum*

*Sources:* Jensen, M. et al., *Microbiology for the Health Sciences*, 4th edn., McGraw Hill, New York, 1997;
Chenault, A.A., *Nutrition and Health*, Holt, Rinehart and Winston, New York, 1984.

## TABLE 2.7
## Antinutrients in Food

| Type of Factors | Effect of Factors | Legumes Containing the Factors |
|---|---|---|
| Antivitamin factors | Interfere with the actions of certain vitamins | Soybeans |
| Antivitamin A | Lipoxidase oxidizes and destroys carotene (provitamin A) | Soybeans |
| Antivitamin $B_{12}$ | Increases requirement for vitamin $B_{12}$ | Soybeans |
| Antivitamin D | Causes rickets unless extra vitamin D is provided | Alfalfa, common beans (*Phaseolus vulgaris*), peas (*Pisum sativum*) |
| Antivitamin E | Damage to the liver and muscles | |
| Cyanide-releasing glucosides | Releases hydrocyanic acid. The poison may also be released by an enzyme in *E. coli*, a normal inhabitant of the human intestine | All legumes contain at least small amounts of these factors; however, certain varieties of lima beans (*Phaseolus lunatus*) may contain much larger amounts |
| Favism factor | Causes the breakdown of red blood cells in susceptible individuals | Fava beans (*Vicia faba*) |
| Gas-generating carbohydrates | Certain indigestible carbohydrates are acted upon by gas-producing bacteria in the lower intestine | Many species of mature dry legume seeds, but not peanuts; the immature (green) seeds contain much lower amounts |
| Goitrogens | Interfere with the utilization of iodine by the thyroid gland | Peanuts and soybeans |
| Inhibitors of trypsin | The inhibitors bind with the digestive enzyme trypsin | All legumes contain trypsin inhibitors; these inhibitors are destroyed by heat |
| Lathyrogenic neurotoxins | Consumption of large quantities of lathyrogenic legumes for long periods (several months) results in severe neurological disorders | Lathyrus pea (*L. sativus*), which is grown mainly in India. Common vetch (*Vicia sativa*) may also be lathyrogenic |
| Metal binders | Bind copper, iron, manganese, and zinc | Soybeans, peas (*P. sativum*) |
| Red blood cell clumping agents (hemagglutinins) | The agents cause the red blood cells to clump together | Occurs in all legumes to some extent |

*Source:* Ensminger et al., *Food and Nutrition Encyclopedia*, 2nd edn., CRC Press, Boca Raton, FL, pp. 2082–2087, 1994.

Phytic acid, or myoinositol hexaphosphate, is a naturally occurring strong acid that binds to many types of bivalent and trivalent heavy metal ions, forming insoluble salts. Consequently, phytic acid reduces the availability of many minerals and essential trace elements. The degree of insolubility of these salts appears to depend on the nature of the metal, the pH of the solution, and for certain metals, on the presence of another metal. Synergism between two metallic ions in the formation of phytate complexes has also been observed. For instance, zinc–calcium phytate precipitates maximally at pH 6, which is also the pH of the duodenum, where calcium and trace metals are absorbed. Phytates occur in a wide variety of foods, such as cereals (e.g., wheat, rye, maize, rice, barley), legumes and vegetables (e.g., bean, soybean, lentil, pea, vetch), nuts and seeds (e.g., walnut, hazelnut, almond, peanut, cocoa bean), and spices and flavoring agents (e.g., caraway, coriander, cumin, mustard, nutmeg). From several experiments in animals and man, it has been observed that phytates exert negative effects on the availability of calcium, iron, magnesium, zinc, and other trace essential elements. These effects may be minimized considerably, if not eliminated, by increased intake of essential minerals. In the case of calcium, intake of cholecalciferol must also be adequate, since the activity of phytates on calcium absorption is enhanced when this vitamin is inadequate or limiting. In many foodstuffs, the phytic acid level can be reduced by phytase, an enzyme occurring in plants, which catalyzes the dephosphorylation of phytic acid.

Oxalic acid is a strong acid that forms water-soluble Na+ and K+ salts but less soluble salts with alkaline earth and other bivalent metals. Calcium oxalate is particularly insoluble at neutral or alkaline pH, whereas it readily dissolves in acid medium. Oxalates mainly exert effects on the absorption of calcium. These effects must be considered in terms of the oxalate/calcium ratio (in milliequivalent/milliequivalent): foods having a ratio greater than 1 may have negative effects on calcium availability, whereas foods with a ratio of 1 or below do not. Examples of foodstuffs having a ratio greater than 1 are rhubarb (8.5), spinach (4.3), beet (2.5–5.1), cocoa (2.6), coffee (3.9), tea (1.1), and potato (1.6). Harmful oxalates in food may be removed by soaking in water. Consumption of calcium-rich foods (e.g., dairy products and seafood), as well as augmented cholecalciferol intake, is recommended when large amounts of high-oxalate food are consumed.

A variety of plants contain a third group of type B antinutritives, the glucosinolates, also known as thioglucosides. Many glucosinolates are goitrogenic. They have a general structure and yield on hydrolysis the active or actual goitrogens, such as thiocyanates, isothiocyanates, cyclic sulfur compounds, and nitriles. Three types of goiter can be identified: (1) cabbage goiter, (2) brassica seed goiter, and (3) legume goiter. Cabbage goiter, also known as struma, is induced by excessive consumption of cabbage. It seems that cabbage goitrogens inhibit iodine uptake by directly affecting the thyroid gland. Cabbage goiter can be treated by iodine supplementation. Brassica seed goiter can result from the consumption of the seeds of Brassica plants

(e.g., rutabaga, turnip, cabbage, rape) that contain goitrogens that prevent thyroxine synthesis. This type of goiter can only be treated by administration of the thyroid hormone. Legume goiter is induced by goitrogens in legumes like soybeans and peanuts. It differs from cabbage goiter in that the thyroid gland does not lose its activity for iodine. Inhibition of the intestinal absorption of iodine or the reabsorption of thyroxine has been shown in this case. Legume goiter can be treated by iodine therapy. Glucosinolates that have been shown to induce goiter, at least in experimental animals, are found in several foods and feedstuffs: broccoli (buds), brussels sprouts (head), cabbage (head), cauliflower (buds), garden cress (leaves), horseradish (roots), kale (leaves), kohlrabi (head), black and white mustard (seed), radish (root), rape (seed), rutabaga (root), and turnips (root and seed). One of the most potent glucosinolates is progoitrin from the seeds of Brassica plants and the roots of rutabaga. Hydrolysis of this compound yields 1-cyano-2-hydroxy-3-butene, 1-cyano-2-hydroxy-3,4-butylepisulfide, 2-hydroxy-3,4-butenylisothiocyanate, and (S)-5-vinyl-oxazolidone-2-thione, also known as goitrin. The latter product interferes, together with its R enantiomer, in the iodination of thyroxine precursors, so that the resulting goiter cannot be treated by iodine therapy.

Type C antinutritives are naturally occurring substances that can inactivate vitamins, form unabsorbable complexes with them, or interfere with their digestive or metabolic utilization. They are also known as antivitamins. The most important type C antinutritives are ascorbic acid oxidase, antithiamine factors, and antipyridoxine factors.

Ascorbic acid oxidase is a copper-containing enzyme that catalyzes the oxidation of free ascorbic acid to diketogluconic acid, oxalic acid, and other oxidation products. It has been reported to occur in many fruits (e.g., peaches, bananas) and vegetables (e.g., cucumbers, pumpkins, lettuce, cress, cauliflowers, spinach, green beans, green peas, carrots, potatoes, tomatoes, beets, kohlrabi). The enzyme is active between pH 4 and 7 (optimum pH 5.6–6.0); its optimum temperature is 38°C. The enzyme is released when plant cells are broken. Therefore, if fruits and vegetables are cut, the vitamin C content decreases gradually. Ascorbic acid oxidase can be inhibited effectively at pH 2 or by blanching at around 100°C. Ascorbic acid can also be protected against ascorbic acid oxidase by substances of plant origin. Flavonoids, such as the flavonols, quercetin, and kaempferol, present in fruits and vegetables, strongly inhibit the enzyme.

A second group of type C antinutritives are the antithiamine factors, which interact with thiamine, also known as vitamin $B_1$. Antithiamine factors can be grouped as thiaminases, catechols, and tannins. Thiaminases, which are enzymes that split thiamine at the methylene linkage, are found in many freshwater and saltwater fish species and in certain species of crab and clam. They contain a nonprotein coenzyme structurally related to hemin. This coenzyme is the actual antithiamine factor. Thiaminases in fish and other sources can be destroyed by cooking. Antithiamine factors of plant origin include catechols and tannins. The most well-known ortho-catechol is found in bracken fern.

## TABLE 2.8
## Toxic Substances in Food (Toxic If Consumed in Excess)

| Poison (Toxin) | Sources | Symptoms and Signs | Distribution | Magnitude | Prevention | Treatment | Remarks |
|---|---|---|---|---|---|---|---|
| Aluminum (Al) | Food additives, mainly presented in such items as baking powder, pickles, and processed cheeses. Aluminum-containing antacids. | Abnormally large intakes of aluminum irritate the digestive tract. Also, unusual conditions have sometimes resulted in the absorption of sufficient aluminum from antacids, causing brain damage. Aluminum may form nonabsorbable complexes with essential trace elements, thereby creating deficiencies of these elements. | Aluminum is widely used throughout the world. | The United States uses aluminum more than any other minerals except iron. However, known cases of aluminum toxicity are rare. | Based on the evidence presented, no preventative measures are recommended. | | Aluminum toxicity has been reported in patients receiving renal dialysis |
| Arsenic (As) | Consumption of contaminated foods and beverages. Arsenical insecticides used in vineyards expose the workers (1) when spraying or (2) by inhaling contaminated dusts and plant debris. Arsenic in the air is from three major sources: smelting of metals, burning of coal, and use of arsenical pesticides. | Burning pain in the throat or stomach, cardiac abnormalities, and the odor of garlic on the breath. Other symptoms may be diarrhea and extreme thirst along with a choking sensation. Small doses of arsenic taken into the body over a long period of time may produce hyperkeratosis (irregularities in pigmentation, especially on the trunk), arterial insufficiency, and cancer. There is strong evidence that inorganic arsenic is a skin and lung carcinogen in humans. | Arsenic is widely distributed, but the amount of the element consumed by humans in food and water, or breathed, is very small and not harmful. | Cases of arsenic toxicity in humans are infrequent. Two noteworthy episodes occurred in Japan in 1955. One involved tainted powdered milk; the other contaminated soy sauce. The toxic milk caused 12,131 cases of infant poisoning, with 130 deaths. The soy sauce poisoned 220 people. | | Induce vomiting, followed by an antidote of egg whites in water or milk. Afterward, give strong coffee or tea, followed by Epsom salts in water or castor oil. | Arsenic is known to partially protect against selenium poisoning. The highest residues of arsenic are generally in the hair and nails. Arsenic in soils may sharply decrease crop growth and yields, but it is not a hazard to people or livestock that eat plants grown in these fields. |
| Chromium (Cr) | Food, water, and air contaminated by chromium compounds in industrialized areas. | Inorganic chromium salt reduces the absorption of zinc; hence, zinc deficiency symptoms may become evident in chronic chromium toxicity. | Chromium toxicity is not common. | Chromium toxicity is not very common. | It is unlikely that people will get too much chromium, because (1) only minute amounts of the element are present in most foods, (2) the body utilizes chromium poorly, and (3) the toxic dose is about 10,000 times the lowest effective medical dose. | | |

*(continued)*

**TABLE 2.8 (continued)**
**Toxic Substances in Food (Toxic If Consumed in Excess)**

| Poison (Toxin) | Sources | Symptoms and Signs | Distribution | Magnitude | Prevention | Treatment | Remarks |
|---|---|---|---|---|---|---|---|
| Copper (Cu) | Diets with excess copper but low in other minerals that counteract its effects. Acid foods or beverages (vinegar, carbonated beverages, or citrus juices) that have been in prolonged contact with copper metal may cause acute gastrointestinal disturbances. | Acute copper toxicity: characterized by headache, dizziness, metallic taste, excessive salivation, nausea, vomiting, stomachache, diarrhea, and weakness. If the disease is allowed to get worse, there may also be racing of the heart, high blood pressure, jaundice, hemolytic anemia, dark-pigmented urine, kidney disorders, and even death. Chronic copper toxicity may be contributory to iron-deficiency anemia, mental illness following childbirth (postpartum psychosis), certain types of schizophrenia, and perhaps heart attacks. | Copper toxicity may occur wherever there is excess copper intake, especially when accompanied by low iron, molybdenum, sulfur, zinc, and vitamin C. | The incidence of copper toxicity is extremely rare in humans. Its occurrence in significant form is almost always limited to (1) suicide attempts by ingestion of large quantities of copper salt or (2) a genetic defect in copper metabolism inherited as an autosomal recessive, known as Wilson's disease. | Avoid foods and beverages that have been in prolonged contact with copper metal. | Administration of copper-chelating agents to remove excess copper. | Copper is essential to human life and health, but as with all heavy metals, it may be toxic in excess. |
| Ergot | Rye, wheat, barley, oats, and triticale carry this mycotoxin. Ergot replaces the seed in the heads of cereal grains, in which it appears as a purplish-black, hard, banana-shaped, dense mass from ¼ to ¾ in. (6 to 9 mm) long. | When a large amount of ergot is consumed in a short period, convulsive ergotism is observed. The symptoms include itching, numbness, severe muscle cramps, sustained spasms and convulsions, and extreme pain. When smaller amounts of ergot are consumed over an extended period, ergotism is characterized by gangrene of the fingertips and toes, caused by blood vessel and muscle contraction stopping blood circulation in the extremities. These symptoms include cramps, swelling, inflammation, alternating burning and freezing sensations ("St. Anthony's fire"), and numbness; eventually the hands and feet may turn black, shrink, and fall off. Ergotism is a cumulative poison, depending on the amount of ergot eaten and the length of time over which it is eaten. | Ergot is found throughout the world wherever rye, wheat, barley, oats, or triticale is grown. | There is considerable ergot, especially in rye. But, normally, screening grains before processing alleviates ergotism in people. | Consists of an ergot-free diet. Ergot in food and feed grains may be removed by screening the grains before processing. In the United States, wheat and rye containing more than 0.3% ergot are classed as "ergoty." In Canada, government regulations prohibit more than 0.1% ergot in feeds. | An ergot-free diet; good nursing; treatment by a doctor. | Six different alkaloids are involved in ergot poisoning. Ergot is used to aid the uterus to contract after childbirth, to prevent loss of blood. Also, another ergot drug (ergotamine) is widely used in the treatment of migraine headaches. |

| | | | | | | | |
|---|---|---|---|---|---|---|---|
| Fluorine (F) (fluorosis) | Ingestion of excessive quantities of fluorine through either the food or water, or a combination of these. Except in certain industrial exposures, the intake of fluoride inhaled from the air is only a small fraction of the total fluoride intake in humans. Pesticides containing fluorides, including those used to control insects, weeds, and rodents. Although water is the principal source of fluoride in an average human diet in the United States, fluoride is frequently contained in toothpaste, tooth powder, chewing gums, mouthwashes, vitamin supplements, and mineral supplements. | Acute fluoride poisoning: abdominal pain, diarrhea, vomiting, excessive salivation, thirst, perspiration, and painful spasms of the limbs. Chronic fluoride poisoning: abnormal teeth (especially mottled enamel) during the first 8 years of life and brittle bones. Other effects, predicted from animal studies, may include loss of body weight and altered structure and function of the thyroid gland and kidneys. Water containing 3–10 ppm of fluoride may cause mottling of the teeth. An average daily intake of 20–80 mg of fluoride over a period of 10–20 years will result in crippling fluorosis. | The water in parts of Arkansas, California, South Carolina, and Texas contains excess fluorine. Occasionally, throughout the United States, high-fluorine phosphates are used in mineral mixtures. | Generally speaking, fluorosis is limited to high-fluorine areas. Only a few instances of health effects in humans have been attributed to airborne fluoride, and they occurred in persons living in the vicinity of fluoride-emitting industries. | Avoid the use of food and water containing excessive fluorine. | Any damage may be permanent, but people who have not developed severe symptoms may be helped to some extent if the source of excess fluorine is eliminated. High dietary levels of calcium and magnesium may reduce the absorption and utilization of fluoride. | Fluorine is a cumulative poison. The total fluoride in the human body averages 2.57 g. Susceptibility to fluoride toxicity is increased by deficiencies of calcium, vitamin C, and protein. Virtually all foods contain trace amounts of fluoride. |
| Lead (Pb) | Consuming food or medicinal products (including health food products) contaminated with lead. Inhaling the poison as a dust by workers in such industries as painting, lead mining, and refining. Inhaling airborne lead discharged into the air from auto exhaust fumes. | Develop rapidly in young children but slowly in mature people. Acute lead poisoning: colic, cramps, diarrhea or constipation, leg cramps, and drowsiness. The most severe form of lead poisoning, encountered in infants and in heavy drinkers of illicitly distilled whiskey, is characterized by profound disturbances of the central nervous system and permanent damage to the brain and damage to the kidneys and shortened life span of the erthrocytes. | Predominantly among children who may eat chips of lead-containing paints, peeled off from painted wood. | The Centers for Disease Control, Atlanta, GA, estimates that (1) lead poisoning claims the lives of 200 children each year and (2) 400,000–600,000 children have elevated lead levels in the blood. Lead poisoning has been reduced significantly with the use of lead-free paint. | Avoid inhaling or consuming lead. | Acute lead poisoning: an emetic (induce vomiting), followed by drinking plenty of milk and ½ oz (14 g) of Epsom salts in half glass of water. | Lead is a cumulative poison. When incorporated in the soil, nearly all the lead is converted into forms that are not available to plants. Any lead taken up by plant roots tends to stay in the roots, rather than move up to the top of the plant. |

(continued)

**TABLE 2.8 (continued)**
**Toxic Substances in Food (Toxic If Consumed in Excess)**

| Poison (Toxin) | Sources | Symptoms and Signs | Distribution | Magnitude | Prevention | Treatment | Remarks |
|---|---|---|---|---|---|---|---|
| | Consuming food crops contaminated by lead being deposited on the leaves and other edible portions of the plant by direct fallout. Consuming food or water contaminated by contact with lead pipes or utensils. Old houses in which the interiors were painted with leaded paints prior to 1945—the chipped wall paint is sometimes eaten by children. Such miscellaneous sources as illicitly distilled whiskey, improperly lead-glazed earthenware, old battery casings used as fuel, and toys containing lead. | Chronic lead poisoning: colic, constipation, lead palsy especially in the forearm and fingers, the symptoms of chronic nephritis, and sometimes mental depression, convulsions, and a blue line at the edge of the gums. | | | | Chronic lead poisoning: remove the source of lead. Sometimes treated by administration of magnesium or lead sulfate solution as a laxative and antidote on the lead in the digestive system, followed by potassium iodide, which cleanses the tracts. Currently, treatment of lead poisoning makes use of chemicals that bind the metal in the body and help in its removal. | Lead poisoning can be diagnosed positively by analyzing the blood tissue for lead content; clinical signs of lead poisoning usually are manifested at blood lead concentrations above 80 mg/100 g. |

| | | | | | | |
|---|---|---|---|---|---|---|
| Mercury (Hg) | Mercury is discharged into air and water from industrial operations and is used in herbicide and fungicide treatments. Mercury poisoning has occurred where mercury from industrial plants has been discharged into water, then accumulated as methylmercury in fish and shellfish. Accidental consumption of seed grains treated with fungicides that contain mercury, used for the control of fungus diseases of oats, wheat, barley, and flax. | The toxic effects of organic and inorganic compounds of mercury are dissimilar. The organic compounds of mercury, such as the various fungicides (1), affect the central nervous system and (2) are not corrosive. The inorganic compounds of mercury include mainly mercuric chloride, a disinfectant; mercurous chloride (calomel), a cathartic; and elemental mercury. Commonly the toxic symptoms are corrosive gastrointestinal effects, such as vomiting, bloody diarrhea, and necrosis of the alimentary mucosa. | Wherever mercury is produced in industrial operations or used in herbicide or fungicide treatments. | Limited. But about 1200 cases of mercury poisoning identified in Japan in the 1950s were traced to the consumption of fish and shellfish from Japan's Minamata Bay contaminated with methylmercury. Some of the offsprings of exposed mothers were born with birth defects, and many victims suffered central nervous system damage. Another outbreak of mercury toxicity occurred in Iraq, where more than 6000 people were hospitalized after eating bread made from wheat that had been treated with methylmercury. | Control mercury pollution from industrial operations. | Mercury is a cumulative poison. Food and Drug Administration prohibits use of mercury-treated grain for food or feed. Grain crops produced from mercury-treated seed and crops produced on soils treated with mercury herbicides have not been found to contain harmful concentrations of this element. |
| Polychlorinated biphenyls (PCBs), industrial chemicals; chlorinated hydrocarbons, which may cause cancer when taken into the food supply. | Sources of contamination to humans include. | Clinical effects on people are eruption of the skin resembling acne, visual disturbances, jaundice, numbness, and spasms. Newborn infants from mothers who have been poisoned show discoloration of the skin, which regresses after 2–5 months. PCBs are fat soluble. | | PCBs are widespread. Their use by industry is declining. | | PCBs have been widely used in dielectric fluids in capacitors and transformers, hydraulic fluids, and heat-transfer fluids. Also, they have more than 50 minor uses including plasticizers and solvents in adhesives, printing ink, sealants, moisture retardants, paints, and pesticide carriers. |

*(continued)*

**TABLE 2.8 (continued)**
**Toxic Substances in Food (Toxic If Consumed in Excess)**

| Poison (Toxin) | Sources | Symptoms and Signs | Distribution | Magnitude | Prevention | Treatment | Remarks |
|---|---|---|---|---|---|---|---|
| | (1) contaminated foods, (2) mammals or birds that have fed on contaminated foods of fish, (3) residues on foods that have been wrapped in papers and plastics containing PCBs, (4) milk from cows that have been fed silage from silos coated with PCB-containing paint, and eggs from layers fed feeds contaminated with PCBs. | | | | | | PCB causes cancer in laboratory animals (rats, mice, and rhesus monkeys). It is not known if it will cause cancer in humans. More study is needed to gauge its effects on the ecological food chain and on human health. When fed, coho salmon from Lake Michigan with 10–15 ppm PCB, mink in Wisconsin, stopped reproducing or their kits died. |
| Salt (NaCl/ sodium chloride) poisoning. | Consumption of high-salt food and beverages. | Salt may be toxic (1) when it is fed to infants or others whose kidneys cannot excrete the excess in the urine or (2) when the body is adapted to a chronic low-salt diet. | Salt is used all over the world. Hence, the potential for salt poisoning exists everywhere. | Salt poisoning is relatively rare. | Drink large quantities of freshwater. | | Even normal salt concentration may be toxic if water intake is low. |

| | | | | | | |
|---|---|---|---|---|---|---|
| Selenium (Se) | Consumption of high levels in food or drinking water. Presence of malnutrition, parasitic infestation, or other factors, which make people highly susceptible to selenium toxicity. | Abnormalities in the hair, nails, and skin. Children in a high-selenium area of Venezuela showed loss of hair, discolored skin, and chronic digestive disturbances. Normally, people who have consumed large excesses of selenium excrete it as trimethyl selenide in the urine or as dimethyl selenide in the breath. The latter substance has an odor resembling garlic. | In certain regions of western United States, especially in South Dakota, Montana, Wyoming, Nebraska, Kansas, and perhaps areas in other states in the Great Plains and Rocky Mountains. Also, in Canada. | Selenium toxicity in people is relatively rare. | Selenium toxicity may be counteracted by arsenic or copper, but such treatment should be carefully monitored. | Confirmed cases of selenium poisoning in people are rare, because (1) only traces are present in most foods, (2) foods generally come from a wide area, and (3) the metabolic processes normally convert excess selenium into harmless substances that are excreted in the urine or breath. |
| Tin (Sn) | From acid fruits and vegetables canned in tin cans. The acids in such foods as citrus fruits and tomato products can leach tin from the inside of the can. Then the tin is ingested with the canned food. In the digestive tract, tin goes through a methylation process in which nontoxic tin is converted to methylated tin, which is toxic. | Methylated tin is a neurotoxin—a toxin that attacks the central nervous system, the symptoms of which are numbness of the fingers and lips followed by a loss of speech and hearing. Eventually, the afflicted person becomes spastic, then coma and death follow. | Worldwide. | The use of tin in advanced industrial societies has increased 14-fold over the last 10 years. | Tin cans are rare. Many tin cans are coated on the inside with enamel or other materials. Most cans are steel. | Currently, not much is known about the amount of tin in the human diet. |

*Sources:* Ensminger et al., *Food and Nutrition Encyclopedia*, 2nd edn., CRC Press, Boca Raton, FL, 1994; Chenault, A.A., *Nutrition and Health*, Holt, Rinehart and Winston, New York, 1984.

**TABLE 2.9**
**Edible Weeds**

| Common Name | Scientific Name | Use |
|---|---|---|
| Maple tree | *Acer* (many varieties) | Sap can be collected and reduced by evaporation into syrup. |
| Sweet flag | *Acorus calamus* | Rootstocks or stems are edible with a sweet taste. Young shoots can be used as salad. |
| Quackgrass | *Agropyron repens* L. (has many other names) | Rootstocks can be chewed or scorched to use as coffee substitute; seeds can be used for breadstuffs and for beer. |
| Water plantain | *Alisma* spp. | Root is starchy and edible; should be dried to reduce acrid taste. Three varieties of this plant can be toxic. |
| Garlic mustard | *Alliaria petiolata* | Leaf, stem, flower, and fruit are spicy and hot. If cooked, some of this spiciness is lost. Several plants that resemble this one are not edible. |
| Wild garlic | *Allium vineale* L. | Used as an herbal seasoning; there are similar plants that are not garlic in aroma; they can be toxic. |
| Pigweed | *Amaranthus* spp. | Leaves from a young plant can be eaten raw as salad or boiled as is spinach. |
| Serviceberry | *Amelanchier* spp. | Berries are rich and sweet; pits and leaves contain cyanide; also called shadbush or juneberry. |
| Hog peanut | *Amphicarpaea bracteata* | Fleshy seedpods found underground are edible. |
| Groundnut | *Apios americana* Medik | Root can be eaten raw or cooked. Seeds can also be used. Europeans use the term groundnut to refer to peanuts. This is not the same plant. |
| Common burdock | *Arctium minus* | Young leaves can be eaten as salad; roots are carrot-like in shape and can be cooked (boiled) and eaten. A little baking soda added to the cooking water improves tenderness and flavor. Scorched roots can be used as a coffee substitute. |
| Giant reed | *Arundo donax* L. | Young shoots and rootstalks are sometimes sweet enough to be used as a substitute for sugar cane. Infusions of the rootstocks can have some herbal properties—local weak anesthetic and in some instances either a hypotensive agent or hypertensive agent (depends on dose). |
| Milkweed | *Asclepias syriaca* L. | Young shoots and flower buds boiled with at least two changes of water. The plant contains cardiac glycosides and can be toxic. |
| Pawpaw | *Asimina triloba* L. | The aromatic fruits are quite tasty. Seeds and bark have pesticide properties and should be handled with caution. |
| Wild oat | *Avena fatua* L. | Seeds are similar to cultivated oats. Useful when dried and ground as a cereal. Seeds can be scorched and used as a coffee substitute. |
| Winter cress/yellow rocket | *Barbarea* spp. (*B. vcma, B. vulgaris*) | Young leaves and stems can be used as a salad. |
| Birches | *Betula* spp. (Betulacea) | Spring sap can be reduced to a syrup; bark can be boiled for tea. |
| Mustard, black, or yellow | *Brassica nigra* | Seeds used to prepare mustard; leaves can be boiled for consumption, as can young stalks. |
| Bromegrass | *Bromus japonicus* | Seeds can be dried, ground, and used as cereal. |
| Shepherd's purse | *Capsella bursa-pastoris* | Seeds are used as a spicy pot herb. Tender young shoots can be eaten raw. Has a peppery taste. |
| Bittercress | *Cardamme bulbosa* | Roots can be ground for a horseradish substitute; leaves and stems can be added to salad. The roots of some species (*C. bulbosa*) can be toxic. |
| Hornbeam | *Carpus caroliniana* | Nuts are edible. |
| Hickory | *Carya* spp. | Nuts are edible. |
| Chestnut | *Castanea* spp. | Nuts are edible but are covered by a prickly coat. Roasting improves flavor and texture. |
| Sandbur | *Cenchrus* spp. | Seeds and burrs can be used as cereal grains. |
| Lambsquarter | *Chenopodium album* L. | Leaves can be eaten raw or cooked as spinach. The Mexican version (Mexican tea, *C. ambrosioides*) is toxic. |
| Oxeye daisy | *Chrysanthemum leucanthemum* | Leaves and flowers can be eaten raw or cooked. |
| Chicory | *Cichorium intybus* L. | Leaves are good salad ingredients. |
| Thistles | *Cirsium* spp. | The taproot is chewy but tasty. |
| Wandering Jew | *Commelina communis* | Leaves can be used as potherbs; flowering shoots can be eaten raw. |
| Hawthorn | *Crataegus* spp. | Berries are edible; thorns can be a problem when gathering the berries. Some species contain heart stimulants. |
| Wild chervil | *Cryptotaenia canadensis* | Roots can be boiled, with a taste like parsnips; young leaves and stems can be eaten as salad; has an herb used in stews and soups. |
| Nut grass | *Cyperus* spp. | Tubers can be eaten or ground up to make a beverage called "chufa" or "horchata". |
| Queen Anne's lace, also called wild carrot | *Daucus carota* L. | Root can be eaten after boiling; however, because it looks like poisonous hemlock, one should be cautious. |
| Crabgrass | *Digitaria sanguinalis* L. | Seeds can be dried and ground for use as a cereal. |
| Persimmon | *Diospyros virginiana* L. | Fruits when ripe are very sweet. |

**TABLE 2.9 (continued)**
**Edible Weeds**

| Common Name | Scientific Name | Use |
|---|---|---|
| Barnyard grass | *Echinochloa crus-galli* L. | Seeds can be dried and used as cereal. |
| Russian olive | *Elaeagnus angustifolia* L. | Fruits are edible though astringent. |
| American burnweed | *Erechtites hieracifolia* | Leaves can be eaten raw as salad or cooked. |
| Redstem filaree | *Erodium cicutarium* | Tender leaves are eaten as salad; can also be used as potherb. |
| Wild strawberry | *Fragaria virginiana* | Fruits are small but delicious. |
| Catchweed bedstraw | *Galium aparine* | Young shoots are good potherbs; leaves and stems can be steamed and eaten as vegetable. |
| Wintergreen | *Gaultheria procumbens* L. | Berries, foliage, and bark can be used to make tea. Berries can be eaten raw. |
| Huckleberry | *Gaylussacia baccata* | Berries can be eaten raw or cooked. |
| Honey locust | *Gleditsia triacanthos* | The pulp around the seeds can be used as a sweetener. (Tender green pods can also be cooked and eaten as a vegetable.) The tree is similar in appearance to the Kentucky coffee tree, and the pods of this tree cannot be eaten. |
| Jerusalem artichoke | *Helianthus tuberosus* | The tubers are crisp and can be used in place of Chinese chestnuts in salads; can also be cooked and mashed. |
| Daylily | *Hemerocallis fulva* L. | Flower buds can be used in salads. Tubers can be cooked and eaten. Can cause diarrhea in sensitive people. |
| Foxtail barley | *Hordeum jubatum* | Seeds can be dried and used as cereal. |
| Touch-me-not | *Impatiens* spp. | Leaves can be used for an herbal tea; leaves can be eaten as salad; pods are also edible. |
| Burning bush | *Kochia scoparia* | Young shoots can be used as a potherb; seeds can be dried and used as cereal. |
| Prickly lettuce | *Lactuca serriola* L. | Young leaves can be used as salad but may have a bitter taste. |
| Virginia peppergrass | *Lepidium virginicum* | Has a pungent mustard-like taste; used as a potherb. |
| Bugleweed | *Lycoris* spp. | Roots can be eaten raw or cooked. |
| Common mallow | *Malva neglecta* | Boiled leaves have a slimy consistency much like okra. Flower buds can be pickled; leaves can be used as a thickener for soup. |
| Black medic | *Medicago lupulina* | Sprouts can be added to salads for texture; leaves can be used as a potherb. |
| Mulberry | *Mortis* spp. | Berries can be eaten out of hand. |
| Watercress | *Nasturtium officinale* R. | Leaves can be eaten raw or used as a potherb. |
| American lotus | *Nelumbo lutea* | Entire plant is edible. |
| Yellow water lily | *Nuphar luteum* L. | Tubers when cooked are a starch substitute. |
| Fragrant water lily | *Nymphaea odorata* | Flower buds and young leaves can be boiled and eaten; seeds can be dried and used as cereal. |
| Evening primrose | *Oenothera biennis* L. | Seeds are a source of g-linolenic acid; taproots can be eaten raw or cooked. |
| Wood sorrel | *Oxalis* spp. | Leaves can be eaten cooked or raw; seedpods can also be eaten. |
| Perilla mint | *Perilla frutescens* L. | Leaves can be eaten cooked or raw. |
| Common reed | *Phragmites communis* | Young shoots are edible. Plant is similar to the poisonous *Arundo*, so the forager should be very careful to correctly identify the plant. |
| Ground-cherry (Chinese lanterns) | *Physalis heterophylla* | Berries can be eaten cooked or raw. |
| Pokeweed | *Phytolacca americana* L. | Young shoots can be used as a potherb; berries and roots may be poisonous. |
| Plantain | *Plantago major* L. | Leaves can be used in salads. |
| Mayapple | *Podophyllum peltatum* | Fruits are edible raw or cooked; rest of the plant may be poisonous. |
| Japanese knotweed | *Polygonum cuspidatum* | Young sprouts can be cooked and eaten like asparagus. |
| Purslane | *Portulaca oleracea* L. | Young leaves can be used as a potherb or salad ingredient. |
| Healall | *Prunella vulgaris* L. | Boiled and used as a potherb. |
| Wild cherry | *Prunus serotina* | Fruits are edible. |
| Kudzu | *Pueraria lobata* | Roots and leaves are edible. |
| Rock chestnut oak | *Quercus prinus* L. | Nuts (acorns) are edible. |
| Sumac | *Rhus glabra* L. | Berries are edible as are the roots; however, some people are allergic to all parts of the plant and will develop skin rash. |
| Multiflora rose | *Rosa multiflora* | The hips are edible in small quantities. |
| Raspberry, blackberry | *Rubus* spp. | Fruits are eaten raw or used to make juice or jam. |
| Red sorrel | *Rumex acetosella* L. | Leaves can be eaten as salad or cooked in water. The leaves contain a lot of oxalic acid, so small quantities would be preferred. |
| Arrowhead | *Sagittaria latifolia* Willd | Roots can be eaten raw or cooked. Plants resemble the poisonous jack-in-the-pulpit plant, so gatherers should beware. |

*(continued)*

**TABLE 2.9 (continued)**
**Edible Weeds**

| Common Name | Scientific Name | Use |
|---|---|---|
| Elderberry | *Sambucus canadensis* | Fruits can be eaten raw or cooked. |
| Hardstem bulrush | *Scirpus acutus* Muhl | Roots can be boiled and eaten. |
| Foxtail grass | *Setaria* spp. | Seed grains can be dried and used as cereal. |
| Tumble mustard | *Sisymbrium altissimum* L. | All parts of the plant are edible but have a strong mustard flavor; better used as a potherb. |
| Roundleaf Catbriar | *Smilax rotundifolia* L. | Young tender shoots can be eaten raw. Young leaves can be eaten as salad; roots can be used for tea. |
| Sow thistle | *Sonchus oleraceus* L. | Leaves are prickly and bitter but can be used as a potherb. |
| Johnson grass | *Sorghum halepense* L. | Young shoots can be eaten raw; seeds can be dried and used as cereal; mature stalks can be ground and the liquid extracted for use as syrup. |
| Chickweed | *Stellaria media* L. | Leaves can be eaten raw or cooked. |
| Dandelion | *Taraxacum officinale* | All parts of the plant are edible. |
| Stinkweed | *Thlaspi arvense* L. | All parts of the plant are edible after cooking. |
| Western salsify | *Tragopogon dubius* Scopoli | Roots can be eaten after boiling; leaves, flowers, and stems can be eaten raw. |
| Red clover | *Trifolium pratense* L. | Flowers can be boiled to make a broth; powdered leaves and flowers can be used as seasoning. |
| Coltsfoot | *Tussilago farfara* L. | Can be used as a potherb in small amounts. |
| Cattail | *Typha* spp. | Roots, stalks, and spears are edible. |
| Stinging nettle | *Urtica dioica* L. | Can be eaten cooked or used as a potherb. |
| Bellwort | *Uvularia perfoliata* L. | Young shoots can be cooked and eaten; leaves are bitter. |
| Blueberry, gooseberry | *Vaccinium stamineum* | Berries can be eaten raw or used to make juice, jam, or jelly. |
| Violet | *Viola papilionacea* Purish | Flowers are edible. |
| Wild grapes | *Vitis* spp. | Fruits can be eaten raw or cooked. |
| Spanish bayonet | *Yucca filamentosa* L. | Flower buds can be eaten raw. |

*Sources:* Duke, J.A., *Handbook of Edible Weeds*, CRC Press, Boca Raton, FL, 1992; Ensminger, A.H. et al., *Food and Nutrition Encyclopedia*, 2nd edn., CRC Press, Boca Raton, FL, 1994.

*Notes:* (1) Persons using this list should be aware that individuals may differ in their responses to these plants. For some consumers, allergic reactions may be elicited. For others, there may be chemicals in the plants that elicit an undesirable physiological effect. Still other plants, especially the water plants, may harbor parasites that may be injurious. The serious forager should consult a plant taxonomist to be sure that the plant gathered is an edible plant. There are many similar plants that may in fact be poisonous, while others are safe to consume. (2) Weeds are plants that grow in places where we humans do not want them to grow. As such, we may not recognize them as food. The aforementioned plants contain edible portions. Not all parts of these plants may be useful as human food. Some varieties, in fact, may contain toxic chemicals that, if consumed in large quantities, may cause problems. A number of the plants have been identified based on their use by Native Americans. These plants can have many different names as common names.

In fact, there are two types of heat-stable antithiamine factors in this fern, one of which has been identified as caffeic acid, which can also by hydrolyzed from chlorogenic acid (found in green coffee beans) by intestinal bacteria. Other ortho-catechols, such as methylsinapate occurring in mustard seed and rapeseed, also have antithiamine activity. The mechanism of thiamine inactivation by these compounds requires oxygen and is dependent on temperature and pH. The reaction appears to proceed in two phases: a rapid initial phase, which is reversible by addition of reducing agents (e.g., ascorbic acid), and a slower subsequent phase, which is irreversible. Tannins, occurring in a variety of plants, including tea, similarly possess antithiamine activity. Thiamine is one of the vitamins likely to be deficient in the diet. Thus, persistent consumption of antithiamine factors and the possible presence of thiaminase-producing bacteria in the gastrointestinal tract may compromise the already marginal thiamine intake.

A variety of plants and mushrooms contain pyridoxine antagonists. These compounds interfere with the use of vitamin $B_6$ and are called antipyridoxine factors. They are hydrazine derivatives. Linseed contains the water-soluble and heat-labile antipyridoxine factor linatine (g-glutamyl-1-amino-D-proline). Hydrolysis of linatine yields the actual antipyridoxine factor 1-amino-proline. Antipyridoxine factors have also been found in wild mushrooms, the common commercial edible mushroom, and the Japanese mushroom shiitake. Commercial and shiitake mushrooms contain agaritine. Hydrolysis of agaritine by g-glutamyl transferase, which is endogenous to the mushroom, yields the active agent 4-hydroxymethylphenylhydrazine. Disruption of the cells of the mushroom can accelerate hydrolysis; careful handling of the mushrooms and immediate blanching after cleaning and cutting can prevent hydrolysis. The mechanism underlying the antipyridoxine activity is believed to be condensation of the hydrazines with the carbonyl

**TABLE 2.10**
**Toxic Plants**

| Common and Scientific Name | Description | Toxic Parts | Geographical Distribution | Poisoning | Symptoms | Remarks |
|---|---|---|---|---|---|---|
| Baneberry and *Actaea* sp. | Perennial growing to 3 ft (1 m) tall from a thick root; compound leaves; small, white flowers; white or red berries with several seeds borne in short, terminal clusters | All parts but primarily roots and berries | Native woodlands of North America from Canada south to Georgia, Alabama, Louisiana, Oklahoma, and the northern Rockies; red-fruited western baneberry from Alaska to central California, Arizona, Montana, and South Dakota | Attributed to a glycoside or essential oil, which causes severe inflammation of the digestive tract | Acute stomach cramps, headache, increased pulse, vomiting, delirium, dizziness, and circulatory failure | As few as six berries can cause symptoms persisting for hours. Treatment may be a gastric lavage or vomiting. Bright red berries attract children. |
| Buckeye (horse chestnut) and *Aesculus* sp. | Shrub or tree; deciduous, opposite, palmately, divided leaves with five to nine leaflets on a long stalk; red, yellow, or white flowers; two- to three-valved, capsule fruit; with thick, leathery husk enclosing one to six brown shiny seeds | Leaves, twigs, flowers, and seeds | Various species throughout the United States and Canada; some cultivated as ornamentals; others grow wild | Toxic parts contain the glycoside, esculin | Nervous twitching of muscles, weakness, lack of coordination, dilated pupils, nausea, vomiting, diarrhea, depression, paralysis, and stupor | By making a "tea" from the leaves and twigs or by eating the seeds, children have been poisoned. Honey collected from the buckeye flower may also cause poisoning. Roots, branches, and fruits have been used to stupefy fish in ponds. Treatment usually is a gastric lavage or vomiting. |
| Buttercup and *Ranunculus* sp. | Annual or perennial herb growing to 16–32 in. (41–81 cm) high; leaves alternate entire to compound and largely basal; yellow flowers borne singly or in clusters on ends of seed stalks; small fruits, single-seeded pods | Entire plant | Widely distributed in woods, meadows, pastures, and along streams throughout temperate and cold locations | The alkaloid protoanemonin, which can injure the digestive system and ulcerate the skin | Burning sensation of the mouth, nervousness, nausea, vomiting, low blood pressure, weak pulse, depression, and convulsions | Sap and leaves may cause dermatitis. Cows poisoned by buttercups produce bitter milk or milk with a reddish color. |
| Castor bean and *Ricinus communis* | Shrub-like herb 4–12 ft (1.2–3.7 m) tall; simple, alternate, long-stalked leaves with 5–11 long lobes, which are toothed on margins; fruits oval, green, or red and covered with spines; three elliptical, glossy, black, white, or mottled seeds per capsule | Entire plant, especially the seeds | Cultivated as an ornamental or oilseed crop primarily in the southern part of the United States and Hawaii | Seeds, pressed cake, and leaves poisonous when chewed; contain the phytotoxin, ricin | Burning of the mouth and throat, nausea, vomiting, severe stomach pains, bloody diarrhea, excessive thirst, prostration, dullness of vision, and convulsions; kidney failure and death 1–12 days later | Fatal dose for a child is one to three seeds and for an adult two to eight seeds. The oil extracted from the seeds is an important commercial product. It is not poisonous and it is used as a medicine (castor oil), for soap, and as a lubricant. |

*(continued)*

## TABLE 2.10 (continued)
## Toxic Plants

| Common and Scientific Name | Description | Toxic Parts | Geographical Distribution | Poisoning | Symptoms | Remarks |
|---|---|---|---|---|---|---|
| Chinaberry and *Melia azedarach* | Deciduous tree 20–40 ft (6–12 m) tall; twice, pinnately divided leaves and toothed or lobed leaflets, purple flowers borne in clusters; yellow, wrinkled, rounded berries that persist throughout the winter | Berries, bark, flowers, and leaves | A native of Asia introduced as an ornamental in the United States; common in the southern United States and lower altitudes in Hawaii; has become naturalized in old fields, pastures, around buildings, and along fence rows | Most result from eating pulp of berries; toxic principal is a resinoid with narcotic effects | Nausea, vomiting, diarrhea, irregular breathing, and respiratory distress | Six to eight berries can cause the death of a child. The berries have been used to make insecticide and flea powder. |
| Death camas and *Zigadenus paniculatus* | Perennial herb resembling wild onions but the onion odor is lacking; long, slender leaves with parallel veins; pale yellow to pink flowers in clusters on slender seed stalks; fruit a three-celled capsule | Entire plant, especially the bulb | Various species occur throughout the United States and Canada; all are more or less poisonous | Due to the alkaloids zygadenine, veratrine, and others | Excessive salivation, muscular weakness, slow heart rate, low blood pressure, subnormal temperature, nausea, vomiting, diarrhea, prostration, coma, and sometimes death | The members of Lewis and Clark Expedition made flour from the bulbs and suffered the symptoms of poisoning. Later some pioneers died when they mistook death camas for wild onions or garlic. |
| Dogbane (Indian hemp) and *Apocynum cannabinum* | Perennial herbs with milky juice and somewhat woody stems; simple, smooth, and oppositely paired leaves; bell-shaped, small, white to pink flowers borne in clusters at ends of axillary stems; paired, long, slender seedpods | Entire plant | Various species growing throughout North America in fields and forests and along streams and roadsides | Only suspected, as it contains the toxic glycoside, cymarin, and is poisonous to animals | In animals, increased temperature and pulse, cold extremities, dilation of the pupils, discoloration of the mouth and nose, sore mouth, sweating, loss of appetite, and death | Compounds extracted from roots of dogbane have been used to make a heart stimulant. |
| Foxglove and *Digitalis purpurea* | Biennial herb with alternate, simple, toothed leaves; terminal, showy raceme of flowers, purple, pink, rose, yellow, or white; dry capsule fruit | Entire plant, especially leaves, flowers, and seeds | Native of Europe commonly planted in gardens of the United States; naturalized and abundant in some parts of the western United States | Due to digitalis component | Nausea, vomiting, dizziness, irregular heartbeat, tremors, convulsions, and possibly death | Foxglove has long been known as a source of digitalis and steroid glycosides. It is an important medicinal plant when used correctly. |
| Henbane and *Hyoscyamus niger* | Erect annual or biennial herb with coarse, hairy stems 1–5 ft (30–152 cm) high; simple, oblong, alternate leaves with a few, coarse teeth, not stalked; greenish-yellow or yellowish with purple vein flowers; fruit a rounded capsule | Entire plant | Along roads, in waste places across southern Canada and northern United States, particularly common in the Rocky Mountains | Caused by the alkaloids, hyoscyamine, hyoscine, and atropine | Increased salivation, headache, nausea, rapid pulse, convulsions, coma, and death | A gastric lavage of 4% tannic acid solution may be used to treat the poisoning. |

| Plant | Description | Parts | Distribution | Toxic constituents | Symptoms | Remarks |
|---|---|---|---|---|---|---|
| Iris (rock mountain iris) and *Iris missouriensis* | Lily-like perennial plants often in dense patches; long, narrow leaves; flowers blue purple; fruit is a three-celled capsule | Leaves but especially the rootstalk | Wetland of meadows, marshes, and along streams from North Dakota to British Columbia, Canada, south of New Mexico, Arizona, and California; scattered over entire Rocky Mountain area; cultivated species also common | An irritating resinous substance, irisin | Burning, congestion, and severe pain in the digestive tract; nausea and diarrhea | Rootstalks have such an acrid taste that they are unlikely to be eaten. |
| Jasmine and *Gelsemium sempervirens* | A woody, trailing, or climbing evergreen vine; opposite, simple, lance-shaped, glossy leaves; fragrant, yellow flowers; flattened two-celled, beaked capsule fruits | Entire plant but especially root and flowers | Native to the southeastern United States; commonly grown in the southwest as an ornamental | Alkaloids, geisemine, gelseminine, and gelsemoidine found throughout the plant | Profuse sweating, muscular weakness, convulsions, respiratory depression, paralysis, and death possible | Jasmine has been used as a medicinal herb, but overdoses are dangerous. Children have been poisoned by chewing on the leaves. |
| Jimmy weed (Rayless goldenrod) and *Haplopappus heterophyllus* | Small, bushy, half-shrub with erect stems arising from the woody crown to a height of 2–4 ft (61–122 cm); narrow, alternate, sticky leaves; clusters of small, yellow flower heads at tips of stems | Entire plant | Common in fields or ranges around watering sites and along streams from Kansas, Oklahoma, and Texas to Colorado, New Mexico, and Arizona | Contains the higher alcohol, tremetol, which accumulates in the milk of cows and causes human poisoning known as "milk sickness" | Other species of *Haplopappus* probably are equally dangerous | White snakeroot also contains tremetol and causes "milk sickness". |
| Jimson wood (thorn apple) and *Datura stramonium* | Coarse, weedy plant with stout stems and foul-smelling foliage; large, oval leaves with wavy margins; fragrant, large, tubular, white to purple flowers; round, nodding or erect prickly capsule | Entire plant, particularly the seeds and leaves | Naturalized throughout North America; common weed of fields, gardens, roadsides, and pastures | Due to the alkaloids hyoscyamine, atropine, and hyoscine (scopolamine) | Dry mouth, thirst, red skin, disturbed vision, pupil dilation, nausea, vomiting, headache, hallucination, rapid pulse, delirium, incoherent speech, convulsion, high blood pressure, coma, and possibly death | Sleeping near the fragrant flowers can cause headache, nausea, dizziness, and weakness. Children using the flowers as trumpets while playing have been poisoned |
| Lantana (red sage) and *Lantana camara* | Perennial shrub with square twigs and a few spines; simple, opposite or whorled oval-shaped leaves with tooth margins; white, yellow, orange, red, or blue flowers occurring in flat-topped clusters; berrylike fruit with a hard, blue-black seed | All parts, especially the green berries | Native of the dry woods in the southeastern United States; cultivated as an ornamental shrub in pots in the northern United States and Canada or a lawn shrub in the southeastern coastal plains, Texas, California, and Hawaii | Fruit contains high levels of an alkaloid, lantanin or lantadene A | Stomach and intestinal irritation, vomiting, bloody diarrhea, muscular weakness, jaundice, and circulatory collapse; death possible but not common | In Florida, these plants are considered a major cause of human poisoning. The foliage of lantana may also cause dermatitis. |

*(continued)*

**TABLE 2.10 (continued)**
**Toxic Plants**

| Common and Scientific Name | Description | Toxic Parts | Geographical Distribution | Poisoning | Symptoms | Remarks |
|---|---|---|---|---|---|---|
| Larkspur and *Delphinium* sp. | Annual or perennial herb 2–4 ft (61–122 cm) high; finely, palmately divided leaves on long stalks; white, pink, rose, blue, or purple flowers each with a spur; fruit a many-seeded, three-celled capsule | Entire plant | Native of rich or dry forest and meadows throughout the United States but common in the West; frequently cultivated in flower gardens | Contains the alkaloids delphinine, delphinidin, ajacine, and others | Burning sensation in the mouth and skin, low blood pressure, nervousness, weakness, prickling of the skin, nausea, vomiting, depression, convulsions, and death within 6 h if eaten in large quantities | Poisoning potential of larkspur decreases as it ages, but alkaloids still concentrated in the seeds. Seeds are used in some commercial lice remedies. |
| Laurel (mountain laurel) and *Kalmia latifolia* | Large evergreen shrubs growing to 35 ft (11 m) tall; alternate leaves dark green on top and bright green underneath; white to rose flowers in terminal clusters; fruit in a dry capsule | Leaves, twigs, flowers, and pollen grains | Found in moist woods and along streams in eastern Canada, southward in the Appalachian Mountains and Piedmont, and sometimes in the eastern coastal plain | Contains the toxic resinoid, andromedotoxin | Increased salivation, watering of eyes and nose, loss of energy, slow pulse, vomiting, low blood pressure, lack of coordination, convulsions, and progressive paralysis until eventual death | The mountain laurel is the state flower of Connecticut and Pennsylvania. Children making "tea" from the leaves or sucking on the flowers have been poisoned. |
| Locoweed (crazyweed) and *Oxytropis* sp. | Perennial herb with erect or spreading stems; pealike flowers and stems—only smaller | Common throughout the southwestern United States | Contains alkaloid-like substances—a serious threat to livestock | In animals, loss of weight, irregular gait, loss of sense of direction, nervousness, weakness, and loss of muscular control | Locoweeds are seldom eaten by humans, and hence, they are not a serious problem | There are more than 100 species of locoweeds. |
| Lupine (bluebonnet) and *Lupinus* sp. | Annual or perennial herbs; digitately divided, alternate leaves; pear-shaped blue, white, red, or yellow flowers borne in clusters at ends of stems; seeds in flattened pods | Entire plant, particularly the seeds | Wide distribution but most common in western North America; many cultivated as ornamentals | Contains lupinine and related toxic alkaloids | Weak pulse, slowed respiration, convulsions, and paralysis | Rarely have cultivated varieties that poisoned children. Not all lupines are poisonous. |
| Marijuana (hashish, Mary Jane, pot, grass) | A tall coarse, annual herb; palmately divided and long-stalked leaves; small, green flowers clustered in the leaf axils | Entire plant, especially the leaves, flowers, sap, and resinous secretions | Widely naturalized weed in temperate North America; cultivated in warmer areas | Various narcotic resins but mainly tetrahydrocannabinol (THC) and related compounds | Exhilaration, hallucinations, delusions, mental confusion, dilated pupils, blurred vision, poor coordination, weakness, and stupor; coma and death in large doses | Poisoning results from drinking the extract, chewing the plant parts, or smoking a so-called reefer (joint). The hallucinogenic and narcotic effects of marijuana have been known for more than 2000 years. |

| | Description | Toxic constituents | Symptoms | Comments |
|---|---|---|---|---|
| Mescal bean (Frijolito) and *Sophora secundiflora* | Evergreen shrub or small tree growing to 40 ft (12 m) tall; stalked, alternate leaves 4–6 in. (10–15 cm) long, which are pinnately divided and shiny, yellow green above, and silky below when young; violet-blue, pealike flowers; bright red seeds | Entire plant, particularly the seed | Contains cytisine and other poisonous alkaloids | Nausea, vomiting, diarrhea, excitement, delirium, hallucinations, coma, and death; deep sleep lasting 2–3 days in nonlethal doses | Native to southwestern Texas and southern New Mexico; cultivated as ornamentals in the southwestern United States | Laws in the United States and Canada restrict the possession of living or dried parts of marijuana. One seed, if sufficiently chewed, is enough to cause the death of a young child. The Indians of Mexico and the Southwest have used the seeds in medicine as a narcotic and as a hallucinatory drug. Necklaces have been made from the seeds. |
| Mistletoe and *Phoradendron serotinum* | Parasitic evergreen plants that grow on trees and shrubs; oblong, simple, opposite leaves, which are leathery; small, white berries | All parts, especially the berries | Contains the toxic amines, β-phenylethylamine and tyrosamine | Gastrointestinal pain, diarrhea, slow pulse, and collapse; possibly nausea, vomiting, nervousness, difficult breathing, delirium, pupil dilation, and abortion; in sufficient amounts, death within a few hours | Common on the branches of various trees from New Jersey and southern Indiana southward to Florida and Texas; other species throughout North America | Mistletoe is a favorite Christmas decoration. It is the state flower of Oklahoma. Poisonings have occurred when people eat the berries or make "tea" from the berries. Indians chewed the leaves to relieve toothache. |
| Monkshood (wolfsbane) and *Aconitum columbianum* | Perennial herb about 2–5 ft (61–152 cm) high; alternate, petioled leaves, which are palmately divided into segments with pointed tips; generally dark blue flowers with a prominent hood; seed in a short-beaked capsule | Entire plant, especially roots and seeds | Due to several alkaloids, including aconine and aconitine | Burning sensation of the mouth and skin; nausea, vomiting, diarrhea, muscular weakness, and spasms; weak, irregular pulse; paralysis of respiration; dimmed vision; convulsions; and death within a few hours | Rich, moist soil in meadows and along streams from western Canada south to California and New Mexico | Small amounts can be lethal. Death in humans reported from eating the plant or extracts made from it. It has been mistaken for horseradish. |

*(continued)*

**TABLE 2.10 (continued)**
**Toxic Plants**

| Common and Scientific Name | Description | Toxic Parts | Geographical Distribution | Poisoning | Symptoms | Remarks |
|---|---|---|---|---|---|---|
| Mushrooms (toadstools) and *Amanita muscaria, Amanita verna, Chlorophyllum molybdites* | Common types with central stalk and cap; flat plates (gills) underneath cap; some with deeply ridged, cylindrical top rather than cap | Entire fungus | Various types throughout North America | Depending on type of mushroom; complex polypeptides such as amanitin and possibly phalloidin; a toxic protein in some; the poisons ibotenic acid, muscimol, and related compounds in others | Vary with type of mushroom but include death-like sleep, manic behavior, delirium, seeing colored visions, feeling of elation, explosive diarrhea, vomiting, severe headache, loss of muscular coordination, abdominal cramps, and coma and death from some types; permanent liver, kidney, and heart damage from other types | Wild mushrooms are extremely difficult to identify and are best avoided. There is no simple rule of thumb for distinguishing between poisonous and nonpoisonous mushrooms—only myths and nonsense. Only one or two bites are necessary for death from some species. During the month of December 1981, three people were killed and two hospitalized in California after eating poisonous mushrooms. |
| Nightshade and *Solanum nigrum, Solanum elaeagnifolium* | Annual herbs or shrub-like plants with simple alternate leaves; small, white, blue, or violet flowers; blackberries or yellow to yellow-orange berries depending on species | Primarily the unripe berries | Throughout the United States and southern Canada in waste places, old fields, ditches, roadsides, fence rows, or edges of woods | Contains the alkaloid solanine; possibly saponin, atropine, and perhaps high levels of nitrate | Headache, stomach pain, vomiting, diarrhea, dilated pupils, subnormal temperature, shock, circulatory and respiratory depression, and possible death | Some individuals use the completely ripe berries in pies and jellies. Young shoots and leaves of the plant have been cooked and eaten like spinach. |
| Oleander and *Nerium oleander* | An evergreen shrub or small tree growing to 25 ft (8 m) tall; short-stalked, narrow, leathery leaves, opposite or in whorls of three; white to pink to red flowers at tips of twigs | Entire plant, especially the leaves | A native of southern Europe but commonly cultivated in the southern United States and California | Contains the poisonous glycosides oleandrin and nerioside, which act similar to digitalis | Nausea, severe vomiting, stomach pain, bloody diarrhea, cold feet and hands, irregular heartbeat, dilation of pupils, drowsiness, unconsciousness, paralysis of respiration, convulsions, coma, and death within a day | One leaf of an oleander is said to contain enough poison to kill an adult. In Florida, severe poisoning resulted when oleander branches were used as skewers. Honey made from oleander flower nectar is poisonous. |

| Plant | Description | Distribution | Poisonous parts | Constituents | Symptoms | Notes |
|---|---|---|---|---|---|---|
| Peyote (mescal buttons) and *Lophophora williamsii* | Hemispherical, spineless member of the cactus family growing from carrot-shaped roots; low, rounded sections with a tuft of yellow-white hairs on top; flower from the center of the plant, white to rose pink; pink berry when ripe; black seeds | Native to southern Texas and northern Mexico; cultivated in other areas | Entire plant, especially the buttons | Contains mescaline, lophophorine, and other alkaloids | Illusions and hallucinations with vivid color, anxiety, muscular tremors and twitching, vomiting, diarrhea, blurred vision, wakefulness, forgetfulness, muscular relaxation, and dizziness | The effects of chewing fresh or dried "buttons" of peyote are similar to those produced by LSD, only milder. In some states, peyote is recognized as a drug. Peyote has long been used by the Indians and Mexicans in religious ceremonies. |
| Poison hemlock (poison parsley) and *Conium maculatum* | Biennial herb with a hairless purple-spotted or lined, hollow stem growing up to 8 ft (2.4 m) tall; turnip-like, long, solid taproot; large, alternate, pinnately divided leaves; small, white flowers in umbrella-shaped clusters, dry; ribbed, two-part capsule fruit | A native of Eurasia, now a weed in meadows and along roads and ditches throughout the United States and southern Canada where moisture is sufficient | Entire plant, primarily seeds and root | The poisonous alkaloid coniine and other related alkaloids | Burning sensation in the mouth and throat, nervousness, dyscoordination, dilated pupils, muscular weakness, weakened and slowed heartbeat, convulsions, coma, and death | Poisoning occurs when the leaves are mistaken for parsley, the roots for turnips, or the seeds for anise. Toxic quantities seldom consumed because the plant has such an unpleasant odor and taste. Assumed by some to be the poison drunk by Socrates. |
| Poison ivy (poison oak) and *Toxicodendron radicans* | A trailing or climbing vine, shrub, or small tree; alternate leaves with three leaflets; flowers and fruits hanging in clusters; white to yellowish fruit (drupes) | An extremely variable native weed throughout southern Canada and the United States with the exception of the west coast; found on floodplains; along lake shores; edges of woods, stream banks, fences; and around buildings | Roots, stems, leaves, pollen, flowers, and fruits | Skin irritation due to an oil–resin containing urushiol | Contact with skin causes itching, burning, redness, and small blisters; severe gastric disturbance and even death by eating leaves or fruit | Almost half of all persons are allergic to poison ivy. Skin irritation may also result from indirect contact such as animals (including dogs and cats), clothing, tools, or sports equipment. |
| Pokeweed (pokeberry) and *Phytolacca americana* | Shrub-like herb with a large fleshy taproot; large, entire, oblong leaves that are pointed; white to purplish flowers in clusters at ends of branches; mature fruit a dark purple berry with red juice | Native to the eastern United States and southeastern Canada | Rootstalk, leaves, and stems | Highest concentration of poison mainly in roots; contains the bitter glycosides, saponin, and glycoprotein | Burning and bitter taste in mouth, stomach cramps, nausea, vomiting, diarrhea, drowsiness, slowed breathing, weakness, tremors, convulsions, spasms, coma, and death if eaten in large amounts | Young tender leaves and stems of pokeweed are often cooked as greens. Cooked berries are used for pies without harm. It is one of the most dangerous poisonous plants because people prepare it improperly. |

*(continued)*

**TABLE 2.10 (continued)**
**Toxic Plants**

| Common and Scientific Name | Description | Toxic Parts | Geographical Distribution | Poisoning | Symptoms | Remarks |
|---|---|---|---|---|---|---|
| Poppy (common poppy) and *Papaver somniferum* | An erect annual herb with milky juice, simple, coarsely toothed, or lobed leaves; showy red, white, pink, or purple flowers; fruit an oval, crowned capsule; tiny seeds in capsule | Unripe fruits or their juice | Introduced from Eurasia and widely grown in the United States until cultivation without a license became unlawful | Crude resin from unripe seed capsule source of narcotic opium alkaloids | From unripe fruit, stupor, coma, shallow and slow breathing, depression of the central nervous system; possibly nausea and severe retching (straining to vomit) | The use of poppy extracts is a double-edged sword—addictive narcotics and valuable medicines. Poppy seeds used as toppings on breads are harmless. |
| Rhododendron, azaleas, and *Rhododendron* sp. | Usually evergreen shrubs; mostly entire, simple, leathery leaves in whorls or alternate; snowy white to pink flowers in terminal clusters; fruit a wood capsule | Entire plant | Throughout the temperate parts of the United States as a native and as an introduced ornamental | Contains the toxic resinoid, andromedotoxin | Watering eyes and mouth, nasal discharge, nausea, severe abdominal pain, vomiting, convulsions, lowered blood pressure, lack of coordination, and loss of energy; progressive paralysis of arms and legs until death, in severe cases | Cases of poisoning are rare in this country, but rhododendrons should be suspected of possible danger. |
| Rosary pea (precatory pea) and *Abrus precatorius* | A twining, more or less woody perennial vine; alternate and divided leaves with small leaflets; red to purple or white flowers; fruit a short pod containing ovoid seeds that are glossy, bright scarlet over three-fourths of their surface and jet black over the remaining one-fourth | Seeds | Native to the tropics but naturalized in Florida and the Keys | Contains the phytotoxin abrin and tetanic glycoside abric acid | Severe stomach pain in 1–3 days, nausea, vomiting, severe diarrhea, weakness, cold sweat, drowsiness, weak, fast pulse, coma, circulatory collapse, and death | The beans are made into rosaries, necklaces, bracelets, leis, and various toys, which receive wide distribution. Seeds must be chewed and swallowed to cause poisoning. Whole seeds pass through the digestive tract without causing symptoms. One thoroughly chewed seed is said to be potent enough to kill an adult or child. |
| Snow on the mountain and *Euphorbia marginata* | A tall annual herb, growing up to 4 ft (122 cm) high; smooth, lance-shaped leaves with conspicuously white margins; whorls of white petallike leaves border flowers; fruit a three-celled, three-lobed capsule | Leaves, stems, milky sap | Native to the western, dry plains and valleys from Montana to Mexico; sometimes escapes in the eastern United States | Toxins causing dermatitis and severe irritation of the digestive tract | Blistering of the skin, nausea, abdominal pain, fainting, diarrhea, possibly death in severe cases | Milky juice of this plant is very caustic. Outwardly resembles a poinsettia. |

| Plant | Description | Toxic part | Distribution | Toxic constituent | Symptoms | Remarks |
|---|---|---|---|---|---|---|
| Skunk cabbage and *Veratrum californicum* | Tall, broad-leaved herbs of the lily family, growing to 6 ft (183 cm) high; large, alternate pleated, clasping, and parallel-veined leaves; numerous whitish to greenish flowers in large terminal clusters; three-lobed, capsule fruit | Entire plant | Various species throughout North America in wet meadows, forests, and along streams | Poisoning; contains such alkaloids as veratridine and veratrine | Nausea, vomiting, diarrhea, stomach pains, lowered blood pressure, slow pulse, reduced body temperature, shallow breathing, salivation, weakness, nervousness, convulsions, paralysis, and possibly death | These plants have been used for centuries as a source of drugs and as a source of insecticide. As the leaves resemble cabbage, they are often collected as an edible wild plant but with unpleasant results. |
| Tansy and *Tanacetum vulgare* | Tall, aromatic herb with simple stems to 3 ft (91 cm) high; alternate, pinnately divided, narrow leaves, flower heads in flat-topped clusters with numerous small, yellow flowers | Leaves, stems, and flowers | Introduced from Eurasia; widely naturalized in North America; sometimes found escarped along roadsides, in pastures, or other wet places; grown for medicinal purposes | Contains an oil, tanacetin, or oil of tansy | Nausea, vomiting, diarrhea, convulsions, violent spasms, dilated pupils, rapid and feeble pulse, and possibly death | Tansy and its oil are employed as an herbal remedy for nervousness, intestinal worms, to promote menstruation and to induce abortion. Some poisonings have resulted from the use of tansy as a home remedy. |
| Water hemlock and *Cicuta* sp. | A perennial with parsley-like leaves; hollow, jointed stems and hollow, pithy roots; flowers in umbrella clusters; stems streaked with purple ridges; 2–6 ft (61–183 cm) high | Entire plant, primarily the roots and young growth | Wet meadows, pastures, and floodplains of western and eastern United States, generally absent in the plains states | Contains the toxic resinlike higher alcohol, cicutoxin | Frothing at the mouth, spasms, dilated pupils, diarrhea, convulsions, vomiting, delirium, respiratory failure, paralysis, and death | One mouthful of the water hemlock root is reported to contain sufficient poison to kill many adults. Children making whistles and peashooters from the hollow stems have been poisoned. The water hemlock is often mistaken for the edible wild artichoke or parsnip. However, it is considered to be one of the poisonous plants of the north temperate zone. |
| White snakeroot and *Eupatorium rugosum* | Erect perennial with stems 1–5 ft (30–152 cm) tall; opposite oval leaves with pointed tips and sharply toothed edges and dull on the upper surface but shiny on the lower surface; showy, snow white flowers in terminal clusters | Entire plant | From eastern Canada to Saskatchewan and south of Texas, Louisiana, Georgia, and Virginia | Contains the higher alcohol, tremetol, and some glycosides | Weakness, nausea, loss of appetite, vomiting, tremors, labored breathing, constipation, dizziness, delirium, convulsions, coma, and death | Recovery from a nonlethal dose is a slow process, due to liver and kidney damage. Poison may be in the milk of cows that have eaten white snakeroot—"milk sickness". |

*Sources:* Ensminger, A.H. et al., *Food and Nutrition Encyclopedia*, 2nd edn., CRC Press, Boca Raton, FL, 1994; Duke, J.A., *Handbook of Edible Weeds*, CRC Press, Boca Raton, FL, 1992.

compounds pyridoxal and pyridoxal phosphate (the active form of the vitamin), resulting in the formation of inactive hydrazones.

In addition to these antinutritives, foods can contain a variety of toxic substances as shown in Table 2.8.[6] Some of these toxic substances are added inadvertently by the food processing methods, but some occur naturally. If consumed in minute quantities, some of these toxic materials are without significant effect, yet other compounds (e.g., arsenic), even in minute amounts, could accumulate and become lethal.

Table 2.9 contains information about plants commonly thought of as weeds.[7] Some of these plants may have toxic components to certain consumers. There can be considerable variability among humans in the plants that can be tolerated. Plants can differ from variety to variety and indeed from one growing condition to another in the content of their certain herbal or nutritive ingredients. Lastly, Table 2.10 provides a list of toxic plants that should not be consumed under any circumstances.[8]

## REFERENCES

1. NLM. http://www.nlm.nih.gov/medlineplus/ency/article/002444htm (accessed October 26, 2011).
2. FDA. http://www.fda.gov/Food/FoodIngredientsPackaging/ucm094211.htm (accessed October 26, 2011).
3. Hosoya, N. (ed.) *Proceedings of International Symposium on Caloric Evaluation of Carbohydrates*, Research Foundation for Sugar Metabolism, Tokyo, Japan, pp. 257, 1990.
4. Helmenstine, A *Food Additives*. http://www.chemistry.about.com/od/foodcookingchemistry/a/additives.htm (accessed October 26, 2011).
5. Jensen, M., Wright, D.N., Robinson, R.A. *Microbiology for the Health Sciences*, 4th edn., McGraw Hill, New York, pp. 495, 1997.
6. Chenault, A.A. *Nutrition and Health*, Holt, Rinehart and Winston, New York, pp. 528, 1984.
7. Ensminger, A.H. et al. *Food and Nutrition Encyclopedia*, 2nd edn., CRC Press, Boca Raton, FL, pp. 2082–2087, 1994.
8. Duke, J.A. *Handbook of Edible Weeds*, CRC Press, Boca Raton, FL, pp. 246, 1992.

# 3 Microbiological Safety of Foods

*Kumar Venkitanarayanan, Anup Kollanoor-Johny, and Michael P. Doyle*

## CONTENTS

## INTRODUCTION

The microbiological safety of foods is a major concern to consumers and to the food industry. Despite considerable progress made in technology, consumer education, and regulations, food safety continues to be a major challenge to our public health and economy. During the last decade, food safety received considerable attention due to the emergence of several new foodborne pathogens and the involvement of foods that traditionally have been considered safe, in many foodborne disease outbreaks. Further, industrialization of the food supply through mass production, distribution, increased globalization, and consumer demands for preservative-free, convenience foods and ready-to-eat meals highlights the significance of the microbial safety of foods. Recently, the U.S. Centers for Disease Control and Prevention (CDC) reported an estimated 48 million cases of foodborne illnesses, with 130,000 hospitalizations and 3000 deaths in the United States annually.[1] Besides the public health impact, outbreaks of foodborne illness impose major economic losses to both the food industry and society. The annual estimated cost of foodborne illnesses accounts for approximately $152 billion with nearly $32 billion attributed to contaminated produce.[2,3] Moreover, isolation of antibiotic-resistant foodborne bacteria as etiologic agents implicated in outbreaks has been increasingly reported. According to the Center for Science in the Public Interest (CSPI), 35 foodborne outbreaks during the last three decades were caused by bacteria resistant to at least one antibiotic.[4] The various microbiological hazards associated with foods can be classified broadly as bacterial, viral, fungal, and parasitic.

### BACTERIAL FOODBORNE PATHOGENS

Bacteria are major agents causing microbial foodborne illnesses and account for an estimated 4.8 million foodborne illnesses annually in the United States (Table 3.1).[5] Bacterial foodborne diseases can be classified into foodborne infections and foodborne intoxications. Foodborne infection is a condition caused by the ingestion of viable cells of a pathogen. Foodborne intoxication is a condition in which preformed toxins in the food produced by a toxigenic pathogen act as the underlying cause of disease.[6] The various bacterial pathogens associated with foodborne diseases are discussed in the following.

### Shiga Toxin Escherichia coli (STEC)

There are six different pathotypes of *E. coli*, including enteropathogenic *E. coli* (EPEC), enterotoxigenic *E. coli* (ETEC), enteroinvasive *E. coli* (EIEC), diffusely adhering *E. coli* (DAEC), enteroaggregative *E. coli* (EAEC), and enterohemorrhagic *E. coli* (EHEC),[7] that have been associated with gastrointestinal illness. Among these, EHEC, which produce Shiga toxins (verotoxins), are most frequently implicated in foodborne disease outbreaks and generally classified into O157 and non-O157 serogroups. EHEC O157:H7 emerged in 1982 as a foodborne pathogen and is now recognized as a major public health concern in the United States.[8] A recent report indicated that *E. coli* O157:H7 causes an estimated 63,000 cases annually in the United States with 2,138 hospitalizations and 20 deaths, accounting for a loss of $607 million.[3] Although approximately 50% of the reported outbreaks in the United States have been associated with consumption of undercooked beef burgers, a wide variety of other foods, including raw milk, roast beef, venison jerky, salami, yogurt, lettuce, unpasteurized apple juice, cantaloupe, alfalfa sprouts, and coleslaw, have been implicated as vehicles of *E. coli* O157:H7 infection.[9,10] Fresh fruits and vegetables are increasingly being identified as vehicles of EHEC infections around the world.[7,11] In the United States, iceberg lettuce and spinach have been implicated in several outbreaks.[7] In addition, outbreaks involving person-to-person and waterborne transmission have been reported.[9] Cattle have been implicated as one of the principal reservoirs of *E. coli* O157:H7.[12–15] In adult cattle, *E. coli* O157:H7 primarily colonizes the terminal rectum, particularly an anatomical area within the terminal rectum referred to as the rectoanal junction.[16] *E. coli* O157:H7 can survive in bovine feces for many months,[17] hence potentially contaminating cattle, food, water, and the environment. Although surveys conducted in the late eighties and nineties estimated a low fecal prevalence of *E. coli* O157:H7 in cattle,[15,18,19] later studies using improved enrichment and isolation procedures have showed that the overall prevalence of *E. coli* O157:H7 in cattle may be significantly higher than originally estimated.[20–23] A survey conducted by Elder et al.[20] indicated that of the 29 feedlots of cattle presented for slaughter in the Midwestern United States, 72% had at least one *E. coli* O157-positive fecal sample and 38% had positive hide samples. The study revealed an overall *E. coli* O157 prevalence of 28% (91 out of 327) in feces and 11% (38 out of 355) in hide. Subsequent research by others estimated that up to 30% of cattle are asymptomatic carriers of EHEC.[24,25] Recently, Woerner et al.[26] observed a relationship between fecal incidence rate (FIR) in cattle and hide contamination by EHEC. When FIR is more than 20%, hides positive for EHEC were about 26%, whereas when FIR was lower than 20%, only 5% of the cattle hides were contaminated. Studies by other researchers revealed that the prevalence of *E. coli* O157 in feedlots in the United States can reach 63%, particularly during the summer, under muddy conditions, or with feeding of barley.[27,28] However, other investigations revealed that EHEC shedding could be as high as 80% during the summer to as low as 5%–10% during winter,[29,30] a factor that could be attributed to the greater occurrence of foodborne outbreaks caused by EHEC during the summer.[31] These results are of particular concern because high fecal shedding and the presence of *E. coli* O157:H7 on hides would lead to contamination of foods of bovine origin with the pathogen during slaughtering and processing operations.[32] In addition, many *E. coli* O157:H7 outbreaks involving nonbovine foods, such as fruits and vegetables, are linked to cross contamination of the implicated food with contaminated bovine manure.[33–36] Direct zoonotic and environmental transmission is a newly recognized mode of *E. coli* O157:H7 spread to humans. Contact with farming

**TABLE 3.1**
**Bacterial Foodborne Pathogens**

| Microorganism | Biochemical and Growth Characteristics | Sources/Reservoirs | Examples of Vehicles | Estimated No. of Foodborne Cases Annually in the United States[2,3] | Incubation Period, Symptoms, and Duration | Detection Methods | Control/Prevention |
|---|---|---|---|---|---|---|---|
| *E. coli* O157:H7 | Gram negative, facultative anaerobe, nonspore-forming, optimum growth at 37°C–40°C, inability to grow at ≥44.5°C in the presence of selective agents, inability to ferment sorbitol within 24 h, does not produce glucuronidase, acid tolerance | Cattle, humans | Raw or undercooked beef, unpasteurized milk and apple juice, lettuce, alfalfa sprouts, water | 63,153 | 3–9 days Severe abdominal cramps, watery diarrhea that can become bloody, absence of fever, kidney failure, seizures, coma Duration is days to weeks | Cultural methods followed by confirmatory biochemical tests[374,375] Latex agglutination assay[376,377] ELISA[378–380] PCR[381–384] Immunomagnetic separation[384] biosensors[385,386] Fourier transform infrared (FT-IR) Spectroscopy and chemometrics[387] Bacteriophage-based assay[388] DNA microarray[389] | Adequate cooking of beef, pasteurization of milk and apple juice, use of potable water for drinking, avoid eating raw alfalfa and vegetable sprouts, good personal hygiene |
| *Salmonella* spp. (nontyphoid) | Gram negative, facultative anaerobe, oxidase negative, catalase positive, nonspore-forming, growth at 5°C–47°C, optimum growth at 37°C, metabolize nutrients by respiratory and fermentative pathways | Cattle, swine, poultry, humans | Raw or undercooked meat, poultry, eggs, and milk, untreated water | 1,027,561 | 6–72 h up to 4 days Abdominal cramps, diarrhea, fever, chills, headache, and vomiting Duration is few days to 1 week, occasionally up to 3 weeks | Cultural methods followed by confirmatory biochemical tests[390–392] Latex agglutination assay[393] ELISA[394] Immunoassay[395] PCR[396–399] | Adequate cooking of food, avoid cross contamination of raw foods of animal origin with cooked or ready-to-eat foods, avoid eating raw or undercooked foods of animal origin, use of potable water, good personal hygiene |
| *Salmonella typhi* | Gram negative, facultative anaerobe, ferment D-xylose | Humans | Raw milk, shellfish, raw salads, undercooked foods | 1,821 | 7–28 days Remittent fever with stepwise increments over a period of days, high temperature of 103°F–104°F, abdominal pain, diarrhea, and headache Duration is up to 3 weeks | Biochemical tests[400] Latex test[401] ELISA[402] PCR[403–405] Quantum dot assay[406] ELISA[407] | Good personal hygiene and food handling practices, proper sewage systems, effective surveillance of known carriers |

(continued)

**TABLE 3.1 (continued)**
**Bacterial Foodborne Pathogens**

| Microorganism | Biochemical and Growth Characteristics | Sources/Reservoirs | Examples of Vehicles | Estimated No. of Foodborne Cases Annually in the United States[2,3] | Incubation Period, Symptoms, and Duration | Detection Methods | Control/Prevention |
|---|---|---|---|---|---|---|---|
| *Campylobacter jejuni* and *C. coli* | Gram negative, microaerophilic, nonspore-forming, optimal growth at 42°C, $CO_2$ is required for good growth, growth optimal in 3%–6% $O_2$, sensitive to dehydration, survives best at refrigeration temperature | Poultry Swine Cattle Sheep Wild birds | Raw or undercooked chicken, pork, and beef and unpasteurized milk | 845,024 | 1–11 days, usually 2–5 days Abdominal pain, diarrhea, malaise, headache, fever Duration is up to 10 days | Cultural methods followed by confirmatory biochemical tests[408,409] Immunoassay[410,411] PCR[412–418] Quantum dot sandwich assay[419] Loop-mediated isothermal amplification (LAMP) assay[420] Biosensor[421] DNA microarray[422] | Adequate cooking of meat; avoid cross contamination of raw foods of animal origin with cooked or ready-to-eat foods; pasteurization of milk |
| *Shigella* spp. | Gram negative, facultative anaerobe, nonspore-forming, does not ferment lactose, growth at 10°C–45°C, optimal growth at 37°C | Humans | Raw foods and water contaminated with human feces, prepared salads | 131,254 | 1–7 days Severe abdominal and rectal pain, bloody diarrhea with mucus, fever, dehydration Duration is few days to few weeks | Cultural methods followed by confirmatory biochemical tests[423] ELISA[424,425] PCR[426–430] Apyrase-based colorimetric test[431] DNA microarray[432] | Good personal hygiene, adequate cooking of food, drinking potable water |
| *Y. enterocolitica* | Gram negative, facultative anaerobe, nonspore-forming, growth at 0°C–44°C, optimal growth at ca. 29°C, growth at pH 4.6–9.0, growth in presence of 5% NaCl but not 7% NaCl | Swine is principal reservoir of pathogenic strains. Humans can also act as a source through contaminated blood transfusion. | Undercooked or raw pork, especially tongue | 97,656 | 1–11 days, usually 24–36 h Severe abdominal pain, nausea, diarrhea, fever, sometimes vomiting Duration is usually 2–3 days but may continue for up to 3 weeks | Cultural methods followed by confirmatory biochemical tests[433] PCR[434–436] Monoclonal antibody-based dot blot assay[437] LAMP assay[438] Mass spectrometry[439] DNA microarray[432] | Adequate cooking of pork, disinfection of drinking water, control of *Y. enterocolitica* in pigs, prevent cross contamination of pig viscera, feces, and hair with food and water |

| Organism | Characteristics | Reservoir | Foods | Cases | Symptoms/Incubation | Detection methods | Prevention/control |
|---|---|---|---|---|---|---|---|
| *V. cholerae* | Gram negative, facultative anaerobe, nonspore-forming, growth at 18°C–42°C with optimal growth at 37°C, growth is stimulated in the presence of 3% NaCl, pH range for growth is 6–11 | Humans, marine waters, especially brackish water and estuaries | Undercooked or raw seafoods, vegetables fertilized with contaminated human feces or irrigated with contaminated water, water | 84 | 1–3 days Profuse watery diarrhea, which can lead to severe dehydration, abdominal pain, vomiting Duration is up to 7 days | Cultural methods followed by confirmatory biochemical tests[440-442] ELISA[443,444] Immunoassay[445] PCR[446-451] Biosensor[450] LAMP assay[420,452] DNA microarray[432,453] | Safe disposal of human sewage, disinfection of drinking water, avoid eating raw seafood, adequate cooking of food |
| *Vibrio parahaemolyticus* | Gram negative, facultative anaerobe, nonspore-forming, growth in presence of 8% NaCl, optimal growth at 37°C with rapid generation time (ca. 10 min), growth at 10°C, sensitive to storage at refrigeration temperature | Coastal seawater, estuarine brackish waters above 15°C, marine fish, shellfish | Raw or undercooked fish and seafoods | 34,664 | 9–25 h, up to 3 days, Profuse watery diarrhea, abdominal pain, vomiting, fever Duration is up to 8 days | Cultural methods followed by confirmatory biochemical tests[440,441] ELISA[454] PCR[455-460] LAMP assay[461] DNA microarray[432,462] | Adequate cooking of seafood, rapid chilling of seafoods, prevent cross contamination from raw seafoods to other foods and preparation surfaces |
| *Vibrio vulnificus* | Gram negative, nonspore-forming, optimal growth at 37°C | Coastal and estuarine waters | Raw seafood, especially raw oysters | 96 | 12 h to 3 days Profuse diarrhea with blood in feces, fulminating septicemia, hypotension Duration is days to weeks | Cultural methods followed by confirmatory biochemical tests[440,441,463] ELISA[464,465] PCR[466-470] LAMP assay[469,471] DNA microarray[432,472] | Avoid eating raw seafood, especially raw oysters when have a history of liver disease or alcoholism |
| *C. sakazakii* | Gram negative, facultative anaerobe, nonspore-forming, α-glucosidase positive, phosphoamidase negative, growth at 5.5°C–37°C, tolerant to high osmotic pressure and desiccation | Not known | Dry, powdered infant formula | Not available | Sepsis, meningitis, meningoencephalitis, brain abscess, ventriculitis, hydrocephalus, necrotizing enterocolitis in infants Bacteremia, osteomyelitis, and pneumonia in elderly adults | Cultural and biochemical methods[473,474] PCR[475-478] DNA-microarray[477,479] | Proper refrigerated storage of reconstituted infant formula Avoid feeding nonrefrigerated formula and formula refrigerated for more than 24 h Prepared infant formula should not be kept warm in bottle heaters or thermoses |

(continued)

**TABLE 3.1 (continued)**
**Bacterial Foodborne Pathogens**

| Microorganism | Biochemical and Growth Characteristics | Sources/Reservoirs | Examples of Vehicles | Estimated No. of Foodborne Cases Annually in the United States[2,3] | Incubation Period, Symptoms, and Duration | Detection Methods | Control/Prevention |
|---|---|---|---|---|---|---|---|
| A. hydrophila | Gram negative, facultative anaerobe, nonspore-forming, oxidase positive, some strains are psychrotrophic (4°C) optimum growth at ca. 28°C | Aquatic environment, freshwater fish (especially salmonids) | Untreated water Undercooked seafoods, especially fish | Very few | 24–48 h Abdominal pain, vomiting, watery stools, mild fever Duration is days to weeks | Cultural methods followed by confirmatory biochemical tests[480–483] ELISA[484] PCR[485–488] Biosensors[489] Indirect fluorescent antibody assay[490] Monoclonal antibody-based dot blot assay[491] LAMP assay[492] DNA microarray[493] | Avoid consumption of raw seafoods, avoid long-term storage of refrigerated foods, adequate cooking of foods, disinfection of drinking water |
| P. shigelloides | Gram negative, facultative anaerobe, nonspore-forming, oxidase positive, some strains are psychrotrophic | Fresh and estuarine waters, fish, and shellfish | Fish, shellfish, oysters, shrimp, and untreated water | Very few | 1–2 days Abdominal pain, nausea, vomiting, diarrhea, chills, headache Duration is days to weeks | Cultural methods followed by confirmatory biochemical tests[480,481] PCR[494] | Avoid consumption of raw seafoods, disinfection of drinking water |
| L. monocytogenes | Gram positive, facultative anaerobe, nonspore-forming, growth at 2°C–45°C, optimal growth at 30°C–35°C, growth in presence of 10% NaCl | Soil, sewage, vegetation, water, and feces of humans and animals | Raw milk, soft cheese, pâté, ready-to-eat cooked meat products (poultry, hot dogs) and cooked seafoods (smoked fish), and raw vegetables | 1,591 | Few days to several weeks Flu-like symptoms such as fever, chills, headache Abdominal pain and diarrhea are present in some cases In pregnant women, spontaneous abortion and stillbirth Duration is days to weeks | Cultural methods followed by confirmatory biochemical tests[495–498] Immunoassay[499–501] PCR[502–507] Biosensors[508] LAMP assay[509] Fluorescent in situ hybridization (FISH)[510] | Proper sanitation of food processing equipment and environments; adequate cooking of meat and meat products; prevent recontamination of cooked products; proper reheating of cooked food; avoid drinking raw milk, avoid certain high-risk foods (e.g., soft cheeses and pâtes) by pregnant women and immunocompromised individuals |

| Organism | Characteristics | Source/reservoir | Foods | Number of cases | Symptoms/incubation | Detection methods | Prevention/control |
|---|---|---|---|---|---|---|---|
| *S. aureus* (staphylococcal enterotoxin) | Gram positive, facultative anaerobe, nonspore-forming, coagulase positive, growth at 7°C–48°C, optimal growth at ca. 37°C, toxin production at $a_w$ of 0.86; toxin is heat stable (can withstand boiling for 1 h) | Humans (nose, throat, and skin) and animals | Ham, chicken and egg salads, cream-filled pastries | 241,148 | 2–6 h. Abdominal cramps, nausea, vomiting, diarrhea, headache, chills, and dizziness. Duration is up to 2 days | Cultural methods followed by confirmatory biochemical tests[511,512]; PCR[513–517]; Immunoassay[518–520]; Detection of toxin by microslide gel double diffusion[521]; FISH[522]; ssDNA aptamer detection[523] | Good personal hygiene in food preparation and handling, adequate cooking of foods, proper refrigeration of cooked foods |
| *C. botulinum* (botulinum neurotoxin) | Gram positive, obligate anaerobe, spore-forming, produce seven potent neurotoxins A–G (only A, B, E, and rarely F associated with human illness); proteolytic strains grow at 10°C–50°C, and nonproteolytic strains can grow at 3.3°C; spores are resistant to normal cooking temperatures and survive freezing and drying | Soil, dust, vegetation, animals, birds, insects, and marine and fresh water sediments and the intestinal tracts of fish (type E) | Beef, pork, fish, vegetables, and honey (infant botulism) | 55 | 12–36 h, can range from few hours to 8 days. Very severe life-threatening intoxication, headache, fixed and dilated pupils, vertigo, blurred or double vision, lack of muscle coordination, dry mouth, difficulty in breathing. Gastrointestinal symptoms include abdominal pain, nausea, vomiting, and constipation. Duration is days to months (8 months) | Cultural methods followed by confirmatory biochemical tests[524]; PCR[525–531]; Detection of toxin by mouse bioassay[532]; immunoaffinity chromatograpgy[533]; mass spectrophotometry[534]; immunodetection kit[535]; LAMP assay[536]; DNA microarray[537] | Boiling of foods will destroy toxin; adequate heat processing of home-canned foods; proper refrigeration of vacuum-packaged fresh or lightly cooked/smoked foods; acid-preserved foods should be below pH 4.6; discard swollen cans; avoid feeding honey to infants |
| *C. perfringens* | Gram positive, anaerobe, spore-forming, optimum growth at 37°C–47°C, grows slowly below 20°C | Soil, sewage, dust, vegetation, feces of humans and animals | Cooked meat and poultry, especially roast beef, turkey, and gravies | 965,958 | 8–24 h. Abdominal pain and diarrhea. Duration is 1–2 days | Cultural methods followed by confirmatory biochemical tests[243]; Latex agglutination test[538]; Colony hybridization assay[539]; ELISA[540,541]; PCR[538,542–545]; FISH[545]; DNA microarray[547] | Adequate cooking of foods; cooked food should be rapidly cooled (<5°C) or held hot (>60°C); proper refrigeration and adequate reheating of stored cooked foods |

*(continued)*

**TABLE 3.1 (continued)**
**Bacterial Foodborne Pathogens**

| Microorganism | Biochemical and Growth Characteristics | Sources/Reservoirs | Examples of Vehicles | Estimated No. of Foodborne Cases Annually in the United States[2,3] | Incubation Period, Symptoms, and Duration | Detection Methods | Control/Prevention |
|---|---|---|---|---|---|---|---|
| C. difficile | Gram positive, spore-forming, anaerobic, showing optimal growth at human body temperature | Water, air, human and animal feces, soil | Ground beef, ground veal, veal chops, ground pork, chicken, vegetables | Not available | Abdominal pain, fever, fulminant colitis, toxic megacolon, sepsis, shock, mild diarrhea in asymptomatic carriers, relapse or reinfection within 2 months | Cultural methods followed by confirmatory biochemical tests[249] ELISA[548] PCR[549-551] LAMP assay[552] PCR ribotyping[553] DNA microarray[554] | Hospital setting: Limit use of antimicrobial drugs, wash hands between contact, use precautions for infected people with diarrhea, clean the environment meticulously Community setting: Proper cooking of meat[555] |
| B. cereus | Gram positive, facultative anaerobe, spore-forming; some strains can grow at 4°C–6°C, optimum growth at 28°C–37°C | Widely distributed in nature, soil, dust, vegetation | Cereals, fried rice, potatoes, cooked meat products, milk and dairy products, spices, dried foods | 63,400 | *Diarrheal syndrome* (toxic infection): 8–16 h Abdominal pain, watery diarrhea Duration is 24–36 h *Emetic syndrome* (preformed, heat-stable toxin): 1–5 h Nausea, vomiting, malaise, sometimes diarrhea Duration is 24–36 h. | Cultural methods followed by confirmatory biochemical tests[556] ELISA[557,558] Colony blot immunoassay[559,560] PCR[561-565] Tecra VIA kit[566] Oxoid BCET-RPLA kit[566] CHO cell culture assay[566] DNA microarray[567] | Adequate cooking of foods; cooked foods should be rapidly cooled (<5°C) or held hot (60°C); avoid leaving cooked foods at room temperature for long time |
| A. butzleri | Fastidious, gram negative, nonspore-forming, motile, spiral organisms, grows microaerobically and aerobically, ability to grow at 15°C differentiating it from *Campylobacter* Preferred temperature for growth is 30°C | Domestic and pet animals, birds including chickens and turkeys, humans | Increased isolation from raw meat products, surface and groundwater, foodborne transmission is not definitive | Unknown | Human enteritis characterized by persistent and watery diarrhea, vomiting, nausea, and fever | Cultural detection by enrichment under aerobic conditions at 25°C[568] Charcoal cefoperazone deoxycholate agar and broth for selective identification Johnson and Murano broth[569] | |

| Organism | Characteristics | Host | Source | Number | Symptoms | Detection methods | Control/Prevention |
|---|---|---|---|---|---|---|---|
| *Brucella* spp. | Gram negative, aerobe, nonspore-forming, optimal growth at 37°C | Cattle, sheep, pig, goat | Raw milk and products made from unpasteurized milk | 839 | Acute form: 3–21 days, infrequently months Pyrexia, profuse sweats, chills, constipation, weakness, malaise, body aches, joint pains, weight loss, anorexia Chronic form: several months Long history of fever, inertia, recurrent depression, sexual impotence, insomnia Duration is weeks | PCR[570] SDS–PAGE[571,572] Random amplification of polymorphic DNA coupled with enterobacterial repetitive intergenic consensus PCR[573] Pulsed-field gel electrophoresis[574] Cultural methods[575] ELISA[576–578] PCR[579–582] LAMP assay[583] Lateral-flow assay[584] | Vaccination of livestock against *Brucella* spp.; avoid contact with infected animals; eradication of diseased animals; pasteurization of milk; avoid eating unpasteurized dairy products |
| *H. pylori* | Gram negative, microaerophile to anaerobe | Humans, cats | Untreated water; foodborne transmission of disease has not been proven | Unknown | Gastritis, dyspepsia, peptic ulcer, gastric carcinoma | Cultural methods[292,585] ELISA[290] Immunoassay[586,587] PCR[588,589] Rapid paper urease test[590] Oligonucleotide-based multiplex PCR[591] | Avoid contact with infected animals; use of chlorinated water for cooking and drinking |

environment, including recreational or occupational visits, has been associated with *E. coli* O157:H7 infections in humans.[37,38] Since reduced fecal shedding of *E. coli* O157:H7 by cattle would potentially decrease foodborne outbreaks of *E. coli* O157:H7, a variety of approaches for decreasing the gastrointestinal carriage of *E. coli* O157:H7 in cattle have been investigated. These approaches have been focused on three important factors, namely, reduction of exposure of cattle to the pathogen, applying the pathogen exclusion principle, and implementing a direct pathogen reduction strategy.[39] *E. coli* O157:H7 can be largely controlled if sufficient hygienic measures are undertaken on farms, including providing good-quality water, feed, and housing for cattle; isolating preweaned calves from the adult herd, because calves can shed the pathogen in large numbers; and excluding nonbovine pathogen sources such as dogs, raccoons, opossums, and wild birds from farms, because they may potentially introduce *E. coli* O157:H7 to farms.[37,39–42] Avoidance of feed ingredients known to increase *E. coli* O157:H7 shedding such as barley, corn silage, and beet pulp and use of probiotics (e.g., Bovamine® that contains a mix of *Lactobacillus acidophilus* and *Propionibacterium freudenreichii*) and prebiotics are other potential strategies to exclude or reduce pathogen colonization in cattle.[39,43] Direct *E. coli* O157:H7 reduction strategies such as feeding of antimicrobial compounds, for example, sodium chlorate,[44] ionophores, neomycin, and bacteriophages, have been investigated. A recent intervention approach has emphasized vaccination of cattle against *E. coli* O157:H7 colonization, targeting intimin[45] of the type III secretion system (Bioniche®), lipopolysaccharide (LPS), and siderophore receptors[46–48] (Epitopix®) in the bacterium. In addition, a variety of postharvest interventions against *E. coli* O157:H7 have been examined, including thermal processing, high-pressure treatment, ultrasound, ionizing radiation, ozone treatment, ultraviolet light, radio waves, chemical antimicrobials, naturally occurring antimicrobial chemicals in plants, electrochemically activated water, and bacteriophages.[7]

Acidification is commonly used in food processing to control survival and growth of spoilage-causing and pathogenic microorganisms in foods. The U.S. Food and Drug Administration does not consider foods with pH ≤ 4.6 (high-acid foods) to be microbiologically hazardous for many foodborne pathogens. However, *E. coli* O157:H7 has been associated with outbreaks attributed to high-acid foods, including apple juice, mayonnaise, fermented sausage, and yogurt,[49] raising concerns about the safety of these foods. Several studies have revealed that many strains of *E. coli* O157:H7 are highly tolerant to acidic conditions, being able to survive for extended periods of time in synthetic gastric juice and in highly acidic foods.[49,50] Further, exposure of *E. coli* O157:H7 to mild or moderate acidic environments can induce an acid tolerance response, which enables the pathogen to survive extreme acidic conditions. For example, acid-adapted cells of *E. coli* O157:H7 survived longer in apple cider, fermented sausage, and hydrochloric acid than nonacid-adapted

cells.[51,52] However, *E. coli* O157:H7 is not unusually heat resistant[53] or salt tolerant[54] unless cells are preexposed to acid to become acid adapted. Acid-adapted *E. coli* O157:H7 cells also have increased heat tolerance.

In humans, two principal manifestations of illness have been reported in *E. coli* O157:H7 infection. These include hemorrhagic colitis (HC) and hemolytic uremic syndrome (HUS).[55] HC is characterized by a watery diarrhea that progresses into grossly bloody diarrhea, indicative of significant amounts of gastrointestinal bleeding. Severe abdominal pain is common, but fever is usually not present. The illness typically lasts from 2 to 9 days. HUS is a severe condition, particularly among the very young and the elderly. Both these manifestations involve damage to kidneys, leading to renal failure and death. Treatment of *E. coli* O157:H7 infections with antibiotics may result in severe outcomes.[56,57] Administration of antibiotics, particularly β-lactams, is risk factor for development of HUS.[58]

The pathogenicity of EHEC is determined by virulence factors encoded by pathogenicity islands, phage chromosomes, and plasmids. The important factors attributed to the pathogenesis of *E. coli* O157:H7 include the ability of the pathogen to adhere to the intestinal mucosa of the host by the locus for enterocyte effacement (LEE) and production of Shiga toxin I (Stx1) and/or Shiga toxin II (Stx2)[35] and the large plasmid pO157.[7] The LEE encodes for an adhesion factor called intimin. Together, these factors are able to produce attaching and effacing lesions on host intestine in EHEC infections.[59] The toxins, both chromosomally and phage encoded, are produced in the colon and have the ability to reach kidneys via blood to cause HUS.[60] STEC isolates capable of producing Stx2, in particular Stx2a, are most often associated with serious disease in affected individuals than isolates that produce only Stx1.[61] The plasmid pO157, which is commonly found in most EHEC isolates, encodes for a hemolysin that is toxic to both human and bovine cells.[62] Retrospective analysis of foods implicated in outbreaks of *E. coli* O157:H7 infection suggests a low oral infectious dose of the pathogen, probably less than a hundred cells.[55]

Although infections caused by non-O157 serogroups were reported as early as 1982, a lack of reliable detection methods hindered the identification of their epidemiologic role in causing disease compared to *E. coli* O157:H7.[63] It is estimated that Shiga toxin-producing non-O157 isolates cause annually 112,750 cases with 271 hospitalizations, which account for an economic loss of $100 million.[3] Among the STEC non-O157 serogroups, serogroups O26, O45, O103, O111, O121, and O145 are leading causes of STEC inflections in the United States.[64] Recent reports suggest that the infections caused by O157 serotypes are more severe, albeit non-O157 serotypes caused significant morbidity.[65] Recently, an Stx2a-producing isolate of enteroaggregative *E. coli* O104:H4 caused a major outbreak of severe HUS and bloody diarrhea in the European Union, particularly Germany.[66] There were more than 4000 cases that included more than 900 cases of HUS and approximately 50 deaths.

## *Salmonella* Species

*Salmonella* spp. are facultatively anaerobic, gram negative, rod-shaped bacteria belonging to the family *Enterobacteriaceae*. Members of the genus *Salmonella* have an optimum growth temperature of 37°C and utilize glucose with the production of acid and gas.[67] *Salmonella* spp. are widely distributed in nature. They colonize the intestinal tract of humans, animals, birds, and reptiles and are excreted in feces, which contaminate the environment, water, and foods.[68] Many food products, especially foods having contact with animal feces, including beef, pork, poultry, eggs, milk, fruits, and vegetables, have been associated with outbreaks of salmonellosis.[69] *Salmonella* spp. can be divided into host-adapted serovars and those without any host preferences. Most of the foodborne serovars are in the latter group.

The ability of many strains of *Salmonella* to adapt to extreme environmental conditions emphasizes the potential risk of these microorganisms as foodborne pathogens. Although salmonellae optimally grow at 37°C, the genus *Salmonella* consists of strains, which are capable of growth from 5°C to 47°C.[70] *Salmonella* spp. can grow at pH values ranging from 4.5 to 7.0, with optimum growth observed near neutral pH.[68] Preexposure of *Salmonella* to mild acidic environments (pH 5.5–6.0) can induce in some strains an acid tolerance response, which enables the bacteria to survive for extended periods of exposure to acidic and other adverse environmental conditions such as heat and low water activity.[71,72] However, most *Salmonella* spp. possess no unusual tolerance to salt and heat. A concentration of 3%–4% NaCl can inhibit the growth of *Salmonella*.[73] Most salmonellae are sensitive to heat; hence, ordinary pasteurization and cooking temperatures are capable of killing the pathogen.[74]

Salmonellosis is one of the most frequently reported foodborne diseases worldwide.[75] The overall incidence of salmonellosis in the United States declined by approximately 8% during the period from 1996 to 2004.[76] However, a recent CDC study revealed that foodborne salmonellosis in the United States during the past decade has not decreased significantly.[1] Food-associated *Salmonella* infections in the United States are estimated by the U.S. Department of Agriculture to cost $3 billion annually.[77] CDC epidemiologists recently estimated 1 million cases of nontyphoidal salmonellosis annually in the United States, resulting in 19,226 hospitalizations and 378 deaths, accounting for an economic loss of $4.4 billion.[3] Among the 7564 foodborne *Salmonella* isolates serotyped in 2010 in the United States, *S.* Enteritidis was most common, followed by *S.* Newport and *S.* Typhimurium.[1] Although the overall incidence of human salmonellosis in 2005 was lower than that in the mid-1990s, the incidence of *S.* Enteritidis infections increased by approximately 25%.[78]

*S.* Enteritidis outbreaks are most frequently associated with the consumption of poultry products, especially undercooked eggs and chicken. Moreover, international travel especially to developing countries has been associated with human infections of *S.* Enteritidis in the United States.[79] A report from the CDC revealed 677 outbreaks of eggborne *S.* Enteritidis with 23,366 illnesses, 1,988 hospitalizations,

and 33 deaths in the United States during the period 1990–2001.[80] Another study reported an estimate of 700,000 cases of eggborne salmonellosis in the United States, which accounted for approximately 47% of total foodborne salmonellosis, costing more than $1 billion annually.[81] In 2010, a nationwide outbreak of *S.* Enteritidis infection consisting of 3578 cases associated with the consumption of shell eggs was reported in the United States during the months from May to November.[82] Given that approximately 65 billion shell eggs are sold annually in the United States,[83] with a per capita consumption of approximately 254 eggs/year, *Salmonella*-contaminated eggs potentially constitute a major health hazard to humans. In light of the mounting evidence linking human salmonellosis with shell eggs, the Food and Drug Administration in 2009 announced that eggs constitute an important source of *S.* Enteritidis infections and issued a final rule that requires shell egg producers to implement measures to prevent *S.* Enteritidis from contaminating eggs on the farm and further growth during storage and transportation.

Apart from eggs, salmonellae are isolated from poultry carcasses and meat. From 1998 through 2003, the U.S. Department of Agriculture-Food Safety Inspection Service (USDA-FSIS) reported isolation of *Salmonella* from 11.2% to 22.5% of broiler and ground chicken samples, respectively.[77] In another study, White et al.[84] reported isolation of *Salmonella* from 26.4% of ground turkey, 22.5% of ground chicken, and 11.2% of broiler samples (N = 12,699/293,938 samples positive for *Salmonella*), with the largest number of *S.* Enteritidis isolates recovered from broiler carcasses.

*S.* Typhimurium is another significant *Salmonella* serotype causing foodborne infections worldwide.[1] A wide variety of foods, including chicken, turkey, beef, pork, peanut butter, and milk, have been associated with outbreaks caused by *S.* Typhimurium. Although the incidence of *S.* Typhimurium infections in the United States has decreased by approximately 40% during 1996–2004,[76] the emergence of *S.* Typhimurium DT 104, a new multidrug-resistant phage type in the 1990s in the United States and Europe, became a major public health concern. This is because *S.* Typhimurium DT 104 is resistant to multiple antibiotics, including ampicillin, chloramphenicol, penicillin, streptomycin, tetracycline, and sulfonamides.[85,86] A major risk factor identified in the development of *S.* Typhimurium DT 104 infection in humans was prior treatment with antimicrobial agents to which the infecting strain was resistant, during four preceding weeks of infection.[87] The CDC reported that 11% of the total *Salmonella* spp. isolated from humans in 2000 were resistant to at least five different antibiotics and a few of the multidrug-resistant strains were also resistant to gentamicin and cephalosporins.[88] These aforementioned reports underscore the prudent use of antibiotics in humans and animal husbandry.

In addition to *S.* Enteritidis and *S.* Typhimurium, several other serotypes of *Salmonella* are linked with foodborne outbreaks. These include *S.* Hadar, *S.* Newport, *S.* Virchow, and *S.* Heidelberg for which poultry meat has been a major vehicle.[89] *S.* Baildon, *S.* Braenderup, *S.* Javiana,

*S*. Montevideo, *S*. Newport, and *S*. Saintpaul have been associated with fresh produce-associated outbreaks.[90] A variety of pre- and postharvest strategies including competitive exclusion bacteria, bacteriophages, organic acids, prebiotic oligosaccharides, and vaccines[91–97] have been determined to help mitigate *Salmonella* contamination of chickens but with varied degrees of success rates. Recently, medium-chain fatty acids and plant-derived antimicrobials reportedly can reduce *S*. Enteritidis colonization of broiler chickens.[98,99]

In the host, *Salmonella* establishes a successful infection utilizing a variety of virulence factors, including motility, adherence to and invasion of host cells, macrophage survival, evasion of the host immune system, systemic dissemination, and finally dissemination to new hosts. Several *Salmonella* pathogenicity islands (SPI), including SPI1 and SPI2, play critical roles in the process. The pathogenicity island SPI1 controls bacterial motility, adherence, and invasion of *Salmonella* in the host's intestinal tract, whereas SPI2 regulates systemic dissemination to reach internal organs, including, for some strains such as *S*. Enteritidis, reproductive organs in chickens.[100] *Salmonella* infection in humans is characterized by fever, headache, abdominal pain, vomiting, and diarrhea and is mostly self-limiting.[101] The incubation period of the disease typically ranges from 12 to 72 h, with the illness lasting for 2–7 days. Patients usually recover within a week without any antibiotic treatment except in cases of severe diarrhea, where intravenous fluid therapy is warranted. However, severe illness caused by antibiotic-resistant strains of *S*. Enteritidis may result in an extended treatment period.[102] Vulnerable populations such as infants, children, the elderly, and immunocompromised are prone to more severe outcomes leading to an invasive disease, characterized by bacteremia and rarely death.[103] In addition, in a small percentage of affected individuals, the lingering effects of disease include chronic reactive arthritis, osteoarthritis, appendicitis, meningitis, and peritonitis.[103]

*S*. Typhi is the causative agent of typhoid (enteric fever), a serious human disease. Typhoid fever has a long incubation period of 7–28 days and is characterized by prolonged and spiking fever, abdominal pain, diarrhea, and headache.[67] The disease can be diagnosed by isolation of the pathogen from urine, blood, or stool specimens of affected individuals. In 2003, a total of 356 cases of typhoid fever were reported in the United States.[104] *S*. Typhi is an uncommon cause of foodborne illness in the United States, and approximately 74% of these cases reported in the United States occurred among persons who traveled internationally, especially South Asia during the preceding 6 weeks of infection.[104]

### *Campylobacter* Species

The genus *Campylobacter* consists of 14 species; however, *C. jejuni* subsp. *jejuni* and *C. coli* are the dominant foodborne pathogens. *C. jejuni* is a slender, rod-shaped, microaerophilic bacterium that requires approximately 3%–6% oxygen for growth. It can be differentiated from *C. coli* by its ability to hydrolyze hippurate.[105] The bacterium does not survive well in the environment, being sensitive to drying, highly acidic conditions, and freezing. It is also readily killed in foods by adequate cooking.[106]

*C. jejuni* is one of the most commonly reported bacterial causes of foodborne infection in the United States[78,106,107] and the European Union.[108] The estimated incidence of campylobacteriosis in the United States is 13.02 per 100,000 population,[109] with an estimated 845,000 cases, 8,463 hospitalizations, and 76 deaths occurring annually.[2] Many animals, including poultry, swine, cattle, sheep, horses, and domestic pets, harbor *C. jejuni* in their intestinal tracts serving as sources of human infection. However, chickens serve as the most common reservoir of *C. jejuni*, where the bacterium primarily colonizes the mucus overlying the epithelial cells in the ceca and small intestine. L-Fucose, the major carbohydrate component present in the mucin of chicken cecal mucus, is used by *C. jejuni* as a sole substrate for growth, which gives the pathogen a competitive advantage over other competing flora for survival in the intestine.[110,111] Hence, the cecal environment in chickens is favorable for the survival and proliferation of *C. jejuni*[110] and selects for colonization of *C. jejuni* in the birds. Although a number of vehicles such as beef, pork, eggs, and untreated water have been implicated as vehicles of outbreaks of campylobacter enteritis, with chicken and unpasteurized milk being the most commonly involved foods,[112,113] epidemiologic investigations have revealed a significant link between human campylobacter infection and handling or consumption of raw or undercooked poultry meat.[113–117] Since colonization of broiler chickens by *C. jejuni* results in horizontal transmission of the pathogen and carcass contamination during slaughter, a variety of approaches for reducing its cecal carriage by chickens have been undertaken. These approaches include competitive exclusion,[94] feeding birds with bacteriophages[118,119] and acidified feed,[120] medium-chain fatty acids,[121,122] and vaccination.[123,124] In the United States, an increasing number of fluoroquinolone-resistant (e.g., ciprofloxacin) human campylobacter infections had been reported,[125] and this was attributed to the use of this antibiotic in food animal production, especially poultry.[126] Besides resistance to fluoroquinolones, strains resistant to tetracyclines and erythromycins have been recently reported.[108]

Usually campylobacter enteritis in humans is a self-limiting illness characterized by abdominal cramps, diarrhea, headache, and fever lasting up to 4 days. However, severe cases, involving bloody diarrhea and abdominal pain mimicking appendicitis, also occur.[105] Guillain–Barré syndrome (GBS) is an infrequent sequel to *Campylobacter* infection in humans.[127] GBS is characterized by acute neuromuscular paralysis[106] and is estimated to occur in approximately one of every 1000 cases of campylobacter enteritis.[128] A few strains of *C. jejuni* reportedly produce a heat-labile enterotoxin similar to that produced by *Vibrio cholerae* and ETEC.[105] Some strains of *C. jejuni* and *C. coli* can also produce a cytolethal distending toxin, which causes a rapid and specific cell cycle arrest in HeLa and Caco-2 cells.[129]

## *Shigella* Species

*Shigella* is a common cause of human diarrhea in the United States. The genus *Shigella* is divided into four major groups: *S. dysenteriae* (group A), *S. flexneri* (group B), *S. boydii* (group C), and *S. sonnei* (group D) based on the organism's somatic (O) antigen. Although all the four groups have been involved in human infections, *S. sonnei* accounts for more than 75% of shigellosis cases in humans[130] and has been linked to persistent infections in community and day-care centers.[131–133] Humans are the natural reservoirs of *Shigella* spp. The fecal–oral route is the primary mode of transmission of Shigellae and proper personal hygiene and sanitary practices of cooks and food handlers can greatly reduce the occurrence of outbreaks of shigellosis. Most foodborne outbreaks of shigellosis are associated with ingestion of foods such as salads and water contaminated with human feces containing the pathogen. Shigellosis is characterized by diarrhea containing bloody mucus, which lasts 1–2 weeks. The infectious dose for *Shigella* infection is low. The $ID_{50}$ of *S. flexneri* and *S. sonnei* in humans is approximately 5000 microorganisms and that of *S. dysenteriae* is a few hundred cells; hence, secondary transmission of *Shigella* by person-to-person contact frequently occurs in outbreaks of foodborne illness. The incidence of shigellosis has decreased significantly during the 1996–2010 surveillance period,[1] although it is estimated to cause an economic loss of $257 million annually.[3] An emerging serotype of *S. boydii*, namely, serotype 20, has been reported in the United States.[134]

## *Yersinia enterocolitica*

*Yersinia enterocolitica* is a gram-negative, rod-shaped, facultative anaerobic bacterium, which was first isolated and described during the 1930s.[135] Swine have been identified as an important reservoir of *Y. enterocolitica*, in which the pathogen colonizes primarily the buccal cavity.[136] Although pork and pork products are considered to be the primary vehicles of *Y. enterocolitica*, a variety of other foods, including milk, ice cream, beef, lamb, seafood, and vegetables, have been identified as vehicles of *Y. enterocolitica* infection.[137] One of the largest outbreaks of yersiniosis in the United States was associated with milk.[138] Water has also been a vehicle of several outbreaks of *Y. enterocolitica* infection.[138] Surveys have revealed that *Y. enterocolitica* is frequently present in foods, having been isolated from 11% of sandwiches, 15% of chilled foods, and 22% of raw milk in Europe.[139] Several serovars of pathogenic *Y. enterocolitica* have been reported, which include O:3, O:5, O:8, and O:9,[140–142] with serovar O:3 (biserotype 4) being the most common causing human disease in the United States.[105–107] Although the incidence of *Yersinia* infection from 1996 to 2010 has decreased by 52% compared to the 1996–1998 surveillance period,[1] the pathogen causes annually an estimated 97,700 cases, 533 hospitalizations, and 29 deaths, accounting for $400 million loss.[3]

In addition to foodborne outbreaks, reports of blood transfusion-associated *Y. enterocolitica* sepsis indicate another potential mode of transmission of this pathogen.[143,144] Among bacteria, *Y. enterocolitica* has emerged as a significant cause of transfusion-associated bacteremia and mortality (53%), with 49 cases reported since this condition was first documented in 1975.[145] A review of these cases revealed that bacteremia may occur in a subpopulation of individuals with *Y. enterocolitica* gastrointestinal infection.[140] The strains of *Y. enterocolitica* responsible for transfusion-acquired yersiniosis are the same serobiotypes as those associated with enteric infections.

An unusual characteristic of *Y. enterocolitica* that influences food safety is its ability to grow at low temperatures, even as low as −1°C.[146] *Y. enterocolitica* readily withstands freezing and can survive in frozen foods for extended periods, even after repeated freezing and thawing.[147] Refrigeration (4°C) is one of the common methods used in food processing to control growth of spoilage and pathogenic microorganisms in foods. However, several studies have revealed growth of *Y. enterocolitica* in foods stored at refrigeration temperature. *Y. enterocolitica* grew on pork, chicken, and beef at 0°C–1°C.[148,149] The psychrotrophic nature of *Y. enterocolitica* also poses problems for the blood transfusion industry, mainly because of its ability to proliferate and release endotoxin in blood products stored at 4°C without manifesting any alterations in their physical appearance. The ability of *Y. enterocolitica* to grow well at refrigeration temperature has been exploited for isolating the pathogen from foods, water, and stool specimens. Such samples are incubated at 4°C–8°C in an enrichment broth for several days to selectively culture *Y. enterocolitica* based on its psychrotrophic nature.

*Y. enterocolitica* is primarily an intestinal pathogen with a predilection for extraintestinal spread under appropriate host conditions such as immunosuppression. In the gastrointestinal tract, *Y. enterocolitica* can cause acute enteritis, enterocolitis, mesenteric lymphadenitis, and terminal ileitis often mimicking appendicitis.[140] In the intestinal tract, the pathogen employs major virulence determinants such as invasins (Inv)—the proteins that mediate binding to host cell integrins, attachment invasion locus (Ail)—an outer-membrane protein associated with adhesion and invasion of the pathogen, a high-pathogenicity island (HPI) that sequesters iron, and a virulence plasmid (pVY) that encodes for YadA and Yop proteins for increased pathogenicity.[142] Infection with *Y. enterocolitica* often leads to secondary, immunologically induced sequelae such as arthritis (most common), erythema nodosum, Reiter's syndrome, glomerulonephritis, and myocarditis.

## *Vibrio* Species

Seafoods form a vital part of the American diet, and their consumption in the United States has risen steadily over the past few decades from an average of 4.5 kg/person in 1960 to about 7 kg in 2002.[150,151] However, according to a recent report published by the CSPI, contaminated seafoods have been recognized as a leading known cause of most foodborne illness outbreaks in the United States.[152] Vibrios, especially *V. parahaemolyticus*, *V. vulnificus*, and *V. cholerae*, which are commonly associated with estuarine and marine waters, represent the major pathogens resulting in disease outbreaks through consumption of seafoods and cause severe infections in cirrhotic patients.[153] The CDC reported a 115% increase in *Vibrio* infections during 1996–2010.[1] In addition, a recent epidemiologic investigation revealed that *Vibrio* spp. cause an estimated 34,800 cases with 195 hospitalizations and 40 deaths annually, accounting for $336 million in losses. However, among the vibrios, *V. vulnificus* caused the greatest economic impact, accounting for a loss of $268 million. *V. parahaemolyticus* and *V. vulnificus* are halophilic in nature, requiring the presence of 1%–3% sodium chloride for optimum growth. *V. cholerae* can grow in media without added salt, although their growth is stimulated by the presence of sodium ions.

Among the three species of *Vibrio*, *V. parahaemolyticus* accounts for the largest number of foodborne disease outbreaks (it was responsible for 34,664 of the total 34,844 cases reported for *Vibrio* spp.).[3] *V. parahaemolyticus* is present in coastal waters of the United States and the world. *V. parahaemolyticus* being an obligate halophile can multiply in substrates with sodium chloride concentrations ranging from 0.5% to 10%, with 3% being the optimal concentration for growth. The ability of *V. parahaemolyticus* to grow in a wide range of salt concentrations reflects on its existence in aquatic environments with various salinities. *V. parahaemolyticus* has a remarkable ability for rapid growth, and generation times as short as 12–18 min in seafoods have been reported at 30°C. Growth rates at lower temperatures are slower, but counts were found to increase from $10^2$ to $10^8$ colony-forming units (CFU)/g after 24 h storage at 25°C in homogenized shrimp and from $10^3$ to $10^8$ CFU/g after 7 days of storage at 12°C in homogenized oysters.[154] Because of its rapid growth, proper refrigeration of cooked seafoods to prevent regrowth of the bacterium is critical to product safety. A survey by the U.S. Food and Drug Administration revealed that 86% of 635 seafood samples contained *V. parahaemolyticus*, being isolated from codfish, sardine, mackerel, flounder, clam, octopus, shrimp, crab, lobster, crawfish, scallop, and oyster.[155] The pathogen has been a major seafood-associated *Vibrio* in Asian countries, including Japan, Taiwan, and China.[156] A new serotype of *V. parahaemolyticus*, O3:K6, that emerged in the Southeast Asia in the 1990s has been implicated in oyster-related outbreaks in the United States in 1997 and 1998.[157] An important virulence characteristic of pathogenic strains of *V. parahaemolyticus* is their ability to produce a thermostable hemolysin (Kanagawa hemolysin).[158] Studies in humans on the infectious dose of pathogenic *V. parahaemolyticus* strains revealed that ingestion of approximately $10^5$–$10^7$ bacteria can cause gastroenteritis.[155]

Among the 206 serogroups of *V. cholerae* identified thus far, serogroups O1 and O139, the causative agents of cholera in humans, are a part of the normal estuarine microflora, and foods such as raw fish, mussels, oysters, and clams have been associated with outbreaks of cholera.[159] The clinical course of cholera, which is a toxin-mediated acute illness, results in severe diarrhea. The bacterium secretes an enterotoxin that binds to receptors on the epithelial cell membrane of the small intestine causing increased levels of cAMP. Subsequently, elevated secretion of fluid and electrolytes results in a characteristic "rice water" diarrhea with large amounts of mucus in the stools.[153] The presence of a type VI secretion system (T6SS) in *V. cholerae* involved in its pathogenesis was recently identified.[160] Infected humans can serve as short-term carriers, shedding the pathogen in feces. Cholera is characterized by profuse diarrhea, potentially fatal in severe cases, and often described as "rice water" diarrhea due to the presence of prolific amounts of mucus in the stools. Gastroenteritis caused by non-O1 and non-O139 serovars of *V. cholerae* is usually mild in nature. During the period from 1996 to 2005, a total of 64 cases of toxigenic *V. cholerae* O1 were reported in the United States, of which 35 (55%) cases were acquired during foreign travel and 29 (45%) cases were domestically acquired.[161] Seven (24%) of the 29 domestic cases were attributed to consumption of Gulf Coast seafood (crabs, shrimp, or oysters). Moreover, seven of the eleven domestic cholera cases in 2005 were reported during October–December, after Hurricanes Katrina and Rita, although no evidence suggests increased risk for cholera among Gulf Coast residents or consumers of Gulf Coast seafood after the hurricanes. In 2003, a total of 111,575 cases of cholera worldwide were reported to the World Health Organization from 45 countries.[162]

*V. vulnificus* is the most serious of the vibrios and is responsible for most of the seafood-associated deaths in the United States, especially in Florida.[155] *V. vulnificus* results in life-threatening bacteremia, septicemia, and necrotizing fasciitis in persons with liver disorders and high iron level in blood, diabetes mellitus, end-stage renal disorders, and immunodeficiency conditions.[163] Although a number of seafoods have been associated with *V. vulnificus* infection, raw oysters are the most common vehicle associated with cases of illness.[164] The major virulence factors responsible for causing sepsis and bacteremia in *V. vulnificus* include its ability to escape acidic conditions in the stomach and its expression of capsular polysaccharide and surface LPSs, cytotoxins, pili, and flagella.[165]

### *Cronobacter sakazakii*

*Cronobacter sakazakii*, formerly *Enterobacter sakazakii*, is a foodborne pathogen that causes severe meningitis, meningoencephalitis, sepsis, and necrotizing enterocolitis in neonates and infants, with a case fatality rate of 40%–80%.[159–163] *C. sakazakii* infections may also result in severe neurological sequelae such as hydrocephalus, quadriplegia, and retarded neural development in survivors.[166] The epidemiology and reservoir of this pathogen are still unknown and most strains have been isolated from clinical specimens such as cerebrospinal fluid, blood, skin, wounds, urine, and respiratory and digestive tract samples.[167] The bacterium has also been isolated from foods such as cheese, eggs, fish, pork, shellfish, sausage, barley, biscuits, cowpea paste, nuts, seeds, rice, soy, sweets, tea, minced beef, sausage, and vegetables, namely, salads and tomato.[168,169] Recently, Kandhai et al.[170,171] isolated *C. sakazakii* from household and food production facility environmental samples, such as scrapings from dust, vacuum cleaner bags, and spilled product near equipment, and proposed that the organism could be more widespread in the environment than previously thought. Although the environmental source of *C. sakazakii* has not been identified, epidemiologic studies implicate dried infant formula as the primary route of transmission to infants.[172–175] The bacterium has been isolated from powdered infant formula by numerous investigators.[174,176–178] Muytjens et al.[178] isolated the pathogen from powdered infant formula from 35 different countries.

*C. sakazakii* possesses several characteristics that enable it to grow and survive in infant formula. For example, the pathogen can grow at temperatures as low as 5.5°C,[179] which is within the temperature range of many home refrigerators.[180] A study on the thermal resistance of *C. sakazakii* in reconstituted infant formula indicated that it is one of most thermotolerant bacteria under *Enterobacteriaceae*.[181] A recent study by Breeuwer et al.[182] reported that *C. sakazakii* also has a high tolerance to osmotic stress and desiccation. In addition, *C. sakazakii* possesses a short lag time and generation time in reconstituted infant formula,[179] raising concerns that improper storage of reconstituted formula may permit its substantial growth. Recently, Iversen and Forsythe[183] reported the isolation of *C. sakazakii* from a variety of foods, including powdered infant formula, dried infant food and milk powder, as well as certain herbs and spices. The first case of neonatal meningitis caused by *C. sakazakii* was reported in 1958,[184] and since then a number of *C. sakazakii* infections have been reported worldwide, including the United States. In the United States, an outbreak of *C. sakazakii* involving four infants occurred in the neonatal intensive care unit of a hospital in Memphis, resulting in sepsis, bloody diarrhea, and intestinal colonization. The source of infection was traced to contaminated infant formula.[174] In 2002, Himelright et al.[185] reported a case of fatal neonatal meningitis caused by *C. sakazakii* in Tennessee, associated with feeding of contaminated infant formula. The infection occurred in the neonatal intensive care unit of a hospital and surveillance studies identified two more cases of suspected infection with positive stool or urine in seven more infants. There were many recalls of *C. sakazakii*-contaminated infant formula in the United States. In November 2002, a nationwide recall of more than 1.5 million cans of dry infant formula contaminated with *C. sakazakii* was reported.[186] Besides survival and growth in several foods including reconstituted infant formula, *C. sakazakii* is a good biofilm former on abiotic surfaces such as latex, silicon and stainless steel, and neonatal nasogastric feeding tubes.[187] The International Commission on Microbiological Specification for Foods classified *C. sakazakii* as "severe hazard for restricted populations, life-threatening or substantial chronic sequelae of long duration." This places *C. sakazakii* in the same category as other serious food- and waterborne pathogens such as *Listeria monocytogenes*, *Clostridium botulinum* types A and B, and *Cryptosporidium parvum*.[188]

The most common clinical manifestations of infections due to *C. sakazakii* are sepsis and meningitis in neonates.

In more than 90% of the cases reported, patients developed meningitis with a very high prevalence for developing brain abscesses and less frequently ventriculitis and hydrocephalus.[189,190] While the reported mortality rates of *C. sakazakii* infections in neonates have declined over time from 50% or more to less than 20% due to advances in antimicrobial chemotherapy, an increasing incidence of resistance to commonly used antibiotic necessitates a reevaluation of existing treatment strategies.[167] Biering et al.[176] indicated that besides the high rate of mortality, the CNS infections due to *C. sakazakii* often lead to permanent impairment in mental and physical capabilities in surviving patients. In addition to meningitis, *C. sakazakii* is also reported to cause necrotizing enterocolitis in neonates and bacteremia, osteomyelitis, and pneumonia in elderly adults.[172,191–193]

### *Aeromonas hydrophila*

Although *Aeromonas* species have been recognized as pathogens of cold-blooded animals, their potential to cause human infections, especially foodborne illness, received attention only recently. *A. hydrophila* has been isolated from drinking water, fresh and saline waters, and sewage.[194] It also has been isolated from a variety of foods such as fish, oyster, shellfish, raw milk, ground beef, chicken, and pork.[194] *A. hydrophila* was isolated from cultured channel catfish, *Ictalurus punctatus*, during a disease outbreak in West Alabama in 2009.[195] Although *A. hydrophila* is sensitive to highly acidic conditions and does not possess any unusual thermal resistance, some strains are psychrotrophic and grow at refrigeration temperature.[196] *A. hydrophila* can grow on a variety of refrigerated foods, including pork, asparagus, cauliflower, and broccoli.[197,198] However, considering the widespread occurrence of *A. hydrophila* in water and food and its relatively infrequent association with human illness, it is likely that most strains of this bacterium are not pathogenic for humans. *A. hydrophila* infection in humans is characterized by watery diarrhea and mild fever. Virulent strains of *A. hydrophila* produce a 52 kDa polypeptide, which possesses enterotoxic, cytotoxic, and hemolytic activities.[199] *A. hydrophila* strains with resistance to multiple antibiotics have been reported.[200]

### *Plesiomonas shigelloides*

*Plesiomonas shigelloides* has been implicated in several cases of sporadic and epidemic gastroenteritis[201] and is regarded as an emerging enteric pathogen in humans.[202] The pathogen is present in fresh and estuarine waters and has been isolated from various aquatic animals.[196] Seafoods such as fish, crabs, and oysters have been associated with cases of *P. shigelloides* infection. The isolation of *P. shigelloides* from vertebrate animals, including swine, cats, dogs, and monkeys, suggests its potential for being a zoonotic pathogen.[202] The most common symptoms of *P. shigelloides* infection include abdominal pain, nausea, chills, fever, and diarrhea. Potential virulence factors of *P. shigelloides* include cytotoxic enterotoxin, invasins, and β-hemolysin.[196] An outbreak of *P. shigelloides* infection associated with drinking well water and involving 30 persons was reported in New York in 1996.[203]

### Listeria monocytogenes

*L. monocytogenes* has emerged into a highly significant and fatal foodborne pathogen throughout the world, especially in the United States. There is an estimated 2500 cases of listeriosis annually in the United States, with a mortality rate of ca. 25%.[204] Further, *L. monocytogenes* is of tremendous economic significance, causing an estimated monetary loss of $2.3 billion annually in the United States.[205] A large outbreak of listeriosis involving more than 100 cases and associated with eating contaminated turkey frankfurters occurred during 1998–1999.[206] During this period of time, there were more than 35 recalls of a number of different food products contaminated with listeriae.[206] In 2002, a large outbreak of listeriosis in the United States involving 46 people, 7 deaths, and 3 miscarriages resulted in a recall of 27.4 million pounds of fresh and frozen ready-to-eat chicken and turkey frankfurters.[88] In 2003, 696 cases of listeriosis were reported in the United States, with more than 50% of the cases occurring in persons above 60 years of age.[104] Contaminated ready-to-eat meat was implicated as the vehicle of two large multiprovince *Listeria* outbreaks that occurred in Canada in 2008.[207] In the same year in Austria, contaminated jellied pork was the vehicle of invasive listeriosis characterized by febrile gastroenteritis.[208] In 2011, a nationwide outbreak of listeriosis in the United States, involving more than 130 people with 30 deaths and one abortion, was associated with consumption of contaminated cantaloupe.[1]

*L. monocytogenes* is widespread in nature, occurring in soil, vegetation, and untreated water. Humans and a wide variety of farm animals, including cattle, sheep, goat, pig, and poultry, are known sources of *L. monocytogenes*.[209] *L. monocytogenes* also occurs frequently in food processing facilities, especially in moist areas such as floor drains, floors, and processing equipment.[210] *L. monocytogenes* can also grow in biofilms attached to a variety of processing plant surfaces such as stainless steel, glass, and rubber.[211] A wide spectrum of foods, including milk, cheese, beef, pork, chicken, seafoods, fruits, and vegetables, has been identified as vehicles of *L. monocytogenes*.[209] However, ready-to-eat cooked foods such as low-acid soft cheese, pâtes, and cooked poultry meat, which can support the growth of listeriae to large populations (>$10^6$ cells/g) when held at refrigeration temperature for several weeks, have been regarded as high-risk foods.[212,213] *L. monocytogenes* possesses several characteristics, which enable the pathogen to successfully contaminate, survive, and grow in foods, thereby resulting in outbreaks. These traits include an ability to grow at refrigeration temperature and in a medium with minimal nutrients; ability to survive in acidic conditions, e.g., pH 4.2; ability to tolerate up to 10% sodium chloride; ability to survive incomplete cooking or subminimal pasteurization treatments; and ability to survive in biofilms on equipment in food processing plants and resist superficial cleaning and disinfection treatments.[206]

Approximately 3%–10% of humans carry listeriae in their gastrointestinal tract with no symptoms of illness.[214] Human listeriosis is an uncommon illness with a high mortality rate. The infection most frequently occurs in people who are older, pregnant, or possess a compromised immune system. Clinical manifestations range from mild influenza-like symptoms to meningitis and meningoencephalitis. Pregnant females infected with the pathogen may not present symptoms of illness or may exhibit only mild influenza-like symptoms. However, spontaneous abortion, premature birth, and stillbirth are frequent sequelae to listeriosis in pregnant females.[213] Although the infective dose of *L. monocytogenes* is not known, published reports indicate that it is likely to be more than 100 CFU per gram of food.[213] However, the infective dose largely depends on the age, condition of health, and immunological status of the host.

*L. monocytogenes* crosses the intestinal barrier in hosts infected by the oral route. However, before reaching the intestine, the bacterium must withstand the adverse environment of the stomach. Gastric acidity may destroy a significant number of *L. monocytogenes* ingested with contaminated food. The site at which intestinal translocation of *L. monocytogenes* occurs is not clearly elucidated. However, both epithelial cells and M cells in the Peyer's patches are believed to be the potential sites of entry.[215] The bacteria are then internalized by macrophages where they survive and replicate. This is followed by the transport of the pathogen via blood to the mesenteric lymph nodes, spleen, and the liver. The primary site of *L. monocytogenes* replication in the liver is the hepatocyte. In the initial phase of infection, the infected hepatocytes are the target for neutrophils and subsequently for mononuclear phagocytes, which aid the control and resolution of the infection.[213] If the immune system fails to contain *L. monocytogenes*, subsequent propagation of pathogen via blood to the brain or uterus takes place.[216] The major virulence factors in *L. monocytogenes* include hemolysin, phospholipases, metalloprotease, Clp proteases and ATPases, internalins, surface protein p104, protein p60, listeriolysin O, and the surface protein *ActA*.[213]

### Staphylococcus aureus

Recent epidemiologic estimates indicate 241,000 cases of *S. aureus*-related illnesses, resulting in 1,064 hospitalizations and 6 deaths annually in the United States, which account for a loss of $130 million.[3] Preformed, heat-stable enterotoxin that can resist boiling for several minutes is the agent responsible for staphylococcal food poisoning. Among these, enterotoxin A is the most common cause of food poisoning episodes.[217] Humans are the principal reservoir of *S. aureus* strains involved in outbreaks of foodborne illness. In addition, a recent study revealed that *S. aureus* can be transmitted between healthy, lactating mothers without mastitis and their infants by breastfeeding.[218] Colonized humans can be long-term carriers of *S. aureus* and thereby contaminate foods and other humans.[219] The organism commonly resides in the throat and nasal cavity and on the skin, especially in boils and carbuncles.[219]

Staphylococcal protein A (*Spa*) typing and DNA microarray have revealed striking similarities between the nasal isolates of food handlers and isolates involved in outbreaks.[220] Protein-rich foods such as ham, poultry, fish, dairy products, custards, cream-filled bakery products, and salads containing cooked meat, chicken, and potatoes are the vehicles most frequently associated with *S. aureus* food poisoning.[221] Additionally, other food vehicles, including hamburgers, milk, pasta salad, and raw milk cheese, have been implicated in *S. aureus* food poisoning.[222] *S. aureus* is usually overgrown by competing bacterial flora in raw foods; hence, raw foods are not typical vehicles of staphylococcal food poisoning. Cooking eliminates most of the normal bacterial flora of raw foods, thereby enabling the growth of *S. aureus*, which can be introduced by infected cooks and food handlers into foods after cooking. The incubation period of staphylococcal food poisoning is very short, with symptoms being observed within 2–6 h after eating toxin-contaminated food. Symptoms include nausea, vomiting, diarrhea, and abdominal pain.

*S. aureus* can grow within a wide range of pH values from 4 to 9.3, with optimum growth occurring at pH 6–7. *S. aureus* has an exceptional tolerance to sodium chloride, being able to grow in foods in the presence of 7%–10% NaCl, with some strains tolerating up to 20% NaCl.[221] *S. aureus* has the unique ability to grow at a water activity as low as 0.83–0.86.[223] *S. aureus* produces nine different enterotoxins, which are quite heat resistant, losing their serological activity at 121°C but not at 100°C for several minutes.[223]

Besides being a foodborne pathogen, *S. aureus* has emerged as an important pathogen in nosocomial infections and community-acquired diseases, because of its toxin-mediated virulence, invasiveness, and antibiotic resistance.[224] This is especially significant due to the emergence of methicillin-resistant strains of *S. aureus* (MRSA), and 50% of healthcare-acquired *S. aureus* isolates in the United States in 1997 were methicillin resistant.[225] Although MRSA are commonly linked to nosocomial infections, the first report of MRSA-associated foodborne disease in a community was reported in 2002.[225] The community-acquired MRSA are particularly virulent, resulting in tissue destructing infections, necrotizing fasciitis, and fulminant pneumonia, and this is attributed to a factor called Panton–Valentine leukocidin (PVL).[226] In addition, the gene responsible for methicillin resistance, *mecA*, encodes a low-affinity penicillin-binding protein called PBP2a that confers resistance to not only methicillin but also to the entire class of β-lactam antibiotics such as cephalosporins, penicillins, and carbapenems.[226] Some clones of MRSA are colonizers of the pig intestinal tract, and recent reports reveal that pig-to-human transmission is possible, highlighting its zoonotic potential.[227,228] Researchers have observed an expanding spectrum of antibiotic resistance in MRSA, with emerging linezolid resistance in MRSA strains.[229]

### *Clostridium botulinum*

Foodborne botulism is an intoxication caused by ingestion of foods containing preformed botulinal toxin, a 150 kDa metalloprotease produced by *C. botulinum* under anaerobic conditions. Botulinal toxin is a neurotoxin, which causes the neuroparalytic disease called botulism. The genes encoding botulinum toxins and other related proteins are located together in a cluster found on the *C. botulinum* chromosome or plasmid. There are two conserved cluster types in *C. botulinum*: the "ha cluster" and the "orf-X cluster."[230] The toxin binds irreversibly to the presynaptic nerve endings of the nervous system, where it inhibits the release of acetylcholine. Unlike botulism in adults, infant botulism results from the colonization and germination of *C. botulinum* spores in the infant's gastrointestinal tract. The disease usually happens in infants during the second month of age and is characterized by constipation, poor feeding or sucking, and decreased muscle tone with a "floppy" head.[231] Although the source of infection is unknown in majority of the cases, most commonly suspected food in infant botulism is honey.[232]

There are seven types of *C. botulinum* (A, B, C, D, E, F, and G) classified on the basis of the antigenic specificity of the neurotoxin they produce.[233] The organism is present in soil, vegetation, and sedimentation under water. Type A strains are proteolytic, whereas type E strains are nonproteolytic.[234] Another classification divides *C. botulinum* into four groups: group 1 (type A strains and proteolytic strains of types B and F), group II (type E strains and nonproteolytic strains of B and F), group III (type C and D strains), and group IV (type G strains). The association of *C. botulinum* types I–III in disease outbreaks in cattle has raised concerns regarding the potential transmission of the toxin to humans via dairy products.[235]

Type A *C. botulinum* occurs frequently in soils of the western United States, whereas type B strains are more often present in the eastern states and in Europe.[234] Type E strains are largely associated with aquatic environments and fish. Type A cases of botulism in the United States are frequently associated with temperature-abused, home-prepared foods. Proteolytic type A, B, and F strains produce heat-resistant spores, which pose a safety concern in low-acid canned foods. In contrast, nonproteolytic type B, E, and F strains produce heat-labile spores, which are of concern in pasteurized or unheated foods.[234] The minimum pH for growth of group I and group II strains is 4.6 and 5, respectively.[233] Group I strains can grow at a minimum water activity of 0.94, whereas group II strains do not grow below a water activity of 0.97.[236] The proteolytic strains of *C. botulinum* are generally more resistant to heat than nonproteolytic strains.

Types of foods associated with cases of botulism include fish, meat, honey, soup, chilli sauce, baked potato, sausage, tofu, and home-canned vegetables.[230,233,237] Several other vehicles such as poultry litter, water, water fowls, silage, brewer's grain, bakery waste, and cat and cattle carcasses have also been implicated in botulism outbreaks during the past three decades.[235] In September 2011, two cases of botulism were associated with ground green olive paste in France.[238]

## Clostridium perfringens

*C. perfringens* is a major bacterial cause of foodborne disease, with 1062 cases reported in the United States in 2004.[8] *C. perfringens* strains are grouped into five types: A, B, C, D, and E, based on the type(s) of toxin(s) produced. *C. perfringens* foodborne illness is almost exclusively associated with type A isolates of *C. perfringens* that carry the plasmid-borne *C. perfringens* enterotoxin (cpe) gene.[239] This toxin type causes gangrene in humans and severe enteric disease in humans and animals.[240] *C. perfringens* is commonly present in soil, dust, water, and in the intestinal tract of humans, animals, and birds.[241] It is frequently present in foods; about 50% of raw or frozen meat and poultry contain *C. perfringens*.[242] Spores produced by *C. perfringens* are quite heat resistant and can survive boiling for up to 1 h.[242] *C. perfringens* spores can survive in cooked foods, and if not properly cooled before refrigerated storage, the spores will germinate and vegetative cells can grow to large populations during holding at growth temperatures. Large populations of *C. perfringens* cells ($>10^6$/g) ingested with contaminated food will enter the small intestine, multiply, and sporulate. During sporulation in the small intestine, *C. perfringens* enterotoxin is produced, which induces a diarrheal response. The enterotoxin is a 35 kDa heat-labile polypeptide that damages the epithelial cells of the gastrointestinal tract to cause fluid and electrolyte loss.[243,244] Although vegetative cells of *C. perfringens* are sensitive to cold temperature and freezing, spores tolerate cold temperature well and can survive in refrigerated foods.

## Clostridium difficile

*Clostridium difficile* is a major cause of enteric disease in humans, and recent evidence indicates that it has emerged into a community-associated pathogen. *C. difficile* has been isolated from the intestinal tract of many food animals,[245,246] and several small-scale studies conducted in different parts of the world have revealed the presence of *C. difficile* in retail meat and meat products.[247,248] This has raised concerns that foods could potentially be involved in the transmission of *C. difficile* to humans.

*C. difficile* is a gram-positive, spore-forming, anaerobic bacterium, which causes a toxin-mediated enteric disease in humans.[249] The total annual number of cases of *C. difficile* infection in the United States is estimated to exceed 250,000,[250] resulting in approximately U.S. $1 billion annually in health-care costs. Among patients diagnosed with *C. difficile* infection, relapse or reinfection occurs in 12%–24% within 2 months.[251] Moreover, the mortality rates of disease associated with *C. difficile* in the United States have increased from 5.7 per million to 23.7 per million from 1999 to 2004, respectively.[252] The symptoms in *C. difficile* disease include abdominal pain, fever, fulminant colitis, toxic megacolon (bowel perforation), sepsis, and shock.[245] In addition, asymptomatic colonization of *C. difficile* causing mild diarrhea has been reported in some patients. *C. difficile* infection has been associated with the use of gastric acid-suppressing agents and

antibiotics, which result in the germination of spores in the stomach and selection for *C. difficile* in the intestine.[253]

Historically, *C. difficile* was considered a nosocomial pathogen that mainly affected the elderly, the severely ill, and the long-term hospital inpatients.[254] However, recently some changes in the epidemiology of *C. difficile* have been reported. For example, an increase in community-acquired *C. difficile*-associated disease (CDAD) has been reported, especially in populations that were not previously considered at risk of infection.[254] Another change in the epidemiology of *C. difficile* is that an increase in morbidity, mortality, and relapse rate in infections has been reported in the United States and elsewhere, which is attributed to the emergence and dissemination of a new hypervirulent strain, classified as North American Pulse type 1(NAP 1) using pulsed-field gel electrophoresis.[245,249] The strain belongs to the toxin type III and ribotype 027.[255] Emerging antimicrobial resistance in *C. difficile* has been reported by many investigators, especially resistance to fluoroquinolones, clindamycin and erythromycin, metronidazole, vancomycin, gatifloxacin, and moxifloxacin.[256]

The major virulence factors of *C. difficile* include two large toxins, namely, toxin A (TcdA, enterotoxin) and toxin B (TcdB, cytotoxin).[257] In addition, a third toxin called *C. difficile* binary toxin (CDT) has been detected in some strains of the pathogen.[258] TcdA and TcdB are encoded by two genes present in a single operon and are highly expressed during late log and stationary phases of growth upon exposure to environmental stimuli.[259] The binary toxin was detected in approximately 6% of clinical *C. difficile* isolates obtained from the United States and Europe,[260] and an increase in the prevalence of binary toxin-producing *C. difficile* strains has been reported during the last decade.[255,261]

The common means of contracting *C. difficile* infection in humans is via the fecal–oral route. The bacterium is ingested in the vegetative form or as spores, which can persist for long periods in the environment and overcome the acidity in the stomach. In the intestine, *C. difficile* spores germinate into the vegetative form, especially if the normal flora has been disrupted by antibiotic therapy. *C. difficile* multiplies in the intestinal crypts, releasing the A and B toxins, causing severe inflammation and disruption of intestinal epithelial cells, thereby leading to colitis, pseudomembrane formation, and watery diarrhea.[251]

Recent studies conducted worldwide have revealed the occurrence of *C. difficile* in a variety of food animals.[246,262] Pigs and calves are among the most common reservoirs of *C. difficile*. Apart from animals serving as reservoirs, foods such as ground beef, ground veal, veal chops, retail chicken (thighs, wings, and legs), raw milk, summer sausage, ground pork, ground turkey, braunschweiger, water, and raw vegetable samples have been identified as potential vehicles of *C. difficile*.[247,248,263]

## Bacillus cereus

*B. cereus* is a spore-forming pathogen present in soil and on vegetation. It is responsible for an increasing number of foodborne diseases in industrial countries,[264] with 103 outbreak associated confirmed cases reported in the United States in 2004.[8] It is reported as the fourth largest cause of foodborne disease in the European Union.[265] It is frequently isolated from foods such as meat, spices, vegetables, dairy products, and cereal grains, especially fried rice.[266] There are two types of foodborne illness caused by *B. cereus*, i.e., a diarrheagenic illness and an emetic syndrome.[264,267] The diarrheal syndrome caused by heat-labile enterotoxins is usually mild and is characterized by abdominal cramps, nausea, and watery stools similar to that observed in *C. perfringens* infection.[268] Types of foods implicated in outbreaks of diarrheal syndrome include cereal food products containing corn and corn starch, mashed potatoes, vegetables, milk, and cooked meat products. The emetic syndrome is caused by a heat-stable dodecadepsipeptide toxin called cereulide that is produced in food[264] and is characterized by severe vomiting. The clinical symptoms are similar to those observed in *S. aureus* poisoning.[269] Refried or rewarmed boiled rice, pasta, noodles, ice cream, and pastry are frequently implicated in outbreaks of emetic syndrome.[270,271] The dose of *B. cereus* required to produce diarrheal illness is estimated at more than $10^5$ cells/g.[272] The toxin-induced pathogenicity of *B. cereus* is regulated by a pleiotropic transcriptional activator, PlcR, that controls the production of enterotoxins—hemolytic Hbl and nonhemolytic Nhe—and the cytotoxin CytK.[273,274]

### *Arcobacter butzleri*

*Arcobacter* species belong to the family of *Campylobacteraceae* and occur primarily as commensals in the gut of animals and humans.[275] Arcobacters are Gram-negative, aerotolerant *Campylobacter*-like organisms that can grow under microaerobic conditions.[276] There are 13 species of *Arcobacter*, of which *A. butzleri*, *A. cryaerophilus*, and *A. skirrowii* are of public health importance.[277] They can grow at 25°C, a differentiating feature from *Campylobacter*, and can hydrolyze indoxyl acetate and reduce nitrate.[278] Although *Arcobacter* can grow at a range of 15°C–37°C, the optimum temperature for growth is 30°C.[279] Among the arcobacters, *A. butzleri* is most commonly associated with human enteritis, characterized by persistent and watery diarrhea, vomiting, nausea, and fever.[280] *A. butzleri* strains resistant to antibiotics such as clindamycin, ciprofloxacin, metronidazole, carbenicillin, cefoperazone, nalidixic acid, and azithromycin have been reported.[277]

*A. butzleri* is the most common *Arcobacter* isolated from livestock species. There is mounting evidence that arcobacters in general, and *A. butzleri* in particular, are efficient colonizers in healthy swine, sheep, horses, and cattle,[281] with poultry being the most significant reservoir. However, there are conflicting reports on the pathogen's role as a commensal in the chicken intestinal tract.[282] Humans may contract *Arcobacter* infection via consumption of contaminated food of animal origin and water,[277] although this is not fully understood.[280] Recent reports have revealed that the pathogen has been isolated from raw beef, pork, and chicken, of which the rate of isolation from chicken was greater compared to

others. The prevalence of *A. butzleri* on broiler carcasses suggests its presence in poultry abattoirs, and that contamination could be processing associated.[783] In addition, *A. butzleri* has been isolated from several water sources, including groundwater, seawater, bays, surface water, and raw sewage.[275] More importantly, the pathogen has been isolated from well water, water treatment plants, and other sources of water storage.[276] It has also been observed that *A. butzleri* can attach to stainless steel, copper, and plastic pipelines[276] that carry water indicating its adherence potential on abiotic surfaces.

Little information is known regarding the virulence mechanisms by which *A. butzleri* infects humans and animals. However, it has been determined that *A. butzleri* is highly adherent, invasive, and cytotoxic to cell cultures. *A. butzleri* is the most invasive species among the arcobacters[284] based on its ability to colonize piglet intestines, although variable results on colonization of chicken and turkeys were observed.

### *Brucella* Species

*Brucella* spp. are pathogens in many animals, causing sterility and abortion. In humans, *Brucella* is the etiologic agent of undulant fever. The genus *Brucella* consists of six species, of which those of principal concern are *B. abortus*, *B. suis*, and *B. melitensis*.[285] *B. abortus* causes disease in cattle and *B. suis* in swine, and *B. melitensis* is the primary pathogen of sheep. *B. melitensis* is the most pathogenic species for humans. Human brucellosis is primarily an occupational disease of veterinarians and meat industry workers. Brucellosis can be transmitted by aerosols and dust. Foodborne brucellosis can be transmitted to humans by consumption of meat and milk products from infected farm animals. The most common food vehicle of brucellosis for humans is unpasteurized milk.[285] Meat is a less common source of foodborne brucellosis because the organisms are destroyed by cooking. Since the National Brucellosis Education program has almost eradicated *B. abortus* infection from U.S. cattle herds, the risk of foodborne infection of brucellosis through consumption of domestically produced milk and dairy products is minimal.[103]

### *Helicobacter pylori*

*H. pylori* is a human pathogen causing chronic gastritis, gastric ulcer, and gastric carcinoma.[286,287] Once colonized in humans, the pathogen could be the predominant species present in the stomach. The infection is mostly acquired early in life (<10 years of age).[288] Although humans are the primary host of *H. pylori*, the bacterium has been isolated from cats.[212] *H. pylori* does not survive well outside its host, but it has been detected in water and vegetables.[289,290] A study on the effect of environmental and substrate factors on the growth of *H. pylori* indicated that the pathogen likely lacks the ability to grow in most foods.[291] However, *H. pylori* may survive for long periods in low-acid environments under refrigerated conditions. *H. pylori* infections spread primarily by person-to-person transmission, especially among children, and contaminated water and food are considered potential vehicles of the pathogen. In the United States, a significant association between *H. pylori* infection and iron-deficiency anemia, regardless of the presence or absence of peptic ulcer, has been reported.[292,293]

## VIRAL FOODBORNE PATHOGENS

Estimates by the CDC of the incidence of foodborne illness in the United States indicate that viruses are responsible for approximately 67% of the total foodborne illnesses of known etiology annually (Table 3.2).[204] Viruses are obligate intracellular microorganisms and most foodborne viruses contain RNA rather than DNA. Since viruses are intracellular organisms requiring a host for multiplication, they cannot grow in foods. Therefore, the number of virus particles on foods will not increase during processing, transport, or storage, causing no deterioration in food quality.[294] Foodborne viruses are generally enteric in nature, causing illness through ingestion of foods and water contaminated with human feces (fecal–oral route). Viruses disseminated through foods also can be spread by person-to-person contact. For example, research with hepatitis A virus has revealed that a few hundred virus particles can readily be transferred from fecally contaminated fingers to foods and surfaces.[295] Fresh produce and shellfish are generally common sources of viral contamination and thus considered as high-risk foods.[296] Hepatitis A virus, norovirus (previously known as Norwalk-like viruses), and possibly rotavirus are among the most significant of the viruses that are foodborne.

### Hepatitis A Virus

Hepatitis A virus is a member of the family *Picornaviridae* and is transmitted by the fecal–oral route. Raw shellfish harvested from waters contaminated by human sewage is among the foods most frequently associated with outbreaks of hepatitis A virus.[297] Besides shellfish, other foods including sandwiches, dairy products, baked products, salads, fruits, and vegetables have also been implicated in various outbreaks of hepatitis A virus.[298,299] A large outbreak in Pennsylvania in 2003 involving more than 500 cases was linked to ingestion of contaminated green onions.[300] Hepatitis A virus is more resistant to heat and drying than other picornaviruses.[297] The incubation period for onset of symptoms of hepatitis A infection ranges from 15 to 45 days, and symptoms include nausea, abdominal pain, jaundice, and fever. The virus is shed in feces by infected humans many days before the onset of symptoms, indicating the importance of good personal hygienic practices of cooks and food handlers who could otherwise contaminate food during the period of asymptomatic fecal shedding. The overall incidence of hepatitis A virus in the United States has decreased since the implementation of routine childhood vaccination against the virus in 1996.[104] In 2007, the CDC reported that the incidence of hepatitis A infections was at their lowest level.[301]

### Norovirus

Norovirus belongs to the family *Caliciviridae* and is often referred to as small, round-structured viruses. Norovirus is recognized as the most common viral cause of foodborne and waterborne acute gastroenteritis in the United States.[1] The virus possesses a low infectious doze of less than 100 virus particles.[302] Raw or undercooked shellfish and other seafoods are common vehicles of norovirus. The incubation period of infection ranges from 24 to 48 h, and symptoms include nausea, vomiting, and diarrhea. The young, immunocompromised, and elderly are considered to be at greatest risk of developing severe illness caused by the pathogen.[303] Infected humans shed the virus in feces for up to a week after symptoms have subsided. The virus survives freezing, heating to 60°C, and chlorine levels up to 10 ppm.[302] Qualitative studies in human volunteers indicate that the viruses are infective for up to 3 h when exposed to a medium at pH 2.2 at room temperature or for 60 min at pH 7 at 60°C.[304]

The impact of norovirus on the U.S. economy is large. A recent study revealed that the virus causes an estimated 5 million cases, resulting in 14,663 hospitalizations and 149 deaths, which accounts for a loss of $2.8 billion.[3] In 2009, the United States launched CaliciNet, an outbreak surveillance network for noroviruses. Of 558 norovirus outbreaks submitted to the CaliciNet since 2009, 14% were associated with foodborne transmission. Of the five genogroups (GI–GV), GI and GII were the most common affecting humans. The genogroup GII has 19 genotypes, of which GII.4 caused more than 85% of the norovirus outbreaks. A GII.4 variant called GII.4 New Orleans emerged as the major disease-causing genotype in October 2009, replacing another variant, GII.4 Minerva, that was the common outbreak strain since 2005.[305]

### Rotavirus

Rotavirus is a nonenveloped, double-shelled virus, with a genome comprised of 11 segments of double-stranded RNA. It is characterized by two surface-expressed neutralizing antigens, a glycosylated outer surface protein (G protein) encoded by the VP7 gene and a protease-cleaved protein (P protein) encoded by the VP4 gene. Rotavirus is the most common cause of diarrhea in children worldwide, especially in developing countries. In the United States and other countries with a temperate climate, infection with rotavirus has been reported to peak during the winter season (November to April). In the United States, there are an estimated 3.9 million cases of rotavirus diarrhea each year; however, only 39,000 cases are estimated to be acquired through contaminated foods.[204] Rotavirus infection has an incubation period of 1–3 days and is characterized by fever, vomiting, and diarrhea. The virus is shed in the feces of infected humans and can survive on vegetables at 4°C or 20°C for many days.[306] It has also been shown to survive the process of making soft cheese.[306] The primary mode of transmission of rotavirus is by fecal-to-oral route. In early 2006, the U.S. Food and Drug Administration approved a new live, oral vaccine (RotaTeq™) for the prevention of rotavirus gastroenteritis in infants. This pentavalent vaccine expresses five different genotypes of the virus, namely, G1, G2, G3, G4, and, the most common P-type, P1A. During the surveillance periods 2005–2006 and 2006–2007, G1 was predominant, and

**TABLE 3.2**
**Viral Foodborne Pathogens**

| Microorganism | Significant Characteristics | Sources/Reservoirs | Examples of Vehicles | Estimated No. of Foodborne Cases Annually in the United States[2,3] | Incubation Period, Symptoms, and Duration | Detection Methods | Control/Prevention |
|---|---|---|---|---|---|---|---|
| Hepatitis A virus | Single-stranded RNA virus, spherical in shape, remains viable for long periods of time in foods stored at refrigeration temperature; virus multiplies in the gut epithelium before being carried by blood to the liver. Virus is shed in feces before symptoms of liver damage become apparent. | Humans, sewage-polluted waters | Raw or undercooked shellfish and seafoods harvested from sewage-polluted water, ready-to-eat foods such as salads prepared by infected food handler | 1,566 | 15–45 days, usually ca. 25 days. Loss of appetite, nausea, abdominal pain, fever, jaundice, dark urine, pale stools. Duration is a few weeks to months. | Cultural methods[592,593] Enzyme immunoassay[594] PCR[595–598] LAMP assay[599] Immunochromatography assay[600] | Avoid consumption of raw seafoods; disinfection of drinking water, good personal hygiene and food handling practices, vaccination of professional food handlers, safe sewage disposal |
| Norovirus | Single-stranded RNA virus, spherical in shape, does not multiply in any known laboratory host. | Humans, sewage-polluted waters | Raw or undercooked shellfish and seafoods harvested from sewage-polluted water, drinking water | 5,461,731 | 1–2 days. Loss of appetite, nausea, abdominal pain, diarrhea, vomiting, headache. Duration is 2 days. | Enzyme immunoassay[601,602] PCR[603–607] Latex agglutination test[608] Third-generation ELISA coupled with immunochromatography[609] DNA microarray[610] | Avoid consumption of raw seafoods, disinfection of drinking water, good personal hygiene and food hand ing practices, hygienic sewage disposal, treatment of wastewater used for irrigation |
| Rotavirus | Double-stranded RNA virus, icosahedral in shape. | Humans | To be determined | 15,433 | 1–3 days. Vomiting, abdominal pain followed by watery diarrhea. Duration is 6–8 days. | Cultural methods[592,593] ELISA[611,612] PCR[612–615] Flow cytometry[310,616] Immunobiosensor[617] | Avoid consumption of raw seafoods Avoid drinking of untreated water Good personal hygiene |
| Avian influenza virus | Single-stranded RNA virus, medium sized, pleomorphic, enveloped. | Chicken, turkey, guinea fowl, and migratory waterfowl | Raw or undercooked contaminated egg and poultry meat | Emerging disease Not reported in the United States 132 cases worldwide (1997–2005) | Typical flu symptoms such as fever, cough, sore throat, and muscle aches. Also eye infections (conjunctivitis), pneumonia, and acute respiratory distress can be present. | Cultural method[310] Rapid antigen detection test[618] PCR[310,619,620] Serological test[310] Resequencing microarray[621] | Avoid consumption of raw or undercooked poultry meat and egg Avoid using raw eggs for preparing foods that are not cooked Avoid handling and slaughtering of infected birds or birds suspected of infection Use hygienic practices during slaughter and postslaughter operations |

during 2007–2008, G3 replaced G1. Currently monitoring of strains for any possible vaccine-pressure-induced changes is underway. Another live attenuated rotavirus vaccine based on genotype G1P, Rotarix, is currently approved for use in the United States.[307]

## Avian Influenza Virus

Avian influenza (bird flu) is a highly contagious viral infection affecting a wide species of birds, including chicken, turkey, guinea fowl, and migratory waterfowl. The disease is of tremendous economic significance to the poultry industry. Recent outbreaks of avian influenza infections in poultry and humans highlight the zoonotic potential of the disease and its impact on public health.[308] During the period from 1997 to 2005, 132 human cases of avian influenza with 64 deaths have been reported worldwide.[309] Based on virulence, avian influenza virus can be classified into the highly pathogenic avian influenza (HPAI) strains that cause a systemic lethal infection, resulting in death of birds as early as 24 h to 1 week postinfection, and the low pathogenic avian influenza (LPAI) viruses that rarely result in fatal disease in birds.[284] The HPAI viruses that cause "fowl plague" are restricted to the subtypes H5 and H7; however, all the viruses of these subtypes do not cause HPAI. H5N1 is the influenza A virus subtype that occurs mainly in birds, causing fatal disease in birds.

Avian influenza viruses, belonging to the family Orthomyxoviridae, are medium-sized, pleomorphic, enveloped viruses with glycoprotein projections from the envelope having hemagglutinating (HA) and neuraminidase (NA) activities.[310] The genome of the virus consists of eight segments of single-stranded RNA of a negative sense, which code for ten viral proteins. Antigenically, three distinct types of influenza viruses are reported, namely, type A, type B, and type C, with the former type causing natural infections in birds. Based on the antigenic properties of hemagglutinin and neuraminidase surface glycoproteins, type A influenza viruses are divided into various subtypes.[311] Currently, 15 HA and 9 NA subtypes have been reported.[284] The ability of these viruses to transform by recombination and assortment enables them to adapt to new hosts, including humans.

The hemagglutinin glycoproteins play a vital role in the pathogenicity by mediating attachment of the virus to host cell receptors followed by release of viral RNA.[308] The HA glycoprotein precursor (HA0) is posttranslationally cleaved into HA1 and HA2 subunits by host proteases, with the HA2 amino terminus mediating fusion between the viral envelope and the endosomal membrane.[312] Klenk et al.[313] reported that proteolytic activation of HA glycoprotein is essential for viral infectivity and dissemination, thus highlighting its role in the pathogenesis of avian influenza virus. The HA precursor proteins of LPAI viruses have a single arginine at the cleavage site; hence, these viruses are limited to cleavage by host proteases such as trypsin-like enzymes. Therefore, replication of LPAI viruses is limited to sites (organs) where such enzymes are found (respiratory and intestinal tracts),

thereby resulting in mild infections. However, the HAs of HPAI viruses contain multiple basic amino acids at the cleavage site, which are cleaved by ubiquitous proteases present in a variety of host cells. These viruses therefore are able to replicate throughout the bird, causing lethal systemic infection and death.[314,315]

The source of infection to poultry in most outbreaks is direct or indirect contact with waterbirds. Once the infection is established in birds, the disease is highly contagious. Fecal-to-oral transmission is the most common mode of spread between birds. Contact with infected material is the most important mode of transmission from bird to bird. In infected birds, the virus is excreted in the droppings and nasal and ocular discharges. Fecal shedding of the virus by infected birds has been documented up to 4 weeks postinfection. Contaminated feed, water, rodents, and insects can also play a role in the spread of virus. Movement of infected birds, contaminated equipment, egg flats, feed truck, and service crew can also spread the virus from flock to flock. Airborne transmission of the virus can potentially occur if birds are kept in close proximity and with air movement. Since lesions have been reported in the ovaries and oviducts of infected egg-laying chickens, avian influenza virus could potentially be transmitted via the egg either through virus in the internal egg contents or on the surface from virus-infected feces.[316] This could potentially lead to hatching of infected chicks and contamination of the hatchery. Implementation of strict biosecurity measures can greatly reduce the risk of secondary spread after an initial outbreak.

Although humans can contract avian influenza virus by handling and slaughtering of infected birds, there is no epidemiologic evidence to suggest transmission of the virus by consumption of properly cooked eggs or other cooked poultry products derived from infected birds. Cooking poultry meat to 160°F (71°C) inactivates the virus.[309] Consumption of raw or partially cooked eggs (runny yolk) or foods containing raw eggs should be avoided. Avian influenza viruses remain viable in contaminated poultry meat and potentially spread through the marketing and distribution of contaminated fresh or frozen poultry meat.

In addition to birds, swine can serve as a critical animal reservoir for the emergence of new influenza A viruses because swine can be infected by both human and avian influenza viruses. For example, the classical H1N1 swine influenza viruses were very similar to the human pandemic influenza isolates of 1918. Moreover, human-associated H3N2 viruses were isolated from pigs shortly after they were identified as disease-causing agents in humans.[317]

## Fungal Foodborne Pathogens

Molds are widely distributed in nature and are an integral part of the microflora of foods. Although molds are major spoilage agents of many foods, many molds also produce mycotoxins of which some are carcinogenic and mutagenic (Table 3.3). Mycotoxins are secondary metabolites produced by molds usually at the end of their exponential phase of growth. Some of the

**TABLE 3.3**

**Fungal Foodborne Pathogens**

| Microorganism/Toxin | Significant Characteristics | Sources/Reservoirs of Fungi | Examples of Vehicles of Toxins | Toxic Effects | Detection Methods | Control/Prevention |
|---|---|---|---|---|---|---|
| A. parasiticus and A. flavus/aflatoxin | Growth at 10°C–43°C, optimal growth at 32°C, produces aflatoxins at 12°C–40°C, growth at pH 3–11 | Environment, soil, vegetation | Corn, peanuts, cottonseed | Effects of aflatoxin in animals: Acute: hemorrhage in the gastrointestinal tract, liver damage, death. Chronic: cirrhosis of liver, liver tumors, immunosuppression | Cultural methods[330,622-624] ELISA[625] Immunoassay[626,627] PCR[628-632] Functionalized-gold nanoparticles[633] Enzyme-linked-immunomagnetic-electrochemical array[634] Near-infrared spectroscopy[635] Monoclonal antibody-based ELISA[636] Electrochemical immunosensor[637] Antibody-based microarray[638] | Proper storage of cereal products, detoxification of mycotoxins in cereal products by treatment with hydrogen peroxide, ammonia |
| P. expansum/patulin, P. citrinum/citrinin | P. expansum is psychrotrophic, capable of growth at −2°C – −3°C and optimal growth at 25°C, | Environment, soil, vegetation | P. expansum: Fruits, especially apples and pears. P. citrinum: Cereals, especially rice, wheat, corn | Effects of patulin: Gastrointestinal, neurological immunological effects in animals. Citrinin: Fatty degeneration and renal necrosis in pigs and dogs; significance in human health is unresolved | Cultural methods[230,623,639] PCR[640-642] Detection of mycotoxin by HPLC[643,644] mass spectrometry[645] Competitive fluorescence assay[646] ELISA[647] | Avoid consumption of rotten apples and pears, proper storage of cereal products |
| F. graminearum/ deoxynivalenol, nivalenol, zearalenone | Growth at 5°C but not at 37°C, optimal growth at 25°C | Environment, soil, vegetation | Cereals, especially wheat, barley, corn | Effects of deoxynivalenol: nausea, vomiting, abdominal pain, diarrhea, headache, fever, chills, throat irritation | Cultural methods followed by morphology[648,649] PCR[642,650-654] Immunoassay[655] ELISA[656] LAMP assay[657] | Proper storage of cereal products |

principal species of molds, which produce mycotoxins in foods, include the following.

## *Aspergillus* Species

*A. flavus and A. parasiticus* are the most important toxigenic foodborne aspergilli. A wide variety of foods such as nuts, corn, oil seeds, and sorghum are potential vehicles of these aspergilli. *Aspergillus* species can cause disease in animals and humans by infection (aspergillosis) or by toxin production (aflatoxicosis). *A. flavus* and *A. parasiticus* produce aflatoxins, which are difuranocoumarin derivatives.[318] The common types of aflatoxins that are produced are $B_1$, $B_2$, $G_1$, and $G_2$.[319] In addition, two other types of aflatoxins, namely, M1 and M2, have also been reported as contaminants in food and feeds. Aflatoxicosis in animals can be acute or chronic. Acute cases are characterized by severe liver damage, whereas liver cirrhosis, liver cancer, and teratogenesis occur in chronic toxicity. Chronic intake of aflatoxins in animals can lead to poor feed conversion and low weight gain. Although fungal toxins cause an estimated economic loss of $1 billion in the United States, most of this is from aflatoxin contamination. The FDA has regulated the concentration of aflatoxin in the milk at not more than 0.5 and 20 ppb in crops.[320] Several outbreaks associated with aflatoxin consumption by humans have been recorded in developing countries.[320–322]

In humans, aflatoxins have been reported to cause hepatic cancer. A significant correlation between aflatoxin exposure and stunted growth has been reported in children exposed to aflatoxin during neonatal stages.[323] Additionally, since aflatoxins can cross the placental barrier, they can potentially lead to genetic defects in the fetus.[324] Following intake, aflatoxins are metabolized into a variety of products such as aflatoxicol, aflatoxin Q1, aflatoxin P1, and aflatoxin M1 in the liver by cytochrome p450 group of enzymes. In addition, another metabolite called aflatoxin 8,9 epoxide can also be formed, which can induce mutations by forming DNA adducts, ultimately leading to hepatic carcinoma.[325–327] Susceptibility of a given species to aflatoxins depends on its liver detoxification systems, genetic makeup, age, and other nutritional factors.[328]

## *Penicillium* Species

The genus *Penicillium* consists of more than 150 species, of which nearly 100 produce known toxins. Three important foodborne toxigenic *Penicillium* species include *P. verrucosum*, *P. expansum*, and *P. citrinum*. *P. verrucosum* is present on grains grown in temperate zones and is commonly associated with Scandinavian barley and wheat.[329] *P. verrucosum* produces ochratoxin A, which has immunosuppressive and potential carcinogenic properties.[329] Ochratoxin A also has been associated with nephritis in pigs in Scandanavia.[330] *Penicillium expansum*, a psychrotrophic mold and one of the most common fruit pathogens, causes a condition known as "blue mold rot" on a variety of fruits, including apples, cherries, nectarines, and peaches.[331–334] Besides its economic impact, *P. expansum* is also of potential public health significance since it produces patulin, a mycotoxin known to

cause immunological, neurological, and gastrointestinal toxic effects in animal models.[329] Exposure to high levels of patulin also results in vomiting, salivation, anorexia, polypnea, weight loss, leukocytosis, erythropenia, and necropsy lesions of hemorrhagic enteritis in piglets.[335] Although the toxic effects of patulin in humans have not been proven conclusively, the presence of patulin has been demonstrated in apple juice[336] and grape juice.[337] This is a major concern since fruit juices, especially apple juice, are commonly consumed by infants and children. *P. expansum* is commonly present in rotten apples and pears and to a lesser extent in cereals. Use of moldy fruits contaminated with *P. expansum* greatly increases the risk of patulin contamination in fruit juices. An unusual characteristic of *P. expansum* is its ability to grow at low temperature, i.e., −2°C to −3°C.[329]

*P. citrinin* is a widely occurring mold commonly present on rice, wheat, and corn. *P. citrinin* produces the metabolite citrinin. Although the toxicological effect of citrinin in humans is not known, it has been reported to cause renal toxicity in pigs and cats.[338]

## *Fusarium graminearum*

*F. graminearum* is a toxigenic mold commonly present in soil and on cereals such as wheat and corn. It causes "head blight" of wheat and barley and "stalk and cob rot" of maize. The head blight condition resulted in an estimated $1 billion loss in 1993 alone and affected cereal farming in the United States significantly.[339] It produces a number of mycotoxins, including deoxynivalenol and zearalenone.[340] Cereals containing high levels of deoxynivalenol are unacceptable for human or animal consumption. Ingestion of foods containing deoxynivalenol produces illness termed scabby grain intoxication, which is characterized by anorexia, nausea, vomiting, diarrhea, dizziness, and convulsions. Foods most frequently implicated as vehicles of deoxynivalenol include cereal grains, wheat, barley, and noodles. Zearalenone, the other *Fusarium* toxin, is an estrogenic compound that causes sterility in animals.[341]

## PARASITIC FOODBORNE PATHOGENS

Parasitic diseases account for 3% of foodborne illnesses and 21% of foodborne illness-related deaths in the United States (Table 3.4).[204] However, the actual number of parasitic diseases could be higher since they are often underdiagnosed and underreported in the United States.[341] Parasites constitute more of a food safety concern now than in the past because of the globalization of our food supply with growing imports of fruits, vegetables, and ethnic foods from countries, where the hygienic and quality control standards in food production may be suboptimal. Foods can be vehicles of several types of parasites, including protozoa, roundworms, and flatworms. Although foodborne transmission of parasites such as *Trichinella spiralis* and *Taenia solium* has been known for many years, the foodborne disease potential of many protozoan parasites such as *Cryptosporidium* and *Cyclospora* has only recently been recognized.

**TABLE 3.4**
**Parasitic Foodborne Pathogens**

| Parasite | Significant Characteristics | Sources/Reservoirs | Vehicles | Estimated No. of Foodborne Cases Annually in the United States[2,3] | Incubation Period, Symptoms, and Duration | Detection Methods | Control/Prevention |
|---|---|---|---|---|---|---|---|
| *G. lamblia* | Flagellate protozoa, produces oval-shaped cysts ranging from 8 to 20 μm in length and 5–12 μm in width; cysts contain four nuclei and are resistant to chlorination used to disinfect water | Humans, animals, especially beavers and muskrats, water | Drinking water, raw fruits and vegetables contaminated with cysts, ready-to-eat foods such as salads contaminated by infected food handlers | 76,840 | 4–25 days, usually 7–10 days. Abdominal cramps, nausea, abdominal distension, diarrhea that can be chronic and relapsing, fatigue, weight loss, anorexia. Duration is weeks to years | Immuno-fluorescence[658] Immunochromatography[659,660] PCR[661-665] ELISA[666] Surface-enhanced resonance spectroscopy[667] Biosensors[668] Flow cytometry[669] | Adequate cooking of foods, filtration of drinking water, good personal hygiene and food handling practices |
| *E. histolytica* | Amoeboid protozoa, anaerobe survives in environment in crypted form, cysts remain viable in feces for several days and in soil for at least 8 days at 30°C and for more than 1 month at 10°C, relatively resistant to chlorine | Humans, dogs, rats | Foods and water contaminated with feces or irrigation water | Unknown | 2–4 weeks. Abdominal pain, fever, vomiting, diarrhea containing blood and mucus, weight loss. Duration is weeks to months | Microscopic examination Line dot hybridization assay[670] ELISA[671,672] PCR[663,673,674] LAMP assay[675] | Good personal hygiene and food handling practices, adequate cooking of foods, filtration of water, hygienic disposal of sewage water, treatment of irrigation water |
| *C. parvum* | Obligate intracellular coccidian parasite; oocysts are spherical to oval in shape with an average size of 4.5–5.0 μm; oocysts are resistant to chlorination used to disinfect water | Humans, wild and domestic animals, especially calves | Contaminated drinking and recreational water, raw milk from infected cattle, fresh vegetables and other foods contaminated with feces from infected humans and animals | 57,616 | 2–14 days. Profuse, watery diarrhea, abdominal pain, nausea, vomiting. Duration is few days to 3 weeks | Immunofluorescence assay[676] PCR[673,677-680] Rapid assay[681] Monoclonal antibody-based dot blot assay[682] Electrochemical-based enzyme-linked biosensor[683] Surface-enhanced resonance spectroscopy[667] Piezoelectric-excited millimeter-sized cantilever sensor[684] | Thorough cooking of food, avoid contact with infected animals, filtration of drinking water, good personal hygiene and food handling practices |

(continued)

**TABLE 3.4 (continued)**
**Parasitic Foodborne Pathogens**

| Parasite | Significant Characteristics | Sources/ Reservoirs | Vehicles | Estimated No. of Foodborne Cases Annually in the United States[2,3] | Incubation Period, Symptoms, and Duration | Detection Methods | Control/Prevention |
|---|---|---|---|---|---|---|---|
| C. cayetanensis | Obligate intracellular coccidian parasite; oocysts are spherical in shape with an average size of 8–10 μm | Humans | Water, fruits, and vegetables contaminated with oocysts | 11,407 | 1 week Watery diarrhea, abdominal pain, nausea, vomiting, anorexia, myalgia, weight loss Duration is a few days to 1 month | Staining and microscopic examination[671] Flow cytometry[685] PCR[686–689] | Good personal hygiene, filtration of drinking water |
| T. gondii | Obligate intracellular coccidian protozoa | Cats, farm animals, transplacental transmission from infected mother to fetus | Raw or undercooked meat, raw goat milk, raw vegetables | 86,686 | 5–23 days Fever, rash, headache, muscle pain, swelling of lymph nodes; transplacental infection may cause abortion Duration is variable | Cell culture and mouse inoculation[690] Immunoassay[691] Serological assay[692] Immunofluorescence[693] PCR[694–698] LAMP assay[699] Oligonucleotide microarray[700] | Prevent environmental contamination with cat feces, avoid consumption of raw meat and milk, safe disposal of cat feces, wash hands after contact with cats |
| T. spiralis | Nematode with no free-living stage in the life cycle; adult female worms are 3–4 mm in length; transmissible form is larval cyst, which can occur in pork muscle | Wild and domestic animals, especially swine and horses | Raw or undercooked meat of animals containing encysted larvae such as swine or horses | 156 | Initial symptoms: 24–72 h Systemic symptoms: 8–21 days Initial phase: Abdominal pain, fever, nausea, vomiting, diarrhea Systemic phase: Periorbital edema, eosinophilia, myalgia, difficulty in breathing, thirst, profuse sweating, chills, weakness, prostration Duration is 2 weeks to 3 months | Microscopic examination ELISA[701,702] Immunoassay[703] PCR[704–707] | Adequate cooking of meat, freezing of meat at –15°C for 30 days or at –35°C, preventing trichinosis in pigs by not feeding swine garbage containing infected meat |

| Organism | Description | Reservoir | Foods | Infective dose | Symptoms | Detection | Prevention |
|---|---|---|---|---|---|---|---|
| *Anisakis* spp. | Nematode, slender threadlike parasite measuring 1.5–1.6 cm in length and 0.1 cm in diameter | Sea mammals | Some undercooked salt water fish, sushi, herring, sashimi, ceviche | Unknown | 4–12 h<br>Epigastric pain, nausea, vomiting, sometimes hematemesis<br>Duration is variable | ELISA[708,709]<br>Immunoblot[710]<br>PCR[711–714]<br>Fluorescence PCR[715] | Adequate cooking of saltwater fish, freezing fish at −23°C for 7 days |
| *T. solium*<br>*T. saginata* | Tapeworm, dependent on the digestive system of the host for nutrition | Humans, cattle, swine | Raw or undercooked beef or pork | Unknown | Few days to >10 years<br>Nausea, epigastric pain, nervousness, insomnia, anorexia, weight loss, digestive disturbances, weakness, dizziness<br>Duration is weeks to months | Detection of eggs or proglottids in feces<br>ELISA[716,717]<br>PCR[718–720] | Adequate cooking of beef and pork, proper disposal of sewage and human wastes, freezing of meat at −10°C for 2 weeks |
| *D. latum* | Largest human tapeworm | Saltwater fish, humans | Raw or undercooked saltwater fish | Unknown | Epigastric pain, nausea, abdominal pain, diarrhea, weakness, pernicious anemia<br>Duration is months to years | Detection of eggs in feces | Adequate cooking of fish, proper disposal of sewage and human waste |

Unlike bacteria, parasites do not multiply in foods. Moreover, parasites need at least one specific host to complete their life cycle. Many of the well-recognized parasites that can be transmitted to humans through foods include the following.

### Giardia lamblia

Giardiasis is the most common parasitic infection reported in the United States, with 21,300 confirmed cases in 1997.[342] However, the numbers have significantly increased over 15 years. A recent study revealed 76,840 cases of *Giardia lamblia* infections causing 225 hospitalizations.[3] *G. lamblia* is a flagellated protozoan parasite that colonizes the intestinal tract of humans and animals. It is commonly present in lakes, rivers, and stagnated waters. The parasite has a very low infective dose, with about 25–100 cysts for causing infection.[343] The life cycle of *G. lamblia* includes flagellated trophozoites, which become pear-shaped cysts.[344] The cysts contaminate water or food through feces of infected animals or humans. Following ingestion of cyst-contaminated water or food, the trophozoites reach the small intestine where they undergo excystation and multiply by binary fission. New trophozoites subsequently become cysts in the distal small intestine, and the encysted trophozoites are shed in the feces. The symptoms of giardiasis include abdominal pain, abdominal distension, nausea, vomiting, and diarrhea. Although water and foods contaminated with cysts are primary vehicles of giardiasis, little is known about the survival characteristics of the cysts in foods. In most cases of foodborne transmission, infected food handlers transfer the cysts to foods they prepare. Humans can also contract giardiasis through the use of contaminated water for irrigating or washing fruits and vegetables.[345] Contaminated water was identified as the source of *Giardia* oocysts in several outbreaks of giardiasis from 1954–2001.[346]

### Entamoeba histolytica

*E. histolytica* is a protozoan parasite that causes amoebiasis or amoebic dysentery in humans. Although the parasite survives in the environment and water, humans are the principal source of amoebiasis. In humans, cysts containing the trophozoites are released, which in turn multiply, and are subsequently excreted in the feces as cysts.[278] Foods and water contaminated with the cysts transmit the disease. Since the fecal–oral route is the principal route of transmission of amoebiasis, personal hygiene of infected food handlers plays a critical role in preventing foodborne amoebiasis. Human amoebiasis can occur in two forms: intestinal amoebiasis and amoebic liver abscess, which is usually a sequel to the intestinal form. Intestinal amoebiasis is characterized by abdominal pain, vomiting, and watery diarrhea containing mucus and blood. Symptoms of the hepatic form of amoebiasis include wasting, painful and enlarged liver, weight loss, and anemia. Amoebiasis is a common cause of diarrhea in tropical and subtropical countries, and most cases in the United States are reported in immigrants and persons returning from endemic areas.[345]

### Cryptosporidium parvum

*C. parvum* is a protozoan parasite that infects a wide range of animals and humans. *C. parvum* is monoxenous in its life cycle, requiring only one host for its development.[344] Infected hosts shed in their feces oocysts of the parasite, subsequently contaminating the environment, food, and water. The life cycle of *C. parvum* can be summarized as follows.[344] Upon ingestion of contaminated water or food, or by inhalation of oocysts, sporozoites are released by excystation of oocysts into the gastrointestinal or respiratory tract. The sporozoites enter the epithelial cells and develop into trophozoites, which in turn differentiate into type I and type II meronts. The merozoites from type I meronts invade new tissues and develop into trophozoites to continue the life cycle. The merozoites from type II meronts invade infected cells and undergo sexual multiplication to give rise to male and female gametes. The zygotes resulting from fertilized gametes become infectious by sporulation, and the sporulated oocysts are excreted in feces. *C. parvum* has an infectious dose of about 9–1042 oocysts.[343]

Cryptosporidiosis is a self-limiting disease with an incubation period of 1–2 weeks and is characterized by profuse, watery diarrhea, abdominal pain, vomiting, and low-grade fever. During the period from 1993 to 1998, seven major outbreaks of cryptosporidiosis have been reported in the United States.[345] Since then, *Cryptosporidium* spp. caused an estimated 57,600 illnesses, 210 hospitalizations, and 4 deaths.[3] Water is the most common source of *C. parvum* for human infections.[212] The largest outbreak of cryptosporidiosis (waterborne) in the United States occurred in Milwaukee, Wisconsin, in 1993 involving more than 400,000 people with 69 deaths.[347,348] In addition to drinking water, water can also potentially contaminate produce when it is used for irrigating plants or washing fruits and vegetables. Oocysts of the pathogen have been detected in fresh vegetables, raw milk, sausage, mussels, oysters, and apple cider.[212] Infected food handlers can also transfer the oocysts to foods.[349,350] *C. parvum* oocysts are sensitive to freezing and freeze-drying. The oocysts lose infectivity in distilled water stored at 4°C.[351] However, the oocysts are quite resistant to chlorine; no loss in infectivity was observed in water containing 1%–3% chlorine for up to 18 h.[352] However, the oocysts are sensitive to ozone, losing more than 90% infectivity in the presence of 1 ppm ozone for 5 min.[353]

Besides affecting humans, *C. parvum* can infect cattle, preweaned calves, sheep and goats, pigs, and horses.[354] *C. parvum* oocysts were responsible for an outbreak of cryptosporidiosis in veterinary students involved in research with cattle,[355] underscoring the pathogen's zoonotic potential.

### Cyclospora cayetanensis

*C. cayetanensis* is a waterborne protozoan pathogen that is also transmitted by contaminated food. The parasite was implicated in several foodborne outbreaks in the United States during 1996 and 1997.[356] The pathogen causes an estimated 11,400 cases, with 11 hospitalizations annually, costing approximately $11 million.[3] Water and foods, especially fruits and vegetables containing oocysts, are common vehicles of human infection.[345,357] During the period from 1996 to 2000, eight major outbreaks of cyclosporidiosis were reported, with imported raspberries as the vehicle of infection in half of the outbreaks.[345] Other types of produce implicated in *C. cayetanensis* outbreaks include lettuce[358] and fresh basil.[359] Humans are the only identified reservoir of *C. cayetanensis*.[357] The symptoms of *C. cayetanensis* infection in humans include watery diarrhea, nausea, abdominal pain, vomiting, and weight loss. Presently, there is very little information on the effects of heat, freezing, and disinfection agents on *Cyclospora* oocysts. Exposure of oocysts to −20°C for 24 h or 60°C for 1 h prevented oocysts from sporulating. Exposing oocysts to 4°C or 37°C for 14 days delayed sporulation.[360]

### Toxoplasma gondii

*T. gondii* is an obligate intracellular protozoan parasite for which cats are the definitive host. A survey on the prevalence of *T. gondii* in cats at spay or neuter clinics in Ohio revealed that 48% of the cats were infected with the parasite.[361] In the intestine of cats, the parasite undergoes sexual reproduction to form oocysts, which are excreted in feces.[362] The oocysts undergo maturation and survive in the environment for months and spread by wind, insects, and tapeworms. Toxoplasmosis in humans results following ingestion of food or water contaminated with oocysts. Raw or undercooked meats contaminated with cysts are potential sources of *T. gondii*. The parasite has been isolated from meat of game, sheep, goats, horses, chickens, and swine.[344,363] Transmission also occurs from an infected pregnant mother to child by transplacental transmission.[364] In the United States, *T. gondii* has been reported to cause about 4000 congenital infections annually, potentially resulting in blindness, learning disabilities, and mental retardation in children.[341] *T. gondii* is also attributed as the leading cause of CNS infection in persons with AIDS.[365] Symptoms in healthy adults are usually mild and include rash, headache, muscle pain, and swelling of lymph nodes. Although the oocysts can survive in refrigerated meat for weeks, they are inactivated by freezing at <12°C.[366] The oocysts are sensitive to irradiation and heat (>67°C). Properly cooked foods are not a vehicle of *T. gondii*.[367] *T. gondii* causes an estimated 86,700 cases, 4,428 hospitalizations, and 327 deaths annually, costing an estimated $3 billion, second only to nontyphoidal salmonellosis.[3]

### Trichinella spiralis

*T. spiralis* is a roundworm that primarily infects wild and domestic animals, especially pigs. Humans contract trichinosis by consumption of raw or undercooked meat containing larvae of the parasite. Pigs are infected by consuming uncooked scraps of infected pork. The encysted larvae upon ingestion are liberated from the cyst in the intestine, where they sexually mature.[368] The mature male and female worms copulate in the lumen of the small intestine, giving rise to a new generation of larvae. The newly born larvae migrate to various tissues in the body. Those larvae that reach the striated muscles penetrate into the sarcolemma of the muscle fibers and develop to maturity as encapsulated cysts.[368] The larvae continue their life cycle when raw or undercooked meat, especially pork containing the larvae, is consumed by humans. Major clinical systems include myalgia, diarrhea, fever, facial edema, conjunctival hemorrhages, and headache.[369]

Trichinosis is a notifiable disease in the United States, with the number of cases progressively decreasing since the 1940s.[345] The decline in trichinosis in the United States has been attributed to changes in swine feeding practices and routine inspections at slaughterhouses. The average number of trichinosis cases reported in the United States in 1997–2001 was 14 per year, down from 400 cases/year in the 1940s.[370] On the other hand, game meat was identified as the most common source of the parasite to humans during 1997–2001.[345] Globally, *Trichinella* spp. cause an estimated 65,818 cases and 42 deaths reported from 41 countries during 1986–2009.[369]

### Anisakis Species

Anisakiasis in humans is caused by two foodborne roundworms. These include *A. simplex*, whose definitive host is whales, and *Pseudoterranova decipiens*, which primarily inhabits seals. The eggs of these roundworms are excreted in feces by their respective hosts. The eggs then undergo molting in suitable intermediate hosts and subsequently develop into larvae, which are ingested by fish.[371] Humans contract anisakiasis by consumption of raw or undercooked fish and seafoods containing the larvae. In noninvasive anisakiasis, the worms released from ingested foods migrate to the pharynx, resulting in "tingling throat syndrome."[371] The worms are ultimately expelled by coughing. In the invasive form of anisakiasis, the worms penetrate the intestinal mucosa, thereby causing symptoms that include epigastric pain, nausea, vomiting, and diarrhea.

### Taenia Species

The genus *Taenia* includes two meatborne pathogenic flatworms, *T. saginata* (beef tapeworm) and *T. solium* (pork tapeworm). The eggs of *T. saginata* survive in the environment, including on pastures, and are ingested by cattle in which they hatch into embryos.[368] The embryos migrate to skeletal muscles or the heart and develop into larvae known as *Cysticercus bovis*. They become infective to humans in approximately 10 weeks.[343] Humans become infected by consuming raw or undercooked beef containing the larvae. Larvae that are released into the small intestine develop into mature, adult worms. Cattle get infected with contaminated human hands or by drinking contaminated feed or water.[372] The symptoms of *T. saginata* infection in humans include decreased appetite, headache, dizziness, diarrhea, and weight loss.

In the normal life cycle of *T. solium*, pigs serve as the intermediate host. Eggs ingested by pigs develop into embryos in the duodenum, penetrate the intestinal wall, migrate through the blood and the lymphatic system, and finally reach the skeletal muscles and myocardium, where they develop into larvae known as *Cysticercus cellulosae*. Humans, the definitive host, consuming raw or undercooked pork are infected with the larvae, which develop into adult worms in the small intestine. The symptoms of *T. solium* infection in humans include discomfort, hunger pains, anorexia, and nervous disorders. Worms are passed in the feces. In the abnormal life cycle of *T. solium*, humans serve as intermediate hosts in which the larvae develop in striated muscles and in subcutaneous tissue. *T. solium* infections are most common in the developing world. However, due to immigration of people from endemic areas, infections have been increasingly diagnosed and reported in developed countries.[373]

### *Diphyllobothrium latum*

*D. latum* is commonly referred to as the broad tapeworm because it is the largest human tapeworm.[371] Humans contract diphyllobothriasis by consuming raw or undercooked fish containing the larval forms called plerocercoids. Upon ingestion, the larvae develop into mature worms in the intestines. Eggs produced by mature worms are excreted in feces. If feces containing the eggs contaminate water, the eggs develop into free-swimming larvae called coricidia. Coricidia are ingested by crustaceans, where they develop into a juvenile stage known as procercoid. Following ingestion of infected crustaceans by fish, procercoids develop into plerocercoids to continue the life cycle. Diphyllobothriasis in humans is characterized by nausea, abdominal pain, diarrhea, weakness, and pernicious anemia.[371] Cases of diphyllobothriasis have been associated with eating foods containing raw salmon such as sushi.

## REFERENCES

1. Anonymous. *Morb Mort Weekly Rep* 60:749;2011.
2. Scharff, RL. URL: http://www.producesafetyproject.org/admin/assets/files/Health-Related-Foodborne-Illness-Costs-Report.pdf-1.pdf (Accessed March 2012).
3. Scharff, RL. *J Food Prot* 75:123;2012.
4. CSPI (Center for Science in the Public Interest). URL: http://cspinet.org/new/pdf/abrfoodbornepathogenswhitepaper.pdf (Accessed March 2012).
5. Buzby, JC, Roberts, T. *Gastroenterology* 136:1851;2009.
6. Kollanoor-Johny, A, Baskaran, SA, Venkitanarayanan, K. In: Oyarzabal, O, Backert, S. eds. *Microbial Food Safety Springer Science Business Media*. Springer Science+Business Media, LLC, NY. p. 44;2012.
7. Viazis, S, Diez-Gonzalez, F. In: Sparks, DL. ed. *Advances in Agronomy*. Academic Press, San Diego, CA. p 111;2011.
8. Anonymous. *Morb Mort Weekly Rep* 53:1;2006.
9. Meng, J, Doyle, MP. In: Kaper, JB, O'Brien, AD. eds. *Escherichia coli O157:H7 and Other Shiga Toxin-Producing E. coli Strains*. ASM Press, Washington, DC. p. 92;1998.
10. Vugia, D, Cronquist, A, Hadler, J. *Morb Mort Weekly Rep* 55:392;2006.
11. Lynch et al. *Epidemiol Infect* 137:307;2009.
12. Laegreid, WW, Elder, RO, Keen, JE. *Epidemiol Infect* 123:291;1999.
13. Shere, JA, Bartlett, KJ, Kaspar, CW. *Appl Environ Microbiol* 64:1390;1998.
14. Zhao, T et al. *Appl Environ Microbiol* 61:1290;1995.
15. Chapman, PA et al. *Epidemiol Infect* 111:439;1993.
16. Naylor, SW et al. *Infect Immun* 71:1505;2003.
17. Wang, GT, Zhao, T, Doyle, MP. *Appl Environ Microbiol* 62:2567;1998.
18. Animal and Plant Inspection Service. National Animal Health Monitoring System Report N182.595;1995. URL: http://www.aphis.usda.gov/vs/ceah/cahm
19. Hancock, DD et al. *Epidemiol Infect* 113:199;1994.
20. Elder, RO et al. *Proc Natl Acad Sci USA* 97:2999;2000.
21. Gansheroff, LJ, O'Brien, AD. *Proc Natl Acad Sci USA* 97:2959;2000.
22. Heuvelink, AE et al. *J Clin Microbiol* 36:3480;1998.
23. Jackson, SG et al. *Epidemiol Infect* 120:17;1998.
24. Callaway, TR et al. *Foodborne Pathog Dis* 3:234;2006.
25. Reinstein, S et al. *Appl Environ Microbiol* 73:1002;2007.
26. Woerner, DR et al. *J Food Prot* 69:2824;2006.
27. Dargatz, DA et al. *J Food Prot* 60:466;1997.
28. Smith, D et al. *J Food Prot* 64:1899;2001.
29. Barkocy-Gallagher, GA et al. *J Food Prot* 66:1978;2003.
30. Naumova, EN et al. *Epidemiol Infect* 135:281;2007.
31. Vugia, D et al. *Morb Mort Weekly Rep* 56:336;2007.
32. Brashears, MM, Jaroni, D, Trimble, J. *J Food Prot* 66:355;2003.
33. Breuer, T et al. *Emerg Infect Dis* 7:977;2001.
34. McLellan, MR, Splittstoesser, DF. *Food Technol* 50:174;1994.
35. Park, GW, Diez-Gonzalez, FJ. *Appl Microbiol* 94:675;2003.
36. Sivapalasingam, S et al. *J Food Prot* 67;2342;2004.
37. Crump, JA et al. *N Engl J Med* 347:555;2002.
38. O'Brien, SJ, Adak, GK, Gilham, C. *Emerg Infect Dis* 7:1049;2001.
39. LeJeune, JT, Wetzel, AN. *J Anim Sci* 85:E73;2007.
40. Davis, MA et al. *Appl Environ Microbiol* 71:6816;2005.
41. Renter, DG, Sargeant, JM, Hungerford, LL. *Am J Vet Res* 65:1367;2004.
42. Cary, WC, Moon, HW. *Appl Environ Microbiol* 61:1586;1995.
43. Zhao, T et al. *J Clin Microbiol* 36:641;1998.
44. Callaway, TR et al. *J Anim Sci* 80:1683;2002.
45. McNeilly, TN et al. *Infect Immun* 76:2594;2008.
46. Thomson, DU et al. *Foodborne Pathog Dis* 6:871;2009.
47. Thornton, AB et al. *J Food Prot* 72:866;2009.
48. Trent Fox, J et al. *Foodborne Pathog Dis* 6:893;2009.
49. Uljas, HE, Ingham, SC. *J Food Prot* 61:939;1998.
50. Arnold, KW, Kaspar, CW. *Appl Environ Microbiol* 61:2037;1995.
51. Leyer, GJ, Wang, LL, Johnson, EA. *Appl Environ Microbiol* 61:3152;1995.
52. Buchanan, RL, Edelson, SG. *Appl Environ Microbiol* 62:4009;1996.
53. Doyle, MP, Schoeni, JL. *Appl Environ Microbiol* 48:855;1984.
54. Glass, KA et al. *Appl Environ Microbiol* 58:2513;1992.
55. Doyle, MP, Zhao, T, Meng, J, Zhao, S. In: Doyle, MP, Beuchat, LR, Montville, TJ. eds. *Food Microbiology: Fundamentals and Frontiers*. ASM Press, Washington, DC, p. 171;1997.
56. Slutsker, L et al. *J Infect Dis* 177:962;1998.
57. Wong, CS et al. *N Engl J Med* 342:1930;2000.
58. Smith, KE et al. *Pediatr Infect Dis J* 31:37;2012.
59. Nataro, JP, Kaper, JB. *Clin Microbiol Rev* 11:142;1998.
60. Kaper, JB. *Int J Med Microbiol* 295:355;2005.
61. Barbieri, J et al. *Infect Immun* 67:6710;1999.
62. Schmidt, H, Beutin, L, Karch, H. *Infect Immun* 63:1055;1995.
63. Bettelheim, KA. *Crit Rev Microbiol* 33:67;2007.
64. Brooks, JT et al. *J Infect Dis* 192:1422;2005.
65. Hedican, EB et al. *Clin Infect Dis* 49:358;2009.

66. Bielaszewska, M et al. *Lancet* 11:671;2011.
67. D'Aoust, J-Y. In: Doyle, MP, Beuchat, LR, Montville, TJ. eds. *Food Microbiology: Fundamentals and Frontiers*. ASM Press, Washington, DC, p. 129;1997.
68. Jay, JM. *Modern Food Microbiology*. Aspen Publishers, Gaithersburg, MD, p. 509;1998.
69. Bean, NH et al. *J Food Prot* 53:711;1983.
70. D'Aoust, J-Y. *Int J Food Microbiol* 13:207;1991.
71. Leyer, GJ, Johnson, EA. *Appl Environ Microbiol* 59:1842;1993.
72. Leyer, GJ, Johnson EA. *Appl Environ Microbiol* 58:2075;1992.
73. D'Aoust, JY. In: Doyle, MP. ed. *Foodborne Bacterial Pathogens*. Marcel Dekker, NY, p. 36;1989.
74. Flowers, RS. *Food Technol* 42:182;1988.
75. Schlundt, J. *Int J Food Microbiol* 78:3;2002.
76. Anonymous. *Morb Mort Weekly Rep* 54:352;2004.
77. United States Department of Agriculture—Economic Research Service. URL: http://www.ers.usda.gov/data/foodborneillness/salm_Intro.asp (Accessed March 2012).
78. Anonymous. *Morb Mort Weekly Rep* 54:352;2005.
79. Kimura, AC et al. *Clin Infect Dis* 38:S244;2004.
80. Anonymous. *Morb Mort Weekly Rep* 51:1149;2003.
81. Frenzen, P et al. *Food Rev* 22:10;1999.
82. Anonymous. *Morb Mort Weekly Rep* 59:418;2010.
83. USDA-NASS. URL: http://usda.mannlib.cornell.edu/usda/nass/ChicEggs/2000s/2009/ChicEggs-12-22-2009.pdf (Accessed March 2012).
84. White, PL et al. *J Food Prot* 70:582;2007.
85. Glynn, MK et al. *N Engl J Med* 338:1333;1998.
86. Cody, SH et al. *J Am Med Assoc* 281:1805;1999.
87. Glynn, MK et al. *Clin Infect Dis* 38:S227;2004.
88. Anonymous. *Morb Mort Weekly Rep* 51:950;2002.
89. Carrasco, E, Morales-Rueda, A, García-Gimeno, RM. *Food Res Int* 45:545;2012.
90. Anonymous. *Morb Mort Weekly Rep* 57:929;2008.
91. Fernandez, F, Hinton, M, Van Gils, B. *Avian Pathol* 31:49;2002.
92. Fernandez, F, Hinton, M, Van Gils, B. *Avian Pathol* 29:575;2000.
93. Spring, P et al. *Poult Sci* 79:20;2000.
94. Stern, NJ et al. *Poult Sci* 80:156;2001.
95. Chadfield, MS, Hinton, MH. *Vet Immunol Immunopathol* 100:81;2004.
96. Fiorentin, L, Vieira, ND, Barioni, W, Jr. *Avian Pathol* 34:258;2005.
97. Inoue, AY et al. *Avian Dis* 52:567;2008.
98. Kollanoor Johny, A et al. *J Food Prot* 72:722;2009.
99. Kollanoor-Johny, A et al. *Appl Environ Microbiol* 78:2981;2012.
100. Bohez, L et al. *Vet Microbiol* 126:216;2008.
101. Anonymous. *Morb Mort Weekly Rep* 56:877;2007.
102. Lee, LA et al. *J Infect Dis* 170;128;1994.
103. Food and Agricultural Organization. URL: http://www.fao.org/docrep/005/y4393e/y4393e00.htm (Accessed March 2012).
104. Hopkins, RS et al. *Morb Mort Weekly Rep* 52:1;2005.
105. Jay, JM. *Modern Food Microbiology*. Aspen Publishers, Gaithersburg, MD, p. 556;1998.
106. Altekruse, SF et al. *Emerg Infect Dis* 5:28;1999.
107. Thormar, H, Hilmarsson, H, Bergsson, G. *Appl Environ Microbiol* 72:522;2006.
108. Silva, J et al. *Front Microbiol* 2:1;2011.
109. Lu, J et al. *Appl Environ Microbiol* 77:5034;2011.
110. Beery, JT, Hugdahl, MB, Doyle, MP. *Appl Environ Microbiol* 54:2365;1988.
111. Hugdahl, MB, Beery, JT, Doyle, MP. *Infect Immun* 56:1560;1988.
112. Stern, NJ, Kazmi, SU. In: Doyle, MP, ed, *Foodborne Bacterial Pathogens*. Marcel Dekker, NY, p. 71;1989.
113. Friedman, CR et al. *Clin Infect Dis* 38:S285;2004.
114. Samuel, MC et al. *Clin Infect Dis* 38:S165;2004.
115. Deming, MS, Tauxe, RV, Blake, PA. *Am J Epidemiol* 126:526;1987.
116. Oosterom, J et al. *J Hygiene* 92:325;1984.
117. Hopkins, RS, Scott, AS. *J Infect Dis* 148:770;1983.
118. Carillo, CL et al. *Appl Environ Microbiol* 71:6554;2005.
119. Wagenaar, JA et al. *Vet Microbiol* 109:275;2005.
120. Heres, LB et al. *Vet Microbiol* 99:259;2004.
121. Solis de los Santos, F et al. *Poult Sci* 87:800;2008.
122. Solis de los Santos, F et al. *Poult Sci* 88:61;2008.
123. Wyszynska, A. et al. *Vaccine*, 22:1379;2004.
124. Scott, DA et al. *New Generation Vaccines*, 2nd edn. Marcel Dekker, Inc., NY, p. 885;1997.
125. Kassenborg, HD et al. *Clin Infect Dis* 38:S279;2004.
126. Smith, KE, Blender, JB, Osterholm, MT. *Am Soc Microbiol* 340:1525;2000.
127. Nachamkin, I, Allos, BM, Ho, T. *Clin Microbiol Rev* 11:555;1998.
128. Allos, BM. *J Infect Dis* 176:S125;1997.
129. Whitehouse, CA et al. *Infect Immun* 66:1934;1998.
130. Gupta, A et al. *Clin Infect Dis* 38:1372;2004.
131. Sobel, J et al. *J Infect Dis* 177:1405;1998.
132. Mohle-Boetani, JC et al. *Am J Public Health* 85:812;1995.
133. Anonymous. *Morb Mort Weekly Rep* 39:509;1990.
134. Woodward, DL et al. *J Med Microbiol* 54:741;2005.
135. Schleifstein, J, Coleman, MB, *NY State J Med* 39:1749;1939.
136. Robins-Browne, RM. In: Doyle, MP, Beuchat, LR, Montville, TJ. eds. *Food Microbiology: Fundamentals and Frontiers*. ASM Press, Washington, DC, p. 192;1997.
137. Jay, JM. *Modern Food Microbiology*. Aspen Publishers, Gaithersburg, MD, p. 555;1998.
138. Shiemann, DA. In: Doyle, MP. ed. *Foodborne Bacterial Pathogens*. Marcel Dekker, NY, p. 631;1989.
139. Schofield, GM. *J Appl Microbiol* 72:267;1992.
140. Bottone, EJ. *Clin Microbiol Rev* 10:257;1997.
141. Schifield, GM. *J Appl Bacteriol* 72:267;1992.
142. Drummond, N et al. *Foodborne Pathog Dis* 9:179;2012.
143. Bottone, JE. *Microbes Infect* 1:323;1999.
144. Wagner, SJ, Friedman, LI, Dodd, RY. *Clin Microbiol Rev* 7:290;1994.
145. Bruining, A, DeWilde-Beekhuizen, CCM. *Medilon* 4:30;1975.
146. Mollaret, HH, Thal, E. *Bergey's Manual of Determinative Bacteriology*. Waverly Press, Baltimore, MD, 8:330;1974.
147. Toora, S et al. *Folia Microbiol (Praha)* 34:151;1989.
148. Hanna, MO et al. *J Food Sci* 42:1180;1977.
149. Palumbo, SA. *J Food Prot* 49:1003;1986.
150. National Oceanic and Atmospheric Administration. Fisheries of the United States. Fisheries Statistics and Economics Division, Silver Springs, MD, p. 86;2003.
151. Eastaugh, J, Shepherd, S. *Arch Intern Med* 149:1735;1989.
152. Anonymous. *Dairy Food Environ Sanit* 22:38;2002.
153. Patel, NM et al. *Transpl Infect Dis* 11:54;2009.
154. Twedt, RM. In: Doyle, MP. ed. *Foodborne Bacterial Pathogens*. Marcel Dekker, Inc., NY, p. 395;1989.
155. Oliver, JD, Kaper, JB. In: Doyle, MP, Beuchat, LR, Montville, TJ. eds. *Food Microbiology: Fundamentals and Frontiers*. ASM Press, Washington, DC, p. 228;1997.
156. Su, YC, Liu, C. *Food Microbiol* 24:549;2007.
157. Daniels, NA et al. *J Am Med Assoc* 284:1541;2000.

158. Miyamato, Y et al. *Infect Immun* 28:567;1980.
159. Mintz, ED, Popovic, T, Blake, PA. *Transmission of Vibrio cholerae O1, Vibrio cholerae and Cholera: Molecular to Global Perspectives*. ASM Press, Washington, DC, p. 345;1994.
160. MacIntyre, DL et al. *Proc Natl Acad Sci USA* 107:19520;2010.
161. Anonymous. *Morb Mort Weekly Rep* 55:31;2006.
162. World Health Organization. *Wkly Epidemiol Rec* 31:281;2003.
163. Tauxe, RV. *Int J Food Microbiol* 78:31;2002.
164. Jay, JM. *Modern Food Microbiology*. Aspen Publishers, Gaithersburg, MD, p. 544;1998.
165. Horseman, MA, Surani, S. *Int J Infect Dis* 15:e157;2011.
166. Forsythe, SJ. *Mater Child Nutr* 1:44;2005.
167. Lai, KK. *Medicine* 80:113;2001.
168. Beuchat, LR et al. *Int J Food Microbiol* 136:204;2009.
169. Leclercq, A, Wanegue, C, Baylac, P. *Appl Environ Microbiol* 68:1631;2002.
170. Kandhai, MC et al. *Lancet* 363:39;2004.
171. Kandhai, MC et al. *J Food Prot* 67:1267;2004.
172. van Acker, J et al. *J Clin Microbiol* 39:293;2001.
173. Bar-Oz, B et al. *Acta Paediatr* 90:356;2002.
174. Simmons, BP et al. *Infect Contr Hosp Epidemiol* 10:398;1989.
175. Weir, E. *Can Med Assoc J* 166:1570;2002.
176. Biering, G et al. *J Clin Microbiol* 27:2054;1989.
177. Postupa, R, Aldova, E. *J Hyg Epidemiol Microbiol Immunol* 28:435;1984.
178. Muytjens, HL, Roelofs-Willemse, H, Jaspar, GHJ. *Clin Microbiol* 26:743;1988.
179. Nazarowec-White, M, Farber, JM. *J Food Prot* 60;226;1997.
180. Harris, RD. *Food Proc* 50:111;1989.
181. Nazarowec-White, M, Farber, JM. *Lett Appl Microbiol* 24:9;1997.
182. Breeuwer, P et al. *J Appl Microbiol* 95:967;2003.
183. Iversen, C, Forsythe, S. *Food Microbiol* 21:771;2004.
184. Urmenyi, AM, Franklin, AW. *Lancet* 1:313;1961.
185. Himelright, I et al. *Morb Mort Weekly Rep* 51:297;2002.
186. FSNET. November 8, 2002. Colorado Department of Public Health and Environment Press Release. URL: http://131.104.232.9/fsnet/2002/11-2002/fsnet_november_8-2. htm#RECALLED%20BABY
187. Murrell, E et al. *Int J Food Microbiol* 136:227;2009.
188. International Commission on Microbiological Specification for Foods. *Microorganisms in Foods*, Vol. 7. Kluwer Academic Press/Plenum Publishers, NY; 2002.
189. Gallagher, PG, Ball, WS. *Pediatr Radiol* 21:135;1991.
190. Kline, MW. *Infect Dis J* 7:891;1988.
191. Sanders, WE, Jr, Sanders, CC. *Clin Microbiol Rev* 10:220;1997.
192. Hawkins, RE, Lissner, CR, Sanford, JP. *South Med J* 84:793;1991.
193. Pribyl, C. *Am J Med* 78:51;1985.
194. Beuchat, LR. *Int J Food Microbiol* 13:217;1991.
195. Pridgeon, JW, Klesius, PH. *Dis Aquat Organ* 94:249;2011.
196. Kirov, SM. In: Doyle, MP, Beuchat, LR, Montville, TJ. eds. *Food Microbiology: Fundamentals and Frontiers*. ASM Press, Washington, DC, p. 265;1997.
197. Berrang, ME, Brackett, RE, Beuchat, LR. *Appl Environ Microbiol* 55:2167;1989.
198. Palumbo, SA. *Int J Food Microbiol* 7:41;1988.
199. Jay, JM. *Modern Food Microbiology*. Aspen Publishers, Gaithersburg, MD, p. 620;1998.
200. Kaskhedikar, M, Chhabra, D. *Vet World* 3:76;2010.
201. Holmberg, SD et al. *Ann Intern Med* 105:690;1986.
202. González-Rey, C et al. *Folia Microbiol* 56:178;2011.
203. Anonymous. *Morb Mort Weekly Rep* 47:394;1998.
204. Mead, P.S. et al. *Emerg Infect Dis* 5:607;1999.
205. Economic Research Service. 2001. URL: http://www.ers. usda.gov/Emphases/SafeFood/features.htm
206. Nickelson, N. *Food Quality* April:28;1999.
207. Gilmour, MW et al. *BMC Genomics* 11:120;2010.
208. Allerberger, F, Wagner, M. *Clin Microbiol Infect* 16:16;2010.
209. Brackett, RE. *Food Technol* 52:162;1998.
210. Cox, LJ et al. *Food Microbiol* 6:49;1989.
211. Jeong, DK, Frank, JF. *J Food Prot* 57:576;1994.
212. Meng, J, Doyle, MP. *Annu Rev Nutr* 17:255;1997.
213. Rocourt, J, Cossart, P. In: Doyle, MP, Beuchat, LR, Montville, TJ. eds. *Food Microbiology: Fundamentals and Frontiers*. ASM Press, Washington, DC, p. 337;1997.
214. Ryser, ET, Marth, EH. *Listeria, Listeriosis and Food Safety*. Marcel Dekker, Inc., NY; 1999.
215. Vázquez-Boland, JA et al. *Clin Microbiol Rev* 14:584;2001.
216. Gaillard, JL. *Infect Immun* 55:2822;1987.
217. Argudin, MA et al. *Toxins* 2:1751;2010.
218. Kwada, M et al. *J Human Lact* 19:411;2003.
219. Jablonski, LM, Bohac, GA. In: Doyle, MP, Beuchat, LR, Montville, TJ. eds. *Food Microbiology: Fundamentals and Frontiers*. ASM Press, Washington, DC, p. 353;1997.
220. Wattinger, L et al. *Eur J Clin Microbiol Infect Dis* 31:455;2012.
221. Newsome, RL. *Food Technol* 42:182;1988
222. Hennekinne, JA, De Buyser, ML, Dragacci, S. *FEMS Microbiol Rev* 36:815;2012.
223. Bergdoll, ML. In: Doyle, MP. ed. *Foodborne Bacterial Pathogens*. Marcel Dekker, NY, p. 463;1989.
224. Le Loir, Y, Baron, F, Gautier, M. *Genet Mol Res* 2:63;2003.
225. Jones, TF et al. *Emerg Infect Dis* 8:82;2002.
226. Chambers, HF, Deleo, FR. *Nat Rev Microbiol* 7:629;2009.
227. Khanna, T et al. *Vet Microbiol* 128:298;2008.
228. Kehrenberg, C et al. *Antimicrob Agents Chemother* 53:779;2009.
229. Garcia, MS, De la Torre, M, Morales, G et al. *J Am Med Assoc* 303:2260;2010.
230. Peck, MW, Stringer, SC, Carter, AT. *Food Microbiol* 28:183;2011.
231. Wilson, R et al. *Pediatr Infect Dis* 1:148;1982.
232. Spika, JS et al. *Am J Dis Child* 143:828;1989.
233. Dodds, KL, Austin, JW. In: Doyle, MP, Beuchat, LR, Montville, TJ. eds. *Food Microbiology: Fundamentals and Frontiers*. ASM Press, Washington, DC, p. 288;1997.
234. Pierson, MD, Reddy, NR. *Food Technol* 42:196;1988.
235. Lindstrom, M et al. *Crit Rev Food Sci Nutr* 50:281;2010.
236. Jay, JM. *Modern Food Microbiology*. Aspen Publishers, Gaithersburg, MD, p. 462;1998.
237. Date, K et al. *J Food Prot* 74:2090;2011.
238. Pingeon, JM et al. *Euro Surveill* 16:20035;2011.
239. Lahti, P et al. *J Clin Microbiol* 46:371;2008.
240. Keyburn, AL et al. *Toxins (Basel)* 2:1913;2010.
241. Hobbs, BC. In: Riemann, H, Bryan, FL. eds. *Clostridium perfringens Gastroenteritis—Foodborne Infections and Intoxications*. Academic Press, NY, p. 131;1979.
242. Labbe, R. In: Doyle, MP. ed. *Foodborne Bacterial Pathogens*. Marcel Dekker, NY, p. 191;1989.
243. Rood, JI et al. *The Clostridia: Molecular Biology and Pathogenesis*. Academic, Press, London, U.K., p. 533;1997.
244. Kokai-Kun JF, McClane, BA. In: Rood, JI, McClane, BA, Songer, JG, Titball, RW. eds. *The Clostridia: Molecular Biology and Pathogenesis*, Academic Press, San Diego, CA, 325;1997.
245. Rupnik, M, Wilcox, MH, Gerding, DN. *Nat Rev Microbiol* 7:526;2009.
246. Indra, A et al. *Middle Eur J Med* 121:91;2009.

247. Rodriguez-Palacios, A et al. *Emerg Infect Dis* 15:802;2009.
248. Weese, JS et al. *Appl Environ Microbiol* 75:5009;2009.
249. Weese, JS, Reid-Smith, RJ, Avery, BP, Rousseau, J *Lett Appl Microbiol* 50:362;2010.
250. Wilkins, TD, Lyerly, DM. *Appl Environ Microbiol* 41:531;2003.
251. Sunenshine, RH, McDonald, LC. *Cleveland Clin J Med* 73:187;2006.
252. Redelings, MD, Sorvillo, F, Mascola, L. *Emerg Infect Dis* 13:1417;2007.
253. Dial, S et al. *J Am Med Assoc* 294:2989;2005.
254. Anonymous. *Morb Mort Weekly Rep* 54:1201;2005.
255. Loo, VG, Poirier, L, Miller, MA. *N Engl J Med* 353:2442;2005.
256. Huang, H, Weintraub, A, Fang, H et al. *Int J Antimicrob Agents* 34:516;2009.
257. Rupnik, M, Dupuy, B, Fairweather, NF et al. *J Med Microbiol* 54:113;2005.
258. Goncalves, C et al. *J Clin Microbiol* 42:1933;2004.
259. Voth, DE, Ballard, JD. *Clin Microbiol Rev* 18:247;2005.
260. Geric, B, Carman, RJ, Rupnik, M et al. *J Infect Dis* 193:1143;2006.
261. Martin, H et al. *J Clin Microbiol* 46:2999;2008.
262. Rupnik, M, Widmer, A, Zimmermann, O et al. *J Clin Microbiol* 46:2146;2008.
263. Jobstl, M et al. *Int J Food Microbiol* 138:172;2010.
264. Ehling-Schulz, M, Fricker, M, Scherer, S. *Mol Nutr Food Res* 48:479;2004.
265. Anonymous. *EFSA J* May:271;2009.
266. Doyle, MP. *Food Technol* 42:199;1988.
267. Kramer, JM. Gilbert, RJ. In: Doyle, MP. eds. *Foodborne Bacterial Pathogens*. Marcel Dekker, NY, p. 327;1989.
268. Granum, PE, Lund, T. *FEMS Microbiol Lett* 157:2203;1997.
269. Ehling-Schulz, M et al. *FEMS Microbiol Lett* 260:232;2006.
270. Messelhausser, U et al. *J Food Prot* 73:395;2010.
271. Johnson, KM. *J Food Prot* 47:145;1984.
272. Hobbs, BC, Gilbert, RJ. *Proc IV Int Cong Food Sci Technol* 3:159;1974.
273. Stenfors Arnesen, LP, Fagerlund, A, Granum, PE. *FEMS Microbiol Rev* 32:579;2008.
274. Cadot, C et al. *J Clin Microbiol* 48:358;2010.
275. Snelling, WJ et al. *Lett App Microbiol* 42:7;2006.
276. Lehner, A., Tasara, T., Stephan, R. *Int J Food Microbiol* 102:127;2005.
277. Shah, AH et al. *Transbound Emerg Dis* 60:9;2013.
278. Speer, CA. In: Doyle, MP, Beuchat, LR, Montville, TJ. eds. *Food Microbiology: Fundamentals and Frontiers*. ASM Press, Washington, DC, p. 478;1997.
279. Hilton, CL et al. *J Appl Microbiol* 91:929;2001.
280. Collado, L., Figueras, M.J. *Clin Microbiol Rev* 24:174;2011.
281. Van Driessche, E et al. *Res Microbiol* 155:662;2004.
282. Eifert, JD et al. *Poult Sci* 82:1898;2003.
283. Gude, A et al. *Lett Appl Microbiol* 41:82;2005.
284. Webster, RG et al. *Microbiol Rev* 56:152;1992.
285. Stiles, ME. In: Doyle, MP. ed. *Foodborne Bacterial Pathogens*. Marcel Dekker, NY, p. 706;1989.
286. Labigne, A, De Reuse, H. *Infect Agents Dis* 5:191;1996.
287. McColl, KEL. *J Infect Dis* 34:7;1997.
288. Cover, TL, Blaser, MJ. *Gastroenterology* 136:1863;2009.
289. Goodman, KJ, Correa, P. *Int J Epidemiol* 24:875;1995.
290. Hopkins, RJ et al. *J Infect Dis* 168:222;1993.
291. Jiang, X, Doyle, MP. *J Food Prot* 61:929;1998.
292. Baggett, HC et al. *Pediatrics* 117:e396;2006.
293. Cardenas, VM et al. *Am J Epidemiol* 163:127;2006.
294. Koopmans, M, Duizer, E. *Int J Food Microbiol* 90:23;2004.
295. Bidawid, S, Farber, JM, Sattar, SA. *Appl Environ Microbiol* 66:2759;2000.
296. Baert, L, Debevere, J, Uyttendaele, M. *Int J Food Microbiol* 131:83;2009.
297. Cromeans, T, Nainan, OV, Fields, HA, Favaorov, MO, Margolis, HA. In:Hui, YH, Gorham, JR, Murrel, KD, Cliver, DO. eds. *Foodborne Diseases Handbook*, Vol. 2. Marcel Dekker, NY, p. 1;1994.
298. Cliver, DO. *World Health Stat Q* 50:91;1997.
299. Feinstone, SM. *Eur J Gastroenterol Hepatol* 8:300;1996.
300. Anonymous. *Morb Mort Weekly Rep* 52:1155;2003.
301. Klevens, RM et al. *Arch Intern Med* 170:1811;2010.
302. Parashar, U. *Morb Mort Weekly Rep* 50:No. RR-9;2001.
303. Wilhelm, CM et al. *Infect Cont Hosp Epidemiol* 31:816;2010.
304. Dolin, R et al. *Proc Soc Exp Biol Med* 140:578;1972.
305. Vega, E et al. *Emerg Infect Dis* 17:1389;2011.
306. Sattar, SA, Springthorpe, VS, Ansari, SA, Hui, YH, Gorham, JR, Murrel, KD, Cliver, DO. *Rotavirus, Foodborne Diseases Handbook*, Vol. 2. Marcel Dekker, NY, p. 81;1994.
307. Hull, JJ et al. *Pediatr Infect Dis J* 30:S42;2011.
308. Horimoto, T, Kawaoka, Y. *Nat Rev Microbiol* 3:591;2005.
309. World Health Organization. *N Engl J Med* 353:1374;2005.
310. Easterday, BC, Hinshaw, VS, Halvorson, DA. *Diseases of Poultry*, 10th edn. Iowa State University Press, Ames, IA, p. 583;1997.
311. Lamb, RA. In: Krug, RM. ed. *The Influenza Viruses*, 1st edn. Plenum Press, NY; 1989.
312. White, J, Kartenbeck, J, Helenius, A. *EMBO J* 1:217;1982.
313. Klenk, H-D et al. *Virology* 68:426;1975.
314. Stieneke-Grober, A et al. *EMBO J* 11:2407;1992.
315. Horimoto, T et al. *J Virol* 68:6074;1994.
316. Swayne, DE, Beck, JR. *Avian Pathol* 33:512;2004.
317. Leibler, JH et al. *Ecohealth* 6:58;2009.
318. Buchi, G, Rae, ID. In: Goldblatt, LA. eds. *Aflatoxins*. Academic Press, NY, p. 55;1969.
319. Hocking, AD. In: Doyle, MP, Beuchat, LR, Montville, TJ. eds. *Food Microbiology: Fundamentals and Frontiers*. ASM Press, Washington, DC, p. 393;1997.
320. Amaike, S, Keller, NP. *Annu Rev Phytopathol* 49:107;2011.
321. Probst, C, Njapau, H, Cotty, PJ. *Appl Environ Microbiol* 73:2762;2007.
322. Probst, C, Schulthless, F, Cotty, PJ. *J Appl Microbiol* 108:600;2010.
323. Gong, YY et al. *BMJ* 325:20;2002.
324. Maxwell, SM et al. *J Toxicol Toxin Rev* 8:19;1998.
325. Mace, K et al. *Carcinogenesis* 18:1291;1997.
326. Smela, ME, Curier, SS. *Carcinogenesis* 22:535;2001.
327. Railey, J et al. *Carcinogenesis* 18:905;1997.
328. Ramdell, HS, Eaton, DL, *Cancer Res* 50:615;1990.
329. Pitt, JI. In: Doyle, MP, Beuchat, LR, Montville, TJ. eds. *Food Microbiology: Fundamentals and Frontiers*. ASM Press, Washington, DC, p. 406;1997.
330. Krogh, P, Hald, B, Perdersen, E. *J Acta Pathol Microbiol Scand* B81:689;1977.
331. Karabulut, OA et al. *Postharvest Biol Tech* 24:103;2002.
332. Karabulut, OA, Baykal, N. *Postharvest Biol Tech* 26:237;2002.
333. Vero, S et al. *Postharvest Biol Tech* 26:91;2002.
334. Venturini, ME, Oria, R, Blanco, D. *Food Microbiol* 19:15;2002.
335. Krogh, P et al. *Dansk vet Tidsskr* 67:123;1984.
336. Scott, PM, Fuleki, T, Harvig, JJ. *Agric Food Chem* 25:434;1977.
337. Moss, MO. *J Appl Microbiol* 84:62S;1998.

338. Friis, P, Hasselager, E, Krogh, P. *Acta Pathol Microbiol Scand* 77:559;1969.
339. Burgess, LW, Bryden, WL. *Microbiol Aust* Mar:22;2012.
340. Bullerman, LB. In: Doyle, MP, Beuchat, LR, Montville, TJ. eds. *Food Microbiology: Fundamentals and Frontiers*. ASM Press, Washington, DC, p. 419;1997.
341. Jones, JL et al. *Clin Infect Dis* 38:S198;2004.
342. Hlavsa, MC, Watson, JC, Beach, MJ. *Morb Mort Weekly Rep* 54:9;2005.
343. Dorny, P et al. *Vet Parasitol* 163:196;2009.
344. Smith, JJ. *Food Prot* 56:451;1993.
345. Doyle, E. *Foodborne Parasites, A Review of the Scientific Literature*, FRI Briefings, University of Wisconsin, Madison, WI, 2003.
346. Karanis, P, Kourenti, C, Smith, H. *J Water Health* 5:1;2007.
347. Fox, KR, Lyte, DAJ. *Am Water Works Assoc* 88:87;1996.
348. Corso, PS et al. *Emerg Infect Dis* 9:426;1993.
349. Hoskin, JC, Wright, REJ. *Food Prot* 54:53;1991.
350. Petersen, C. *Lancet* 345:1128;1995.
351. Tzipori, S. *Microbiol Rev* 47:84;1983.
352. Reduker, DW, Speer, CA. *J Parasitol* 71:112;1985.
353. Korich, DG et al. *Appl Environ Microbiol* 56:1423;1990.
354. Xiao, L. *Exp Parasitol* 124:80;2010.
355. Gait, R et al. *Vet Rec* 162:843;2008.
356. Sterling, CR, Ortega, YR. *Emerg Infect Dis* 5:48;1999.
357. Rose, JB, Slifko, TR. *J Food Prot* 62:1059;2000.
358. Anonymous. *Morb Mort Weekly Rep* 47:782;1997.
359. Lopez, AS, Dodson, DR, Arrowood, MJ et al. *Clin Infect Dis* 32:1010;2001.
360. Smith, HV et al. *Appl Environ Microbiol* 63:1631;1997.
361. Dubey, JP et al. *J Parasitol* 32:99;2002.
362. Casemore, DP. *Lancet* 336:1427;1990.
363. Tenter, AM, Heckeroth, AR, Weiss, LM. *Int J Parasitol* 30:1217;2000.
364. Fayer, R, Dubey, JP. *Food Technol* 39:57;1985.
365. Anonymous. *Morb Mort Weekly Rep* 48:1;1999.
366. Lindsay, DS, Blagburn, BL, Dubey, JP. *Vet Parasitol* 103:309;2002.
367. Fleck, DG. *PHLS Microbiol Digest* 6:69;1989.
368. Kim, CW. In: Doyle, MP, Beuchat, LR, Montville, TJ. eds. *Food Microbiology: Fundamentals and Frontiers*. ASM Press, Washington, DC, p. 449;1997.
369. Murrell, KD, Pozio, E. *Emerg Infect Dis* 17:2194;2011.
370. Anonymous. Surveillance summaries. *Morb Mortal Weekley Rep* 52:1;2003.
371. Hayunga, EG. In: Doyle, MP, Beuchat, LR, Montville, TJ. eds. *Food Microbiology: Fundamentals and Frontiers*. ASM Press, Washington, DC, p. 463;1997.
372. Dorny, P, Praet, N. *Vet Parasitol* 149:22;2007.
373. Garcia, HH et al. *Lancet* 362:547;2003.
374. March, SB, Ratnam, S. *J Clin Microbiol* 23:869;1986.
375. Kleanthous, H et al. *Epidemiol Infect* 101:327;1988.
376. Doyle, MP, Schoeni, JL. *Appl Environ Microbiol* 53:2394;1987.
377. March, SB, Ratnam, S. *J Clin Microbiol* 27:1675;1989.
378. Okrend, AJG, Rose, BE, Matner, R. *J Food Prot* 53:936;1990.
379. Padhye, NV, Doyle, MP. *Appl Environ Microbiol* 57:2693;1991.
380. Zhao, ZJ, Liu, XM. *Biomed Environ Sci* 18:254;2005.
381. Pollard, DR et al. *J Clin Microbiol* 28:540;1990.
382. Nguyen, LT et al. *Foodborne Pathog Dis* 1:231;2004.
383. Johnston, LM et al. *J Food Prot* 68:2256;2005.
384. Fedio, WM et al. *Int J Food Microbiol* 48:87;2011.
385. Eum, N et al. *Sens Actuator B* 143:784;2010.
386. Burr, MD, Nocker, A, Camper, AK. *Handbook Water Wastewater Syst Prot* 2:205;2011.
387. Davis, R et al. *J Food Sci* 75:M340;2010.
388. Kannan, P et al. *Foodborne Path Dis* 7:551;2010.
389. Soderlund, R et al. *Epidemiol Infect* 1;2011.
390. Cox, NA et al. *J Food Prot* 47:74;1984.
391. Cox, NA et al. *Dairy Food Environ Sanit* 7:628;1987.
392. Maciorowski, KG. et al. *Vet Res Commun* 30:127;2006.
393. Feng, PJ, *Food Prot* 55:927;992.
394. Tietjen, M, Fung, DYC. *Crit Rev Microbiol* 21:53;1995.
395. Kim, U, Su, XL, Li, Y. *J Food Prot* 68:1799;2005.
396. Nguyen, AV, Khan, MI, Lu, Z. *Avian Dis* 38:119;1994.
397. Bansal, NS, Gray, V, McDonell, F. *J Food Prot* 69:282;2006.
398. Seo, KH et al. *J Food Prot* 67:864;2004.
399. Bolton, LF et al. *J Clin Microbiol* 37:1348;1999.
400. Le Minor, L, Craige, J, Yen, C. *Can Publ Health J* 29:484;1938.
401. Lim, P et al. *J Clin Microbiol* 36:2271;1998.
402. Chaicumpa, W et al. *J Clin Microbiol* 30:2513;1992.
403. Kumar, S, Balakrishna, K, Batra, HV. *Lett Appl Microbiol* 42:149;2006.
404. Farrell, JJ et al. *Am J Clin Pathol* 123:339;2005.
405. Pui, CF et al. *Food Contr* 22:337e;2011.
406. Jackeray, R et al. *Talanta* 84:952;2011.
407. Jain, S et al. *Biosens Bioelectron* 31:37;2012.
408. Stern, NJ, Kazmi, SU. In: Doyle, MP. ed. *Foodborne Bacterial Pathogens*. Marcel Dekker, NY, p. 71;1989.
409. Park, CE et al. In: Speck, ML et al. eds. *Compendium of Methods for the Microbiological Examination of Foods*, 2nd edn. American Public Health Association, Washington, DC, p. 386;1984.
410. Rice, BE et al. *Clin Diagn Lab Immunol* 3:669;1996.
411. Endtz, HP et al. *Eur J Clin Microbiol Infect Dis* 19:794;2000.
412. Linton, D et al. *J Clin Microbiol* 35:2568;1997.
413. Ng, LK et al. *Appl Environ Microbiol* 63:4558;1997.
414. Oliveira, TC, Barbut, S, Griffiths, MW. *Int J Food Microbiol* 104:105;2005.
415. Sails, AD et al. *Appl Environ Microbiol* 69:1383;2003.
416. Bolton, FJ et al. *J Food Prot* 65;760;2002.
417. Keramas, G et al. *J Clin Microbiol* 42:3985;2004.
418. Bui, XT et al. *Res Microbiol* 163:64;2011.
419. Bruno, JG et al. *J Fluoresc* 19:427;2009.
420. Yamazaki, W. *Methods Mol Biol* 739:13;2011.
421. Huang, J et al. *Biosens Bioelectron* 25:1204;2010.
422. Marotta, F et al. *Mol Biotechnol* 53:182;2013.
423. Morris, GK. In: Speck, ML et al. eds. *Compendium of Methods for the Microbiological Examination of Foods*, 2nd edn. American Public Health Association, Washington, DC, p. 343;1984.
424. Pal, T et al. *J Clin Microbiol* 35:1757;1997.
425. Rahman, SR, Stimson, WH. *Hybridoma* 20:85;2001.
426. Lampel, KA et al. *Appl Environ Microbiol* 56:1536;1990.
427. Theron, J et al. *Water Res* 35:869;2001.
428. Lindqvist, RJ, *Appl Microbiol* 86:971;1999.
429. Achi-Berglund, R, Lindberg, AA. *Clin Microbiol Infect* 2:55;1996.
430. Wiemer, D et al. *Int J Med Microbiol* 301:577;2011.
431. Sankaran, K et al. *Diagn Microbiol Infect Dis* 63:243;2009.
432. Kim, DH et al. *J Microbiol* 48:682;2010.
433. Restaino, L et al. *J Food Prot* 42:120;1979.
434. Kapperud, G et al. *Appl Environ Microbiol* 59:2938;1993.
435. Wolffs, P et al. *J Clin Microbiol* 42:1042;2004.
436. Wannet, WJ et al. *J Clin Microbiol* 40:739;2002.
437. Khamjing, W, Khongchareonporn, N, Rengpipat, S. *Microbiol Immunol* 55:605;2011.
438. Gao, H et al. *J Microbiol Methods* 77:198;2009.

439. Wittwer, M et al. *Syst Appl Microbiol* 34:12;2011.
440. Farmer, JJ, III, Hickmann-Brenner, FW, Kelly, MT, In: Lennette, EH, Balows, A, Hausler, WJ, Jr., Jean-Shadomy, H. eds. *Manual of Clinical Microbiology*, 4th edn. American Society for Microbiology, Washington, DC, p. 282;1985.
441. Twedt, RM., Madden, JM, Colwell, RR. In: Speck, ML et al. eds. *Compendium of Methods for the Microbiological Examination of Foods*, 2nd edn. American Public Health Association, Washington, DC, p. 368;1984.
442. Choopun, N et al. *Appl Environ Microbiol* 68:995;2002.
443. Castillo, L et al. *Hybridoma* 14:271;1995.
444. Martinez-Govea, A et al. *Clin Diagn Lab Immunol* 8:768;2001.
445. Goel, AK et al. *Folia Microbiol (Praha)* 450:448;2005.
446. Miyagi, K et al. *J Med Microbiol* 48:883;199.
447. Varela, P et al. *J Clin Microbiol* 32:1246;1994.
448. Panicker, G et al. *Appl Environ Microbiol* 70:7436;2004.
449. Lyon, WJ. *Appl Environ Microbiol* 67:4685;2001.
450. Yu, CY et al. *J Microbiol Methods* 86:277;2011.
451. Koskela, KA et al. *Diagn Microbiol Infect Dis* 65:339;2009.
452. Yamazaki, W et al. *BMC Microbiol* 8:94;2008.
453. Chen, W et al. *Appl Microbiol Biotechnol* 89:1979;2011.
454. Honda, T et al. *J Clin Microbiol* 22:383;1985.
455. Kim, YB et al. *J Clin Microbiol* 37:1173;1999.
456. Ward, LN, Bej, AK. *Appl Environ Microbiol* 72:2031;2006.
457. Cai, T et al. *FEMS Immunol Med Microbiol* 46:180;2006.
458. Pinto, AD et al. *Lett App Microbiol*, 54:494;2012.
459. Rizvi, AV, Bej, AK. *Antonie Van Leeuwenhoek* 98:279;2010.
460. Kang, MH et al. *Diagn Microbiol Infect Dis* 69:21;2011.
461. Nemoto, J et al. *J Food Prot* 72:748;2009.
462. Wang, R et al. *J Genet Genomics* 38:129;2011.
463. Cerda-Cuellar, M, Jofre, J, Blanch, AR. *Appl Environ Microbiol* 66:855;2000.
464. Parker, RW, Lewis, DH. *Appl Environ Microbiol* 61:476;1995.
465. Marco-Noales, E et al. *J Appl Microbiol* 89:599;2000.
466. Campbell, MS, Wright, AC. *Appl Environ Microbiol* 69:7137;2003.
467. Chase, E, Harwood, VJ. *Appl Environ Microbiol* 77:4200;2011.
468. Baker-Austin, C et al. *Environ Microbiol Rep* 2:76;2010.
469. Han, F, Ge, B. *Lett Appl Microbiol* 51:234;2010.
470. Warner, EB, Oliver, JD. *Foodborne Pathog Dis* 5:691;2008.
471. Yongjun, LI et al. *Acta Oceanol* 29:93;2010.
472. Zheng, Z et al. *Mar Environ Sci* 28:211;2009.
473. Guillaume-Gentil, O et al. *J Food Prot*, 68:64;2005.
474. U.S. Food and Drug Administration, 2002. URL: http://www.fda.gov/food/scienceresearch/laboratorymethods/ucm114665.htm (Accessed February 2013).
475. Nair, MKM, Venkitanarayanan, K. *Appl Environ Microbiol*, 72:2006;2539–2546.
476. Seo, KH, Brackett, RE. *J Food Prot* 68:59;2005.
477. Wang, M et al. *J Clin Microbiol* 47:3178;2009.
478. Chiang, YC et al. *J Microbiol Methods* 88:110;2012.
479. Lu, X et al. *Mod Food Sci Tech* 26:540;2010.
480. Janda, JM, Abott, SL, Carnahan, AM. In: Murray, PR, Baron, EJ, Pfaller, MA, Tenover, FC, Yolken, RH. eds. *Manual of Clinical Microbiology*, 6th edn. American Society for Microbiology, Washington, DC, p. 477;1995.
481. Jeppesen, C. *Int J Food Microbiol* 26:25;1995.
482. Joseph, SE, Carnahan, A. *Annu Rev Fish Dis* 4:315;1994.
483. Kannan, S et al. *Int J Med Microbiol* 19:190;2001.
484. Delamare, AP et al. *J Appl Microbiol* 92:936;2002.
485. Borrel, N et al. *J Clin Microbiol* 35:1671;1997.
486. Chu, WH, Lu CP. *J Fish Dis* 28:437;2005.
487. Peng, X et al. *J Microbiol Methods* 49:335;2002.
488. Wang, HB et al. *Zhonghua Yu Fang Yi Xue Za Zhi* 43:611;2009.
489. Tichoniuk, M et al. *Biosens Bioelectron* 26:1618;2010.
490. Xue-Mei, B et al. URL: http://en.cnki.com.cn/Article_en/CJFDTotal-CHAN201010010.htm (Accessed March 2012).
491. Longyant, S et al. *J Fish Dis* 33:973;2010.
492. Chang, W et al. *Sens Actuators B*, URL: http://dx.doi.org/10.1016/j.snb.2011.12.054 (Accessed February 2013).
493. Lee, DY et al. *Sci Total Environ* 398:203;2008.
494. Gonzalez-Rey, C et al. *FEMS Immunol Med Microbiol* 29:107;2000.
495. Jones, GL. *Isolation and Identification of Listeria monocytogenes*. U.S. Department of Health and Human Services Public Health Service; 1989.
496. McClain, D, Lee, WH. *J Assoc Off Anal Chem* 71:876;1988.
497. VanNetten, P et al. *Int J Food Microbiol* 8:299;1989.
498. Gasanov, U, Hughes, D, Hansbro, PM. *FEMS Microbiol Rev* 29:851;2005.
499. Fliss, I et al. *Appl Environ Microbiol* 59:2698;1993.
500. Kim, SH et al. *J Vet Sci* 6:41;2005.
501. Garrec, N et al. *J Microbiol Methods* 55:763;2003.
502. Amagliani, G et al. *J Appl Microbiol* 100:375;2006.
503. Oravcova, K et al. *Lett Appl Microbiol* 42:15;2006.
504. Rodriguez-Lazaro, D et al. *J Food Prot* 68:1467;2005.
505. O'Grady, J et al. *Food Microbiol* 26:4;2009.
506. D'Urso, OF et al. *Food Microbiol* 26:311;2009.
507. Kawasaki, S et al. *Foodborne Pathog Dis* 7:549;2010.
508. Wang, R et al. *Nano Lett* 8:2625;2008.
509. Tang, MJ et al. *Curr Microbiol* 63:511;2011.
510. Moreno, Y et al. *Water Res* 45:4634;2011.
511. Bennett, RW. In: Pierson, MD, Stern, NJ. eds. *Foodborne Microorganisms and Their Toxins: Developing Methodology*. Marcel Dekker, NY, p. 345;1986.
512. Taitini, SR, Hoover, DG, and Lachicha, RVF. In: Speck, ML et al. eds. *Compendium of Methods for the Microbiological Examination of Foods*, 2nd edn. American Public Health Association, Washington, DC, p. 411;1984.
513. Van der Zee, A et al. *J Clin Microbiol* 37:342;1999.
514. Alarcon, B, Vicedo, B, Aznar, RJ. *Appl Microbiol* 100:352;2006.
515. Cremonesi, P. *Mol Cell Probes* 19:299;2005.
516. Fusco, V et al. *Int J Food Microbiol* 144:528;2011.
517. Fosheim, GE et al. *J Clin Microbiol* 49:3071;2011.
518. Sapsford, KE et al. *Appl Environ Microbiol* 71:5590;2005.
519. Ruan, C et al. *Biosens Bioelectron* 20:585;2004.
520. Vernozy-Rozand, C et al. *Lett Appl Microbiol* 39:490;2004.
521. Bennett, RW. *Bacteriological Analytical Manual*, 6th edn. U.S. Food and Drug Administration Association of Official Analytical Chemists, Arlington, VA, p. 15.01;1984.
522. Lawson, TS et al. *Clin Lab* 57:789;2011.
523. Cao, X et al. *Nucleic Acids Res* 37:4621;2009.
524. Dowell, VR et al. *Media for Isolation Characterization and Identification of Obligate Anaerobic Bacteria*. CDC, Atlanta, GA; 1981.
525. Aranda, E et al. *Lett Appl Microbiol* 25:186;1997.
526. Fach, P et al. *Appl Environ Microbiol* 61:389;1995.
527. Braconnier, A et al. *J Food Prot* 64:201;2001.
528. Lindstrom, M et al. *Appl Environ Microbiol* 67:5694;2001.
529. Dahlenborg, M, Borch, E, Radstrom, P. *Appl Environ Microbiol* 67:4781;2001.
530. Anniballi, F et al. *Vet Microbiol* 154:332;2012.
531. Satterfield, BA et al. *J Med Microbiol* 59:55;2010.
532. Kautter, DA, Lynt, RK, Solomon, HM. *Bacteriological Analytical Manual*, 6th edn. U.S. Food and Drug Administration Association of Official Analytical Chemists, Arlington, VA, p. 18.01;1984.

533. Gessler, F, Hampe, K, Bohnel, H. *Appl Environ Microbiol* 71:7897;2005.
534. Barr, JR et al. *Emerg Infect Dis* 11:1578;2005.
535. Sharma, SK et al. *Appl Environ Microbiol* 71:3935;2005.
536. Sakuma, T et al. *J Appl Microbiol* 106:1252;2009.
537. Raphael, BH et al. *Mol Cell Probes* 24:146;2010.
538. Fach, P, Popoff, MR. *Appl Environ Microbiol* 63:4232;1997.
539. Baez, LA, Juneja, VK. *Appl Environ Microbiol* 61:807;1995.
540. Asha, NJ, Wilcox, MH. *J Med Microbiol* 51:891;2002.
541. Hale, ML, Stiles, BG. *Toxicon* 37:471;1999.
542. Wise, MG, Siragusa, GR. *Appl Environ Microbiol* 7:3911;2005.
543. Augustynowicz, E., Gzyl, A., Slusarczyk, J. *J Med Microbiol* 51:169;2002.
544. Albini, S et al. *Vet Microbiol* 127:179;2008.
545. Gurjar, AA et al. *Mol Cell Probes* 22:90;2008.
546. Shimizu, S et al. *Food Microbiol* 26:425;2009.
547. Janvilisri, T et al. *Diagn Microbiol Infect Dis* 66:140;2010.
548. Quinn, CD et al. *J Clin Microbiol* 48:603;2010.
549. Barbut, F et al. *J Clin Microbiol* 47:1276;2009.
550. Stamper, PD et al. *J Clin Microbiol* 47:3846;2009.
551. Huang, H et al. *J Clin Microbiol* 47:3729;2009.
552. Noren, T et al. *J Clin Microbiol* 49:710;2011.
553. Janežič, S, Štrumbelj, I, Rupnik, MJ. *Clin Microbiol* 49:3024;2011.
554. Janvilisri, T et al. *J Bacteriol* 191:3881;2009.
555. Worsley, MA. *J Antimicrob Chemother* 41:59;1998.
556. Harmon, SM, Goepfert, JM. In: Speck, ML et al. eds. *Compendium of Methods for the Microbiological Examination of Foods*, 2nd edn. American Public Health Association, Washington, DC, p. 458;1984.
557. Chen, CH, Ding, HC, Chang, TC. *J Food Prot* 64:348;2001.
558. Charni, N et al. *Appl Environ Microbiol* 66:2278;2000.
559. Chen, CH, Ding, HC. *J Food Prot* 67:387;2004.
560. Moravek, M et al. *FEMS Microbiol Lett* 238:107;2004.
561. Mantynen, V, Lindstrom, K. *Appl Environ Microbiol* 64:1634;1998.
562. Nakano, S et al. *J Food Prot* 67:1694;2004.
563. Hansen, BJ, Hendriksen, NB. *Appl Environ Microbiol* 67:185;2001.
564. Fricker, M et al. *Appl Environ Microbiol* 73:1892;2007.
565. Kim, K et al. *FEMS Immunol Med Microbiol* 43:301;2005.
566. Buchanan, RL, Schultz, FJ. *Lett Appl Microbiol* 19:353;1994.
567. Sergeev, N et al. *J Microbiol Methods* 65:488;2006.
568. Corry, JEL, Atabay, HI, Forsythe, SJ, Mansfield, LP. In: Corry, JEL, Curtis, GDW, Baird, RM. eds. *Progress in Industrial Microbiology*. Elsevier, Amsterdam, the Netherlands. p. 271;2003.
569. Johnson, LG, Murano, EA. *J Food Prot* 62:456;1999.
570. Fera, MT et al. *Appl Environ Microbiol* 70:1271;2004.
571. Atabay, HI, Corry, JE, On, SLJ. *Appl Microbiol* 84:1007;1998.
572. Atabay, HI et al. *Int J Food Microbiol* 25:21;2003.
573. Atabay, HI et al. *Lett Appl Microbiol* 35:142;2002.
574. Hume, ME et al. *J Food Prot* 64:645;2001.
575. Ruiz, J et al. *J Clin Microbiol* 35:2417;1997.
576. Luccero, NE et al. *J Clin Microbiol* 37:3245;1999.
577. Romero, C et al. *J Clin Microbiol* 33:3198;1995.
578. Batra, HV, Agarwal, GS, Rao, PV. *J Commun Dis* 35:71;2003.
579. Probert, WS et al. *J Clin Microbiol* 42:1290;2004.
580. Al Dahouk, S et al. *Clin Lab* 50:387;2004.
581. Tantillo, GM, Di Pinto, A, Buonavoglia, CJ. *Dairy Res* 70:245;2003.
582. Schmoock, G et al. *Diagn Microbiol Infect Dis* 71:341;2011.
583. Lin, GZ et al. *Mol Cell Probes* 25:126;2011.
584. Qu, Q et al. *J Microbiol Methods* 79:121;2009.
585. Kabir, SJ. *Med Microbiol* 50:1021;2001.
586. Hauser, B et al. *Acta Paediatr* 95:297;2006.
587. Koletzko, S et al. *Gut* 52:804;2003.
588. Shahamat, M et al. *J Clin Microbiol* 42:3613;2004.
589. Smith, SI et al. *World J Gastroenterol* 10:1958;2004.
590. Mousavi, S et al. *Med Sci Monit* 12:I15;2006.
591. Woo, HY et al. *Helicobacter* 14:22;2009.
592. Smith, EM, Gerba, CP, Goyal, SM. In: *Methods in Environmental Virology*. Marcel Dekker, NY. p. 15;1982.
593. Williams, FP, Jr, Fout, GS. *Environ Sci Technol* 26:689;1992.
594. Polish, LB et al. *J Clin Microbiol* 37:3615;1977.
595. Perelle, S et al. *J Virol Methods* 157:80;2009.
596. Yang, N et al. *Marine Poll Bull* 62:2654;2011.
597. Abd el-Galil, KH et al. *Appl Environ Microbiol* 71:7113;2005.
598. Sincero, TC et al. *Water Res* 2006.
599. Yoneyama, T et al. *J Virol Methods* 145:162;2007.
600. Lee, HJ et al. *Virol J* 7:164;2010.
601. Herrmann, JE et al. *J Clin Microbiol* 33:2511;1995.
602. Dimitriadis, A, Marshall, JA. *Eur J Clin Microbiol Infect Dis* 24:615;2005.
603. Jothikumar, N et al. *Appl Environ Microbiol* 71:1870;2005.
604. Tian, P, Mandrell, R. *J Appl Microbiol* 100:564;2006.
605. Schmid, M et al. *BMC Infect Dis* 4:15;2004.
606. Tonelli, A et al. *Mol Biosyst* 7:1684;2011.
607. Suffredini, E et al. *New Microbiol* 34:9;2011.
608. Lee, H et al. *J Microbiol* 48:419;2010.
609. Geginat, G, Kaiser, D, Schrempf, S. *Eur J Clin Microbiol Infect Dis* 31:733;2011.
610. Pagotto, F et al. *J Food Prot* 71:1434;2008.
611. Tsunemitsu, H, Jiang, B, Saif, LJ. *J Clin Microbiol* 30:2129;1992.
612. Adler, M et al. *Biochem Biophys Res Commun* 333:1289;2005.
613. Kittigul, L et al. *J Virol Methods* 124:117;2005.
614. Reynolds, KA. *Methods Mol Biol* 268:69;2004.
615. Grassi, T et al. *Eur J Clin Microbiol Infect Dis* 31:575;2011.
616. Bosch, A et al. *Methods Mol Biol* 268:61;2004.
617. Jung, JH et al. *Angew Chem Int Ed Engl* 49:5708;2010.
618. Nicholson, KG, Wood, JM, Zambon, M. *Lancet* 362:1733;2003.
619. Mahony, JB et al. *J Clin Virol* 45:200;2009.
620. Poon, LL et al. *Clin Chem* 55:1555;2009.
621. Lin, B et al. *J Clin Microbiol* 47:988;2009.
622. Pitt, JI, Hocking, AD, Glenn, DRJ. *Appl Bacteriol* 54:109;1983.
623. Samson, RA, Hoekstra, ES, Frisvad, JC, Filtenborg, O. *Introduction to Foodborne Fungi*, 4th edn. Centraalbureau voor Schimmelcultures, Baarn, the Netherlands; 1995.
624. McClenny, N. *Med Mycol* 43:S125;2005.
625. Shapira, R et al. *Appl Environ Microbiol* 63:990;1997.
626. Yong, RK, Cousin, MA. *Int J Food Microbiol* 65:27;2001.
627. Fenelon, LE et al. *J Clin Microbiol* 37:1221;1999.
628. Passone, MA et al. *Int J Food Microbiol* 138:276;2010.
629. Shapira, R et al. *Appl Environ Microbiol* 62:3270;1996.
630. Yang, ZY et al. *J Food Prot* 67:2622;2004.
631. Zachova, I et al. *Folia Microbiol (Praha)* 48:817;2003.
632. Chen, RS et al. *J Food Prot* 65:840;2002.
633. Sharma, A et al. *Thin Solid Films* 519:1213;2010.
634. Piermarini, S et al. *Food Control* 20:371;2009.
635. Fernández-Ibañez, V et al. *Food Chem* 113:629;2009.
636. Pei, SC et al. *Food Contr* 20:1080;2009.
637. Parker, CO et al. *Anal Chem* 81:5291;2009.
638. Lamberti, I et al. *Mycotox Res* 25:193;2009.
639. King, AD, Pitt, JI, Beuchat, LR, Corry, JEL. *Methods for the Mycological Examination of Food*. Plenum Press, NY; 1986.

640. Marek, P, Annamalai, T, Venkitanarayanan, K. *Int J Food Microbiol* 89.139,2003.
641. Pedersen, LH et al. *Int J Food Microbiol* 35:169;1997.
642. Suanthie, Y, Cousin, MA, Wolozshuk, CPJ. *Stored Prod Res* 45:139;2009.
643. Watanabe, M, Shimizu, HJ. *Food Prot* 68:610;2005.
644. Franco, CM et al. *J Chromatogr A* 723:69;1996.
645. Ito, R et al. *J Agric Food Chem* 52:7464;2004.
646. Champdore, M et al. *Anal Chem* 79:751;2007.
647. Duan, ZH et al. *Biomed Environ Sci* 22:237;2009.
648. Nelson, PE, Tousoun, TA, Marasas, WFO. *Fusarium Species: An Illustrated Manual for Identification.* The Pennsylvania State University Press, University Park, PA; 1983.
649. Trane, U et al. In: Hocking, AD, Pitt, JI, King, AD. eds. *Modern Methods in Food Microbiology.* Elsevier Science Publishers, NY, p. 285;1992.
650. Demeke, T et al. *Int J Food Microbiol* 103:271;2005.
651. Jurado, M et al. *Syst Appl Microbiol* 28:562;2005.
652. Bluhm, BH, Cousin, MA, Woloshuk, CP. *J Food Prot* 67:36;2004.
653. Reischer, GH et al. *J Microbiol Methods* 59:141;2004.
654. Knoll, S, Vogel, RF, Niessen, L. *Lett Appl Microbiol,* 34:144;2002.
655. Maragos, CM, Plattner, RDJ. *Agric Food Chem* 50:1827;2002.
656. Iyer, MS, Cousin, MAJ. *Food Prot* 66:451;2003.
657. Niessen, L, Vogel, RF. *Int J Food Microbiol* 140:183;2010.
658. Deng, MQ, Cliver, DO. *Parasitol Res* 85:733;1999.
659. Pillai, DR, Kain, KC. *J Clin Microbiol* 37:3017;1999.
660. Garcia, LS et al. *J Clin Microbiol* 43:1256;2003.
661. Ng, CT et al. *J Clin Microbiol* 43:1256;2005.
662. Guy, RA, Xiao, C, Horgen, PA. *J Clin Microbiol* 42:3317;2004.
663. Verweij, JJ et al. *J Clin Microbiol* 42:1220;2004.
664. Guy, RA et al. *Appl Environ Microbiol* 69:5178;2003.
665. Yu, X et al. *Ecotoxicology* 18:661;2009.
666. Christy, NCV et al. *J Clin Microbiol* 50:1762;2012.
667. Rule, KL, Vikesland, PJ. *Environ Sci Technol* 43:1147;2009.
668. Xu, S, Mutharasan, R. *Environ Sci Technol* 44:1736;2010.
669. Keserue, H, Füchslin, HP, Egli, T. *Appl Environ Microbiol* 77:5420;2011.
670. Verweij, JJ et al. *J Clin Microbiol* 41:5041;2003.
671. Zengzhu, G et al. *J Clin Microbiol* 37:3034;1999.
672. Tanyuksel, M. *Exp Parasitol* 110:322;2004.
673. Haque, R et al. *J Clin Microbiol* 48:2798;2010.
674. Roy, SJ, *Clin Microbiol* 43:2168;2005.
675. Liang, Z, Keeley, A. *Appl Environ Microbiol* 77:6476;2011.
676. Sterling, CR, Arrowood, M. *J Pediatr Infect Dis* 5:139;1986.
677. Coupe, SJ, *Clin Microbiol* 43:1017; 2005.
678. Miller, WA et al. *J Microbiol Methods* 65:367;2006.
679. Xiao, L, Lal, AA, Jiang, *J Methods Mol Biol* 268:163;2004.
680. Ripabelli, G et al. *Foodborne Pathog Dis* 4:216;2004.
681. Muccio, JL. *J Am Vet Assoc* 225:7;2004.
682. Jenkins, MC, O'Brien, CN, Trout, JM. *J Parasitol* 94:94;2008.
683. Thiruppathiraja, C et al. *J Environ Monit* 13:2782;2011.
684. Xu, S, Mutharasan, R. *Anal Chim Acta* 669:81;2010.
685. Dixon, BR et al. *J Clin Microbiol* 43:2375;2005.
686. Chu, DM et al. *Am J Trop Med Hyg* 71:373;2004.
687. Shields, JM, Olson, BH. *Appl Environ Microbiol* 69:4662;2003.
688. Verma, M et al. *J Microbiol Methods* 53:27;2003.
689. Lee, S et al. *Korean J Parasitol* 48:297;2010.
690. Hitt, JA, Filice, GA. *J Clin Microbiol* 30:3181;1992.
691. Hofgartner, WT et al. *J Clin Microbiol* 35:3313;1997.
692. Roux-Buisson, N et al. *Diagn Microbiol Infect* 53:79;2005.
693. Abdel Hameed, DM, Helmy, HJ. *Egypt Soc Parasitol* 34:893;2004.
694. Switaj, K et al. *Clin Microbiol Infect* 11:170;2005.
695. Kourenti, C, Karanis, P. *Water Sci Technol* 50:287;2004.
696. Matsuo, J et al. *Southeast Asian J Trop Med Public Health* 35:270;2004.
697. Schwab, KJ, McDevitt, J. *J Appl Environ Microbiol* 69:5819;2003.
698. Montoya, A et al. *Res Vet Sci* 89:212;2010.
699. Zhang, H et al. *Exp Parasitol* 122:47;2009.
700. Bahl, A et al. *BMC Genomics* 11:603;2010.
701. Boulos, LM et al. *Parasite* 8:136;2001.
702. Yepez-Mulia, L et al. *Vet Parasitol* 81:57;1999.
703. Gamble, HR. *J Food Prot* 59:295;1996.
704. Wu, Z et al. *Parasitology* 118:211;1999.
705. Sohn, W et al. *Korean J Parasitol* 41:125;2003.
706. Kapel, CM et al. *Parasite* 8:S39;2001.
707. Atterby, H et al. *Vet Parasitol* 161:92;2009.
708. Yagihashi, A et al. *J Infect Dis* 161:995;1990.
709. Campos, M et al. *Parasitol Res* 93:433;2004.
710. Caballero, ML, Moneo, I. *Ann Allergy Asthma Immunol* 89:74;2002.
711. Zhu, X et al. *Int J Parasitol* 28:1911;1998.
712. Szostakowska, B, Myjak, P, Kur, J. *Mol Cell Probes* 16:111;2002.
713. Kijewska, A et al. *Mol Cell Probes* 14:349;2000.
714. Zhang, SL et al. *Zhongguo Ji Sheng Chong Xue Yu Ji Sheng Chong Bing Za Zhi* 28:194;2010.
715. Fang, W et al. *Exp Parasitol* 127:587;2011.
716. D'Souza, PE, Hafeez, M. *Vet Res Commun* 23:293;1999.
717. Dorny, P et al. *Acta Trop* 87:79;2003.
718. Gottstein, B et al. *Trans R Soc Trop Hyg* 85:248;1991.
719. Nunes, CM et al. *Exp Parasitol* 104:67;2003.
720. Gonzalez, LM et al. *J Clin Microbiol* 38:737;2000.

# 4 Safe Food Handling for the Consumer

*Susan Bowerman*

## CONTENTS

## INTRODUCTION

Foodborne illness is a major public health problem, and the home kitchen is believed to be a point of origin for many cases of foodborne disease. The importance of proper food handling in the home cannot be overstated. Pathogens are associated with a wide range of foods that are brought into the home, which means that consumer food storage and preparation practices are the final link to ensuring that home-prepared foods are safe to eat.

The chief cause of foodborne illness is pathogenic microorganisms—bacteria, viruses, and parasites. Since bacteria and other infectious organisms are pervasive in the environment, the contamination of food can occur at any point between the farm and the plate. Some organisms are naturally present in food-producing animals—such as *Salmonella* Enteritidis bacteria present in eggs and *Escherichia coli* normally present in the intestines of cattle. Exposure to animal manure or sewage runoff can contaminate crops or spill into rivers and streams and contaminate the fish that live there.

With food production becoming more global and more centralized and food being mass produced or processed at central locations prior to wide distribution, the patterns and incidence of foodborne illness have increased. Food production systems that involve large-scale farming and intensive animal farming practices have increased over the past several decades in the United States in order to meet increasing demand for food. On the other hand, these practices have been blamed for the evolution of new pathogens.[1]

Globalization of the food supply is likely to impact food safety as well. More than 50% of fresh vegetables in the developed world marketplace are imported from developing countries.[2] Imported food accounted for 15% (based on volume) of food consumed in the United States in 2005,[3] with fresh produce, tree nuts, and fish and shellfish being the most commonly imported food items.

Health-care providers are encouraging consumers to eat more fruits and vegetables to promote health, but at the same time the number of foodborne illness outbreaks related to fresh raw produce is on the rise.[4] Water contamination is a significant public health issue in many developing countries, and contaminated water is one of the most common sources of contamination in fresh produce.[5,6] Imported produce has been implicated in a number of large outbreaks of foodborne illness and has introduced unique pathogens into the food supply.[7]

The importation of food from other countries that may have inferior food safety standards can increase the risk of foodborne illness in the United States. Billions of people travel globally by air annually, so that those who have contracted gastroenteric illness while abroad could bring these agents into the home, providing an opportunity for further spread.[2]

## INCIDENCE AND COST OF FOODBORNE ILLNESS

The Centers for Disease Control (CDC) estimates that each year roughly 1 in 6 Americans (or 48 million people) gets sick, 128,000 are hospitalized, and 3,000 die of foodborne diseases.[8] However, it is believed that the actual incidence may be much higher, since many illnesses may only cause short-term discomfort that does not require medical attention, and only the more severe cases are reported. Outbreak data demonstrate that foods once considered low risk, such as fruits and vegetables, cause a surprising number of outbreaks.[7] By far, the majority of reported foodborne outbreaks are associated with foods that are prepared or consumed in the home.[9]

Certain populations are more vulnerable, particularly the elderly, the young, the immunocompromised, and those who are pregnant. Due to better health care and advances in medicine, older adults and people with weakened immune systems are living longer, so these subpopulations are growing, which suggests that more people will be vulnerable to foodborne illness.

Even though most cases are mild, foodborne illness places significant burdens on the economy, in terms of lost productivity, medical expenses, and lawsuits resulting in compensation for loss of income, medical expenses, legal fees, and other damages.[10] The annual estimated cost of foodborne illness in the United States, including medical costs, loss in productivity, pain, suffering, and disability, has been estimated at $77.7 billion.[8]

In the United States, numerous programs and campaigns are designed to improve consumer education about food safety. One of the main educational tools is the "*Fight* BAC!™" campaign, which is supported by a partnership among the food industry, government, and consumer organizations.[11]

Recent improvements, such as the introduction of Hazard Analysis and Critical Control Point (HACCP) systems in seafood, meat, and poultry plants and greatly expanded food testing programs, have reduced the disease burden from some food products. Intensified surveillance by the CDC indicates a declining incidence of foodborne disease in most areas of the United States.[12]

## ROLE OF THE HOME IN FOODBORNE DISEASE

The home is multifunctional setting, which impacts the need for good hygiene and proper food handling. The home kitchen may serve as not only a food preparation area but a gathering place for family members and household pets. Enteropathogens can be transmitted from domestic cats and dogs to humans, as well as to contact surfaces or directly to foods via carriage on the hands. Additional hazards can come from the presence of dirty laundry in the kitchen or use of kitchen sinks to clean gardening implements or tools. In addition, foods prepared at home not only are eaten by those residing there but are often distributed outside, such as for bake sales or school events.

Due to shifts in health-care delivery, the home plays an extension of traditional care that is generally provided outside the home. There is a growing population of elderly and others who are immunocompromised living in the home, and these individuals are more vulnerable to the impact of foodborne disease. Additionally, in the United States, more than half of children under 5 years of age receive home-based day care,[13] which increases the potential for outbreaks of foodborne illness via home-prepared food.

## BACTERIAL CONTAMINATION IN THE KITCHEN

The entry of potential pathogens to the home kitchen can begin at many points in the process from food production to food consumption. Consider, for example, the preparation of a chicken meal at home. The poultry could have been contaminated on the farm, at the processing plant, or during transportation to the supermarket. Once at the grocery store, it could be improperly refrigerated or held too long before purchase. As it is transported into the home, it may not be refrigerated promptly, or cross contamination could occur through the use of an unclean reusable grocery bag, or the home refrigerator temperature could be too warm for the food to be stored safely. In preparing the raw poultry, there is the possibility of cross contamination to fresh foods, such as a salad, if hands and cutting boards are not properly washed. Finally, the poultry may not be cooked adequately to ensure that it is safe to eat. Foodborne illness could result from improper handling at any point in this process, and since pathogens generally cannot be seen, smelled, or tasted, it is important for consumers to be knowledgeable about food safety practices in the home.

Studies have shown that bacterial contamination in the kitchen can be higher than in bathrooms.[14] The locations that tend to harbor the most contamination are sites that are wet or moist, including dishcloths, cleaning cloths, sponges, sinks, and towels. The rough texture of sponges and cloths are particularly problematic, in that they are almost always moist and contaminated with food scraps.[15] In addition, pathogens can survive on tap handles, refrigerator handles, cutting boards, trash cans, and other work surfaces.

## CONSUMER KNOWLEDGE AND PRACTICE OF FOOD SAFETY

There is limited information on consumer food-handling and preparation behavior, and most of the information is based on anecdotal evidence or self-report.[16–18] But self-reported data can be flawed, since there is often a difference between what people say they do at home with regard to safe food handling and what they actually do. Beyond food handling, risky food consumption practices have also been widely observed, including the consumption of raw eggs, undercooked hamburgers, and raw fish.[19]

Several surveys have been conducted to determine food safety practices in the home. Although survey respondents might be somewhat biased in their answers and indicate that they follow recommended procedures, there is still evidence that a significant number of adults do not follow recommendations.[17,19] Knowledge, attitudes, intentions, and self-reported practices often do not correspond to observed behaviors,[17] so that observational studies provide a more realistic indication of the food hygiene actions actually used in domestic food preparation.

In a national mail survey that focused on consumer handling of fresh fruits and vegetables in the United States,[20] 2000 households were asked about food safety behaviors related to the purchase, transport, storage, and preparation of fresh produce. Almost half said that they do not routinely wash their hands before handling fresh produce, and 6% responded that they seldom or never wash fresh produce. Twenty-three percent of the respondents said that they stored raw meat, poultry, and fish on a refrigerator shelf above other foods, increasing the risk for contamination from meat juices to other foods and surfaces. Ninety-seven percent of respondents reported that they always wash their food preparation surfaces after contact with meat products, but 5% only dry-wiped the surface, and 24% washed with water only.[20]

In a study of 153 young adults attending a major U.S. university,[21] students completed an online survey about food safety knowledge and practices and then were observed preparing a meal in a lab setting as well as at home. Despite reporting high self-efficacy with regard to food safety, the students engaged in less than half of the recommended safe food-handling practices that were evaluated and incorrectly answered a third of the food safety knowledge items.[21]

In a study in the United Kingdom that examined the food safety practices of a small sample of older people living at home,[22] it was found that most participants had not measured their refrigerator temperature and did not know what it should be and that while "use-by" dates on food packages were generally understood, not all participants adhered to the dates and were often kept for up to a month before consumption.[22]

Several studies have used videotaping as a way to observe and evaluate food preparation in the home. In one study,[23] researchers placed video cameras in the kitchens of 100 families and observed them preparing a meal. Among those families who tended to be confident in their food safety habits, cooks were "caught on tape" undercooking meals and making other food-handling mistakes during preparation, including improper refrigerator storage of raw meat and seafood and improper or nonexistent hand washing, countertop cleansing, and fruit and vegetable washing.[23]

Foodborne illness has been linked to the unsafe preparation of ground beef, leading one group[24] to videotape 199 individuals while preparing hamburgers and a salad to observe their compliance with established safe food-handling practices. While the majority cooked ground meat to the recommended internal temperature of 155°F, 22% concluded that the burger patty was adequately cooked when the internal temperature was below 155°F. Only 13% knew the recommended internal temperature for cooked ground beef, and only 4% used a meat thermometer. The average hand-washing time was only 8 s, well below the recommended 20 s, which was

observed in only 7% of volunteers, and inadequate hand washing was the most commonly observed vehicle for potential cross contamination.[24]

In another study of 99 U.S. consumers[23] who were videotaped in their homes while preparing a meal, numerous food-handling errors were observed. Only a third of subjects washed hands with soap, and the average hand-wash length was significantly lower than the 20 s recommendation. Surface cleaning was found to be inadequate with only a third of surfaces thoroughly cleaned, and one-third of subjects made no attempt to clean surfaces during food preparation. Nearly all subjects cross contaminated raw meat, poultry, seafood, eggs, and/or unwashed vegetables with ready-to-eat foods multiple times during food preparation, many undercooked meat and poultry, and almost none used a food thermometer.[23]

An Australian study using video observation in 40 home kitchens found similar lapses in food safety practices.[25] In this case, kitchens were continuously video monitored for 1–2 weeks. Infrequent hand washing; poor hand-washing technique; lack of hand washing prior to food preparation; inadequate cleaning of kitchen surfaces; involvement of pets in the kitchen; touching of the face, mouth, nose, and/or hair during food preparation; and lack of separate hand and dish towels were the most common unhygienic practices observed.[25]

Several pathogens can be transmitted from animals to humans via uncooked or undercooked meat and poultry products, which is why it is so important that foods be cooked to a safe minimum internal temperature to destroy harmful pathogens. The use of a food thermometer is the only reliable method for ensuring that this temperature has been reached, and is considered one of the most important food-handling behaviors in the home.[26] This message is apparently reaching consumers, as the percentage of consumers who own food thermometers has jumped from 49% in 1998 to 70% in 2010.[27]

One study has reported a substantial improvement in food-handling practices and an increase in perceived risk from foodborne illness between 1993 and 2010.[19] During the same time period, the number of media stories related to food safety increased as well, suggesting that consumers became more attentive to food safety in the home. Women are reported to have safer food-handling and consumption practices than men, while the least safe food-handling behaviors are seen in the oldest and youngest consumers and those with the most education.[28] Changes in the safety of practices are consistent with change in number of media stories about food safety, suggesting that increased media attention to food safety issues may be raising awareness of hazards and improving the safety of food handling in the home.[19]

## PROPER FOOD HANDLING

The most common mistakes in home food handling and preparation involve inappropriate food storage and refrigeration, failure to attain the required cooking or reheating temperature, and cross contamination. The Partnership for Food Safety Education's Fight BAC! program[11] was created and endorsed by the U.S. Departments of Agriculture, Education, and Health and Human Services in 1997. The campaign was designed to reduce the incidence of foodborne illness in the home by educating Americans about safe food-handling practices. There are four pillars of the campaign—clean, separate, cook, and chill—and specific recommendations for each step are delineated.

## FOOD PURCHASING

When purchasing foods, the selling area or facility should be clean and sanitary, and foods should be kept at the appropriate temperature. Cross contamination can occur at the grocery store, such as at meat, seafood, or poultry counter, where raw and cooked products may be displayed next to one another. Foods that are stored hot, such as cooked poultry, should be held at temperatures of at least 135°F, and cold foods that are stored in refrigerated cases should be at 40°F or below.[29]

Many consumers find food-dating systems on packages confusing but should be encouraged to understand what they mean. Perishable foods such as meat, fish, poultry, yogurt, and milk have "sell-by" dates, after which time retailers should pull these items from their shelves. However, if consumers store perishables properly in the home, they do not necessarily need to discard them once the sell-by date has passed. Milk that is stored at the proper temperature, for example, can remain sweet and safe to drink for a week past the sell-by date if it has been properly stored. Even ground beef, which is highly perishable, is safe to eat for a day or two after purchase, even if the "sell-by" date has passed, as long as it is properly refrigerated.[30]

A "Best if Used By (or Before)" date on foods such as canned goods is not an indicator of food safety. "Best By" indicates the date by which foods should be consumed for best flavor or quality but does not mean that the product must be purchased or consumed before that date. Similarly, "use-by" dates that are often seen on nonperishable items are the last dates of recommended use of the product for peak quality, and the date is determined by the manufacturer.

Canned goods should be free of dents, cracks, or bulging lids, and any food packages that are torn, crushed, or open should also be avoided. In grocery stores where frozen goods are displayed in open, chest-type freezers, item should be displayed below the frost line to ensure that they have been kept at 0°F. If frozen food packages have visible contents, those containing heavy frost or ice crystals should be avoided, since it may indicate a long storage time or that the product has thawed and refrozen.

The most perishable items should be purchased last. To avoid cross contamination, packaged meat, poultry, and seafood should be placed into plastic bags before placing into the cart, to prevent juices from dripping onto other food items. Foods such as fresh meats, poultry, seafood, and any items purchased hot or cold should be the last foods to be purchased, so they will have the shortest possible time from the point of purchase to the home, and should be placed in the coolest part of the car. In hot weather, it is further recommended that perishable foods be transported to the home in a cooler with ice to keep them safe.

## REUSABLE GROCERY BAGS

Reusable bags for the transport of groceries from the store to the consumer's home have become popular in recent years. Since these bags are often reused and are often used for multiple purposes, there exists the possibility for contamination of food products as well as the hands. Although the majority of reusable bags are used for food, consumers report using reusable bags for other shopping purposes, to carry lunches, snacks, or clothing or to carry books and papers to work or school. Further, few people report carrying vegetables and raw meats in separate reusable bags, and only 3% of users report ever cleaning reusable bags.[31]

Reusable bags, if not properly washed between uses, create the potential for cross contamination of foods. This potential exists when raw meat products and foods traditionally eaten uncooked, such as fruits and vegetables, are carried in the same bags, either together or between uses. In one study, reusable bags were randomly collected from consumers as they entered grocery stores and tested for bacterial contamination. Large numbers of bacteria were found in almost all bags, and when meat juices were added to bags and stored in the trunks of cars for 2 h, the number of bacteria increased 10-fold, indicating the potential for significant bacterial growth in the bags. At the same time, hand or machine washing, even in the absence of bleach, was found to reduce the bacteria in bags by more than 99.9%.[31]

## SAFE FOOD STORAGE

Once food is brought into the home, proper storage is key in keeping foods safe to eat. Aside from keeping food safe, proper storage helps preserve food quality and also decreases food waste.

### COLD STORAGE

Consumers are advised to monitor the temperature of the refrigerator with an appliance thermometer and to maintain the temperature at 40°F or colder. Further, they are advised to consider the capacity of their refrigerators to avoid overloading, since cold air needs to freely circulate in order to keep foods at a safe temperature. The refrigerator should be cleaned on a regular basis to remove spills and spoiled food, which can be breeding grounds for bacteria.

Perishable foods should be refrigerated as soon as possible after purchase. Raw meats, poultry, fish, and eggs, as well as fresh dairy products, prepared foods, and cut fruits and vegetables should not remain at room temperature longer than 2 or 1 h when the ambient temperature is above 90°. The most perishable items—meats, fish, poultry, eggs, and dairy products—should be stored in the coldest area of the refrigerator, which is usually the area closest to the freezer compartment.

Meats, fish, and poultry should also be securely wrapped and, ideally, placed on a plate or in a separate container, to avoid leakage of any juices onto other fresh foods. Eggs are best kept in their original carton, rather than on the door, which is often warmer than the rest of the refrigerator.

The temperature of the freezer compartment should also be monitored and maintained at 0°F or below. While freezer temperatures may stop the growth of bacteria, it does not extinguish them, and foods may become unsafe as they thaw if conditions allow the pathogens to reproduce. For this reason, foods should be thawed in the refrigerator, rather than at room temperature. Foods that are to be cooked immediately can be safely thawed in the microwave or tightly wrapped and submerged in cold water. Partially thawed foods that still retain ice crystals can be safely refrozen, although refreezing can reduce food quality.

## PANTRY STORAGE

Ideal pantry storage conditions are cool, dry, and dark. If possible, temperatures should range between 50° and 70°, as higher temperatures can lead to more rapid deterioration of food. The coolest areas will generally be away from appliances such as stoves, refrigerators, hot water heaters, and dishwashers. The area under the sink may be warm due to the presence of hot water pipes and is also unsuitable since leakage from sink pipes could contaminate foods, or they could come in contact with cleaning products that are often stored there. Containers should be checked regularly for any signs of vermin, and shelves should be routinely wiped down to keep them clean. Information on suggested food storage times is widely available online.

## SAFE FOOD PREPARATION

All foods should be handled with care to ensure their safety, but certain foods carry a relatively high risk for foodborne illness. The highest risk is associated with foods that are the least processed such as raw milk; raw or lightly cooked eggs (or dishes that contain them); raw or undercooked meat, fish, poultry, and shellfish; and, to a lesser extent, fresh produce. Among produce-associated outbreaks, the food items most frequently implicated have been salad blends, lettuce, juice, melon, sprouts, and berries.[32]

The Partnership for Food Safety Education[11] promotes the following four key steps to safe food preparation:

1. Clean: Wash hands and surfaces often.
2. Separate: Don't cross contaminate.
3. Cook: Cook foods to the proper temperatures.
4. Chill: Refrigerate promptly.

## CLEAN

Washing hands and surfaces often helps reduce bacterial spread throughout the kitchen. Hands should be washed in warm, soapy water for at least 20 s before and after handling any food. Those preparing foods in the home are often engaged in other household activities, and therefore it is imperative that they also wash their hands after using the restroom, caring for children, handling pets, doing laundry, or gardening.

In addition, cutting boards, dishes, utensils, and countertops should be cleaned with hot soapy water between the preparation of raw meat, poultry, or seafood and the preparation of any foods that will be consumed uncooked, such as fruit or salads. As an added precaution, cutting boards and countertops can be sanitized by rinsing them with a liquid bleach solution. Cloth towels retain moisture that can encourage bacterial growth, so consideration should be given to using paper towels as an alternative. If cloth towels are used, it is recommended that home cooks keep three clean cloths available: one for hands, one for dishes, and one for countertops,[33] and they should be washed frequently in the washing machine using the hottest water available.

## SEPARATE

Cross contamination occurs when disease-causing microorganisms are transferred from one food to another, most commonly between raw meats, fish, or poultry and ready-to-eat items such as fresh produce. While cooking these foods usually destroys pathogens, they can be transferred to other foods during preparation via cutting boards, kitchen countertops, by the hands, or through improper practices during the preparation process. Raw meat products, for example, are often contaminated with foodborne bacteria such as *Salmonella* and *Campylobacter*, which could be spread to a fresh salad if the same cutting board is used to prepare the raw meat and the raw vegetables. For this reason, separate cutting boards are advised: one for fresh produce and one for raw meats, fish, and poultry.

Cutting boards are one of the top five sites most contaminated with bacteria in the home kitchen.[34] In general, wood is said to dull knives less than plastic, and plastic is seen as less porous than wood, and these factors can affect cross contamination. Many consumers believe that plastic cutting surfaces are superior to wood for cutting raw meats, but studies suggest otherwise.

New plastic cutting surfaces are relatively easy to clean, but, depending on the plastic that is used, some plastics can become heavily knife-scarred, leaving a rough surface that is very difficult to clean and disinfect.[34,35] Small plastic cutting boards, and some specially treated wooden boards, can be cleaned in a dishwasher, but the dishwasher may distribute the bacteria onto other food-contact surfaces.[34]

Wood, on the other hand, is intrinsically porous, which allows food juices and bacteria to penetrate the wood. Although the bacteria are not killed instantly, they do not return to the surface, which renders them unavailable for cross contamination to other foods.[35] Cleaning with hot water and detergent generally removes these bacteria, regardless of bacterial species, wood species, and whether the wood was new or used.

Raw meats, fish, and poultry are often seasoned or marinated before cooking. These foods should always be placed in the refrigerator while marinating, and marinades should never be used to baste meats while they are cooking unless they have first been brought to a full boil. Cooked foods should never be placed on plates or dishes that have held raw meats, fish, poultry, or eggs unless they have been thoroughly washed in hot soapy water, again, to reduce the risk of cross contamination between raw and cooked foods.

## Cook

Foods are considered safely cooked when they are heated to the USDA-FDA recommended safe minimum internal temperatures[36] necessary to kill potential foodborne pathogens. As noted earlier, the percentage of consumers who own food thermometers has jumped significantly in the last decade, and the use of food thermometers has also increased but varies by food type.[27] Of those who own thermometers, a higher percentage use them for roasts than for chicken parts or hamburgers.

Internal temperature is an important gauge when cooking meats, as the color of food is not a reliable indicator of safety.[37] The thermometer should be inserted into the food in several places to ensure even heating. Even heating is a potential problem in microwave cooking as well, so foods should be stirred and rotated frequently during the cooking process. When reheating foods such as soups, stew, and sauces, foods should be simmered for 10 min before eating.

Table 4.1 shows the recommended safe minimum internal temperatures for common foods.

### Low-Temperature Cooking

Countertop slow cookers are convenient, since they allow home cooks to prepare meals long in advance. Foods cook slowly at low temperatures, generally between 170°F and 280°F. The combination of direct heat from the pot, long cooking times, and steam created during the cooking process works to destroy foodborne bacteria, thus making slow cooking a safe process for preparing meals. However,

consumers are advised to heed a few precautions to avoid cross contamination.

Since several hours may be required for the slow cooker to reach a high enough temperature to kill bacteria, cut meats and vegetables should be kept refrigerated until just before they are added to the slow cooker. If these ingredients are cut in advance, they should be refrigerated separately. In addition, meats and poultry should be thoroughly thawed before placing in the slow cooker so that these foods can reach safe cooking temperatures throughout within an acceptable time frame.

"Sous vide" is a precise method for cooking foods in vacuum-sealed plastic bags at low temperatures for long periods of time. It is a method generally applied to meats, and the vacuum process excludes all air and provides a barrier between the food and the surrounding liquid in which it is cooked. However, the combination of anaerobic conditions and relatively low cooking temperatures creates an atmosphere in which *Clostridium botulinum* thrives. For this reason, the method is more suitable to restaurants than home kitchens, since the method also calls for a quick pasteurization of the food in a hot bath (185°F) or by passing the flame of a blow torch over the surface of the meat before it is vacuum sealed.[38] While there are instructions for home cooks to prepare foods using this method,[39] it is a technique that should be used only by trained professionals who can maintain hygienic, precise conditions on a consistent basis.

## Chill

In addition to the recommendations for cold storage earlier, proper chilling of prepared foods is also important in reducing the risk of foodborne illness. Bacteria grow rapidly between the so-called danger zone of 40°F and 140°F degrees, which is why it is recommended that foods be kept below or above this range. Once foods have been prepared, they should be refrigerated promptly. Again, foods should not remain at room temperature for longer than 2 h or longer than 1 h if the outside temperature is above 90°F. Ideally, storage containers should be shallow so that the depth of food in the container is 2 in. or less. This ensures that foods will cool quickly. Containers should be dated so that consumers can

### TABLE 4.1
### Safe Minimum Internal Temperatures for Foods

| Food Item | Steaks, Roasts, and Chops (Beef, Pork, Veal, Lamb) | Fish | Ground Meats (Beef, Pork, Veal, Lamb) | Egg Dishes | Poultry (Turkey, Chicken, Duck) Whole, Pieces, or Ground |
|---|---|---|---|---|---|
| Safe minimum internal temperature | 145°F with 3 min rest time | 145°F | 160°F | 160°F | 165°F |

determine how long food can safely stay in the refrigerator. Comprehensive cold storage information for various foods is available from the USDA-FDA at http://www.foodsafety.gov/keep/charts/storagetimes.html.

## CONCLUSION

The traditional focus on meat, eggs, poultry, and milk dishes as the major targets of prevention of foodborne disease must now be expanded to include produce such as lettuce, alfalfa and bean sprouts, watermelons, cantaloupe, and strawberries. Careful selection, washing, and avoidance of cross contamination are all needed to prevent potential foodborne illness. Prompt and appropriate cooling/chilling procedures are also essential to keeping bacterial and viral growth to a minimum in home kitchens.

Consumer education can help raise awareness of food safety by addressing how pathogens cause foodborne illness and how illness can be prevented. Consumers themselves bear significant burden in avoiding foodborne illness by handling food safely, following food preparation recommendations, and avoiding foods commonly associated with foodborne illness.

## REFERENCES

1. Nyachuba, DG, *Nutr Rev* 68: 257; 2010.
2. Scott, E, *Can J Infect Dis* 14: 277; 2003.
3. USDAS-ERS, What share of U.S. consumed food is imported? http://www.ers.usda.gov/amberwaves/february08/datafeature/ (Accessed May 1, 2012).
4. Lynch, MF, Tauxe, RV, Hedberg, CW, *Epidemiol Infect* 137: 307; 2009.
5. USDHHS-FDA, Guide to minimize microbial food safety hazards of fresh-cut fruits and vegetables. http://www.fda.gov/food/guidancecomplianceregulatoryinformation/guidancedocuments/produceandplanproducts/ucm064458.htm (Accessed May 1, 2012).
6. Gerba, CP, In: Fan, X, Niemira, BA, Doona, CJ. et al., eds, *Microbial Safety of Fresh Produce*. Wiley-Blackwell, Ames, IA, 2009.
7. CSPI (Center for Science in the Public Interest). Global and local: Food safety around the world. http://www.cspinet.org/new/pdf/global.pdf (Accessed May 1, 2012).
8. Scharff, RL, *J Food Prot* 75: 123; 2012.
9. vanAsselt, ED, deJong, AEI, deJonge, R, Nauta MJ, *J Appl Microbiol* 105: 1392; 2008.
10. Buzby, JC, Roberts T, Jordan Lin CT. et al., *Bacterial Foodborne Disease: Medical Costs and Productivity Losses*. USDA-ERS Agricultural Economics Report No. (AER741). http://www.ers.usda.gov/publications/aer741/AER741fm.PDF (Accessed May 1, 2012).
11. Partnership for Food Safety Education, Four steps to fight BAC! http://www.fightbac.org (Accessed May 1, 2012).
12. Centers for Disease Control (CDC), *MMWR* 54: 352; 2005.
13. U.S. Census Bureau, Who's minding the kids? http://www.census.gov/prod/2010pubs/p70-121.pdf (Accessed May 24, 2011).
14. Ojima, M, Toshima, Y, Koya, E. et al., *Int J Environ Health Res* 12: 41; 2002.
15. Mattick, K, Durham, K, Domingue, G. et al., *Int J Food Microbiol* 25: 213; 2003.
16. Williamson, DM, Gravani, RB, Lawless, HT, *Food Technol* 46: 94; 1992.
17. Redmond, EC, Griffith, CJ, *J Food Prot* 66: 130; 2003.
18. Altekruse, SF, Street, DA, Fein, SB, Levy, AS, *J Food Prot* 59: 287; 1996.
19. Fein, SB, Lando, AM, Levy, AS. et al., *J Food Prot* 74: 1513; 2011.
20. Li-Cohen, AE, Bruhn, CM, *J Food Prot* 65: 1287; 2002.
21. Abbot, JM, Byrd-Bredbenner, C, Schaffner, D. et al., *Eur J Clin Nutr* 63: 572; 2009.
22. Hudson, PK, Hartwell, HJ, *J Soc Promot Health* 122: 165; 2002.
23. Anderson, JB, Shuster, TA, Hansen, KE. et al., *J Am Diet Assoc* 104: 186; 2004.
24. Phang, HS, Bruhn, CM, *J Food Prot* 74: 1708; 2011.
25. Jay, LS, Comar, D, Govenlock, L, *J Food Prot* 62: 1285; 1999.
26. Hillers, VN, Medeiros, L, Kendall P. et al., *J Food Prot* 66: 1893; 2003.
27. Lando, AM, Chen, CC, *J Food Prot* 75: 556; 2012.
28. Wilcock, A, Pun, M, Khanona, J, Aung, M, *Trends Food Sci Technol* 15: 56; 2004.
29. USDA, Managing food safety. http://www.fda.gov/Food/FoodSafety/RetailFoodProtection/ManagingFoodSafetyHACCPPrinciples/Operators/default.htm (Accessed June 1, 2012).
30. USDA-FSIS, Food product dating http://www.fsis.usda.gov/Factsheets/Food_Product_dating/#5 (Accessed June 13, 2011).
31. Williams, DL, Gerba, CP, Maxwell, S, Sinclair, RG, *Food Protection Trends* 31: 508; 2011.
32. Sivapalasingam, S, Friedman, CR, Cohen, L, Tauxe, RV, *J Food Prot* 67: 2342; 2004.
33. Dols, CL, Bowers, JM, Copfer, AE, *Am J Nursing* 101: 24AA; 2001.
34. Ak, N, Cliver, D, Kaspari, CW, *J Food Prot* 57: 23; 1994.
35. Cliver, DO, *J AOAC Int* 89: 538; 2006.
36. Carpentier, B, *Food Microbiol* 14: 31; 1997.
37. USDA-FSIS, Is it done yet? http://www.fsis.usda.gov/is_it_done_yet/brochure_text/index.asp#5 (Accessed June 25, 2012).
38. Hyytiä-Trees, E, Skyttä, E, Mokkila, M. et al., *Appl Environ Microbiol* 66: 223; 2000.
39. Los Angeles Times, *Sous vide* cooking gives chefs an option. http://www.latimes.com/features/food/la-fo-master-class-thomas-keller-20110908,0,3863290.htmlstory (Accessed June 27, 2012).

# 5 Food Labeling
## Foods and Dietary Supplements

*Constance J. Geiger*

## CONTENTS

## OVERVIEW

### DEFINITION OF FOOD LABELING

Food labeling includes all the information present on food packages. Nutrition labeling is one component of the food label. Other components include the principal display panel; the information panel; the identity of the food; the list of ingredients; the name and place of business of the manufacturer, packer, or distributor; and any claims made.[1]

This chapter reviews the regulatory history of food labeling, required sections of the nutrition label, labeling of restaurant and fresh foods, definitions of allowed nutrient content claims, and requirements for allowed health claims and structure/function claims. The chapter also provides information on front-of-package (FOP) and allergen labeling. Lastly, additional resources for food labeling are listed.

## HISTORY OF FOOD LABELING

### MAJOR FOOD AND NUTRITION LABELING LAWS AND REGULATIONS

Food labeling laws have progressed from merely protecting consumers from economic harm (Pure Food and Drug Act of 1906)[2] to reducing consumers' risk of chronic disease (Nutrition Labeling and Education Act [NLEA] of 1990).[3] NLEA amended the Federal Food, Drug, and Cosmetic Act (FFDCA) of 1938[4] and required nutrition information be conveyed to consumers, so they can readily understand the information and its significance in the context of a total daily diet. NLEA[3] mandated major revisions in the Food and Drug Administration's (FDA) food labeling regulations, including requiring nutrition labeling on almost all processed foods, a revised list of nutrients to be labeled, standardized serving sizes, nutrient content

**TABLE 5.1**

**Major Food and Nutrition Labeling Laws/Selected Regulations**

| Law | Primary Provisions |
| --- | --- |
| Pure Food and Drug Act, 1906 | Barred false and misleading statements on food and drug labels.[2] |
| FFDCA, 1938 | Replaced the Pure Food and Drug Act of 1906. Created distinct food labeling requirements. Required "common and usual name" of food, ingredient declarations, net quantity information, and name and address of manufacturer/distributor. Defined misbranding.[4] |
| Fair Packaging and Labeling Act, 1966 | Provided FDA with authority to regulate provision of label information and package size.[33] |
| Regulations for the Enforcement of the FFDCA and the Fair Packaging and Labeling Act, 1972, 1973 | Merged existing regulations into one entity. Required nutrition labeling on processed foods that were fortified or that carried claims. Provided for labeling of fat and cholesterol. Established standards for dietary supplements (DS). Established regulations for artificially flavored foods and imitation foods per serving. Disallowed nutrient claims unless food contained 10% or more of the U.S. recommended dietary allowance (RDA). Incorporated label information: number of servings/container; calories, protein, carbohydrate, and fat content; and percentage of adult U.S. RDA for protein and seven vitamins and minerals. Provided for sodium labeling without requirement of a full nutrition label panel.[34–36] |
| Nutrition Labeling and Education Act, 1990 | Provided for mandatory nutrition labeling on almost all food products, expanded required nutrition information in a new format, created standardized serving sizes, provided consistent definitions of nutrient content claims, and delineated permissible health claims.[3] |
| Dietary Supplement Health and Education Act (DSHEA), 1994 | Defined DS, provided for nutrition labeling in a new format, required the name and quantity of every active ingredient, provided for structure/functions claims and good manufacturing practices, encouraged research on DS, and created two new government entities: Commission on DS Labels and the Office of Dietary Supplements.[26] |
| FDA Modernization Act (FDAMA), 1997 | Expanded procedures by which FDA can authorize health claims and nutrient contents, for example, provided for a notification process.[20] |
| Food Allergen Labeling and Consumer Protection Act (FALCPA), 2004 | Expanded ingredient labeling. Labels must clearly identify the food source names of all ingredients that are—or contain any protein derived from—the eight most common food allergens.[32] |
| Patient Protection and Affordable Care Act, 2010 | Required restaurants and similar retail food establishments with 20 or more locations to list calorie content information for standard menu items on restaurant menus and menu boards, including drive-through menu boards. Other nutrient information has to be made available in writing upon request. The Act also required vending machine operators who own or operate 20 or more vending machines to disclose calorie content for certain items.[15] |

claims, and, for the first time, health claims. In the interest of harmony and uniformity, the U.S. Department of Agriculture's (USDA) Food Safety and Information Service (FSIS) issued similar regulations for meat and poultry products.[5] Table 5.1 summarizes the major laws and selected regulations dealing with food labeling (for further details, see Ref. [6,7]).

## REGULATORY OVERSIGHT FOR LABELING

A number of regulatory agencies have jurisdiction over food labeling, including the FDA, FSIS, Federal Trade Commission (FTC), and Bureau of Alcohol, Tobacco and Firearms (BATF). Table 5.2 outlines their responsibilities.

## REQUIRED SECTIONS OF THE FOOD LABEL

Those sections of the "Nutrition Facts panel" that are required are illustrated in Figure 5.1. The "Nutrition Facts" information is normally based on a serving of the product as packaged.

**TABLE 5.2**

**Agencies Having Jurisdiction over Food Labeling**

| Agency | Responsibility |
| --- | --- |
| FDA: Department of Health and Human Services | Mandatory labeling of most packaged foods, except products containing certain amounts of meat and poultry and beverages with certain amounts of alcohol. Voluntary labeling of fresh fruits and vegetables, fresh fish, game, and restaurant foods, except those containing certain amounts of meat and poultry. |
| FSIS: USDA | Mandatory labeling on most fresh and processed meat and poultry products (e.g., hot dogs and chicken noodle soup). |
| FTC | Claims made in food advertising. |
| BATF | Voluntary labeling of alcoholic beverages. |

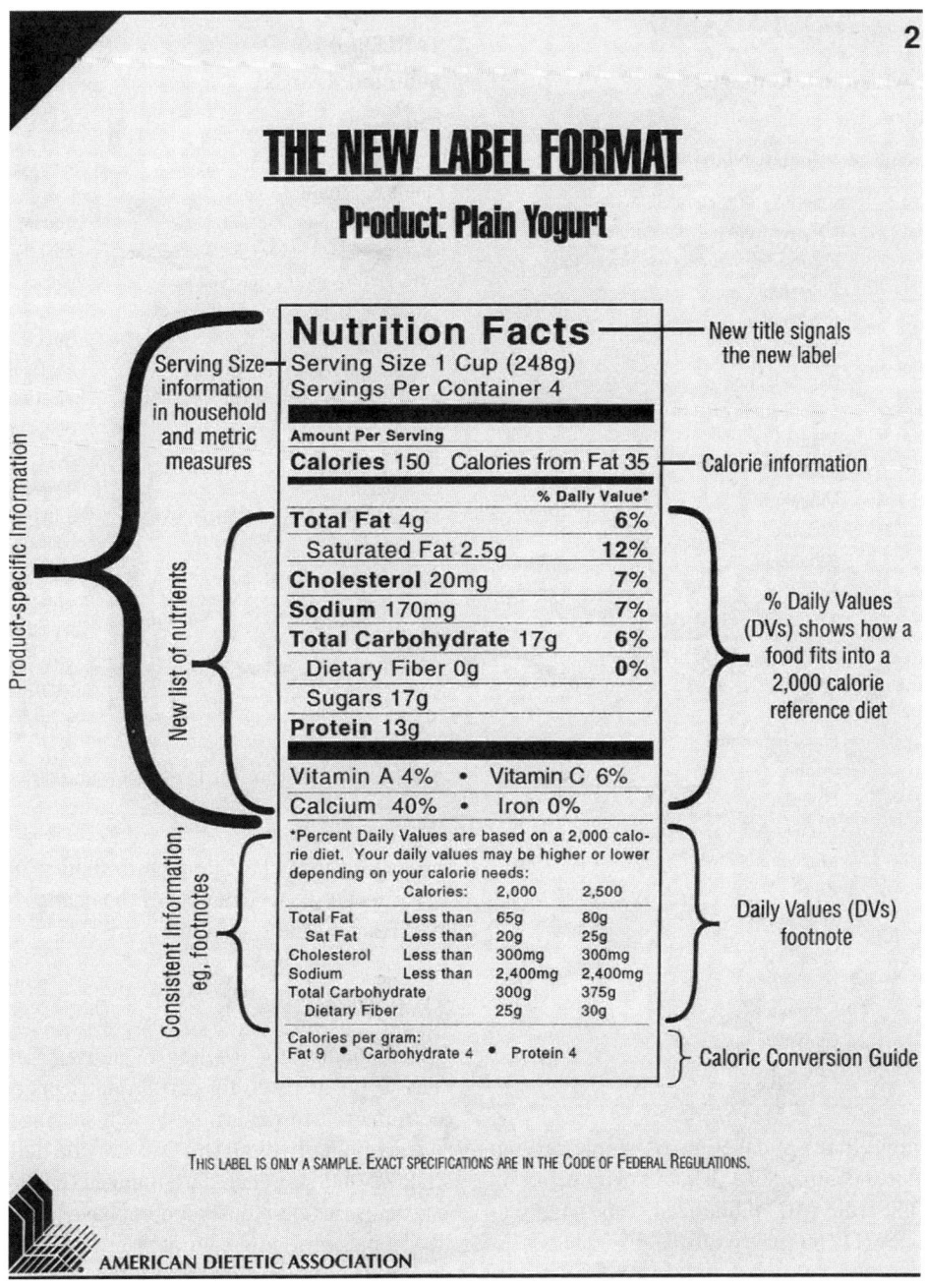

**FIGURE 5.1** Nutrition Facts panel format.

## REQUIRED NUTRIENTS

The nutrients required to be listed on the Nutrition Facts panel are detailed in Table 5.3. If a product is fortified or a claim is made about a voluntary nutrient, that nutrient also is to be listed. Other nutrients (voluntary nutrients) that may be included on the Nutrition Facts panel are found in Table 5.3.

## SERVING SIZE

Standardized serving sizes, known as reference amounts customarily consumed (RACCs), are established for many categories of foods. RACCs are based on average amounts people usually eat at one time as determined by the USDA survey data. The basis of using typical consumption data for the standardized serving sizes was mandated by NLEA.[3] The RACCs are not based on what is recommended by government agencies or health professional associations. These uniform serving sizes help consumers compare similar products. See Table 5.4 for selected RACCs.

In April 2005, FDA published an advance notice of proposed rule making (ANPRM) entitled "Food labeling: Serving sizes of products that can reasonably be consumed at one eating occasion; updating of reference amounts customarily consumed; approaches for recommending smaller portion sizes."[8] The FDA requested comments on serving-size

## TABLE 5.3
### Labeling of Nutrients: Required and Voluntary

| Required Nutrients | Voluntary Nutrients |
|---|---|
| Total calories | Calories from saturated fat |
| Calories from fat | Calories from polyunsaturated fat |
| Total fat | Calories from monounsaturated fat |
| Saturated fat | Potassium |
| *Trans* fat | Soluble fiber |
| Cholesterol | Insoluble fiber |
| Sodium | Sugar alcohol |
| Total carbohydrate | Other carbohydrates |
| Dietary fiber | Vitamin D |
| Sugars | Vitamin E |
| Protein | Vitamin K |
| Vitamin A | Thiamin |
| Vitamin C | Riboflavin |
| Calcium | Niacin |
| Iron | Vitamin $B_6$ |
| | Folate |
| | Vitamin $B_{12}$ |
| | Biotin |
| | Pantothenic acid |
| | Choline |
| | Phosphorus |
| | Iodine |
| | Magnesium |
| | Zinc |
| | Selenium |
| | Copper |
| | Manganese |
| | Chromium |
| | Molybdenum |
| | Chloride |

## TABLE 5.4
### Selected RACCs[a]

| Category | RACC |
|---|---|
| *Bakery products*: biscuits, bagels, tortillas, and soft pretzels | 55 g |
| *Beverages*: carbonated and noncarbonated beverages, wine coolers, water, coffee or tea (flavored and sweetened), juice, and fruit drinks | 240 mL |
| *Breads* | 50 g |
| *Cereals and other grain products* | Varies from 25 g for dry pasta to 140 g for prepared rice |
| *Cheese* | 30 g |
| *Eggs* | 50 g |
| *Fats and oils* | 1 tbsp |
| *Fruits*: fresh, canned, or frozen, except watermelon | 140 g |
| *Meat*: entrees without sauce | 85 g cooked; 110 g uncooked |
| *Nuts and seeds* | 30 g |
| *Soups* | 245 g |
| *Vegetables*: fresh, canned, or frozen | 85 g fresh or frozen 95 g for vacuum packed 130 g for canned in liquid |

[a] See Ref. [1] (21 CFR 101.12) for further details.

information, updating RACCs, labeling of single-serving containers, and caloric comparisons of foods with different serving amounts. This rule will be finalized with the updating of the daily values (DVs) (see section "Daily Values").

### CALORIES AND CALORIES FROM FAT

Calories and calories from fat are required because of public health authorities' concern with fat in the diet. In 2004, FDA released the Report of the Working Group on Obesity.[9] The working group recommended that the calorie information on the food label be made more prominent and that realistic serving sizes be used. The working group also recommended that restaurants be encouraged to display nutrition information and that a consumer education program be launched focusing on a "calorie count" message.

In June 2005, FDA published an ANPRM requesting comments on whether calorie information should be more prominent by use of bold print, whether calories from fat should be replaced with % DV from calories, how consumers use calories, and how to reformulate foods or redesign

packaging to make calorie information more prominent by other means.[10] An example of the change in calorie information format can be seen in Figure 5.2.

### DAILY VALUES

The standards for labeling of nutrients are known as DVs. The % DV is listed for certain nutrients on the label so that consumers can determine how a serving of a food fits into their total daily diet. The DVs include daily reference values (DRVs) and reference daily intakes (RDIs). DRVs are set for nutrients that previously did not have label standards, such as fat, cholesterol, and saturated fat (see Table 5.5). DRVs are based on a daily intake of 2000 calories, which is a reasonable reference number for adults and children over 4 years, and are calculated based on current nutrition recommendations. The term RDIs replaced the term U.S. recommended dietary allowances (RDAs), but the values are currently the same as the U.S. RDAs, which represent the highest recommended levels of the 1968 RDAs (see Table 5.6).

The DVs for labeling are being updated. The Committee on Use of DRIs in Nutrition Labeling, Food and Nutrition Board, Institute of Medicine, National Academy of Science, developed a report to assist the U.S. FDA, the USDA, and Health Canada by "providing guiding principles for selecting reference values for labeling the nutritive value of foods based on the DRIs and for discretionary fortification of foods including meat and poultry products."[11] The committee's report was published in December 2004.[11] The committee recommended that a population-weighted

Possible changes in calorie
information

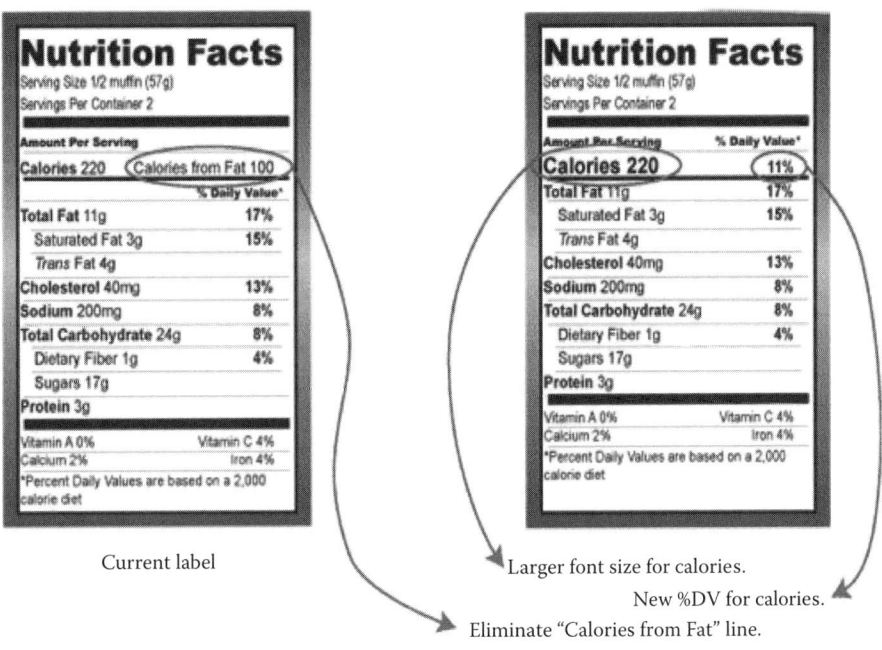

Current label

Larger font size for calories.
New %DV for calories.
Eliminate "Calories from Fat" line.

FIGURE 5.2 Possible changes in calorie information.

## TABLE 5.5
### DRVs for Adults: Calculations and Values[a]

| Nutrient | Derivation/Calculation | Label Value |
|---|---|---|
| Fat | 30% of 2000 cal from fat = 600 cal/9 cal/g | 65 g |
| Saturated fat | 10% of calories from saturated fat = 200 cal/9 cal/g | 20 g |
| Carbohydrate | 60% of calories from carbohydrate = 1200 cal/4 cal/g | 300 g |
| Protein | 10% of calories from protein = 200 cal/4 cal/g | 50 g |
| Fiber | 11.5 g/1000 cal | 25 g (rounded up) |
| Cholesterol[a] | NA | Less than 300 mg |
| Sodium[a] | NA | Less than 2400 mg |
| Potassium[a] | NA | 3500 mg |

[a] Based on the 1989 National Research Council's Diet and Health Report.[37]

## TABLE 5.6
### RDIs for Adults and Children over 4 Years of Age[a]

| Nutrient | RDI |
|---|---|
| Vitamin A | 5000 IU |
| Vitamin C | 60 mg |
| Calcium | 1000 mg |
| Iron | 18 mg |
| Vitamin D | 400 IU |
| Vitamin E | 30 IU |
| Vitamin K | 80 µg |
| Thiamin | 1.5 mg |
| Riboflavin | 1.7 mg |
| Niacin | 20 mg |
| Vitamin $B_6$ | 2.0 mg |
| Folate | 400 µg |
| Vitamin $B_{12}$ | 6 µg |
| Biotin | 300 µg |
| Pantothenic acid | 10 mg |
| Phosphorus | 1000 mg |
| Iodine | 150 µg |
| Magnesium | 400 µg |
| Zinc | 15 mg |
| Selenium | 70 µg |
| Copper | 2 mg |
| Manganese | 2 mg |
| Chromium | 120 µg |
| Molybdenum | 75 µg |
| Chloride | 3400 mg |

[a] See Ref. [1] (21 CFR 101.9) for further detail.

Estimated Average Requirement (EAR) be used for labeling or, if one does not exist, that the adequate intake (AI) be used.

On November 2, 2007, FDA published an ANPRM for Food Labeling: Revision of Reference Values and Mandatory Nutrients. FDA requested comments on which nutrients should be required on the Nutrition Facts panel and the appropriate reference value to use for each nutrient.[12] The agency requested information about the approach for setting DVs, populations for which the DVs are intended, and labeling of individual nutrients. FDA has evaluated the comments and will publish a proposed rule. Once the proposed rule is published, comments are again solicited, compiled, and evaluated. Then a final rule implementing the revisions will be published. The food industry will probably have 2 years to implement these changes. The final rule is not likely to come into effect until 2016 or later.

The DVs, calorie information, and serving-size information will be finalized and implemented together. The change in DVs may affect nutrient content claim and health claim requirements.[13] For example, to carry an "excellent source of folate" claim today, a food would need to provide 20% of the DV for folate, or 80 µg/RACC. If a population-weighted EAR were used as the basis of the claim instead of the RDA, the amount required for a food to carry a health claim could drop to 62 µg. Therefore, using a population-weighted EAR versus an RDA has important implications for dietary adequacy, educational programs and messaging, and consumer purchase selections.

A footnote is provided at the bottom of the Nutrition Facts panel to inform consumers of the DVs for both 2000 and 2500 calorie levels. The calorie information at the very bottom of the label is voluntary (see Figure 5.1).

### SUBSTANCES WITHOUT DVs

Those substances without DVs, such as sugars, *trans* fats, and soluble and insoluble fibers, do not carry a % DV.

## LABELING OF RESTAURANT FOODS AND FRESH FOODS

### RESTAURANT FOODS

Labeling of restaurant foods is voluntary. Nutrition labeling becomes mandatory if a nutrient content claim or health claim is made. However, a full Nutrition Facts panel is not required. Only the amount of the nutrient that is the subject of the claim is required to be labeled, for example, "low fat" contains 3 g of fat (21 CFR 101.10).[1] Because Americans spend almost half of their food budget on food prepared away from home, FDA commissioned the Keystone Group to hold a forum on away-from-home foods.[14] The group recommended consumers be provided with nutrition information at the point of purchase.

With the signing of the Patient Protection and Affordable Care Act of 2010, Section 4205[15] requires restaurants and similar retail food establishments with 20 or more locations to list calorie content information for standard menu items on restaurant menus and menu boards, including drive-through menu boards. Other nutrient information—total calories, fat, saturated fat, cholesterol, sodium, total carbohydrates, sugars, fiber, and total protein—would have to be made available in writing upon request. The Act also requires vending machine operators who own or operate 20 or more vending machines to disclose calorie content for certain items.

The FDA has issued two Federal Register notices that address implementation of the menu labeling provisions of the Patient Protection and Affordable Care Act of 2010.

The proposed rules are entitled "Food labeling: Nutrition labeling of standard menu items in restaurants and similar retail food establishments," and "Food labeling: Calorie labeling of articles of food in vending machines" (21 CFR 101.11).[16,17] FDA also published a notice[14] that explains how restaurants and similar retail food establishments with fewer than 20 locations and vending machine operators with fewer than 20 vending machines can voluntarily register to become subject to new federal menu labeling requirements.[18]

### FRESH FRUITS, VEGETABLES, AND SEAFOOD

FDA recommends food retailers provide nutrition information for raw fruits, vegetables, and fish at the point of purchase. Charts, brochures, or signs can be used to depict the nutrition information for the 20 most commonly consumed fruits, vegetables, and raw fish. FDA provides the data for retailers in the Code of Federal Regulations (CFR)[1] (21 CFR 101.45 and Appendix C to Part 101). The data are updated periodically to reflect current analyses.

### MEATS AND POULTRY

Previously, FSIS recommended food retailers provide point-of-purchase information for fresh meat and poultry.[5] As with fresh produce and fish, charts, brochures, or signs could be used to depict nutrition information. As of January 2012, fresh meat and poultry labeling is no longer voluntary. In 2010, FSIS published a final rule requiring nutrition labeling on single-ingredient, fresh meat, and poultry products. The rule calls for packages of ground or chopped meat and poultry, such as hamburger or ground turkey, to feature Nutrition Facts panels on their labels.[19] Additionally, 40 of the most popular whole, raw cuts of meat and poultry, such as chicken breast or steak, also have nutritional information either on the package labels or on display at the store.

## NUTRIENT CONTENT CLAIMS ALLOWED FOR FOODS AND DIETARY SUPPLEMENTS

### OVERVIEW

FDA and USDA have issued regulations for uniform definitions for nutrient content claims as a result of NLEA.[1,5] Current nutrient content claims have been authorized either by (1) FDA and FSIS as a result of NLEA,[3] which also allowed for petitions for new nutrient content claims, or (2) notification of FDA through the FDA Modernization Act (FDAMA).[20] A nutrient content claim characterizes the level of a nutrient in a food (e.g., "high fiber"). Nutrient content claims include two types of claims: absolute (free, low, good source, high, lean, or extra lean) and comparative claims (reduced, light, less, or more). The regulations establish the allowed terms and the criteria/requirements for their use (see Table 5.7). For additional details, see 21 CFR 101.13[1] and

**TABLE 5.7**
**Allowed Nutrient Content Claims with Definitions[a,b]**

| Claim | Calories | Fat | Saturated Fat | Cholesterol | Sodium | Fiber | Sugar | Protein | Vitamins/Minerals |
|---|---|---|---|---|---|---|---|---|---|
| "Free," "no," "zero," or "without" | Less than 5 cal | 0.5 g or less | 0.5 g or less | Less than 2 mg cholesterol and 2 g or less saturated fat and *trans* fat | Less than 5 mg | NA | Less than 0.5 g | NA | NA |
| "Very low" | NA | NA | NA | NA | Less than 35 mg | NA | NA | NA | NA |
| "Low" | 40 cal or less | 3 g or less | 1 g or less | 20 mg or less cholesterol and 2 g or less saturated fat | 140 mg or less | NA | NA | NA | NA |
| "Reduced" | 25% lower in calories than the comparable food | 25% lower in calories than the comparable food | 25% lower in calories than the comparable food | 25% lower in calories than the comparable food | 25% lower in calories than the comparable food | NA | 25% lower in calories than the comparable food | NA | NA |
| "Light" | ⅓ fewer calories than the reference foods, only if the reference food contains less than 50% cal from fat | 50% less fat than the reference food | NA | NA | 50% less sodium than the reference food; food also is "low fat" and "low calorie" | NA | NA | NA | NA |
| "Good source," "provides," or "contains" | NA | NA | NA | NA | NA | 2.5–4.9 g | NA | 5 g or more | 10%–19% of the DV |
| "High," "excellent source of," or "rich in" | NA | NA | NA | NA | NA | 5 g or more | NA | 10 g or more | 20% or more of the DV |
| "More," "added," "enriched," or "fortified" | NA | NA | NA | NA | NA | NA | NA | 10% more of the DV (5 g or more) | 10% more of the DV |

[a] Definitions vary for meal and main dishes.
[b] Complete definitions are found in Ref. [1] (21 CFR 101.13 and 21 CFR 101.54–101.69) and Ref. [5] (9 CFR 317.313–317.363).

**TABLE 5.8**
**Other Nutrient Content Claims[a,b]**

| Claim | Definition |
|---|---|
| "% Fat-free" | Must be "low fat" or "fat-free." Must indicate the amount of fat present in 100 g of food. |
| "Healthy" | Must be "low fat" and "low saturated fat" or "extra lean." Must not exceed disclosure levels for sodium or cholesterol 21 CFR 101.13(h). Must contain 10% DV for vitamin A, vitamin C, iron, calcium, protein, or fiber. (*Exceptions*: fruits and vegetables; frozen or canned single-ingredient fruits and vegetables, except those ingredients whose addition does not change the nutrient profile of the fruit or vegetable may be added; enriched cereal-grain products that conform to a standard of identity). |
| "Lean" | Less than 10 g fat, less than 4 g saturated fat, less than 95 mg cholesterol per RACC and per 100 g. |
| "Extra lean" | Less than 5 g fat, less than 2 g saturated fat, less than 95 mg cholesterol per RACC and per 100 g. |
| "High potency" | Food must contain individual vitamins or minerals that are present at 100% or more of the RDI per reference amount or a multi-ingredient food product that contains 100% or more of the RDI for at least 2/3 of the vitamins and minerals with DVs and that are present in the product at 2% or more of the RDI (e.g., "High potency multivitamin, multimineral DS tablets"). |
| "Antioxidant" | Food must contain a nutrient that has an RDI. The nutrient must have recognized antioxidant activity. The level of the nutrient in the food must meet the requirement for "high", "good source" or "more". |

[a] Definitions vary for main dish and meal products and may differ for meat, poultry, seafood, and game.

[b] Complete definitions are found in Ref. [1] (21 CFR 101.13 and 21 CFR 101.54–101.69) and Ref. [5] (9 CFR 3177.313–317.363).

101.54–101.69[1] and 9 CFR 317.360–317.362[5] (Table 5.8). FDA allowed FDAMA nutrient content claims notifications to pass through for choline and omega-3 fatty acids. The labeling page of the FDA's website provides detail on the choline notification.[21] The omega-3 fatty acid notifications can be found on the dockets page of FDA's website using their docket numbers.[22]

# HEALTH CLAIMS ALLOWED FOR FOODS AND DIETARY SUPPLEMENTS

## OVERVIEW

NLEA allowed health claims to be carried on qualified food products. Prior to this time, these claims were considered unauthorized drug claims. A health claim describes the relationship between a food, a nutrient, or other substance in a food and the risk of a health-related condition or disease (21 CFR 101.14).[1]

Health claims can be made through third-party references, such as the American Heart Association, and with the use of symbols such as a heart, statements, and vignettes or descriptions. Regardless of the manner of presentation, the requirements for the claim must be met in order for a food or supplement to carry the claim on its product packaging or in its advertising. Health claims carry general and specific requirements. General requirements include not exceeding certain amounts of fat (13 g), saturated fat (1 g), cholesterol (60 mg), and sodium (480 mg)/RACC and serving size. The food must be a "good source" of fiber, protein, vitamin A, vitamin C, calcium, or iron prior to fortification. The specific requirements for each health claim are listed in the CFR

(21 CFR 101.72–101.83),[1] except for those authorized through FDAMA[20] or by the courts and enforcement discretion. The requirements for those health claims authorized through FDAMA[20] can be found on FDA's website.[21]

A listing of the requirements for health claims authorized by (1) FDA as a result of NLEA,[3] which also allowed for petitions for new health claims, is found in (Table 5.9); (2) notification of FDA through FDAMA[20] (Table 5.10); or (3) court action as a result of the Pearson Decision,[23] which provided for qualified health claims (QHCs) for which FDA exercises enforcement discretion (Table 5.11). QHC petitions follow a similar procedure as other health claim petitions.

FDAMA[20] allowed notification of FDA about a health claim. FDAMA health claims, unlike the other claims, allow no opportunity for public comment. A company must compile the data and use an authoritative statement. If FDA takes no action within 120 days of the notification, then the health claim can be made on the foods qualifying for the claim.

The Pearson Decision[23] was brought about by a lawsuit filed by Durk Pearson, Sandy Shaw, and the American Preventive Medical Association to allow four previously denied health claims to be made on dietary supplements (DS). The court decision mandated that FDA (1) reconsider whether to authorize the four previously denied health claims, (2) determine if the weight of the scientific evidence in support of the claims is greater than that against it, and (3) if so, determine if qualifying language would not mislead consumers. FDA was also required to define significant scientific agreement (SSA).

As a result, FDA now provides enforcement discretion for health claims that are not supported by SSA. A procedure for approving these claims resulted from

## TABLE 5.9
## Health Claims Authorized through the Regulations Implementing NLEA[a]

| Health Claim | Model Language | Requirements | Can Be Made on Qualified |
|---|---|---|---|
| *Cancer* | | | |
| Fruits and vegetables and cancer | Development of cancer depends on many factors. A diet low in fat and high in fruits and vegetables, such as oranges, which are fat-free and high in vitamin C, vitamin A, and fiber, may reduce the risk of some cancers. | Food product must be or must contain a fruit or vegetable. Product is "low fat" and is a "good source" of at least one of the following: vitamin A, vitamin C, or fiber. | Foods |
| Fiber-containing grain products, fruits and vegetables, and cancer | Low-fat diets rich in fiber-containing grain products, fruits, and vegetables may reduce the risk of some types of cancer, a disease associated with many risk factors. | Food product must be or must contain a grain product, fruit, or vegetable. Food product is "low fat" and is (prior to fortification) a "good source of dietary fiber". | Foods |
| Fat and cancer | Development of cancer depends on many factors. A diet low in total fat may reduce the risk for some cancers. | Food product is "low fat." Fish and game meats must be "extra lean". | Foods |
| *Coronary heart disease (CHD)* | | | |
| Fruits, vegetables, and grain products that contain fiber, especially soluble fiber, and risk of CHD | Diets low in saturated fat and cholesterol and rich in fruits, vegetables, and grain products that contain some types of dietary fiber, particularly soluble fiber, may reduce the risk of heart disease, a disease associated with many factors. | Food product contains greater than 0.6 g soluble fiber. Soluble fiber is listed on Nutrition Facts panel. Food product must be "low fat," "low saturated fat," and "low cholesterol." Food is, or must contain, a vegetable, fruit, or grain product. | Foods |
| Soluble fiber from certain foods (oats, psyllium, and barley) and CHD | Diets low in saturated fat and cholesterol that include ( ) g of soluble fiber per day from (name of food) may reduce the risk of heart disease. One serving of (name of food) supplies ( ) g of the ( ) g necessary to have this effect. | *Oats and barley*: Food contains β-glucan soluble fiber from whole oats or barley and beta-fiber from barley. Food contains greater than 0.75 g whole-oat soluble fiber or whole-grain barley and dry milled barley. Soluble fiber is listed on the Nutrition Facts panel. Food is "low saturated fat," "low cholesterol," and "low fat". *Psyllium*: Food contains greater than 1.7 g soluble fiber from psyllium husk. Food is "low saturated fat," "low cholesterol," and "low fat." Soluble fiber is listed on the Nutrition Facts panel. | Foods |
| Soy protein and CHD | Diets low in fat and cholesterol that include 25 g of soy protein a day may reduce the risk of heart disease. One serving of (name of food) provides ( ) g of soy protein. | Food contains greater than 6.25 g soy protein. Food is "low saturated fat" and "low cholesterol." Food is "low fat," unless it consists of or is derived from whole soybeans and contains no fat in addition to the fat inherently present in the whole soybeans it contains or from which it is derived. | Foods |
| Saturated fat and cholesterol and CHD | While many factors affect heart disease, diets low in saturated fat and cholesterol may reduce the risk of this disease. | Food must be "low saturated fat," "low fat," and "low cholesterol." Fish and game meats must be "extra lean". | Foods |
| Plant sterols/stanol esters and CHD | *Plant stanol esters*: Diets low in saturated fat and cholesterol that include two servings of foods that provide a daily total of at least 3.4 g of vegetable oil stanol esters in two meals may reduce the risk of heart disease. A serving of (name of food) supplies ( ) g of vegetable oil stanol esters. | Food contains 0.65 g of plant sterol esters/RACC (spreads and salad dressings) or 1.7 g of plant stanol esters/RACC (spreads, salad dressings, snack bars, and DS in softgel form). Food is "low saturated fat" and "low cholesterol." Food must not exceed the fat disqualifying levels of health claims unless it is a spread or a salad dressing. Those products (spreads or salad dressings) that exceed 13 g of fat must carry a disclosure statement referring consumers to the Nutrition Facts panel for information about fat content. Food contains 10% or more of the DV for vitamin A, vitamin C, iron, calcium, protein, or fiber unless the product is a salad dressing. | Foods and DS |

*(continued)*

**TABLE 5.9 (continued)**

**Health Claims Authorized through the Regulations Implementing NLEA[a]**

| Health Claim | Model Language | Requirements | Can Be Made on Qualified |
|---|---|---|---|
| | *Plant sterol esters*: Foods containing at least 0.65 g per serving of plant sterol esters, eaten twice a day with meals for a daily total intake of at least 1.3 g, as part of a diet low in saturated fat and cholesterol, may reduce the risk of heart disease. A serving of (name of food) supplies ( ) g of vegetable oil sterol esters. | The final rule may be updated. Go to the following link for further details for a new proposed rule: http://www.gpo.gov/fdsys/pkg/FR-2010-12-08/pdf/2010-30386.pdf. | |
| *Other health claims* | | | |
| Calcium and osteoporosis | Regular exercise and a healthy diet with enough calcium help teen and young adult white and Asian women maintain good bone health and may reduce their high risk of osteoporosis later in life. Adequate calcium intakes are important, but daily intakes above 2000 mg are not likely to provide any additional benefit. | Food or DS must be "high" calcium. | Foods and DS |
| Sodium and hypertension | Diets low in sodium may reduce the risk of high blood pressure, a disease caused by many factors. | Food must be "low sodium". | Foods |
| Dietary noncariogenic carbohydrate sweeteners and dental caries | Frequent eating of foods high in sugars and starches as between-meal snacks can promote tooth decay. The sugar alcohol (name, optional) used to sweeten this food may reduce the risk of dental caries. Frequent between-meal consumption of foods high in sugars and starches promotes tooth decay. (Name of sugar from paragraph (c) (2) (ii) (B) of this section), the sugar in (name of food), unlike other sugars, does not promote tooth decay. | Food must contain less than 0.5 g sugar. Food product contains (1) sugar alcohols xylitol, sorbitol, mannitol, maltitol, isomalt, lactitol, hydrogenated starch hydrolysates, hydrogenated glucose syrups, and erythritol or a combination of these; (2) the sugars D-tagatose and isomaltulose; or (3) sucralose. | Foods |
| Folic acid and neural tube defects | Healthful diets with adequate folate may reduce a woman's risk of having a child with a brain or spinal cord defect. | Food or supplements must be a "good source" of folate. Health claim cannot be made on foods that contain more than 100% RDI for vitamin A or D. | Foods and DS |

[a] See Ref. [1] (21 CFR101.14 and 101.72–101.83) for complete requirements.

FDA's Consumer Health Information for Better Nutrition Initiative.[24] In July 2003, FDA published the Task Force Report and Guidance on Qualified Health Claims.[24] Key components included the following:

1. An evidence-based rating system from the Agency for Health Care Research. The strength of the evidence is assigned a rating, and the corresponding language now appears on product packages. The four levels and related qualified statements are as follows:
   "A": SSA (no qualifier).
   "B": "Although there is scientific evidence supporting the claim, the evidence is not conclusive."

   "C": "Some scientific evidence suggests …. However, FDA has determined that this evidence is limited and not conclusive."
   "D": "Very limited and preliminary scientific research suggests …. FDA concludes that there is little scientific evidence supporting this claim."
2. A proposed regulatory framework for QHCs.
3. Consumer studies research agenda.
4. Resources for the review of scientific data.

The final QHC guidance was published in spring 2009.[25] The guidance further details the process for submitting QHC petitions and the language that is used. The process of submitting QHC petitions is similar to that for health claims based on

## TABLE 5.10
## Health Claims Allowed to Pass Through FDAMA[a]

| Health Claim | Model Language | Requirements per RACC | Can Be Made on Qualified |
|---|---|---|---|
| Whole grains and risk of heart disease and certain cancers and CHD | Diets rich in whole grains and other plant foods and low in total fat, saturated fat, and cholesterol may help reduce the risk of heart disease and certain cancers. | Food contains at least 51% whole-grain ingredient(s) by weight, and whole grain is the first ingredient listed. Food must be "low fat," "low saturated fat," and "low cholesterol." Food must provide at least 16 g of whole grain. Food contains a minimum amount of dietary fiber related to RACC size: 3 g for 55 g RACC, 2.8 g for 50 g RACC, 2.5 g for 45 g RACC, and 1.7 g for 35 g RACC. | Foods |
| Whole-grain foods with moderate fat content and CHD and certain cancers | Diets rich in whole grains and other plant foods and low in total fat, saturated fat, and cholesterol may help reduce the risk of heart disease and certain cancers. | Food contains at least 51% whole-grain ingredient(s) by weight, and whole grain is the first ingredient listed. Food must be "low saturated fat" and "low cholesterol" and contain less than 6.5 g total fat and 0.5 g or less trans fat. Food contains a minimum amount of dietary fiber related to RACC size: 3 g for 55 g RACC, 2.8 g for 50 g RACC, 2.5 g for 45 g RACC, and 1.7 g for 35 g RACC. Food contains at least 7% of fiber DV if the product does not contain at least 10% DV for protein, calcium, iron, and vitamin A or C. | Foods |
| Potassium containing foods and blood pressure and stroke | Diets containing foods that are good sources of potassium and low in sodium may reduce the risk of high blood pressure and stroke. | Food contains at least 10% DV for potassium. Potassium is listed on the Nutrition Facts panel. Food is "low sodium," "low cholesterol," "low saturated fat," and "low fat". | Foods |
| Fluoridated water and reduced risk of dental caries | Drinking fluoridated water may reduce the risk of (dental caries or tooth decay). In addition, the health claim is not intended for use on bottled water products specifically marketed for use by infants. | Eligible food is bottled water meeting the standards of identity and quality set forth in 21 CFR 165.110. Bottled must contain greater than 0.6 and up to 1.0 mg/L *total* fluoride and meet all general requirements for health claims (21 CFR 101.14) with the exception of minimum nutrient contribution (21 CFR 101.14 (e)(6)). | Foods |
| Saturated fat, cholesterol and *trans* fat and reduced risk of heart disease | Diets low in saturated fat and cholesterol, and as low as possible in *trans* fat, may reduce the risk of heart disease. | Food must be "low saturated fat" (1 g or less) and "low cholesterol" (20 mg or less)/RACC. Food must contain <0.5 g of *trans* fat/RACC or meet any FDA definition of "low *trans* fat" if a definition is established. Food must contain <6.5 g total fat/RACC. | Foods |
| Substitution of saturated fat in the diet with unsaturated fatty acids and reduced risk of heart disease | Replacing saturated fat with similar amounts of unsaturated fats may reduce the risk of heart disease. To achieve this benefit, total daily calories should not increase. | Food should contain 80% of fat from unsaturated fat/RACC and meet the requirements of 21 CFR 101.14. Food should be "low fat," "low saturated fat," and "low cholesterol". | Foods |

[a] See http://www.fda.gov/Food/LabelingNutrition/LabelClaims/FDAModernizationActFDAMAClaims/default.htm

SSA petitions. However, as mentioned, the SSA requirement is not enforced. QHCs need to meet all general health claim requirements unless enforcement discretion is provided. These exceptions are noted in the QHC table (Table 5.11). The guidance also represents the agency's current thinking on (1) the evidence-based review system for evaluating the scientific evidence for a health claim, (2) the meaning of the SSA standard 21 CFR 101.14(c), and (3) credible scientific evidence to support a QHC.

FDA authorized seven claims as a result of NLEA.[3] Since that time, FDA has approved numerous other claims submitted as petitions and notifications. The health claim model language and requirements are indicated in Tables 5.9 through 5.11: those resulting from NLEA[3] and petitions (Table 5.9), those not prohibited by FDA through FDAMA[20] (Table 5.10), and those allowed by court decision[23] (enforcement discretion is applied[24]) and accompanied by extensive qualifying language (Table 5.11).

**TABLE 5.11**

**QHC Allowed by the Pearson Decision and FDA Enforcement Discretion[a–d]**

| Health Claim | Model Language | Requirements per RACC | Can Be Made on Qualified |
|---|---|---|---|
| *Atopic dermatitis* | | | |
| 100% Whey-protein partially hydrolyzed infant formula and reduced risk of atopic dermatitis: *Docket No. FDA-2009-Q-0301* | Very little scientific evidence suggests that, for healthy infants who are not exclusively breastfed and who have a family history of allergy, feeding a 100% whey-protein partially hydrolyzed infant formula from birth up to 4 months of age instead of a formula containing intact cow's milk proteins may reduce the risk of developing atopic dermatitis throughout the 1st year of life and up to 3 years of age. Partially hydrolyzed formulas should not be fed to infants who are allergic to milk or to infants with existing milk allergy symptoms. If you suspect your baby is already allergic to milk, or if your baby is on a special formula for the treatment of allergy, your baby's care and feeding choices should be under a doctor's supervision. | 100% Whey-protein partially hydrolyzed infant formula. | *Foods Formula* |
| *Cancer* | | | |
| Tomatoes or tomato sauce and prostate, ovarian, gastric, and pancreatic cancers: *Docket No. 2004Q-0201* | *Prostate cancer*: Very limited and preliminary scientific research suggests that eating 1/2–1 cup of tomatoes or tomato sauce a week may reduce the risk of prostate cancer. FDA concludes that there is little scientific evidence supporting this claim. *Ovarian cancer*: One study suggests that consumption of tomato sauce two times per week may reduce the risk of ovarian cancer, while this same study shows that consumption of tomatoes or tomato juice had no effect on ovarian cancer risk. FDA concludes that it is highly uncertain that tomato sauce reduces the risk of ovarian cancer. *Gastric cancer*: Four studies did not show that tomato intake reduces the risk of gastric cancer, but three studies suggest that tomato intake may reduce this risk. Based on these studies, FDA concludes that it is unlikely that tomatoes reduce the risk of gastric cancer. *Pancreatic cancer*: One study suggests that consuming tomatoes does not reduce the risk of pancreatic cancer, but one weaker, more limited study suggests that consuming tomatoes may reduce this risk. Based on these studies, FDA concludes that it is highly unlikely that tomatoes reduce the risk of pancreatic cancer. | Food is cooked, raw, dried, or canned tomatoes. Tomato sauces must contain at least 8.37% salt-free tomato solids. | Foods |
| Calcium and colon/rectal cancer and calcium and recurrent colon/rectal polyps: *Docket No. 2004Q-0097* | *Colon/rectal cancer*: Some evidence suggests that calcium supplements may reduce the risk of colon/rectal cancer; however, FDA has determined that this evidence is limited and not conclusive. *Recurrent colon polyps*: Very limited and preliminary evidence suggests that calcium supplements may reduce the risk of colon/rectal polyps. FDA concludes that there is little scientific evidence to support this claim. | DS is "high" calcium. DS contains bioavailable calcium that meets the U.S. Pharmacopeia (USP) standards for disintegration and dissolution applicable to their component calcium salts. For DS for which no USP standards exist, the DS must be bioavailable under conditions of use. | DS |
| Green tea and cancer: *Docket No. 2004Q-0083* | *Breast cancer*: Two studies do not show that drinking green tea reduces the risk of breast cancer in women, but one weaker, more limited study suggests that drinking green tea may reduce this risk. Based on these studies, FDA concludes that it is highly unlikely that green tea reduces the risk of breast cancer. *Prostate cancer*: One weak and limited study does not show that drinking green tea reduces the risk of prostate cancer, but another weak and limited study suggests that drinking green tea may reduce this risk. Based on these studies, FDA concludes that it is highly unlikely that green tea reduces the risk of prostate cancer. | Food or DS must contain green tea. Food or DS do not need to contain 10% minimum nutrient content requirement. | Foods and DS |

**TABLE 5.11 (continued)**

**QHC Allowed by the Pearson Decision and FDA Enforcement Discretion[a–d]**

| Health Claim | Model Language | Requirements per RACC | Can Be Made on Qualified |
|---|---|---|---|
| Selenium and cancer: *Docket No. 02P-0457* | Selenium may reduce the risk of certain cancers. Some scientific evidence suggests that consumption of selenium may reduce the risk of certain forms of cancer. However, FDA has determined that this evidence is limited and not conclusive. | DS must be "high selenium." DS labeling cannot recommend daily intake exceeding 400 g. | DS |
| Antioxidant vitamins and cancer: *Docket No. 91N-0101* | Some scientific evidence suggests that consumption of antioxidant vitamins may reduce the risk of certain forms of cancer. However, FDA has determined that this evidence is limited and not conclusive. | DS must be "high vitamin C" or "high vitamin E." DS labeling cannot recommend daily intake more than 2000 mg vitamin C or more than 1000 mg vitamin E. | DS |
| *Cardiovascular disease risk* | | | |
| Omega-3 fatty acids and CHD: *Docket No. 2003Q-0401* | Supportive but not conclusive research shows that consumption of EPA and DHA omega-3 fatty acids may reduce the risk of CHD. One serving of (name of the food) provides ( ) g of EPA and DHA omega-3 fatty acids. (See nutrition information for total fat, saturated fat, and cholesterol content). *Note*: DS may declare the amount of EPA and DHA per serving in "supplement facts," instead of making the declaration in the claim. | *Fish*: Fish (i.e., "products that are essentially all fish") must have 16 g or less fat/RACC. Fish with fat content greater than 13 g/RACC must include disclosure statement. Fish may not exceed saturated fat disqualifying level and must contain less than 95 mg cholesterol/RACC/100 g. If fish contains more than 60 mg, claim must carry disclosure statement. *Foods other than fish*: Foods other than fish may not exceed fat disqualifying levels and must be "low saturated fat" and "low cholesterol". *DS*: DS should not recommend daily intake exceeding 2 g of EPA and DHA. DS weighing 5 g or less /RACC are exempted from total fat disqualifying level, but if DS exceed fat disqualifying level, must include disclosure statement. DS that weigh more than 5 g/RACC must not exceed fat disqualifying level. DS must meet the criterion for "low" saturated fat, but not with regard to the no more than 15% calories from saturated fat criterion. DS that weigh 5 g or less/RACC are exempt from the cholesterol disqualifying level (60 mg/50 g), but those that exceed cholesterol disqualifying level must include disqualifying statement. DS that weigh more than 5 g/RACC must meet the criterion for "low cholesterol". | Foods and DS |
| Folic acid, vitamin $B_6$, and vitamin $B_{12}$ and vascular disease: *Docket No. 99P-3029* | As part of a well-balanced diet that is low in saturated fat and cholesterol, folic acid, vitamin $B_6$, and vitamin $B_{12}$ may reduce the risk of vascular disease. FDA evaluated the aforementioned claim and found that, while it is known that diets low in saturated fat and cholesterol reduce the risk of heart disease and other vascular diseases, the evidence in support of the aforementioned claim is inconclusive. | DS cannot state the daily dietary intake necessary to achieve a claimed effect because the evidence is not definitive. Products greater than 100% DV folic acid must state safe upper limit of 1000 µg. DS containing folic acid must meet USP standards for disintegration and dissolution, except that, if there are no applicable USP standards, folate must be bioavailable under conditions of use. | DS |

*(continued)*

**TABLE 5.11 (continued)**
**QHC Allowed by the Pearson Decision and FDA Enforcement Discretion[a-d]**

| Health Claim | Model Language | Requirements per RACC | Can Be Made on Qualified |
|---|---|---|---|
| Walnuts and heart disease: *Docket No. 02P-0292* | Supportive but not conclusive research shows that eating 1.5 oz/day of walnuts, as part of a low-saturated-fat and low-cholesterol diet and not resulting in increased caloric intake, may reduce the risk of CHD. | Food must be whole or chopped walnuts. Food may exceed disqualifying level for fat and is not required to contain 10% minimum nutrient content requirement. | Foods |
| Nuts and heart disease: *Docket No. 02P-0505* | Scientific evidence suggests but does not prove that eating 1.5 oz/day of most nuts (such as *name of specific nut*) as part of a diet low in saturated fat and cholesterol may reduce the risk of heart disease.<br><br>*Notes*: The bracketed phrase naming a specific nut is optional. The bracketed fat content disclosure statement is applicable to a claim made for whole or chopped nuts, but not a claim made for nut-containing products. | Food must be whole or chopped nuts or nut-containing products that contain at least 11 g of one or more of almonds, hazelnuts, peanuts, pecans, some pine nuts, pistachio nuts, and walnuts.<br>*Nuts*: Nuts must not exceed 4 g saturated fat/50 g.<br>Nuts may exceed fat disqualifying level. Walnuts do not need to contain 10% minimum nutrient content requirement.<br>*Nut-containing products*: Nut-containing products must be "low saturated fat" and "low cholesterol". | Foods |
| Monounsaturated fatty acids from olive oil and CHD: *Docket No. 2003Q-0559* | Limited and not conclusive scientific evidence suggests that eating about 2 tablespoons (23 g) of olive oil daily may reduce the risk of CHD due to the monounsaturated fat in olive oil. To achieve this possible benefit, olive oil is to replace a similar amount of saturated fat and not increase the total number of calories you eat in a day. One serving of this product contains ( ) g of olive oil.<br><br>*Note:* The last sentence of the claim "One serving of this product contains ( ) g of olive oil" is optional when the claim is used on the label or in the labeling of olive oil. | *Olive oil*: Food must be pure olive oil<br>*Salad dressing*: Salad dressing must contain at least 6 g olive oil, be "low cholesterol," and not contain more than 4 g of saturated fat/50 g.<br>*Vegetable oil spreads*: Vegetable oil spreads must contain at least 6 g olive oil, be "low cholesterol," and not contain more than 4 g saturated fat.<br>*Olive oil-containing foods*: Olive oil-containing foods must provide at least 6 g olive oil, be "low cholesterol," and contain 10% DV vitamin A, vitamin C, iron, calcium, protein, or dietary fiber. If the RACC of the olive oil-containing food is greater than 30 g, the food cannot contain more than 4 g of saturated fat/RACC, and if the RACC of the olive oil-containing food is 30 g or less, the food cannot contain more than 4 g of saturated fat/50 g.<br>*Shortenings*: Shortenings must contain at least 6 g olive oil, be "low cholesterol," and not contain more than 4 g of saturated fat/RACC. | Foods |
| Unsaturated fatty acids from canola oil and reduced risk of CHD: *Docket No. 2006Q-0091* | Limited and not conclusive scientific evidence suggests that eating about 1 1/2 tablespoons (19 g) of canola oil daily may reduce the risk of CHD due to the unsaturated fat content in canola oil. To achieve this possible benefit, canola oil is to replace a similar amount of saturated fat and not increase the total number of calories you eat in a day. One serving of this product contains (x) grams of canola oil. | *Canola oil*: Food must contain ≥4.75 g canola oil/RACC (19 g canola oil minimum effective dose [or 17.7 g UFA]) and must have ≤1 g saturated fat/RACC and be "low cholesterol" (has no *trans* fat/RACC requirement).<br>*Other foods*: Vegetable spreads, dressing for salads, and shortenings, canola oil-containing foods must contain ≥4.75 g canola oil/RACC. Canola oil-containing foods do not need to be "low fat"; | |

**TABLE 5.11 (continued)**
**QHC Allowed by the Pearson Decision and FDA Enforcement Discretion[a–d]**

| Health Claim | Model Language | Requirements per RACC | Can Be Made on Qualified |
|---|---|---|---|
| | | enforcement discretion provided for products ≥4.75 g canola oil/RACC. If food contains >13 g total fat/RACC, must use disclosure statement. Food must be "low saturated fat"/RACC and be "low cholesterol" (no *trans* fat/RACC requirement). | |
| | | Margarines, margarine products, spreads, and other foods must provide ≥10% DV of vitamin A, vitamin C, iron, calcium, protein, or dietary fiber. | |
| Corn oil and corn oil-containing products and reduced risk of CHD: *Docket No. 2006P-0243* | Very limited and preliminary scientific evidence suggests that eating about 1 tablespoon (16 g) of corn oil daily may reduce the risk of heart disease. FDA concludes that there is little scientific evidence supporting this claim. To achieve this possible benefit, corn oil is to replace a similar amount of saturated fat and not increase the total number of calories you eat in a day. One serving of this product contains ( ) grams of corn oil. | *Corn oil and vegetable oil blends*: Must contain ≥4 g corn oil/RACC (minimum effective dose, 16 g corn oil/d with 13.3 g UFAs). | |
| | | If product ≥13 g/RACC, per label serving size and per 50 g if the RACC is ≤30 g or 2 T or less), product must carry the disclosure statement. | |
| | | Oil must contain ≤4 g/RACC but not per 50 g saturated fat. If product is not "low saturated fat" (≤1 g/RACC and ≤15% calories from saturated fatty acids) product must carry disclosure statement. | |
| | | Food must be "low cholesterol. | |
| | | *Corn oil-containing foods* (vegetable oil spreads, dressings for salads, shortenings, and other corn oil-containing foods): The requirements vary, but include food that must contain ≥4 g corn oil/RACC. Contain ≤4g/RACC but not per 50 g saturated fat. If product is not "low saturated fat," product must carry disclosure statement. However, salad dressings and corn oil-containing foods must comply with all requirements of the saturated fat disqualifying level. | |
| | | If product fat content is ≥13 g/RACC, per label serving size and per 50 g if the RACC is ≤30 g (or 2 T or less), product must carry the disclosure statement. | |
| | | Food must be "low cholesterol". | |
| | | Margarines and corn oil-containing products must provide ≥10% DV of vitamin A, vitamin C, iron, calcium, protein, or dietary fiber. | |
| *Hypertension* | | | |
| Calcium and hypertension, pregnancy-induced hypertension and preeclampsia: *Docket No. 2004Q-0098* | *Hypertension*: Some scientific evidence suggests that calcium supplements may reduce the risk of hypertension. However, FDA has determined that the evidence is inconsistent and not conclusive.<br>*Pregnancy-induced hypertension*: Four studies, including a large clinical trial, do not show that calcium supplements reduce the risk of pregnancy-induced hypertension during pregnancy. However, three other studies suggest that | Must be "high calcium." DS calcium content must be bioavailable and must meet USP standards for disintegration and dissolution applicable to their component calcium salts. For DS for which no USP standards exist, the DS must exhibit appropriate assimilability under the conditions of use. | DS |

*(continued)*

**TABLE 5.11 (continued)**
**QHC Allowed by the Pearson Decision and FDA Enforcement Discretion[a–d]**

| Health Claim | Model Language | Requirements per RACC | Can Be Made on Qualified |
|---|---|---|---|
| | calcium supplements may reduce the risk. Based on these studies, FDA concludes that it is highly unlikely that calcium supplements reduce the risk of pregnancy-induced hypertension. *Preeclampsia*: Three studies, including a large clinical trial, do not show that calcium supplements reduce the risk of preeclampsia during pregnancy. However, two other studies suggest that calcium supplements may reduce the risk. Based on these studies, FDA concludes that it is highly unlikely that calcium supplements reduce the risk of preeclampsia. | | |
| *Cognitive function*<br>Phosphatidylserine and cognitive dysfunction and dementia: *Docket No. 02P-0413* | *Dementia*: Consumption of phosphatidylserine may reduce the risk of dementia in the elderly. Very limited and preliminary scientific research suggests that phosphatidylserine may reduce the risk of dementia in the elderly. FDA concludes that there is little scientific evidence supporting this claim. *Cognitive dysfunction*: Consumption of phosphatidylserine may reduce the risk of cognitive dysfunction in the elderly. Very limited and preliminary scientific research suggests that phosphatidylserine may reduce the risk of cognitive dysfunction in the elderly. FDA concludes that there is little scientific evidence supporting this claim. | The claim may not suggest level of phosphatidylserine as being useful in achieving the claimed effect. The soy-derived phosphatidylserine must be of very high purity. | DS containing soy-derived phosphatidylserine |
| *Diabetes*<br>Chromium picolinate and diabetes: *Docket No. 2004Q-0144* | One small study suggests that chromium picolinate may reduce the risk of insulin resistance and therefore possibly may reduce the risk of type 2 diabetes. FDA concludes, however, that the existence of such a relationship between chromium picolinate and either insulin resistance or type 2 diabetes is highly uncertain. | DS must be "high chromium". | DS |
| *Neural tube defects*<br>0.8 mg folic acid and neural tube birth defects: *Docket No. 91N-100H* | 0.8 mg folic acid in a DS is more effective in reducing the risk of neural tube defects than a lower amount in foods in common form. FDA does not endorse this claim. Public health authorities recommend that women consume 0.4 mg folic acid daily from fortified foods or DS or both to reduce the risk of neural tube defects. | There also is a folic acid/neural tube defect health claim authorized by regulation (see 21 CFR 101.79). | DS |

[a] For all QHC requirements, the claim meets the general requirements for health claims in Ref. 1 (21 CFR 101.14) (unless otherwise noted), *except* for the requirement that the evidence for the claim meet the SSA standard and be made in accordance with an authorizing regulation Ref. [1] (21 CFR 101.14(c).

[b] All conventional foods must meet the 10% minimum nutrient requirement (vitamin A 5000 IU, vitamin C 6 mg, iron 1.8 mg, calcium 100 mg, protein 5 g, fiber 2.5 g/RACC), prior to any nutrient addition. The 10% minimum nutrient requirement does not apply to DS (21 CFR 101.14(e) (6)).

[c] If disclosure levels of fat, saturated fat, or cholesterol are exceeded, the appropriate disclosure statements must be included immediately adjacent to the claims, for example, "See nutrition information for total fat content" with the health claim.

[d] Further detail for all claims can be found on the FDA website: http://www.fda.gov/Food/LabelingNutrition/LabelClaims/QualifiedHealthClaims/default.htm

The qualifying language (an appropriate disclaimer, i.e., "some scientific evidence suggests ...") must be placed immediately adjacent to and directly beneath the claim, with no intervening material, and in the same size, typeface, and contrast as the claim itself.

Again, the requirements for the FDAMA[20] and court-mandated health claims[23] or those allowed through enforcement discretion[24] are not published in the CFR.[1] These requirements can be found on FDA's website, www.fda.gov

## STRUCTURE/FUNCTION CLAIMS

### OVERVIEW

Structure/function claims can be made on DS.[26] A structure/function claim describes "the role of a nutrient or dietary ingredient intended to affect the structure or function in humans or that characterizes the documented mechanism by which a nutrient or dietary ingredient acts to maintain such structure of function, provided that such statements are not disease claims" (21 CFR 101.93).[1] "Calcium helps build strong bones" is an example of a structure/function claim.

### REQUIREMENTS

The general requirements for structure/function claims include (1) statement be truthful and not misleading, (2) the manufacturer of the DS product carrying the claim notify the FDA within 90 days of entering the product into commerce, and (3) DS carry the following disclaimer: "This product is not meant to prevent, treat, mitigate, or cure any disease."

Specific requirements for structure/function claims are not found in the CFR. Individual claims are not approved by the FDA.

## FRONT-OF-PACKAGE LABELING

### OVERVIEW

With the increased public interest in identifying healthier foods, U.S. food processors have been adding nutrition information and icons to the FOPs in addition to nutrient content or health claims. This type of labeling also is being used in other countries.[27]

The FDA held a public hearing on the Use of Symbols to Communicate Nutrition Information that addressed the number of different profiles on product packages and emphasized the need for a consistent, consumer-tested format.[28] The agency also partially supported two Institute of Medicine reports on FOP labeling.[29,30]

The FDA is developing a proposed regulation that would define the nutrition criteria that would need to be met by manufacturers making broad FOP or shelf label claims concerning the nutrition quality of a food, whether the claim is made in text or in symbols. The FDA's intent is to provide standardized, science-based criteria on which FOP nutrition

labeling must be based. The agency has also conducted consumer research to determine the most effective format for portraying FOP information.[31]

Notably, while currently voluntary, nutrition-related FOP and shelf labeling is subject to the provisions of the FFDCA that prohibit false or misleading claims and restrict nutrient content claims to those defined in FDA regulations.

## ALLERGEN LABELING

The Food Allergen Labeling and Consumer Protection Act of 2004 (FALCPA) (Public Law 108-282)[32] was enacted in August 2004 and addresses, among other issues, the labeling of foods that contain certain food allergens. It was passed in part because the common or usual name of an ingredient may be unfamiliar to consumers and many consumers do not recognize that certain ingredients contain or are derived from a food allergen. This new requirement for food helps allergic consumers to identify foods or ingredients that they may be allergic to, so they can more easily avoid them.

FALPCA requires that labels must clearly identify the food source names of all ingredients that are—or contain any protein derived from—the eight most common food allergens, which FALCPA defines as "major food allergens." These are milk, eggs, fish, crustacean shellfish, tree nuts, peanuts, wheat, and soybeans.

The law applies to all foods whose labeling is regulated by FDA, both domestic and imported. (FDA regulates the labeling of all foods, except for poultry, most meats, certain egg products, and most alcoholic beverages.)

FALCPA requires that food labels identify the food source names of all major food allergens used to make the food. This requirement is met if the common or usual name of an ingredient (e.g., buttermilk) that is a major food allergen already identified that allergen's food source name (i.e., milk). Otherwise, the allergen's food source name must be declared at least once on the food label in one of two ways.

The name of the food source of a major food allergen must appear in parentheses following the name of the ingredient in the ingredient list. For example, lecithin (soy) must be placed immediately after or next to the list of ingredients in a "contains" statement, for example, "Contains Wheat, Milk, and Soy."

The law also required that proposed and final rules be issued to define, and permit use of, the term "gluten-free" on the labeling of foods.

## RESOURCES

**Food and Drug Association:** http://www.fda.gov/ (Accessed June 8, 2012)

The FDA website provides a wealth of information about FDA labeling activities, regulatory actions and positions, and industry guidance. The site provides FDA organizational structure and a telephone and e-mail directory so that staff contacts can be made. One can check out the "What's New" section for the FDA's latest actions. Links are provided to other regulatory agencies such as the FTC and the FSIS.

**Food Safety and Inspection Service:** http://www.fsis.usda.gov (Accessed June 8, 2012)

The USDA's FSIS is responsible for overseeing labeling of meat and poultry foods. The agency allows health claims on a case-by-case basis. (FSIS requires label approval prior to use on a product.) The FSIS website provides regulatory guidelines and current information.

**CFR:** http://www.accessdata.fda.gov/scripts/cdrh/cfdocs/cfcfr/cfrsearch.cfm (Accessed June 8, 2012)

The CFR codifies all of the general and permanent rules published in the Federal Register by FDA and FSIS, USDA, FTC, and BATF. The CFR is divided into 50 titles, each representing an area of federal regulation, for example, 21 CFR is Food and Drugs, and 9 CFR is USDA. The titles are then divided into chapters that usually bear the name of the responsible agency. Those most pertinent to the food label include 21 CFR 100–169[1] (FDA, food labeling), 21 CFR 170–199[1] (FDA, food additives), and 9 CFR 200 to end[5] (FSIS, food labeling). The CFR can be accessed online through the FDA website. The CFR is updated annually.

**Federal Register:** http://www.fda.gov/RegulatoryInformation/Dockets/FR/default.htm (Accessed June 8, 2012)

The federal government, FDA and FSIS, publishes regulations in the Federal Register to implement food and DS laws in various forms (notice, proposed rule, and final rule) on a daily basis. Once a final rule is published, it is incorporated into the CFR. The Federal Register can be accessed through the FDA's website. It can be searched by agency, date, date range, or topic.

## REFERENCES

1. Food and Drug Administration, U.S. Department of Health and Human Services. Code of federal regulations, Title 21, Parts 100–169. Washington, DC: Superintendent of Documents, U.S. Government Printing Office, 2012. http://www.accessdata.fda.gov/scripts/cdrh/cfdocs/cfcfr/cfrsearch.cfm (Accessed August 6, 2012).
2. Federal Food and Drug Act of 1906. 34 USC § 768. http://www.fda.gov/opacom/laws/wileyact.htm (Accessed August 6, 2012).
3. Nutrition Labeling and Education Act. 1990/Pub L No. 101-535, 104 Stat 2353. http://thomas.loc.gov/cgi-bin/bdquery/z?d101:HR03562:@@@D&summ2=3&|TOM:/bss/d101query.html (Accessed August 6, 2012).
4. Federal Food, Drug and Cosmetic Act of 1938. 52 USC § 1040. http://www.fda.gov/opacom/laws/fdcact/fdctoc.htm (Accessed August 6, 2012).
5. U.S. Department of Agriculture, Food Safety and Information Service. Code of federal regulations, Title 9, Parts 200 to end. Washington, DC: Superintendent of Documents, U.S. Government Printing Office, 2012.
6. Geiger, CJ, Parent, CRM, Wyse, BW. *JADA*. 91: 808; 1991.
7. Geiger, CJ. *JADA*. 98: 1312; 1998.
8. Food and Drug Administration. Food labeling: Serving sizes of products that can reasonably be consumed at one eating occasion; updating of reference amounts customarily consumed; approaches for recommending smaller portion sizes: Advance notice of proposed rulemaking. *Federal Register*. 2005; 70: 17010. http://www.fda.gov/OHRMS/DOCKETS/98fr/05-6644.pdf (Accessed August 6, 2012).
9. Food and Drug Administration, Working Group on Obesity. Counting calories: Report of the working group on obesity. 2004. http://www.fda.gov/Food/LabelingNutrition/ReportsResearch/ucm081696.htm (Accessed August 6, 2012).
10. Food and Drug Administration. Food labeling; prominence of calories. Advance notice of proposed rulemaking. *Federal Register*. 2005; 70: 1708–1710. http://www.fda.gov/OHRMS/DOCKETS/98fr/05-6643.pdf (Accessed August 6, 2012).
11. Committee on Use of Dietary Reference Intake in Nutrition Labeling. *Dietary Reference Intakes: Guiding Principles for Nutrition Labeling and Fortification*. Washington, DC: National Academy Press, 2003.
12. Food and Drug Administration. Food labeling; revision of reference values and mandatory nutrients. Advance notice of proposed rulemaking. *Federal Register*. 2007; 72: 62149–62175.
13. Geiger, CJ. *IFT Annual Meeting Technical Program*. Book of Abstracts. No. 103-05, p. 245, 2006.
14. Keystone Center. *Keystone Forum on Away-From-Home Foods: Opportunities for Preventing Weight Gain and Obesity*. Final Report. Washington, DC: The Keystone Center, 2006. www.keystone.org (Accessed August 6, 2012).
15. Patient Protection and Affordable Care Act, 2010 (Public Law 111–148) http://housedocs.house.gov/energycommerce/ppacacon.pdf (Accessed August 3, 2012).
16. Food and Drug Administration. Food labeling; nutrition labeling of standard menu items in restaurants and similar retail food establishments; proposed rule. *Federal Register*. 2011; 76: 1919.
17. Food and Drug Administration. Food labeling; calorie labeling of articles of food in vending machines; proposed rule. *Federal Register*. 2011; 76: 19237–19255.
18. Food and Drug Administration. Food labeling; notice. Voluntary registration by authorized officials of non-covered retail food establishments and vending machine operators electing to be subject to the menu and vending machine labeling requirements established by the patient protection and affordable care act of 2010. *Federal Register*. 75; 43182–43184.
19. Food Safety and Inspection Service. Nutrition labeling of single-ingredient products and ground of chopped meat and poultry products. Final rule. *Federal Register*. 2010; 75: 82147–82167. http://www.gpo.gov/fdsys/pkg/FR-2010-12-08/pdf/2010-30386.pdf (Accessed August 6, 2012).
20. Food and Drug Administration Modernization Azlic Law 105–115. http://www.fda.gov/RegulatoryInformation/Legislation/FederalFoodDrugandCosmeticActFDCAct/SignificantAmendmentstotheFDCAct/FDAMA/default.htm (Accessed August 6, 2012).
21. Food and Drug Administration. Label claims: FDA Modernization Act of 1997 (FDAMA) Claims. http://www.cfsan.fda.gov/~dms/labfdama.html. http://housedocs.house.gov/energycommerce/ppacacon.pdf (Accessed August 3, 2012).
22. Food and Drug Administration. Dockets Management. Omega-3 Fatty Acids. Docket Nos. 2003Q-0401, 2005P-0189 and 2006 P-0137. http://www.fda.gov/ohrms/dockets/default.htm (Accessed August 6, 2012).
23. Pearson V. Shalala, 164 F.3d at 661 (DC Cir. 1999).

24. Food and Drug Administration. Consumer health information for better nutrition initiative: Task force. Final Report. 2003. http://www.fda.gov/Food/LabelingNutrition/LabelClaims/QualifiedHealthClaims/QualifiedHealthClaimsPetitions/ucm096010.htm (Accessed August 6, 2012).

25. Food and Drug Administration. Guidance for industry: Evidence-based review system for the scientific evaluation of health claims—Final 2009 http://www.fda.gov/Food/GuidanceComplianceRegulatoryInformation/GuidanceDocuments/FoodLabelingNutrition/ucm073332.htm (Accessed August 6, 2012).

26. Dietary Supplement Health and Education Act of 1994. 108 Stat 4325, 4322. http://www.fda.gov/opacom/laws/dshea.html. Public Law 103–417.

27. Food and Drug Administration. New front-of-package labeling initiative. www.fda.gov/Food/LabelingNutrition/ucm202726.htm (Accessed August 11, 2012).

28. Food and Drug Administration. Food labeling: Use of symbols to communicate nutrition information, consideration of consumer studies and nutritional criteria. Public hearing; Request for comments. *Federal Register*. 2007; 72: 39815–39818.

29. Institute of Medicine. *Examination of Front-of-Package Nutrition Rating Systems and Symbols: Promoting Healthier Choices*: *Phase II Report*. Washington, DC: National Academies Press, 2011.

30. Institute of Medicine, Committee on Examination of Front-of-Package Nutrition Ratings Systems and Symbols. *Examination of Front-of-Package Nutrition Ratings Systems and Symbols: Phase I Report*. Washington, DC: National Academies Press, 2010.

31. Food and Drug Administration. Experimental study on consumer responses to labeling statements on food packages. *Comment Request*. 2012; 77: 21779–21782.

32. Food Allergen Labeling and Consumer Protection Act of 2004 (Public Law 108-282, Title II). http://www.fda.gov/Food/LabelingNutrition/FoodAllergensLabeling/GuidanceComplianceRegulatoryInformation/ucm106187.htm (Accessed August 6, 2012).

33. Federal Fair Packaging and Labeling Act 1966. 80 USC § 1966. http://www.fda.gov/opacom/laws/fplact.htm (Accessed August 6, 2012).

34. Food and Drug Administration. Nutrition labeling: Proposed criteria for food label information panel. *Federal Register*. March 30, 1972; 37: 6493–6497.

35. Food and Drug Administration. Nutrition labeling. *Federal Register*. January 19, 1973; 38: 2124–2164.

36. Food and Drug Administration. Nutrition labeling. *Federal Register*. March 14, 1973; 38: 6950–6975.

37. National Research Council. *Diet and Health: Implications for Reducing Chronic Disease Risk*. Washington, DC: National Academy Press, 1989.

# 6 A Primer on Food Law

*Ricardo Carvajal*

## CONTENTS

The term "food law" generally refers to the body of laws that govern the production, distribution, and marketing of food. Particularly in developed economies, the business of producing food and making it available to the consumer has become the preoccupation of relatively few hands. The vast majority of consumers no longer grow their own food or know much about food production, but instead choose and purchase their food based on individual preferences shaped by social and economic circumstances, marketing efforts, and government policy. Those consumers rely on a complex, interwoven system of laws intended to ensure that the information they receive about foods is truthful, not misleading, and accurate and that the food is safe to eat. In turn, the businesses that provide foods must successfully navigate that system of laws to prosper or at least remain viable.

In the United States, there are many laws that govern the production, distribution, and marketing of food, and these are administered by an array of federal and state agencies. For the sake of simplicity and brevity, this chapter focuses primarily on the laws administered by the U.S. Food and Drug Administration (FDA),* the U.S. Department of Agriculture (USDA),[†] and the Federal Trade Commission (FTC).[‡] For the sake of completeness, a brief discussion of state and local laws is included.

## FEDERAL LAW

At a federal level, foods other than meat, poultry, and egg products are governed by the Federal Food, Drug, and Cosmetic Act (FDCA), which is administered by FDA.[§] FDA regulates the safety of food, which includes food ingredients, substances used in the manufacture of food, and food packaging. Although certain uses of substances in food or in its packaging must be authorized by FDA before marketing, FDA generally exercises its authority through post-market inspections of food manufacturers. If FDA detects serious problems in a facility, FDA can take administrative action to prevent the food from proceeding in commerce and can also ask the U.S. Department of Justice to initiate judicial proceedings to seize the food (referred to as seizure) and enjoin the manufacturer from further distribution (referred to as injunction). Because of the cumbersome nature of these proceedings and the very large number of food manufacturers that fall under FDA's jurisdiction, FDA focuses its resources on manufacturers and foods associated with higher food safety risks.

FDA also regulates food labeling.[¶] Labeling includes any written, printed, or graphic matter on the food's containers or wrappers, and any such matter that "accompanies" the food. Thus, FDA has deemed labeling to include product brochures and, under certain circumstances, product websites. With limited exceptions, FDA has no authority to review or approve labeling prior to marketing.

Meat, poultry, and egg products are governed by the Federal Meat Inspection Act (FMIA),[**] Poultry Products Inspection Act (PPIA),[††] and Egg Products Inspection Act (EPIA),[‡‡] which are administered by USDA. Generally, USDA regulates the safety of foods under its jurisdiction through a system that relies on the continuous presence of inspectors in production facilities, referred to as continuous inspection. If a USDA inspector detects serious problems in a facility, the inspector can withdraw inspection, thereby shutting down the facility.

USDA also regulates the labeling of foods under its jurisdiction.[§§] Unlike FDA, USDA reviews and approves labeling prior to marketing. In addition, USDA administers certain

---

* www.fda.gov
[†] www.usda.gov
[‡] www.ftc.gov
[§] The full text of the FDCA is available at http://www.fda.gov/RegulatoryInformation/Legislation/FederalFoodDrugandCosmeticActFDCAct/default.htm

[¶] FDA publishes a guide to food labeling, available at http://www.fda.gov/Food/GuidanceComplianceRegulatoryInformation/GuidanceDocuments/FoodLabelingNutrition/FoodLabelingGuide/default.htm
[**] The full text of the FMIA is available at http://www.fsis.usda.gov/regulations/federal_meat_inspection_act/index.asp
[††] The full text of the PPIA is available at http://www.fsis.usda.gov/Regulations_&_Policies/Poultry_Products_Inspection_Act/index.asp
[‡‡] The full text of the EPIA is available at http://www.fsis.usda.gov/Regulations_&_Policies/Egg_Products_Inspection_Act/index.asp. Although USDA has jurisdiction over egg products, note that FDA has jurisdiction over whole eggs in the shell.
[§§] USDA publishes a guide to its labeling requirements, available at http://www.fsis.usda.gov/PDF/Labeling_Requirements_Guide.pdf

marketing claims that are used on foods otherwise under FDA's jurisdiction, most notably the claim of "organic." Given the overlap in the functions of FDA and USDA, periodically, there is talk of unifying USDA and the food-related organizational units of FDA into a single food agency. However, there are political, organizational, and logistical obstacles that render unification unlikely.

Food advertising is governed by the FTC Act,* which is administered by the FTC.† Although there is no statutory definition of advertising, the term is understood to encompass labeling, as well as other promotional materials that fall outside the definition of labeling (e.g., television and radio ads). Because there is overlap in FDA and FTC's jurisdiction, the two agencies have agreed to divide up their responsibilities such that FDA exercises jurisdiction over labeling and FTC generally exercises jurisdiction over promotional materials other than labeling. Nonetheless, it is sometimes the case that a particular promotional activity will draw the scrutiny of both FDA and FTC, and the two agencies occasionally undertake joint enforcement activities that target specific products and promotional practices deemed to be unlawful under both the FDCA and the FTC Act.

## SUMMARY OF MAJOR AMENDMENTS TO THE FDCA

The history of federal food law is largely captured in the evolution of the FDCA. The FDCA was preceded by the 1906 Pure Food and Drug Act, which marked the birth of federal food and drug law.‡ The 1906 Act was intended to deal with products and practices that were obviously unsafe or fraudulent and thus was relatively narrow in scope. As the limitations of that law became apparent, support grew for a more comprehensive federal law that took the form of the FDCA, enacted in 1938.

The FDCA established a range of circumstances under which a food is deemed adulterated. For example, a food is adulterated if it bears or contains a poisonous or deleterious substance in an amount that may render it injurious to health or if it has been produced under insanitary conditions whereby it may have been contaminated with filth or rendered injurious to health. The FDCA also established a range of circumstances under which a food is deemed misbranded. For example, a food is misbranded if its label fails to declare the ingredients in descending order of predominance. The distribution in interstate commerce of a food that is adulterated or misbranded is prohibited by law and is punishable by civil and criminal penalties.

FDA has been resourceful in its interpretation and application of the FDCA. Not long after the passage of the FDCA, FDA began to recognize that it was inefficient to undertake

individual seizure actions against foods alleged to be adulterated or misbranded under general provisions of the FDCA such as those discussed earlier. FDA therefore began to establish more detailed requirements through the issuance of regulations.§ For example, FDA interpreted the FDCA's adulteration provisions to authorize the issuance of regulations to require adherence to good manufacturing practices (GMPs) in the manufacture of foods.¶ For certain types of foods, namely juice and seafood, FDA issued additional regulations requiring implementation of hazard analysis and critical control points (HACCP), a systematic approach to identification and prevention of potential food safety hazards.**

Notwithstanding FDA's resourcefulness, the U.S. Congress has seen the need to amend the FDCA numerous times since its passage in 1938. The following is a summary of a few of those amendments, most of which FDA implemented through the issuance of detailed regulations.

1. *1958 Food Additives Amendment*: Prior to 1958, the use of a substance in food generally was prohibited only if the substance was poisonous or deleterious, and if it was added in an amount that gave rise to a reasonable possibility of injury to health. Concerns about the increasing use of various substances in food in the aftermath of World War II prompted passage of the Food Additives Amendment. That law amended the FDCA to require premarket approval by FDA of the use of any substance in food that is not generally recognized as safe (GRAS). If a particular use of a substance is not GRAS, then that use is deemed a food additive use that is subject to premarket approval.††

   Because the focus of the law is on the safety of the use of a substance (and not on the substance itself), the same substance might have some uses that are considered GRAS and other uses that are considered food additive uses. Both GRAS and food additive uses are subject to the same safety standard (i.e., reasonable certainty that no harm will result under the intended conditions of use). What distinguishes a GRAS use from a food additive use is not the safety of the use, but rather whether the safety of that use is generally recognized by appropriately qualified experts, oftentimes on the basis of peer-reviewed scientific publications.

2. *1960 Color Additives Amendment*: This amendment gave FDA the authority to review and approve the use of any color additive prior to marketing, regardless of whether the color additive is synthesized or

---

\* The full text of the FTC Act is available at http://www.law.cornell.edu/uscode/text/15/41. Also see FTC's Enforcement Policy Statement on Food Advertising, available at http://www.ftc.gov/bcp/policystmt/ad-food.shtm

† www.ftc.gov

‡ The full text of the 1906 Act is available at http://www.ncbi.nlm.nih.gov/books/NBK22116/

§ FDA's regulations are published in Title 21 of the Code of Federal Regulations (CFR), available at http://www.accessdata.fda.gov/scripts/cdrh/cfdocs/cfcfr/cfrsearch.cfm

¶ The GMP regulations are found in 21 CFR Part 110.

\** The juice and seafood HACCP regulations are found in 21 CFR Parts 120 and 123.

†† FDA maintains a web page on its regulation of food ingredients at http://www.fda.gov/Food/FoodIngredientsPackaging/default.htm

derived from a natural source. Synthetic color additives are subject to certification, and each batch must be tested to ensure that it meets the specifications established by FDA. Certified color additives must be individually declared in the ingredient statement that is required to be provided on a food label. Color additives derived from natural sources are exempt from certification and need not be individually declared unless individual declaration is required due to a potential safety risk (e.g., if the color additive can provoke an allergic reaction in sensitized individuals). FDA does not recognize any distinction between "artificial" and "natural" color additives; from the FDA's perspective, all color additives are "artificial" regardless of source.*

3. *1990 Nutrition Labeling and Education Act (NLEA)*: Through the 1970s and 1980s, pressure began building for the provision of accurate, comprehensible nutrition information on the labels of packaged foods. Among other things, the NLEA authorized FDA to issue regulations requiring the provision of nutrition information in a specified format and establishing requirements for the use of nutrient content claims and health claims. These requirements are addressed in detail elsewhere in this volume. It suffices to say that NLEA ushered in the modern era of nutrition labeling. Nearly 20 years later, some of its provisions, such as those governing health claims, are still being fleshed out in judicial decisions. Recent developments in the marketplace, such as the increasing use of nutrition symbols on the principal display panels of food labels, could test the limits of FDA's authority under the NLEA.

4. *1994 Dietary Supplement Health and Education Act (DSHEA)*: Prior to 1994, FDA regulated products marketed as dietary supplements as either foods or drugs. DSHEA amended the FDC Act to establish a separate regulatory framework for dietary supplements. Although dietary supplements are subject to many of the same general requirements as conventional foods, they are also subject to specific requirements that govern their manufacture, labeling, and introduction to the marketplace.†

The legal definition of "dietary supplement" is broad and includes the following dietary ingredients: vitamins, minerals, herbs and other botanicals, amino acids, and any dietary substance for use by man to supplement the diet by increasing the total dietary intake. All dietary ingredients used in dietary supplements must be safe (i.e., they must not present a significant or unreasonable risk of injury under their recommended conditions of use, or in the absence thereof, under ordinary conditions of use). However, dietary ingredients that were not marketed prior to October 15, 1994, are "new dietary ingredients" (NDIs) that are subject to additional requirements. For any NDI, there must be adequate information to provide reasonable assurance that the NDI does not present a significant or unreasonable risk of illness or injury. In the absence of such information, any dietary supplement containing the NDI is deemed adulterated. In addition, an NDI must be the subject of a premarket notification submitted to FDA unless the NDI has been present in the food supply as an article used for food in a form in which the food has not been chemically altered.

Dietary supplements must be manufactured in compliance with comprehensive GMP regulations.‡ In addition, a manufacturer must report any serious adverse events to FDA.

Dietary supplements must be labeled to provide information on the dietary and other ingredients that they contain. At the option of the manufacturer or distributor, the label of a dietary supplement can also bear certain types of claims, namely, (1) claims of a benefit related to a classical nutrient deficiency disease, (2) claims that describe the role of a nutrient or dietary ingredient intended to affect the structure or function in humans, or that characterize the documented mechanism by which a nutrient or dietary ingredient acts to maintain such structure or function, and (3) claims that describe general well-being from the consumption of a nutrient or dietary ingredient.

5. *2004 Food Allergen Labeling and Consumer Protection Act (FALCPA)*: Since 1938, food labels have been required to bear a declaration of their ingredients by common or usual name, except that flavors and colors can be declared collectively. In some instances, this requirement failed to ensure that information on the presence of a food allergen was adequately conveyed to consumers with food allergies. The common or usual name of an ingredient might or might not readily reveal that the ingredient was derived from a food allergen such as milk or peanut, and the exception for collective declaration of flavors meant that food allergens present as flavors would remain undisclosed (declaration of allergenic colors can be required as a condition of premarket approval). FALCPA amended the FDC Act to require disclosure of the presence of a major food allergen (i.e., peanut, tree nut, soy, wheat, fish, Crustacean shellfish, milk, and egg) either in parentheses after the name of the ingredient (e.g., "casein [milk]") or in a separate "contains" statement

---

* FDA maintains a web page on its regulation of color additives at http://www.fda.gov/ForIndustry/ColorAdditives/default.htm

† FDA maintains a web page on its regulation of dietary supplements at http://www.fda.gov/Food/DietarySupplements/default.htm

‡ The dietary supplement GMP regulations are found in 21 CFR Part 111.

(e.g., "Contains milk").* Although this requirement is of clear benefit to food-allergic consumers, it has proven challenging for industry to implement on a consistent basis. Allergen-related labeling errors have become one of the principal causes of food recalls.[†]

6. *2010 Patient Protection and Affordable Care Act (PPACA)*: The nutrition labeling requirements ushered in by NLEA did not extend to restaurants. In the 20 years since, three trends emerged that prompted Congress to revisit the issue. First, government estimates of the percentage of consumers believed to be obese increased significantly. Second, consumers increased their reliance on so-called away-from-home foods to fulfill their dietary needs. Third, municipalities began imposing their own disparate requirements for restaurants to provide nutrition information. PPACA therefore amended the FDCA to require that restaurants with 20 or more locations provide certain nutrition information on their menus or menu boards, informally referred to as "menu labeling." At present, FDA is working on regulations to implement menu labeling requirements.[‡]

7. *2011 FDA Food Safety Modernization Act (FSMA)*: The passage of the FSMA marked the first comprehensive overhaul of the food safety requirements in the FDCA since 1938. Recurring outbreaks of foodborne illness and greater reliance on imported foods led Congress to conclude that the existing emphasis on responsive measures was no longer adequate to ensure food safety and that the FDCA needed to be amended to place greater emphasis on preventive practices and controls.

For our purposes, it is most useful to highlight two major changes made by the FSMA. First, the FSMA took the systemic, preventive approach embodied in FDA's HACCP regulations for juice and seafood, and extended it to virtually the entire food industry. The FSMA eschews the term "HACCP" in favor of Hazard Analysis and Risk-Based Preventive Controls (HARBPC). Once the HARBPC requirements take effect, an owner, operator, or agent in charge of a facility engaged in manufacturing, processing, packing, or holding food will be required to take the following actions:

a. Develop a written analysis that identifies and evaluates a wide range of known or reasonably foreseeable hazards, including those that may be intentionally introduced

b. Implement preventive controls, including at critical control points, to assure that the identified hazards are significantly minimized or prevented

c. Monitor the effectiveness of the preventive controls

d. Establish procedures to ensure that corrective action is taken in instances where preventive controls are not properly implemented or proven ineffective

e. Verify the adequacy of preventive controls, monitoring, and corrective actions

f. Prepare a written plan that documents the procedures used to comply with the earlier requirements

g. Keep records documenting the earlier activities

Second, in recognition of the fact that the manufacture and the distribution of food are increasingly a global enterprise, the FSMA imposed the obligation on food importers to develop and implement a Foreign Supplier Verification Program (FSVP). The goal of an importer's FSVP is to ensure that its suppliers comply with processes and procedures that provide the same level of public health protection as HARBPC and that the foods that the importer introduces into domestic commerce are as safe as domestically produced foods. Examples of verification activities that an importer may be expected to perform include annual on-site inspection, checking of the HARBPC plan of the foreign supplier, periodic testing and sampling of shipments, and lot-by-lot certification of compliance.

At present, FDA is working on regulations and guidance documents to implement the HARBPC and FSVP requirements—an endeavor that could take years to finalize.[§]

Comparatively speaking, the laws administered by USDA have seen less change over time. In instances where the FDCA was amended in ways that affected USDA's programs, such as through the requirement of nutrition labeling and allergen labeling, USDA made conforming changes in its regulations or policies to maintain overall consistency in the two agencies' regulatory approaches. Similarly, the FTC's approach to regulation of food advertising has largely tracked FDA's approach to regulation of food labeling.

## STATE AND LOCAL LAWS

Many states have enacted laws that largely mirror the FDCA, such as California's Sherman Food, Drug, and Cosmetic Act.[¶] Further, state regulatory agencies generally try to coordinate their activities with those of FDA so as to minimize the waste of federal and state resources that would result from the conduct of duplicative activities. In point of fact, most FDA inspections of manufacturers are conducted by state officials under contract with FDA.

---

* Guidance on food allergen labeling is available at http://www.fda.gov/Food/LabelingNutrition/FoodAllergensLabeling/default.htm

[†] Information on FDA's implementation of menu labeling is available at http://www.fda.gov/Food/LabelingNutrition/ucm217762.htm

[‡] Information on FDA's implementation of menu labeling is available at http://www.fda.gov/Food/LabelingNutrition/ucm217762.htm

[§] Information on FDA's implementation of FSMA is available at http://www.fda.gov/Food/FoodSafety/FSMA/default.htm

[¶] The full text of the Sherman Law is available at http://www.cdph.ca.gov/services/Documents/fdb%20Sher%20Law.pdf

Ensuring consistency in the requirements of federal and state agencies is a significant preoccupation of food manufacturers, whose ability to efficiently and profitably manufacture and distribute foods can be compromised by the need to comply with differing and potentially conflicting requirements. When state and local authorities enact requirements that go beyond federal requirements or that differ from one another, the stage is often set for the passage of new federal laws intended to achieve uniformity and thereby facilitate interstate commerce. In one recent example described earlier, the adoption by some localities of requirements that restaurants provide certain nutrition information to their customers prompted the inclusion of such a requirement in recently enacted national healthcare legislation (PPACA).

FDA does not exercise its jurisdiction over retail food establishments such as restaurants. Instead, FDA sponsors development and maintenance of the FDA Model Food Code.* The Model Food Code is used by the state and local regulators to develop their own requirements for the retail food sector. As of 2005, 48 of 56 states and territories were reported to have adopted food codes that are "patterned after" some version of the Model Food Code, of which a new version is released every 4 years. There has been renewed interest in the regulation of the retail food sector, given consumers' increasing consumption of so-called away-from-home foods.

In addition to the laws administered by state agencies, food manufacturers must contend with lawsuits filed by consumers under various causes of action provided under state law. In cases of illness or injury believed to result from food contamination, the lawsuit typically alleges negligence on the part of the manufacturer and/or breach of express or implied warranty. In cases where the veracity of marketing claims is at stake, the lawsuit typically alleges false advertising and/or unlawful, unfair, or fraudulent business acts or practices. The potential losses associated with such lawsuits are believed to provide an additional incentive to manufacturers to comply with all applicable federal and state requirements.

## FURTHER READING

As is hopefully evident from this brief summary, food law is a discipline that rewards the intellectually curious. Readers may wish to consult the following texts for a more in-depth treatment of the subject: *Food Regulation: Law, Science, Policy, and Practice*, Neal J. Fortin, J.D.; *Food and Drug Law*, 3rd edn., Peter B. Hutt, Richard A Merrill, Lewis A. Grossman, I. Nelson Rose (especially Chapter III); and *FDA's Creative Application of the Law: Not Merely A Collection of Words*, 2nd edn., Frederick H. Degnan. The author helps maintain a blog on current developments in food and drug law at www.fdalawblog.net

---

* Information on FDA's Retail Food Protection Program, including the Model Food Code, is available at http://www.fda.gov/Food/FoodSafety/RetailFoodProtection/default.htm

# 7 Computerized Nutrient Analysis Systems

*Judith Ashley and Doina Kulick*

## CONTENTS

## INTRODUCTION

Since the early 1980s, the incorporation of microcomputer technology into nutrient analysis has resulted in the advent of computerized nutrient analysis systems. These software systems offer an effective and time-saving method for calculating the nutrient composition of foods and beverages for a variety of applications.[1–5] Health professionals can use computerized dietary analyses to provide clients with specific information about their current food/beverage choices and healthful alternatives, with the goal of fostering positive dietary changes. For nutrition educators, the hands-on application of these software programs is an integral part of student education. For researchers and government agencies, nutrient analysis software is an essential tool for analyzing and documenting the usual food intake of individuals, groups, or populations for a variety of uses (e.g., identifying diet–disease relationships). Nutrient analysis software is also important for recipe and menu development by food service managers, chefs, and caterers, and for calculating nutrient information for food labels.

Several companies and organizations offer nutrient analysis software. To be competitive in the market and to stay abreast of changes in scientific knowledge and food production, software vendors must frequently update their programs and the quality and scope of their services. In general, nutrient analysis software programs provide information about the nutrient composition of foods and beverages using government and academic databases, as well as food industry information and the scientific literature. Specific information about foods/beverages (e.g., type or quantity) is entered into the program and assigned a code. The software then uses these codes to locate and store information about the nutrient composition of the specific food items selected and, eventually, to sum across all foods for each nutrient or nutrient component. Programs vary considerably in cost, ease of use, capabilities, size, and available features.[6–8] For the prospective user, the choice of software requires careful consideration of needs and available resources, and financial support for computer hardware and peripherals.

## FEATURES OF NUTRIENT ANALYSIS SOFTWARE

Primary features of nutrient analysis software include (1) food descriptions, (2) food portions and weights, (3) nutrients and food components, (4) a user interface, and (5) output options.

Commonly, programs include reference standards for evaluating dietary quality (e.g., Dietary Reference Intakes [DRI] and Dietary Guidelines for Americans 2010) and allow users to enter tracking or contact information (e.g., case number, name, address, telephone number, and email address) and data about physiological characteristics (e.g., gender, age, height, and weight; for women, pregnancy or lactation status) specific to individual subjects or clients. This latter feature makes it possible to tailor reference standards to reflect client profiles (e.g., energy needs or targeted weight goals). Refer to Table 7.1 for contact information, program applications, and database characteristics of some of the programs currently available and Table 7.2 for a comprehensive list of nutrients and food components included in such programs.

Programs vary considerably in the number and types of available output options, with some offering both electronic and printed reports, and textual and graphical data displays (e.g., 2D and 3D pie and bar charts). Report contents also vary by vendor and may include simple nutrient summaries, lists of foods in descending or ascending order by nutrient contribution, or recommendations for enhancing dietary quality.

Additional software features include mechanisms for comparing food/beverage choices with food exchange lists; assessing nutrient intake by meal, food item, or food category; and classifying foods according to the glycemic index or glycemic load. Programs are also available that allow data to be collected and averaged for individuals or groups or for a specified time period, ranging from a single eating occasion to several days' worth of meals and snacks.

**TABLE 7.1**
**Selected Nutrition Analysis Software Systems**

| Software Name | Company/ Organization | Web Address | Food Database/s | Number of Foods in Database | Number of Nutrients/Food Components | General Software Uses[a] |
|---|---|---|---|---|---|---|
| ASA24[b] | National Cancer Institute | www.riskfactor.cancer.gov/ tools/instruments/asa24 | USDA NDB SR, FNDDS, MPED, (NHANES) Dietary Supplement Database | 7,000 | 97 | Nutrient analysis Nutrition assessment |
| Food Intake Analysis System (FIAS) | University of Texas School of Public Health | www.sph.uth.tmc.edu/ research/centers/dell/ fias-food-intake-and- analysis-system/ | USDA NDB SR, CSFII/FNDDS, other | 7,300 | 64 | Nutrient analysis Nutrition assessment Recipe calculations |
| Food Processor SQL | ESHA Research | www.esha.com | USDA NDB SR, CSFII/FNDDS, Canadian Nutrient File, other | 40,000 | 144 | Client management Exercise tracking Nutrition analysis Menu management NLEA food labels |
| Foodworks[14] | The Nutrition Company | www.nutritionco.com | USDA NDB SR, CSFII/FNDDS, Canadian Nutrient File, other | >30,000 | 113 | Nutrient analysis Nutrition assessment Recipe calculations |
| NutriGenie[c] | NutriGenie | www.nutrigenie.biz/ | USDA NDB SR, other | 8,000 | 30 | Menu management Nutrient analysis Nutrition assessment |
| Nutrition Data System for Research (NDS-R) | Nutrition Coordinating Center, University of Minnesota | www.ncc.umn.edu | USDA NDB SR, CSFII/FNDDS, other | 18,000 | 140 | Nutrient analysis Nutrition assessment Recipe Calculations Menu management |
| Nutritionist Pro™[c] | Axxya Systems | www.nutritionistpro.com | USDA NDB SR, CSFII/FNDDS, Alaskan foods, Canadian Nutrient File, Mexifoods database, Malaysian foods database, other | >32,000 | 90 | Nutrient analysis of diets, recipes, and menus Nutrient analysis Corporate wellness consulting NLEA food labels |
| Nutrition Service Suite®[c] | The CBORD Group, Inc. | http://hcl.cbord.com/ products/product_193 | USDA NDB SR, CSFII/FNDDS, Canadian Nutrient, other | 20,000 | 143 | Food service management Menu management Nutrient analysis Nutrition assessment NLEA food labels |

*Source:*   Stein, K., *J. Am. Diet Assoc.*, 111, 214, 2011; *35th National Nutrient Databank Conference*, International Nutrient Databank Directory, Software Vendors, www.nutrientdataconf.org/indd/, accessed on March 1, 2012.

[a]   For complete software uses access the product website.

[b]   Free software system.

[c]   Multiple products available; product characteristics vary.

**TABLE 7.2**
**Dietary Components Available in Computerized Nutrient Analysis Systems**

*Energy sources*
  Energy (kcal)
  Energy (kJ)
  Total protein
    Animal protein
    Vegetable protein
  Total fat
  Total carbohydrate
  Alcohol
  Percentage of calories from
    Protein
    Fat
    *Trans* fat
    Carbohydrate
    Alcohol
*Fat and cholesterol*
  Cholesterol
  Total saturated FA[a] (SFA)
  Total monounsaturated FA[a] (MUFA)
  Total polyunsaturated FA[a] (PUFA)
  Total *trans* FA[a] (TFA)
  Total omega-3 FA[a]
    Eicosapentaenoic acid 20:5
    Docosahexaenoic acid 22:6
  Total omega-6 FA[a]
    Docosapentaenoic acid 22:5
*Percentage of calories from*
  SFA
  MUFA
  PUFA
  PUFA:SFA
  Cholesterol to SFA index
*Fatty acids*
  SFA: 4:0–22:0
  MUFA: 14:1–22:1
  PUFA: 18:2–22:6
  *Trans* FA: 16:1–18:2
  *CLA cis-9,trans-11*
  *CLA trans-10,cis-12*
*Carbohydrates*
  Starch
  Total sugar
  Added sugar
  Fructose
  Galactose
  Glucose
  Lactose
  Maltose
  Sucrose
*Fiber*
  Total dietary fiber
  Soluble fiber
  Insoluble fiber
  Pectins

**TABLE 7.2 (continued)**
**Dietary Components Available in Computerized Nutrient Analysis Systems**

*Vitamins*
  Total vitamin A activity (RE[b] and IU)
  Beta–carotene equivalents
  Vitamin E, IU[c]
  Vitamin E, total alpha-tocopherol
  Natural alpha-tocopherol
  Synthetic alpha-tocopherol
  Total alpha–tocopherol equivalents
  Beta-tocopherol
  Gamma-tocopherol
  Delta-tocopherol
  Vitamin C
  Vitamin D (IU and micrograms)
  Vitamin K
  Thiamin ($B_1$)
  Riboflavin ($B_2$)
  Niacin ($B_3$)
  Niacin equivalents
  Folate
  Dietary folate equivalents
  Natural folate
  Synthetic folate (folic acid)
  Vitamin $B_6$
  Vitamin $B_{12}$
  Pantothenic acid
  Biotin
*Carotenoids*
  Beta-carotene (provitamin A carotenoid)
  Alpha-carotene (provitamin A carotenoid)
  Beta-cryptoxanthin (provitamin A carotenoid)
  Lutein + Zeaxanthin
  Lycopene
*Minerals*
  Calcium
  Chloride
  Chromium
  Copper
  Iodine
    Fluoride
  Iron
  Magnesium
  Manganese
  Molybdenum
  Phosphorous
  Potassium
  Selenium
  Sodium
  Zinc
*Amino acids*
  Tryptophan
  Threonine
  Isoleucine
  Leucine
  Lysine

*(continued)*

**TABLE 7.2 (continued)**
**Dietary Components Available in Computerized Nutrient Analysis Systems**

Methionine
Cystine
Phenylalanine
Tyrosine
Valine
Arginine
Histidine
Alanine
Aspartic acid
Glutamic acid
Glycine
Proline
Serine
*Isoflavones*
  Daidzein
  Genestein
  Glycitein
  Coumestrol
  Biochanin A
  Formononetein
*Sugar alcohols, total*
  Erythritol
  Inositol
  Isomalt
  Lactitol
  Maltitol
  Pinitol
  Sorbitol
  Xylitol
*Sweeteners*
  Acesulfame potassium
  Aspartame
  Saccharine
  Suclarose
  Tagatose
*Other*
  Betaine
  Caffeine
  Choline
  Glycemic index
  Glycemic load
  3-Methylhistidine
  Nitrogen
  Oxalic acid
  Phytic acid
  Sucrose polyester

ᵃ FA, fatty acids.
ᵇ RE, retinol equivalents.
ᶜ IU, International Units.

Some programs allow users to export data into statistical analysis software packages or word-processing programs or to enter data by scanning questionnaires (e.g., food frequency checklists). The latter would be useful for entering large data sets or calorie-count data for patients who are hospitalized or institutionalized. Alternatively, nutrient analysis software might support multiuser platforms, interface with food service management software, provide information about potential food–drug interactions, contain recipe databases, and include nutrient information for nutrition support regimens. Programs are available that allow users to add or modify foods, nutrients, and recipes; scale or cost recipes; plan meals; generate sample menus; or customize nutrition support regimens.

## BASIC QUESTIONS WHEN CONSIDERING DIFFERENT SOFTWARE SYSTEMS

Depending on the projected use of nutrient analysis software, many or all of the following questions may apply when evaluating individual programs:

- What are the operating system and hardware requirements? Are these requirements compatible with existing equipment and peripherals? If not, are funds available to purchase new hardware?
- How many food items are included in the database? What types of foods are included? For example, does the database contain information about baby foods, convenience foods, fast foods, regional specialties, ethnic specialties, fortified/enriched foods, fat-modified foods, sugar-free foods, or nutritional supplements? Can foods, beverages, or recipes be added?
- What specific nutrients and nutritional components are in the database? Does this list include the nutrients and food components or values (e.g., glycemic index or glycemic load) of interest to you? Is the number of nutrients in the database at the low-end, middle, or high-end range of available nutrients? Can information about nutrients and food components be added?
- How complete is the nutrient information? What are the origins of nutrient values? What is the extent of missing values? When data for specific nutrients are missing, are these estimated or left as zero? Are missing nutrient values identified in reports so that findings are not misleading? (*Note*: Methods for estimating and reporting missing values dramatically affect the accuracy of nutrient reports.)
- What dietary reference standards are available for use? Are these standards up-to-date (e.g., vitamin D)? Are standards included for subpopulations (e.g., children, pregnant or lactating women)?
- How is the quality of the database maintained? How often is the software upgraded to reflect changes in the market or advances in scientific knowledge?

- How easy or difficult is it to enter dietary information? Do data entry options include numeric code, food name, brand name, and search features? Can users store or copy frequently used food or meal categories for ready access? Is technical support available to assist users in distinguishing among food listings?

- Can data related to portion sizes be entered using weight, volume, dimensions, or all three measures? Can data be entered in common household measures?

- Does the software allow data from standard food frequency forms to be entered? Can data from such forms be scanned? Is this option included in the usual cost of the software or available for a price?

- Are reports available for a variety of criteria such as reference standards (e.g., RDA), dietary recommendations (e.g., MyPlate Food Guidance System), and meal planning methods (e.g., food exchange lists)? Can reports be customized to reflect specific nutrients?

- Are reports available that summarize intake data from several days or weeks for comprehensive analysis? Are reports available that summarize intake data by eating occasion? Are reports available that summarize intake data by days of the week? Are reports available that compare data from several points in time to allow for longitudinal comparisons?

- Are reports available that identify key sources of nutrients from the data entered? Can lists of food sources of nutrients be generated?

- Are on-screen reports available in a form that is suitable for use with clients? Can dietary choices be manipulated to demonstrate the effects of dietary changes on nutrient intake or dietary quality? Is this feedback provided instantaneously?

- Are printed reports available? How many options for reference criterion and nutrient content are available for printed reports? Can additional information or comments be added to printed reports?

- Are reports available that use easy-to-understand graphics (e.g., bar graphs and pie charts) and tables to compare intake with designated standards? Are these graphical comparisons available for a variety of reference criterion (see aforementioned text) and nutrients?

- Are reports accurate, descriptive, and attractive? Are key findings or recommendations readily apparent and concise?

- What formulas are used to calculate energy requirements? If healthy or ideal body weights are suggested, how are these determined? Are such recommendations based on current and reasonable standards?

- Can exercise data be incorporated into caloric requirements? Do reports include exercise recommendations?

- Are there system utilities for backing up valuable data and reports? Are there mechanisms in place to maintain the confidentiality of client information?

- What is the quality of software documentation, online help, and tutorials? Are these easy to understand and specific to user needs? Are these comprehensive in scope?

- What is the quality of customer service, product support, and ongoing maintenance? Is there sufficient technical support provided to answer user needs? Is training available or required?

- What does the complete system, with updates and service, cost? Are there additional costs for multiple users or stations?

- How often are upgrades offered? Is there an additional cost for upgrades?

- Who is the target audience of the output? Are appropriate output options available for consumers, health professionals, medical centers or hospitals, or researchers?

## IMPORTANCE OF FOOD COMPOSITION DATABASES

Nutrient analysis software relies heavily on existing food composition databases for nutrient information. Importantly, multiple factors affect the accuracy of these databases, such as the sources of nutrient composition information, the number of foods and nutrients in the database, the number of missing values, the methods by which missing values are handled, and the frequency with which databases are updated.[9–13] Several published reports have compared the accuracy of nutrient calculations among a limited number of database systems.[14–25] When these calculations were compared with a standard,[20–22] or tested against chemical analyses from a single source,[23–25] findings indicated that most nutrients were within 15% of reference values. For example, after comparing calculations from four different computerized nutrient databases to chemical composition analysis of 36 menus used in the Dietary Approaches to Stop Hypertension (DASH) trial, researchers found that the database values for the nutrients examined had relatively good accuracy and precision: seven nutrients deviated by values <10%; five, by 10%–15%; and only one, by 15%–20%.[25] While these findings are positive, it is important to note that no standardized benchmarks have been established for comparing the different methods used to determine the nutrient content of foods/beverages. In addition to the quality of nutrient composition databases, other factors affect the accuracy of nutrient analyses (e.g., see Table 7.3).

Most nutrient analysis systems in the United States are based primarily on USDA Nutrient Database for Standard Reference (NDSR) which is available to the public and scientific community on the Internet at no cost.[26] Data can be viewed or downloaded for use on computers with various software packages. An online search is provided to look up

## TABLE 7.3
### Factors That May Affect Consistency of Nutrient Analysis Outputs

Data entry errors (e.g., misidentification of foods or incorrect food substitutions)
Nutrient variability in the food supply
Frequent changes in the nutrient content of processed foods
Margin of error allowed for nutrient information from food labels
Estimated or imputed values for missing nutrient information
Constraints of chemically determined nutrient values used for comparison (e.g., sample collection or assayed values)

## TABLE 7.4
### Nutrient Analysis Software Reports: Discussion Topics for Patient Counseling

Comments that explain and clarify results
Synopsis of the limitations of the analysis
Suggestions to improve dietary intake (e.g., information about good food sources of specific nutrients)
Information about dietary supplements (if warranted)
Information about supplementary resources, as appropriate

the nutrient content of different foods as well as nutrient lists for selected foods and nutrients. Included are details about all of the foods in the database (e.g., scientific name and nutrient content), nutrient lists for selected foods and nutrients, and documentation (e.g., content of files, weights and measures, and data sources). The Nutrient Data Laboratory also provides access to additional special interest databases for some nutrients (i.e., choline and fluoride) and specific dietary components (i.e., flavonoids, isoflavones, proanthocyanidins, and oxalic acid). The NDSR database is routinely updated and increases in size with each new release. For example, the most recent version, NDSR-24, contains data for over 7906 foods for up to 146 nutrients and food components, including an updated flavonoid data for 500 food items as well as new nutrient datasets for retail cuts of beef and pork.

## LIMITATIONS OF NUTRIENT ANALYSIS SOFTWARE

Nutrient analysis software programs have unique limitations.[6] For example, calculations of nutrient intakes may lack precision because of the multiple variables involved, including the size and quality of the databases, calculation methods, and extent of missing values. However, these software-related variables are minor when compared with the human challenges to accuracy. Food intake reports from clients and subjects (e.g., food records and food frequencies) may be inaccurate. Data entry errors may occur if operators misinterpret food descriptions or do not select the correct matches from the database. In other cases, results may be misinterpreted. For example, computer-generated printouts might appear authoritative, giving the impression that reports are extremely precise, but this may not always be the case (e.g., database may contain multiple missing values). Additionally, individuals unfamiliar with DRI/RDA comparisons may misinterpret these values as minimal nutrient needs and assume that intake levels should be over 100% to avoid deficiencies. Even professionals may have difficulty drawing specific conclusions for individuals when using the DRI/RDA as reference standards.

With regard to these and other limitations, health professionals who use nutrient analysis software to evaluate dietary

intake of clients and patients are advised to provide counseling along with software-generated reports (see Table 7.4 for suggestions).

## TRENDS IN NUTRIENT ANALYSIS SOFTWARE

Continual advances in scientific knowledge and technology, changes in dietary guidance, and variations in the needs and interests of researchers, educators, and health professionals present constant challenges and multiple opportunities for the development and maintenance of and applications for nutrient analysis software. Mobile technologies including mobile phones/smartphones, handheld personal digital assistants (PDAs), and tablet computer (iPad) are increasingly employed in the computerized nutrition analysis. Mobile phones/smartphones are the most commonly used mobile devices. Digital photograph capability of these devices provide a real-time method of capturing food consumption that is fast, flexible, and easily accessible at any time. These features may overcome some of the barriers related to self-report.[27] The expanded marketing and adoption of smartphones and mobile-friendly website applications will allow for convenient access to nutrition information, instruction, and behavior change support systems.[28]

## CONCLUSION

Nutrient analysis software can be a useful tool for individuals, agencies, or organizations interested in assessing the dietary intake of individuals and populations. Output from these programs can be used to provide specific guidance or develop interventions that may ultimately improve dietary intake and health among individuals and populations. It is important to keep abreast of the ongoing improvements in nutrient analysis technology and potential uses of the available software, Internet, and wireless programs in order to use them effectively in a variety of practice settings.

## REFERENCES

1. Youngwirth, J., *J Am Diet Assoc*, 82: 62–67; 1983.
2. Hoover, L.W., *Clin Nutr*, 6: 198; 1987.
3. Feskanich, D., Buzzard, I.M., Welch, B.T. et al., *J Am Diet Assoc*, 88: 1263; 1988.

4. Harrison, G.G., *J Food Compost Anal*, 17: 259; 2004.

5. Stumbo, P.J. and Murphy, S.P., *J Food Compost Anal*, 17: 485; 2004.

6. Grossbauer, S., in *Communicating as Professionals*, 2nd edn., Chernoff, R., Ed., The American Dietetic Association, Chicago, IL, 1994, p. 56.

7. Prestwood, E., *Today's Dietitian*, December: 44; 2005.

8. Pennington, J.A.T., Stumbo, P.J., Murphy, S.P. et al., *J Am Diet Assoc*, 107: 2105; 2007.

9. Dwyer, J.T., Picciano, M.F., Betz, J.M. et al., *J Food Compost Anal*, 17: 493; 2004.

10. Stumbo, P., *J Food Compost Anal*, 21(Suppl 1): S13; 2008.

11. Adelman, M.O., Dwyer, J.T., Woods, M. et al., *J Am Diet Assoc*, 83: 421; 1983.

12. Buzzard, I.M., Price, K.S., and Warren, R.A., *Am J Clin Nutr*, 54: 7; 1991.

13. Hoover, L.W., *J Am Diet Assoc*, 83: 501; 1983.

14. Frank, G.C., Farris, R.P., Hyg, M.S. et al., *J Am Diet Assoc*, 84: 818; 1984.

15. Taylor, M.L., Kozlowski, B.W., and Baer, M.T., *J Am Diet Assoc*, 85: 1136; 1985.

16. Shanklin, D., Endres, J.M., and Sawicki, M., *J Am Diet Assoc*, 85: 308; 1985.

17. Eck, L.H., Klesges, R.C., Hanson, C.L. et al., *J Am Diet Assoc*, 88: 602; 1988.

18. Stumbo, P.J., *J Am Diet Assoc*, 92: 57; 1992.

19. LaComb, R.P., Taylor, M.L., and Noble, J.M., *J Am Diet Assoc*, 92: 1391; 1992.

20. Nieman, D.C. and Nieman, C.N., *J Am Diet Assoc*, 81: 930; 1987.

21. Nieman, D.C., Butterworth, D.E., Nieman, C.N. et al., *J Am Diet Assoc*, 92: 48; 1992.

22. Lee, R.D., Nieman, D.C., and Rainwater, M., *J Am Diet Assoc*, 95: 858; 1995.

23. Pennington, J.A.T. and Wilson, D.B., *J Am Diet Assoc*, 90: 375; 1990.

24. McKeown, N.M., Rasmussen, H.M., Charnley, J.M. et al., *J Am Diet Assoc*, 100: 1201; 2000.

25. McCullough, M.L., Karanja, N.M., Lin, P.H. et al., *J Am Diet Assoc*, 99: 545; 1999.

26. U.S. Department of Agriculture (USDA) National Nutrient Database for Standard, http://ndb.nal.usda.gov/, accessed: April 1, 2012.

27. Zhu, F., Bosch, M., Woo, I. et al., *IEEE J Sel Topics Signal Process*, 4: 756; 2010.

28. Free, C., Phillips, G., Felix, L. et al., *BMC Res Notes*, 3: 250; 2010.

29. Stein, K., *J Am Diet Assoc*, 111: 214; 2011.

30. Steering Committee of the 35th National Nutrient Databank Conference, Bethesda, MD, International Nutrient Databank Directory, Software Vendors, www.nutrientdataconf.org/indd/, accessed: March 1, 2012.

# Part II

Nutrition Science

# 8 Food Intake Regulation

*Lynda M. Brown and Deborah J. Clegg*

## CONTENTS

## INTRODUCTION

In its simplest form, the regulation of body weight involves a negative feedback loop where factors generated in proportion to body fat act centrally to control energy intake and expenditure.[1,2] It involves hormones secreted in proportion to body fat that are able to communicate with the brain by binding to their receptors within the central nervous system (CNS),[3] which is a confirmation of the lipostatic hypothesis proposed by Kennedy.[4] This review will focus on the regulation of food intake by adiposity signals that begin as peripheral circulating factor that communicate with the brain in a negative feedback loop.

## CRITICAL CNS CIRCUITS FOR THE REGULATION OF BODY WEIGHT

Leptin and insulin act centrally through receptors in the hypothalamus to control food intake and energy balance.[5–9] The hypothalamus is a complex structure of nuclei, pathways, and neurotransmitter systems that control food intake.[7,8,10,11] Early interest in the hypothalamus stemmed from findings that dramatic changes in food intake and energy homeostasis were produced by lesioning specific hypothalamic nuclei. This led to the dual-center hypothesis.[12] Stellar eloquently argued that the hypothalamus is the central neural structure involved in the control of food intake more specifically and that this "control" is represented by two separate hypothalamic nuclei. The first was the "satiety" in the ventromedial hypothalamus (VMH). Hetherington and colleagues provided strong evidence for this hypothesis with experiments that bilaterally lesioned the VMH. VMH-lesioned rats ate more than controls and became obese.[13,14] These rats were thought to have a defect in satiety, and as a result, the VMH was termed the "satiety" center.[15,16] Second, electrical stimulation of the VMH caused animals to stop eating, i.e., to demonstrate

enhanced satiety.[17] In contrast to the VMH, lesions of the lateral hypothalamic area (LHA) resulted in rats that stopped eating and lost body weight.[18] Additionally, electrical stimulation of the LHA caused sated rats to eat.[19] As a consequence, the LHA was considered to be the brain's hunger center.[20] The dual-center hypothesis was the dominant theory of how the CNS controlled food intake for many years.[12,21,22]

## ANABOLIC AND CATABOLIC CIRCUITS FOR THE REGULATION OF BODY WEIGHT

Hypothalamic effector systems that respond to hormonal adiposity signals have been identified and potently influence food intake and energy balance.[23–25] On functional grounds, hypothalamic effector systems can be described as anabolic or catabolic. Anabolic effectors increase food intake, decrease energy expenditure, and consequently increase adipose tissue. They are activated when energy stores are low (negative energy balance) as signaled by reduced levels of insulin and leptin. Catabolic effectors do just the opposite and are activated by positive energy balance. These pathways decrease food intake, increase energy expenditure, and decrease the amount of adipose tissue. A critical aspect of this negative feedback model is that hormones responsive to increasing levels of adiposity are proposed to inhibit anabolic pathways while activating catabolic pathways, and the balance of these pathways that ultimately determines food intake and energy balance.[23–25]

## REGULATION OF FOOD INTAKE

Most adult mammals, including humans, maintain a relatively constant level of adiposity over long intervals.[26–29] This occurs despite the variability of daily food intake, variations in energy expenditure, and differences in physical activity.

There is a level of homeostasis in the body weight, and it is often explained in thermodynamic terms, i.e., energy balance, which is measured through basal metabolism, heat production, and physical activity. The accuracy of body weight regulation has several features. First, the amount of body weight/fat is regulated under strict feedback control, such that when there are changes to body weight due to fat loss, processes are employed to restore equilibrium by restoring body weight. Second, there is coordination of peripheral signals that alert the CNS when body weight changes. This homeostatic system suggests that the brain senses the amount of body weight/body. When changes in energy balance occur, the brain takes corrective action and generates signals that will restore homeostasis.

This makes teleological sense as the body would defend against changes in body weight in the downward direction, protecting the species from weight loss. However, this could also explain why dieters have such a difficult time maintaining weight loss—the body has a homeostatic tendency to defend against negative energy balance. Importantly, not only does the brain regulate food intake during this process, but also it regulates the number of calories burned or energy expenditure, and therefore can adapt or make changes to facilitate body weight restoration.[27,30,31]

This homeostatic mechanism is represented in Figure 8.1, in which signals from the periphery, adiposity signals, are released into circulation and cross the blood–brain barrier (BBB). They then bind to receptors within the CNS, and food intake is increased or decreased to restore body

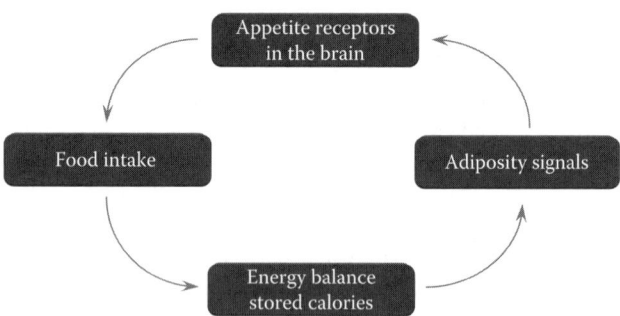

**FIGURE 8.1** Hormone regulation of body weight: a simple model. The hormone regulation of body weight is modeled in this figure. There are signals from the periphery, which are called appetite (adiposity) signals, which are released into circulation in proportion to the amount of body fat. The adiposity signals cross the BBB and bind to receptors that are located in critical regions within the CNS. Once these signals are initiated, food intake is driven in an attempt to maintain energy balance. The stored calories then impact the adiposity signals that begin the process again. Given that the brain is thought to control hunger and appetite, this homeostatic system would suggest that the brain is able to sense the amount of body weight/body fat. When changes in energy balance occur, the brain takes corrective action and generates signals that will restore homeostasis. Importantly, not only does the brain regulate food intake during this process, but it also regulates the number of calories stored, represented by energy balance, and therefore can make changes in metabolic rate in concert with changes in food intake to facilitate body weight restoration.

weight homeostasis. An example would be that when there is a reduction in body weight/body adiposity, a signal to be released from the now smaller fat stores, which alerts the CNS to increase food intake and body weight. The precision of the body weight regulatory system is further illustrated when adipose tissue is surgically removed and the suddenly "below-body weight homeostasis individual" will consume extra calories to regain the lost weight.[32–34] In contrast, when there is an increase in body weight/adiposity, this causes signals from the expanded adipose tissue to be released and received in the CNS resulting in lower food intake and eventually reduced body weight.

## INSULIN AND LEPTIN AS ADIPOSITY SIGNALS

Adiposity signals transmit information related to the size of adipose mass, and they potently influence energy balance.[35,36] While insulin is released from pancreatic beta cells following glucose stimulation, the magnitude of the response is tightly coupled to total adipose mass.[37,38] While peripheral administration of insulin results in increased food intake, when delivered in small amounts directly into the CNS, insulin decreases food intake.[39–41] This observation is consistent with the homeostatic theory of body weight regulation in that insulin regulates meal size, total food intake, and body weight.[9,42–45] Reduced insulin signaling caused by the administration of insulin antibodies[46] or by genetic disruption of the insulin receptors in the CNS[47] increases food intake and body weight.

First described in 1994, leptin is a key metabolic protein.[48] Leptin provides a powerful catabolic signal to the brain, resulting in the inhibition of food intake and increasing energy expenditure.[21,23,49–55] Leptin is secreted from adipose tissue in direct proportion to fat content, and it crosses the BBB to interact with leptin receptors in the hypothalamus.[49,50,52,56–58] Although there are several splice variants of the leptin receptor, the long form (termed OB-Rb) is the critical variant for regulating energy balance.[59] Ob-Rb is localized in several brain areas including the ventromedial nucleus (VMN) and the arcuate (ARC), and Ob-Rb is colocalized with several neuropeptides believed to be involved in controlling food intake.[60–62] Leptin has the ability to activate or inhibit discrete hypothalamic neurons,[62–64] which makes leptin ideally suited to link metabolic status and the amount of body fat.

Two critical features are required for a hormone to be considered an adiposity signal. The first feature is the need for circulating signals to have access to the CNS. Importantly, insulin crosses the BBB,[65] where it can interact with specific receptors for insulin that are found in the ARC.[66,67] The relationship between CNS and plasma levels of insulin is saturable (nonlinear), consistent with a receptor-mediated transport process. Like insulin, leptin crosses the BBB with kinetics that is consistent with active transport by a saturable receptor-mediated process.[68,69] Importantly, and consistent with these hormones' critical involvement in body weight homeostasis, relative levels of both leptin and insulin in the

CNS are decreased in association with obesity.[10,70–74] The functional implication is that in circumstances of chronic hyperinsulinemia and hyperleptinemia, such as obesity, leptin and insulin resistance would result in a disruption of regulation and obesity would result.

The second critical factor for these hormones to be adiposity signals is that their receptors must be located in key brain regions known to regulate food intake and body weight. Receptors for both insulin[47,75–77] and leptin[23,49,56,60–62,78] are expressed throughout the CNS. The medial hypothalamus, which is a key center for the regulation of energy homeostasis, is a major target for both insulin and leptin action.[6–10,79–81] Reduced leptin signaling produced by genetic disruption of the leptin receptor as in the *db/db* mouse or *fa/fa* rat results in dramatic increases in food intake and body weight.

While leptin and insulin have received considerable attention as afferent adiposity signals, there are other potential humoral factors as well. For example, growing evidence points to the possibility that amylin, a peptide hormone that is co-secreted with insulin from pancreatic beta cells, also acts as a negative feedback signal to the CNS.[82] Considerable evidence also implicates a role for adrenal glucocorticoids as potentially positive feedback signals in the control of food intake and energy balance.[22,83] However, the precise role of glucocorticoids in the control of energy homeostasis is complex and controversial.[81] The ultimate picture of how several circulating factors contribute to CNS regulation of energy homeostasis is far from complete and will likely involve complex interactions among many hormones and their receptors.

## ANABOLIC FACTORS

*NPY*: Neuropeptide Y (NPY) is a highly expressed peptide in the mammalian CNS.[84,85] When administered into the CNS, NPY induces a robust feeding response.[86–88] Repeated administration of NPY results in sustained hyperphagia and rapid body weight gain.[89,90] In the ARC, food deprivation, food restriction, or exercise-induced negative energy balance upregulate NPY expression.[91–96] The response of the NPY system to negative energy balance is accompanied by reduced insulin and leptin signaling[97–100] (Table 8.1).

*MCH*: There are two peptide systems that operate in the LHA to control food intake. The first is melanin concentrating hormone (MCH). MCH is an orexic hormone that is increased in the leptin-deficient *ob/ob* mice.[101] In wild-type mice, MCH expression is inhibited by leptin and elevated by food deprivation. Consistent with a proposed role as an anabolic effector transmitter in the CNS, when delivered into the lateral ventricle, MCH increases food intake.[102,103] However, unlike what happens with NPY, repeated administration of MCH does not result in increased body weight.[104] Mice with targeted deletion of MCH have reduced food intake and decreased body weight and body adiposity.[105]

*Orexins*: Another LHA peptide system was simultaneously identified by two groups of investigators. One termed these peptides "hypocretins"[106] and the other "orexins."[107] Both terms continue to be used, but hypocretins are the more common name in circles studying sleep/waking cycles while orexin is more commonly used when referring to the control of food intake. The orexins are comprised of two peptides (ORX-A and ORX-B) and two receptors, and while the cell bodies are located in close proximity to MCH-expressing neurons in the LHA, the two systems do not co-localize to any significant extent.[108] Considerable evidence indicates that central administration of ORX-A increases food intake.[109,110] Orexin expression in the LHA is inhibited by leptin[107] and increased by decreased glucose utilization,[111] suggesting that it is tied to energy homeostasis as well. Interestingly, there appear to be significant interactions between the ARC and the LHA involving these neuropeptide systems. While there are few leptin or insulin receptors in the LHA, information concerning the levels of adiposity signals can be transmitted to the LHA via projections from the ARC.

*Ghrelin*: Ghrelin is the endogenous ligand for the growth hormone secretagogue receptor.[112,113] Ghrelin is made primarily in endocrine cells of the stomach, and circulating levels are increased during fasting and rapidly decline after nutrients are provided to the stomach[112,113] (for review see Ref. [114]). Consistent with a role as an anabolic effector, endogenous ghrelin infusion increases food intake in rats[115] and humans.[116] Sustained ghrelin infusions result in dramatic obesity.[117] Clinical evidence points to elevated levels of ghrelin in weight-reduced patients.[118]

## CATABOLIC FACTORS

As opposed to the anabolic systems described earlier, catabolic systems are those that are activated during positive rather than negative energy balance. Homeostatic regulation of food intake suggests that when overfed, voluntary food intake drops to near zero, facilitating return of body weight homeostasis. Animals not only have potent regulatory responses to

**TABLE 8.1**
**Anabolic and Catabolic Factors**

*Anabolic Factors*

| | |
|---|---|
| NPY | Increases food intake and body weight |
| MCH | Increases food intake |
| ORX-A | Increases food intake |
| Ghrelin | Increases food intake and body weight |
| AgRP | Increases food intake |

*Catabolic Factors*

| | |
|---|---|
| αMSH | Reduces food intake and increases energy expenditure |
| GLP-1 | Reduces food intake and insulin secretion |

Anabolic and catabolic factors that affect food intake, body weight, and energy expenditure.

NPY, neuropeptide Y; MCH, melanin concentrating hormone; ORX-A, orexin-A; AgRP, agouti-related peptide; αMSH, α melanocyte-stimulating hormone; GLP-1, glucogon-like peptide-1.

being in negative energy balance, but also possess regulatory responses to positive energy balance. Catabolic systems are activated during positive energy balance, and they act to reduce energy intake and increase energy expenditure.

*Melanocortin System*: The ARC has been well investigated with regard to central leptin action.[8,9] OB-Rb is expressed by two populations of ARC neurons, those expressing pro-opiomelanocortin (POMC)[119,120] and those expressing NPY and agouti-related peptide (NPY/AgRP neurons).[121] NPY is an effective anabolic peptide. Central administration of NPY potently increases food intake and decreases energy expenditure and fat oxidation.[122–125] ARC neurons co-express NPY mRNA and OB-Rb protein. Leptin administration decreases NPY (and AgRP) mRNA, demonstrating that leptin is a critical determinant of ARC NPY function.[121] POMC neurons secrete the catabolic melanocortin neuropeptide, α melanocyte-stimulating hormone (αMSH), which acts in the PVN and the LHA on melanocortin 3 and melanocortin 4 (MC3/MC4) receptors to reduce food intake and increase energy expenditure.[21,52,63,126] If administered chronically, MC3/4 agonists reduce body weight and adiposity.[127] Leptin stimulates POMC neurons to synthesize and release αMSH.[128,129] AgRP antagonizes MC3/MC4 receptors, and its administration increases food intake. Leptin elicits a powerful catabolic effect by activating αMSH and simultaneously inhibiting anabolic NPY/AgRP production and release. This results in reduced feeding and increased energy expenditure.[21]

*GLP-1*: Preproglucagon is a peptide made both in the periphery and in the CNS. Preproglucagon encodes two peptides: glucagon-like-peptide 1 (GLP-1) and glucagon-like-peptide 2 (GLP-2). Both peptides are made in the L-cells of the distal intestine and have well-described functions in the periphery with GLP-1 critical for enhancing nutrient-induced insulin secretion[130] and GLP-2 playing an important role in the maintenance of the gut mucosa.[131] When administered centrally, GLP-1 produces a profound reduction in food intake and antagonists to the GLP-1 receptor increase food intake.[132,133]

## OBESITY

Anabolic and catabolic signals and areas in the hypothalamus that are identified as targets for hormonal and neuropeptide signals are extensively studied because of the growing prevalence of obesity and obesity-related health problems in the developed world.[81,134,135] One could argue that if body weight is tightly regulated, why then do individuals gain weight and become obese? Or another question is why is the incidence of obesity increasing, even in the face of exquisite biological controls?

Obesity is associated with an imbalance of regulatory hormones that normally act to maintain stable energy balance and body weight. However, after an enormous amount of research, spanning a period of at least 45 years, the causes of the current obesity epidemic remain elusive. Much of this work attempted to link the cause of obesity with failures in hypothalamic signaling systems (e.g., leptin, melanocortins) and/or if there is something in the diet (e.g., dietary fat) that

may impart "resistance" to signals that normally regulate food intake and body weight.[136] Consistently, elevations in dietary fat, either directly or indirectly, confers an insensitivity to hormones or peptides that would otherwise reduce body weight;[136,137,138] therefore, obesity could result from continued consumption of food even in the presence of elevated energy stores because the brain becomes resistant to the effects of inhibitory mechanisms.

Additionally, the role of environmental factors, such as the increased availability of highly palatable, energy dense foods and beverages,[136,139] must be considered when referring to homeostatic regulation of body weight. With the modernization of society, highly palatable and energy dense food is abundant, and marketing practices keep thoughts of these foods almost constantly in mind. Does increased access to food and exposure to food-related environmental cues actually facilitate overeating and dysregulation in the homeostatic model?

There are data to suggest that the regulation of food intake relies on learning and memory processes that exist between food cues and their postingestive sensory consequences. Impairment of the ability to use such learning processes results in energy and body weight dysregulation. Humans typically do not eat in response to hunger or to other internal signals of energy deficit, but rather meals are initiated in response to environmental stimuli (e.g., time of day; advertising) that have been associated previously with food and the consequences of eating. These conditioned environmental cues will evoke eating behavior until those behaviors give rise to signals referred to as satiety signals that tell the brain to stop eating and terminate the meal. That is, energy regulation depends not only on hunger signals, but also on the generation of physiological satiety signals that act to terminate meals.

## CONCLUSION

In this chapter, we present a basic outline of some of the homeostatic systems involved in the control of food intake and energy balance. One review can no longer capture all of the current knowledge on this subject. Many other CNS systems, including those utilizing serotonin, neurotensin,[140] histamine,[141] or norepinephrine[142] (or many others), have not been discussed here. Likewise, hypothalamic neurons that are involved in direct nutrient sensing and that play a prominent role in the control of food intake[123] have also been ignored. What has been included is a review of the pathways important in integrating body adiposity with food intake.

The pace of research on energy homeostasis has been extraordinary over the last decade. This explosion in our knowledge has been driven in part by the multitude of new tools now available to investigators and in part by the crushing clinical need to address the epidemic of obesity that confronts the developed world. In many ways, the explosion of knowledge around these systems reflects the application of powerful molecular tools to pick the lowest hanging fruit by identifying peptide systems whose activity is somehow regulated by energy balance. The hard work remains in front of us, which is to understand the interactions of these systems whose combined output doggedly defends the level of stored fuel in the body with incredible precision.

A key challenge therefore is to understand the independent contribution of specific receptor populations to the maintenance of energy balance. To address this, we not only have to understand the neuroscience of how food intake and energy expenditure are controlled, but how the body weight regulatory system interfaces with other critical functions such as arousal, reward, sensation, emotion, and memory. The important point is that the control of energy balance is not an isolated function but rather an integrated part of how an animal survives. The hypothalamic systems described in this chapter must also be understood in the context of how they interface with other CNS circuits inside and outside the hypothalamus.

Stellar's dual-center hypothesis dominated our view of how food intake was controlled for decades.[12] The conceptualization offered in this chapter emphasizes the regulation of long-term energy balance rather than the initiation and termination of individual bouts of ingestion. It also emphasizes neurochemical effector pathways over specific hunger and satiety centers.[8] These changes in emphasis provide a new context in which to interpret the mountain of data concerning these hypothalamic systems.[11,81] However, this chapter can hardly be considered the final word. Our ability to meet the next challenges in understanding the regulation of energy balance and the interaction of multiple systems will not rest solely upon developing better tools for collecting data but will require that we advance our theoretical perspectives as well.

## REFERENCES

1. Obici, S, *Endocrinology* **150**: 2512; 2009.
2. Berthoud, HR, Morrison, C, *Ann Rev Psychol.* **59**: 55; 2008.
3. Cone, RD, *Trends Endocrinol Metab.* **10**: 211; 1990.
4. Kennedy, GC, *Proc R Soc Lond (Biol).* **140**: 579; 1953.
5. Milanski, M, Degasperi, G, Coope, A et al., *J Neurosci.* **29**: 359; 2009.
6. Niswender, KD, Morrison, CD, Clegg, DG et al., *Diabetes* **52**: 227; 2003.
7. Grill, HJ, Kaplan, JM, *Front Neuroendocrinol.* **23**: 2; 2002.
8. Williams, G, Bing, C, Cai, XJ et al., *Physiol Behav.* **74**: 683; 2001.
9. Woods, SC, Seeley, RJ, *Nutrition* **16**: 894; 2000.
10. Zhang, X, Zhang, G, Zhang, H et al., *Cell* **135**: 61; 2008.
11. Xu, Y, Nedungadi, TP, Zhu, L et al., *Cell Metab.* **14**: 453; 2011.
12. Stellar, E, *Psychol Rev.* **61**: 5; 1954.
13. Hetherington, AW, Ranson, SW, *Am J Physiol.* **136**: 609; 1942.
14. Hetherington, R, Ranson, S, *Anat Rec.* **78**: 149; 1940.
15. Weingarten, HP, Chang, PK, McDonald, TJ, *Brain Res Bull.* **14**: 551; 1985.
16. Vilberg, TR, Keesey, RE, *Am J Physiol.* **247**: R183; 1984.
17. Saito, M, Minokoshi, Y, Shimazu, T, *Brain Res.* **481**: 298; 1988.
18. Anand, BK, Brobeck, JR, Yale, *J Biol Med.* **24**: 123; 1951.
19. Bernardis, LL, Bellinger, LL, *Neurosci Biobehav Rev.* **20**: 189; 1996.
20. Ungan, P, Karakas, S, *Int J Psychophysiol.* **8**: 73; 1989.
21. Elmquist, JK, Elias, CF, Saper, CB, *Neuron* **22**: 221; 1999.
22. Jeanrenaud, B, Rohner-Jeanrenaud, F, *Int J Obes Relat Metab Disord.* **24(Suppl 2)**: S74; 2000.
23. Schwartz, MW, Woods, SC, Porte, DJ et al., *Nature* **404**: 661; 2000.
24. Benoit, SC, Clegg, DJ, Seeley, RJ et al., *Recent Prog Horm Res.* **59**: 267–285; 2004.
25. Woods, SC, Seeley, RJ, Porte, DJ et al., *Science* **280**: 1378; 1998.
26. Bray, GA, *The Obese Patient.* 1976, Philadelphia, PA: Saunders.
27. Keesey, RE, Hirvonen, MD, *J Nutr.* **127**: 1875S; 1997.
28. Schwartz, MW, Seeley, RJ, *JADA.* **97**: 54; 1997.
29. Stallone, DD, Stunkard, AJ, *Ann Behav Med.* **13**: 220; 1991.
30. Kirchner, H, Hofmann, SM, Fischer-Rosinsky, A et al., *Diabetes* 2012.
31. Woods, SC, Ramsay, DS, *Physiol Behav.* **104**: 4; 2011.
32. Coelho, DF, Gualano, B, Artioli, GG et al., *Endocr Regul.* **43**: 107; 2009.
33. Schreiber, JE, Singh, NK, Shermak, MA, *Plast Reconstr Surg.* **117**: 1829; 2006.
34. Faust, IM, Johnson, PR, Hirsch, J, *Proc Soc Exp Biol Med.* **161**: 111; 1979.
35. Coleman, DL, *Diabetologia.* **9**: 294; 1973.
36. Hervey, GR, *J Physiol.* **145**: 336; 1952.
37. Polonsky, KS, Given, BD, Hirsch, L et al., *J Clin Invest.* **81**: 435; 1988.
38. Polonsky, KS, Given, E, Carter, V, *J Clin Invest.* **81**: 442; 1988.
39. Chavez, M, Seeley, RJ, Woods, SC, *Behav Neuro.* **109**: 547; 1995.
40. Chavez, M, Kaiyala, K, Madden, LJ et al., *Behav Neurosci.* **109**: 528; 1995.
41. Woods, SC, Lotter, EC, McKay, LD et al., *Nature* **282**: 503; 1979.
42. Asarian, L, Geary, N, *Philos Trans R Soc Lond B Biol Sci.* **361**: 1251; 2006.
43. Moran, TH, Kinzig, KP, *Am J Physiol Gastrointest Liver Physiol.* **286**: G183; 2004.
44. Halford, JC, Cooper, GD, Dovey, TM, *Curr Drug Targets* **5**: 221; 2004.
45. Asarian, L, Geary, N, *Horm Behav.* **42**: 461; 2002.
46. McGowan, MK, Andrews, KM, Grossman, SP, *Physiol Behav.* **51**: 753; 1992.
47. Brüning, JC, Gautam, D, Burks, DJ et al., *Science* **289**: 2122; 2000.
48. Zhang, Y, Proenca, R, Maffei, M et al., *Nature* **372**: 425; 1994.
49. Ahima, RS, Kelly, J, Elmquist, JK et al., *Endocrinology* **140**: 4923; 1999.
50. Schwartz, MW, Porte, Jr. D, *Science* **307**: 375; 2005.
51. Seeley, RJ, Woods, SC, *Nat Rev Neurosci.* **4**: 901; 2003.
52. Elias, CF, Aschkenasi, C, Lee, C et al., *Neuron* **23**: 775; 1999.
53. Morton, GJ, Niswender, KD, Rhodes, CJ et al., *Endocrinology* **144**: 2016; 2003.
54. Woods, SC, Schwartz, MW, Baskin, DG et al., *Ann Rev Psychol.* **51**: 255; 2000.
55. Balthasar, N, Coppari, R, McMinn, J et al., *Neuron* **42**: 983; 2004.
56. Ahima, RS, Prabakaran, D, Mantzoros, C et al., *Nature* **382**: 250; 1996.
57. Tartaglia, LA, Dembski, M, Weng, X et al., *Cell* **83**: 1263; 1995.
58. Seeley, RJ, van Dijk, G, Campfield, LA et al., *Horm Metab Res.* **28**: 664; 1996.
59. Chen, H, Charlat, O, Tartaglia, LA et al., *Cell* **84**: 491; 1996.

60. Van Dijk, G, Thiele, TE, Donahey, JC et al., *Am J Physiol.* **271**: R1096; 1996.
61. Elmquist, JK, Ahima, RS, Maratos-Flier, E et al., *Endocrinology* **138**: 839; 1997.
62. Elmquist, JK, Bjorbaek, C, Ahima, RS et al., *J Comp Neurol.* **395**: 535; 1998.
63. Elmquist, JK, Ahima, RS, Elias, CF et al., *Proc Natl Acad Sci USA.* **95**: 741; 1998.
64. Elmquist, JK, Maratos-Flier, E, Saper, CB et al., *Nature Neurosci.* **1**: 445; 1998.
65. Baura, G, Foster, D, Porte, Jr. D et al., *J Clin Invest.* **92**: 1824; 1993.
66. Baskin, DG, Sipols, AJ, Schwartz, MW et al., *Endocrinology* **134**: 1952; 1994.
67. Baskin, DG, Marks, JL, Schwartz, MW et al., in *Endocrine and Nutritional Control of Basic Biological Functions*, H. Lehnert et al, (Eds.), Stuttgart, Germany: Hogrefe & Huber, pp. 202, 1990.
68. Banks, WA, Kastin, AJ, Huang, WEA, *Peptides* **17**: 305; 1996.
69. Banks, WA, DiPalma, CR, Farrell, CL, *Peptides* **20**: 1341; 1999.
70. Kim, JY, van de Wall, E, Laplante, M et al., *J Clin Invest.* **117**: 2621; 2007.
71. Clegg, DJ, Brown, LM, Woods, SC et al., *Diabetes* **55**: 978; 2006.
72. Havel, PJ, *Diabetes* **53(Suppl 1)**: S143; 2004.
73. Woods, SC, Seeley, RJ, Rushing, PA et al., *J Nutr.* **133**: 1081; 2003.
74. Havel, PJ, *Curr Opin Lipid* **13**: 51; 2002.
75. Ozcan, U, Cao, Q, Yilmaz, E et al., *Science* **306**: 457; 2004.
76. van Dijk, G, de Vries, K, Benthem, L et al., *Eur J Pharmacol.* **480**: 31; 2003.
77. Air, EL, Strowski, MZ, Benoit, SC et al., *Nat. Med.* **8**: 179; 2002.
78. Woods, SC, Seeley, RJ, *Int J Obes Relat Metab Disord.* **25 (Suppl 5)**: S35; 2001.
79. Klockener, T, Hess, S, Belgardt, BF et al., *Nat Neurosci.* **14**: 911; 2011.
80. Trayhurn, P, Hoggard, N, Mercer, JG et al., *Arch Tierernahr.* **51**: 177; 1998.
81. Bray, G, York, D, *Recent Prog Horm Res.* **53**: 95; 1998.
82. Rushing, PA, Hagan, MM, Seeley, RJ et al., *Endocrinology* **141**: 850; 2000.
83. Strack, AM, Sebastian, RJ, Schwartz, MW et al., *Am J Physiol.* **268**: 142; 1995.
84. Allen, YS, Adrian, TE, Tatemoto, K et al., *Science* **221**: 877; 1983.
85. Minth, CD, Andrews, PC, Dixon, JE, *J Biol Chem.* **261**: 11975; 1986.
86. Clark, JT, Kalra, PS, Crowley, WR et al., *Endocrinology* **115**: 427; 1984.
87. Stanley, BG, Leibowitz, SF, *Proc Natl Acad Sci USA* **82**: 3940; 1984.
88. Seeley, RJ, Payne, CJ, Woods, SC, *Am J Physiol.* **268**: R423; 1995.
89. Stanley, BG, Kyrkouli, SE, Lampert, S et al., *Peptides* **7**: 1189; 1986.
90. McMinn, JE, Seeley, RJ, Wilkinson, CW et al., *Regul Pept.* **75**: 425; 1998.
91. Mizuno, TM, Makimura, H, Silverstein, J et al., *Endocrinology* **140**: 4551; 1999.
92. Sahu, A, Sninsky, CA, Phelps, CP et al., *Endocrinology* **131**: 2979; 1992.
93. Marks, JL, Mu, L, Schwartz, MW et al., *Mol Cell Neurosci.* **3**: 199; 1992.
94. Sahu, A, Sninsky, CA, Kalra, PS et al., *Endocrinology* **126**: 192; 1990.
95. Kalra, SP, Dube, MG, Sahu, A et al., *Proc Natl Acad Sci USA.* **88**: 10931; 1991.
96. Sahu, A, Kalra, PS, Kalra, SP, *Peptides* **9**: 83; 1988.
97. Sipols, AJ, Baskin, DG, Schwartz, MW, *Diabetes* **44**: 147; 1995.
98. Sipols, AJ, Baskin, DG, Schwartz, MW, *Diabetes* **42(Suppl 1)**: 152; 1993.
99. Stephens, TW, Bashinski, M, Bristow, PK et al., *Nature* **377**: 530; 1995.
100. Schwartz, MW, Baskin, DG, Bukowski, TR et al., *Diabetes* **45**: 531; 1996.
101. Qu, D, Ludwig, DS, Gammeltoft, S et al., *Nature* **380**: 243; 1996.
102. Ludwig, D, Mountjoy, K, Tatro, J et al., *Am J Physiol.* **274**: E627; 1998.
103. Sanchez, M, Baker, B, Celis, M, *Peptides* **18**: 393; 1997.
104. Rossi, M, Choi, SJ, O'Shea, D et al., *Endocrinology* **138**: 351; 1997.
105. Shimada, M, Tritos, N, Lowell, B et al., *Nature* **396**: 670; 1998.
106. de Lecea, L, Kilduff, TS, Peyron, C et al., *Proc Natl Acad Sci USA.* **95**: 322; 1998.
107. Sakurai, T, Amemiya, A, Ishii, M et al., Cell **92**: 573; 1998.
108. Broberger, C, De Lecea, L, Sutcliffe, JG et al., *J Comparat Neurol.* **402**: 460; 1998.
109. Yamanaka, A, Kunii, K, Nambu, T et al., *Brain Res.* **859**: 404; 2000.
110. Rauch, M, Riediger, T, Schmid, HA et al., *Pflugers Arch.* **440**: 699; 2000.
111. Sergeyev, V, Broberger, C, Gorbatyuk, O et al., *Neuroreport* **11**: 117; 2000.
112. Kojima, M, Hosoda, H, Date, Y et al., *Nature* **402**: 656; 1999.
113. Kojima, M, Hosoda, H, Kangawa, K, *Horm Res.* **56**: S93; 2001.
114. Horvath, TL, Diano, S, Sotonyi, P et al., *Endocrinology* **142**: 4163; 2001.
115. Tschöp, M, Smiley, DL, Heiman, ML, *Nature* **407**: 908; 2000.
116. Wren, AM, Seal, LJ, Cohen, MA et al., *J Clin Endocrinol Metab.* **86**: 5992; 2001.
117. Horvath, TL, Diano, S, Tschop, M, *Curr Top Med Chem.* **3**: 921; 2003.
118. Tschöp, M, Weyer, C, Tataranni, PA et al., *Diabetes* **50**: 707; 2001.
119. Cheung, CC, Clifton, DK, Steiner, RA, *Endocrinology* **138**: 4489; 1997.
120. Thornton, JE, Cheung, CC, Clifton, DK et al., *Endocrinology* **138**: 5063; 1997.
121. Baskin, DG, Breininger, JF, Schwartz, MW, *Diabetes* **48**: 828; 1999.
122. Chavez, M, van Dijk, G, Arkies, BJ et al., *Obes Res.* **3**: 335s; 1995.
123. Levin, BE, *Am J Physiol.* **276**: R382; 1999.
124. Cone, RD, Cowley, MA, Butler, AA et al., *Int J Obes Relat Metab Disord.* **25**: S63; 2001.
125. Herzog, H, *Eur J Pharmacol.* **480**: 21; 2003.
126. Elias, CF, Kelly, JF, Lee, CE et al., *J Comp Neurol.* **423**: 261; 2000.
127. Pierroz, DD, Ziotopoulou, M, Ungsunan, L et al., *Diabetes* **51**: 1337; 2002.
128. Seeley, R, Yagaloff, K, Fisher, S et al., *Nature* **390**: 349; 1997.

129. Korner, J, Chua, Jr. SC, Williams, JA et al., *Neuroendocrinology* **70**: 377; 1999.
130. D'Alessio, DA, Vogel, R, Prigeon, R et al., *J Clin Invest.* **97**: 133; 1996.
131. Drucker, DJ, Boushey, RB, Wang, F et al., *J Parenter Enteral Nutr.* **23**: S98; 1999.
132. Turton, MD, O'Shea, D, Gunn, I et al., *Nature* **379**: 69; 1996.
133. Tang-Christensen, M, Larsen, PJ, Goke, R et al., *Am J Physiol.* **271**: R848; 1996.
134. Pi-Sunyer, X, *Postgrad Med.* **121**: 21; 2009.
135. Kleinridders, A, Schenten, D, Konner, AC et al., *Cell Metab.* **10**: 249; 2009.
136. Clegg, DJ, Gotoh, K, Kemp, C et al., *Physiol Behav.* **103**: 10; 2011.
137. Benoit, SC, Kemp, CJ, Elias, CF et al., *J Clin Invest.* **119**: 2577; 2009.
138. Clegg, DJ, Benoit, SC, Reed, JA et al., *Am J Physiol. Regul Integr Comp Physiol.* **288**: R981; 2005.
139. Woods, SC, D'Alessio, DA, Tso, P et al., *Physiol Behav.* **83**: 573; 2004.
140. Watts, AG, *Horm Behav.* **37**: 261; 2000.
141. Sakata, T, Yoshimatsu, H, Kurokawa, M, *Nutrition* **13**: 403; 1997.
142. Wellman, PJ, *Nutrition* **16**: 837; 2000.

# 9 Nutrition and Genetics

*Carolyn D. Berdanier*

## CONTENTS

Nutrition science is concerned with the many factors that influence the need and use of macro- and micronutrients. Among these factors is the genetic heritage of the consumer. This heritage is conferred by the base sequence of the genetic material, deoxyribonucleic acid (DNA). DNA is found in both the nucleus and mitochondria of the cell and dictates the characteristics of every living cell in every living creature. Nuclear DNA is organized into units called chromosomes. The chromosomes are found in pairs and contain the individual units called genes. Although all cells contain the same DNA, not all genes are expressed in every cell; some are specific to specific cell types.

DNA is a double-stranded helix composed of four bases: two pyrimidines (cytosine and thymine) and two purines (adenine and guanine) that are joined together by ribose and phosphate groups (Figure 9.1). DNA is formed when the bases are joined through phosphodiester bonds using ribose as the common linkage. The phosphodiester linkage is between the 5′ phosphate group of one nucleotide and the 3′ OH group of the adjacent nucleotide. This provides a direction (5′ to 3′) to the chain. The bases are hydrophobic and contain charged polar groups. These features are responsible for the helical shape of the nuclear DNA chain. A double helix forms when the bases of each chain interact through hydrogen bonding.

The DNA base sequence dictates the amino acid sequence in every protein and peptide in the body. This base sequence determines the *genotype* of the individual for each gene product. While only a few bases are used for the DNA, it is the sequence of these bases that determine the product being produced. Each gene is unique to each gene product and determines not only the particular characteristics of the individual but also the properties of each cell through the provision of a multitude of genes, each coded for a particular protein found in that cell. Thus, DNA functions to transmit genetic information from one generation to the next in a given species and ensures the identity of specific cell types.

Much of the overall base sequence of DNA has been identified, yet there are individual differences that characterize the unique features of every living creature. It is these differences that make each individual unique. The identification of each gene and its corresponding controls of expression have not been completely elucidated. Some of these controls are nutrient related.[1–13] While the nuclear genome has been sequenced, it has not been completely mapped. By mapping we mean the identification, base sequence and location, within the DNA, of each gene (and its promoter region), and the protein it encodes. In addition, we do not know all the details of the regulation of gene expression.

Nutrients interact with genes at several levels. Some nutrients affect the function of specific gene products by influencing the environment in which the gene product functions. Some have specific effects on the synthesis of messenger RNA, i.e., transcription.[14–21] Some affect the synthesis of the pyrimidine and purine bases used for DNA and RNA syntheses. Some nutrients have an overall effect on protein synthesis while others influence the translation of the messenger RNA into protein or the posttranslational modification of the newly synthesized protein.[22–24]

## GENE EXPRESSION

By definition, gene expression includes all those steps (transcription, translation, and post translation processing) involved in the synthesis and activation of a specific gene product, a protein or peptide. It is a highly controlled process producing a product that has a specific function in the cell, tissue, organ, and indeed the whole body. Some of the operative controls or signals involve the nutrients. These signals can be specific nutrients or simply a dietary change that results in a change in cell constituents or in the metabolism of the whole body through changes in gene expression. In some instances, the metabolic change is that of an increase (or decrease) in specific enzymes of a specific metabolic pathway. In others, the change in gene product might be a change in a hormone or the release of a metabolic signal that in turn could involve a change in behavior or a change in energy balance. The gene product itself might be affected should there be a substitution, deletion, or rearrangement of the bases in the gene or its

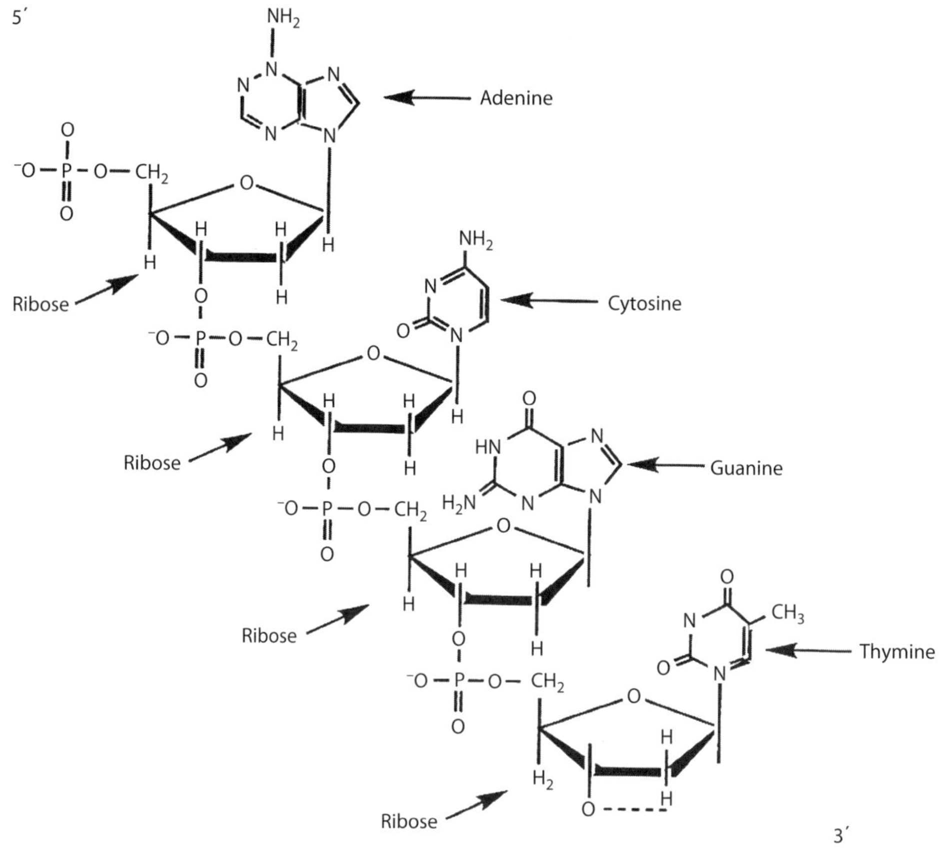

**FIGURE 9.1** The bases that make up the DNA polynucleotide chain are joined together by phosphodiester bonds using ribose as the common link between the bases.

promoter region. If there is a change in the sequence of bases that comprise the genetic code for a given protein, the amino acid sequence generated in that protein might be incorrect. Some amino acids are encoded by more than one triplet of bases in the DNA. Thus, a change in the base sequence might or might not result in a change in the amino acid being dictated. Whether this substitution of one amino acid for another affects the functionality of the protein being generated depends entirely on the protein and amino acid in question. Some amino acids can be replaced without affecting the secondary, tertiary, or quaternary structures of the protein (and hence, its chemical and physical properties) whereas others cannot. In addition, genetically dictated changes in amino acid sequence may pose no threat to the individual if the protein in question is of little importance in the maintenance of health and well-being. Conversely, it can have large effects on health if the protein is a critical one. The functionality of the protein or gene product gives the individual a certain characteristic. This characteristic is then called the *phenotype* of the individual.

## MUTATION VERSUS POLYMORPHISM

The DNA in the nucleus is very stable with respect to the base sequence and content. Chemicals that generate free radicals can damage it. In Figure 9.1, arrows point to vulnerable spots in the DNA where such damage can occur. Free radical attack results in DNA strand breaks and a possible loss of a base. Replacement of that base can occur and the strand repaired. However, in some instances, the base used for the repair might not be identical to the one lost and a base substitution will be made. If the base substitution affects the amino acid sequence of the gene product and this substitution is in a critical area that affects function, then a *mutation* is said to have occurred. Otherwise the difference in base sequence is referred to as a *polymorphism* rather than a mutation. Mutation can also be the result of a deletion of bases or a rearrangement of bases. A few or many bases can be destroyed by free radicals, for example, leaving the cell less able to produce a given protein. In turn, this affects the function of the cell. It should be noted that a single affected cell is not a lethal event except for that particular cell. It becomes a problem when many cells have their DNA damaged in the same way and the loss of cell function is significant. In most instances, DNA repair will occur so well that there is little noticeable effect of the initial insult. However, over time, mismatch repair or cumulative assaults on the DNA can have cumulative effects on DNA and cellular function. This cumulative effect of assault has been suggested to explain aging. Aging as a result of cumulative effects of free radical attack on DNA as well as on the vulnerable membranes within and around the cell has been used to explain the gradual loss in cell function that occurs with age. Some nutrients protect cells against free radical attack. Such nutrients as vitamin E,

## TABLE 9.1
### Nutrients That Have a Role in Free Radical Suppression

| Nutrient | Role |
|---|---|
| Carotene | Serves as a $H^+/e^-$ donor acceptor |
| Vitamin K | Serves as a $H^+/e^-$ donor acceptor |
| Ascorbic acid | Serves as a $H^+/e^-$ donor acceptor |
| Copper and zinc | Essential cofactors for the enzyme, superoxide dismutase |
| Manganese | Essential cofactor for mitochondrial superoxide dismutase |
| Selenium | Essential for glutathione peroxidase |
| Vitamin E | Quenches free radicals |

ascorbic acid, carotene, selenium, and others serve to suppress free radical formation or serve to promote the synthesis of enzymes that function in the free radical suppression system. Table 9.1 lists these nutrients and their roles in free radical protection.

While the nucleus has a very efficient DNA repair process, the mitochondrion does not. However, while there is only one nucleus in each cell, there are many mitochondria in that same cell. If one or two are damaged, there are many in that cell to compensate. Disease develops only when damage occurs to a large majority of the mitochondria.[25,26] A certain threshold of damage must be approached for such damage to have a physiological effect. Again, nutrients that function as free radical suppressants or that enhance the synthesis of enzymes of the free radical suppression system function to protect mitochondria from free radical damage.

In the nucleus, the DNA is protected from free radical attack by histone and nonhistone proteins.[27–33] Histones are highly basic proteins varying in molecular weight from ~11,000 to ~21,000. The histones keep the DNA in a very compact form. In contrast, the mitochondrial DNA does not have this protective histone coat. It is "naked" and much more vulnerable to damage. In addition, ~90% of oxygen free radicals are generated in the mitochondria providing the means for such damage should the enzyme superoxide dismutase, a manganese-dependent enzyme found in this compartment, not suppress these radicals. The damage can be quite severe, yet because each mitochondrion contains 8–10 copies of its genome and there are so many mitochondria in each cell (up to 20,000), the effects of this damage might not be apparent. There is another superoxide dismutase found in the cytosol that has a similar function. It is a copper–zinc-dependent enzyme.

The deletion or substitution of bases in the DNA of a particular gene could occur in a noncoding region of the DNA or be a base substitution that does not affect the amino acid sequence of the gene product. If any of these occur, there will be little discernible effect on the gene product. Such changes in base sequence are not mutations per se but polymorphisms. The resultant gene product retains its pre-mutation function, yet has a slightly different amino acid sequence. Such polymorphisms are useful tools because they allow population geneticists to track mutation and evolutionary events through related family members.

Particularly useful in this respect are the polymorphisms in mitochondrial DNA and in the Y chromosome DNA. Mitochondrial DNA is inherited from the mother almost exclusively while Y chromosome DNA is passed from father to son.

## TRANSCRIPTION

Messenger RNA synthesis using DNA as the template is called transcription.[34,35] This is illustrated in Figure 9.2. The mRNA carries genetic information from the DNA of the chromosomes in the nucleus to the surface of the ribosomes in the cytosol. It is synthesized as a single strand. Chemically, RNA is similar to DNA. It is an unbranched linear polymer in which the monomeric subunits are the ribonucleoside 5′ monophosphates. The bases are the purines, adenine and guanine, and the pyrimidines, uracil and cytosine. Thymine, used in DNA synthesis, is not used in mRNA. Instead, uracil is used. Messenger RNA is much smaller than DNA and is far less stable. It has a very short half-life (from seconds to minutes to hours) compared to that of nuclear DNA (years). Because it has a short half-life, the purine and pyrimidine bases that are used to make mRNA must be continually resynthesized. This synthesis requires a number of micronutrients (niacin, riboflavin, pyridoxine, folacin, $B_{12}$, copper, iron, sulfur, zinc, magnesium, and phosphorus) as well as energy. Should any of these be in short supply, symptoms of malnutrition will be observed especially in those cell types that have very short half-lives, i.e., red blood cells (half-life: 60 days) and epithelial cells (half-life: 7 days). All the components of the new cells must be synthesized in order to form the new red cell or skin cell.

The synthesis of mRNA from DNA involves three steps: initiation, elongation, and termination.[4,34–37] Initiation is the process whereby basal transcription factors recognize and bind the start point for transcription on DNA and form a complex with RNA polymerase II. Most of gene expression can be defined as *trans*-acting factors or proteins binding *cis*-acting elements (base sequences). Upstream of the transcription start site on DNA is a region called the promoter. Within the promoter, approximately 25 base pairs upstream of the start site, is a consensus sequence called the TATA box, which contains A–T base pairs. One of the basal transcription factors, the TATA binding protein (TBP), recognizes this sequence of DNA and binds there. This begins the process of transcription initiation as the *trans*-acting TBP binds the *cis*-acting TATA box and a large complex of basal transcription factors, RNA polymerase II, and DNA is formed. Elongation is the actual process of RNA formation using a DNA template in the 5′–3′ direction. Shortly after elongation begins, the 5′ end of mRNA is capped by 7-methylguanosine triphosphate. This cap stabilizes the mRNA and is necessary for processing and translation. The third step is the termination of the chain.

The regulation of transcription occurs at the initiation step. The promoter region contains many *cis*-acting elements, each named for the factor that binds to them.

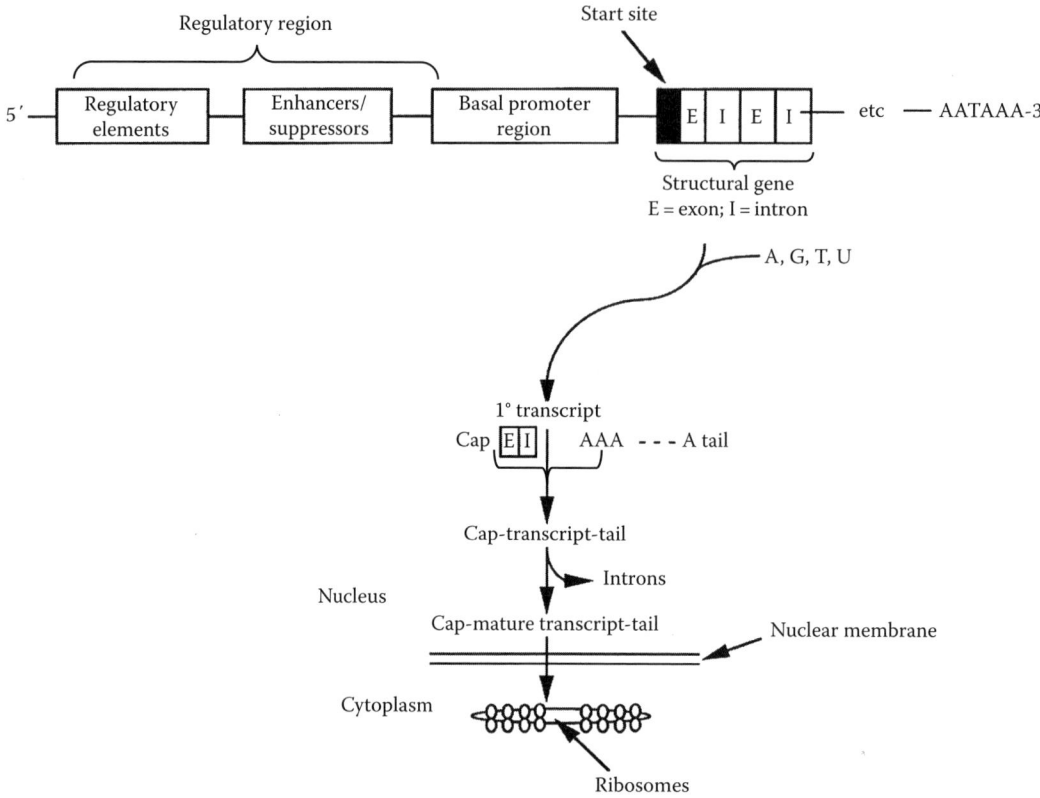

**FIGURE 9.2**    Synthesis of messenger RNA and its processing and migration to the ribosomes in the cytoplasm.

In general, these regions are called enhancers, silencers, or more recently named response elements. Examples include the retinoic acid response element, heat shock element, and cAMP response element. The *trans*-acting factors that bind these elements are in general called transcription factors. They are proteins with at least two domains, a DNA-binding domain and a transcription activation domain. Recently, it has been shown that coactivators are needed to bind transcription factors and increase transcription by both interacting with basal transcription factors and altering chromatin structure. Corepressors act to decrease transcription at the level of both basal transcription factors and chromatin structure. Coactivators and corepressors are proteins.

The true regulation of transcription occurs by the regulation of transcription factors. Transcription factors can be regulated by (1) their rates of synthesis or degradation; (2) phosphorylation or dephosphorylation; (3) ligand binding; (4) cleavage of a protranscription factor; or (5) release of an inhibitor. One class of transcription factors important for nutrition is the nuclear hormone receptor superfamily, which is regulated by ligand binding. Ligands for these transcription factors include retinoic acid (the acid form of vitamin A), fatty acids, vitamin D, thyroid hormone, and steroid hormones. All members of this superfamily of receptors contain two zinc fingers in their DNA-binding domains. Zinc is bound to histidine- and cysteine-rich regions of the protein that envelops the DNA in a shape that looks like a finger. The zinc ion plays an enormous

role in gene expression because of its central use in the zinc finger. The nuclear hormone receptor superfamily is divided into four groups according to their dimerization potential, their site specificity, and their localization. Group I receptors bind the steroid hormones and bind DNA as homodimers. Group I response elements are palindromes of either AGAACA or AGGTCA spaced by three nucleotides. The specificity occurs by interactions between the specific nucleotide sequence and the protein sequence of the first zinc finger.

The RXRαβγ receptor that binds 9-*cis* retinoic acid binds to either the DR-1 or the IR-O response element. The DR1 response element also binds the PPARα, β or γ) receptor that in turn binds fatty acids. The PPARγ receptor binds prostaglandin $E_2$. All three of these receptors bind to the same element. If only one were to bind, the process would be called homodimerization. If more than one receptor binds to the same element, we would have heterodimerization.

Group II receptors, also called the retinoid/thyroid subfamily, bind nutrients and metabolites such as retinoic acid, vitamin D, and fatty acids. All of these receptors form heterodimers with the retinoid X receptor (RXR). 9-*cis* Retinoic acid binds RXR and has a synergistic effect on transcription when dimerized with most receptors in this group. Generally, these receptors bind to direct repeats of degenerative AGGTCA sequences spaced by (1) (RXR, LXR, PPAR), (2) (alternative RAR, TR), (3) (VDR), (4) (TR, LXR), or (5) (RAR) nucleotides. Specificity occurs due to the spacing between the consensus sequence

## TABLE 9.2
### Some Nutrient Effects on Transcription

| Nutrient | Gene | Effect |
|---|---|---|
| Manganese | Superoxide dismutase | ↑ Transcription and translation[43] |
| Vitamin D | Vitamin D receptor | ↑ Transcription[18] |
| Vitamin E | Adiponectin, leptin | ↑ Transcription and translation[19] |
| DHA | Apolipoprotein A-1 | ↑ Transcription[44] |
| Copper | Hepcidin | ↑ Transcription[45] |
| Iron | Hepcidin | ↑ Transcription[46] |
| Selenium | Glutathione peroxidase | ↑ Transcription[17] |
| Retinoic acid | RAR | ↑ Transcription[47] |
| PUFA | Fatty acid synthetase | ↓ Transcription[48] |
| Sodium | Aldosterone synthetase | ↑ Transcription[49] |
| Potassium | " | " |

*Sources:* Berdanier, C.D. and Hargrove, J.L., eds., *Nutrition and Gene Expression*, CRC Press, Boca Raton, FL, 579p., 1993; Berdanier, C.D., ed., *Nutrients and Gene Expression: Clinical Aspects*, CRC Press, Boca Raton, FL, 216p., 1996; 16. Moustaid-Moussa, N. and Berdanier, C.D., ed., *Nutrient-Gene Interactions in Health and Disease*, CRC Press, Boca Raton, FL, 472p., 2001.

DHA, docosahexaenoic acid; PUFA, polyunsaturated fatty acids.

half sites. In the case of the retinoic acid receptor (RAR) and thyroid receptor (TR), unliganded receptor can bind DNA and repress transcription.

There are numerous proteins aside from those of the steroid receptor superfamily that bind to specific base sequences in the promoter region. Some of these bind minerals, some bind other hormones, and some are, by themselves, transcription factors that have control properties.

In addition to the receptor proteins that bind to certain base sequences in the promoter region, we also have smaller molecules that similarly serve to stimulate or suppress transcription. One such is the glucose molecule. It serves to stimulate the transcription of glucokinase that has a glucose-sensitive promoter region. Only the β cell and the hepatocyte DNA have this region exposed and only these cell types express the glucokinase gene. Other cells have the gene but do not express it probably because their glucose promoter site is unexposed. Instead, these other cell types express a similar (but different) gene that encodes hexokinase. There are a number of instances in the nutrition science literature where specific nutrients influence the transcription of genes that encode enzymes or receptors or carriers that are important to the use of that nutrient. Shown in Table 9.2 are examples of these influences. All of the earlier examples serve to control transcription, a vital step in controlling gene expression.

Once the bases are joined together in the nucleus to form messenger RNA, the nucleus must edit and process it. Processing it includes capping, nucleolytic and ligation reactions that shorten it, and terminal additions of nucleosides and nucleoside modifications (Figure 9.3). Through this processing, less than 25% of the original RNA migrates from the nucleus to the ribosomes where it attaches prior to translation. Editing and processing are needed because immature RNA contains all those bases corresponding to the DNA introns. Introns are those groups of bases that are not part of the structural gene. Introns are intervening sequences that separate the exons or coding sequences of the structural gene. The removal of these segments is a cut-and-splice process whereby the intron is cut at its 5' end, pulled out of the way, and cut again at its

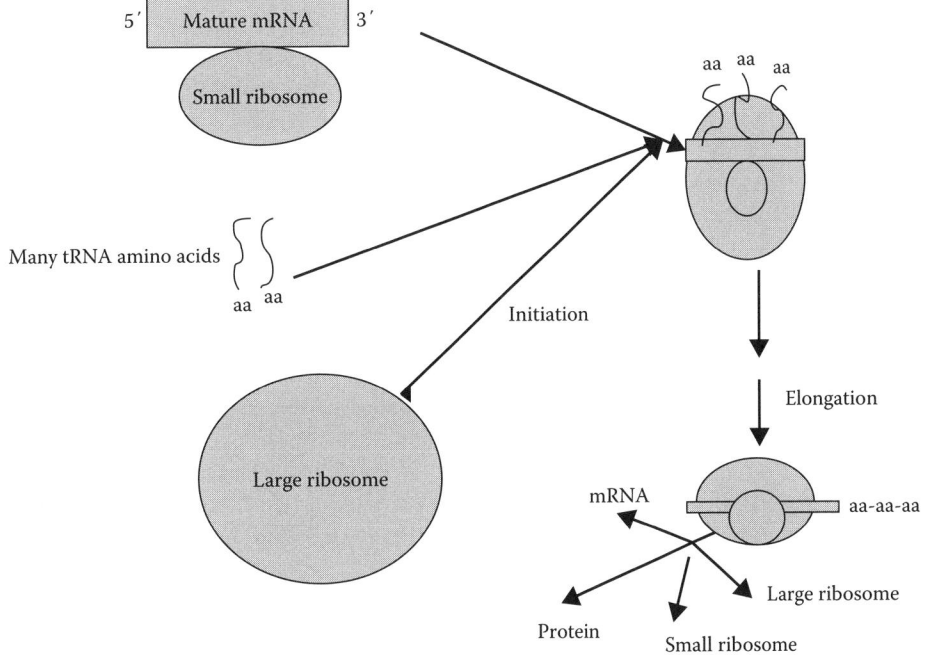

**FIGURE 9.3** Overview of translation involving mRNA, tRNA amino acids, and small and large ribosomal units.

3′ end; at the same time, the two exons are joined. This cut-and-splice routine is continued until all the introns are removed and the exons joined. Some editing of the RNA also occurs with base substitutions made as appropriate. Finally, a 3′ terminal poly A tail is added.

The editing and processing step is now complete. The mature messenger RNA now leaves the nucleus and moves to the cytoplasm for translation. The nucleotides that have been removed during editing and processing are either reused or totally degraded. Of note is the fact that editing and processing also are mechanisms used to degrade the whole message unit. This serves to control the amount and half-life of messenger RNA. The endonucleases and exonucleases used in the cut-and-splice processing also come into play in the regulation of mRNA stability. Some mRNAs have very short half-lives (seconds to minutes) while others have longer half-lives (hours). This is important because some gene products are needed for only a short time. Hormones and cell signals must be short lived and, therefore, the body needs to control/counterbalance their synthesis and action. One of the ways to do this is by regulating the amount of mRNA (number of copies of mRNA for each gene product) that leaves the nucleus. Thus, this regulation is a key step in metabolic control.

## TRANSLATION

Following transcription is translation shown in Figure 9.3. Translation is the synthesis of the protein using mRNA to dictate the order with which the amino acids are assembled. This process is also influenced by specific nutrients. The translation of the ferritin gene, for example, is influenced by the amount of iron available in the cell. In iron deficiency, the messenger RNA start site for ferritin translation is covered up by an iron-responsive protein. This protein binds the 3′UTR and inhibits the movement of the 40s ribosome from the cap to the translation start site. When iron status is improved, the start site is uncovered and translation proceeds.

The actual site of translation is on the ribosomes; some ribosomes are located on the membrane of the endoplasmic reticulum, and some are free in the cell matrix. Ribosomes consist almost entirely of ribosomal RNA and ribosomal protein. RNA is synthesized via RNA polymerase I in the cell nucleus as a large molecule; there, it is cleaved and leaves the nucleus as two subunits, a large one and a small one. The ribosome is reformed in the cytoplasm by the reassociation of the two subunits; the subunits, however, are not necessarily derived from the same precursor.

Ribosomal RNA makes up a large fraction of the total cellular RNA. It serves as the "docking" point for the activated amino acids bound to the transfer RNA and the mRNA that dictates the amino acid polymerization sequence. Transfer RNA (tRNA) is used to bring an amino acid to the polysome (ribosome), the site of protein synthesis. Each amino

acid has a specific tRNA. Each tRNA molecule is thought to have a cloverleaf arrangement of nucleotides. With this arrangement of nucleotides, there is the opportunity for the maximum number of hydrogen bonds to form between base pairs. A molecule that has many hydrogen bonds is very stable. Transfer RNA also contains a triplet of bases known, in this instance, as the anticodon. The amino acid carried by tRNA is identified by the codon of mRNA through its anticodon; the amino acid itself is not involved in this identification.

A few general statements can be made about the distribution of ribosomes in cells that have different capacities for the synthesis of proteins. (1) Cells that synthesize large numbers of proteins have numerous ribosomes; conversely, cells that synthesize small numbers of proteins contain few. (2) Of the proteins synthesized by a cell to be secreted from that cell for use elsewhere, most of the ribosomes are attached to the endoplasmic reticulum. (3) Those cells that synthesize protein primarily for intracellular use have relatively few ribosomes attached to the endoplasmic reticulum membrane. Small groups of ribosomes called *polysomes* are involved in protein synthesis; under physiological conditions, polysomes are bound to the endoplasmic reticulum. The ribosome is bound to the membrane through its large subunit; the small subunit is involved in the binding of mRNA to the ribosome. The ribosomes have two binding sites used in protein synthesis: the amino-acyl site and the peptidyl site. These two sites have specific functions in protein synthesis.

Translation takes place in four stages, as illustrated in Figure 9.3. Each stage requires specific cofactors and enzymes. In the first stage, which occurs in the cytosol, the amino acids are activated by esterifying each one to its specific tRNA. This requires a molecule of ATP. In addition to a specific tRNA, each amino acid requires a specific enzyme for this reaction.

During the second stage, the initiation of the synthesis of the polypeptide chain occurs. Initiation requires that mRNA bind to the ribosome. An initiation complex is formed by the binding of mRNA cap and the first activated amino acid–tRNA complex to the small ribosomal subunit. The ribosome finds the correct reading frame on the mRNA by "scanning" for an AUG codon. The large ribosomal unit then attaches, thus forming a functional ribosome. A number of specific protein initiation factors are involved in this step.

In the third stage of protein synthesis, the peptide chain is elongated by the sequential addition of amino acids from the tRNA complexes. The amino acid is recognized by base pairing of the codon of mRNA to the bases found in the anticodon of tRNA, and a peptide bond is formed between the peptide chain and the newly arrived amino acid. The ribosome then moves along the mRNA; this brings the next codon in the proper position for attachment of the next activated amino-acyl–tRNA complex. The mRNA and nascent polypeptide appear to "track" through a groove in the ribosomal subunits. This protects them from attack by enzymes in the surrounding environment.

The final stage of protein synthesis is the termination of the chain. The termination is signaled by one of three special codons (stop codons) in the mRNA. After the carboxy terminal amino acid is attached to the peptide chain, it is still covalently attached to tRNA, which is, in turn, bonded to the ribosome. A protein release factor promotes the hydrolysis of the ester link between the tRNA and the amino acid. Once the polypeptide chain is generated and free of the ribosome, it assumes its characteristic three-dimensional structure.

After translation is complete, the primary structure is complete. At this point, some posttranslational modification can occur, and again specific nutrients can influence the process. For example, after the translation of osteocalcin and prothrombin, two proteins that have glutamic-acid-rich regions, these glutamate residues are carboxylated. This posttranslational carboxylation requires vitamin K. Should vitamin K be in short supply, this carboxylation will not occur (or will occur in only a limited way), and these proteins will not be able to bind calcium. Both must bind calcium in order to function; osteocalcin in bone can neither bind calcium nor prothrombin. Hence, bone will be more fragile, and blood will not clot as needed.

As the chain of amino acids is produced, the amino acids in that chain begin to interact to form the protein's secondary structure. Then, as the chain twists and turns, more global interactions occur and the tertiary structure becomes apparent. All of these interactions, i.e., hydrogen bonding, disulfide bridges, etc., serve to stabilize the protein. Lastly, as these tertiary structures are synthesized, they assemble as subunits of more complex structures (quaternary structures) in the functional protein. Some proteins are very complex and have many subunits; for example, the cytochromes in the mitochondrial respiratory chain, whereas others are not as complex.

## EPIGENETICS

Epigenetics is the study of heritable changes in gene expression that occur without a change in the sequence of the DNA. Epigenetic regulation of gene expression occurs at the chromatin level, for example, DNA methylation and histone modification. Chromatin is a complex of DNA, the $H_1$, $H_{2A}$, $H_{2B}$, $H_3$, and $H_4$ histones, and nonhistone proteins.[38–42] DNA and histones form repetitive nucleoprotein units called nucleosomal core particles. Each particle consists of 146 base pairs of DNA wrapped around an octamer of core histones (one $H_3$–$H_3$–$H_4$–$H_4$ tetramer and two $H_{2A}$–$H_{2B}$ dimers). The DNA located between nucleosomal core particles is associated with histone $H_1$. This 11 nm histone fiber is then further packed into an irregular 30 nm chromatin fiber structure, which is coiled into even more complex structures to form a chromosome.

The amino terminal tails of histones protrude from the nucleosomal surface; covalent modifications of these tails affect the structure of chromatin and form the basis for the epigenetic regulation of chromatin structure and gene function. Epigenetics is defined as the study of heritable changes of gene function that occur without a change in the nucleotide sequence of DNA. For example, amino acid residues in histone tails are modified by covalent acetylation, biotinylation, methylation, phosphorylation, and ubiquitination, and these serve to regulate gene transcription, mitotic condensation of chromatin, and DNA replication/repair. These modifications are deciphered by proteins containing motifs that target them to chromatin. Indeed, some transcription factors contain bromodomains with an affinity for acetylated histones that then serve to increase gene expression.

Modifications of distinct amino acid residues in histones have unique functions. For example, tri-methylation of lysine (K)-4 in histone $H_3$ is associated with transcriptional activation of surrounding DNA, whereas di-methylation of $K_9$ is associated with transcriptional silencing. Covalent modifications of histones can be reversed by a large variety of enzymatic processes. Nutrients and nutritional status can affect these processes.[34] Several vitamins have been shown to modify histones. These include the binding of biotin to lysine residues in histones; folate-dependent methylation of lysine residues; and the niacin-dependent poly(ADP-ribosylation) of glutamate residues. Acetylation of histones also represents a vitamin-dependent form of chromatin structure regulation, based on the fact that pantothenate-derived coenzyme A is a building block in the formation of acetyl-CoA, which is the substrate for acetylation of histones. The methylation of histones can alter acetylation patterns, and deacetylation of histones is dependent on dietary niacin status via the size of the nicotinamide adenine dinucleotide pool.

Finally, another folate-dependent epigenetic event has captured the scientific interest for decades: covalent binding of methyl groups (derived from folate) to produce 5-methylcytosine in mammalian DNA. This modification of DNA also depends on a number of other nutrients, including S-adenosyl methionine, cobalamin (vitamin $B_{12}$), pyridoxine, methionine, betaine, riboflavin, zinc, and choline. Methylation of cytosine residues in DNA is associated with repression of transcription. Table 9.3 lists a few epigenetic events.

## TABLE 9.3
## Nutrients and Epigenetic Response

| Nutrient | Response |
|---|---|
| Folate | ↑ DNA methylation[34,50,51] |
| γ-Tocopherol | Inhibition of DNA methylation[52] |
| $B_{12}$ | ↑ DNA methylation[34] |

**TABLE 9.4**

**Examples of Different Polymorphisms and Responses to a Nutrient Variable**

| Gene | Polymorphism | Nutrient | Result |
|---|---|---|---|
| β-2-Adrenoceptor | Gln27Glu | Carbohydrate | ↑ Insulin levels; ↑ obesity[53] |
| Hepatic lipase | 480C>T | Fat | Higher enzyme activity in CT and TT genotypes than CC genotypes[54] |
| PPARα | 162L>V | PUFA | V had lower apoC-III[55] |
| MTHFR | C677T | Folate, $B_{12}$ | TT genotypes had higher serum homocysteine levels, lower RBC folate, and needed more dietary folate[56–59] |
| MTHFR | 677 +/+ vs. +/− | Folate and choline | Increased choline turnover[60] |
| MTHFR | 1298A→C | PUFA | Assoc. with hypertension; interacts with PUFA intake; ↓homocysteine[61] |
| IL2 | 330A→C | Vitamin E | Respiratory tract (RI) infection was lower in C |
| IL10 | 819G→C | Vitamin E | RI was lower in C |
|  | 1982C→T | Vitamin E | RI was lower in T |
| ANGPTL4 | A→G | Fat intake | A had higher HDL-C and lower TG |
| TCN267 | A→G vs. AA | Vitamin $B_{12}$ | Holotranscarbamylase was lower in TCN267A→G[62] |
| GST | M1 vs. T1 | Vitamin C | GSTM1 had higher vitamin C and lower malondialdehyde, higher iron and total LDL cholesterol levels than GSTT1[63] |

## NUTRIENT–POLYMORPHISM INTERACTIONS

It is generally assumed that polymorphisms in the structural genes have little immediate effect on the gene products. However, there are indications that there can be some long-term differences in health and well-being due to interactions between diet variables and these polymorphisms. Table 9.4 lists some reports of such nutrient–polymorphism interactions. That such polymorphisms could have long-term effects suggests that these polymorphisms could serve as important indicators of individual needs and tolerances for the individual nutrients. This, in turn, may set the stage for recommending nutrient intakes based on the genetic signature of the individual. This is a very active area of research that holds much promise for the future.

## REFERENCES

1. Kunkel, TA, *J. Biol. Chem.* 267: 18251; 1992.
2. Clarke, SD, Abraham, S, *FASEB J.* 6: 3146; 1992.
3. Freedman, LP, Luisi, BF, *J. Cell. Biochem.* 51: 140; 1993.
4. Kollmar, R, Farnham, PJ, *PSEBM* 203: 127; 1993.
5. Lea, MA, *Int. J. Biochem.* 25: 457; 1993.
6. Reichel, RR, Jacob, ST, *FASEB J.* 7: 427; 1993.
7. Semenza, GL, *Hum. Mutat.* 3: 180; 1994.
8. Johnson, PF, Sterneck, E, Williams, SC, *J. Nutr. Biochem.* 4: 386; 1993.
9. Klug, A, Rhodes, D, *Trends Biochem. Sci.* 12: 464; 1987.
10. Bray, P, Lichter, HJ, Ward, DC, Dawid, IB, *Proc. Natl. Acad. Sci. USA* 88: 9563; 1991.
11. Miller, SG, DaVos, P, Guerre-Mills, M et al., *Proc. Natl. Acad. Sci. USA* 93: 5507; 1996.
12. Hastings, KEM, Emerson, CD, In: *Recombinant DNA and Cell Proliferation*, Stein, GS, Stein, JL, eds., Academic Press, Orlando, FL, p. 219, 1984.
13. Tsai, M-J, O'Malley, BW, *Ann. Rev. Biochem.* 63: 451; 1994.
14. Berdanier, CD, Hargrove, JL, eds., *Nutrition and Gene Expression*, CRC Press, Boca Raton, FL, 579pp., 1993.
15. Berdanier, CD, ed., *Nutrients and Gene Expression: Clinical Aspects*, CRC Press, Boca Raton, FL, 216pp., 1996.
16. Moustaid-Moussa, N, Berdanier, CD, ed., *Nutrient-Gene Interactions in Health and Disease*, CRC Press, Boca Raton, FL, 472pp., 2001.
17. Huang, J-Q, Li, D-L, Zhao, L-H et al., *J. Nutr.* 141: 1605; 2011.
18. Kamei, KY, Kawada, T, Kazuki, R et al., *BBRC* 193: 948; 1993.
19. Shen, X-H, Tang, Q-Y, Huang, J, Cai, W, *Exp. Biol. Med.* 235: 47; 2010.
20. Everts, HB, Classen, DO, Hermoyian, CL, Berdanier, CD, *IUBMB-Life* 53: 295; 2002.
21. Berdanier, CD, *Proc. Exp. Biol. Med.* 231: 1593; 2006.
22. Falvey, E, Schibler, U, *FASEB J.* 5: 309; 1991.
23. Griffin, JB, Rodriguez-Melendez, R, Zempleni, J, *J. Nutr.* 133: 3409; 2003.
24. Rodriguez-Melendez, R, Schwab, LD, Zempleni, J, *Int. J. Vitam. Nutr. Res.* 74: 209; 2004.
25. Wallace, DC, *Ann. Rev. Biochem.* 61: 1175; 1992.
26. Taanman, JW, Williams, SL, In: *Mitochondria in Health and Disease*, Berdanier, CD, ed., CRC Press, Boca Raton, FL, p. 95, 2005.
27. Robyr, D, Wolfe, AP, *Life Sci.* 54: 113; 1998.
28. Wolffe, A, *Chromatin*, 3rd edn., Academic Press, San Diego, CA, 300pp., 2001.
29. Camporeale, G, Zempleni, J, In: *Present Knowledge in Nutrition*, 9th edn., Bowman, BA, Russell, RM, eds., ILSI Press, Washington, DC, p. 314, 2006.
30. Espino, PS, Drobic, B, Dunn, KL, Davie, JR, *J. Cell Biochem.* 94: 1088; 2005.
31. Jenuwein, T, Allis, CD, *Science* 293: 1074; 2001.
32. Fischle, W, Wang, Y, Allis, CD, *Curr. Opin. Cell Biol.* 215: 172; 2003.
33. Shilatifard, A, *FASEB J.* 12: 1437; 1998.
34. Choi, S-W, Friso, S, eds., *Nutrition and Epigenetics*, CRC Press, Boca Raton, FL, 245pp., 2009.
35. Aso, T, Conaway, JW, Conaway, RC, *FASEB J.* 9: 1419; 1995.
36. Ren, H, Stiles, GL, *Proc. Natl. Acad. Sci. USA* 91: 4864; 1994.

37. Weiss, L, Reinberg, D, *FASEB J.* 6: 3300; 1992.

38. Camporeale, G, Shubert, EE, Sarath, G et al., *Eur. J. Biochem.* 271: 2257; 2004.

39. Kobza, K, Camporeale, G, Rueckert, B, *FEBS J.* 272: 4249; 2005.

40. Chew, YC, Camporeale, G, Kothapalli, N et al., *J. Nutr. Biochem.* 17: 225; 2006.

41. Dey, A, Chitsaz, F, Abbasi, A et al., *Proc. Natl. Acad. Sci. USA* 100: 8758; 2003.

42. Christman, JK, In: *Molecular Nutrition*, Zempleni, J, Daniel, H, eds., CAB International, Wallingford, U.K., p. 237; 2003.

43. Li, S, Lu, L, Hao, S et al., *J. Nutr.* 141: 189; 2011.

44. Kuang, Y-L, Paulson, KE, Lichtenstein, AH et al., *J. Clin. Nutr.* 94: 594; 2011.

45. Jenkitkasemwong, S, Broderius, M, Nam, H et al., *J Nutr.* 140: 723; 2010.

46. Hansen, SL, Trakooljul, N, Spears, JW, Lin, H-C, *J. Nutr.* 140: 271; 2010.

47. Jump, DB, Lepar, GJ, MacDougald, OA, In: *Nutrition and Gene Expression*, Berdanier, CD, Hargrove, JL, eds., CRC Press, Boca Raton, FL, p. 431, 1993.

48. Blake, WL, Clarke, SD, *J. Nutr.* 120: 1727; 1990.

49. Holland, OB, Carr, B, *Endocrinology* 132: 2666; 1993.

50. Kotsopoulos, J, Sohn, K-J, Kim, Y-I, *J. Nutr.* 138: 703; 2008.

51. Friso, S, Choi, SW, *Curr. Drug Metab.* 6: 37; 2005.

52. Huang, Y, Khor, TO, Shu, L et al., *J. Nutr.* 142: 818; 2012.

53. Martinez, JA, Calaban, MS, Sanchez-Villegas, A et al., *J. Nutr.* 133: 2549; 2003.

54. Bos, G, Dekker, JM, Feskens, EJ et al., *Am. J. Clin. Nutr.* 81: 911; 2005.

55. Tai, ES, Corella, D, Demissie, S et al., *J. Nutr.* 135: 397; 2005.

56. Huh, HJ, Chi, HS, Shim, EH et al., *Thromb. Res.* 117: 501; 2006.

57. Robitaille, J, Hammer, HC, Cogswell, ME, Yang, Q, *Am. J. Clin. Nutr.* 89: 1269; 2009.

58. Tsai, MY, Loria, CM, Cao, J et al., *J. Nutr.* 139: 33; 2009.

59. Crider, KS, Zhu, J-H, Hao, Q-H et al., *Am. J. Clin. Nutr.* 93:1365; 2011.

60. Chew, TW, Jiang, X, Yan, J et al., *J. Nutr.* 141: 1475; 2011.

61. Huang, T, Tucker, KL, Lee, YY et al., *J. Nutr.* 141: 654; 2011.

62. Riedel, BM, Molloy, AM, Meyer, K et al., *J. Nutr.* 141: 1784; 2011.

63. Block, G, Shaikh, N, Jensen, CD et al., *Am. J. Clin. Nutr.* 94: 929; 2011.

# 10 Nutrition Terminology

*Carolyn D. Berdanier*

## CONTENTS

As with any discipline, nutrition science has its own vocabulary and terminology. It uses many of the same words as do biochemists, physiologists, and medical practitioners. This chapter gives the reader several tables providing this terminology. The first is a table giving the factors for converting the results of laboratory analysis to standard units called SI units. Many scientific journals require the use of these units in manuscripts reporting the results of laboratory investigations. The result, or common component from clinical laboratory assessment, is given in its common form with reference interval and present unit, followed by the conversion factor that is used to convert the result into SI units, its reference intervals, significant digits, and suggested minimum increment. These standard units for expressing biological data are listed in Table 10.1.[1]

Over the years, there has been some confusion over the names of the vitamins. Vitamins were named according to (a) their function; (b) their location; (c) the order in which they were discovered; or (d) combinations of (a), (b), or (c). Some of these names became obsolete as their proposed functions or their isolated structures were found to duplicate already named and described compounds. Obsolescence also occurred as research showed that certain of these compounds were not needed dietary factors, but were synthesized by the body in needed amounts. Table 10.2 provides a list of vitamin names (both obsolete and current), and it is hoped that the reader will find this useful. Following this is a list (Table 10.3) of all the compounds having vitamin A activity. This is a fairly lengthy list, as this vitamin is found in a variety of foods, both of animal origin and of plant origin. The body can convert these forms to its useful and most active form, all-*trans* retinol. These conversions are not 100% efficient, and correction factors must be applied to determine vitamin A activity.

In the area of energy research, there are a number of terms that the workers in this area assume that the reader knows. These are listed with their definitions in Table 10.4.

## BODY COMPOSITION ESTIMATION AND TERMINOLOGY

Normal bodies usually consist of 16%–20% protein, 3%–5% ash (mineral matter), 10%–12% fat, and 60%–70% water. Age, diet, genetic background, physical activity, hormonal status, and gender can affect not only the proximate composition of the whole body, that is, the magnitude of each of these components, but also their distribution. Body composition can be measured directly or estimated indirectly using a variety of techniques. Direct measurement involves the analysis of the major body components: fat, water, protein, and ash (mineral matter). Direct measurements are usually impractical for large species, including man. The equations used for the calculation of body components from direct analysis are given in Table 10.5.

Sophisticated techniques using ultrasound, neutron activation analysis, infrared interactance, dual-energy x-ray absorptiometry, computer-assisted tomography, magnetic resonance imaging, or bioelectrical impedance are available for the indirect estimation of body composition. The equations for converting data obtained using these sophisticated techniques are available.[2]

There are locations in the body where subcutaneous fat can be assessed using calipers to measure skin-fold thickness and thereby estimate body fatness. The fold below the upper arm (triceps fold) and the fold at the iliac crest are frequently used locations. Other locations include the abdominal fold and the thigh fold. Equations have been derived (Table 10.6) to calculate body fatness using these measurements.[3,4] Knowing the composition of the body, particularly its fat content, suggests that there should be ways of estimating body energy need. Some of these equations are shown in Table 10.7.[4]

Perhaps more popular now is the use of body mass index (BMI). This is a useful term in that it is an index of the body weight (kg) divided by the height (m) squared (weight/height$^2$). BMI correlates with body fatness and with the risk of obesity-related disease or diseases for which obesity is a compounding factor. Overweight is defined as a BMI between 25 and 30, and obesity is a BMI over 30. The BMI varies with age. A desirable BMI for people of age 19–24 is between 19 and 24, while that for people of age 55–64 is between 23 and 28. While simple in concept, this term does not assess body composition per se. It only provides a basis for assessing the health risks associated or presumed to be associated with excess body fatness. BMI applies only to normal individuals, and not the superathlete or the bodybuilder, who may be quite heavy yet have little body fat.

**TABLE 10.1**

**Conversion Factors for Values in Clinical Chemistry (SI Units)**

| Component Present | Reference Intervals (Examples) | Present Unit | Conversion Factor | SI Reference Intervals | SI Unit | Symbol | Significant Digits | Suggested Minimum Increment |
|---|---|---|---|---|---|---|---|---|
| Acetaminophen (P) toxic | >5.0 | mg/dL | 66.16 | >330 | mmol/L | XXO | 10 | mmol/L |
| Acetoacetate (S) | 0.3–3.0 | mg/dL | 97.95 | 30–300 | mmol/L | XXO | 10 | mmol/L |
| Acetone (B.S) | 0 | mg/dL | 172.2 | 0 | mmol/L | XXO | 10 | mmol/L |
| Acid phosphatase (S) | 0–5.5 | U/L | 16.67 | 0–90 | nkat/L | XX | 2 | nkat/L |
| Adrenocorticotropin (ACTH) (P) | 20–100 | pg/mL | 0.2202 | 4–22 | pmol/L | XX | 1 | pmol/L |
| Alanine aminotransferase (ALT) (S) | 0–35 | U/L | 0.01667 | 0–0.58 | mkat/L | X.XX | 0.02 | mkat/L |
| Albumin (S) | 4.0–6.0 | g/dL | 10.0 | 40–60 | g/L | XX | 1 | g/L |
| Aldolase (S) | 0–6 | U/L | 16.67 | 0–100 | nkat/L | XXO | 20 | nkat/L |
| Aldosterone (S) | | | | | | | | |
|   Normal salt diet | 8.1–15.5 | ng/dL | 27.74 | 220–430 | pmol/L | XXO | 10 | pmol/L |
|   Restricted salt diet | 20.8–44.4 | ng/dL | 27.74 | 580–1240 | pmol/L | XXO | 10 | pmol/L |
| Aldosterone (U): sodium excretion | | | | | | | | |
|   = 25 mmol/day | 18–85 | mg/24 h | 2.774 | 50–235 | nmol/day | XXX | 5 | nmol/day |
|   = 75–125 mmol/day | 5–26 | mg/24 h | 2.774 | 15–70 | nmol/day | XXX | 5 | nmol/day |
|   = 200 mmol/day | 1.5–12.5 | mg/24 h | 2.774 | 5–35 | nmol/day | XXX | 5 | nmol/day |
| Alkaline phosphatase (S) | 0–120 | U/L | 0.01667 | 0.5–2.0 | mkat/L | X.X | 0.1 | mkat/L |
| $\alpha_1$-Antitrypsin (S) | 150–350 | mg/dL | 0.01 | 1.5–3.5 | g/L | X.X | 0.1 | g/L |
| $\alpha$-Fetoprotein (S) | 0–20 | ng/mL | 1.00 | 0–20 | mg/L | XX | 1 | mg/L |
| $\alpha$-Fetoprotein (Amf) | Depends on gestation | mg/dL | 10.0 | Depends on gestation | mg/L | XX | 1 | mg/L |
| $\alpha_2$-Macroglobulin (S) | 145–410 | mg/dL | 0.01 | 1.5–4.1 | g/L | X.X | 1 | mg/L |
| Aluminum (S) | 0–15 | mg/L | 37.06 | 0–560 | nmol/L | XXO | 10 | nmol/L |
| Amino acid fractionation (P) | | | | | | | | |
|   Alanine | 2.2–4.5 | mg/dL | 112.2 | 245–500 | mmol/L | XXX | 5 | mol/L |
|   $\alpha$-Aminobutyric acid | 0.1–0.2 | mg/dL | 96.97 | 10–20 | mmol/L | XXX | 5 | mmol/L |
|   Arginine | 0.5–2.5 | mg/dL | 57.40 | 30–145 | mmol/L | XXX | 5 | mmol/L |
|   Asparagine | 0.5–0.6 | mg/dL | 75.69 | 35–45 | mmol/L | XXX | 5 | mmol/L |
|   Citrulline | 0.2–1.0 | mg/dL | 75.13 | 0–20 | mmol/L | XXX | 5 | mmol/L |
|   Cystine | 0.2–2.2 | mg/dL | 57.08 | 15–55 | mmol/L | XXX | 5 | mmol/L |
|   Glutamic acid | 0.2–2.8 | mg/dL | 67.97 | 15–190 | mmol/L | XXX | 5 | mmol/L |
|   Glutamine | 6.1–10.2 | mg/dL | 68.42 | 420–700 | mmol/L | XXX | 5 | mmol/L |
|   Glycine | 0.9–4.2 | mg/dL | 133.2 | 120–560 | mmol/L | XXX | 5 | mmol/L |
|   Histidine | 0.5–1.7 | mg/dL | 64.45 | 30–110 | mmol/L | XXX | 5 | mmol/L |
|   Hydroxyproline | 0–trace | mg/dL | 76.26 | 0–trace | mmol/L | XXX | 5 | mmol/L |
|   Isoleucine | 0.5–1.3 | mg/dL | 76.24 | 40–100 | mmol/L | XXX | 5 | mmol/L |

| Analyte | Reference range (conventional) | Conventional unit | Factor | SI reference range | SI format | SI significance | SI unit |
|---|---|---|---|---|---|---|---|
| Leucine | 1.2–3.5 | mg/dL | 76.24 | 75–175 | XXX | 5 | mmol/L |
| Lysine | 1.2–3.5 | mg/dL | 68.40 | 80–240 | XXX | 5 | mmol/L |
| Methionine | 0.1–0.6 | mg/dL | 67.02 | 5–40 | XXX | 5 | mmol/L |
| Ornithine | 0.4–1.4 | mg/dL | 75.67 | 30–400 | XXX | 5 | mmol/L |
| Phenylalanine | 0.6–1.5 | mg/dL | 60.54 | 35–90 | XXX | 5 | mmol/L |
| Proline | 1.2–3.9 | mg/dL | 86.86 | 105–340 | XXX | 5 | mmol/L |
| Serine | 0.8–1.8 | mg/dL | 95.16 | 75–170 | XXX | 5 | mmol/L |
| Taurine | 0.9–2.5 | mg/dL | 79.91 | 25–170 | XXX | 5 | mmol/L |
| Threonine | 0.9–2.5 | mg/dL | 83.95 | 75–210 | XXX | 5 | mmol/L |
| Tryptophan | 0.5–2.5 | mg/dL | 48.97 | 25–125 | XXX | 5 | mmol/L |
| Tyrosine | 0.4–1.6 | mg/dL | 55.19 | 20–90 | XXX | 5 | mmol/L |
| Valine | 1.7–3.7 | mg/dL | 85.36 | 145–315 | XXX | 5 | mmol/L |
| Amino acid nitrogen (P) | 4.0–6.0 | mg/dL | 0.7139 | 2.9–4.3 | X.X | 0.1 | mmol/L |
| Amino acid nitrogen (U) | 50–200 | mg/24 h | 0.07139 | 3.6–14.3 | X.X | 0.1 | mmol/day |
| δ-Aminolevulinate (as levulinic acid) (U) | 1.0–7.0 | mg/24 h | 7.626 | 8–53 | XX | 1 | mmol/day |
| Amitriptyline (P,S) therapeutic | 50–200 | ng/mL | 3.605 | 180–270 | XO | 10 | nmol/L |
| Ammonia (vP) as | | | | | | | |
| Ammonia ($NH_3$) | 10–80 | mg/dL | 0.5872 | 5–50 | XXX | 5 | mmol/L |
| Ammonium ion ($NH_4^+$) | 10–85 | mg/dL | 0.5543 | 5–50 | XXX | 5 | mmol/L |
| Nitrogen (N) | 10–65 | mg/dL | 0.7139 | 5–50 | XXX | 5 | mmol/L |
| Amylase (S) | 0–130 | U/L | 0.01667 | 0–2.17 | XXX | 0.01 | mkat/L |
| Androstenedione (S) | | | | | | | |
| Male >18 years | 0.2–3.0 | mg/L | 3.492 | 0.5–10.5 | XX.X | 0.5 | nmol/L |
| Female >18 years | 0.8–3.0 | mg/L | 3.492 | 3.0–10.5 | XX.X | 0.5 | nmol/L |
| Angiotensin converting as | | | | | | | |
| Enzyme (S) | <40 | nmol/mL/min | 16.67 | <670 | XXO | 10 | nkat/L |
| Arsenic (H) (as As) | <1 | mg/g (ppm) | 13.35 | <13 | XX.X | 0.5 | nmol/g |
| Arsenic (U) (as As) | 0–5 | mg/24 h | 13.35 | 0–67 | XX | 1 | nmol/day |
| $As_2O_3$ | <25 | | 0.05055 | <1.3 | XX.X | 0.1 | mmo/L |
| Ascorbate (P) (as ascorbic acid) | 0.6–2.0 | mg/dL | 56.78 | 30–110 | XO | 10 | mmo/L |
| Aspartate aminotransferase (AST) (S) | 0–35 | U/L | 0.0167 | 0–0.58 | O.XX | 0.01 | mkat/L |
| Barbiturate (S) overdose total expressed as | Depends on composition of mixture usually not known | | | | | | |
| Phenobarbital | | mg/dL | 43.06 | — | XX | 5 | mmol/L |
| Sodium phenobarbital | | mg/dL | 39.34 | — | XX | 5 | mmol/L |
| Barbitone | | mg/dL | 54.29 | — | XX | 5 | mmol/L |

(continued)

**TABLE 10.1 (continued)**
**Conversion Factors for Values in Clinical Chemistry (SI Units)**

| Component Present | Reference Intervals (Examples) | Present Unit | Conversion Factor | SI Reference Intervals | SI Unit | Symbol | Significant Digits | Suggested Minimum Increment |
|---|---|---|---|---|---|---|---|---|
| Barbiturate (S) therapeutic | See phenobarbital, pentobarbital, thiopental | | | | | | | |
| Bile acids, total (S) | | | | | | | | |
| As chenodeoxycholic acid | Trace–3.3 | mg/mL | 2.547 | Trace–8.4 | mmol/L | X.X | 0.2 | mmol/L |
| Cholic acid | Trace–1.0 | mg/mL | 2.448 | Trace–2.4 | mmol/L | X.X | 0.2 | mmol/L |
| Chenodeoxycholic acid | Trace–1.3 | mg/mL | 2.547 | Trace–3.4 | mmol/L | X.X | 0.2 | mmol/L |
| Deoxycholic acid | Trace–1.0 | mg/mL | 2.547 | Trace–2.6 | mmol/L | X.X | 0.2 | mmol/L |
| Lithocholic acid | Trace | mg/mL | 2.656 | Trace | mmol/L | X.X | 0.2 | mmol/L |
| Bile acids (Df) (after cholecystokinin stimulation) total as | | | | | | | | |
| Chenodeoxycholic acid | 14.0–58.0 | mg/mL | 2.547 | 35–148 | mmol/L | XX.X | 0.2 | mmol/L |
| Cholic acid | 2.4–33.0 | mg/mL | 2.448 | 6.8–81.0 | mmol/L | XX.X | 0.2 | mmol/L |
| Chenodeoxycholic acid | 4.0–24.0 | mg/mL | 2.547 | 10.0–61.4 | mmol/L | XX.X | 0.2 | mmol/L |
| Deoxycholic acid | 0.8–6.9 | mg/mL | 2.547 | 2–18 | mmol/L | XX.X | 0.2 | mmol/L |
| Lithocholic acid | 0.3–0.8 | mg/mL | 2.656 | 0.8–2.0 | mmol/L | XX.X | 0.2 | mmol/L |
| Bilirubin, total (S) | 0.1–1.0 | mg/dL | 17.10 | 2–18 | mmol/L | XX | 2 | mmol/L |
| Bilirubin, conjugated (S) | 0–0.2 | mg/dL | 17.10 | 0–4 | mmol/L | XX | 2 | mmol/L |
| Bromide (S) toxic | | | | | | | | |
| As bromide ion | >120 | mg/dL | 0.1252 | >15 | mmol/L | XX | 1 | mmol/L |
| As sodium bromide | >150 | mg/dL | 0.09719 | >15 | mmol/L | XX | 1 | mmol/L |
| | >15 | mEq/L | 1.00 | >15 | mmol/L | XX | 1 | mmol/L |
| Cadmium (S) | <3 | mg/dL | 0.08897 | <0.3 | mmol/L | X.X | 0.1 | mmol/L |
| Calcitonin (S) | <100 | pg/mL | 1.00 | <100 | ng/L | XXX | 10 | ng/L |
| Calcium (S) | | | | | | | | |
| Male | 8.8–10.3 | mg/dL | 0.2495 | 2.20–2.58 | mmol/L | X.XX | 0.02 | mmol/L |
| Female <50 years | 8.8–10.0 | mg/dL | 0.2495 | 2.20–2.50 | mmol/L | X.XX | 0.02 | mmol/L |
| Female >50 years | 8.8–10.2 | mg/dL | 0.2495 | 2.20–2.56 | mmol/L | X.XX | 0.02 | mmol/L |
| | 4.4–5.1 | mEq/L | 0.500 | 2.20–2.56 | mmol/L | X.XX | 0.02 | mmol/L |
| Calcium ion (S) | 2.00–2.30 | mEq/L | 0.500 | 1.00–1.15 | mmol/L | X.XX | 0.01 | mmol/L |
| Calcium (U), normal diet | <250 | mg/24 h | 0.02495 | <6.2 | mmol/day | X.X | 0.1 | mmol/day |
| Carbamazepine (P) therapeutic | 4.0–10.0 | mg/L | 4.233 | 17–42 | mmol/L | XX | 1 | mmol/L |
| Carbon dioxide content (B,P,S) (bicarbonate + $CO_2$) | 22–28 | mEq/L | 1.00 | 22–28 | mmol/L | X | 1 | mmol/L |
| Carbon monoxide (B) (proportion of Hb that is COHb) | <15 | % | 0.01 | <0.15 | 1 | O.XX | 0.01 | |
| β Carotenes (S) | 50–250 | mg/dL | 0.01863 | 0.9–4.6 | mmol/L | X.X | 0.1 | mmol/L |
| Catecholamines, total (U) (as norepinephrine) | <120 | mg/24 h | 5.911 | <675 | nmol/day | XXO | 10 | mg/day |
| Ceruloplasmin (S) | 20–35 | mg/dL | 10.0 | 200–350 | mg/L | XXO | 10 | mg/L |

|  | | | | | | | | |
|---|---|---|---|---|---|---|---|---|
| Chlordiazepoxide (P) | | | | | | | | |
|   Therapeutic | mg/L | 0.5–5.0 | 3.336 | 2–17 | mmol/L | XX | 1 | mmol/L |
|   Toxic | mg/L | >10.0 | 3.336 | >33 | mmol/L | XX | 1 | mmol/L |
| Chloride (S) | mEq/L | 95–105 | 1.00 | 95–105 | mmol/L | XXX | 1 | mmol/L |
| Chlorimipramine (P) (includes desmethyl metabolite) | ng/mL | 50–400 | 3.176 | 150–1270 | nmol/L | XXO | 10 | nmol/L |
| Chlorpromazine (P) | ng/mL | 50–300 | 3.136 | 150–950 | nmol/L | XXO | 10 | nmol/L |
| Chlorpropamide (P) therapeutic | mg/L | 75–250 | 3.613 | 270–900 | mmol/L | XXO | 10 | mmol/L |
| Cholestanol (P) (as a fraction of total cholesterol) | % | 1–3 | 0.01 | 0.01–0.03 | 1 | O.XX | 0.01 |  |
| Cholesterol (P) | | | | | | | | |
|   <29 years | mg/dL | <200 | 0.02586 | <5.20 | mol/L | X.XX | 0.05 | mmol/L |
|   30–39 years | mg/dL | <225 | 0.02586 | <5.85 | mmol/L | X.XX | 0.05 | mmol/L |
|   40–49 years | mg/dL | <245 | 0.02586 | <6.35 | mmol/L | X.XX | 0.05 | mmol/L |
|   >50 years | mg/dL | <265 | 0.02586 | <6.85 | mmol/L | X.XX | 0.05 | mmol/L |
| Cholesterol esters (P) (as a fraction of total cholesterol) | % | 60–75 | 0.01 | 0.60–0.75 | 1 | O.XX | 0.01 |  |
| Cholinesterase (S) | U/L | 620–1370 | 0.01667 | 10.3–22.8 | mkat/L | XX.X | 0.1 | mkat/L |
| Chorionic gonadotropin (P) (β HCG) | mIU/mL | 0 if not pregnant | 1.00 | 0 if not pregnant | IU/L | XX | 1 | IU/L |
| Citrate (B) (as citric acid) | mg/dL | 1.2–3.0 | 52.05 | 60–160 | mmol/L | XXX | 5 | mmol/L |
| Complement, C3 (S) | mg/dL | 70–160 | 0.01 | 0.7–1.6 | g/L | X.X | 0.1 | g/L |
| Complement, C4 (S) | mg/dL | 20–40 | 0.01 | 0.2–0.4 | g/L | X.X | 0.1 | g/L |
| Copper (S) | mg/dL | 70–140 | 0.1574 | 11.0–22.0 | mmol/L | XX.X | 0.2 | mmol/L |
| Copper (U) | mg/24 h | <40 | 0.01574 | <0.6 | mmol/day | X.X | 0.2 | mmol/L |
| Coproporphyrins (U) | mg/24 h | <200 | 1.527 | <300 | nmol/day | XXO | 10 | nmol/day |
| Cortisol (S) | | | | | | | | |
|   800 h | mg/dL | 4–19 | 27.59 | 110–520 | nmol/L | XXO | 10 | nmol/L |
|   1,600 h | mg/dL | 2–15 | 27.59 | 50–410 | nmol/L | XXO | 10 | nmol/L |
|   2,400 h | mg/dL | 5 | 7.59 | 140 | nmol/L | XXO | 10 | nmol/L |
| Cortisol, free (U) | mg/24 h | 10–110 | 2.759 | 30–300 | nmol/day | XXO | 10 | nmol/day |
| Creatine (S) | | | | | | | | |
|   Male | mg/dL | 0.17–0.50 | 76.25 | 10–40 | mmol/L | XO | 10 | mmol/L |
|   Female | mg/dL | 0.35–0.93 | 76.25 | 30–70 | mmol/L | XO | 10 | mmol/L |
| Creatine (U) | | | | | | | | |
|   Male | mg/24 h | 0–40 | 7.625 | 0–300 | mmol/day | XXO | 10 | mmol/day |
|   Female | mg/24 h | 0–80 | 7.625 | 0–600 | mmol/day | XXO | 10 | mmol/day |

(continued)

**TABLE 10.1 (continued)**
**Conversion Factors for Values in Clinical Chemistry (SI Units)**

| Component Present | Reference Intervals (Examples) | Present Unit | Conversion Factor | SI Reference Intervals | SI Unit | Symbol | Significant Digits | Suggested Minimum Increment |
|---|---|---|---|---|---|---|---|---|
| Creatine kinase (CK) (S) | | | | | | | | |
| Creatine kinase | | | | | | | | |
|   Isoenzymes (S) | 0–130 | U/L | 0.01667 | 0–2.16 | mkat/L | X.XX | 0.01 | mkat/L |
|   MB fraction | >5 in myocardial infarction | % | 0.01 | >0.05 | 1 | O.XX | 0.01 | |
| Creatinine (S) | 0.6–1.2 | mg/dL | 88.40 | 50–110 | mmol/L | XXO | 10 | mmol/L |
| Creatinine (U) | Variable | g/24 h | 8.840 | Variable | mmol/day | XX.X | 0.1 | mmol/day |
| Creatinine clearance (S,U) | 75–125 | mL/min | 0.01667 | 1.24–2.08 | mL/A (where A is the body surface area in square meters [m²]) | X.XX | 0.02 | mL/s |
| Cyanide (B) | | | | | | | | |
|   Lethal | >0.10 | mg/dL | 384.3 | >40 | mmol/L | XXX | 5 | mmol/L |
| Cyanocobalamin (S) | | | | | | | | |
|   (Vitamin B₁₂) | 100–200 | pg/mL | 0.7378 | 150–750 | pmol/L | XXO | 10 | pmol/L |
| Cyclic AMP (S) | 2.6–6.6 | mg/L | 3.038 | 8–20 | nmol/L | XXX | 1 | nmol/L |
| Cyclic AMP (U) | | | | | | | | |
|   Total urinary | 2.9–5.6 | mmol/g creatinine | 113.1 | 330–630 | nmol/mmol creatinine | XXO | 10 | nmol/mmol creatinine |
|   Renal tubular | <2.5 | mmol/g creatinine | 113.1 | <280 | nmol/mmol creatinine | XXO | 10 | nmol/mmol creatinine |
| Cyclic GMP (S) | 0.6–3.5 | mg/L | 2.897 | 1.7–10.1 | nmol/L | XX.X | 0.1 | nmol/L |
| Cyclic GMP (U) | 0.3–1.8 | mmol/g creatinine | 113.1 | 30–200 | nmol/mmol creatinine | XXO | 10 | nmol/mmol creatinine |
| Cystine (U) | 10–100 | mg/24 h | 4.161 | 40–420 | mmol/day | XXO | 10 | mmol/day |
| Dehydroepiandrosterone (DHEA) (P,S) | | | | | | | | |
|   1–4 years | 0.2–0.4 | mg/L | 3.467 | 0.6–1.4 | nmol/L | XX.X | 0.2 | nmol/L |
|   4–8 years | 0.1–1.9 | mg/L | 3.467 | 0.4–6.6 | nmol/L | XX.X | 0.2 | nmol/L |
|   8–10 years | 0.2–2.9 | mg/L | 3.467 | 0.6–10.0 | nmol/L | XX.X | 0.2 | nmol/L |
|   10–12 years | 0.5–9.2 | mg/L | 3.467 | 1.8–31.8 | nmol/L | XX.X | 0.2 | nmol/L |
|   12–14 years | 0.9–20.0 | mg/L | 3.467 | 3.2–69.4 | nmol/L | XX.X | 0.2 | nmol/L |
|   14–16 years | 2.5–20.0 | mg/L | 3.467 | 8.6–69.4 | nmol/L | XX.X | 0.2 | nmol/L |
|   Premenopausal female | 2.0–15.0 | mg/L | 3.467 | 7.0–52.0 | nmol/L | XX.X | 0.2 | nmol/L |
|   Male | 0.8–10.0 | mg/L | 3.467 | 2.8–34.6 | nmol/L | XX.X | 0.2 | nmol/L |
| DHEA (U) | See steroids | Fractionation | | | | | | |

| | Conventional range | Conversion factor | Conventional unit | SI range | SI unit | Sig. figures | Round | SI unit |
|---|---|---|---|---|---|---|---|---|
| DHEA sulfate (DHEA-S) (P,S) | | | | | | | | |
| Newborn | 1,670–3,640 | 0.002714 | ng/mL | 4.5–9.9 | µmol/L | XX.X | | µmol/L |
| Prepubertal children | 100–600 | 0.002714 | ng/mL | 0.3–1.6 | µmol/L | XX.X | | µmol/L |
| Male | 2,000–3,500 | 0.002714 | ng/mL | 5.4–9.1 | µmol/L | XX.X | | µmol/L |
| Female (premenopausal) | 820–3,380 | 0.002714 | ng/mL | 2.2–9.2 | µmol/L | XX.X | | µmol/L |
| Female (postmenopausal) | 110–610 | 0.002714 | ng/mL | 0.3–1.7 | µmol/L | XX.X | | µmol/L |
| Pregnancy (term) | 0–1,170 | 0.002714 | ng/mL | 0.6–3.2 | µmol/L | XX.X | | µmol/L |
| 11-Deoxycortisol (S) | 0–2 | 28.86 | µg/dL | 0–60 | nmol/L | XXO | 10 | nmol/L |
| Desipramine (P) therapeutic | 50–200 | 3.754 | ng/mL | 170–700 | nmol/L | XXO | 10 | nmol/L |
| Diazepam (P) | | | | | | | | |
| Therapeutic | 0.10–0.25 | 3512 | mg/L | 350–900 | nmol/L | XXO | 10 | nmol/L |
| Toxic | >1.0 | 3512 | mg/L | >3510 | nmol/L | XXO | 10 | nmol/L |
| Dicoumarol (P) therapeutic | 8–30 | 2.974 | mg/L | 25–90 | µmol/L | XX | 5 | µmol/L |
| Digoxin (P) | | | | | | | | |
| Therapeutic | 0.5–2.2 | 1.281 | ng/mL | 0.6–2.8 | nmol/L | X.X | 0.1 | nmol/L |
| | 0.5–2.2 | 1.281 | mg/L | 0.6–2.8 | nmol/L | X.X | 0.1 | nmol/L |
| Toxic | >2.5 | 1.281 | ng/mL | >3.2 | nmol/L | X.X | 0.1 | nmol/L |
| Dimethadione (P) therapeutic | <1.00 | 7.745 | g/L | <7.7 | mmol/L | X.X | 0.1 | mmol/L |
| Disopyramide (P) therapeutic | 2.0–6.0 | 2.946 | mg/L | 6–18 | µmol/L | XX | 1 | µmol/L |
| Doxepin (P) therapeutic | 50–200 | 3.579 | ng/mL | 180–720 | nmol/L | XO | 10 | nmol/L |
| Electrophoresis, protein (S) | | | | | | | | |
| Albumin | 60–65 | 0.01 | % | 0.60–0.65 | 1 | O.XX | 0.01 | 1 |
| α$_1$-Globulin | 1.7–5.0 | 0.01 | % | 0.02–0.05 | 1 | O.XX | 0.01 | 1 |
| α$_2$-Globulin | 6.7–12.5 | 0.01 | % | 0.07–0.13 | 1 | O.XX | 0.01 | 1 |
| β-Globulin | 8.3–16.3 | 0.01 | % | 0.08–0.16 | 1 | O.XX | 0.01 | 1 |
| γ-Globulin | 10.7–20.0 | 0.01 | % | 0.11–0.20 | 1 | O.XX | 0.01 | 1 |
| Albumin | 3.6–5.2 | 10.0 | g/dL | 36–52 | g/L | XX | 1 | g/L |
| α$_1$-Globulin | 0.1–0.4 | 10.0 | g/dL | 1–4 | g/L | XX | 1 | g/L |
| α$_2$-Globulin | 0.4–1.0 | 10.0 | g/dL | 4–10 | g/L | XX | 1 | g/L |
| β-Globulin | 0.5–1.2 | 10.0 | g/dL | 5–12 | g/L | XX | 1 | g/L |
| γ-Globulin | 0.6–1.6 | 10.0 | g/dL | 6–16 | g/L | XX | 1 | g/L |
| Epinephrine (P) | 31–95 (at rest for 15 min) | 5.458 | pg/mL | 170–520 | pmol/L | XXO | 10 | pmol/L |
| Epinephrine (U) | <10 | 5.458 | µg/24 h | <55 | nmol/day | XX | 5 | nmol/day |
| Estradiol (S) male >18 years | 15–40 | 3.671 | pg/mL | 55–150 | pmol/L | XX | 1 | pmol/L |
| Estriol (U) (nonpregnant) | | | | | | | | |
| Onset of menstruation | 4–25 | 3.468 | mg/24 h | 15–85 | nmol/day | XXX | 5 | nmol/day |
| Ovulation peak | 28–99 | 3.468 | mg/24 h | 95–345 | nmol/day | XXX | 5 | nmol/day |
| Luteal peak | 22–105 | 3.468 | mg/24 h | 75–365 | nmol/day | XXX | 5 | nmol/day |
| Menopausal woman | 1.4–19.6 | 3.468 | mg/24 h | 5–70 | nmol/day | XXX | 5 | nmol/day |
| Male | 5–18 | 3.468 | mg/24 h | 15–60 | nmol/day | XXX | 5 | nmol/day |

(continued)

**TABLE 10.1 (continued)**
**Conversion Factors for Values in Clinical Chemistry (SI Units)**

| Component Present | Reference Intervals (Examples) | Present Unit | Conversion Factor | SI Reference Intervals | SI Unit | Symbol | Significant Digits | Suggested Minimum Increment |
|---|---|---|---|---|---|---|---|---|
| Estrogens (S) (as estradiol) | | | | | | | | |
| Female | 20–300 | pg/mL | 3.671 | 70–1100 | pmol/L | XXXO | 10 | pmol/L |
| Peak production | 200–800 | pg/mL | 3.671 | 750–2900 | pmol/L | XXXO | 10 | pmol/L |
| Male | <50 | pg/mL | 3.671 | <180 | pmol/L | XXO | 10 | pmol/L |
| Estrogens, placental (U) (as estriol) | Depends on period of gestation | mg/24 h | 3.468 | Depends on period of gestation | mmol/day | XXX | 1 | mmol/day |
| Estrogen receptors (T) | | | | | | | | |
| Negative | 0–3 | fmol estradiol bound/mg cytosol protein | 1.00 | 0–3 | fmol estradiol/mg cytosol protein | XXX | 1 | fmol/mg protein |
| Doubtful | 4–10 | fmol estradiol bound/mg cytosol protein | 1.00 | 4–10 | fmol estradiol/mg cytosol protein | XXX | 1 | fmol/mg protein |
| Positive | >10 | fmol estradiol bound/mg cytosol protein | 1.00 | >10 | fmol estradiol/mg cytosol protein | XXX | 1 | fmol/mg protein |
| Estrone (P,S) | | | | | | | | |
| Female 1–10 days of cycle | 43–180 | pg/mL | 3.699 | 160–665 | pmol/L | XXX | 5 | pmol/L |
| Female 11–20 days of cycle | 75–196 | pg/mL | 3.699 | 275–725 | pmol/L | XXX | 5 | pmol/L |
| Female 20–39 days of cycle | 131–201 | pg/mL | 3.699 | 485–745 | pmol/L | XXX | 5 | pmol/L |
| Male | 29–75 | pg/mL | 3.699 | 105–275 | pmol/L | XXX | 5 | pmol/L |
| Estrone (U) female | 2–25 | mg/24 h | 3.699 | 5–90 | nmol/day | XXX | 5 | mmol/day |
| Ethanol (P) | | | | | | | | |
| Legal limit (driving) | <80 | mg/dL | 0.2171 | <17 | mmol/L | XX | 1 | nmol/L |
| Toxic | >100 | mg/dL | 0.2171 | >22 | mmol/L | XX | 1 | mmol/L |
| Ethchlorvynol (P) toxic | >40 | mg/L | 6.915 | >280 | mmol/L | XXO | 10 | mmol/L |
| Ethosuximide (P) therapeutic | 40–110 | mg/L | 7.084 | 280–780 | mmol/L | XXO | 10 | mmol/L |
| Ethylene glycol (P) toxic | >30 | mg/dL | 0.1611 | >5 | mmol/L | XX | 1 | mmol/L |
| Fat (F) (as stearic acid) | 2.0–6.0 | g/24 h | 3.515 | 7–21 | mmol/day | XXXX | 1 | mmol/day |
| Fatty acids, nonesterified (P) | 8–20 | mg/dL | 10.00 | 80–200 | mg/L | XXO | 10 | mg/L |
| Ferritin (S) | 18–300 | ng/mL | 1.00 | 18–300 | mg/L | XXO | 10 | mg/L |
| Fibrinogen (P) | 200–400 | mg/dL | 0.01 | 2.0–4.0 | g/L | X.X | 0.1 | g/L |
| Fluoride (U) | <1.0 | mg/24 h | 52.63 | <50 | mmol/day | XXO | 10 | mmol/day |
| Folate (S) (as pteroylglutamic acid) | 2–10 | ng/mL | 22.66 | 4–22 | nmol/L | XX | 2 | nmol/L |
| | | mg/dL | 2.266 | | nmol/L | XX | 2 | nmol/L |
| Folate (Erc) | 140–960 | ng/mL | 2.266 | 550–2200 | nmol/L | XXO | 10 | nmol/L |
| Follicle-stimulating hormone (FSH) (P) | | | | | | | | |
| Female | 2.0–15.0 | mIU/mL | 1.00 | 2–15 | IU/L | XX | 1 | IU/L |
| Peak production | 20–50 | mIU/mL | 1.00 | 20–50 | IU/L | XX | 1 | IU/L |
| Male | 1.0–10.0 | mIU/mL | 1.00 | 1–10 | IU/L | XX | 1 | IU/L |

| Analyte | Conventional reference range | Conventional units | Conversion factor | SI reference range | SI units | Format | Minimum increment | SI units |
|---|---|---|---|---|---|---|---|---|
| Follicle-stimulating hormone (FSH) (U) | | | | | | | | |
| Follicular phase | 2–15 | IU/24 h | 1.00 | 2–15 | IU/day | XXX | 1 | IU/day |
| Midcycle | 8–40 | IU/24 h | 1.00 | 8–40 | IU/day | XXX | 1 | IU/day |
| Luteal phase | 2–10 | IU/24 h | 1.00 | 2–10 | IU/day | XXX | 1 | IU/day |
| Menopausal women | 35–100 | IU/24 h | 1.00 | 35–100 | IU/day | XXX | 1 | IU/day |
| Male | 2–15 | IU/24 h | 1.00 | 2–15 | IU/day | XXX | 1 | IU/day |
| Fructose (P) | <10 | mg/dL | 0.05551 | <0.6 | mmol/L | X.XX | 0.1 | mmol/L |
| Galactose (P) (children) | <20 | mg/dL | 0.05551 | <1.1 | mmol/L | X.XX | 0.1 | mmol/L |
| Gases (aB) | | | | | | | | |
| pO$_2$ (= Torr) | 75–105 | mm Hg | 0.1333 | 10.0–14.0 | kPa | XX.X | 0.1 | kPa |
| pCO$_2$ (= Torr) | 33–44 | mm Hg | 0.1333 | 4.4–5.9 | kPa | X.X | 0.1 | kPa |
| γ-Glutamyltransferase (GGT) (S) | 0–30 | U/L | 0.01667 | 0–0.50 | mkat/L | X.XX | 0.01 | mkat/L |
| Gastrin (S) | 0–180 | pg/mL | 1.00 | 0–180 | ng/L | XXO | 10 | ng/L |
| Globulins (S) | See immunoglobulins | | | | | | | |
| Glucagon (S) | 50–100 | pg/mL | 1.00 | 50–100 | ng/L | XXO | 10 | ng/L |
| Glucose (P) fasting | 70–110 | mg/dL | 0.05551 | 3.9–6.1 | mmol/L | XX.X | 0.1 | mmol/L |
| Glucose (Sf) | 50–80 | mg/dL | 0.05551 | 2.8–4.4 | mmol/L | XX.X | 0.1 | mmol/L |
| Glutethimide (P) | | | | | | | | |
| Therapeutic | <10 | mg/L | 4.603 | <46 | mmol/L | XX | 1 | mmol/L |
| Toxic | >20 | mg/L | 4.603 | >92 | mmol/L | XX | 1 | mmol/L |
| Glycerol, free (S) | <1.5 | mg/dL | 0.1086 | <0.16 | mmol/L | X.XX | 0.01 | mmol/L |
| Gold (S) therapeutic | 300–800 | mg/dL | 0.05077 | 15.0–40.0 | mmol/L | XX.X | 0.1 | mmol/L |
| Gold (U) | <500 | mg/24 h | 0.005077 | <2.5 | mmol/day | X.X | 0.1 | mmol/day |
| Palmitic acid (Amf) | Depends on gestation | mmol/L | 1000 | Depends on gestation | mmol/L | XXX | 5 | mmol/L |
| Pentobarbital (P) | 20–40 | mg/L | 4.419 | 90–170 | mmol/L | XX | 5 | mmol/L |
| Phenobarbital (P) therapeutic | 2–5 | mg/L | 43.06 | 85–215 | mmol/L | XXX | 5 | mmol/L |
| Phensuximide (P) | 4–8 | mg/L | 5.285 | 20–40 | mmol/L | XX | 5 | mmol/L |
| Phenylbutazone (P) therapeutic | <100 | mg/L | 3.243 | <320 | mmol/L | XXO | 10 | mmol/L |
| Phenytoin (P) | | | | | | | | |
| Therapeutic | 10–20 | mg/L | 3.964 | 40–80 | mmol/L | XX | 5 | mmol/L |
| Toxic | >30 | mg/L | 3.964 | >120 | mmol/L | XX | 5 | mmol/L |
| Phosphate (S) (as phosphorus, inorganic) | 2.5–5.0 | mg/dL | 0.3229 | 0.80–1.60 | mmol/L | X.XX | 0.05 | mmol/L |
| Phosphate (U) (as phosphorus, inorganic) | Diet dependent | g/24 h | 32.29 | Diet dependent | mmol/day | XXX | 1 | mmol/day |
| Phospholipid phosphorus, total (P) | 5–12 | mg/dL | 0.3229 | 1.60–3.90 | mmol/L | X.XX | 0.05 | mmol/L |
| Phospholipid phosphorus, total (Erc) | 1.2–12.0 | mg/dL | 0.3229 | 0.40–3.90 | mmol/L | X.XX | 0.05 | mmol/L |

*(continued)*

**TABLE 10.1 (continued)**
**Conversion Factors for Values in Clinical Chemistry (SI Units)**

| Component Present | Reference Intervals (Examples) | Present Unit | Conversion Factor | SI Reference Intervals | SI Unit | Symbol | Significant Digits | Suggested Minimum Increment |
|---|---|---|---|---|---|---|---|---|
| Phospholipids (P) substance fraction of total phospholipid | | | | | | | | |
| Phosphatidyl choline | 65–70 | %/total | 0.01 | 0.65–0.70 | 1 | O.XX | 0.01 | |
| Phosphatidyl ethanolamine | 4–5 | %/total | 0.01 | 0.04–0.05 | 1 | O.XX | 0.01 | |
| Sphingomyelin | 15–20 | %/total | 0.01 | 0.15–0.20 | 1 | O.XX | 0.01 | |
| Lysophosphatidyl choline | 3–5 | %/total | 0.01 | 0.03–0.05 | 1 | O.XX | 0.01 | |
| Phospholipids (Erc) substance fraction of total phospholipid | | | | | | | | |
| Phosphatidyl choline | 28–33 | %/total | 0.01 | 0.28–0.33 | 1 | O.XX | 0.01 | |
| Phosphatidyl ethanolamine | 24–31 | %/total | 0.01 | 0.24–0.31 | 1 | O.XX | 0.01 | |
| Sphingomyelin | 22–29 | %/total | 0.01 | 0.22–0.29 | 1 | O.XX | 0.01 | |
| Phosphatidyl serine + Phosphatidyl inositol | 12–20 | %/total | 0.01 | 0.12–0.20 | 1 | O.XX | 0.01 | |
| Lysophosphatidyl choline | 1–2 | %/total | 0.01 | 0.01–0.02 | 1 | O.XX | 0.01 | |
| Phytanic acid (P) | Trace–0.3 | mg/dL | 32.00 | <10 | mmol/L | XX | 5 | mmol/L |
| Human placental lactogen SO (HPL) | >4.0 after 30 weeks gestation | mg/mL | 46.30 | >180 | nmol/L | XXO | 10 | nmol/L |
| Porphobilinogen (U) | 0–2 | mg/24 h | 4.420 | 0–9 | mmol/day | X.X | 0.5 | mmol/day |
| Porphyrins | | | | | | | | |
| Coproporphyrin (U) | 45–180 | mg/24 h | 1.527 | 68–276 | nmol/day | XXX | 2 | nmol/day |
| Protoporphyrin (Erc) | 15–50 | mg/dL | 0.0177 | 0.28–0.90 | mmol/L | X.XX | 0.02 | mmol/L |
| Uroporphyrin (U) | 5–20 | mg/24 h | 1.204 | 6–24 | nmol/day | XX | 2 | nmol/day |
| Uroporphyrinogen synthetase (Erc) | 22–42 | mmol/mL/h | 0.2778 | 6.0–11.8 | mmol/(L s) | X.X | 0.2 | mmol/(L s) |
| Potassium ion (S) | 3.5–5.0 | mEq/L | 1.00 | 3.5–5.0 | mmol/L | X.X | 0.1 | mmol/L |
| | | mg/dL | 0.2558 | | mmol/L | X.X | 0.1 | mmol/L |
| Potassium ion (U) (diet dependent) | 25–100 | mEq/24 h | 1.00 | 25–100 | mmol/day | XX | 1 | mmol/day |
| Pregnanediol (U) | | | | | | | | |
| Normal | 1–6 | mg/24 h | 3.120 | 3.0–18.5 | mmol/day | XX.X | 0.5 | mmol/day |
| Pregnancy | Depends on gestation | | | | | | | |
| Pregnanetriol (U) | 0.5–2.0 | mg/24 h | 2.972 | 1.5–6.0 | mmol/day | XX.X | 0.5 | mmol/day |
| Primidone (P) | | | | | | | | |
| Therapeutic | 6–10 | mg/L | 4.582 | 25–46 | mmol/L | XX | 1 | mmol/L |
| Toxic | >10 | mg/L | 4.582 | >46 | mmol/L | XX | 1 | mmol/L |

| | Conventional reference interval | Conventional units | Conversion factor | SI reference interval | SI units | | Significant digits | SI units |
|---|---|---|---|---|---|---|---|---|
| Procainamide (P) | | | | | | | | |
| Therapeutic | 4–8 | mg/L | 4.249 | 17–34 | mmol/L | XX | 1 | mmol/L |
| Toxic | >12.0 | mg/L | 4.249 | >50 | mmol/L | XX | 1 | mmol/L |
| N-Acetyl procainamide (P) therapeutic | 4–8 | mg/L | 3.606 | 14–29 | mmol/L | XX | 1 | mmol/L |
| Progesterone (P) | | | | | | | | |
| Follicular phase | <2 | ng/mL | 3.180 | <6 | nmol/L | XX | 2 | nmol/L |
| Luteal phase | 2–20 | ng/mL | 3.180 | 6–64 | nmol/L | XX | 2 | nmol/L |
| Progesterone receptors (T) | | | | | | | | |
| Negative | 0–3 | fmol progesterone bound/mg cytosol protein | 1.00 | 0–3 | fmol progesterone bound/mg cytosol protein | XX | 1 | fmol/mg protein |
| Doubtful | 4–10 | fmol progesterone bound/mg cytosol protein | 1.00 | 4–10 | fmol progesterone bound/mg cytosol protein | XX | 1 | fmol/mg protein |
| Positive | >10 | fmol progesterone bound/mg cytosol protein | 1.00 | >10 | fmol progesterone bound/mg cytosol protein | XX | 1 | fmol/mg protein |
| Prolactin (P) | <20 | ng/mL | 1.00 | <20 | mg/L | XX | 1 | mg/L |
| Propoxyphene (P) toxic | >2.0 | mg/L | 2.946 | >5.9 | mmol/L | X.X | 0.1 | mmol/L |
| Propranolol (P) (Inderal) therapeutic | 50–200 | ng/mL | 3.856 | 190–770 | nmol/L | XXO | 10 | nmol/L |
| Protein, total (S) | 6.0–8.0 | g/dL | 10.0 | 60–80 | g/L | XX | 1 | g/L |
| Protein, total (Sf) | <40 | mg/dL | 0.01 | <0.40 | g/L | X.XX | 0.1 | g/L |
| Protein, total (U) | <150 | mg/24 h | 0.001 | <0.15 | g/day | X.XX | 0.01 | g/day |
| Protriptyline (P) | 100–300 | ng/mL | 3.797 | 380–1140 | nmol/L | XXO | 10 | nmol/L |
| Pyruvate (B) (as pyruvic acid) | 0.30–0.90 | mg/dL | 113.6 | 35–100 | mmol/L | XXX | 1 | mmol/L |
| Quinidine (P) | | | | | | | | |
| Therapeutic | 1.5–3.0 | mg/L | 3.082 | 4.6–9.2 | mmol/L | X.X | 0.1 | mmol/L |
| Toxic | >6.0 | mg/L | 3.082 | >18.5 | mmol/L | X.X | 0.1 | mmol/L |
| Renin (P) normal sodium diet | 1.1–4.1 | ng/mL/h | 0.2778 | 0.30–1.14 | ng/(L s) | X.XX | 0.2 | ng/(L s) |
| Restricted sodium diet | 6.2–12.4 | ng/mL/h | 0.2778 | 1.72–3.44 | ng/(L s) | X.XX | 0.02 | ng/(L s) |
| Salicylate (S) (salicylic acid) toxic | >20 | mg/dL | 0.07240 | >1.45 | mmol/L | X.XX | 0.05 | mmol/L |
| Serotonin (B) (5 hydroxytryptamine) | 8–21 | mg/dL | 0.05675 | 0.45–1.20 | mmol/L | X.XX | 0.05 | mmol/L |
| Sodium ion (S) | 135–147 | mEq/L | 1.00 | 135–147 | mmol/L | XXX | 1 | mmol/L |
| Sodium ion (U) | Diet dependent | mEq/24 h | 1.00 | Diet dependent | mmol/day | XXX | 2 | mmol/day |
| Steroids 17-hydroxy-corticosteroids (U) (as cortisol) | | | | | | | | |
| Female | 2.0–8.0 | mg/24 h | 2.759 | 5–25 | mmol/day | XX | 1 | mmol/day |
| Male | 3–10 | mg/24 h | 2.759 | 10–30 | mmol/day | XX | 1 | mmol/day |
| 17-Ketogenic steroids (U) (as DHEA) | | | | | | | | |
| Female | 7–12 | mg/24 h | 3.467 | 25–40 | mmol/day | XX | 1 | mmol/day |
| Male | 9–17 | mg/24 h | 3.467 | 30–60 | mmol/day | XX | 1 | mmol/day |

(continued)

**TABLE 10.1 (continued)**
## Conversion Factors for Values in Clinical Chemistry (SI Units)

| Component Present | Reference Intervals (Examples) | Present Unit | Conversion Factor | SI Reference Intervals | SI Unit | Symbol | Significant Digits | Suggested Minimum Increment |
|---|---|---|---|---|---|---|---|---|
| 17-Ketosteroids (U) (as DHEA) | | | | | | | | |
| Female | 6–17 | mg/24 h | 3.467 | 20–60 | mmol/day | XX | 1 | mmol/day |
| Male | 6–20 | mg/24 h | 3.467 | 20–70 | mmol/day | XX | 1 | mmol/day |
| Ketosteroid fractions (U) androsterone | | | | | | | | |
| Female | 0.5–2.0 | mg/24 h | 3.443 | 1–10 | mmol/day | XX | 1 | mmol/day |
| Male | 2.0–5.0 | mg/24 h | 3.443 | 7–17 | mmol/day | XX | 1 | mmol/day |
| Dehydroepiandrosterone | | | | | | | | |
| Female | 0.2–1.8 | mg/24 h | 3.467 | 1–6 | mmol/day | XX | 1 | mmol/day |
| Male | 0.2–2.0 | mg/24 h | 3.467 | 1–7 | mmol/day | XX | 1 | mmol/day |
| Etiocholanolone | | | | | | | | |
| Female | 0.8–4.0 | mg/24 h | 3.443 | 2–14 | mmol/day | XX | 1 | mmol/day |
| Male | 1.4–5.0 | mg/24 h | 3.443 | 4–17 | mmol/day | XX | 1 | mmol/day |
| Sulfonamides (B) (as sulfanilamide) therapeutic | 10–15 | mg/dL | 58.07 | 580–870 | mmol/L | XXO | 10 | mmol/L |
| Testosterone (P) | | | | | | | | |
| Female | 0.6 | ng/mL | 3.467 | 2.0 | nmol/L | XXX.X | 0.5 | nmol/L |
| Male | 4.6–8.0 | ng/mL | 3.467 | 14–28 | nmol/L | XX.X | 0.5 | nmol/L |
| Theophylline (P) therapeutic | 10–20 | mg/L | 5.550 | 55–110 | mmol/L | XX | 1 | mmol/L |
| Thiocyanate (P) (nitroprusside toxicity) | 10.0 | mg/dL | 0.1722 | 1.7 | mmol/L | X.XX | 0.1 | mmol/L |
| Thiopental (P) | Individual | mg/L | 4.126 | Individual | mmol/L | XX | 5 | mmol/L |
| Thyroid tests | | | | | | | | |
| Thyroid-stimulating hormone (TSH) (S) | 2–11 | mU/mL | 1.00 | 2–11 | mU/L | XX | 1 | mU/L |
| Thyroxine (T4) (S) | 4–11 | mg/dL | 12.87 | 51–142 | nmol/L | XXX | 1 | nmol/L |
| Thyroxine-binding globulin (TGB) (S) (as thyroxine) | 12–28 | mg/dL | 12.87 | 150–360 | nmol/L | XXO | 1 | nmol/L |
| Thyroxine, free (S) | 0.8–2.8 | ng/dL | 12.87 | 10–36 | pmol/L | XX | 1 | pmol/L |
| Triiodothyronine (T3) (S) | 75–220 | ng/dL | 0.01536 | 1.2–3.4 | nmol/L | X.X | 0.1 | nmol/L |
| T3 uptake (S) | 25–35 | % | 0.01 | 0.25–0.35 | 1 | O.XX | 0.01 | |
| Tolbuamide (P) therapeutic | 50–120 | mg/L | 3.699 | 180–450 | mmol/L | XXO | 10 | mmol/L |
| Transferrin (S) | 170–370 | mg/dL | 0.01 | 1.70–3.70 | g/L | X.XX | 0.01 | g/L |

| | | | | | | | | |
|---|---|---|---|---|---|---|---|---|
| Triglycerides (P) (as triolein) | mg/dL | <160 | 0.01129 | <1.80 | mmol/L | X.XX | 0.02 | mmol/L |
| Trimethadione (P) therapeutic | mg/L | <50 | 6.986 | <350 | mmol/L | XXO | 10 | mmol/L |
| Trimipramine (P) therapeutic | ng/mL | 50–200 | 3.397 | 170–680 | nmol/L | XXO | 10 | nmol/L |
| Urate (S) (as uric acid) | mg/dL | 2–7 | 59.48 | 120–420 | mmol/L | XXO | 10 | mmol/L |
| Urate (U) (as uric acid) | g/24 h | Diet dependent | 5.948 | Diet dependent | mmol/day | XX | 1 | mmol/day |
| Urea nitrogen (S) | mg/dL | 8–18 | 0.3570 | 3.0–6.5 | mmol/L UREA | X.X | 0.5 | mmol/L |
| Urea nitrogen (U) | g/24 h | 2–20 diet dependent | 35.700 | 450–700 | mmol/day UREA | XXO | 10 | mol/day |
| Urobilinogen (U) | mg/24 h | 0–4 | 1.693 | 0.0–6.8 | mmol/day | X.X | 0.1 | mmol/day |
| Valproic acid (P) therapeutic | mg/L | 50–100 | 6.934 | 350–700 | mmol/L | XO | 10 | mmol/L |
| Vanillylmandelic acid (VMA), urine | mg/24 h | <6.8 | 5.046 | <35 | mmol/day | XX | 1 | mmol/day |
| Vitamin A (retinol) (P,S) | mg/dL | 10–50 | 0.03491 | 0.35–1.75 | mmol/L | X.XX | 0.05 | mmol/L |
| Vitamin B$_1$ (thiamine hydrochloride) (U) | mg/24 h | 60–500 | 0.002965 | 0.18–1.48 | mmol/day | ZX.XX | 0.01 | mmol/day |
| Vitamin B$_2$ (riboflavin) (S) | mg/dL | 2.6–3.7 | 26.57 | 70–100 | nmol/L | XXX | 5 | nmcl/L |
| Vitamin B$_6$ (pyridoxal) (B) | ng/mL | 20–90 | 5.982 | 120–540 | nmol/L | XXX | 5 | nmcl/L |
| Vitamin B$_{12}$ (cyanocobalamin) (P,S) | pg/mL | 200–1000 | 0.7378 | 150–750 | pmol/L | XO | 10 | pmcl/L |
| Vitamin C | See ascorbate (B,P,S) | | | | | | | |
| Vitamin D$_3$ (cholecalciferol) (P) | mg/mL | 24–40 | 2.599 | 60–105 | nmol/L | XXX | 5 | nmol/L |
| 25 OH-cholecalciferol | ng/mL | 18–36 | 0.496 | 45–90 | nmol/L | XXX | 5 | mmol/L |
| Vitamin E (α-tocopherol) (P,S) | mg/dL | 0.78–1.25 | 23.22 | 18–29 | mmol/L | XX | 1 | mmcl/L |
| Warfarin (P) therapeutic | mg/L | 1–3 | 3.243 | 3.3–9.8 | mmol/L | XX.X | 0.1 | mmcl/L |
| Xanthine (U) Hypoxanthine | mg/24 | 5–30 | 6.574 | 30–200 | mmol/day | XXO | 10 | mmcl/day |
| | hmg/24 h | | 7.347 | | mmol/day | XXO | 10 | mmcl/day |
| D-Xylose (B) (25 g dose) | mg/dL | 30–40 (30–60 min) | 0.06661 | 0–2.7 (30–60 min) | mmol/L | X.X | 0.1 | mmcl/L |
| D-Xylose excretion (U) (25 g dose) | % | 21–31 | 0.01 | 0.21–0.31 (excreted in 5 h) | 1 | O.XX | 0.01 | |
| Zinc (S) | mg/dL | 75–120 | 0.1530 | 11.5–18.5 | mmol/L | XX.X | 0.1 | mmol/L |
| Zinc (U) | mg/24 h | 150–1200 | 0.01530 | 2.3–18.3 | mmol/day | XX.X | 0.1 | mmol/day |

**TABLE 10.2**
**Vitamin[a] Terminology**

| Name | Comment |
| --- | --- |
| Vitamin A | A number of compounds have vitamin A activity but differ in biopotency. All-*trans* retinol is the standard, and the activity of other compounds can be stated as retinol equivalents. This includes the aldehyde (retinal), acid (retinoic acid), and provitamin (carotene) forms. |
| Vitamin B | Although originally thought to be a single compound, researchers have found that eight major compounds comprised this "vitamin." |
| Vitamin B complex | A group of vitamins; includes thiamin, riboflavin, niacin, pyridoxine (three forms), pantothenic acid, biotin, cyanocobalamin ($B_{12}$), and folacin. |
| Vitamin $B_1$ | Aneurin; antineuritic factor. Obsolete synonym for thiamin. |
| Vitamin $B_2$ | Lactoflavin, ovoflavin. Obsolete synonym for riboflavin. |
| Vitamin $B_3$ | Antipellagra factor. Obsolete synonym for niacin. |
| Vitamin $B_4$ | Not proven to have vitamin activity; thought to be a mixture of arginine, glycine, riboflavin, and pyridoxine. |
| Vitamin $B_5$ | Probably identical to niacin. |
| Vitamin $B_6$ | Synonym for pyridoxine, pyridoxal, and pyridoxamine. |
| Vitamin $B_7$ | Not proven to have vitamin activity; sometimes referred to as vitamin I, a factor that improves food digestibility in pigeons. |
| Vitamin $B_8$ | Not proven to have vitamin activity; found to be adenylic acid. |
| Vitamin $B_{10}$, $B_{11}$ | An unrefined mixture of folacin and cyanocobalamin; obsolete term. |
| Vitamin $B_{12}$ | Cyanocobalamin; $B_{12a}$ is aquacobalamin; $B_{12b}$ is hydroxocobalamin; $B_{12c}$ is nitritocobalamin. |
| Vitamin $B_{13}$ | Orotic acid; a metabolite of pyrimidine metabolism; not considered a vitamin. |
| Vitamin $B_{15}$ | Synonym for "pangamic acid," a compound of no known biologic value; not a vitamin. |
| Vitamin $B_{17}$ | Synonym for laetrile; a cyanogenic glycoside of no known biologic value; not a vitamin. |
| Vitamin Bc | Obsolete term for pteroylglutamic acid; a component of folacin. |
| Vitamin Bp | A compound that prevents perosis in chicks; can be replaced by choline and manganese. |
| Vitamin Bf | Shown to be carnitine. |
| Vitamin Bx | Probably a mixture of pantothenic acid and *p*-aminobenzoic acid. |
| Vitamin C | Synonym for ascorbic acid. |
| Vitamin $C_2$ | Unrecognized, unconfirmed compound purported to have antipneumonia activity; also called vitamin J. |
| Vitamin D | Antirachitic factor; a group of sterols (the calciferols) that serve to enhance bone calcification. |
| Vitamin $D_2$ | Ergocalciferol; one of the D vitamins from plant sources. |
| Vitamin $D_3$ | Cholecalciferol; one of the D vitamins from animal sources. |
| Vitamin E | A group of tocopherols that have an important function in the antioxidant system; suppresses free radical formation. |
| Vitamin F | Obsolete term for the essential fatty acids (linoleic and linolenic acids). |
| Vitamin G | Obsolete term for riboflavin before riboflavin and niacin were recognized as separate vitamins. |
| Vitamin H | Obsolete term for biotin. |
| Vitamin I | Obsolete term for a mixture of B vitamins. |
| Vitamin K | A group of fat-soluble compounds that function in the posttranslational carboxylation of the glutamic acid residues of prothrombin and osteocalcin. |
| Vitamin $K_1$ | Phylloquinone; vitamin K of plant origin. |
| Vitamin $K_2$ | Menaquinone; vitamin K of animal origin. |
| Vitamin $K_3$ | Menadione; synthetic vitamin K. |
| Vitamin $L_1$ | Unrecognized factor that may be related to anthranitic acid and that has been proposed to be important for lactation; not proven to have vitamin activity. |
| Vitamin $L_2$ | See earlier text. |
| Vitamin M | Obsolete term for pteroylglutamic acid (folacin). |
| Vitamin N | Obsolete term used to designate an anticancer compound mixture; undefined and unrecognized. |
| Vitamin P | Not a vitamin; but is a metabolite of citrin. |
| Vitamin Q | Not a vitamin; but is probably a synonym for coenzyme Q. |
| Vitamin R | Obsolete term for folacin. |
| Vitamin S | Not a vitamin; but does act to enhance chick growth; related to the peptide "streptogenin" and also to biotin. |
| Vitamin T | Not a vitamin; reported to improve protein utilization in rats; an extract from termites. |

**TABLE 10.2 (continued)**
**Vitamin[a] Terminology**

| Name | Comment |
|---|---|
| Vitamin U | Not a vitamin; an extract from cabbage that has been reported to suppress gastric acid production; may be important to folacin activity. |
| Vitamin V | Not a vitamin. |
| Bioflavonoids | Not a vitamin. |
| Carnitine | Not a vitamin; except in preterm infants and in severely traumatized persons. |
| Choline | Can be synthesized by the body but some conditions interfere with adequate synthesis. |
| Citrovorum factor | Synonym for folacin; a B vitamin. |
| Extrinsic factor | Obsolete term for vitamin $B_{12}$, cyanocobalamin. |
| Factors U, R, X | Obsolete terms for folacin. |
| Filtrate factor | Obsolete term for riboflavin. |
| Flavin | A general term for the riboflavin-containing coenzymes, FMN, and FAD. |
| Hepatoflavin | Obsolete term for riboflavin. |
| Intrinsic factor | Not a vitamin; an endogenous factor needed for vitamin $B_{12}$, cyanocobalamin, absorption. |
| LLD factor | Obsolete term for vitamin $B_{12}$, cyanocobalamin. |
| Lipoic acid | Not a vitamin, but does serve as a cofactor in oxidative decarboxylation. |
| Myoinositol | Sometimes a vitamin when endogenous synthesis is inadequate. |
| Norite eluate | Not a vitamin. |
| P–P factor | Obsolete term for niacin. |
| Pyrroloquinoline quinone | Not a vitamin; component of metallo-oxido-reductases. |
| Rhizopterin | Obsolete term for folacin. |
| SLR factor | Obsolete term for folacin. |
| Streptogenin | Not a vitamin. |
| Wills factor | Obsolete term for folacin. |
| Zoopherin | Obsolete term for vitamin $B_{12}$, cyanocobalamin. |

[a] A vitamin is an organic compound required in small amounts for the maintenance of normal biochemical and physiological function of the body. These compounds must be present in food, and if absent, well-defined symptoms of deficiency will develop. An essential nutrient such as a vitamin cannot be synthesized in amounts sufficient to meet needs.

**TABLE 10.3**
**Nomenclature of Compounds with Vitamin A Activity**

| Recommended Name | Synonyms |
|---|---|
| Retinol | Vitamin A alcohol |
| Retinal | Vitamin A aldehyde, retinene, retinaldehyde |
| Retinoic acid | Vitamin A acid |
| 3-Dehydroretinol | Vitamin $A_2$ (alcohol) |
| 3-Dehydroretinal | Vitamin $A_2$ aldehyde, retinene2 |
| 3-Dehydroretinoic acid | Vitamin $A_2$ acid |
| Anhydroretinol | Anhydrovitamin A |
| Retro retinal | Rehydrovitamin A |
| 5,6-Epoxyretinol | 5,6-Epoxyvitamin A alcohol |
| Retinyl palmitate | Vitamin A palmitate |
| Retinyl acetate | Vitamin A acetate |
| Retinyl β-glucuronide | Vitamin A acid β-glucuronide |
| 11-*cis*-Retinaldehyde | 11-*cis* or neo γ vitamin A aldehyde |
| 4-Ketoretinol | 4-Keto vitamin A alcohol |
| Retinyl phosphate | Vitamin A phosphate |
| β-Carotene | Provitamin A |
| α-Carotene | Provitamin A |
| γ-Carotene | Provitamin A |

**TABLE 10.4**

**Terminology Used in Energy Assessment of Humans and Animals**

| | |
|---|---|
| Anabolism | The totality of reactions that account for the synthesis of the body's macromolecules; heat is a by-product of these reactions. |
| Android obesity | A form of obesity in which fat distribution is mainly in the shoulders and abdomen; sometimes referred to as the "apple" type of obesity. |
| Anthropometry | Measurements of body features, that is, height, weight, skin-fold thickness, etc. |
| Apparent digestible energy (DE) | Energy of the consumed food (IE) less the energy of the feces (FE); $DE = IE - FE$. |
| Archimedes principle | An object's volume, when submerged in water, equals the volume of the water displaced. If the mass of the body is known, then the density can be calculated. Less dense bodies have more body fat than very dense bodies. |
| Balance | Intake = expenditure. |
| BMI | $BMI = (Body\ weight\ (kg)/Height\ (cm)^2)$. Used as a general index of body fatness; however, it does not apply to persons with high muscle mass such as elite athletes. |
| Basal metabolic rate (BMR) | The minimal amount of energy needed to sustain the body's metabolism. Frequently expressed in terms of the amount of oxygen used to sustain this metabolism, because of the constancy between energy flux and oxygen use. |
| Body cell mass | The metabolically active, energy—requiring mass of the body. |
| Body density | Mass/unit volume. |
| Calorie | A unit of energy; a calorie is the amount of heat needed to raise the temperature of 1 kg of water 1°C; also referred to as a kilocalorie. Can be converted to kilojoules (kJ): $kcal \times 4.184 = kJ$. |
| Calorimetry | The measurement of heat production by the body. This measurement can be either direct (using a whole-body calorimeter) or indirect using measurements of oxygen consumed and carbon dioxide produced. |
| Catabolism | The totality of those reactions that reduce macromolecules to usable metabolites, $CO_2$, and water. Heat is a by-product of these reactions. |
| Digestive energy (DE) | The energy of food after the energy losses of digestion is subtracted. Similar to apparent ingestive energy (see earlier text). |
| Gaseous products of digestion (GE) | The energy of the combustible gases produced in the digestive tract incident to the fermentation of food by microorganisms. In ruminants, this is a substantial component of the energy balance equation; in humans, this is much smaller and perhaps negligible. |
| Gynoid obesity | Excess body fat deposited mainly on the hips, abdomen, and thighs. Sometimes called "pear-shaped" obesity. |
| Heat of activity (HiE) | The heat produced through muscular activity. |
| Heat of digestion and absorption (HdE) | The heat produced in the digestive tract as a result of the activity of the digestive enzymes and the energy of the absorptive processes. Sometimes referred to as diet-induced thermogenesis (DIT). |
| Heat of fermentation (HfE) | Heat produced in the digestive tract due to the action of microbial action. |
| Heat of product formation (HrE) | The heat produced associated with the production of a product, that is, milk or eggs, etc. |
| Heat of thermic regulation (HcE) | The heat needed to maintain the body temperature. |
| Heat of waste formation and excretion (HwE) | The heat associated with the production of waste products such as urea in urine. |
| Heat increment (HI) | The increase in heat production following the consumption of food. |
| IDW | Ideal body weight. |
| Indirect calorimetry | The calculation of energy (heat) production through the measurement of oxygen consumed and carbon dioxide released. |
| Metabolizable energy (ME) | The energy in food minus that is lost through digestion, absorption, and excretion. $ME = IE - (FE + UE + GE)$. |
| N-corrected metabolizable energy (MnE) | ME adjusted for total nitrogen retained or lost by the body tissue. $MnE = ME - (k \times TN)$ where TN = nitrogen retained in the body tissue. |
| NPU | Net protein use. |
| NDp Cal% | Net protein calories percent; the percent of the total energy value of the diet provided by protein. |
| Nutrient density | The nutrient composition of food expressed in terms of nutrient quantity/100 kcal. |
| Nutritional assessment | Measurement of indicators of dietary status and nutrition-related health status of individuals or population groups. |
| Obesity | Excess fat stores. |
| Postprandial | After a meal. |
| Quantitative computed tomography | An imagine technique that allows for the calculation of body fatness and body composition. |
| Respiratory quotient | The ratio of carbon dioxide produced to oxygen consumed. |

**TABLE 10.4 (continued)**
**Terminology Used in Energy Assessment of Humans and Animals**

| | |
|---|---|
| Skin-fold thickness | A double fold of skin and underlying tissue that can be used to estimate body fatness. |
| Thermic effect of food | Same as heat increment. |
| Total heat production (HE) | The energy lost as heat from the body as a result of its metabolism. |
| True digestive energy (TDE) | The intake of energy in food minus that lost through the feces, HfE, and digestive gases. |
| True metabolizable energy (TME) | Food energy minus energy lost through feces and urine. |
| Urinary energy | The gross energy of the urine. |

**TABLE 10.5**
**Equations for Calculating Body Components Using Direct Analysis**

$$\% \text{ body fat} = \frac{\text{Body weight} - \text{Fat solvent extracted body weight}}{\text{Body weight}}$$

$$\% \text{ body water} = \frac{\text{Body weight} - \text{Dried body weight}}{\text{Body weight}}$$

$$\% \text{ body ash} = \frac{\text{Body weight after complete oxidation in a muffle furnace}}{\text{Body weight}}$$

$$\% \text{ body protein} = \frac{\text{Nitrogen content} \times 6.25}{\text{Body weight}}$$

**TABLE 10.6**
**General Formulas for Calculating Body Fatness from Skin-Fold Measurements**

| | |
|---|---|
| Males | $\% \text{ body fat} = 29.288 \times 10^{-2} (X) - 5 \times 10^{-4} (X)^2 + 15.845 \times 10^{-2} (\text{Age})$ |
| Females | $\% \text{ body fat} = 29.699 \times 10^{-2} (X) - 43 \times 10^{-5} (X)^2 + 29.63 \times 10^{-3} (\text{Age}) + 1.4072$ |

where X = sum of abdomen, suprailiac, triceps, and thigh skin-folds and age is in years

**Other equations for the estimation of body fat**

1. $\% \text{ fat} = \dfrac{2.118 - 1.354 - 0.78}{\text{Density}} \cdot \dfrac{\% \text{ TBW}}{\text{Body weight}}$

   where 2.118, 1.354, and 0.78 are constants and the density (g/cc), body weight (kg), and total body weight (TBW) (kg) are determined

2. $\% \text{ fat} = \dfrac{100(5.548 - 5.044)}{\text{Specific gravity}}$

3. $\% \text{ fat} = \dfrac{100 - \text{TBW}}{0.732}$

*Source:* Malina, R.M., *Am. J. Human Biol.*, 11, 141, 1999.

**TABLE 10.7**
**Methods and Equations Used for Calculating Basal**
**Energy Need**

| | |
|---|---|
| 1. Heat production, direct measurement (calorimetry) | kcal (kJ)/m$^2$ (surface area) |
| 2. Oxygen consumption; indirect | $O_2$ cons/w$^{0.75}$ |
| 3. Heat production; indirect | Insensible water loss (IW) = insensible weight loss (IWL) + ($CO_2$ exhaled – $O_2$ inhaled) |
| | Heat production = IW × 0.58 (0.58 = kcal to evaporate 1 g water) |
| 4. Estimate (energy need not be measured) | BMR = 66.4730 + 13.751 W + 5.0033 L – 6.550 A (males) |
| | BMR = 655.0955 + 9.463 W + 1.8496 L – 4.6756 A (females) |
| 5. Estimate (energy need not be measured) | BMR = 71.2 W$^{0.75}$ [1 – 0.004 (30–A) +0.010(L/W$^{0.33}$ – 43.4)] (men) |
| | BMR = 65.8 W$^{0.75}$ [1 + 0.004(30 – A) + 0.018(L/W$^{0.33}$ – 42.1)] (women) |

W, weight in kg; L, height in cm; A, age in years.

**TABLE 10.8**
**Adipokines (Cytokines), Their Receptors, and Function**

| Adipokine | Receptor Distribution | Function |
|---|---|---|
| Resistin | Vascular tissue, adipose tissue | Promotes insulin resistance; induced by glucocorticoids, prolactin, testosterone, growth hormone; appears to be involved in inflammatory response. |
| NPY | Found in most neural cells; released by the GI tract | Signals hunger. |
| Leptin | Found in brain cells as well as other cell types | Signals satiety; involved in apoptosis. |
| Ghrelin | Synthesized in stomach Receptors are in hypothalamus | Transfers information from stomach to hypothalamus and influences growth hormone release in response to changes in energy homeostasis. Stimulates satiety in response to protein/low-carbohydrate feeding. |
| Cholecystokinin | Receptors are in brain, gallbladder, and endocrine pancreas | Stimulates bile release and pancreatic exocrine enzyme release; signals satiety. |
| Adiponectin | Released by adipose tissue; receptors in insulin target tissues | Increases insulin sensitivity. |
| Galanin | Pancreas | Inhibits release of insulin, pancreatic polypeptide, somatostatin, and neurotensin; stimulates food intake. |
| Neurotensin | Brain | Suppresses appetite. |

**TABLE 10.9**
**Prefixes and Suffixes Used in Medical Terms**

| Prefix/Suffix | Example | Meaning |
|---|---|---|
| Pre—before | Prenatal | Period before birth |
| Peri—around | Perinatal | Period around birth |
| Epi—above, upon | Epidermis | Outer most layer of skin |
| Hypo—under, below | Hypodermic | Under the skin |
| Hyper—above | Hyperglycemia | Above normal blood glucose |
| Infra—under, below | Infracostal | Below the ribs |
| Sub—under, below | Subdural | Below the dura mater |
| Inter—between | Intercostal | Between the ribs |
| Post—behind | Posteria | Back part of anatomical part |
| Retro—backward, behind | Retroversion | Tipping backward |
| Bi—two | Bilateral | Two sides |
| Diplo—two | Diplococcus | Two attached cells |
| Hemi—one half | Hemiplegia | Paralysis on one side |
| Macro—large | Macrophage | Large cell |
| Micro—small | Micronemia | Small blood cells |
| Ab—from, away | Abduction | Movement away from center line |
| Ad—toward | Adduction | Movement toward the center line |
| Circum—around | Circumduction | Movement in a circular direction |
| A—without, not | Aphagia | Not eating |
| Anti—against | Antibacterial | Against bacteria |
| Contra—not | Contraindicated | Not recommended |
| Brady—slow | Bradycardia | Slow heart rate |
| Tachy—rapid | Tachycardia | Rapid heart rate |
| Dys—bad, painful | Dystocia | Difficult birth |
| Homeo—same | Homeostasis | Maintenance of sameness |
| Eu—good, normal | Eupnea | Normal breathing |
| Mal—bad | Malnutrition | Poor nutrient intake |
| Pseudo—false | Pseudostratified cells | False appearance of cell layers |

Listed in Table 10.8 are some small proteins (adipokines or cytokines) that influence feeding and that are thought to be related to body fat regulation.

Nutrition has always been related to health and thus much of medical terminology has infiltrated nutrition terminology. Hence, Table 10.9 provides a list of prefixes and suffixes used in medical terms used to describe body parts.

## REFERENCES

1. Young, D.S., *Ann. Int. Med.*, 106, 20, 1987.
2. Malina, R.M., *Am. J. Hum. Biol.*, 11, 141, 1999.
3. Jackson, A.S., Pollack, M.L., *Phys. Sport Med.*, 13, 76, 1985.
4. Berdanier, C.D., Zempleni, J., *Advanced Nutrition: Macronutrients, Micronutrients and Metabolism*, CRC Press, Boca Raton, FL, 2009, p. 23.

# 11 Nutritional Biochemistry

*Carolyn D. Berdanier*

## CONTENTS

Nutrition science is based on concepts of biochemistry and physiology. It is an integration of knowledge about living systems. In part, the knowledge about how nutrients are used depends on an understanding of how cells work. The pathways of intermediary metabolism show how the dietary macromolecules, proteins, fats, and carbohydrates are used. They also show how the micronutrients work in facilitating the use of the macronutrients. With an understanding of the physiology and endocrinology of the consumer, we have the basis for integrating the systems that comprise the science. This chapter reviews the pathways of intermediary metabolism and provides some basic information about the use of the macro- and micronutrients found in food.

## PHYSIOLOGY OF DIGESTION

Before the nutrients in food can be metabolized, they must first be ingested, chewed, swallowed, digested, and absorbed. With each of the macronutrients, the macromolecules must be broken down to their simpler components. In addition, the micronutrients that are part of the food matrix must be made available for absorption. In the mouth, the food is chewed and mixed with saliva before it is swallowed. The saliva contains an α-amylase that begins the digestion of the carbohydrates and a lipase that begins the digestion of lipid. With swallowing, the food moves down the esophagus and enters the stomach. In the stomach, the food is mixed with the gastric acid (hydrochloric acid), pepsin, and intrinsic factor (necessary for the absorption of vitamin $B_{12}$) and moved into the small intestine. The protein in the food stimulates the release of ghrelin, a hormone that signals satiety. The stomach contents that move into the duodenum are called chyme. The movement of chyme into the duodenum stimulates cholecystokinin release. This gut hormone acts on the exocrine pancreas stimulating it to release pancreatic juice into the duodenum and on the gallbladder to release bile. Cholecystokinin is secreted by the epithelial endocrine cells of the small intestine, particularly the duodenum. Its release is stimulated by amino acids in the lumen and by the acid pH of the stomach contents as it passes into the duodenum. The low pH of the chyme also stimulates the release of secretin, which, in turn, stimulates the exocrine pancreas to release bicarbonate and water so as to raise the pH of the chyme. This is necessary to maximize the activity of the digestive enzymes located in and on the surface of the absorptive luminal cell. The digestive enzymes are listed in Table 11.1.

As mentioned, cholecystokinin stimulates the release of bile from the gallbladder. Bile contains the primary bile acids, cholic and chenodeoxycholic acids, that are produced from cholesterol by the liver. They are secreted into the intestine, where they serve as emulsifying agents for the digestion and absorption of fat. Bile that is not immediately used is acted on by the intestinal flora. These flora convert the bile acids to their conjugated forms by dehydroxylating carbon-7. Further metabolism occurs at the far end of the intestinal tract, where lithocholate is sulfated and excreted in the feces. The dehydroxylated and unhydroxylated bile acids are recirculated via the enterohepatic system such that very little of the bile acids are lost. It has been estimated that the bile acid lost in the feces (~0.8 g/day) equals that newly synthesized by the liver such that the total pool remains between 3 and 5 g. The amount secreted per day is on the order of 16–70 g. As the pool size is only 3–5 g, this means that these acids are recirculated as many as 14 times a day.

## CARBOHYDRATE DIGESTION/ABSORPTION

Once a carbohydrate-rich food is consumed, digestion begins. As the food is chewed, it is mixed with saliva, which contains α-amylase. This amylase begins the digestion of starch by attacking the internal α-1,4-glucosidic bonds. It will not attack the branch points having α-1,4- or α-1,6-glucosidic bonds, and hence, the salivary α-amylase will produce molecules of glucose, maltose, α-limit dextrin, and maltotriose. The α-amylase in saliva is an isozyme with the same function as that in the pancreatic juice. The salivary α-amylase is denatured in the stomach as the food is mixed and acidified with the gastric hydrochloric acid. The limit dextrins are further hydrolyzed by α-glucosidases on the surface of the luminal cells. The glycosidic bonds of the disaccharides are attacked by the disaccharidases, maltase, lactase, or sucrase (Table 11.1). This results in absorbable monosaccharides, glucose, fructose, and galactose. Glucose, once absorbed, stimulates the endocrine β-cells of the pancreas to release insulin, an important hormone for glucose use. Carbohydrates having bonds that are not attacked by the glycosidic enzymes are passed to the lower part of the intestine, where they are

**TABLE 11.1**

**Enzymes of Importance to Digestion**

| Enzyme | Substrate | Products |
|---|---|---|
| α-amylase | Starch and amylopectin | Glucose, maltose, maltotriose, and α-limit dextrin |
| α-Glucosidase | α-Limit dextrin | Glucose |
| Lactase | Lactose | Galactose and glucose |
| Maltase | Maltose | Glucose |
| Sucrase | Sucrose | Glucose and fructose |
| Lipase | Triacylglycerides | Fatty acids, DGs, and MGs |
| Colipase | Triacylglycerides | Fatty acids, DGs, and MGs |
| Lipid esterase | Cholesterol esters | Cholesterol and fatty acids |
| | Vitamin A esters | Vitamin A and glycerol |
| Pepsin | Peptide bonds involving aromatic amino acids | Phenylalanine, tyrosine peptide fragments |
| Trypsin | Peptide bonds involving arginine and lysine | Arginine, lysine, and peptide fragments |
| Chymotrypsin | Peptide bonds involving tyrosine, phenylalanine, methionine tryptophan, and leucine | Tyrosine, leucine, tryptophan, phenylalanine, methionine, and peptide fragments |
| Elastase | Peptide bonds involving alanine, serine, and glycine | Alanine, serine, glycine, and peptide fragments |
| Carboxypeptidase A | Peptide bonds involving valine, leucine, isoleucine, and alanine | Valine, leucine, isoleucine, alanine, and peptide fragments |
| Carboxypeptidase B | Peptide bonds involving lysine and arginine | |
| Endopeptidase | Peptide fragments | Amino acids |
| Aminopeptidase | Peptide fragments | Amino acids |
| Dipeptidase | Dipeptides | Amino acids |

attacked by the enzymes of the intestinal flora. Most of the products of this digestion are used by the flora themselves, but some of metabolic products (short-chain fatty acids) may be of use. The flora produce lactate, methane gas, carbon dioxide, water, and hydrogen gas. Gas production (flatus) can be uncomfortable if large amounts of undigestible carbohydrates are consumed. The carbohydrates of legumes typify the substrates these flora use. Raffinose, an α-galactose 1 → 6 glucose 1 → 2 β-fructose, and trehalose, an α-glucose 1 → 1 α-glucose, are the typical substrates from legumes for these flora. The flora will also attack portions of the fibers and celluloses that are the structural elements in fruits and vegetables. Again, some useful products may be produced, but the bulk of these complex polysaccharides having β-linkages and perhaps other substituent groups as part of their structure are largely untouched by both intestinal and bacterial enzymes. These undigested unavailable carbohydrates provide bulk to the diet, which, in turn, helps to regulate the rate of food passage from the mouth to the anus. They also act as adsorbants of noxious or potentially noxious materials in the food, and they assist in the excretion of cholesterol and several minerals, thereby protecting the body from overload. Populations consuming high-fiber diets have a lower incidence of colon cancer, fewer problems with constipation, and lower serum cholesterol levels.

## LIPID DIGESTION/ABSORPTION

Food lipids (fats and oils) are digested initially in the mouth and then in the stomach and intestine. The digestion of lipid begins in the mouth with the mastication of food and its mixing with the acid-stable lingual lipase. The food is then swallowed and, through the churning action of the stomach, is mixed with the various digestive juices and hydrochloric acid. This action separates the lipid particles from the proteins, thus exposing more lipid surface area for emulsion formation. These changes in physical state are essential steps that precede absorption. Little degradation of fat occurs in the stomach except that catalyzed by lingual lipase. Lingual lipase originates from glands in the back of the mouth and under the tongue. This lipase is active in the acid environment of the stomach. However, because of the tendency of lipid to coalesce and form a separate phase, this lipase has limited opportunity to attack triacylglycerols. Those that are attacked release a single fatty acid, usually a short- or medium-chain one. The remaining diacylglycerol is subsequently hydrolyzed in the duodenum. In adults consuming a mixed diet, lingual lipase is relatively unimportant. However, in infants having an immature duodenal lipase, lingual lipase is quite important. In addition, this lipase has its greatest activity on the triacylglycerols commonly present in whole milk. Milk fat has more short- and medium-chain fatty acids than fats from other food sources.

Although the action of lingual lipase is slow relative to lipases found in the duodenum, its action to release diacylglycerol and short- and medium-chain fatty acids serves another function—these fatty acids serve as surfactants.

Surfactants spontaneously adsorb to the water–lipid interface, conferring a hydrophilic surface to lipid droplets and thereby provide a stable interface with the aqueous environment. The dietary surfactants are the free fatty acids, lecithin, and phospholipids. The action of acid-stable lingual lipase provides more fatty acids to supplement the dietary supply. Altogether these surfactants plus the churning action of the stomach produce an emulsion, which is then expelled into the duodenum as chyme.

Once the chyme enters the duodenum, it is mixed with bile. This is an additional surfactant or emulsifying agent and serves to further disperse the lipid droplets at the lipid–aqueous interface, facilitating the hydrolysis of the glycerides (triglycerides [TGs], diglycerides [DGs], and monoglycerides [MGs]) by the pancreatic lipases. Pancreozymin stimulates the exocrine pancreas to release pancreatic juice, which contains three lipases (lipase, lipid esterase, and colipase) that act at the water–lipid interface of the emulsion particles. One lipase acts on the fatty acids esterified at positions 1 and 3 of the glycerol backbone, leaving a fatty acid esterified at carbon 2. This 2-monoacylglyceride can isomerize, and the remaining fatty acid can move to carbon 1 or 3. The pancreatic juice contains another less specific lipase (called a lipid esterase), which cleaves the fatty acid from cholesterol esters, MGs, or esters such as vitamin A ester. Its action requires the presence of the bile salts. The lipase that is specific for the ester linkage at carbons 1 and 3 does not have a requirement for the bile salts and, in fact, is inhibited by them. The inhibition of pancreatic lipase by the bile salts is relieved by the third pancreatic enzyme, colipase. The products of the lipase-catalyzed reaction, a reaction that favors the release of fatty acids having 10 or more carbons, are these fatty acids and MG. The products of the lipid esterase–catalyzed reaction are cholesterol, vitamins, fatty acids, and glycerol. Phospholipids present in food are attacked by phospholipases specific to each of the phospholipids. The pancreatic juice contains these lipases as prephospholipases, which are activated by the enzyme trypsin.

The bile salts impart a negative charge to the lipids that in turn attracts the pancreatic enzyme, colipase (see Table 11.1). Colipase binds to both the water–lipid interface and to lipase, thereby anchoring and activating the lipase. As the pH of the chyme rises, aggregates, called micelles, are formed. The micelles are much smaller in size than the emulsified lipid droplets. Micelle sizes vary depending on the ratio of lipids to bile acids but typically range from 40 to 600 Å, and it is from these structures that the products of lipid digestion are absorbed.

## CHOLESTEROL ABSORPTION

Only 30%–40% of the dietary cholesterol is absorbed; it is absorbed by diffusion with the other lipid components of the diet. Absorption requires the emulsification step with the bile acids as emulsifiers. Absorbed cholesterol passes into the lacteals and thence into the thoracic duct. The percentage of cholesterol absorbed depends on a number of factors including the fiber content of the diet, the gut passage time, and the total amount of cholesterol present for absorption. At higher intake levels, less is absorbed and vice versa at lower intake levels. Compared with fatty acids and the acylglycerides, the rate of cholesterol absorption is very low. It is estimated that the half-life of cholesterol in the enterocyte is 12 h. With high fiber intakes, less cholesterol is absorbed because the fiber (cellulose and lignins) acts as an adsorbent, reducing cholesterol availability. These carbohydrates also shorten the residence time of the ingesta in the intestine. Thus, high-fiber diets reduce gut passage time, which, in turn, results in less time for cholesterol absorption. The mode of action of pectins and gums in lowering cholesterol absorption is different. These carbohydrates also affect transit time, but rather than acting as adsorbants, they lower serum cholesterol levels by giving chyme a gel-like consistency, rendering the cholesterol in the chyme less available for absorption.

## LIPID TRANSPORT

Short-chain fatty acids (fatty acids having fewer than 10 carbon atoms) are absorbed directly into the portal blood system and carried by albumin. Longer-chain fatty acids and cholesterol are taken up by the lacteals of the lymphatic system that drains the intestine. They are formed into chylomicrons (a very-low-density lipid–protein complex) and then enter the blood via the thoracic duct. Once absorbed, the lipids are transported through the circulatory system by proteins in a complex called lipoprotein. Lipoproteins carry not only the absorbed food lipids but also the lipids synthesized or mobilized from organs and fat depots. Nine different lipid-carrying proteins have been identified, and each plays a specific role in the lipid-transport process. In addition, there are several minor proteins that may be involved in some aspects of lipid cycling and uptake. The proteins involved in lipid transport are listed in Table 11.2. The hepatic and intestinal apolipoproteins can be distinguished using electrophoresis, a technique of separating proteins based on their electrophoretic mobility. Mutations in the genes that encode these proteins can lead to aberrant lipid transport, and the individual may have either abnormally high or low blood lipid values.

The intestinal cell has three apolipoproteins called A-1, A-IV, and B-48. Apolipoprotein B-48 (apo B-48) is unique to the enterocyte and is essential for chylomicron release by the intestinal cell. Apo A-1 is synthesized in the liver. Apo B-48 is actually an edited version of the hepatic apo B-100. It is the result of an apo B mRNA editing process that converts codon 2153 to a translational stop codon. Apo B-48 is thus an edited form of apo B-100, and this editing is unique to the intestinal cell.

As chylomicrons circulate, they acquire an additional protein, apo C-II. This additional protein is an essential cofactor

### TABLE 11.2
### Proteins Involved in Lipid Transport

| Protein | Function |
|---|---|
| Apo A-II | Transport protein in HDL. |
| Apo B-48 | Transport protein for chylomicrons; synthesized in the enterocyte in the human. |
| HDl-binding protein (HDLBP) | Binds HDL and functions in the removal of excess cellular cholesterol. |
| Apo D | Transport protein similar to retinol-binding protein. |
| Apo (a) | Abnormal transport protein for LDL. |
| Apo A-I | Transport protein for chylomicrons and HDL; synthesized in the liver and its synthesis is induced by retinoic acid. |
| Apo C-III | Transport protein for VLDL. |
| Apo A-IV | Transport protein for chylomicrons. |
| CETP | Participates in the transport of cholesterol from peripheral tissue to liver; reduces HDL size. |
| LCAT | Synthesized in the liver and is secreted into the plasma, where it resides on the HDL Participates in the reverse transport of cholesterol from peripheral tissues to the liver; esterifies the HDL cholesterol. |
| Apo E | Mediates high affinity binding of LDLs to the LDL receptor and the putative chylomicron receptor; required for clearance of chylomicron remnant; synthesized primarily in the liver. |
| Apo C-I | Transport protein for VLDL. |
| Apo C-II | Chylomicron-transport protein required cofactor for LPL activity. |
| Apo B-100 | Synthesized in the liver and is secreted into the circulation as part of the VLDL. Also serves as the ligand for the LDL-receptor-mediated hepatic endocytosis. |
| Lipoprotein lipase | Catalyzes the hydrolysis of plasma TG into free fatty acids. |
| Hepatic lipase | Catalyzes the hydrolysis of TG and phospholipids of the LDL and HDL. It is bound to the surfaces of both hepatic and nonhepatic tissues. |

for the recognition and hydrolysis of the chylomicron by the capillary endothelial enzyme, lipoprotein lipase (LPL). LPL hydrolyzes most of the core TG in the chylomicron, leaving a remnant that is rich in cholesterol and cholesterol esters. During the LPL-catalyzed hydrolytic process, the excess surface compounds, that is, the phospholipids and apolipoproteins B, A-I, and A-IV are transferred to high-density lipoproteins (HDL) and, in exchange, apo E is transferred from the HDL to the cholesterol-ester-rich chylomicron remnant. These remnants are then cleared from the blood by the liver. On the hepatocyte is a lipoprotein receptor that recognizes apo E, and this receptor plays an important role in remnant clearance.

The chylomicron is a relatively stable way of ensuring the movement, in an aqueous medium (blood), of hydrophobic molecules such as cholesterol and triacylglycerols from their point of origin, the intestine, to their point of use or storage. As mentioned, there are several unique proteins that facilitate this movement. These lipid-transporting proteins determine which cells of the body receive which lipids. At the target cell, the particles lose their lipid through hydrolysis facilitated by an interstitial LPL, which is found in the capillary beds of muscle, fat cells, and other tissues using lipid as a fuel. This LPL is synthesized by these target cells but is anchored on the outside of the cells by a polysaccharide chain on the endothelial wall of the surrounding capillaries.

## PROTEIN DIGESTION/ABSORPTION

Upon consumption, food protein is degraded into its component amino acids which are then absorbed (Table 11.1). In the stomach, food proteins are denatured by gastric hydrochloric acid and attacked by the proteases (pepsin, parapepsin I, and parapepsin II). The hydrochloric acid makes the protein more vulnerable to attack by pepsin, an endopeptidase. Actually, pepsin is not a single enzyme. It consists of pepsin A, which attacks peptide bonds involving phenylalanine or tyrosine, and several other enzymes, which have specific attack points. The pepsins are released into the gastric cavity as pepsinogen. Food entering the stomach stimulates HCl release, and the pH of the gastric contents falls below 2. Through the action of the acid environment, the pepsinogen loses a 44-amino-acid sequence. This happens through one of two mechanisms: the first, called autoactivation, occurs when the pH drops below 5. At low pH the bond between the 44th and 45th amino acid residue falls apart and the 44-amino-acid residue (from the amino terminus) is liberated. The liberated residue acts as an inhibitor of pepsin by binding to the catalytic site until pH 2 is achieved. The inhibition is then relieved when this fragment is acid degraded, as happens at pH 2 or below or when it is attacked by pepsin. As the fragment binds at the catalytic site of pepsin, this can happen. The other process is called autocatalysis and occurs when already active pepsin attacks the precursor pepsinogen. This is a self-repeating process and serves to ensure ongoing catalysis of the resident protein. The cleavage of the

44-amino-acid residue, in addition to providing activated pepsin, has another purpose. That is, it serves as a signal peptide for cholecystokinin release in the duodenum. This then sets the stage for the subsequent pancreatic phase of protein digestion. As described in the sections on lipid and carbohydrate digestion, cholecystokinin stimulates both the exocrine pancreas and the intestinal mucosal epithelial cells to release its digestive enzymes. The intestinal cell releases an enzyme, enteropeptidase or enterokinase, which serves to activate the protease, trypsin, released as trypsinogen by the exocrine pancreas. This trypsin not only acts on food proteins but also acts on other preproteases, released by the exocrine pancreas, activating them. Thus, trypsin acts as an endoprotease on chymotrypsinogen, releasing chymotrypsin, on proelastase, releasing elastase, and on procarboxypeptidase, releasing carboxypeptidase. Trypsin, chymotrypsin, and elastase are all endoproteases each having specificity for particular peptide bonds. Each of these three proteases have serine as part of their catalytic site, so any compound that ties up the serine will inhibit the activity of these proteases.

The daily protein intake of about 100 g in addition to that protein appearing in the gut as enzymes, sloughed epithelial gut cells, and mucins, is almost completely digested and absorbed. This is a very efficient process that ensures a continuous supply of amino acids to the whole-body amino acid pool. Less than 1% of the total protein that passes through the gastrointestinal tract appears in the feces. If the food contributes between 70 and 100 g of protein and the endogenous protein contributes another 100 g (range: 35–200 g), then one might expect to see about 1–2 g of nitrogen in the feces. This is equivalent to 6–12 g protein. Of the dietary protein, the fecal protein might include the hard-to-chew/digest tough fibrous connective tissue of meat or nitrogen-containing indigestible kernel coats of grains or particles of nuts that are not attacked by the digestive enzymes. Peanuts, for example, eaten whole have a structure that is difficult to broach by the digestive enzymes. Unless chewed very finely, much of the nutritive value of this food may be lost. Peanut butter, on the other hand, is very well digested because the preparation of the peanut butter ensures that its particle size is very small and is thus quite digestible.

The protein hydrolases, called peptidases, fall into two categories. Those that attack internal peptide bonds and liberate large peptide fragments for subsequent attack by other enzymes are called the endopeptidases. Those that attack the terminal peptide bonds and liberate single amino acids from the protein structure are called exopeptidases. The exopeptidases are further subdivided according to whether they attack at the carboxy end of the amino acid chain (carboxypeptidases) or the amino end of the chain (aminopeptidases). The initial attack on an intact protein is catalyzed by endopeptidases, while the final digestive action is catalyzed by the exopeptidases. The final products of digestion are free amino acids and some di- and tripeptides that are absorbed by the intestinal epithelial cells.

**TABLE 11.3**

**Carriers for Amino Acids**

| Carrier | Amino Acids Carried |
| --- | --- |
| 1 | Serine, threonine, alanine |
| 2 | Phenylalanine, tyrosine, methionine, valine, leucine, isoleucine |
| 3 | Proline, hydroxyproline |
| 4 | Taurine, β-alanine |
| 5 | Lysine, arginine, cysteine–cysteine |
| 6 | Aspartatic and glutamic acids |

## AMINO ACID ABSORPTION

Although single amino acids are liberated in the intestinal contents, there is insufficient power in the enzymes of the pancreatic juice to render all of the amino acids singly for absorption. The brush border of the absorptive cell therefore not only absorbs the single amino acids but also di- and tripeptides. In the process of absorbing these small peptides, it hydrolyzes them to their amino acid constituents. There is little evidence that peptides enter the bloodstream. There are specific transport systems for each group of functionally similar amino acids, di- and tripeptides. These carriers are listed in Table 11.3.

Most of the biologically important L-amino acids are transported by an active carrier system against a concentration gradient. This active transport involves the intracellular potassium ion and the extracellular sodium ion. As the amino acid is carried into the enterocyte, sodium also enters in exchange for potassium. This sodium must be returned (in exchange for potassium) to the extracellular medium. This return uses the sodium–potassium ATP pump. In several instances, the carrier is a shared carrier. That is, the carrier will transport more than one amino acid. Such is the case with the neutral amino acids and those with short or polar side chains (serine, threonine, and alanine). The mechanism whereby these carriers participate in amino acid absorption is similar to that described for glucose uptake. Once amino acids are absorbed and in circulation, they will either be used to synthesize body proteins and essential nitrogenous compounds (thyroxine or epinephrine) or catabolized.

## CARBOHYDRATE METABOLISM

### GLYCOLYSIS

Once absorbed, glucose travels to the liver and other tissues via the portal bloodstream. At the target tissue, it enters the glycolytic sequence. The glycolytic pathway for the anaerobic catabolism of glucose can be found in all cells in the body (Figure 11.1). The pathway begins with glucose, a six-carbon unit, and through a series of reactions produces two molecules of ATP and two molecules of pyruvate. The control of glycolysis is vested in several key steps. The first step is the activation of glucose through the formation of glucose-6-phosphate. In the liver and pancreatic β-cells,

this step is catalyzed by the enzyme glucokinase. A molecule of ATP is used and magnesium is required. Glucose-6-phosphate is a key metabolite. It can proceed down the glycolytic pathway or move through the hexose monophosphate shunt (see hexose monophosphate shunt) or be used to make glycogen. How much glucose-6-phosphate is oxidized directly to pyruvate depends on the nutritional state of the animal, cell type, the genetics of the animal, and its hormonal state. Some cell types, the brain cell, for example, do not make glycogen. Some people do not have shunt activity in the red cell because the code for glucose-6-phosphate dehydrogenase has mutated such that the enzyme is not functional. Insulin-deficient animals likewise have little glycolytic and shunt activity because of the lack of insulin's effect on the synthesis of key enzymes of these pathways. All these factors determine how much glucose-6-phosphate goes in which direction.

Two enzymes are used for the activation of glucose: glucokinase and hexokinase. In the liver, both enzymes are present. While hexokinase activity is product inhibited, glucokinase is not. The hexokinase in the nonhepatic tissues must be product inhibited to prevent the hexokinase from tying up all the inorganic phosphate (Pi) in the cells as glucose-6-phosphate. The Km for glucokinase is greater than that for hexokinase, so the former is the main enzyme for the conversion of glucose to glucose-6-phosphate in the liver. The other enzyme will phosphorylate not only glucose but other six-carbon sugars such as fructose. However, the amount of fructose phosphorylated to fructose-6-phosphate is small in comparison to the phosphorylation of fructose at the carbon 1 position catalyzed by fructokinase. Both kinase reactions require magnesium as a cofactor.

Glucose-6-phosphate is isomerized to fructose-6-phosphate and is then phosphorylated once again to form fructose-1,6-bisphosphate. Another molecule of ATP is used, and again magnesium is an important cofactor. Both kinase reactions are rate-controlling reactions in that their activity determines the rate at which subsequent reactions proceed. The phosphofructokinase reaction is unique to the glycolytic sequence, while the glucokinase or hexokinase step provides substrates for either the shunt or the glycogenic sequences. Thus, one could argue that the formation of fructose-1,6-bisphosphate is the first committed step in glycolysis. Glycolysis is inhibited when phosphofructokinase is inhibited. This occurs when levels of fatty acids in the cytosol rise as in the instance of high rates of lipolysis and fatty acid oxidation. Phosphofructokinase activity is increased when levels of fructose-6-phosphate rise or when cyclic adenosine monophosphate (cAMP) levels rise. Stimulation occurs also when fructose-2,6-bisphosphate levels rise. In any event, glycolysis then proceeds with the splitting of fructose-1,6-bisphosphate to dihydroxyacetone phosphate (DHAP) and glyceraldehyde-3-phosphate. At this point, another rate-controlling step occurs. This step is one which shuttles reducing equivalents into the mitochondria for use by the respiratory chain. This is the α-glycerophosphate shuttle (Figure 11.2). This shuttle carries reducing equivalents from the cytosol

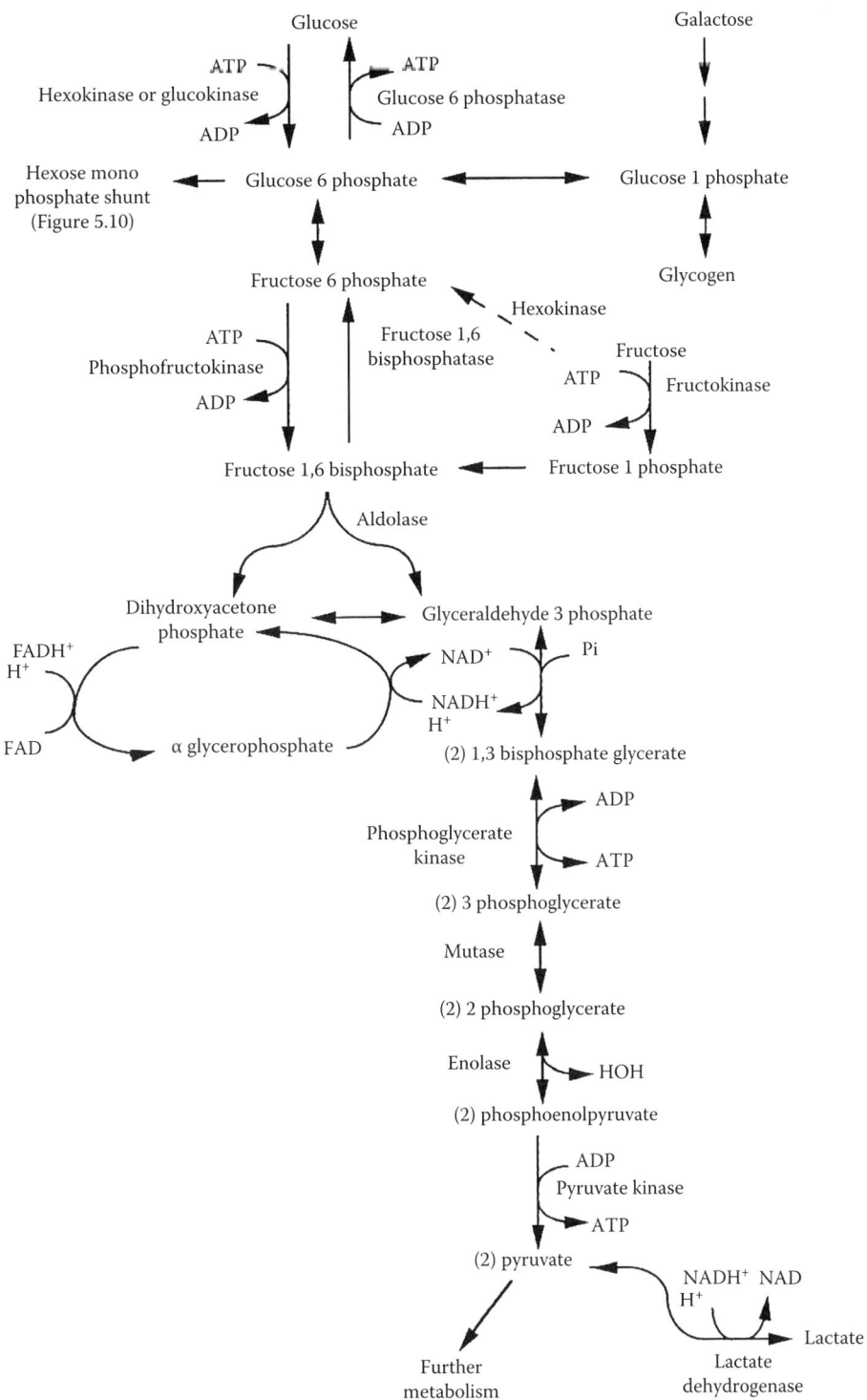

**FIGURE 11.1**  The glycolytic pathway.

to the mitochondria. DHAP picks up reducing equivalents when it is converted to α-glycerol phosphate. These reducing equivalents are produced when glyceraldehyde-3-phosphate is oxidized in the process of being phosphorylated to 1,3-diphosphate glycerate. The α-glycerophosphate enters the inner mitochondrial membrane, whereupon it is converted back to DHAP, releasing its reducing equivalents to FAD (a riboflavin-containing coenzyme) that in turn transfers the reducing equivalents to the mitochondrial respiratory

chain. The reason why this shuttle is rate limiting is the need to regenerate NAD⁺. Without NAD⁺ the glycolytic pathway ceases. NADH⁺ (a niacin-containing coenzyme) is produced during glycolysis when reducing equivalents are accepted by NAD⁺. NADH⁺ itself cannot pass through the mitochondrial membrane, so substrate shuttles are necessary. Another means of producing NAD⁺ is by converting pyruvate to lactate. This is a nonmitochondrial reaction catalyzed by lactate dehydrogenase. It occurs when an oxygen debt is developed as

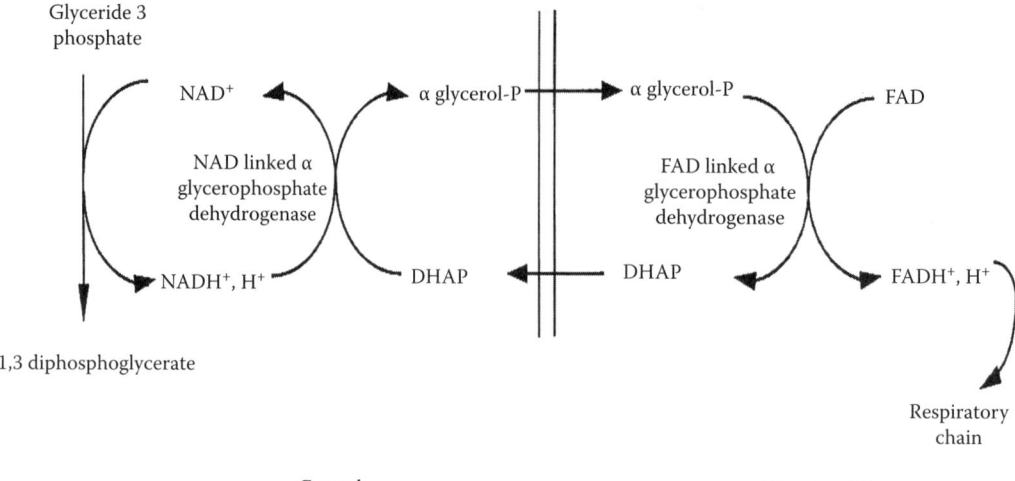

**FIGURE 11.2**  The α-glycerophosphate shuttle.

happens in exercising muscle. In these muscles, more oxygen is consumed than can be provided. Glycolysis occurs at a rate higher than can be accommodated by the respiratory chain that joins the reducing equivalents transferred to it by the shuttles to molecular oxygen, making water. If more reducing equivalents are generated than can be used to make water, the excess are added to pyruvate to make lactate. Thus, rising lactate levels are indicative of oxygen debt.

There are other shuttles that also serve to transfer reducing equivalents into the mitosol. These are the malate–aspartate shuttle (Figure 11.3) and the malate–citrate shuttle. Neither of these is rate limiting with respect to glycolysis. The malate–aspartate shuttle has rate-controlling properties with respect to gluconeogenesis, while the malate–citrate shuttle is important to lipogenesis.

Once 1,3-bisphosphate glycerate is formed, it is converted to 3-phosphoglycerate with the formation of one ATP. The 3-phosphoglycerate then goes to 2-phosphoglycerate and then to phosphoenolpyruvate (PEP). These are all bidirectional reactions that are also used in gluconeogenesis. The PEP is dephosphorylated to pyruvate with the formation of another ATP. Because of the great energy lost to ATP formation at this step, this reaction is not reversible. Gluconeogenesis uses another enzyme, PEP carboxykinase (PEPCK), to reverse this step. Glycolysis uses pyruvate kinase to catalyze the reaction. At any rate, pyruvate can now be converted to acetyl CoA via pyruvate dehydrogenase or carboxylated to oxalacetate via pyruvate carboxylase. Oxalacetate is the beginning substrate for the citric acid cycle.

The citric acid cycle is the central cycle in intermediary metabolism. All the major macromolecules produce substrates that in one way or another enter the citric acid cycle. This cycle is shown in Figure 11.4. The purpose of this cycle is to produce reducing equivalents that can be used to make

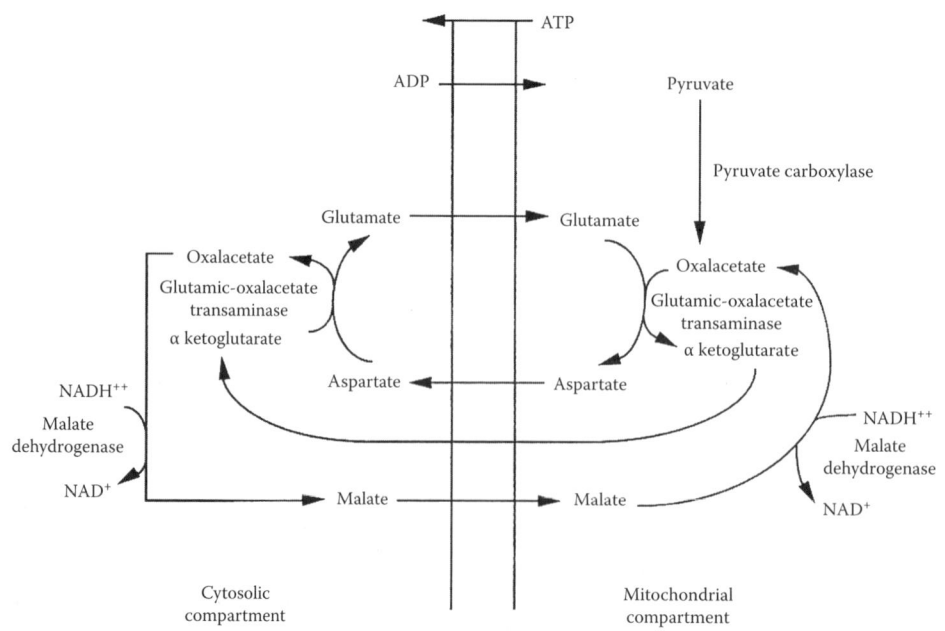

**FIGURE 11.3**  The malate aspartate shuttle.

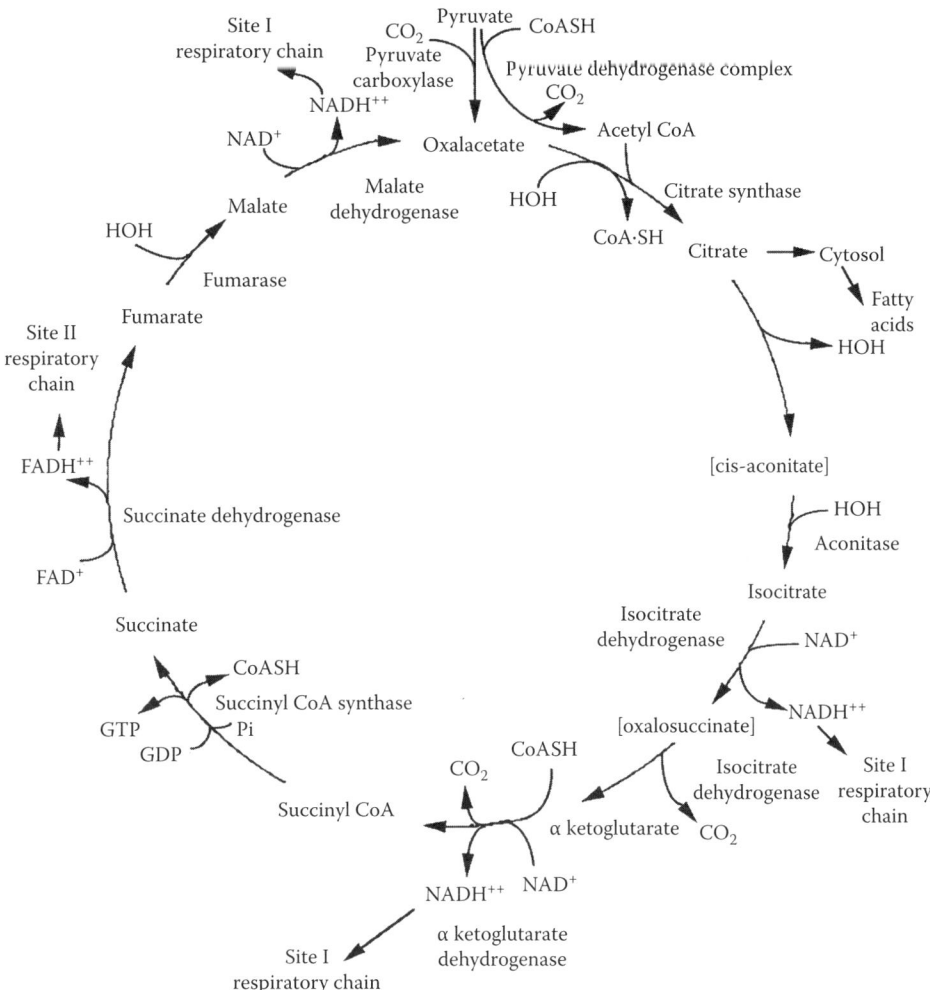

**FIGURE 11.4** Krebs citric acid cycle in the mitochondria. This cycle is also called the tricarboxylate cycle (TCA). Abbreviations used: HOH, water; FAD, flavin adenine nucleotide; FADH$^{++}$, flavin adenine nucleotide, reduced; NAD, niacin adenine dinucleotide; NADH$^{++}$, niacin adenine dinucleotide reduced; GTP, guanosine triphosphate; GDP, guanosine diphosphate; CoA, coenzyme A; CO$_2$, carbon dioxide.

water by the respiratory chain (Figure 11.5) and CO$_2$. In the process of making water, substantial energy is released. Some of this is captured in the high-energy bond of ATP, while the majority is released as heat. The citric acid cycle begins with joining of a two-carbon group (acetyl CoA) to oxalacetate to form citrate. The CoA is lost in the reaction and a molecule of water is added. The CoA is a pantothenic-acid-containing reactive group that plays an important role not only in the citric acid cycle but also in the many reactions of lipid metabolism. Citrate then loses a molecule of water, becoming the unstable compound, *cis*-aconitate. Water is added back, and isocitrate is formed. Reducing equivalents are then lost (picked up by NAD$^+$) and sent to the respiratory chain at site 1. Another unstable compound is formed, which in turn loses a CO$_2$ to become α-ketoglutarate. Another CO$_2$ is lost as are reducing equivalents (again picked up by NAD$^+$ and again sent to site 1 of the respiratory chain), and succinyl CoA is formed. Succinyl CoA loses its CoA group to become succinate and in turn loses reducing equivalents (picked up by FAD and sent to site 2 of the respiratory chain) to become fumarate. Water is added to fumarate, and malate is produced.

This malate can leave the mitochondrial compartment in the malate–citrate shuttle and become oxalacetate, the starting point of gluconeogenesis. In the citric acid cycle, malate loses reducing equivalents (picked up by NAD$^+$ and sent to site 1 of the respiratory chain), and once again oxalacetate is produced. The cycle has now returned to its starting point.

The glycolytic pathway is dependent on both ATP for the initial steps of the pathway, the formation of glucose-6-phosphate and fructose-1,6-bisphosphate, and on the ratio of ATP to ADP and inorganic phosphate, Pi. In working muscle, the continuance of work and the continuance of glycolysis depend on the cycling of the adenine nucleotides and the export of lactate to the liver. ATP must be provided at the beginning of the pathway, and ADP as well as Pi must be provided in the latter steps. If the tissue runs out of ATP, ADP, or Pi or accumulates lactate and H$^+$, glycolysis will come to a halt and work cannot continue. This is what happens to the working skeletal muscle. Exhaustion sets in when glycolytic rate is downregulated by an accumulation of lactate.

Many diets contain carbohydrates in addition to starch and glucose. These carbohydrates are metabolized to their primary

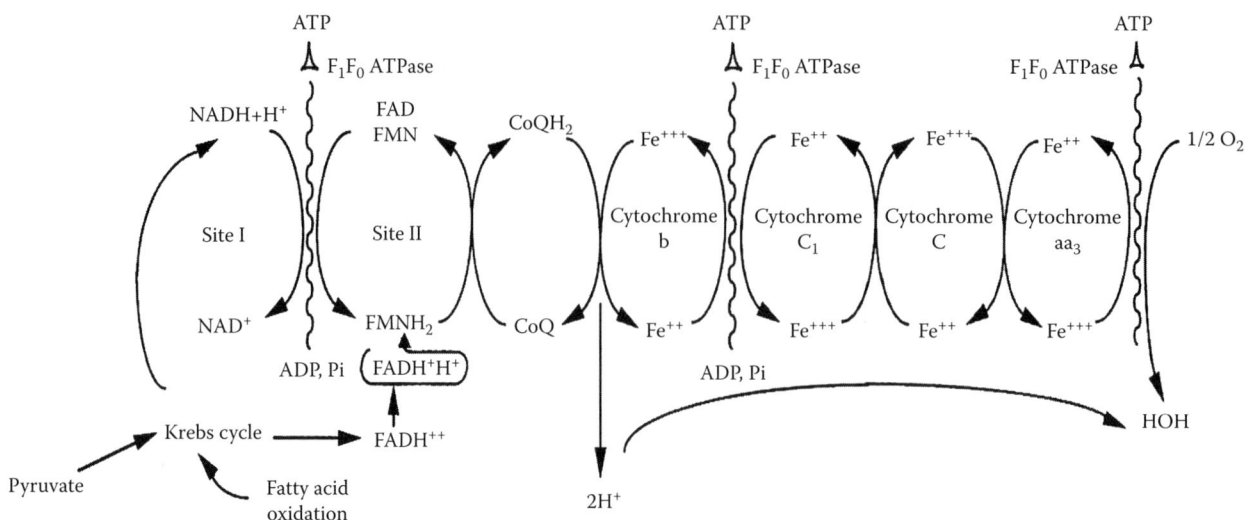

**FIGURE 11.5** The respiratory chain showing the points where sufficient energy has been generated to support the synthesis of 1 molecule of ATP from ADP and Pi. Each of the segments generates a proton gradient. This energy is captured by the $F_0$ portion of the ATPase and transmitted to the $F_1$ portion of the ATPase. If uncouplers are present, the proton gradient is dissipated and all of the energy is released as heat.

monosaccharides and used. Of these monosaccharides, two are most important: fructose and galactose. Fructose is converted to glucose after phosphorylation (Figure 11.6). Although two enzymes are available for the phosphorylation of fructose, one of these, fructokinase, is present only in the liver. Hexokinase can catalyze the phosphorylation of fructose. However, fructokinase is a much more active enzyme. Its activity is so high that, in fact, most of the dietary fructose whether as the free sugar or

as a component of sucrose is metabolized in the liver. This is in contrast to glucose, which is metabolized by all the cells in the body. As a result, fructose- or sucrose-rich diets fed to rats or mice will result in a fatty liver. This occurs because the dietary overload of fructose or sucrose exceeds the capacity of the liver to oxidize it, and so it uses the sugar metabolites as substrate for fatty acid and triacylglyceride synthesis. Until the hepatic lipid export system increases sufficiently to transport this lipid to the storage depots, the lipid accumulates, hence resulting in the fatty liver. Adaptation to a high fructose intake can and does occur in normal individuals, and the fatty liver disappears.

Galactose, a component of the milk sugar, lactose, is converted to glucose and eventually enters the glycolytic sequence as glucose-6-phosphate (Figure 11.7). Galactose is phosphorylated at carbon 1 in the first step of its conversion to glucose. It can be isomerized to glucose-1-phosphate or converted to uridune diphosphate (UDP)-galactose by exchanging its phosphate group for a UDP group. This UDP-galactose can be joined with glucose to form lactose in the adult mammary tissue under the influence of the hormone prolactin. However, usually the UDP-galactose is converted to UDP-glucose and thence used to form glycogen.

## PENTOSE PHOSPHATE SHUNT

The pentose phosphate shunt is an alternative pathway for the metabolism of glucose (Figure 11.8). The shunt uses glucose-6-phosphate and generates phosphorylated ribose for use in DNA and RNA synthesis. It also produces reducing equivalents for use by the microsomal P450 enzymes and the lipogenic pathway. It is estimated that approximately 10% of the glucose-6-phosphate generated from glucose is metabolized by the shunt.

The shunt contains two NADP-linked dehydrogenases, glucose-6-phosphate dehydrogenase and 6-phosphogluconate dehydrogenase. These two enzymes catalyze the rate-limiting steps in the reaction sequence. In the instance where there is an active lipogenic state, these reactions provide about 50% of the

**FIGURE 11.6** Metabolism of fructose.

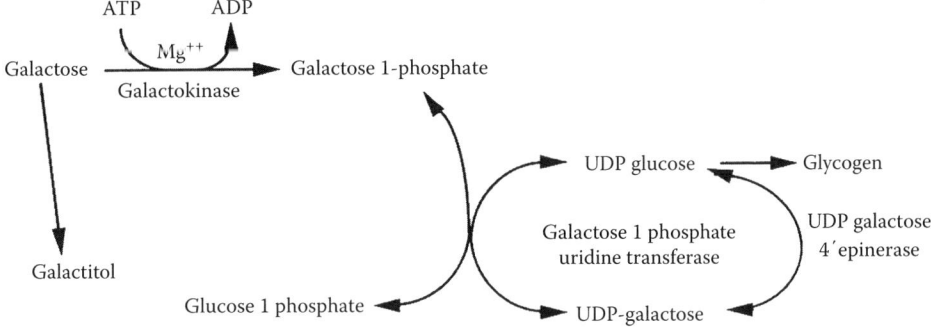

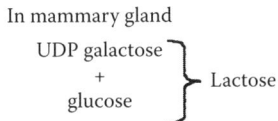

**FIGURE 11.7**  Conversion of galactose to glucose.

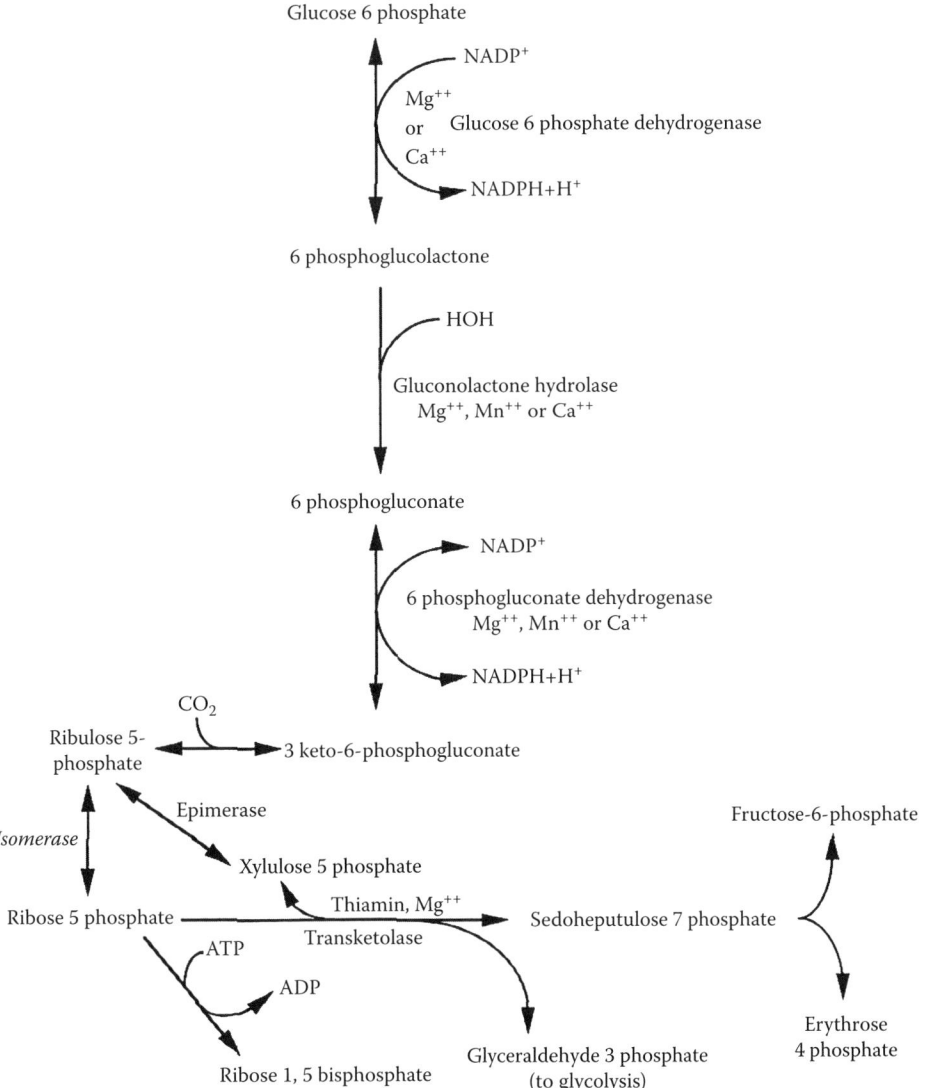

**FIGURE 11.8**  The reaction sequence of the hexose monophosphate shunt commonly referred to as the "shunt."

reducing equivalents needed by the lipogenic process. There is an excellent correlation between this dehydrogenase activity and lipogenesis. The microsomal P450 enzymes also use the reducing equivalents carried by NADP⁺ as does the red blood cell in the maintenance of glutathione in the reduced state. The glutathione system in the red blood cell maintains the redox state and integrity of the cell membrane. If sufficient reducing equivalents are not produced by the shunt dehydrogenase reactions to reduce glutathione, the red blood cell membrane integrity is lost and hemolytic anemia results. This is important to the red blood cell function of carrying oxygen and exchanging it for carbon dioxide. In any event, glucose-6-phosphate proceeds to 6-phosphogluconolactone, a very unstable metabolite, which is in turn reduced to 6-phosphogluconate. 6-Phosphogluconate is decarboxylated and dehydrogenated to form ribulose 5-phosphate with an unstable intermediate (keto-6-phosphogluconate) forming between the 6-phosphogluconate and ribulose 5-phosphate. Ribulose 5-phosphate can be isomerized to ribose 5-phosphate or epimerized to xylulose 5-phosphate. Xylulose and ribose 5-phosphate can reversibly form sedoheptulose 7-phosphate with release of glyceraldehyde 3-phosphate. If glucose does not proceed down the glycolytic sequence or through the pentose shunt, it can be used to make glycogen.

## GLYCOGENESIS

Glycogen synthesis begins with glucose-1-phosphate formation from glucose-6-phosphate through the action of phosphoglucomutase (Figure 11.9). Glucose-1-phosphate then is converted to UDP-glucose, which can then be added to the glycogen already in storage (the glycogen primer). UDP-glucose can be added through α 1,6 linkage or α 1,4 linkage. Two high-energy bonds are used to incorporate each molecule of glucose into

the glycogen. The straight-chain glucose polymer is comprised of glucoses joined through the 1,4 linkage and is less compact than the branched-chain glycogen, which has both 1,4 and 1,6 linkages. The addition of glucose to the primer glycogen with a 1,4 linkage is catalyzed by the glycogen synthase enzyme, while the 1,6 addition is catalyzed by the so-called glycogen branching enzyme, amylo (1 → 4, 1 → 6) transglucosidase. Once the liver and muscle cell achieve their full storage capacity, these enzymes are product inhibited and glycogenesis is "turned off." Glycogen synthase is inactivated by a cAMP-dependent kinase and activated by a synthase phosphatase enzyme that is stimulated by changes in the ratio of ATP to ADP. Glycogen synthesis is stimulated by the hormone insulin and suppressed by the catabolic hormones. The process does not fully cease but operates at a very low level. Glycogen does not accumulate appreciably in cells other than liver and muscle although all cells contain a small amount of glycogen. Note that a glycogen primer is required for glycogen synthesis to proceed. This primer is carefully guarded so that some is always available for glycogen synthesis. This means that glycogenolysis never fully depletes the cell of its glycogen content. When glucose is needed by the body, it can generate glucose either from glycogenolysis or through gluconeogenesis.

## GLYCOGENOLYSIS

Glycogenolysis is a carefully controlled series of reactions referred to as the glycogen cascade (Figure 11.10). It is called a cascade because of the stepwise changes in activation states of the enzymes involved. To release glucose for oxidation by the glycogenolytic pathway, the glycogen must be phosphorylated. This is accomplished by the enzyme glycogen phosphorylase. Glycogen phosphorylase exists in the cell in an inactive form

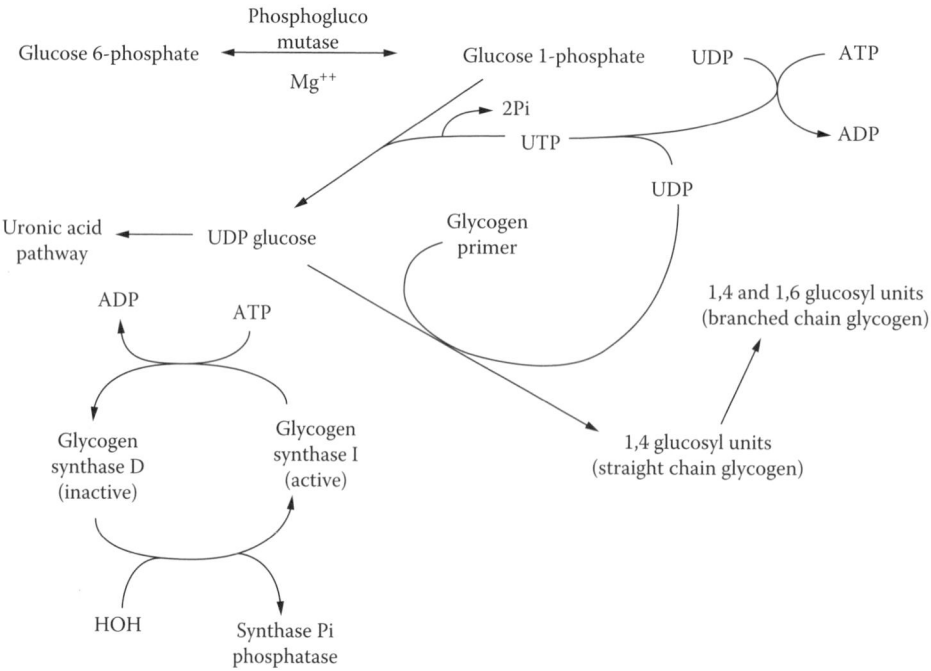

**FIGURE 11.9**  Glycogen synthesis (glycogenesis).

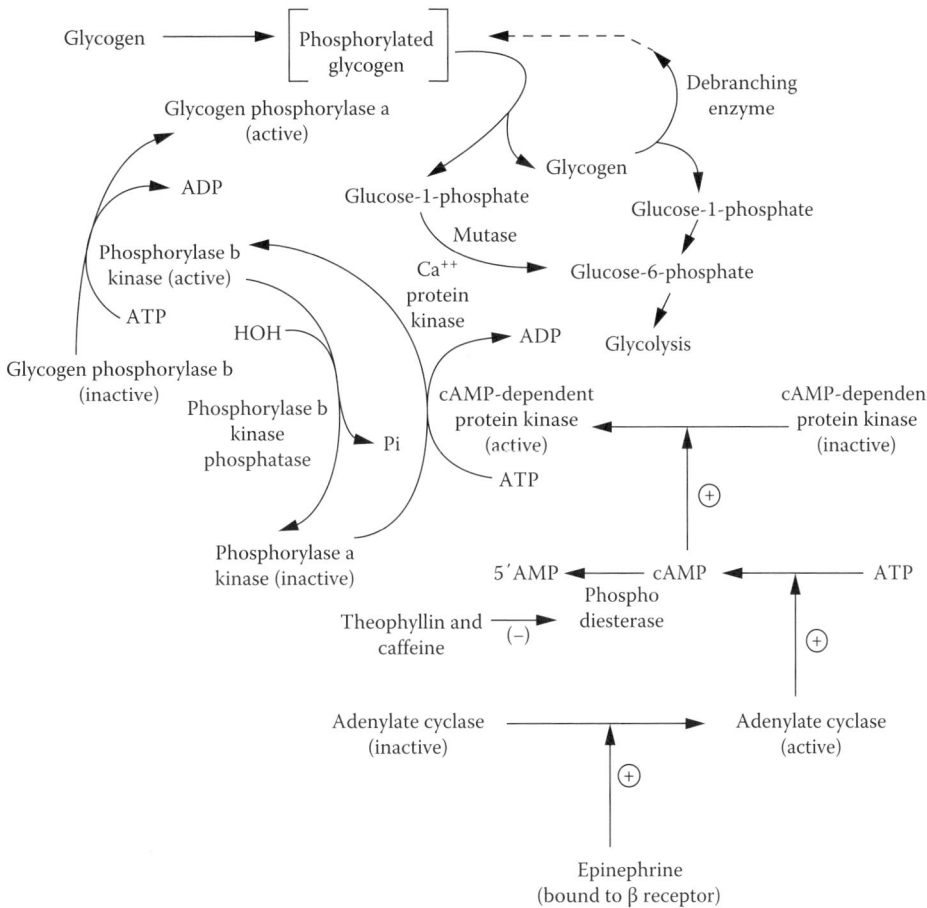

**FIGURE 11.10**  Glycogen breakdown (glycogenolysis).

(glycogen phosphorylase b) and is activated to its active form (glycogen phosphorylase a) by the enzyme phosphorylase b kinase. In turn, this kinase also exists in an inactive form, which is activated by the calcium-dependent enzyme, protein kinase, and active cAMP-dependent protein kinase. These activations each require a molecule of ATP. Lastly, the cAMP-dependent protein kinase must have cAMP for its activation. This cAMP is generated from ATP by the enzyme adenylate cyclase, which, in itself, is inactive unless stimulated by a hormone such as epinephrine, thyroxine, or glucagon. As can be seen, this cascade of activation is energy dependent with three molecules of ATP needed to get the process started. Once started, the glycolytic pathway will replenish the ATP needed initially as well as provide a further supply of ATP to provide needed energy. As mentioned, the liver and muscle differ in the use of glycogen. This also affects how ATP is generated within the glycogen-containing cell and how much is generated by cells that do not store glycogen.

Glycogenolysis is stimulated by the catabolic hormones, glucagon, epinephrine, glucocorticoids, and thyroxine, and/or by the absence of food in the digestive tract. Because the glycogen molecule has molecules of water as part of its structure, it is a very large molecule and cumbersome to store in large amounts. The average 70 kg man has only an 18 h fuel supply stored as glycogen, while that same individual might have up to a 2-month supply of fuel stored as fat. Muscle and

liver glycogen stores have very different functions. Muscle glycogen is used to synthesize ATP for muscle contraction, whereas hepatic glycogen is the glucose reserve for the entire body particularly the central nervous system. The amount of glycogen in the muscle is dependent on the physical activity of the individual. After bouts of strenuous exercise, the glycogen store will be depleted only to be rebuilt during the resting period following exercise. Hepatic glycogen stores are dependent on nutritional status. They are virtually absent in the 24 h starved animal while being replenished within hours of feeding. Clusters of glycogen molecules with an average molecular weight of $2 \times 10^7$ form quickly when an abundance of glucose is provided to the liver. The amount of glycogen in the liver is diet and time dependent. There is a 24 h rhythmic change in hepatic glycogen that corresponds to the feeding pattern of the animal. In nocturnal animals such as the rat, the peak hepatic glycogen store will be found in the early morning hours, while the nadir will be found in the evening hours just before the nocturnal feeding begins. In humans accustomed to eating during the day, the reverse pattern will be observed.

## GLUCONEOGENESIS

Gluconeogenesis occurs primarily in the liver and kidney (Figure 11.11). Except under conditions of prolonged starvation, the kidneys do not contribute appreciable amounts of

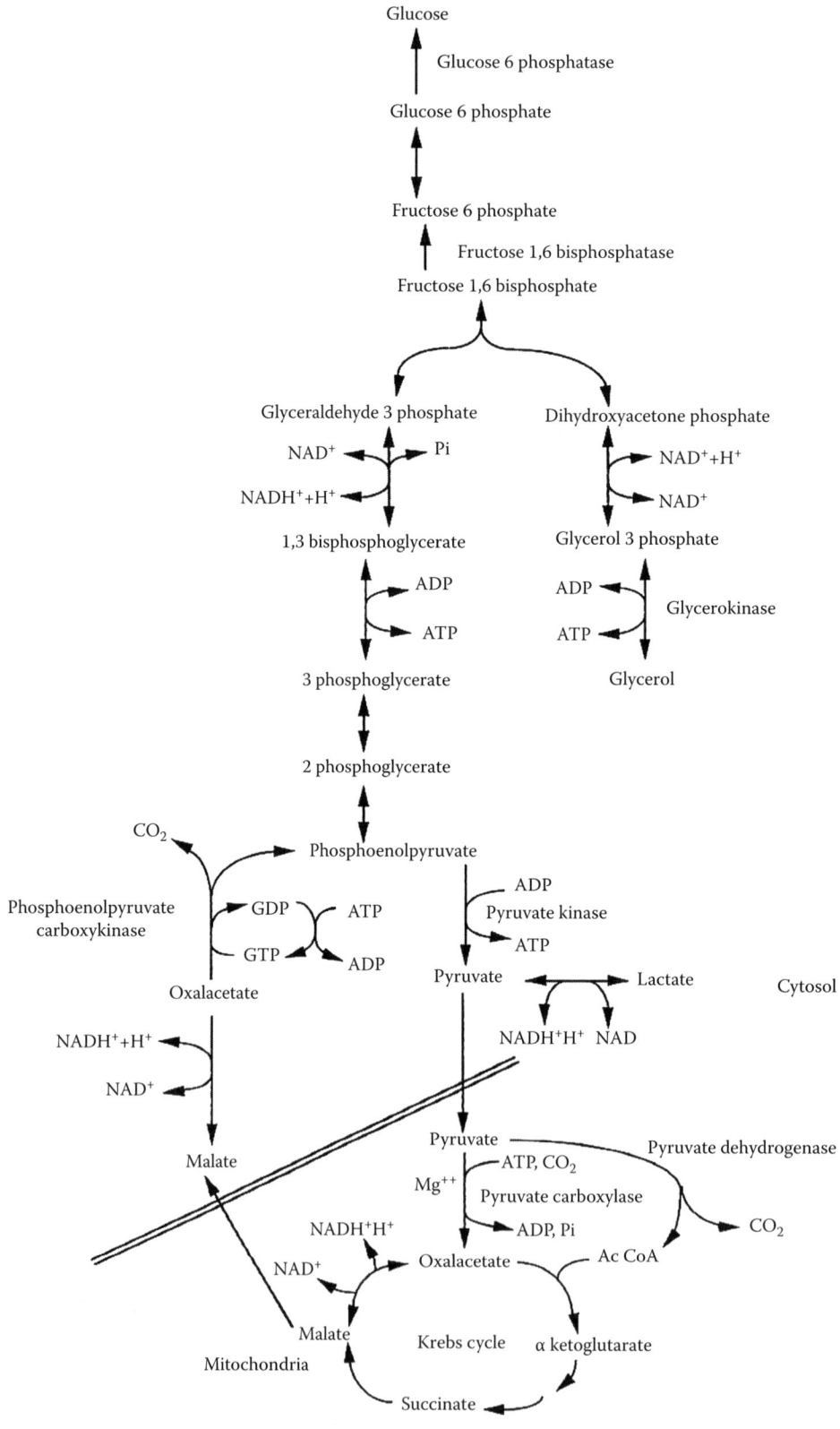

**FIGURE 11.11** Pathway for gluconeogenesis.

glucose to the circulation. Most tissues lack the full complement of enzymes needed to run this pathway. In particular, the rate-limiting enzyme PEPCK is not found to be active in tissues other than liver and kidney. The other reactions use the same enzymes as glycolysis and do not have control properties with respect to gluconeogenesis. The rate-limiting enzymes are glucose-6-phosphatase, fructose-1,6-bisphosphatase, and PEPCK. Pyruvate kinase and pyruvate carboxylase are also of interest because their control is a coordinated one with respect to the regulation of PEPCK.

Oxalacetate in the cytosol is essential to gluconeogenesis because it is the substrate for PEPCK that catalyzes its conversion to PEP. This is an energy-dependent conversion that overcomes the irreversible final glycolytic reaction catalyzed by pyruvate kinase. The activity of PEPCK is closely coupled with that of pyruvate carboxylase. Whereas the pyruvate kinase reaction produces one ATP, the formation of PEP uses two ATPs—one in the mitochondria for the pyruvate carboxylase reaction and one in the cytosol for the PEPCK reaction. PEPCK requires guanosine triphosphate (GTP) provided via the nucleoside diphosphate kinase reaction that uses ATP. ATP transfers one high-energy bond to GDP to form ADP and GTP.

In starvation or uncontrolled diabetes, PEPCK activity is elevated as is gluconeogenesis. Starvation elicits a number of catabolic hormones that serve to mobilize tissue energy stores as well as precursors for glucose synthesis. Uncontrolled diabetes elicits similar hormonal responses. In both instances, the synthesis of the PEPCK enzyme protein is increased. Unlike other rate-limiting enzymes, PEPCK is not regulated allosterically or by phosphorylation–dephosphorylation mechanisms. Instead, it is regulated by changes in gene transcription of its single-copy gene from a single promoter site. This regulation is unique because all of the known factors (hormones, vitamins, and metabolites) act in the same place. They either turn on the synthesis of the messenger RNA for PEPCK or they turn it off. What is also unique is the fact that liver and kidney cells translate this message into sufficient active enzyme protein that catalyzes PEP formation. Other cells and tissues have the code for PEPCK in their nuclear DNA but do not usually synthesize the enzyme. Instead, these cell types synthesize the enzyme that catalyzes glycerol synthesis. In effect then, only the kidney and liver have active gluconeogenic processes.

The next few steps in gluconeogenesis are identical to those of glycolysis but are in the reverse direction. When the step for the dephosphorylation of fructose-1,6-bisphosphate occurs, there is another energy barrier and, instead of a bidirectional reaction catalyzed by a single enzyme, there are separate forward and reverse reactions. In the synthesis of glucose, this reaction is catalyzed by fructose-1,6-bisphosphatase and yields fructose-6-phosphate. No ATP is involved, but a molecule of water and an inorganic phosphate are produced. Rising levels of fructose-2,6-bisphosphatase allosterically inhibits gluconeogenesis, while it stimulates glycolysis. AMP likewise inhibits gluconeogenesis at this step.

Lastly, the removal of the phosphate from glucose-6-phosphate via the enzyme complex glucose-6-phosphatase completes the pathway to yield free glucose. This is an irreversible reaction that does not involve ATP. The glucose-6-phosphate moves to the endoplasmic reticulum, where the phosphatase is located and glucose is released for use.

## LIPID METABOLISM

### FATTY ACID ESTERIFICATION

In course of lipid absorption, the glycerides are hydrolyzed only to be reesterified for transport. This process of hydrolysis and reesterification happens every time a glyceride crosses a membrane. The resultant product of esterification is a MG, DG, or TG. The TG is hydrolyzed by interstitial LPL, and the fatty acids are transported into the target cell and reesterified to glycerol-3-phosphate. In the fat cell, this glycerol-3-phosphate usually is a product of glycolysis rather than the glycerol liberated when stored TG is hydrolyzed. The liberated glycerol usually passes back to the liver, which has a very active glycerokinase to phosphorylate it. In the liver, the phosphorylated glycerol is either used as a substrate for glucose synthesis or recycled into hepatic phospholipids or TG or oxidized to $CO_2$ and water.

Triacylglycerides are formed in a stepwise fashion (Figure 11.12). First, a fatty acid (usually a saturated fatty acid) is attached at carbon 1 of the glycerophosphate. The phosphate group at carbon 3 is electronegative, and because it pulls electrons toward it, it leaves carbon 1 more reactive than carbon 2. The fatty acid (as acyl CoA) is transferred to carbon 1 through the action of a transferase. The attachment uses the carboxy end of the fatty acid chain and makes an ester linkage releasing the CoA. Now the molecule has electronegative forces at each end—the phosphate group on carbon 3 and the oxygen plus carbon chain at carbon 1. Now carbon 2 is vulnerable and reactive, and another carbon chain can be attached. In this instance the fatty acid is usually an unsaturated fatty acid. At this point, the 1,2-diacylglyceride-phosphate loses its phosphate group so that carbon 3 is now reactive. The 1,2-diacylglyceride can either be esterified with another fatty acid to make triacylglyceride or can be used to make the membrane phospholipids, phosphatidylcholine, phosphatidylethanolamine, phosphatidylinositol, cardiolipin, and phosphatidylserine. In the stored triacylglycerides and in membranes, most unsaturated fatty acids are found at carbon 2. In the membrane phospholipids, the unsaturated fatty acid at carbon 2 is usually arachidonic acid. This arachidonic acid, produced by elongation and desaturation of dietary linoleic acid, is preferentially used in the membrane phospholipid. It can either be attached to the glycerol backbone when the phospholipid is made or exchanged for another fatty acid as the lipids in and around the cells remodel themselves. There is constant hydrolysis and reesterification in the cell, and there is a rapid exchange of fatty acids between those in the membranes and those inside the cell.

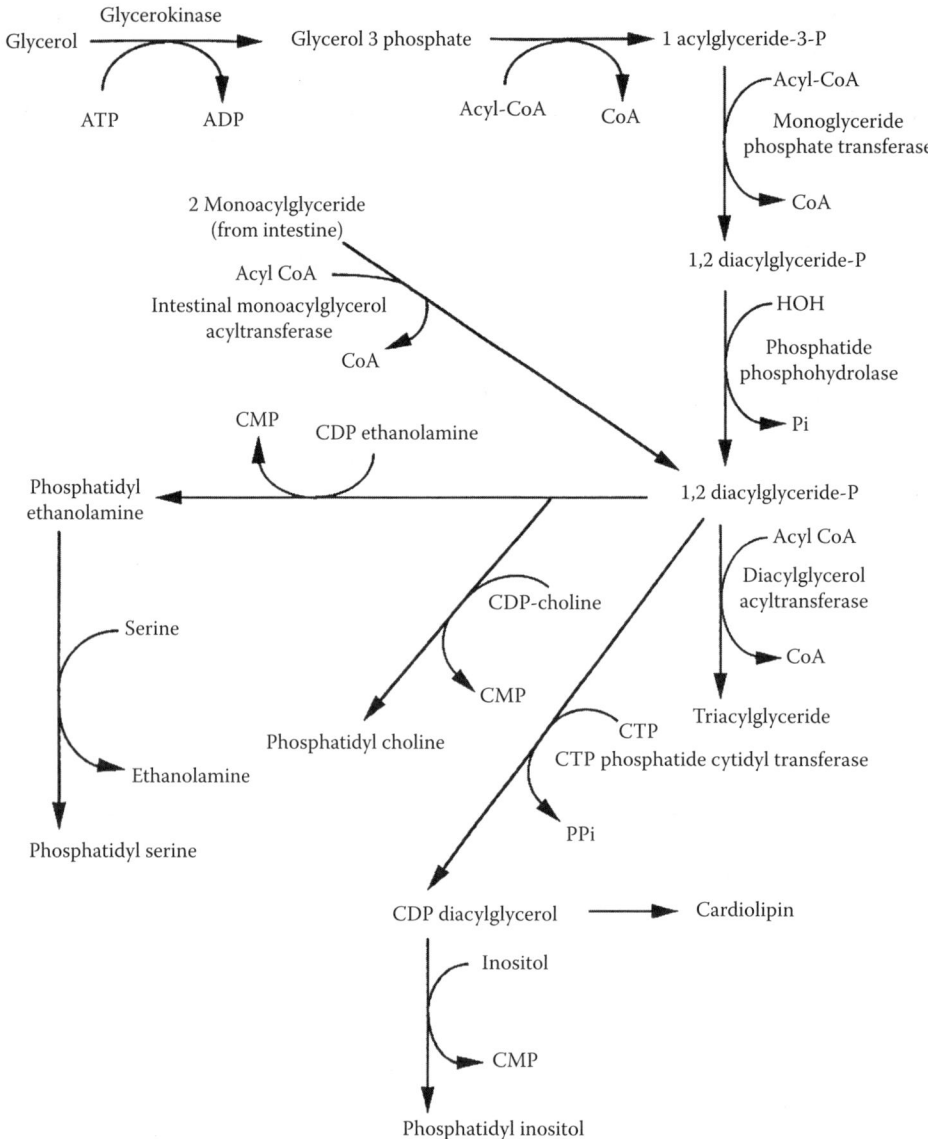

**FIGURE 11.12** Pathways for the synthesis of triacylglycerides and phospholipids.

## ENDOGENOUS LIPID TRANSPORT

Fatty acids, TG, cholesterol, cholesterol esters, and phospholipids are synthesized in the body and are transported from sites of synthesis to sites of use and storage. While the transport of these lipids is, in many instances, similar to that of the dietary lipids, there are differences in the processing and in some of the proteins involved. Endogenous fat transport involves the production and secretion of very-low-density lipoproteins (VLDL) by the liver. These lipid–protein complexes are rich in TG and contain cholesterol. The polypeptides that transport these lipids comprise approximately 10% of the weight of the VLDL. They include the polypeptides apo B, B-100, apo C-I, C-II, C-III, and apo E. As mentioned, several of these polypeptides are also involved in exogenous lipid transport. Once the VLDLs are released by the hepatocyte, they are hydrolyzed by the interstitial LPL, and intermediate-density lipoproteins (IDL) are formed. These are cleared from the circulation as they are recognized and bound to hepatic

IDL receptors. The hepatic receptors recognize the apo E that is part of the IDL. Any of the IDL that escapes hydrolysis at this stage is available for hydrolysis by the hepatic LPL. This hydrolysis leaves a cholesterol-rich particle of low-density lipoprotein (LDL). The LDL has apo B-100 as its polypeptide carrier, and both hepatic and extrahepatic cells have receptors that recognize this polypeptide. Normally, about 70% of LDL is cleared by the LDL receptors, and most of this is cleared by the liver. From the foregoing, it is apparent that considerable lipid recycling occurs in the liver. The VLDLs originate in the liver, and the liver is the primary site for LDL disposal. However, other organs and tissues also participate in disposal, but their participation is minor compared with that of the liver.

## FATTY ACID OXIDATION

Fatty acids are a source of metabolic fuel. They are available for oxidation once they are released from the gylcerides by hydrolysis. This oxidation occurs via the β-oxidation

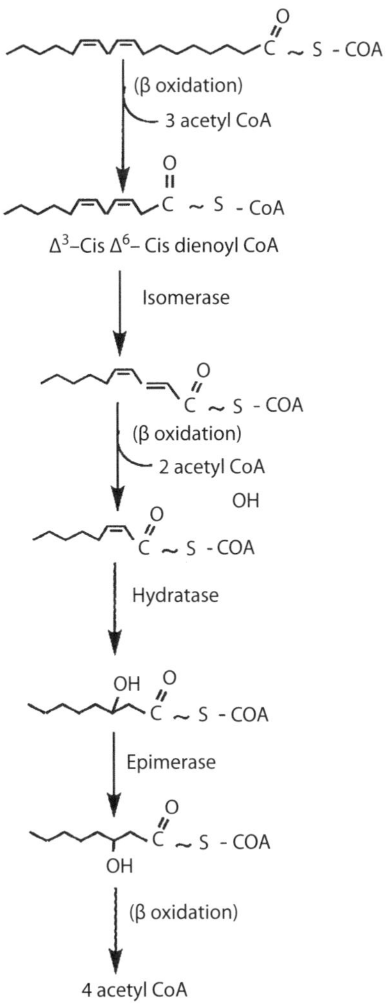

**FIGURE 11.13** Pathway for β-oxidation of fatty acids in the mitochondria.

pathway and occurs in the mitochondria (Figure 11.13). Prior to oxidation, the fatty acids must be transported into the mitochondria via the acylcarnitine transport system (Figure 11.14). The fatty acids are activated by conversion to their CoA thioesters. This activation requires ATP and the enzyme, acyl CoA synthase or thiokinase. There are several thiokinases, which differ with respect to their specificity for the different fatty acids. The activation step is dependent on the release of energy from ATP. Once the fatty acid is activated, it is bound to carnitine with the release of CoA. The acylcarnitine is then translocated through the mitochondrial membranes into the mitochondrial matrix via the carnitine acylcarnitine translocase. As one molecule of acylcarnitine is passed into the matrix, one molecule of carnitine is translocated back to the cytosol, and the acylcarnitine is converted back to acyl CoA. The acyl CoA can then enter the β-oxidation pathway. Without carnitine, the oxidation of fatty acids, especially the long-chain fatty acids, cannot proceed. Acyl CoA cannot traverse the membrane into the mitochondria and thus requires a translocase for its entry. The translocase requires carnitine. Carnitine is synthesized from lysine and methionine (Figure 11.15). While most of

the fatty acids that enter the β-oxidation pathway are completely oxidized via the citric acid cycle and respiratory chain to $CO_2$ and HOH, some of the acetyl CoA is converted to the ketones, acetoacetate, and β-hydroxybutyrate. The condensation of two molecules of acetyl CoA to acetoacetyl CoA occurs in the mitochondria via the enzyme β-ketothiolase. Acetoacetyl CoA then condenses with another acetyl CoA to form HMG CoA. At last, the HMG CoA is cleaved into acetoacetic acid and acetyl CoA. The acetoacetic acid is reduced to β-hydroxybutyrate, and this reduction is dependent on the ratio of $NAD^+$ to $NADH^+H^+$. The enzyme for this reduction, β-hydroxybutyrate dehydrogenase, is tightly bound to the inner aspect of the mitochondrial membrane. Because of its high activity, the product (β-hydroxybutyrate) and substrate (acetoacetate) are in equilibrium.

HMG CoA is also synthesized in the cytosol, where it serves as a starting point for the synthesis of cholesterol (Figure 11.16). The ketones can ultimately be used as fuel but may appear in the blood, liver, and other tissues at a level of less than 0.2 mM. In starving individuals or in people consuming a high-fat diet, blood and tissue ketone levels may rise above normal (3–5 mM). However, unless these levels greatly exceed the body's capacity to use them as fuel (as is the case in uncontrolled diabetes mellitus with levels up to 20 mM), a rise in ketone levels is not a cause for concern. Ketones are choice metabolic fuels for muscle and brain. Although both tissues may prefer to use glucose, the ketones can be used when glucose is in short supply. Ketones are used to spare glucose wherever possible under these conditions.

The oxidation of unsaturated fatty acids follows the same pathway as the saturated fatty acids until the double-bonded carbons are reached (Figure 11.17). At this point, a few side steps must be taken that involve a few additional enzymes. Linoleate has two double bonds in the *cis* configuration. β-Oxidation removes three acetyl units, leaving a CoA attached to the terminal carbon just before the first *cis* double bond. At this point an isomerase enzyme, Δ3 *cis* Δ6 *trans* enoyl CoA isomerase, acts to convert the first *cis* bond to a *trans* bond. Now, this part of the molecule can once again enter the β-oxidation sequence and two more acetyl CoA units are released. The second double bond is then opened and a hydroxyl group is inserted. In turn, this hydroxyl group is rotated to the L position, and the remaining product can then reenter the β-oxidation pathway. Other unsaturated fatty acids can be similarly oxidized. Each time the double bond is approached, the isomerization and hydroxyl group addition takes place until all of the fatty acid is oxidized.

While β-oxidation is the main pathway for the oxidation of fatty acids, some fatty acids undergo α oxidation so as to provide the substrates for the synthesis of sphingolipids. These reactions occur in the endoplasmic reticulum and mitochondria and involve the mixed function oxidases because they require molecular oxygen, reduced NAD, and specific cytochromes. The fatty acid oxidation that occurs in organelles other than the mitochondria is an energy-wasteful reaction because these other organelles do not have the citric acid cycle nor do they have the respiratory chain, which takes

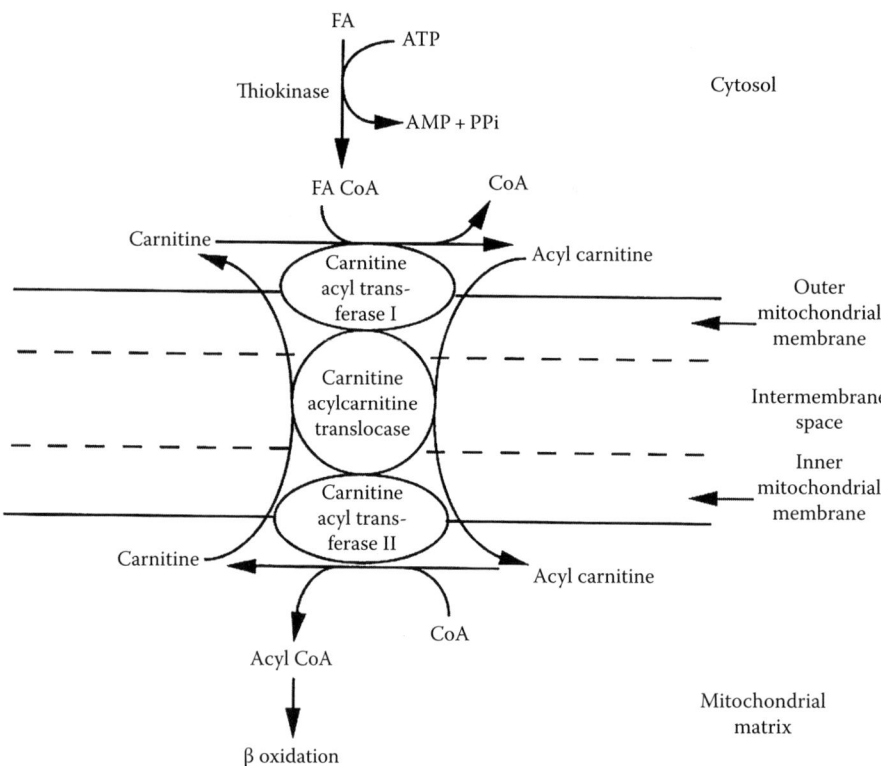

**FIGURE 11.14** Mechanism for the entry of fatty acids into the mitochondrial compartment fatty acid is activated, it is bound to carnitine with the release of CoA. The acylcarnitine is then translocated through the mitochondrial membranes into the mitochondrial matrix via the carnitine acylcarnitine translocase. As one molecule of acylcarnitine is passed into the matrix, one molecule of carnitine is translocated back to the cytosol and the acylcarnitine is converted back to acyl CoA. The acyl CoA can then enter the β-oxidation pathway shown in Figure 11.13.

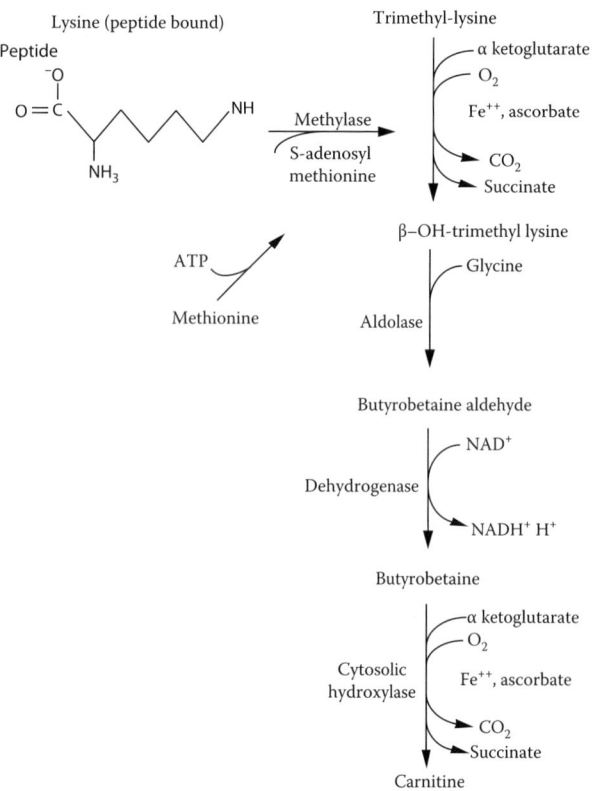

**FIGURE 11.15** Synthesis of carnitine from lysine and methionine.

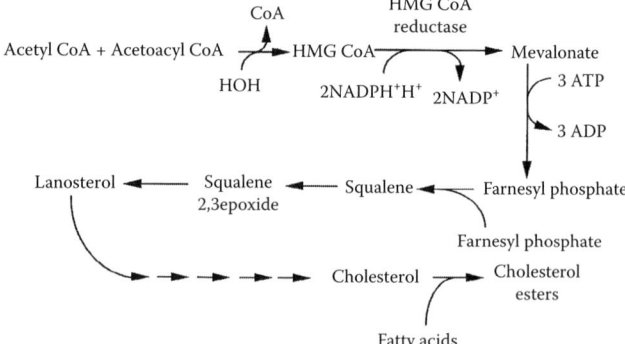

**FIGURE 11.16** Cholesterol biosynthesis.

the reducing equivalents released by the oxidative steps and combines them with oxygen to make water-releasing energy that is then trapped in the high-energy bonds of the ATP.

Peroxisomal oxidation in the kidney and liver is an important aspect of drug metabolism. The peroxisomes are a class of subcellular organelles that are important in the protection against oxygen toxicity. They have a high level of catalase activity, which suggests their importance in the antioxidant system. The peroxisomal fatty acid oxidation pathway differs in three important ways from the mitochondrial pathway. First, the initial dehydrogenation is accomplished by a cyanide-insensitive oxidase that

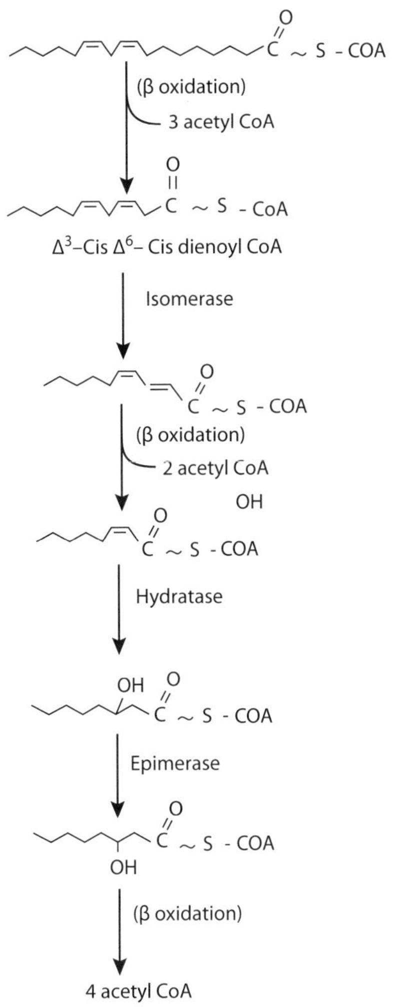

**FIGURE 11.17** Modification of β-oxidation for unsaturated fatty acid.

produces $H_2O_2$. This $H_2O_2$ is rapidly extinguished by catalase. Second, the enzymes of the pathway prefer long-chain fatty acids and are slightly different in structure from those (with the same function) of the mitochondrial pathway. Third, β-oxidation in the peroxisomes stops at eight carbons rather than proceeding all the way to acetyl CoA. The peroxisomes also serve in the conversion of cholesterol to bile acids and in the formation of ether lipids (plasmalogens).

## Fatty Acid Synthesis

Fatty acid synthesis occurs in the cytosol of the living cell using two-carbon units (acetyl units) that are the result of glucose oxidation or amino acid degradation (Figure 11.18). Fatty acid synthesis begins with acetyl CoA. Acetyl CoA arises from the oxidation of glucose or the carbon skeletons of deaminated amino acids. Acetyl CoA is converted to malonyl CoA with the addition of one carbon (from bicarbonate) in the presence of the enzyme acetyl CoA carboxylase. The reaction uses the energy from one molecule of ATP and biotin as a coenzyme. This reaction is the first committed step in the reaction sequence that results in the synthesis of a

fatty acid. The activated $CO_2$ attached to the biotin–enzyme complex is transferred to the methyl end of the substrate. Although most fatty acids synthesized in mammalian cells have an even number of carbons, this first committed step yields a three-carbon product. This results in an asymmetric molecule that becomes vulnerable to attack (addition) at the center of the molecule with the subsequent loss of the terminal carbon. The vulnerability is conferred by the fact that both the carboxyl group at one end and the group at the other end are both powerful attractants of electrons from the hydrogen of the middle carbon. This leaves the carbon in a very reactive state, and a second acetyl group carried by a carrier protein with the help of phosphopantetheine, which has a sulfur group connection, can be joined to it through the action of the enzyme, malonyl transferase. Subsequently, the "extra" carbon is released via the enzyme β-ketoacyl enzyme synthase, leaving a four-carbon chain still connected to a sulfhydryl (SH) group at the carboxyl end. This SH group is the docking end for all the enzymes that comprise the fatty acid synthase complex. These enzymes catalyze the addition of two-carbon acetyl groups in sequence to the methyl end of the carbon chain until the final product palmityl CoA and then palmitic acid is produced. Members of this fatty acid synthase complex include the aforementioned malonyl transferase and β-ketoacyl synthase; β-ketoacyl reductase, which catalyzes the addition of reducing equivalents carried by FMN; and an acyl transferase. Upon completion of these six steps, the process is repeated until the chain length is 16 carbons long. At this point, the SH-acyl carrier protein is removed through the action of the enzyme palmityl-$S$-enzyme deacylase and the palmitic acid is available for esterification to glycerol to form a mono-, di-, or triacylglyceride (see Section "Fatty Acid Esterification").

## Fatty Acid Elongation

Elongation or the lengthening of fatty acids by the addition of two-carbon units (acetyl groups), occurs in either the endoplasmic reticulum or the mitochondria (Figure 11.19). The reaction differs depending on where it occurs. In the endoplasmic reticulum, the reaction sequence is similar to that described for the cytosolic fatty acid synthase complex. The source of the two-carbon unit is malonyl CoA, and $NADPH^+H^+$ provides the reducing power. The intermediates are CoA esters, not the acyl carrier protein (ACP) 4′-phosphopantetheine. The reaction sequence produces stearic acid (18:0) in all tissues that make fatty acids except the brain. In the brain, elongation can proceed further producing fatty acids containing up to 24 carbons. In the mitochondria, elongation uses acetyl CoA rather than malonyl CoA as the source of the two-carbon unit. It uses either $NADH^+H^+$ or $NADPH^+H^+$ as the source of reducing equivalents and uses, as substrate, carbon chains of less than 16 carbons. Mitochondrial elongation is the reversal of fatty acid oxidation, which also occurs in this organelle. Not all species can make all of the fatty acids found in the body tissues. Some of these fatty acids are therefore essential. In mammals the essential fatty acids are linoleic

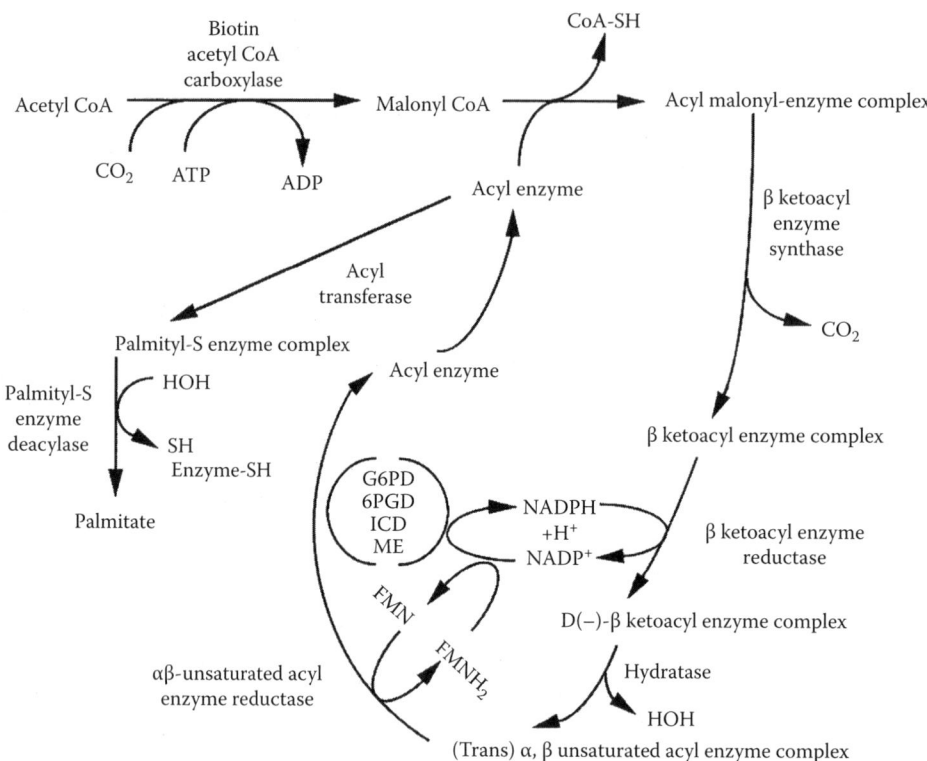

**FIGURE 11.18**  Fatty acid synthesis from acetyl CoA.

and linolenic acids. In felines, the essential fatty acids include these two and arachidonic acid. Table 11.4 gives the structures and names of the important fatty acids.

## FATTY ACID DESATURATION

Desaturation occurs in the endoplasmic reticulum and microsomes (Figure 11.20). The enzymes that catalyze this are the Δ4, Δ5, or Δ6 desaturases. Desaturation is species specific. Mammals, for example, lack the ability to desaturate fatty acids in the n-6 or n-3 position. They cannot make linoleic or linolenic acid, and in addition, felines cannot convert linoleic to arachidonic acid. Only plants can desaturate fatty acids at the n-6 or n-3 position, and even among plants, there are species differences. Cold water plants can desaturate at the n-3 position, while land plants of warmer regions cannot. The cold water plants are consumed by cold water creatures in a food chain that includes fish as well as sea mammals. The fatty acids of these plants then enter the human food supply and become sources of the n-3, or omega-3, fatty acids in the marine oils. In animals desaturation of de novo synthesized fatty acids usually stops with the production of a monounsaturated fatty acid with the double bond in the 9–10 position counting from the carboxyl end of the molecule. Hence, palmitic acid (16:0) becomes palmitoleic acid (16:1), and stearic acid (18:0) becomes oleic acid (18:1). In the absence of dietary EFA, most mammals will desaturate eicosenoic acid to produce eicosatrienoic acid. Increases in this fatty acid with unsaturations at the n-7 and n-9 positions characterize the tissue lipids of EFA-deficient animals. The enzymes are sometimes called mixed function oxidases

because two substrates (fatty acid and NADPH) are oxidized simultaneously. These desaturases prefer substrates with a double bond in the n-6 position but will also act on n-3 fatty acids bonds and on saturated fatty acids. Desaturation of de novo synthesized stearic acid to form oleic acid results in the formation of a double bond at the omega-9 position. This is the first committed step of this desaturation/elongation reaction sequence. Oleic acid can also be formed by the desaturation and elongation of palmitic acid. Fatty acid desaturation can be followed by elongation and repeated such that a variety of mono- and polyunsaturated fatty acids (PUFA) can be formed. The body can convert the dietary saturated fatty acids to unsaturated fatty acids, thus maintaining an optimal P:S ratio in the tissues.

## AUTOXIDATION

Unsaturated fatty acids, particularly the PUFA, are more reactive than saturated fatty acids. The double bonds can be attacked by oxygen radicals in a process called autoxidation. In food, autoxidation occurs and is responsible for the deterioration of food quality. The discoloration of red meat upon exposure to air at room temperature is an indication of the autoxidation process. The off odor that accompanies this discoloration is the result of the autoxidation of the fatty acids in the meat fat. In living systems, the process of autoxidation is suppressed to a large extent. This is essential because the products of this oxidation, fatty acid peroxides, can be very damaging. Peroxides denature proteins, rendering them inactive, and attack the DNA in the nucleus and mitochondria, resulting in base pair deletions

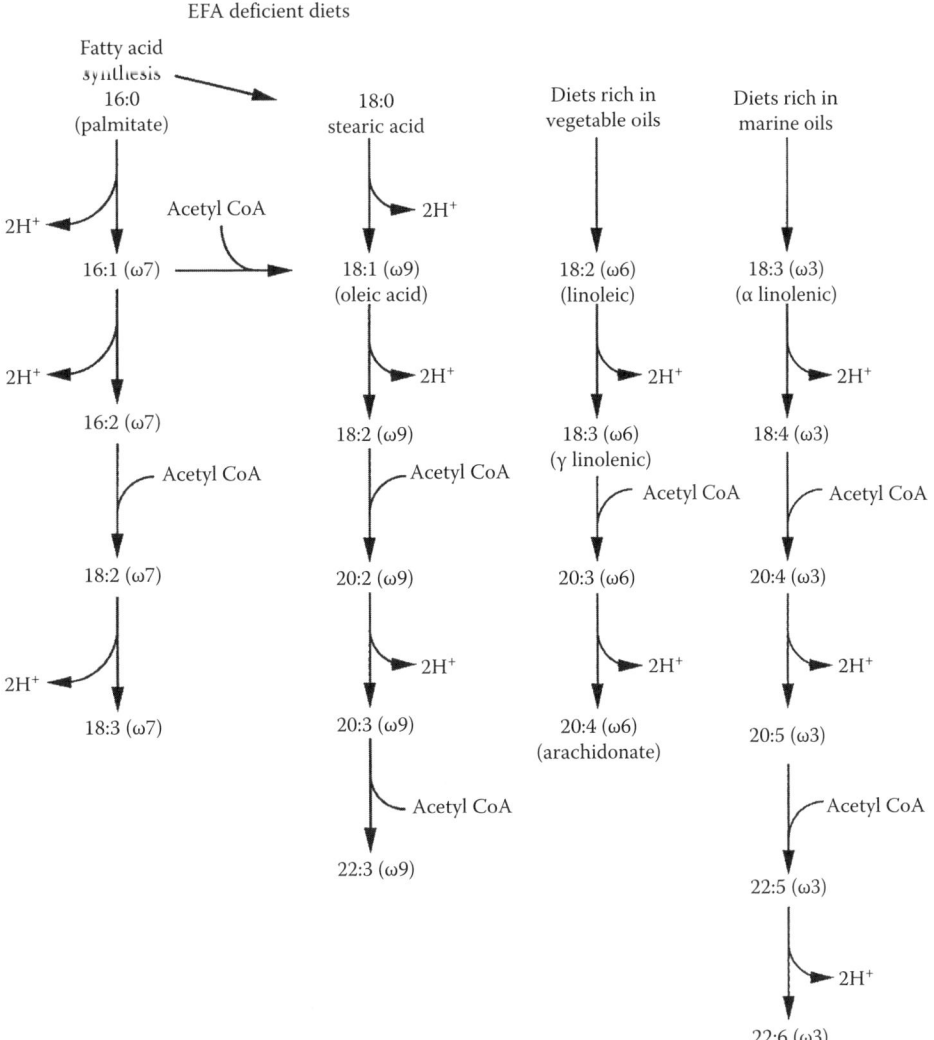

**FIGURE 11.19** Pathways for synthesis of long-chain PUFA through elongation and desaturation. Not all of these reactions occur in all species. Cold water ocean plants and simple cell organisms, for example, can synthesize (through desaturation and elongation) long-chain PUFA. These become part of the food chain and end up in the lipid components of marine fish and mammals consumed by humans. The ω symbol is the same as the n symbol. Thus, 18:2ω6, linoleic acid, could also be written 18:2n6.

**TABLE 11.4**

**Free Radical Suppression Enzymes Found in Mammalian Cells**

| Enzyme | Required Mineral Cofactors | Reaction Catalyzed |
|---|---|---|
| SOD | Cu, Zn, Mn | $2O \ 2O_2^- + 2H^+ \rightarrow + H_2O_2$ |
| Glutathione peroxidase | Se | $H_2O_2 + 2GSH \rightarrow GSSG + 2H_2O$ |
| | | $ROOH + 2GSH \rightarrow GSSG + ROH + H_2O$ |
| Catalase | Fe | $2H_2O_2 \rightarrow 2H_2O + O_2$ |
| Glutathione-S-transferases | — | $ROOH + 2GSH \rightarrow GSSG + ROH + H_2O$ |

or breaks in the DNA, which, in turn, result in mutations or errors. In the nucleus, these breaks or deletions can be repaired. In the aging animal, the repair mechanism loses its efficiency, and one of the characteristics of aged cells is the loss of its DNA repair ability. To prevent widespread damage to cellular proteins and DNA by these radicals, there is a potent antioxidation system. This antioxidation system includes the selenium-containing enzyme, glutathione peroxidase, catalase, and superoxide dismutase (SOD). These enzymes are found in the peroxisomes. SOD is also found in the mitochondria. All of these components serve to suppress free radical formation.

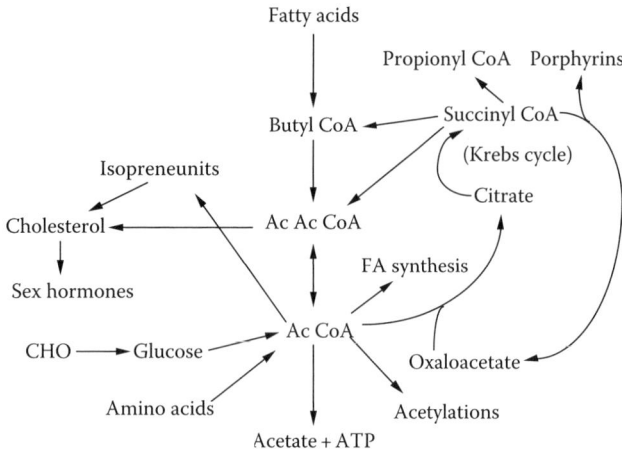

**FIGURE 11.20**  Integration of cholesterol and fatty acid synthesis.

The free radical chain reaction occurs when the oxygen atom is excited by a variety of drugs and contaminants or by ultraviolet light. The excited oxygen atom is called singlet oxygen $(O_2^-)$. Pollutants such as the oxides of nitrogen or carbon tetrachloride can provoke this reaction. In vivo, the detoxification reactions catalyzed by the cytochrome P450 enzymes generate free radicals. In the respiratory chain of the mitochondria, the possibility of oxygen radical production exists, and it is for this reason the mitochondria possess a particularly potent peroxide suppressor, SOD. SOD in the mitochondria requires the manganese ion as a cofactor. The cytosol also has SOD, but this enzyme requires the copper and zinc ions. Both forms of the enzyme catalyze the reaction,

$$O_2^- + O_2^- + 2H^+ \rightarrow H_2O_2 + O_2$$

Two superoxides and two hydrogen ions are joined to form one molecule of hydrogen peroxide and a molecule of oxygen. In turn, the peroxide can be converted to water through the action of the enzyme catalase. Peroxides can also be "neutralized" through the action of glutathione-*S*-transferase. This reaction requires two molecules of reduced glutathione and produces two molecules of oxidized glutathione and two molecules of water. Fatty acid radicals can also be neutralized by glutathione peroxidase producing a molecule of an alcohol with the same chain length as the fatty acid. Glutathione-*S*-transferase can duplicate the action of glutathione peroxidase. These enzymes and the reactions they catalyze are listed in Table 11.4. In addition to the reactions that counteract the in vivo formation of oxygen radicals or fatty acid peroxides, certain of the vitamins have this role as well. Ascorbic acid has antioxidant function as it can donate reducing equivalents to a peroxide converting it to an alcohol. β-Carotene can quench singlet oxygen and thus convert it into $O_2$. Vitamin E is perhaps the best known antioxidant vitamin, and its action is similar to that of ascorbic acid. It donates reducing equivalents to a peroxide converting it to an alcohol.

Although the foregoing has emphasized the negative aspects of the partial reduction products of oxygen, there is some evidence that peroxide formation has some benefit.

For example, leukocytes produce peroxides as a means of killing invading bacteria. Other examples, no doubt, will emerge as scientists continue in their efforts to understand the role of peroxidation (and the peroxisomes) in mammalian metabolism.

## CHOLESTEROL SYNTHESIS

The body synthesizes nearly 90% of the cholesterol that is in the circulation. The starting point for cholesterol synthesis is the joining of acetyl CoA to acetoacetyl CoA to form HMGCoA (Figure 11.16). HMGCoA through the action of HMGCoA reductase (the rate-limiting step in this pathway) is converted to mevalonate. Cholesterol-lowering drugs such as the statin drugs, act on this step inhibiting in vivo cholesterol synthesis. Mevalonate is phosphorylated to farnesyl phosphate, which in turn is converted to squalene and then, through a series of reactions, to cholesterol. Cholesterol serves as the beginning substrate for the synthesis of a variety of hormones, active vitamin D, and the bile acids. Cholesterol is also an important component of cellular membranes.

## EICOSANOID SYNTHESIS

Eicosanoids are 20 carbon molecules having hormone-like activity. They are produced in their various forms and released by many different mammalian cells. When each of these compounds is produced, their site of action is local. That is, whereas insulin may be transported from the pancreas to peripheral target cells, the eicosanoids are produced, released, and have as their targets the surrounding cells. For this reason, the eicosanoids are called local hormones. They have a variety of actions. Table 11.5 lists the major eicosanoids and their functions.

The eicosanoids fall into three general groups of compounds: the prostaglandins (compounds of the PG series), the thromboxanes (compounds of the TBX series), and the leukotrienes (compounds of the LKT series). All of these compounds arise from a 20-carbon PUFA (Figure 11.21). This fatty acid is usually arachidonic acid (20 carbons; 4 double bonds at 5, 8, 11, and 14). However, in instances where the diet is rich in n-3 fatty acids, the precursor may be a 20-carbon 5-double-bond fatty acid, eicosapentaenoic acid (double bonds at 5, 8, 11, 14, and 17). Other eicosanoids can be synthesized from a 20-carbon fatty acid, dihomo-γ-linoleic acid, which has only three double bonds at carbons 8, 11, and 14. Each of these precursors yields a particular set of eicosanoids. During their synthesis, they take up oxygen and are cyclized. Dihomo-γ-linoleic acid is the precursor of prostaglandin $E_1$ (PGE₁), prostaglandin $E_{1\alpha}$ (PGE₁ₐ), and subsequent prostaglandins. Arachidonic acid is the precursor of prostaglandins of the 2 series (PGE₂, PGF₂ₐ, etc.), and eicosapentaenoic acid is the precursor of prostaglandins of the 3 series (PGE₃, PGF₃ₐ, etc.).

The cyclization of these 20-carbon fatty acids is accomplished by a complex of enzymes called the prostaglandin synthesis complex. The first step is the cyclooxygenase step,

**TABLE 11.5**
**Functions of Eicosanoids**

| Eicosanoid | Function |
|---|---|
| $PGG_2$ | Precursor of $PGH_2$ |
| $PGH_2$ | Precursor of $PGD_2$, $PGE_2$, $PGI_2$, $PGF_{2a}$ |
| $PGD_2$ | Promotes sleeping behavior |
| | Precursor of $PGF_2$ |
| $PGE_2$ | Enhances perception of pain when histamine or bradykinin is given |
| | Induces signs of inflammation |
| | Promotes wakefulness |
| | Precursor of $PGF_{2a}$ |
| | Reduces gastric acid secretion, induces parturition |
| | Vasoconstrictor in some tissues |
| | Vasodilator in other tissues |
| | Maintains the patency of the ductus arteriosus prior to birth |
| $PGF_{2a}$ | Bronchial constrictor |
| | Vasoconstrictor especially in coronary vasculature |
| | Increases sperm motility |
| | Induces parturition, stimulates steroidogenesis corpus luteum, induces luteolysis |
| $PGI_2$ | Inhibits platelet aggregation |
| $PGE_1$ | Inhibits motility of nonpregnant uterus increases motility of pregnant uterus |
| | Bronchial dilator |
| $TXA_2$ | Stimulates platelet aggregation |
| | Potent vasoconstrictor |
| $TXB_2$ | Metabolite of $TXA_2$ |
| $LTA_4$ | Precursor of $LTB_4$ |
| $LTB_4$ | Potent chemotaxic agent |

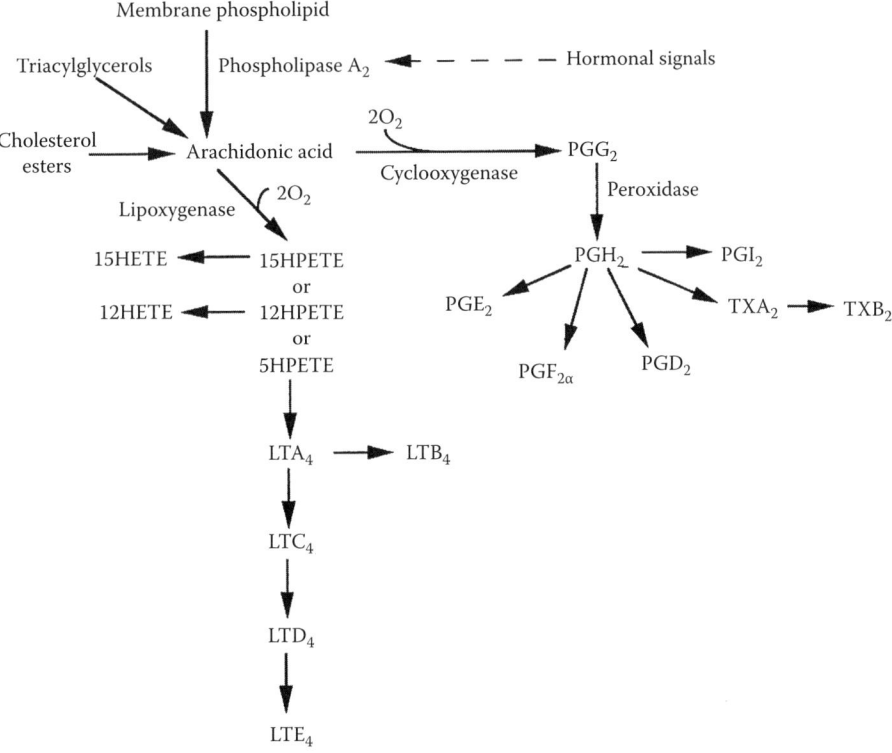

**FIGURE 11.21** Overall pathway for the synthesis of the major eicosanoids.

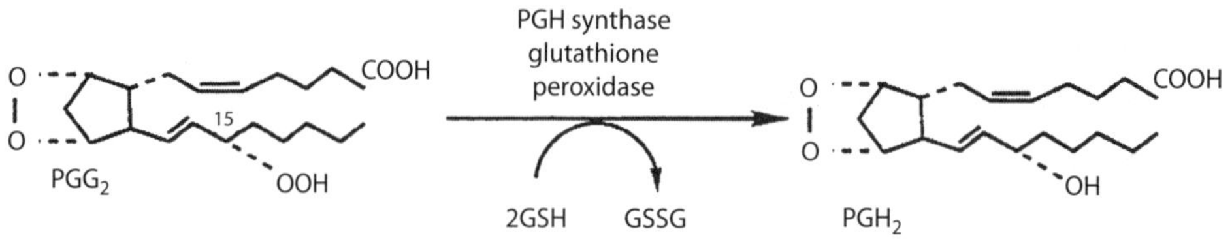

**FIGURE 11.22**  Formation of PGH$_2$.

which involves the cyclization of C-9–C-12 of the precursor to the cyclic form 9,11-endoperoxide 15-hydroperoxide (PGG$_2$). PGG$_2$ is then used to form prostaglandin H$_2$ (PGH$_2$) through the removal of one oxygen from the carbonyl group at carbon 15. Glutathione peroxidase and prostaglandin H synthase catalyze the reaction shown in Figure 11.22. Prostaglandin H synthase is a very unstable short-lived enzyme with a messenger RNA that is one of the shortest-lived species so far found in mammalian cells. The expression of genes for this enzyme is under the control of polypeptide growth factors such as interleukin-1α and colony-stimulating factor-1. Interferon-α and interferon-β inhibit expression and prostanoid production by the macrophages. Glutathione peroxidase is a selenium-containing enzyme. PGH$_2$ is then converted through the action of a variety of isomerases to PGD$_2$, PGE$_2$, prostacylin I$_2$ (PGI$_2$), or prostaglandin F$_{2\alpha}$ (PGF$_{2\alpha}$). These are the primary precursors of the prostaglandins of the D, E, and F series and PGI or thromboxane. The conversion to subsequent prostaglandins is mediated by enzymes that are specific to a certain cell type and tissue. Not all of these subsequent compounds are formed in all tissues. Thus, PGE$_2$ and PGF$_{2\alpha}$ are produced in the kidney and spleen. PGF$_{2\alpha}$ and PGE are also produced in the uterus only when signals from the pituitary induce their production and so stimulate parturition. PGI$_2$ is primarily produced by endothelial cells lining the blood vessels. This prostaglandin inhibits platelet aggregation and thus is important to maintaining a blood flow free of clots. It is counteracted by thromboxane A$_2$, which is produced by the platelets when these cells contact a foreign surface. PGE$_2$, PGF$_{2\alpha}$, and PGI$_2$ are formed by the heart in about equal amounts. All of these prostaglandins have very short half-lives. No sooner are they released than they are inactivated. The thromboxanes are highly active metabolites of the prostaglandins. As mentioned earlier, they are formed when PGH$_2$ has its cyclopentane ring replaced by a six-membered oxane ring shown in Figure 11.23.

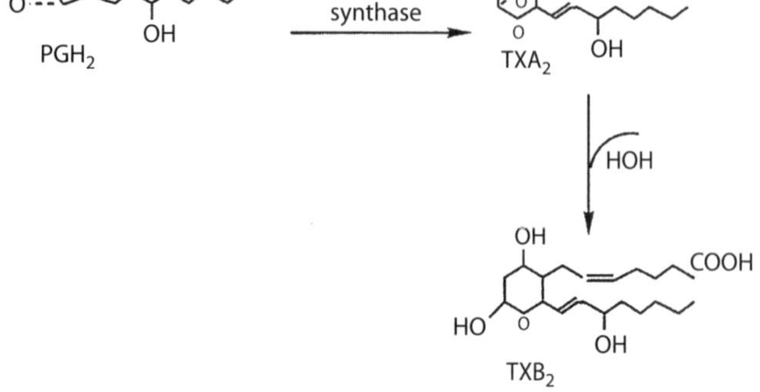

**FIGURE 11.23**  Reaction sequence that produces TXA$_2$ and TXB$_2$.

Imidazole is a potent inhibitor of thromboxane A synthase and is used to block TXA$_2$ production and platelet aggregation.

Thromboxane A$_2$ has a role in clot formation, and the name thromboxane comes from this function (thrombus means clot). The half-life of TXA$_2$ is less than 1 min. TXB$_2$ is its metabolic end product and has little biological activity. Measuring TXB$_2$ levels in blood and tissue can give an indication of how much TXA$_2$ had been produced. PGD$_2$ and PGE$_2$ are involved in the regulation of sleep–wake cycles in a variety of species.

Although the cyclooxygenase pathway is quite important in the production of prostaglandins, equally important is the lipoxygenase pathway. This pathway is catalyzed by a family of enzymes called the lipoxygenase enzymes. These enzymes differ from the cyclooxygenase enzymes in its catalytic site for oxygen addition to the unsaturated fatty acid. One lipoxygenase is active at the double bond at carbon 5, while a second is active at carbon 11, and a third is active at carbon 15. The products of these reactions are monohydroperoxy-eicosatetraenoic acids (HPETEs) and are numbered according to the location of the double bond to which the oxygen is added. 5HPETE is the major lipoxygenase product in basophils, polymorphonuclear leukocytes, macrophages, mast cells, and any organ undergoing an inflammatory response. 12HPETE is the major product in platelets, pancreatic endocrine cells, vascular smooth muscle, and glomerular cells. 15HPETE predominates in reticulocytes, eosinophils, T-lymphocytes, and tracheal epithelial cells. The HPETEs are not in themselves active hormones; rather, they serve as precursors for the leukotrienes. The leukotrienes are the metabolic end products of the lipoxygenase reaction. These compounds contain at least three conjugated double bonds. The unstable 5HPETE is converted to either an analogous alcohol (hydroxy fatty acid) or is reduced by a peroxide or converted to leukotriene. The peroxidative reduction of 5-HPETE to the stable 5-HETE (5-hydroxyeicosatetraenoic acid) is similar to that of 12-HPETE to 12-HETE and of 15-HPETE to 15-HETE. In each instance, the carbon–carbon double bonds are unconjugated, and the geometry of the double bonds is *trans* and *cis*, respectively. In contrast to the active thromboxanes, which have very short half-lives, the leukotrienes can persist as long as 4 h. These compounds comprise a group of substances known as the slow-acting anaphylaxis substances. They cause slowly evolving but protracted contractions of smooth muscles in the airways and gastrointestinal tract. Leukotriene C$_4$ is rapidly converted to LTD$_4$, which in turn is slowly converted to LTE$_4$. Enzymes in the plasma are responsible for these conversions.

The products of the lipoxygenase pathway are potent mediators of the response to allergens, tissue damage (inflammation), hormone secretion, cell movement, cell growth, and calcium flux. Within minutes of stimulation, lipoxygenase products are produced. In an allergy attack, for example, an allergen can instigate the release of leukotrienes, which are the immediate mediators of response. The leukotrienes are more potent than histamine in stimulating the contraction of the bronchial nonvascular smooth muscles. In addition, $LTD_4$ increases the permeability of the microvasculature. The mono-HETEs and $LTB_4$ stimulate the movement of eosinophils and neutrophils, making them the first line of defense in injury resulting in inflammation.

As mentioned, when dihomo-γ-linoleic acid or eicosapentaenoic acid serves as the substrate for eicosanoid production, the products are either of the 1 series or 3 series. The products they form may be less active than those formed from arachidonic acid and this decrease in activity can be of therapeutic value. Hence, ingestion of n-3 fatty acids leads to the decreased production of prostaglandin $E_2$ and its metabolites, a decrease in the production of thromboxane $A_2$, a potent platelet aggregator and vasoconstrictor, and a decrease in leukotriene $B_4$, a potent inflammatory hormone and a powerful inducer of leukocyte hemotaxis and adherence. Counteracting these decreases are an increase in thromboxane $A_3$ ($TXA_3$), a weak platelet aggregator and vasoconstrictor; an increase in the production of $PGI_3$ without an increase in $PGI_2$, which stimulates vasodilation and inhibits platelet aggregation; and an increase in leukotriene $B_5$, which is a weak inducer of inflammation and a weak chemotoxic agent.

## PROTEIN METABOLISM

The protein in the diet provides the essential and nonessential amino acids that are used to synthesize body proteins. Dietary amino acids fall into two categories: essential and nonessential (Table 11.6). There are species differences in the

### TABLE 11.6
### Essential and Nonessential Amino Acids

| Essential | Nonessential |
|---|---|
| Valine | Hydroxyproline |
| Leucine | Cysteine |
| Isoleucine | Glycine |
| Threonine | Alanine |
| Phenylalanine | Serine |
| Methionine | Proline |
| Tryptophan | Glutamic acid |
| Lysine | Aspartic acid |
| Histidine | Glutamine |
| Arginine[a] | Asparagine |
| | Hydroxylysine |
| | Tyrosine |

[a] Not essential for maintenance of most adult mammals.

amino acids that are considered essential. An essential amino acid is one that the body cannot synthesize in sufficient quantities to meet the body's need for that amino acid. Sometimes the physiological state of the animal determines essentiality. Persons with renal disease, for example, have a greater need for arginine than healthy people. People who have been severely burned may need more essential amino acids than healthy people. Felines require taurine in their diets, while other animals do not. Good food proteins are those proteins that provide sufficient quantities of essential amino acids. Poor-quality proteins might have one or two of these essential amino acids in short supply. With careful blending of poor-quality proteins, a good array of amino acids is possible. These proteins must be consumed at or nearly at the same time in order to allow for optimal use.

### PROTEIN DENATURATION

One of the most striking characteristics of proteins is the response to heat, alcohol, and other treatments that affect their quaternary, tertiary, and secondary structures. This characteristic response is called denaturation. Denaturation results in the unfolding of a protein molecule, thus breaking its hydrogen bonds and the associations between functional groups; as a result, the 3D structure is lost. Denaturation affects many of the properties of the protein molecule. Its physical shape is changed, its solubility in water is decreased, and its reactivity with other proteins may be lost. When denatured, the protein loses its biological activity. Heating will denature most proteins. As low a temperature as 15°C can denature some proteins, while the majority of food proteins are denatured at temperatures in excess of 60°C. Some proteins are very heat stable (those found in thermophilic bacteria, for example), while others are quite labile. Heat denaturation, unless extreme, does not affect the amino acid composition of protein and, indeed, may make these amino acids more available to the body because heating provokes the unfolding or uncoiling of the protein and exposes more of the amino acid chain to the action of the proteolytic digestive enzymes. If only mild denaturation occurs, it can be reversed. This process is called renaturation. If a protein is renatured, it will resume its original shape and biological activity.

### PROTEIN TURNOVER

Protein turnover consists of two processes: synthesis and degradation. In synthesis, amino acids are joined together to form peptides and proteins. Amino acids in the circulation enter a vast array of cell types, and each cell type has many uses for the amino acids brought to it by the circulation. As mentioned, small, medium, and large molecules can be made. The largest of these molecules are the proteins. Protein synthesis is dependent on the simultaneous presence of all the amino acids necessary for the protein being synthesized and on the provision of energy. If there is an insufficient supply of either, protein biosynthesis will not proceed at its normal pace. Chemically, the polymerization of amino acids into

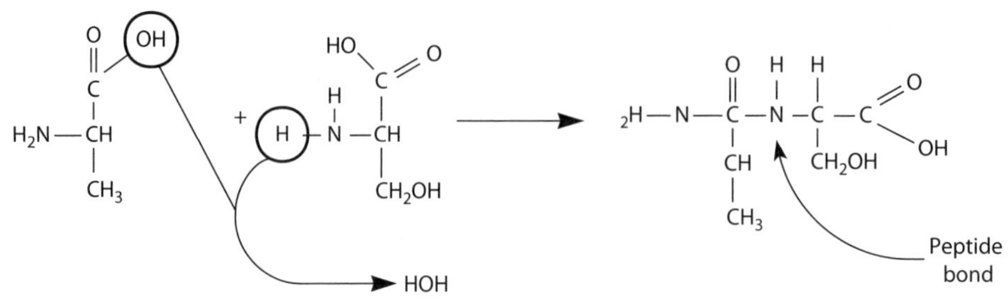

**FIGURE 11.24** Formation of the peptide bond. Example: L-alanine + L-Serine → Alanyl-serine (a dipeptide).

protein is a dehydration reaction between two amino acids that are joined together by a peptide bond.

The peptide bond is the most common amide bond and is formed when two amino acids are joined together as illustrated in Figure 11.24. The two amino acids when joined together form a dipeptide, three form a tripeptide, and so on. Each amino acid in a chain is referred to as an amino acid residue. A chain of up to 100 amino acids joined together is called a polypeptide. If many more amino acids are involved, then the compound is called a protein. Proteins have been identified that have as many as 300,000 amino acids residues and molecular weights in excess of $4 \times 10^7$.

The amino acid sequence of a given peptide or protein can vary, and its variation is controlled genetically. Proteins are complex molecules having characteristic primary, secondary, tertiary, and quaternary structures. The primary structure is determined genetically as the particular sequence of amino acids in a given protein. Protein conformation is usually divided into two categories: secondary and tertiary. The secondary and tertiary structures of a protein result from interactions between the reactive groups on the amino acids in the protein.

The process whereby proteins are synthesized provides the basis for understanding genetic differences. It is also the basis for understanding how the unique properties of each cell type are conferred by the proteins within them. Some of these proteins are the structural elements of the cell. Others are enzymes that catalyze specific reactions and processes that characterize the cell in question. Still other proteins confer a particular biochemical function on the cell. The amino acid sequence of a particular protein is genetically controlled. This control is exerted through the polynucleotide, deoxyribonucleic acid (DNA). DNA is found in both the nucleus and the mitochondria.

The proteins synthesized by the body have a finite existence. They are subject to a variety of insults and modifications. Some of these modifications have already been described: A prohormone is converted to an active hormone, an enzyme is activated or inactivated with the addition or removal of a substituent, and so forth. Thus, a dynamic state within the body exists with respect to its full complement of peptides and proteins. Some proteins have very short lifetimes and very rapid turnover times; other proteins are quite stable and long lived. Their turnover time is quite long. The estimate of the life of a protein, that is, how long it will exist in the body, is its half-life. A half-life is that time interval that occurs when half of

the amount of a compound synthesized at time X will have been degraded. Given the dynamic state of metabolism, some of these time estimates will be very short. Half-lives of biologically active compounds are very difficult to estimate.

## AMINO ACID CATABOLISM

Protein degradation results in amino acids that are usually recycled. There are some exceptions to this general rule; histidine in the muscle protein is methylated and excreted as 3-methyl histidine. This 3-methyl histidine cannot be reused and thus is an indication of muscle breakdown. Most of the products of protein degradation (the liberated amino acids) join the body amino acid pool from which the synthetic processes withdraw their needed supply. It is estimated that 75%–80% of the liberated amino acids are reused.

Different proteins are degraded at different rates, and these rates are determined not only by the physiological status of the individual but also by the amino acid composition of the protein in question. High rates of degradation of the structural proteins mean that considerable structural rearrangement is occurring. Short-lived proteins such as enzymes or receptors have in common regions that are rich in proline, glutamate, serine, and threonine. These amino acids, when clustered, provide a target for rapid degradation.

The process of degradation first reduces the protein to peptides and then reduces these peptides to their constituent amino acids. Two major pathways are used for this process. Extracellular, membrane, and long-lived intracellular proteins are degraded in the lysosomes by an ATP-independent pathway. Short-lived proteins as well as abnormal proteins are degraded in the cytosol using ATP and ubiquitin. Proteins that are degraded via the ubiquitin-dependent pathway are derivatized by several molecules of ubiquitin. The ubiquitin is attached by nonpeptide bonds between the carboxy terminus of ubiquitin and the δ-amino groups of lysyl residues in the protein. This requires ATP.

Although the proteases of digestion are important to the degradation of dietary protein, they have no role in the intracellular protein degradation. Intracellular proteases hydrolyze internal peptide bonds. This is followed by the action of carboxy- and aminopeptidases, which remove single amino acids from the carboxy end or the amino end of the peptides.

Proteins in the extracellular environment are brought into the cell by endocytosis. This is a process similar to pinocytosis, where the cell membrane engulfs and encapsulates the extracellular material. Endocytosis occurs at indentations in the plasma membrane that are internally coated with a protein called clathrin. As in pinocytosis, the extracellular protein is surrounded by the plasma membrane to form an intracellular vesicle, which, in turn, fuses with a lysosome. Degradation then occurs via calcium-dependent proteases called calpains or cathepsin. Both the Golgi and the endoplasmic reticulum are involved in providing proteases that degrade peptide fragments that arise during the maturation of proteins in the secretory pathway.

The rate of degradation varies from protein to protein, and this rate is determined by the amino acid at the amino end of the protein amino acid chain. Proteins with short half-lives have regions rich in proline, glutamate, serine, and threonine. Proteins without these regions are degraded slowly and therefore have slower turnover times and longer half-lives.

Those amino acids in the body's amino acid pool that are not used for peptide or protein synthesis and that are not used to synthesize metabolically important intermediates are deaminated, and the carbon skeletons are either oxidized or used for the synthesis of glucose or fatty acids. There are three general reactions for the removal of $NH_3$ from the amino acids: (1) transamination with the amino group transferred to another carbon chain via amino transaminases, (2) oxidative deamination to yield $NH_3$, or (3) deamination through the activity of an amino acid oxidase.

The amino acids can be loosely grouped in terms of their catabolism. Valine, leucine, and isoleucine, the branched-chain amino acids, are similar in that each has a methyl group on its carbon chain. They can be transaminated with $\alpha$-ketoglutarate to form $\alpha$-keto acids. These acids are considered homologues of pyruvate and are oxidized by a series of enzymes that are similar to those that catalyze the oxidation of $\alpha$-ketoglutarate and pyruvate. The degradative steps are shown in Figure 11.25. Valine ultimately is converted to succinyl CoA, whereas isoleucine ends up as either acetyl CoA or propionyl CoA, and leucine catabolism results in HMG CoA. HMG CoA is split to acetyl CoA and acetoacetate. The HMG CoA produced in the catabolism of leucine is not used for cholesterol synthesis because it is produced in the mitochondria and does not travel to the cytosol, where cholesterol is synthesized. Instead, HMG CoA is further metabolized to acetoacetate and acetyl CoA.

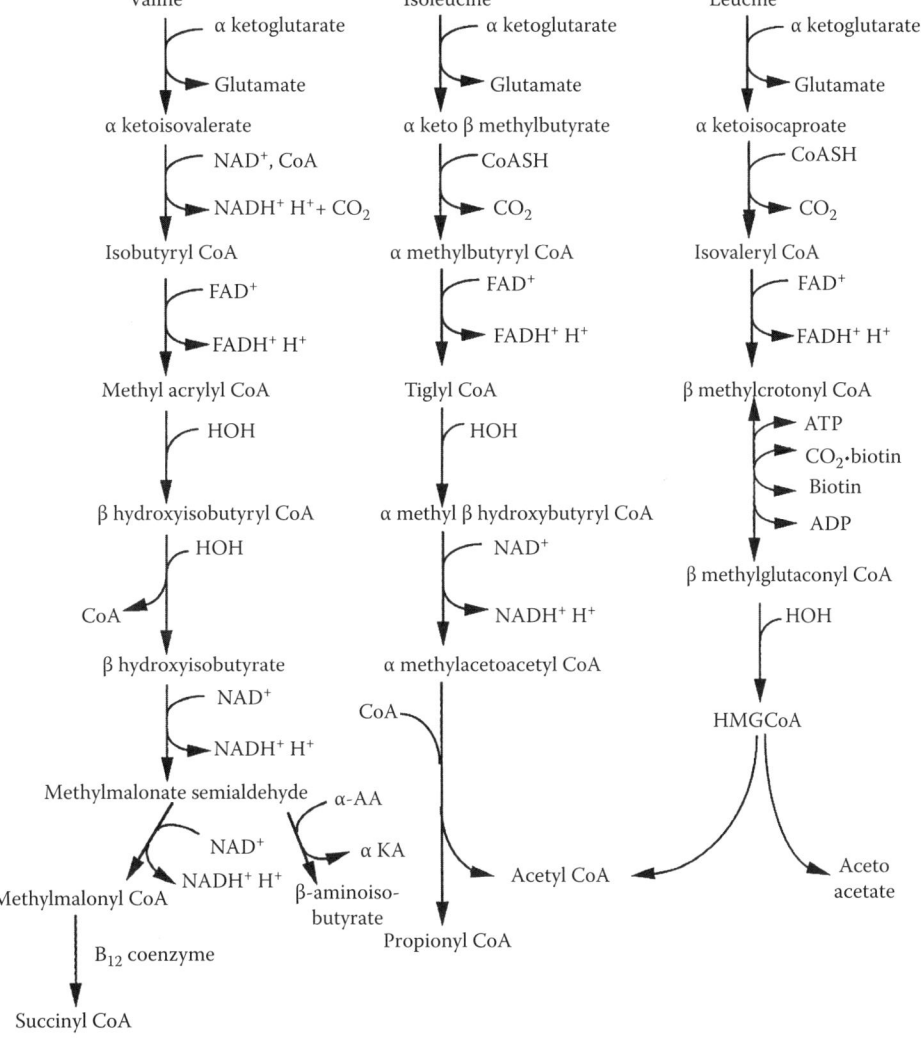

**FIGURE 11.25** Catabolism of branched-chain amino acids showing their use in the production of metabolites that are either lipid precursors or metabolites that can be oxidized via the Krebs cycle.

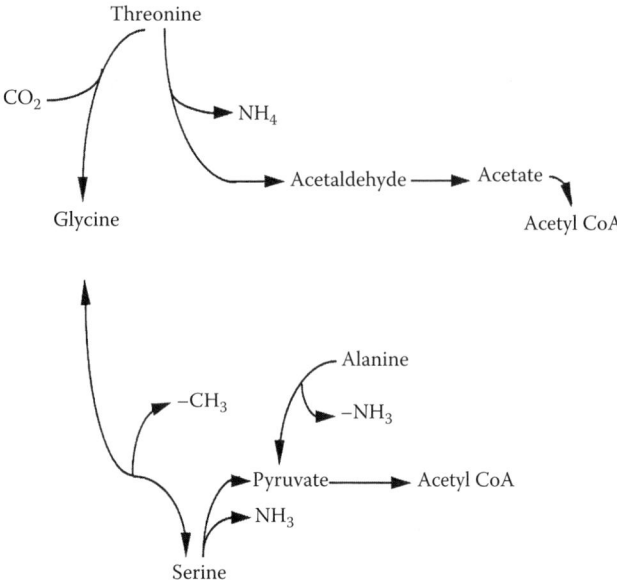

**FIGURE 11.26** Catabolism of threonine showing its relationship to that of serine and glycine.

Serine, threonine, and glycine are hydroxyamino acids. All three are gluconeogenic precursors. Serine can be deaminated to pyruvate, which then can be transaminated to alanine. Serine can also be demethylated to form glycine, releasing a methyl group useful in one-carbon metabolism. Threonine is degraded to acetyl CoA after deamination as shown in Figure 11.26. Glutamate may be converted to glutamine via the enzyme glutamine synthetase. This enzyme is a mitochondrial enzyme and serves to fix the ammonia released in this compartment. Rat renal tissue is particularly rich in this enzyme; however, human renal tissue is not. In birds and alligators, this enzyme is a cytosolic enzyme rather than a mitochondrial enzyme. Although the brain has some urea cycle activity, it uses glutamine formation primarily to reduce its ammonia level. In order to do this, it must also synthesize glutamate from α-ketoglutarate. If it did not also convert pyruvate to oxalacetate, this synthesis of α-ketoglutarate would deplete the brain of citric acid cycle intermediates. Fortunately, carboxylation of pyruvate is very active in brain tissue.

Glutamate is converted to and formed from ornithine and arginine. These two amino acids are essential components of the urea cycle (Figure 11.27). The urea cycle consists of the synthesis of carbamoyl phosphate, citrulline, and then argininosuccinate, arginine, and finally urea. Ornithine and citrulline are shuttled back and forth as the cycle turns to get rid of the excess ammonia via urea release from arginine. The cycle functions to reduce the potentially toxic amounts of ammonia that arise when the ammonia group is removed from amino acids. Most of the ammonia released reflects the coupled action of the transaminases and L-glutamate dehydrogenase. The glutamate dehydrogenase is a bidirectional enzyme that plays a pivotal role in nitrogen metabolism. It is present in kidney, liver, and brain. It uses either $NAD^+$ or $NADP^+$ as a reducing equivalent receiver. It operates close to equilibrium using ATP,

GTP, NADH, and ADP depending on the direction of the reaction. In catabolism, it channels $NH_3$ from glutamate to urea. In anabolism, it channels ammonia to α-ketoglutarate to form glutamate. In the brain, glutamate can be decarboxylated to form γ-aminobutyrate (GABA), an important neurotransmitter. The decarboxylation is catalyzed by the enzyme L-glutamate decarboxylase. Putrescine also can serve as a precursor of GABA either by deamination or via N-acetylated intermediates. The urea cycle is, energetically speaking, a very expensive process. The synthesis of urea requires three molecules of ATP for every molecule of urea formed. The urea cycle is very elastic. That is, its enzymes are highly conserved, readily activated, and readily deactivated. Adaptation to a new level of activity is quickly achieved. While urea cycle activity can be high when protein-rich diets are consumed and low when low-protein diets are consumed, the cycle never shuts down completely. The cycle, shown in Figure 11.27, is fine-tuned by the first reaction, the synthesis of carbamoyl phosphate. This reaction, which occurs in the mitochondria, is catalyzed by the enzyme carbamoyl phosphate synthetase. The enzyme is inactive in the absence of its allosteric activator, N-acetylglutamate, a compound synthesized from acetyl CoA and glutamate in the liver. As arginine levels increase in the liver, N-acetylglutamate synthetase is activated, which results in an increase in N-acetylglutamate. The urea cycle is initiated in the hepatic mitochondria and finished in the cytosol. The urea is then liberated from arginine via arginase and released into the circulation, whereupon it is excreted from the kidneys in the urine. Ornithine, the other product of the arginase reaction, is recycled back to the mitochondrion only to be joined once again to carbamoyl phosphate to make citrulline. Rising levels of arginine turn on mitochondrial N-acetylglutamate synthetase, which provides the N-acetylglutamate, which, in turn, activates carbamoyl phosphate synthetase, and the cycle goes on.

Arginine has many uses in metabolism. Not only is it an essential component of the urea cycle, it is precursor for nitric oxide (NO), the polyamines, proline, glutamate, and creatine. When citrulline is produced from arginine, NO is produced. This occurs not only in the liver but also in other vital organs and the vascular tree. NO production by endothelial cells is a vasodilator and thus plays a role in the regulation of smooth muscle tone. Many vasodilators such as the widely prescribed drug for angina pain, nitroglycerine, work by increasing the production of NO.

Phenylalanine is the precursor of tyrosine, and tyrosine can be used for the synthesis of thyroxine in the thyroid gland or for the synthesis of epinephrine, norepinephrine, or dopamine (see Figure 11.28). Phenylalanine is converted to tyrosine via the hepatic enzyme, phenylalanine hydroxylase. Tyrosine, if not used to make one of several hormones, is then deaminated and, through a series of reactions, ends up as fumarylacetate, which is split to provide acetoacetate and fumarate. Tryptophan catabolism shows no similarity to the catabolic pathways of any of the other amino acids (Figure 11.29). Tryptophan can be converted to niacin, one of the B vitamins. This conversion

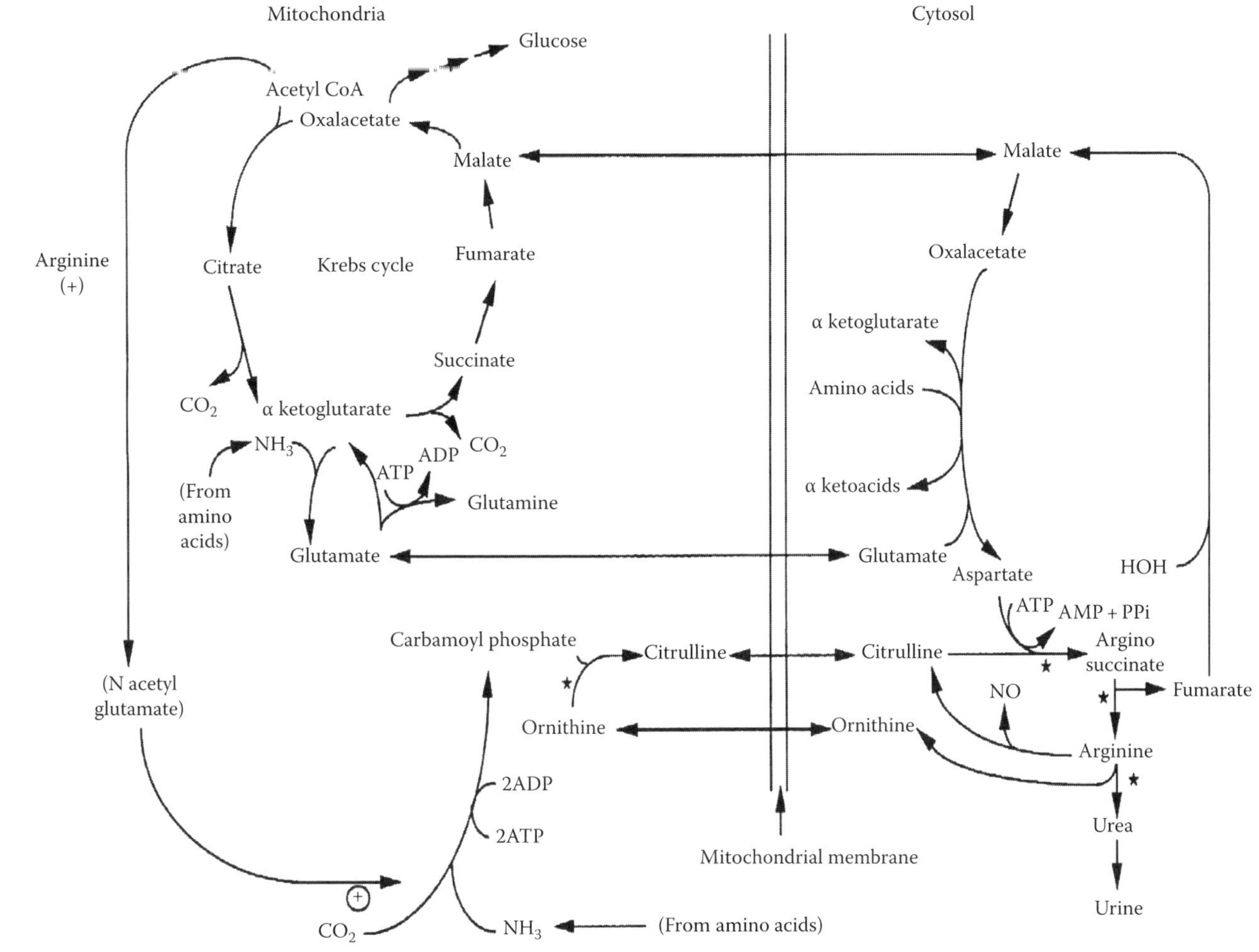

Mitochondria
Cytosol
Glucose
Acetyl CoA
Oxalacetate
Malate
Malate
Arginine
(+)
Citrate
Krebs cycle
Fumarate
Oxalacetate
α ketoglutarate
Succinate
Amino acids
$CO_2$
α ketoglutarate
$NH_3$
ADP
$CO_2$
ATP
(From
amino
acids)
Glutamine
α ketoacids
Glutamate
Glutamate
Aspartate
HOH
ATP
AMP + PPi
Carbamoyl phosphate
Citrulline
Citrulline
Argino
succinate
(N acetyl
glutamate)
NO
Fumarate
Ornithine
Ornithine
Arginine
2ADP
2ATP
Urea
Mitochondrial membrane
Urine
$CO_2$
$NH_3$
(From amino acids)

**FIGURE 11.27** The urea cycle.

DOPA
Dopamine
Norepinephrine
Phenylalanine
Tyrosine
Epinephrine
thyroxine
$NH_3$
Phenylethanolamine
Phenylacetate
Phenylpyruvate
p-hydroxyphenylpyruvate
Phenylacetylglutamine
Homogentisate
Maleylacetoacetate
Fumarylacetoacetate
Acetate
Fumarate
Acetoacetate
Acetyl CoA

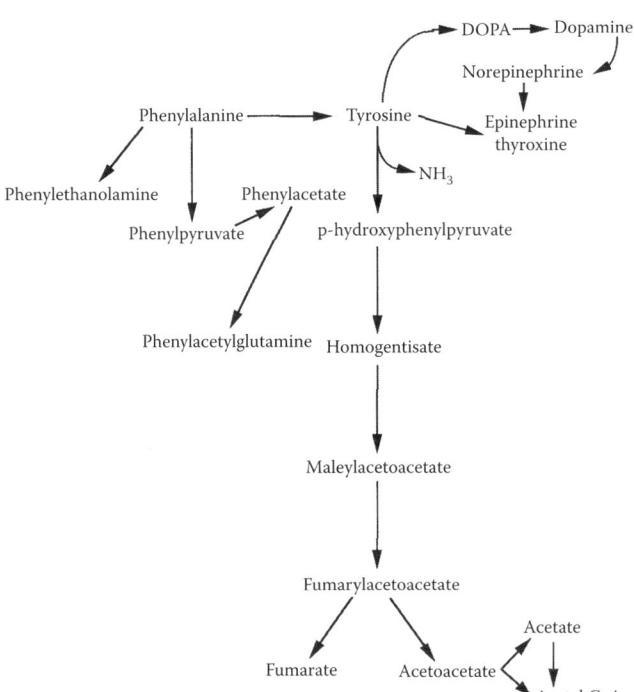

**FIGURE 11.28** Phenylalanine and tyrosine catabolism.

is not very efficient. There is considerable product feedback inhibition of this reaction sequence by niacin. The metabolism of tryptophan is dependent on adequate intakes of vitamin $B_6$, pyridoxine. In pyridoxine deficiency, hydroxyanthranilate formation via the enzyme kynureninase is impaired, resulting in a characteristic increase in urinary levels of xanthurenic acid. This is used as a test of vitamin $B_6$ sufficiency. If subjects are deficient and are given a load dose of tryptophan, these subjects will excrete abnormal amounts of xanthurenate in their urine. Tryptophan is the precursor of serotonin, an important neurotransmitter, that serves a variety of functions in the regulation of smooth muscle tone especially those smooth muscles of the vascular tree. Histidine, an amino acid especially important for muscle protein biosynthesis, is also of great importance in one-carbon metabolism. The principle pathway of histidine catabolism leads to glutamate formation and is shown in Figure 11.30 (as well as in other figures where glutamate and α-ketoglutarate act in transamination). Glutamate is an important component of the urea cycle (Figure 11.27). The decarboxylation of histidine yields histamine. This amine serves to stimulate gastric hydrochloric acid production and to stimulate vasoconstriction. A number of cold remedies and sinus remedies contain substances known as antihistamines, which interfere with the vasoconstrictor action of histamine.

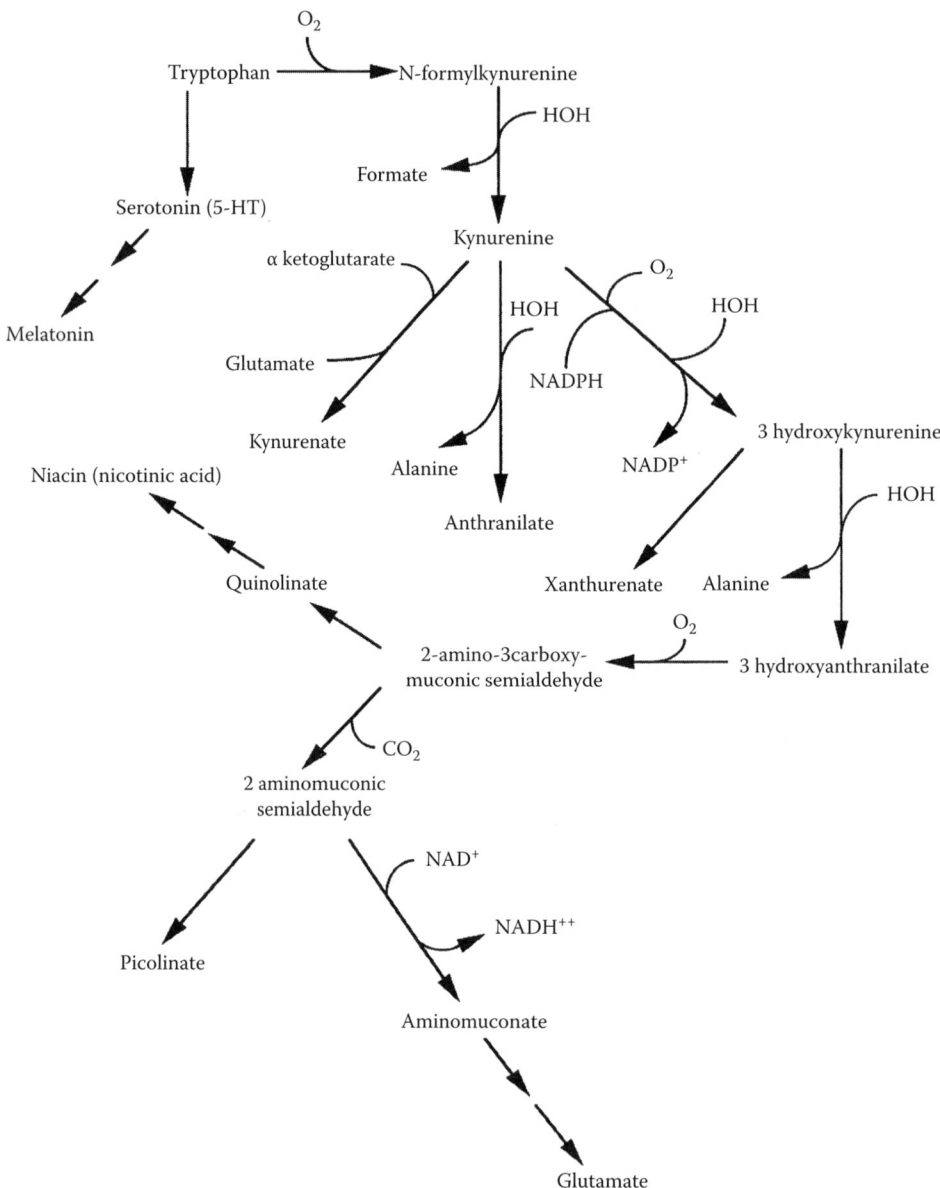

**FIGURE 11.29** Catabolism of tryptophan showing conversion to the vitamin niacin. This conversion is not very efficient. Tryptophan catabolism also results in picolinate, which is believed by some to play a role in trace-mineral conservation.

Histidine in muscle can be methylated and the end product 3-methyl histidine can be measured in the urine and used as a measure of muscle protein turnover.

Lysine is one of the two essential amino acids whose amino group does not contribute to the total body amino group pool; the other is threonine. Although lysine can donate its amino group to other carbon chains, the reverse does not occur. Lysine is catabolized to acetoacetyl CoA, which then enters the Krebs cycle as acetyl CoA.

Methionine, cysteine, and cystine are important sulfur group donors. Sulfur groups are essential to the formation of disulfide bridges, an essential structure for proteins. Methionine is important for carnitine synthesis. The pathway for methionine and cysteine is shown in Figure 11.31. Propionate is also the result of methionine catabolism. Should there be a defect in propionyl CoA carboxylase,

propionate will accumulate. This is not the usual situation, for propionate is usually carboxylated to form succinyl CoA. Accumulations of methyl malonate are characteristic of vitamin $B_{12}$ deficiency. Propionate can serve as the substrate for long-chain odd-numbered fatty acids that are incorporated into myelin, the fatty covering of nerves. For some unknown reason, this myelin is abnormal in its function and fails to protect the peripheral nerve endings, which then die. This may explain the peripheral paresia that characterizes $B_{12}$ deficiency.

## Amino Acid Derivatives

Creatine phosphate is one of the amino acid derivatives that function in muscle contraction by providing energy for this process. Creatine is formed from glycine, arginine, and

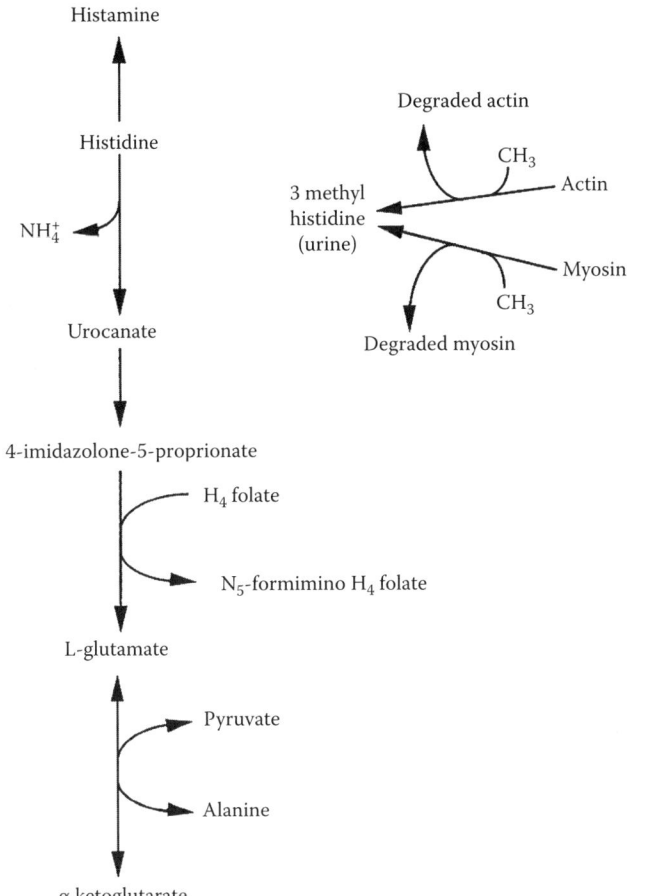

**FIGURE 11.30** Catabolism of histidine. Note that 3-methyl histidine is not part of the pathway. This metabolite is formed in the muscle when the contractile proteins actin and myosin are methylated.

$S$-adenyl methionine in a reaction sequence (Figure 11.32). The creatine circulates in the blood and can be found in measurable quantities in brain and muscle. The creatine is phosphorylated to form creatine phosphate via the enzyme creatine kinase. Creatine is also converted to creatinine by an irreversible nonenzymatic dehydration. Upon hydrolysis, creatine phosphate will provide sufficient energy for muscle contraction. This hydrolysis yields creatine and inorganic phosphate. Some of the creatine is enzymatically rephosphorylated, while the remainder is converted to creatinine that then is excreted in the urine. Creatine phosphate has the same free energy of hydrolysis as ATP. Creatine phosphate is found primarily in the muscle and provides the quick burst of energy needed each time a muscle contracts. Because the muscle activity produces the end product, creatinine, measuring creatinine allows for the estimation of the muscle mass.

Choline is a highly methylated compound synthesized from serine. Choline is an essential component of the neurotransmitter acetylcholine as well as an essential ingredient of the phospholipid, phosphatidylcholine. Certain amino acids can be decarboxylated to form the polyamines. Some polyamines are very-short-lived compounds that are neurotransmitters. They are quickly broken down so as to limit

their effects. The catecholamines fall into this category of polyamines. Other polyamines, putrescine and spermine, bind nucleic acids and other polyanions. They have a role in cell division.

## ROLE OF VITAMINS AND MINERALS IN INTERMEDIARY METABOLISM

Vitamins (Table 11.7) and minerals (Table 11.8) are essential to life. As described earlier, several of the vitamins as well as minerals are needed for the reaction sequences of intermediary metabolism. Niacin, thiamin, riboflavin, pyridoxine, and pantothenic acid (as part of the CoA molecule) all serve as coenzymes in these reactions. Ascorbic acid, vitamin E, and selenium function in the free radical suppression system. Magnesium, manganese, and other divalent ions serve as cofactors in a variety of reactions. Iron and copper function in the cytochromes and hemoglobin, both of which are essential to the use of oxygen. In the former, oxygen is used to make water by the respiratory chain, and in the latter, oxygen is transported to the cells for exchange for carbon dioxide. The synthesis of the purines and pyrimidines, components of DNA and RNA, likewise demands that adequate micronutrients be present for this synthesis.

### SYNTHESIS OF PURINES AND PYRIMIDINES

Before pyrimidines and purines can be incorporated into DNA and RNA, they must be synthesized. This synthesis requires a number of micronutrients as well as sufficient energy to support this synthesis. The purines are adenine and guanine, whereas the pyrimidines are cytosine, uracil, and thymine. Uracil is used for RNA synthesis, whereas thymine is used mainly for DNA synthesis. The purines and pyrimidines form glycosidic bonds to ribose. The purine pathway is shown in Figure 11.33, and the pyrimidine pathway is shown in Figure 11.34. Shown in these figures are the vitamins and minerals needed at each step in the pathway. Where ATP is involved in a reaction step, all of the vitamins that serve as coenzymes in intermediary metabolism are needed. This includes niacin, thiamin, riboflavin, lipoic acid, pantothenic acid, biotin, folacin, vitamin $B_{12}$, pyridoxine, choline, and inositol. Also needed are the minerals of importance to the redox reactions of oxidative phosphorylation (OXPHOS), that is, iron, copper, and, of course, the iodine-containing hormone thyroxine, which regulates OXPHOS and the selenium-containing enzyme (5′-deiodinase), which converts thyroxine to its active form, triiodothyronine.

### MICRONUTRIENTS AS STABILIZERS

Although vitamins and minerals serve in gene expression, certain of the micronutrients have a unique role in assuring that cells and tissues continue to function as intact structures and that these cells continue to reproduce themselves faithfully. This role is that of protection from insult by peroxides. Peroxides are a normal product of metabolism. They are

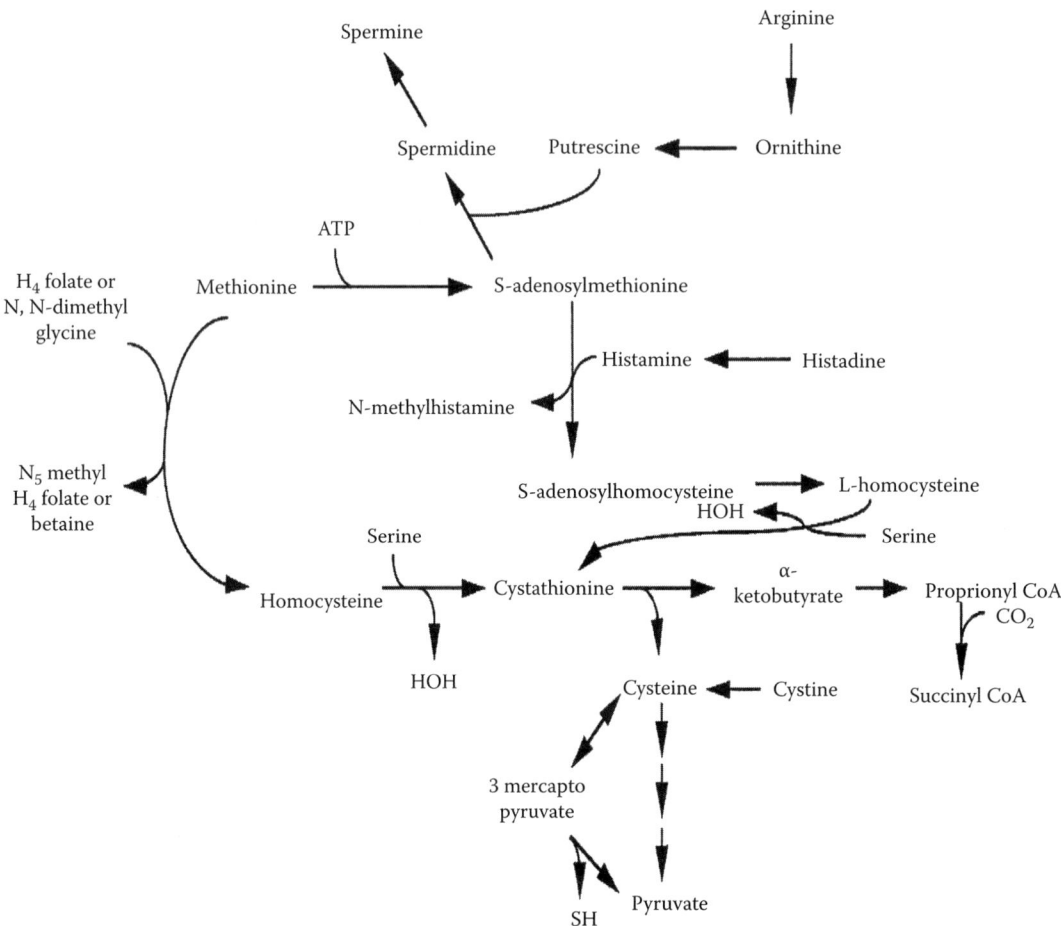

**FIGURE 11.31** Catabolism of methionine and the conservation of SH groups via methionine–cysteine interconversion. Spermine, putrescine, and spermidine are polyamines that are important in cell and tissue growth.

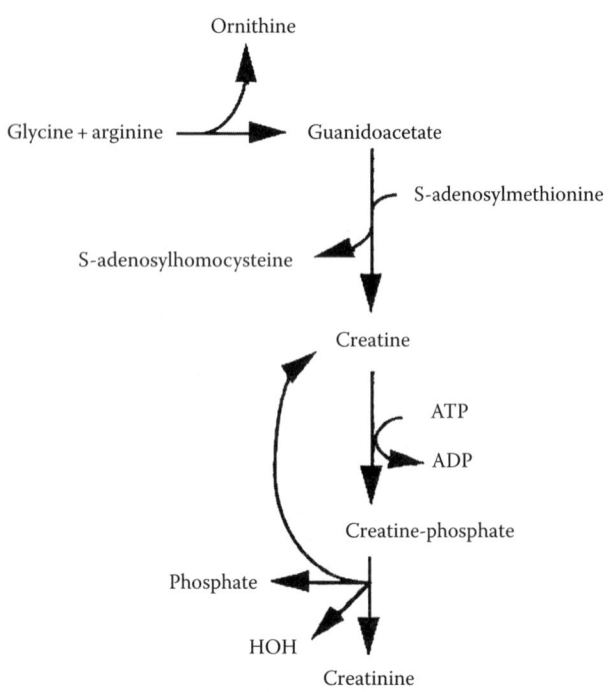

**FIGURE 11.32** Formation of creatine phosphate.

useful agents in the defense against pathogens. However, peroxides are very reactive substances. They can damage the membranes that are the physical barriers to the cells and the organelles within the cell. They can react with DNA. The DNA, enclosed within the nucleus, can repair itself. Occasionally there is a missense repair, and very occasionally this results in a mutation that is random. That is, the damage and subsequent missense repair can occur anywhere in the nuclear DNA, and the resultant gene product could be one of more than a million products encoded by the nuclear genome. Peroxide or free radical damage to the nuclear genome is nowhere as serious on an individual genomic basis as damage to the mitochondrial genome. This genome encodes only 13 products, but these products are important components of the mitochondrial respiratory chain and ATP synthesis. The mitochondrial DNA does not have the repair capacity of the nuclear genome. In fact, its repair capacity is quite limited. When added to the fact that the mitochondria consume about 90% of all the oxygen consumed by the cell, the potential for free radical damage is quite large. Fortunately each cell has many hundred mitochondria, and so the loss of a few has little impact on the overall health and well-being of the cell or organ or whole animal. Nonetheless, should wholesale destruction of the genome occur, the results could be quite devastating.

**TABLE 11.7**
**Summary of Vitamin Function**

| Vitamin | Functions |
|---|---|
| *Fat-soluble vitamins* | |
| Vitamin A | As retinaldehyde, is essential in the visual cycle. |
| | Essential for body growth. |
| | As retinoic acid, plays an important role in the expression of genes that encode a wide variety of body proteins that play roles in metabolism, growth, and development. |
| | Downregulates uncontrolled cell growth. |
| Vitamin D | Increases calcium and phosphorus absorption from the small intestine, thus promoting the growth and mineralization of bones. |
| | Increases resorption of phosphates from the kidney tubules. |
| | Maintains normal level of citrate in the blood. |
| | Protects against the loss of amino acids through the kidneys. |
| | Serves in gene regulation. |
| Vitamin E | Serves as an antioxidant that protects body cells from free radical damage. |
| | Has a role in cellular respiration. |
| Vitamin K | Essential for the posttranslational carboxylation of glutamic acid residues in osteocalcin and in four blood-clotting proteins: Factor II, prothrombin; Factor VII, proconvertin; Factor IX, Christmas factor; and Factor X, Stuart–Prower. The carboxylation of glutamic acid residues increases calcium-binding activity of these proteins. |
| *Water-soluble vitamins* | |
| Biotin | Functions as a coenzyme mainly in decarboxylation–carboxylation and in deamination reactions. |
| Folacin/folate (folic acid) | Serves as a coenzyme in synthesis of purines, pyrmidines, hemoglobin, and in the metabolism of several amino acids and vitamins: Serine to glycine, tyrosine from phenylalanine, glutamic acid from histadine, choline from ethanolamine, $N$-metylnicotinamide from nicotinamide. |
| Niacin (nicotinic acid or nicotinamide) | Serves as a coenzyme (NAD and NADP) in intermediary metabolism. These coenzymes function as reducing equivalent ($H^+$) acceptors or donors. |
| Pantothenic acid | Functions as part of two enzymes—coenzyme A (CoA) and ACP. Both of these are important in intermediary metabolism. |
| Riboflavin | Serves as coenzymes FAD and FMN. These coenzymes accept or donate reducing equivalents. |
| Thiamin | As a coenzyme in transketolase reactions also has a role in the maintenance of normal appetite, muscle tone, and normal mental function. |
| Vitamin $B_6$ | Serves as a coenzyme (pyridoxal phosphate) in transamination. |
| Pyridoxine; alamine | Decarboxylation and *trans*-sulfuration reactions; also is a coenzyme in the conversion of tryptophan to niacin, the absorption of amino acids, glycogenolysis, and the elongation of linoleic acid to arachidonic acid. |
| Vitamin $B_{12}$ (cobalamins) | Synthesis or transfer of single-carbon units, in the biosynthesis of methyl groups (–CH3) and in reduction reactions such as the conversion of disulfide (S–S) to the sulfhydryl group (–SH). |
| Vitamin C (ascorbic acid) | Functions in redox systems and aids in the regulation of redox states. This function is due to its interconversion between a reduced and oxidized state and plays a role in collagen synthesis (hydroxylation of proline to hydroxyproline). |

See Chapter 14 for more information on vitamins and vitamin deficiencies.

Fortunately, there is a very active antioxidant system in place that protects the cells from such damage. Some of the vitamins and minerals play an important role in this system. Vitamin E quenches free radicals as they form via the conversion of tocopherol to the tocopheroxyl radical, which is then converted to its quinone. Vitamin K, although not truly an antioxidant, does serve as an $H^+/e^-$ donor/acceptor in its role to facilitate the carboxylation of the peptide glutamyl residues of certain proteins to their epoxide form. Vitamin C and vitamin A are both good $H^+/e^-$ donor/acceptors in the suppression of free radical formation. Of course, indirectly, all those vitamins that serve as coenzymes are involved as well. Shown in Table 11.4 is the free radical suppression system. Note that selenium is complimentary to the role of vitamin E in the suppression of free radicals. Some of the antioxidant role for vitamin E could be met if there is a sufficient intake of selenium. This mineral is important to the glutathione peroxidase enzyme that is an important component of the free radical suppression system. Selenium plays a role in both the synthesis of this enzyme and as a required cofactor.

**TABLE 11.8**
**Essential Minerals and Their Functions**

| Mineral | Function |
|---|---|
| *Macrominerals* | |
| Sodium (Na⁺) | Participates in the regulation of osmotic pressure |
| | Functions in nerve conduction (depolarization/repolarization) |
| | Participates in active transport mechanisms as part of the plasma membrane Na⁺K⁺ ATPase |
| | Part of the mineral apatite of bones and teeth |
| Calcium (Ca⁺⁺) | Important part of the mineral apatite of bones and teeth |
| | Important cell signal with respect to metabolic regulation and the transport of metabolites (and some hormones) from one compartment to another or from one cell to the bloodstream |
| | Key mineral in cell death and in muscle contraction |
| Potassium (K⁺) | Participates in the regulation of osmotic pressure |
| | Participates in active transport mechanisms as part of the Na⁺K⁺ATPase |
| | Has a role in muscle contraction |
| Chloride (Cl⁺) | Participates in the regulation of osmotic pressure |
| | Part of gastric acid (HCl) |
| | Good oxidizing agent |
| | Participates in the exchange of oxygen for carbon dioxide |
| | Important to B$_{12}$ absorption |
| Phosphorus | As a component of high-energy compounds (ATP, ADP, AMP, UTP [P as PO$_4^{3-}$], etc.) and phosphorylated metabolites |
| | Component of bones and teeth |
| | Serves as a component of nucleic acids (RNA and DNA) |
| Magnesium (Mg⁺⁺) | Constituent of bones and teeth |
| | Essential element of cellular metabolism, often as an activator of enzymes involved in phosphorylated compounds and of high-energy phosphate transfer of ADP and ATP |
| | Involved in activating certain peptidases in protein digestion |
| | Relaxes nerve impulse, functioning antagonistically to calcium, which is stimulatory |
| Cobalt (Co⁺⁺⁺) | Serves as an integral part of Vitamin B$_{12}$ |
| Copper (Cu⁺⁺) | Facilitates the absorption and use of iron |
| | Essential for the formation of hemoglobin, although it is not a part of hemoglobin as such |
| | Cofactor for several enzymes |
| | Important for the development and maintenance of the vascular and skeletal structures (blood vessels, tendons, and bones) |
| | Structure and function of the central nervous system |
| | Required for normal pigmentation of hair |
| | Component of important copper-containing proteins |
| Fluorine (F⁻) | Constitutes 0.02 to 0.05% of the bones and teeth |
| | Necessary for sound bones and teeth |
| | Assists in the prevention of dental caries |
| Iodine (I⁻) | Serves as an important component of the thyroid hormones |
| Iron (Fe⁺⁺ and Fe⁺⁺⁺) | Iron (heme) combines with protein (globin) to make hemoglobin and the iron–sulfur components of the respiratory chain |
| Manganese (Mn⁺⁺) | Formation of bone and the growth of other connective tissues |
| | Serves as a cofactor for SOD |
| Molybdenum (Mo) | Cofactor for iron and flavin-containing enzymes |
| Selenium (Se²⁺,⁴⁺,⁶⁺) | Component of the enzyme glutathione peroxidase |
| Zinc (Zn⁺⁺) | Component of the zinc fingers of transcription agents |
| | Serves as a cofactor for more than 70 enzymes |

See Chapters 12 and 13 for more information about minerals.

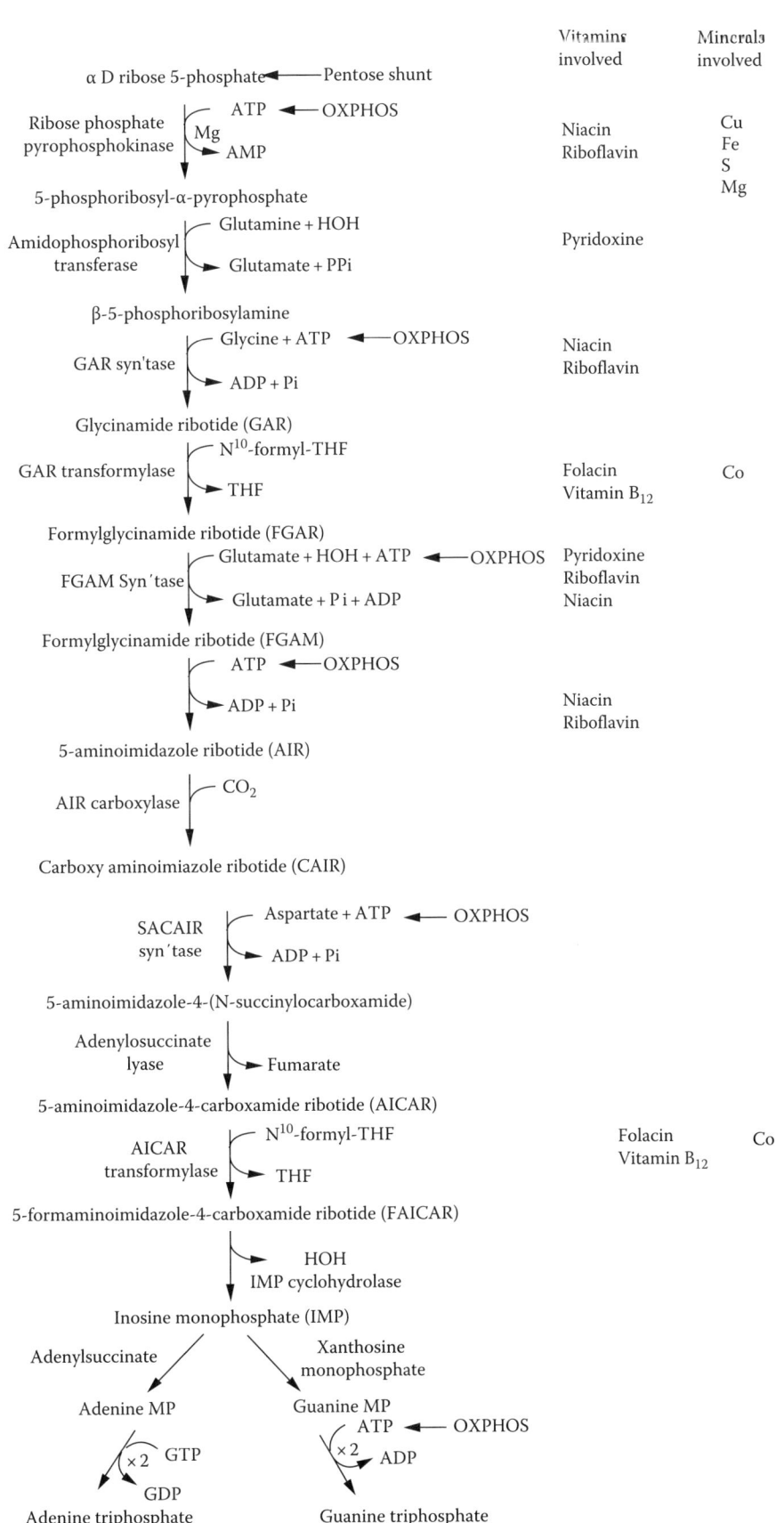

**FIGURE 11.33** Purine synthesis. In this pathway, the addition of ribose occurs prior to ring closure and phosphorylation.

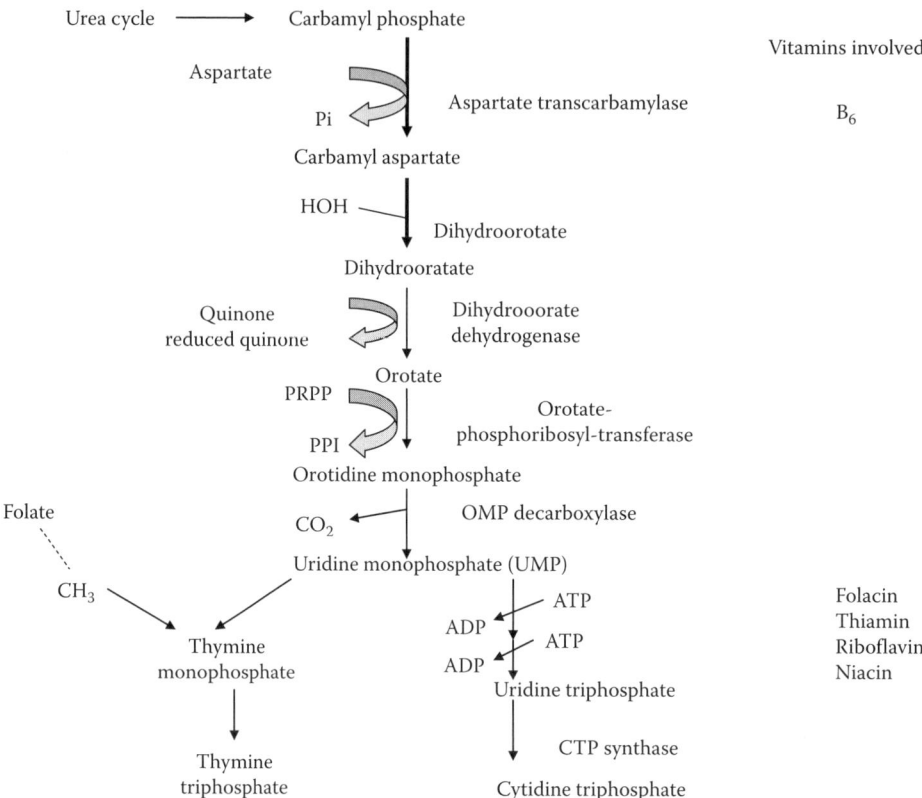

**FIGURE 11.34** Pyrimidine synthesis. In this pathway the pyrimidine ring is formed before it is attached to ribose and phosphorylated.

## SUMMARY

From the forgoing brief review of intermediary metabolism, it can be seen that nutrients in the diet function collectively and individually to maintain the health and well-being of the consumer. Subsequent chapters in this book will provide further information on particular aspects of the roles nutrition plays in a variety of situations from conception to death.

## FURTHER READINGS

Bender, DA. *Introduction to Nutrition and Metabolism*, 3rd edn. CRC Press, Boca Raton, FL, 2002, 450pp.

Berdanier, CD, Zempleni, J. *Advanced Nutrition: Macronutrients, Micronutrients, and Metabolism*. CRC Press, Boca Raton, FL, 2009, 530pp.

Brody, T. *Nutritional Biochemistry*, Academic Press, San Diego, CA, 1994, 658pp.

# 12 Macromineral Nutrition

*Forrest H. Nielsen*

## CONTENTS

## INTRODUCTION

The macrominerals are mineral elements required in gram quantities on a daily basis by humans. The macrominerals include calcium, magnesium, phosphorus, potassium, and sodium. These elements are needed for critical functions that include electrolyte balance, signal transduction, enzyme function, energy metabolism, and bone formation and maintenance. These elements also can have detrimental effects when intakes exceed homeostatic control mechanisms. Thus, intakes of these nutrients that are neither too low nor excessive are needed for health and well-being.

## CALCIUM

Calcium is the most abundant mineral element in the body. Calcium accounts for 1%–2% of body weight, or 920–1000 g in an adult female and ~1.22 kg in adult male.[1] Approximately 1% of total body calcium is found in extracellular fluids, intracellular structures, and cell membranes. Extracellular $Ca^{2+}$ concentrations are about 10,000 times higher than intracellular $Ca^{2+}$ concentrations (about 100 nM).[1] Bones and teeth contain the other 99% of body calcium.

The properties of $Ca^{2+}$ (ionic radius of 0.99 Å and ability to form coordination bonds with up to 12 oxygen atoms) have made $Ca^{2+}$ the ion of choice to fit into the folds of peptide chains for maintenance of tertiary structure. The ionic size of $Ca^{2+}$ and its ability to bind reversibly to cell proteins have made $Ca^{2+}$ the most common signal transmitter across cell membranes and an activator of numerous enzymes. In the role as a signaling or messenger ion, $Ca^{2+}$ mediates vascular contraction and vasodilatation, muscle contraction, nerve transmission, and hormone action. In response to a chemical, electrical, or physical stimulus, extracellular $Ca^{2+}$ enters the cell or increases intracellularly through release from internal stores (e.g., endoplasmic or sarcoplasmic reticulum).[1,2] Increased intracellular $Ca^{2+}$ stimulates a specific cellular response, such as activation of a kinase to phosphorylate a protein, that results in a physiological response.[1] A number of enzymes, including several proteases and dehydrogenases, are activated or stabilized by bound calcium independent of changes in intracellular $Ca^{2+}$.[3] These enzymes include glyceraldehyde phosphate dehydrogenase, pyruvate dehydrogenase, and α-ketoglutarate dehydrogenase.[3]

Most of the calcium in bone exists as crystals with a composition similar to hydroxyapatite $[Ca_{10}(PO_4)_6(OH)_2]$, which contains about 39% calcium. The crystals, which have the ability to resist compression, are arrayed in a protein matrix, which has the ability to withstand tensile loads. Alterations in either the inorganic (hydroxyapatite) or organic (protein matrix) components can result in changes in bone strength.[4] The skeleton undergoes continuous remodeling throughout life (it is replaced every 10–12 years) to adapt its internal microstructure to changes in its mechanical and physiological environment. Additionally, bone is renewed continuously to repair microdamage to minimize the risk of fracture.

The maintenance of extracellular $Ca^{2+}$ by mobilization of skeletal calcium stores means that nutritional calcium deficiency almost never is manifested as a shortage $Ca^{2+}$ in critical cellular or physiological processes.[5] However, a deficient calcium intake might increase circulating 1,25(OH)$_2$-vitamin D to a level that opens calcium channels in some cells, such as adipocytes, resulting in increased intracellular $Ca^{2+}$.[3] The increased intracellular $Ca^{2+}$ might contribute to the development or severity of chronic diseases such as those associated with obesity and characterized by chronic inflammatory stress. However, for most healthy individuals, the main concern about calcium intake is an amount that will maintain bone health. If bone renewal during remodeling or turnover is slower than bone loss, osteoporosis may occur. If bone repairing is slower than microdamage accumulation, stress fractures may occur. In a large case-controlled study of hip fracture risk in European women, fracture risk declined until calcium intake rose to an estimated 500 mg/day.[6] Calcium supplementation alone of individuals consuming more than 500 mg/day apparently does not decrease fracture risk.[6–9] A meta-analysis of prospective cohort studies and randomized controlled trials found that calcium supplementation did not decrease hip fracture risk, but suggested instead an increased fracture risk.[10] Studies with adults showing a positive influence of high dietary calcium in decreasing bone loss or fracture risk usually have supplemental vitamin D as an experimental co-variable. Coadministration of calcium and vitamin D also has been associated with decreased risk of total, breast, and colorectal cancers.[11]

There is no good biochemical indicator of nutritional calcium deficiency. As indicated earlier, the skeleton assures adequate calcium for critical cellular functions and maintains extracellular fluid concentrations. Thus, serum calcium is not useful as an indicator of nutritional calcium deficiency. If serum calcium is more than 10% away from the population mean, diseases (e.g., hypo- or hyperthyroidism) probably are the cause.[3] Determination of the amount of bone mineral is the best current method for assessing calcium status, but this determination may be affected by other factors such as weight, hormones, and other dietary factors (e.g., vitamin D and magnesium). Total body bone minerals can be estimated by using dual x-ray absorptiometry, microcomputed tomography, and peripheral quantitative computed tomography.[12] Numerous blood and urine tests indicate whether bone is being lost or formed after a dietary modification or pharmacologic intervention. However, these tests do not indicate calcium status well.

There are some studies that suggest excessive intakes of calcium can be detrimental. Nephrolithiasis (kidney stones) has been associated with excessive calcium intake.[9,13] However, numerous other factors have been associated with nephrolithiasis, including high intakes of oxalate, protein, and phosphorus and low intakes of magnesium.[13] Thus, excess calcium might be only a contributing factor to the development of nephrolithiasis. Some studies suggest that high calcium intakes might affect the metabolism of some minerals, particularly magnesium and zinc. High calcium intakes decreased zinc balance in one study,[14] but another study found that increased milk consumption and calcium phosphate supplementation did not decrease zinc absorption.[15] A high calcium intake has been found to decrease magnesium absorption in animals and humans[16] and reduce the magnesium status of rats.[17] Recently, high calcium supplementation was found to be associated with an increased risk of cardiovascular disease.[18–20] This association might be related to an effect on metabolism of some other nutrient such as magnesium because more complex forms of calcium, such as that in dairy products, apparently can prevent the adverse finding.[20] In addition, the increased risk for cardiovascular disease resulting from high calcium intakes has not been corroborated by other analyses.[21]

A summary of biological, clinical, and nutritional aspects of calcium, including that discussed earlier, is provided in Table 12.1.

---

## TABLE 12.1
## Biological, Clinical, and Nutritional Aspects of Calcium

| | |
|---|---|
| *Biological function* | Calcium is a second messenger that couples intracellular responses to extracellular signals, an activator of some functional proteins, and indispensable for bone and tooth formation and maintenance |
| *Signs and symptoms of deficiency* | |
| Biochemical | Increased circulating $1,25(OH)_2$-vitamin D |
| Physiological | Bone loss and osteoporosis |
| *Pathological consequences of deficiency* | |
| Established | Increased fracture risk |
| Suggested | Increased risk for hypertension;[22] total, breast, and colorectal cancers;[11] cardiovascular disease;[23,24] total mortality[24] |
| *Pathological consequences of excessive intake* | |
| Established | None firmly established |
| Suggested | Increased risk of cardiovascular disease and kidney stones |
| | Increased risk of magnesium and zinc deficiencies |
| *Predisposing factors for deficiency* | Factors that reduce bioavailability such as oxalate and phytate[25,26] |
| | Factors that increase urinary loss such as high dietary sodium,[1,27] phosphorus,[28] and protein[28] and aluminum antacids[27,29] |
| *Recommended intakes* | |
| Prevention of deficiency | RDAs and AIs (in parenthesis) set by the Food and Nutrition Board[30] (mg/day): infants 0–0.5 year, (200), and 0.5–1 year, 260; children 1–3 years, 700, and 4–8 years, 1000; males 9–18 years, 1300, 19–70 years, 1000, and >70 years, 1200; females 9–18 years, 1300, 19–50 years, 1000, ≥51 years, 1200; pregnancy 14–18 years, 1300, and ≥19 years, 1000; lactation, 1000 |
| | The values for adults are similar to those suggested by others[31–33] |
| Therapeutic or beneficial | In combination with vitamin D, intakes higher than the RDA have been found to reduce the risk for osteoporosis |
| | Increased intakes of calcium help in weight loss[34–36] |
| Tolerable upper intake level (UL) | ULs set by the Food and Nutrition Board[30] (mg/day): infants 0–0.5 year, 1000, and 0.5–1 year, 1500; children 1–8 years, 2500; males 9–18 years, 3000 and ≥19 years, 2500; females 9–18 years, 3000, 19–50 years, 2500, and ≥51 years, 2000; pregnancy and lactation 14–18 years, 3000, and ≥19 years, 2500 |
| *Food sources* | Milk and milk products, soybeans, nuts, *Brassica* vegetables (e.g., broccoli, bok choy, and kale)[1,26,37] |

# MAGNESIUM

Magnesium as $Mg^{2+}$ is the fourth most abundant cation in the body[38] and is second to potassium as the most abundant cellular cation. The adult human body contains about 25 g of magnesium, which is about equally divided between bone and soft tissue.[39] Less than 1% of the total body magnesium is in blood. About one-third of skeletal magnesium is exchangeable and acts as a pool for maintaining normal concentrations of extracellular magnesium. The ratio of extracellular to intracellular $Mg^{2+}$ is 0.33, which contrasts markedly with the ratio of 10,000 for $Ca^{2+}$. Thus, unlike calcium, magnesium is not commonly used to transmit signals from the outside to the inside of cells. However, magnesium through affecting cell membrane receptors and protein phosphorylation is a critical cation for cell signaling. Magnesium at the cell membrane level regulates intracellular calcium and potassium and thus is a controlling factor in nerve transmission, skeletal and smooth muscle contraction, cardiac excitability, vasomotor tone, blood pressure, and bone turnover.

$Mg^{2+}$, although chemically similar to $Ca^{2+}$, does not bond as well as $Ca^{2+}$ to proteins, but still is involved in over 300 enzyme reactions through binding enzyme substrates or directly with enzymes.[38] Magnesium is needed for enzymatic reactions vital to every metabolic pathway.[13,38,39] These reactions include those involving DNA, RNA, protein, and adenylate cyclase syntheses; cellular energy production and storage; glycolysis; and preservation of cellular electrolyte composition. Magnesium has two functions in enzymatic reactions. It binds directly to some enzymes to alter their structure or to serve in a catalytic role (e.g., exonuclease, topoisomerase, RNA polymerase, and DNA polymerase). Magnesium also binds to enzyme substrates to form complexes with which enzymes react. The predominant role of magnesium is involvement in ATP utilization (e.g., the reaction of kinases with MgATP to phosphorylate proteins). Magnesium exists primarily as MgATP in all cells.

Based on dietary intake recommendations, subclinical or marginal magnesium deficiency (intakes of 50% to <100% of requirement) commonly occurs throughout the world.[40] Yet pathological disorders attributed specifically to dietary magnesium deficiency alone are considered rare. However, epidemiological and correlation studies indicate that subclinical magnesium deficiency and subnormal plasma or serum magnesium concentrations (<0.75 mmol/L) are associated with numerous pathological conditions associated with aging and obesity, including cardiovascular disease,[41–44] hypertension,[41,45,46] osteoporosis,[47] metabolic syndrome,[48–51] diabetes mellitus, [52–54] and some cancers.[55–58] In addition, subclinical magnesium deficiency and subnormal plasma or serum magnesium concentrations have been associated with asthma,[59] migraine headaches,[60] preeclampsia,[60] and increased kidney stones.[61]

The pathological conditions most often associated with subclinical magnesium deficiency and subnormal plasma or serum magnesium concentration have been characterized as having a chronic inflammatory and/or oxidative stress component.[62,63] Human studies indicate that subclinical magnesium deficiency and subnormal plasma or serum magnesium concentrations often are associated with increased inflammatory and oxidative stress.[51,54,64–72] Animal experiments, however, suggest that subclinical or marginal magnesium deficiency in humans more often has a contributory rather than a primary causative role in pathological disorders characterized by chronic inflammatory and oxidative stress.[40] Although severe magnesium deficiency (feeding less than 10% of requirement) results in an inflammatory response,[73] a moderate magnesium deficiency alone (~50% of requirement) apparently does not markedly affect variables associated with chronic inflammatory stress in animal models.[74,75] However, animal experiments indicate that moderate magnesium deficiency can enhance the inflammatory oxidative stress induced by other factors.[40] Thus, magnesium deficiency might be a significant nutritional concern under conditions that cause oxidative or inflammatory stress (e.g., obesity and high fructose or sucrose intakes) that lead to chronic diseases associated with aging.[40]

In addition to contributing to the risk for some chronic diseases, controlled metabolic ward studies indicate that magnesium deficiency also can affect physical performance and heart function. Heart rate and oxygen consumption increased significantly during submaximal exercise when untrained postmenopausal women were fed about 150 mg compared to 320 magnesium per day.[76] Postmenopausal women fed with magnesium-deficient diets also exhibited heart arrhythmias and changes in potassium metabolism.[77–79]

Efforts to find an indicator of subclinical magnesium status (also called chronic latent magnesium deficiency[80]) have not yielded a cost-effective one that has been well validated. At present, the magnesium load test is considered the best test to diagnose a total body deficit of magnesium. This test determines the percentage of magnesium retained over a given period of time after parenteral administration of a magnesium load.[38,80] Retention of greater than 22% to 25% (amount usually retained by magnesium-adequate individuals) indicates some whole-body magnesium depletion.[38]

The magnesium load test is invasive, time-consuming, and expensive; requires hospitalization or close supervision for about 24 h after magnesium infusion; and requires careful urine collection for laboratory analysis. Thus, serum magnesium is most commonly used to determine magnesium status. Low serum magnesium (<0.75 mmol/L) is useful for diagnosing a significant magnesium deficiency, often caused by factors other than a deficient intake (e.g., disease and drugs). However, plasma or serum magnesium is a poor indicator of subclinical magnesium deficiency because exchangeable skeletal magnesium and urinary excretion responses to changes in magnesium intake maintain extracellular magnesium at a rather constant concentration even while tissue magnesium is decreasing. Thus, serum or plasma magnesium concentrations have been found to be in the normal range (0.75–1.0 mmol/L) in individuals with low tissue magnesium.[38,80]

Hypermagnesemia between >1.0 and <1.5 mmol/L is clinically latent, but ≥1.5 mmol/L causes lethargy, confusion, nausea, diarrhea, appetite loss, muscle weakness, breathing difficulty, low blood pressure, and irregular heart rhythm.[38,39] Hypermagnesemia is most commonly associated with the combination of impaired renal function and high intakes

**TABLE 12.2**
**Biological, Clinical, and Nutritional Aspects of Magnesium**

| | |
|---|---|
| *Biological function* | Magnesium is a cofactor for more than 300 enzymes in humans. The cofactor role is either as a direct allosteric activator of enzymes or as part of a substrate (e.g., MgATP and MgGTP) in enzyme reactions. Magnesium also has functions at the cell membrane level that regulates intracellular calcium and potassium and thus is a controlling factor in nerve transmission, skeletal and smooth muscle contraction, cardiac excitability, vasomotor tone, blood pressure, and bone turnover. |
| *Signs and symptoms of deficiency* | |
| Biochemical | Excessive renal potassium excretion; low blood calcium, magnesium, and potassium; impaired parathyroid secretion and vitamin D metabolism; renal and skeletal resistance to parathyroid hormone; decreased intracellular potassium.[38] |
| Physiological | Neuromuscular symptoms (e.g., positive Trousseau's signs, tremors, fasciculations, muscle spasms, cramps and weakness, seizures, dizziness, and disequilibrium); electrocardiographic abnormalities and cardiac dysrhythmias, which include tachycardia, premature beats, and fibrillation.[38] |
| *Pathological consequences of deficiency* | |
| Established | Severe deficiency results in cardiac arrhythmias, seizures, cramps, depression, and psychosis. |
| Suggested | Based on numerous epidemiological studies and magnesium supplementation trials, subclinical magnesium deficiency or chronic latent magnesium deficiency is associated with, and might contribute to, numerous disorders including coronary heart disease, stroke, hypertension, diabetes, osteoporosis, asthma, migraine headaches, and some cancers. |
| *Pathological consequences of excessive intake* | Diarrhea, nausea, and abdominal cramping. Hypermagnesemia usually caused by high intakes of nonfood sources by individuals with impaired renal function can result in lethargy, confusion, nausea, diarrhea, appetite loss, muscle weakness, breathing difficulty, low blood pressure, and irregular heart rhythm. |
| *Predisposing factors for deficiency* | Factors interfering with absorption and utilization or promoting excretion including alcoholism, kidney failure, malabsorption syndromes, extensive bowel resection, gastroileal bypass, severe or prolonged diarrhea, protein–calorie malnutrition, acute pancreatitis, hyperaldosteronism, diabetes mellitus, thyroid gland disease, hyperparathyroidism, vitamin D resistance or deficiency, burns, and drugs (e.g., diuretics and proton pump inhibitors).[38] |
| | High calcium,[16,81] phosphorus,[16] and zinc[82,83] and low protein intakes.[84,85] |
| *Recommended intakes* | |
| Prevention of deficiency | RDAs and AIs (in parenthesis) set by the Food and Nutrition Board[13] (mg/day): infants 0–0.5 year, (30), and 0.5–1 year, 75; children 1–3 years, 80, 4–8 years, 130, and 9–13 years, 240; males 14–18 years, 410, 19–30 years, 400, and ≥31 years, 420; females 14–18 years, 360, 19–30 years, and 310, ≥31 years, 320; pregnant, +40 for each age group. |
| | The official RDA values for adults are higher than that recently estimated to meet the requirement of most adults (265 mg/day) by the use of balance data from controlled metabolic ward experiments.[86] |
| Therapeutic or beneficial | Infusion of magnesium has been indicated as a means to quickly overcome symptoms of magnesium deficiency. For example, a reported effective treatment is intravenous administration of 24 mmol of magnesium as a 50% solution over 24 h for 3–7 days.[87] Patients who are hypomagnesemic and have seizures or acute dysrhythmia may be given 4–8 mmol of magnesium over 5–10 min followed by the same regimen. |
| | Supra nutritional magnesium has been suggested to be an enhancer of antihypertensive medications[88] and a reducer of menopausal hot flashes.[89] |
| Tolerable UL | ULs (supplemental amounts to intakes from food and water) set by the Food and Nutrition Board[13] (mg/day): infants 0–1.0 year, not determined; children 1–3 years, 65, and 4–8 years, 110; individuals >9 years, 350. |
| *Food sources* | Whole grains, nuts, legumes, and green leafy vegetables.[37,39] |

of nonfood sources of magnesium such as magnesium-containing laxatives and antacids. Thus, hypermagnesemia is not an issue for healthy individuals. The major effect of excessive magnesium intake without hypermagnesemia is diarrhea.[13,39] Nausea and abdominal cramping may also occur.

A summary of biological, clinical, and nutritional aspects of magnesium, including those discussed above, is provided in Table 12.2.

## PHOSPHORUS

The adult human body contains about 850 g of elemental phosphorus (about 1.1% of total body weight) with about 85% in the skeleton, 14% in the soft tissues, and 1% in the extracellular fluids, intracellular structures, and cell membranes.[90] Phosphate is the most abundant anion in the cell. The predominant species of inorganic phosphate in all biological fluids and tissues is the divalent anion, $HPO_4^{2-}$. At normal blood pH, the ratio of $HPO_4^{2-}$ to $H_2PO_4^{1-}$ is 4:1. Hydroxyapatite, $[Ca_{10}(PO_4)_6(OH)_2]$, in bone crystals has a constant calcium/phosphate ratio of about 2:1. Bone acts as a reservoir for exchangeable phosphate ions.

Phosphorus is involved in virtually every aspect of metabolism.[90–92] Phosphorus is an integral part of structural molecules including phospholipids and phosphoproteins. Membranes that surround all cells and separate intracellular organelles from cytoplasm are primarily a bilayer of phospholipids. Glucose, the ultimate energy source for most cellular activities, must be phosphorylated before entering the glycolytic pathway. Energy storage and use is in the form of phosphorus-containing compounds ATP and creatine phosphate. Cyclic AMP and cyclic GMP are intracellular second messengers regulating many biochemical processes including the actions of many hormones. DNA and RNA contain phosphate groups linking the deoxyribose and ribose along the backbone of these molecules, respectively. Phosphate is a critical component of almost all enzyme reactions, often in the form of enzymatic cofactor such as MgATP and nicotinamide adenine dinucleotide (NAD) and through changing catalytic activity by its addition or removal from the enzyme. Phosphate ions (about 30% in blood) serve as a buffer of blood pH and as a regulator of whole-body acid–base balance through facilitating the renal excretion of hydrogen ions by shifting from $HPO_4^{2-}$ to $H_2PO_4^{1-}$. The highly anionic organic phosphate, 2,3-diphosphoglycerate, binds to hemoglobin to facilitate the release of oxygen to tissues. In bones and teeth, over 50% of the mineral mass is the phosphate ion as a component of crystalline hydroxyapatite.

When inorganic phosphorus concentrations in extracellular fluid are deficient, cellular dysfunction occurs. The consequences of hypophosphatemia include anorexia, anemia, muscle weakness, bone pain, osteomalacia, increased susceptibility to infection, paresthesias, ataxia, confusion, and even death.[93] However, the typical abundance of phosphorus in the diet and the ability of the body to avidly retain phosphorus minimize the risk of hypophosphatemia and its consequences in healthy individuals.[91] Near-total starvation is required to produce phosphorus deficiency by only dietary deprivation.[13]

Serum phosphorus concentration is generally used as an indicator of phosphorus status. However, the concentration of phosphorus in serum can be falsely elevated or depressed, which results in concentrations that appear normal when body stores are low or concentrations that appear deficient when body stores are adequate. For example, phosphate loading for ergogenic purposes elevates serum phosphate concentrations.[94] Exercise, which results in the redistribution of phosphate from extracellular fluids to intracellular sites, decreases serum phosphate concentrations.[90] Other factors that decrease serum phosphorus concentrations include respiratory alkalosis, various disease states, and changes in hormonal status.[91] For example, individuals with insulin-dependent diabetes mellitus have fluctuating serum phosphorus concentrations because insulin decreases serum phosphorus concentrations. Thus, assessing phosphorus status by using serum phosphorus concentrations requires awareness of possible factors, especially the large number that can cause hypophosphatemia without phosphorus deficiency,[91] affecting the values obtained.

Excessive phosphorus intake from any source is expressed as hyperphosphatemia[13] (>1.6 mmol/L). Essentially all toxic effects of phosphorus are caused by elevated inorganic phosphate in the extracellular fluid.[13] Hyperphosphatemia can induce changes in the hormonal regulation of calcium metabolism and utilization. Hyperphosphatemia induced by phosphate loading results in decreased ionized calcium in the extracellular fluid (decreased calcium/phosphorus ratio) and increased circulating parathyroid hormone and 1, 25-dihydroxy vitamin D concentrations.[95,96] If these changes continue for an extended period, bone loss might occur. Clinical evidence for such bone loss is lacking, but support for this decreased calcium/phosphorus ratio effect is provided by animal and epidemiological findings.[95] Although calcium intakes in the United States are often low, the U.S. Food and Nutrition Board concluded that current phosphorus intakes in the United States are unlikely to be high enough to change the calcium/phosphorus ratio such that it adversely affects bone health.[13] This conclusion has been disputed.[97]

Another potential concern about excessive phosphorus intake is nonskeletal tissue calcification (ectopic or metastatic calcification), particularly of the kidney. This has been found in animal studies.[98] Metastatic calcification of the kidney has not been reported to occur through dietary means alone in persons with adequate renal function but occurs often in patients with end-stage renal and other diseases and is associated with increased all-cause and cardiovascular mortality and vascular calcification.[99,100] High serum phosphorus also has been associated with increased cardiovascular disease in individuals without chronic kidney disease.[101]

A summary of biological, clinical, and nutritional aspects of phosphorus, including those discussed earlier, is provided in Table 12.3.

## POTASSIUM

Potassium is the second most abundant cation in the body. The body of a 70 kg person contains about 140 g of potassium.[104] About 2% of potassium is in the extracellular fluid with circulating potassium concentrations about 136–196 mg/L (3.5–5.0 mmol/L).[105] Intracellular potassium is maintained at 5.46–5.85 g/L (140–150 mmol/L). The largest fraction of body potassium, about 60%–70%, is in skeletal muscle.[104] Virtually all body potassium is labile and exchangeable.[105]

Potassium is an activator or cofactor in some enzymatic reactions. These reactions include pyruvate kinase in carbohydrate metabolism that yields ATP and $Na^+, K^+$-ATPase that is responsible for the active transport or pumping of $Na^+$ and $K^+$ in opposite directions across plasma membranes.[104] The pumping results in potassium being the major intracellular cation and sodium the major extracellular cation. Potassium is the ion that neutralizes high concentrations of intracellular anions (e.g., proteins, phosphates, and $Cl^-$). In addition, a major function of potassium is membrane polarization, which depends upon the concentrations of

**TABLE 12.3**
**Biological, Clinical, and Nutritional Aspects of Phosphorus**

| | |
|---|---|
| *Biological function* | Phosphorus as phosphate has a structural role in DNA and RNA and is a component of structural molecules such as phospholipids and phosphoproteins. Energy storage and use is in the form of ATP and creatine phosphate. Cyclic AMP and cyclic GMP are intracellular second messengers. Phosphate is critical to almost all enzyme reactions, often in the form of ATP or NAD(H). Phosphorus needed for bone mineralization, serves as a blood pH buffer, facilitates the release of oxygen from hemoglobin, and regulates whole-body acid–base balance. |
| *Signs of deficiency* | |
| Biochemical | Low serum phosphorus (hypophosphatemia). |
| Physiological | Anorexia, anemia, muscle weakness, bone pain, and bone loss. |
| *Pathological consequences of deficiency* | |
| Established | Increased susceptibility to infection, paresthesia, ataxia, confusion, and even death. |
| Suggested | Increased fracture risk.[102,103] |
| *Pathological consequences of excessive intake* | |
| Established | In persons with diseases causing hyperphosphatemia, such as impaired renal function, rhabdomyolysis and tumor lysis syndrome, metastatic calcification of tissue, and increased all-cause and cardiovascular mortality and vascular calcification. |
| Suggested | Bone loss and increased cardiovascular disease risk. |
| *Predisposing factors for deficiency* | Vitamin D deficiency, phosphate-binding antacids, licorice ingestion, and drugs such as diuretics, corticosteroids, and aminophylline.[91] |
| *Recommended intakes* | |
| Prevention of deficiency | RDAs and AIs (in parenthesis) set by the Food and Nutrition Board[13] (mg/day): infants 0–0.5 year, (100), and 0.5–1 year, (275); children 1–3 years, 460, and 4–8 years, 500; males 9–18 years, 1250, and ≥19 years, 700; females 9–18 years, 1250, and ≥19 years, 700; pregnancy 14–18 years, 1250, and ≥19 years, 700; lactation 14–18 years, 1250, and ≥19 years, 700. |
| Therapeutic or beneficial | Phosphate loading suggested as an ergogenic aid.[94] |
| Tolerable UL | ULs set by the Food and Nutrition Board[13] (g/day): infants 0–1 year, not determined; children 1–8 years, 3; males 9–70 years, 4, and >70 years, 3; females 9–70 years, 4, and >70 years, 3; pregnancy, 3.5; lactation, 4. |
| *Food sources* | Protein-rich foods and cereal grains are rich sources of phosphorus.[9,10] |

intracellular and extracellular potassium.[105] The biochemical functions of potassium result in it being involved in acid–base regulation, osmotic pressure maintenance, nerve impulse transmission, muscle contraction, and carbon dioxide and oxygen transport.[105,106]

Because of its role in membrane polarization, the major effects of both hypokalemia (<3.5 mmol/L plasma) and hyperkalemia (>5.5 mmol/L) involve changes in membrane function, which are particularly significant in neuromuscular and cardiac conduction systems.[104,105] Adverse effects of hypokalemia include cardiac arrhythmias, muscle weakness, and glucose intolerance. Because potassium is the principal intracellular cation in animals and plants, it is widely distributed in foods. Thus, severe potassium deficiency is not common because potassium is usually consumed in amounts required for obligatory losses and maintenance of tissue levels. However, intakes of potassium higher than those needed to prevent hypokalemia, which might not be commonly achieved, have been reported to be beneficial. Chronic low potassium intakes (e.g., <2.0 mg/day) not resulting in hypokalemia have been associated with hypertension, cardiovascular disease (stroke and coronary heart disease), and cardiovascular mortality.[107,108] Numerous studies have shown

that potassium supplementation may lower blood pressure, especially in salt-sensitive individuals, and decrease cardiovascular mortality.[106,108–110]

Chronic low potassium intakes not causing hypokalemia also have been associated with bone loss.[111,112] This association is thought to occur through a disordered acid–base metabolism.[113] Modern diets generally are high in acid-producing sodium chloride, phosphorus, and proteins (contain acid-producing sulfur amino acids) and low in fruits and vegetables containing acid-balancing potassium and bicarbonate, which results in a metabolic acidosis.[113] This acid–base imbalance has been associated with bone loss that may lead to osteoporosis.[113–115] The suggestion that chronic low potassium intake adversely affects bone maintenance is supported by the finding that potassium citrate prevented increased urine calcium excretion and bone resorption induced by a high sodium chloride diet.[116] However, some potassium supplementation trials have not shown significant positive effects on bone maintenance in older men and women.[117,118] These conflicting findings indicate that further studies are needed to determine the significance of potassium intake in the relationship between metabolic acidosis and bone maintenance.[119]

Plasma potassium concentration is used as an indicator of potassium status. However, because only a small percentage of potassium is in the extracellular fluid, the plasma concentration of potassium is often poor indicator of tissue potassium stores.[105]

Hyperkalemia occurs when potassium intake exceeds the capacity of the kidneys to excrete potassium. This rarely happens when the kidneys are functioning because their capacity to excrete potassium is substantial.[104] Hyperkalemia also can occur in the absence of potassium retention caused by such things renal disease or a lack of aldosterone secretion.[104] A shift of intracellular potassium into the plasma to cause hyperkalemia also can occur in metabolic acidosis and from tissue damage such as hemolysis, burns, major trauma, or lysis of tumor cells.[104] Symptoms of hyperkalemia include paresthesia, muscle weakness, and cardiac dysrhythmia, which ranges from sinus bradycardia to ventricular tachycardia, ventricular fibrillation, and ultimately cardiac arrest.[104]

A summary of biological, clinical, and nutritional aspects of potassium, including those discussed earlier, is provided in Table 12.4.

# SODIUM

Sodium is the third most abundant cation in the body. The body of a 70 kg person contains about 100 g of sodium.[104] The distribution of sodium in the body is about 50% in the extracellular fluid, 40% associated with bone, and 10% intracellularly.[105] The concentration of sodium is about 145 mmol/L in plasma and only about 12 mmol/L in intracellular fluid.[104] Sodium exists in both the exchangeable and non-exchangeable forms.[105] Intracellular sodium, extracellular sodium, and about half of bone sodium are exchangeable. Essentially all non-exchangeable sodium is buried in bone structure.[105]

Sodium is an activator of $Na^+$, $K^+$-ATPase, which hydrolyzes one molecule of ATP to transport three $Na^+$ ions and two $K^+$ ions in opposite directions across cell membranes to maintain or restore the normally high $K^+$ and low $Na^+$ concentrations inside the cell.[104] This transport results in a net movement of cations out of the cell and a negative charge inside the cell relative to the outside, and thus is called an electrogenic pump.[104] This electrogenic pump is involved in the transport of many nutrients across cell membranes, including

## TABLE 12.4
## Biological, Clinical, and Nutritional Aspects of Potassium

| | |
|---|---|
| *Biological function* | Potassium is an enzyme activator or cofactor (e.g., pyruvate kinase and $Na^+$, $K^+$-ATPase), neutralizes high concentrations of intracellular anions (e.g., proteins, phosphates, and chloride), and polarizes membranes. In these roles, potassium is involved in acid–base regulation, osmotic pressure maintenance, nerve impulse transmission, muscle contraction, and carbon dioxide and oxygen transport. |
| *Signs of deficiency* | |
| Biochemical | Hypokalemia or low plasma potassium (<3.5 mmol/L). |
| Physiological | Cardiac arrhythmias and glucose intolerance. |
| *Pathological consequences of deficiency* | |
| Established | Muscle weakness, fatigue, and cramps. |
| Suggested | Hypertension, cardiovascular disease (e.g., stroke and coronary heart disease), and mortality; bone loss; insulin resistance, glucose intolerance, and diabetes.[104,120] |
| *Pathological consequences of excessive intake* | |
| Established | Paresthesia, muscle weakness, flaccid paralysis, and cardiac arrhythmias ranging from sinus bradycardia to ventricular tachycardia, ventricular fibrillation, and cardiac arrest. |
| Suggested | None suggested. |
| *Predisposing factors for deficiency* | High intakes of sodium chloride,[104–106] acidogenic foods (e.g., proteins high in sulfur amino acids and phosphorus),[106] and magnesium deficiency.[38] |
| *Recommended intakes* | |
| Prevention of deficiency | To replace obligatory loss of potassium, an adult should consume 0.8 mg/day.[104] The Food and Nutrition Board set only AIs for potassium because of insufficient dose–response data to establish estimated average requirements (EAR) to determine RDAs.[106] The AIs set (g/day) were as follows: infants 0–0.5 year, 0.4, and 0.5–1 year, 0.7; children 1–3 years, 3, and 4–8 years, 3.8; males and females 9–13 years, .45, and ≥14 years, 4.7; pregnancy, 4.7; lactation, 5.1. |
| Therapeutic or beneficial | Only 10% of men and 1% of women consume at least the AI for potassium.[104] The high AIs were set to achieve beneficial effects on blood pressure and cardiovascular and bone health. |
| Tolerable UL | The Food and Nutrition Board did not set ULs for potassium.[106] However, individuals with impaired renal function should avoid high intakes of potassium from foods and supplemental potassium[104]. |
| *Food sources* | Milk, meat, grains, nuts, potatoes, pulses, and soybeans.[37] |

the absorption chloride, amino acids, glucose, galactose, and water.[104] Another role of Na$^+$ and its accompanying anions, Cl$^-$ and HCO$_3^-$, is the regulation of the osmolarity of plasma and extracellular fluid.[104] The amount of osmotic particles in the extracellular fluid compartment (interstitial fluid and plasma) is the primary determinant of its volume. Changes in extracellular fluid volume alter cardiac filling pressure, cardiac output, and arterial pressure.[104]

Individuals with chronic low intakes of sodium chloride do not normally exhibit any sodium deficiency signs because the body efficiently conserves sodium.[104] However, a very low intake of sodium (<700 mg/day) in short-term clinical studies increased serum total and LDL cholesterol and changed carbohydrate metabolism,[121,122] which suggests a chronic deficiency might increase the risk for cardiovascular disease. In addition, sodium deficits may occur with profuse sweating, prolonged diarrhea and vomiting, diuretic therapy, and diseases affecting renal sodium excretion.[104] Deficits caused by

these factors can result in hypovolemia, dehydration, hypotension, increased pulse rate, dizziness and syncope, muscle weakness and cramps, and circulatory shock.[104]

Chronic high intakes of sodium are of more nutritional concern than low intakes. High sodium or salt intakes have been implicated in the development of hypertension, hypertension-related cardiovascular diseases, renal diseases unrelated to blood pressure, gastric mucosal damage, gastric cancer, and bone demineralization that can result in osteoporosis.[104] In addition, water and sodium retention can occur in some pathological conditions (e.g., congestive heart failure, renal failure, and excessive production of aldosterone), which may result in the accumulation of excess fluid in the body or edema.[104,105] Accumulation of fluid in the lungs results in difficulty in breathing.[105]

A summary of biological, clinical, and nutritional aspects of sodium, including those discussed earlier, is provided in Table 12.5.

## TABLE 12.5
### Biological, Clinical, and Nutritional Aspects of Sodium

| | |
|---|---|
| *Biological function* | Sodium is an activator of Na$^+$, K$^+$-ATPase that hydrolyzes ATP to transport Na$^+$ and K$^+$ in opposite directions across cell membranes. The transport is called an electrogenic pump because it results in a negative charge inside the cell relative to the outside. The electrogenic pump is involved in the transport of many nutrients across cell membranes (e.g., chloride, amino acids, glucose, galactose, and water). Sodium also is involved in the regulation of the osmolarity of plasma and extracellular fluid. |
| *Signs of deficiency* | |
| Biochemical | Low plasma sodium or hyponatremia (<135 mmol/L).[106] |
| Physiological | Hypovolemia, dehydration, hypotension, increased pulse rate, dizziness and syncope, muscle weakness, and cramps. |
| *Pathological consequences of deficiency* | |
| Established | Circulatory shock. |
| Suggested | Increased risk for cardiovascular disease.[121–123] |
| *Pathological consequences of excessive intake* | |
| Established | Water and sodium retention can occur in some pathological conditions (e.g., congestive heart failure, renal failure, and excessive production of aldosterone), which can cause the accumulation of excess fluid in the body or edema. |
| Suggested | High sodium or salt intake has been implicated in the development of hypertension, hypertension-related cardiovascular diseases, renal diseases unrelated to blood pressure, gastric mucosal damage, gastric cancer, and bone demineralization that can result in osteoporosis. |
| *Predisposing factors for deficiency* | Sodium deficits that result in signs of deficiency listed earlier are primarily caused by profuse sweating, prolonged diarrhea, diuretic therapy, or diseases that increase renal sodium excretion. |
| *Recommended intakes* | |
| Prevention of deficiency | The daily minimum requirement needed to replace obligatory losses of sodium when substantial sweating does not occur is not more than 0.18 mg/day.[106] The Food and Nutrition Board set only AIs for sodium because of insufficient dose–response data to establish EAR to determine RDAs.[106] The AIs set (g/day) were as follows: infants 0–0.5 year, 0.37, and 0.5–1 year, 0.7; children 1–3 years, 1.0, and 4–8 years, 1.2; males and females 9–50 years, 14.5, 51–70 years, 1.3, and >70 years, 1.2; pregnancy and lactation, 1.5. |
| Therapeutic or beneficial | None reported. |
| Tolerable UL | The Food and Nutrition Board set ULs, based on the association between salt intake and the development of hypertension; the AIs are (g/day) as follows: infants 0–1.0 year, not determined; children 1–3 years, 1.5, 4–8 years, 1.9, and 9–13 years, 2.2; individuals ≥14 years, 2.3. |
| *Food sources* | Sodium in the diet comes mainly from sodium chloride, which is high in cured meat products, processed foods, and canned vegetables. Fresh fruits and vegetables are low in sodium. |

## SUMMARY

Deficient dietary intakes resulting in pathological disorders are not likely for phosphorus because of its typical abundance in foods and for sodium because of efficient mechanisms for conservation in the body. Potassium deficiency causing hypokalemia-related pathology is not likely because of its abundance in foods. However, chronic low potassium intake not causing hypokalemia has been associated with hypertension, cardiovascular disease (stroke and coronary heart disease), cardiovascular mortality, and bone loss. Calcium deficiency causing pathological disorders related to its critical cellular functions is unlikely, but a chronic low intake is associated with decreased bone mineral density and osteoporosis. Deficient intakes of magnesium apparently are common, but the pathological consequences of these deficient intakes have not been clearly established. Subclinical magnesium deficiency and subnormal serum or plasma magnesium concentrations have been associated with an increased risk for pathological conditions characterized by chronic inflammatory and/or oxidative stress, including cardiovascular disease, hypertension, osteoporosis, metabolic syndrome, and some cancers.

Excessive dietary intakes of sodium, phosphorus, and perhaps calcium have been associated with some pathological disorders. Sodium has been implicated in hypertension, hypertension-related cardiovascular diseases, renal diseases unrelated to blood pressure, gastric mucosal damage, gastric cancer, and bone mineralization that can result in osteoporosis. Excessive phosphorus intake has been associated with bone loss, kidney calcification, and increased all-cause and cardiovascular mortality and vascular calcification. High calcium intakes have been associated with an increased risk of cardiovascular disease, but this association has been disputed. Excessive magnesium intakes that cause pathological disorders are unlikely because diarrhea and abdominal cramping occur with intakes that are only a few times higher than the RDAs. High dietary potassium causing pathology is unlikely and is considered more as a therapeutic agent for such things as lowering blood pressure.

Calcium, magnesium, phosphorus, potassium, and sodium are essential nutrients for humans. Dietary recommendations for these nutrients for these foods should be followed because material summarized here indicates that intakes that are neither too low nor excessive are needed for health and well-being.

## REFERENCES

1. Weaver, CM, In: Bowman, BA, Russell, RM eds., *Present Knowledge in Nutrition*, 9th edn., Vol. 1, ISLI Press, Washington, DC, p. 373; 2006.
2. Awumey, EM, Bukoski, RD, In: Weaver, CM, Heaney, RP eds., *Calcium in Human Health*, Humana Press, Totowa, NJ, p. 13; 2006.
3. Weaver, CM, Heaney, RP, In: Shils, MP, Shike, M, Ross, AC, Caballero, B, Cousins, RJ eds., *Modern Nutrition in Health and Disease*, 10th edn., Lippincott Williams & Wilkins, Baltimore, MD, p. 194; 2006.
4. Rubin, C, Rubin, J, In: Favus, MJ ed., *Primer on the Metabolic Bone Diseases and Disorders of Mineral Metabolism*, 6th edn., American Society for Bone and Mineral Research, Washington, DC, p. 36; 2006.
5. Heaney, RP, In: Weaver, CM, Heaney, RP eds., *Calcium in Human Health*, Humana Press, Totowa, NJ, p. 7; 2006.
6. Dawson-Hughes, B, In: Holick, MF, Dawson-Hughes, B eds., *Nutrition and Bone Health*, Humana Press, Totowa, NJ, p. 197; 2004.
7. Cumming, RG, Nevitt, MC, *J Bone Miner Res* 12:1321;1997.
8. Shea, B, Wells, G, Cranny, A et al., *Endocr Rev* 23:552;2002.
9. Jackson RD, LaCroix, AZ, Gass, M et al., *N Engl J Med* 354:669;2006.
10. Bischoff-Ferrari, HA, Dawson-Hughes, B, Baron, JA et al., *Am J Clin Nutr* 86:1780;2007.
11. Bolland, MJ, Grey, A, Gamble, GD, Reid, IR, *Am J Clin Nutr* 94:1144;2011.
12. MacNeil, JA, Boyd, SK, *Med Eng Phys* 29:1096;2007.
13. Food and Nutrition board, Institute of Medicine, *Dietary Reference Intakes for Calcium, Phosphorus, Magnesium, Vitamin D, and Fluoride*, National Academy Press, Washington, DC, 432pp; 1997.
14. Wood, RJ, Zheng, JJ, *Am J Clin Nutr* 65:1803;1997.
15. Wood, RJ, Zheng, JJ, *J Nutr* 120:398;1990.
16. Hardwick, LL, Jones, MR, Brautbar, N, Lee, DBN, *J Nutr* 121;13;1991.
17. Kubena, KS, McIntosh, WA, Conboy-Downs, J et al., In: Halpern, MJ, Durlach, J eds., *Current Research in Magnesium*, John Libbey & Company, London, U.K., p. 343; 1996.
18. Bolland MJ, Barber PA, Doughty, RN et al., *BMJ* 336:262;2008.
19. Reid, IR, Bolland, MJ, Avenell, A, Grey, A, *Osteoporos* 22:1649;2011.
20. Bolland MJ, Avenell, A, Baron, JA et al., *BMJ* 341:c3691;2010.
21. Wang, L, Manson, JE, Song, Y, Sesso, HD, *Ann Intern Med* 152:315;2010.
22. McCarron, DA, *Am J Clin Nutr* 65(suppl):712S;1997.
23. Bostick, RM, Kushi, LH, Wu, Y et al., *Am J Epidemiol* 149:151;1999.
24. Kaluza, J, Orsini, N, Levitan, EB et al., *Am J Epidemiol* 171:801;2010.
25. Weaver, CM, Proulx, WR, Heaney R, *Am J Clin Nutr* 70(suppl):543S;1999.
26. Weaver, CM, Heaney, RP, In: Weaver, CM, Heaney, RP eds., *Calcium in Human Health*, Humana Press, Totowa, NJ, p. 129; 2006.
27. Heaney, RP, In: Marcus, R, Feldman, D, Nelson, DA, Rosen, CJ eds., *Osteoporosis*, Elsevier, Amsterdam, the Netherlands, p. 799; 2008.
28. Cao, J, Nielsen, FH, *Cur Opin Clin Nutr Metab Care* 13:698;2010.
29. Spencer, H, Kramer, L, Norris, C, Osis, D, *Am J Clin Nutr* 36:32;1982.
30. Food and Nutrition Board, Institute of Medicine, *Dietary Reference Intakes for Calcium and Vitamin D*, National Academies Press, Washington, DC, 1132pp.; 2011.
31. Uenishi, K, Ishida, H, Kamei, A et al., *Osteoporos Int* 12:858;2001.
32. Hunt, CD, Johnson, LK, *Am J Clin Nutr* 86:1054;2007.
33. Nordin BEC, Morris, HA, *Am J Clin Nutr* 93:442;2011.
34. Zhou, J, Zhao, L-J, Watson, P et al., *Nutr Metab* 7:62;2010.
35. Shahar, DR, Schwarzfuchs, D, Fraser, D et al., *Am J Clin Nutr* 92:1017;2010.

36. Onakpoya, IJ, Perry, R, Zhang, J, Ernst, E, *Nutr Rev* 69:335;2011.
37. Nielsen, FH, In: Bruulsema, T, Heffer, P, Welch, R, Cakmak, I, Moran, K eds., *Fertilizing Crops to Improve Human Health: A Scientific Review*, Vol. 2, *Functional Foods*, IFA-IPNI Scientific Publications, Paris, France, p. 123; 2012.
38. Rude, RK, Shils, ME, In: Shils, MP, Shike, M, Ross, AC, Caballero, B, Cousins, RJ eds., *Modern Nutrition in Health and Disease*, 10th edn., Lippincott Williams & Wilkins, Baltimore, MD, p. 223; 2006.
39. Volpe, SL, In: Bowman, BA, Russell, RM eds., *Present Knowledge in Nutrition*, 9th edn., Vol. 1, ISLI Press, Washington, DC, p. 400; 2006.
40. Nielsen, FH, *Nutr Rev* 68:333;2010.
41. Ma, J, Folsom, AR, Melnick, SL et al., *J Clin Epidemol* 48:927;1995.
42. Abbott, RD, Ando, F, Masaki, KH et al., *Am J Cardiol* 92:665;2003.
43. Chiuve, SE, Korngold, EC, Januzzi, JL et al., *Am J Clin Nutr* 93:253;2011.
44. Zhang, W, Iso, H, Ohira, T et al., *Atherosclerosis* 221:587;2012.
45. Touyz, RM, *Mol Aspects Med* 24:107;2003.
46. Kass, L, Weekes, J, Carpenter, L, *Eur J Clin Nutr* 66:411;2012.
47. Rude, RK, Singer, FR, Gruber, HE, *J Am Coll Nutr* 28:131;2009.
48. He, K, Liu, K, Daviglus, ML, *Circulation* 113:1675;2006.
49. Belin, RJ, He, K, *Magnes Res* 20:107;2007.
50. Bo, S, Pisu, E, *Curr Opin Lipidol* 19:50;2008.
51. Rayssiguier, Y, Libako, P, Nowacki, W, Rock, E, *Magnes Res* 23:73;2010.
52. Barbagallo, M, Dominguez, LJ, Galioto, A et al., *Mol Aspects Med* 24:39;2003.
53. Chaudhary, DP, Sharma, R, Bansal, DD, *Biol Trace Elem Res* 134:119;2010.
54. Kim, DJ, Xun, P, Liu, K et al., *Diabetes Care* 33:2604;2010.
55. Larsson, SC, Bergkvist, L, Wolk, A, *J Am Med Assoc* 293:86;2005.
56. Leone, N, Courbon, D, Ducimetiere, P, Zureik, M, *Epidemiology* 17:308;2006.
57. Dai, Q, Shrubsole, MJ, Ness, RM et al., *Am J Clin Nutr* 86:743;2007.
58. Kesavan, Y, Giovannucci, E, Fuchs, CS, Michaud, DS, *Am J Epidemiol* 171:233;2010.
59. Landon, RA, Young, EA, *J Am Diet Assoc* 93:674;1993.
60. Beckstrand, RL, Pickens, JS, *J Evid Based Complementary Altern Med* 16:181;2011.
61. Reungjui, S, Prasongwatana, V, Premgamone, A et al., *BJU Int* 90:635;2002.
62. Hotamisligil, GS, *Nature* 444:860;2006.
63. Libbey, P, *Nutr Rev* 65(suppl):S140;2007.
64. King, DE, Mainous, AG III, Geesey, ME, Woolson, RF, *J Am Coll Nutr* 24:166;2005.
65. King, DE, Mainous, AG III, Geesey, ME, Ellis, T, *Magnes Res* 20:32;2007.
66. Bo, S, Durazzo, M, Guidi, M et al., *Am J Clin Nutr* 84:1062;2006.
67. Song, Y, Li, TY, van Dam, RM et al., *Am J Clin Nutr* 85:1068;2007.
68. Chacko, SA, Song, Y, Nathan, L et al., *Diabetes Care* 33:304;2010.
69. Nielsen, FH, Johnson, LK, Zeng, H, *Magnes Res* 23:158;2010.
70. Rodriguez-Morán, M, Guerrero-Romero, F, *Arch Dis Child* 93:676;2008.
71. Almozino-Sarafian, D, Berman, S, Mor, A et al., *Eur J Nutr* 46:230;2007.
72. Chacko, SA, Sul, J, Song, Y et al., *Am J Clin Nutr* 93:463;2011.
73. Mazur, A, Maier, JAM, Rock, E et al., *Arch Biochem Biophys* 458:48;2007.
74. Vormann, J, Günther, T, Höllriegl, V, Schümann, K, *Z Ernährungswiss* 37(suppl 1):92;1998.
75. Kramer, JH, Mak, IT, Phillips, TM, Weglicki, WB, *Exp Biol Med* 228:665;2003.
76. Lukaski, HC, Nielsen, FH, *J Nutr* 132:930;2002.
77. Nielsen, FH, *Magnes Res* 17:197;2004.
78. Nielsen, FH, Milne, DB, Klevay, LM et al. *J Am Coll Nutr* 26:121;2007.
79. Klevay, LM, Milne, DB, *Am J Clin Nutr* 75:550;2002.
80. Elin, RJ, *Magnes Res* 23:1;2010.
81. Matsuzaki, H, Katsumata, S-I, Uehara, M et al., *Magnes Res* 18:97;2005.
82. Spencer, H, Norris, C, Williams, D, *J Am Coll Nutr* 13:479;1994.
83. Nielsen, FH, Milne, DB, *Eur J Clin Nutr* 58:703l;2004.
84. Hunt, MS, Schofield, FA, *Am J Clin Nutr* 22:367;1969.
85. Schwarz, R, Walker, G, Linz, MD, MacKellar, I, *Am J Clin Nutr* 26:510;1973.
86. Hunt, CD, Johnson, LK, *Am J Clin Nutr* 84:843;2006.
87. Tong, GM, Rude, RK, *Intensive Care Med* 20:3;2005.
88. Rosanoff, A, *Magnes Res* 23:27;2010
89. Park, H, Parker, GL, Boardman, CH et al., *Support Care Cancer* 19:859;2011.
90. Anderson, JJB, Klemmer, PJ, Watts, ML et al., In: Bowman, BA, Russell, RM eds., *Present Knowledge in Nutrition*, 9th edn., Vol. 1, ISLI Press, Washington, DC, pp. 383; 2006.
91. Knochel, JP, In: Shils, MP, Shike, M, Ross, AC, Caballero, B, Cousins, RJ eds., *Modern Nutrition in Health and Disease*, 10th edn., Lippincott Williams & Wilkins, Baltimore, MD, p. 211; 2006.
92. Shapses, SA, In: Stipanuk, MH, Caudill, MA eds., *Biochemical, Physiological, and Molecular Aspects of Human Nutrition*, 3rd edn., Elsevier Saunders, St. Louis, MO, p. 721; 2013.
93. Lotz, M, Zisman, E, Bartter, FC, *N Engl J Med* 278:409;1968.
94. Kreider, RB, In: Driskell, J, Wolinsky, I eds., *Macroelements, Water, and Electrolytes in Sports Nutrition*, CRC Press, Boca Raton, FL, p. 29; 1999.
95. Calvo, MS, Park YK, *J Nutr* 126:1168S;1996.
96. Anderson, JJB, *J Nutr Biochem* 2:300;1991.
97. Sax, L, *J Am Coll Nutr* 20:271;2001.
98. Matsuzaki, H, Uehara, M, Suzuki, K et al., *J Nutr Sci Vitaminol* 43:627; 1997.
99. Kooienga, L, *Semin Dial* 20:342;2007.
100. Razzaque, MH, *Clin Sci (Lond)* 120:91;2011.
101. Dhingra, R, Sullivan, LM, Fox, CS et al., *Arch Intern Med* 167:879;2007.
102. Elmstähl, S, Gullberg, B, Janson, L et al., *Osteoporos Int* 8:333;1998.
103. Huesa, C, Yadav, MC, Jinnilä, MAJ, *Bone* 48:1066;2011.
104. Sheng, H-P, In: Stipanuk, MH, Caudill, MA eds., *Biochemical, Physiological, and Molecular Aspects of Human Nutrition*, 3rd edn., Elsevier Saunders, St. Louis, MO, p. 759; 2013.
105. Preuss, HG, In: Bowman, BA, Russell, RM eds., *Present Knowledge in Nutrition*, 9th edn., Vol. 1, ISLI Press, Washington, DC, p. 409; 2006.
106. Food and Nutrition Board, Institute of Medicine, *Dietary Reference Intakes for Water, Potassium, Sodium, Chloride, and Sulfate*, National Academies Press, Washington, DC, 617pp.; 2005.
107. Krishna, GG, Kapoor, SC, *Ann Int Med* 115:77;1991.

108. He, F, MacGregor G, *Physiol Plant* 133:725;2008.

109. Chang, H-Y, Hu, Y-W, Yue, C-SJ et al., *Am J Clin Nutr* 83:1289;2006.

110. Braschi A. Naismith DJ, *Br J Nutr* 99;1284;2008.

111. Sasaki, S, Yanagibori, R, *J Nutr Sci Vitaminol* 47:289;2001.

112. Tucker, KL, Hannan, MT, Kiel, DP, *Eur J Nutr* 40:231;2001.

113. Morris, RC Jr, Frassetto, LA, Schmidlin O et al., In: Burckhardt, P, Dawson-Hughes, B, Heaney, RP eds., *Nutritional Aspects of Osteoporosis*, Academic Press, San Diego, CA, p. 357; 2001.

114. New, SA, MacDonald, HM, Campbell, MK et al., *Am J Clin Nutr* 79:131;2004.

115. MacDonald, HM, New, SA, Fraser, MK et al., *Am J Clin Nutr* 81:923;2005.

116. Sellmeyer, DS, Schloetter, M, Sebastian, A, *J Clin Endocrinol Metab* 87:2008;2002.

117. Dawson-Hughes, B, Harris, SS, Palermo, NJ et al., *J Clin Endocrinol Metab* 94:96;2009.

118. Macdonald, HM, Black, AJ, Aucott, L et al., *Am J Clin Nutr* 88:465;2008.

119. Lanham-New, SA, *J Nutr* 138:172S;2008.

120. Chatterjee, R, Yeh, H-C, Shafi, T et al., *Am J Clin Nutr* 93:1087;2011.

121. Fliser, D, Nowack, R, Allendorf-Ostwald, N et al. *Am J Hypertens* 6:320;1993.

122. Egan, BM, Lackland, DT, *Am J Med Sci* 320:233;2000.

123. Stolarz-Skrzypek, K. Kuznetsova, T, Thijs, L et al., *J Am Med Assoc* 305:1777;2011.

# 13 Trace Mineral Deficiencies

*Forrest H. Nielsen*

## CONTENTS

## INTRODUCTION

By 1940, the concept of essential nutrients was well established. They were defined as chemical substances found in food that could not be synthesized by the body to perform functions necessary for life. In the 1960s and 1970s, the standard for essentiality was liberalized for mineral elements because it was hypothesized that diets could not be made low enough in some elements to cause death or interrupt the life cycle (interfere with growth, development, or maturation such that procreation is prevented). Thus, during this time period, an accepted definition of an essential mineral element was one whose dietary deficiency consistently and adversely changed a biological function from optimal, and this change was preventable or reversible by physiological or nutritional amounts of the element. This definition of essentiality became less acceptable when numerous elements were suggested to be essential based on small physiological or biochemical differences in experimental models fed low and supplemental (some possibly supra nutritional) amounts of the elements.

These differences were regularly questioned to be indicative of a suboptimal function and alternatively suggested to be the consequence of a pharmacologic action, a toxic response, or an effect on intestinal organisms. This resulted in the present conviction that a mineral element cannot be considered essential unless it has a defined biochemical function if its lack cannot be shown to cause death or interrupt the life cycle. However, some elements (e.g., chromium) that do not meet the current definition of essentiality are occasionally still indicated as essential in current literature because they were ingrained as so by using the older definition of essentiality in the 1960s and 1970s. Some mineral elements have defined biochemical functions in lower species (e.g., nickel) or have been found to interrupt the life cycle in only a limited number of vertebrates (e.g., boron) and thus are occasionally designated as essential. Some elements (e.g., vanadium) have beneficial actions when supplemented in supra nutritional amounts. These findings suggest that some mineral elements other than those firmly established as essential might be of nutritional importance. Thus, changes in both higher animals and humans consuming low and apparently nutritional amounts (amounts normally found in food) of these elements will be described here.

## BIOLOGICAL ROLES OF TRACE MINERALS

Trace elements have at least five roles in living organisms. In close association with enzymes, some trace elements are integral parts of catalytic centers at which the reactions for life occur. Working in concert with a protein, and frequently with other organic coenzymes, trace elements are involved in attracting substrate molecules and converting them into specific end products. Some trace elements donate or accept electrons in reactions of reduction or oxidation. In addition to the generation and utilization of metabolic energy, redox reactions frequently involve the chemical transformation of molecules. One trace element, iron, is involved in binding, transporting, and releasing oxygen. Some trace elements have structural roles, that is, imparting stability and 3D structure to important biological molecules. Some trace elements have regulatory roles. They control important biological processes through actions such as making hormones active, facilitating the binding of molecules to receptor sites on cell membranes, altering the structure or ionic nature of membranes to prevent or allow specific molecules to enter a cell, and inducing gene expression.

## HOMEOSTATIC REGULATION OF TRACE MINERALS

*Homeostasis* is the term used to describe the ability to maintain the content of a specific substance within a certain range in the body despite varying intakes. Homeostasis involves the processes of absorption, storage, and excretion. The relative importance of each of these processes varies among the trace elements. The amount absorbed from the gastrointestinal tract often is a primary controlling factor for trace elements needed in the cationic state such as copper, iron, and zinc. Trace elements absorbed as negatively charged anions (e.g., boron, fluoride, and selenium) are usually absorbed quite freely and completely from the gastrointestinal tract. Excretion through the urine, bile, sweat, and breath becomes the primary homeostatic control mechanism for these elements. By being stored in inactive sites, some trace elements are prevented from causing adverse effects when absorbed in high amounts. Examples of this homeostatic mechanism include the storage of iron as ferritin and fluoride in bone. Release of a trace element from a storage site also can help prevent deficiency.

## FACTORS AFFECTING THE MANIFESTATION OF DEFICIENCY SIGNS

Although trace elements play key roles in a variety of processes necessary for life, except for iodine, iron, and zinc, the occurrence of overt, simple, or uncomplicated deficiency of any trace element does not commonly occur in humans. Homeostatic mechanisms and consumption of diets with different types of foods from different sources are primary reasons for the low occurrence. However, impaired health and well-being caused by a suboptimal status for some trace elements probably are not uncommon because other factors may affect their metabolism or utilization. Deficiencies of several trace elements can be of concern when their metabolism or utilization is impaired or need is increased by nutritional, metabolic, hormonal, or physiological stressors. In addition, genetic errors or missense variants, diseases, and drugs that affect absorption, retention, or excretion of a trace element can result in a deficiency, even though intake meets dietary guidelines set for healthy people.

## TREATMENT OF TRACE MINERAL DEFICIENCIES

The preferred method to treat or prevent trace element deficiencies is by consuming a variety of nutrient-dense foods. A diet based on the USDA MyPlate[1] is an example of one that is likely to provide trace minerals in adequate amounts. If it is decided that a mineral supplement is needed to overcome a deficiency or for "insurance" to prevent deficiency, consuming those that supply is the recommended dietary allowance (RDA) or adequate intake (AI) of minerals[2-4] should be adequate. Such an intake will not result in one that exceeds the upper intake level (UL), which is the maximum level of daily intake likely to pose no risk of adverse effects. The UL is attestation that all mineral elements are toxic when ingested in excessive amounts. Intakes higher than the RDA might be indicated if a deficiency is caused by a factor that induces malabsorption or excessive excretion of a mineral. These intakes should be adjusted to maintain normal status after indicators of deficiency have abated.

## ESSENTIAL TRACE ELEMENTS

The evidence for essentially for humans is substantial and noncontroversial for the elements included in this section. Specific biochemical functions have been found for each of these elements. Because magnesium has many characteristics of a trace element, it will be included in this group of elements.

### COBALT

Ionic cobalt is not an essential nutrient for humans. However, vitamin $B_{12}$, in which cobalt is an integral component, is an essential nutrient for humans. In the nineteenth century, a megaloblastic anemia was described that was called pernicious anemia because it was invariably fatal. The first effective treatment for this disease was one pound of raw liver daily. In 1948, the antipernicious anemia factor, vitamin $B_{12}$, in liver was isolated and found to contain 4% cobalt. Severe dietary deficiency of vitamin $B_{12}$ causing anemia and neurological disorders is rare because of the widespread consumption of foods of animal origin or meat substitutes that often contain supplemental vitamin $B_{12}$. However, mild vitamin $B_{12}$ deficiency is recognized as highly prevalent in countries where the availability of foods of animal origin is limited. Otherwise, vitamin $B_{12}$ deficiency

## TABLE 13.1
### Biochemical, Clinical, and Nutritional Aspects of Cobalt

| | |
|---|---|
| *Biological function* | Vitamin $B_{12}$ is a cofactor for two enzymes, methionine synthase that methylates homocysteine to form methionine and methylmalonyl CoA mutase that converts L-methylmalonyl CoA, formed by the oxidation of odd-chain fatty acids, to succinyl CoA |
| *Signs and symptoms of deficiency* | |
| Biochemical | Decreased erythrocyte and plasma folate and plasma vitamin $B_{12}$ and increased plasma homocysteine and urinary formiminoglutamate and methylmalonate |
| Physiological | Megaloblastic anemia; spinal cord demyelination and peripheral neuropathy |
| *Pathological consequences of deficiency* | |
| Established | Pernicious anemia, memory loss, dementia, depression, irreversible neurological disease called subacute combined degeneration of the spinal cord; death |
| Suggested | Cardiovascular disease associated with elevated plasma homocysteine |
| *Predisposing factors for deficiency* | Factors causing malabsorption including atrophic gastritis, *Helicobacter pylori* infection, GI bacteria overgrowth, achlorhydria, total or partial gastric resection or bypass, ileal disease or resection, chronic inflammatory disease of the ileum (e.g., Crohn's disease, tropical sprue), pancreatic insufficiency, and celiac disease |
| | Factors inhibiting utilization including drugs such as histamine $H_2$-receptor antagonists, proton-pump inhibitors, oral biguanides (used in the treatment of type II diabetes), and nitrous oxide anesthesia |
| *Recommended intakes* | |
| Prevention of deficiency | RDAs and AIs (in parenthesis) set by the Food and Nutrition Board[79] (µg/day): infants 0–0.5 year, (0.4) and 0.5–1 year, (0.5); children 1–3 years, 0.9, 4–8 years, 1.2, and 9–13 years, 1.8; males ≥14 years, 2.4; females ≥14 years, 2.4; pregnant, 2.6; and lactating, 2.8 |
| Therapeutic or beneficial | Milligram doses are used to treat vitamin $B_{12}$ malabsorption and deficiency; a common dose is 1 mg/day of cobalamin |
| *Food sources* | Meat, dairy products, some seafoods, and fortified cereals |

most commonly occurs through a defect in its absorption caused by such factors as gastric or ileal disease or resection. Most of the information in Table 13.1 was obtained from reviews by Stabler[5] and Caudill et al.[6]

## COPPER

Although copper is well established as an essential trace element, the prevalence of its dietary deficiency causing pathology in otherwise healthy people has not been resolved. Well-established consequences of copper deprivation in humans have come mainly from special populations whose sources of intake contained limited amounts of copper (e.g., parenteral nutrition solutions, milk, or formulas with no supplemental copper), consuming drugs (e.g., penicillamine), undergoing dialysis resulting in excessive loss of copper, gastric bypass surgery, or having a genetic disorder (e.g., Menkes' disease) that results in defective copper metabolism. Other consequences of inadequate copper intakes for humans such as cardiovascular disease have been hypothesized from epidemiological, animal, and short-term copper deprivation studies. Most of the information in Table 13.2 was obtained from reviews by Uauy et al.,[7] Beshgetoor and Hambidge,[8] Cordano,[9] Saari and Schuschke,[10] Klevay,[11] Prohaska,[12] and Harvey et al.[13]

## IODINE

Recognition that iodine is nutritionally important began in 1907 when it was found that iodine prevented goiter. In the 1920s, goiter prophylaxis through salt iodization began, which eventually resulted in a marked reduction in iodine

deficiency worldwide. However, iodine deficiency is still one of the largest public health problems in the world today. Iodine deficiency is most prevalent in areas of high new mountains (e.g., Himalayas, Andes, and Alps); areas of frequent flooding, rainfall, and sublimation (e.g., Ganges river plain of northeastern India, Taklamakan desert of western China, and central sub-Saharan Africa); and inland areas of central and Eastern Europe. Most of the information in Table 13.3 was obtained from reviews by Zimmerman[14] and Pearce and Freake.[15]

## IRON

Iron has the longest and best-documented history among the mineral elements. Despite extensive and effective intervention activities, iron deficiency is the most prevalent mineral deficiency in the United States and the world. Table 13.4 only briefly outlines some of the important aspects of iron nutrition that was obtained from reviews by Beard[16] and Crichton.[17]

## MAGNESIUM

Magnesium is the fourth most abundant cation in the human body and is second only to potassium in intracellular concentration. This concentration reflects that magnesium is critical for a large number of cellular functions including oxidative phosphorylation, glycolysis, DNA transcription, fatty acid degradation, and protein synthesis. Although it is critically important, reported signs and symptoms of magnesium deficiency attributed to dietary restriction alone are surprisingly limited. Described cases of clinical magnesium

**TABLE 13.2**
**Biochemical, Clinical, and Nutritional Aspects of Copper**

| | |
|---|---|
| *Biological function* | Copper is an essential cofactor for the enzymes amine oxidase, ceruloplasmin, cytochrome *c* oxidase, dopamine-β-monooxygenase, extracellular superoxide dismutase, hephaestin, lysyl oxidase, peptidylglycine-α-amidating monooxygenase, superoxide dismutase 1, and tyrosinase. Thus, copper is essential for several fundamental processes including angiogenesis, neuropeptide signaling, iron metabolism, oxygen transport, energy production, antioxidant defense, and immune function |
| *Signs and symptoms of deficiency* | |
| Biochemical | Decreased serum copper and, in severe deficiency, decreased ceruloplasmin |
| | Other potential markers include copper chaperone for superoxide dismutase (CCS)/superoxide dismutase ratio in erythrocytes and cytochrome *c* oxidase in platelets |
| Physiological | Signs of copper deficiency in premature and malnourished infants and infants with Menkes' disease include hematologic changes characterized by hypochromic, normocytic, or macrocytic anemia accompanied by reduced reticulocyte count, neutropenia count, and thrombocytopenia count; bone abnormalities mimicking those found with scurvy, including osteoporosis, bone fractures, spur formation, subperiosteal new bone formation; hypopigmentation of hair; and impaired growth, immunity, and neurological function |
| *Pathological consequences of deficiency* | |
| Established | *Premature and malnourished infants*: anemia, osteoporosis, bone fractures, poor growth, and increased infections |
| | *Menkes' disease*: "kinky" steely hair, progressive neurological disorder, and death |
| Suggested | *Fetus and children*: impaired brain development |
| | *Adults*: osteoporosis, ischemic heart disease, and increased susceptibility to infections |
| *Predisposing factors for deficiency* | |
| Impaired absorption | High intakes of zinc, celiac disease, short bowel syndrome, cystic fibrosis, diarrhea, and jejunoileal bypass surgery |
| Excessive loss | Peritoneal dialysis, burn trauma, penicillamine therapy, dexamethasone treatment, and excessive use of antacids |
| Increased oxidative stress | High iron intake or iron overload and marginal zinc deprivation |
| *Recommended intakes* | |
| Prevention of deficiency | RDAs and AIs (in parenthesis) set by the Food and Nutrition Board[4] (mg/day): infants 0–0.5 year, (0.20), and 0.5–1 year, (0.22); children 1–3 years, 0.34, and 4–8 years, 0.44; adolescents 9–13 years, 0.70, and 14–18 years, 0.89; adults, 0.90; pregnancy, 1.0; lactation, 1.3 |
| Therapeutic or beneficial | Increased intakes of copper (e.g., 3 mg/day for adults) might be beneficial for overcoming the adverse effects of high zinc intake and more quickly overcoming copper deficiency |
| *Food sources* | Legumes, whole grains, nuts, organ meats (e.g., liver), seafood (e.g., oysters, crab), peanut butter, chocolate mushrooms, and ready-to-eat cereal |

deficiency generally have been conditioned deficiencies where factors interfering with absorption or promoting excretion were present. However, short-term human magnesium deprivation experiments suggest that low magnesium intakes similar to those consumed by a significant number of people might induce heart arrhythmias and cause soft tissue calcium retention that could exacerbate disorders induced by chronic inflammatory and/or oxidative stress.[18,19] Table 13.5 briefly outlines some of the important aspects of magnesium deficiency, most of which were obtained by reviews by Leone et al.,[20] Beckstrand and Pickens,[21] Larsson et al.,[22] and Vormann.[23]

## MANGANESE

The essentiality of manganese for animals has been known for over 80 years. Deficiency causes testicular degeneration (rats), slipped tendons (chicks), osteodystrophy, severe glucose intolerance (guinea pig), ataxia (mice, mink), depigmentation of hair, and seizures.[24] Manganese activates numerous enzymes and is a constituent of several metalloenzymes.

One enzyme, manganese superoxide dismutase is essential for life; a deletion mutation in mice results in death within 5–21 days of birth.[25] The neonatal mice exhibit myocardial injury, neurodegeneration, lipid peroxidation, fatty liver, anemia, and severe mitochondrial damage. Descriptions of signs of manganese deficiency in humans are very limited. The most convincing case of manganese deficiency is that of a child with a postoperative short bowel on long-term parenteral nutrition with low manganese content. The child developed short stature and diffuse bone demineralization resulting in brittle bones.[26] However, a low manganese status has been associated with osteoporosis, diabetes, epilepsy, atherosclerosis, impaired wound healing, and cataracts.[27] Recently, decreased plasma manganese and associated increased nitric oxide have been associated with childhood asthma[28] and Alzheimer's disease.[29] In addition, low maternal blood manganese concentration has been associated with increased risk of low birth weight and fetal intrauterine growth retardation.[30] Most of the information in Table 13.6 was obtained from reviews by Freeland-Graves and Llanes,[24] Leach and Harris,[31] and Nielsen.[32]

## TABLE 13.3
## Biochemical, Clinical, and Nutritional Aspects of Iodine

| | |
|---|---|
| *Biological function* | Iodine is a component of thyroid hormones, which have an impact on a wide range of metabolic and developmental functions. |
| *Signs and symptoms of deficiency* | |
| Biochemical | Decreased plasma or serum thyroxine ($T_4$) and triiodothyronine ($T_3$) and urinary iodine and increased plasma or serum thyroid stimulating hormone (TSH) and cholesterol. |
| Physiological | Decreased metabolic rate; increased heart rate, size, stroke volume, and output; reduced muscle mass and delayed skeletal maturation; abnormal production of glial cells and myelinogenesis and goiter. |
| *Pathological consequences of deficiency* | |
| Established | The large spectrum of deficiency disorders include fetal congenital anomalies and perinatal mortality; neurological cretinism characterized by mental deficiency, deaf-mutism, spastic diplegia, and squint; psychomotor defects; fatigue and slowing of bodily and mental functions; weight increase and cold intolerance caused by slowing of the metabolic rate. |
| Suggested | Increased risk for mammary dysplasia and fibrocystic breast disease, impaired immune response, and increased risk of gastric cancer. |
| *Predisposing factors for deficiency* | Residence in an area with low soil iodine. |
| *Recommended intakes* | |
| Prevention of deficiency | RDAs and AIs (in parenthesis) set by the Food and Nutrition Board[4] (µg/day): infants 0–0.5 year, (110), and 0.5–1 year, (130); children 1–8 years, 90, and 9–13 years, 120; males ≥14 years, 150; females ≥14 years, 150; pregnant, 220; lactating, 290. |
| Therapeutic or beneficial | Iodized oil, which has fatty acids chemically modified by iodination, slowly releases iodine over a period of month or years in the body. In populations with a high prevalence of severe iodine-deficiency disorders, iodized oil providing 200–400 mg of iodine administered orally or by injection provides long-term protection against deficiency. A dose of potassium iodide or iodate providing 30 mg monthly or 8 mg biweekly is an effective prophylaxis for deficiency. |
| *Food sources* | Iodized salt has been the major method for assuring adequate iodine intake since the 1920s. Other sources are seafoods and foods from plants grown in high-iodine soils. |

## TABLE 13.4
## Biochemical, Clinical, and Nutritional Aspects of Iron

| | |
|---|---|
| *Biological function* | Iron is involved in oxygen transport and storage, in electron transport, and in numerous enzymatic reactions. The classes of enzymes dependent on iron for activity include the oxidoreductases (e.g., xanthine oxidase/dehydrogenase), monooxygenases (e.g., cytochrome P450), dioxygenases (e.g., amino acid or amine dioxygenases), lipoxygenases, peroxidases, fatty acid desaturases, nitric oxide synthases, and miscellaneous enzymes such as aconitase. |
| *Sign and symptoms of deficiency* | |
| Biochemical | Decreased tissue and blood iron enzymes, myoglobin, hemoglobin, ferritin, transferrin saturation, and iron and increased erythrocyte protoporphyrin. |
| Physiological | Anemia, glossitis, angular stomatitis, spoon nails (koilonychia), blue sclera, lethargy, apathy, listlessness, and fatigue. |
| *Pathological consequences of deficiency* | |
| Established | Impaired thermoregulation, immune function, mental function, and physical performance and complications in pregnancy including increased risk of premature delivery, low birth weight, infant mortality, and impaired brain development. |
| Suggested | Osteoporosis.[80–82] |
| *Predisposing factors for deficiency* | Blood loss (e.g., menstruation, gastrointestinal disease, and nonsteroidal anti-inflammatory drug use) and inhibitors of iron absorption (vegetarian diets high in phytates, polyphenols, calcium, and fiber). |
| *Recommended intakes* | |
| Prevention of deficiency | RDAs and AIs (in parenthesis) set by the Food and Nutrition Board[4] (mg/day): infants 0.05 year, (0.27), and 0.5–1 year, 11; children 1–3 years, 7, and 4–8 years, 10; adolescents 9–13 years, 8; males 14–18 years, 11, and females 14–18 years, 15; males ≥19 years, 8; females 19–50 years, 18, and >50 years, 8; pregnant, 27; lactating ≤18 years, 10, and ≥19 years, 9. |
| Therapeutic or beneficial | Short-term higher doses than the RDAs may be given to more quickly overcome iron deficiency, usually caused by blood loss; doses used include 50–60 mg/day or 120 mg/week. Long-term high intakes of iron have been associated with increased risk of cardiovascular disease and cancer. |
| *Food sources* | Red meat, organ meats (e.g., liver), seafood (e.g., oysters, shrimp), fortified cereals, potatoes with skin, and tofu; some whole grains and vegetables (e.g., spinach) are high in iron, but the bioavailability of this iron may be low. |

**TABLE 13.5**

**Biochemical, Clinical, and Nutritional Aspects of Magnesium**

| | |
|---|---|
| *Biological function* | Magnesium is a cofactor for more than 300 enzymes in the body. This cofactor role is either as a direct allosteric activator of enzymes or as a part of a substrate (e.g., MgATP and MgGTP) in enzyme reactions. Magnesium also has functions that affect membrane properties and thus influences potassium and calcium channels and nerve conduction |
| *Signs and symptoms of deficiency* | |
| Biochemical | Excessive renal potassium excretion; low blood calcium, magnesium, and potassium; impaired parathyroid hormone secretion and vitamin D metabolism; renal and skeletal resistance to parathyroid hormone; decreased intracellular potassium |
| Physiological | Neuromuscular symptoms (e.g., positive Trousseau's signs, tremors, fasciculations, muscle spasms, cramps and weakness, seizures, dizziness, disequilibrium); electrocardiographic abnormalities and cardiac dysrhythmias, which include tachycardia, premature beats, and fibrillation |
| *Pathological consequences of deficiency* | |
| Established | Conditioned deficiencies result in cardiac arrhythmias, seizures, cramps, depression, and psychosis |
| Suggested | Based on numerous epidemiological studies and magnesium supplementation trials, low magnesium status is associated with numerous disorders including coronary heart disease, stroke, hypertension, diabetes, osteoporosis, asthma, migraine headaches, preeclampsia, and some cancers |
| *Predisposing factors for deficiency* | Factors interfering with absorption and utilization or promoting excretion including alcoholism, kidney failure, malabsorption syndromes, extensive bowel resection, gastroilieal bypass, severe or prolonged diarrhea, protein–calorie malnutrition, acute pancreatitis, hyperaldosteronism, diabetes mellitus, thyroid gland disease, hyperparathyroidism, vitamin D resistance or deficiency, burns, drugs (e.g., diuretics, proton-pump inhibitors), and high calcium and phosphorus intakes |
| *Recommended intakes* | |
| Prevention of deficiency | RDAs and AIs (in parenthesis) set by the Food and Nutrition Board[2] (mg/day): infants 0.5 year, (30) and 0.5–1 year, 75; children 1–3 years, 80, 4–8 years, 130, and 9–13 years, 240; males 14–18 years, 410, 19–30 years, 400, and ≥31 years, 420; females 14–18 years, 360, 19–30 years, 310, ≥31 years, 320; pregnant +40 for each age group |
| Therapeutic or beneficial | Infusion of magnesium has been indicated as a means to quickly overcome symptoms of magnesium deficiency. For example, a reported effective treatment is intravenous administration of 24 mmol of magnesium as a 50% solution over 24 h for 3–7 days.[83] Patients who are hypomagnesemic and have seizures or acute dysrhythmia may be given 4–8 mmol of magnesium over 5–10 min followed by the same regimen |
| *Food sources* | Whole grains, nuts, legumes, green leafy vegetables |

## MOLYBDENUM

Because molybdenum is a cofactor for some enzymes, its essentiality is well established. However, molybdenum deficiency has not been unequivocally identified in humans other than in an individual nourished by total parenteral nutrition and in individuals with inborn errors of metabolism that affect the synthesis of the molybdenum cofactor present in molybdoenzymes. Thus, molybdenum is not considered a practical concern in human nutrition. The information in Table 13.7 was obtained primarily from reviews by Nielsen[32,33] and Novotny.[34]

## SELENIUM

Although selenium was first suggested to be essential in 1957, it was not firmly established as so until a biochemical role was identified in 1972. The first report of human selenium deficiency appeared in 1979; the subject resided in an area with low-selenium soil and, after surgery, was receiving total parenteral nutrition low in selenium. Subsequent findings of selenium-responsive disorders, including Keshan disease and cancer, suggest that some people might benefit from an increased intake of selenium. The information earlier and in Table 13.8 was obtained primarily from reviews by Sunde[35] and Combs.[36]

## ZINC

Signs of zinc deficiency in humans were first described in the 1960s. However, the prevalence of zinc deficiency is still not well established, but is thought to be one of the most common trace element deficiencies in the world. Zinc supplementation studies indicate that a mild zinc deficiency that results in growth retardation, diarrhea, and/or impaired immune function might be quite prevalent.[37] Unquestionable zinc deficiency has been induced by zinc-deficient total parenteral nutrition, by short-term experimental human deprivation experiments, and by feeding cow's milk to infants who have a genetic inability to absorb zinc from this source. The information in Table 13.9 primarily comes from reviews by Prasad,[38] Dibley,[39] Bray and Levy,[40] and Cousins.[41]

## BENEFICIAL BIOACTIVE TRACE ELEMENTS

In humans and higher animals dietary deprived of these elements, supplements in nutritional or physiological amounts result in beneficial effects. In addition, beneficial bioactivity of some of these elements is supported by being found essential in lower forms of life or being a component of known biologically important molecules in some life form.

## TABLE 13.6
## Biochemical, Clinical, and Nutritional Aspects of Manganese

| | |
|---|---|
| *Biological function* | Manganese is a cofactor for enzymes involved in protein and energy metabolism, antioxidant action, and mucopolysaccharide synthesis. These enzymes include the metalloenzymes, superoxide dismutase 2, pyruvate carboxylase and arginase, and the manganese-activated enzymes, phosphoenolpyruvate carboxykinase, glycosyl transferase, glutamine synthetase, and farnesyl pyrophosphate synthetase. Manganese also can activate numerous other enzymes including oxidoreductases, lyases, ligases, hydrolases, kinases, decarboxylases, and transferases; these enzymes are activated by other metals, especially magnesium. |
| *Signs and symptoms of deficiency* | |
| Biochemical | Possible signs are decreased cholesterol and increased serum alkaline phosphatase activity. |
| Physiological | Impaired growth and brittle bones (found in one child); another possible sign is fleeting dermatitis. |
| *Pathological consequences of deficiency* | |
| Established | Osteoporosis (one case report in a child). |
| Suggested | Low dietary manganese or low blood manganese and low tissue manganese have been associated with osteoporosis, diabetes, epilepsy, atherosclerosis, cataracts, asthma, Alzheimer's disease, impaired wound healing, low birth weight, and retarded intrauterine growth. |
| *Predisposing factors for deficiency* | High dietary intakes of calcium, phosphorus, iron, fiber, phytate, and polyphenols (based on human absorption experiments and animal studies). |
| *Recommended intakes* | |
| Prevention of deficiency | AIs set by the Food and Nutrition Board[4] (mg/day): infants 0–0.5 year (0.003) and 0.5–1 year (0.6); children 1–3 years (1.2) and 4–8 years (1.5); males age 9–13 years (1.9), 14–18 years (2.2), and ≥19 years (2.3); females 9–18 years (1.6), ≥19 years (1.8); pregnant (2.0); and lactating (2.6). |
| Therapeutic or beneficial | Caution is indicated against high intakes of manganese because of potential neurotoxicological effects, especially in people with compromised homeostatic mechanisms or infants whose homeostatic control of manganese is not fully developed. |
| *Food sources* | Unrefined grains, nuts, green leafy vegetables, and tea. |

## TABLE 13.7
## Biochemical, Clinical, and Nutritional Aspects of Molybdenum

| | |
|---|---|
| *Biological function* | For humans, molybdenum exists as a small nonprotein factor containing a pterin nucleus in at least four enzymes; these are aldehyde oxidase, xanthine oxidase/dehydrogenase, sulfite oxidase, and mitochondrial amidoxime-reducing component. Molybdoenzymes oxidize and detoxify various pyrimidines, purines, and pteridines; catalyze the transformation of hypoxanthine and xanthine to uric acid; and catalyze the conversion of sulfite to sulfate and might play a role in the detoxification of *N*-hydroxylated substrates. |
| *Signs and symptoms of deficiency* | |
| Biochemical | A patient on total parenteral nutrition exhibited hypermethioninemia, hypouricemia, hyperoxypurinemia, hypouricosuria, and low urinary sulfate excretion. |
| | Patients with inborn errors of molybdenum cofactor synthesis exhibit increased plasma and urine sulfite, sulfate, thiosulfate, *S*-sulfocysteine, taurine, and xanthine; increased serum *S*-sulfonated transthyretin; and decreased urine and serum uric acid. |
| Physiological | A total parenteral nutrition patient exhibited mental disturbances progressing to coma. Genetic errors patients exhibit seizures, brain atrophy/lesions, and failure to thrive. |
| *Pathological consequences of deficiency* | |
| Established | Patients with inborn errors of molybdenum cofactor synthesis exhibit mental retardation, dislocated lenses, and death at early age. |
| Suggested | Increased susceptibility to cancer,[84] diabetes,[85] and hypertension.[86] |
| *Predisposing factors for deficiency* | A high sulfur amino acid intake may increase the need for molybdenum. |
| *Recommended intakes* | |
| Prevention of deficiency | RDAs and AIs (in parenthesis) set by the Food and Nutrition Board[4] (μg/day): infants 0–0.5 year, (2) and 0.5–1 year (3); children and adolescents 1–3 years, 17, 4–8 years, 22, 9–13 years, 34, and 14–18 years, 43; adults, 45; pregnant and lactating females, 50. |
| Therapeutic or beneficial | High doses of tetrathiomolybdate inhibited some advanced and metastatic cancers dogs and humans[87] and hyperglycemia induced by streptozotocin in rats,[85] and sodium molybdate prevented hyperinsulinemia and hypertension induced by fructose in rats.[86] |
| *Food sources* | Milk and milk products, pulses, organ meats (e.g., liver and kidney) cereals, nuts. |

**TABLE 13.8**

**Biochemical, Clinical, and Nutritional Aspects of Selenium**

| | |
|---|---|
| *Biological function* | Selenium is a component of some 26 enzymes that catalyze redox reactions; these enzymes include various types of glutathione peroxidases, iodothyronine 5′-deiodinases, thioredoxin reductases, and methionine-*R*-sulfoxide reductase. Selenium as selenocysteine is also present in numerous other proteins, some of which might have enzymatic functions |
| *Signs and symptoms of deficiency* | |
| Biochemical | Decreased plasma or serum selenium, glutathione peroxidase-3 and selenoprotein P, and buccal cell selenium and glutathione peroxidase-1 |
| Physiological | Bilateral muscular discomfort, muscle pain, dry flaky skin, and wasting |
| *Pathological consequences of deficiency* | |
| Established | In the presence of other factors, Keshan disease, a multiple focal myocardial necrosis resulting in acute or chronic heart function insufficiency, heart enlargement, arrhythmia, pulmonary edema, and death; other consequences include impaired immune function and increased susceptibility to viral infections |
| Suggested | Increased susceptibility to certain types of cancer, Kashin–Beck disease (an endemic osteoarthritis), and mood disturbances[88] |
| *Predisposing factors for deficiency* | Viral infections and increased oxidative stress (e.g., vitamin E deficiency) |
| *Recommended intakes* | |
| Prevention of deficiency | RDAs and AIs (in parenthesis) set by the Food and Nutrition Board[3] (μg/day): infants 0.0–0.5 year, 15 and 0.5–1 year, 2; children 1–3 years, 20, 4–8 years, 30, and 9–13 years, 40; males ≥14 years, 55; females ≥14 years, 55; and lactating, 70 |
| Therapeutic or beneficial | A supra nutritional amount (e.g., 200 μg/day) was found to have cancer-protective effects, especially in men with low (<106 ng/mL) or suboptimal (<121 ng/mL) plasma selenium concentrations |
| *Food sources* | Fish, eggs, and meat from animals fed luxuriant selenium; grains grown on high-selenium soil |

**TABLE 13.9**

**Biochemical, Clinical, and Nutritional Aspects of Zinc**

| | |
|---|---|
| *Biological function* | Zinc has catalytic, structural, and regulatory functions. Zinc has essential roles in >200 enzymes in all six classes (oxidoreductases, ligases, lyases, isomerases, transferases, and hydrolases). Zinc stabilizes the tertiary structure of some enzymes and has a role in cellular signal transduction and in maintaining DNA integrity. Zinc is a component of transcription factors known as zinc finger proteins that bind to DNA and activate transcription of a message. |
| *Signs and symptoms of deficiency* | |
| Biochemical | Decreased plasma, urinary, and hair zinc concentrations. Suggested biomarkers needing further confirmation include salivary zinc, plasma extracellular superoxide dismutase, and erythrocyte and monocyte metallothionein.[89] |
| Physiological | Depressed growth; anorexia; parakeratotic skin lesions; diarrhea; and impaired development, immune function, and cognitive function. |
| *Pathological consequences of deficiency* | |
| Established | Dwarfism, delayed puberty, failure to thrive (acrodermatitis enteropathica in infants), mental lethargy and impaired neuropsychological function, hypogeusia (poor taste), impaired dark adaptation, impaired wound healing, and increased susceptibility to infectious disease. |
| Suggested | Osteoporosis,[90] atherosclerosis,[91] infertility, diabetes, cancer, Alzheimer's disease, rheumatoid arthritis. |
| *Predisposing factors for deficiency* | Factors causing impaired absorption including phytate; vegetarianism; intestinal infestation by bacteria, protozoa, and helminthes; gastric and intestinal resection; inflammatory bowel disease; exocrine pancreatic insufficiency; biliary obstruction; and high intakes of copper and iron. |
| | Factors causing excessive loss including protein-losing enteropathies, renal failure, renal dialysis, chronic blood loss (e.g., sickle cell disease), and exfoliative dermatoses. |
| *Recommended intakes* | |
| Prevention of deficiency | RDAs and AIs (in parenthesis) set by the Food and Nutrition Board[4] (mg/day): infants 0–0.5 year, (2) and 0.5–1 year, 3; children 1–3 years, 3 and 4–8 years, 5; males 9–13 years, 8 and ≥14 years, 11; females 9–13 years, 8, 14–18 years, 9 ≥19 years, 8; pregnant ≤18 years, 12 and ≥19 years, 11; lactating ≤18 years, 13 and ≥19 years, 12. |
| Therapeutic or beneficial | Supra nutritional amounts of zinc have been used for the alleviation and prevention of colds and treatment of macular degeneration, acute diarrhea, and Wilson's disease; doses have ranged from 20 mg/day for children with diarrhea to 150 mg/day for treatment of Wilson's disease. |
| *Food sources* | Red meats, organ meats (e.g., liver), shellfish, nuts, legumes. |

**TABLE 13.10**

**Arsenic: Biological Function in Lower Forms of Life, Deficiency Signs in Animals, and Speculated Importance and Postulated AI for Humans**

| | |
|---|---|
| *Biological function in lower forms of life* | The bacterium *Chrysiogenes arsenatis* reduces $As^{5+}$ to $As^{3+}$ to gain energy for growth. There are enzymes in higher animals and humans that methylate arsenic with *S*-adenosylmethionine as the methyl donor. For example, arsenite methyltransferase methylates arsenite to monomethylarsenic acid, which is methylated by monomethylarsenic acid methyltransferase to yield dimethylarsinic acid, the major form of metabolized arsenic in urine. |
| *Possible biological function in humans* | The beneficial bioactivity of arsenic might occur through the methylation of metabolically or genetically important molecules. |
| *Deficiency signs in selected experimental animals* | |
| Goat | Depressed growth and serum triglycerides, abnormal reproduction characterized by impaired fertility and elevated perinatal mortality, and death during lactation with myocardial damage.[92] |
| Pig | Depressed growth and abnormal reproduction characterized by impaired fertility and elevated perinatal mortality.[92] |
| Rat | Depressed growth and hepatic putrescine, spermine, and *S*-adenosylmethionine; elevated hepatic *S*-adenosylhomocysteine; abnormal reproduction.[93,94] |
| *Speculated importance for humans* | Deficient intakes might increase the risk for some types of cancers. |
| *Predisposing factors for deficiency* | Stressors that affect the utilization of labile methyl groups including high dietary arginine and high dietary taurine and low dietary methionine and low dietary choline. |
| | Stressors that affect arsenic metabolism including low dietary zinc and high dietary selenium. |
| *Postulated AI for humans* | Based on hypothesized requirements for experimental animals, 12–25 μg/day might be beneficial or adequate for humans.[95] |
| *Food sources* | Shellfish, fish, grains, and cereal products. |

## ARSENIC

Arsenic is unquestionably a bioactive element in higher animals and humans. Most studies of this bioactivity have been directed toward demonstrating that amounts sometimes found in food and water are toxic. However, several animal and epidemiological studies suggest that arsenic has beneficial effects when ingested in low microgram or nanogram quantities. For example, compared with exposure to drinking water containing about 50 μg/L, a low exposure (<50 μg/L) was associated with a higher number of cancers.[42] A similar finding was obtained in an animal study that determined the effect of arsenic on dimethylhydrazine-induced aberrant crypts in rats.[43] In addition, low versus physiological amounts of arsenic have been found to decrease global DNA methylation in cultured Caco-2 cells.[44] Much information in Table 13.10 comes from reviews by Nielsen.[32,33]

## BORON

Boron possibly could be included in the list of essential trace elements because it has been shown to be required by zebra fish and frogs to complete their life cycle. However, boron has not been definitively established to be needed to complete the life cycle of any mammal and does not have an established biochemical function in higher animals and humans. Nonetheless, there is substantial evidence indicating that nutritional versus low intakes of boron are beneficial for bone health, brain function, and immune response. The diverse responses reported for low intakes of boron in higher animals have made it difficult to identify a primary mechanism responsible for the bioactivity of boron. The wide range of responses is probably secondary to boron influencing a cell signaling system or the formation and/or activity of an entity that is involved in many biochemical processes. The findings earlier and the information in Table 13.11 have been described in reviews by Nielsen[32,33,45,46] and Nielsen and Meacham.[47]

## CHROMIUM

Over 50 years ago, trivalent chromium was reported to be the active component of the "glucose tolerance factor" in rats fed torula yeast–sucrose diets.[48] This resulted in chromium being accepted as essential for higher animals. Essentiality for humans gained acceptance when it was reported between 1977 and 1986 that chromium supplementation alleviated glucose tolerance and neuropathy exhibited by three patients on long-term total parenteral nutrition.[49] Since then, no reports of chromium supplementation helping patients on long-term parenteral nutrition have appeared. In addition, efforts to induce consistent signs of chromium deficiency in animals have not produced convincing findings,[50] and a clearly defined in vivo biochemical function has not been established for chromium.[51] Thus, chromium should no longer be classified as an essential nutrient because it does not fulfill the criteria that currently define essentiality. There is no question, however, about chromium being a bioactive beneficial element. Supra nutritional amounts of chromium have been found to enhance insulin sensitivity or action in some people, especially insulin-resistant individuals with type 2 diabetes and highly elevated fasting plasma glucose and hemoglobin $A_{1c}$ concentrations.[52] The information in Table 13.12 comes primarily from reviews by Nielsen,[32,33] Cefalu and Hu,[53] and Vincent and Stallings.[54]

**TABLE 13.11**
**Biochemical, Clinical, and Nutritional Aspects of Boron**

| | |
|---|---|
| *Biological function* | |
| Established | None |
| Hypothesized | The diverse actions of boron might occur through its reactions with biomolecules containing adenosine or formed from adenosine precursors, including S-adenosylmethionine, diadenosine phosphates, cyclic adenosine diphosphate ribose, and nicotinamide adenine dinucleotide |
| | Boron also might be bioactive through forming diester borate complexes with phosphoinositides, glycoproteins, and glycolipids, which contain *cis* hydroxyl groups in membranes and thus affect membrane integrity and function |
| *Signs and symptoms of deficiency* | |
| Biochemical | The wide range of responses to boron deprivation probably is secondary to an influence on a cell signaling system or the formation and/or activity of an entity that is involved in many biochemical processes. These responses in humans include decreased serum 25-hydroxycholecalciferol, triglycerides and creatinine, urinary hydroxyproline, and erythrocyte superoxide dismutase; increased blood urea nitrogen, urinary urea, and serum glucose; and, in women on estrogen therapy, decreased 17β-estradiol and increased plasma copper |
| Physiological | Because boron deprivation causes a variety of biochemical responses, it also results in a variety of physiological effects including altered electroencephalograms suggesting impaired behavior activation (e.g., increased drowsiness) and decreased mental alertness, impaired psychomotor skills and cognitive processes (e.g., attention and memory), and increased erythrocyte and decreased white blood cell numbers |
| | Several physiological signs in boron-deprived animals might have counterparts in humans. These include impaired bone development, decreased bone strength, and impaired inflammatory and immune response |
| *Pathological consequences of deficiency* | |
| Established | None |
| Suggested | Increased susceptibility to osteoporosis, arthritis, and cancer and impaired cognitive and psychomotor function and impaired bone development and wound healing |
| *Predisposing factors for deficiency* | Stressors that affect hormone action or signal transduction including vitamin D and magnesium deficiencies |
| | Increased oxidative or inflammatory stress |
| *Recommended intakes* | |
| Postulated AI for humans | Based human and animal experiments, 1.0 mg/day has been suggested as a safe AI |
| Therapeutic or beneficial | Luxuriant intakes (e.g., ≥3 mg/day) might have therapeutic action in conditions characterized by increased inflammatory or oxidative stress such as arthritis and osteoporosis |
| *Food sources* | Food and drink of plant origin, especially non-citrus fruits, leafy vegetables, nuts, pulses, wine, and cider |

## NICKEL

By 1984, extensive signs of nickel deprivation had been reported for six animal species. Unfortunately, many of the reported signs might have been misinterpreted manifestations of pharmacologic actions because nickel was provided in relatively high amounts to supplemented controls fed nutritionally suboptimal diets in some experiments. Thus, many of the early reported nickel deprivation findings are not shown in Table 13.13. Recent animal experiments have indicated that nickel might be needed for optimal reproductive function, bone composition and strength, and sensory function. Additional evidence for possible essentiality is that nickel is essential for some lower forms of life, where it participates in hydrolysis and redox reactions, regulates gene expression, and stabilizes certain structures. Interestingly, the substrates or products for all the nickel-requiring enzymes are dissolved gases: hydrogen, carbon monoxide, carbon dioxide, methane, oxygen, and ammonia. The gene function of nickel is involved in the diffusion of oxygen and hydrogen into the cell. The information earlier and in Table 13.13 primarily comes from reviews by Nielsen[32,33,55] and Eder and Kirchgessner.[56]

## SILICON

Silicon is nutritionally essential for some lower forms of life. Silicon has a structural role in diatoms, radiolarians, and some sponges. Diatoms, which are unicellular microscopic plants, have a silicon requirement for normal cell growth. Silicon also might be essential for some higher plants (e.g., rice). Other findings supporting possible essentiality for silicon include its localization in the active growth areas, or osteoid layer, and within osteoblasts of bone in young experimental animals; its consistent presence in collagen and glycosaminoglycan fractions from several types of connective tissue; and its increased intake associated with increased cortical bone mineral density in men and premenopausal women. In addition, orthosilicic acid at physiological concentrations was found to stimulate collagen type I synthesis in human osteoblast-like cells and enhance osteoblast differentiation in culture. The information earlier and in Table 13.14 primarily comes from reviews by Nielsen,[32,33,55] Carlisle,[57] and Jugdaohsingh.[58]

## TABLE 13.12
## Biochemical, Clinical, and Nutritional Aspects of Chromium

| | |
|---|---|
| *Biological function* | |
| Established | None |
| Hypothesized | In vitro findings have resulted in the hypothesis that a low-molecular-weight chromium-binding organic complex (LMWCr or chromodulin) acts in a unique auto-amplification system for insulin signaling. Chromodulin is an oligopeptide of about 1500 Da that binds four chromic ions. |
| | Another hypothesized role is the activation of glucose transporter, GLUT 4, trafficking via a cholesterol-dependent mechanism. |
| *Signs and symptoms of deficiency* | |
| Biochemical | Based on the response to relatively high amounts of parenteral chromium by some patients, suggested biochemical signs of deprivation include elevated serum glucose, cholesterol, triglycerides, and insulin. |
| Physiological | Based on the response to relatively high amounts of parenteral chromium by a few patients, physiological signs of chromium deprivation might be impaired glucose tolerance, weight loss, neuropathy, and encephalopathy. |
| *Pathological consequences of deficiency* | |
| Established | None. |
| Suggested | Impaired glucose tolerance, diabetes, and atherosclerosis. |
| *Predisposing factors for deficiency* | Factors that promote urinary excretion including acute strenuous exercise, physical trauma, and high dietary sugar. |
| *Recommended intakes* | |
| Prevention of deficiency | AIs set by the Food and Nutrition Board[4] (µg/day): infants 0–0.5 year (0.2) and 0.5–1 year (5.5); children 1–3 years (11), 4–8 years (15); males 9–13 years (25), 14–50 years (35), and ≥51 years (30); females 9–13 years (21), 14–50 years (25), ≥51 years (20); pregnant ≤18 years (29) and ≥19 years (30); lactating ≤44 years and ≥19 years (45). |
| Therapeutic or beneficial | Doses of 200–1000 µg/day, especially as an organic complex (e.g., chromium picolinate), have been shown to improve the efficacy of insulin and decrease plasma glucose and hemoglobin $A_{1c}$ (glycosylated hemoglobin) in some persons with type I, type II, gestational, and steroid-induced diabetes. |
| *Food sources* | Whole grains, pulses (e.g., dried beans), some vegetables such as broccoli and mushrooms, liver, processed meats, ready-to-eat cereals, and spices. |

## TABLE 13.13
## Nickel: Biological Function in Lower Forms of Life, Deficiency Signs in Animals, and Speculated Importance and Postulated AI for Humans

| | |
|---|---|
| *Biological function in lower forms of life* | Nickel has been identified as an essential component of eight enzymes:[96] urease, hydrogenase, carbon monoxide dehydrogenase, acetyl-CoA synthase, methyl-S-coenzyme-M reductase, Ni-superoxide dismutase, glyoxalase 1, and acireductone dioxygenase. Nickel has been reported to be required for the expression of the hydrogenase gene in *Bradyrhizobium japonicum.* |
| *Possible functions in humans* | Nickel bioactivity might involve the function of gaseous molecules such as oxygen and carbon monoxide. Nickel might be needed for the stabilization of hypoxia-inducible factor 1 or influence the activation of hypoxia-inducible expression of genes that are involved in such things as glucose transport, glycolysis, erythropoiesis, and osteogenesis. Carbon monoxide activates guanylyl cyclase, resulting in cGMP production. Thus, nickel might influence the cGMP signal transduction system, which has a crucial role in vision, taste, smell, blood pressure control, and sperm motility. Nickel also might be bioactive through altering methyl metabolism involving vitamin $B_{12}$. |
| *Deficiency signs in selected experimental animals* | |
| Goat | Depressed growth, hematocrit, and reproductive performance. |
| Pig | Depressed growth. |
| Rat | Altered iron metabolism, brain and erythrocyte fatty acid composition, long bone shape, and taste preference to saccharin; diminished sperm quantity and movement; and decreased long bone strength and circulating thyroid hormone concentration. |
| Sheep | Depressed growth, total serum protein, erythrocyte counts, ruminal urease activity, total hepatic lipids and cholesterol, and altered tissue distribution of copper and iron. |
| *Speculated importance for humans* | Deficient intakes might impair sensory functions, bone strength, and fertility. |
| *Predisposing factors for deficiency* | Stressors that affect labile methyl metabolism (e.g., folic acid, vitamin $B_6$, and vitamin $B_{12}$ deficiencies and homocysteine supplementation), iron metabolism (e.g., iron deficiency), and signaling (e.g., high dietary sodium chloride). |
| *Postulated AI for humans* | Based on hypothesized requirements for animals, 25–35 µg/day might be beneficial or adequate. |
| *Food sources* | Nuts, pulses, grains, and chocolate. |

**TABLE 13.14**

**Silicon: Biological Function in Lower Forms of Life, Deficiency Signs in Animals, and Speculated Importance and Postulated AI for Humans**

| | |
|---|---|
| *Biological function in lower forms of life* | Silicon has a structural role in some primitive classes of organisms including diatoms (unicellular microscopic plants), radiolarians, and some sponges. Diatoms have an absolute requirement for monomeric silicic acid for normal growth. |
| *Possible biological function in humans* | Silicon easily forms stable complexes with polyols that have at least four hydroxyl groups (e.g., hexosamines and ascorbic acid),[97] which may be the basis for hypothesis that silicon is involved in connective tissue stabilization or formation. In addition, silicon also apparently binds hydroxyl groups of proteins involved in signal transduction,[98] which might be the basis for its effect on the inflammatory or immune response and cognitive function, and in the stimulation of gene expression of factors involved in osteoblastogenesis and suppressed osteoclastogenesis. Silicon also has been hypothesized to alter the absorption or utilization of other mineral elements(e.g., aluminum, copper, iron, and magnesium) that affect bone metabolism, immune or inflammatory response, or cognitive function. |
| *Deficiency signs in experimental animals* | |
| Chick | Bone abnormalities characterized by defective endochondral bone growth with increased chondrocyte density and associated with decreased articular cartilage, water, hexosamine, and collagen. |
| Rat | Bone abnormalities characterized by reduced bone growth plate thickness, increased chondrocyte density, and decreased hydroxyproline. |
| | Increased urinary helical peptide (collagen breakdown product) excretion. |
| | Mild chronic inflammation and altered immune response. |
| *Beneficial supra nutritional effects in animals* | Alleviates bone loss in ovariectomized rats and stimulates gene expression of factors involved in osteoblastogenesis and suppresses expression of factors involved in osteoclastogenesis in mice. |
| *Human studies of health benefits* | |
| Epidemiological | Dietary silicon positively associated with bone mineral density in men and premenopausal women. |
| | Silicon intake positively associated with bone mineral density at the spine and femur in premenopausal women and postmenopausal women on hormone therapy. |
| | Silicon in drinking water associated with decreased incidence of Alzheimer's disease and associated disorders. |
| Supplementation trials | Increased bone mineral density in women with low bone mass. |
| | Improved photodamaged skin surface and mechanical properties and decreased hair and nail brittleness in women. |
| In vitro studies | Stimulates collagen type I synthesis and osteoblastic differentiation in human osteoblast-like cells. |
| | Silica-based bioactive glass and ceramics improve the efficiency of bone implants. |
| *Speculated importance for humans* | Deficient intakes might impair bone growth and remodeling resulting in an increased risk for osteoporosis, impair collagen metabolism resulting in impaired wound healing, and impair immune function. |
| *Predisposing factors for deficiency* | Stressors that affect the metabolism of silicon including high dietary fiber and aluminum. |
| | Stressors that affect silicon utilization such as low dietary calcium and conditions causing an immune or inflammatory response. |
| *Postulated AI for humans* | Based on animal findings and human urinary excretion data, suggested beneficial or AIs range from 5 to 25 mg/day. On the basis of weak balance data, a silicon intake of 30–35 mg/day was suggested for athletes, which was 5–10 mg higher than that suggested for nonathletes. |
| *Food sources* | Unrefined grains of high fiber content, cereal products, seafood, and some vegetables. |

## STRONTIUM

Strontium in supra nutritional or pharmacological amounts has beneficial effects on bones and teeth. In 1993, it was found that strontium ranelate (a compound containing the organic acid, ranelic acid, and two atoms of strontium) decreased bone resorption and maintained bone formation in ovariectomized rats.[59] Since then, strontium ranelate has become a promising pharmaceutical for the treatment of postmenopausal osteoporosis. Moderate doses of strontium (e.g., 315–525 mg/L drinking water) were found to stimulate bone formation and volume in rats,[60] and a supplemental 50 mg strontium/kg to a corn–soybean-based diet enhanced

breaking strength, mineral content, and mineral density of metatarsals and femurs in young pigs.[61] The information in Table 13.15 primarily comes from reviews by Nielsen,[32,62] Marie et al.,[63] and Marie.[64]

## VANADIUM

Vanadium is essential for some lower forms of life (algae, seaweeds, a lichen, and a fungus) where it is a component of various haloperoxidases. Vanadium in pharmacological or supra nutritional amounts has been repeatedly found to have beneficial bioactivity. The ability of vanadium to selectively inhibit protein tyrosine phosphatases probably

## TABLE 13.15
### Strontium: Deficiency Signs in Animals, Possible Biological Function, and Speculated Importance for Humans

| | |
|---|---|
| *Biological function in lower forms of life* | None established. |
| *Possible biological function or mechanism of action of supra nutritional or pharmacological intakes* | In vitro studies suggest that strontium as strontium ranelate both increases bone formation by osteoblasts and decreases bone resorption by osteoclasts. One suggested mechanism for the anti-catabolic effect is that strontium acts on the calcium-sensing receptor to induce osteoclast apoptosis[99] and/or to activate extracellular signal-related kinase 1/2 phosphorylation, which stimulates osteoblast replication.[64] Another suggested mechanism is that strontium ranelate upregulates osteoprotegerin and decreases bone resorption by modulating the RANK/RANK-ligand/osteoprotegerin system, which is essential for osteoclastogenesis.[64] |
| *Possible signs of deficiency in experimental animals* | |
| Guinea pigs and rats | Depressed growth, impaired mineralization of bones and teeth, and increased dental caries. |
| Pig | Decreased breaking strength, mineral content, and mineral density in bone. |
| Chick | Decreased bone volume and increased bone porosity.[100] |
| *Speculated importance for humans* | Strontium ranelate has been found to be an effective pharmaceutical for the treatment of postmenopausal osteoporosis. |
| *Postulated AI for humans* | None suggested, but the typical dietary intake of strontium is 1.5–3 mg/day. |
| *Food sources* | Whole grains and unpeeled fruits and vegetables. |

## TABLE 13.16
### Vanadium: Biological Function in Lower Forms of Life, Deficiency Signs in Animals, and Speculated Importance and Postulated AI for Humans

| | |
|---|---|
| *Biological function in lower forms of life* | Vanadium is an essential cofactor for some nitrogenases that reduce nitrogen to ammonia in bacteria and for bromoperoxidase, iodoperoxidase, and chloroperoxidase in algae, lichens, and fungi, respectively. The haloperoxidases catalyze the oxidation of halide ions by hydrogen peroxide, thus facilitating the formation of a carbon–halogen bond. |
| *Possible biological function in humans* | Vanadium might have a role that promotes phosphorylation and/or inhibits dephosphorylation such that a regulatory cascade is altered. Vanadium might have a role that affects the iodine metabolism and thus thyroid hormone production or utilization. |
| *Deficiency signs in selected experimental animals* | |
| Goat | Depressed milk production and life span; increased rate of spontaneous abortion; death, sometimes preceded by convulsions, between ages 7 and 91 days; skeletal deformations in the forelegs; and thickened forefoot tarsal joints. |
| Rat | Impaired reproduction and altered thyroid hormone metabolism and bone morphology. |
| *Speculated importance for humans* | Low intakes might impair thyroid hormone function (e.g., its role in proper bone development[101]). |
| *Predisposing factors for deficiency* | Stressors of thyroid or iodine metabolism and factors that reduce vanadium absorption including high dietary iron, aluminum hydroxide, and chromium. |
| *Postulated AI for humans* | Based on animal data, a daily intake of 10 μg/day probably would be adequate for humans. |
| *Therapeutic or beneficial intake for humans* | Doses used to experimentally treat diabetes have been in the range of 40–50 mg/day in both inorganic and organic forms. This is much higher than the tolerable UL of 1.8 mg/day for male adults set by the Food and Nutrition Board.[4] |
| *Food sources* | Shellfish, mushrooms, prepared foods, whole grains. |

explains the broad range of effects reported for supra nutritional intakes of vanadium; these effects include having insulin-like actions at the cellular level and stimulating cellular proliferation and differentiation. Effects on phosphorylation/dephosphorylation might be the basis for the findings that vanadium deprivation altered the response to low and high dietary iodine, impaired reproduction, and induced abnormal bone morphology in experimental animals. The earlier information and that shown in Table 13.16 come from reviews by Nielsen,[32,33,65,66] Anke et al.,[67] Marzan and McNeill,[68] Hulley and Davison,[69] and Sakurai.[70]

### OTHER ELEMENTS WITH BENEFICIAL OR BIOLOGICAL ACTIONS

There are several elements that have limited circumstantial evidence suggesting that they might beneficial actions in nutritional amounts. This evidence is generally limited to a few gross suggested signs of deficiency in one or two animals species observed by one or two research groups. Some of these elements have beneficial pharmacological actions (fluoride and lithium). In addition, bromide has been associated with insomnia,[71] and lithium has been associated with decreased all-cause mortality.[72] The information in Table 13.17 comes from reviews by Nielsen[32,33,55,73] and Anke et al.[74–78]

**TABLE 13.17**

**Reported Deficiency Signs in Experimental Animals and Usual Human Dietary Intakes of Apparently Bioactive Beneficial Mineral Elements**

| Element | Deficiency Signs (Experimental Animals) | Usual Daily Dietary Intake (Humans) | Food Sources |
|---|---|---|---|
| Aluminum | *Chick*: depressed growth<br>*Goat*: depressed growth and insemination success, increased abortion and kid mortality, and uncoordinated and weak hind legs | 2–25 mg | Processed cheese, foods containing baking powder, grains, vegetables, herbs, and tea |
| Bromine | *Goat*: depressed feed intake, growth, conception rate, hematocrit, and hemoglobin and increased abortions and kid mortality | 2–5 mg | Grains, nuts, and fish |
| Cadmium | *Goat*: muscular weakness, degenerative changes in liver and kidney mitochondria, decreased insemination success and milk production, and increased mortality<br>*Rat*: depressed growth | 10–20 µg | Shellfish, grains, and leafy vegetables grown in high-cadmium soils |
| Fluorine | *Goat*: decreased feed efficiency and growth, kid mortality, and skeletal deformations<br>*Rat*: depressed growth and incisor pigmentation | 0.3–1.0 mg without fluoridated water<br>1.4–3.4 mg with fluoridated water | Fish, tea, and foods produced in high-fluoride areas |
| Germanium | *Rat*: decreased tibial DNA and altered bone and liver mineral composition | 0.4–1.5 mg | Wheat bran, vegetables, and pulses |
| Lead | *Pig*: depressed growth and elevated serum cholesterol and phospholipids<br>*Rat*: depressed growth and liver glucose and lipids, increased liver cholesterol and serum ceruloplasmin, and anemia | 5–50 µg | Seafood, foods grown on high-lead soils |
| Lithium | *Goat*: depressed conception rate, birth weight, milk production, serum citric acid cycle enzyme, and liver monoamine oxidase activities and increased mortality and serum creatine kinase activity<br>*Rat*: depressed fertility, birth weight, litter size, and weaning weight | 0.2–0.6 mg | Meat, eggs, fish, milk products, potatoes, and vegetables (content varies with geographic region) |
| Rubidium | *Goat*: depressed growth, food intake, conception rate, milk production, and plasma progesterone and estradiol and increased abortions and kid mortality<br>*Rat*: altered tissue mineral concentrations | 1–5 mg | Fruits, vegetables (especially asparagus), poultry, fish, coffee, and tea |
| Tin | *Rat*: depressed growth, feed efficiency, and response to sound and altered mineral composition of heart, tibia, muscle, spleen, kidney, and lung | 1–40 mg | Canned foods |

## SUMMARY

Except for iodine and iron, the full extent of the pathological consequences of marginal or deficient intakes of the trace elements has not been well established. In addition, it is quite likely that not all the essential mineral elements for humans have been identified, and the mechanisms for the beneficial effects of many bioactive mineral elements have not been clearly defined. Thus, it is difficult to tabulate trace mineral deficiency signs and symptoms for humans. The tables in this section are works in progress, and the presented information can change because of ongoing research. However, findings to date indicate that many trace elements are of more practical nutritional concern than currently acknowledged.

## REFERENCES

1. US Department of Agriculture. www.choosemyplate.gov, accessed on May 30, 2012.
2. Food and Nutrition Board, Institute of Medicine, *Dietary Reference Intakes of Calcium, Phosphorus, Magnesium, Vitamin D, and Fluoride*, National Academy Press, Washington, DC, p. 190, 288; 1997.
3. Food and Nutrition Board, Institute of Medicine, *Dietary Reference Intakes for Vitamin C, Vitamin E, Selenium, and Carotenoids*, National Academy Press, Washington, DC, p. 284; 2000.
4. Food and Nutrition Board, Institute of Medicine, *Dietary Reference Intakes for Vitamin A, Vitamin K, Arsenic, Boron, Chromium, Copper, Iodine, Iron, Manganese, Molybdenum,*

*Nickel, Silicon, Vanadium, and Zinc*, National Academy Press, Washington, DC, p. 197, 224, 258, 290, 394, 420, 442, 502, 2001.

5. Stabler, SP. In: Bowman, BA, Russell, RM, eds., *Present Knowledge in Nutrition*, 9th edn., Vol. 1, ILSI Press, Washington, DC, p. 302; 2006.

6. Caudill, MA, Miller, JW, Gregory, JF III, Shane, B. In: Stipanuk, MH, Caudill, MA, eds., *Biochemical, Physiological, and Molecular Aspects of Human Nutrition*, 3rd edn., Elsevier Saunders, St. Louis, MO, p. 565; 2013.

7. Uauy, R, Olivares, M, Gonzalez, M, *Am J Clin Nutr*, 67(Suppl): 952S; 1998.

8. Beshgetoor, D, Hambidge, MH, *Am J Clin Nutr*, 67(Suppl): 1017S; 1998.

9. Cordano, A, *Am J Clin Nutr*, 67(Suppl): 1021S; 1998.

10. Saari, JT, Schuschke, DA, *Biofactors*, 10: 359; 1999.

11. Klevay, LM, *J Nutr*, 130: 489S; 2000.

12. Prohaska, JR, In: Bowman, BA, Russell, RM, eds., *Present Knowledge in Nutrition*, 9th edn., Vol. 1, ILSI Press, Washington, DC, p. 458; 2006.

13. Harvey, LJ, Ashton, K, Hooper, L, Casgrain, A, Fairweather-Tait, SJ, *Am J Clin Nutr*, 89(Suppl): 2009S; 2009.

14. Zimmerman, MB, In: Bowman, BA, Russell, RM, eds., *Present Knowledge in Nutrition*, 9th edn., Vol. 1, ISLI Press, Washington, DC, p. 471; 2006.

15. Pearce, EN, Freake, HC, In: Stipanuk, MH, Caudill, MA, eds., *Biochemical, Physiological, and Molecular Aspects of Human Nutrition*, 3rd edn., Elsevier Saunders, St. Louis, MO, p. 849; 2013.

16. Beard, J, In: Bowman, BA, Russell, RM, eds., *Present Knowledge in Nutrition*, 9th edn., Vol. 1, ILSI Press, Washington, DC, p. 430; 2006.

17. Crichton, RR, In: Stipanuk, MH, Caudill, MA, eds., *Biochemical, Physiological, and Molecular Aspects of Human Nutrition*, 3rd edn., Elsevier Saunders, St. Louis, MO, p. 801; 2013.

18. Nielsen, FH, *Magnes Res*, 17: 197; 2004.

19. Nielsen, FH, Milne, DB, Klevay, LM et al., *J Am Coll Nutr*, 26: 121; 2007.

20. Leone, N, Courbon, D, Ducimettiere, P, Zureik, M, *Epidemiology*, 17: 308; 2006.

21. Beckstrand, RL, Pickens, JS, *J Evid Based Complement Alternat Med*, 16: 181; 2011.

22. Larsson, SC, Orsini, N, Wolk, A, *Am J Clin Nutr*, 95: 362; 2012.

23. Vormann, J, In: Stipanuk, MH, Caudill, MA, eds., *Biochemical, Physiological, and Molecular Aspects of Human Nutrition*, 3rd edn., Elsevier Saunders, St. Louis, MO, p. 747; 2013.

24. Freeland-Graves, J, Llanes, C, In: Klimis-Tavantzis, DJ, ed., *Manganese in Health and Disease*, CRC Press, Boca Raton, FL, p. 59; 1994.

25. Macmillan-Crow, LA, Cruthirds, DL, *Free Radic Res*, 34: 325; 2001.

26. Norose, N, Arai, K, *Jpn J Parent Ent Nutr*, 9: 978; 1987.

27. Klimis-Tavantzis, DJ, *Manganese in Health and Disease*, CRC Press, Boca Raton, FL, pp. 88, 115, 133, 141; 1994.

28. Kocyigit, A, Zeyrek, D, Keles, H et al., *Biol Trace Elem Res*, 102: 11; 2004.

29. Vural, H, Sirin, B, Yilmaz, N et al., *Biol Trace Elem Res*, 129: 58; 2009.

30. Wood, RJ, *Nutr Rev*, 67: 416; 2009.

31. Leach, RM Jr, Harris, ED, In: O'Dell, BL, Sunde, RA, eds., *Handbook of Nutritionally Essential Mineral Elements*, Marcel Dekker, New York, p. 335; 1997.

32. Nielsen, FH, In: Erdman, JW, Macdonald, IA, Zeisel, SH, eds., *Present Knowledge in Nutrition*, 10th edn., Wiley–Blackwell, Ames, IA, p. 586; 2012.

33. Nielsen, FH, In: Stipanuk, MH, Caudill, MA, eds., *Biochemical, Physiological, and Molecular Aspects of Human Nutrition*, 3rd edn., Elsevier Saunders, St. Louis, MO, p. 899; 2013.

34. Novotny, JA, *J Evid Based Complement Alternat Med*, 16: 164; 2011.

35. Sunde, RA, In: Bowman, BA, Russell, RM, eds., *Present Knowledge in Nutrition*, 9th edn., Vol. 1, ILSI Press, Washington, DC, p. 480; 2006.

36. Combs, GF Jr, In: Stipanuk, MH, Caudill, MA, eds., *Biochemical, Physiological, and Molecular Aspects of Human Nutrition*, 3rd edn., Elsevier Saunders, St. Louis, MO, p. 867; 2013.

37. Hambidge, KM, Krebs, NF, *J Nutr*, 137: 1101; 2007.

38. Prasad, AS, *J Trace Elem Exp Med*, 11: 63; 1998.

39. Dibley, MJ, In; Bowman, BA, Russell, RM, eds., *Present Knowledge in Nutrition*, 8th edn., ILSI Press, Washington, DC, p. 329; 2001.

40. Bray, TM, Levy, MA, In: Lieberman, HR, Kanarek, RB, Prasad, C, eds., *Nutritional Neuroscience*, CRC Press, Boca Raton, FL, p. 275; 2005.

41. Cousins, RJ, In: Bowman, BA, Russell, RM, eds., *Present Knowledge in Nutrition*, 9th edn., Vol. 1, ILSI Press, Washington, DC, p. 445; 2006.

42. Kayajanian, G, *Ecotoxicol Environ Saf*, 55: 139; 2003.

43. Uthus, EO, Davis, CD, *Biol Trace Elem Res*, 103: 133; 2005.

44. Davis, CD, Uthus, EO, Finley, JW, *J Nutr*, 130: 2903; 2000.

45. Nielsen, FH, *J Trace Elem Exp Med*, 9: 215; 1996.

46. Nielsen, FH, *Nutr Rev*, 66: 183; 2008.

47. Nielsen, FH, Meacham, SL, *J Evid Based Complement Alternat Med*, 16: 169; 2011.

48. Schwarz, K, Mertz, W, *Arch Biochem Biophys*, 85: 292; 1959.

49. Moukarzel, A, *Gastroenterology*, 137: S18; 2009.

50. Di Bona, KR, Love, S, Rhodes, NR et al., *J Biol Inorg Chem*, 16: 381; 2011.

51. Vincent, JB, Bennett, R, In: Vincent, JB, ed., *The Nutritional Biochemistry of Chromium (III)*, Elsevier, Amsterdam, the Netherlands, p. 139; 2007.

52. Cefalu, WT, Rood, J, Pinsonat, P et al., *Metabolism*, 59: 755; 2010.

53. Cefalu, WT, Hu, FB, *Diabetes Care*, 27: 2741; 2004.

54. Vincent, JB, Stallings, D, In: Vincent, JB, ed., *The Nutritional Biochemistry of Chromium (III)*, Elsevier, Amsterdam, the Netherlands, p. 1; 2007.

55. Nielsen, FH, In: Bowman, BA, Russell, RM, eds., *Present Knowledge in Nutrition*, 9th edn., Vol. 1, ILSI Press, Washington, DC, p. 506; 2006.

56. Eder, K, Kirchgessner, M, In: O'Dell, BL, Sunde, RA, eds., *Handbook of Nutritionally Essential Mineral Elements*, Marcel Dekker, New York, p. 439; 1997.

57. Carlisle, EM, In: O'Dell, BL, Sunde, RA, eds., *Handbook of Nutritionally Essential Mineral Elements*, Marcel Dekker, New York, p. 603; 1997.

58. Jugdaohsingh, R, *J Nutr Health Aging*, 11: 99; 2007.

59. Marie, PJ, Hott, M, Modrowski, D et al., *J Bone Miner Res*, 8: 607; 1993.

60. Marie, PJ, Garba, MT, Hott, M, Miravet, L, *Miner Electrolyte Metab*, 11: 5; 1985.

61. Pagano, AR, Yasuda, K, Roneker, KR et al., *J Nutr*, 137: 1795; 2007.

62. Nielsen, FH, In: Mertz, W, ed., *Trace Elements in Human and Animal Nutrition*, 5th edn., Vol. 2, Academic Press, New York, p. 415; 1986.

63. Marie, PJ, Ammann, P, Boivin, G, Rey, C, *Calcif Tissue Int*, 69: 121; 2001.
64. Marie, PJ, *Bone*, 40: S5; 2007.
65. Nielsen, FH, In: Tracey, AS, Crans, DC, eds., *Vanadium Compounds: Chemistry, Biochemistry, and Therapeutic Applications*, ACS Series 711, American Chemical Society, Washington, DC, p. 297; 1998.
66. Nielsen, FH, In: O'Dell, BL, Sunde, RA, eds., *Handbook of Nutritionally Essential Mineral Elements*, Marcel Dekker, New York, p. 619; 1997.
67. Anke, M, Illing-Günther, H, Schäfer, U, *Biomed Res Trace Elem*, 16: 208; 2005.
68. Marzban, L, McNeill, JH, *J Trace Elem Exp Med*, 16: 253; 2003.
69. Hulley, P, Davison, A, *J Trace Elem Exp Med*, 16: 281; 2003.
70. Sakurai, H, *Biomed Res Trace Elem*, 18: 241; 2007.
71. Oe, PL, Vis, RD, Meijer JH et al., In: McHowell, J, Gawthorne, JM, White, CL, eds., *Trace Element Metabolism in Man and Animals, TEMA-4*, Australian Academy of Science, Canberra, Australia, p. 526; 1981.
72. Zarse, K, Terao, T, Tian, J et al., *Eur J Nutr*, 50: 387; 2011.
73. Nielsen, FH, In: Bogden, JD, Klevay, LM, eds., *Clinical Nutrition of the Essential Trace Elements and Minerals, The Guide for Health Professionals*, Humana Press, Totowa, NJ, p. 11; 2000.
74. Anke, M, Arnhold, W, Schäfer, U, Müller, R, *Biomed Res Trace Elem*, 16: 169; 2005.
75. Anke, M, Groppel, B, Masaoda, T, *Biomed Res Trace Elem*, 16: 177; 2005.
76. Anke, M, Müller, M, Hoppe, C, *Biomed Res Trace Elem*, 16: 183; 2005.
77. Anke, M, Dorn, W, Müller, M, Seifert, M, *Biomed Res Trace Elem*, 16: 198; 2005.
78. Anke, M, Angelow, L, Müller, R, Anke, S, *Biomed Res Trace Elem*, 16: 203; 2005.
79. Food and Nutrition Board, Institute of Medicine, *Dietary Reference Intakes for Thiamin, Riboflavin, Niacin, Vitamin $B_6$, Folate, Vitamin $B_{12}$, Pantothenic Acid, Biotin, and Choline*, National Academy Press, Washington, DC, p. 306; 1998.
80. Harris, MM, Houtkooper, LB, Stanford, VA et al., *J Nutr*, 33:3598; 2003.
81. Medeiros, DM, Stoecker, B, Plattner, A et al., *J Nutr*, 134: 3061; 2004.
82. Maurer, J, Harris, MM, Stanford, VA et al., *J Nutr*, 135: 863; 2005.
83. Tong, GM, Rude, RK, *Intensive Care Med*, 20: 3; 2005.
84. Seaborn, CD, Yang, SP, *Biol Trace Elem Res*, 39: 245; 1993.
85. Zeng, C, Hou, G, Dick, R et al., *Exp Biol Med*, 233: 1021; 2008.
86. Güner, S, Tay, A, Altan, VM et al., *Trace Elem Electrolytes*, 18: 39; 2001.
87. Brewer, GJ, *J Trace Elem Exp Med*, 16: 191; 2003.
88. Finley, JW, Penland, JG, *J Trace Elem Exp Med*, 11: 11; 1998.
89. Lowe, NM, Fekete, K, Decsi, T, *Am J Clin Nutr*, 89(Suppl): 2040S; 2009.
90. Yamaguchi, M, *Biomed Res Trace Elem*, 18: 346; 2007.
91. Bao, B, Prasad, AS, Beck, FWJ et al., *Am J Clin Nutr*, 91: 1634; 2010.
92. Anke, M, *Biomed Res Trace Elem*, 16: 177; 188.
93. Uthus, EO, *Environ Geochem Health*, 14: 55; 1992.
94. Uthus, EO, In: Chappell, WR, Abernathy, CO, Cothern, CR, eds., *Arsenic: Exposure and Health*, Science and Technology Letters, Northwood, London, U.K., p. 199; 1994.
95. Uthus, EO, In: Mertz, W, Abernathy, CO, Olin, SS, eds., *Risk Assessment of Essential Elements*, ILSI Press, Washington, DC, p. 273; 1994.
96. Ragsdale, SW, *J Biol Chem*, 284: 18571; 2009.
97. Kinrade, S, Del Nin, JW, Schach, AS et al., *Science*, 285: 1542; 1999.
98. Řezanka, T, Sigler, K, *Phytochemistry*, 69: 585; 2007.
99. Hurtel-Lemaire, AS, Mentaverri, R, Caudrillier, A et al., *J Biol Chem*, 284: 575; 2009.
100. Shahnazari, M, Lang, DH, Fosmire, GJ et al., *Calcif Tissue Int*, 80: 160; 2007.
101. Bassett, JHD, Boyde, A, Howell, PGT et al., *Proc Natl Acad Sci USA*, 107: 7604; 2010.

# 14 Vitamin Deficiencies

*Richard S. Rivlin*

## CONTENTS

## GENERAL COMMENTS ON VITAMIN DEFICIENCIES

In general, vitamin deficiencies arise when the diet is inadequate in its content of one or more of the vitamins or when the body is unable to utilize those consumed adequately. Impaired intestinal absorption or defects in metabolic processes, storage, or excretion can each result in vitamin deficiency. Single-nutrient deficiencies are rare, because a diet that is suboptimal in one vitamin is nearly always suboptimal in others. Thus, a poor diet tends to have multiple inadequacies. Furthermore, some vitamins are involved in the metabolism of other vitamins, and therefore deficiencies may be interconnected.

A number of exogenous factors may serve to intensify the biological effects of a poor diet. For example, excess alcohol consumption has specific and selective effects on vitamin metabolism, interfering with the absorption of some vitamins (e.g., thiamin and riboflavin) and accelerating the metabolic degradation of another pyridoxine (see Chapter 51). In addition, a number of medications may affect vitamin metabolism at multiple sites. From a practical point of view, laxatives and diuretics, often used for minimal indications and prolonged periods by vulnerable elderly patients, are probably among the most common causes of drug-induced vitamin deficiencies.

The concept of risk factors, utilized effectively in the evaluation and prevention of heart disease, needs to be applied to the assessment of vitamin deficiency. Thus, a patient who abuses alcohol, requires several medications chronically, and suffers from malabsorption due to alcohol will have a greatly enhanced risk of becoming vitamin deficient.

A much greater understanding is needed of the effects of herbal products and the so-called alternative/complementary remedies on vitamin metabolism (see Chapters 56 and 57). Many prescription drugs are known to affect vitamin metabolism. With large numbers of people consuming a wide variety of unregulated products about which there is little information, a potential exists for developing significant forms of malnutrition. There is a need for more information on drug–herbal and food–herbal interactions and their implications for vitamin metabolism. Several comments about the patterns of vitamin deficiencies currently emerging in the United States are summarized in Table 14.1.

While the effects of full-blown vitamin deficiencies are well known and have been thoroughly described, the effects of lesser or marginal deficiencies are not as well appreciated by health professionals. In recent years, both scientists and the general public have been paying more attention to marginal vitamin and mineral deficiencies in

---

### TABLE 14.1
### Some Features of Vitamin Deficiencies[1–17]

1. Dietary vitamin deficiencies tend to be multiple, not single.

2. Clinical evidence of vitamin deficiencies develops gradually, and early symptoms, such as fatigue and weakness, may be vague, ill-defined, and nonspecific.

3. The physical examination cannot be relied upon to make a diagnosis of early vitamin deficiency; classic features of vitamin deficiencies, such as the corkscrew hairs of scurvy, are only detectable after a profound deficiency state has been attained.

4. The rate of development of vitamin deficiencies is highly variable. In general, most water-soluble vitamins may be depleted within several weeks; longer periods are needed for significant depletion of fat-soluble vitamins. Several years are required for clinical manifestations of vitamin B$_{12}$ deficiency unless there are complicating factors, such as ileal resection or inflammatory bowel disease involving the ileum.

5. The impact of dietary deficiencies of vitamins is greatly augmented by the long-term chronic use of certain medications that may affect absorption, utilization, or excretion of vitamins. Chief among these are laxatives and diuretics. These considerations are particularly relevant to older individuals, who use the largest number of drugs and remedies, for the longest duration, and may have marginal diets to begin with.

6. The concept of "risk factors" may be helpful in assessing factors, such as drugs and alcohol, that contribute to accelerating the clinical presentation of a given dietary inadequacy.

attempting to gain maximal benefits from diet for health. Recent findings suggest that the concept of so-called normal needs to be carefully reconsidered, inasmuch as there may be different risks for disease within the range considered "normal."

For example, individuals with serum folic acid levels in the lower part of the normal range have been shown to have significantly elevated serum concentrations of homocysteine compared with those whose folic acid concentrations are in the upper range of normal. With elevated serum homocysteine concentrations emerging as a risk factor for heart disease, these observations suggest that perhaps we should set higher standards and more defined expectations for the "normal" range.

In the prevention and treatment of vitamin deficiencies, one must approach the patient in a logical fashion and proceed in an orderly direction. Medical history is of greatest importance, and one needs to know details of food intake, portion size supplement use, remedies, and drugs. The physical examination only rarely reveals pathognomonic signs of specific vitamin deficits. Laboratory tests, appropriately utilized, may be helpful in documenting vitamin deficiencies. Long-term compliance with an appropriate diet and the use of supplements, if indicated, is the goal, but may be difficult to achieve. Some of the points regarding correction of vitamin deficiencies are summarized in Table 14.2.

---

## TABLE 14.2
### Some Considerations in the Correction of Vitamin Deficiencies[10,11]

1. Approach the clinical setting in its entirety; ask yourself how could a vitamin deficiency develop in the first place. Ask whether there are complicating conditions, that is, other risk factors, in addition to the poor diet.
2. Unless there are specific indications of a single-nutrient deficiency, such as vitamin $B_{12}$ in pernicious anemia, most malnourished patients will have multiple deficiencies and require rehabilitation with multiple nutrients. Repletion is best accomplished primarily with diet and additionally with specific supplementation, if necessary.
3. Simple steps can often improve a diet significantly, such as discarding old produce, avoiding "fast food" meals on a regular basis, and increasing the intake of fresh fruits and vegetables. In modern nutrition, one speaks of "junk diets" rather than single "junk foods," and of the necessity of moderation and variety in one's daily diet.
4. Learn how to read a label from a nutritional supplement bottle so that you can properly instruct your patients. The array of choices of nutritional supplements is bewildering, and patients must learn that more is not necessarily better.
5. Remember that vitamins may behave like drugs and have a defined toxic: therapeutic ratio. Some vitamins, such as vitamins A and D, have a real potential for causing toxicity. B vitamins may also cause problems, as exemplified by the sensory neuropathy resulting from large doses of vitamin $B_6$.
6. A multivitamin supplement containing all nutrients at the levels of the RDI is safe to take by nearly everyone and may help to alleviate deficiencies and prevent them in the future.

---

## VITAMIN A

### FUNCTIONS

Vitamin A has a wide variety of functions, including specific roles in vision, embryogenesis, cellular differentiation, growth, reproduction, immune status, taste sensations, and, increasingly, in disease prevention and treatment.

### DEFICIENCY

Deficiency of vitamin A is of crucial importance as a worldwide nutritional problem. The resultant xerophthalmia is a cause of blindness in at least half a million preschool children each year in the developing countries. In these areas, the diet is composed primarily of such items as rice, wheat, maize, and tubers, which contain far from adequate amounts of vitamin A precursors. The World Health Organization (WHO) and other groups have made great efforts to plan programs that identify people at risk and to institute appropriate preventive measures on a broad scale. It is now recognized that dietary deficiency of vitamin A is a clear risk factor for severe cases of measles. Many of the deaths that result from measles in young children could be greatly reduced by large doses of vitamin A given parenterally. The diet prevailing in these areas simply does not contain enough vitamin A precursors or vitamin A itself to prevent a deficient state from developing.

Clinical deficiency of vitamin A may be overt or subclinical. One of the earliest signs of vitamin A deficiency is night blindness, observed in both children and adults. The development of xerophthalmia follows a defined sequence, leading eventually to keratomalacia, in which perforation of the cornea occurs. A characteristic sign that is observed later in advanced vitamin A deficiency is Bitot's spots, collections of degenerated cells in the outer aspects of the conjunctivae that appear white in color. Vitamin-A-deficiency eye disease in its end stages is irreversible, but if abnormalities are detected earlier and treated vigorously, they may be potentially preventable.

Vitamin A deficiency also causes skin disorders in the form of follicular hyperkeratosis. Although characteristic skin changes occur in response to a deficiency of vitamin A, in practical terms, one should remember that skin lesions of some kind may be caused by other nutrient deficiencies such as zinc, biotin, niacin, and riboflavin.

Children significantly deficient in vitamin A manifest increased incidence of serious and life-threatening infections and elevated mortality rates. It has been recognized that deficient vitamin A status is a risk factor for the maternal-to-fetal transmission of human immunodeficiency virus; the relative risk of transmission of the virus is fourfold greater in vitamin-A-deficient than in vitamin-A-sufficient mothers.

Vitamin A deficiency in the United States is identified largely with certain risk groups: the urban poor, elderly persons (particularly those living alone), abusers of alcohol, patients with malabsorption disorders, and persons with poor diets. Vitamin A deficiency is generally found in a setting in which there are multiple vitamin and mineral deficits. Special attention must be paid to the deficiency of zinc, a frequent finding in alcoholism, as depletion of zinc interferes with the mobilization of vitamin A from its storage sites in liver. This effect is achieved by blocking the release of holo-retinol-binding protein from the liver. Even in Western countries, severe cases of measles have been found in children with borderline vitamin A stores, suggesting that perhaps parenteral vitamin A should be administered in this setting as well.

Health professionals must keep in mind that a deficiency of vitamin A in the United States may develop after the long-term use of several medications. Drug-induced nutritional deficiencies, in general, particularly those involving vitamin A, occur most frequently among elderly persons, because they use medications in the largest number for the most prolonged duration, and they may have borderline nutritional status to begin with. Among the drugs most relevant to compromising vitamin A status are mineral oil, which dissolves this nutrient; other laxatives, which accelerate intestinal transit and may diminish the magnitude of vitamin A absorption; cholestyramine and colestipol, which bind vitamin A; and, under certain conditions, neomycin and colchicines. Olestra may possibly interfere with the absorption of a number of vitamins, including A: patients using this agent have been advised to take a multivitamin supplement regularly.

## Laboratory Diagnosis of Vitamin A Deficiency

The laboratory diagnosis of vitamin A deficiency is based on the finding of a low plasma retinal; levels below 10 µg/dL signify severe or advanced deficiency. Interpretation of plasma retinal concentrations may be confounded, however, by a number of other factors, such as generalized malnutrition and weight loss. Some authorities have preferred to utilize a form of retinal tolerance test, measuring the increment in serum vitamin A levels over 5 h following an oral load of vitamin A.

## Prevention

Deficiency of vitamin A can be prevented by a diet high in carotenes, which serve as precursors to vitamin A. The carotenes, particularly β-carotene, are derived exclusively from plant sources, the richest of which are palm oil, carrots, sweet potatoes, dark green leafy vegetables, cantaloupe, oranges, and papaya. Preformed vitamin A is derived only from animal sources, such as dairy products, meat, and fish. The commercial preparations of fish oils are rich, sometimes too rich, as sources of preformed vitamin A.

The nutritional value of dietary sources of vitamin A may be compromised when food items are subject to oxidation, particularly in the presence of light and heat. Antioxidants, such as vitamin E, may prevent the loss of vitamin A activity under these conditions.

## Treatment

Vitamin A deficiency has been treated worldwide with single intramuscular injections of massive amounts (100,000–200,000 IU) of vitamin A, repeated at intervals of approximately 6 months to 1 year. WHO has recommended that doses of 200,000 IU of vitamin A be given initially and at 2 days to children admitted to hospitals in those areas of the world where the case fatality rate is very high. Such doses have been effective and are associated with remarkably little toxicity, perhaps because body stores are markedly depleted at the time of therapy. These doses, however, may produce some acute toxic symptoms in well-nourished persons.

Clinical vitamin A deficiency in the United States can be treated with either β-carotene if there is normal body conversion to vitamin A or vitamin A itself. Daily doses in the range of 25,000 IU of β-carotene are being consumed by many healthy individuals. The yellowish discoloration of the skin associated with prolonged use of β-carotene is not believed to be harmful. Vitamin A, in contrast, is quite toxic when ingested in amounts considerably higher than the RDI, especially for prolonged periods. It is probably advisable not to exceed two to three times the RDI for vitamin A when planning a domestic treatment program involving vitamin A administration.

Congenital malformations, a particularly disturbing consequence of vitamin A overdosage, have been reported in women consuming 25,000–50,000 IU daily during pregnancy. The lowest dose of vitamin A that would be completely safe as a supplement for pregnant women is not known definitely. Therefore, it is not a good idea for pregnant women to take supplementary vitamin A unless there are specific indications, such as malabsorption, or proven dietary deficiency. Many advisory groups caution that the maximal intake of preformed vitamin A consumed during pregnancy should not exceed 10,000 IU/day.

At present, there is widespread interest in newer therapeutic applications of vitamin A and its derivatives. Certain forms of leukemia have been found to respond to derivatives of vitamin A. The therapeutic potential of this vitamin is being expanded greatly in studies of chemoprevention and treatment of cancer. The toxicity of large doses of vitamin A places important limits on its feasibility in cancer prevention. Attention has turned to β-carotene and related agents, which, in addition to their role as precursors of vitamin A, have strong antioxidant activity and other effects as well. β-Carotene, however, may possibly pose a risk in heavy smokers—two studies in this population have shown an actual increase in the prevalence of lung cancer when β-carotene was administered for several years.

Diminished prevalence of certain cancers has been found among people whose intake of fruits and vegetables is high; this finding has been attributable at least in part to the high content of carotenoids in the diet. However, many phytochemicals in addition to carotenoids have been found in fruits and vegetables with potential health benefits. Some data show that a combination of antioxidants (i.e., vitamin E, vitamin C, and β-carotene) may be more effective than any of these single agents, providing more evidence in favor of moderation and variety in the diet.

## VITAMIN D

Just as night blindness was recognized as a disease treatable by diet (vitamin A), the classical disease of vitamin D deficiency, rickets, has been evident since ancient times. Historians do not agree as to when the first symptoms of vitamin D deficiency were recorded. Some suggest that the stooped appearance of the Neanderthal man (ca. 50,000 BC) was due to an inadequate vitamin D intake rather than being characteristic of a low evolutionary status. Evidence of rickets in skeletons from humans of the Neolithic age, the first settlers of Greenland, the ancient Egyptians, Greeks, and Romans has been reported by anthropologists.

The first detailed descriptions of rickets are found in the writings of Dr. Daniel Whistler of Leiden, Netherlands, and Professor Francis Glisson in the mid-1600s. Beyond these descriptions and the acceptance of rickets as a disease entity, little progress was made until the late 1800s when it was suggested that the lack of sunlight and perhaps a poor diet were related to the appearance of bone malformation. Funk, in 1914, suggested that rickets was a nutrient deficiency disorder. This was verified by Edward Mellanby. Mellanby constructed a grain diet which produced rickets in puppies. When he gave cod-liver oil, the disease did not develop. At that time, Mellanby did not know that there were two fat-soluble vitamins (A and D) in cod-liver oil, and he thought that he was studying the antirachitic properties of vitamin A. Not until the two vitamins were separated and identified was it realized that Mellanby's antirachitic factor was vitamin D. The recognition of vitamin D as a separate entity from vitamin A came from the work of McCollum and associates in 1922. Although the importance of sunlight had long been recognized in the prevention and treatment of rickets, the relationship of ultraviolet light to the dietary intake of vitamin D was not appreciated until Steenbeck and also Goldblatt et al. demonstrated that ultraviolet light gave antirachitic properties to sterol-containing foods if these foods were incorporated into diets previously shown to produce rickets. The body, if exposed to sunlight, can convert the 7-dehydrocholesterol at the skin's surface to cholecalciferol, and this compound is then further metabolized in the kidney producing the active principle, 1,25-dihydroxy cholecalciferol. The body, under the right conditions, can synthesize all the vitamins it needs. However, in the person with renal disease or in persons using excessive amounts of sun blocker and who does not have sufficient ultraviolet light exposure, the synthesis of 1,25-dihydroxy cholecalciferol is impaired, and in this individual, a dietary supplement of vitamin $D_3$ is essential.

### DEFICIENCY

Bone deformities are the hallmarks of the vitamin D-deficient child while porous brittle bones are indications

of the deficiency in the adult. Prior to the enrichment of milk and other food products with vitamins $D_{2 \text{ and } 3}$, vitamin D deficiency was common. In the early part of the twentieth century, the vitamin D deficiency disorders developed in part because of the custom of wearing heavy clothing that shielded the skin from the ultraviolet rays of the sun. Ultraviolet light is essential for the in vivo synthesis of the active vitamin. Today, with the heavy emphasis on the use of sunscreen to prevent skin cancer, there is concern that the people who follow this recommendation may be at greater risk for developing vitamin D deficiency disorders. Lacking ultraviolet light exposure, the only source is food. Very few foods contain significant quantities of the vitamin unless they are enriched. Without this source of dietary vitamin, a deficiency state could develop. A recent population study of children in the northeastern part of the United States revealed low serum levels of 25(OH)D, and these low levels were associated with reduced bone mass. Today, osteoporosis develops not only because of these reasons mentioned but also maybe due to disease or damage to either the liver or kidney. Both of these organs are essential for the conversion of cholecalciferol to the active vitamin form, 1,25-dihydroxy $D_3$. If either organ is nonfunctional in this respect, the deficient state will develop. On rare occasions, the deficient state will develop not because of any lack of dietary D or sunlight or because of kidney or liver damage, but because through a genetic error, the 1,25-hydroxylase enzyme is missing and the 1,25-dihydroxy $D_3$ cannot be synthesized. In individuals so afflicted, 1,25-dihydroxy $D_3$ must be supplied as an essential nutrient. 1,25-Dihydroxy $D_3$ must also be provided to the anephritic patient, since these patients cannot synthesize this hormone. Until the realization that the kidney served as the endocrine organ for 1,25-dihydroxy $D_3$ synthesis, renal disease was almost always accompanied by a disturbed calcium balance and osteoporosis. See www.ods.od.nih.gov/ Health_Information/Dietary Reference Intakes for intake recommendations.

See Chapter 59, hypertension and renal disease, Chapter 71 on calcium in bone health, and Chapter 56 on calcium and vitamin D in dietary supplements for additional information on vitamin D.

## VITAMIN E

Vitamin E functions as a scavenger of free radicals, and in this capacity, it protects cell membranes from free radical damage. Vitamin E is also essential for the immune system, particularly T-lymphocytes, and has a role in DNA repair. Vitamin E inhibits the oxidation of low-density lipoprotein (LDL); oxidized LDL becomes more atherogenic. The neuromuscular system and the retina also require vitamin E for optimal function. This vitamin protects the sulfhydryl groups in enzymes and other proteins from oxidation. Stores of vitamin E may be conserved by the glutathione-S-transferase system, which utilizes reduced glutathione and serves similar antioxidant functions.

## Need

Because of the interacting effects of vitamin E with selenium and other antioxidants, the requirement for the vitamin has been difficult to ascertain. It has been estimated that the average adult consumes approximately 15 mg/day, but the range of intake is very large. The dietary reference intakes (DRIs) are periodically reviewed, and updates can be found on the DRI website: www.ods.od.nih.gov/Health_Information/Dietary Reference_Intakes

## Deficiency

One of the first deficiency symptoms recorded for the tocopherols was infertility. This was followed by the discovery that the white muscle disease or a peculiar muscle dystrophy could be reversed if vitamin E was provided. Later it was recognized that selenium also played a role in the muscle symptom. Listed in Table 14.3 are the many symptoms attributed to inadequate vitamin E intake. All of these symptoms are related either primarily to the level of peroxides in the tissue or to peroxide damage to the membranes and/or the DNA.

Dietary vitamin E deficiency is relatively unusual in the United States under ordinary circumstances, as sources of

### TABLE 14.3
### Vitamin E Deficiency Disorders

| Disorder | Species Affected | Tissue Affected |
| --- | --- | --- |
| Reproductive failure | | |
| Female | Rodents, birds | Embryonic vascular tissue |
| Male | Rodents, dog, birds, monkey, rabbit | Male gonads |
| Hepatic necrosis[a] | Rat, pig | Liver |
| Fibrosis[a] | Chicken, mouse | Pancreas |
| Hemolysis[b,c] | Rat, chick, premature infant | Erythrocytes |
| Anemia | Monkey | Bone marrow |
| Encephalomalacia[b,c] | Chick | Cerebellum |
| Exudative diathesis[a] | Birds | Vascular system |
| Kidney degeneration[a,b] | Rodents, monkey, mink | Kidney tabular epithelium |
| Steatitis[b,c] | Mink, pig, chick | Adipose tissue |
| Nutritional myopathies | | |
| Type A muscular dystrophy | Rodents, monkey, duck, mink | Skeletal muscle |
| Type B white muscle disease[a] | Lamb, calf, kid | Skeletal and heart muscle |
| Type C myopathy[a] | Turkey | Gizzard, heart |
| Type D myopathy | Chicken | Skeletal muscle |

[a]  Can be reversed by addition of selenium to the diet.

[b]  Increased intake of polyunsaturated acids potentiate deficiency.

[c]  Antioxidants can be substituted for vitamin E to cure condition.

vitamin E are widely available from the food supply. The recognizable cases of vitamin E deficiency tend to arise in debilitated patients who have had severe and prolonged periods of fat malabsorption. Vitamin E is incorporated into chylomicrons with other products of fat digestion during the process of intestinal absorption. Any illness that interferes with fat digestion, absorption, or metabolism may also impair absorption of vitamin E. Disorders in which symptomatic vitamin E deficiency develops include cystic fibrosis, celiac disease, cholestatic liver disease, and short-bowel syndrome from any cause.

Major abnormalities of neurological function are observed in a severe and prolonged vitamin E deficiency state. Patients display areflexia, ophthalmoplegia, and disturbances of gait, proprioception, and vibration. In premature infants, vitamin E deficiency results in hemolytic anemia, thrombocytosis, edema, and intraventricular hemorrhage. There is increased risk of retrolental fibroplasia and bronchopulmonary dysplasia under these circumstances.

In hemolytic anemia, such as that caused by glucose-6-phosphate dehydrogenase deficiency and sickle-cell anemia, vitamin E levels in blood tend to be decreased. Inborn errors of vitamin metabolism have been identified, but are rare. There are severe neurological abnormalities in this category. In abetalipoproteinemia, there is a defect in the serum transport of vitamin E. A hallmark of this disease is the finding of extremely low serum cholesterol levels together with very low serum levels of vitamin E.

## Laboratory Diagnosis of Deficiency

Ideally, the diagnosis of vitamin E deficiency should be made by detailed chromatographic analysis of the various E isomers. In practice, such a procedure is not realistic, and the clinical evaluation usually depends on the measurement of total plasma E alone. Plasma concentrations of vitamin E below 0.50 μg/mL are generally regarded as indicative of deficiency. It has been observed that despite a wide range of dietary intake, the serum variations in vitamin E levels often tend to be in a much more limited range.

It is important to keep in mind that vitamin E is transported in blood bound to lipoproteins, particularly LDL. In any condition in which the serum cholesterol is abnormally high or low, the vitamin E level will vary accordingly. Therefore, before concluding that anyone is vitamin-E-deficient or has an excess of vitamin E, the plasma level of this vitamin should be evaluated in relation to the prevailing cholesterol concentrations. Furthermore, an α-tocopherol transport protein has been identified recently; its physiological role is at present under study.

## Prevention

Deficiency of vitamin E can be avoided by regular consumption of the many sources of this vitamin in the food supply. The richest sources of vitamin E in the U.S. diet are vegetable oils, including corn, cottonseed, safflower, and soybean oils, and the margarines and other products made from these oils.

Green leafy vegetables are also good sources of vitamin E. In evaluating the adequacy of any given dietary regimen, one should keep in mind the losses of the vitamin that often occur during storage, cooking, and food processing, particularly with exposure to high temperatures and oxygen.

Because vitamin E deficiency frequently occurs as a result of severe intestinal malabsorption, it is essential to identify this condition early and avoid measures that may intensify the degree of malabsorption of vitamin E and other fat-soluble vitamins. Specific supplementation with vitamin E and other vitamins may be needed. The usual multivitamin supplement containing 400 IU should be adequate for this purpose.

There is evidence that dietary zinc is necessary in order for vitamin E to achieve adequate concentrations in peripheral blood. The relationship has been shown in both experimental animals and patients.

There is a wide margin of safety in the therapeutic administration of the vitamin. Daily doses of vitamin E in the range of 100–800 IU can be given safely to nearly all-deficient patients. This dosage is higher than that usually found in multivitamin supplements. This dose range can be used appropriately in those patients with vitamin E deficiency diagnosed in association with celiac disease, inflammatory bowel disease, or other chronic and prolonged forms of intestinal malabsorption. In such instances, many other nutrient deficiencies are likely to be found in association with that of vitamin E, and they, too, necessitate treatment.

In the genetic disorders of vitamin E metabolism, such as isolated vitamin E deficiency, doses in the range of 800–1000 IU or higher must be taken. Large doses of vitamin E given therapeutically under these conditions appear to be generally safe. Some investigators have suggested that pharmacologic doses of vitamin E may interfere with the intestinal absorption of vitamins A and K. In addition, there are suggestive reports that doses of vitamin E in excess of 1200 IU/day may possibly interfere with the action of vitamin K and intensify the effects of anticoagulant drugs. Further information is needed on this subject.

# VITAMIN K

## FUNCTIONS

Vitamin K is a cofactor for posttranslational modification in a diverse group of calcium-binding proteins, whereby selective glutamic acid (Glu) residues are transformed into gamma-carboxyglutamic acid (Gla). The vitamin-K-dependent proteins that are best known include the four classic vitamin procoagulants (factors II, VII, IX, and X) and two feedback anticoagulants (proteins C and S), all synthesized by the liver. Therefore, severe liver disease leads to extensive abnormalities in vitamin K metabolism and frequent disturbances in blood coagulation.

Gla proteins also occur in several other tissues besides liver. Actions of vitamin K in bone have assumed greater importance in recent years. Osteocalcin, which contains three Gla residues, is synthesized by the osteoblasts of bone.

It is one of the 10 most abundant proteins in the body and may play a role in regulating bone turnover. A second protein isolated from bone that is related structurally to osteocalcin is matrix Gla protein. This protein is more widely distributed, and there is now evidence that this protein is an important inhibitor of calcification of arteries and cartilage. Gla residues provide efficient chelating sites for calcium ions that enable vitamin-K-dependent proteins to bind to other surfaces (e.g., procoagulants to platelet and vessel wall phospholipids, and osteocalcin to the hydroxyapatite matrix of bone). The carboxylation reaction is catalyzed by a microtome vitamin-K-dependent gamma-glutamyl carboxylase, which requires the dietary quinone form of vitamin K to be first reduced to the active cofactor vitamin K hydroquinone, vitamin $KH_2$.

In bone, vitamin K achieves gamma-carboxylation of osteocalcin. In addition, vitamin K regulates interleukin-6 production, synthesis of prostaglandin $E_2$, and urinary excretion of calcium. It is not surprising, therefore, that in patients with long-term low dietary intake of vitamin K, the risk for hip fractures is increased.

## DEFICIENCY

Isolated deficiency of vitamin K due entirely to inadequate dietary intake tends to be unusual in adults in the United States, because this vitamin is widely distributed in the food supply. Overt deficiency of vitamin K is more likely to be observed in conditions in which there are significant complicating factors, such as long-term use of broad-spectrum antibiotics, or illnesses and drugs associated with fat malabsorption. It is essential to recognize that vitamin K is synthesized by intestinal bacteria. Antibiotic treatment will largely eliminate these bacterial sources of vitamin K and may have some clinical impact, particularly when treatment is prolonged. One class of antibiotics, the cephalosporins, causes vitamin K deficiency by an entirely different mechanism, namely, by inhibiting the vitamin-K-dependent hydroxylase. The extent to which the bacterial source of vitamin K provides a significant contribution to the bodily supply of the vitamin is a subject of debate among experts.

Fat malabsorption is regularly observed as a feature of severe regional enteritis, nontropical sprue, cystic fibrosis, ulcerative colitis, and a number of other disorders. Following extensive intestinal resection, patients are left with a short-bowel syndrome, in which fat malabsorption is prominent because of the reduction in intestinal surfaces available for absorption and transport. In a recent study of more than 100 patients with cystic fibrosis, evidence of insufficient vitamin K nutrition was found in 70% of the sample. The clinical severity of deficiency was highly individualized.

Vitamin K deficiency with the most serious consequences is that associated with the hemorrhagic disease of the newborn. The pathogenesis of this syndrome derives from (1) the poor placental transport of vitamin K combined with (2) lack of fetal production of vitamin K by intestinal bacteria as the intestinal tract is sterile, and (3) diminished synthesis by an immature liver of prothrombin and its precursors. In adults with vitamin K deficiency, multiple purpuric lesions may be noted.

As noted earlier, dietary sources of vitamin K are widespread in the food supply in the United States. The highest amounts are found in green leafy vegetables, such as broccoli, brussel sprouts, spinach, turnip greens, and lettuce. Interestingly, the risk of hip fracture is reported to be the highest in women who have the lowest consumption of lettuce, which contributes significantly to vitamin K nutrition. Some vitamin K at lower amounts can be found in meat, dairy products, coffee, and certain teas. Green leafy vegetables contain vitamin K largely as phylloquinone. Meat, cheese, and certain fermented foods contain vitamin K in the form of menaquinone.

## LABORATORY DIAGNOSIS OF DEFICIENCY

Vitamin K in body fluids and in foods can be measured by biological and chemical methods. The vitamin is light sensitive and must be shielded from light during storage and analysis. In practice, functional vitamin K status is assessed indirectly by measurements of serum prothrombin. Clinical vitamin K deficiency should be suspected wherever there is an unusual hemorrhagic tendency. In assessing vitamin K deficiency clinically, it is important to remember that adequate carboxylation of proteins in bone requires higher doses of vitamin K than the carboxylation of proteins in liver. Thus, in repleting deficient patients, the blood coagulation profile could be normalized early but bone metabolism still compromised. Due to the fact that intestinal synthesis of vitamin K usually provides sufficient amounts of the vitamin to the body, primary vitamin K deficiency is rare. However, secondary deficiency states can develop as a result of biliary disease that results in an impaired absorption of the vitamin. Deficiency can also occur as a result of long-term broad spectrum antibiotic therapy that may kill the vitamin K-synthesizing intestinal flora, or as a result of anticoagulant therapy using coumadin (warfarin), which interferes with the metabolism and function of the vitamin. The primary characteristic of the deficiency state is a delayed or prolonged clotting time. Deficient individuals may have numerous bruises indicative of subcutaneous hemorrhaging in response to injury. Studies of human populations have shown that low intakes of vitamin K (dihydrophylloquinone) are associated with low bone mineral density. Newborn infants, because they do not yet have established their K-synthesizing intestinal flora, have delayed coagulation times.

## PREVENTION

For healthy individuals, dietary vitamin K deficiency should be preventable by maintaining a diet high in green leafy vegetables. When antibiotics are prescribed long term, they should be kept to the minimal time period and doses necessary. Efforts should be initiated early to recolonize the gastrointestinal tract by providing live-culture yogurt or other sources of normal flora. Similar guidelines should

be followed in cases in which drugs causing malabsorption of vitamin K are required. Vitamin supplements containing vitamin K may be advisable. Effective treatment of an underlying disorder of the gastrointestinal tract should be undertaken in a specific fashion where possible, such as a gluten-free diet for nontropical sprue. All of these measures should help to prevent vitamin K deficiency.

## THIAMIN (VITAMIN B₁)

### FUNCTIONS

Dietary thiamin functions as precursor of the coenzyme thiamin pyrophosphate, which by the process of oxidative decarboxylation converts α-ketoacids to aldehydes. These reactions are an important source of generating energy and are widely distributed throughout intermediary metabolism. Thiamin pyrophosphate is also the coenzyme for transketolase, which converts xylulose-5-$PO_4$ and ribose-5-$PO_4$ to sedoheptulose-7-$PO_4$ and glyceraldehyde. The efficient generation of energy from oxidation of glucose requires adequate concentrations of thiamin pyrophosphate in the tissues.

More recent evidence suggests that thiamin has a role beyond that of coenzyme in regulating transmission of impulses in peripheral nerves. Some patients with peripheral neuropathy have been improved by thiamin administration. The metabolic role of thiamin in this proposed function is not well understood.

### DEFICIENCY

Initial clinical presentations of thiamin deficiency are often subtle and nonspecific, comprising anorexia, general malaise, and weight loss. The typical Western diet is high in carbohydrate and may not be adequately matched in its thiamin content. An increase in carbohydrate content of the diet lowers the plasma and urinary levels of thiamin. Nonspecific symptoms of thiamin deficiency as it progresses are often followed by more intense weakness, peripheral neuropathy, headache, and tachycardia. When thiamin deficiency is far advanced, the patient usually exhibits prominent cardiovascular and neurological features. The thiamin deficiency disease is called beriberi. The clinical condition includes cardiac and central nervous symptoms. The cardiac findings include an enlarged heart, tachycardia, edema, and ST-segment and T-wave changes. There is high-output failure due, at least in part, to peripheral vasodilatation. This clinical syndrome has a number of similarities to that of apathetic hyperthyroidism, with which it is often confused.

The central nervous system findings in advanced thiamin deficiency are those of the Wernicke–Korsakoff syndrome with vomiting, horizontal nystagmus, ataxia, weakness of the extraocular muscles, mental impairment, memory loss, and confabulation. There may be significant peripheral neuropathy as well. It is important to remember that the Wernicke–Korsakoff syndrome is not restricted to alcohol abuse and occurs with severe malnutrition, gastrointestinal disorders, and congestive heart failure. Some investigators have suggested that the reduction of thiamin pyrophosphate concentrations in brains of patients with Alzheimer's disease may have functional significance. Treatment of these patients with thiamin has been reported to be beneficial in some instances.

Beriberi is classified into several types: acute, mixed, wet, or dry (Table 14.4). The acute, mixed type is characterized by neural and cardiac symptoms producing neuritis and heart failure. In wet beriberi, the edema of heart failure is the most striking sign; digestive disorders and emaciation are additional symptoms. In dry beriberi, loss of functions of the lower extremities or paralysis predominates; it is often called polyneuritis.

A most serious level of thiamin deficiency is seen in malnourished alcoholics. It is known as alcoholic beriberi. It is seen in those individuals who consume alcohol in preference to food and thus have a minimal intake of thiamin. It is characterized by symmetrical foot and wrist drop associated with a great deal of muscle tenderness. It may also affect cardiac muscle metabolism and may result in congestive heart failure.

The mildest and most common form of thiamin deficiency is the polyneuropathy affecting only the lower extremities of the chronic alcoholic. The signs and symptoms of thiamin deficiency are listed in Table 14.4. All forms of thiamin deficiency respond to thiamin treatment unless the pathology is irreversible, a situation not infrequently found with pathological changes in the nerve tracts (polyneuropathy).

Red cell transketolase activity seems to be a sensitive index of thiamin nutritional status. Transketolase catalyzes two reactions of the pentose phosphate shunt. One takes ribulose-5-phosphate and ribose-5-phosphate and makes sedoheputulose-7-phosphate plus glyceraldehyde-3-phosphate. The other takes xyulose-5-phosphate and erythrose-4-phosphate and makes fructose-6-phosphate and glyceraldehyde-3-phoshate. Both reactions require thiamin pyrophosphate (TPP) as a coenzyme. An in vitro test can be used to differentiate thiamin deficiency from other enzymatic defects. This test consists of the stimulation of red cell transketolase activity using glyceradehyde-3-phosphate as the substrate in the presence of saturating amounts of TPP. This is coupled with an NADH indicator reaction. The reaction results in the so-called TPP effect (TPPE) and is claimed to be a good indicator of thiamin nutritional status.

In addition to the enzymatic test, a measure of urinary thiamin in relation to dietary intake has been the basis for balance studies to assess the adequacy of intake. When thiamin excretion is low, a larger portion of the test dose is retained, indicating a tissue need for thiamin. A high excretion indicates tissue saturation. On low intakes, excretion drops to zero.

## NEEDS

Thiamin needs of an individual are influenced by many factors: age, caloric intake, carbohydrate intake, body weight. The presence of infection may drive up the need for thiamin. Periodically, the DRIs are reexamined, and sometimes the recommendations are changed. The reader should visit the NIH website for these updates: www.ods.od.nih.gov/Health_information/Dietary Reference Intakes

## RIBOFLAVIN (VITAMIN B₂)

### FUNCTIONS

To fulfill its metabolic functions, dietary riboflavin must be converted to its flavin coenzymes, flavin mononucleotide (FMN; riboflavin-5′-phosphate) and flavin adenine dinucleotide (FAD). In addition, several flavins, such as monoamine oxidase, sarcosine dehydrogenase, and succinate dehydrogenase, are bound covalently to tissue proteins. The flavin coenzymes as a group catalyze many different types of reactions, particularly oxidation–reduction reactions, dehydrogenations, and oxidative decarboxylation. Most importantly, flavin coenzymes are involved in the respiratory chain, lipid metabolism, the cytochrome P-450 system, and drug metabolism.

Riboflavin has antioxidant activity in its role as precursor to FAD, the coenzyme required by glutathione reductase. The glutathione redox cycle provides major protection against lipid peroxides. Glutathione reductase generates reduced glutathione (GSH) from glutathione (GSSG), which is the substrate required by glutathione peroxidase to inactivate hydrogen peroxide and other lipid peroxides. Thus, increased lipid peroxidation is a feature of riboflavin deficiency, and one that is not widely appreciated.

**TABLE 14.4**
**Clinical Features of Thiamin Deficiency**

| | |
|---|---|
| Wet and dry beriberi | Malaise |
| | Heaviness and weakness of legs |
| | Calf muscle tenderness |
| | "Pins and needles" and numbness in legs |
| | Anesthesia of skin |
| | Increased pulse rate and heart palpitations |
| Wet beriberi | Edema of legs, face, trunk, and serous cavities |
| | Tense calf muscles |
| | Fast pulse |
| | Distended neck veins |
| | High blood pressure |
| | Decreased urine volume |
| Dry beriberi | Polyneuritis |
| | Difficulty walking |
| | Wernicke–Korsakoff syndrome: |
| | Encephalopathy; disorientation; short-term memory loss |
| | Jerky movements of eyes |
| | Staggering gait |

Some flavoproteins contain both FMN and FAD as coenzymes. Included in this category of biflavin enzymes are microsomal NADPH-cytochrome P450-reductase, nitric oxide synthase, and methionine synthase.

## DEFICIENCY

Clinically, patients with advanced riboflavin deficiency exhibit seborrheic dermatitis, severe burning and itching of the eyes, abnormal vascularization of the cornea leading to cataract, cheilosis, angular stomatitis, anemia, and neuropathy. A smooth red tongue is classically observed in riboflavin deficiency, but is not pathognomonic of this deficiency.

The clinical features of human riboflavin deficiency are not unique compared with the specificity of some aspects of vitamin C deficiency such as scurvy. The earliest symptoms of riboflavin deficiency include weakness and fatigue, mouth pain, itching eyes, and occasionally personality disorders.

The evolution of dietary riboflavin deficiency may be intensified by diseases, drugs, and endocrine disorders that block riboflavin utilization. The conditions in which such effects are observed include thyroid and adrenal insufficiency, treatment with the psychotropic drugs, chlorpromazine, imipramine, and amitriptyline; the antimalarial, quinacrine; and the cancer chemotherapeutic drug, adriamycin. Alcohol ingestion may be a significant cause of riboflavin deficiency by its interference with both its digestion from food sources and its intestinal absorption.

Riboflavin deficiency seldom occurs as an isolated entity and is nearly always detected in association with deficiencies of other B vitamins.

## LABORATORY DIAGNOSIS OF DEFICIENCY

Riboflavin and its derivatives can be analyzed precisely by high-performance liquid chromatography (HPLC). Other available techniques are not generally utilized in clinical practice. Urinary riboflavin excretion is reduced with long-term dietary deficiency, but may rise abruptly after recent intake of the vitamin. Therefore, the test must be run in the truly basal state. Collections have to be made carefully in subdued light and stored in dark bottles because of the light sensitivity of the vitamin.

A functional test, the erythrocyte glutathione reductase activity coefficient (EGRAC), measures saturation of the enzyme with its coenzyme (FAD) by the same principle as that developed earlier to assess thiamin status with transketolase. The larger the increase in EGRAC noted after the addition of FAD in vitro, the greater the degree of unsaturation of the apoenzyme with its cofactor and the more severe the deficiency of riboflavin.

## NEEDS

As mentioned, there is almost no riboflavin reserve. Thus, a daily intake of riboflavin is essential. The DRIs are periodically reviewed, and updates can be found on the NIH website: www.ods.od.nih.gov/Health_information/Dietary Reference_Intakes

## PREVENTION

Riboflavin deficiency can be prevented by maintaining a diet high in meat and dairy products, the major sources of the vitamin in the United States. Certain green vegetables, including broccoli, asparagus, and spinach, also contain significant quantities of riboflavin, as do fortified cereals. In developing countries, vegetables constitute the major sources of riboflavin.

It should be recalled that because of its heat and light sensitivity, considerable amounts of the vitamin can be lost when liquids are stored in clear bottles, when fruits and vegetables are sun-dried, and when baking soda is added to fresh vegetables to maintain color and texture. Under the latter conditions, riboflavin loss is accelerated by photodegradation.

Riboflavin has been reported to decrease the frequency of migraine attacks, the severity of lactic acidosis in AIDS patients undergoing therapy, and in rare genetic defects of the respiratory chain. The utilization of dietary folate requires adequate FAD, and for this reason, riboflavin ($B_2$) as well as $B_6$, $B_{12}$, and folic acids are needed to regulate homocysteine metabolism optimally.

## TREATMENT

Treatment of clinical deficiency can be accomplished by oral intake of the vitamin. Levels greater than 25 mg cannot be completely absorbed as a single dose. This dose level is certainly safe to administer. The parenteral administration of riboflavin is limited by its low solubility. FMN is more soluble than riboflavin, but is not usually available for clinical use.

A theoretical risk involved in treatment with riboflavin lies in its photosensitizing properties. In vitro, phototherapy results in DNA degradation and increased formation of lipid peroxides. Riboflavin forms an adduct with tryptophan and accelerates its photodegradation. The extent to which these observations have implications for conditions prevailing in vivo in humans needs to be elucidated.

# NIACIN

## FUNCTIONS

Niacin is the dietary precursor of two important coenzymes, nicotinamide adenine dinucleotide (NAD) and nicotinamide adenine dinucleotide phosphate. Both coenzymes catalyze oxidation–reduction reactions and are involved in a wide variety of reactions in intermediary metabolism. These reactions include glycolysis and lipid, amino acid, and protein metabolism.

## DEFICIENCY

As with the other B vitamins, dietary deficiency of niacin generally occurs together with other vitamin deficiencies.

The deficiency disorder is called pellagra. Pellagra is characterized by skin lesions that are blackened and rough especially in areas exposed to sunlight and abraided by clothing. The typical skin lesions of pellagra are accompanied by insomnia, loss of appetite, weight loss, soreness of mouth and tongue, indigestion, diarrhea, abdominal pain, burning sensations in various parts of the body, vertigo, headache, numbness, nervousness, apprehension, mental confusion, and forgetfulness. Many of these symptoms can be related to niacin deficiency-induced deficits in the metabolism of the central nervous system. This system has, as its choice metabolic fuel, glucose. Glycolysis with its attendant need for NAD as a coenzyme is appreciably less active. As the deficient state progresses, numbness followed by a paralysis of the extremities occurs. The more advanced cases are characterized by tremor and a spastic or ataxic movement that is associated with peripheral nerve inflammation. Death from pellagra ensues if the patient remains untreated.

Early indications of niacin deficiency include reductions in the levels of urinary niacin metabolites especially those that are methylated ($N'$-methyl-nicotinamide and $N'$-methyl-2-pyridone-5-carboxamide). Since the discovery early in this century of the curative power of nicotinic acid and nicotinamide, pellagra is very rare. The exception is in the alcoholic population. This population frequently substitutes alcoholic beverages for food and thereby is at risk for multiple nutrient deficiencies including pellagra. The metabolism of ethanol is NAD dependent. This dependency drives up the need for niacin in the face of inadequate intake setting the stage for alcoholic pellagra. In part, the CNS symptoms of alcoholism are those of pellagra (see Chapter 51).

An unusual aspect of niacin compared with other vitamins is that it is not obtained entirely from the diet. Niacin is formed from dietary tryptophan, an essential amino acid. Thus, high-quality protein sources tend to protect against niacin deficiency, and poor protein sources that are inadequate in tryptophan, such as corn, tend to accelerate niacin deficiency. For this reason, in parts of the world where the diet is based primarily on corn or maize as the dietary staple without other varied sources of protein, pellagra can develop readily.

In addition to alcoholism, some drugs, such as isonicotinic acid hydrazide (isoniazid; INH), can induce niacin deficiency. The anticancer agent 6-mercoptopurine may produce severe niacin deficiency. One may also find niacin deficiency in the rare inborn error of Hartnup's disease and in cancer. In cancer, dietary tryptophan is diverted to the synthesis of serotonin at the expense of niacin.

## NEED

Age, gender, and protein intake affect the DRI for niacin. Low-protein diets increase the need for niacin in the diet since there is little excess tryptophan available for conversion to niacin. The need for niacin is related to energy intake as well, particularly the carbohydrate intake. However, the DRI takes into account varying diet composition as well as individual differences in nutrient need. The DRIs are periodically updated, and these updates are posted on the NIH website: www.ods.od.nih.gov/Health_information/ Dietary Reference_Intakes

## LABORATORY DIAGNOSIS AND DEFICIENCY

In practice, the diagnosis of niacin deficiency can be established by assay of the urinary excretion of niacin metabolites, specifically $N$-methylnicotinamide, and, less commonly, 2-pyridone. Accurate determinations can be made by HPLC.

## PREVENTION

As noted earlier, the diet needs to be adequate in protein of high biological value that contains tryptophan. Intake of meat and dairy products tends to assure adequate intake of tryptophan. A vegetarian diet may contain adequate amounts of niacin if it is sufficiently balanced and varied.

## TREATMENT

The syndrome of niacin deficiency can be treated rapidly and effectively with oral administration of the vitamin. Doses in the range of 50–150 mg/day of nicotinamide are recommended to treat severe deficiency and need to be maintained during the initial treatment period. Improvement is usually noted clinically after only a few days of treatment. The patient usually reports relief of pain and pruritus.

Niacin as a drug in the form of nicotinic acid is a first-line agent for the management of an abnormal serum lipid profile. Doses in the range of 1.5–6.0 g are administered daily. Niacin may be effective alone and in combination with other agents in lowering LDL-cholesterol, raising HDL-cholesterol, and reducing serum triacylglycerols (triglycerides). There may, however, be significant side effects noted at this dose range, including worsening of diabetes, abnormalities in liver function tests, elevation of the serum uric acid, and ocular abnormalities. Flushing may be troublesome to the patient, but is often transient. In most instances, the flushing can be minimized by taking a tablet of aspirin shortly before the niacin, taking a long-acting preparation of niacin, or taking the niacin at bedtime so that the flushing occurs as the patient sleeps.

The form of niacin selected for the improvement of the serum lipid profile is crucial. Nicotinic acid is the only form that is effective. Often patients choose niacinamide on their own from a health food store because it does not cause a flush. Unfortunately, it also does not benefit the abnormal serum lipid concentrations.

## PYRIDOXINE (VITAMIN B₆)

### FUNCTIONS

The role of vitamin $B_6$ is primarily that of precursor to pyridoxal phosphate. This coenzyme participates in a large number of reactions in intermediary metabolism, particularly transamination and decarboxylation. In addition, pyridoxal phosphate is involved in side-chain cleavage, dehydratase activity, and racemization of amino aids. These reactions relate to gluconeogenesis, lipid metabolism, immune function, cerebral metabolism, nucleic acid synthesis, and steroid hormone action. Deficiency of vitamin $B_6$ can lead to secondary deficiencies of other vitamins because it plays a role in the metabolic pathway leading to the synthesis of niacin from tryptophan. Vitamin $B_6$, together with $B_{12}$, folic acid, and probably $B_2$, is involved in synthetic and degradative pathways of homocysteine metabolism.

Although some $B_6$ is present in the diet in the form of pyridoxal, the majority is in other forms. In plants, $B_6$ is present largely as pyridoxine, whereas animal sources comprise pyridoxamine as well as pyridoxal phosphate, and other forms.

## DEFICIENCY

As with other B vitamins, isolated pyridoxine deficiency entirely on a dietary basis is seldom found. In some instances, a marginal diet may result in overt deficiency if there are other complicating factors, such as the long-term use of specific pyridoxine antagonists. Two common examples of this effect are isoniazid and cycloserine, used to treat tuberculosis and generally prescribed for an extended period to eradicate the organism. In some individuals, a genetic trait leads to delays in inactivating isoniazid; as a result, these patients become unusually susceptible to developing $B_6$ deficiency.

Pyridoxine deficiency is a common feature of chronic alcoholism, found in association with overall malnutrition and inadequate intake of many other vitamins and minerals. An unusual feature of the pathogenesis of $B_6$ deficiency in alcoholism is that the major effect of alcohol appears to be that of accelerating the rate of degradation of pyridoxal into its inactive metabolites, particularly pyridoxic acid.

$B_6$ deficiency is not recognizable as a distinct, pathogenomic clinical syndrome. Patients develop degrees of dermatitis, glossitis, cheilosis, and weakness. In more severe deficiency, patients may progress to have dizziness, depression, peripheral neuropathy, and seizures. The risk of kidney stones is increased because of hyperoxaluria. In children, $B_6$ deficiency is an important cause of anemia and seizures. Deficiency of $B_6$ causes a hypochromic, microcytic anemia that resembles the anemia due to iron deficiency. The diagnosis of $B_6$-deficiency anemia is suggested when a bone marrow aspiration reveals that stainable iron, instead of being reduced as in iron deficiency, is normal or even increased in amounts.

In laboratory animals, dermatitis (acrodynia) is the chief symptom. Lesions occur on paws, ears, nose, chin, head, and upper thorax. This skin disorder resembles EFA deficiency. A high-fat diet protects somewhat against a $B_6$ deficiency. Other symptoms include poor growth; muscular weakness; fatty livers; convulsive seizures; anemia; reproductive impairment; edema; nerve degeneration; enlarged adrenal glands; increased excretion of xanthurenic acid, urea, and oxalate; decreased transaminase activity; synthesis of ribosomal RNA, mRNA,

DN;, and impaired immune response. High-protein intakes accelerate the development of the deficiency.

In man, the deficiency syndrome is ill defined. If it occurs, it is accompanied by other deficiency disorders as well. The exception to this is in patients treated with the pantothenic acid antagonist, ω methyl pantothenic acid. In these patients, neurological symptoms (paresthesia of toes and feet) depression, fatigue, insomnia, vomiting, and muscle weakness have been reported. Changes in glucose tolerance, increased sensitivity to insulin, and decreased antibody production have also been noted. Cheilosis (cracks at the corners of the mouth) that is not responsive to biotin or riboflavin may also be a sign of deficiency. Infants consuming $B_6$-deficient milk formula have convulsive seizures, which can be corrected almost immediately with intravenously administered vitamin. There is a deranged tryptophan metabolism and evidence of increased excretion of xanthurenic acid. In $B_6$ deficiency, the conversion of tryptophan to niacin is impaired, and thus skin lesions develop, which resemble those of pellagra and riboflavin deficiency.

Hypochromic, sideroblastic anemia is a common finding and is due to the role $B_6$ plays in hemoglobin synthesis. While $B_6$ is found in a wide variety of foods, $B_6$ deficiency can be observed when antivitamin drugs are used. For example, isoniazid, a drug used in the treatment of tuberculosis, results in excessive $B_6$ loss. Penicillamine, a drug used in the treatment of Wilson's disease, has antivitamin activity.

There are several congenital diseases of importance to $B_6$ status. Homocysteinuria due to a defect in the enzyme cystathione β synthase is characterized by dislocation of the lenses in the eyes, thromboses, malformation of skeletal and connective tissue, and mental retardation. Pyridoxal phosphate is a coenzyme for this synthase. Cystathioninuria due to a defect in cystathione γ lyase is characterized by mental retardation, also drives up the need for $B_6$. GABA deficiency due to mutation in glutamate decarboxylase is manifested by a variety of neuropathies and sideroblastic anemia due to a mutation in δ-aminolevulinate synthetase is characterized by anemia, cystathioninuria, and xanthurenic aciduria. All of these genetic disorders can be ameliorated somewhat by massive doses of the vitamin. Why this works is not known, but patients with these disorders do not have any symptoms of $B_6$ deficiency.

## LABORATORY DIAGNOSIS OF DEFICIENCY

Vitamin $B_6$ can be measured directly in blood, with levels less than 50 ng/mL generally considered to represent deficiency. The measurement needs to be interpreted in light of the patient's diet, as exceptionally high dietary protein intake depresses plasma pyridoxal phosphate levels, probably because of increased utilization of the coenzyme in protein and amino acid metabolism.

Urinary tests measure the excretion of metabolites of pyridoxine, most commonly 4-pyridoxic acid. Indirect assessments of vitamin $B_6$ deficiency can be made using functional assays of the enzymes aspartate or alanine aminotransferase with and without the addition of their cofactors in vitro. The principle of these assays is similar to that discussed earlier for thiamin and riboflavin deficiency. Activity coefficients greater than 1.2 for alanine aminotransferase and 1.5 for aspartate aminotransferase are generally considered as diagnostic of a deficient state.

At one time, a specific diagnosis of $B_6$ deficiency was made by measuring xanthurenic acid after a tryptophan load, inasmuch as $B_6$ is the coenzyme involved in the metabolic transformation. This procedure, although theoretically sound, is very laborious and has largely been abandoned in routine clinical diagnosis.

## PREVENTION

Vitamin $B_6$ is widely available in the food supply and is found in vegetables, beans (especially soybeans), meat, nuts, seeds, and cereals. A diet that is adequate and diversified in these dietary items will generally prevent vitamin $B_6$ deficiency. It is evident that this kind of diet will prevent deficiencies of the other B vitamins as well. Certain kinds of food processing, particularly heat sterilization, can result in significant losses of activity of vitamin $B_6$.

## TREATMENT

Once vitamin $B_6$ deficiency is diagnosed, it can be satisfactorily managed at a level of 2–10 mg/day, which represents doses several times those of the DRI. Vitamin $B_6$ deficiency during pregnancy should be treated with higher doses in the 10–20 mg range because of the increased requirement at this time.

Vitamin $B_6$ is routinely advised during prolonged treatment with isoniazid, which is a pyridoxine antagonist. In doses of 50–100 mg/day, vitamin $B_6$ has been noted to reduce peripheral neuropathy without apparently lessening efficacy of INH against tuberculosis. In patients with Parkinson's disease receiving treatment with L-DOPA, too much pyridoxine will interfere with drug action; therefore, as a general rule, these large doses should not be taken unless there is a specific indication.

It is important not to exceed certain limits in therapeutic administration of vitamin $B_6$. Cases of sensory neuropathy have been occasionally noted in patients taking 1–2 g/day and noted rarely when taking only 500 mg/day. The genetic $B_6$ dependency syndromes can be managed on doses of 100–200 mg/day. There have been some encouraging reports that $B_6$ supplementation may be beneficial in managing premenopausal young women with depression. These findings require confirmation and extension in larger groups of depressed young women.

## NEED

The need for $B_6$ depends on the composition of the diet and on the age and gender of the individual. Aging and diabetes both may have effects on vitamin need. In both instances, an increase in intake is warranted. The DRIs are periodically reviewed and updated. Visit the NIH website: www.ods.od.nih.gov/Health_information/dietary Reference_Intakes for the latest recommendations for the intakes of this vitamin.

## PANTOTHENIC ACID

Deficiency symptoms are not specific.

### NEED

An acceptable intake has been developed for pantothenic acid. Age has an effect on pantothenic need. Check the NIH website for updates to this recommendation: www.ods.od.nih.gov/Health_information/Dietary Reference_Intakes

## BIOTIN

### DEFICIENCY

In man, the symptoms of severe deficiency include dermatitis, skin rash, hair loss (alopecia), developmental delay, seizures, conjunctivitis, visual and auditory loss, metabolic ketolactic acidosis, hyperammonemia, and organic academia. Biotin deficiency results in reproductive failure and impairs the growth and development of the fetus. Abnormal plasma fatty acid profiles are also observed in biotin deficiency. These symptoms have been reported in persons lacking normal biotinidase activity through a genetic error. In a genetically normal human population, a true biotin deficiency is extremely rare; however, in persons that are suffering from protein-energy malnutrition, biotin deficiency may develop secondarily. Only a few instances have been reported. In one, the deficient state was caused by the chronic consumption of 30 raw eggs/day for several months. In this individual, the symptoms were primarily related to the skin.

## FOLIC ACID

### NEED

Because the vitamin is present in a wide variety of foods and because it can be synthesized by the intestinal flora, a fixed intake figure has been difficult to determine. However, the National Academy of Sciences Food and Nutrition Board has published an adequate dietary intake (AI) for this vitamin. However, as mentioned in the preceding section, women contemplating pregnancy should increase their intake twofold. There are racial and ethnic differences in the usual folic acid intake, and it has been suggested that despite food fortification, every woman of childbearing age should take a folic acid supplement. Since folate is not toxic, this is probably a good idea, with the caveat that $B_{12}$ status is normal. If this is not the case, excess folate could mask a $B_{12}$ deficiency somewhat until the irreversible neurological features of $B_{12}$ deficiency appears. Excess folate intake leads to specific and significant downregulation of intestinal and renal folate uptake.

## DEFICIENCY

While anemia, dermatitis, and impaired growth are the chief symptoms of folate deficiency in the human, scientists are now beginning to recognize the importance of adequate folate intake in early embryonic development. Inadequate intake by the mother prior to and/or during the early stages of development can have teratogenic effects on the embryo. Embryonic development, particularly the neural tube, is impaired in folate deficiency. As a result, infants with spina bifida and other neural tube defects are born. It is estimated that about 2500 infants/year are born with these defects. Available evidence indicates that women contemplating pregnancy should consume 400 µg/day as a prophylactic measure. Low folate intake has been suggested as a factor in the development of colon cancer as well as in the bronchial squamous metaplasia (premalignant lesions) of smokers, and cervical dysplasia (another premalignant lesion) in women. Folate antagonists serve important roles as anti-infective, antineoplastic, and anti-inflammatory drugs. These antagonists work by inhibiting dihydrofolate reductase, a key enzyme in the synthesis of thymidylate and therefore DNA. Low zinc intake compromises folate status by negatively affecting intestinal folate uptake. Other symptoms of deficiency are leukopenia (low white cell count), general weakness, depression, and polyneuropathy. The latter sign is probably related to the folate–$B_{12}$ interaction. Alcoholism drives up the need for folacin as well as that of vitamin $B_{12}$.

In rats, folate deficiency has been shown to result in an increased rate of mitochondrial DNA deletion, decreased mitochondrial DNA content, and decreased mitogenesis. These changes were accompanied by an increase in the expression of nuclear encoded genes that regulate mitochondrial gene expression as well as biogenesis. Folate deprivation induced aberrant mitochondrial function via aberrations in mitochondrial DNA, and the cell tried to compensate for this by increasing the synthesis of nuclear factors that upregulate mitochondrial gene expression. Whether this decrease in expression ultimately impinged upon mitochondrial oxidative phosphorylation has not been determined. Studies have not been performed in humans to determine whether folate status affects mitochondrial DNA or mitochondrial function yet; there is every indication that folate may play an important role in mitochondrial health.

## VITAMIN $B_{12}$

### DEFICIENCY

The deficiency state has as its main characteristic, pernicious anemia. While inadequate $B_{12}$ intake can result in this anemia, this is a rather unusual nutritional state

because most foods of animal origin contain $B_{12}$, and so little is needed. More common as a cause of pernicious anemia is a genetically determined deficiency of intrinsic factor. This trait is inherited as an autosomal dominant trait and occurs in about 1 in 1000. It can be treated with monthly $B_{12}$ injections (~60 to 100 µg per dose). In the absence of this trait, the people most at risk for pernicious anemia are those who abstain from eating foods of animal origin. In addition to these are those who have had one of the illnesses described earlier that impair absorption. Humans who have had a gastrectomy or some disease of the gastric mucosa or some disease resulting in malabsorption are in this category.

Following the development of pernicious anemia (which is reversible) is the irreversible loss of peripheral sensation. This is due to the degenerative changes in these nerves including demyelination or loss of the lipid protective coat that surrounds the nerve tracts. Once the myelin is lost, the nerve dies. Neural loss begins in the feet and hands and progresses upward to the major nerve trunks such that a progressive neuropathy can be followed. Because both folate and $B_{12}$ are interactively involved in DNA and RNA synthesis, it used to be difficult to segregate one deficiency anemia from the other. However, given the presence of methylmalonicaciduria and differential analysis of the red cell, one can determine the cause of the anemia. In addition to folacin and $B_{12}$, deficient intakes of iron, copper, and zinc can also explain anemia (see Chapter 13).

### NEED

Updates to the DRIs for vitamin $B_{12}$ can be found on the NIH website: www.ods.od.nih.gov/health_information/dietary Reference Intakes

Daily requirements for $B_{12}$ are very small. The normal turnover rate is about 2.5 µg/day, thus the recommendation for adults is close to this turnover rate or 2 µg/day. For updates to this recommendation, visit the NIH website: www.ods.od.nih.gov/Health_information/Dietary Reference_Intakes. The need for $B_{12}$ is also related to the intake of ascorbic acid, thiamin, carnitine, and fermentable fiber. Each of these nutrients affect the production of proprionate, and in their absence or relative deficiency, proprionate production is increased, and this, in turn, drives up the need for $B_{12}$. As already mentioned, the needs for $B_{12}$ and folate are related. Compromised cobalamin status during pregnancy may put both mother and child at risk for further deterioration of vitamin $B_{12}$ status during lactation compromising the growth and the development of the infant.

## VITAMIN C (ASCORBIC ACID)

### FUNCTIONS

Ascorbic acid serves in both oxidation and reduction reactions, based on the prevailing environmental conditions. Therefore, depending on circumstances, ascorbic acid may act as either an antioxidant or a prooxidant. An important function of ascorbic acid is that of preventing oxidation of tetrahydrofolate. Ascorbic acid is involved in collagen biosynthesis, wound healing, immune function, and drug metabolism. It enhances the intestinal absorption of non-heme iron. This vitamin is involved in the biosynthesis of neurotransmitters and carnitine.

Ascorbic acid concentrations in plasma are inversely related to markers of inflammation, such as C-reactive protein. Recent findings suggest that ascorbic acid may have anti-inflammatory effects in addition to its other actions.

## DEFICIENCY

Dietary deficiency develops when the diet does not contain adequate amounts of citrus fruits, vegetables, and tomatoes, most commonly among the elderly and the urban poor. Vitamin C deficiency may also arise when there is food faddism or very limited food choices, behaviors that are commonly observed these days. The classical "tea and toast" diet, followed by some elderly people, is particularly deficient in vitamin C. The macrobiotic diet may lead to scurvy because of both poor dietary sources and the practice of pressure-cooking food, which destroys ascorbic acid.

In infancy and childhood, a diet composed exclusively of unsupplemented cow's milk is deficient in vitamin C and may lead to scurvy. Chronic alcoholism at any age is associated with poor ascorbic acid intake and, if prolonged, will greatly increase the risk for development of scurvy.

The clinical symptoms of vitamin C deficiency develop slowly and, as with other vitamins, are often vague and nonspecific. Patients complain of weakness and fatigue, progressing to dyspnea and lethargy. The characteristic features of scurvy are not observed until the deficiency syndrome is well advanced. Bone and joint pain may occur because of hemorrhages in the subperiosteum. Perifollicular hemorrhages, especially in relation to hair follicles, are observed. Hairs may show a recognizable corkscrew pattern. Swollen bleeding gums are observed in advanced deficiency followed by loss of teeth. Pallor may be due to bleeding or reduced hematopoiesis. Scurvy results in poor wound healing and secondary breakdown of wounds that had healed previously. It is generally believed that clinical features of scurvy become evident after about 3 months without adequate intake of vitamin C, usually because of failure to consume fruits or vegetables.

Estimates of the prevalence of vitamin C deficiency in the United States were released in 2004, based upon the results of the Third National Health and Nutrition Examination Survey, conducted from 1988 to 1994. Evidence of early vitamin C depletion was found in 13%–23% of the individuals surveyed and evidence of frank ascorbic acid deficiency in 5%–17% of them. The highest risks for deficiency were found among smokers, non-Hispanic Black males, and persons who did not use nutritional supplements of any kind.

## LABORATORY DIAGNOSIS OF DEFICIENCY

Ascorbic acid can be measured directly in the blood serum or plasma by a variety of chemical methods, most commonly spectrophotometric or fluorometric. Levels of 0.1 mg/dL or lower are generally indicative of vitamin C deficiency. Serum levels may be reduced in many chronic digestive disorders in smokers and in some women taking oral contraceptive drugs. Vitamin C concentrations may be measured accurately in leukocytes, but this assay is not commonly available.

Blood levels tend to segregate in a relatively narrow range in the face of very large differences in dietary intake. Megadoses of ascorbic acid remain almost entirely unabsorbed in the gastrointestinal tract, and what little is absorbed is rapidly metabolized by an efficient hepatic drug-metabolizing enzyme system. With its low renal threshold, ascorbic acid is excreted rapidly in the urine.

## PREVENTION

Vitamin C deficiency can be prevented simply by consuming a diet adequate in citrus fruits and vegetables. Consuming orange juice with meals may be a healthy habit that increases the intestinal absorption of nonheme iron severalfold. Avoiding heating or prolonged storage of foods containing vitamin C can also help maintain adequate concentrations. Educating people about the potential hazards of a macrobiotic diet, food faddism, and sharply limited food choices should also help to prevent scurvy in the general population.

The prevention of scurvy may be accomplished by ingestion of very small amounts of ascorbic acid. Some authorities believe that doses as low as 10 mg/day may be effective. The maintenance of an adequate vitamin C status has generally been considered to be in the 40–60 mg range, as reflected in the RDI.

Recently, it has been proposed that the optimal intake of ascorbic acid should be one that not only prevents deficiency but also achieves full concentrations in tissue stores. Based on these assumptions, daily doses of 100–200 mg/day may be needed. To achieve this level of intake, major public health efforts will need to be made, particularly to reach the urban poor.

## TREATMENT

Doses of ascorbic acid as low as 10 mg/day, as noted earlier, may prevent scurvy and can achieve benefits in treatment. In advanced cases, a dose range of 100–200 mg/day orally may be administered safely and effectively, with therapeutic benefit evident within a few days. As noted earlier, it has been proposed that these larger doses need to be maintained to achieve tissue saturation. Meat sources containing heme iron are more bioavailable than the nonheme iron present in vegetables. As noted, the efficiency of absorption of nonheme iron can be greatly improved by simultaneous consumption of orange juice.

There is some risk for toxicity in doses greater than 1–2 g/day in a highly individual fashion. Gastrointestinal upset may occur. Inasmuch as oxalic acid is a direct metabolite of ascorbic acid, the risk of kidney stones theoretically should be increased with large doses of ascorbic acid. The exact prevalence of symptomatic stone formation after ingestion of variable doses of vitamin C is not known with certainty.

Caution in administering vitamin C should be followed when giving it to individuals with hemochromatosis or those at risk for this disorder, as the intestinal absorption and tissue storage of iron may be increased excessively. As the gene for hemochromatosis is one of the most common genetic abnormalities known, there may be risk associated with indiscriminate use of megadoses of ascorbic acid supplements by the general population.

## REFERENCES

1. Adams J, Pepping J. *Am. J. Health Syst. Pharm.* 62:1574; 2005.
2. Agus DB, Vera JC, Golde DW. *Cancer Res.* 59:4555; 1999.
3. Carr A, Frei B. *FASEB J.* 13:1007; 1999.
4. Conway SP, Wolfe SP, Brownlee KG et al. *Pediatrics* 115:1325; 2005.
5. D'Souza RM, D'Souza R. *J. Trop. Pediatr.* 48:323; 2002.
6. Fontana M. *Compendium* 15:916; 1994.
7. Hampl JS, Taylor CA, Johnston CS. The Third National Health and Nutrition Examination Survey, 1988 to 1994. *Am. J. Public Health* 94:870; 2004.
8. Levine M, Padayatty SJ, Katz A, Kwon O et al. In: *Vitamin C: Functions and Biochemistry in Animals and Plants.* Asard H, May JM, Smirnoff N, Eds. B105 Scientific Publishers, London, U.K., 2004, p. 291.
9. Lonsdale D. *eCAM* 3:49; 2006.
10. Rivlin RS. In: *Present Knowledge in Nutrition.* Russell R, Bowman B, Eds. ILSI Press, Washington, DC, 2007, pp. 1114–1120.
11. Rivlin RS. In: *Cecil Textbook of Medicine*, 19th edn. Wyngaarden JH, Smith LH, Jr, Bennett JC, Plum F, Eds. WB Saunders, Philadelphia, PA, 1991, pp. 1170–1183.
12. Sommer A, Davidson FR. *J. Nutr.* 132:2845S; 2002.
13. Standing Committee on the Scientific Evaluation of Dietary References Intakes, Food and Nutrition Board, Institute of Medicine. *Dietary Reference Intakes for Thiamin, Riboflavin, Niacin, Vitamin B_6, Folate, Vitamin B_{12}, Pantothenic Acid, Biotin and Choline.* National Academy Press, Washington, DC, 1999.
14. Underwood BA. *J. Nutr.* 134:231S; 2004.
15. Wannamethee SG, Lowe GDO, Rumley A et al. *Am. J. Clin. Nutr.* 83:567; 2006.
16. Weber P. *Int. J. Vitam. Nutr. Res.* 69:194; 1999.
17. Williams AL, Cotter A, Sabina A et al. *Fam. Pract.* 5:532; 2005.

# 15 Nutrient Interactions

*Carolyn D. Berdanier*

## CONTENTS

Food contains a variety of nutrients either naturally or added as enrichment or supplements. Within a food matrix, nutrients can interact. Most of these interactions are beneficial, but there can be some concerns when the intake of nutrients is unbalanced. This chapter addresses these interactions and describes their effects within the body.

## MINERAL INTERACTIONS

Minerals are found in every cell, tissue, and organ. They are important constituents of essential molecules such as thyroxine ($T_4$), hemoglobin, and vitamin $B_{12}$. They serve as critical cofactors in numerous enzymatic reactions (see Chapters 11 through 13) and form the hard mineral complexes that comprise bone. Minerals serve in the maintenance of pH, osmotic pressure, nerve conductance, and muscle contraction and in almost every aspect of life. Minerals interact such that bioavailability or use is affected.[1,2] The ratios of calcium to phosphorus, iron to copper to zinc, and calcium to magnesium, and other factors are examples of such interactions. Some of these interactions are mutually beneficial, while others are antagonistic. Most of these interactions occur at the level of the gut, in that many are concerned with mineral absorption. For example, zinc absorption is impaired by high iron intakes; high zinc intake impairs copper absorption. High iron intakes impair manganese absorption.[3] Molybdenum and sulfur antagonize copper, and tungsten (not an essential nutrient) interferes with molybdenum absorption. These antagonisms contribute to the relative inefficiency of absorption of minerals that are poorly absorbed and just as poorly lost once absorbed.

Many of the trace minerals have more than one charged state, and living cells have preferences for these states. For example, the uptake of iron is much greater when the iron is in the ferrous (+2) state than when in the ferric (+3) state. Minerals that keep iron in the ferric state will interfere with iron absorption and use. Minerals that do the reverse will enhance iron uptake. Such is the beneficial action of copper on iron. The cuprous ion keeps the ferrous ion from losing electrons and becoming the ferric ion. The interactions of essential minerals are best illustrated in Figure 15.1.

The availability of iron from food depends on its source. Soybean protein, for example, contains an inhibitor of iron uptake. Diets such as those in Asia contain numerous soybean products, and iron absorption is adversely affected by this soybean inhibitor. Tannins, phytates, certain fibers (not cellulose), carbonates, phosphates, and low-protein diets also adversely affect the apparent absorption of iron. In contrast, ascorbic acid, fructose, citric acid, high-protein foods, lysine, histidine, cysteine, methionine, and natural chelates (i.e., heme) all enhance the apparent absorption of iron.[4,5] Zinc and manganese reduce iron uptake by about 30%–50% and 10%–40%, respectively. Excess iron reduces zinc uptakes by 13%–22%. Stearic acid, one of the main fatty acids in meat, enhances iron uptake.

Two types of iron are present in the food, namely, heme iron, which is found principally in animal products, and nonheme iron, which is inorganic iron bound to various proteins in the plant. Most of the iron in the diet, usually greater than 85%, is present in the nonheme form. The absorption of nonheme iron is strongly influenced by its solubility in the upper part of the intestine. Absorption of nonheme iron depends on the composition of the meal and is subject to enhancers of absorption such as animal protein and by reducing agents such as vitamin C. On the other hand, heme iron is absorbed more efficiently. It is not subject to these enhancers. Although heme iron accounts for a smaller proportion of iron in the diet, it provides quantitatively more iron to the body than dietary nonheme iron.

Carcinogenesis can be instigated by some minerals. Nickel subsulfide, for example, is a potent carcinogen, having the renal tissue as its target. In the presence of high to moderate iron levels, the activity of the nickel compound (with respect to carcinogenesis) is increased. In copper excess due to a genetic disorder involving the protein that transports copper, hepatic cancer develops, and this cancer is potentiated by high iron levels. It would appear in these last examples that

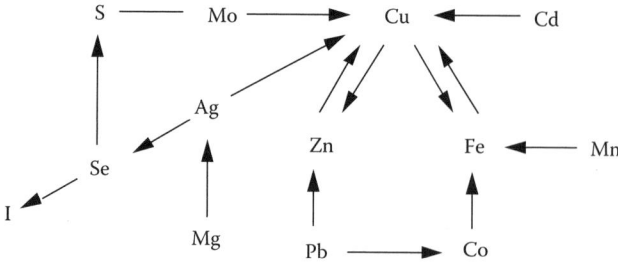

**FIGURE 15.1** Trace mineral interactions.

the role of iron is that of a cancer promoter rather than that of an initiator as described for colon cancer.

Although high iron intakes can be harmful, it should be noted that optimal iron intakes can protect against lead toxicity. Lead competes with iron for uptake by the enterocyte. If the transporter is fully saturated by its preferred mineral, iron, then the lead will be poorly absorbed and get excreted in the feces. Well-nourished individuals with respect to iron nutriture are at lesser risk for lead toxicity than are those whose iron intake is marginal or deficient.

As with iron, zinc absorption is relatively poor. Of the approximately 4–14 mg/day consumed, only 10%–40% is absorbed.[6,7] Absorption is decreased by the presence of binding agents or chelating agents, which bind the mineral making it unavailable. Zinc binds to ligands that contain sulfur, nitrogen, or oxygen. Zinc will form complexes with phosphate groups ($PO_4^-$), chloride ($Cl^-$), and carbonate groups ($HCO_3^-$) as well as with cysteine and histidine. Low zinc status impairs the absorption of calcium.[7]

Zinc can sometimes be displaced on the zinc fingers of DNA-binding proteins (receptors) by other divalent metals.[8] Iron, for example, has been used to displace zinc on the DNA-binding protein that also binds estrogen. This protein binds to the estrogen response element of the DNA promoter region encoding the estrogen-responsive gene products. When this occurs in the presence of $H_2O_2$ and ascorbic acid, damage to the proximate DNA, the estrogen response element, occurs. It has been suggested that, in this circumstance of an iron-substituted zinc finger, free radicals are more readily generated with the consequence of genomic damage. This suggestion has been offered as an explanation of how excess iron (iron toxicity) could instigate the cellular changes that occur in carcinogenesis.

In excess, cadmium can also substitute for zinc in the zinc fingers. In this substitution, the resultant zinc fingers are nonfunctional. Because of the importance of these fingers in cell survival and renewal, a cadmium substitution is lethal. Cadmium toxicity is an acute illness with little lag time needed for the symptom of cell death to manifest itself.

Excess zinc intake can adversely affect copper and iron absorption. Further, excess zinc can interfere with the function of iron as an antioxidant and can interfere with the action of cadmium and calcium as well. Ferritin, the iron storage protein, can also bind zinc. In zinc excess, zinc can replace iron on this protein.[9] Other interactions include a copper–zinc interaction. Copper in excess can interfere

with the uptake and binding of zinc by metallothionine in the enterocyte. In humans consuming copper-rich diets, the apparent absorption of zinc is markedly reduced. In part, this is due to a copper–zinc competition for enterocyte transport and in part due to a copper effect on metallothionine gene expression. Metallothionine has a greater affinity for copper than for zinc, and thus, zinc is left behind while copper is transported to the serosal side of the enterocyte for export to the plasma, whereupon the copper rather than the zinc is picked up by albumin and transported to the rest of the body. Fortunately, excess copper in the normal diet is not common. Zinc is usually present in far greater amounts, and this interaction is of little import in the overall scheme of zinc metabolism. The metallothionine proteins, in addition to binding zinc and copper, also bind other heavy metals such as mercury and cadmium. This occurs when the individual is acutely exposed to toxic levels of these metals.

Selenium is an integral part of the enzyme, type 1 iodothyronine deiodinase, which catalyzes the deiodination of the iodothyronines, notably the deiodination of thyroxine ($T_4$) to triiodothyronine ($T_3$), the most active of the thyroid hormones.[10] This deiodination is also catalyzed by type II and type III deiodinases, which are not selenoproteins. While all the deiodinases catalyze the conversion of $T_4$ to $T_3$, there are differences in the tissue distribution of these enzymes. The pituitary, brain, central nervous system, and brown adipose tissue contain types II and III, whereas type I is found in liver, kidney, and muscle. These two isozymes (II and III) contribute very little $T_3$ to the circulation except under conditions (i.e., starvation) that enhance reverse triiodothyronine ($rT_3$) production. In selenium-deficient animals, type I synthesis is markedly impaired, and this impairment is reversed when selenium is restored to the diet. Under these same conditions, the ratio of $T_3$ to $T_4$ is altered. There is more $T_4$ and less $T_3$ in selenium-deficient animals, and the ratio of the two is reversed when selenium is restored. Because type II and III deiodinases also exist, these enzymes should increase in activity so as to compensate for the selenium-dependent loss of function. However, they do not do this because their activity is linked to that of the type I. When $T_4$ levels rise (as in selenium deficiency), this rise feeds back to the pituitary, which in turn alters (reduces) thyroid-stimulating hormone (TSH) release. The conversion of $T_4$ to $T_3$ in the pituitary is catalyzed by the type II deiodinase, yet TSH release falls. $T_4$ levels are high because the type I deiodinase is less active. Whereas the deficient animal might have a $T_3/T_4$ ratio of 0.01, the selenium-sufficient animal has a ratio of 0.02, a doubling of the conversion of $T_4$ to $T_3$. The effect of selenium supplementation on the synthesis and activity of the type I deiodinase probably explains the poor growth of deficient animals. Bermano et al.[11] have reported significant linear growth in deficient rats given a single selenium supplement, and this growth was directly related to the supplement-induced increase in type I deiodinase activity. In turn, the observations of changes in selenium status coincident with changes in thyroid hormone status provided the necessary background for establishing the selenium–iodine interaction that today is taken for granted. The role of selenium in the synthesis of type I deiodinase clearly explains the lack of goiter (enlarged thyroid gland) in cretins who lack both iodine and selenium in their diet. Thus, low selenium intakes impair thyroid hormone activity, and there is a selenium–iodine interaction.

Other trace mineral interactions also exist. Copper-deficient rats and mice have been shown to have reduced glutathione peroxidase activity.[12] Glutathione peroxidase is a selenium-containing enzyme. Copper deficiency increases oxidative stress, yet oxidative stress affects all of the enzymes involved in free-radical suppression. Even though glutathione peroxidase does not contain copper, the expression of the genes for this enzyme and for catalase is reduced in the copper-deficient animal. There are numerous nutrient interactions required for the maintenance of the optimal redox state in the cell. This is important not only because it stabilizes the lipid portion of the membranes within and around the cells but also because it optimizes the functional performance of the many cellular proteins. Copper, zinc, magnesium, and manganese are part of the anti-oxidant system as are $NADPH^+$ and $NAD^+$ (niacin-containing coenzymes). The $NAD^+$, although not usually shown as part of the system, is involved because it transfers reducing equivalents via the transhydrogenase cycle to $NADP^+$. Excess selenium intake interferes with zinc absorption and use, reduces tissue iron stores, and increases copper level in heart, liver, and kidney.[13] Manganese and calcium share a uniport mechanism for mitochondrial transport.[14] Manganese can accumulate in this organelle because it is cleared very slowly. Mitochondrial manganese efflux is not sodium dependent and in fact appears to inhibit both sodium-dependent and sodium-independent calcium effluxes. This manganese effect on calcium is not reciprocal; calcium has no effect on manganese efflux.

As already mentioned, cobalt in excess can block iron absorption. Cobalt together with manganese and iodine is involved in the synthesis of $T_4$. Whether they interact or are merely essential cofactors in $T_4$ synthesis has not been satisfactorily resolved.[15]

As ions, minerals react with charged amino acid residues of intact proteins and peptides. Table 15.1 provides a list of minerals and the amino acids with which they react. Depending on their valence state, these electrovalent bonds can be very strong or very weak associations or anything in between. The marginally charged ion (either an electron acceptor or an electron donor) will be less strongly attracted to its opposite number than will an ion with a strong charge.

### TABLE 15.1
### Minerals–Amino Acid Interactions

| Minerals | Amino Acid |
| --- | --- |
| Calcium | Serine, carboxylated glutamic acid (GLA) |
| Magnesium | Tyrosine, sulfur-containing amino acids |
| Copper | Histidine |
| Selenium | Methionine, cysteine |
| Zinc | Cysteine, histidine |

The formation of mineral–organic compound bonds is also seen when one examines the roles of minerals in gene expression. Almost every mineral is involved in one or more ways. Zinc–cysteine or zinc–histidine linkages form the zinc fingers that bond with certain base sequences of DNA, thereby affecting transcription. Mineral–protein complexes serve as *cis*- or *trans*-acting elements that enhance or inhibit promoter activity and/or RNA polymerase II activity. Minerals can bond either by themselves or in complexes with proteins to inhibit or enhance translation. Lastly, minerals by themselves or in a complex can influence posttranslation protein modification. Additional information regarding the trace minerals can be found in Chapter 13.

## INTERACTIONS OF VITAMINS WITH MINERALS

The uptake of both calcium and phosphorus by bone as well as the regulation of flux of these two minerals by vitamin D is well known. In this instance, vitamin D acts as a hormone in the regulation of calcium homeostasis. Already mentioned is the interaction of ascorbic acid and iron with respect to iron uptake by the intestinal mucosa. There is the interaction of vitamin E and selenium, as well; each of these nutrients plays a role in the maintenance of the free-radical suppression system. One can replace the other to a certain extent, and so both are considered partners in this important system. If there is a deficiency of intake of selenium, for example, the effects of this deficiency can be ameliorated to some extent by an adequate intake of vitamin E. Although each of these nutrients has a different role in the maintenance of the redox state, their roles are both complementary and substitutive. Additional information on the vitamins can be found in Chapters 13 and 57. Divalent minerals have been reported to impair the uptake of the carotenoids in vitro.[16]

### VITAMIN INTERACTIONS

A number of vitamin interactions have been reported. Table 15.2 summarizes these reports. In the chapter on nutritional biochemistry (Chapter 10), the interacting and complementary roles of the B vitamins were described. These vitamins serve as coenzymes in many reactions of intermediary metabolism. Other interacting and complementary vitamin interactions include that of vitamin C and vitamin E. Both have roles in the regulation of the redox state in the cell. In species that synthesize their own vitamin C (i.e., in rats, mice), vitamin E deficiency leads to vitamin C deficiency because the former plays a role in ascorbic acid synthesis from glucose. Vitamin E also interacts with vitamin $B_{12}$ and zinc. Vitamin-E-deficient animals, although furnished with adequate vitamin $B_{12}$, have been found to have $B_{12}$-deficiency symptoms. Probably this is due to a role of vitamin E on the use of $B_{12}$ as a coenzyme for the enzyme, methylmalonyl-coenzyme-A mutase. With respect to zinc, the interaction has to do with the complementary roles of both nutrients as membranes stabilizers.

**TABLE 15.2**
**Vitamin–Vitamin Interactions**

| Vitamins | Effect |
|---|---|
| $B_6$–$B_{12}$ | Optimizes absorption of both; together both optimize absorption of thiamin |
| E–K | One interferes with the absorption of the other |
| $B_6$–niacin | One interferes with the absorption of the other |
| $B_6$–thiamin | $B_6$ protects against excess thiamin intake |
| $B_{12}$–thiamin | $B_{12}$ deficiency results in increased urinary loss of thiamin |
| $B_{12}$–pantothenic acid | $B_{12}$ spares pantothenic acid |
| Biotin and folacin–pantothenic acid | Biotin and folacin optimize the use of pantothenic acid |
| Thiamin–riboflavin | One interferes with the absorption of the other |
| Riboflavin–$B_6$–niacin | One needed for the metabolism of the other |
| $B_6$–niacin | $B_6$ needed for the synthesis of niacin from tryptophan |
| C–$B_6$ | C protects $B_6$ from excess catabolism and urinary excretion |
|  | A deficiency of $B_6$ reduces blood C levels |
| E–A | E protects A from oxidative destruction |
| C–E | C protects E from oxidative destruction |
| C–A | When A is consumed in excess, tissue C levels fall |
| A–D | A protects against some of the signs of D excess |
| A–E | When A is consumed in excess, E requirement is increased |
| A–K | When A is consumed in excess, K requirement increases |
| A–C | C can increase the conversion of β-carotene to retinol |
| E–C | Both are synergistic in maintaining redox state in the cell |
| Folacin–thiamin | Folacin optimizes thiamin absorption |
| Folacin–$B_{12}$ | If $B_{12}$ is deficient, folacin can mask deficiency signs |
| Riboflavin–folacin | Riboflavin needed for conversion of folic acid to its coenzyme |

*Source:* Biehler, E. et al., *J. Nutr.*, 141, 1769, 2011.

The fat-soluble vitamins A and D can be toxic if consumed in excess over a period of time. The toxicity of vitamin A can be ameliorated by vitamin E. Vitamin E can downregulate the conversion of the carotenes to retinol and thereby reduce the toxicity of vitamin A. Vitamin E can also ameliorate the cellular responses to excess vitamin A through its actions on membrane stability and its function in the free-radical suppression system.

Vitamin D represses the retinoic acid–dependent transactivation of the $RAR\beta_2$ promoter.[17,18] Vitamin A antagonizes the calcium response to vitamin D.[19,20] High intakes of vitamin A result in decreases in bone lipid, while high intakes of vitamin D have the opposite effect. Together, high vitamin A ameliorates the effect of high intakes of vitamin D.[21] Lastly, when intakes of vitamins A, D, and K are considered, vitamin A reduces the vitamin D–induced renal calcification by altering the K-dependent γ-carboxylation of matrix γ-carboxyglutamic acid protein.[22]

## MACRONUTRIENT INTERACTIONS

The need for an adequate energy intake to support growth and development is a long-established principle of nutrition science. The energy intake is primary, for, without sufficient energy, protein synthesis cannot take place at a normal rate. This meets the definition of a nutrient interaction. However, having this as a principle, there are other interactions that are important in intermediary metabolism.

Students of intermediary metabolism have long recognized that these macronutrients share some of the pathways of metabolism. Excess carbohydrate intake results in carbohydrate being converted to lipid. Inadequate energy intake means a depletion of the fat stores, with a subsequent rise in fatty acid oxidation and an increase in glucose production from gluconeogenesis and glycogenolysis (see Chapter 11). The composition of the diet can affect these pathways. Rats fed a 65% sucrose (as compared with those fed starch) have a heightened rate of hepatic lipogenesis. If the fat source is fish oil rather than corn oil or beef tallow, lipogenesis is reduced. If the fat source is coconut oil, lipogenesis is increased.[23–25] In humans, a similar interacting effect of carbohydrate and fat sources has been reported.[26] In this human study, serum cholesterol levels were lower, and triglyceride levels were higher in humans fed a sucrose-saturated fat diet vs. a starch-saturated fat diet compared with humans fed a sucrose-unsaturated or starch-saturated fat diet. Thus, there is an interaction between the two energy sources with respect to lipogenesis and overall lipid dynamics.

## AMINO ACID INTERACTIONS

It has long been recognized that interactions and competitions exist between amino acids in the small intestine. The amino acid carriers (carriers that transport amino acids from the lumen into the absorptive cell) will transport more than one amino acid.[27] Neutral amino acids share a common carrier, as do those with short or polar side chains (serine, threonine, and alanine). There is also a carrier for phenylalanine and methionine and a specific one for proline and hydroxyproline. Similarly, there are carriers that transport amino acids across the blood–brain barrier, and there is some competition among amino acids for these carriers. For example, tryptophan competes with tyrosine for entry through the blood–brain barrier. Both tryptophan and aromatic amino acids (phenylalanine and tyrosine) serve as precursors of neurotransmitters, and a competition between them for transport may have a role in the regulation of the balance of these transmitters in the body. Sulfur-containing amino acids are spared by each other, that is, methionine is spared by cysteine.[28]

In intermediary metabolism, there appears to be an interaction between leucine, isoleucine, and valine.[29] All are branched-chain amino acids and share the same enzymes for their metabolism. All are needed for appropriate rates of protein synthesis. Should one be in short supply, the rate of protein synthesis will fall. Thus, amino acid interactions occur as part of the overall body amino acid economy to ensure appropriate body protein homeostasis.

## SUMMARY

Components of the diet can interact sometimes with beneficial and sometimes with deleterious effects. So much depends on the dietary mixture consumed and the physiological status of the consumer. Where the consumer is marginally nourished, the interacting nutrients can have unexpected results. However, in the well-nourished individual consuming a wide variety of foods and not consuming an excess of any one nutrient or class of nutrients, such interactions are probably insignificant. It is only when individuals restrict their food selections and consume unbalanced supplements should there be concern over deleterious nutrient interactions.

## REFERENCES

1. Fairweather-Tait, B., *Food Chem*, 43: 213; 1992.
2. Frieden, E.J., *Chem Educ*, 62: 917; 1985.
3. Hansen, R. et al., *J Nutr*, 139: 1474; 2009.
4. Johnson, M.A., *J Nutr*, 120: 1486; 1990.
5. Herbert, V. et al., *Stem Cells*, 12: 289; 1994.
6. Reyes, J.G., *Am J Physiol*, 270: C401; 1996.
7. Emery, M.P., Boyd, B.L., *Proc Soc Exp Biol Med*, 203: 480; 1993.
8. Conte, D., Narindrasorasak, S., Sarkar, B., *J Biol Chem*, 271: 5125; 1996.
9. Price, D., Joshi, J.G., *Proc Natl Acad Sci USA*, 79: 3116; 1982.
10. Arthur, J.R., Nicol, F., Beckett, G.J., *Am J Clin Nutr*, 57: 236S; 1993.
11. Bermano, G. et al., *Biol Trace Element Res*, 51: 211; 1996.
12. Lai, C.C. et al., *J Nutr Biochem*, 6: 256; 1995.
13. Chen, S.Y., Collipp, P.J., Hsu, J.M., *Biol Trace Element Res*, 7: 169; 1985.
14. Gavin, C.E., Gunter, K.K., Gunter, T.E., *Biochem J*, 266: 329; 1990.
15. Maberly, G.F., *J Nutr*, 124: 1473S; 1994.
16. Biehler, E. et al., *J Nutr*, 141:1769; 2011.
17. Jimenez-Lara, A.M., Aranda, A., *Endocrinology*, 140: 2898; 1999.
18. Jimenez-Lara, A.M., Aranda, A., *Horm Res*, 54: 301; 2000.
19. Johansson, S., Melhies, H., *J Bone Min Res*, 16: 1899; 2001.
20. Rohde, C.M. et al., *J. Nutr*, 129: 2246; 1999.
21. Cruess, R.L., Clark, I., *Biochem J*, 96: 262; 1965.
22. Fu, X. et al., *J Nutr* 138: 2337; 2008.
23. Machlin, L.J., Langseth, L., In: *Nutrient Interactions*, Bodwell, C.E., Erdman, J.W., eds., Marcel Dekker, New York, 1988, p. 287.
24. Baltzell, J.K., Berdanier, C.D., *J Nutr*, 115: 104; 1985.
25. Berdanier, C.D., In: *Nutrient Interactions*, Bodwell, C.E., Erdman, J.W., eds., Marcel Dekker, New York, 1988, p. 265.
26. Berdanier, C.D., Johnson, B.J., Buchanan, M., *Nutr Res*, 9: 1167; 1989.
27. Antar, M.A. et al., *Atherosclerosis* 11: 191; 1970.
28. Murray, R.K., Granner, D.K., Mayes, P.A., Rodwell, V.W., *Harper's Biochemistry*, Lange Medical, Stamford, CT, 1996, p. 643.
29. Ball, R.D., Courtney Martin, G., Pencharz, P.B., *J Nutr*, 136: 1682S; 2006.

# 16 Finding Mouse Models of Human Disease for Use in Nutrition Research

*Edward H. Leiter and Andrew J. Schile*

## CONTENTS

## INTRODUCTION

Developments in molecular genetics have made the mouse the premier platform for modeling disease in humans. Although there are points of divergence between mice and humans in the regulation of metabolic, immunologic, behavioral, and reproductive functions, overall, there is remarkable conservation of genomic organization and physiologic processes.[1] Many murine pathology-producing monogenic mutations, either spontaneous or induced, currently exist that reflect their human disease syndromic counterparts. An ambitious international project (Knockout Mouse Project, or KOMP) is now under way to functionally characterize the mouse genome by knocking out the entire repertoire of expressed genes. Indeed, the new technologies for mouse genetic manipulation permit the generation of "humanized" mouse models wherein a known human disease-producing mutation is introduced into the mouse genome either by transgenesis or by replacing the wild-type allele in the mouse with the human mutation by locus-specific homologous recombination. The purpose of this chapter is to acquaint food and nutrition scientists with the various information resources available to assist them in matching their research questions with the large collection of mouse models available.

## GENERAL TYPES OF MOUSE MODELS

### INBRED STRAINS

The oldest inbred strains now widely used in biomedical research originated in the beginning of the twentieth century and represent a mosaic of wild house mouse species.[2] If maintained by brother × sister matings over many generations (most inbred mouse strains produce on average three to four generations per year), each inbred strain represents a unique and homogeneous germplasm that carries strain-specific allelic variants (e.g., mutations). These independent collections of allelic variation are reflected by strain-specific development of a variety of constitutive anomalies or differential responses to a variety of experimental modalities. These include differential responsiveness to diet-induced obesity, as well as to drugs and carcinogens, etc. Indeed, some inbred strains are known primarily for their development of complex diseases, such as diabesity in NZO/HlJ and TALLYHO/JngJ males or type 1 autoimmune diabetes in NOD/ShiLtJ mice of both sexes. In addition to the "classical" inbred strains like C57BL/6, DBA/2, BALB/c, 129, CBA, C3H, SWR, SJL, NZO, NZB, NZW, and FVB, new inbred strains continue to be generated. Some of these newer inbreds are derived from relatively recent-trapped wild mice (e.g., CAST, MOLF, PWK, POHN). A large collection of more recent inbred strains produced by inbreeding of outbred ICR stock further expands the spectrum of disease-relevant phenotypes (examples reposited at The Jackson Laboratory include ICR/HaJ, NOD/ShiLtJ, NON/ShiLtJ, ALR/LtJ, and ALS/LtJ). It is standard practice to refer to inbred mouse strains by their letter string abbreviations rather than by full names (e.g., NOD rather than nonobese diabetic; NZO rather than New Zealand obese). Additional types of genetically characterized inbred strains are represented by a variety of Recombinant Inbred (RI) lines, Chromosome Substitution Strains (CSSs), and Collaborative Cross (CC) strains. The latter represent different combinations of the genomes of eight progenitor inbred strains.[3]

At the present time, The Jackson Laboratory, the world's largest repository of inbred strains (http://jaxmice.jax.org/), currently lists over 200 inbred strains or substrains. The important issue of substrains will be discussed later. The website that locates extant inbred strains worldwide is the International Mouse Strain Resource (IMSR) (http://www.findmice.org/). This site identifies not only the availability and supplier or holder of the strain but also the state in which the strain is maintained (live or cryopreserved [embryo in the case of inbred strains]). The site also provides strain information and links for contacting the supplier or holder of the strain and lists all mutations (spontaneous or targeted) available on that strain background. The Jackson Laboratory also maintains an extensive body of phenotypic information for those strains it distributes. Most of this information is available online and will be discussed in more detail below. A publication from The Jackson Laboratory containing useful descriptions of the most popular strains of JAX®Mice is available.[4] Specific strains can be searched using the following link: http://jaxmice.jax.org/query/. Datasheets in the JAX Mice strain database contain valuable information regarding strain origin, husbandry, genotypic and phenotypic characteristics,

and, when relevant to a specific disease phenotype, recommended control strains. Another source of strain-specific information may be found in Festing's inbred strains of mice and rats (http://www.informatics.jax.org/external/festing/search_form.cgi). Some of the information in the Festing listing is dated, however, and thus may not precisely reflect phenotypes of the currently distributed strains. The food/nutrition scientist needs to be aware that a given phenotype is contingent not only on genotype but also on a variety of critical environmental factors extant in the vivarium (including season, enteric flora, diet and diet treatment, temperature, light cycle, bedding, water purity, and treatment) and the specific pathogen-free status of the colony. The NOD/ShiLtJ mouse model of spontaneous autoimmune diabetes provides an excellent example; semidefined diets lacking the complex xenobiotic factors in chow-based diets suppress diabetogenesis.[5] In a model of type 2 diabetes, concentrations of refined carbohydrates are the more important diabetogenic catalysts.[6] Table 16.1 lists relevant website information for locating specific inbred mouse strains as well as contact information for the major suppliers of inbred strains. Table 16.2 provides additional web links relevant to inbred strains of mice.

**TABLE 16.1**
**Websites for Finding an Inbred Mouse Strain**

| Organization | Web Address |
| --- | --- |
| IMSR | www.findmice.org/ |
| The Jackson Laboratory (vendor) JAX®Mice strain database | www.jaxmice.jax.org/query |
| Taconic (vendor) | www.taconic.com |
| Harlan Laboratories (vendor) | www.harlan.com |
| Charles River (vendor) | www.criver.com |
| Central Laboratory for Experimental Animals (Japan, vendor) | www.clea-japan.com |

**TABLE 16.2**
**Other Public Websites: Information about Mouse Strains**

| Organization | Web Address |
| --- | --- |
| National Institutes of Health (NIH) | www.nih.gov |
| Trans-NIH Mouse Initiatives | www.nih.gov/science/models/mouse/ |
| European mutant mouse pathology database | www.pathbase.net |
| Organizations related to specific research areas, for example, | |
|     National Cancer Institute | www.cancer.gov |
|     American Society of Hematology | www.hematology.org |
| Literature search engines, for example, the PubMed service provided by the National Library of Medicine and the NIH | www.pubmed.gov |
| Institute for Laboratory Animal Research (ILAR), U.S. National Academy of Sciences | http://dels.nas.edu/ilar |
| Deltagen Mouse Histology Atlas | www.deltagen.com/target/histologyatlas/HistologyAtlas.html |
| Ensembl Genome Browser | www.ensembl.org |
| University of California, Davis (UCDavis) Mouse Biology Program | mouse.ucdavis.edu |

*Source:* Flurkey, K. et al. *The Jackson Laboratory Handbook on Genetically Standardized Mice,* The Jackson Laboratory, Bar Harbor, ME, 2009.

To the food scientist interested in a specific mouse phenotype tractable to dietary manipulation (e.g., blood HDL cholesterol or fasting blood glucose) but who may be unaware of the variation in that phenotype among inbred strains, the Mouse Phenome Database (MPD) maintained at The Jackson Laboratory (http://phenome.jax.org) can be of great value in comparing well-characterized inbred strains (up to 46 priority strains contained in the database).

Figure 16.1a shows an example of how the MPD can be utilized to survey strain variation in a specific phenotype (in this example, HDL cholesterol of mice fed a high-fat diet). Figure 16.1b provides another MPD example of hepatotoxic

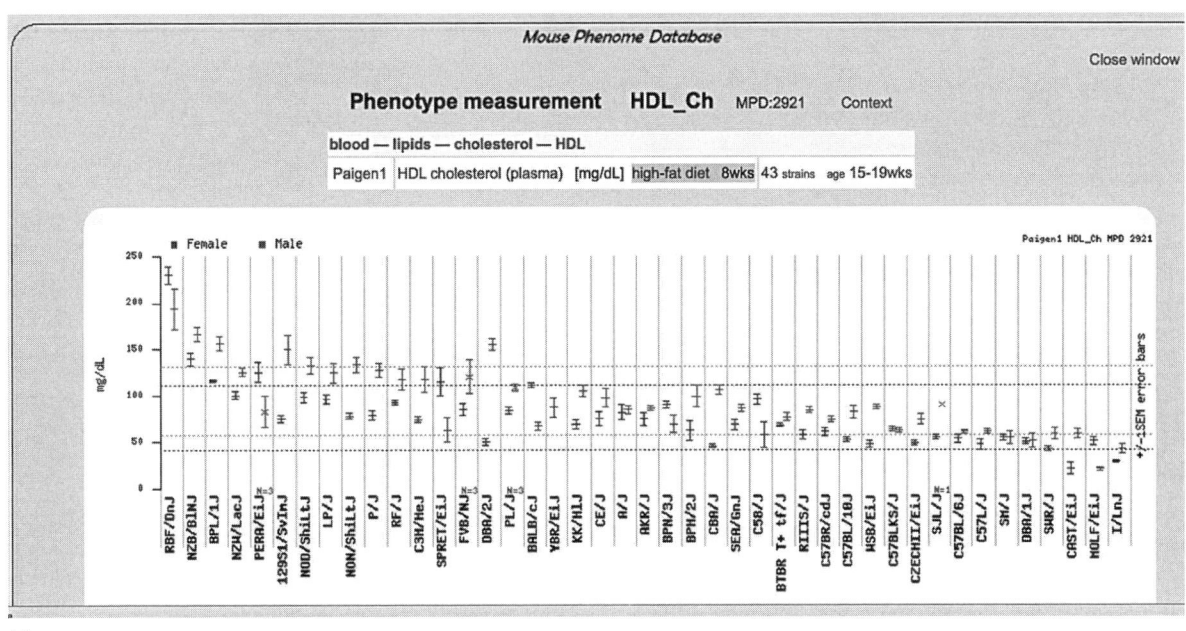

(a)

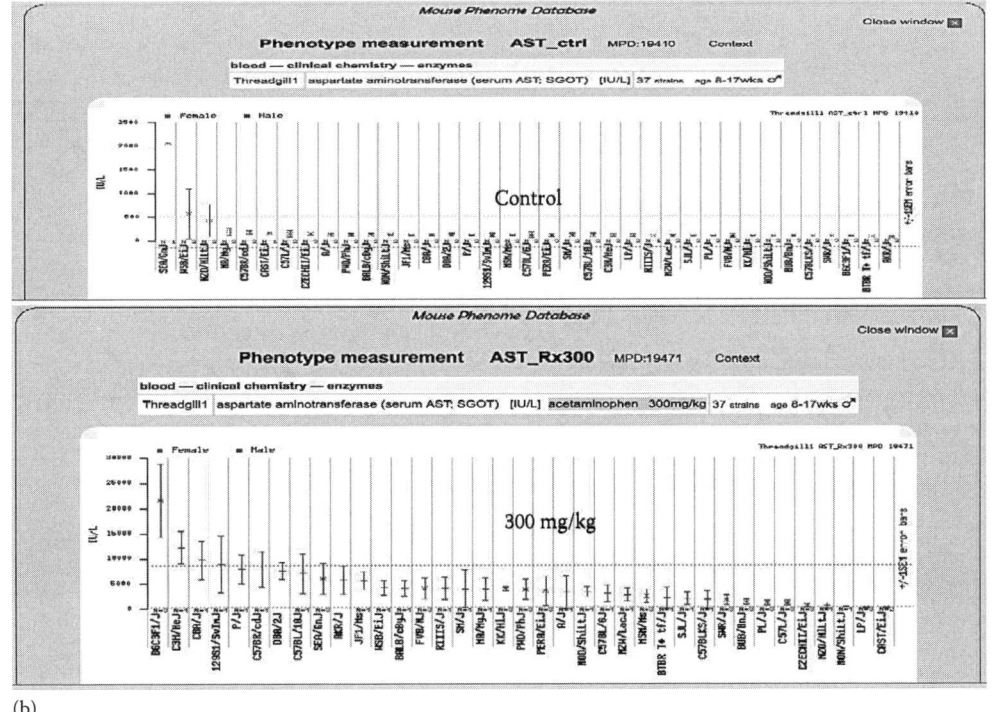

(b)

**FIGURE 16.1** (a) Example of strain distribution pattern for a phenotype (HDL cholesterol) generated from the MPD. (b) Strain distribution pattern of male hepatotoxic to acetaminophen.

(continued)

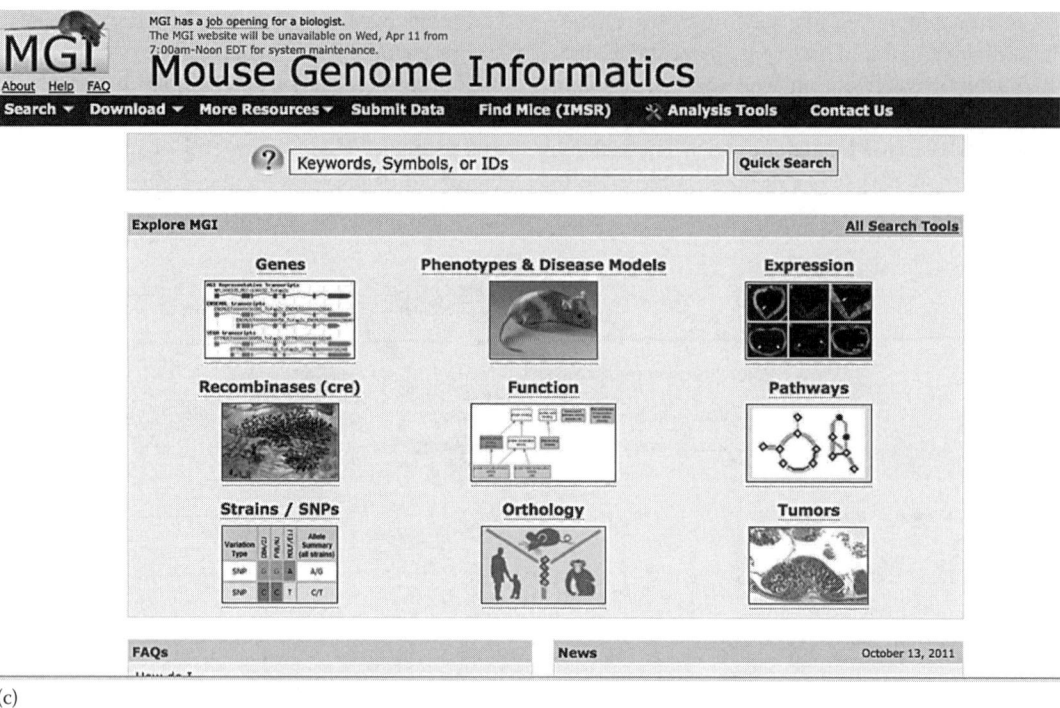

(c)

**FIGURE 16.1 (continued)**   (c) MGI home page options.

responses to acetaminophen as measured by a liver marker enzyme, serum aspartate aminotransferase. Each inbred strain is denoted by the approved letter string descriptor. Since all 32 strains depicted in these illustrations are JAX Mice, details pertaining to each strain listed (origins, salient characteristics, substrains, and genetic mutations/modifications available from JAX) can be obtained at the JAX Mice Database website (http://jaxmice.jax.org/query/). Virtually all MPD data come from ad libitum fed mice. The ad libitum fed laboratory mouse has recently been criticized as "metabolically morbid" as a result of being overfed, with the suggestion that diet restriction produces a more "normal" physiological baseline.[7]

## MICE WITH SPONTANEOUS MUTATIONS

It has been estimated that three spontaneously occurring mouse mutations are fixed to homozygosity with each generation of sib mating.[8] Most of these are silent, but when they produce an altered or deviant phenotype, they can be readily mapped to a chromosome with the genetic tools currently available. Spontaneous mutations may result from single base changes, deletions, or insertions. At least 10% of spontaneous mutations are associated with insertional mutagenesis produced by transposition of endogenous retroviral components. Spontaneous mutations may produce complete loss of function, reduction of function (hypomorphs), or gain of function (hypermorphs).

Table 16.3 provides useful links for locating spontaneous mutations or relevant information regarding a specific gene. The IMSR (http://www.findmice.org/) is an excellent starting point. The Mouse Mutant Resource (MMR) at The Jackson Laboratory (http://mousemutant.jax.org/index.html)

is that institution's primary repository for strains and stocks carrying spontaneous mutations. Mouse Mutant Regional Resource Centers in the United States (queried at http://www.mmrrc.org and summarized at http://dpcpsi.nih.gov/orip/cm/rodent_resource_researchers.aspx) are an additional source of spontaneous mutants. The European Mouse Mutant Archive (http://www.emmanet.org/) serves a similar repository function. The Mouse Genome Informatics (MGI) database (www.informatics.jax.org/) maintained at The Jackson Laboratory provides a seamless link to multiple databases providing a rich source of detailed information regarding a specific gene, including nomenclature, map coordinates, sequence information, alleles, SNP polymorphisms, phenotypes, gene expression and relevant pathways, and mammalian orthologies. Figure 16.1c depicts the home page of this invaluable resource and shows its major components.

Whether affecting only a single gene product or multiple other gene products (e.g., loss of a transcription factor and its downstream target genes), a spontaneous gene mutation will be coisogenic on the inbred strain background on which it occurs. Therefore, any deviation in phenotype from wild type on that specific inbred background can be ascribed to the mutation and not to other complications potentially introduced when the same gene is targeted using embryonal stem cells derived from a different inbred strain than the one eventually carrying the targeted gene. The importance of inbred strain genetic background in influencing a mutation-associated phenotypic deviation was powerfully illustrated by the spontaneous recessive mutations *obese* (*ob*) and *diabetes* (*db*) that are mutations in the leptin (*Lep*) and leptin receptor (*Lepr*) genes, respectively. On the C57BL6/J background, both the *Lep*[ob] and *Lepr*[db] mutations produce

**TABLE 16.3**

**Information Sources Relevant to Mutant Mouse Strains and Stocks (Spontaneous and Induced) and Useful Research Tools**

| Organization | Web Address |
|---|---|
| IMSR | www.nih.gov |
| Trans-NIH Mouse Initiatives | www.nih.gov/science/models/mouse/ |
| NIH Office of Infrastructure Mouse Resources | dpcpsi.nih.gov/orip/cm/rodent_resource_researchers.aspx |
| The Jackson Laboratory Mouse Mutant Gene Resource | mousemutant.jax.org/index.html |
| JAX Cre Repository | cre.jax.org/ |
| European Mouse Mutant Archive | www.emmanet.org |
| Mouse Mutant Regional Resource Centers | www.mmrrc.org |
| KOMP | www.komp.org |
| EUCOMM/International Mouse Knockout Project | www.eucomm.org |
| NorCOMM | www.norcomm.org |
| MGI | www.informatics.jax.org |
| European mutant mouse pathology database | www.pathbase.net |
| Taconic Transgenic Exchange | www.taconic.com/wmspage.cfm?parm1=898 |
| Literature search engines, for example, the PubMed service provided by the National Library of Medicine and the NIH | www.pubmed.gov |
| ILAR, U.S. National Academy of Sciences | dels.nas.edu/ilar |
| Deltagen Mouse Histology Atlas | www.deltagen.com/target/histologyatlas/HistologyAtlas.html |
| Ensembl Genome Browser | www.ensembl.org |
| UCDavis Mouse Biology Program | mouse.ucdavis.edu |

an obesity syndrome uncomplicated by chronic diabetes. In contrast, both mutations on the related C57BLKS/J inbred strain background produce an obesity syndrome accompanied by an early and chronic diabetes syndrome.[9] This is but one of many examples where genetic modifiers of mutant genes in different inbred strain backgrounds produce differential outcomes. This is true regardless of whether the mutation is spontaneous or induced.

## INDUCED MUTATIONS

### Mice with Mutations Generated by Chemical Agents or X-Irradiation

Point mutations in single DNA bases in male mice are generated at random by treatment with chemical mutagens, most notably $N$-ethyl-$N$-nitrosourea (ENU). Isolation and identification of a single gene mutation producing a strong deviant phenotype requires extensive breeding, high-throughput phenotypic screens, and eventually, high-throughput sequencing across a linkage region to identify the altered base pair. X-irradiation of males produces chromosomal deletions, inversions, and aneuploidy; specific screens can produce mouse models of human diseases entailing aneuploidy, for example, Down syndrome.[10] However, the bulk of mouse mutations today are generated by the more recent molecular techniques permitting transgenesis and gene targeting.

### Transgenic Mice

Gene cloning has allowed generation of specific cDNAs coupled to a variety of ubiquitous or cell type-specific promoters or of larger genomic fragments containing endogenous

regulatory elements. Isolated from the mouse genome or genomes of other genera, notably humans, these DNA constructs, sometimes engineered to contain "reporter" genetic elements such as fluorophores, are injected into fertilized mouse zygotes. Integration is random and often entails multiple transgene copies integrated in tandem. In some cases, the integration event itself can functionally inactivate an endogenous gene or otherwise alter normal physiology. To avoid such unwanted side effects, most transgenes are analyzed in hemizygous state (1 copy). An ever-increasing battery of transgenic mouse resources are currently being generated to produce cell-specific conditional "knockout" mice described below.

### Gene-Targeted "Knockouts" and Conditionally Targeted Models

The genomic manipulation of mouse embryonic stem (ES) cells by homologous recombination permits either knockout or knock-in of "designer" alleles altered to contain elements for selection of transduced clones in vitro and then either germ line (global) or conditional (cell-specific) excision. Additional genetic elements responsive to antibiotics or hormones, either within the targeting construct or introduced separately as transgenes, permit postpartum temporal activation or repression. Such alleles designed to be activated or repressed by exogenous stimuli are referred to as "conditional" alleles.

Until quite recently, 129/Sv substrains were the primary source of ES cells used in targeting. For ease of identifying chimeras arising from these ES cells by coat color, they have been commonly injected into C57BL/6 (B6) blastocysts. Because C57BL/6 has become widely accepted as the "standard" background for comparison of knockout/knock-in mice with wild-type controls, multiple backcrosses (five at a minimum) are required to produce C57BL/6 congenic stocks fixed for the chromosomal 129/Sv segment carrying the targeted allele. In this case, investigators need to be aware that other donor strain alleles are being introduced in addition to the targeted allele. With the advent of germ line-competent C57BL/6N ES cells now available, homologous recombination can be effected directly into the B6 genetic background. Newer technologies only now being introduced (zinc finger nucleases, TALENs) will allow gene targeting directly in zygotes of any inbred strain of mice or rats,[11] thereby circumventing this complication. Mice are also being "humanized" by inserting human transgenes or by knocking in a human allele in place of the mouse ortholog.[12] An excellent illustration is represented by transgenic mouse models of Lou Gehrig's disease (amyotrophic lateral sclerosis) expressing the human disease-associated glycine to alanine mutation at residue 93 of the superoxide dismutase 1 (SOD1) gene. As is the case for spontaneous mutations, the phenotype elicited is very sensitive to inbred strain background.[13]

Table 16.3 lists web addresses helpful in locating genetically engineered mouse models and research tools for generating them. Gene knockouts in specific cell types generally entail flanking of the exon(s) to be deleted by *loxP* sites (34 nucleotide sequence). These sites are excised in the presence of separately introduced transgenes expressing a bacteriophage cyclization recombination enzyme (Cre) that mediates recombination between the *loxP* sites and removes the sequence between them. Coupling cell-specific promoters to the Cre gene leads to cells specific deletion. However, cell mosaic expression of the Cre driver may produce incomplete knockdown of the gene product in the tissue, and the promoter itself may be "leaky," that is, expressed in multiple other tissues. The JAX Cre Repository (http://cre.jax.org/) provides a useful website describing the Cre-*lox* technology and characterizing the various Cre-driver stocks maintained in the large repository. The MGI

database can be queried for more than 1000 stocks relevant to Cre recombinase (http://www.creportal.org/). Other web addresses in Table 16.3 provide access to sources of targeted ES cell lines as well as mice generated from them. The International Knockout Mouse Consortium, encompassing KOMP, North American Conditional Mouse Mutagenesis Project (NorCOMM), and European Conditional Mouse Mutagenesis Program (EUCOMM) and Regeneron Pharmaceuticals, is an ambitious initiative to generate C57BL/6N ES cells containing null and conditional mutations in every expressed gene in the mouse.

## FINDING MICE MODELING A SPECIFIC HUMAN DISORDER

A search of the scientific literature is an obvious place to begin (http://www. Pubmed.gov); with the large numbers of genetically engineered mouse mutations being generated, there is likely to be a mouse counterpart for most monogenic human syndromes in the database (over 3600 mouse genotypes modeling a human disease are currently listed in MGI [http://www.informatics.jax.org/orthology.shtml]). The Jackson Laboratory's Genetics Resource Sciences unit assembles collections of mutant mice modeling for specific human illnesses (http://research.jax.org/grs/disease-specific.html). These include Alzheimer's disease, Parkinson's disease, type 1 diabetes, amyotrophic lateral sclerosis, and craniofacial, hearing, ocular, and smooth muscle deficiencies, as well as a large collection of cancer and metabolic disease models, especially obesity and type 2 diabetes. The Jackson Laboratory's JAX Mice and Services database also provides a link to mice by research area (http://jaxmice.jax.org/research/index.html). The major suppliers of mice all maintain technical staff that can handle inquiries and guide model selection. Given the complexities of mouse nomenclature, especially of mice carrying combinations of gene knockouts and transgenes, it is important that the investigator makes the correct selection before ordering mice. Table 16.4 provides useful links by specific disease area of the mouse models maintained at The Jackson Laboratory.

**TABLE 16.4**
**Resources for Mouse Disease Models at The Jackson Laboratory**

| Disease | Web Address |
| --- | --- |
| Alzheimer's disease | http://research.jax.org/grs/alzheimers.html |
| Parkinson's disease | http://research.jax.org/grs/parkinsons.html |
| Type 1 diabetes | http://type1diabetes.jax.org/index.html |
| Amyotrophic lateral sclerosis | http://jaxmice.jax.org/research/neurobiology/als.html |
| Craniofacial | http://www.jax.org/facebase/index.html |
| Hearing | http://hearingimpairment.jax.org/index.html |
| Ocular | http://eyemutant.jax.org/index.html |
| Cancer | http://jaxmice.jax.org/cancer/index.html |
| Obesity and type 2 diabetes | http://jaxmice.jax.org/diabetes/index.html |

## GENETIC NOMENCLATURE AND SUBSTRAIN DESIGNATIONS

Some scientists new to working with mice sometimes view this complex organism as a generic reagent, much as they would a chemical compound on the shelf. In fact, it is critical to pay attention to the genetic nomenclature on the shipping tag of any mouse received from a supplier or a colleague. MGI contains a link (http://www.informatics.jax.org/mgihome/nomen/index.shtml) that helps interpret what, to the uninitiated, appears to be arcane symbology applied to genetically manipulated mouse strains. When searching for mutant alleles, it is helpful to know the formal abbreviation (also called the gene symbol) for the affected gene because the worldwide repositories are categorized using formal gene nomenclature. The MGI can be used to identify gene symbols; for example, a query using common shorthand (the tumor suppressor gene p53) returns the formal gene abbreviation (*Trp53*). Mouse gene symbols are italicized and begin with a capital letter followed by lowercase letters.

In addition to understanding the information contained in a nomenclature string, it also is very important to understand that multiple substrains of the standard inbred strains may exist and that substrain divergence leads to important genotypic and phenotypic distinctions. For example, in PubMed, there are over 100,000 "hits" for "BALB/c," but only about 10% specify which BALB/c substrain is used. This is unfortunate—the two major BALB/c substrains maintained at The Jackson Laboratory, BALB/cJ and BALB/cByJ, differ markedly in multiple behavioral and physiologic parameters (the interested reader may compare the two in MPD). In another example of substrain divergence, C57BL/6J males show a differential weight gain response to a low-fat diet compared to the C57BL/6NJ substrain fed the same diet in the same vivarium.[14] At the level of ES cells used to target a gene, there are important differences in 129/Sv substrains that could impact phenotype independently of a given genetic manipulation. Additional resources to aid investigators in interpreting strain names are available from The Jackson Laboratory's website (http://jaxmice.jax.org/support/nomenclature/index.html).

## ACKNOWLEDGMENT

The author thanks Dr. James Yeadon (Technical Information Services, The Jackson Laboratory) for his critical review.

## REFERENCES

1. Paigen, K, *Nat. Med.* 1: 215; 1995.
2. Silver, LM, *Mouse Genetics Concepts and Applications.* Oxford University Press, New York, 1995; 351p.
3. Threadgill, DW and Churchill, GA, *G3 (Bethesda)* 2: 153; 2012.
4. Flurkey, K, Currer, JM, Leiter, EH, and Witham, B, *The Jackson Laboratory Handbook on Genetically Standardized Mice.* The Jackson Laboratory, Bar Harbor, ME, 2009; 380p.
5. Coleman, DL, Kuzava, JE, and Leiter, EH, *Diabetes* 39: 432; 1990.
6. Leiter, EH, Coleman, DL, Ingram, DK, and Reynolds, MA, *J. Nutr.* 113: 184; 1983.
7. Martin, B, Ji, S, Maudsley, S, and Mattson, MP, *Proc. Natl. Acad. Sci. USA* 107: 6127; 2010.
8. Bailey, D, *Immunol. Today* 3: 210; 1982.
9. Coleman, DL, *Diabetologia* 14: 141; 1978.
10. Costa, AC, Stasko, MR, Schmidt, C, and Davisson, MT, *Behav. Brain Res.* 206: 52; 2010.
11. Jacob, HJ, Lazar, J, Dwinell, MR, Moreno, C, and Geurts, AM, *Trends Genet.* 26: 510; 2010.
12. Ito, R, Takahashi, T, Katano, I, and Ito, M, *Cell. Mol. Immunol.* 9: 208; 2012.
13. Heiman-Patterson, TD, Sher, RB, Blankenhorn, EA, Alexander, G, Deitch, JS, Kunst, CB, Maragakis, N, and Cox, G, *Amyotroph. Lateral Scler.* 12: 79; 2011.
14. Nicholson, A, Reifsnyder, PC, Malcolm, RD, Lucas, CA, MacGregor, GR, Zhang, W, and Leiter, EH, *Obesity (Silver Spring)* 18: 1902; 2010.

# 17 Nutrient Needs of Man and Animals

*John P. McNamara*

## CONTENTS

## INTRODUCTION

### NUTRITIONAL REQUIREMENTS FOR DIFFERENT SPECIES

The nutritional requirements for different species of animals, including mammals, birds, and fish, vary markedly. Some of the factors affecting nutritional requirements are age, gender, stage of maturity, level of activity (work); body size, type, and level of production (i.e., lean or adipose body tissue, milk, eggs, wool, bone growth, etc.); environment (temperature, wind speed, moisture); physiological function (i.e., maintenance, pregnancy, lactation); and health status (presence of disease). The basic nutrient requirements for glucose, amino acids, fatty acids, vitamins, and minerals are quite universal among species, with some important differences. However, the dietary feedstuffs used to supply those requirements vary widely.

Differing species have adapted over time to their nutritional environment, and this has led to a tremendous variety in the type of gastrointestinal tract and the present-day diet. For example, ruminants (cattle, sheep, goats, and deer), as a result of microbial fermentation in the rumen and reticulum, prior to the stomach, usually consume diets high in forages and dietary fiber. Higher producing animals, such as dairy cattle, can tolerate more grain in the diet if it is well-mixed and fed properly. Many nonruminants (humans, swine, dogs, cats, nonhuman primates) by definition are omnivores and can consume a wide variety of animal and vegetable matter and, other than dogs and cats, can utilize some dietary fiber in the large intestine. Nonruminant herbivores such as horses and rabbits and some ruminants utilize a primarily fiber diet, but can use and are often fed grain sources as well. Clearly, the benefits of using ruminant animals are that they can convert plant biomass (fiber, consisting of primarily cellulose and hemicellulose) to food and power for human use.

There are species differences in lipid and amino acid digestion and use as well. Most herbivores cannot tolerate diets with more than a few percent of fat unless they are high producing or highly active. Although all species require 20 or so amino acids, the source and ability to make them vary, and care needs to be taken when formulating rations. Mammals excrete excess nitrogen resulting from amino acid metabolism as urea, whereas birds excrete uric acid and fish simply ammonia. This alters their kidney function and their energy requirement as well, and in modern agriculture, how we manage their manure.

Animals are used for food production, companionship and pleasure, and for research into basic biology or human disease or function. Nutritionists must be aware of differences in the nutritional requirements of different species, or erroneous conclusions could be drawn. For example, vitamin C is required for humans, guinea pigs, and monkeys but not for swine and rats, which are frequently used as animal models.

It is essential for livestock, poultry, and aquatic food producers as well as veterinarians, animal caretakers, biomedical research scientists, and others involved in caring for and feeding animals to know what types of dietary ingredients are appropriate, variation in nutrients required, and the effects of different factors on the efficiency of nutrient utilization. Because of the economic importance of this knowledge, scientists throughout the world have conducted research with different species of animals, birds, and fish, and feeding standards based on this research have been developed to formulate diets and rations for domestic livestock, poultry, companion animals, laboratory animals, and other species.

For more than 150 years, scientists worldwide have worked intensively to identify the specific nutritional requirements of numerous species of animals, including the chemistry of available feedstuffs. Although in many ways nutrition is a "completed" field (we likely will not discover new nutrients or metabolic pathways), modern nutritional research includes asking questions on the interactions of genetics and nutrition (nutri-genetics and nutri-genomics); nutrition and longevity or disease, including cancer, heart disease, immunity, and inflammation. For example, research in just the last 20 years or so has clearly shown that even within a species, there is variation in how nutrition and genetics interact to affect diabetes, food allergies, obesity, and other problems. The use of specific fatty acid molecules (omega-3 fatty acids) is widespread and shown to affect brain development and inflammatory responses throughout the body.

The data presented in this section are based on research summarized by groups of scientists who are most knowledgeable on that particular species. In the United States, the National Academy of Sciences, National Research Council (NRC), Board on Agriculture, and Committee on Animal Nutrition (National Academy Press, 2101 Constitution Avenue NW, Washington, DC 20055) have been responsible for appointing committees of expert animal scientists to publish periodical reports that summarize the most up-to-date information on

**TABLE 17.1**

**Nutrient Requirements of Various Species**

*Companion Animals (Cats and Dogs)*

Cats

*Nutrient Requirements of Dogs and Cats*, 2006. National Research Council, National Academy Press (NAP), 424pp. ISBN-10: 0-309-08628-0.

Mink and Foxes

*Nutrient Requirements of Mink and Foxes*, Second Revised Edition, 1982. National Research Council, National Academy Press (NAP), 72 pp. ISBN 0-309-03325-X. Subcommittee on Furbearer Nutrition, 1982.

Rabbits

*Nutrient Requirements of Rabbits*, Second Revised Edition, 1977. National Research Council, National Academy Press (NAP), Subcommittee on Rabbit Nutrition, 1977.

*Laboratory Animals*

Rat, mouse, guinea pigs, hamster, gerbils, voles

*Nutrient Requirements of Laboratory* Animals, Fourth Revised Edition, 1995. National Research Council, National Academy Press (NAP).

*Nutrient Requirements of Domestic Animals*, National Research Council, National Academy Press, Washington, DC, 1995, 173pp. ISBN 0-309-05126-6 (SF 406.2.N88 1995). Subcommittee on Laboratory Animal Nutrition.

Fish

*Nutrient Requirements of Fish and Shrimp*. National Research Council, National Academy Press (NAP), 128pp. ISBN-0-309-16338-2, 2011.

*Avian Species*

Poultry (chickens, turkeys, geese, ducks, pheasants, Japanese quail, bobwhite quail)

*Nutrient Requirements of Poultry*, Ninth Revised Edition, 1994 (BOA), 176pp. ISBN 0-309-04892-3.

*Domestic Livestock*

Nonruminant Species

Swine

*Nutrient Requirements of Swine*, Eleventh Revised Edition, 2012. National Research Council, National Academy Press (NAP), 400pp. ISBN 10: 0-309-22423-3.

Horses

*Nutrient Requirements of Horses*, Sixth Revised Edition, 2007. National Research Council, National Academy Press (NAP), 360pp. ISBN-10: 0-309-10212-X.

Ruminant Species

Beef cattle

*Nutrient Requirements of Beef Cattle*, Seventh Revised Edition, update 2000. National Research Council, National Academy Press (NAP), Note: The 7th Revised Edition Update 2000 was released and is on the website. 242pp. ISBN 0-309-05426-5.

Dairy cattle

*Nutrient Requirements of Dairy Cattle*, Seventh Revised Edition, 2001. National Research Council, National Academy Press (NAP), 408pp. ISBN 10: 0-309-06997-1.

Sheep, Goats, Carved, New World Camelids

*Nutrient Requirements of Small Ruminants: Sheep, Goats, Carved, New World Camelids*, 1007, 384pp. ISBN 10: 0-309-10213-8.

Nonhuman Primates

*Nutrient Requirements of Nonhuman Primates*, Second Revised.

nutritional requirements of various species. The nutrient composition of feeds usually consumed by these animals is also included in each of the publications, because the feed evaluation system used to express the nutritional value of feeds determines the manner in which the nutritional requirements of the animal are expressed. Specific information on each species may be obtained in the most recent NRC publication (Table 17.1) on that species and visiting the website www.nap.edu. Many of the publications are now free for download.

The health and well-being of animals are affected markedly by their nutritional status. It is important to know how to properly provide feed that contains the nutrients animals need to meet their nutritional requirements. This applies to companion animals such as dogs, cats, birds, and fish as well

as recreational animals such as horses, ponies, donkeys, and camels. The efficient and economical production of food and fiber by domestic livestock and poultry requires good management practices and especially balanced rations that contain adequate supplies of protein, minerals, vitamins, and energy.

The most recent National Academy Press publications on Nutrient Requirements of Domestic Animals are listed in Table 17.1. Publications on the nutrient requirements of a variety of species are available online at http://books.nap.edu.[1] To locate each publication, type "Nutrient Requirements" in the box labeled SEARCH ALL TITLES. Tables with specific information on the nutrient requirements of each species as well as the composition of diet ingredients (feedstuffs) may be accessed by clicking on OPEN BOOK Searchable READ.

# Part III

## Nutrition throughout Life

# 18 Nutrition during Pregnancy and Lactation

*Kathryn M. Kolasa and David G. Weismiller*

## CONTENTS

## RECOMMENDATIONS FOR WOMEN BEFORE PREGNANCY

It seems logical that the nutritional status of a woman prior to pregnancy as well as maternal nutrition should affect fetal development and subsequent pregnancy outcome. However, many confounding variables are common to the investigation of maternal nutrition and fetal development.[1] This section briefly summarizes recommendations for maternal nutrition.[2–11] It also includes comments about lactation, because maternal diet plays a central role in the transfer of nutrients to the infant. Table 18.1 includes special recommendations for women during childbearing years. Suggestions for counseling and treatment during preconception care office visits based on recommendations from the Center for

Disease Control (CDC)[12] and others[13] are given in Table 18.2. Evidence supporting the value of preconception counseling continues to grow.

## RISK FACTORS FOR PRENATAL NUTRITION RISK AND INDICATIONS FOR REFERRAL

Table 18.2 includes nutrition assessment, counseling, and treatment strategies for women seeking care in both the prenatal and postnatal stages. Fetal growth is affected by the quality and quantity of the maternal diet, the ability of the mother to digest and absorb nutrients, maternal cardiorespiratory function, uterine blood flow, placental transfer, placental blood flow, and appropriate distribution and handling of nutrients and oxygen by the fetus. Factors that

**TABLE 18.1**

**Special Recommendations for Women before Pregnancy**

Maintain a healthy weight.

Engage in physical activity regularly.

If you need to gain or lose weight, do so gradually (no more than 1–2 lb/week).

If trying to become pregnant and ordinarily drink alcoholic beverages, stop drinking or cut back on the amount you drink.

If you smoke, quit. Cutting back does not suggest overall improvement in outcomes.

To minimize risk of having an infant with an NTD, eat a highly fortified breakfast cereal that provides 100% of the Daily Value for folate or take a vitamin supplement that provides 600 μg/day of folic acid (4 weeks preconception through 12 weeks postconception). Folic acid, the synthetic form of folate, is obtained only from fortified foods or vitamin supplements. It is not yet known whether naturally occurring folate is as effective folic acid in the prevention of NTDs. For secondary prevention, the dosage is 4 mg/day.

put women at nutritional risk for pregnancy are listed in Table 18.3.[6,14] Patients at high nutritional risk should be provided professional nutritional counseling and/or referral to a nutrition intervention program (Table 18.4)[13,14] The Women, Infants, and Children (WIC) program is a food prescription program designed and proven to reduce poor pregnancy outcomes. Major changes to the program were made in 2011 to align the food packages with the Dietary Guidelines for Americans and promote breast-feeding (www.fns.usda.gov/wic, accessed April 5, 2012).

## WEIGHT GAIN AND PREGNANCY

### Pregnancy Weight Goals

A growing body of research is providing a better understanding of findings concerning relationships of birth interval, parity, prepregnancy weight or body mass index (BMI), height, and physical activity to maternal weight or weight gain. What remains elusive is a prospective, longitudinal study that follows a sufficiently large cohort of women from before pregnancy through each trimester and into the puerperium, measuring the quality and the quantity of women's food intake, and correlating the diet with maternal and newborn outcomes. The Cochrane Pregnancy and Childbirth Group[15] summarized the findings on the effects of advising pregnant women to increase their energy and protein intakes, on gestational weight gain, and on the outcome of pregnancy. The main results in five trials including 1135 women was that nutritional advice to increase energy and protein intakes was successful in achieving those goals, but no consistent benefit was observed on pregnancy outcomes. The authors conclude that dietary advice appears effective in increasing pregnant women's energy and protein intakes but is unlikely to confer major benefits on infant or maternal health. The Dietary Reference Intake (DRI) for protein in pregnancy is 71 g/day.

Less than 50% of pregnant women gain in the outlined weight ranges. Some researchers question the notion that African-American women gain more weight than

Caucasian women, suggesting that the data only showed questionable benefit in reducing risks for low-birth-weight babies.[7] Some experts believe that the weight-gain guidelines are too high for all and that it should be individualized.

Maternal obesity is a major risk factor in pregnancy for maternal and fetal complications, including maternal and fetal mortality, miscarriages, gestational diabetes mellitus (GDM), and hypertensive disorders of pregnancy, infection, thromboembolic disease, induction of labor, macrosomia, cesarean delivery, and stillbirth.[4] Infants of obese women may be at greater risk for perinatal mortality and prematurity, and low birth weight is associated with diabetes mellitus, hypertension, and heart disease in adulthood.[15,16]

The recommendations in Table 18.5 were established by the Institute of Medicine of the National Academies in 2009.[4] In developing these guidelines, the institute considered not only the welfare of the infant, but also the welfare of the mother. The 2009 guidelines differ from the 1990 guidelines[7] in two important ways. First, they are based on the World Health Organization (WHO) BMI categories* rather than the previous categories from the Metropolitan Life Insurance tables. While the prepregnancy BMI is a relatively weak proxy for a woman's nutritional status, one of the most important modifiers of pregnancy weight gain and its impact on a mother's and her baby's health is a woman's weight at the start of pregnancy. Weight-gain goals have been determined to provide optimal risk reduction for delivering a low-birth-weight baby while avoiding adverse effects on the mother's health. Second, the 2009 guidelines[4] include a specific and relatively narrow range of recommended gain for obese women. Excessive weight gain in pregnancy, on top of baseline obesity, significantly increases the risk of fetal macrosomia and pregnancy complications.[4,20,21] Because positive outcomes are achieved within a range of weight gains, the guidelines are

---

* http://apps.who.int/bmi/index.jsp?introPage=intro_3.html (accessed April 5, 2012).

**TABLE 18.2**

**Nutritional Care at Preconception, Prenatal, and Postnatal Visits**

| Visit | Assessment | Counseling/Treatment |
|---|---|---|
| Preconception care | Determine body mass index | If <18 or >25, counsel on appropriate weight |
| | Evaluate diet/supplement intake | Develop a concrete plan for eating enough food to achieve/maintain a healthy weight |
| | | Begin prenatal vitamin/mineral supplement |
| | | Prescribe calcium supplement if intake <1000 mg |
| | | Prescribe synthetic folic acid supplement of 400 µg/day |
| | Botanical use | Discontinue those with known or potential toxicities |
| | Evaluate for anemia | If Hgb <12 g/dL, start therapeutic regimen of approximately 60–120 mg/day of ferrous iron; give multivitamin/ mineral supplement that contains ~15 mg of zinc and ~2 mg of copper |
| | | When anemia has resolved, discontinue high-dose iron |
| Prenatal | Use of harmful substances | Reinforcement for any constructive steps already taken; provide assistance with quitting and refer for further evaluation |
| | Evaluate diet | Utilize dietary intake questionnaire, for example, Diet Score, and food frequency questionnaires |
| | Optimal weight gain during pregnancy is controversial | BMI     <18.5         28–40 lb |
| | |           18.5–24.9     25–35 lb |
| | |           25.0–29.9     15–25 lb |
| | |           >30             11–20 lb |
| | Optimal weight gain for women carrying twins | Weekly weight gain of 0.75 kg during second and third trimesters to a total of 37–54 lb if normal-weight prepregnancy; 31–50 lb if overweight; 25–42 lb if obese |
| | Rate of weight gain, singleton pregnancy | First trimester: none |
| | | Second and third trimesters: BMI, 18.5—1 lb; BMI 25.0–29.9—0.6 lb; BMI >30—0.5 lb; BMI 18.5–24.0—1 lb |
| | | Intensive assessment and counseling |
| | | The additional calories needed are 340 kcal/day and 452 kcal/day in patients second third trimesters |
| | Poor weight gain <br> <2 lb/month <br> <10 lb by midpregnancy | If patient is economically unable to meet nutritional needs—referral to federal food and nutrition programs (WIC) |
| | Nutritional needs/barriers | Increase knowledge with dietary counseling |
| | Vitamin/mineral supplementation | No requirement for routine supplementation except folate (400 µg/day) and iron (30–60 mg elemental iron/day) |
| | | Dietary supplements should be given if the adequacy of a patient's diet is questionable or if she is at high nutritional risk |
| | | Excessive vitamin and mineral intake (more than twice the Recommended Dietary Allowance [RDA]) should be avoided |
| | Prophylaxis for iron deficiency | Supplement of ferrous iron is 30 mg elemental iron daily |
| | | Zinc supplements are recommended if taking high doses of iron |
| | Calcium supplementation | 60–120 mg elemental iron daily |
| | Evaluate use of alcohol, tobacco, and drugs | Recommended for women who have diet deficient in calcium, have prepregnancy hypertension, history of eclampsia or chronic use of heparin or steroids, and adolescents |
| | Caffeine intake | Effects of substance use/abuse on perinatal outcomes |
| | | Abstinence from alcoholic beverages |
| | Lactose intolerance | Consumption of two to three servings of caffeinated beverages is unlikely to have adverse effects; in general, caffeinated beverages provide few essential nutrients and often crowd out better sources of nutrients |
| | | *Moderate intake* is <300 mg/day—5 oz |
| | |     Cup of coffee = 115 mg |
| | |     Iced tea = 40 mg |
| | |     Cola = 15 mg |
| | |     Hot chocolate = 4 mg |
| | | *High intake* (>500 mg/day) |
| | |     Increased risk (2.2 ×) of first-trimester spontaneous abortions |
| | GDM | May result in insufficient calcium intake |
| | | Supplemental calcium necessary if insufficient calcium consumed from food sources |

*(continued)*

## TABLE 18.2 (continued)
## Nutritional Care at Preconception, Prenatal, and Postnatal Visits

| Visit | Assessment | Counseling/Treatment |
|---|---|---|
| | Nausea and vomiting during pregnancy | Referral for nutrition assessment and counseling. Generally, diet is 40% carbohydrate, 30% fat, 30% protein |
| | Constipation | Eat crackers before getting out of bed in the morning; eat frequent small meals; eat low-fat, bland foods; eat ginger (soda, tea, or ginger snaps); suck on hard candy; eat salty/tart foods combined (e.g., potato chips with lemonade); supplement with vitamin $B_6$ (25 mg three times daily); wear Sea Band® (an elastic band worn on wrists to counter nausea caused by seasickness) |
| | | Strong evidence for taking a multivitamin at the time of conception decreasing the severity |
| Postpartum diet | | Foods high in dietary fiber, including cereals, bread fruits, and vegetables; adequate fluids; moderate exercise; soluble fiber (e.g., Metamucil, Citrucel, or Benefiber); docusate; change the brand of iron supplement |
| | | DRI for water is 3.0 L/day |
| | | DRI for dietary fiber is 28 g/day |
| | Caloric requirement | Utilize dietary intake questionnaire |
| | | Dietary guidelines are similar to those established during pregnancy |
| | | Continue multiple vitamin–mineral supplements |
| | Vitamin/mineral supplement | Balanced, nutritious diet will ensure both the quality and the quantity of milk produced without depletion of maternal stores. Increased need of 300–500 cal. At least three servings of milk daily. The adequate intakes (AI) for water for lactating women is 3.8 L/day |
| | Weight retention | Not needed routinely although recommended for the 400 µg/day folic acid; mothers at nutritional risk should be given a multivitamin supplement with particular emphasis on calcium and vitamins $B_{12}$ and D |
| | Residual postpartum weight retention | The relationship between BMI or total weight gain and weight retention is unclear. It appears that women who gain more than the Institute of Medicine (ION) guidelines retain twice as much weight as those who gain within the guidelines |
| | | Aging, rather than parity, is the major determinant of increases in a woman's weight over time |
| | | Special attention to lifestyle including exercise and eating habits |

## TABLE 18.3
## Risk Factors for Prenatal Nutritional Risk

| Risk Factor | Low Risk | High Risk |
|---|---|---|
| Is the patient pre- or adolescent or <3 years postmenarche? | No | Yes |
| Is the patient economically disadvantaged or have limited income for food? | No | Yes |
| Does the patient have history of anemia or is anemic (hematocrit <32 mg/% during pregnancy)? | No | Yes |
| Is the patient's BMI <19.8 or >26.1? | No | Yes |
| Does the patient have history of fad dieting or restrictive eating? | No | Yes |
| Does the patient have illness or medication that will interfere with absorption; is she HIV+? | No | Yes |
| Does the patient use tobacco, alcohol, or drugs? | No | Yes |
| Does the patient practice pica (consume ice, starch, clay, or other substances in large amounts)? | No | Yes |
| Does the patient experience nausea and/or vomiting? | No | Yes |
| Is the patient lactose intolerant? | No | Yes |
| Is the weight gain 0.8–1.0 lb/week? | No | Yes |
| Does the patient stay within the weight gain range recommended for her prepregnancy BMI? | Yes | No |
| Weight gain <15 lb or >45 lb? | No | Yes |
| Prior bariatric surgery | No | Yes |

## TABLE 18.4
### Indications for Referral of Pregnant Patients for Nutrition Assessment and Counseling

Patient has interest in and desire to see a nutritionist

Patient has inappropriate weight gain: patient has a BMI <18.5 or >30.0

Patient has food intolerances, aversions, or has pica (e.g., dirt, ice, clay, starch)

Patient has conceived three or more times in the last 2 years

Patient is currently breast-feeding

Patient has gestational diabetes

Patient has chronic condition managed with diet (e.g., diabetes or hyperlipidemia)

Patient has a history of anemia

Patient has inadequate or inappropriate food supply

Patient has a history of prepregnancy anorexia or bulimia

Patient has significant discomforts of pregnancy (e.g., heartburn, nausea, or vomiting)

Patient has multiple gestation

Patient is adolescent or older than 35 years

Patient is vegetarian

Patient has prior bariatric surgery

Patient is interested in or undecided about breast-feeding

formulated as a range of weight gain for each category of prepregnancy BMI. A single number cannot accommodate differences such as age, race/ethnicity, or other factors that may affect pregnancy outcomes. The recommended weight gain ranges for short women and for racial or ethnic groups are the same as those for the whole population. In addition, teenagers who are pregnant should use the adult BMI categories to determine their weight gain range pending additional research to determine whether special categories are needed for them.

### RATE OF WEIGHT GAIN

In 1996, the Maternal and Weight Gain Expert Group[22] suggested a weight gain of 1 lb/week for normal-weight women during the second and third trimesters of a singleton pregnancy. These recommendations are reinforced in the 2009 IOM guidelines on Weight Gain During Pregnancy[4] and further clarified for those women classified as overweight (BMI 25.0–29.9) and obese (BMI ≥ 30.0). Weight gain is the single most reliable indicator of pregnancy outcome.[23,24] Weight status should be routinely assessed for amount and rate. Figure 18.1 depicts an example of a graph for tracking weight.[25] Weight charts should be shown to

## TABLE 18.5
### Recommendations for Total and Rate of Weight Gain during Pregnancy, by Prepregnancy BMI

| Prepregnancy BMI | BMI (kg/m²) (WHO) | Total Weight Gain Range (lb) | Rates of Weight Gain[a] Second and Third Trimesters (Mean Range in lb/week) |
|---|---|---|---|
| Underweight | <18.5 | 28–40 | 1 (1–1.3) |
| Normal weight | 18.5–24.9 | 25–35 | 1 (0.8–1) |
| Overweight | 25.0–39.9 | 15–25 | 0.6 (0.5–0.7) |
| Obese (includes all classes) | ≥30.0 | 11–20 | 0.5 (0.4–0.6) |

[a] Calculations assume a 0.5–2 kg (1.1–4.4 lb) weight gain in the first trimester.[17–19]

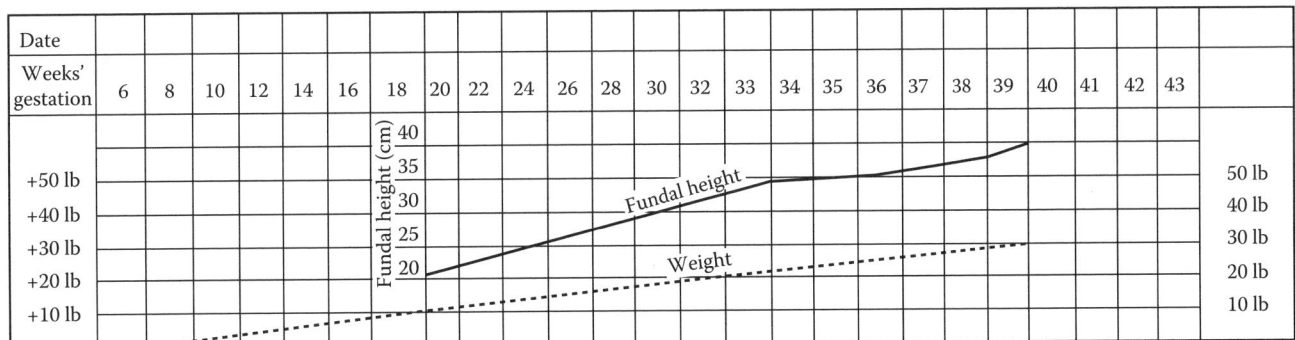

**FIGURE 18.1** Graph for tracking weight and fundal height. (With permission from Kolasa, K.M. and Weismiller, D.G., *Am. Fam. Phys.*, 56(1), 206, July 1997.)

women and their support partners.* Table 18.5 gives recommended rates of weight gain. The optimal weight for a newborn infant of 39–41 weeks gestation is 6.6–8.8 lb.[15]

Women with inadequate weight gain should eat more frequently, be referred to a dietitian for nutrient assessment and counseling, choose more nutrient-dense foods, avoid alcohol and tobacco use, limit activity, and avoid caffeine or other appetite depressants. Women with excessive gain should reduce portion sizes, limit intake of sweets and foods high in fat, increase activity, and be evaluated by a registered dietitian.

The guidelines and supporting recommendations are to be used in conjunction with sound clinical judgment and should include a discussion between the woman and her care provider about nutrition and physical activity. The types of services needed to meet women's needs include recording prepregnancy height and weight, charting women's weight gain throughout pregnancy, and sharing the results with them so they are aware of their progress toward their weight gain goal. A healthful diet and greater physical activity are associated with reduced risk for excessive gestational weight gain.[26] Special attention should be given to low-income and minority women who are more likely to be in higher BMI categories, consume diets of poor nutritional quality, and get less physical activity before pregnancy.

## WEIGHT GAIN DISTRIBUTION DURING PREGNANCY

Weight gain by pregnant women consists of water, protein, and fat. Measurements of maternal water gain may predict birth weight better than measurements of composite weight gain. The total amount of weight gained, the composition of gain, and the rate of energy metabolism all differ among healthy pregnant women. Table 18.6 is a typical teaching tool about weight-gain distribution.

## Nutritious Snacks

Pregnant women may need suggestions for healthy snacks. Table 18.7 includes snacks of about 100 cal.

### TABLE 18.6
### Weight-Gain Distribution during Pregnancy (lb)

| Source | lb |
| --- | --- |
| Amniotic fluid | 2–2.6 |
| Baby | 7–8.5 |
| Fat/breast tissue stores for breast-feeding | 1–4 |
| Increased blood volume | 4–5 |
| Increased weight of uterus | 2 |
| Maternal fat stores | 4–7 |
| Placenta | 0.7–1.0 |
| Tissue fluid | 3–5 |
| Total | 25–35 |

### TABLE 18.7
### Nutritious Snacks of 100 kcal or Less

| Food Item | Serving Size |
| --- | --- |
| Applesauce | ⅔ cup |
| Bagel | ½ |
| Carrot, raw | 1 cup or 1 large |
| Cheese, low fat | 1 oz |
| Cottage cheese, low fat | ⅓ cup |
| Entenmann's fat-free cakes/pastries | 1 small slice |
| Figs, low fat, or other Newton cookies | 1–½ tsp |
| Fruit, dried (like apricots, raisins, prunes) | 4 tsp |
| Fruit, fresh | 1 medium |
| Graham crackers | 2 |
| Grits | 1 package |
| Milk, skim | 1 cup |
| Pretzels | 15 |
| Pudding made with skim milk | ⅓ cup |
| Rice cakes, flavored | 2 |
| Tortilla chips, baked, low-fat, and with salsa | 12 |
| Tuna | ½ cup |
| Yogurt, frozen | ½ cup |
| Yogurt, low fat | ½ cup |

## Sugar Substitutes

Rebaudioside A is considered generally recognized as safe. Acesulfame Potassium and Aspartame consumed at a moderate level are considered safe by the Food and Drug Administration (FDA). Sucralose has no effect on blood sugar, offers no calories, and is considered safe for consumption during pregnancy.

## DIETARY REQUIREMENTS FOR PREGNANCY AND LACTATION

### DIETARY REFERENCE INTAKE

DRIs are the levels of intake of essential nutrients considered adequate to meet or exceed known nutritional needs of practically all healthy people. The National Agricultural Library maintains a link† to the DRI tables developed and published by the Institute of Medicine.‡ These levels are set by the Food and Nutrition Board of the National Academy of Sciences. Not all nutrient requirements increase in pregnancy; those that do include energy, protein, choline, chromium, copper, folate, iodine, iron, magnesium, manganese, molybdenum, niacin, pantothenic acid, riboflavin, selenium, thiamin zinc, vitamins A, $B_6$, and C. The amounts may vary by trimester. Energy needs are also increased by 340 kcal/day (recommend 200–300 kcal/day) in the second trimester of pregnancy and by

---

* An example of one state's health department's translation of the weight guidelines into tracking graphs is found at http://www.nal.usda.gov/wicworks/Sharing_Center/NY/prenatalwt_charts.pdf (accessed April 5, 2012).

† http://fnic.nal.usda.gov/nal_ display/index.php?info_center=4&tax_ level=3&tax_subject=256&topic_id=1342&level3_id=5140&level4_ id=0&level5_id=0&placement_default=0 (accessed April 5, 2012).

‡ http://www.iom.edu/Activities/ Nutrition/SummaryDRIs/~/media/ Files/Activity%20 Files/Nutrition/DRIs/5_Summary%20Table%20 Tables%20-4.pdf (accessed April 5, 2012).

## TABLE 18.8
## Dietary Sources of Folate (DRI = 500–600 μg/day of Dietary Folate Equivalents [DFE])

| Food Item | Serving Size |
|---|---|
| *Excellent >100 μg* | |
| Asparagus | ½ cup or four spears |
| Baked beans | 1 cup |
| Bean burritos | 2 |
| Black-eyed peas | 1 cup |
| Fortified grain, rice, pasta and cereal products | Varies, read label or ½ cup |
| Kidney beans, Great White northern | 1 cup |
| Lentils | 1 cup |
| Liver and other organ meats | 6 oz |
| Beef | 3.5 oz |
| Chicken | 3.5 oz |
| Orange juice | 1 cup |
| Peanuts | 4 oz |
| Spinach | ½ cup |
| *Good: 15–99 μg* | |
| Almonds | 4 oz |
| Avocado | 1/2 cup |
| Banana | 1 medium |
| Bread, fortified | 1 slice |
| Beets | ½ cup |
| Broccoli, cooked | ½ cup |
| Cantaloupe/Honeydew melon | 1 cup |
| Cauliflower | ½ cup |
| Egg | 1 large order |
| French fries | ½ cup |
| Green peas | 1/2 cup |
| Lettuce (romaine) | 1 cup |
| Orange | 1 medium |
| Papaya | 1 cup |
| Strawberries | 1 cup |
| Tomato juice | 1 cup |
| Turnip greens | 1/2 cup |
| Yellow corn | 1/2 cup |

452 kcal/day (recommend 200–500 kcal/day) during lactation so that adequate breast milk supply is produced. Most pregnant women will need between 2200 and 2900 kcal/day unless giving birth to more than one baby. If multiples, the range is 3000–4000 kcal/day.

The 2010 Dietary Guidelines for Americans and ChooseMyPlate[27] (www.myplate.gov, accessed April 5, 2012) include some recommendations for pregnant women. Women are encouraged to obtain adequate nutrients within calorie needs. During the first trimester, they should consume adequate synthetic folic acid daily (from fortified foods or supplements) in addition to food forms of folate from a varied diet. Table 18.8 lists food sources for folic acid. Alcoholic beverages should not be consumed.

### Prevention of Listeriosis Caused by Bacteria

*Listeria monocytogenes* includes avoiding contact with wild and domestic animals and consumption of soft cheese, deli meats, and cold salads from salad bars. Foods should always be adequately cooked. Avoid raw fish or sushi that includes raw fish, raw or unpasteurized milk or products made from unpasteurized milk, raw or partially cooked eggs, and alfalfa sprouts. The prevention of Toxoplasmosis caused by a parasite called *Toxoplasma gondii* is done by cooking foods to safe temperatures and ensuring meat is cooked to 160°F by testing with a food thermometer. Only deli meats and frankfurters that have been reheated to steaming hot can be eaten. Women are advised to avoid some types of fish and shellfish and to avoid fish and shellfish that are higher in mercury such as shark, swordfish, king mackerel, and tile fish.* Fresh fruits and vegetables should be washed or peeled before eating. Cutting boards, dishes, counters, utensils, and hands that are in contact with raw foods should be washed with warm soapy water.

Personalized plans showing food groups and amounts of foods from each food group, based on calorie needs, can be downloaded from www.choosemyplate.gov (accessed April 5, 2012). Pregnant women should drink at least 3.0 L of water each day.

### Dietary Assessment of the Pregnant Woman

Individualized nutrition assessment and planning is important because of the strong associations between extremes in pre-pregnancy BMI, extremes in weight gain, and adverse pregnancy outcomes.[3,7,14,25] Many electronic resources are available to monitor dietary intake.†,‡ There are special nutrition implications for pregnant women who have had bariatric surgery; especially the Roux-en-Y procedure.[16] Adequate weight gain to promote fetal growth is advised. There are no published weight-gain criteria for post-gastric bypass. Serum iron and TIBC, CBC, folate, and vitamin $B_{12}$ levels should be monitored.

### BEHAVIOR-CHANGE TOOL

Assessment relies on the woman's medical record, history, and physical examination. Nutritional factors of importance include previous nutritional challenges, eating disorders, pica, fad dieting, botanicals and teas, strict vegetarian diet, medications, and quantity and quality of current diet. The Institute of Medicine provides a sample dietary history tool (Table 18.9).[3] Systematic assessment of the diet is preferable to questions such as "How are you eating?" The 24 h dietary recall method is commonly used to recall the types and amounts of foods and beverages consumed during the previous day. The food frequency questionnaire has been demonstrated to detect pregnancy-related changes in diet.

---

* The FDA maintains toll-free information at 1-888-SAFEFOOD or http://www.fda.gov/food/foodsafety/product-specificinformation/seafood/foodbornepathogenscontaminants/methylmercury/ucm115662.htm (accessed April 5, 2012).

† https://www.choosemyplate.gov/SuperTracker/default.aspx (accessed April 5, 2012).

‡ http://www.myfitnesspal.com/mobile (accessed April 5, 2012).

**TABLE 18.9**

**Behavior-Change Dietary Assessment Tool**

*Eating behavior*

1. Are you frequently bothered by any of the following? (circle all that apply)

| Nausea | Vomiting | Heartburn | Constipation |

2. Do you skip meals at least three times a week? — No  Yes
3. Do you try to limit the amount or kind of food you eat to control your weight? — No  Yes
4. Are you on a special diet now? — No  Yes
5. Do you avoid any foods for health or religious reasons? — No  Yes

*Food sources*

6. Do you have a working stove? — No  Yes
   Do you have a working refrigerator? — No  Yes
7. Do you sometimes run out of food before you are able to buy more? — No  Yes
8. Can you afford to eat the way you should? — No  Yes
9. Are you receiving any food assistance now? (circle all that apply)

| Food stamps | School breakfast | School lunch |
| Donated food | Commodity Supplemental | Food program |
| Food from a food pantry, soup kitchen, or food banks | | |

10. Do you feel you need help in obtaining food? — No  Yes

*Food and drink*

11. Which of these did you drink yesterday? (circle all that apply)

| Soft drinks | Coffee | Tea | Fruit drink |
| Orange juice | Grapefruit juice | Other juices | Milk |
| Kool-Aid | Beer | Wine | Alcoholic drinks |
| Water | Other beverages (list) | | |

12. Which of these foods did you eat yesterday? (circle all that apply)

| Cheese | Pizza | Macaroni and cheese |
| Yogurt | Cereal with milk | |

13. Other foods made with cheese (such as tacos, enchiladas, lasagna, and cheeseburgers)

| Corn | Potatoes | Sweet potatoes | Green salad |
| Carrots | Collard greens | Spinach | Turnip greens |
| Broccoli | Green beans | Green peas | Other vegetables |
| Apples | Bananas | Berries | Grapefruit |
| Melon | Oranges | Peaches | Other fruit |
| Meat | Fish | Chicken | Eggs |
| Peanut butter | Nuts | Seeds | Dried beans |
| Cold cuts | Hot dog | Bacon | Sausage |
| Cake | Cookies | Doughnut | Pastry |
| Chips | French fries | Deep fried foods, such as fried chicken or egg rolls | |
| Bread | Rolls | Rice | Cereal |
| Noodles | Spaghetti | Tortillas | |

Were any of these whole grains? — No  Yes

Is the way you ate yesterday the way you usually eat? — No  Yes

*Lifestyle*

14. Do you exercise for at least 30 min on a regular basis—three times a week or more? — No  Yes
15. Do you ever smoke cigarettes or use smokeless tobacco? — No  Yes
16. Do you ever drink beer, wine, liquor, or any other alcoholic beverages? — No  Yes
17. Which of these do you take? (circle all that apply)
   Prescribed drugs or medications
   Any OTC products (such as aspirin, acetaminophen, antacids, or vitamins)

*Source:* Institute of Medicine, Subcommittee for a Clinical Application Guide. *Nutrition during Pregnancy and Lactation: An Implementation Guide*, National Academy Press, Washington, DC, 1992.

## COMPLICATIONS OF PREGNANCY THAT MAY IMPACT NUTRITIONAL STATUS

A number of complications of pregnancy may impact nutritional status. Some of these include nausea and vomiting, constipation, caffeine intake, and alcohol intake as well as hypertension and gestational diabetes.

### NAUSEA AND VOMITING

Up to 80% of pregnant women report nausea during the first 14–16 weeks of pregnancy, and 37%–58% experience vomiting. The etiology is unknown. The remedies include diet, fluids, and reassurance.[28,29] Table 18.10 is a collection of remedies.

### HYPEREMESIS GRAVIDARUM

Vomiting that produces weight loss, dehydration, acidosis from starvation, alkalosis from loss of hydrochloric acid in vomitus, and/or hypokalemia may be treated pharmacologically. Management is to correct dehydration, fluid and electrolyte deficits, acidosis, and alkalosis. Table 18.11 includes some pharmacological approaches.[28]

### CONSTIPATION

Up to 25% of women experience constipation in pregnancy, in part due to decreased motility of the gastrointestinal (GI) tract. Constipation can be exacerbated by iron supplementation. Constipation is often related to low dietary fiber intake and low fluid intake. Table 18.12 includes foods rich in dietary fiber. The recommended intake is 28 g of dietary fiber daily during pregnancy and 29 g during lactation.

### CAFFEINE DURING PREGNANCY AND LACTATION

The literature is mixed on the effects of caffeine during pregnancy. The official FDA position advises pregnant women

## TABLE 18.10
### Nonpharmacological Remedies for Nausea and Vomiting

Eat small, frequent meals
Eat dry foods/cold foods
Take dietary supplements after meals
Suck on candy
Switch brands of iron supplements
Eat combinations of foods that are salty and tart
Eat vitamin-$B_6$-rich foods
Try seabands or acupressure bands
Avoid beverages with meat
Avoid caffeine
Avoid fried, spicy, acidic foods, and strong odors
Sniff lemon
Drink ginger root tea, ginger ale; eat ginger snaps; take ginger tablets (250 mg tablets four times daily for 4–5 days)
Drink plenty of fluids to avoid dehydration; take small sips

## TABLE 18.11
### Hyperemesis Gravidarum

| Medication | Dosage |
|---|---|
| Vitamin $B_6$ | 25 mg–50 mg TID along with doxylamine |
| Doxylamine | 12.5–25 mg TID along with Vitamin $B_6$ |
| *Antiemetic/anti-nausea medications* | |
| Promethazine (Phenergan) | 12.5–25 mg PO, per rectum or IV every 4–6 h as needed |
| Trimethobenyamine (Tigan) | 200 mg per rectum every 8 h as needed |
| Ondansetron (Zofran) | 4–8 mg PO or 4 mg IV every 12 h as needed |
| Emetrol (OTC) | 15–30 cc ipo q 15 min until vomiting stops; not to exceed 5 doses/h |

## TABLE 18.12
### Dietary Sources of Fiber

| Serving Size | Food | Grams of Fiber |
|---|---|---|
| *Breads, cereals, pastas* | | |
| 3 cups | Air-popped popcorn | 4 |
| 1 medium | Bran muffin | 3 |
| ⅔ cup | Brown rice | 3 |
| 1 slice | Whole wheat bread | 3 |
| ½ cup | Cooked legumes | 5 |
| ½ cup | Baked beans | 10 |
| ½ cup | Great northern beans | 7 |
| ½ cup | Lima beans | 7 |
| ½ cup | Selected fiber cereals (read label) | 14 |
| *Fruit* | | |
| 1 cup | Raisins | 6 |
| 3 | Dried prunes | 5 |
| 1 medium | Pear with skin | 4 |
| 1 medium | Apple with skin | 3 |
| 1 cup | Strawberries | 3 |
| 1 medium | Banana | 3 |
| 1 medium | Orange | 3 |
| *Vegetables* | | |
| ½ cup | Cooked frozen peas | 4 |
| 1 medium | Baked potato with skin | 4 |
| ½ cup | Brussels sprouts | 3 |
| ½ cup | Cooked broccoli tops | 3 |
| ½ cup | Cooked carrots | 3 |
| ½ cup | Cooked corn | 3 |

to avoid caffeine or consume it sparingly. Most experts agree that caffeine should be limited to less than two servings per day. Caffeine is known to decrease the availability of calcium, iron, and zinc. It is known to exert effects on the fetus. The relationship of caffeine to spontaneous abortion remains controversial, although increasingly data support an association with caffeine

**TABLE 18.13**

**Caffeine Quiz and Caffeine Values for Popular Beverages**

| Source of Caffeine | Column A Number of Servings per Day | Column B Amount of Caffeine per Serving (mg) | Column C Total Caffeine (mg) |
|---|---|---|---|
| *Coffee (6 oz)* | _____ | | |
| Automatic drip | _____ | × 180 | = _____ |
| Automatic perk | _____ | × 135 | = _____ |
| Instant | _____ | × 125 | = _____ |
| Decaffeinated | _____ | × 5 | = _____ |
| Coffee Grande, Starbucks (16 oz) | _____ | × 550 | |
| Coffee flavored ice cream (1/2 cup) | | | |
| *Soft drinks (12 oz)* | | | |
| Regular colas | _____ | × 37 | = _____ |
| Diet colas | _____ | × 50 | = _____ |
| Mt Dew × 55 | | × 5 | |
| 7 Eleven Big Gulp (64 oz) | | × 190 | |
| *Energy drinks* | | | |
| Rockstar (16 oz) × 240 | | | |
| Monster (16 oz) × 140 | | | |
| Chaser 5 (2 oz) × 250 | | | |
| Enviga (12 oz) × 100 | | | |
| *Cocoa products* | | | |
| Chocolate candy (2 oz) | _____ | × 45 | = _____ |
| Baking chocolate (1 oz) | _____ | × 30 | = _____ |
| Milk chocolate (2 oz) | _____ | × 10 | = _____ |
| South American cocoa (6 oz) | _____ | × 40 | = _____ |
| *Drugs (one tablet or capsule)* | | | |
| Dexatrim (not caffeine free) | _____ | × 200 | = _____ |
| NoDoz | _____ | × 100 | = _____ |
| Anacin | _____ | × 35 | = _____ |
| Midol | _____ | × 30 | = _____ |
| Coricidin | _____ | × 30 | = _____ |
| *Tea (6 oz)* | | | |
| Iced tea | _____ | × 36 | = _____ |
| Hot tea (moderate steeping time) | _____ | × 65 | = _____ |
| Chai tea × 50 | _____ | | |
| Decaf tea × 5 | | | |
| Total | | | = _____ |

intake and late miscarriage and still birth. One report suggests that risk increases with the consumption in the range of 6–18 cups of coffee per day (>450 mg/day of caffeine).[30]

Caffeine does pass into breast milk, and, therefore, consumption during lactation should be limited. Table 18.13 lists caffeine values for popular beverages. Some suggestions for reducing caffeine consumption include (1) switching to decaffeinated coffee or soft drinks, (2) cutting down on caffeinated beverages, (3) mixing caffeinated and decaffeinated coffee grounds together before making coffee, and (4) limiting consumption of caffeinated beverages to a preselected number and then switching to decaffeinated beverages over time.

## ALCOHOL

Consumption of alcohol during pregnancy and lactation is controversial. The Society of Obstetricians and Gynecologists of Canada issued a clinical practice guideline in 2010.[31] ACOG describes at-risk drinking and alcohol dependence and its implications for women's health.[32] Together with the CDC, ACOG hosts the Women and Alcohol website (www.womenandalcohol.org, accessed April 5, 2012).

A safe lower limit of alcohol during pregnancy is not known. Therefore, the only sure way to avoid the possible harmful effects of alcohol on the fetus is to abstain. Women of childbearing ages should be aware of potential negative outcomes including fetal alcohol syndrome, growth restriction, and physical and neurological delays.[31,32] Binge drinking or excessive drinking during pregnancy can result in fetal alcohol syndrome. However, even small amounts of alcohol can temporarily alter fetal function. Adverse outcomes have not been found with daily consumption of fewer than two standard drinks. The danger from light drinking should not be overstated.

**TABLE 18.14**

**Effects of Alcohol, Tobacco, and Drug Use on Nutritional Status and Pregnancy Outcomes and Lactation**

| Effect | Cause |
|---|---|
| Increased nutrient requirements/impaired nutrient absorption | Smokers have reduced vitamin C levels. Drinkers have reduced serum folate and vitamin C levels. |
| Impaired growth of the fetus/stunted growth of child | Drinkers of one to two alcoholic beverages/day associated with LBW, slow weight gain, and failure to thrive Smokers. |
| Infant sleep disruption/increased arousal | Consumption of one drink/day in the first trimester. |
| Delayed development/mental retardation | Drinkers have children who are more at risk for hyperactivity, poor attention span, language dysfunction. |
| Reduced fertility | Chronic drinking and smoking associated with lower fertility in men and women. |
| Transfer to baby during lactation disrupted sleep pattern of infant | Alcohol is concentrated in breast milk. An occasional small drink is acceptable, but breast-feeding should be avoided for 2 h. |

However, this may cause undue stress in some patients who had a few drinks before realizing they were pregnant (Table 18.14).

Alcohol does not increase milk volume. Chronic consumption can inhibit milk production. The American Academy of Pediatrics does suggest that an occasional celebratory single, small alcoholic drink is acceptable, but breast-feeding should be avoided for 2 h after the drink as alcohol is concentrated in breast milk.[33,34]

## Hypertension

The Seventh Report of the Joint National Committee on Prevention, Detection, Evaluation, and Treatment of High Blood Pressure (JNC 7)[35] outlines five classifications of hypertension in pregnancy. Treatment includes lifestyle modification for women with stage 1 hypertension. Data are sparse, but many experts recommend restricting sodium intake to 2.4 g/day. Pharmacological management is described.[36]

A Cochrane Review[37] examining the risk of hypertensive disorders during pregnancy looked at randomized trials comparing at least 1 g daily of calcium intake during pregnancy with placebo. The review included 13 studies of good quality (involving 15,730 women). The average risk of high blood pressure was reduced with calcium supplementation rather than placebo (12 trials, 15,470 women: risk ratio [RR] 0.65, 95% confidence interval [CI] 0.53–0.81). There was also a reduction in the average risk of preeclampsia associated with calcium supplementation (13 trials, 15,730 women: RR 0.45, 95% CI 0.31–0.65). The effect for the prevention of preeclampsia was greatest for women with low baseline calcium intake (eight trials, 10,678 women: RR 0.36, 95% CI 0.20–0.65), that is, communities with low dietary calcium intake (mean intake < 900 mg/day) and those selected as being at high risk for gestational hypertension (five trials, 587 women: RR 0.22, 95% CI 0.12–0.42), that is, teenagers, previous preeclampsia, women with increased sensitivity to angiotensin II, and preexisting hypertension. The variable methods

of selecting women as being at high risk limit the clinical usefulness of these pooled results. The authors conclude that calcium supplementation appears to approximately halve the risk of preeclampsia, to reduce the risk of preterm birth, and to reduce the occurrence of the composite outcome "death or serious morbidity." There were no other clear benefits or harms. Table 18.15 shows dietary sources of calcium. None of the following supplements have been shown to prevent preeclampsia: magnesium, zinc, fish oil, or antioxidant therapy (vitamins C or E). The adequate intake (AI) for sodium in pregnancy and lactation is 1.5 g/day with an upper limit of 2.3 g/day. The AI for potassium in pregnancy is 4.7 g/day and 5.1 during lactation.

## Gestational Diabetes

GDM, carbohydrate intolerance first diagnosed or recognized during pregnancy, represents a heterogeneous group of metabolic disorders, which result in varying degrees of maternal hyperglycemia and pregnancy-associated risk.[38] The definition applies whether insulin or only diet modification is used for treatment and whether the condition persists after pregnancy. There is an ongoing debate as to the benefit to the treatment of GDM. The 2008 guidelines of the U.S. Preventive Services Task Force concluded that there is insufficient evidence to assess the benefits and harms of screening and treatment of GDM.[39] This group acknowledged that their review did not consider intermediate outcomes such as macrosomia, cesarean delivery, and shoulder dystocia. More recently, a systematic review and meta-analysis evaluated the effects of treatment in women with GDM. The authors concluded that compared with routine care, treatment of GDM is associated with a reduction in the incidence of shoulder dystocia and macrosomia.[40] The mainstay of treatment of GDM remains nutritional counseling and dietary intervention. The optimal diet should provide caloric and nutrient needs to sustain pregnancy without resulting in significant postprandial hyperglycemia. A dietary program of 2000–2500 kcal daily is typically recommended.[41] This represents approximately

## TABLE 18.15
### Dietary Sources of Calcium (DRI = 1000–1300 mg/day)

| Food Item | Serving Size |
|---|---|
| *Good > 200 mg* | |
| Broccoli/greens | 2 cups |
| Calcium fortified foods (juice, cereal, soy beverage, instant breakfast drinks) | Varies, read label |
| Canned salmon with bones | 3 oz |
| Canned sardines with bones | 3 oz |
| Cheese (cheddar, edam, Monterey jack, mozzarella, Parmesan, provolone, ricotta) | 1 oz |
| Ice cream | 1 cup |
| Ice milk | 1 cup |
| Milk (skim, 2%, whole, buttermilk) | 1 cup |
| Yogurt | 6–8 oz |
| Tofu made with calcium sulfate | 1/2 cup |

35 kcal/kg of present pregnancy weight. It has been suggested that carbohydrate intake be limited to 33%–40% of calories.[42] Complex carbohydrates are preferred to simple carbohydrates because they are less likely to produce significant postprandial hyperglycemia. In practice, three meals and two to three snacks are recommended to distribute glucose intake and to minimize postprandial glucose excursions. In light of the 2009 IOM recommendations[4] concerning weight gain during pregnancy, it is not clear if caloric restriction, limited weight gain, or both advisable in obese women with GDM. A specified carbohydrate-limited diet in obese women with GDM improves glycemic control and reduces weight gain. Regular physical activity improves insulin sensitivity and may therefore be a useful adjunct in the treatment of GDM.

Once the woman with GDM is placed on an appropriate diet, surveillance of blood glucose levels is necessary to be certain that glycemic control has been established. Target thresholds of a fasting glucose less than 95 mg/dL and 1 h postprandial glucose less than 140 mg/dL as well as 2 h postprandial glucose less than 120 mg/dL have been suggested by the Fifth International Workshop Conference on GDM.[43] Until data are available from controlled trials to identify ideal glycemic targets for the prevention of fetal risk for women with GDM, the recommended target thresholds (Table 18.16) are suggested for clinical use.

## TABLE 18.16
### Target Plasma Glucose Levels in Pregnancy

| Time | mg/dL |
|---|---|
| Before breakfast | 60–90 |
| Before lunch, supper, bedtime snack | 60–105 |
| 2 h after meals | At or below 120 |
| 2–6 AM | Above 60 |

*Source:* Landon, M.B. and Gabbe, S.G., *Obstet. Gynecol.*, 118, 1379, 2011.

## VITAMIN AND MINERAL REQUIREMENTS, FOOD SOURCES, AND SUPPLEMENTATION

In the United States, vitamin and mineral supplementation is common among pregnant women. During pregnancy, maternal requirements for most increase. For some nutrients, the evidence indicates a direct link between chronic maternal deficiency and poor outcome for the mother and the infant. Excessive intake (usually defined as more than twice the Recommended Dietary Allowance [RDA]) of some nutrients may be harmful to the fetus, especially very early in the pregnancy.[44] Supplementation, with the exception of folic acid, is recommended only after the assessment of dietary practices of pregnant women. Table 18.8 lists dietary sources of folate. The Institute of Medicine does not recommend routine use of prenatal vitamins; however, many physicians prescribe them because of the marginal nutritional status of their patients or because it is difficult to be completely sure of their patients' nutritional status.[3] Indications for vitamin and mineral supplementation are shown in Table 18.17, which lists nutrient dose and indication for use. The contents of typical prenatal vitamin–mineral supplements change and the Supplement Facts label on over-the-counter (OTC) products should be read. Prescription prenatal vitamins have 1 mg folic acid and may have higher dosages of other nutrients than typically found in an OTC. Prenatal vitamins and minerals are indicated for high-risk populations and those with an obstetric history of high parity, previous delivery of a low-birth-weight infant, a short interval between births, and smokers, drug or alcohol abusers, and those with multiple pregnancies. Supplementation with herbals or other natural products should be done only with the knowledge of physician as some herbals are contraindicated during pregnancy, and the safety of many products is not assured.[45]

### Vitamin A

Most pregnant women in developed countries do not need supplemental vitamin A, the teratogenic threshold of which may be lower than previously thought. Vitamin A is essential for embryogenesis, growth, and epithelial differentiation. The RDA in pregnancy is only slightly increased to 770 mg/day.* Case reports have suggested an association between high doses of vitamin A (>25,000 IU) during pregnancy and birth defects. The American College of Obstetricians and Gynecologists established 10,000 IU (or 3000 μg RAE) as the cutoff for supplemental vitamin A (retinol) prior to or during pregnancy. WHO provides guidelines for those requiring supplementation to prevent and treat vitamin A deficiencies,† especially to reduce the risk of mother-to-infant transmission of HIV.‡ There is no concern about β-carotene intake.

---

* http://fnic.nal.usda.gov/nal_display/index.php?info_center=4&tax_level=3&tax_subject=256&topic_id=1342&level3_id=5140&level4_id=0&level5_id=0&placement_default=0 (accessed April 5, 2012).
† http://www.who.int/nutrition/events/guideline_dev_vas/en/index.html (accessed April 5, 2012).
‡ http://whqlibdoc.who.int/publications/2011/9789241501804_eng.pdf (accessed April 5, 2012).

## TABLE 18.17
## Indications for Vitamin and Mineral Supplementation

| Indication | Nutrient | Dose |
|---|---|---|
| Inadequate diet; during first two trimesters for women at risk for preterm labor or low-birth-weight baby | Prenatal supplements | Read label |
| Up to 1,200 mg/day if dairy or fortified foods not consumed | Calcium | 250–300 mg |
| For women receiving supplemental iron | Copper | 2 mg |
| For all women of childbearing age | Folate | 400 µg |
| Inadequate diet; anemia | Iron[a] | 30–60 mg elemental |
| Inadequate diet | Vitamin $B_6$ | 2 mg |
| Inadequate diet | Vitamin C | 50 mg |
| Inadequate diet; no exposure to sunlight | Vitamin D | 10 µg |
| For women receiving supplemental iron | Zinc | 15 mg |

[a] Supplements containing high levels of folate or iron negatively affect zinc metabolism. Supplementary forms of folic acid are better absorbed than folate occurring in food.

## CALCIUM, MAGNESIUM, AND VITAMIN D

About 99% of calcium in pregnant women and their fetus is located in their bones and teeth. Pregnancy and lactation are associated with increased bone turnover to meet needs. If dietary deficiencies occur, maternal bone will supply the calcium to the fetus. Calcium supplementation during pregnancy has been shown to lead to an important reduction in systolic and diastolic blood pressure.[37] Controlled clinical trials to test the hypothesis that calcium supplements during pregnancy reduce the incidence of pregnancy-induced hypertension have had mixed results. The DRI for calcium in pregnant and lactating women less than 18 years is 1300 mg/day and 1000 mg/day for those over 18 years.* In pregnant women who have diets deficient in calcium, are adolescent, have prepregnancy hypertension, history of preeclampsia, or chronic use of heparin and/or steroids, supplemental calcium is recommended.[46]

The fetus absorbs 6 mg of magnesium each day. Maternal magnesium levels remain constant during pregnancy despite reported inadequate intakes. The RDA for most pregnant women is increased to 350 mg/day.† Magnesium supplementation has been associated with fewer hospitalizations, fewer preterm births, and more perinatal hemorrhages compared with placebo-supplemented women. Thus, further study is needed before routine supplementation is recommended.

Vitamin D is critical in the absorption, distribution, and storage of calcium. Relatively few foods, except those fortified, are good sources of vitamin D. The RDA is unchanged in pregnancy.‡ Vitamin D deficiency in pregnancy has been

linked with preeclampsia, low birth weight, and other complications such as neonatal rickets and asthma. African American and Hispanic women are more likely to have vitamin D insufficiency than white women. Since 25 (OH) D readily crosses the placenta, fetal and newborn vitamin D status is almost entirely dependent on vitamin D from the mother. Further research is required to establish need, safety, and efficacy of supplementation during pregnancy.

## FOLATE AND IRON

The available data from controlled trials provide clear evidence of an improvement in hematological indices in women receiving routine iron and folate supplementation during pregnancy. Iron supplementation with and without folic acid results in substantial reduction of women with hemoglobin levels <100 g/L late in pregnancy, at delivery, and 6 weeks postpartum.[46] The Cochrane Pregnancy and Childbirth Group recommends iron supplementation.[47] Both folate intake from food and synthetic folic acid should be included in assessing and planning diet. The DRI is higher than that usually obtained from food. The current recommendation during pregnancy is 600 µg/day of folic acid.§ It is well established that periconceptional use of folic acid supplementation and fortification reduces the risk of first occurrence and recurrence of neural tube defect (NTD)-affected pregnancies by 70%. The CDC recommends supplementation of 400 µg/day for all women of childbearing age and 4 mg/day for women who have had an NTD-affected pregnancy starting 1–3 months prior to conception and to continue through the first 3 months of pregnancy. Additional iron is needed by many pregnant women in the United States. A substantial amount of iron is required, given the amount of erythropoiesis. For example, a term infant contains an average

* http://fnic.nal.usda.gov/nal_display/index.php?info_center=4&tax_level=3&tax_subject=256&topic_id=1342&level3_id=5140&level4_id=0&level5_id=0&placement_default=0 (accessed April 5, 2012).

† http://fnic.nal.usda.gov/nal_display/index.php?info_center=4&tax_level=3&tax_subject=256&topic_id=1342&level3_id=5140&level4_id=0&level5_id=0&placement_default=0 (accessed April 5, 2012).

‡ http://fnic.nal.usda.gov/nal_display/index.php?info_center=4&tax_level=3&tax_subject=256&topic_id=1342&l evel3_id=5140&level4_id=0&level5_id=0&placement_default=0 (accessed April 5, 2012).

§ http://fnic.nal.usda.gov/nal_display/index.php?info_center=4&tax_level=3&tax_subject=256&topic_id=1342&level3_id=5140&level4_id=0&level5_id=0&placement_default=0 (accessed April 5, 2012).

of 225 mg of iron and the placenta and cord contain 50 mg of iron through the pregnancy, and the maternal red blood count volume increases by 500 mL. The RDA for iron is increased to 27 mg/day (assuming 75% is heme iron). It is suggested that vegetarians require twice the amount of non-heme iron. Although maternal absorption of iron from the GI tract is increased by about 15%, it remains difficult to meet the increased iron need through diet alone. Table 18.18 lists dietary sources of iron. Iron absorption is increased in the presence of ascorbic acid. Adverse pregnancy outcomes are associated with hemoglobin levels below 10.4 g/dL or above 13.2 g/dL. Clinical diagnosis of anemia is made based on hemoglobin below 10.5 g/dL, a low MCV, and a serum ferritin level below 12 µg/dL. Supplementation of 30–60 mg/day of elemental iron is usually prescribed. A 2009 Cochrane Review concluded that universal prenatal supplementation with iron or iron + folic acid provided either daily or weekly is effective to prevent anemia and iron deficiency at term[47], and the 2010 USPSTF Guide to Clinical Preventive Services states that there is insufficient evidence to make a recommendation for or against routine iron supplementation in non-anemic pregnant women.[48] Healthy Canada states that an iron supplement of 16 mg/day throughout pregnancy is justified as both efficacious and safe.[49]

## TABLE 18.18
### Dietary Sources of Iron (DRI = 15–30 mg/day)

| Food Item | Serving Size |
| --- | --- |
| *Excellent >4 mg* | |
| Beef liver,[a] Chicken liver[a] | 3 oz |
| Clams,[a] Oysters[a] | ½ cup |
| Figs (dried) | 10 |
| Iron-fortified infant cereal | ½ cup |
| Lima beans, navy beans | ½ cup |
| Kidney beans, black-eyed peas | 1 cup |
| Molasses (blackstrap) | 3 tbsp |
| Peaches (dried) | 10 halves |
| Pinto beans | 1 cup |
| Ready-to-eat, fortified cereals (such as Product 19®, Total®) | ¾ cup |
| Sunflower seeds (dried, hulled) | ⅔ cup |
| *Good: 2–4 mg* | |
| Beef[a] | 3 oz |
| Egg yolks | 3 |
| Iron-fortified infant formula | 4 oz |
| Lamb[a] | 3 oz |
| Tofu | ½ cup |
| Spinach | ½ cup |
| Peas | 1 cup |
| Pork | 3 oz |
| Prune juice | 1 cup |
| Raisins | ⅔ cup |
| Soybeans | ½ cup |

[a] Indicates heme iron.

Common side effects include stomach upset, nausea, and constipation. These effects may be relieved by reducing the dosage or switching the brand of iron supplement. Some, but not all, sustained release preparations have been clinically shown to be associated with fewer discomforts. Researchers suggest that excess iron may lead to zinc depletion, which is associated with intrauterine growth retardation.

## FATTY ACIDS

Long-chain polyunsaturated fatty acids appear important for healthy lifestyle and may be critical for the developing fetus and young infant. The DRI (adequate intake) for omega 6 fatty acids is 13 g/day in pregnancy and lactation. For omega 3 fatty acids, it is 1.4 g/day in pregnancy and 1.3 g/day in lactation. Dietary sources for omega n-3 are fish (DHA, EPA): tuna, Pollock, salmon, cod, catfish, flounder, grouper, halibut, red snapper, shark, swordfish, tilefish, and king mackerel; krill; seed oil (LNA): chia, kiwifruit, perilla, flax linseed oil, lingonberry, camelina, purslane, black raspberry, butternuts, hempseed, walnuts, pecan nuts, and hazel nuts. There is growing evidence that adequate omega-3 fatty acid intake, in particular DHA, should be consumed during pregnancy to ensure optimal cognitive, eye, and brain development of the infant. Fish should be consumed during pregnancy, at least 12 oz a week, while avoiding fish known to have high levels of mercury such as shark, swordfish, king mackerel, tilefish, bowfin, and bass, wild catfish, South Atlantic grouper, orange roughy, shark, and tuna (fresh or frozen). See www.epa.gov/ost/fish for warnings (accessed April 5, 2012). Fish low in mercury are canned tuna, cod, flounder, halibut, lobster, mahimahi, oysters, salmon, scallops, shrimp, white fish, tilapia, and trout. There are no standard recommendations for supplementation,[50] although many prenatal vitamin preparations contain DHA and EPA. Some experts recommend that the DHA requirement is 200 mg/day, which can come from two fish meals per week or dietary supplements.

## PHYSICAL ACTIVITY DURING PREGNANCY

Several factors influence physical activity during pregnancy, including prepregnancy exercise levels, current levels, personal preferences, risk, limitations, and contraindications.[51] In the absence of medical or obstetric complications, the 2008 Physical Activity Guidelines for Americans[52] specify healthy women who are not already highly active or doing vigorous-intensity activity should get at least 150 min (2 h and 30 min), preferably spread over the week of moderate-intensity aerobic activity per week during pregnancy and the postpartum period. Those who have habitually engaged in vigorous-intensity aerobic activity or are highly active can continue through pregnancy and the postpartum period, provided that they remain healthy and discuss with their health-care provider how and when activity should be adjusted over time. Activities with a high risk of falling or abdominal trauma should be avoided as well as lying on back to exercise after the first trimester. Tables 18.19 through 18.23 include guidelines for physical activity.

## POSTPARTUM WEIGHT LOSS

While a great deal of attention is given to counseling women about appropriate weight gain for pregnancy, clinicians have typically given less assistance in achieving postpartum weight loss. Researchers have linked failure to return to pre-pregnancy weight with increased risks for chronic disease later in life. One in five retains substantial weight postpartum.

### TABLE 18.19
### Benefits of Physical Activity during Pregnancy and Postpartum

Improvement in circulation

Improved posture

Improved or maintained cardiovascular fitness

Reduced risk for discomforts of pregnancy (e.g., back pain, swelling, constipation, sleeping difficulties), excessive gestational weight gain

Reduced risk of preeclampsia, preterm birth, cesarean section, decreased labor time, and decreased use of epidural and forceps

Positive effects on mood, energy level; reduced physical and mental fatigue

Release of tension and reduction of stress

Prevention of injury

Primary prevention of gestational diabetes, especially in women with BMI > 33

After pregnancy, associated with decreased incidence of postpartum depression, reduced risk for long-term obesity

### TABLE 18.20
### Contraindications to Physical Activity

Active myocardial disease, congestive heart failure, and rheumatic heart disease

Thrombophlebitis

Risk of premature labor, incompetent cervix, uterine bleeding, and ruptured membranes

Intrauterine growth restriction

Severe hypertensive disease

Suspected fetal intolerance

### TABLE 18.21
### Warning Signs to Stop Physical Activity

Vaginal bleeding

Uterine contractions

Nausea, vomiting

Dizziness or faintness

Difficulty walking

Decreased fetal activity

Palpitations or rapid heart rate

Numbness in any part of the body

Problems with vision

### TABLE 18.22
### Guidelines for Physical Activity

| Activity | Guideline |
|---|---|
| Intensity | Reduce the intensity of exercise by 25% |
| Heart rate | Not to exceed 140 beats/min |
| Temperature | Not to go above 101°F |
| Time | Moderate activity of 30 min or more |
| Position | Avoid supine positions and motionless standing |
| Frequency | Exercise should be performed on most, if not all days of the week |
| Duration | Physiological and morphologic changes of pregnancy persist 4–6 weeks postpartum |

### TABLE 18.23
### Guidelines for Recreational Activity

| Activity | Guideline |
|---|---|
| General conditioning exercises | Kegel, breathing, calf pumping, abdominal, bridging, lower trunk rotation, tail wagging |
| Jogging | May be continued moderately, but should not be started as a new activity after pregnancy; watch out for joint pain and decrease overall distance—recommendation is 2 mi or less per day |
| Aerobics | Avoid high-impact or step aerobics; as for jogging, look out for joint pain or signs of over exertion; avoid exercises that involve lying on the back for more than 5 min |
| Bicycling | In the third trimester, it may be necessary to switch to a stationary bike due to problems with balance |
| Weight lifting | Can be continued during pregnancy—use lightweights and moderate repetitions; avoid heavy resistance |
| Avoid during pregnancy | Downhill skiing, gymnastics, horseback riding, scuba diving, and any contact sports |

Weight loss can safely occur by diet alone or diet and physical activity.[53] There are insufficient data to suggest breast-feeding women restrict calorie intake. Table 18.24 includes recommended strategies for postpartum weight loss.

## NUTRITION AND LACTATION

The National Agricultural Library maintains a link* to the DRI tables developed and published by the Institute of Medicine.† These levels are set by the Food and Nutrition Board of the National Academy of Sciences. In lactation, requirements for carbohydrates, dietary fiber, water, biotin,

* http://fnic.nal.usda.gov/nal_display/index.php?info_center=4&tax_level=3&tax_subject=256&topic_id=1342&level3_id=5140&level4_id=0&level5_id=0&placement_default=0 (accessed April 5, 2012).
† http://www.iom.edu/Activities/Nutrition/SummaryDRIs/~/media/Files/Activity%20Files/Nutrition/DRIs/5_Summary%20Table%20Tables%201-4.pdf (accessed April 5, 2012).

**TABLE 18.24**

**Strategies for Postpartum Weight Loss**

Encourage exclusive breast-feeding

Encourage a healthy diet based on current dietary guidelines

Make energy intake less than energy expenditure

Reduce portion size but do not restrict kilocalories to <1800/day

Determine foods high in fats and calories and substitute with fruits, vegetables, lean meats and fish, skinless poultry

Avoid cooking in oil, butter, margarine

Drink 8–10 glasses of no/low-calorie fluids per day

Discuss feasible physical activity

Monitor women who

    Restrict intake to <1800 kcal/day

    Are vegans (avoid all animal products including dairy, eggs, and meats)

    Avoid foods enriched with vitamin D and have limited exposure to sunlight

    Have severe iron deficiency in last trimester

choline, chromium, copper, manganese, pantothenic acid, riboflavin, selenium, zinc, vitamin A, vitamin $B_6$, vitamin $B_{12}$, vitamin E, vitamin C, iodine, and potassium are increased over the increased pregnancy needs. In lactation, the iron requirements are reduced. Suggestions for maternal nutrition to meet the increased energy and nutrient needs are listed in Table 18.25. Until relatively recently, breast-feeding has been considered too imprecise to study. A wealth of information is being developed about lactation and breast milk.[54] Table 18.26 lists some of the benefits of unrestricted nursing for the infant. Many women and their clinicians still are concerned about ways to identify whether an infant is obtaining enough nutriture. Table 18.27 lists signs of insufficient milk intake. The social history of infant feeding from the late 1800s to the 1950s in the United States shows a transition from breast-feeding to scientific feeding of infants. As a result of that, much cultural knowledge and support

**TABLE 18.25**

**Maternal Nutrition during Breast-Feeding**

Encourage a healthy diet based on current dietary guidelines

Reinforce that milk quality is generally not affected by the mother's diet

Suggest eating meals and snacks that are easy to prepare

Provide patient with information on normal postpartum weight loss in a breast-feeding woman

Drink enough fluids to keep from getting thirsty

Eat at least 1800 kcal/day

Use appetite as a guide to the amount of food eaten in first 6 weeks

Keep intake of coffee, cola, or other sources of caffeine to two servings or less per day. Caffeine accumulates in the infant and use should be discontinued if infant becomes wakeful, hyperactive, or has disturbed sleep patterns. This reaction is intensified with a smoking mother

**TABLE 18.26**

**Benefits of Frequent, Early, Unrestricted Nursing**

Helps establish early, exclusive breast-feeding by stimulating mother's milk supply

Provides colostrum that the baby needs

Helps decrease newborn jaundice because of the laxative effect of colostrums

Provides a period of practice time before milk volume increases

Stimulates uterine contractions, lessening chances of maternal postpartum hemorrhage

Prevents infant hypoglycemia

**TABLE 18.27**

**Signs of Insufficient Milk Intake in the Newborn**

Evaluate weight gain (body weight loss no more than 7%) from birth and no further weight loss by day 5. Assess feeding and consider more frequent follow-up.

The American Academy of Pediatrics breast-feeding policy[a] details the strategies for breast-feeding management of the healthy infant (see Table 18.5)

[a] http://pediatrics.aappublications.org/content/129/3/e827.full?sid=5afa31f8-2d37-497f-89b3-3be84d4386a9 (accessed April 5, 2012).

for breast-feeding was lost. Guidebooks are important for women and clinicians.[33–34,54] Tables 18.28 and 18.29 include common concerns and recommended actions to support breast-feeding.

## RESOURCE MATERIALS

Academy of Nutrition and Dietetics. www.eatright.org; Also Evidence Analysis Library (EAL). www.adaevidencelibrary.com

Agency for Healthcare Research and Quality. Guide to Clinical Preventive Services. http://www.ahrq.gov

American Academy of Family Physicians. http://www.aafp.org/online/en/home.html

American Congress of Obstetricians and Gynecologists, PO Box 70620 Washington, DC 20024-9988, 1-800-673-8444. http://www.acog.org

Environmental Protection Agency. Fish advisories. http://www.epa.gov/mercury/advisories.htm

Food and Nutrition Information Center, National Agricultural Library, ARS, USDA, Beltsville, MD 20705–2351. http://fnic.nal.usda.gov

La Leche League International, 957 N Plum Grove Rd, Schaumburg IL 60173. http://www.llli.org. 1-800-525-3243

March of Dimes Birth Defects Foundation Resource Center. http://www.marchofdimes.org

National Maternal and Child Health Clearinghouse, 1-888-275-4772.

Partnership for Food Safety Education. http://www.fightbac.org

**TABLE 18.28**

**Breast-Feeding Tips: Common Concerns about the Infant**

| Concern | Recommended Action |
|---|---|
| Jaundice | Continue to breast-feed at least every 2 h around the clock. Pump breasts to maintain milk supply. Avoid water or formula feeding. |
| Latch-on | Latch-on is necessary for baby to begin sucking at the breasts. Poor latch-on is a major cause of sore nipples. Baby's mouth should be at nipple level. Support the breast by placing the thumb on the top and four fingers underneath. Tickle baby's bottom lip with nipple until baby opens mouth very wide. Center nipple quickly and bring baby very close. Baby's nose and chin should be touching breast. Ear, shoulder, and hip should be in alignment. |
| Leaking | Leaking is a sign of normal letdown in the early weeks of breast-feeding. Use pads in bra between feedings. Avoid pads with plastic lining. During sexual activity, leaking may occur; breast-feed baby first. |
| Duration of breast-feeding: how long and how often? | Feed on demand, frequently and unrestricted. Read baby's hunger cues not the clock. Baby should empty one breast, be burped, and offered the second breast. Watch baby for signs that he or she is full, such as falling asleep, losing interest in feeding, or stopping breast-feeding. |
| Early first feeding | Put baby to breast soon after delivery, within 1 h. Cuddling, licking, and brief sucking are good signs that baby is learning to breast-feed. Offer breast often to let baby practice. Ask a supportive nurse or lactation consultant for help. Offer breast whenever infant shows signs of early hunger. In general, there should be 8–12 feedings per 24 h. |
| Extra feedings | Healthy breast-fed newborns do not need formula, water, or juice. Breast-feed at least every 2–3 h during the first month. Complementary foods should be added at 6 months of age. |

**TABLE 18.29**

**Breast-Feeding Tips: Common Discomforts That Lead to Breast-Feeding Termination**

| Concerns | Recommended Action |
|---|---|
| Hospital survival skills | "Rooming in" with the baby is a consumer right. Keep baby with mother as much as possible to facilitate breast-feeding often. Do not give bottles of formula or water, but if supplementation is necessary, use cup or syringe feeding. Do not limit feeding time at a breast. Ask a supportive nurse or lactation consultant for help. Do not offer/accept formula gift packs. Delay circumcision. |
| Mastitis | Mastitis is a swollen, inflamed, or infected area in the breast. Watch for flu-like symptoms such as fever above 101°F, chills and muscle aches, and a reddened, hot, tender, or swollen area in the breasts. Rest, breast-feed often, and drink more fluids. Avoid tight bra or clothing. Apply warm water soaks or cold packs (whichever gives relief). Massage affected area. Antibiotics may be needed. Not a reason to stop breast-feeding. |
| Myths and misconceptions | Breast sagging is not a result of breast-feeding. Breast size does not affect ability to breast-feed. Drinking beer, manzanilla tea, or large amounts of fluids does not make more milk. |
| Nipples, flat or inverted (before birth) | Flat or inverted nipples retract or move in toward the breast. Air-dry nipples if leaking occurs. Breast shells should not be used by women at risk for preterm labor. There is no evidence of harm or benefit for breast shells. |
| Nipples, flat or inverted (after birth) | Begin breast-feeding as soon as possible after birth. Breast-feed frequently to avoid engorgement. Pump breasts for a short period before breast-feeding or apply ice wrapped in a cloth and place on the nipple before feeding. Breast shells (milk cups) may be used between feedings. Refer to lactation consultant to learn how to use a nipple shield as a temporary tool for the initial latch. Remove the breast shell just before placing baby at breast. Reverse pressure softening helps. |
| Engorgement | Engorgement may occur when milk first comes in or when feeding are missed or delayed. Use cold compresses or shower before feedings. Hand-express to soften areola, making it easier for baby to latch on. Breast-feed every 1–2 h for 10–30 min/breast. Gently massage breast toward nipple. Take nonaspirin pain reliever. Reverse pressure softening helps. |
| Breast care | Nipple pulling, tugging, or rolling during pregnancy is not necessary to prepare for breast-feeding. Avoid soaps or lotions to the nipples. Air-dry nipples after breast-feeding. |
| Breast creams | Vitamin E, breast creams, or ointments are not recommended. No evidence exists that they heal the nipple. May make soreness worse by keeping the nipple moist. Use pure lanolin. Can massage drops of breast milk on nipples. Use hydrogel dressings |
| Breast surgery | Any type of breast surgery can interfere with milk supply. Referral to lactation consultant is appropriate. |
| Operative delivery | Breast-feed baby as soon as possible after delivery, preferably in the recovery room. Hold baby in a comfortable position. Use pillows across abdomen to protect the incision and support baby. Use side lying position. |

The National Academies Press. The Complete Dietary Reference Intakes Set. http://www.nap.edu/catalog/dri/?gclid=CP3i49m Ho68CFUKQ7Qod4Bi1YQ

Vegetarian Resource Group. http://www.vrg.org/nutrition/vegan-pregnancy.php

Womenshealth.org. Pregnancy and Healthy Diet. http://womenshealth.org

## REFERENCES

1. Am Coll OB-GYN. ACOG Committee Opinion. No. 313. September 2005, Reaffirmed 2012.
2. American Academy of Pediatrics, American College of Obstetricians and Gynecologists and March of Dimes Birth Defects Foundation. *Guidelines for Perinatal Care,* American Academy of Pediatrics, EIK Grove Village, IL, 2007.
3. Institute of Medicine, Subcommittee for a Clinical Application Guide. *Nutrition during Pregnancy and Lactation: An Implementation Guide*, National Academy Press, Washington, DC, 1992.
4. Institute of Medicine. Weight gain during pregnancy: Reexamining the guidelines. Report Brief. National Academy Press, Washington, DC, 2009.
5. Villar, J, Merialdi, M, and Gulmezoglu, AM et al. *J Nutr.* 5:1606s, 2003.
6. Newton, E. Maternal nutrition. In: Queenan's Management of High Risk Pregnancy. (Queenan, JT, Spong Y, Lakewood C, Eds.) Blackwell Science, Victoria, Australia, 6th edn., 2012.
7. Suitor, CW. Update for nutrition during pregnancy and lactation: An implementation guide. National Center for Education in Maternal and Child Health. Maternal and Child Health Bureau, Health Resources and Services, 1998.
8. ACOG. Nausea and vomiting of pregnancy. ACOG Practice Bulletin No. 52. 2004. Reaffirmed 2011.
9. Cox JT and Phelan ST. *Minerva Ginecol.* 61:373–400, 2009.
10. Kuhlmann AKS, Dietz PM, Galavotti C and England LJ. *Am J Prev Med.* 34:523–528, 2008.
11. Phelan S, Phipps MC, Abrams B et al. *Am J Clin Nutr.* 93:772–779, 2011.
12. Johnson K, Posnter SF, Biermann J et al. *MMWR.* 55(RR06):1–23, 2006.
13. Lum KJ, Sundaram R, Buck Louis GM. *Am J Obstet Gynecol.* 205:203.e1–203.e7, 2011.
14. Siega-Riz AM, King JC. *J Am Diet Assoc.* 109:918–927, 2009.
15. Kramer MS, Kakuma R. *Cochrane Database Syst Rev.* 8, 2010.
16. ACOG. Committee on Obstetric Practice. No. 315, September 2005.
17. Abrams, B, Altman, SL, and Pickett, KE. *Am J Clin Nutr.* 71: 233s, 2000.
18. Carmichael, S, Abrams, B, and Selvin, S. *Am J Public Health* 87:1984–1988, 1997.
19. Siega-Riz, AM, Adair, LS, and Hobel, CJ. *Nutrition* 126:146, 1996.
20. Streuling, I, Beyerlein, A, Rosenfeld, E et al. *BJOG* 118:278–284, 2011.
21. Dodd JM, Grivell RM, Crowther CA, and Robinson JS. *BJOG* 117:1316–1326, 2010.
22. Suitor, CW. Maternal weight gain: A report of an expert work group, National Center for Education in Maternal and Child Health, Arlington, VA, 1997.
23. Abrams, B, Carmichael, S, and Selvin, S. *Obstet Gynecol.* 86:170, 1995.
24. Taffel, SM, Keppel, KG, and Jones, GK. *Ann N Y Acad Sci.* 678: 93, 1993.
25. Kolasa, KM and Weismiller, D. *Am. Fam. Phys.* 56:205, 1997.
26. Stuebe AM, Oken E, and Gillman MW. *Am J Obstet Gynecol.* 201:58.e1–58.e 8, 2001.
27. U.S. Dept. Health and Human Services and USDA. 7th edn., www.healthierus.gov/dietaryguidelines, 2010 (accessed April 5, 2012).
28. ACOG. ACOG Practice Bulletin No. 52. 103:803, 2004.
29. Jewell, D. and Young, G. Cochrane pregnancy and childbirth group. *Cochrane Database Syst Rev.* (9):CD000145, 2010.
30. ACOG. Committee on Obstetric Practice. No. 464. September 2005, Reaffirmed August 2010.
31. SOG. Alcohol use and pregnancy consensus clinical guidelines. *J Obstet Gynaecol Can.* 245:s1, 2010.
32. ACOG. Bulletin No. 496, August 2011.
33. Am Acad Pediatrics. Breastfeeding and the use of human milk. *Pediatrics* 129:3e827–e841, 2012.
34. Mohrbacher, N and Stock, J. *The Breastfeeding Answer Book*, La Leche League International. Bartlett, Boston, MA, 2003.
35. NHLBI. JNC7. NIH Publication No. 04–5230, 2004.
36. NIH. Working group report on high blood pressure in pregnancy. NIH Publication No. 00–3029, July 2000.
37. Hofmeyr GJ, Lawrie TA, Atallah ÁN, and Duley L. *Cochrane Database Syst Rev.* 8:CD001059, 2010. DOI: 10.1002/14651858.CD001059.pub3.
38. Landon MB and Gabbe SG. *Obstet Gynecol.* 118:1379–1393, 2011.
39. USPSTF U.S. preventive services task force recommendations statement. *Ann Intern Med.* 148:759–766, 2008.
40. Horvath K, Koch K, Jeitler K et al. *BMJ.* 340:c1395, 2010.
41. Mumford MI, Jovanovic-Peterson L, Peterson CM. *Clin Perinatol.* 20:619–634, 1993.
42. Moses RG, Barker M, Winter M Petocz P, Brand-Miller JC. *Diabetes Care* 32:996–1000, 2009.
43. Metzger BE, Buchanan TA, Coustan DR et al. *Diabetes Care* 30 (Suppl. 2):S251–S260, 2007.
44. Keppel, KG and Taffel, SM. *Am J Public Health* 83:1100, 1993.
45. Marcus DM, Snodgrass WR. *Obstet Gynecol.* 105:1119–1122, 2005.
46. National Academy of Sciences, Institute of Medicine, Food and Nutrition Board, Committee on Nutritional Status during Pregnancy and Lactation. *Nutrition Services in Perinatal Care*, 2nd edn., National Academy Press, Washington, DC, 1992.
47. Peña-Rosas JP, Viteri FE. *Cochrane Database Syst. Rev.* 4:CD004736, 2009. DOI: 10.1002/14651858.CD004736.pub3.
48. USPSTF. Guide to clinical preventive services, http://www.ahrq.gov/clinic/pocketgd1011/gcp10s2d.htm (accessed April 5, 2012).
49. Cockell KA, Miller DC, Lowell H. *Am J Clin Nutr.* 90:1023–1028, 2009.
50. Forchielli MS, Walker WA. *Nutr Today* 46:224–234, 2011.
51. ACOG Committee Opinion No. 267. January 2002, Reaffirmed 2009.
52. USDA. 2008 Physical activity guidelines for Americans, http://www.health.gov/paguidelines (accessed April 5, 2012).
53. Amorim Adegboye AR, Linne YM, Lourenco PMC. *Cochrane Database Syst. Rev.* 3:CD005627, 2007. DOI: 10.1002/14651858.CD005627.pub 2.
54. Lawrence, RA. *Breastfeeding: A Guide for the Medical Profession*, C.V. Mosby, St. Louis, MO, 7th edn., 2010.

# 19 Feeding the Premature Infant

*Cynthia Mundy and Jatinder Bhatia*

## CONTENTS

Approximately 4 million neonates are born annually in the United States, and the prematurity rate has remained stable at approximately 12% over the past 10 years.[1,2] Advances in perinatal and neonatal medicine have allowed the age of viability to decrease although morbidity rates for these extremely premature infants remain significant.[3] Since the majority of somatic growth occurs in the final trimester of pregnancy, neonatal caregivers are challenged with providing adequate nutrition to simulate these later stages of pregnancy so understanding the principles of nutritional therapy becomes all the more important. Additionally, evidence supports adequate nutrition, and appropriate growth is directly related to improved neurodevelopmental outcomes[4] so the comprehension and implementation of proper nutritional management cannot be understated. This chapter will review the nutritional goals, nutrient requirements, and enteral and parenteral routes of nutritional therapy for this unique population.

## NUTRITIONAL GOALS FOR THE PREMATURE INFANT

A premature infant is an infant born before the completion of 37 weeks of gestation. A post-term infant is one whose birth occurs from the beginning of the first day of week 43

(>42 weeks). Classifying infants as preterm, term, or post-term assists in establishing the level of risk for neonatal morbidity, nutritional needs, and long-term sequelae. Assessment of gestational age is based on maternal dates, obstetrical dating by ultrasonography, and by physical examination.[5] The New Ballard Score is used to estimate the gestational age of infants and is appropriate for use in very small premature infants.[5] Items of neuromuscular maturity and physical maturity are scored from −1 to 5, a total score obtained and gestational age estimated based on maturity rating score. However, in the case of the very-low-birth-weight infant, early estimation of gestational age is more accurately obtained by obstetrical dating versus the Ballard exam.[6]

Infants are considered low birth weight if birth weight is less than 2500 g regardless of gestational age. Very low birth weight defines infants with weight less than 1500 g with an additional classification of extremely low birth weight describing infants less than 1000 g.

Crown–heel length performed by two examiners is measured by achieving full extension of the infant on a measuring board with a fixed head piece and movable foot piece. The infant needs to be supine, head held in the Frankfurt plane vertical, legs extended, ankles flexed, and the movable foot piece is brought to rest firmly against the infant's heels. An average of two measurements documents

Name ______________________ Date of exam ______________ Length ______________

Hospital no. ______________________ Sex ______________ Head circ. ______________

Race ______________________ Birth weight ______________ Gestational age ______________

Date of birth ______________________

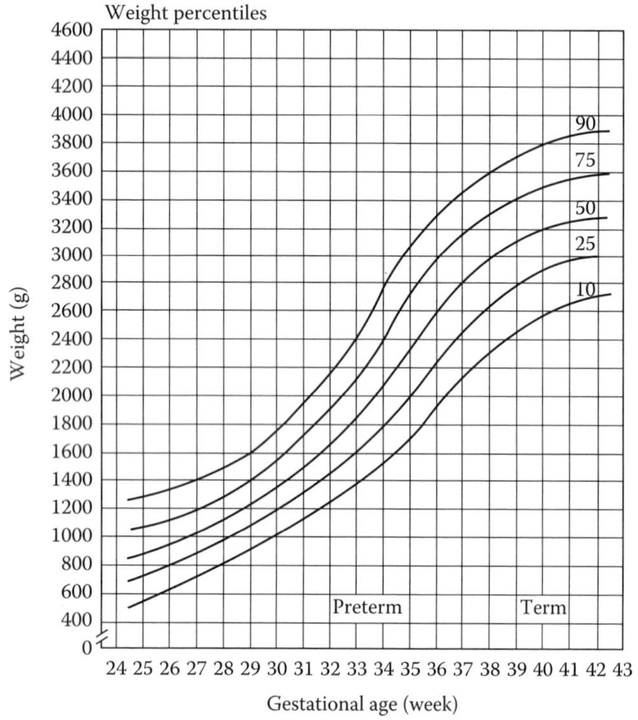


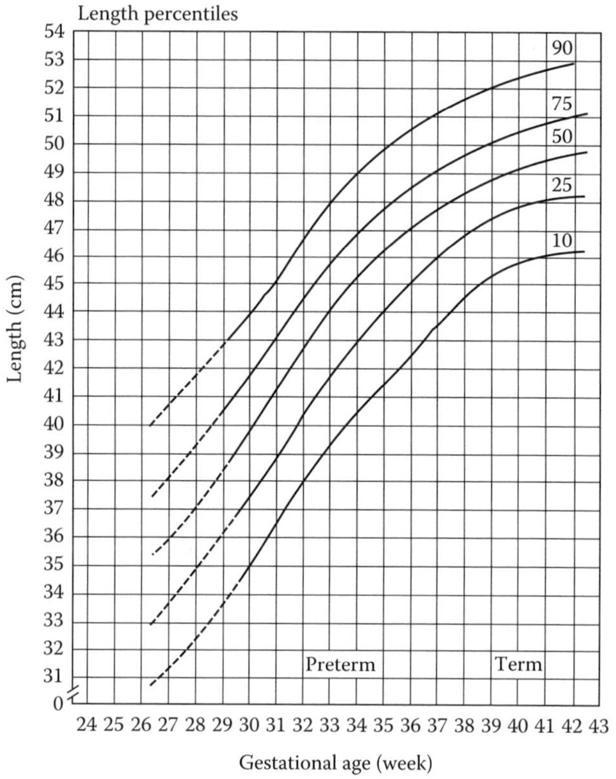


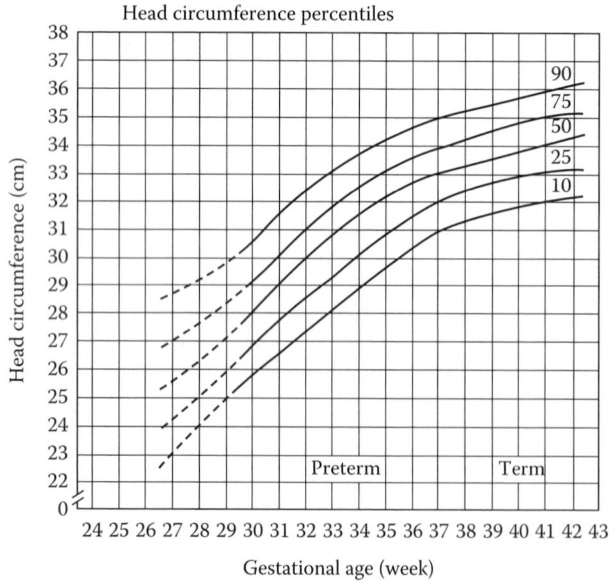


| Classification of infant* | Weight | Length | Head circ. |
|---|---|---|---|
| Large for gestational age (LGA) (>90th percentile) | | | |
| Appropriate for gestational age (AGA) (10th–90th percentile) | | | |
| Small for gestational age (SGA) (<10th percentile) | | | |

* Place an "X" in the appropriate box (LGA, AGA, or SGA) for weight, for length, and for head circumference.

**FIGURE 19.1** Classification of newborns (both sexes) by intrauterine growth and gestational age. (From Ballard, J.L. et al., *J. Pediatr.*, 119(3), 417, 1991.)

the length. If crown–heel length cannot be measured due to limb anomalies or if there is a discrepancy between weight and length, a crown–rump length is sometimes measured. In preterm infants, this measurement is fraught with error even when performed by a trained team. In addition, measurement in an open bed or on a ventilator or with multiple intravenous lines makes accurate measurements difficult to achieve.

Head circumference measured with a non-stretchable tape is the largest of three measurements around the head with the tape held snugly above the ears.

Weight, length, and head circumference are then plotted on standard curves to classify an infant as appropriate, small, or large for gestational age for each measurement. Most measurements define appropriate for age as measurements that fall within the 10th–90th percentiles or 3rd–97th, ideally based on charts constructed for similar race and length above sea level. Infants who are appropriate for age on the three measures are at the lowest risk, within that gestational age grouping, for problems associated with neonatal morbidity and mortality.

An example of growth curves commonly used in neonatal nurseries is depicted in Figure 19.1.

## GROWTH AND NUTRIENT REQUIREMENTS

Estimation of nutrient requirements in premature infants is based on the goals for growth of this cohort of infants. The common goal has been to achieve growth similar to that of the "reference fetus" as described.[7] These growth standards serve as a reference to judge the adequacy of growth; however, postnatal changes in energy requirements as well as environmental stresses are likely to be different, and the ideal growth of these infants remains to be defined. An alternative approach may be to achieve the best possible growth without adverse metabolic consequences. In a recent NICHD evaluation of more than 1600 preterm infants, most had not achieved the growth rates of the reference fetus of the same post-menstrual age by the time they were discharged.[8]

Nutrient requirements for preterm infants have been estimated by various methods including the factorial method based on the reference fetus, nitrogen balance studies, turnover studies, or based on nutrient values in the serum. For example, Table 19.1 provides nutrient intake estimates to achieve growth similar to that in utero.[9] In a more recent publication, Ziegler[10] provides estimated nutrient intakes needed to achieve fetal weight gain, representing the current best estimates. This approach serves not only as a basis for the calculation of nutrient needs, but also as a measure of sufficiency of particular nutrients as discussed (Table 19.1). The factorial approach is based on the assumption that the requirement for a nutrient is the sum of losses (fecal, urine, dermal, etc.) and the amount required for growth. Advisable intakes of protein are obtained by adding 8%–10% of the estimated requirement.

## TABLE 19.1
### Estimated Nutrient Intakes and Fetal Weight Gain

| Body Weight (g) | 500–700 | 700–900 | 900–1,200 | 1,200–1,500 |
|---|---|---|---|---|
| Fetal weight gain (g/kg/day) | 21 | 20 | 19 | 18 |
| Protein intake required, parenteral | 3.5 | 3.5 | 3.5 | 3.4 |
| Protein intake required, enteral | 4.0 | 4.0 | 4.0 | 3.9 |
| Energy intake required, parenteral | 89 | 92 | 101 | 108 |
| Energy intake required, enteral | 105 | 108 | 119 | 127 |

*Source:* Modified from Ziegler, E.E. et al., *Growth*, 40(4), 329, 1976.

## PROVISION OF NUTRIENTS

### Energy Needs

Energy needs are based on basal metabolic rate, cost of growth, and losses in stool and urine. The factorial method cannot be used to estimate energy requirements. It is generally recognized that preterm infants have higher energy requirements compared to their term counterparts.[11] To gain the predicted growth in weight for premature infants (15–20 g/kg/day), it is estimated that premature infants would need between 110 and 130 kcal/kg/day, an estimate higher than the usually held notion that infants need 120 kcal/kg/day regardless of size or age. Energy requirements must take into account the route of administration, enteral versus parenteral, since 90–95 kcal/kg/day may satisfy energy requirements by the parenteral route. Disease states such as sepsis, chronic lung disease,[12,13] and concomitant use of corticosteroids will increase energy needs. The mainstay of energy support should be balanced between carbohydrates, fat, and amino acids.

### Amino Acid Needs

The factorial approach is commonly used to estimate protein requirements. The protein need will be greater if catch-up growth is also to be produced. It is generally accepted that the newborn infant will lose up to 10% of their body weight within the first 2 weeks of life. In sick premature infants where nutrition cannot be provided or is not tolerated, the amount of catch-up growth will be greater. Several studies suggest that endogenous protein losses in the absence of exogenous protein intake are at least 1 g/kg/day.[14,15] When fed in the conventional manner, premature infants run the risk of undernutrition. Therefore, strategies to optimize amino acid intakes to include provision for catch-up growth need to be developed since early initiation of parenteral nutrition results in positive nitrogen balance and has been shown to be safe.[14–19] The more traditional method is to start with 0.5 mg/kg/day of amino acids and slowly increase by 0.5 mg/kg to reach a goal of 3–3.5 mg/kg/day. However, with improvements in amino acid solutions and preterm formulas, recent studies have demonstrated that preterm infants can safely tolerate up to 3.5 mg/kg/day of protein in just a few days after birth.[19,20] In one randomized controlled trial, infants <1500 g on day of life 1 were given glucose only and protein added in a stepwise fashion or glucose and 2.4 g/kg/day of amino acid solution from the first day of life, and this trial showed that high amino acid concentrations could be safely tolerated from birth.[21] Based on this new evidence, the traditional method is not supported, and amino acids should be started at a minimum of 2.5 g/kg/day on the first day of life and advanced to 3.5 g/kg/day within the first 3 days of life.

Cysteine and tyrosine are provided as cysteine hydrochloride (40 mg/g/amino acid, not to exceed 100 mg/kg/day) and N-acetyl-L-tyrosine (0.24 g%).[22] It has been demonstrated that infants receiving cysteine retain significantly more nitrogen than do infants receiving an isonitrogenous amino acid intake without cysteine.[15]

Carnitine is an essential amino acid that transports long-chain fatty acids into mitochondrial cells so they can be broken down as a source of energy. Low plasma concentrations of carnitine and its decline with postnatal age have been demonstrated in infants receiving carnitine-free nutrition.[23,24] Although fatty acid metabolism has not been shown to be impaired in short-term parenteral nutrition, carnitine is an accepted additive for infants requiring parenteral nutrition for longer periods.[25–27] Carnitine is provided at doses of 8.0–20 mg/kg/day.

Glutamine is the most abundant amino acid in the human body and is the most important "nitrogen shuttle," accounting for 30%–35% of all amino acid nitrogen transported in the blood.[28] Glutamine concentrations in blood and tissue fall following starvation, surgery, infection, and trauma.[29,30] In addition, glutamine plays an important role in protein and energy metabolism, nucleotide synthesis, and lymphocyte function.[31] Glutamine is known to be an important fuel for small intestinal enterocytes[32]; however, an absolute need of glutamine for gut growth has not been demonstrated with either detrimental or negligible effects reported in the literature.[33,34] A recent review of six randomized controlled trials of glutamine supplementation in preterm infants did not show significant decreases in mortality and no significant effect on the incidence of necrotizing enterocolitis (NEC), sepsis, days to full feeds, or length of hospitalization.[35]

Taurine is considered to be an essential amino acid in preterm infants. Premature infants fed formulas enriched with the nutrient had better Bayley scores at 18 months than those fed term formula without taurine.[36]

## Carbohydrate Needs

It is generally accepted that infants receiving between 80 and 90 kcal/kg/day from parenteral nutrition with an adequate amino acid intake should gain weight similar to the intrauterine rate.[37] Most of this energy intake is provided by glucose and lipid. The glucose utilization rate of a preterm infant is 5–8 mg/kg/min. Carbohydrates, most readily available as glucose, should provide approximately 35% of the daily kilocalories. However, premature and sick infants may not tolerate increasing glucose concentrations/delivery without concomitant hyperglycemia, making the goal of achieving adequate energy intake difficult in the first week of life.

## Lipid Needs

Lipid emulsions are used in conjunction with glucose and amino acid solutions. Generally, lipids are started at 0.5 g/kg/day intravenously increasing by 0.5 g/kg to a maximum of 3.0 g/kg/day. The goal is to provide 50% of the daily caloric intake as fat. Infusion rates are maintained between 0.15 and 0.25 g/kg/h in order to avoid hypertriglyceridemia (triglycerides > 175 mg/dL). Essential fatty acid deficiency may be prevented by lipid intakes as low as 0.5–1.0 g/kg/day.

Clearance of lipids by premature infants may be limited thereby requiring frequent assessment of tolerance. Emulsions of 20% are preferred due to lower total phospholipid and liposome content per gram of triglyceride.[38]

## PARENTERAL NUTRITION

It is common practice to provide the initial nutrient requirements, especially in a sick neonate, by the parenteral route. A typical parenteral regimen is depicted in Table 19.2. It is generally recommended that parenteral nutrition be started within the first hours of life in preterm infants and advanced in a systematic fashion to achieve 3–3.5 g/kg/day of amino acids, 90–100 kcal/kg/day of energy. Most preterm infants do not achieve these intakes until well into the second week of life because of issues such as glucose and lipid intolerance.

## Mineral Requirements

Mineral requirements have also been estimated based on body composition and the reference fetus.[7,9] Daily needs for sodium, potassium, and chloride are based on serum measurements while calcium and phosphorus are based on the factorial method.[7,9] Requirements are listed in Table 19.2. It should be noted that premature infants in general, and very-low-birth weight infants in particular, receive large amounts of sodium inadvertently.[39] Therefore, sodium should not be added to parenteral nutrition regimens until the sodium is below 130 mEq/L.

Feeding the Premature Infant

283

## TABLE 19.2
### Parenteral Nutrition Regimen

| Component | Amount/kg/day |
|---|---|
| Amino acids (g) | 3–3.5 |
| Glucose (g) | 15–25 |
| Lipid (g) | 0.5–3.0 |
| Sodium (mEq)[a] | 2–5 |
| Potassium (mEq)[b] | 2–4 |
| Calcium (mg) | 80–100 |
| Magnesium (mg) | 3–6 |
| Chloride (mEq) | 2–3 |
| Phosphorus (mg)[b] | 40–60 |
| Zinc (μg) | 200–400 |
| Copper (μg) | 20 |
| Other trace minerals[c] | |
| Iron (μg) | 100–200 |
| Vitamins[d] | |
| Total volume | 120–150 mL |

[a] Sodium requirements may vary between infants and within the same infant and should be tailored to serum values.

[b] Phosphorus intakes are maintained in a ratio of 1:2–1:2.6 with calcium (mEq:mM) and may be limiting in parenteral nutrition because of insolubility; in general, more acidic the TPN, more calcium and phosphorus can be dissolved in the solution without precipitation. Care must be taken to avoid hyperphosphatemia with its resultant hypocalcemia.

[c] Amount/kg/day.

| Nutrient | <14 Day | >14 Day |
|---|---|---|
| Manganese (μg) | 0.0–0.75 | 1.0 |
| Chromium (μg) | 0.0–0.05 | 0.2 |
| Selenium (μg) | 0.0–1.3 | 2.0 |
| Iodide (μg) | 0.0–1.0 | 1.0 |
| Molybdenum (μg) | 0 | 0.25 |

[d] Provided as MVI-Pediatric[R]; each 5 mL provides (MVI is to be provided in amounts not exceeding 2.0 mL/kg/day.).

| | |
|---|---|
| C (mg) | 80 |
| A (mg) | 0.7 |
| D (μg) | 10 (= 400 μ) |
| $B_1$ (mg) | 1.2 |
| $B_2$ (mg) | 1.4 |
| $B_6$ (mg) | 1 |
| Niacin (mg) | 17 |

In general, the preterm infant has higher requirements of most minerals compared to term infants. During total parenteral nutrition, requirements for calcium and phosphorus may not be met because of the insolubility of calcium salts. Human milk may not provide adequate amounts of sodium, and hyponatremia has been reported.[40] Calcium and phosphorus needs of preterm infant cannot be met by human milk, if from mothers delivering preterm or term infants, and will need to be supplemented.[41] Since calcium transfer across the placenta occurs in the third trimester, the very premature infant is relatively "osteopenic," and prolonged parenteral nutrition and/or unfortified human milk feedings put the infant at great risk for further osteopenia and metabolic bone disease.

Iron is accumulated in the fetus in the third trimester with an iron content of 75 mg/kg at term. Small-for-gestational-age infants, preterm infants, and infants of diabetic mothers have low iron stores at birth. Coupled with the need for frequent blood sampling, the premature infant is at great risk for the development of iron-deficiency anemia, and the exact time for supplementation remains controversial. However, given that the criteria for blood transfusion have become more stringent,[41] iron should be supplemented as early as 2 weeks. If recombinant erythropoietin is used to stimulate endogenous iron production,[42] iron requirements may be 6.0 mg/kg/day or higher.

### Nutrient Delivery

Delivery of enteral nutrients is based on gestational age. In general, infants of 33 weeks of gestation and beyond can be fed orally soon after birth. However, if medical or surgical illness precludes enteral feedings, parenteral nutrition is indicated. Parenteral nutrition can be considered as total (where all nutrients are delivered, e.g., in an infant with a surgical condition precluding enteral nutrition: gastroschisis) or supplemental (to complement enteral nutrition). It can be further described as peripheral parenteral nutrition (provided by a peripheral intravenous line) or central (where the tip of the catheter is in a central location or deep vein). The latter should be the route if long-term parenteral nutrition (e.g., greater than 2 weeks) or the need for >12.5% dextrose in water is anticipated.

A typical nutrition plan for a very-low-birth-weight infant is depicted in Table 19.3.

Parenteral nutrition is indicated in the following conditions:

| Medical | Inadequate enteral nutrition |
|---|---|
| | Necrotizing enterocolitis |
| | Feeding intolerance/difficulty |
| | Ileus |
| | Prematurity |
| Surgical | Omphalocele |
| | Gastroschisis |
| | Tracheo-esophageal fistula |
| | Atresias of the intestine (duodenal/jejunal/ileal) |
| | Diaphragmatic hernia |
| | Hirschsprung's disease |

**TABLE 19.3**

**Initiation and Advancement of Parenteral and Minimal Enteral Feedings in an Infant with a Birth Weight of <1000 g**

| | Parenteral | | | | |
|---|---|---|---|---|---|
| Age, Day | Amino Acid (g/kg) | Glucose | Lipids (g/kg) | Electrolytes | Enteral mL/h[c] |
| 1 | 2.5–3.0 | $D_5W$–$D_{10}W$ | 0.0–0.5 | 0.0 | 0.0 |
| 2 | 3.0–3.5 | $D_5W$–$D_{10}W$ | 0.5–1.0 | Add if Na <130 mEq/L | 0.25 |
| 3 | 3.0–3.5 | Increments of 2.5% | 1.0–1.5[a] | Standard | 0.25 |
| 4 | Same | Increase as tolerated | 1.5–2.0[a] | Standard | 0.5 |
| 5 | Same | Increase as tolerated | 2.0–2.5[a] | Standard | 0.5 |
| 6 | Same | Increase as tolerated | 2.5[a] | Standard | 0.75 |
| 7 | 3.0 or higher[b] | Same or higher | 3.0[a] | Standard | 0.75 |

[a] Monitor triglycerides to assess lipid tolerance.

[b] Optional; infants requiring catch-up growth, on corticosteroids, or demonstrating low BUN despite adequate protein intakes may need higher amino acid intakes at later stages.

[c] In larger infants, studies have demonstrated that feeding of 20 mL/kg/day and advancing at that rate are safe[43] while other studies have demonstrated an increased incidence of NEC when feeds are advanced at that rate.[44]

Complications of parenteral nutrition include the following:

| Metabolic | Hypo- or hyperglycemia |
|---|---|
| | Electrolyte imbalance |
| | Metabolic bone disease |
| | Hepatic dysfunction |
| Infectious | Bacterial sepsis |
| | Fungal sepsis |
| Mechanical | Extravasation |
| | Thrombosis |
| | Pericardial effusion |
| | Diaphragmatic palsy |
| | Pleural effusion |

The metabolic complications can be avoided by careful assessment of tolerance to the macronutrients as nutrition delivery is advanced. Premature infants do not tolerate high concentrations of glucose or rapid advances in glucose delivery; similarly, rates of fat infusion of greater than 2.0 g/kg/day may result in hypertriglyceridemia particularly in the small or ill preterm infant (triglycerides > 175 mg/dL). A suggested regimen of monitoring parenteral nutrition is depicted in Table 19.4. A multidisciplinary approach with physicians, pharmacists, nutritionists, and nursing staff who are knowledgeable in parenteral nutrition and monitoring should be involved in the care of such infants. Early recognition of metabolic effects (pharmacist or nutritionist) or catheter-related effects (nursing) could assist in minimizing the potential complications of parenteral nutrition. The most common metabolic complications observed are hepatic dysfunction and metabolic bone disease.

Hepatic dysfunction is defined as an increase in serum bile acids, followed by an increase in direct bilirubin, alkaline phosphatase, and gamma-glutamyl transferase. The hepatocellular enzymes, ALT and AST, are late to

**TABLE 19.4**

**Suggested Monitoring during Parenteral Nutrition**

| Component | Initial | Later[a] |
|---|---|---|
| Weight | Daily | Daily |
| Length | Weekly | Weekly |
| Head circumference | Weekly | Weekly |
| Na, K, Cl, $CO_2$ | Daily until stable | Weekly |
| Glucose | Daily | PRN |
| Triglycerides | With every lipid change | Weekly or biweekly |
| Ca, $PO_4$ | Daily until stable | Weekly or biweekly |
| Alkaline phosphatase | Initial | Weekly or biweekly |
| Bilirubin | Initial | Weekly or biweekly |
| Mg | Initial | Weekly or biweekly |
| Ammonia | PRN | PRN |
| Gamma GT | Initial | Weekly or biweekly |
| ALT/AST | Initial | Weekly or biweekly |
| Complete blood count | Initial | Weekly or PRN |

[a] A practical way to monitor parenteral nutrition may simply include measurement of direct bilirubin and alkaline phosphatase at 2–4 weeks of age. If they are increased, a comprehensive metabolic panel may be ordered to evaluate the traditional "liver function tests" and calcium and phosphorus. This may achieve the same end point as monitoring the parameters routinely.

increase and often seen in the more severe cases. Gamma-glutamyl transferase is probably the most sensitive but least specific indicator, whereas elevation in direct bilirubin is the most specific and least sensitive indicator of hepatic dysfunction. The etiology is multifactorial,[45–47] but the incidence appears to be declining as a result of both specialized amino acid solutions and early provision of enteral nutrients. Limiting the use of lipids to 1 g/kg/day has also shown reduction and possible prevention of hepatic dysfunction.[48]

Premature infants are at high risk for the development of metabolic bone disease most commonly due to inadequate intakes of calcium and phosphorus during parenteral nutrition. Infants born before 32 weeks of gestation have some degree of hypomineralization, which is worsened during the subsequent period of hospitalization especially coupled with inadequate intakes of calcium and phosphorus. In general, both calcium and phosphorus levels are maintained in serum while the bones appear more osteopenic on radiographs, and ultimately hypophosphatemia with increasing alkaline phosphatase is observed. Rising alkaline phosphatase in the absence of elevated "liver" enzymes is a strong indicator of metabolic bone disease. Incidence of rickets (metabolic bone disease) is inversely proportional to birth weight and has been reported to be as high as 50%–60% in very-low-birth-weight infants.[49] Diagnosis is made by routine radiographs, which in the initial stages would demonstrate bone undermineralization, especially in the ribs and scapula, subsequently showing the classic forms of rickets in the wrists and long bones. Strategies to increase calcium and phosphorus delivery should be considered.

Unfortunately, the very small preterm infant is more often at risk for these complications given the duration of parenteral nutrition and the coexistence of hepatic dysfunction.

## ENTERAL NUTRITION

Even if enteral nutrition is started in the first days after birth, it is suggested that supplemental parenteral nutrition be started because immaturity, feeding intolerance, and GI motility may affect the rate of advancement of enteral nutrition. Further, intakes are also dictated by the feedings used: human milk or formula. Composition of human milk (Table 19.5), especially from a mother delivering a preterm infant, is different from that of mothers delivering at term; further, differences between and within the same woman makes the average content difficult to estimate. Breast milk does appear to provide the best protection from infection and the development of NEC. However, it may not provide adequate amounts of calcium, phosphorus, protein, and sodium for the growing premature infant. Various fortifiers are available and appear to enhance short-term weight gain and to be safe (described later). Whether the content is mostly in the form of carbohydrates or fat, the result is increased fat deposition.[50,51] The route of enteral nutrition is dictated not only by the gestational age of the infant, but also by the coexistence or medical or surgical morbidity. Routes and types of delivery are depicted in Table 19.6.

Motor responses to feedings are similar whether feedings are provided by the gastric or transpyloric route.[52] However, when feeds are provided slowly over 120 min as compared to 15 min, gastric emptying is better, suggesting that in the smaller premature infant, slow infusions may be better tolerated.[53,54]

## Oral Feeding

Term and preterm infants greater than 34 weeks of gestation may be fed soon after birth by the oral route. This should be

## TABLE 19.5
## Composition of Human Milk

| | | Human Milk (2 Weeks Postpartum) | |
| | | Term | Preterm |
|---|---|---|---|
| Volume | (mL) | 147–161 | 139–150 |
| Water | (mL) | 133–145 | 125–135 |
| *Protein* | | | |
| Content | (g) | 1.8–2.5 | 2.4–3.1 |
| Percent of energy | | 7–11 | 9.6–12 |
| Whey/casein ratio | | 80: 20 | 80: 20 |
| *Lipid* | | | |
| Content | (g) | 4.4–6 | 4.9–6.3 |
| Percent of energy | | 44–56 | 42–55 |
| *Composition* | | | |
| Saturated | (%) | 43 | 41–47 |
| Monosaturated | (%) | 42 | 39–40 |
| Polyunsaturated | (%) | 15 | 12–14 |
| *Carbohydrate* | | | |
| Content | (g) | 9–10.6 | 8–9.8 |
| Percent of energy | | 38–44 | 31–38 |
| Lactose | (%) | 100 | 100 |
| *Minerals and trace elements* | | | |
| Calcium | (mg) | 39–42 | 31–40 |
| | (mmol) | 0.9–1 | 0.7–1 |
| Chloride | (mg) | 69–76 | 76–127 |
| | (mmol) | 1.9–2.1 | 2.1–3.6 |
| Copper | (mg) | 37–85 | 107–111 |
| Iodine | (μg) | 16 | — |
| Iron | (mg) | 0.04–0.12 | 0.13–0.14 |
| Magnesium | (mg) | 3.9–4.5 | 4.3–4.7 |
| | (mmol) | 0.16–0.18 | 0.17–0.2 |
| Manganese | (μg) | 0.9 | — |
| Phosphorus | (mg) | 22–25 | 20–23 |
| | (mmol) | 0.7–0.9 | 0.6–0.7 |
| Potassium | (mg) | 90–91 | 81–93 |
| | (mmol) | 2.2–2.4 | 2.1–2.4 |
| Sodium | (mg) | 37–43 | 44–77 |
| | (mmol) | 1.6–1.9 | 1.9–3.3 |
| Zinc | (mg) | 0.18–0.50 | 0.61–0.69 |
| *Vitamins* | | | |
| Fat-soluble | | | |
| Vitamin A | (IU) | 155–333 | 72–357 |
| Vitamin D | (IU) | 0.7–3.3 | 0.7–12 |
| Vitamin E | (IU) | 0.45–0.75 | 0.42–1.42 |
| Vitamin K | (μg) | 0.29–3 | 0.29–3 |
| Water-soluble | | | |
| Vitamin $B_6$ | (μg) | 15–119 | 9–129 |
| Vitamin $B_{12}$ | (μg) | 0.01–1.2 | 0.01–0.07 |
| Vitamin C | (mg) | 6.6–7.8 | 6.3–7.4 |
| Biotin | (μg) | 0.01–1.2 | 0.01–1.2 |
| Folic acid | (μg) | 7.5–9 | 5–8.6 |
| Niacin | (mg) | 0.2–0.25 | 0.24–0.3 |
| Pantothenic acid | (mg) | 0.26 | 0.33 |
| Riboflavin | (μg) | 15–104 | 14–79 |
| Thiamin | (μg) | 3–31 | 1.4–31 |
| *Other* | | | |
| Carnitine | (mg) | 1.04 | — |
| Choline | (mg) | 13.4 | 10–13 |
| Inositol | (mg) | 22.2–83.5 | 21.3 |

**TABLE 19.6**
**Routes of Feeding Preterm Infants**

| Route | <34 weeks | >34 weeks |
|---|---|---|
| Per os | No | Yes |
| Continuous gastric | <1250 g | Failure to tolerate bolus gastric, significant GER |
| Bolus gastric (every 3 h) | >1250 g; infants <1250 g not tolerating continuous | Failure to tolerate per os |
| Transpyloric, continuous | Failure to tolerate gastric feeds, gastric distention due to positive pressure, poor gastric emptying | Same as <34 weeks |

attempted in the delivery room in healthy infants or initiated soon after birth. Breast-feeding should be encouraged and all steps taken by the medical team and hospital staff to encourage breast-feeding once the decision is made. If breast-feeding is precluded due to craniofacial anomalies such as cleft clip or palate, feeding devices are available and speech therapy and/or feeding teams may need to be involved. Lactation consultation should be sought for mothers who have difficulty in either initiation or maintenance of breast-feeding.

Often, mothers delivering preterm infants have not made a decision about breast-feeding and should be counseled appropriately. All delivery sites should have facilities to pump breast milk if actual breast-feeding is not possible and the mother wishes to breast-feed. Teaching should include appropriate techniques for pumping and storing milk.

## Nutrient Delivery

For infants born at or after 34 weeks of gestation, enteral feedings may be started per os. Although it is recognized that infants at this gestational age can coordinate their suck, swallow and respiratory activities thus enabling feedings, not all infants respond in such a fashion, and careful assessment is warranted. In the event oral feedings are not achieved, the infant may require feedings through a feeding tube.

Tube feedings can be delivered by gastric or transpyloric routes. Gastric feedings can be further described as bolus provided intermittently every 2–3 h or continuous where the feeds are provided by a pump at a constant hourly rate. Transpyloric feeds are provided continuously with the tip of the feeding tube in the second part of the duodenum. General indications for the latter include failure to tolerate gastric feeding due to delayed gastric emptying, gastric distention due to positive pressure ventilation, or gastroesophageal reflux. In a review of transpyloric versus gastric feeds, no difference in the incidence of NEC, aspiration, or perforation was found. However, an increased incidence of feeding difficulties was noted with the transpyloric route. No differences were noted in weight or head circumference at 3 and 6 months of chronological age.[55]

Feeding routes can also be initiated based on birth weight. In general, infants below 1250 g are fed by the continuous gastric method, whereas larger infants by the intermittent method.

A further concern with preterm infants is the amount needed to start feedings and how fast to increase feeds. This concern arises from observations that advancing too

quickly or initiation of feedings with larger volumes can increase the incidence of NEC and feeding intolerance. In neonatal dogs, as little as 10% of the total daily intake induced mature gastric motor patterns.[56] Advancement of the feeds by 20 mL/kg/day appears to be well tolerated by most preterm infants. Full-strength formula given slowly (over longer than 15 min) appears to induce the best duodenal motor response.[57]

## SPECIAL CONSIDERATIONS

### Essential Fatty Acids

Vegetable oils contain the parent essential fatty acids linoleic acid (18:2w-6) and in most cases alpha-linolenic acid (18:3w-3). Linoleic and linolenic acids serve as precursors for the synthesis of long-chain polyunsaturated fatty acids (LC-PUFAs) including arachidonic (20:4w-6) and docosahexaenoic (22:6w-3) acids. Human milk lipids contain preformed LC-PUFA; LC-PUFAs are essential components of membrane systems and are incorporated in membrane-rich tissues such as the brain during early growth.[58,59] The fetus and the fully breast-fed infant do not depend on the active synthesis of LC-PUFA since the placenta and human milk provide LC-PUFA in amounts considered appropriate.[60–63] Preterm birth halts the transfer of DHA and ARA, 80% of which is transferred during the third trimester. Preterm infants have high cord blood levels of DHA, ARA, and other LC-PUFAs, but these levels decline rapidly.[64] Premature infants fed formulas without LC-PUFA develop depletion of LC-PUFA in plasma and red cell membranes indicating limited endogenous LC-PUFA synthesis.[65]

DHA and ARA are important for growth and development and visual acuity. Addition of DHA and ARA to preterm formulas leads to levels similar to human milk in North America. This can be achieved with DHA between 0.24% and 0.76% and ARA between 0.32% and 1.1%[66] from single oils. Both are required for effective growth and development. Supplementation with DHA alone led to decreased growth in preterm infants in most studies.[67] Supplementation with the precursor ALA did not sustain DHA levels found in breast milk or confer the benefits on growth and visual acuity. Furthermore, ALA supplementation appeared to lower AA levels possibly secondary to competition between ARA and DHA for precursor enzymes or the previously mentioned inability of preterm infants to synthesize DHA and ARA from precursors.[68–70]

Early trials of DHA and ARA supplementation did not show sustained significant differences in weight, length, or head circumference in larger healthy preterm infants,[71] but more recent studies including younger sicker infants have shown improvement in growth.[66,72] DHA is found in large amounts in the photoreceptor outer segment of the retina. In studies of visual acuity using Teller acuity cards or ERG or VEP, transient improvements in visual acuity were seen in infants fed the supplemented formula, but they were not sustained.[71,73] While some trials showed improvement in Bayley scores of infant development, others did not. Individual studies have shown better vocabulary comprehension at 14 months[73] and improvement in development.[74] However, a 2004 Cochrane review of the literature did not find benefit in supplementation.[71] DHA and ARA supplementation appears to be safe, and blood levels equal to those in breast milk can be achieved. Large differences in the numbers of patients studied, birth weights, and gestational ages, and doses of DHA and ARA make comparisons between studies difficult.

## Fish Oil Emulsions

There has been recent research focused on the reduction of cholestatic liver disease, or intestinal failure-associated liver disease (IFALD), due to the use of long-term parenteral nutrition. IFALD is most associated with birth weights less than 1 kg and having short bowel syndrome.[75,76] One of the nutrients that may lead to the development of IFALD is the use of parenteral lipids. Currently, two safflower and/or soybean-based lipid preparations are available for use in the United States. Soybean oils have been shown to produce lipid peroxidation and inflammatory mediators that play a role in the development of IFALD.[77] In animal and pediatric studies, fish oils containing omega-3 fatty acids may decrease inflammation and stimulate biliary flow.[77] Two research studies have documented reduction in direct bilirubin levels in children who received fish compared to the standard soybean oil preparations.[78,79] The only adverse effect of fish oils that has been documented is an isolated case of Burr cell anemia that resolved after discontinuation of the fish oil.[80]

While early research may show beneficial effects of fish oils, no studies are available documenting the prevention of cholestatic liver disease. Additionally, two studies have documented histological evidence demonstrating progression of liver fibrosis in children with normal direct bilirubin levels receiving fish oils.[81,82] The growth and neurodevelopment of patients receiving fish oils have not been investigated.[77]

Research on the use of fish oils in the premature population is limited, and preparations have not been approved for use by the Food and Drug Administration except for research and compassionate use protocols.[77] Currently, two randomized controlled trials are in progress investigating the prevention of IFLAD in neonates.[77]

## Donor Breast Milk

Breast milk continues to be the gold standard when feeding term and preterm neonates. However, some mothers are unable to supply enough breast milk to meet the needs of their growing premature infant. The American Academy of Pediatrics has recognized that donor breast milk is recommended when maternal milk is not available.[83] Studies have shown various benefits to the use of donor milk including prevention against NEC,[84,85] less generalized feeding intolerance,[84] and long-term health benefits including lower blood pressure and lower cholesterol levels.[86,87] Presumptive immunological benefits are also recognized since donor milk contains some immune components that are not impacted by pasteurization.[88] When donor milk is used, basic quality control guidelines should be followed.

Although the benefits are documented, there are some limitations in the use of donor human milk. Most of the supply is from women who delivered term infants and therefore is not adequate to meet the nutritional needs of a premature infant. Use of donor milk has shown slower growth even if fortified.[89,90] While the pasteurization process does not alter some immune components (oligosaccharides, vitamins A, D, E, lactose LC-PUFAs, and epidermal growth factor), others become less active or are destroyed.[88]

## Human Milk Fortification

Studies have consistently shown that preterm infants who receive human milk continue to display poor growth due to inadequate nutrient intake, with decreased protein intake being one of the most significant factors. Poor growth is directly related to poor neurocognitive outcomes.[91] Fortification of human milk is necessary to improve nutrient acquisition. Most commercially available fortifiers contain various amounts of protein, carbohydrate, calcium, phosphorus, and other vitamins and minerals.

The amount of protein in human milk is variable and decreases as lactation continues thus making standardization of human milk fortification difficult. Mean human milk protein concentrations are estimated to be 1.5 g/dL, but it is known that milk protein concentrations are often much less than this, especially if term donor milk is being used. Commercially available fortifiers add 0.8–1.1 g/dL of protein to human milk for a total of approximately 2.5 g/dL, which is inadequate for postnatal growth. To address this issue, new strategies of individualized fortification are now being adopted.

Two methods of individualized fortification have been implemented: targeted and adjustable fortification.[91] Targeted fortification requires the analysis of the human milk being used to determine protein content. Supplementation is then added to ensure achieve an intake of 3.5 gm/kg/day. This method requires equipment and the use of trained personnel, which may inhibit its use. Adjustable fortification examines the infant's metabolic needs through the interpretation of blood urea nitrogen levels. Adjustments are made to the protein fortification based on these values. This method has been shown to be effective in providing appropriate protein intake, increasing growth at rates similar to intrauterine growth, and avoiding excessive protein intake.[91]

## POSTNATAL GROWTH

The plotting of growth, as previously discussed in the gestational age assessment, facilitates the assessment of trends in growth as the infant progresses. It has been shown that infants at the time of discharge or at 36 weeks of post-menstrual age plot at less than the 10th percentile when compared to infants born at that gestation.[8] In-hospital growth velocity has a direct effect of neurodevelopmental and growth outcomes at 18–22 months corrected age.[4] The rate of weight gain and head circumference were associated with lower rates of cerebral palsy, lower incidence of low Bayley Mental Developmental Index and Psychomotor Developmental Index scores, and less neurodevelopmental impairment.[4] Therefore, maximizing nutrition in high-risk infants to achieve appropriate postnatal weight gain should be a major focus of neonatal care.

## CONCLUSION

Despite the many questions that remain regarding optimal nutritional management of the neonate, it is nonetheless important to develop rational protocols for the management of nutritional issues that arise. This chapter has provided some guidelines and framework from which these guidelines arose. There are numerous different approaches to feeding a neonate. The ultimate goal should be to optimize nutrition and hence growth and ultimately development in this ever-increasing population of small premature infants.

## REFERENCES

1. Martin JA, Hamilton BE, Ventura SJ, Osterman MJ, Kirmeyer S, Mathews TJ, Wilson EC. *Natl Vital Stat Rep* 60:1;2011.
2. March of Dimes. *Peristats*. Retrieved March 10, 2012 from www.marchofdimes.com/peristats
3. Stephens BE, Tucker R, Vohr BR. *Pediatrics* 125:1152;2010.
4. Ehrenkranz RA, Dusick AM, Vohr BR. *Pediatrics* 117:1253;2006.
5. Ballard JL, Khoury JC et al. *J Pediatr* 119(3):417;1991.
6. Jeanty P, Romero R. *Seminars in Ultrasound* (5):121;1984.
7. Widdowson EM, Spray CM. *Arch Dis Child* 26:205;1951.
8. Ehrenkranz RA, Younes AN et al. *Pediatrics* 104(2 Pt 1):280; 1999.
9. Ziegler EE, O'Donnell AM et al. *Growth* 40(4):329;1976.
10. Ziegler EE. *Clin Perinatol* 29:225;2002.
11. Weinstein MR, Oh W. *J Pediatr* 99(6):958;1981.
12. Billeaud C, Piedbouef B et al. *J Pediatr* 120(3):461;1992.
13. Kashyap S, Hierd WC, in Neils CR Raiha (ed.) *Protein Metabolism during Infancy*. Nestle' Nutrition Workshop Series. V. 33, Raven Press, 1994.
14. Rivera AJ, Bell EF et al. *J Pediatr* 115(3):465;1989.
15. Mitton SG, Garlick PJ. *Pediatr Res* 32(4):447;1992.
16. Saini J, MacMahon P et al. *Arch Dis Child* 64(10 Spec No):1 362;1989.
17. van Lingen RA, van Goudoever JB et al. *Clin Sci* (Lond) 82(2):199;1992.
18. Van Goudoever JB, Sulkers EJ et al. *JPEN J Parenter Enteral Nutr* 18(5):404;1994.
19. Ibrahim HM, Jeroudi MA et al. *J Perinatol* 24(8):482;2004.
20. Thureen PJ, Melara D et al. *Pediatr Res* 53(1):24;2003.
21. te Braake FW, van den Akker CH et al. *J Pediatr* 147(4):457; 2005.
22. Zlotkin SH, Bryan MH et al. *Am J Clin Nutr* 34(5):914;1981.
23. Penn D, Schmidt-Summerfield E et al. *Early Hum Dev* 4:23;1979.
24. Shenai JP, Borum PR. *Pediatr Res* 18(7):679;1984.
25. Orzali A, Donzelli F et al. *Biol Neonate* 43:186;1983.
26. Schmidt-Sommerfeld E, Penn D et al. *J Pediatr* 102:931;1983.
27. Orzali A, Maetzke G et al. *J Pediatr* 104:436;1984.
28. Souba WW. *J Parent Enteral Nutr* 11:569;1987.
29. Askanazi J, Carpentier YA et al. *Ann Surg* 192:78;1980.
30. Roth E, Funovics J et al. *Clin Nutr* 1:25;1982.
31. Neu J, Shenoy V et al. *FASEB J* 10 829;1996.
32. Souba WW, Herskowitz K et al. *J Parent Enteral Nutr* 14: 458;1990.
33. Burrin DG, Shulam RJ et al. *J Parent Enteral Nutr* 15:262;1991.
34. Vanderhoof JA, Blackwood DJ et al. *J Am Coll Nutr* 11:223;1992.
35. Tubman TR, Thompson SW et al. *Cochrane Database Syst Rev* (1):CD001457;2005.
36. Wharton BA, Morley R et al. *Arch Dis Child Fetal Neonatal Ed* 89(6):F497;2004.
37. Haumont D, Deckelbaum RJ et al. *J Pediatr* 115(5 Pt 1):787; 1989.
38. Wu PY, Edwards N et al. *J Pediatr* 109(2):347;1986.
39. Bartley JH, Nagy S et al. *J Perinatol* 25:593;2004.
40. Schanler RJ, Lau C et al. *Pediatrics* 116(2):400;2005.
41. Widness JA, Seward VJ et al. *J Pediatr* 129(5):680;1996.
42. Shannon KM, Keith JF, 3rd et al. *Pediatrics* 95(1):1;1995.
43. Caple J, Armentrout D et al. *Pediatrics* 114(6):1597;2004.
44. Berseth CL, Bisquera JA et al. *Pediatrics* 111(3):529;2003.
45. Grant JP, Cox CE et al. *Surg Gynecol Obstet* 145(4):573;1977.
46. Balistreri WF, Bove KE. *Prog Liver Dis* 9:567;1990.
47. Bhatia J, Moslen T et al. *Pediatr Res* 33(5):487;1993.
48. Rollins M, Scaife ER, Jackson D. *Nutr Clin Pract* 25:199;2010.
49. Greer FR *Acta Paediatr Suppl* 405:20–24;1994.
50. Moro G, Minoli I et al. *Acta Paediatr Scand* 73(1):49;1984.
51. Romero G, Figueras J et al. *J Pediatr Gastroenterol Nutr* 38:407;2004.
52. Koenig WJ, Amarnath AP et al. *Pediatrics* 95(2):203;1995.
53. Berseth CL, *Pediatrics* 117(5):777;1990.
54. Berseth CL, Ittman PI J. *Pediatr Gastroenterol Nutr* 14(2):182;1992.
55. McGuire W, Anthony MY. *Arch Dis Child Fetal Neonatal Ed* 88(1):F1;2002.
56. Owens L, Burrin DG et al. *J Nutr* 132(9):2717;2002.
57. Baker JH, Berseth CL. *Pediatr Res* 42(5):618;1997.
58. Clandinin MT, Chappell JE et al. *Early Hum Dev* 4(2):131;1980.
59. Martinez M, Ballabriga A. *Lipids* 22(3):133;1987.
60. Sanders TA, Naismith DJ. *Proc Nutr Soc* 38(2):94A;1979.
61. Putnam JC, Carlson SE et al. *Am J Clin Nutr* 36(1):106;1982.
62. Koletzko B, Thiel I et al. *Eur J Clin Nutr* 46:S45–S55;1992.
63. Jensen RG *The Lipids of Human Milk*. Academic Press, San Diego, CA, 1995.
64. Carlson SE, Rhodes PG et al. *Am J Clin Nutr* 44(6):708;1986.
65. Koletzko B, Schmidt E et al. *Eur J Pediatr* 148(7):669;1989.
66. Clandinin MT, Van Aerde JE et al. *J Pediatr* 146(4):461;2005.
67. Lapillone A, Clarke SD et al. *J Pediatr* 143(4 Suppl):S9;2003.
68. Jensen CL, Prager TC et al. *J Pediatr* 131(2):200;1997.
69. Makrides M., Neumann MA et al. *Am J Clin Nutr* 71(1):120;2000.
70. Udell T, Gibson RA et al. *Lipids* 40(1):1;2005.
71. Simmer K, Patole S. *Cochrane Database Syst Rev* (1):CD000 375;2004.
72. Groh-Wargo S, Jacobs J et al. *Pediatrics Res* 57(5 Pt 1):712;2005.
73. O'Connor DL, Hall R et al. *Pediatrics* 108(2):359;2001.

74. Fleith M, Clandinin MT. *Crit Rev Food Sci Nutr* 45(3):205;2005.
75. Teitelbaum DH. *Curr Opin Pediatr* 9:270;1997.
76. Kelley DA. *Gastroenterology* 130:S70;2006.
77. Venick RS, Calkins K. *Curr Opin Org Trans* 16:306;2011.
78. Puder M, Valim C, Meisel JA et al. *Ann Surg* 250:395;2009.
79. Diamond IR, Sterescu A, Pencharz PB et al. *J Periatr Gastroenterol Nutr* 48:209;2009.
80. Mallah HS, Brown MR, Rossi TM et al. *J Pediatr* 156:324;2010.
81. Soden JS, Lovell MA, Brown K et al. *J Pediatr* 156:327;2010.
82. Fitzgibbons SC, Jones BA, Hull MA et al. *J Pediatr Surg* 45:95;2010.
83. American Academy of Pediatrics. Policy statement. Section of breastfeeding. *Pediatrics* 115:496;2005.
84. Boyd CA, Quigley MA, Brocklehurst P *Arch Dis Child Fetal Neonatal Ed* 92:F169;2007.
85. Quigley MA, Henderson G, Anthony MY et al. *Cochrane Database Syst Rev* 4:CD002971;2007.
86. Singhal A, Cole TJ, Lacas A. *Lancet* 357:413;2001.
87. Singhal A, Lovelady CA, Dillard RG et al. *J Perinatol* 27:428;2007.
88. Arslanoglu S, Moro GE, Ziegler E. *J Perinat Med* 38:233;2010.
89. Wight NE. *J Perinatol* 21(4):249;2001.
90. McGuire W, Anthony MY. *Arch Dis Child Fetal Neonatol Ed* 88(1):F11;2003.
91. Arslanoglu S, Ziegler E, Moro G. *J Perinat Med* 38:347;2010.

# 20 Nutrition for Healthy Children and Adolescents Ages 2–18 Years

*Suzanne Domel Baxter*

## CONTENTS

## PHYSICAL GROWTH AND DEVELOPMENT

A child's first year of life is marked by rapid growth, with birth weight tripling and birth length increasing by 50%. After the rapid growth of the first year, physical growth slows down considerably during the preschool and school years, until the pubertal growth spurt of adolescence. Birth weight does not quadruple until 2 years of age, and birth length does not double until 4 years of age. A 1-year-old child has several teeth, and his or her digestive and metabolic systems are functioning at or near adult capacity. By 1 year of age, most children are walking or beginning to walk; with improved coordination over the next few years, activity increases dramatically. Although increased activity in turn increases energy needs, a child's rate of growth decreases. Growth patterns vary in individual children, but each year children from 2 years to puberty gain an average of 4.5–6.5 lb (2–3 kg) in weight and 2.5–3.5 in. (6–8 cm) in height. As the growth rate declines during the preschool years, a child's appetite decreases and food intake may become unpredictable and erratic. Parents and other caregivers need to know that these changes are normal so that they can avoid struggles with children over food and eating behaviors.

After the first year of life, more significant development occurs in fine and gross motor, cognitive, and social–emotional areas than during the first year of life. During the second year of life, children learn to feed themselves independently. By 15 months of age, children can manage a cup, but with some spilling. At 18–24 months of age, children learn to tilt cups by manipulating their fingers. Children are able to transfer food from bowls to their mouths with less spilling by 16–17 months of age when well-defined wrist rotation develops. Two-year-old children often prefer foods that can be picked up with their fingers without having to use utensils to chase foods across their plates.

Puberty and the simultaneous growth spurt are the primary influences on nutritional requirements during the second decade of life. During puberty, height and weight increase, many organ systems enlarge, and body composition is altered due to increased lean body mass and changes in the quantity and distribution of fat. The timing of the growth spurt is influenced by genetic as well as environmental factors. Children who weigh more than average for their height tend to mature early, and vice versa. Although stature tends to increase most rapidly during the spring and summer, weight either tends to increase at a fairly steady rate over the entire year or undergoes a more rapid increase during the autumn. The most rapid linear growth spurt for an average American boy occurs between 12 and 15 years of age. For the average American girl, the growth spurt occurs about 2 years earlier, between 10 and 13 years of age. The growth spurt during adolescence contributes about 15% to final adult height and approximately 50% to adult weight. During adolescence, boys tend to gain more weight than girls do and at a faster rate. Furthermore, the skeletal growth of boys continues for a longer time than that of adolescent girls. Adolescent boys deposit more muscle mass,

and adolescent girls deposit relatively more total body fat. Menarche, which is closely linked to the growth process, has a lasting impact on nutritional requirements of adolescent girls.

Adolescence is a period of various cognitive challenges. For example, when an adolescent realizes that his or her body is in the process of maturing, he or she may begin to assess changes in his or her own body size and shape, compare them with those of others, and form opinions about any differences. Adolescent girls and boys may be very self-conscious, especially during early and mid-adolescence. According to Piaget's developmental levels, it is usually during adolescence that abstract thinking supersedes concrete thinking. Thus, an adolescent may consider his or her body not just as it is, but also as it *might* be. In addition, an adolescent can contemplate new or different ways of combining or eating food. Furthermore, an adolescent can more easily conceptualize nutrients such as calories and fat and skillfully manipulate his or her dietary intake.

## ENERGY AND NUTRIENT NEEDS

### DIETARY REFERENCE INTAKES

The Dietary Reference Intakes (DRIs) were published in several reports between 1997 and 2005,[1–12] and in 2006, an essential guide was published.[13] Discussions in 2004 through 2008 to evaluate the DRI development process resulted in the process being placed more clearly in the context of the risk assessment approach.[14,15] The 2011 report on calcium and vitamin D is the first DRI report to be completed subsequent to the 2004–2008 evaluation.[16] The DRI publications are available online at *www.nap.edu*.

The DRI component values include *Estimated Average Requirement* (EAR), *Recommended Dietary Allowance* (RDA), *Adequate Intake* (AI), *Tolerable Upper Intake Level* (UL), and *Acceptable Macronutrient Distribution Range* (AMDR). The EAR is the level of intake for which the risk of inadequacy would be 50%. The RDA is 2 standard deviations above the EAR; it covers 97% of the population. The AI is used when an EAR/RDA cannot be developed; it is based on observed or experimental intakes. The UL is the highest level of daily intake that poses no risk of an adverse effect to almost any individual in the general population; as intake increases above the UL, the potential risk of adverse effects may increase. The AMDR is an intake range for an energy source associated with decreased risk of chronic disease.[15]

Table 20.1 provides reference heights, weights, and body mass indexes (BMIs) for children and adolescents in the United States. Table 20.2 provides RDAs and AIs for children and adolescents. Table 20.3 provides AMDRs for children and adolescents. Table 20.4 provides additional macronutrient recommendations for children and adolescents. Table 20.5 provides ULs for children and adolescents. Table 20.6 provides EARs for groups of children and adolescents.

**TABLE 20.1**

**DRIs: New Reference Heights, Weights, and BMIs for Children and Adolescents in the United States**

| | Children | | Boys | | Girls | |
|---|---|---|---|---|---|---|
| | 1–3 Years | 4–8 Years | 9–13 Years | 14–18 Years | 9–13 Years | 14–18 Years |
| Median reference height,[a] cm (in.) | 86 (34) | 115 (45) | 144 (57) | 174 (68) | 144 (57) | 163 (64) |
| Reference weight,[b] kg (lb) | 12 (27) | 20 (44) | 36 (79) | 61 (134) | 37 (81) | 54 (119) |
| Median BMI[a] (kg/m²) | — | 15.3 | 17.2 | 20.5 | 17.4 | 20.4 |

*Source:* Adapted from: National Research Council, *Dietary Reference Intakes for Energy, Carbohydrate, Fiber, Fat, Fatty Acids, Cholesterol, Protein, and Amino Acids,* The National Academies Press, Washington, DC, 2002/2005. This report may be accessed via www.nap.edu.

[a] Taken from height-for-age data and median BMI data for boys and girls from the CDC/NCHS growth charts from Kuczmarski et al., *Adv Data,* 314, 1–28, 2000

[b] Calculated CDC/NCHS growth charts from Kuczmarski et al., *Adv Data,* 314, 1–28, 2000; median BMI and median height for ages 4–19 years

## ENERGY

Energy is needed to maintain the various functions of the body including respiration, circulation, physical work, and protein synthesis. Energy is supplied in the diet by carbohydrates, proteins, fats, and alcohol. An individual's energy balance depends on his or her intake of dietary energy and expenditure of energy. Within the DRIs, Estimated Energy Requirements (EERs) were established at various levels of energy expenditure, and recommendations were provided for levels of physical activity associated with a normal BMI range.[9] The EER is the average dietary energy intake predicted to maintain energy balance in a healthy individual of a defined age, sex, weight, height, and level of physical activity, consistent with good health.[9] Table 20.7 provides estimated calorie needs per day by age, gender, and physical activity level for children and adolescents.

Components of energy expenditure include basal and resting metabolism, thermic effect of food, thermoregulation, physical activity, physical activity level, and total energy requirement.[9] Factors that affect energy expenditure and requirements include body composition and body size (i.e., effects on basal and resting metabolic rate, effects on total energy expenditure, and obesity), physical activity (i.e., effect of exercise on postexercise energy expenditure and spontaneous nonexercise activity), sex, growth, older age, genetics, ethnicity, environment (i.e., climate, altitude), and adaptation and accommodation.[9]

Energy needs for children and adolescents vary depending on basal metabolism, rate of growth, physical activity, body size, gender, and onset of puberty. Many nutrient requirements are dependent on energy needs and intake. An accepted and practical method for assessing the adequacy of a child or adolescent's energy intake is to monitor growth by tracking height and weight on growth charts developed by the National Center for Health Statistics (NCHS); these Centers for Disease Control and Prevention (CDC) growth charts may be accessed via http://www.cdc.gov/growthchart.

## PROTEIN

Protein is essential for growth, development, and maintenance of the body; it also provides energy. Protein yields 4 kcal/g. Food sources of protein include meat, fish, poultry, milk, cheese, yogurt, dried beans, peanut butter, nuts, and grain products. Protein from animal sources is called "complete protein" because it contains all nine indispensable amino acids. (The nine indispensable amino acids must be provided in the diet.) Protein from plant sources is called "incomplete protein" because it tends to be deficient in one or more of the indispensable amino acids. A vegetable protein may be paired with another vegetable protein or with a small amount of animal protein to provide adequate amounts of all the indispensable amino acids. For example, black-eyed peas can be paired with rice, peanut butter with wheat bread, pasta with cheese, or cereal with milk.

Proteins in the body are continuously being degraded and resynthesized. Because the process is not entirely efficient and some amino acids are lost, a continuous supply of amino acids is needed to replace these losses, even after growth has stopped. The primary factor that influences protein needs is energy intake because when energy intake is insufficient, protein is used for energy. Thus, all protein recommendations are based on the assumption that energy needs are adequately met. In addition, protein recommendations are based on intakes of complete protein; appropriate corrections must be made for diets that customarily provide incomplete proteins.

Protein content of foods varies. For example, 3 oz of poultry or lean meat provides about 25 g of protein. Three ounces of fish or 1 cup of soybeans provides about 20 g of protein. One cup of yogurt provides about 8 g of protein. One cup of milk provides about 8 g of protein. One egg provides

**TABLE 20.2**
**DRIs: RDAs and AIs for Children and Adolescents[a]**

|  | Children | | Boys | | Girls | |
|---|---|---|---|---|---|---|
|  | 1–3 Years | 4–8 Years | 9–13 Years | 14–18 Years | 9–13 Years | 14–18 Years |
| *Vitamins* | | | | | | |
| **Vitamin A (µg/day)[b]** | 300 | 400 | 600 | 900 | 600 | 700 |
| **Vitamin C (mg/day)** | 15 | 25 | 45 | 75 | 45 | 65 |
| **Vitamin D (µg/day)[c,d]** | 15 | 15 | 15 | 15 | 15 | 15 |
| **Vitamin E (mg/day)[e]** | 6 | 7 | 11 | 15 | 11 | 15 |
| **Vitamin K (µg/day)** | 30* | 55* | 60* | 75* | 60* | 75* |
| **Thiamin (mg/day)** | 0.5 | 0.6 | 0.9 | 1.2 | 0.9 | 1.0 |
| **Riboflavin (mg/day)** | 0.5 | 0.6 | 0.9 | 1.3 | 0.9 | 1.0 |
| **Niacin (mg/day)[f]** | 6 | 8 | 12 | 16 | 12 | 14 |
| **Vitamin B$_6$ (mg/day)** | 0.5 | 0.6 | 1.0 | 1.3 | 1.0 | 1.2 |
| **Folate (µg/day)[g]** | 150 | 200 | 300 | 400 | 300 | 400[h] |
| **Vitamin B$_{12}$ (µg/day)** | 0.9 | 1.2 | 1.8 | 2.4 | 1.8 | 2.4 |
| **Pantothenic acid (mg/day)** | 2* | 3* | 4* | 5* | 4* | 5* |
| **Biotin (µg/day)** | 8* | 12* | 20* | 25* | 20* | 25* |
| **Choline (mg/day)[i]** | 200* | 250* | 375* | 550* | 375* | 400* |
| *Elements* | | | | | | |
| **Calcium (mg/day)** | 700 | 1000 | 1300 | 1300 | 1300 | 1300 |
| **Chromium (µg/day)** | 11* | 15* | 25* | 35* | 21* | 24* |
| **Copper (µg/day)** | 340 | 440 | 700 | 890 | 700 | 890 |
| **Fluoride (mg/day)** | 0.7* | 1* | 2* | 3* | 2* | 3* |
| **Iodine (µg/day)** | 90 | 90 | 120 | 150 | 120 | 150 |
| **Iron (mg/day)** | 7 | 10 | 8 | 11 | 8 | 15 |
| **Magnesium (mg/day)** | 80 | 130 | 240 | 410 | 240 | 360 |
| **Manganese (mg/day)** | 1.2* | 1.5* | 1.9* | 2.2* | 1.6* | 1.6* |
| **Molybdenum (µg/day)** | 17 | 22 | 34 | 43 | 34 | 43 |
| **Phosphorus (mg/day)** | 460 | 500 | 1250 | 1250 | 1250 | 1250 |
| **Selenium (µg/day)** | 20 | 30 | 40 | 55 | 40 | 55 |
| **Zinc (mg/day)** | 3 | 5 | 8 | 11 | 8 | 9 |
| **Potassium (g/day)** | 3.0* | 3.8* | 4.5* | 4.7* | 4.5* | 4.7* |
| **Sodium (g/day)** | 1.0* | 1.2* | 1.5* | 1.5* | 1.5* | 1.5* |
| **Chloride (g/day)** | 1.5* | 1.9* | 2.3* | 2.3* | 2.3* | 2.3* |
| *Total water and macronutrients* | | | | | | |
| **Total water (L/day)[j]** | 1.3* | 1.7* | 2.4* | 3.3* | 2.1* | 2.3* |
| **Carbohydrate (g/day)** | 130 | 130 | 130 | 130 | 130 | 130 |
| **Total fiber (g/day)** | 19* | 25* | 31* | 38* | 26* | 26* |

| | | | | | | |
|---|---|---|---|---|---|---|
| Fat (g/day) | $ND^k$ | ND | ND | ND | ND | ND |
| Linoleic acid (g/day) | 7* | 10* | 12* | 16* | 10* | 11* |
| α-Linolenic acid (g/day) | 0.7* | 0.9* | 1.2* | 1.6* | 1.0* | 1.1* |
| **Protein (g/day)** | **$13^l$** | **$19^m$** | **$34^n$** | **$52^o$** | **$34^n$** | **$46^p$** |
| **Protein (g/kg/day)** | **1.05** | **0.95** | **0.95** | **0.85** | **0.95** | **0.85** |

*Source:* Adapted from National Research Council, The National Academies Press, Washington, DC: *Dietary Reference Intakes for Calcium, Phosphorus, Magnesium, Vitamin D, and Fluoride*, 1997; *Dietary Reference Intakes for Thiamin, Riboflavin, Niacin, Vitamin $B_6$, Folate, Vitamin $B_{12}$, Pantothenic Acid, Biotin, and Choline*, 1998; *Dietary Reference Intakes for Vitamin C, Vitamin E, Selenium, and Carotenoids*, 2000; *Dietary Reference Intakes for Vitamin A, Vitamin K, Arsenic, Boron, Chromium, Copper, Iodine, Iron, Manganese, Molybdenum, Nickel, Silicon, Vanadium, and Zinc*, 2001; *Dietary Reference Intakes for Water, Potassium, Sodium, Chloride, and Sulfate*, 2005; *Dietary Reference Intakes for Energy, Carbohydrate, Fiber, Fat, Fatty Acids, Cholesterol, Protein, and Amino Acids*, 2002/2005; and *Dietary Reference Intakes for Calcium and Vitamin D*, 2011. These reports may be accessed via www.nap.edu.

a   RDAs are presented in **bold type** and AIs in ordinary type followed by an asterisk (*). RDAs and AIs may both be used as goals for individual intake. The RDAs cover 97% of the population. The AI for life stage and sex groups is believed to cover needs of all individuals in the group, but lack of data or uncertainty in the data prevent being able to specify with confidence the percentage of persons covered by this intake.

b   As retinol activity equivalents (RAEs). 1 RAE = 1 μg retinol, 12 μg β-carotene, 24 μg α-carotene, or 24 μg β-cryptoxanthin. The RAE for dietary provitamin A carotenoids is twofold greater than retinol equivalents (RE), whereas the RAE for preformed vitamin A is the same as RE.

c   As cholecalciferol. 1 μg cholecalciferol = 40 IU vitamin D.

d   Under the assumption of minimal sunlight.

e   As α-Tocopherol. α-Tocopherol includes *RRR*-α-tocopherol, the only form of α-tocopherol that occurs naturally in foods, and the 2*R*-stereoisomeric forms of α-tocopherol (*RRR*-, *RSR*-, *RRS*-, and *RSS*-α-tocopherol) that occur in fortified foods and supplements. It does not include the 2*S*-stereoisomeric forms of α-tocopherol (*SRR*-, *SSR*-, *SRS*-, and *SSS*-α-tocopherol), also found in fortified foods and supplements.

f   As niacin equivalents (NE). 1 mg niacin = 60 mg tryptophan.

g   As dietary folate equivalents (DFE). 1 DFE = 1 μg food folate = 0.6 μg folic acid from fortified food or as a supplement consumed with food = 0.5 μg of a supplement taken on an empty stomach.

h   In view of evidence linking folate intake with neural tube defects in the fetus, it is recommended that all women capable of becoming pregnant consume 400 μg from supplements or fortified foods in addition to intake of food folate from a varied diet. It is assumed that females will continue consuming 400 μg from supplements or fortified food until their pregnancy is confirmed and they enter prenatal care.

i   Although AIs have been set for choline, there are few data to assess whether a dietary supply of choline is needed at all stages of the life cycle, and it may be that the choline requirement can be met by endogenous synthesis at some of these stages.

j   Total water includes all water contained in drinking water, food, and beverages.

k   ND, not determined.

l   13 g/day of protein or 1.05 g protein/kg of body weight.

m   19 g/day of protein or 0.95 g protein/kg of body weight.

n   34 g/day of protein or 0.95 g protein/kg of body weight.

o   52 g/day of protein or 0.85 g protein/kg of body weight.

p   46 g/day of protein or 0.85 g protein/kg of body weight.

**TABLE 20.3**
**DRIs: AMDRs for Children and Adolescents**

| | Range (Percent of Energy) | |
|---|---|---|
| | 1–3 Years | 4–18 Years |
| *Macronutrient* | | |
| Fat | 30–40 | 25–35 |
| *n*–6 Polyunsaturated fatty acids[a] (linoleic acid) | 5–10 | 5–10 |
| *n*–3 Polyunsaturated fatty acids[a] (α-linolenic acid) | 0.6–1.2 | 0.6–1.2 |
| Carbohydrate | 45–65 | 45–65 |
| Protein | 5–20 | 10–30 |

*Source:* Adapted from: National Research Council, *Dietary Reference Intakes for Energy, Carbohydrate, Fiber, Fat, Fatty Acids, Cholesterol, Protein, and Amino Acids*, The National Academies Press, Washington, DC, 2002/2005. This report may be accessed via www.nap.edu.

[a] Approximately 10% of the total can come from longer-chain *n*–3 or *n*–6 fatty acids.

**TABLE 20.4**
**DRIs: Additional Macronutrient Recommendations for Children and Adolescents**

| Macronutrient | Recommendation |
|---|---|
| Added sugars[a] | Limit to no more than 25% of total energy |
| Dietary cholesterol | As low as possible while consuming a nutritionally adequate diet |
| Saturated fatty acids | As low as possible while consuming a nutritionally adequate diet |
| *Trans* fatty acids | As low as possible while consuming a nutritionally adequate diet |

*Source:* Adapted from: National Research Council, *Dietary Reference Intakes for Energy, Carbohydrate, Fiber, Fat, Fatty Acids, Cholesterol, Protein, and Amino Acids*, The National Academies Press, Washington, DC, 2002/2005. This report may be accessed via www.nap.edu.

[a] Not a recommended intake. A daily intake of added sugars that individuals should achieve for a healthful diet was not set.

about 6 g of protein. One ounce of cheese provides about 6 g of protein. One cup of legumes provides about 15 g of protein. Cereals, grains, nuts, and vegetables provide about 2 g of protein per serving.[9]

The RDAs for protein for children and adolescents are provided in Table 20.2 in g/day and g/kg/day. The EARs for protein for children and adolescents are provided in Table 20.6 in g/kg/day. The EARs and RDAs for indispensable amino acids for children and adolescents are provided in Table 20.8. As Table 20.2 indicates, protein requirements slowly decline relative to weight during the preschool to mid-elementary school years and during the upper elementary to high-school years. A 14-year-old adolescent boy who weighs 61 kg (134 lb) needs 52 g of protein each day; assuming that

energy needs are met, this protein need can be met by eating a hamburger (3 oz meat patty on a bun for a total of 29 g of protein) and two slices of pizza topped with meat and cheese (for a total of 23 g of protein).

Children ages 1–3 years should get 5%–20% of their daily energy from protein; children and adolescents ages 4–18 years should get 10%–30% of their daily energy from protein[9] (see Table 20.3).

## CARBOHYDRATES

Carbohydrates (starches and sugars) provide energy to cells in the body, especially the brain, which is a carbohydrate-dependent organ. Carbohydrate yields 4 kcal/g. The RDA for carbohydrate for children, adolescents, and adults is set at 130 g/day based on the average amount of glucose utilized by the brain[9] (see Table 20.2). This level of intake is typically exceeded to meet energy needs while consuming acceptable intake levels of protein and fat.[9]

Children and adolescents should get 45%–65% of their daily energy from carbohydrates[9] (see Table 20.3). Complex carbohydrates (starchy foods such as pasta, breads, cereals, rice, and legumes) should provide the majority of energy from carbohydrates, and simple carbohydrates (naturally occurring sugars in fruits and vegetables) should provide the rest. The 2010 Dietary Guidelines for Americans[17] recommend that at least half of all grains consumed should consist of whole-grain sources such as whole-wheat breads, whole-grain cereals, and brown rice. Added sugars should be limited to no more than 25% of total energy[9] (see Table 20.4). Added sugars include white sugar, brown sugar, high-fructose corn syrup, corn syrup, corn syrup solids, raw sugar, malt sugar, maple syrup, pancake syrup, fructose sweetener, liquid fructose, honey, molasses, anhydrous dextrose, and crystal dextrose.[17] The major sources of added sugars in the diets of Americans are soda, energy drinks, and sports drinks (36% of added sugar intake), grain-based desserts (13%), sugar-sweetened fruit drinks (10%), dairy-based desserts (6%), and candy (6%).[17] An active 6-year-old boy who needs about 1750 kcal/day would need about 788–1138 kcal (or 197–284 g) from carbohydrates daily. An active 11-year-old girl who needs about 2075 kcal/day would need about 934–1349 kcal (or 233–337 g) from carbohydrates daily.

## FAT AND CHOLESTEROL

Fat is a major source of energy for the body and helps in the absorption of fat-soluble vitamins and carotenoids. Fat yields 9 kcal/g. Neither an AI nor RDA was set for total fat because there are insufficient data to determine a defined level of fat intake at which risk of inadequacy or prevention of chronic disease occurs.[9] Likewise, an UL was not set for total fat because there is no defined intake level of fat at which an adverse effect occurs.[9] However, the AMDR for total fat was set at 30%–40% of energy for children ages 1–3 years and 25%–35% of energy for children and adolescents ages 4–18 years[9] (see Table 20.3). In the 2010 Dietary Guidelines

**TABLE 20.5**
**DRIs: ULs for Children and Adolescents[a]**

| | 1–3 Years | 4–8 Years | 9–13 Years | 14–18 Years |
|---|---|---|---|---|
| *Vitamins* | | | | |
| Vitamin A (µg/day)[b] | 600 | 900 | 1700 | 2800 |
| Vitamin C (mg/day) | 400 | 650 | 1200 | 1800 |
| Vitamin D (µg/day) | 63 | 75 | 100 | 100 |
| Vitamin E (mg/day)[c,d] | 200 | 300 | 600 | 800 |
| Vitamin K | ND[e] | ND | ND | ND |
| Thiamin | ND | ND | ND | ND |
| Riboflavin | ND | ND | ND | ND |
| Niacin (mg/day)[d] | 10 | 15 | 20 | 30 |
| Vitamin B$_6$ (mg/day)[d] | 30 | 40 | 60 | 80 |
| Folate (µg/day)[d] | 300 | 400 | 600 | 800 |
| Vitamin B$_{12}$ | ND | ND | ND | ND |
| Pantothenic acid | ND | ND | ND | ND |
| Biotin | ND | ND | ND | ND |
| Choline (g/day) | 1.0 | 1.0 | 2.0 | 3.0 |
| Carotenoids[f] | ND | ND | ND | ND |
| *Elements* | | | | |
| Arsenic[g] | ND | ND | ND | ND |
| Boron (mg/day) | 3 | 6 | 11 | 17 |
| Calcium (mg/day) | 2500 | 2500 | 3000 | 3000 |
| Chromium | ND | ND | ND | ND |
| Copper (µg/day) | 1000 | 3000 | 5000 | 8000 |
| Fluoride (mg/day) | 1.3 | 2.2 | 10 | 10 |
| Iodine (µg/day) | 200 | 300 | 600 | 900 |
| Iron (mg/day) | 40 | 40 | 40 | 45 |
| Magnesium (mg/day)[h] | 65 | 110 | 350 | 350 |
| Manganese (mg/day) | 2 | 3 | 6 | 9 |
| Molybdenum (µg/day) | 300 | 600 | 1100 | 1700 |
| Nickel (mg/day) | 0.2 | 0.3 | 0.6 | 1.0 |
| Phosphorus (g/day) | 3 | 3 | 4 | 4 |
| Potassium | ND | ND | ND | ND |
| Selenium (µg/day) | 90 | 150 | 280 | 400 |
| Silicon[i] | ND | ND | ND | ND |
| Sulfate | ND | ND | ND | ND |
| Vanadium (mg/day)[j] | ND | ND | ND | ND |

(continued)

**TABLE 20.5 (continued)**
**DRIs: ULs for Children and Adolescents[a]**

| | 1–3 Years | 4–8 Years | 9–13 Years | 14–18 Years |
|---|---|---|---|---|
| Zinc (mg/day) | 7 | 12 | 23 | 34 |
| Sodium (g/day) | 1.5 | 1.9 | 2.2 | 2.3 |
| Chloride (g/day) | 2.3 | 2.9 | 3.4 | 3.6 |

*Source:* Adapted from National Research Council, The National Academies Press, Washington, DC: *Dietary Reference Intakes for Calcium, Phosphorus, Magnesium, Vitamin D, and Fluoride,* 1997; *Dietary Reference Intakes for Thiamin, Riboflavin, Niacin, Vitamin B6, Folate, Vitamin B12, Pantothenic Acid, Biotin, and Choline,* 1998; *Dietary Reference Intakes for Vitamin C, Vitamin E, Selenium, and Carotenoids,* 2000; *Dietary Reference Intakes for Vitamin A, Vitamin K, Arsenic, Boron, Chromium, Copper, Iodine, Iron, Manganese, Molybedenum, Nickel, Silicon, Vanadium, and Zinc,* 2001; *Dietary Reference Intakes for Water, Potassium, Sodium, Chloride, and Sulfate,* 2005; and *Dietary Reference Intakes for Calcium and Vitamin D,* 2011. These reports may be accessed via www.nap.edu.

[a] UL: The maximum level of daily nutrient intake that is likely to pose no risk of adverse health effects to almost all individuals in the general population. Unless otherwise specified, the UL represents total intake from food, water, and supplements.

[b] As preformed vitamin A only.

[c] As α-tocopherol; applies to any form of supplemental α-tocopherol.

[d] The ULs for vitamin E, niacin, and folate apply to synthetic forms obtained from supplements, fortified foods, or a combination of the two.

[e] ND: Not determinable due to lack of data of adverse effects in these age groups and concern with regard to lack of ability to handle excess amounts. In the absence of ULs, extra caution may be warranted in consuming levels above recommended intakes. Sources of intake should be from food only to prevent high levels of intake.

[f] β-Carotene supplements are advised only to serve as a provitamin A source for individuals at risk of vitamin A deficiency.

[g] Although the UL was not determined for arsenic, there is no justification for adding it to food or supplements.

[h] The ULs for magnesium represent intake from a pharmacological agent only and do not include intake from food and water.

[i] Although silicon has not been shown to cause adverse effects in humans, there is no justification for adding it to supplements.

[j] Although vanadium in food has not been shown to cause adverse effects in humans, there is no justification for adding it to food, and vanadium supplements should be used with caution. The UL for adults is 1.8 mg/day of elemental vanadium; the UL for adults is based on adverse effects in laboratory animals, but these data could not be used to set an UL for children and adolescents.

## TABLE 20.6
## DRIs: EARs for Groups of Children and Adolescents[a]

|  | Children | | Boys | | Girls | |
| --- | --- | --- | --- | --- | --- | --- |
|  | 1–3 Years | 4–8 Years | 9–13 Years | 14–18 Years | 9–13 Years | 14–18 Years |
| Calcium (mg/day) | 500 | 800 | 1100 | 1100 | 1100 | 1100 |
| Carbohydrate (g/day) | 100 | 100 | 100 | 100 | 100 | 100 |
| Protein (g/kg/day) | 0.87 | 0.76 | 0.76 | 0.73 | 0.76 | 0.71 |
| Vitamin A ($\mu$g/day)[b] | 210 | 275 | 445 | 630 | 420 | 485 |
| Vitamin C (mg/day) | 13 | 22 | 39 | 63 | 39 | 56 |
| Vitamin D ($\mu$g/day) | 10 | 10 | 10 | 10 | 10 | 10 |
| Vitamin E (mg/day)[c] | 5 | 6 | 9 | 12 | 9 | 12 |
| Thiamin (mg/day) | 0.4 | 0.5 | 0.7 | 1.0 | 0.7 | 0.9 |
| Riboflavin (mg/day) | 0.4 | 0.5 | 0.8 | 1.1 | 0.8 | 0.9 |
| Niacin (mg/day)[d] | 5 | 6 | 9 | 12 | 9 | 11 |
| Vitamin $B_6$ (mg/day) | 0.4 | 0.5 | 0.8 | 1.1 | 0.8 | 1.0 |
| Folate ($\mu$g/day)[e] | 120 | 160 | 250 | 330 | 250 | 330 |
| Vitamin $B_{12}$ ($\mu$g/day) | 0.7 | 1.0 | 1.5 | 2.0 | 1.5 | 2.0 |
| Copper ($\mu$g/day) | 260 | 340 | 540 | 685 | 540 | 685 |
| Iodine ($\mu$g/day) | 65 | 65 | 73 | 95 | 73 | 95 |
| Iron (mg/day) | 3.0 | 4.1 | 5.9 | 7.7 | 5.7 | 7.9 |
| Magnesium (mg/day) | 65 | 110 | 200 | 340 | 200 | 300 |
| Molybdenum ($\mu$g/day) | 13 | 17 | 26 | 33 | 26 | 33 |
| Phosphorus (mg/day) | 380 | 405 | 1055 | 1055 | 1055 | 1055 |
| Selenium ($\mu$g/day) | 17 | 23 | 35 | 45 | 35 | 45 |
| Zinc (mg/day) | 2.5 | 4.0 | 7.0 | 8.5 | 7.0 | 7.3 |

*Source:* Adapted from National Research Council, The National Academies Press, Washington, DC: *Dietary Reference Intakes for Calcium, Phosphorus, Magnesium, Vitamin D, and Fluoride*, 1997; *Dietary Reference Intakes for Thiamin, Riboflavin, Niacin, Vitamin B₆, Folate, Vitamin B₁₂, Pantothenic Acid, Biotin, and Choline*, 1998; *Dietary Reference Intakes for Vitamin C, Vitamin E, Selenium, and Carotenoids*, 2000; *Dietary Reference Intakes for Vitamin A, Vitamin K, Arsenic, Boron, Chromium, Copper, Iodine, Iron, Manganese, Molybedenum, Nickel, Silicon, Vanadium, and Zinc*, 2001; *Dietary Reference Intakes for Energy, Carbohydrate, Fiber, Fat, Fatty Acids, Cholesterol, Protein, and Amino Acids*, 2002/2005; and *Dietary Reference Intakes for Calcium and Vitamin D*, 2011. These reports may be accessed via www.nap.edu.

[a] EARs serve two purposes: for assessing adequacy of population intakes and as the basis for calculating RDAs for individuals. EARs have not been established for vitamin K, pantothenic acid, biotin, choline, chromium, fluoride, manganese, or other nutrients not yet evaluated via the DRI process.

[b] As RAEs. 1 RAE = 1 $\mu$g retinol, 12 $\mu$g β-carotene, 24 $\mu$g α-carotene, or 24 $\mu$g β-cryptoxanthin. The RAE for dietary provitamin A carotenoids is twofold greater than RE, whereas the RAE for preformed vitamin A is the same as RE.

[c] As α-tocopherol. α-Tocopherol includes *RRR*-α-tocopherol, the only form of α-tocopherol that occurs naturally in foods, and the *2R*-stereoisomeric forms of α-tocopherol (*RRR*-, *RSR*-, *RRS*-, and *RSS*-α-tocopherol) that occur in fortified foods and supplements. It does not include the *2S*-stereoisomeric forms of α-tocopherol (*SRR*-, *SSR*-, *SRS*-, and *SSS*-α-tocopherol), also found in fortified foods and supplements.

[d] As niacin equivalents (NE). 1 mg niacin = 60 mg tryptophan.

[e] As DFE. 1 DFE = 1 $\mu$g food folate = 0.6 $\mu$g folic acid from fortified food or as a supplement consumed with food = 0.5 $\mu$g of a supplement taken on an empty stomach.

for Americans, the level for total fat intake is between 30% and 40% of energy for children ages 1–3 years and between 25% and 35% of energy for children and adolescents ages 4–18 years, with most fats coming from sources of polyunsaturated and monounsaturated fatty acids, such as fish, nuts, and vegetable oils.[17] The American Academy of Pediatrics recommends that children's fat intake (averaged over several days) provides approximately 30% of total energy, with a lower limit of 20% of energy from fat.[18]

For saturated fatty acids, neither an AI nor RDA was set because they have no known role in preventing chronic diseases and because they are synthesized by the body to provide adequate levels needed for their physiological and structural functions.[9] An UL was not set because any incremental increase in saturated fatty acid intake increases risk of coronary heart disease.[9] Intake of saturated fatty acids should be as low as possible while consuming a nutritionally adequate diet.[9] According to the 2010 Dietary Guidelines for

**TABLE 20.7**

**Estimated Calorie Needs per Day by Age, Gender, and Physical Activity Level for Children and Adolescents[a]**

| Gender/Activity Level[b] | Boy | | | Girl | | |
|---|---|---|---|---|---|---|
| | Sedentary | Moderately Active | Active | Sedentary | Moderately Active | Active |
| Age (Years) | Estimated Calorie Needs per Day | | | | | |
| 2 | 1000 | 1000 | 1000 | 1000 | 1000 | 1000 |
| 3 | 1200 | 1400 | 1400 | 1000 | 1200 | 1400 |
| 4 | 1200 | 1400 | 1600 | 1200 | 1400 | 1400 |
| 5 | 1200 | 1400 | 1600 | 1200 | 1400 | 1600 |
| 6 | 1400 | 1600 | 1800 | 1200 | 1400 | 1600 |
| 7 | 1400 | 1600 | 1800 | 1200 | 1600 | 1800 |
| 8 | 1400 | 1600 | 2000 | 1400 | 1600 | 1800 |
| 9 | 1600 | 1800 | 2000 | 1400 | 1600 | 1800 |
| 10 | 1600 | 1800 | 2200 | 1400 | 1800 | 2000 |
| 11 | 1800 | 2000 | 2200 | 1600 | 1800 | 2000 |
| 12 | 1800 | 2200 | 2400 | 1600 | 2000 | 2200 |
| 13 | 2000 | 2200 | 2600 | 1600 | 2000 | 2200 |
| 14 | 2000 | 2400 | 2800 | 1800 | 2000 | 2400 |
| 15 | 2200 | 2600 | 3000 | 1800 | 2000 | 2400 |
| 16 | 2400 | 2800 | 3200 | 1800 | 2000 | 2400 |
| 17 | 2400 | 2800 | 3200 | 1800 | 2000 | 2400 |
| 18 | 2400 | 2800 | 3200 | 1800 | 2000 | 2400 |

*Source:* Adapted from U.S. Department of Agriculture and U.S. Department of Health and Human Services, *Dietary Guidelines for Americans, 2010*, 7th edn., Washington, DC, U.S. Government Printing Office, 2010. Available online at www.healthierus. gov/dietaryguidelines.

[a] Estimated amounts of calories (rounded to the nearest 200 calories) needed to maintain calorie balance for various gender and age groups of children and adolescents at three different levels of physical activity. An individual's calorie needs may be higher or lower than these average estimates, which are based on EER equations, using reference heights (average) and reference weights (healthy) for each age–gender group. For children and adolescents, reference height and weight vary. The EER equations are from the National Research Council; *Dietary Reference Intakes for Energy, Carbohydrate, Fiber, Fat, Fatty Acids, Cholesterol, Protein, and Amino Acids*; the National Academies Press, Washington, DC, 2002/2005 (which is available online at www.nap.edu).

[b] Sedentary means a lifestyle that includes only the light physical activity associated with typical day-to-day life. Moderately active means a lifestyle that includes physical activity equivalent to walking about 1.5–3 miles/day at 3–4 miles/h, in addition to the light physical activity associated with typical day-to-day life. Active means a lifestyle that includes physical activity equivalent to walking more than 3 miles/day at 3–4 miles/h, in addition to the light physical activity associated with day-to-day life.

Americans,[17] consuming less than 10% of energy from saturated fatty acids, and replacing them with monounsaturated and polyunsaturated fatty acids, is associated with a lower risk of cardiovascular disease.

Linoleic acid serves as a precursor to eicosanoids; it is the only n–6 polyunsaturated fatty acid that is an essential fatty acid.[9] n–3 Polyunsaturated fatty acids (α-linolenic acid) play an important role as structural membrane lipids, especially in nerve tissue and the retina, and are precursors to eicosanoids.[9] AIs and AMDRs are found in Tables 20.2 and 20.3, respectively, for linoleic acid and α-linolenic acid for children and adolescents. There was insufficient evidence to set an UL for n–6 polyunsaturated fatty acids or n–3 polyunsaturated fatty acids.[9]

No AI or RDA was set for trans fatty acids because they are not essential and provide no known benefit to human health.[9] An UL was not set because any incremental increase in intake of trans fatty acids increases risk of coronary heart disease. Intake of trans fatty acids should be as low as possible while consuming a nutritionally adequate diet.[9,17] "Natural" or "ruminant" trans fatty acids are produced by grazing animals, so small quantities are found in meat and milk products. "Synthetic" or "industrial" trans fatty acids are produced by the process of hydrogenation used by food manufacturers to make products more resistant to spoilage or rancidity. Since 2006 (when the declaration of the amount of trans fatty acids on Nutrition Facts labels became mandatory), synthetic trans fatty acids in the U.S. food supply have decreased dramatically.[17]

Although cholesterol plays an important role in steroid hormone and bile acid biosynthesis and is an integral component of cell membranes, there is no evidence for a biological requirement for dietary cholesterol because all tissues are capable of synthesizing sufficient amounts of cholesterol. Thus, neither an AI nor an RDA was set for dietary cholesterol.[9] An UL was not set because any incremental

**TABLE 20.8**

**EARs and RDAs for Indispensable Amino Acids for Children and Adolescents**

| | Children | | Boys | | Girls | |
|---|---|---|---|---|---|---|
| | 1–3 Years | 4–8 Years | 9–13 Years | 14–18 Years | 9–13 Years | 14–18 Years |
| *EAR* (mg/kg/day) | | | | | | |
| Histidine | 16 | 13 | 13 | 12 | 12 | 12 |
| Isoleucine | 22 | 18 | 18 | 17 | 17 | 16 |
| Leucine | 48 | 40 | 40 | 38 | 38 | 35 |
| Lysine | 45 | 37 | 37 | 35 | 35 | 32 |
| Methionine + cysteine | 22 | 18 | 18 | 17 | 17 | 16 |
| Phenylalanine + tyrosine | 41 | 33 | 33 | 31 | 31 | 28 |
| Threonine | 24 | 19 | 19 | 18 | 18 | 17 |
| Tryptophan | 6 | 5 | 5 | 5 | 5 | 4 |
| Valine | 28 | 23 | 23 | 22 | 22 | 20 |
| *RDA* (mg/kg/day) | | | | | | |
| Histidine | 21 | 16 | 17 | 15 | 15 | 14 |
| Isoleucine | 28 | 22 | 22 | 21 | 21 | 19 |
| Leucine | 63 | 49 | 49 | 47 | 47 | 44 |
| Lysine | 58 | 46 | 46 | 43 | 43 | 40 |
| Methionine + cysteine | 28 | 22 | 22 | 21 | 21 | 19 |
| Phenylalanine + tyrosine | 54 | 41 | 41 | 38 | 38 | 35 |
| Threonine | 32 | 24 | 24 | 22 | 22 | 21 |
| Tryptophan | 8 | 6 | 6 | 6 | 6 | 5 |
| Valine | 37 | 28 | 28 | 27 | 27 | 24 |

*Source:* Adapted from National Research Council, *Dietary Reference Intakes for Energy, Carbohydrate, Fiber, Fat, Fatty Acids, Cholesterol, Protein, and Amino Acids,* The National Academies Press, Washington, DC, 2002/2005. This report may be accessed via www.nap.edu.

increase in intake of dietary cholesterol increases risk of coronary heart disease.[9] Intake of dietary cholesterol should be as low as possible while consuming a nutritionally adequate diet.[9] According to the 2010 Dietary Guidelines for Americans, intake of cholesterol should be less than 300 mg/day.[17]

Dietary sources of fat include oils, margarine, butter, fried foods, egg yolks, mayonnaise, salad dressings, ice cream, hard cheese, cream cheese, nuts, fatty meats, chips, and doughnuts. Most fats with a high percentage of saturated or trans fatty acids are solid at room temperature and referred to as "solid fats." Fats with more unsaturated fatty acids are usually liquid at room temperature and referred to as "oils." Solid fats are found in most animal foods but can also be made from vegetable oils through the process of hydrogenation. To keep saturated fat intake low, limit intake of animal fats (e.g., full-fat dairy products such as cheese, milk, butter, and ice cream; fatty meat; bacon; sausage; and poultry skin and fat). To keep trans fat intake low, limit intake of foods made with partially hydrogenated vegetable oils. To keep cholesterol intake low, limit egg yolks and organ meats especially, as well as meat, shellfish, and poultry, and dairy products that contain fat. Table 20.9 provides the total fat, saturated fat, and cholesterol content of various foods.

## FIBER

Because a variety of definitions of dietary fiber existed worldwide, the National Research Council convened a special panel to develop a proposed definition of fiber.[8] Based on the panel's deliberations, along with consideration of public comments and subsequent modifications, the following definitions were developed:[9]

- *Dietary fiber* consists of nondigestible carbohydrates and lignin that are intrinsic and intact in plants.
- *Functional fiber* consists of isolated, nondigestible carbohydrates that have beneficial physiological effects in humans.
- *Total fiber* is the sum of dietary fiber and functional fiber.[9]

Separate definitions were developed for dietary fiber and functional fiber.[9] One definition concerns dietary fiber because many other substances in high-fiber foods (including vitamins and minerals) often have made it challenging to demonstrate a significant health benefit specially attributable to the fiber in foods. In other words, it has been difficult to separate out the effect of fiber per se from the high-fiber food. Having a separate definition for functional fiber means that when isolated nondigestible carbohydrates are added as

**TABLE 20.9**

**Total Fat, Saturated Fat, and Cholesterol Content of Various Foods**

| Food | Serving Size | Total Fat (g) | Saturated Fat (g) | Cholesterol (mg) |
|---|---|---|---|---|
| Almonds, dry roasted | 1 oz (~22 nuts) | 14.8 | 1.1 | 0 |
| Bacon, cured, broiled/pan fried | 3 med. slices | 7.9 | 2.6 | 21 |
| Bread, white | 0.88 oz slice | 0.8 | 0.2 | 0 |
| Butter | 1 T | 11.4 | 7.2 | 30 |
| Cheese, American processed | 1 oz | 8.8 | 5.5 | 26 |
| Cheese, cheddar | 1 oz | 9.3 | 5.9 | 29 |
| Chicken breast with skin, roasted | ½ breast (3.5 oz) | 7.6 | 2.1 | 82 |
| Chicken breast without skin, roasted | ½ breast (3 oz) | 3.1 | 0.9 | 73 |
| Coconut, dried, sweetened, flaked, packaged | 1 oz | 7.8 | 7.4 | 0 |
| Corn oil | 1 T | 14.0 | 1.8 | 0 |
| Cottonseed oil | 1 T | 14.0 | 3.6 | 0 |
| Egg (chicken), boiled, hard | 1 large | 5.3 | 1.6 | 212 |
| Egg (chicken), white, raw | 1 large | 0.1 | 0.0 | 0 |
| Egg (chicken), yolk, raw | 1 large | 4.5 | 1.6 | 210 |
| Flatfish, flounder/sole, cooked by dry heat | 3 oz | 1.3 | 0.3 | 58 |
| Ground beef, 25% fat, patty, broiled | 3 oz patty | 15.9 | 6.2 | 76 |
| Ground beef, 5% fat, patty, broiled | 3 oz patty | 5.6 | 2.5 | 65 |
| Ice cream, vanilla, regular (10% fat) | ½ c | 7.3 | 4.5 | 29 |
| Lard (pork fat), raw | 1 oz | 19.9 | 7.0 | 22 |
| Margarine, corn and soy, stick | 1 T | 11.3 | 2.1 | 0 |
| Margarine, liquid | 1 T | 11.3 | 1.8 | 0 |
| Milk (cow), whole, 3.25% fat | 8 fl oz | 7.9 | 4.6 | 24 |
| Milk (cow), reduced fat, 2% fat | 8 fl oz | 4.8 | 3.1 | 20 |
| Milk (cow), low fat, 1% fat | 8 fl oz | 2.4 | 1.5 | 12 |
| Milk (cow), nonfat | 8 fl oz | 0.2 | 0.1 | 5 |
| Olive oil | 1 T | 14.0 | 1.9 | 0 |
| Peanut butter, chunk style/crunchy | 2 T | 16.0 | 2.6 | 0 |
| Peanuts, dry roasted, salted | 1 oz (~28 nuts) | 13.9 | 1.9 | 0 |
| Pecans, dried | 1 oz (20 halves) | 20.2 | 1.7 | 0 |
| Pork, tenderloin, lean, roasted | 3 oz | 3.0 | 1.0 | 62 |
| Safflower oil, >70% linoleic acid | 1 T | 14.0 | 0.9 | 0 |
| Shrimp, cooked by moist heat | 3 oz (15 ½ large) | 0.9 | 0.2 | 166 |
| Soy oil (salad/cooking) | 1 T | 14.0 | 2.2 | 0 |
| Tuna, light, canned in oil | 3 oz | 7.0 | 1.3 | 15 |
| Tuna, light, canned in water | 3 oz | 0.7 | 0.2 | 26 |
| Turkey, breast with skin, roasted | 3 oz | 2.7 | 0.7 | 76 |
| Yogurt, frozen, soft serve, vanilla | ½ c | 4.0 | 2.5 | 1 |

*Source:* Adapted from Pennington, J.A.T. and Spungen, J., *Bowes & Church's Food Values of Portions Commonly Used*, 19th edn., Lippincott Williams & Wilkins, Philadelphia, PA, 2010.

a fiber source to a food, researchers and practitioners may draw conclusions about functional fiber itself with regard to its physiological role rather than that of the food in which it is found.[9]

The different properties of fibers result in different physiological effects.[9] For example, viscous fibers may delay gastric emptying; this results in a sensation of fullness, which may contribute to weight control. In addition, delayed gastric emptying may reduce postprandial blood glucose concentrations and potentially have a beneficial effect on insulin sensitivity. Viscous fibers may reduce blood cholesterol concentrations by interfering with the absorption of

dietary fat and cholesterol, as well as with the enterohepatic recirculation of cholesterol and bile acids. Fecal bulk, laxation, and constipation are improved by consumption of dietary fiber and certain functional fibers, especially those that are poorly fermented. Normal laxation can be a problem for many children. The AIs for total fiber in foods for children and adolescents are found in Table 20.2; ULs were not set for dietary fiber or functional fiber due to insufficient evidence.[9]

According to the 2010 Dietary Guidelines for Americans, foods that provide more dietary fiber should be chosen because fiber is a nutrient of concern in American diets.[17]

The American Health Foundation recommends that children older than 2 years of age consume a minimal amount of fiber equal to their age plus 5 g/day, and a maximum amount of age plus 10 g/day, to achieve intakes of a maximum of 35 g/day after the age of 20 years.[19,20] These recommendations were endorsed at a conference held in May 1994 about dietary fiber in childhood.[21] This range is thought to be safe, reasonable, and practical.[22,23] The "age plus 5" recommendation results in a gradual increase in fiber intake over time with a 3-year-old eating 8 g/day and an 18-year-old eating 23 g/day.

Fiber intake should be increased gradually through consumption of a variety of fruits, vegetables, legumes, cereals, and other whole-grain products such as breads and crackers. Fiber supplements for children are not recommended as a means of meeting dietary fiber goals.[20] Increased intakes of dietary fiber should be accompanied by increased intakes of water because dietary fiber increases water retention in the colon, which leads to bulkier and softer stools.[20] For most children and adolescents, dietary fiber goals can be met if the daily diet includes two servings of vegetables, three servings of fruits, two slices of whole-wheat bread, and one serving of breakfast cereal containing 3 or more g of fiber.[19] Table 20.10 provides the fiber content of foods that most U.S. children and adolescents will eat.

High-fiber diets have the potential for reduced energy density, reduced energy intake, and poor growth, especially in very young children. Furthermore, high-fiber diets may reduce the bioavailability of minerals such as iron, calcium, and zinc. However, the potential health benefits of a moderate increase in dietary fiber intake in childhood (e.g., adhering to the "age plus 5" recommendation) are thought to significantly outweigh the potential risks, especially in highly industrialized countries such as the United States.[20]

## WATER

Water is the largest single constituent of the human body; it is essential for cellular homeostasis and life.[12] A low intake of total water (from drinking water, water in beverages, and food) has been associated with some chronic diseases, but this evidence is insufficient to establish water intake recommendations in order to reduce the risk of chronic diseases; thus, an AI for total water (see Table 20.2) was set to prevent deleterious (mainly acute) effects of dehydration, which include metabolic and functional abnormalities.[12] Higher intakes of total water are required for individuals who are physically active or exposed to hot environments.[12]

About 80% of total water intake comes from drinking water and other beverages.[12] Although diuretic effects have been shown in some studies from consumption of caffeinated beverages, available information indicates that this may be transient in nature, and thus, such beverages do contribute to total water intake similar to that contributed by noncaffeinated beverages.[12] Deficits in body water

**TABLE 20.10**

**Fiber Content of Foods That Most U.S. Children and Adolescents Will Eat[a]**

| Food | Serving Size | Dietary Fiber (g) |
|---|---|---|
| Baked beans, canned with pork | 1 c | 13.9 |
| Chili with beans | 9 oz/1 c | 11.3 |
| Refried beans, canned | 1 c | 12.9 |
| Brown rice, boiled | 1 c | 3.5 |
| Peanuts, dry roasted, salted | 1 oz | 2.2 |
| Strawberries, whole | 1 c | 2.9 |
| Bread, whole wheat | 1 oz slice | 1.9 |
| Potato, baked, with skin | 1 medium | 3.8 |
| Apple | 1 medium | 3.3 |
| Banana | 1 medium | 3.1 |
| Carrot, raw | 1 (7.5 in. long) | 2.0 |
| Carrot, baby, raw | 1 medium | 0.3 |
| Corn, frozen, boiled, drained | 1 c | 3.9 |
| Corn, canned, drained | 1 c | 3.1 |
| Kiwi | 1 medium | 2.3 |
| Raisins, seeded | 1/2 c | 5.0 |
| Cracker, whole wheat | 0.5 oz (~3.5 crackers) | 1.5 |
| Cereal, ready to eat | 1 c | 2–3[a] |
| Applesauce, canned/bottled, sweetened | 1 c | 3.1 |
| Broccoli, raw | 1 c (pieces) | 2 |
| Broccoli, boiled, drained | 1 medium stalk | 5.9 |
| Oatmeal, instant, prepared | 1 c | 4.0 |
| Orange | 1 medium | 3.1 |
| Peanut butter, smooth | 2 T | 1.9 |
| Peanut butter, chunk style/crunchy | 2 T | 2.6 |

*Sources:* Adapted from Williams, C.L., *J. Am. Diet. Assoc.*, 95, 1140, 1995; Pennington, J.A.T. and Spungen, J., *Bowes & Church's Food Values of Portions Commonly Used*, 19th edn., Lippincott Williams & Wilkins, Philadelphia, PA, 2010.

[a] Dietary fiber content of cereal varies widely. Best fiber choice for children has 3 + g/cup.

can occur over the course of a few hours due to decreased intake or increased water losses from physical activity and environmental factors (e.g., heat, exposure). However, on a daily basis, fluid intake, which is driven by a combination of thirst and consumption of beverages at meals and snacks, allows for hydration status and for normal levels of total body water to be maintained.[12]

An UL was not set for water because healthy individuals have considerable ability to excrete excess water and thus maintain water balance.[12] However, there have been reports of acute water toxicity due to rapid consumption of large quantities of fluids that greatly exceeded the kidney's maximal excretion rate of about 0.7–1.0 L/h.[12]

## Selected Vitamins and Minerals

### Vitamin D and Calcium

Vitamin D and calcium are essential nutrients long known for their role in bone health. During the past decade, there have been conflicting messages about other possible health benefits of these nutrients—especially vitamin D—such as preventing cancer and diabetes. Calcium has been increasingly added to foods, and calcium supplement use is widespread, especially among the elderly. Thus, the DRIs for vitamin D and calcium published in 1997[1] were updated in 2011.[16] To update the DRIs for vitamin D and calcium, more than 1000 studies were thoroughly reviewed. The review found a strong body of evidence from rigorous testing that substantiated the importance of vitamin D and calcium in promoting bone health; however, the current evidence did not support other health benefits for vitamin D or calcium intake. An assumption in developing the DRIs for calcium was that they are predicated on intakes that meet requirements for vitamin D; similarly, DRIs for vitamin D rest on the assumption of intakes that meet requirements for calcium. The DRIs for vitamin D assume minimal sun exposure. No amount of vitamin D is able to compensate for inadequate total calcium intake. For vitamin D and calcium for children and adolescents, the RDAs are provided in Table 20.2, the EARs are provided in Table 20.6, and the ULs are provided in Table 20.5.

Throughout the world, the major source of vitamin D for humans is the exposure of the skin to sunlight; vitamin D that is synthesized in the skin during the summer and fall months can be stored in the body's fat for use in the winter, which minimizes requirements for vitamin D. In nature, very few foods contain vitamin D; thus, children and adolescents who live in far northern latitudes (e.g., northern Canada, Alaska) may need vitamin D supplements. Food sources of vitamin D include fish liver oil, fatty fish, and egg yolk. Foods fortified with vitamin D include milk products and other foods such as margarine and breakfast cereals; the majority of human intake of vitamin D is from fortified foods.[16]

Over 99% of total body calcium is found in teeth and bones. Approximately 45% of adult skeletal mass is accounted for by skeletal growth during adolescence; thus, achieving and maintaining adequate calcium intake during adolescence are necessary for the development of a maximal peak bone mass, which may help reduce the risk of osteoporosis later in adulthood.

Major food sources of calcium include milk, yogurt, cheese, and green leafy vegetables. Calcium-fortified orange juice is also an excellent source of calcium, as is tofu. Table 20.11 provides the calcium content of various common foods. Vitamin D is needed for the body to absorb calcium.

The percent of calcium present in foods that is absorbed by humans varies with the type of food consumed. Calcium absorption from dairy and fortified foods is good. Calcium may be poorly absorbed from foods high in oxalic acid (e.g., spinach, collard greens, beans, sweet potatoes, rhubarb) or foods high in phytic acid (e.g., fiber-containing whole-grain products and wheat bran, beans, seeds, nuts, soy isolates).[16]

According to the 2011 updated DRIs for vitamin D and calcium, there were inadequate data to conclude significant levels of vitamin D deficiency in the population; however, calcium remained a nutrient of concern because median intakes from foods are close to the EAR values for most groups.[16] According to the 2010 Dietary Guidelines for Americans[17], children ages 9 years and older and adolescent girls are among the age groups of particular concern due to low calcium intake.

The exclusion of dairy products (all of which are rich sources of calcium and some of which are fortified with vitamin D) because of lactose intolerance can be a risk factor for inadequate intakes of calcium and vitamin D.[16] Lactose intolerance is more common in Black, Hispanic, and Asian individuals than in White individuals.[24] Many individuals with lactose intolerance or lactose malabsorption are able to tolerate up to 12 g of lactose (the equivalent of 1 cup of milk) in a single dose and may be able to tolerate larger amounts if consumed in smaller doses spread over the day and with other foods. Consumption of larger amounts of reduced-lactose dairy products (e.g., certain yogurts, certain fluid milks) and virtually unrestricted amounts of reduced-fat hard cheeses with very low amounts of lactose can ensure adequate calcium intake. Consumption of nondairy sources of calcium, such as low-oxalate vegetables (e.g., broccoli, kale, bok choy, Chinese cabbage), calcium-containing tofu, and fortified plant-based foods (e.g., cereals, fruit juice), can also ensure adequate calcium intake.[16] Over-the-counter lactase can help the body digest foods that contain lactose. Also, lactose-free or lactose-reduced milk and other dairy products are available.

### Folate

Folate is important during periods of increased cell replication and growth due to its role in DNA synthesis and the formation of healthy red blood cells; thus, the RDAs for folate are 1.5 times greater for children ages 9–13 years than for children ages 4–8 years[2] (see Table 20.2). There is strong evidence that the risk of having a fetus with a neural tube defect decreases with increased intake of folate during the periconceptional period. Therefore, it is recommended that all females capable of becoming pregnant take 400 µg of synthetic folic acid daily, from fortified foods or supplements, in addition to consuming food folate from a varied diet. Folate fortification became mandatory for enriched grain products in the United States as of January 1998. Besides fortified grains and cereals, other food sources of folate include leafy green vegetables, orange juice, liver, cantaloupe, yeast, and seeds.[2]

### Iron

According to the American Academy of Pediatrics,[25] iron deficiency is the most common nutritional deficiency in the United States. Children ages 1–2 years are the most susceptible to iron deficiency due to increased iron needs related

### TABLE 20.11
### Calcium Contents of Various Common Foods[a]

| Food | Serving Size | Calcium (mg) |
|---|---|---|
| Milk, whole/3.25%, 1%, or 2% | 8 oz | 276–290 (whole = 276; 1% = 290; 2% = 285) |
| Buttermilk, cultured, reduced fat | 8 oz | 350 |
| Yogurt, low fat, plain | 8 oz | 415 |
| Yogurt, nonfat, plain | 8 oz | 452 |
| Cheese, Swiss | 1 oz | 221 |
| Cheese, cheddar | 1 oz | 202 |
| Cheese, mozzarella, part skim | 1 oz | 219 |
| Cheese, American processed | 1 oz | 155 |
| Cheese, provolone | 1.5 oz | 325 |
| Orange juice, calcium fortified | 8 oz | 350 |
| Canned salmon, with bones | 3 oz | 181 |
| Collard greens, boiled, drained | 1 c chopped | 266 |
| Vanilla pudding, from regular mix with 2% milk | ½ c | 151 |
| Spinach, cooked, boiled, drained | 1 c | 245 |
| Frozen yogurt, vanilla, soft serve | ½ c | 103 |
| Ice cream, vanilla, 10% fat | ½ c | 84 |
| Mustard or kale greens, boiled, drained | 1 c | 94–104 (mustard = 104; kale = 94) |
| Cottage cheese, 1% fat | 1 c | 138 |
| Cottage cheese, 2% fat | 1 c | 206 |
| Spinach, raw | 1 c | 30 |
| Orange | 1 medium | 52 |
| Kidney beans, all types, mature, canned | 1 c | 87 |
| Pinto beans, mature, canned | 1 c | 103 |
| Lima beans, mature, large, canned | 1 c | 51 |
| Sweet potato, baked | 1 medium | 43 |
| Sweet potatoes, canned, mashed | 1 c | 76 |
| Sweet potato, canned in light syrup, drained | 1 c | 33 |
| Broccoli, boiled, drained | 1 medium stalk | 72 |
| Cheese pizza, regular crust | 3.6 oz slice | 182 |

*Source:* Adapted from Pennington, J.A.T. and Spungen, J., *Bowes & Church's Food Values of Portions Commonly Used*, 19th edn., Lippincott Williams & Wilkins, Philadelphia, PA, 2010.

to rapid growth during the first 2 years of life and a relatively low iron content in most infant diets when iron is not added by supplementation or fortification. Children ages 3–11 years are at less risk for iron deficiency until the rapid growth of puberty. Adolescent girls are at greater risk for iron deficiency anemia due to blood losses during menstruation. Adolescent athletes have a higher rate of iron deficiency. A major consequence of iron deficiency is that significant iron deficiency adversely affects child development and behavior. Furthermore, iron deficiency leads to enhanced lead absorption, and childhood lead poisoning is a well-documented cause of neurological and developmental deficits. These consequences, along with evidence that dietary intake during infancy is a strong determinant of iron status for older infants and younger children, emphasize the importance of a dietary approach for the primary prevention of iron deficiency in younger children.[25]

Dietary iron is classified as "heme" or "nonheme" iron. Heme iron is found in foods from animals such as meat, fish, and poultry. Nonheme iron is provided by plants; good sources include dark-green leafy vegetables, tofu, lentils, white beans, dried fruits, and iron-fortified breads and cereals. On average, healthy people absorb about 5%–10% of the iron consumed, and people who are iron deficient absorb about 10%–20%. Heme iron is more easily absorbed than nonheme iron. About 20% of heme iron consumed is absorbed regardless of how it is prepared and served; however, the absorption rate of nonheme iron can be increased by eating nonheme iron foods with either meat, foods rich in vitamin C, or foods that contain some heme iron at the same meal. Nonheme iron absorption can be hindered by as much as 50% when tannins, phytates, and calcium (which are found in foods such as tea, bran, and milk, respectively) are eaten at the same meal.

The RDAs for iron for children and adolescents are included in Table 20.2. Because the amount of iron available in the U.S. diet is estimated to be about 5–7 mg/1000 kcal, it may be difficult for adolescent girls to obtain 15 mg of iron from dietary sources alone if their caloric intake is between 2000 and 2400 kcal/day. Groups of adolescents who are at special risk of iron deficiency include (1) older adolescent girls due to increased iron need and low dietary intake, (2) pregnant adolescents, and (3) female athletes such as runners who may lose iron through occult gastrointestinal bleeding.

### Zinc

Zinc is needed for protein synthesis, wound healing, and sexual maturation; thus, zinc is especially important during adolescence due to the rapid rate of growth and sexual maturation (see Table 20.2 for the RDAs for zinc for children and adolescents). Adolescents undergoing rapid growth are at risk for inadequate zinc levels and should be encouraged to include zinc-rich foods in their daily diet. Foods high in zinc include red meats, certain seafood, and whole grains; many breakfast cereals are fortified with zinc. The bioavailability of zinc in foods varies widely. Zinc from whole-grain products is less available than zinc from meat, liver, eggs, and seafood (especially oysters). Furthermore, consumption of phytate-rich foods limits absorption and maintenance of zinc balance.[7]

### Potassium

Potassium is required for normal cellular function. The level of potassium from dietary intake according to the AI (see Table 20.2) should maintain lower blood pressure levels, reduce adverse effects of sodium chloride intake on blood pressure, decrease the risk of recurrent kidney stones, and possibly decrease bone loss.[12] Currently, dietary intake of potassium by all groups in the United States and Canada is much lower than the AI.[12] Black individuals would especially benefit from an increased intake of potassium due to their relatively low intake and high prevalence of elevated blood pressure and salt sensitivity.[12]

Fruits and vegetables are good sources of potassium. Relatively high amounts of potassium are found in spinach, cantaloupe, dry roasted almonds, Brussels sprouts, mushrooms, bananas, oranges, grapefruit, and potatoes. An UL was not set because potassium intake from foods above the AI poses no potential for increased risk as excess potassium is readily excreted in the urine in generally healthy populations with normal kidney function.[12]

## 2010 DIETARY GUIDELINES FOR AMERICANS AND *MYPLATE*

The 2010 Dietary Guidelines for Americans are for healthy Americans over 2 years of age.[17] The intent of the Dietary Guidelines is to summarize and synthesize knowledge about individual nutrients and food components into an inter-related set of recommendations for healthy eating that the public can adopt. The Dietary Guidelines recommendations encompass two overarching concepts. The first concept is to maintain calorie balance over time to achieve and sustain a healthy weight. The second concept is to focus on consuming nutrient-dense foods and beverages.[17]

Table 20.7 provides estimated calorie needs per day by age, gender, and physical activity for children and adolescents ages 2–18 years from the 2010 Dietary Guidelines for Americans. Table 20.12 shows food patterns by food group for calorie levels ranging from 1000 to 3200 from the 2010 Dietary Guidelines for Americans.

An example of an eating pattern that exemplifies the 2010 Dietary Guidelines for Americans and is appropriate for children and adolescents is the Dietary Approaches to Stop Hypertension (DASH) eating plan.[17] Specifically, the DASH eating patterns from 1200 to 1800 kcal meet the nutritional needs of children ages 4–8 years, and the DASH eating patterns from 1600 to 3100 kcal meet the nutritional needs of children ages 9 years and older and adults.[17] Table 20.13 shows the DASH eating plan by food groups for calorie levels ranging from 1200 to 3100.

In June 2011, the U.S. Department of Agriculture (USDA) released *MyPlate*[26,27] (replacing *MyPyramid*) as a new-generation icon to prompt consumers to think about building a healthy plate at mealtimes and to seek more information online at http://www.ChooseMyPlate.gov. *MyPlate* promotes the messages of the 2010 Dietary Guidelines for Americans[17] to help consumers build and visualize healthy diets. The *MyPlate* image was designed to be a simple and familiar representation of five food groups (fruits, vegetables, grains, protein, and dairy). *MyPlate* depicts a plate divided into sections, and each section represents the portion of space on a plate that each of the five food groups should occupy at every meal. The emphasis on food groups is to help consumers think about their entire meal as opposed to components or ingredients of a meal. The key consumer message is to "Make half your plate fruits and vegetables." A SuperTracker is available online at https://www.choosemyplate.gov/SuperTracker/default.aspx to help consumers plan, analyze, and track their diet and physical activity. Materials are available online at http://www.ChooseMyPlate.gov for children, parents, educators, and health-care professionals. For example, the online section for children ages 6–11 years* includes coloring pages and an interactive computer game called "Blast Off Game." In the game, children can reach Planet Power by fueling their rocket with food and physical activity; "fuel" tanks for each food group help children keep track of their choices. For parents, the "10 Tips Nutrition Education Series" covers several topics such as making vegetables and fruits child friendly (see Figure 20.1),† decreasing added sugars (see Figure 20.2),‡ and being a healthy role model for children (see Figure 20.3).§

---

* http:// www.choosemyplate.gov/children-over-five.html
† Available at http://www.choosemyplate.gov/food-groups/downloads/TenTips/DGTipsheet11KidFriendlyVeggiesAndFruits.pdf
‡ Available at http:// www.choosemyplate.gov/food-groups/downloads/TenTips/ DGTipsheet13CutBackOnSweetTreats.pdf
§ Available at http://www.choosemyplate.gov/food-groups/downloads/TenTips/DGTipsheet12BeAHealthyRoleModel.pdf

## TABLE 20.12
## Food Patterns by Food Group for Calorie Levels from 1000 to 3200 from the 2010 Dietary Guidelines for Americans

For each food group or subgroup,[a] recommended average daily intake amounts[b] at all calorie levels. Recommended intakes from vegetable and protein foods subgroup are per week. For information and tools for application, go to www.ChooseMyPlate.gov

| Daily Calorie Level of Pattern[c] | 1000 | 1200 | 1400 | 1600 | 1800 | 2000 | 2200 | 2400 | 2600 | 2800 | 3000 | 3200[c] |
|---|---|---|---|---|---|---|---|---|---|---|---|---|
| Fruits | 1 c | 1 c | 1½ c | 1½ c | 1½ c | 2 c | 2 c | 2 c | 2 c | 2½ c | 2½ c | 2½ c |
| Vegetables[d] | 1 c | 1½ c | 1½ c | 2 c | 2½ c | 2½ c | 3 c | 3 c | 3½ c | 3½ c | 4 c | 4 c |
| Dark-green vegetables | ½ c/week | 1 c/week | 1 c/week | 1½ c/week | 1½ c/week | 1½ c/week | 2 c/week | 2 c/week | 2½ c/week | 2½ c/week | 2½ c/week | 2½ c/week |
| Red and orange vegetables | 2½ c/week | 3 c/week | 3 c/week | 4 c/week | 5½ c/week | 5½ c/week | 6 c/week | 6 c/week | 7 c/week | 7 c/week | 7½ c/week | 7½ c/week |
| Beans and peas (legumes) | ½ c/week | ½ c/week | ½ c/week | 1 c/week | 1½ c/week | 1½ c/week | 2 c/week | 2 c/week | 2½ c/week | 2½ c/week | 3 c/week | 3 c/week |
| Starchy vegetables | 2 c/week | 3½ c/week | 3½ c/week | 4 c/week | 5 c/week | 5 c/week | 6 c/week | 6 c/week | 7 c/week | 7 c/week | 8 c/week | 8 c/week |
| Other vegetables | 1½ c/week | 2½ c/week | 2½ c/week | 3½ c/week | 4 c/week | 4 c/week | 5 c/week | 5 c/week | 5½ c/week | 5½ c/week | 7 c/week | 7 c/week |
| Grains[e] | 3 oz-eq | 4 oz-eq | 5 oz-eq | 5 oz-eq | 6 oz-eq | 6 oz-eq | 7 oz-eq | 8 oz-eq | 9 oz-eq | 10 oz-eq | 10 oz-eq | 10 oz-eq |
| Whole grains | 1½ oz-eq | 2 oz-eq | 2½ oz-eq | 3 oz-eq | 3 oz-eq | 3 oz-eq | 3½ oz-eq | 4 oz-eq | 4½ oz-eq | 5 oz-eq | 5 oz-eq | 5 oz-eq |
| Enriched grains | 1½ oz-eq | 2 oz-eq | 2½ oz-eq | 2 oz-eq | 3 oz-eq | 3 oz-eq | 3½ oz-eq | 4 oz-eq | 4½ oz-eq | 5 oz-eq | 5 oz-eq | 5 oz-eq |
| Protein foods[d] | 2 oz-eq | 3 oz-eq | 4 oz-eq | 5 oz-eq | 5 oz-eq | 5½ oz-eq | 6 oz-eq | 6½ oz-eq | 6½ oz-eq | 7 oz-eq | 7 oz-eq | 7 oz-eq |
| Seafood | 3 oz/week | 5 oz/week | 6 oz/week | 8 oz/week | 8 oz/week | 8 oz/week | 9 oz/week | 10 oz/week | 10 oz/week | 11 oz/week | 11 oz/week | 11 oz/week |
| Meat, poultry, eggs | 10 oz/week | 14 oz/week | 19 oz/week | 24 oz/week | 24 oz/week | 26 oz/week | 29 oz/week | 31 oz/week | 31 oz/week | 34 oz/week | 34 oz/week | 34 oz/week |
| Nuts, seeds, soy products | 1 oz/week | 2 oz/week | 3 oz/week | 4 oz/week | 4 oz/week | 4 oz/week | 4 oz/week | 5 oz/week | 5 oz/week | 5 oz/week | 5 oz/week | 5 oz/week |
| Dairy[f] | 2 c | 2½ c | 2½ c | 3 c | 3 c | 3 c | 3 c | 3 c | 3 c | 3 c | 3 c | 3 c |
| Oils[g] | 15 g | 17 g | 17 g | 22 g | 24 g | 27 g | 29 g | 31 g | 34 g | 36 g | 44 g | 51 g |
| Maximum SoFAS[h] limit, calories (% of calories) | 137 (14%) | 121 (10%) | 121 (9%) | 121 (8%) | 161 (9%) | 258 (13%) | 266 (12%) | 330 (14%) | 362 (14%) | 395 (14%) | 459 (15%) | 596 (19%) |

Source: Adapted from U.S. Department of Agriculture and U.S. Department of Health and Human Services, *Dietary Guidelines for Americans, 2010*, 7th edn., Washington, DC, U.S. Government Printing Office, 2010. Available online at www.healthierus.gov/dietaryguidelines.

a　All foods are assumed to be in nutrient-dense forms, lean, or low fat and prepared without added fats, sugars, or salts. SoFAS may be included up to the daily maximum limit identified in the table. Food items in each group and subgroup are

Fruits: Fresh, frozen, canned, and dried fruits and fruit juices (e.g., oranges and orange juice, apples and apple juice, bananas, grapes, melons, berries, raisins).

Vegetables: Dark-green vegetables: fresh, frozen, and canned dark-green leafy vegetables and broccoli, cooked or raw (e.g., broccoli, spinach, romaine, collard, turnips, mustard greens).

　　Red and orange vegetables: fresh, frozen, and canned red and orange vegetables, cooked or raw (e.g., tomatoes, red peppers, carrots, sweet potatoes, winter squash, pumpkin).

　　Beans and peas (legumes): cooked beans and peas (e.g.: kidney beans, lentils, chickpeas, pinto beans); does not include green beans or green peas; see additional comment under protein foods group.

　　Starchy vegetables: fresh, frozen, and canned starchy vegetables (e.g., white potatoes, corn, green peas).

　　Other vegetables: fresh, frozen, and canned other vegetables, cooked or raw (e.g., iceberg lettuce, green beans, onions).

(continued)

**TABLE 20.12 (continued)**
**Food Patterns by Food Group for Calorie Levels from 1000 to 3200 from the 2010 Dietary Guidelines for Americans**

*Grains:* Whole grains: whole-grain products and whole grains used as ingredients (e.g., whole-wheat bread, whole-grain cereals and crackers, oatmeal, brown rice).

Enriched grains: enriched refined-grain products and enriched refined grains used as ingredients (e.g., white breads, enriched grain cereals and crackers, enriched pastas, white rice).

*Protein foods:* Meat, poultry, seafood, eggs, nuts, seeds, and processed soy products. Meat and poultry should be lean or low fat and nuts should be unsalted. Beans and peas are considered part of this group as well as the vegetables group but should be counted in one group only.

*Dairy:* Milks, including lactose-free and lactose-reduced products and fortified soy beverages, yogurts, frozen yogurts, dairy desserts, and cheeses. Most choices should be fat-free or low fat. Cream, sour cream, and cream cheese are not included due to their low calcium content.

b Food group amounts are shown in cup (c) or ounce-equivalents (oz-eq). Oils are shown in grams (g). Quantity equivalents for each food group are:

Grains, 1 oz-eq is: 1 one-oz slice bread; 1 oz uncooked pasta or rice; ½ c cooked rice, pasta, or cereal; 1 tortilla (6 in. diameter); 1 pancake (5 in. diameter); 1 oz ready-to-eat cereal (about 1 c cereal flakes).

Vegetables and fruits, 1 c equivalent is: 1 c raw or cooked vegetable or fruit; ½ c dried vegetable or fruit; 1 c vegetable or fruit juice; 2 c leafy salad greens.

Protein foods, 1 oz-eq is: 1 oz lean meat, poultry, seafood; 1 egg; 1 tbsp peanut butter; 1.2 oz nuts or seeds. Also, ¼ c cooked beans or peas may also be counted as 1 oz-eq.

Dairy, 1 c equivalent is: 1 c milk, fortified soy beverage, or yogurt; 1½ oz natural cheese (e.g., cheddar); 2 oz processed cheese (e.g., American).

c See Table 20.7 for estimated calorie needs per day by age, gender, and physical activity level. Food intake patterns at 1000, 1200, and 1400 calories meet the nutritional needs of children ages 2–8 years. Patterns from 1600 to 3200 calories meet the needs of children ages 9 and older. If a child between the ages of 4–8 years needs more calories and, therefore, is following a pattern at 1600 calories or more, the recommended amount from the dairy group can be 2½ c/day. Children ages 9 years and older should not use the 1000, 1200, or 1400 calorie patterns.

d Vegetable and protein food subgroup amounts are shown in this table as weekly amounts because it would be difficult for consumers to select food from all subgroups daily.

e Whole-grain subgroup amounts shown in this table are minimums. More whole grains up to all of the grains recommended may be selected, with offsetting decreases in the amounts of enriched refined grains.

f The amount of dairy foods in the 1200 and 1400 calorie patterns has increased to reflect new RDAs for calcium that are higher than previous recommendations for children ages 4–8 years.

g Oils and soft margarines include vegetable, nut, and fish oils and soft vegetable oil table spreads that have no *trans* fats.

h SoFAS are calories from solid fats and added sugars. The limit of SoFAS is the remaining amount of calories in each food pattern after selecting the specified amounts in each food group in nutrient-dense forms (forms that are fat-free or low fat and with no added sugars). The number of SoFAS is lower in the 1200, 1400, and 1600 calorie patterns than in the 1000 calorie patterns. The nutrient goals for the 1300–1600 calorie patterns are higher and require that more calories be used for nutrient-dense foods from the food groups.

**TABLE 20.13**
**DASH Eating Plan by Food Group for Calorie Levels from 1200 to 3100[a]**

| Food Group | Daily Calorie Levels | | | | | | | Examples | Serving Sizes | Notes |
|---|---|---|---|---|---|---|---|---|---|---|
| | 1200 | 1400 | 1600 | 1800 | 2000 | 2600 | 3100 | | | |
| | Number of servings per day (unless specified otherwise) | | | | | | | | | |
| *Grains* | 4–5 | 5–6 | 6 | 6 | 6–8 | 10–11 | 12–13 | Whole-wheat bread and rolls; whole-wheat pasta, English muffin, pita bread, bagel, cereals; grits, oatmeal, brown rice; unsalted pretzels and popcorn | 1 slice bread; 1 oz dry cereal[c]; ½ c cooked rice, pasta, or cereal[a] | Major source of energy and fiber. Whole grains are recommended for most grain sources as a food source of fiber and nutrients. |
| *Vegetables* | 3–4 | 3–4 | 3–4 | 4–5 | 4–5 | 5–6 | 6 | Broccoli, carrots, collards, green beans, green peas, kale, lime beans, potatoes, spinach, squash, sweet potatoes, tomatoes | 1 c raw leafy vegetable; ½ c cut-up raw or cooked vegetable; ½ c vegetable juice | Rich sources of potassium, magnesium, and fiber. |
| *Fruits* | 3–4 | 4 | 4 | 4–5 | 4–5 | 5–6 | 6 | Apples, apricots, bananas, dates, grapes, oranges, grapefruit juice, mangoes, melons, peaches, pineapple, raisins, strawberries, tangerines | 1 medium fruit; ¼ c dried fruit; ½ c fresh frozen or canned fruit; ½ c fruit juice | Important sources of potassium magnesium, and fiber. |
| *Fat-free or low-fat milk and milk products* | 2–3 | 2–3 | 2–3 | 2–3 | 2–3 | 3 | 3–4 | Fat-free milk or buttermilk; fat-free, low-fat or reduced-fat cheese; fat-free/low-fat regular or frozen yogurt | 1 c milk or yogurt; 1½ oz cheese | Major source of calcium and protein. |
| *Lean meats, poultry, and fish* | 3 or less | 3–4 or less | 3–4 or less | 6 or less | 6 or less | 6 or less | 6–9 | | 1 oz cooked meats, poultry, or fish 1 egg | Rich sources of protein and magnesium. Select only lean; trim away visible fats; broil, roast, or poach; remove skin from poultry. As eggs are high in cholesterol, limit egg yolk intake to no more than 4/week; two egg whites have the same protein content as 1 oz meat. |
| *Nuts, seeds, and legumes* | 3/week | 3/week | 3/week | 4/week | 4–5/week | 1 | 1 | Almonds, filberts, mixed nuts, peanuts, walnuts, sunflower seeds, peanut butter, kidney beans, lentils, split peas | 1/3 c or 1½ oz nuts; Two tbsp peanut butter; Two tbsp or ½ oz seeds; ½ c cooked legumes (dried beans, peas) | Rich sources of energy, magnesium, protein, and fiber. |

*(continued)*

**TABLE 20.13 (continued)**
**DASH Eating Plan by Food Group for Calorie Levels from 1200 to 3100[a]**

| Daily Calorie Levels / Food Group | 1200 | 1400 | 1600 | 1800 | 2000 | 2600 | 3100 | Examples | Serving Sizes | Notes |
|---|---|---|---|---|---|---|---|---|---|---|
| *Fats and oils* | 1 | 1 | 2 | 2–3 | 2–3 | 3 | 4 | Soft margarine, vegetable oil (canola, corn, olive, safflower), low-fat mayonnaise, light salad dressing | One tsp soft margarine<br>One tsp vegetable oil<br>One tbsp mayonnaise<br>One tbsp salad dressing | DASH study had 27% of calories as fat, including fat in or added to foods. Fat content changes serving amount for fats and oils. One tbsp regular salad dressing = 1 serving; two tbsp low-fat dressing = 1 serving; one tbsp fat-free dressing = 0 servings. |
| *Sweets and added sugars* | 3 or less per week | 3 or less per week | 3 or less per week | 5 or less per week | 5 or less per week | <2 | <2 | Fruit-flavored gelatin, fruit punch, hard candy, jelly, maple syrup, sorbet and ices, sugar | One tbsp sugar<br>One tbsp jelly or jam<br>½ c sorbet, gelatin dessert<br>One c lemonade | Sweets should be low in fat. |
| *Maximum sodium limit[b] (mg/day)* | 2300 | 2300 | 2300 | 2300 | 2300 | 2300 | 2300 | | | |

*Source:* Adapted from U.S. Department of Agriculture and U.S. Department of Health and Human Services, *Dietary Guidelines for Americans, 2010*, 7th edn., Washington, DC, U.S. Government Printing Office, 2010. Available online at www.healthierus.gov/dietaryguidelines.

[a] The number of daily servings in a food group varies depending on caloric needs. The DASH eating patterns from 1200 to 1800 calories meet the nutritional needs of children 4–8 years old. Patterns from 1600 to 3100 calories meet the nutritional needs of children 9 years and older. See Table 20.7 for estimated calorie needs per day by age, gender, and physical activity level.

[b] The DASH eating plan consists of patterns with a sodium limit of 2300 mg and 1500 mg/day.

[c] Cereal serving sizes vary by type between ½ and 1¼ c; check product's nutrition facts label.

**10 tips**
*Nutrition Education Series*

# kid-friendly veggies and fruits

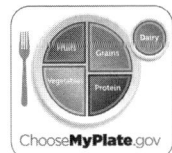

**10 tips** for making healthy foods more fun for children

**Encourage children to eat vegetables and fruits by making it fun.** Provide healthy ingredients and let kids help with preparation, based on their age and skills. Kids may try foods they avoided in the past if they helped make them.

**1 smoothie creations**
Blend fat-free or low-fat yogurt or milk with fruit pieces and crushed ice. Use fresh, frozen, canned, and even overripe fruits. Try bananas, berries, peaches, and/or pineapple. If you freeze the fruit first, you can even skip the ice!

**2 delicious dippers**
Kids love to dip their foods. Whip up a quick dip for veggies with yogurt and seasonings such as herbs or garlic. Serve with raw vegetables like broccoli, carrots, or cauliflower. Fruit chunks go great with a yogurt and cinnamon or vanilla dip.

**3 caterpillar kabobs**
Assemble chunks of melon, apple, orange, and pear on skewers for a fruity kabob. For a raw veggie version, use vegetables like zucchini, cucumber, squash, sweet peppers, or tomatoes.

**4 personalized pizzas**
Set up a pizza-making station in the kitchen. Use whole-wheat English muffins, bagels, or pita bread as the crust. Have tomato sauce, low-fat cheese, and cut-up vegetables or fruits for toppings. Let kids choose their own favorites. Then pop the pizzas into the oven to warm.

**5 fruity peanut butterfly**
Start with carrot sticks or celery for the body. Attach wings made of thinly sliced apples with peanut butter and decorate with halved grapes or dried fruit.

**6 frosty fruits**
Frozen treats are bound to be popular in the warm months. Just put fresh fruits such as melon chunks in the freezer (rinse first). Make "popsicles" by inserting sticks into peeled bananas and freezing.

**7 bugs on a log**
Use celery, cucumber, or carrot sticks as the log and add peanut butter. Top with dried fruit such as raisins, cranberries, or cherries, depending on what bugs you want!

**8 homemade trail mix**
Skip the pre-made trail mix and make your own. Use your favorite nuts and dried fruits, such as unsalted peanuts, cashews, walnuts, or sunflower seeds mixed with dried apples, pineapple, cherries, apricots, or raisins. Add whole-grain cereals to the mix, too.

**9 potato person**
Decorate half a baked potato. Use sliced cherry tomatoes, peas, and low-fat cheese on the potato to make a funny face.

**10 put kids in charge**
Ask your child to name new veggie or fruit creations. Let them arrange raw veggies or fruits into a fun shape or design.

USDA United States Department of Agriculture Center for Nutrition Policy and Promotion

Go to www.ChooseMyPlate.gov for more information.

DG TipSheet No. 11
June 2011
*USDA is an equal opportunity provider and employer.*

**FIGURE 20.1** Kid-friendly veggies and fruits—10 tips for making healthy foods more fun for children. (Available at http://www.choosemyplate.gov/food-groups/downloads/TenTips/DGTipsheet11KidFriendlyVeggiesAndFruits.pdf.)

## VITAMIN–MINERAL SUPPLEMENTS

A basic premise of the 2010 Dietary Guidelines for Americans is that nutrient needs should be met primarily through consuming foods. Foods in nutrient-dense and mostly intact forms contain not only the essential vitamins and minerals often contained in supplements but also dietary fiber and other naturally occurring substances that may have positive effects on health.[17] In certain cases, fortified foods and supplements may be useful in providing one or more nutrients that otherwise might be consumed in less than recommended amounts. Dietary supplements may be recommended in some cases, but they cannot replace a healthful diet.[17]

According to the American Academy of Pediatrics, routine supplementation is not necessary for healthy growing children who consume a varied diet.[18] If parents wish to give supplements to their children, a standard pediatric vitamin–mineral product with nutrients in amounts no larger than the DRI (EAR or RDA) poses no risk; however, megadose levels should be discouraged due to potential toxic effects. Parents should be cautioned to keep vitamin–mineral supplements out of the reach of children because the taste, shape, and color of most pediatric preparations make them quite appealing to children.[18]

Although the American Academy of Pediatrics advocates that routine vitamin–mineral supplementation is *not* necessary for healthy growing children who eat a varied

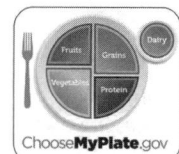

**10 tips**
*Nutrition*
*Education Series*

# cut back on your kid's sweet treats

**10 tips** to decrease added sugars

ChooseMyPlate.gov

**Limit the amount of foods and beverages with added sugars your kids eat and drink.** If you don't buy them, your kids won't get them very often. Sweet treats and sugary drinks have a lot of calories but few nutrients. Most added sugars come from sodas, sports drinks, energy drinks, juice drinks, cakes, cookies, ice cream, candy, and other desserts.

**1 serve small portions**
It's not necessary to get rid of all sweets and desserts. Show kids that a small amount of treats can go a long way. Use smaller bowls and plates for these foods. Have them share a candy bar or split a large cupcake.

**2 sip smarter**
Soda and other sweet drinks contain a lot of sugar and are high in calories. Offer water, 100% juice, or fat-free milk when kids are thirsty.

**3 use the check-out lane that does not display candy**
Most grocery stores will have a candy-free check-out lane to help moms out. Waiting in a store line makes it easy for children to ask for the candy that is right in front of their faces to tempt them.

**4 choose not to offer sweets as rewards**
By offering food as a reward for good behavior, children learn to think that some foods are better than other foods. Reward your child with kind words and comforting hugs, or give them non-food items, like stickers, to make them feel special.

**5 make fruit the everyday dessert**
Serve baked apples, pears, or enjoy a fruit salad. Or, serve yummy frozen juice bars (100% juice) instead of high-calorie desserts.

**6 make food fun**
Sugary foods that are marketed to kids are advertised as "fun foods." Make nutritious foods fun by preparing them with your child's help and being creative together. Create a smiley face with sliced bananas and raisins. Cut fruit into fun and easy shapes with cookie cutters.

**7 encourage kids to invent new snacks**
Make your own snack mixes from dry whole-grain cereal, dried fruit, and unsalted nuts or seeds. Provide the ingredients and allow kids to choose what they want in their "new" snack.

**8 play detective in the cereal aisle**
Show kids how to find the amount of total sugars in various cereals. Challenge them to compare cereals they like and select the one with the lowest amount of sugar.

**9 make treats "treats," not everyday foods**
Treats are great once in a while. Just don't make treat foods an everyday thing. Limit sweet treats to special occasions.

**10 if kids don't eat their meal, they don't need sweet "extras"**
Keep in mind that candy or cookies should not replace foods that are not eaten at meal time.

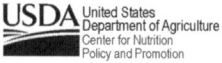

USDA United States Department of Agriculture Center for Nutrition Policy and Promotion

Go to www.ChooseMyPlate.gov for more information.

DG TipSheet No. 13
June 2011
*USDA is an equal opportunity provider and employer.*

**FIGURE 20.2** Cut back on your kid's sweet treats—10 tips to decrease added sugars. (Available at http://www.choosemyplate.gov/food-groups/downloads/TenTips/DGTipsheet13CutBackOnSweetTreats.pdf.)

diet, it does identify groups of children at nutritional risk who may benefit from supplementation;[18] these groups are identified in Table 20.14. Dietary intake over several days should be assessed by a registered dietitian to determine if an individual child from one of these groups needs to take a supplement.

## LEARNING TO EAT

Widespread evidence indicates that the nutrition guidelines are not being followed by most Americans.[28–31] Furthermore, the prevalence of obesity among children and adolescents increased dramatically between 1976–1980 and 1999–2000 (although between 1999–2000 and 2007–2008, there was no significant trend in obesity prevalence for any age group).[32–35] To help understand why children eat less of what is recommended by nutrition guidelines and more of what is not recommended, Birch and Fisher[36] recommend that consideration be given to factors that impact children's food preferences and consumption patterns. Extensive evidence suggests that children's food preferences are shaped by early experience with food and eating and that family environment and practices used by parents and other adults (e.g., school staff and caregivers) may permanently affect dietary practices of children.[37]

## 10 tips
*Nutrition Education Series*

# be a healthy role model for children

**10 tips** for setting good examples

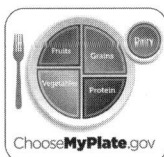

ChooseMyPlate.gov

**You are the most important influence on your child.** You can do many things to help your children develop healthy eating habits for life. Offering a variety of foods helps children get the nutrients they need from every food group. They will also be more likely to try new foods and to like more foods. When children develop a taste for many types of foods, it's easier to plan family meals. Cook together, eat together, talk together, and make mealtime a family time!

**1 show by example**
Eat vegetables, fruits, and whole grains with meals or as snacks. Let your child see that you like to munch on raw vegetables.

**2 go food shopping together**
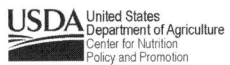
Grocery shopping can teach your child about food and nutrition. Discuss where vegetables, fruits, grains, dairy, and protein foods come from. Let your children make healthy choices.

**3 get creative in the kitchen**
Cut food into fun and easy shapes with cookie cutters. Name a food your child helps make. Serve "Janie's Salad" or "Jackie's Sweet Potatoes" for dinner. Encourage your child to invent new snacks. Make your own trail mixes from dry whole-grain, low-sugar cereal and dried fruit.

**4 offer the same foods for everyone**
Stop being a "short-order cook" by making different dishes to please children. It's easier to plan family meals when everyone eats the same foods.

**5 reward with attention, not food**
Show your love with hugs and kisses. Comfort with hugs and talks. Choose not to offer sweets as rewards. It lets your child think sweets or dessert foods are better than other foods. When meals are not eaten, kids do not need "extras"—such as candy or cookies—as replacement foods.

**6 focus on each other at the table**
Talk about fun and happy things at mealtime. Turn off the television. Take phone calls later. Try to make eating meals a stress-free time.

**7 listen to your child**
If your child says he or she is hungry, offer a small, healthy snack—even if it is not a scheduled time to eat. Offer choices. Ask "Which would you like for dinner: broccoli or cauliflower?" instead of "Do you want broccoli for dinner?"

**8 limit screen time**
Allow no more than 2 hours a day of screen time like TV and computer games. Get up and move during commercials to get some physical activity.

**9 encourage physical activity**
Make physical activity fun for the whole family. Involve your children in the planning. Walk, run, and play with your child—instead of sitting on the sidelines. Set an example by being physically active and using safety gear, like bike helmets.

**10 be a good food role model**
Try new foods yourself. Describe its taste, texture, and smell. Offer one new food at a time. Serve something your child likes along with the new food. Offer new foods at the beginning of a meal, when your child is very hungry. Avoid lecturing or forcing your child to eat.

USDA United States Department of Agriculture Center for Nutrition Policy and Promotion

Go to www.ChooseMyPlate.gov for more information.

DG TipSheet No. 12
June 2011
*USDA is an equal opportunity provider and employer.*

**FIGURE 20.3** Be a healthy role model for children—10 tips for setting good examples. (Available at http://www.choosemyplate.gov/food-groups/downloads/TenTips/DGTipsheet12BeAHealthyRoleModel.pdf.)

Birch et al.[38] have repeatedly found that exposure to novel foods, as well as the social environment in which food is eaten, are crucial in the development of preschool children's food preferences and consumption patterns. Children's food preferences are important because research indicates they are major determinants of consumption;[39–44] therefore, not eating certain items (such as vegetables) is related to low preferences. Parents, caregivers, and school staff need to expose children to a variety of healthful foods, provide opportunities for children to learn to like rather than dislike a variety of healthful foods, encourage children to respect their own feelings of hunger and satiety, and reduce the extent to which learning and experience potentiate children's liking for high-sugar and/or high-fat foods.[45] The two subsections that follow highlight research regarding the influence of learning on children's food preferences and consumption patterns.

## NEOPHOBIA (REJECTION OF NOVEL FOODS)

During pregnancy, flavors from a pregnant woman's diet are transmitted to amniotic fluid and swallowed by the fetus; thus, the types of food eaten by women during pregnancy and, hence, the flavor principles of their culture may be experienced by infants before birth and well before their first exposure to solid foods.[46] After birth and during the first years of life, an enormous amount of learning about food and eating occurs as infants transition from consuming only milk (i.e., breast milk or formula) to consuming a variety

**TABLE 20.14**

**Groups of Children at Nutritional Risk Who May Benefit from Vitamin–Mineral Supplementation**

Children from deprived families or who suffer parental neglect or abuse

Children with anorexia or an inadequate appetite or who consume fad diets

Children with chronic disease (e.g., cystic fibrosis, inflammatory bowel disease, and hepatic disease)

Children who participate in a dietary program to manage obesity

Children who consume a vegetarian diet without adequate dairy products

Children with failure to thrive

*Source:* Adapted from American Academy of Pediatrics (Committee on Nutrition), Feeding the Child, *Pediatric Nutrition Handbook*, 6th edn., Kleinman, R.E., ed., American Academy of Pediatrics, Elk Grove Village, IL, 2009, p. 145.

of foods[36] and from eating when hungry to eating due to a variety of social, cultural, environmental, or physiological cues.[47] According to Birch and Fisher,[36] this transition from univore to omnivore is shaped by the infant's innate preference for sweet and salty tastes and the rejection of sour and bitter tastes[48] and by the predisposition of infants and children to be neophobic or to reject novel foods.[49] In addition, a child's experience with food and flavors is shaped by the parents' decision to breastfeed or formula feed.[36] In a study by Sullivan and Birch,[50] 4- to 6-month-old infants were randomly assigned and fed one vegetable (either salted or unsalted peas or green beans) on 10 occasions over a 10-day period. Results showed that after 10 opportunities to consume the vegetable, all infants significantly increased their intake. Furthermore, although they did not differ initially, breastfed infants had greater increases in intake of the vegetable after exposure and an overall greater level of intake of the vegetable than formula-fed infants.

Table 20.15 provides an overview of three studies by Birch et al.[51–53] indicating that preschool children's neophobia (or rejection of novel [i.e., new, unfamiliar] foods) can be overcome by exposure. Results from these studies indicate that preschool children's food preferences, which are major determinants of consumption, are learned through repeated exposure to foods. Thus, although children may reject novel foods initially, parents and caregivers should continue to make them available to children.

Children's age is a factor when considering exposure to novel foods. Loewen and Pliner[54] found that for older (10- to 12-year-old) children, exposure to novel-good-tasting foods increased their willingness to taste novel foods compared to the familiar-good-tasting control, but exposure to novel-bad-tasting foods had no effect. In contrast, for younger (7- to 9-year-old) children, exposure to both novel-good-tasting and novel-bad-tasting foods decreased willingness to taste novel foods.[54]

Reluctance to try novel foods can be decreased by adding the familiar flavor principle (the distinctive combinations of seasonings that characterize many cuisines) to the unfamiliar food. For example, Pliner and Stallberg-White[55] found that 10- to 12-year-old children were more willing to try a novel food when it was accompanied by a familiar flavor principle than when it was served alone.

### SOCIAL ENVIRONMENT

The social environment of eating is crucial because children learn about what to eat and why to eat, and receive reinforcements and incentives for eating, from their families and the larger environment.[56] Most of this learning occurs during routine mealtime experiences, in the absence of formal teaching.[38] This section provides an overview of several studies that investigated various aspects of the social environment (e.g., rewards, choice offerings, modeling by adults, modeling by peers, and class challenges); Table 20.16 provides details for several of these studies in chronological order by year of publication.

**TABLE 20.15**

**Research Concerning Exposure to Novel Foods and Preschool Children's Food Preferences and Consumption**

| Year, Authors, and Reference No. | Subjects | Study Design | Results |
|---|---|---|---|
| 1982, Birch and Marlin [51] | 14 children age 2 years | Each child received 2–20 exposures to five novel fruits or cheeses over 25–26 days. | Children ate more of items with higher exposures when given pairs of items, tasted both, and picked one to consume. |
| 1987, Birch et al. [52] | 43 children in 3 age groups: 26, 38, or 64 months | Each child received 5, 10, or 15 exposures to seven new fruits and was asked to taste some and look at others. | For all age groups, preferences increased significantly only when foods were tasted. |
| 1990, Sullivan and Birch [53] | 39 children, ages 4–5 years | Each child tasted one of three versions of tofu (sweetened, salty, or plain) 15 times over several weeks. | Preferences increased with exposure regardless of added sugar, salt, or plain; 10 exposures were needed. |

**TABLE 20.16**

**Research (in Chronological Order by Year of Publication) Concerning the Social Environment and Children's Food Preferences and Consumption**

| Year, Authors, and Reference No. | Subjects | Description of Study | Results |
|---|---|---|---|
| 1980, Birch et al. [57] | 64 children ages 3–4 years; 16 per context | Children given sweet or nonsweet foods (of neutral preferences initially) over several weeks in one of four contexts: (1) as reward for behavior, (2) paired with adult greeting, (3) as nonsocial behavior (put in child's locker), or (4) at snack time. | Preferences increased when foods presented as rewards or paired with adult greeting; effects lasted longer than 6 weeks after contexts ended. Suggested positive social contexts can be used to increase preferences for foods not liked but more nutritious. |
| 1982, Birch et al. [58] | 12 children ages 3–5 years | Children told if they drank juice, then they could play. | Instrumental ("if") use of juice reduced preferences for it. |
| 1984, Birch et al. [59] | 31 children ages 3–5 years | Children told if they drank milk drink, then they received verbal praise or a movie. | Instrumental ("if") use of milk beverage reduced preferences for it. |
| 1992, Newman and Taylor, [60] | 86 children ages 4–7 years | Children told that if they ate one snack, then they could eat another snack (with both of neutral preference initially). | "If" snacks became less preferred and "then" snacks became more preferred. |
| 1999, Hendy [61] | 64 preschool children | To encourage acceptance of four new fruits and vegetables during three preschool lunches, teachers used one of five actions: (1) choice offering ("Do you want any of this?"), (2) reward (special dessert), (3) insisting children try one bite, (4) modeling by teacher, or (5) simple exposure. | Choice offering and reward were more effective than other actions. Hendy concluded that dessert rewards are not needed because the less expensive and more nutritious action of choice offering works as well. |
| 2000, Hendy and Raudenbush [69] | Study 1: 58 teachers of preschool children | Study 1: Teacher questionnaire to rate effectiveness of five teacher actions to encourage children's food acceptance. | Study 1: Teachers rated modeling as most effective over choice offering, insist, tangible reward, and exposure. |
| | Study 2: 18 boys, 16 girls (preschool) | Study 2: Familiar foods presented under silent teacher modeling or exposure. | Study 2: Silent teacher modeling ineffective to encourage acceptance of familiar foods. |
| | Study 3: 13 boys, 10 girls (preschool) | Study 3: Novel foods presented under silent teacher modeling or exposure. | Study 3: Silent teacher modeling ineffective to encourage acceptance of novel foods. |
| | Study 4: 12 boys, 14 girls (preschool) | Study 4: Novel foods presented under enthusiastic teacher modeling ("Mmm! I love mangos!") or exposure. | Study 4: Enthusiastic teacher modeling maintained novel food acceptance across five meals. |
| | Study 5: six boys, eight girls (preschool) | Study 5: Novel foods presented under enthusiastic teacher modeling versus peer modeling versus exposure. Preschool lunch was setting for Studies 2–5. Preferences assessed only for Study 5 and after 1-month delay. | Study 5: Boys ate and liked novel foods equally under all three conditions. Girls ate and liked novel foods most when modeled by peers. Enthusiastic teacher modeling ineffective if peer models were present; peer modeling more effective for girls than boys. |
| 2002, Hendy [70] | 38 preschool children | Three novel foods presented to eight tables of 38 children during five preschool lunches. After three baseline lunches, 16 of 38 children were trained to serve as peer models of food acceptance for one novel food in exchange for small toy rewards; each novel food was assigned to either girl model, boy model, or no model conditions for next two lunches. Remaining 22 of 38 children were observed, and their food bites were recorded during baseline and modeled lunches. | For children of either gender, girl models were more effective than boy models at increasing food acceptance by observed children from baseline to modeled lunches. One month later, neither food preferences nor consumption decreased for trained peer models, but both decreased for observed children. |

(continued)

**TABLE 20.16 (continued)**

**Research (in Chronological Order by Year of Publication) Concerning the Social Environment and Children's Food Preferences and Consumption**

| Year, Authors, and Reference No. | Subjects | Description of Study | Results |
|---|---|---|---|
| 2003, Wardle et al. [65] | 49 children ages 5–7 years | Randomized controlled design with children from three primary schools in London assigned to one of two intervention groups (exposure, reward) or no-treatment control group for a 2-week period with liking for, and consumption of, red pepper assessed before and after 2-week period. Children in each intervention group had eaten daily, individual sessions with those in exposure group offered a taste of red pepper and told they could eat as much as they liked, and those in reward group shown cartoon stickers and told they could pick one if they ate at least one piece of pepper. | Liking and consumption were increased for the exposure group compared to the control group. For the reward group, the outcomes were intermediate, lying between, and not significantly different from the exposure and control groups. Contrary to results from previous studies by others, the promise of a reward did not decrease liking. |
| 2003, Wardle et al. [62] | 156 children (mean age = 53 months; range from 34 to 82 months) and parents (95% mothers) who had participated in larger study (n = 564) of predictors of children's fruit and vegetable intake | Randomized controlled trial with parents of children assigned to one of three groups: exposure (offer child taste of target vegetable daily for 14 consecutive days; encourage tasting without offering rewards; keep "vegetable" diary with space for children to record liking using small "face" stickers after each tasting; modeling "taste" was suggested), information (nutritional advice and leaflet), or control (no treatment). | Only the exposure group had significant increases in liking, ranking, and consumption of the target vegetable from pre- to postintervention. The authors concluded that a parent-led, exposure-based intervention involving daily tasting of a vegetable, along with a daily vegetable "sticker" diary, holds promise for improving children's acceptance of vegetables. |
| 2004, Perry et al. [66] | Baseline—1668 children (in first or third grade); end (2 years later)—1168 of same children (in third or fifth grade); 26 schools (13 intervention, 13 delayed-program control); data collected on ~23 children per grade per school | Randomized controlled trial of school cafeteria-based intervention, which lasted two school years and included daily activities (increased availability, appeal, and encouragement of fruits and vegetables in lunch program and changes in lunch line and school snack cart) and special events (2-week kickoff campaign with posters, monthly samplings served at lunch by peers with help from parents, theater production, two challenge weeks when students competed to eat three fruit and vegetable daily lunch servings and classes rewarded at week's end with frozen fruit yogurt, final meal demonstration). | Students in intervention schools significantly increased total fruit intake by 0.14–0.17 servings at lunch with no differences for vegetables. Process measures indicated that verbal encouragement by food service staff was associated with outcomes. Authors concluded that environmental interventions alone may have limited impact without classroom and home (parental) activities, and interventions are needed that focus solely on vegetable intake among children. |
| 2005, Hendy et al. [67] | 188 children in first, second, or fourth grade at baseline | School cafeteria-based intervention. For 18 lunches (3/week), children (in classes) randomly assigned to receive token reinforcement for eating either fruits or vegetables. Lunch observers recorded intake and punched holes into nametags each day for children who ate assigned foods. Weekly during lunch, children traded token "punches" for small prizes. Preferences assessed with individual interviews at baseline and follow-up at 2 weeks and 7 months after program. | Fruit and vegetable consumption increased for all grades and lasted throughout the program. Preferences increased 2 weeks after the program for both fruits and vegetables but returned to baseline levels 7 months after the program. |

| | | | |
|---|---|---|---|
| 2005, Addessi et al. [71] | 27 children ages 2 to 5 years | Children's behaviors toward novel foods (cooked semolina, colored and flavored as yellow cumin, green caper, or red anchovy) were assessed when an adult model (1) was not eating (*presence* condition), (2) was eating food of different color (*different color* condition), and (3) was eating food of same color (*same color* condition). Adult models given same colored semolina but flavored with sugar so they would eat it enthusiastically. | Children accepted and ate novel food more in *same color* condition than in *different color* and in *presence* conditions. Children ate less food in first trial than in second and third trials. Authors concluded that "*social influences— together with repeated experiences with novelty—are a powerful instrument to promote the acceptance of novel foods in young children.*" |
| 2007, Johnson et al. [63] | 4 Head Start preschool centers (2 experimental [26 children], 2 control [20 children]) | Experimental sites received a 12-week social marketing intervention program to increase preschoolers' willingness to try new foods. Program consisted of child-driven nutrition activities, food-related children's storybooks, repeated opportunities to try new foods, activity outline to guide teachers, and parent newsletters. | Children at the experimental sites had increased preference for and willingness to try new foods. Authors concluded that "*a social marketing campaign is an effective method to reduce children's neophobia.*" |
| 2011, Cooke et al. [68] | 422 children ages 4–6 years in 16 classes at 8 schools | Cluster-randomized trial to examine children's acceptance of a disliked vegetable over 12 daily taste exposures. Exposures were paired with a tangible reward (sticker), social reward (praise), or no reward, and findings were compared with a no-treatment control condition immediately after the intervention and 1 and 3 months later. | Liking increased more in the three intervention conditions than in the control condition and with no significant differences between the intervention conditions; these effects were maintained 1 and 3 months later. Intake increased for both reward conditions and was maintained for 3 months. Intake increased for exposure with no reward but became nonsignificant by 3 months. Authors concluded that "*this large study demonstrated that rewarding children for tasting an initially disliked food produced sustained increases in acceptance, with no negative effects on liking.*" |
| 2012, Remington et al. [64] | 173 children ages 3–4 years | Families with children randomly assigned to exposure plus tangible reward (sticker), exposure plus social reward (praise), or no-treatment control. In intervention groups, parents offered their children 12 daily tastes of an initially liked vegetable and gave either sticker or praise for tasting. Researchers assessed liking and intake immediately after intervention and 1 and 3 months later. | Intake and liking of target vegetable increased significantly more for children in exposure plus tangible reward group than in control group, and differences were maintained at 3 months. Increases in intake and liking for exposure plus social reward group were not significantly different from control group. Authors concluded that "*a parent-delivered program combining repeated taste exposures with small rewards increases the acceptance of an initially disliked vegetable.*" |

The use of rewards to encourage children to eat healthily is controversial. For example, a 1980 study by Birch et al.[57] (see Table 20.16) found that when specific foods were used as rewards with preschool children, preferences for those "reward" foods were enhanced. In contrast, providing rewards to preschool children for consuming specific foods may result in later decreases in preferences for the foods that had to be consumed to obtain rewards, as illustrated in a 1982 study by Birch et al.,[58] a 1984 study by Birch et al.,[59] and a 1992 study by Newman and Taylor[60] (all described in Table 20.16). In a 1999 study by Hendy[61] (see Table 20.16), modeling by the teacher, insisting that children try a bite, and simple exposure were less effective than choice offering and reward of a special dessert to encourage acceptance of new fruits and vegetables during preschool lunches. A 2003 study by Wardle et al.[62] (see Table 20.16) found that preschool children's preferences for and consumption of vegetables can be enhanced if parents offer children daily tastes for 14 days and keep a daily vegetable "sticker" diary with children. A 2007 study by Johnson et al.[63] (see Table 20.16) found that a social marketing campaign was an effective method to increase preschool children's preference for and willingness to try new foods. A 2012 home-based study by Remington et al.[64] (see Table 20.16) found that parental use of tangible rewards (stickers) with repeated taste exposures (for 12 days) increased children's preferences and intake of initially disliked vegetables immediately after the intervention as well as 1 and 3 months later.

For elementary school children, research indicates that rewards, if used appropriately, may enhance consumption without negatively affecting preferences. A 2003 study by Wardle et al.[65] (see Table 20.16) found that exposure increased elementary school children's preferences and consumption more than rewards (stickers) but that the promise of a reward did not decrease preferences. A 2004 study by Perry et al.[66] (see Table 20.16) found that a 2-year, elementary school, cafeteria-based lunch intervention with daily activities (such as increased availability during lunch and encouragement by food service staff to select foods) and special events (including class competitions) increased fruit but not vegetable intake. A 2005 study by Hendy et al.[67] (see Table 20.16) indicated that token reinforcements (small prizes) provided to elementary school children for eating fruits or vegetables during school lunch did not result in decreased preferences during the program or 2 weeks after it ended. According to Hendy et al.,[67] the token reinforcement used in their program avoided the "overjustification effects" of later decreases in food preferences because it included three recommended components: (1) small and delayed reinforcement, (2) food choice along with the requirement to eat only a small amount, and (3) conditions that encourage peer participation and modeling. A 2011 study by Cooke et al.[68] (see Table 20.16) indicated that external rewards (stickers, praise) do not necessarily produce negative effects and may be useful in promoting healthful eating among children ages 4–6 years.

Research studies provide insight into the effect of modeling by adults and peers on young children's consumption. A series of small studies in 2000 by Hendy and Raudenbush[69] (see Table 20.16) suggest that to encourage preschool children's acceptance of novel foods, teachers should provide enthusiastic modeling, (Mmm! I love mangos!) rather than silent modeling, and avoid placing competing peer models at the same table with fussy eaters, especially girls. A small 2002 study by Hendy[70] (see Table 20.16) indicated that teachers may train preschool girls as peer models to encourage acceptance of novel foods by other preschool-age children during preschool meals; however, the modeling effects on novel food acceptance of observing children may not be present a month later. A small but well-controlled 2005 study by Addessi et al.[71] (see Table 20.16) demonstrated that adult modeling can positively impact preschool children's acceptance of "unusual" and novel foods (e.g., cooked semolina, colored red and flavored with anchovy). According to Nahikian-Nelms,[72] although caregivers may believe they positively influence children's eating behaviors, observed behaviors of caregivers at mealtimes were inconsistent with expert recommendations in a study of influential factors of caregiver behavior at lunch in early child-care programs.

Research indicates that infants are born with the ability to self-regulate their caloric intake by adjusting their formula intake when the caloric level of the formula changes[73] and when solid foods are added.[74] Preschool children are able to adjust the calories eaten in a snack or meal, based on the calories eaten in a preload snack.[75,76] Furthermore, preschool children are able to adjust the calories eaten at various meals and snacks during the day, so that the number of calories consumed in a 24 h period is relatively constant.[77]

Although children have the ability to self-regulate their caloric intake, well-conducted laboratory studies[78,79] indicate that this ability may be negatively impacted by child-feeding practices that encourage or restrict children's eating. Using observations of family mealtimes, Klesges et al.[80] found that parental prompts, especially encouragements to eat, were highly correlated to preschool children's relative weight and increased the probability that a child would eat. Furthermore, a child's refusal to eat usually led to a parental prompt to eat more food, whereas a child's food request was not likely to elicit either a parental prompt to eat or subsequent eating by the child. Results from a small but well-controlled study by Fisher and Birch[44] indicated that preschool children's preferences for dietary fat were positively related to their own triceps' skin-fold measurements, as well as to the composite BMI of their parents. Laboratory experiments with preschool children indicate that restricting access to palatable foods can sensitize children to external rather than internal eating cues and increase children's desire to obtain and consume the restricted foods.[81] For preschool girls (but not boys), child and maternal reports of restricting access were predictive of girls' snack food intake, with higher levels of snack food intake predicted by higher levels of restriction.[82] Child-feeding practices have been found to be key behavioral variables that explain more of the variance in children's total fat mass than energy intake.[83] Among girls, longitudinal data provide evidence that maternal restriction can promote over-eating in the absence of hunger.[84]

The feeding style used by parents or adults is associated with children's intake and weight. Authoritative feeding is characterized by adults encouraging children to eat healthy foods and allowing children limited choices but not pressuring or forcing intake. Authoritarian feeding is characterized by adults attempting to control children's eating, for example, by telling children to clean their plates. Permissive feeding is characterized by adults providing little structure in feeding. An authoritative feeding style is recommended.[85] According to a 2011 review by Blissett,[86] evidence suggests that an authoritative feeding style is associated with better fruit and vegetable consumption in the childhood years. A 2008 review by Venture and Birch[87] reveals some well-established associations between aspects of parenting and children's eating and weight but limited evidence for the influence of parenting and feeding practices on children's eating and weight status. A 2004 study by Faith et al.[88] found that the relationship between parental feeding styles and BMI of children ages 5–7 years depended on child obesity predisposition, which suggests a gene–environment interaction. In other words, among children predisposed to obesity, elevated child weight appeared to elicit parental restrictive feeding practices, which in turn appeared to produce additional weight gain in children. According to a 2007 review by Savage et al.,[89] feeding strategies that are responsive to children's hunger and satiety cues, and which encourage children's attention to hunger and fullness, are needed to support self-regulation and thus promote healthy weight instead of excessive consumption.

Portion sizes have increased (see http://hin.nhlbi.nih.gov/portion/index.htm), and supersizing has happened with serving sizes at restaurants and in homes and with package sizes in grocery stores.[90,91] This is a problem because research indicates that adults consume more from large containers than medium containers.[92] According to Wansick and Van Ittersum,[90] the answer to this problem is not simply education, but the elimination of large packages, large servings, and large dinnerware from our lives.

Research indicates interesting insight into the relationship between portion sizes and young children's intake. In a study by Rolls et al.,[93] 16 younger (3 years of age) and 16 older (5 years of age) preschool children participated in three lunches during their usual lunchtime at day care. Each lunch consisted of macaroni and cheese served in small, medium, or large portion sizes, along with set portion sizes of carrot sticks, applesauce, and milk. Results indicated that older preschoolers consumed more macaroni and cheese when served the large portion compared to the small portion. However, portion sizes did not significantly affect food intake among younger preschoolers. These results indicate the important role of portion size in shaping children's dietary intake and imply that portion size can either promote or prevent the development of overweight among older preschool children. Furthermore, these results indicate the importance of encouraging preschool children to focus on their own internal cues of hunger and satiety instead of "eating everything to clean the plate."[93]

Fisher et al.[94] extended the previous investigation in a study with 30 children ages 3–5 years who participated in a series of lunches once a week for 12 weeks during their usual lunchtime at day care. Each lunch consisted of an entrée of macaroni and cheese served either as an age-appropriate portion, a large portion that was double the size of the age-appropriate one, or a portion self-served by the child, along with standard portion sizes of carrots, applesauce, milk, and sugar cookies. Results indicated that doubling an age-appropriate portion of the entrée increased entrée and total lunch energy intakes by 25% and 15%, respectively. Changes were attributable to increases in children's average bite size of the entrée without compensatory decreases in the intake of other foods served at the lunch. Children's average self-served portion size did not differ significantly from the size of the age-appropriate portion served to them. Furthermore, when the children served their own entrée, they ate 25% less of it than when they were served a large entrée portion. According to the authors, their results "provide initial evidence that allowing children to self-select portion sizes can affect the amount consumed and may play an important role in reducing the effects of exposure to large portion sizes on children's intake."[94]

McConahy et al.[95] analyzed data from 1994 to 1996 and 1998 of the Continuing Survey of Food Intakes by Individuals for children ages 2–5 years to evaluate the relationship of portion size for 10 commonly eaten foods, number of eating occasions per day, and number of foods consumed per day with children's total energy intake. Results indicated that body weight accounted for only 4% of the variability in energy intake in contrast to food portion size, number of eating occasions, and number of foods that accounted for 17%–19%, 9%, and 6%–8%, respectively. The authors concluded that feeding recommendations for children should focus on moderation in portion sizes as well as frequent feeding.[95]

## DIVISION OF FEEDING RESPONSIBILITY

Satter advocates a division of feeding responsibility in which parents (or adults) present a variety of nutritious and safe foods at regular snack- and meal-times and provide the physical and emotional setting of eating, and children ultimately decide how much and whether to eat on a given eating occasion.[96–98] The American Academy of Pediatrics endorses the division of feeding responsibility as a sound basis for implementing appropriate child-feeding practices.[18] The following seven points summarize the American Academy of Pediatrics' feeding guidance for parents (or adults): First, choose foods and offer them repeatedly (up to 10 times) and patiently to establish children's acceptance of the foods. Second, set mealtime routines (because children need a daily routine of three meals and two snacks). Third, create positive mealtime environments that are free of distractions (such as television and loud music) with appropriate physical components (such as tables, chairs, utensils, and cups). Fourth, model behaviors for children to learn (such as consuming a varied and healthy diet). Fifth, regard mealtime as a time of learning and mastery with respect to eating and social skills as well as respect to family and community time. Sixth, let children decide which of the foods (that are provided by parents) that they will consume and how much they will eat. Seventh, pressuring children to eat or rewarding children for eating certain foods is ultimately counterproductive.[18]

## CAFFEINE, SPORTS DRINKS, AND ENERGY DRINKS

Caffeine is a stimulant for the central nervous system; it tends to decrease drowsiness and reduce the sense of fatigue, but too much can cause palpitations, stomach upset, insomnia, and anxiety. Its effects vary among individuals, depending on the amount ingested, body size of the individual, and personal tolerance. Some people are able to build up a tolerance to caffeine through regular use; others are more sensitive to it. If someone who has regularly consumed caffeine suddenly stops using it, mild withdrawal symptoms (e.g., headaches and craving for caffeine) may occur. Substantial amounts of caffeine are found in several soft drinks, coffee, tea, and some pain relievers; smaller amounts are found in chocolate and foods with cocoa.

Consumption of caffeine increases during adolescence with greater intakes of soft drinks, tea, and coffee. This can be a concern because the stimulating effect of caffeine may set the stage for needing stimulation; although caffeine is classified as a drug, society is very accepting of this stimulant and has not considered it a nuisance.[99]

A clinical report published in 2011 by the American Academy of Pediatrics[100] addresses the appropriateness of sports drinks and energy drinks for children and adolescents. Key points in this report include the following: (1) sports drinks and energy drinks are significantly different products, (2) sports drinks and energy drinks are being marketed to children and adolescents for a wide variety of inappropriate uses, (3) caffeine and other stimulant substances contained in energy drinks have no place in the diet of children and adolescents, and (4) frequent or excessive intake of caloric sports drinks can substantially increase the risk of overweight or obesity in children and adolescents.[100]

## NUTRITIVE AND NONNUTRITIVE SWEETENERS

Although there are widespread beliefs that both sugar (i.e., sucrose) and nonnutritive sweeteners (e.g., aspartame) produce hyperactivity and other behavioral problems in children, both dietary challenge and dietary replacement studies have demonstrated that sugar has little if any adverse effects on behavior.[101] For example, Wolraich et al.[102] conducted a double-blind controlled trial with 23 primary-school children (6–10 years of age) reported by their parents as sensitive to sugar and 25 normal preschool children (3–5 years of age) reported by their parents as *not* sensitive to sugar. The different diets that children and their families followed for each of three consecutive 3-week periods were high either in sucrose, aspartame, or saccharin (placebo). Children's behavior and cognitive performance were evaluated weekly. Results strongly indicated that even when intake exceeded typical dietary levels, neither sucrose nor aspartame had discernible cognitive or behavioral effects in normal

preschool children or in school-age children who were believed to be sensitive to sugar. Furthermore, the few differences associated with the ingestion of sucrose were more consistent with a slight calming effect than with hyperactivity.[102] Results from a 1995 meta-analytic synthesis of 16 reports containing 23 controlled double-blind challenge studies found that sugar did not affect the behavior or cognitive performance of children; however, due to the small number of studies, power was low to detect a small effect of sugar or to detect differential effects of sugar on subsets of children.[103] A review published in 2004 stated that sugar does not affect behavior or cognition in children with or without attention-deficit/hyperactivity disorder.[104]

According to Kanarek,[101] the strong belief of parents, educators, and medical professionals that sugar has adverse effects on children's behavior may be attributed to several factors. First, adults may misconceive the relationship between sugar and behavior. Children in general have difficulty altering their behavior in response to changing environmental conditions, such as shifting from the unstructured nature of a party or snack time at school to the more rigorous demands of class work. If the party or snack included foods with high-sugar content, adults may relate the child's sugar intake with behavioral problems as the child tries to adapt from an unstructured activity to one with structure. Second, sugar-containing foods such as candy are often forbidden or given to children in very limited amounts; the prohibited nature of these foods may contribute to the belief that associates them with increased activity. Finally, expectations of both adults and children could promote the idea that sugar leads to hyperactivity. Children hear adults comment that "too much sugar makes children hyper" and children believe them and act accordingly to fulfill the prophecy.[101]

Although experimental evidence fails to indicate that sugar affects children's behavior and cognition, children should not have unlimited access to sugar because undernutrition may occur if foods with essential nutrients are replaced by calories from sugar; furthermore, sugar (and starch) can promote tooth decay. According to *MyPlate*,[105] the major food and beverage sources of added sugars for Americans are regular soft drinks, energy drinks, and sports drinks; candy; cakes; cookies; pies and cobblers; sweet rolls, pastries, and donuts; fruit drinks such as fruitades and fruit punch; and dairy desserts such as ice cream. The 2010 Dietary Guidelines for Americans[17] acknowledge that the body metabolizes added sugars and natural sugars found in fruits and dairy foods the same but that typically foods high in added sugars are higher in energy and lower in essential nutrients or dietary fiber. Recommendations related to added sugars from 2010 Dietary Guidelines for Americans[17] include the following: (1) reduce calories from solid fats and added sugars (SoFAS) and (2) limit the consumption of foods that contain refined grains, especially refined grain foods that contain SoFAS and sodium. According to the DRIs, added sugars should be limited to no more than 25% of total energy, after which dietary quality might be reduced.[9]

Nutritive sweeteners contain carbohydrate and provide energy, while nonnutritive sweeteners are sweetened with minimal or no carbohydrate or energy. Seven nonnutritive sweeteners approved for use in the United States are acesulfame K, aspartame, luo han guo fruit extract, neotame, saccharin, stevia, and sucralose; they have different functional properties that may affect perceived taste or use in different food applications. The position of the Academy of Nutrition and Dietetics concerning the use of nutritive and nonnutritive sweeteners is that "consumers can safely enjoy a range of nutritive and nonnutritive sweeteners when consumed within an eating plan that is guided by current federal nutrition recommendations, such as the Dietary Guidelines for Americans and the Dietary Reference Intakes, as well as individual health goals and personal preference."[106]

The 2010 Dietary Guidelines for Americans[17] contain few statements concerning the use of nonnutritive sweeteners. A key recommendation related to the use of nonnutritive sweeteners is to control total energy intake and increase physical activity to manage body weight; although substituting nonnutritive sweeteners for higher-energy foods and beverages can decrease energy intake, evidence of their effectiveness for weight management is limited.[17]

## MEDIA INFLUENCES

Children's food preferences and consumption patterns can be altered either positively or negatively by media and advertising. Youth are the target of intense and specialized food marketing and advertising efforts via television advertising, in-school marketing, the Internet, toys and products with brand logos, product placements, kids clubs, and youth-targeted promotions.[107] However, foods marketed to youth are predominantly high in fat and sugar, which is inconsistent with dietary recommendations. For example, a 2005 study by Harrison and Marske[108] found that snacks, convenience foods, fast foods, and sweets dominated food advertisements aired during television programs heavily viewed by children. Furthermore, advertised foods exceeded recommended daily values for total fat, saturated fat, and sodium but failed to provide recommended daily values for fiber, vitamin A, vitamin C, calcium, and iron.[108] A review by Story and French[107] examined the food advertising and marketing channels used to target youth in the United States, the impact on eating behavior of food advertising, and current regulations and policies. A 2004 Kaiser Family Foundation issue brief reviewed more than 40 studies and explored what is and is not known about the role of media in the dramatically increasing rates of childhood obesity in the United States.[109] It outlines media-related policy options that have been proposed to help address this important public health problem, such as decreasing the time children spend with media to reducing their exposure to food advertising. In addition, it identifies ways in which media could play a positive role in helping address childhood obesity, such as increasing the number of media messages that promote fitness and sound nutrition.[109] A 2006 study by Wiecha et al.[110] found that increases in television viewing were associated with increased caloric intake among youth; the association was mediated by increased consumption of calorie-dense, low-nutrient foods frequently advertised on television. In 2006, the Kaiser Family Foundation released the first comprehensive analysis of the nature and scope of online food advertising to children; the

report found that 85% of the top food brands that target children through television advertising also use branded websites to market to children online.[111] A 2007 Kaiser Family Foundation report concerning television food advertising to children found that children ages 2–7 years, 8–12 years, and 13–17 years see an average of 12, 21, and 17 food ads per day on television, respectively, which, over the course of a year, translates to an average of more than 4400, 7600, and 6000 food ads per year, respectively.[112] A 2010 report of a national survey by the Kaiser Family Foundation found that with technology allowing almost 24 h media access, the amount of time children and teens spend with entertainment media has risen dramatically, especially among minority youth.[113] According to the 2010 Dietary Guidelines for Americans,[17] a strategy to help create and promote healthy lifestyles for children is to develop and support effective policies to limit food and beverage marketing to children.

## VEGETARIAN DIETS

There is considerable variation in the eating patterns of vegetarians. For the lacto–ovo vegetarian, the eating pattern is based on grains, vegetables, fruits, legumes, seeds, nuts, dairy products, and eggs; meat, fish, and fowl are excluded. For the vegan or total vegetarian, the eating pattern is similar to the lacto–ovo vegetarian pattern except for the additional exclusion of eggs, dairy, and other animal products. However, considerable variation may exist in the extent to which animal products are avoided within both of these patterns.[114]

The position of the American Dietetic Association (the Academy of Nutrition and Dietetics as of January 2012) concerning vegetarian diets is that "appropriately planned vegetarian diets, including total vegetarian or vegan diets, are healthful, nutritionally adequate, and may provide health benefits in the prevention and treatment of certain diseases. Well-planned vegetarian diets are appropriate for individuals during all stages of the life cycle, including pregnancy, lactation, infancy, childhood, and adolescence, and for athletes."[114] Vegetarian children can be helped to meet energy and nutrient needs by eating frequent meals and snacks, as well as by using some refined foods (e.g., fortified breakfast cereals, breads, pasta) and foods higher in unsaturated fat.[114] Food guides for vegetarian children have been published.[115] For adolescent vegetarians, key nutrients of concern include calcium, vitamin D, iron, zinc, and vitamin $B_{12}$.[114]

## FEEDING TODDLERS AND PRESCHOOL CHILDREN

Children depend on adults to offer them a variety of nutritious and developmentally appropriate foods. Many parents become anxious about the adequacy of their young child's diet or frustrated with their child's unpredictable eating behavior, which may include refusals to eat certain foods and food jags (i.e., when children want to eat only a few foods day after day). Table 20.17 contains suggestions for concerns that parents may commonly encounter when feeding young children.

**TABLE 20.17**

**Suggestions for Concerns Parents Commonly Encounter when Feeding Young Children**

*If a child refuses to try new foods or refuses to eat what is served …*

Remember, this is normal! Continue to offer each new food 10–12 times, twice per week.

Serve a new food with familiar ones.

Ask the child if she or he would like to try some of the new food. Be an effective role model and enthusiastically eat some of the new food yourself; comment to the child about how much you like it.

Involve the child in shopping for and preparing food, and in setting and clearing the table.

Remember, a child may have strong likes and dislikes, but this does *not* mean that she or he needs to be served different foods than the rest of the family.

Allow the child to choose what she or he will eat from the foods available at a meal, but avoid forcing or bribing him or her to eat.

Include at least one food at each meal that you know the child will eat, but do not cater to a child's likes or dislikes. Avoid becoming a short-order cook. The less attention paid to this behavior, the better.

Avoid pressuring, coaxing, bribing, or nagging the child to eat.

Attempt to have family meals be as pleasant as possible by avoiding arguments and criticism. Use the child's developmental stage to determine expectations for manners and neatness while at the same time setting limits on inappropriate behaviors (such as throwing food).

Let the child determine when she or he is full and has had enough instead of insisting that she or he clean the plate.

Schedule meals at regular times. Avoid having a child get too hungry or too tired before mealtime. Snacks should be 1.5–2 h before meals.

*If a child is stuck on a food jag or wants to eat the same food over and over …*

A child may want to eat only one or two foods day after day, meal after meal; common food jags occur with peanut butter and jelly sandwiches, pizza, macaroni and cheese, and dry cereal with milk.

Relax, and realize this is normal and temporary. Refuse to call attention to the behavior.

Continue to offer regular meals, but do not force or bribe the child to eat them.

Serve the food jag item as you normally would (maybe once or twice a week).

*If a child refuses to eat meat …*

Tough meat is often difficult for a child to chew. Offer bite-size pieces of tender, moist meat, poultry, or boneless fish.

Use meat in casseroles, meatloaf, soup, spaghetti sauce, pizza, or burritos.

Try other high-protein foods such as eggs, legumes, and peanut butter.

*If a child refuses to drink milk or drinks too little milk…*

Offer cheese, cottage cheese, yogurt, or pudding either alone or in combination dishes (such as macaroni and cheese, pizza, cheese sauce, banana pudding).

Use milk when cooking hot cereals, scrambled eggs, macaroni and cheese, soup, and other recipes.

Offer flavored milks.

Use calcium-fortified juices.

*If a child drinks too much milk or juice …*

Offer water between meals to quench thirst.

Limit milk to one serving with meals or at the end of meals, and offer water for seconds.

*If a child refuses to eat vegetables and fruits …*

Offer more fruits if a child refuses vegetables, and vice versa.

Avoid overcooking vegetables; serve vegetables steamed or raw (if appropriate). Include dips or sauces (e.g., applesauce with broccoli or carrots).

Include vegetables in soups, casseroles, and pizza.

Add fresh or dried fruit to cold and hot cereals.

Continue to offer a variety of fruits and vegetables.

*If a child eats too many sweets …*

Avoid using sweets as a bribe or reward.

Limit the purchase and preparation of sweet foods in the home.

Incorporate sweets into meals instead of snacks for better dental health. Also, by serving desserts (if any) with the meal, they become less important and cannot be used as a reward.

Decrease sugar by half in recipes for muffins, quick breads, cookies, etc.

Try using fruit as dessert.

*Source:* Adapted from Lucas, B. and Ogata, B. Normal Nutrition from Infancy through Adolescence, *Handbook of Pediatric Nutrition*, 3rd edn., Samour, P.Q. and, King, K., eds., Jones and Bartlett, Boston, MA, 2005, pp. 107–130.

Most young children fare best when fed four to six times a day due to their smaller stomach capacities and fluctuating appetites. Snacks should be considered as mini-meals that contribute to the total day's nutrient intake. Snacks generally accepted by many children include fresh fruit, cheese, whole-grain crackers, breads (e.g., bagels and tortillas), low-fat milk, raw vegetables, 100% fruit juices, sandwiches on whole-grain breads, peanut butter on crackers or whole-grain bread, and yogurt.

Chewing and swallowing functions are not fully developed until 8 years of age; thus, precautions should be followed to avoid choking.[18] Foods most likely to become easily lodged in the esophagus, and, thus, to avoid, include round candy, nuts, raw carrots, and popcorn. Other potentially problematic foods (e.g., hot dogs, grapes, and string cheese) may be modified by cutting them into small strips. Any food can cause choking if the child is not supervised while eating, if the child runs while eating, or if too much food is stuffed in the mouth. Thus, an adult should always be present when children are eating; children should sit down while eating; and the mealtime environment, ideally, should be free of distractions such as television, loud music, and activities. Allowing children to eat in the car is discouraged because it can be difficult to help a choking child if the only adult present is driving.[18]

Children's consumption of fruit juice and other sweetened beverages should be monitored to avoid excess. The American Academy of Pediatrics recommends an upper limit per day of fruit juice of 4–6 oz for children ages 1–6 years, and 8–12 oz for children ages 7–18 years, and encourages children to eat whole fruits (instead of drinking fruit juice) to meet their recommended levels of daily fruit intake.[18]

## FEEDING SCHOOL-AGE CHILDREN AND ADOLESCENTS

During the school-age years (ages 6–12), steady growth is paralleled by increased food intake. Although children tend to eat fewer times a day, after-school snacks are common. Key eating and activity concerns for school-aged children include fruit and vegetable acceptance, high-energy snacks, beverages and foods with added sugar, low fiber intake, decreased milk consumption, television and screen time, and dieting and body image.[18]

Breakfast consumption plays an important role in general health and well-being of children and adolescents and is associated with nutritional adequacy, body weight, and cognitive and academic performance.[116] Studies indicate that eating breakfast is positively related to cognitive function and school performance, especially for undernourished children.[117,118] For example, schoolchildren who had fasted both overnight and in the morning, particularly children who were nutritionally at risk, demonstrated slower stimulus discrimination, increased errors, and slower memory recall.[119] Although eating breakfast is important, research indicates that between 6% and 16% of elementary school children skip breakfast.[120–122] Furthermore,

between 1965 and 1991, breakfast consumption declined significantly for each age group of children (1–4, 5–7, and 8–10 years) and adolescents (11–14 and 15–18 years), especially for older adolescents ages 15–18 years; breakfast was consumed by 90% of boys and 84% of girls in 1965 and by 75% and 65%, respectively, in 1991.[123] Children who skip breakfast tend to have a lower energy intake and consume fewer nutrients than children who eat breakfast.[120,122] During the second decade of life, breakfast skipping tends to increase, perhaps due to time constraints or lack of appetite in the morning.

Adolescents have unique nutritional needs because they grow and develop at a different rate than children. Adolescents experience newly found independence, busy schedules, search for self-identification, dissatisfaction with body image, difficulty accepting existing values, a desire for peer acceptance, and a need to conform to the adolescent lifestyle.[124] Each of these events may help explain changes in food habits of adolescents. Common characteristics of food habits of adolescents include an increased tendency to skip meals (especially breakfast and lunch), eating more meals outside the home, increased snacking (especially on candy), consumption of fast foods, and dieting.[124] Aspects of poor nutrition that are related to the adolescent's diet include (1) energy intake needs, which vary with physical activity levels and stage of maturation; (2) protein needs, which correlate more closely with growth pattern than chronologic age; (3) increased calcium needs due to accelerated muscular and skeletal growth; (4) increased iron needs to sustain increasing lean body mass and hemoglobin mass, as well as menstrual losses in female adolescents; (5) zinc needs for growth and sexual maturation; (6) vegetarianism, which excludes all animal products, that can increase vulnerability to deficiencies of several nutrients, especially vitamin D, vitamin $B_{12}$, riboflavin, protein, calcium, iron, zinc, and possibly other trace minerals; (7) dental caries; and (8) obesity.[124] Teen pregnancy causes additional stress on the nutritional status of the growing and maturing adolescent.[124]

With regard to long-term bone health, adolescence is of utmost importance. Factors that influence bone growth and mineral accretion during adolescence include genetics, hormonal status, exercise, adequacy of dietary calcium, adequacy of vitamin D, and general nutrition and health. Trends during adolescence that are detrimental to good bone health include a general decline in dairy intake, decreased physical activity, and increased screen time.[124]

Evidence of a strong positive association between frequency of family meals and quality of dietary intake among adolescents was provided by a 2003 study that included 4746 middle- and high-school students of diverse racial and socioeconomic backgrounds who attended public schools in Minneapolis/St. Paul.[125] Variability in the frequency of family meals during the previous week was wide and ranged from never (14%), one or two times (19%), three or four times (21%), five or six times (19%), seven times (9%), and more than seven times (18%). Sociodemographic characteristics associated with more frequent family meals included socio-economic status (high), mother's employment status (not employed), race (Asian American), school level (middle), and sex (boy). Frequency of family meals was negatively associated with soft drink consumption and positively associated with intake of calcium-rich foods, grains, fruits, and vegetables. Because of the important role family meals appear to play in promoting healthful dietary intake among adolescents, feasible ways of increasing the frequency of family meals need to be explored with adolescents and their families.[125]

Story et al.[126] proposed an ecological model to help understand and explain the numerous and interacting influences on adolescent eating behavior. Four levels of influence described include individual or intrapersonal (such as biological and psychosocial), social environmental or interpersonal (such as peers and family), physical environmental or community settings (such as school, fast-food restaurants, and convenience stores), and macrosystem or societal (such as social and cultural norms, mass media, marketing, and advertising). Interventions that address factors at these different levels of influence, as well as complement and build on each other, are needed to improve eating behaviors of youth.[126]

## GROUP FEEDING

Many young children spend some or most days away from home in child-care centers, preschools, Head Start programs, or home child-care centers where they may eat up to two meals and two snacks daily. Federal and state regulations or guidelines exist for food service in child-care centers, Head Start programs, and preschool programs in public schools. Some centers participate in USDA-sponsored child nutrition programs. When choosing a child-care center or preschool, parents should be encouraged to consider the feeding program, including food variety, quality, safety, cultural aspects, and developmental appropriateness. It is the position of the American Dietetic Association (the Academy of Nutrition and Dietetics as of January 2012) concerning benchmarks in nutrition for child care that "child-care programs should achieve recommended benchmarks for meeting children's nutrition needs in a safe, sanitary, and supportive environment that promotes optimal growth and development."[127] That position statement provides guidance for food and nutrition practitioners, health professionals, and child-care providers regarding recommendations (which target children ages 2–5 years attending child-care programs) for nutritional quality of foods and beverages served; menus, meal patterns, and portion sizes; food preparation and service; physical and social environment; nutrition training; nutrition consultation; physical activity and active play; and working with families.[127]

Children have acquired knowledge about eating and have developed food preferences by the time they enter school; however, their food preferences and consumption patterns are continually modified because they eat daily.[128] More than 95% of children in the United States are enrolled in school,

where they may eat one or two meals per school day.[129] One in 10 children gets two of their three major meals in school, and more than half get one of their three major meals in school.[130] Thus, schools play a critical role in shaping children's food acceptance patterns and can, therefore, help improve their dietary intake.[131] No other public institution has as much continuous and intensive contact with children during their first two decades of life than public schools.[132] School staff have a greater potential influence on a child's health than any other group outside of the home.[133] School-based programs offer a systematic and efficient means to improve the health of youth in the United States by promoting positive lifestyles.[134] Health promotion programs in schools have the potential to help prevent chronic diseases in U.S. adults.[133] Although school-based health programs may promote healthful lifestyles, classroom lessons are not sufficient to produce lasting changes in students' eating behaviors.[56] In fact, curriculum-based nutrition education in schools has had minimal effects on student's eating behavior.[135] Children's food preferences and consumption are influenced by the school environment through familiarity and reinforcement.[136] Children in public schools generally attend for 7 h a day, 180 days a year. Although students have options for obtaining food in schools, the most prominent federally supported programs are the National School Lunch Program (NSLP) and the School Breakfast Program (SBP).

Concerning child and adolescent nutrition assistance programs, the position of the American Dietetic Association (the Academy of Nutrition and Dietetics as of January 2012) is that "children and adolescents should have access to an adequate supply of healthful and safe foods that promote optimal physical, cognitive, and social growth and development. Nutrition assistance programs, such as food assistance and meal service programs and nutrition education initiatives, play a vital role in meeting this critical need."[137]

### NATIONAL SCHOOL LUNCH PROGRAM AND SCHOOL BREAKFAST PROGRAM

The NSLP is a federally assisted meal program that operates in more than 101,000 public and nonprofit private schools and residential child-care institutions; it provides nutritionally balanced, free, low-cost, or full-price lunches to more than 31 million children each school day.[138] In 1998, Congress expanded the NSLP to include reimbursement for snacks served to children in after-school educational and enrichment programs.[138]

The SBP is a federally assisted meal program that operates in more than 88,000 public and nonprofit private schools and residential child-care institutions.[139] It provides nutritionally balanced, free, low-cost, or full-price breakfasts to more than 11.6 million children each school day.[139]

Regulations stipulate that NSLP lunches and SBP breakfasts meet the applicable recommendations of the Dietary Guidelines for Americans, which recommend no more than 30% of energy from fat and less than 10% of energy from saturated fat.[138,139] In addition, regulations stipulate that an

NSLP lunch provides one-third, and that an SBP breakfast provides one-fourth, of the RDAs for energy, protein, iron, calcium, and vitamins A and C.[130,139] Although NSLP lunches and SBP breakfasts must meet federal nutrition requirements, decisions about what specific foods to serve and how they are prepared are made by local school food authorities.[138,139]

Any child at a participating school may purchase an NSLP lunch or an SBP breakfast.[138,139] Children from families with incomes at or below 130% of the poverty level are eligible for free breakfasts and lunches. Children from families with incomes between 130% and 185% of the poverty level are eligible for reduced-price meals, for which students can be charged no more than 30 cents for breakfast and 40 cents for lunch. Children from families with incomes over 185% of the poverty level pay a full price, but their meals are still subsidized to some extent. Although local school food authorities set their own prices for full-price meals, they must operate their meal services as nonprofit programs. The majority of the support provided by the USDA to schools in the NSLP and SBP comes in the form of a cash reimbursement for each lunch or breakfast served that meets NSLP and SBP requirements, respectively; in addition, schools participating in the NSLP receive donated commodities from the USDA for each meal served.[138,139]

## SCHOOL MEALS INITIATIVE FOR HEALTHY CHILDREN AND TEAM NUTRITION

The USDA issued the final School Meals Initiative (SMI) for Healthy Children regulations in 1995 after the Healthy Meals for Healthy Americans Act of 1994 (P. L. No. 103–448, sec. 106, 1994) was passed; the SMI requires that meals in the NSLP and SBP meet the Dietary Guidelines for Americans, and thus SMI regulations define how the Dietary Guidelines are applied to school meals.[140]

Team Nutrition is USDA's integrated, behavior-based, comprehensive plan for promoting the nutritional health of the nation's children; the plan involves schools, parents, and communities in efforts to continuously improve school meals and to promote the health and education of 50 million school children in more than 96,000 schools nationwide.[141] The goal of Team Nutrition is "to improve children's lifelong eating and physical activity habits by using the principles of the Dietary Guidelines for Americans and MyPlate."[141] Schools are the focal point for Team Nutrition, and emphasis is placed on working through state agencies for training and technical assistance for healthy school meals, nutrition education, and partners and support. The focus of training and technical assistance is on planning and preparing healthy meals that appeal to children's ethnic/cultural taste preferences, linking meal programs to other educational activities, providing nutrition expertise and awareness to the school, and using sound business practices. Through interactive nutrition education, children are encouraged to eat a variety of foods; eat more fruits, vegetables, and whole grains; eat lower-fat foods more often; get calcium-rich foods; and be physically active. Team Nutrition is implemented through behavior-oriented

strategies that help school and community leaders adopt and implement school policies that promote healthy eating and physical activity, provide school resources adequate to achieve success, and foster school and community environments that support healthy eating and physical activity. A network of public and private organizations is used to promote Team Nutrition, develop and disseminate materials, leverage resources, expand the reach of messages, and build a broad base of support; the network includes private sector companies and nonprofit and advocacy organizations including nutrition, health, education, entertainment, and industry groups.[141]

Team Nutrition has developed resources to help foster healthy school nutrition environments. For example, Changing the Scene—Improving the School Nutrition Environment is a tool kit that addresses the entire school nutrition environment from a commitment to nutrition and physical activity, pleasant eating experiences, quality school meals, other healthy food options, nutrition education, and marketing the issue to the public.[142] The HealthierUS School Challenge was established in 2004 as a voluntary initiative to recognize schools participating in the NSLP that have created healthier school environments by promoting nutrition and physical activity.[143] In February 2010, First Lady Michelle Obama introduced the Let's Move! campaign and incorporated the HealthierUS School Challenge into her campaign to help raise a healthier generation of children.[144]

## SCHOOL NUTRITION DIETARY ASSESSMENT STUDIES

During the 1991–1992 school year, the first School Nutrition Dietary Assessment Study (SNDAS-I) collected information on school meals from a nationally representative sample of schools (n = 545) and 24 h recalls from approximately 3350 students from these schools.[145] Results from SNDAS-I regarding dietary intakes of NSLP participants and nonparticipants[146] indicated that (1) NSLP participants had higher lunch intakes of vitamin A, calcium, and zinc and lower intakes of vitamin C than nonparticipants who ate lunch; (2) NSLP participants' lunches provided a higher percentage of kcal from fat and saturated fat and a lower percentage of carbohydrate than nonparticipants' lunches; (3) NSLP participants were more than twice as likely as nonparticipants to consume milk and milk products at lunch; and (4) NSLP participants also consumed more meat, poultry, fish, and meat mixtures than nonparticipants. Results from SNDAS-I regarding dietary intakes of SBP participants and nonparticipants[146] indicated that (1) SBP participants had higher average breakfast intakes of kcal, protein, and calcium and derived a greater proportion of kcal from fat and saturated fat than nonparticipants; (2) SBP participants were three times more likely than nonparticipants to consume meat, poultry, fish, or meat mixtures at breakfast; and (3) SBP participants were also more likely than nonparticipants to consume milk or milk products at breakfast. The most surprising finding from SNDAS-I was that the presence of the SBP in schools did not affect the likelihood that a child ate breakfast before starting school.

Results from SNDAS-I indicated that approximately 42% of children who were eligible for free or reduced-price school breakfast did not eat it.[121]

During the 1998–1999 school year, SNDAS-II was conducted to provide information about how schools are progressing toward meeting nutrition standards of the SMI for Healthy Children (discussed previously in this chapter) and to provide information about menu planning practices used in school food service programs.[147] Data collection was primarily a mail survey completed by 1075 cafeteria managers who each provided data for meals served during a single week; in addition, a telephone interview was completed by 430 school food service directors, who provided supplementary information about district and school characteristics.[147] Results from SNDAS-II indicated that more than one in five elementary schools served lunches, which met the SMI standard for ≤30% of calories from fat, and about one in seven met the SMI standard for <10% of calories from saturated fat; for secondary schools, about one in seven schools met each of the SMI standards. Even when the average lunch served to (i.e., selected by) students did not meet the SMI standards for fat and saturated fat, 82% of elementary schools and 91% of secondary schools offered options that were consistent with these SMI standards. Lunches served in elementary and secondary schools provided more than a third of the recommended levels for all targeted nutrients, except in secondary schools where they fell short of providing one-third of the recommended level for calories. Breakfasts served were consistent with the SMI standard for calories from fat and came very close to meeting the SMI standard for calories from saturated fat. Breakfasts served in both elementary and secondary schools provided one-fourth or more of the recommended levels for all targeted nutrients but fell short of providing one-fourth of the recommended level of calories.[148] Results from SNDAS-II confirm the important role that school meals have toward helping youth achieve nutritional recommendations and that more research is needed to determine how to encourage more youth to actually select the healthful options available in schools.

During the 2004–2005 school year, SNDAS-III data were collected with a national sample of 129 school food authorities, 398 schools, and 2314 children.[149] School food authority directors provided information on district-wide policies. School food service managers completed a menu survey and a brief interview (telephone or in person). School principals were interviewed about school schedules, rules about student mobility, nutrition education, and availability of competitive foods outside the food service area. Study staff completed checklists based on observations of competitive foods. Children participated in a 24 h recall, responded to questions about their views of school meals, and had their weight and height measured. Key findings from SNDAS-III about school meals and competitive foods indicated that (1) NSLP lunches offered and served by most schools met USDA goals for target nutrients over a typical week and were lower in saturated fat than meals offered and served for SNDAS-II; (2) most schools offered and served SBP

breakfasts that met USDA standards; and (3) foods sold in competition with USDA school meals were widely available on campus, particularly in secondary schools. Key findings from SNDAS-III about students' dietary intake included the following: (1) NSLP participants consumed more nutrients at lunch and were more likely to have adequate usual daily intakes of key nutrients than nonparticipants; (2) breakfast intakes of SBP participants and nonparticipants were generally similar, as was the prevalence of inadequate usual daily intakes; and (3) competitive foods were consumed by fewer NSLP participants than nonparticipants, and the most popular choices for both groups were energy dense and relatively low in nutrients.[149]

Research is identifying methods to increase children's participation in the SBP.[150] A promising practice is district-wide "universal" school breakfast (which allows all students to eat school breakfast at no charge); this removes the stigma for low-income children to participate in the SBP. Another promising practice is making breakfast part of the school day (such as breakfast in the classroom); when breakfast is part of the school day, instead of a before-school activity, it is convenient and accessible to all, irrespective of tight bus schedules and how students arrive at school.[150]

## CHILDHOOD OBESITY AND PARTICIPATION IN SCHOOL-MEAL PROGRAMS

There is growing concern that childhood obesity may be related to participation in school-meal programs.[151–153] The growing body of literature on this topic has provided conflicting results, possibly because different studies have relied on different sources of participation information. For example, four studies of elementary school children that based participation on parental reports have found (1) a positive association between participation in the NSLP and BMI,[154] (2) no association between participation in the NSLP and overweight status,[155] (3) an inverse association between participation in the SBP and BMI and no association between participation in the NSLP and BMI,[156] and (4) a positive association between participation in the SBP and BMI but an inverse association between participation in the NSLP and BMI.[157] One study with fourth-grade children that based participation on school-district administrative daily records found no association between BMI and participation in the SBP and/or NSLP.[158] Another study with fourth-grade children that based participation on nametag records (compiled by research staff for school-meal observations) found no association between BMI and participation in the SBP and/or NSLP.[159]

Research on the accuracy of parental reports concerning their children's participation in school-provided meals is rather sparse; four studies that have investigated this topic warrant caution when using parental reports. For a 2002 article,[160] parental responses of fourth-grade children's usual participation in the SBP were compared to nametag records (compiled by research staff for direct meal observations); results showed that 24% of parents gave incorrect responses.

For a 2009 article,[161] when compared to school-district administrative records, parental responses concerning children's school-meal participation were more accurate for 1 day or 1 week's participation than for annual participation and more accurate for participation in the NSLP than for participation in the SBP. For a 2012 article, data from four cross-sectional studies conducted from fall 1999 to spring 2003 with fourth-grade children in Augusta, Georgia, were analyzed.[157] Those results showed that, compared to nametag records (compiled by research staff for direct observations of school-provided meals), although parental report accuracy was 74% for participation in the SBP and 92% for participation in the NSLP, there were disparate effects by children's age and race, with better parental report accuracy for older children for participation in the SBP and the NSLP and for Black than White children for participation in the NSLP.[157] For a submitted article,[162] misclassification of children's school-meal participation using parental reports was investigated relative to school-district administrative records; parental reports were fairly accurate for NSLP participation but not for SBP participation. As parents are usually not present when their children are at school, the use of parental reports concerning children's participation in school-provided meals may contribute to the conflicting results on the relationship between childhood obesity and school-meal participation.

Results from two studies[158,159] have suggested that children's energy intake at school-provided meals, rather than participation in them, may be related to obesity. For both studies, subjects were fourth-grade children, and weight and height were measured; also, for a subset of children, energy intake was assessed from direct observations of school-provided meals. The following paragraphs briefly summarize these two studies.

For one study,[158] Baxter and colleagues analyzed data collected from a dietary-reporting validation study with children in Columbia, South Carolina, to examine the relationship between BMI and school-meal participation (for 1571 children) and the relationship between BMI and energy intake at school-provided meals (for a subset of 465 children). The school district had implemented offer-versus-serve food service, so children could refuse meal components. Those results, published in 2010, showed that children's BMI was not significantly related to school-meal participation (assessed via daily administrative records from the school district), but energy intake at school meals was significantly and positively related to BMI.[158] To help explain that positive relationship, another article[163] investigated seven outcome variables concerning aspects of school-provided meals—energy content of items selected, number of meal components selected, number of meal components eaten, amounts eaten of standardized school-meal portions, energy intake from flavored milk, energy intake received in trades, and energy content given in trades. Results showed that BMI was (1) positively related to amounts eaten of standardized school-meal portions, (2) positively related to energy intake from flavored milk, and (3) negatively related to energy intake received in trades; there were no significant relationships with BMI for the other four outcome variables.[163]

In the other study,[159] Paxton et al. analyzed data collected from four cross-sectional dietary-reporting validation studies with children in Augusta, Georgia, to examine the relationship between BMI and school-meal participation (for 1535 children) and the relationship between BMI and energy intake at school-provided meals (for a subset of 342 children). The school district had not implemented offer-versus-serve food service, so children could not refuse meal components. Those results, published in 2012, showed that children's BMI was not significantly related to school-meal participation (assessed via nametag records compiled by research staff for direct meal observations); however, energy intake at school meals was significantly and positively related to BMI.[159] To help explain that positive relationship, an article[164] investigated the relationship between BMI and six aspects of school-provided meals—amounts eaten of standardized portions, energy content given in trades, energy intake received in trades, energy intake from flavored milk, energy intake from á la carte ice cream, and breakfast type (cold [i.e., ready-to-eat cereal, graham or animal crackers, milk, and juice or fruit] or hot [e.g., sausage biscuit, milk, and juice]). Results showed that BMI was positively related to amounts eaten of standardized portions and negatively related to energy content given in trades; there were no significant relationships with BMI for the other four aspects of school-provided meals.[164]

Additional studies are needed to provide further insight toward explaining the positive relationship between children's BMI and energy intake at school-provided meals.

## LOCAL WELLNESS POLICIES IN SCHOOL DISTRICTS

Federal legislation mandates that all school districts participating in the NSLP have local wellness policies.[165] Sample school wellness plans have been developed by the National Alliance for Nutrition and Activity,[166] and Action for Healthy Kids has a wellness policy tool with eight steps;[167] these resources can serve as guides for local school systems.

The position of the American Dietetic Association (the Academy of Nutrition and Dietetics as of January 2012) concerning local support for nutrition integrity in schools is that "schools and communities have a shared responsibility to provide students with access to high-quality, affordable, nutritious foods and beverages. School-based nutrition services, including the provision of meals through the NSLP and the SBP, are an integral part of the total education program. Strong wellness policies promote environments that enhance nutrition integrity and help students to develop lifelong healthy behaviors."[165] That position statement includes a summary of initiatives to improve school eating environments.[165]

Concerning comprehensive school nutrition services, the joint position of the American Dietetic Association (the Academy of Nutrition and Dietetics as of January 2012), School Nutrition Association, and Society for Nutrition Education is that "comprehensive integrated nutrition services in schools, kindergarten through grade 12, are an essential component of coordinated school health programs that will improve the nutritional status, health, and academic performance of our nation's children. Local school wellness policies may strengthen comprehensive nutrition services in schools by providing opportunities for multidisciplinary teams to identify and address local school needs."[168]

## HEALTH PROMOTION AND DISEASE PREVENTION

### HEALTHY PEOPLE 2020

Several objectives for Healthy People 2020 concern nutrition for children and adolescents. These nutrition objectives address healthier food access, health care, weight status, food insecurity, food and nutrient consumption, and iron deficiency. The objectives, along with baseline and target details, are available online at http://www.healthypeople.gov.

### FRUITS & VEGGIES—MORE MATTERS®

The Produce for Better Health Foundation (a nonprofit organization to achieve increased daily consumption of fruits and vegetables by leveraging private industry and public sector resources [http://www.pbhfoundation.org]), the CDC, and other national partners launched a new national health initiative known as the Fruits & Veggies—More Matters® program in 2007 to replace the previous 5 A Day for Better Health campaign. The brand for the Fruits & Veggies—More Matters program was developed based on comprehensive formative research that included interviews, focus groups, and an online survey conducted in 2005 to inspire or create a desire to serve and eat more fruits and vegetables.[169] The Fruits & Veggies—More Matters program's concept of "fill half your plate with fruits and vegetables at each meal or eating occasion" is supported by MyPlate developed by the USDA. The website for the Fruits & Veggies—More Matters program (http://www.fruitsandveggiesmorematters.org) contains information about the benefits of eating more fruits and vegetables, planning and shopping, cooking, and getting children involved.

### KIDS EAT RIGHT

Kids Eat Right is a joint effort of the Academy of Nutrition and Dietetics and the Academy of Nutrition and Dietetics Foundation, launched in November 2010. (Prior to January 2012, the Academy and its Foundation were known as the American Dietetic Association.) Kids Eat Right is a member-driven campaign that is dedicated to supporting the efforts of the White House to end the childhood obesity epidemic within a generation. The initiative encourages the involvement of both Academy members and consumers. Members can opt to become Kids Eat Right campaign volunteers and take part in various actions to educate families, communities, and policy makers about the importance of quality nutrition

for children. Consumers can visit the Kids Eat Right website at http://www.kidseatright.org to access information (including articles, tips, recipes, and videos), to help their kids and family eat right (including articles, tips, recipes, and videos).

### FUEL UP TO PLAY 60

Fuel Up to Play 60 is the in-school nutrition and physical activity program founded by the National Dairy Council® and the National Football League, based on a mutual commitment to the health of the next generation. The USDA has joined the effort along with many businesses and industry leaders. The focus of the comprehensive program is to promote healthier eating and more physical activity opportunities schoolwide. Students and adults work together to select and implement a series of "plays" that result in long-term changes in these two important areas. Along the way, students become empowered to lead—by making healthy decisions, taking action for change, and encouraging their friends to do the same. Since launching nationally in 2009, more than 70,000 schools that serve more than 36 million students nationwide have enrolled. Fuel Up to Play 60 supports national recommended standards for nutrition and physical education/physical activity for grades 5 through 12. The free program also helps schools meet their wellness goals by complementing existing wellness efforts and a coordinated school health approach. Information about resources and funding opportunities is available online at http://www.fueluptoplay60.com.

### FOOD SAFETY

Food safety is an important principle for building healthy eating patterns. A key recommendation of the 2010 Dietary Guidelines for Americans is to follow food safety recommendations when preparing and eating foods to decrease the risk of foodborne illnesses. In the United States each year, foodborne illness affects more than 76 million people.[17] Behaviors most likely to prevent food safety problems are washing hands, rinsing vegetables and fruits, preventing cross contamination, cooking foods to safe internal temperatures, and storing foods safely in the home kitchen. Four food safety principles—clean, separate, cook, and chill—work together to reduce the risk of foodborne illness; these four principles are the cornerstones of Fight Bac!® (discussed briefly in the next paragraph). Foods that pose high risk of foodborne illness and, thus, should be avoided include raw or partially cooked eggs or foods containing raw eggs; raw (unpasteurized) milk and products made from unpasteurized milk; unpasteurized juice; raw or undercooked seafood, meat, poultry, fish, or shellfish; and raw sprouts.[17]

Fight Bac! is a multifaceted, national food safety education campaign of the Partnership for Food Safety Education that combines resources of the federal government, industry, and consumer organizations to conduct broad-based food safety education.[170] Fight Bac! has a website (http://www.fightbac.org) and materials for educators, the media, and

**TABLE 20.18**

**Details Regarding the Four Principles of Fight Bac!®**

*Clean: Wash hands and surfaces often.*

Wash hands with warm water and soap for at least 20 sec before and after handling food and after using the bathroom, changing diapers, and handling pets or animals.

Wash cutting boards, dishes, utensils, and countertops with hot soapy water after preparing each food item and before preparing the next food item.

Consider using paper towels to clean up kitchen surfaces. If cloth towels are used, wash them often in the hot cycle of the washing machine.

Rinse fresh fruits and vegetables under running tap water, including those with skins and rinds that are not eaten.

Rub firm-skin fruits and vegetables under running tap water or scrub with a clean vegetable brush while rinsing with running tap water.

*Separate: Do not cross contaminate!*

Keep raw meat, poultry, seafood, and eggs separate from other foods in grocery carts, grocery bags, and the refrigerator.

Use one cutting board for fresh produce and another cutting board for raw meat, poultry, and seafood.

Never place cooked food on a plate or dish that previously held raw meat, poultry, seafood, or eggs.

*Cook: Cook to proper temperatures.*

Use a food thermometer that measures the internal temperature of cooked meat, poultry, and egg dishes to make sure that the food is cooked to a safe internal temperature.

Cook roasts and steaks to a minimum of 145°F; all poultry should reach a safe minimum internal temperature of 165°F.

Cook ground meat to at least 160°F; color is not a reliable indicator of doneness.

Cook eggs until the yolk and white are firm, not runny.

Do not use recipes or eat foods in which eggs remain raw or only partially cooked.

Cook fish to 145°F or until the flesh is opaque and separates easily with a fork.

When microwaving foods, make sure there are no cold spots by covering, stirring, and rotating food for even heating.

Bring sauces, soups, and gravies to a boil when reheating. Heat other leftovers thoroughly to 165°F.

*Chill: Refrigerate promptly!*

Refrigerate or freeze meat, poultry, eggs, and other perishables as soon as possible.

Never let raw meat, poultry, eggs, cooked food, or cut fresh fruits or vegetables sit at room temperature more than 2 h before putting them in the refrigerator or freezer (1 h when the temperature is above 90°F).

Never defrost food at room temperature; three safe ways to defrost food are in the refrigerator, in an airtight package in cold water, and in the microwave.

Marinate food in the refrigerator.

Divide large amounts of leftovers into small, shallow containers for quicker cooling in the refrigerator.

Use or discard refrigerated food on a regular basis.

*Source:* Adapted from *Fight Bac!*® Partnership for Food Safety Education, www.fightbac.org (accessed on June 16, 2012).

consumers. Table 20.18 provides details concerning the four principles (clean, separate, cook, and chill) of Fight Bac!.

Children, adolescents, and adults of all ages need to understand the important role they play in decreasing the incidence of foodborne illnesses through proper hand washing as well as safe food preparation and storage.

## DENTAL HEALTH

The risk of dental caries is increased by naturally occurring sugars (found in fruit [fructose] and fluid milk and milk products [lactose]) as well as by added sugars (such as high-fructose corn syrup, white sugar, brown sugar, corn syrup, fructose sweetener, honey, and molasses added during processing, preparation, or at the table). To help reduce the risk of dental caries, drink fluoridated water and/or use fluoride-containing dental products. (Note: Most bottled water is not fluoridated.) The length of time that sugars and starches are in contact with teeth also contributes to dental caries. According to the 2010 Dietary Guidelines for Americans, the most effective way to reduce dental caries is a combined approach of reducing the amount of time sugars and starches

are in the mouth, drinking fluoridated water, and brushing and flossing teeth.[17]

The risk of dental caries increases as the frequency of eating and drinking increases. Children who are constantly snacking and drinking sugar-containing substances are at greater risk of developing dental caries than children who eat three meals and few snacks each day.[171]

Early childhood caries are thought to result from the inappropriate use of a bottle or sippy cup while children sleep or its unsupervised use during the day, with liquids other than water. It is best for parents to limit sweetened drinks for children to meal and snack times only.[171]

## ASSESSING CHILDREN'S DIETARY INTAKE

Assessment of dietary intake is challenging, especially among children who eat several meals and snacks at school or day care when their parents are not present. Nevertheless, parents are often asked to provide information about their children's intake; unfortunately, several studies underscore concerns that these parents' reports cannot be taken as truth.[172–174] In addition, parents are often asked to provide joint reports with their children about their children's intake. A 1989 study by Eck et al.[175] found that consensus recalls provided by mother, father, and child yielded better estimates of observed intake of a single cafeteria meal by 34 children ages 4–9.5 years than did recalls from either the mother or father alone. Unfortunately, the Eck et al.[175] study is often incorrectly cited as the rationale for obtaining joint recalls from parents and children. However, for that study, children by themselves did not provide recalls, so no comparison could be made of the accuracy of child-only recalls, parent-only recalls, and joint parent–child recalls of the child's intake. Furthermore, consensus recalls were always obtained after the mother and father had each provided separate recalls, but having the mother and father provide two back-to-back recalls about the child's intake could have altered reporting accuracy during the second recall, which was always the consensus parent–child recall. Sobo et al.[176,177] provided recommendations to improve the accuracy of data about children's intake obtained during parent-assisted dietary recalls based on a study with 34 children ages 7–11 years. Sobo et al. found that parents "contributed primarily by adding food details and, secondarily, by prompting children;" in addition, "children rejected a notable proportion of items added" by parents, and "children's knowledge of food details was considerable."[176,177] Unfortunately, their study did not validate the children's actual intake, and unassisted children's dietary recalls were not obtained. Dietary-reporting studies with adults have found interesting relationships between reported intake and various characteristics of adults such as BMI, sex, social desirability, body image, and self-esteem. There is some concern that these adult characteristics could affect dietary intake reported during joint parent–child recalls about children's intake. Validation studies are needed to determine the impact on accuracy of dietary information obtained from joint parent–child dietary recalls about children's intake.

Children in upper elementary school are able to verbally recall their dietary intake. Methodological research by Baxter and colleagues, including validation studies that use observations of school meals to compare to elementary school children's verbal recalls (obtained without parental assistance), is providing insight to improve recall accuracy;[178,179] the following paragraphs summarize results from this methodological research by Baxter et al.

Among first-grade children, specific prompting (preference, food category, or visual) after free recall hurt more than helped recall accuracy; in contrast, among fourth-grade children, prompting for food category after free recall yielded small gains in recall accuracy with minimal losses.[180] When interviewed in the morning about the previous day's intake, individual fourth-grade children were inconsistent in recall accuracy from one interview to the next (with approximately 1 month between any two recalls for an individual child), but overall accuracy improved slightly between the first and third recalls.[181] Fourth-grade boys were more accurate when prompted to report meals and snacks in reverse order (evening to morning), while girls were more accurate in forward order (morning to evening).[182] When interviewed in the evening about that day's intake, fourth-grade children's recall accuracy did not depend significantly on whether interviews were conducted in person or by telephone.[183] Accuracy by meal component for school lunch recalls was less when the lunch recalls were obtained in the context of a 24 h dietary recall than as a single meal.[184] Providing meal cues elevated false reports compared to allowing fourth-grade children to report using an open interview format.[185]

Fourth-grade children were less accurate in recalling intake for school breakfast than school lunch.[186] Secondary analyses of data from five studies found asymmetry in fourth-grade children's misreports of school breakfast; specifically, children observed eating a cold breakfast (i.e., ready-to-eat cereal) almost never misreported having eaten a hot breakfast (i.e., non-ready-to-eat-cereal entrée), but children observed eating a hot breakfast often misreported having eaten a cold breakfast.[187] Thus, children reported eating ready-to-eat cereal at more school breakfasts than were observed.

Research has shown that retention interval (i.e., elapsed time between the to-be-reported meals and the interview) substantially influences children's accuracy for reporting school meals during 24 h dietary recalls. Specifically, fourth-grade children's accuracy depended systematically on target period (with better accuracy when interviewed about the prior 24 h [e.g., between 3:00 p.m. on Monday and 3:00 p.m. on Tuesday for an interview on Tuesday at 3:00 p.m.] than the previous day [e.g., from midnight to midnight on Monday for an interview anytime on Tuesday]) and on the target period by interview-time interaction (with accuracy best for prior 24 h recalls in the afternoon and evening and worst for previous-day recalls in the afternoon and evening).[188,189]

Several studies have found that when children recalled the *correct* food items (i.e., matches), the amounts children recalled eaten were fairly accurate in terms of servings (e.g., within one-fourth serving); however, when children omitted (i.e., forgot) food items and when children intruded (i.e., falsely recalled) food items, amounts were almost one-half to full servings.[181–183,188] This suggests that efforts to improve children's recall accuracy should focus first on helping children recall the correct food items.

Two studies[190,191] have found that being observed eating school meals (breakfast and lunch) did not influence fourth-grade children's 24 h dietary recalls. Thus, conclusions about 24 h dietary recalls by fourth-grade children observed eating school meals in validation studies can be generalized to 24 h dietary recalls by comparable but unobserved children in nonvalidation studies (such as national surveys and epidemiological studies).

Several studies have found a relationship between fourth-grade children's dietary recall accuracy and BMI.[192–194] Some studies have found a relationship between fourth-grade children's dietary recall accuracy and social desirability.[194,195]

One study has found a relationship between fourth-grade children's dietary recall accuracy and cognitive ability.[196] Several studies have demonstrated a relationship between children's dietary recall accuracy and liking ratings for foods; specifically, studies have found that children's liking ratings were better for matches (food observed eaten and reported eaten) than for omissions (foods observed eaten but not reported eaten) and intrusions (foods not observed eaten but reported eaten).[197,198]

Although children (and adults) recall their intake as food, it is common for validation studies to investigate accuracy of reported energy and nutrients. Most validation studies do this by utilizing the *conventional approach*, which was not designed to capture errors of reported foods and amounts. Several studies have found that the conventional approach was problematic for reasons such as it misrepresented reporting accuracy, masked effects of manipulated aspects of 24 h dietary recalls, or did not permit adequate assessment of the relationship of dietary recall accuracy with correlates of recall accuracy such as BMI and social desirability. When analyzing validation study data to investigate accuracy for reporting energy and nutrients, the analytic approach used should be sensitive to reporting errors for foods and amounts.[194,199–203]

Additional validation studies are needed to continue to improve the accuracy of dietary recalls from youth of various ages.

## SUMMARY

In summary, the childhood and adolescent years are marked by growth, change, and learning. The DRIs, 2010 Dietary Guidelines for Americans, and *MyPlate*, along with recommendations from the American Academy of Pediatrics and the Academy of Nutrition and Dietetics, provide key nutritional guidance for children and adolescents. By following a division of feeding responsibility, exposing children to a variety of healthful foods, providing opportunities and social environments for children to learn to like a variety of healthful foods, and encouraging children and adolescents to respect their own feelings of hunger and satiety, parents, caregivers, and school staff have important roles in helping children and adolescents establish healthful eating habits and healthy weights.

## ACKNOWLEDGMENTS

Revisions to this chapter were supported in part via several grants (R21HL88617, R21HL96035, and R01HL103737 with Suzanne D. Baxter, PhD, RD, LD, FADA, as principal investigator) funded by the National Heart, Lung, and Blood Institute of the National Institutes of Health. Grateful appreciation is expressed to Kathleen L. Collins; Caroline H. Guinn, RD, LD; Amy Paxton-Aiken, RD, LD; Megan Puryear, RD, LD; Alyssa L. Smith; and Kate Vaadi, RD, LD (all with the Institute for Families in Society in the College of Social Work at the University of South Carolina) for their help in revising an earlier version of this chapter.

## REFERENCES

1. National Research Council. *Dietary Reference Intakes for Calcium, Phosphorus, Magnesium, Vitamin D, and Fluoride*, The National Academies Press, Washington, DC. 1997; 448pp. Available online at www.nap.edu
2. National Research Council. *Dietary Reference Intakes for Thiamin, Riboflavin, Niacin, Vitamin $B_6$, Folate, Vitamin $B_{12}$, Pantothenic Acid, Biotin, and Choline*, The National Academies Press, Washington, DC. 1998; 592pp. Available online at www.nap.edu
3. National Research Council. *Dietary Reference Intakes: Proposed Definition and Plan for Review of Dietary Antioxidants and Related Compounds*, The National Academies Press, Washington, DC. 1998; 24pp. Available online at www.nap.edu
4. National Research Council. *Dietary Reference Intakes: A Risk Assessment Model for Establishing Upper Intake Levels for Nutrients*, The National Academies Press, Washington, DC. 1998; 82pp. Available online at www.nap.edu
5. National Research Council. *Dietary Reference Intakes for Vitamin C, Vitamin E, Selenium, and Carotenoids*, The National Academies Press, Washington, DC. 2000; 529pp. Available online at www.nap.edu
6. National Research Council. *Dietary Reference Intakes: Applications in Dietary Assessment*, The National Academies Press, Washington, DC. 2000; 306pp. Available online at www.nap.edu
7. National Research Council. *Dietary Reference Intakes for Vitamin A, Vitamin K, Arsenic, Boron, Chromium, Copper, Iodine, Iron, Manganese, Molybdenum, Nickel, Silicon, Vanadium, and Zinc*, The National Academies Press, Washington, DC. 2001; 800pp. Available online at www.nap.edu
8. National Research Council. *Dietary Reference Intakes: Proposed Definition of Dietary Fiber*, The National Academies Press, Washington, DC. 2001; 74pp. Available online at www.nap.edu
9. National Research Council. *Dietary Reference Intakes: Energy, Carbohydrate, Fiber, Fat, Fatty Acids, Cholesterol, Protein, and Amino Acids (Macronutrients)*, National Academies Press, Washington, DC. 2002/2005; 1357pp. Available online at www.nap.edu
10. National Research Council. *Dietary Reference Intakes: Guiding Principles for Nutrition Labeling and Fortification*, The National Academies Press, Washington, DC. 2003; 224pp. Available online at www.nap.edu
11. National Research Council. *Dietary Reference Intakes: Applications in Dietary Planning*, The National Academies Press, Washington, DC. 2003; 248pp. Available online at www.nap.edu
12. National Research Council. *Dietary Reference Intakes for Water, Potassium, Sodium, Chloride, and Sulfate*, The National Academies Press, Washington, DC. 2005; 640pp. Available online at www.nap.edu
13. National Research Council. *Dietary Reference Intakes: The Essential Guide to Nutrient Requirements*, The National Academies Press, Washington, DC. 2006; 560pp. Available online at www.nap.edu
14. National Research Council. *Dietary Reference Intakes Research Synthesis: Workshop Summary*, The National Academies Press, Washington, DC. 2006; 310pp. Available online at www.nap.edu
15. National Research Council. *The Development of DRIs 1994–2004: Lessons Learned and New Challenges: Workshop Summary*, The National Academies Press, Washington, DC. 2008; 198pp. Available online at www.nap.edu

16. National Research Council. *Dietary Reference Intakes for Calcium and Vitamin D*, The National Academies Press, Washington, DC. 2011; 1132pp. Available at www.nap.edu

17. U.S. Department of Agriculture and U.S. Department of Health and Human Services. *Dietary Guidelines for Americans, 2010*, 7th edn., U.S. Government Printing Office, Washington, DC. 2010; 112pp. Available online at www.healthierus.gov/dietaryguidelines (accessed June 16, 2012).

18. American Academy of Pediatrics (Committee on Nutrition). In: *Pediatric Nutrition Handbook*, 6th edn., Kleinman, RE ed. American Academy of Pediatrics, Elk Grove Village, IL. pp. 145; 2009.

19. Williams, CL. *J Am Diet Assoc* 95:1140;1995.

20. Williams, CL, Bollella, M, Wynder, EL. *Pediatrics* 96:985;1995.

21. American Academy of Pediatrics. *Pediatrics* 96(5 Pt 2): S1023;1995.

22. Dwyer, JT. *Pediatrics* 96:1019;1995.

23. Williams, CL, Bollella, M. *Pediatrics* 96:1014;1995.

24. American Academy of Pediatrics (Committee on Nutrition). In: *Pediatric Nutrition Handbook*, Kleinman, RE ed. American Academy of Pediatrics, Elk Grove Village, IL. pp. 387; 2009.

25. American Academy of Pediatrics (Committee on Nutrition). In: *Pediatric Nutrition Handbook*, 6th edn., Kleinman, RE ed. American Academy of Pediatrics, Elk Grove Village, IL. pp. 403; 2009.

26. U.S. Department of Agriculture. *MyPlate background*. http://www.cnpp.usda.gov/Publications/MyPlate/Backgrounder.pdf (accessed June 16, 2012).

27. U.S. Department of Agriculture. *MyPlate FAQs*. http://www.choosemyplate.gov/faqs.html (accessed June 16, 2012).

28. Enns, CW, Mickle, SJ, Goldman, JD. *Fam Econ Nutr Rev* 14:56;2002.

29. Harnack, L, Walters, SH, Jacobs, DR. *J Am Diet Assoc* 103:1015;2003.

30. Krebs-Smith, SM, Guenther, PM, Subar, AF et al. *J Nutr* 140:1832;2010.

31. U.S. Department of Agriculture (Agricultural Research Service). *Food and Nutrient Intakes by Children 1994–96, 1998*. ARS Food Surveys Research Group. 1999. http://www.ars.usda.gov/SP2UserFiles/Place/12355000/pdf/scs_all.PDF (accessed June 16, 2012).

32. Ogden, C, Carroll, M. *Prevalence of Obesity among Children and Adolescents: United States, Trends 1963–1965 through 2007–2008*. http://www.cdc.gov/nchs/data/hestat/obesity_child_07_08/obesity_child_07_08.htm (accessed June 16, 2012).

33. Ogden, CL, Carroll, MD, Curtin, LR et al. *J Am Med Assoc* 303:242;2010.

34. Ogden, CL, Carroll, MD, Curtin, LR et al. *J Am Med Assoc* 295:1549;2006.

35. Ogden, CL, Flegal, KM, Carroll, MD, Johnson, CL. *J Am Med Assoc* 288:1728;2002.

36. Birch, LL, Fisher, JO. *Pediatrics* 101:539;1998.

37. Hill, JO, Trowbridge, FL. *Pediatrics* 101:570;1998.

38. Birch, LL, Johnson, SL, Fisher, JA. *Young Child* 50:71;1995.

39. Baxter, SD, Thompson, WO, Davis, HC. *Nutr Res* 20:439;2000.

40. Birch, LL. *J Nutr Educ* 11:189;1979.

41. Calfas, KJ, Sallis, JF, Nader, PR. *J Dev Behav Pediatr* 12:185;1991.

42. Domel, SB, Baranowski, T, Davis, H et al. *Prev Med* 22:866;1993.

43. Domel, SB, Thompson, WO, Davis, HC et al. *Health Educ Res* 11:299;1996.

44. Fisher, JO, Birch, LL. *J Am Diet Assoc* 95:759;1995.

45. Birch, LL. *Nutr Rev* 50:249;1992.

46. Mennella, JA, Jagnow, CP, Beauchamp, GK. *Pediatrics* 107:e88;2001.

47. Birch, LL. *Bull Psychon Soc* 29:265;1991.

48. Cowart, BJ. *Psychol Bull* 90:43;1981.

49. Birch, LL. *J Am Diet Assoc* 87:S36;1987.

50. Sullivan, SA, Birch, LL. *Pediatrics* 93:271;1994.

51. Birch, LL, Marlin, DW. *Appetite* 3:353;1982.

52. Birch, LL, McPhee, L, Shoba, BC et al. *Appetite* 9:171;1987.

53. Sullivan, SA, Birch, LL. *Dev Psychol* 26:546;1990.

54. Loewen, R, Pliner, P. *Appetite* 32:351;1999.

55. Pliner, P, Stallberg-White, C. *Appetite* 34:95;2000.

56. Lytle, L, Achterberg, C. *J Nutr Educ* 27:250;1995.

57. Birch, LL, Zimmerman, SI, Hind, H. *Child Dev* 51:856;1980.

58. Birch, LL, Birch, D, Marlin, DW, Kramer, L. *Appetite* 3:125;1982.

59. Birch, LL, Marlin, DW, Rotter, J. *Child Dev* 55:431;1984.

60. Newman, J, Taylor, A. *J Exp Child Psychol* 53:200;1992.

61. Hendy, HM. *Ann Behav Med* 21:20;1999.

62. Wardle, J, Cooke, LJ, Gibson, EL et al. *Appetite* 40:155;2003.

63. Johnson, SL, Bellows, L, Beckstrom, L, Anderson, J. *Am J Health Behav* 31:44;2007.

64. Remington, A, Anez, E, Croker, H et al. *Am J Clin Nutr* 95:72;2012.

65. Wardle, J, Herrera, M-L, Cooke, L, Gibson, EL. *Eur J Clin Nutr* 57:341;2003.

66. Perry, CL, Bishop, DB, Taylor, GL et al. *Health Educ Behav* 31:65;2004.

67. Hendy, HM, Williams, KE, Camise, TS. *Appetite* 45:250;2005.

68. Cooke, LJ, Chambers, LC, Anez, EV et al. *Psychol Sci* 22:190;2011.

69. Hendy, HM, Raudenbush, B. *Appetite* 34:61;2000.

70. Hendy, HM. *Appetite* 39:217;2002.

71. Addessi, E, Galloway, AT, Visalberghi, E, Birch, LL. *Appetite* 45:264;2005.

72. Nahikian-Nelms, M. *J Am Diet Assoc* 97:505;1997.

73. Fomon, SJ. *Nutrition of Normal Infants*, Mosby-Yearbook, St. Louis, MO. 1993; pp. 114.

74. Adair, LS. *J Am Diet Assoc* 84:543;1984.

75. Birch, LL, Deysher, M. *Learn Motiv* 16:341;1985.

76. Birch, LL, Deysher, M. *Appetite* 7:323;1986.

77. Birch, LL, Johnson, SL, Andresen, G et al. *N Engl J Med* 324:232;1991.

78. Birch, LL, Mcphee, L, Shoba, BC et al. *Learn Motiv* 18:301;1987.

79. Johnson, SL, Birch, LL. *Pediatrics* 94:653;1994.

80. Klesges, RC, Coates, TJ, Brown, G et al. *J Appl Behav Anal* 16:371;1983.

81. Fisher, JO, Birch, LL. *Am J Clin Nutr* 69:1264;1999.

82. Fisher, JO, Birch, LL. *Appetite* 32:405;1999.

83. Spruijt-Metz, D, Lindquist, CH, Birch, LL et al. *Am J Clin Nutr* 75:581;2002.

84. Birch, LL, Fisher, JO, Davison, KK. *Am J Clin Nutr* 78:125;2003.

85. Patrick, H, Nicklas, TA, Hughes, SO, Morales, M. *Appetite* 44:243;2005.

86. Blissett, J. *Appetite* 57:826;2011.

87. Ventura, AK, Birch, LL. *Int J Behav Nutr Phys Act* 5:15;2008.

88. Faith, MS, Berkowitz, RI, Stallings, VA et al. *Pediatrics* 114:e429;2004. http://pediatrics.aappublications.org/cgi/content/full/114/4/e429 (accessed June 16, 2012).
89. Savage, JS, Fisher, JO, Birch, LL. *J Law Med Ethics* 35:22;2007.
90. Wansick, B, Van Ittersum, K. *J Am Diet Assoc* 107:1103;2007.
91. Wansick, B, Wansink, CS. *Int J Obesity* 34:943;2010.
92. Wansick, B, Kim, J. *J Nutr Educ Behav* 37:242;2005.
93. Rolls, BJ, Engell, D, Birch, LL. *J Am Diet Assoc* 100:232;2000.
94. Fisher, JO, Rolls, BJ, Birch, LL. *Am J Clin Nutr* 77:1164;2003.
95. McConahy, KL, Smiciklas-Wright, H, Mitchell, DC, Picciano, MF. *J Am Diet Assoc* 104:975;2004.
96. Satter, E. *How to Get Your Kids to Eat But Not Too Much*, Bull Publishing, Palo Alto, CA. 1987.
97. Satter, E. *Child of Mine: Feeding with Love and Good Sense*, Bull, Palo Alto, CA. 2000.
98. Satter, EM. *J Am Diet Assoc* 86:352;1986.
99. Frank, G. In: *Promoting Teen Health: Linking Schools, Health Organizations and Community*, Henderson, A, Champlin, S, Evashwick, W eds. Sage Publications, Thousand Oaks, CA. pp. 28; 1998.
100. American Academy of Pediatrics (Committee on Nutrition and the Council on Sports Medicine and Fitness). *Pediatrics* 127:1182;2011.
101. Kanarek, RB. *Nutr Rev* 52:173;1994.
102. Wolraich, ML, Lindgren, SD, Stumbo, PJ et al. *N Engl J Med* 330:301;1994.
103. Wolraich, ML, Wilson, DB, White, JW. *J Am Med Assoc* 274:1617;1995.
104. Bellisle, F. *Br J Nutr* 92(suppl 2):S227;2004.
105. U.S. Department of Agriculture. *What are Added Sugars?* http://www.choosemyplate.gov/weight-management-calories/calories/added-sugars.html (accessed June 16, 2012).
106. Academy of Nutrition and Dietetics. *J Acad Nutr Diet* 112:739;2012.
107. Story, M, French, S. *Int J Behav Nutr Phys Act* 1:3;2004.
108. Harrison, K, Marske, AL. *Am J Public Health* 95:1568;2005.
109. Henry J. Kaiser Family Foundation. *The Role of Media in Childhood Obesity (Issue Brief; publication #7030)*. 2004. http://www.kff.org/entmedia/7030.cfm (accessed June 16, 2012).
110. Wiecha, JL, Peterson, KE, Ludwig, DS et al. *Arch Pediatr Adolesc Med* 160:436;2006.
111. Henry J. Kaiser Family Foundation. *It's Child's Play: Advergaming and the Online Marketing of Food to Children—Report (Report; publication #7536)*. 2006. http://www.kff.org/entmedia/7536.cfm (accessed June 16, 2012).
112. Henry J. Kaiser Family Foundation. *Food for Thought—Television Food Advertising to Children in the United States*. 2007. http://www.kff.org/entmedia/upload/7618.pdf (accessed June 16, 2012).
113. Henry J. Kaiser Family Foundation. *Generation M²: Media in the Lives of 8- to 18-Year-Olds (Report; publication #8010)*. 2010. http://www.kff.org/entmedia/8010.cfm (accessed June 16, 2012).
114. American Dietetic Association. *J Am Diet Assoc* 109:1266;2009.
115. Mangels, R, Messina, V, Messina, M. *The Dietitian's Guide to Vegetarian Diets: Issues and Applications*, 3rd edn., Jones and Bartlett Publishers, Sudbury, MA. 2010; 596pp.
116. Rampersaud, GC, Pereira, MA, Girard, BL et al. *J Am Diet Assoc* 105:743;2005.
117. Mahoney, CR, Taylor, HA, Kanarek, RB, Samuel, P. *Physiol Behav* 85:635;2005.
118. Pollitt, E. *J Am Diet Assoc* 95:1134;1995.
119. Pollitt, E, Cueto, S, Jacoby, ER. *Am J Clin Nutr* 67:779S;1998.
120. Dwyer, JT, Ebzery, MK, Nicklas, TA et al. *Fam Econ Nutr Rev* 11:3;1998.
121. Gleason, PM. *Am J Clin Nutr* 61:213S;1995.
122. Nicklas, TA, Bao, W, Webber, LS, Berenson, GS. *J Am Diet Assoc* 93:886;1993.
123. Siega-Riz, AM, Popkin, BM, Carson, T. *Am J Clin Nutr* 67:748S;1998.
124. American Academy of Pediatrics (Committee on Nutrition). In: *Pediatric Nutrition Handbook*, 6th edn., Kleinman, RE ed. American Academy of Pediatrics, Elk Grove Village, IL. pp. 175; 2009.
125. Neumark-Sztainer, D, Hannan, PJ, Story, M et al. *J Am Diet Assoc* 103:317;2003.
126. Story, M, Neumark-Sztainer, D, French, SA. *J Am Diet Assoc* 102:S40;2002.
127. American Dietetic Association. *J Am Diet Assoc* 111:607;2011.
128. Birch, LL. *Dev Psychol* 26:515;1990.
129. Kennedy, E. *Prev Med* 25:56;1996.
130. Dwyer, J. *Am J Clin Nutr* 61:173S;1995.
131. Centers for Disease Control and Prevention. *Guidelines for School Health Programs to Promote Lifelong Healthy Eating. MMWR* 45:1;1996. http://www.cdc.gov/mmwr/preview/mmwrhtml/00042446.htm (accessed June 16, 2012).
132. Resnicow, K. *Ann N Y Acad Sci* 699:154;1993.
133. Berenson, GS, Arbeit, ML, Hunter, SM et al. *Ann N Y Acad Sci* 623:299;1991.
134. Kolbe, LJ. *Prev Med* 22:544;1993.
135. Contento, IR, Manning, AD, Shannon, B. *J Nutr Educ* 24:247;1992.
136. Contento, IR, Balch, GI, Bronner, YL et al. *J Nutr Educ* 27:298;1995.
137. American Dietetic Association. *J Am Diet Assoc* 110:791;2010.
138. U.S. Department of Agriculture (Food and Nutrition Service). *National School Lunch Program*. http://www.fns.usda.gov/cnd/lunch/AboutLunch/NSLPFactSheet.pdf (accessed June 16, 2012).
139. U.S. Department of Agriculture (Food and Nutrition Service). *The School Breakfast Program*. http://www.fns.usda.gov/cnd/Breakfast/AboutBFast/SBPFactSheet.pdf (accessed June 16, 2012).
140. U.S. Department of Agriculture (Food and Nutrition Service). *Road to SMI Success—A Guide for School Foodservice Directors*. http://www.fns.usda.gov/tn/Resources/roadtosuccess.html (accessed June 16, 2012).
141. U.S. Department of Agriculture (Food and Nutrition Service). *Team Nutrition*. http://www.fns.usda.gov/tn (accessed June 16, 2012).
142. U.S. Department of Agriculture (Food and Nutrition Service). *Changing the Scene—Improving the School Nutrition Environment*. http://teamnutrition.usda.gov/Resources/changing.html (accessed June 16, 2012).
143. U.S. Department of Agriculture (Food and Nutrition Service). *HealthierUS School Challenge*. http://www.fns.usda.gov/tn/HealthierUS/index.html (accessed June 16, 2012).
144. U.S. White House, U.S. Department of Health and Human Services, U.S. Department of Agriculture et al. *Let's Move!* http://www.letsmove.gov (accessed June 16, 2012).
145. Burghardt, JA. *Am J Clin Nutr* 61:182S;1995.

146. Burghardt, JA, Devaney, BL, Gordon, AR. *Am J Clin Nutr* 61:252S;1995.

147. U.S. Department of Agriculture, Food and Nutrition Service, Office of Analysis Nutrition and Evaluation. *School Nutrition Dietary Assessment Study-II Final Report*, Fox, MK et al. eds. Alexandria, VA. 2001. http://www.fns.usda.gov/ora/menu/Published/CNP/FILES/sndaII.pdf (accessed June 16, 2012).

148. U.S. Department of Agriculture, Food and Nutrition Service, Office of Analysis Nutrition and Evaluation. *School Nutrition Dietary Assessment Study-II Summary of Findings*, ed. Fox, MK et al. Alexandria, VA. 2001. http://www.fns.usda.gov/ora/menu/Published/CNP/FILES/SNDAIIfind.pdf (accessed June 16, 2012).

149. U.S. Department of Agriculture, Food and Nutrition Service, Office of Research Nutrition and Analysis. *School Nutrition Dietary Assessment Study-III Summary of Findings*. 2007. http://www.fns.usda.gov/ora/MENU/Published/CNP/FILES/SNDAIII-SummaryofFindings.pdf (accessed June 16, 2012).

150. Food Research and Action Center. *School Breakfast in America's Big Cities: School Year 2010–2011*. 2012. http://frac.org/pdf/urban_school_breakfast_report_2012.pdf (accessed June 18, 2012).

151. Story, M, Kaphingst, KM, Robinson-O'Brien, R, Glanz, K. *Annu Rev Public Health* 29:253;2008.

152. U.S. Department of Agriculture, Economic Research Service. *The National School Lunch Program: Background, Trends, and Issues (Report No. EER-61)*. 2008. http://www.ers.usda.gov/Publications/ERR61/ (accessed June 16, 2012).

153. U.S. Department of Agriculture, Food and Nutrition Service, Office of Research Nutrition and Analysis. *Obesity, Poverty, and Participation in Nutrition Assistance Programs (FSP-04-PO; Project Office, S Cristofar)*, Alexandria, VA. 2004. http://www.fns.usda.gov/ora/MENU/Published/NutritionEducation/Files/ObesityPoverty.pdf (accessed June 16, 2012).

154. Wolfe, WS, Campbell, CC, Frongillo, EAJ et al. *Am J Public Health* 84:807;1994.

155. Melnik, TA, Rhoades, SJ, Wales, KR et al. *Int J Obesity* 22:7;1998.

156. Gleason, PM, Dodd, AH. *J Am Diet Assoc* 109:S118;2009.

157. Paxton-Aiken, AE, Baxter, SD, Tebbs, JM et al. *Int J Behav Nutr Phys Act* 9:30;2012.

158. Baxter, SD, Hardin, JW, Guinn, CH et al. *Int J Behav Nutr Phys Act* 7:24;2010.

159. Paxton, AE, Baxter, SD, Tebbs, JM et al. *J Acad Nutr Diet* 112:104;2012.

160. Guinn, CH, Baxter, SD, Thompson, WO et al. *J Nutr Educ Behav* 34:159;2002.

161. Moore, Q, Hulsey, L, Ponza, M. *Factors Associated with School Meal Participation and the Relationship Between Different Participation Measures (Report No. 53)*. 2009. http://naldc.nal.usda.gov/catalog/35701 (accessed June 16, 2012).

162. Paxton-Aiken, AE, Baxter, SD, Royer, JA et al. (submitted).

163. Guinn, CH, Baxter, SD, Royer, JA, Hitchcock, DB. *J Sch Health* 83:328;2013.

164. Baxter, SD, Paxton-Aiken, AE, Tebbs, JM, et al. *Nutr Res* 32:659;2012.

165. American Dietetic Association. *J Am Diet Assoc* 110:1244;2010.

166. National Alliance for Nutrition and Activity. *Model Local School Wellness Policies*. http://www.schoolwellnesspolicies.org/WellnessPolicies.html (accessed June 16, 2012).

167. Action for Healthy Kids. *Wellness Policy Tool*. http://www.actionforhealthykids.org/for-schools/wellness-policy-tool/ (accessed June 16, 2012).

168. American Dietetic Association, School Nutrition Association, Society for Nutrition Education. *J Am Diet Assoc* 110:1738;2010.

169. Pivonka, E, Seymour, J, McKenna, J et al. *J Am Diet Assoc* 111:1570;2011.

170. Partnership for Food Safety Education. *Fight Bac!* http://www.fightbac.org (accessed June 16, 2012).

171. American Academy of Pediatrics (Committee on Nutrition). In: *Pediatric Nutrition Handbook*, 6th edn., Kleinman, RE ed. American Academy of Pediatrics, Elk Grove Village, IL. pp. 1041; 2009.

172. Emmons, L, Hayes, M. *J Am Diet Assoc* 62:409;1973.

173. Mack, K, Blair, J, Presser, S. Measuring and improving data quality in children's reports of dietary intake. In: *Proceedings of the 6th Conference on Health Survey Methods,* Warnecke, RB, ed. DHHS Publication No. (PHS), 96–1013, Hyattsville, MD, pp. 51–55; 1996.

174. Presser, S, Blair, J, Mack, K et al. Final report on the University of Maryland-USDA cooperative agreement to improve reporting for children in the Continuing Survey of Food Intakes by Individuals. Survey Research Center, University of Maryland, 1993.

175. Eck, L, Klesges, R, Hanson, C. *J Am Diet Assoc* 89:784;1989.

176. Sobo, E, Rock, C. *Med Anthropol Q* 15:222;2001.

177. Sobo, E, Rock, C, Neuhouser, M et al. *J Am Diet Assoc* 100:428;2000.

178. Baxter, SD. *Eur J Clin Nutr* 63:S19;2009.

179. Baxter, SD, Guinn, CH, Hardin, JW et al. In: *Appetite and Nutritional Assessment*, Ellsworth, SJ, Schuster, RC eds. Nova Science Publishers, Inc, New York. pp. 197; 2010. Link to open access chapter: https://www.novapublishers.com/catalog/product_info.php?products_id=16499

180. Baxter, SD, Thompson, WO, Davis, HC. *J Am Diet Assoc* 100:911;2000.

181. Baxter, SD, Thompson, WO, Litaker, MS et al. *J Am Diet Assoc* 102:386;2002.

182. Baxter, SD, Thompson, WO, Smith, AF et al. *Prev Med* 36:601;2003.

183. Baxter, SD, Thompson, WO, Litaker, MS et al. *J Nutr Educ Behav* 35:124;2003.

184. Baxter, SD, Thompson, WO. *Nutr Res* 22:679;2002.

185. Baxter, SD, Smith, AF, Guinn, CH et al. *Nutr Res* 23:1537;2003.

186. Baxter, SD, Royer, JA, Hardin, JW et al. *J Nutr Educ Behav* 39:126;2007.

187. Baxter, SD, Hardin, JW, Royer, JA et al. *Appetite* 51:489;2008.

188. Baxter, SD, Hardin, JW, Guinn, CH et al. *J Am Diet Assoc* 109:846;2009.

189. Baxter, SD, Smith, AF, Litaker, MS et al. *Ann Epidemiol* 14:385;2004.

190. Baxter, SD, Hardin, JW, Smith, AF et al. *J Clin Epidemiol* 62:878;2009.

191. Smith, AF, Baxter, SD, Hardin, JW et al. *Public Health Nutr* 10:1057;2007.

192. Baxter, SD, Smith, AF, Litaker, MS et al. *J Am Diet Assoc* 106:1656;2006.

193. Baxter, SD, Smith, AF, Nichols, MN et al. *Nutr Res* 26:241;2006.

194. Guinn, CH, Baxter, SD, Royer, JA et al. *J Health Psychol* 15:505;2010.

195. Guinn, CH, Baxter, SD, Hardin, JW et al. *Obesity* 16:2169;2008.

196. Smith, AF, Baxter, SD, Hardin, JW et al. *Am J Epidemiol* 173:103;2011.

197. Baxter, SD, Hardin, JW, Smith, AF et al. *Appl Cogn Psychol* 22:1038;2008.

198. Baxter, SD, Thompson, WO, Davis, HC, Litaker, MS. *Nutrition* 15:848;1999.

199. Baxter, SD, Guinn, CH, Royer, JA et al. *Eur J Clin Nutr* 63:1394;2009.

200. Baxter, SD, Guinn, CH, Royer, JA et al. *J Am Diet Assoc* 110:1178;2010.

201. Baxter, SD, Smith, AF, Hardin, JW, Nichols, MN. *Prev Med* 44:34;2007.

202. Baxter, SD, Smith, AF, Hardin, JW, Nichols, MN. *J Am Diet Assoc* 107:595;2007.

203. Smith, AF, Baxter, SD, Hardin, JW, Nichols, MN. *Public Health Nutr* 10:1247;2007.

# 21 Healthy Diet through Adulthood*

*Joan G. Fischer*

## CONTENTS

## INTRODUCTION

Dietary and nutrient recommendations for healthy adults are designed not only to meet basic nutrient needs and prevent nutrient deficiencies, but also to prevent chronic disease. The first Surgeon General's Report on Nutrition and Health in 1988[2] brought together a substantial body of research documenting that diet was a key factor in the development of chronic diseases and conditions such as coronary heart disease, cancer, diabetes, and obesity. The following sections describe the most recent nutrient recommendations and dietary guidelines and provide information on current nutrient and food intake of adults as compared to those recommendations.

## DIETARY RECOMMENDATIONS AND GUIDELINES

### DIETARY REFERENCE INTAKES

The Dietary Reference Intakes are recommendations for nutrient intake for healthy people of all age groups.[3] These standards are revised periodically and are based on current research on nutrient intakes needed to prevent nutrient deficiencies as well as chronic disease. They can be used to assess whether nutrient intake is likely to be adequate. The reference values include the estimated average requirement (EAR), the recommended dietary allowance (RDA), adequate intake (AI), and the tolerable upper intake level (UL) for nutrients. The EAR is the average daily nutrient intake level that will meet the needs of half of a population group. The RDA is the daily nutrient intake level that will meet the needs of most, or to be more specific, 97%–98% of a population. The AI is used for nutrients when research is not sufficient to establish an EAR and RDA, and is the amount of a nutrient that is assumed to meet nutrient needs for healthy people. The UL is defined as "the highest average daily nutrient intake level that is likely to pose no risk of adverse health effects."[3] The acceptable macronutrient distribution ranges (AMDRs) are also useful when determining whether adults are consuming appropriate amounts of macronutrients. The AMDRs provide guidance on the range of intakes for carbohydrate, protein, and fat that are associated with reduced risk for chronic disease.[3] Individuals who are undernourished and who have certain diseases may have a greater need for some nutrients.[4]

An adult can use the RDAs and AIs as goals for their nutrient intake. However, since these standards are set at levels that are intended to meet the needs of almost all of the population, it cannot be assumed that a person who does not consume that amount has developed a nutrient deficiency.[4] If a nutrient deficiency is suspected, appropriate nutrition assessment techniques, such as observation of clinical signs and laboratory tests, should be used to determine whether a person has a nutrient deficit and needs supplementation. The EAR can be used to determine nutrient adequacy of a population. The complete and updated tables of the Dietary Reference Intakes can be found at http://www.iom.edu/Activities/Nutrition/SummaryDRIs/~/media/Files/Activity%20Files/Nutrition/DRIs/5_Summary%20Table%20Tables%201-4.pdf

---

* This chapter is an update of a chapter written by Marsha Read in the 2007 version of this book.[1]

## DIETARY GUIDELINES

Dietary guidelines for Americans have been issued by the federal government since 1980[5] and were last revised in 2010. Table 21.1 provides a summary of some of the current Dietary Guidelines for Americans, 2010.[6] The complete document is available at www.dietaryguidelines.gov. The purpose of the dietary guidelines is to provide recommendations that will not only help people meet basic nutrient requirements, but also prevent chronic disease. Guidance to select foods that are high in nutrients and low in total fat, saturated fat, sodium, and sugar has remained consistent throughout the past several decades.[5]

The dietary and physical activity behaviors of adults have a major impact upon the risk of chronic disease. The 2010 Dietary Guidelines have two major messages: (1) to balance energy intake and physical activity to achieve a healthy weight and (2) to consume nutrient-dense foods and beverages.[6,7] However, there are a number of specific recommendations provided to help the consumer meet these broad goals. In addition, the U.S. Department of Agriculture (USDA) has developed food intake patterns for a wide range of energy intake levels. These food intake patterns provide guidance on the number of servings of each food group that should be consumed. Emphasis is placed on meeting nutrient needs through food, but supplements may be needed by some to achieve nutritional adequacy.[6,7]

Additional guidance to help the consumer meet the dietary guidelines is provided by the MyPlate educational materials (http://www.choosemyplate.gov/), which were introduced by the USDA Center for Nutrition Policy and Promotion in 2011. MyPlate provides a visual representation of recommended foods from the Dietary Guidelines for Americans, 2010, using a plate with spaces for fruits, vegetables, grains, protein-containing foods, and dairy products. Some of the major messages conveyed with this graphic are to build a healthy plate with more fruits, vegetables, whole grains, and low-fat milk, to reduce foods high in solid fats, added sugars and salt, to eat the right amount of calories, and to be physically active. One of the areas of focus in the dietary guidelines is to increase the intake of fruits and vegetables,[6] and the plate graphic communicates the concept that half the plate should be fruits and vegetables.

## FOOD LABELS

Food labeling became mandatory in 1993 with the enactment of the Nutrition Labeling and Education Act.[8] The legislation required food labeling on most foods, with the exceptions of low-nutrient-dense foods such as coffee, spices, and ready-to-eat food prepared on site. Nutrition information remains voluntary on many raw foods. The nutrition facts panel on food labels provides information to help the consumer make more informed choices, including information on calories per serving, calories from fat, saturated fat and cholesterol, and protein, among other nutrients (Table 21.2).

The daily values (DVs) are used as standards in food labeling. DVs provide reference intake standards for vitamins and minerals called the reference daily intakes (RDIs). Daily reference values (DRVs) are established for total fat, saturated fat, cholesterol, carbohydrate, dietary fiber, sodium, potassium, and protein. As a rule, the RDIs are greater than the RDA for specific nutrients and provide a large margin of safety.[8]

## TABLE 21.1
### Selected Recommendations from the Dietary Guidelines for Americans, 2010

Prevent and/or reduce overweight and obesity through improved eating and physical activity behaviors.

Reduce daily sodium intake to <2300 mg and to 1500 mg for some persons

Consume <10% of calories from saturated fatty acids by replacing them with monounsaturated and polyunsaturated fatty acids

Consume less than 300 mg/day of dietary cholesterol

Keep trans fatty acid consumption as low as possible

Reduce the intake of calories from solid fats and added sugars

Limit consumption of foods that contain refined grains

If alcohol is consumed, it should be consumed in moderation

Increase vegetable and fruit intake and eat a variety of vegetables

Consume at least half of all grains as whole grains

Increase intake of fat-free or low-fat milk and milk products

Choose a variety of protein foods and increase seafood consumption

Use oils to replace solid fats where possible

*Source:* U.S. Department of Agriculture and U.S. Department of Health and Human Services, *Dietary Guidelines for Americans, 2010*, 7th edn., U.S. Government Printing Office, Washington, DC, 2010, available at www.dietaryguidelines.gov

## TABLE 21.2
### Nutrition Facts Label Information

Serving size (based on amounts commonly used)

Number of servings per container

Calories per serving

Calories from fat

Percent DV of total fat, saturated fat, trans fat, cholesterol, sodium, total carbohydrate, dietary fiber, sugars, protein, vitamin A, vitamin C, calcium, and iron

Reference values for total fat, saturated fat, cholesterol, sodium, total carbohydrate, and fiber

A complete description of the Nutrition Facts Label can be accessed at: http://www.fda.gov/Food/ResourcesForYou/Consumers/NFLPM/ucm274593.htm#twoparts

## DIETARY RECOMMENDATIONS FROM OTHER ORGANIZATIONS TO PREVENT CHRONIC DISEASE

The World Health Organization (WHO) has also published dietary recommendations to reduce chronic disease risk that are similar to the Dietary Guidelines for Americans.[9] These guidelines are found in Table 21.3.

The American Heart Association has issued diet and lifestyle recommendations to reduce cardiovascular risk.[10] These guidelines are available at the association's website www.heart.org and are also very similar to the Dietary Guidelines for Americans, 2010, except that it is advised to reduce saturated fat intake to less than 7% of energy and trans fat intake to less than 1% of energy.

The American Cancer Society has developed nutrition and physical activity guidelines to reduce the risk of cancer.[11] It has been estimated that one-third of cancer deaths may be the result of dietary and physical activity patterns. The primary recommendations are to achieve and maintain a healthy weight throughout life, to adopt a physically active lifestyle, to consume a healthy diet with an emphasis on plant foods, and for those who do drink alcoholic beverages, to limit consumption. Specific recommendations for physical activity are included in the guidelines. There is an emphasis on the consumption of fruits and vegetables (at least 2.5 cups/day) and whole grains, and a recommendation to limit the consumption of processed meat and red meat. Selecting foods that are low in salt is also advised.[11] Guidelines are available at http://www.cancer.org/Healthy/EatHealthyGetActive/ACSGuidelinesonNutritionPhysicalActivityforCancerPrevention/index. Organizations that have similar diet and physical activity recommendations to reduce cancer risk are the American Institute for Cancer Research (www.aicr.org) and the National Cancer Institute (www.cancer.gov).

### TABLE 21.3
### WHO Dietary Recommendations

Achieve energy balance and a healthy weight

Limit energy intake from total fats and shift fat consumption away from saturated fats to unsaturated fats and toward the elimination of trans-fatty acids

Increase consumption of fruits and vegetables, and legumes, whole grains, and nuts

Limit the intake of free sugars

Limit salt (sodium) consumption from all sources and ensure that salt is iodized

*Source:* World Health Organization. Global strategy on diet, physical activity and health. Available at http://www.who.int/dietphysicalactivity/diet/en/index.html, accessed March 11, 2012.

## DETERMINING ENERGY REQUIREMENTS

Total energy requirements include the sum of basal energy needs, energy needs for physical activity, and the energy needed for the thermic effect of foods.[12] Energy needs tend to decrease with age due to reductions in lean body mass, particularly after age 40 for men and age 50 for women. Men have higher energy needs than women. The Dietary Reference Intakes include equations to determine the estimated energy requirement (EER) for adults of a normal weight (BMI of 18.5 up to 25 kg/m$^2$).[12] The equations use age in years, weight in kilograms (kg), height in meters (m), and a physical activity coefficient (PA). To obtain weight in kilograms, divide weight in pounds by 2.2. To obtain height in meters, multiply height in inches by 0.0254.

Equations are as follows:

- Men

$$EER = 662 - (9.53 \times age\,[year]) + PA$$
$$\times (15.91 \times weight\,[kg] + 539.6 \times height\,[m])$$

The physical activity coefficient (PA) to use will be 1.00, 1.11, 1.25, or 1.48 for men that are sedentary, low active, active, or very active, respectively.

- Women

$$EER = 354 - (6.91 \times age[year]) + PA$$
$$\times (9.36 \times weight\,[kg] + 726 \times height\,[m])$$

The physical activity coefficient (PA) to use will be 1.00, 1.12, 1.27, or 1.45 for women that are sedentary, low active, active, or very active, respectively.

Different equations have been developed for adults who are overweight and obese, and these equations are available in the Dietary Reference Intakes for energy.[12]

## ENERGY INTAKE AND OBESITY

Excess consumption of calories and insufficient physical activity result in positive energy balance and weight gain. Overweight and obesity are associated with increased risk for coronary heart disease, hypertension, stroke, heart failure, type II diabetes mellitus, osteoarthritis, gallstones, gastroesophageal reflux disease, gallstones, and cancer at many sites including the colon and rectum, endometrium, kidney, esophagus, pancreas, breast, and gall bladder.[11,13] Obesity in midlife may increase the risk of mortality by two- to threefold.[14] A body mass index (BMI) of 25–29.99 is classified as overweight, while a BMI of 30 and above is classified as obese. The prevalence of overweight and obesity has increased for the past several decades.[6]

Table 21.4 provides data on the prevalence of overweight and obesity in the United States.[15] Seventy-four percent of men and 64% of women had a BMI of 25 and over in 2009–2010. More

**TABLE 21.4**

**Prevalence of Overweight and Obesity among U.S. Adults, 2009–2010**

| Age (Years) | Overweight and Obesity BMI[a] ≥ 25 | | Obesity BMI ≥ 30 | |
|---|---|---|---|---|
| | M[b] (%) | W | M (%) | W |
| 20–39 | 67.1 | 55.8 | 33.2 | 31.9 |
| 40–59 | 79.5 | 66.0 | 37.2 | 36.0 |
| ≥60 | 76.5 | 73.5 | 36.6 | 42.3 |
| ≥20 | 73.9 | 63.7 | 35.5 | 35.8 |

*Source:* Flegal, K.M. et al., *JAMA*, 307, 491, 2012.

[a] BMI, body mass index.

[b] M, men; W, women.

than one-third of adults (35.7%) were obese. The prevalence of obesity was essentially the same for men and women.[15,16] Between 1999–2000 and 2009–2010, the prevalence of obesity in the United States increased in men from 27.5% to 35.5% but remained the same in women at 35.8%.[16] The increase in obesity is a worldwide trend, as well. The WHO estimated that the international prevalence of obesity has more than doubled since 1980.[17] The medical costs of obesity in the United States were estimated at $147 billion for 2008.[18]

With this rise in obesity, the 2010 Dietary Guidelines recommended the consumption of nutrient-dense foods that contribute essential nutrients with relatively few calories.[6] Nutrient-dense foods include fruits and vegetables, whole grains, low-fat milk and milk products, and lean meats, poultry, and fish. In contrast, it is recommended that consumption of energy-dense foods, or those that are high in calories and provide few essential nutrients, be minimized. Adults tend to consume lower amounts of fruit, vegetables, whole grains, low-fat milk and milk products, and seafood, but more sugars, solid fats, refined grains, and sodium than recommended.[7]

Foods high in solid fats and added sugars provide most of the excess calories in the adult diet and contribute about 35% of the energy consumed in the United States.[7] In comparison, it is recommended that a maximum of 5%–15% of calories come from solid fats and added sugars. Grain-based desserts such as cakes and cookies, regular cheese, sausage, frankfurters, bacon, pizza, fried potatoes, and dairy-based desserts are some of the sources of solid fats frequently consumed in the United States. High-calorie, low-nutrient beverages contribute to excess consumption of calories. Among beverages, regular soda contributes the greatest amount of energy to the average adult diet (114 kcal/day) and is a major source of added sugar. Other sources of added sugars are regular energy and sports drinks, grain and dairy-based desserts, sugar-sweetened fruit drinks, and candy.[7]

Regular physical activity is also essential to maintain a healthy weight. The 2010 Dietary Guidelines have provided specific physical activity recommendations for adults aged 18–64 that are derived from the 2008 Physical Activity Guidelines for Americans.[6,19]

## ESTIMATES OF ACTUAL INTAKES OF ADULTS FOR MACRONUTRIENTS

The National Nutrition Monitoring and Related Research Program uses surveys and other means to monitor food and nutrient intake in the United States.[20] Tables 21.5 and 21.6 include data on energy intake and sources of energy for U.S. adults in 2007–2008.[21] Adult men consumed an average of about 2510 kcal/day while women consumed about 1770 kcal/day. Energy requirements decrease with age beginning in the fourth decade of life. Thus, mean calorie intakes for men and women decreased with each decade of life above age 50. Both men and women obtained an average of 16% of their energy from protein and 34% of their energy

**TABLE 21.5**

**Mean Energy Intake for Adult Men and Women (1 Day), United States, 2007–2008**

| Age (Years) | M[a] | W |
|---|---|---|
| | kcal | |
| 20–29 | 2756 | 1828 |
| 30–39 | 2654 | 1858 |
| 40–49 | 2692 | 1879 |
| 50–59 | 2493 | 1793 |
| 60–69 | 2140 | 1597 |
| ≥70 | 1837 | 1491 |
| ≥20 | 2507 | 1766 |

*Source:* U.S. Department of Agriculture, Agricultural Research Service, Nutrient intakes from food: Mean amounts consumed per individual, by gender and age, what we eat in America, NHANES 2007–2008, http://www.ars.usda.gov/ba/bhnrc.fsrg, 2010.

[a] M, men; W, women.

**TABLE 21.6**

**Sources of Energy Intake (% of Total Energy) for Adult Men and Women (1 Day), United States, 2007–2008**

| Age (Years) | Protein | | Fat | | Carbohydrate | |
|---|---|---|---|---|---|---|
| | M[a] | W | M | W | M | W |
| | % kcal | | | | | |
| 20–29 | 16 | 15 | 31 | 32 | 50 | 52 |
| 30–39 | 16 | 15 | 34 | 33 | 47 | 50 |
| 40–49 | 16 | 15 | 34 | 34 | 47 | 50 |
| 50–59 | 16 | 16 | 35 | 34 | 47 | 49 |
| 60–69 | 16 | 16 | 35 | 35 | 47 | 49 |
| ≥70 | 16 | 16 | 34 | 33 | 49 | 52 |
| ≥20 | 16 | 16 | 34 | 34 | 48 | 50 |

*Source:* U.S. Department of Agriculture, Agricultural Research Service, Nutrient intakes from food: Mean amounts consumed per individual, by gender and age, what we eat in America, NHANES 2007–2008, http://www.ars.usda.gov/ba/bhnrc.fsrg, 2010.

[a] M, men; W, women.

## TABLE 21.7
### Total Protein, Carbohydrate, and Fat Intakes (1 Day), United States, 2007–2008

| Age (Years) | Protein M[a] | Protein W | Carbohydrate M | Carbohydrate W | Fat M | Fat W |
|---|---|---|---|---|---|---|
| | | | g/day | | | |
| 20–29 | 105 | 68 | 342 | 231 | 96 | 68 |
| 30–39 | 102 | 69 | 309 | 232 | 103 | 70 |
| 40–49 | 105 | 71 | 317 | 231 | 103 | 72 |
| 50–59 | 100 | 68 | 281 | 218 | 100 | 70 |
| 60–69 | 85 | 61 | 246 | 195 | 84 | 63 |
| ≥70 | 73 | 57 | 225 | 193 | 70 | 56 |
| ≥20 | 98 | 67 | 296 | 220 | 95 | 67 |

Source: U.S. Department of Agriculture, Agricultural Research Service, Nutrient intakes from food: Mean amounts consumed per individual, by gender and age, what we eat in America, NHANES 2007–2008, http://www.ars.usda.gov/ba/bhnrc.fsrg, 2010.

[a] M, men; W, women.

from fat. Those aged 20–29 consumed the lowest percent of calories from fat, 31%–32%. Carbohydrate provided 48% and 50% of calories, respectively, for men and women. A small percentage of energy intake, about 4% for men and 2% for women, was provided by alcoholic beverages.

Table 21.7 provides information on the total amount of carbohydrate, protein, and fat consumed by U.S. adults in grams.[21] Adults require 0.8 g of protein per kilogram of body weight per day, which equates to 46 g/day for a typical woman and 56 g/day for a typical man.[3] Animal sources of protein include meat, poultry, fish, eggs, milk, and milk products, while plant sources include beans, peas, and nuts. In 2007–2008, average intakes of protein were about 98 g for adult men and 67 g for adult women. Since protein intake is correlated with calorie intake, average protein intake decreased with age and was greater for men than for women. Most adult men and women consume recommended amounts of protein or more. However, about 7%–8.5% of women aged 51 and above may not meet protein needs.[22]

Carbohydrates are the major energy source for adults, and men consume a greater amount of carbohydrate (about 80 g/day) than women, due to their higher caloric needs. It is recommended that adults obtain 45%–65% of their energy as carbohydrate.[3] Thus average carbohydrate intake for adults, as a percent of calories, is within this range. Nutrient-dense sources of carbohydrate include fruits, vegetables, grains, dried beans and peas, and low-fat dairy products. Carbohydrate intake also includes added sugars, defined as sugar added to foods during processing or preparation. Intake of added sugars declined between 1999–2000 and 2007–2008 in the United States, primarily due to a decline of soft drink consumption during this time period.[23]

Fat also serves as an energy source, and total intake increases as caloric need increases. Men and women consumed an average of 95 and 67 g of fat per day, respectively. Total fat intake should account for 20%–35% of calories for

adults.[3] Since average intake of total fat for adults is 34% of calories, this suggests that many are consuming more fat than recommended. Research studies suggest that the quality of fat consumed may have more impact on cardiovascular disease than the quantity of fat intake.[7] Table 21.8 provides data on the intake of saturated, monounsaturated, and polyunsaturated fatty acids and cholesterol by adults.[21] High saturated fat intake is associated with the elevation of serum low-density lipoprotein (LDL) cholesterol, a risk factor for coronary heart disease. Hence, the 2010 Dietary Guidelines recommend that adults consume less than 10% of their calories as saturated fat.[6,24] In comparison, adults in the U.S. currently consume an average of 11% of energy as saturated fat.[21] Replacement of saturated fat with mono- and polyunsaturated fatty acids, found in higher amounts in oils, is associated with reduced serum LDL cholesterol.[24] Men and women currently consume an average of 7% of their calories as polyunsaturated fatty acids and 12%–13% as monounsaturated fatty acids.[21] In comparison, the USDA food patterns suggest for an adult consuming 2000 cal that 9% of calories be polyunsaturated fat and 12% be monounsaturated fat.[7] Thus, the average intake of polyunsaturated fat is well below the recommended amounts. Consumption of total and saturated fat by U.S. adults has not changed over the past several decades, even with consistent recommendations to make these changes.[7] To achieve a decrease in saturated fat intake and increase in unsaturated fats, one of the recommendations in the Dietary Guidelines for Americans, 2010, is to consume oils in place of solid fats.[6] Fatty fish, such as salmon and trout, are a good source of omega-3 fatty acids, a type of polyunsaturated fatty acid. Consumption of eight ounces of fish that is high in omega-3 fatty acids (eicosapentaenoic and docosahexaenoic acids) per week has been linked to reduced mortality from coronary heart disease.[10]

## TABLE 21.8
### Mean Daily Intake of Saturated Fatty Acids (SFA), Monounsaturated Fatty Acids (MUFA), Polyunsaturated Fatty Acids (PUFA), and Cholesterol (CHOL) (1 Day), United States, 2007–2008

| Age (Years) | SFA M[a] | SFA W | MUFA M | MUFA W | PUFA M | PUFA W | CHOL M | CHOL W |
|---|---|---|---|---|---|---|---|---|
| | | | | g/day | | | | |
| 20–29 | 32.6 | 22.5 | 34.9 | 24.3 | 20.1 | 14.6 | 355 | 216 |
| 30–39 | 33.6 | 23.6 | 39.2 | 25.4 | 21.0 | 15.3 | 377 | 248 |
| 40–49 | 35.2 | 24.1 | 37.9 | 26.2 | 20.6 | 15.3 | 406 | 256 |
| 50–59 | 32.4 | 22.9 | 37.7 | 25.3 | 21.5 | 16.2 | 375 | 227 |
| 60–69 | 27.1 | 20.6 | 31.8 | 23.0 | 17.7 | 13.8 | 319 | 228 |
| ≥70 | 22.8 | 18.2 | 26.1 | 20.1 | 15.0 | 12.5 | 285 | 192 |
| ≥20 | 31.6 | 22.3 | 35.6 | 24.4 | 19.8 | 14.8 | 362 | 230 |

Source: U.S. Department of Agriculture, Agricultural Research Service, Nutrient intakes from food: Mean amounts consumed per individual, by gender and age, what we eat in America, NHANES 2007–2008, http://www.ars.usda.gov/ba/bhnrc.fsrg, 2010.

[a] M, men; W, women.

**TABLE 21.9**

**Mean Dietary Fiber Intake (1 Day), United States, 2007–2008**

| Age (Years) | M[a] | W |
|---|---|---|
| | g/day | |
| 20–29 | 16.9 | 13.3 |
| 30–39 | 18.7 | 13.8 |
| 40–49 | 17.6 | 14.1 |
| 50–59 | 18.4 | 15.6 |
| 60–69 | 17.4 | 14.9 |
| ≥70 | 17.0 | 14.1 |
| ≥20 | 17.7 | 14.3 |

*Source:* U.S. Department of Agriculture, Agricultural Research Service, Nutrient intakes from food: Mean amounts consumed per individual, by gender and age, what we eat in America, NHANES 2007–2008, http://www.ars.usda.gov/ba/bhnrc.fsrg, 2010.

[a] M, men; W, women.

Trans fatty acids, also associated with enhanced risk of cardiovascular disease, are found in foods high in solid fats. Higher intakes of trans fatty acids increase serum LDL cholesterol, but decrease the levels of the beneficial high-density lipoprotein (HDL) cholesterol in blood.[24] Trans fatty acids are found naturally in some animal foods, and current recommendations focus on minimizing the intake of industrial trans fatty acids that are produced through hydrogenation of oils. The current intake of trans fatty acids by U.S. adults is estimated to be 2% of calorie intake.[25] It is also recommended that healthy adults consume less than 300 mg of cholesterol per day.[6] Average cholesterol intake for men was 362 mg and for women was 230 mg/day in 2007–2008.

Average fiber intake for adults is shown in Table 21.9.[21] It is recommended that adults consume 14 g of fiber for every 1000 cal.[3] This means that younger men and women (aged 20–49) should consume about 38 and 25 g of fiber per day, respectively, while men aged 50 and over should eat about 30 g and women 50 years and over should eat 21 g. However, men in the United States consume on average only about 18 g of fiber, while women consume only about 14 g of fiber per day. Less than 3% of men and only 6% of women consume the recommended amount of dietary fiber, and thus it is considered to be a nutrient of concern.[7] Fruits, vegetables, and whole grains provide dietary fiber, and diets high in these foods tend to be low in caloric density that helps prevent weight gain.

Some vitamins and minerals are consumed in less than recommended amounts by a significant proportion of the adult population. National nutrient intake data collected in 2003–2006 showed that many adults consumed less than the established EAR for vitamins A, C, D, and E and the minerals calcium and magnesium.[26] Of note, 68% of adults did not consume the EAR for vitamin D. Another mineral consumed in less than recommended amounts by a significant proportion of the adult population is potassium.[7,26] Even though

these data suggest that many adults consumed low amounts of vitamins A, C, and E, only small percentages of the U.S. population have low blood levels of these three nutrients.[7] In contrast, many adults have low blood levels of vitamin D. In addition, bone density, which reflects calcium status, is low in many adults. Vitamin D and calcium are both essential for bone health and prevention of osteoporosis.[7] Thus, the 2010 Dietary Guidelines for Americans included calcium and vitamin D, as well as potassium, as nutrients of concern.[6] While nutrient-dense foods are good sources of these nutrients, some adults need to consume vitamin and/or mineral supplements to achieve nutritional adequacy. For example, foods fortified with vitamin D such as milk and fatty fish are good sources of vitamin D, and milk and milk products are good sources of calcium. However, some adults will not be able to meet daily recommendations for 1000 mg of calcium (1200 mg for women aged 51 and over) and 15 µg of vitamin D[27] without taking supplements. Calcium supplements were taken by 34%–51% of men and 39%–67% of women aged 19–70 in 2003–2006.[28] Use of vitamin D supplements has increased during recent decades for both men and women, and 27%–45% of adults aged 20–59 took vitamin D supplements.[29]

There are specific recommendations for supplement use for some segments of the adult population. Adults aged 50 and over are advised to obtain the recommended amount of vitamin $B_{12}$, 2.4 µg/day, from foods fortified with $B_{12}$ or vitamin supplements that contain $B_{12}$.[3,6] This is because a significant portion of the population aged 50 and over is unable to absorb the $B_{12}$ naturally found in foods. Additionally, it is recommended that women of childbearing age consume 400 µg/day of folic acid from fortified foods or supplements to prevent neural tube defects. Over 34% of women aged 20–39 reported taking a dietary supplement with folic acid in 2003–2006.[29]

Total dietary supplement use is high in the adult population. Fifty-three percent used dietary supplements in 2003–2006. The most common supplements taken were multivitamin/multimineral supplements, with 39% reporting the use of these preparations.[29] There is a concern that some adults who need to take supplements to meet nutrient needs do not take them, while other adults may consume unneeded supplements.[4] While multivitamin/multimineral supplements may be needed by some individuals to meet nutrient needs, these preparations have not been found to be effective in reducing chronic disease mortality in healthy populations.[4,7]

The combination of nutrients naturally found in foods, food enrichment and fortification, and use of nutrient supplements can sometimes lead to nutrient intakes that exceed the UL of intake.[26] Small percentages of adults (3% or less) consumed more than the UL for zinc, vitamin A, and folate in 2003–2006. However, a greater percentage exceeded the UL for niacin.

Adults in the United States tend to consume too much sodium, which has an impact on blood pressure regulation. High sodium intakes are associated with higher blood pressure. In contrast, potassium intake is inversely related to blood pressure.[7] With adults consuming less than adequate levels of potassium along with high sodium levels, this has generated concern because hypertension is a leading risk factor for the development of coronary heart disease, stroke, and renal disease.[30] Further, a higher dietary sodium to potassium ratio has been associated with increased risk for cardiovascular mortality.[31] One-third of U.S. adults have hypertension.[30] Thus, current recommendations are to limit sodium intake to less than 2300 mg/day. In addition, adults who are over 50 years and those who are African American or who have hypertension, diabetes, or chronic kidney disease are advised to reduce sodium intake even further to no more than 1500 mg/day.[6] In comparison, adult men in the United States consumed an average of 4043 mg of sodium per day, while women consumed an average of 2884 mg/day according to national data from 2007–2008.[32] As calorie intake increases, so does sodium intake, which is why men tend to have higher intakes of sodium than women. Despite the continuous recommendations to reduce sodium intake, intake has not changed during the past decade. The majority of sodium in foods comes from the salt added during processing. Meat (particularly cured meats), poultry, fish, eggs, mixed dishes, cheese, soups, yeast breads, and some condiments provide the majority of sodium in the U.S. diet.[7,32]

Much of the research linking diet and chronic disease risk has focused on the intake of foods rather than specific nutrients. Consumption of five or more servings of fruits and vegetables per day is associated with reduced risk for cardiovascular disease and some cancers.[11,24] Fruits and vegetables are nutrient dense, with high concentrations of nutrients and relatively low levels of calories.[6] Higher consumption of fruits and vegetables has been associated with lower risk for weight gain.[33] The USDA food patterns recommend daily consumption of 2.5 cups of a variety of vegetables and two cups of fruits for an adult consuming 2000 cal/day. Most adults do not consume the recommended amounts of fruits and vegetables.[7]

Greater consumption of whole grains has been associated with reduced risk for cardiovascular disease, type 2 diabetes, lower body weight, and possibly reduced risk for some gastrointestinal cancers.[7,11,34] The dietary guidelines indicate that at least 50% of grains consumed should be whole grains.[6] Only 15% of all Americans consume recommended amounts of whole grains, and adults eat, on average, less than one serving per day.[7,34,35] In addition, adults overconsume refined grains.

Low-fat milk products are good sources of calcium, vitamin D, potassium, and protein. There is evidence that consumption of low-fat dairy products may lower blood pressure and reduce the risk for cardiovascular disease and type 2 diabetes.[7,24,36] Three servings of low-fat dairy products per day is recommended for a person consuming 2000 cal.[6] This includes low-fat milk, yogurt, and cheese. Only 52% of Americans consume recommended amounts of milk and milk products.[7] Lactose intolerance, either diagnosed or self-perceived, contributes to lower intakes of dairy foods and calcium.[37] People who are lactose intolerant are often able to consume a limited amount of regular milk with food, but other options such as lactose-free milk, low-fat cheese, and yogurt can contribute to dairy product intake.

Meat, poultry, fish, eggs, nuts, seeds, legumes, and soy products are major sources of protein and micronutrients in the adult diet. Choosing a wide variety of protein-containing foods is recommended.[6] Selection of lean meats and poultry will help reduce consumption of saturated fatty acids, which are associated with elevated risk for cardiovascular disease. Eating about 8 oz of seafood per week is associated with reduced cardiovascular disease mortality. Since eggs are high in cholesterol, to meet recommendations for total cholesterol intake of less than 300 mg/day, no more than moderate consumption is suggested. However, consumption of one egg per day by a healthy adult does not result in elevated risk for cardiovascular disease.[24] Consumption of 100 g (3.5 oz) of red meat or 50 g (1.8 oz) of processed meat per day has been linked to about a 15%–20% increase in the risk for cancers of the colon and rectum.[11] Thus, American Cancer Society guidelines to reduce cancer risk suggest that intake of red and processed meat should be limited. Intake of processed meats has also been associated with increased risk for cardiovascular disease and diabetes.[38] Processed meats are high in saturated fat and sodium, two of the nutrients consumed in higher amounts than recommended. For a person consuming 2000 cal/day, the USDA food pattern for people that consume meat, poultry, and/or fish suggests an average of 1.8 oz of meat, 1.5 oz of poultry, and 1.2 oz of fish per day. In contrast, average daily intake of meat, poultry, and fish by U.S. adults, based on 2000 cal of intake, is 2.5 oz of meat, 1.2 oz of poultry, and 0.5 oz of fish.[6] Thus average meat intake is higher than the recommended levels. Americans consume only 44% of the recommended amounts of fish.[6,7] Plant-based diets and vegetarian diets are associated with lower risk for cardiovascular disease and obesity.[6,7,24] Vegetarian dietary patterns that include eggs, milk, beans and peas, processed soy products, and/or nuts and seeds as protein sources are also provided as a component of the Dietary Guidelines for Americans, 2010.[6]

While moderate alcohol intake has been associated with reduced risk for cardiovascular disease, higher amounts are associated with increased risk for cardiovascular disease and some cancers.[11,24] Moderate consumption is no more than two drinks for men and no more than one drink per day for women. This level is associated with reduced all-cause mortality risk. One drink is 12, 5, or 1.5 fluid ounces of beer, wine, or distilled spirits, respectively, and is 14 g of alcohol. It has been estimated that 9% of men and 4% of women consume more than recommended levels.[6]

## FOOD ENVIRONMENT AND FOOD CONSUMPTION PATTERNS

Table 21.10 provides data on the contribution of breakfast, snacks, and food eaten away from home to caloric intake. Food consumption patterns can impact a person's ability to consume a healthy diet. Dietary behaviors that

## TABLE 21.10

### Contribution of Breakfast, Snacks, and Foods Consumed Away from Home to Total Energy Intake (1 Day), United States, 2007–2008

|              | Breakfast | | Snacks | | Foods Away from Home | |
|--------------|-----------|----|--------|----|------|----|
| Age (Years)  | M[a]      | W  | M      | W  | M    | W  |
|              | % kcal    |    |        |    |      |    |
| 20–29        | 14        | 14 | 26     | 25 | 40   | 39 |
| 30–39        | 18        | 17 | 22     | 25 | 46   | 35 |
| 40–49        | 16        | 15 | 23     | 25 | 35   | 34 |
| 50–59        | 16        | 16 | 23     | 23 | 37   | 35 |
| 60–69        | 18        | 19 | 24     | 23 | 29   | 26 |
| ≥70          | 23        | 20 | 20     | 19 | 19   | 17 |
| ≥20          | 17        | 16 | 23     | 24 | 37   | 33 |

*Sources:* U.S. Department of Agriculture, Agricultural Research Service, Breakfast: Percentages of selected nutrients contributed by foods eaten at breakfast, by gender and age, what we eat in America, NHANES 2007–2008, 2010; U.S. Department of Agriculture, Agricultural Research Service, Snacks: Percentages of selected nutrients contributed by foods eaten at snack occasions, by gender and age, what we eat in America, NHANES 2007–2008, 2010; U.S. Department of Agriculture, Agricultural Research Service, Snacks: Percentages of selected nutrients contributed by foods eaten away from home, by gender and age, what we eat in America, NHANES 2007–2008, www.ars.usda.gov/ba/bhnrc.fsrg, 2010.

[a] M, men; W, women.

may be associated with weight gain, overweight, and obesity in adults include skipping breakfast, eating out at fast-food restaurants, and snacking on energy-dense foods.[7] Breakfast, on average, provides about 16%–17% of energy for adults. The age group with the lowest percent of calories from breakfast (14%) was adults in their 20s. Some studies suggest that consumption of breakfast may be inversely related to body weight in adults, although this research is not conclusive.[7] Most U.S. adults eat at least one snack per day, and snacks provide an average of almost 25% of adult energy intake. Snacks contribute to intakes of fruits, vegetable, grains, protein-containing foods, and dairy products, but also provide 41% of added sugars and 17% of the solid fats consumed by adults.[39] The percent of food purchased away from home in the United States has increased for the past four decades.[40] Men consumed 37%, while women consumed 33% of their calories away from home in 2007–2008. Younger adults consumed the greatest percent of their calories away from home, and as age increased, the percent of calories consumed away from home was reduced. Eating meals away from home is associated with consumption of larger portion sizes and increased energy intake, which can contribute to excess weight gain.[10,41] Many foods eaten away from home also are high in specific food components associated with increased disease risk such as saturated fat, trans fat, added sugars, and sodium.[10] Making healthy food choices and selecting smaller portion sizes when selecting snacks and consuming foods away from home will result in lower risk for weight gain and subsequent chronic diseases.

## SUMMARY

Adulthood is a time not only to focus on meeting basic nutrient requirements, but also to engage in dietary and physical activity behaviors that will result in the lowest risk for chronic diseases. The prevention of overweight and obesity is critical to reducing the risk for chronic diseases that become more prevalent with age. Achieving a balance of energy intake and energy expenditure is necessary to maintain a healthy weight. As recommended in the Dietary Guidelines for Americans, 2010, adults should increase intakes of fruits, vegetables, whole grains, and low-fat dairy products, without consuming more energy than needed. Oils should be consumed in place of solid fats. A variety of protein-containing foods such as lean meat, poultry, fish, beans, and nuts should be consumed in moderation. Finally, engaging in regular physical activity is essential to prevent weight gain.

## REFERENCES

1. Read, M. In: Berdanier, CD, Dwyer, J, Feldman, EB eds., *Handbook of Nutrition and Food*, 2nd edn. CRC Press, Boca Raton, FL. 2007, 1288pp.
2. U.S. Department of Health and Human Services, Public Health Service, No. 88–50210, Surgeon General's Report on Nutrition and Health. U.S. Government Printing Office, Washington, DC, 1988.
3. Institute of Medicine, Food and Nutrition Board. *Dietary Reference Intakes: The Essential Guide to Nutrient Requirements.* National Academies Press, Washington, DC, 2006, 543pp.
4. American Dietetic Association. *J Am Diet Assoc* 109:2073;2009.
5. Watts, ML, Hager, MH, Toner, CD, Weber, JA. *Nutr Rev* 69:404;2011.
6. U.S. Department of Agriculture and U.S. Department of Health and Human Services. *Dietary Guidelines for Americans, 2010*, 7th edn. U.S. Government Printing Office, Washington, DC, 2010. Available at www.dietaryguidelines.gov, Accessed on March 11, 2012.
7. Dietary Guidelines Advisory Committee, 2010. Report of the Dietary Guidelines Advisory Committee on the Dietary Guidelines for Americans, 2010 to the Secretary of Agriculture and the Secretary of Health and Human Services. U.S. Department of Agriculture, Agricultural Research Service, Washington, DC. Available at http://www.cnpp.usda.gov/Publications/DietaryGuidelines/2010/DGAC/Report/2010DGACReport-camera-ready-Jan11-11.pdf, Accessed on March 11, 2012.
8. Food and Drug Administration, Focus on Food Labeling. Special Issue of FDA Consumer Magazine, May 1993, DHHS Publication No. (FDA) 93-2262, U.S. Government Printing Office, Washington, DC, 1993.
9. World Health Organization. Global strategy on diet, physical activity and health. Available at http://www.who.int/dietphysicalactivity/diet/en/index.html, Accessed March 11, 2012.

10. Lichtenstein, AH, Appel, LJ, Brands, M et al. *Circulation* 114:82;2006.

11. Kushi, LH, Doyle, C, McCullough, M et al. *Cancer J Clin* 62:30;2012.

12. Institute of Medicine, Food and Nutrition Board. *Dietary Reference Intakes for Energy, Carbohydrate, Fiber, Fat, Fatty Acids, Cholesterol, Protein, and Amino Acids.* National Academies Press, Washington, DC, 2005.

13. Kumanyika, SK, Obarzanek, E, Stettler, N et al. *Circulation* 118:428:2008.

14. Adams, KF, Schatzkin, A, Harris, TB et al. *N Engl J Med* 355;763:2006.

15. Flegal, KM, Carroll, MD, Kit, BK, Ogden, CL. *JAMA* 307:491;2012.

16. Ogden, CL. Prevalence of obesity in the United States. Data brief. Available at http://www.cdc.gov/nchs/data/databriefs/db82.pdf, Accessed March 10, 2012.

17. World Health Organization. Available at www.who.int/mediacentre/factsheets/fs311/en/index.html, Accessed March 11, 2012.

18. Finkelstein, EA, Trogdon, JG, Cohen, JW, Dietz, W. *Health Aff* 28:w822;2009, doi:10.1377/hlthaff.28.5.w822.

19. U.S. Department of Health and Human Services. 2008 Physical Activity Guidelines for Americans. Washington DC. 2008. Available at http://www.health.gov/paguidelines

20. Interagency Board for Nutrition Monitoring and Related Research. Bialostosky, K, ed. *Nutrition Monitoring in the United States: The directory of Federal and State Nutrition Monitoring and Related Research Activities.* National Center for Health Statistics, Hyattsville, MD, 2000.

21. U.S. Department of Agriculture, Agricultural Research Service. Nutrient intakes from food: Mean amounts consumed per individual, by gender and age, what we eat in America, NHANES 2007–2008. 2010. Available at www.ars.usda.gov/ba/bhnrc/fsrg, Accessed March 11, 2012.

22. Fulgoni, VL. *Am J Clin Nutr* 87:1554S;2008.

23. Welsh, JA, Sharma, AJ, Grellinger, L, Vos, MB. *Am J Clin Nutr* 94:726;2011

24. Flock, MR, Kris-Etherton, PM. *Curr Atheroscler Rep* 13:499;2011.

25. Remig, V, Franklin, B, Margolis, S et al. *J Am Diet Assoc* 110:585;2010.

26. Fulgoni, VL, Keast, DR, Bailey, RL, Dwyer, J. *J Nutr* 141:1847;2011.

27. Institute of Medicine, Food and Nutrition Board. *Dietary Reference Intakes for Calcium and Vitamin D.* The National Academies Press, Washington, DC, 2011.

28. Bailey, RL, Dodd, KW, Goldman, JA et al. *J Nutr* 140:817:2010.

29. Gahche, J, Bailey, R, Burt, V et al. Dietary supplement use among U.S. adults has increased since NHANES III (1988–1994). NCHS Data Brief No. 61. National Center for Health Statistics, Hyattsville, MD, 2011.

30. Roger, VL, Go, AS, Lloyd-Jones, DM et al. *Circulation* 125:e2;2012.

31. Yang, Q, Liu, T, Kuklina, EV et al. *Arch Intern Med* 171:1183;2011.

32. Hoy MK, Goldman JD, Murayi T et al. Sodium intake of the U.S. population: What we eat in America, NHANES 2007–2008. Food Surveys Research Group Dietary Data Brief No. 8 October 2011. Available at http://www.ars.usda.gov/SP2UserFiles/Place/12355000/pdf/DBrief/8_sodium_intakes_0708.pdf, Accessed March 10, 2012.

33. Mozaffarian, D, Hao, T, Rimm, EB et al. *N Engl J Med* 364:2392;2011.

34. O'Neil, CE, Zanovec, M, Cho, SS, Nicklas, TA. *Nutr Res* 30:815;2010.

35. Wells, HF, Buzby, JC. Dietary Assessment of Major Trends in U.S. Food Consumption, 1970–2005, Economic Information Bulletin No. 33. Economic Research Service, U.S. Dept. of Agriculture. March 2008. Available at http://www.ers.usda.gov/publications/eib33/eib33.pdf, Accessed March 10, 2012.

36. Tremblay, A, Gilbert, JA. *J Am Coll Nutr* 28:91S;2009.

37. Nicklas, TA, Qu, H, Hughes, SO et al. *Am J Clin Nutr* 94:191;2011.

38. Micha, R, Wallace, SK, Mozaffarian, D. *Circulation* 121:2271;2010.

39. Sebastian, RS, Wilkinson Enns, C, Goldman, JD. MyPyramid intakes and snacking patterns of U.S. adults. What we eat in America, NHANES 2007–2008. Food Surveys Research Group, Agricultural Research Service, U.S. Department of Agriculture. Dietary Data Brief No. 5, June 2011.

40. U.S. Department of Agriculture, Economic Research Service. Diet quality and food consumption: Food away from home, 2008. Available at http://www.ers.usda.gov/Briefing/DietQuality/FAFH.htm, Accessed March 10, 2012.

41. Todd, JE, Mancino, L, Lin, B-H. The impact of food away from home on adult diet quality, ERR-90. U.S. Department of Agriculture, Economic Research Service, February 2010. Available at http://www.ers.usda.gov/publications/err90/, Accessed March 10, 2012.

42. U.S. Department of Agriculture, Agricultural Research Service, Breakfast: Percentages of selected nutrients contributed by foods eaten at breakfast, by gender and age, what we eat in America, NHANES 2007–2008, 2010. Available at: www.ars.usda.gov/ba/bhnrc.fsrg

43. U.S. Department of Agriculture, Agricultural Research Service, Snacks: Percentages of selected nutrients contributed by foods eaten at snack occasions, by gender and age, what we eat in America, NHANES 2007–2008, 2010. Available at: www.ars.usda.gov/ba/bhnrc.fsrg

44. U.S. Department of Agriculture, Agricultural Research Service, Snacks: Percentages of selected nutrients contributed by foods eaten away from home, by gender and age, what we eat in America, NHANES 2007–2008, 2010. Available at: www.ars.usda.gov/ba/bhnrc.fsrg

# 22 Nutrition in the Later Years

*Mary Ann Johnson and Alyson Haslam*

## CONTENTS

## INTRODUCTION

Older adults are a diverse and growing population. They range in age from 65 to more than 100 years and include the very fit and the very frail. Older adults vary in ethnicity, culture, income, mobility, knowledge of nutrition and health, health behaviors, and health status. The main nutritional problems are poor food patterns and nutrient intake, as well as a high prevalence of overweight and obesity. The requirements for most essential vitamins and minerals do not change with advanced age, with only a few exceptions. Requirements for calcium and vitamin D are increased and the recommended chemical form of vitamin $B_{12}$ changes to crystalline. Decreased lean body mass and low physical activity are the main determinants of the low energy requirements of older people. Paradoxically, older adults are at increased risk for both overnutrition (overweight and obesity) and undernutrition, with the accompanying problems of nutritional deficiencies and weight loss. This chapter will review the primary nutritional problems associated with aging and recommend ways to improve the nutritional status of older people.

## DEMOGRAPHICS OF AGING

The growth rate of the older population (over 65 years) has rapidly increased during the last few decades and will continue to increase for the next 50 years in the United States.[1] The number of people over 65 years was greater than 40 million in 2010 and is expected to increase to nearly 55 million in 2020 and to more than 88 million in 2050.[1,2] The number of people over 85 years was approximately 5.4 million in 2010 and is expected to increase to 19 million in 2050.[1,2] About 84% of older adults were between the ages of 65 and 84 and 16% were 85 and older in 2010.[1] The majority of people aged 65 and older are white followed by black and Hispanic (Figure 22.1).[3] Over 96% of older adults live in the community rather than in long-term care facilities.[3] Human life expectancy has increased dramatically during the past century. Those who are 65 years old today can expect to live more than 18 additional years and those who are 85 years old today can expect more than 6 additional years.[3]

Aging is an inevitable process. The efficiencies of cell function and homeostatic mechanisms decrease with advanced age. In some organs, new cells replace old cells.[4] However, during each replication, the telomeres are shortened

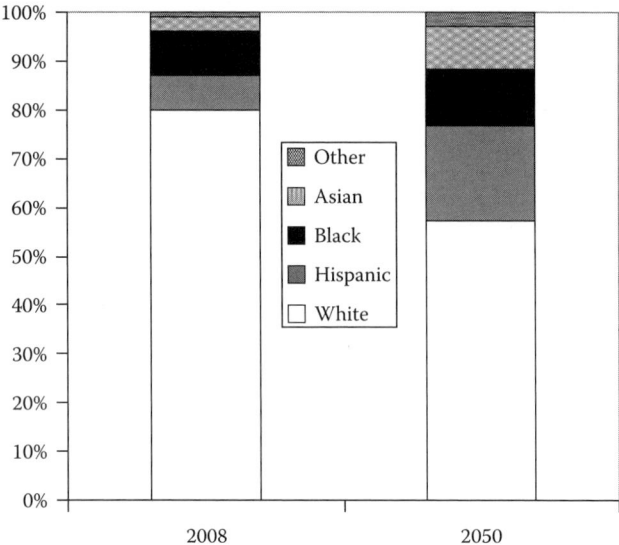

**FIGURE 22.1** Projected population aged 65 and older in the United States by race/ethnicity: 2008 and 2050. (From Federal Interagency Forum on Aging and Related Statistics, *Older Americans 2010: Key Indicators of Well-Being*, 2010; From Martinez-Gonzalez, M.A. et al., *BMJ*, 336, 1348, 2008.)

in chromosomes. This incomplete replication is a part of the aging process and results in diminished cell functions.[5] The number of cells decreases as part of the natural aging process. However, aging itself may not cause visible diminished cell function. For example, physically and emotionally active older adults have better body function than less active older adults.[4]

Most older adults have one or more age-related diseases. Common diseases are memory loss, cognitive impairment, depression, chronic disability, hearing impairment, visual impairment, osteopenia, osteoporosis, Parkinson's disease, dental and oral health problems, gastrointestinal disorders, neoplasms, kidney disease, and paralysis (Table 22.1).

**TABLE 22.1**

**Selected Chronic Health Conditions in Adults 65 and Older (2007–2008)**

|  | Men (%) | Women (%) |
| --- | --- | --- |
| Hypertension | 53 | 58 |
| Heart disease | 38 | 27 |
| Arthritis symptoms | 42 | 55 |
| Any cancer | 24 | 21 |
| Diabetes | 20 | 18 |
| Stroke | 9 | 9 |
| Asthma | 9 | 12 |
| Chronic bronchitis or emphysema | 9 | 9 |

*Source:* Federal Interagency Forum on Aging and Related Statistics, *Older Americans 2010: Key Indicators of Well-Being*, 2010.

Nutrition is an important component in the prevention and/or management of most of these health conditions.[6] With increased human longevity, healthy aging and well-being are important issues. Although certain age-related diseases are common in older adults, healthy diet and lifestyle may delay the onset of diseases and diminish the severity of symptoms.[5,7]

## NUTRITION ASSESSMENT

As will be discussed throughout this chapter, overnutrition and undernutrition are serious and prevalent problems in older people. Undernutrition and overnutrition can impair many aspects of the quality of life.[8] However, nutrition assessment is not routinely considered in geriatric assessments.[9] Nutrition assessments help to prevent or address health risks caused by malnutrition.[10] Most nutritional assessment tools are questionnaires that collect information about age, food intake, ingestion and digestion, alcohol intake, mobility, presence of diseases, medical history, mental condition, family history, anthropometric measures, biochemical measures, and functional impairment.[11] Some tools are developed for hospital patients or for fragile older adults[11] and may not provide useful information for healthy, community-dwelling older adults who may have different nutrition problems and goals than frail individuals.[12] Nutritional assessment tools that meet criteria for reliability, validity, sensitivity, and specificity are recommended and are described elsewhere.[11]

## DIET, LIFESTYLE, MORBIDITY, AND MORTALITY

Similar to other age groups, the older adult population does not consume the recommended amounts of key nutrients and food groups such as fruits, vegetables, whole grains, and milk products (Table 22.2). Healthy diets and body weight, along with other healthy lifestyle practices, delay disability, improve quality of life, and compress morbidity—that is, shorten the period of poor health and disability prior to death.[13–16] Abundant intakes of fruits, vegetables, and whole grains with adequate protein and essential fats are associated with the lowest risk of chronic diseases.[16–20] In midlife, for example, controlling body weight and cardiovascular disease risk factors, both of which are profoundly affected by food patterns and portion sizes, leads to better quality of life in the domains of physical and mental limitations, bodily pain, energy and fatigue, social functioning, and mental health later in life.[13,14] The combination of a healthy lifestyle and a "Mediterranean diet"—a diet that focuses on whole grains, legumes, and fruits and vegetables—has been shown to reduce mortality from cardiovascular diseases, coronary heart disease, and cancer.[16–20] The combination has also been shown to lower blood pressure and lower the risk of cardiovascular disease, diabetes, and Parkinson's and Alzheimer's disease.[21–23] For example, men in the Baltimore Longitudinal Study of Aging who consumed more than or equal to five servings of fruits and vegetables daily and ≤12%

**TABLE 22.2**

**Nutrient and Food Recommendations versus Intake among Older Adults**

| | Recommendations | Intakes from Food (Not Including Supplements) |
|---|---|---|
| *Nutrients* | | |
| Calcium (mg/day) | | |
| Men (51–70 years) | 1000[79] | 991[111] |
| Women(51–70 years) | 1200 | 795 |
| Men and women 70 years | 1200 | 759–878 |
| Vitamin D (IU/day) | | |
| Men and women (51–70 years) | 600[79] | 160–204[111] |
| Men and women >70 years | 800 | 180–224 |
| Vitamin $B_{12}$ (μg of crystalline/day) | | |
| Men | 2.4[112] | 5.4 (1.14 crystalline)[113] |
| Women | 2.4 | 4.4 (0.94 crystalline) |
| Sodium (mg/day) | | |
| Men | <1500[114] | 3012[113] |
| Women | <1500 | 2364 |
| Potassium (mg/day) | | |
| Men | 4700[114] | 2728[113] |
| Women | 4700 | 2189 |
| Protein (g/day) | | |
| Men | 56[115] | 73[113] |
| Women | 46 | 57 |
| Fiber (g/day) | | |
| Men | 30[115] | 17[113] |
| Women | 21 | 14 |
| Saturated fat (% energy) | | |
| Men | 10[115] | 11[113] |
| Women | 10 | 11 |
| *Food groups* | | |
| Milk and milk products as a source of calcium and other key nutrients (cups/day) | 3[20] | ~1.8[116] |
| Whole grains (ounce equivalents/day) | 3[20] | 0.9[116] |
| Fruits and vegetables (cups/day) | 4[20] | 2.6[116] |

*Sources:* USDHHS & USDA, *2010 Dietary Guidelines for Americans*, 2010; Institute of Medicine, *Dietary Reference Intakes for Calcium and Vitamin D*, National Academy of Sciences, National Academy Press, Washington, DC, 2011; U.S. Department of Agriculture, What we eat in America, NHANES 2005–2006, 2009; Institute of Medicine, *Dietary Reference Intakes for Thiamin, Riboflavin, Niacin, Vitamin $B_6$, Folate, Vitamin $B_{12}$, Pantothenic Acid, Biotin, and Choline*, National Academy of Sciences, National Academy Press, Washington, DC, 1998; U.S. Department of Agriculture, What we eat in America, NHANES 2007–2008, 2009; Food and Nutrition Board, *Dietary Reference Intakes for Water, Potassium, Sodium, Chloride, and Sulfate*, National Academy of Sciences, National Academy Press, Washington, DC, 2004; Food and Nutrition Board, *Dietary Reference Intakes for Energy, Carbohydrate, Fiber, Fat, Fatty Acids, Cholesterol, Protein, and Amino Acids (Macronutrients)*, National Academy of Sciences, National Academy Press, Washington, DC, 2005; Wells, H.F. and Buzby, J.C., U.S. Department of Agriculture, Dietary assessment of major trends in U.S. food consumption, 1970–2005, 2008.

of energy from saturated fat were 76% less likely to die of cardiovascular disease and 31% less likely to die of any cause.[24]

Increasing health-care costs and the personal burdens of chronic diseases caused by the global obesity epidemic are prompting serious evaluation of the roles of nutrition and other lifestyle factors in preventing and managing chronic diseases.[25] The Institute of Medicine (IOM) evaluated the role of nutrition in maintaining health for the Medicare population.[26] They emphasized that poor nutrition, inadequate nutrient intakes, and obesity are major problems and the vast majority (86%) of older Americans have chronic conditions in which nutrition interventions have been shown to improve both health and quality of life. As part of a comprehensive management and treatment approach, nutrition therapy was recommended for dyslipidemia (high blood cholesterol and triglycerides), hypertension, heart failure, diabetes, and kidney failure. The IOM recognized the registered dietitian (RD) as the most qualified health professional to provide medical

nutrition therapy, which includes individualized nutrition services and procedures to treat an illness, injury, or condition.

## WEIGHT CONCERNS IN OLDER ADULTS

Older adults comprise a segment of the population that spans a wide range of ages and, consequently, present a wide range of health conditions. Overnutrition and undernutrition are both concerns for this age group. The prevalence of overweight (BMI $\geq 25$ to $<30\,kg/m^2$) and obesity (BMI $\geq 30\,kg/m^2$) among those aged $\geq 60$ is 76.5% in men and 73.5% in women (National Health and Nutrition Examination Survey, NHANES, 2009–2010). The prevalence of obesity among those aged $\geq 60$ in men is 36.6% and in women is 42.3%.[27] In contrast, the prevalence of malnourished individuals over 70 years, residing in the community, is about 5%–10% but is estimated to be as high as 70% among those who are older and/or hospitalized or institutionalized (Figures 22.2 and 22.3).[28]

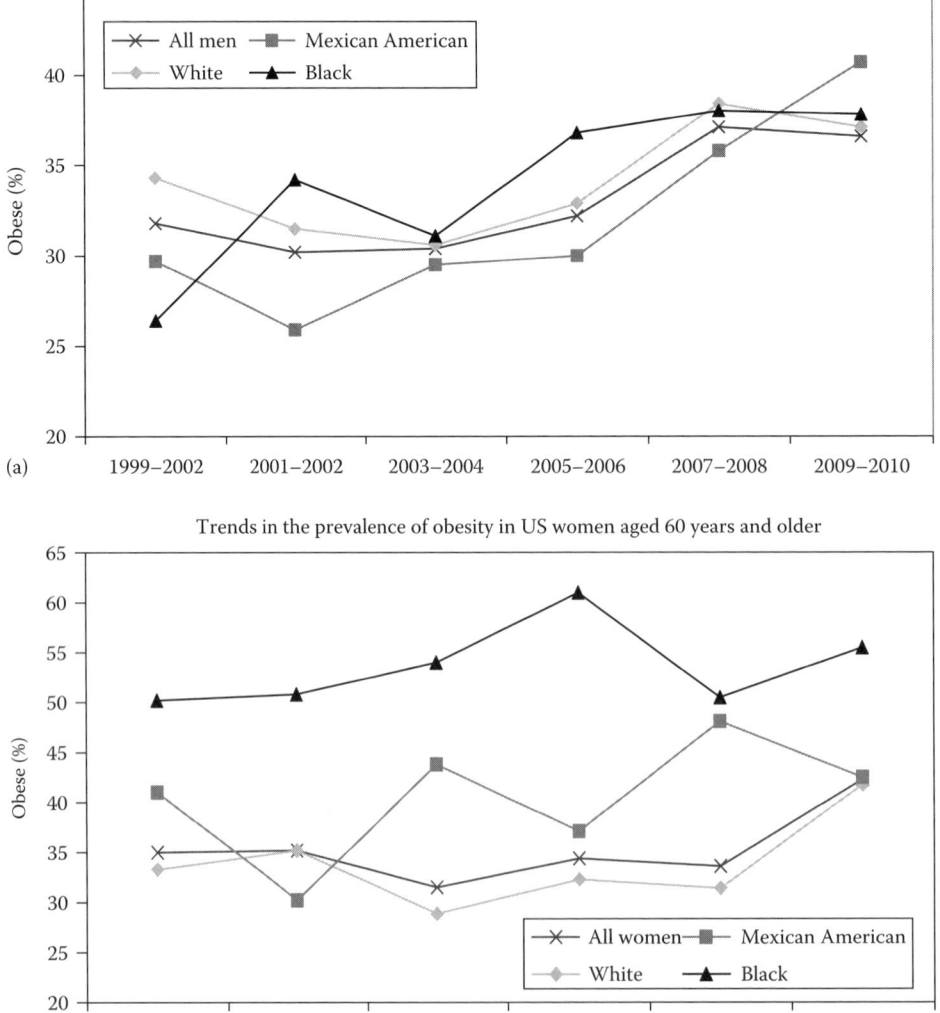

**FIGURE 22.2**  Trends in the prevalence of obesity among U.S. (a) men and (b) women by race/ethnicity (1999–2010). (From Flegal, K.M. et al., *JAMA*, 307(5), 491, 2012; Flegal, K.M. et al., *JAMA*, 303, 235, 2010.)

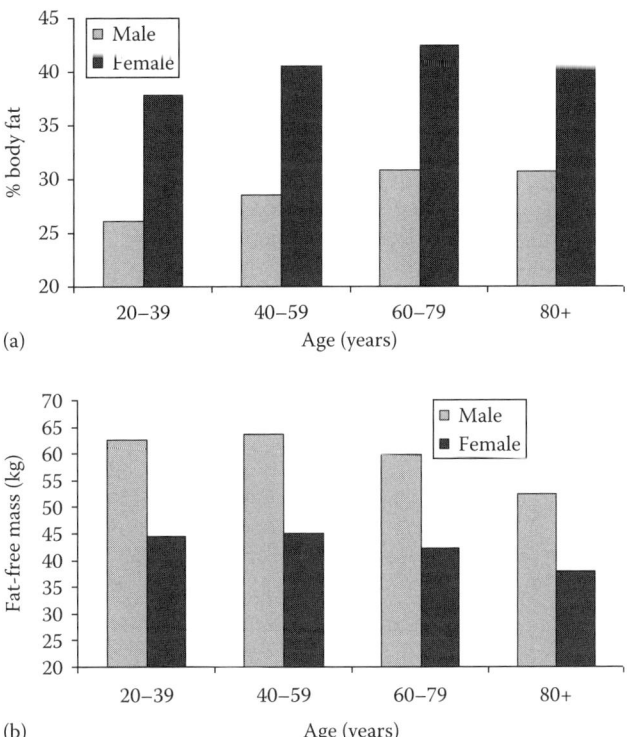

**FIGURE 22.3**   (a) Changes in percent of body fat by age and gender. (b) Changes in fat-free mass (kg) by age and gender. (From Borrud, L.G. et al., *Body Composition Data for Individuals 8 Years of Age and Older: U.S. Population, 1999–2004*, Vital and Health Statistics Series 11, U.S. Department of Health and Human Services, Centers for Disease Control and Prevention, Hyattsville, MD, 2010.)

## BODY COMPOSITION, OBESITY, OVERWEIGHT, AND CHRONIC DISEASE

Overweight and obesity are associated with increased health-care costs and numerous chronic disorders in older adults including hypertension, diabetes mellitus, metabolic syndrome, dyslipidemia, coronary artery disease, respiratory disease, and some types of cancer.[29–33] Of particular significance are the physical disabilities associated with overweight and obesity, such as impaired walking, traveling, shopping, and preparing food. Obesity may cause premature aging. For example, the prevalence of severe disability (having three or more impairments in activities of daily living) was 6% in those aged 51–60, which was similar to non-obese people aged 70 and older (7%).[30]

Although obesity can be influenced by genetic predisposition, there are several modifiable risk factors for obesity such as environment, lifestyle, and behavioral issues. During middle age, many people experience weight gain that is associated, at least in part, with a sedentary lifestyle. Weight gain and a sedentary lifestyle might be accepted as a normal part of the aging process, which might cause older adults to make few efforts toward prevention.[29]

In the older adult, obesity appears to be associated with poor food choices, high intakes of fat and saturated fat, low intakes of fiber and micronutrients, and low blood levels of micronutrients.[34,35] Obesity also has been associated with poor vitamin D status, perhaps because of low vitamin D intakes and redistribution or sequestration of vitamin D into

the fat mass,[36] or perhaps because of altered endocrine function that accompanies low vitamin D levels.[37] Thus, obese older adults are at risk for nutrient excesses (energy, fat, and carbohydrate) as well as nutrient deficiencies (protein, vitamins, and minerals).[34–36]

The American Society for Nutrition (ASN) and the North American Association for the Study of Obesity (NAASO), The Obesity Society, provided a technical review and position statement regarding obesity in older adults.[31] They note that appropriate treatment for obesity in older adults is controversial, but current research shows that voluntary weight-loss therapy in obese older people improves physical function, quality of life, and the medical complications associated with obesity. It is widely agreed that overweight or obese older adults should not gain additional weight, but weight loss cannot be broadly recommended or attempted without medical evaluation and supervision.[29,37–39] Thus, ASN and NAASO emphasize the importance of a thorough medical history, physical examination, medication review, and assessment of readiness to lose weight before initiating weight-loss therapy.[31]

## SARCOPENIC OBESITY

Aging is associated with increases in weight, total body fat, and visceral fat and decreases in skeletal muscle.[31,40] The loss of skeletal muscle is called sarcopenia and may be caused by low physical activity, changes in hormone function, insulin resistance, decreased protein consumption, and increased protein requirements and may be accelerated by weight loss.[40,41] "Sarcopenic obesity" is a condition in which low muscle mass and/or poor functioning muscle and high fat mass coexist.[42] High fat mass promotes a biochemical imbalance that promotes insulin resistance, inflammatory cytokines, and altered hormone production, leading to muscle loss and eventually disability and obesity-related disorders.[42] In order to preserve fat-free mass and minimize the effects of aging, older adults are encouraged to participate in both aerobic and strength training exercises.[43] Increased protein consumption may also be encouraged in older adults, as higher intakes of protein have been associated with smaller losses of lean mass.[44]

## UNDERNUTRITION, POOR APPETITE, AND WEIGHT LOSS

A physiological decrease in food intake called "anorexia of aging" occurs even in healthy older adults.[45,46] Weight loss is common and is associated with frailty, functional impairment, immune disorders, pressure ulcers, hip fractures, cognitive impairment, low quality of life, and increased mortality. Weight loss results in loss of muscle mass, which decreases energy needs. Physical activity helps maintain muscle mass, so physically active older people experience less decline in muscle mass. The digestion process in the stomach diminishes with advanced age, which leads to faster feelings of satiety and lower food intake. Also, changes in some hormones that sense satiety and changes in energy expenditure contribute to decreased food intake. The ability to adjust subsequent food intake after under- or overeating is impaired with advanced age. Sensing and responding to thirst is impaired, increasing the risk of dehydration.

People who are institutionalized are more likely to be undernourished, largely because of poor physical or mental conditions among these individuals.[47] Some chronic diseases are associated with negative energy balance (e.g., more energy is expended than is taken in) and weight loss.[46] Weight loss associated with low food intake is common in Alzheimer's disease. Energy needs are increased with congestive heart failure, chronic obstructive pulmonary disease, Parkinson's disease, and infections. Infectious diseases can increase energy needs and at the same time interfere with appetite.

Many social, mental, physical, financial, and individual choice factors contribute to poor nutritional status (Table 22.3).[12,48,49] Hearing and visual impairments may cause social segregation due to difficulty in communicating with others. Physical disability may decrease mobility and limit daily activities, such as shopping for groceries and cooking meals.[9,49] Oral health disorders may limit food intakes and choices because of chewing and swallowing difficulties. Therefore, diminished quantity and quality of food are concerns.[46,50–52] Changes in taste and smell associated with aging, chronic health problems, and medications can interfere with appetite and the ability to enjoy food.[46] Low income,[53,54]

## TABLE 22.3
### Lifestyle and Socioeconomic Changes Affecting the Nutritional Status of the Older Population

Changes with aging include
  Reduced income with retirement
  Insufficient funds for purchase of food
  Skipping meals
  Illness and increased medical expenses
  Loss of mobility
  Diminished acuity in sensory perceptions (hearing, vision, and taste)
  Inability to drive to doctor's appointments or to the grocery store
  Inability to prepare or store food
  Loss of balance
  Diminished self-esteem
  Social isolation

Diseases and health problems that are common in older adults and impact their nutritional status include
  Alzheimer's disease and other dementias, with cognitive impairment and memory loss
  Arthritis, with pain and joint deformities
  Osteoporosis, with pain, bone fractures, and spinal compression
  Parkinson's disease, with rigidity and tremor
  Dental and oral health problems, including problems with chewing
  Gastrointestinal disorders, including swallowing and digestive difficulties
  Neoplasms, with hypercatabolism, anorexia, and cachexia
  Diabetes mellitus, with restrictive diets and medication interactions
  Renal insufficiency, with restrictive diets and dialysis treatment
  Paralysis, limiting mobility
  Depression and other mental health conditions, leading to anorexia or emotional eating

*Source:*  Adapted from Feldman, E.B., in *Handbook of Nutrition and Food*, Berdanier, C.D., Ed., CRC Press, Boca Raton, FL, pp. 319–336, 2002.

taking several medications,[55] alcoholism,[45,56] eating alone, loneliness, bereavement, depression, and cognitive impairment[45,57] cause poor nutritional status in older people. In addition, being homebound, residing in a nursing home, or being hospitalized may also impair nutrition status,[49] as lack of transportation may become an issue.[58]

Treatment for poor appetite, weight loss, and undernutrition is guided by a medical evaluation and recommendations and should involve the older adult as well as their family members and caregivers.[5,29,57,59] Poor appetite and eating habits are not a normal part of aging. The goal is to improve oral intake, which can be facilitated by honoring food preferences at meals and snacks, using stronger flavorings and seasonings, and/or substituting higher calorie versions of familiar foods. Taste tests by the older individual can help identify nutritional supplements, such as liquids and bars that are most palatable and best tolerated in addressing poor appetite, weight loss, and undernutrition.

Families, caregivers, and the health-care team need to find a balance between the benefits and risks of therapeutic diets for older people experiencing poor appetite and weight loss.

When medically appropriate, therapeutic diets should be liberalized for the undernourished older adult. Overly restrictive diets, such as those low in cholesterol, fat, salt, and sugar, may take much of the enjoyment out of eating. Therefore, these restrictions should be used with caution in those with poor appetite and unintentional weight loss. To maintain muscle mass and energy levels, it is vitally important that those with poor appetite and weight loss ingest adequate proteins, vitamins, and minerals from a variety of foods in so far as is possible. Failure to consume protein will result in further deterioration of muscle mass, loss of strength, and poor recovery from illness.

## HUNGER AND FOOD SECURITY

Although older adults are less likely to be in poverty than children, poverty rates are notable among older adults (10% vs. 18%).[3] Incomes below the poverty level increase the risk of food insufficiency, food insecurity, hunger, low intakes of calories, vitamins, and minerals, and low body weight.[53,54,60,61] For example, compared to older adults with sufficient food, those experiencing food insufficiency were four times more likely to have a low body weight, consumed nearly 300 fewer calories each day, and consumed less protein, meat, and vegetables.[54] Food insecurity has also been associated with a higher prevalence of abdominal obesity, chronic disease, and disability compared to food-secured individuals.[62,63] Older adults have relatively low participation rates in the Supplemental Nutrition Assistance Program (SNAP) and other federal, state, and local assistance programs[53] due to lack of awareness of the programs, perception that the benefits are too low to be worth the effort of applying, reluctance to accept food assistance because of stigma associated with receiving public assistance, and a lack of transportation and/or physical mobility to reach the site of the program, especially if they reside in rural or urban areas.[53] Elder abuse or neglect also can interfere with the ability to obtain adequate food.

There are several ways to address the problem of food security,[60] which has been found in about 8% of older adult households.[64] Screening for food insecurity with tools that assess all the dimensions of food insecurity in older adults will improve identification of those in need. Screening and information about local food resources and food budgeting can be provided in many settings such as senior centers, public health programs, faith-based organizations, physician's offices, and hospitals.

## NUTRIENT REQUIREMENTS AND INTAKES

The authoritative sources of nutrient recommendations for older adults are the Dietary Reference Intakes (DRIs)[65] and the Dietary Guidelines for Americans.[20] Recommended intakes vary with age and gender (Tables 22.2 and 22.4). The low intake of several key nutrients and food groups shows a great need for nutrition education and health promotion targeted to older adults (Table 22.2). Compared to younger people, nutrient requirements are not uniformly increased or decreased. Aging decreases energy needs because of the loss of muscle mass and low physical activity. Iron needs are decreased in women because of the cessation of menstruation. The increased need for calcium is related to decreased absorption efficiency, and the increased recommendation for vitamin D in very late life is related to decreased sun exposure and skin synthesis.

## DIETARY SUPPLEMENTS

Dietary supplements include vitamins, minerals, herbs and other botanicals, amino acids, and other substances. Dietary supplement use is high among older adults over 70 years—about 75% in women and 66% in older men.[66] Obese and Mexican Americans are less likely to use dietary supplements than normal weight individuals or non-Hispanic whites.[66]

Some nutrient-containing dietary supplements are recommended for older adults by the Dietary Guidelines and other reliable sources.[67] Recommended supplements include vitamin $B_{12}$[20] and vitamin D[20,65] from fortified foods and/or supplements. Calcium supplements may also be recommended for those not consuming adequate calcium from dietary sources.[67] While typical foods can be consumed to meet the dietary requirements for vitamin $B_{12}$ and calcium, it is unlikely that those foods will be fortified to the high levels needed to meet the daily recommendation of 600–800 IU of vitamin D. It is generally accepted that older adults are particularly vulnerable to deficiencies of vitamin $B_{12}$, vitamin D, and calcium,[68] so these three nutrients will be discussed in the next sections.

### VITAMIN $B_{12}$

Vitamin $B_{12}$ is essential for cognition, the nervous system, vascular health, and red blood cell synthesis.[69] Vitamin $B_{12}$ deficiency among older adults has been associated with poor cognition, depression, and anemia[70–73]; however, poor vitamin $B_{12}$ status is not consistently associated with anemia.[74] Poor vitamin $B_{12}$ status is prevalent among older adults in general (5%–20%)[69] and is particularly high in some vulnerable subgroups of older adults, such as recipients of home-delivered or congregate meals[71] and centenarians.[75] The prevalence of vitamin $B_{12}$ deficiency increases with age, mainly because of decreased ability to digest the natural chemical form of vitamin $B_{12}$ found in meat, poultry, fish, and dairy foods.[69] About 10%–30% of older adults have atrophic gastritis, which is caused by infection of the stomach with *Helicobacter pylori* and subsequent atrophy of the cells in the stomach that secrete acid and digestive enzymes needed for the digestion and absorption of vitamin $B_{12}$.[69] Protein-bound vitamin $B_{12}$ from animal foods requires these digestive enzymes, while the crystalline form does not. Crystalline vitamin $B_{12}$ from fortified foods and dietary supplements is believed to be normally absorbed in those with atrophic gastritis.[76] About 1%–2% of older adults have pernicious anemia, which is a loss of the intrinsic factor

**TABLE 22.4**

**Vitamin and Mineral Recommendations for Older Individuals (Recommended Dietary Allowances or Adequate Intakes)**

| | Males | | Females | |
|---|---|---|---|---|
| | 51–70 Years | >70 Years | 51–70 Years | >70 Years |
| Vitamin A, retinol (μg/day) | 900 | 900 | 700 | 700 |
| Vitamin C (mg/day) | 90 | 90 | 75 | 75 |
| Vitamin D (IU/day)[a] | 600 | 800 | 600 | 800 |
| Vitamin E (mg/day) | 15 | 15 | 15 | 15 |
| Vitamin K (μg/day) | 120 | 120 | 90 | 90 |
| Thiamin (mg/day) | 1.2 | 1.2 | 1.1 | 1.1 |
| Riboflavin (mg/day) | 1.3 | 1.3 | 1.1 | 1.1 |
| Niacin (mg/day) | 16 | 16 | 14 | 14 |
| Vitamin B$_6$ (mg/day) | 1.7 | 1.7 | 1.5 | 1.5 |
| Folate (μg/day) | 400 | 400 | 400 | 400 |
| Vitamin B$_{12}$, crystalline (μg/day)[b] | 2.4 | 2.4 | 2.4 | 2.4 |
| Pantothenic (mg/day) | 5 | 5 | 5 | 5 |
| Biotin (μg/day) | 30 | 30 | 30 | 30 |
| Choline (mg/day) | 550 | 550 | 425 | 425 |
| Calcium (mg/day) | 1000 | 1200 | 1200 | 1200 |
| Chromium (μg/day) | 30 | 30 | 20 | 20 |
| Copper (μg/day) | 900 | 900 | 900 | 900 |
| Fluoride (mg/day) | 4 | 4 | 3 | 3 |
| Iodine (μg/day) | 150 | 150 | 150 | 150 |
| Iron (mg/day) | 8 | 8 | 8 | 8 |
| Magnesium (mg/day) | 420 | 420 | 320 | 320 |
| Manganese (mg/day) | 2.3 | 2.3 | 1.8 | 1.8 |
| Molybdenum (μg/day) | 45 | 45 | 45 | 45 |
| Phosphorus (mg/day) | 700 | 700 | 700 | 700 |
| Selenium (μg/day) | 55 | 55 | 55 | 55 |
| Zinc (mg/day) | 11 | 11 | 8 | 8 |

*Sources:* Food and Nutrition Board, Institute of Medicine, National Academies, *Dietary Reference Intakes (DRIs): Recommended Intakes for Individuals, Vitamins, Elements,* National Academy of Sciences, National Academy Press, Washington, DC, 2004; USDHHS & USDA, *Dietary Guidelines for Americans, 2010,* U.S. Government Printing Office, Washington, DC, 2011.

[a] Vitamin D recommendations can also be expressed in μg/day (15 μg/day for males and females 51–70 years; 20 μg/day for males and females over 70 years).

[b] The majority of vitamin B$_{12}$ consumed by older adults should come from crystalline sources.

needed for intestinal absorption of vitamin B$_{12}$. Under medical supervision, vitamin B$_{12}$ status in these individuals is maintained by monthly injections of vitamin B$_{12}$ or daily oral doses of 500–2000 μg.[77]

Similar to the DRIs, the Dietary Guidelines recommends that the intake of vitamin B$_{12}$ (2.4 μg/day) be met from crystalline sources such as vitamin B$_{12}$-containing fortified foods or supplements. Crystalline vitamin B$_{12}$ is in many, but not all, fortified breakfast cereals and multivitamin supplements. The daily value for vitamin B$_{12}$ is 6 μg[78]; therefore, a single serving of a vitamin B$_{12}$-containing food and supplement with at least 40% of the daily value would meet the recommended dietary allowance (RDA) for vitamin B$_{12}$. Several studies show that older adults consuming between 9 and 50 μg of vitamin B$_{12}$ daily, often found in multivitamins

marketed to older adults, have improved vitamin B$_{12}$ status.[61] There is no upper level for vitamin B$_{12}$, and it is generally considered nontoxic.

## Vitamin D

In 2010, a new RDA for vitamin D was established, which is 600 IU from ages 51 to 70 and 800 IU for those aged 70+.[79] However, some researchers and health professionals suggest that individuals at higher risk may need increased intake levels, as much as 2000 IU/day (50 μg/day).[80] Risk factors that may warrant a higher intake of vitamin D include obesity, limited sun exposure (institutionalized), osteoporosis, malabsorption problems, and having darker skin.[79,80] Adequate vitamin D status is needed for optimal calcium absorption.[20]

Although not conclusive and research is ongoing, poor vitamin D status has been associated with numerous health conditions, such as an increased risk of falling, and increased incidence and mortality of certain types of cancers, type 2 diabetes, and cardiovascular disease.[79,81,82]

Vitamin D comes from diet, supplements, and skin synthesis. Older adults, as well as people with dark pigmented skin or people who use sunscreen properly, have low synthesis of vitamin D precursors in the skin, even in sunny areas of the United States such as southern Florida.[83,84] People living at higher latitudes in the northern United States are particularly at risk for vitamin D deficiency. In addition to low skin synthesis, darker-skinned ethnic/racial groups may be at increased risk of poor vitamin D status because of low intakes of dairy foods and vitamin D-containing supplements.[84] Obese individuals may also be at greater risk because of the sequestration of vitamin D by adipose tissue or because of increased vitamin D catabolism or decrease vitamin D synthesis.[85]

The best marker of vitamin D status from oral intake and skin synthesis is serum 25-hydroxyvitamin D. According to the DRIs, the optimal serum 25-hydroxyvitamin D concentration is at least 50 nmol/L. Concentrations below this could be inadequate for bone and overall health.[80] Mean concentrations of serum 25-hydroxyvitamin D generally decline with increasing age and are lower in blacks than in whites.[86,87] In one study of well-functioning older adults, aged 70–81, 54% of blacks and 18% of whites were found to have 25-hydroxyvitamin D concentrations less than 50 nmol/L (20 ng/mL).[86]

Food sources of vitamin D include salmon, tuna, and other vitamin D-fortified milk products and foods. As it is difficult to meet vitamin D recommendations from food alone and increased time spent in the sun increases a person's risk of deseloping certain types of cancers, supplements are recommended. The upper level of vitamin D is 4000 IU daily, so older adults should carefully read the labels on supplements to ensure staying below the upper level.

## CALCIUM

Calcium is most well known for its role in bone health and is required for many other essential functions.[20,80] Food provides only 55%–66% of the recommended amounts of calcium (Table 22.2). The Dietary Guidelines recommend food sources of calcium, but does not mention calcium supplements.[20] The surgeon general's report on bone health and osteoporosis provides an algorithm to calculate calcium intake from the diet[67] that can then be used to determine the amount of calcium, if any, needed from supplements. For older adults, they suggest starting with a baseline amount of calcium of 290 mg, which is the average of amount of calcium from non-calcium-rich foods, then adding 300 mg for each 8 oz serving of milk or equivalent serving of other calcium-rich foods (e.g., yogurt, cheese, calcium-fortified juice). The shortfall can be obtained from supplements. Careful label reading should ensure that the upper level for calcium 2500 mg daily is not exceeded.

## ANTIOXIDANT SUPPLEMENTS

The U.S. Preventive Services Task Force (USPSTF)[88] concluded that there is insufficient evidence to recommend for or against the use of vitamin A, C, or E supplements, multivitamins with folic acid, or antioxidant combinations for prevention of cancer or cardiovascular disease. The USPSTF did recommend against using supplements of beta-carotene for prevention of cancer or cardiovascular disease because of adverse outcomes in some people such as heavy smokers.

## NON-NUTRIENT SUPPLEMENTS

The most commonly used non-nutrient supplements in the United States in 2007 were fish oil or omega-3, or DHA, glucosamine, Echinacea, flaxseed oil (pills included), ginseng, ginkgo biloba, chondroitin, garlic supplements, and coenzyme Q-10.[89] Only a few supplements have been recently and systematically reviewed for safety and efficacy, such as by the Agency for Healthcare Research and Quality or the Cochrane Reviews system. Fish oil supplements were associated with a significant reduction in deaths from cardiac causes, but the optimal formulation of DHA and EPA is not yet clear.[90] There is limited evidence indicating a decreased requirement for rheumatoid drugs with the use of omega-3 (fish oil).[91] Another review has shown that glucosamine is no more effective at relieving some symptoms of osteoarthritis than a placebo.[92] While Echinacea is widely used to treat and prevent common colds, randomized control trials have failed to show any preventative benefits from taking Echinacea and have shown mixed results in symptom improvement, as compared to those taking a placebo.[93] Flaxseed is a rich source of alpha-linolenic acid, which is thought to help reduce the risk of cardiovascular disease. However, data are very limited and more research is needed to further investigate this association.[94] Ginseng has been thought to help with cognition, but again, studies showing improvement are limited.[95]

## CAUTIONS ABOUT DIETARY SUPPLEMENTS

Older adults must use dietary supplements carefully, treat them like any other medication, and inform their physicians about the products they are using.[96] Most supplements contain active ingredients that may interfere with several medications making them stronger or weaker. For example, garlic, ginkgo, Echinacea, ginseng, St. John's wort, and kava are all suspected of interacting with medications, especially anticancer drugs and blood thinners.[96–99] Some supplements promote bleeding or interfere with other aspects of surgery and recovery.

## FOOD SAFETY

Although the most important food safety problem is microbial food-borne illness from bacteria and viruses, there are also food safety risks from parasites, toxins, and chemical and physical contaminants in foods. The food safety recommendations in the 2010 Dietary Guidelines are based on the FightBAC principles of safe food-handling practices (clean, separate, cook, and chill). Foods posing a high risk of food-borne illness that should be avoided include raw (unpasteurized) milk, cheeses, and juices; raw or under-cooked animal foods, such as seafood, meat, poultry, and eggs; and raw sprouts.[20] Hotdogs and deli and luncheon meats should also be reheated to steaming hot to kill certain bacteria, which pose a greater risk of disease among older individuals.[20] Other reliable sources of information on food safety and food-borne illness are the FightBAC Partnership for Food Safety Education (www.fightbac.org), the American Dietetic Association,[100,101] and the medical profession.[102] Risk of food-borne illness may be decreased by education targeted to older adults, caregivers, and food service staff in nursing homes, cafeterias, restaurants, assisted living facilities, congregate meal sites, and home-delivered meals programs.[101–103] Chapter 3 provides information on the various organisms causing food-borne illness.

Food-borne illness can cause mild to fatal reactions involving diarrhea, vomiting, and other symptoms. The Centers for Disease Control and Prevention reported that compared to younger people, older adults have safer food-handling and food-consumption behaviors and lower rates of infection from several food-borne illnesses.[103] However, along with children and immune-compromised people, older adults are at high risk for severe complications from food-borne illness, such as death from gastroenteritis. These high complication rates may result from poor nutritional status, age-related decreases in stomach acid that allow more microorganisms to survive in the gastrointestinal tract, dehydration related to impaired sense of thirst, increased intestinal transit time, age-related impairments in immunity, and surgery or other illnesses that may also impair immunity. People in nursing homes are particularly vulnerable to food-borne illness, with fatality rates 10–100 times higher than the general population.[103] Risk factors include illness, impaired immunity, and close confinement with others. Proactive steps that nursing homes take in preventing food-borne illness include thoroughly cooking eggs and meat and using pasteurized eggs and irradiated meats with decreased bacterial loads. Older adults living in assisted living facilities, receiving home-delivered meals, and/or receiving meals at congregate meal sites may also be at higher risk for food-borne illness than other older adults because of their advanced age and higher prevalence of frailty.

## PHYSICAL ACTIVITY

Along with a healthy diet, physical activity can extend years of active life, help maintain healthy body weight, decrease risk of cardiovascular disease and other chronic diseases, reduce disability, relieve symptoms of depression, help maintain independent living, and enhance overall quality of life.[20,104,105] An alarming 78% of older Americans do not engage in at least 30 min of physical activity five times a week,

and only 14% of older people reported engaging in strength exercises.[3] The American College of Sports Medicine recommends a well-rounded physical activity program encompassing aerobic, strength, balance, and flexibility exercises for overall health, fitness, and well-being.[43] In addition, older adults with health conditions should participate in activities that meet their abilities.[106]

## CONCLUSION

A growing body of evidence shows that nutrition promotes health and quality of life as people age. To reap the full benefits, nutrition needs to be integrated into all aspects of health promotion, disease prevention, and disease management. This can be accomplished in a variety of ways including nutrition screening, assessment and referral to registered dietitians and other appropriate health professionals in routine physician visits, as well as community-based nutrition education and wellness programs that target older adults, families, caregivers, and health professionals. Key recommendations from the 2005 White House Conference on Aging that are relevant to nutrition include reauthorizing the Older Americans Act; supporting geriatric education and training for all health-care professionals, paraprofessionals, health profession students, and direct care workers; attaining adequate numbers of health-care personnel in all professions who are skilled, culturally competent, and specialized in geriatrics; and improving state- and local-based integrated delivery systems to meet twenty-first-century needs of older people.[107] Many of these issues were also raised in the 2011 IOM's Workshop on Nutrition and Healthy Aging in the Community, which emphasized the need for research into how to expand and integrate the broad array of medical and supportive services, including nutrition, that are needed to address the range of health and functional status among older adults.[108] Such strategies will improve the quality and availability of nutrition services for older people.

## REFERENCES

1. U.S. Census Bureau, U.S. Interim projections by age, sex, race, and Hispanic origin, 2012.
2. U.S Census Bureau. Resident population projections by race, Hispanic-origin status, and age: 2010–2015, 2010.
3. Federal Interagency Forum on Aging and Related Statistics, *Older Americans 2010: Key Indicators of Well-Being*, 2010.
4. Beers, M.H. et al., *The Merck Manual of Health & Aging*, Merck Research Laboratories, Whitehouse Station, NJ, 2004.
5. Norman, R.A. and Henderson, J.N., *Dermatol. Ther.*, 16(3), 181, 2003.
6. American Dietetic Association, *J. Am. Diet. Assoc.*, 105, 616, 2005.
7. World Health Organization, Keep fit for life: Meeting the nutritional needs of older persons, World Health Organization, Geneva, Switzerland, 2002.
8. Amarantos, E., Martinez, A., and Dwyer, J., *J. Gerontol.*, 56A, 54, 2001.
9. Sahyoun, N.R., *Nutr. Clin. Care*, 2, 155, 1999.

10. Green, S. and McDougall, T., *Nurs. Older People*, 14(6), 31, 2002.
11. Green, S.M. and Watson, R., *J. Adv. Nurs.*, 50(1), 69, 2005.
12. Callen, B.L. and Wells, T.J., *Public Health Nurs*, 22(2), 138, 2005.
13. Daviglus, M.L. et al., *Arch. Intern Med.*, 163(20), 2460, 2003.
14. Daviglus, M.L. et al., *Arch. Intern Med.*, 163(20), 2448, 2003.
15. Fries, J.F., *Ann. Intern. Med.*, 139(5 Pt 2), 455, 2003.
16. Knoops, K.T. et al., *JAMA*, 292, 1433, 2004.
17. Cerhan, J.R. et al., *Cancer Epidemiol. Biomarkers Prev.*, 13(7), 1114, 2004.
18. Hu, F.B., *Am. J. Clin. Nutr.*, 78(3 Suppl.), 544S, 2003.
19. Kant, A.K., *J. Am. Diet. Assoc.*, 104(4), 615, 2004.
20. U.S. Department of Health and Human Services and U.S. Department of Agriculture, *Dietary Guidelines for Americans, 2010*, U.S. Government Printing Office, Washington, DC, 2011.
21. Writing Group of the PREMIER, Collaborative Research Group, *JAMA*, 289(16), 2083, 2003.
22. Sofi, F. et al., *BMJ*, 337, a1344, 2008.
23. Martinez-Gonzalez, M.A. et al., *BMJ*, 336, 1348, 2008.
24. Tucker, K.L. et al., *J. Nutr.*, 135(3), 556, 2005.
25. Yach, D. et al., *J. Am. Med. Assoc.*, 291(21), 2616, 2004.
26. Institute of Medicine, *The Role of Nutrition in Maintaining Health in the Nation's Elderly: Evaluating Coverage of Nutrition Services for the Medicare Population*, National Academy of Sciences, National Academy Press, Washington, DC, 2000.
27. Flegal, K.M. et al., *JAMA*, 307(5), 491, 2012.
28. Guigoz, Y, *J. Nutr. Health Aging*, 10, 466, 2006.
29. Callahan, E. and Jensen, G.L., *Generations*, 28, 39, 2004.
30. Center on an Aging Society, *Obesity among Older Americans*, Georgetown University, Washington, DC, 2003.
31. Villareal, D.T. et al., *Obes. Res.*, 13(11), 1849, 2005.
32. Finkelstein, E.A., Fiebelkorn, I.C., and Wang, G., *Health Aff. (Millwood)*, Suppl Web Exclusives, W3-219–W3-226, 2003.
33. Finkelstein, E.A., Fiebelkorn, I.C., and Wang, G., *Obes. Res.*, 12(1), 18, 2004.
34. Ledikwe, J.H. et al., *Am. J. Clin. Nutr.*, 77(3), 551, 2003.
35. Ledikwe, J.H. et al., *J. Am. Geriatr. Soc.*, 52(4), 589, 2004.
36. Jacques, P.F. et al., *Am. J. Clin. Nutr.*, 66, 929, 1997.
37. National Institutes of Health, Clinical guidelines on the identification, evaluation, and treatment of obesity in adults: The evidence report, NIH Publication Number 98-4083, 1998.
38. National Institutes of Health, The practical guide: Identification, evaluation, and treatment of overweight and obesity in adults, NIH Publication Number 00-4084, 2000.
39. Jensen, G.L. et al., *Obes. Res.*, 12, 1814, 2004.
40. Evans, W.J., *J. Am. Coll. Nutr.*, 23(6 Suppl), 601S, 2004.
41. Stenholm, S., *Curr. Opin. Clin. Nutr. Metab. Care*, 11, 693, 2008.
42. Roubenoff, R., *Obes. Res.*, 12, 887, 2004.
43. Chodzko-Zajjko, W.J. et al., *Med. Sci. Sports Exerc.*, 41(7), 1510, 2009.
44. Houston, D.K. et al., *Am. J. Clin. Nutr.*, 87, 150, 2008.
45. Morley, J.E., *Nutrition*, 17, 660, 2001.
46. Wilson, M.M. and Morley, J.E., *J. Appl. Physiol.*, 95, 1728, 2003.
47. Kvamme, J.M. et al., *Psychiatry*, 11, 112, 2011.
48. Holmes, S., *Nurs. Stand.*, 15(2), 42, 2000.
49. Feldman, E.B., in *Handbook of Nutrition and Food*, Berdanier, C.D., Ed. CRC Press, Boca Raton, FL, 2002, pp. 319–336.
50. Sheiham, A. et al., *Community Dent. Oral. Epidemiol.*, 29, 195, 2001.
51. Bailey, R.L. et al., *J. Am. Diet. Assoc.*, 104, 1273, 1276, 2004.
52. Sahyoun, N.R., Pratt, C.A., and Anderson, A., *J. Am. Diet. Assoc.*, 104, 58, 2004.
53. Food Security Institute, Center on Hunger and Poverty, the Heller Graduate School for Social Policy and Management, Brandeis University, *Hunger Issue Brief*, February 2003.
54. Sahyoun, N.R. and Basiotis, P.P., *Nutrition Insights*, U.S. Department of Agriculture, Center for Nutrition Policy and Promotion, 2000.
55. Fick, D.M. et al., *Arch. Intern. Med.*, 163, 2716, 2003.
56. Knauer, C., *Geriatr. Nurs.*, 24, 152, 2003.
57. Elsner, R.J.F., *Eat. Behav.*, 3, 15, 2002.
58. American Association for Retired Persons, *The Impact of Federal Programs on Transportation for Older Adults*, Koffman, D., Raphael, D., and Weiner, R., Nelson/Nygaard Consulting Associates, San Francisco, CA, December 2004.
59. Johnson, M.A. and Fischer, J.G., *Generations*, 28(3), 11, 2004.
60. Frongillo, E.A. and Horan, C.M., *Generations*, 28, 28, 2004.
61. Johnson, M.A., *Generations*, 28(3), 45, 2004.
62. Brewer, D.P. et al., *J. Nutr. Elder.*, 29, 150, 2010.
63. Seligman, H.K., Laraia, B.A., and Kushel, M.B., *J. Nutr.*, 140, 304, 2010.
64. Coleman-Jensen, A. et al., U.S. Department of Agriculture. *Household Food Security in the United States in 2010*, 2011.
65. Food and Nutrition Board, Institute of Medicine, National Academies, *Dietary Reference Intakes (DRIs): Recommended Intakes for Individuals, Vitamins, Elements,* National Academy of Sciences, Washington DC, National Academy Press, 2004.
66. Bailey RL. et al., *J. Nutr.*, 141, 261, 2011.
67. U.S. Department of Health and Human Services, Bone health and osteoporosis: A report of the surgeon genera, Rockville, MD, U.S. Department of Health and Human Services, Office of the Surgeon General, 2004.
68. Russell, R.M., Rasmussen, H., and Lichtenstein, A.H., *J. Nutr.*, 129, 751, 1999.
69. Baik, H.W. and Russell, R.M., *Ann. Rev. Nutr.*, 19, 357, 1999.
70. Coppen, A. and Bolander-Gouaille, C., *J. Psychopharmacol.*, 19(1), 59, 2005.
71. Johnson, M.A. et al., *Am. J. Clin. Nutr.*, 77, 211, 2003.
72. Lewis, M.S. et al., *J. Nutr. Elder.*, 24(3), 47, 2005.
73. Morris, M.S. et al., *Am. J. Clin. Nutr.*, 85, 193, 2007.
74. Haslam, A. et al., *J. Gerontol. A Biol. Sci. Med. Sci.*, 67, 100, 2011.
75. Johnson M.A. et al., *J. Nutr. Health Aging*, 14(5), 339, 2010.
76. Campbell, A. et al., *J. Nutr.*, 133, 2770, 2003.
77. Kuzminski, A.M. et al., *Blood*, 92, 1191, 1998.
78. Code of Federal Regulations, Title 21. Vol. 2, Pt. 101, 2003.
79. Institute of Medicine, *Dietary Reference Intakes for Calcium and Vitamin D*, National Academy of Sciences, National Academy Press, Washington, DC, 2011.
80. Dawson-Hughes, B. et al., *Osteoporos. Int.*, 21, 1151, 2010.
81. Vitamin D and calcium: Systematic review of health outcomes. Evidence Report/Technology Assessment: Number 183, AHRQ Publication No. 09-E015, 2009.
82. Adams, J.S. and Hewison M., *J. Clin. Endocrinol. Metab.*, 95, 471, 2010.
83. Levis, S. et al., *J. Clin. Endocrinol. Metab.*, 90(3), 1557, 2005.
84. Tseng, M., Giri, V., and Bruner, D.W., *BMC Public Health*, 9, 191, 2009.
85. Earthman, C.P. et al., *Int. J. Obes.*, 21, June 2011.
86. Shea, M.K. et al., *J. Am. Geriatr. Soc.*, 59, 1165, 2011.
87. Zadshir, A. et al., *Ethn. Dis.*, 15, 97, 2005.

88. U.S. Preventive Services Task Force, *Ann. Intern. Med.*, 139(1), 51, 2003.

89. U.S. Department of Health and Human Services. National Health Statistics Reports. Complementary and alternative medicine use among adults and Children: United States, 2007, Number 12, 2008.

90. Hooper, L. et al., *Cochrane Database Syst. Rev.*, 4, CD003177, 2004. DOI: 10.1002/14651858.CD003177.pub2. 2004.

91. Agency for healthcare research and quality, summary, Evidence Report/Technology Assessment: Number 89. AHRQ Publication Number 04-E012-1, March 2004.

92. León, H. et al., *BMJ*, 337, a2931, 2008.

93. Linde, K. et al., *Cochrane Database Syst. Rev.*, 1, CD000530, 2006. DOI: 10.1002/14651858.CD000530. 2007.

94. Rodriguezz-Leyva, D. et al., *Can. J. Cardiol.*, 26, 489, 2010.

95. Geng, J. et al., *Cochrane Database Syst. Rev.*, 12, CD007769, 2010. DOI: 10.1002/14651858.CD007769.pub2. 2010.

96. U.S. Food and Drug Administration, Center for Food Safety and Applied Nutrition, Office of Nutritional Products, Labeling, and Dietary Supplements, Dietary Supplements, Tips for Older Dietary Supplement Users, 2003.

97. Ernst, E., *Complement. Altern. Med. Ser.*, 136(1), 42, 2002.

98. Sparreboom, A. et al., *J. Clin. Oncol.*, 22(12), 2489, 2004.

99. Memorial Sloan-Kettering Cancer Center, Information Resource: About Herbs, Botanicals & Other Products.

100. Kendall, P. et al., *J. Am. Diet. Assoc.*, 103(12), 1646, 2003.

101. McCabe-Sellers, B.J. and Beattie, S.E., *J. Am. Diet. Assoc.*, 104(11), 1708, 2004.

102. Mao, Y., Zhu, C., and Boedeker, E.C., *Curr. Opin. Gastroenterol.*, 19(1), 11, 2003.

103. Buzby, J.C., *Food Rev.*, 25(2), 30, 2002.

104. Kennedy, R.L., Chokkalingham, K., and Srinivasan, R., *Curr. Opin. Clin. Nutr. Metab. Care*, 7, 3, 2004.

105. Cress, M.E. et al., *J. Aging Phys. Act.*, 13(1), 61, 2005.

106. U.S. Department of Health and Human Services. *2008 Physical Activity Guidelines for Americans*, 2008.

107. White House Conference on Aging, 50 Resolutions, As Voted by 2005 WHCoA Delegates, 2005.

108. Institute of Medicine, *Nutrition and Healthy Aging in the Community: A Workshop*, Washington, DC, October 5–6, 2011.

109. Flegal, K.M. et al. *JAMA*, 303, 235, 2010.

110. Borrud, L.G. et al., *Body Composition Data for Individuals 8 Years of Age and Older: U.S. Population, 1999–2004*, Vital and Health Statistics Series 11. U.S. Department of Health and Human Services, Centers for Disease Control and Prevention, Hyattsville, MD, 2010.

111. U.S. Department of Agriculture. What we eat in America, NHANES 2005–2006, 2009.

112. Institute of Medicine, *Dietary Reference Intakes for Thiamin, Riboflavin, Niacin, Vitamin $B_6$, Folate, Vitamin $B_{12}$, Pantothenic Acid, Biotin, and Choline*, National Academy of Sciences, National Academy Press, Washington, DC, 1998.

113. U.S. Department of Agriculture. What we eat in America, NHANES 2007–2008, 2009.

114. Food and Nutrition Board, *Dietary Reference Intakes for Water, Potassium, Sodium, Chloride, and Sulfate*, National Academy of Sciences, National Academy Press, Washington, DC, 2004.

115. Food and Nutrition Board, *Dietary Reference Intakes for Energy, Carbohydrate, Fiber, Fat, Fatty Acids, Cholesterol, Protein, and Amino Acids (Macronutrients)*, National Academy of Sciences, National Academy Press, Washington, DC, 2005.

116. Wells, H.F. and Buzby, J.C., U.S. Department of Agriculture. Dietary assessment of major trends in U.S. food consumption, 1970–2005, 2008.

# 23 Exercise and Nutrient Needs

*Emma M. Laing*

## CONTENTS

## INTRODUCTION

Nutrition supports exercise and training across the continuum of activity whether the goal is to attain a desired peak competition echelon or maintain an existing level of health and fitness. Achieving the appropriate combination of energy, macronutrients, micronutrients, and fluids will support the regulation of metabolism, maintenance of normal endocrine function, and the provision of adequate fuel during exercise participation. Together, these factors can significantly impact an individual's body size, body weight and composition, level of fatigue (both physical and cognitive) during exercise, recovery from exercise, and overall risk for illness and injury. Appropriate selection of foods and fluids can determine the intensity or duration of physical activity, and by the same token, the type, intensity, and volume of physical activity can affect daily energy expenditure and fuel-type utilization, which ultimately enhance or reduce success in one's sport or activity. Indeed, according to the most recent (2009) Nutrition and Athletic Performance position paper[1] issued by the Academy of Nutrition and Dietetics (formerly the American Dietetic Association), Dietitians of Canada and the American College of Sports Medicine, "physical activity, athletic performance, and recovery from exercise are enhanced by optimal nutrition." The collective organizations recommend "appropriate selection of food and fluids, timing of intake and supplement choices for optimal health and exercise performance." This chapter highlights the basic principles outlined in the Nutrition and Athletic Performance position paper,[1] while integrating contemporary national recommendations for healthy adults such as those from the Institute of Medicine's Dietary Reference Intakes (DRIs)[2–7] and the 2010 Dietary Guidelines for Americans.[8]

This chapter begins by summarizing energy intake requirements for Americans categorized by physical activity level (PAL) (shown in Table 23.1). Tables 23.2 and 23.3 outline the recommendations for macronutrients and micronutrients,

respectively. "Nutrient/Exercise Considerations" are presented for each nutrient (in Table 23.3) to provide additional recommendations based on existing information supporting the role of nutrition in exercise performance (e.g., nutrient functions in the metabolic processes of exercise, nutrient recommendations for physically active individuals, groups at risk for nutrient deficiency, and possible effects of dietary/supplemental interventions on exercise performance). Table 23.4 lists the number of daily servings within each food group for adults according to varying levels of energy intake needs. Finally, Table 23.5 highlights recommendations for the timing of foods and fluids, including water and electrolytes, for optimal exercise performance.

Whereas exercising versus inactive persons generally require higher fluid and energy (and in some cases, macronutrient) intakes, the need for most nutrients to support exercise participation can be met by consuming an adequate, well-balanced diet while considering the timing and frequency of food intake to optimize nutrient metabolism and availability. Therefore, national dietary recommendations should be considered appropriate for all athletic individuals, including both elite and recreational, unless otherwise stated (see Chapter 23 for specific recommendations for the elite athlete as well as International Olympic Committee Medical Commission consensus statements, available at: http://www.olympic.org/medical-commission?tab=Statements [accessed April 1, 2012]). The recommendations presented here should be specially modified by a qualified health-care professional, such as a registered and licensed dietitian or a Board-certified specialist in sports dietetics, to combine evidence-based principles in preparing nutrition prescription with exercise, in order to meet the individual's goals and translate them into practical recommendations. The nutrition professional will target variations in age, sex, fitness level, mode of activity, intensity and duration of training, time between exercise sessions, as well as body weight and composition goals (see Chapter 23 for expansion on the role of a qualified sports dietitian in providing nutrition services to athletes).

**TABLE 23.1**

**Energy Intake Recommendations Based on the DRIs and the Dietary Guidelines for Americans**

Energy Intake

| DRI[7] Estimated Energy Requirement (EER)[a–c] | | | Dietary Guidelines for Americans[8] Estimated Kilocalorie Requirements[d–f] | | |
|---|---|---|---|---|---|
| Height (m)/ Activity Level | EER Males BMI 18.5–24.99 | EER Females BMI 18.5–24.99 | Age (Years)/ Activity Level | Males Average BMI 22.1 | Females Average BMI 21.6 |
| *1.50* | | | *19–30* | | |
| Sedentary | 1848–2080 | 1625–1762 | Sedentary | 2400–2600 | 1800–2000 |
| Low active | 2009–2267 | 1803–1956 | Moderately active | 2600–2800 | 2000–2200 |
| Active | 2215–2506 | 2025–2198 | Active | 3000 | 2400 |
| Very active | 2554–2898 | 2291–2489 | | | |
| *1.65* | | | *31–50* | | |
| Sedentary | 2068–2349 | 1816–1982 | Sedentary | 2200–2400 | 1800 |
| Low active | 2254–2566 | 2016–2202 | Moderately active | 2400–2600 | 2000 |
| Active | 2490–2842 | 2267–2477 | Active | 2800–3000 | 2200 |
| Very active | 2880–3296 | 2567–2807 | | | |
| *1.80* | | | *51+* | | |
| Sedentary | 2301–2635 | 2015–2211 | Sedentary | 2000–2200 | 1600 |
| Low active | 2513–2884 | 2239–2459 | Moderately active | 2200–2400 | 1800 |
| Active | 2782–3200 | 2519–2769 | Active | 2400–2800 | 2000–2200 |
| Very active | 3225–3720 | 2855–3141 | | | |

[a] *DRIs represent requirements for males and females 30 years of age; for each year below/above 30, add/subtract 7 kcal/day for females and add/subtract 10 kcal/day for males, respectively.*

[b] EER is the average energy intake that is predicted to maintain energy balance in healthy normal-weight individuals of a defined age, sex, weight, height, and level of physical activity consistent with good health (based on body mass index [BMI; $kg/m^2$] values of 18.5 and 24.99).

[c] Regression equations based on doubly labeled water data:
- Female EER = $354 - 6.91 \times$ age (year) + PA $\times$ [$9.36 \times$ weight (kg) + $726 \times$ height (m)]
- Male EER = $662 - 9.53 \times$ age (year) + PA $\times$ [$15.91 \times$ weight (kg) + $539.6 \times$ height (m)]

PA represents physical activity, which differs depending on PAL (the ratio of total energy expenditure/basal energy expenditure):
- PA = 1.0 for both males and females if PAL 1.0–1.39; *sedentary* (typical daily living activities).
- PA = 1.11 (males) 1.12 (females) if PAL 1.4–1.59; *low active* (typical daily living activities +30 to 60 min of daily moderate activity).
- PA = 1.25 (males) 1.27 (females) if PAL 1.6–1.89; *active* (typical daily living activities +at least 60 min of daily moderate activity).
- PA = 1.48 (males) 1.45 (females) if PAL 1.9–2.5; *very active* (Typical daily living activities +at least 60 min of daily moderate activity +60 min of vigorous activity; or 120 min of moderate activity).

[d] Dietary Guideline recommendations are used when no quantitative DRI value is available and are applied to ages 2 years and older.

[e] Values are rounded to the nearest 200 cal; an individual's calorie needs may be higher or lower than these average estimates.

[f] Values are based on EER and the reference size of median height and weight for that height; for adults, the reference man is 5 ft 10 in. tall and weighs 154 lb, and the reference woman is 5 ft 4 in. tall and weighs 126 lb.
- Sedentary is a lifestyle that includes only the light physical activity associated with typical day-to-day life.
- Moderately active is a lifestyle that includes physical activity equivalent to walking ~1.5–3 miles/day at 3–4 miles/h, in addition to the light physical activity associated with typical day-to-day life.
- Active is a lifestyle that includes physical activity equivalent to walking more than 3 miles/day at 3–4 miles/h, in addition to the light physical activity associated with typical day-to-day life.
- The kilocalorie ranges shown are to accommodate the needs of different ages within the group; fewer calories are needed at older ages.
- Estimates for females do not include women who are pregnant or breast-feeding.

## TABLE 23.2

## Macronutrient Recommendations Based on the DRIs and the Position on Nutrition and Athletic Performance

| Macronutrient/Function | DRIs[7] Recommendations | Position on Nutrition and Athletic Performance[1] Recommendations |
|---|---|---|
| *Carbohydrate*: Important for maintaining normal levels of glucose in the brain and in circulation; needed to supply fiber, a key nutrient for reducing blood cholesterol and maintaining blood glucose levels; excess amounts can result in low intakes of essential fatty acids and indispensable amino acids, and could lead to surplus body fat storage, body weight gain, and associated chronic diseases | *AMDR[a] (percent of total energy)* <br> Adults aged 19 to >70 years: 45–65 <br> *Carbohydrate RDA[b] (g/day)* <br> Males aged 19 to >70 years: 130 <br> Females aged 19 to >70 years: 130 <br> *Total Fiber AI[c,d] (g/day)* <br> Males aged 19–50 years: 38 <br> Females aged 19–50 years: 25 <br> Males aged 51 to >70 years: 30 <br> Females aged 51 to >70 years: 21 <br> *Added sugars[e]* <br> Limit to no more than 25% of energy | • Range for exercising adults: 6–10 g/kg body weight/day <br> • Caution is recommended in using specific percentages of carbohydrates (e.g., 60% energy intake) as a basis for meal plans |
| *Protein*: Needed to maintain body nitrogen and supply indispensable amino acids for the synthesis of protein (during growth, repair of damaged tissues, muscle hypertrophy, and enzyme synthesis); provides indispensable amino acids, which are found in high-quality protein foods in the diet; excess protein can interfere with maintaining sufficient dietary carbohydrates to replenish muscle glycogen as well as maintaining proper hydration; excess protein ingestion could lead to the progression of renal function impairments, surplus body fat storage, and associated chronic diseases | *AMDR (percent of total energy)* <br> Adults aged 19 to >70 years: 10–35 <br> *Protein RDA[f] (g/day)* <br> Males aged 19 to >70 years: 56 <br> Females aged 19 to >70 years: 46 <br> *Indispensable amino acids RDA (mg/kg/day)* <br> Adult males and females <br> Histidine: 14 <br> Isoleucine: 19 <br> Leucine: 42 <br> Lysine: 38 <br> Methionine + cysteine: 19 <br> Phenylalanine + tyrosine: 33 <br> Threonine: 20 <br> Tryptophan: 5 <br> Valine: 24 | • Most individuals should aim to follow the current RDA, 0.8 g/kg body weight/day <br> • Range for endurance athletes is often recommended in practice as 1.2–1.4 g/kg body weight/day <br> • Range for strength-trained athletes is often recommended in practice as 1.2–1.7 g/kg body weight/day <br> • The amount of protein needed to maintain muscle mass may be lower for those who routinely engage in resistance training due to more efficient protein utilization <br> • The amount of protein needed to maintain muscle mass may be higher for those in the early phase of training when significant gains in muscle size occurs <br> • Protein recommendations can generally be met through diet alone, without the use of protein or amino acid supplements <br> • Because vegetarian athletes may be at risk for low-protein intake, consultation with a sports dietitian is recommended |
| *Fat*: Provides energy, essential fatty acids, and fat-soluble vitamins (vitamins A, D, E, and K); assists in the absorption of these vitamins; serves as a structural component for the development of tissues and as a precursor to numerous compounds; excess dietary fat could lead to alterations in carbohydrate and protein intakes and ultimately body weight gain; linoleic acid is an essential component of structural membrane lipids; α-linolenic acid is involved in neurological development and growth; both of these fatty acids are precursors of eicosanoids | *AMDR (percent of energy) for fat[g]* <br> Adults aged 19 to >70 years: 20–35 <br> *AMDR (percent of energy) for n − 6 polyunsaturated fatty acids[h]* <br> Adults aged 19 to >70 years: 5–10 <br> *AMDR (percent of energy) for n − 3 polyunsaturated fatty acids[i]* <br> Adults aged 19 to >70 years: 0.6–1.2 <br> *Linoleic acid AI (g/day)* <br> Males aged 19–50 years: 17 <br> Females aged 19–50 years: 12 <br> Males aged 51 to >70 years: 14 <br> Females aged 51 to >70 years: 11 <br> *α-Linolenic acid AI (g/day)* <br> Males aged 19 to >70 years: 1.6 <br> Females aged 19 to >70 years: 1.1 | • Recommendations for 20%–35% fat intake should be followed <br> • Fat composition should be 10% saturated, 10% polyunsaturated, and 10% monounsaturated <br> • A trained individual uses a greater percentage of fat than an untrained person does at the same workload <br> • There is no physical performance benefit in consuming a fat-restricted diet (less than 15% of energy from fat) <br> • Diets that supply fat as ≥70% of energy intake do not support national recommendations and should be carefully evaluated |

[a] AMDR, Acceptable macronutrient distribution range; a range of intakes associated with reduced risk of chronic diseases while providing AIs of essential nutrients; values are expressed as percentages of total energy intake.

[b] RDA, Recommended dietary allowances; values are set to meet the needs of almost all (97%–98%) individuals in a group.

[c] AI, Adequate intake; values are set to cover the needs of all individuals in a group, but lack of data or uncertainty in the data prevent being able to specify with confidence the percentage of individuals covered by this intake.

[d] AI for fiber is based on 14 g total fiber/1000 kcal.

[e] Added sugars are defined as sugars and syrups that are added to food during processing and preparation.

[f] RDA for protein is based on 0.8 g protein/kg body weight/day.

[g] No RDA or AI was set due to insufficient data linking a defined level of dietary fat to prevention of chronic disease; however, the recommendation states that intakes of dietary cholesterol, trans-fatty acids, and saturated fatty acids should be "as low as possible while consuming a nutritionally adequate diet."

[h] Linoleic acid.

[i] α-Linolenic acid, eicosapentaenoic acid, and docosahexaenoic acid.

**TABLE 23.3**

**Micronutrient Recommendations Based on the DRIs and the Position on Nutrition and Athletic Performance**

| Micronutrient/Function | DRI[2,3,5] Recommendations | Nutrient/Exercise Considerations |
|---|---|---|
| *B-Complex Vitamins* | | |
| Overall function | | The B-complex vitamins are involved in energy production during exercise and are required for the production of red blood cells, protein synthesis, as well as tissue repair and maintenance. Thiamin, riboflavin, niacin, vitamin $B_6$, pantothenic acid, and biotin are involved in energy production during exercise. Folate and vitamin $B_{12}$ are involved in the production of red blood cells for protein synthesis and in tissue repair. |
| Position on Nutrition and Athletic Performance[1] Recommendation | | Consuming the RDA for B-vitamins is recommended for athletes; however, exercise may increase the need for the B-complex vitamins, perhaps up to twice the current recommended amounts. These increased needs can generally be met via the higher energy intakes required by exercising individuals to maintain body weight. Of the B-vitamins, riboflavin, vitamin $B_6$, folate, and vitamin $B_{12}$ are often low in the diets of female athletes, particularly among those who practice vegetarian diets or have disordered eating. Short-term deficiencies have not been shown to affect exercise performance. However, severe deficiency of vitamin $B_{12}$ and/or folate can result in anemia, which can negatively impact exercise performance. |
| *Thiamin*: plays a role in carbohydrate and amino acid metabolism; acts as a coenzyme in the conversion of pyruvate to acetyl CoA and α-ketoglutarate to succinyl CoA; participates in the decarboxylation of branched-chain amino acids | *RDA[a] (mg/day)*<br>Males aged 19 to >70 years: 1.2<br>Females aged 19 to >70 years: 1.1 | • 0.5 mg thiamin/1000 kcal has been recommended for physically active individuals who have increased energy needs[3,73]<br>• A temporary thiamin insufficiency can lead to pyruvate accumulation and an increase in circulating lactate during exercise, which may result in muscle fatigue[74]<br>• Thiamin supplementation has been shown to improve perceived recovery from exercise fatigue but has not been shown to alter metabolic or other physical performance indices[75,76] |
| *Riboflavin*: required for oxidative energy production; functions specifically in the mitochondrial electron transport system as the coenzymes flavin mononucleotide and flavin adenine dinucleotide | *RDA (mg/day)*<br>Males aged 19 to >70 years: 1.3<br>Females aged 19 to >70 years: 1.1 | • 0.6 mg riboflavin/1000 kcal has been recommended for physically active individuals who have increased energy needs[3]<br>• For exercising women who may be restricting energy intake or choosing to omit certain food groups, 1.4–1.6 mg riboflavin/day has been suggested for those engaging in moderate exercise and 2–3 mg riboflavin/day for those participating in high-intensity competitive activities[66,73,77] |
| *Niacin*: an electron carrier in many oxidative reactions; a precursor of electron (nicotinamide adenine nucleotide) and proton (nicotinamide adenine dinucleotide) acceptors | *RDA (as NE[b] mg/day)*<br>Males aged 19 to >70 years: 16<br>Female aged 19 to >70 years: 14 | • While niacin supplementation has been shown to decrease circulating free fatty acid concentrations and reduce excess postexercise oxygen consumption, supplementation does not appear to improve overall performance outcomes during exercise[78,79] |
| *Vitamin $B_6$*: a cofactor for transferases, transaminases, decarboxylases, and cleavage enzymes used in transformations of amino acids; needed for gluconeogenesis and glyconeogenesis processes | *RDA (mg/day)*<br>Males aged 19–50 years: 1.3<br>Females aged 19–50 years: 1.3<br>Males aged 51 to >70 years: 1.7<br>Female aged 51 to >70 years: 1.5 | • Because vitamin $B_6$ is involved in the process of muscle glycogen breakdown, exercise may increase the turnover and urinary losses of vitamin $B_6$[80–82]<br>• Physically active females may need up to 2–3 mg vitamin $B_6$/day, in proportion to increased energy needs[66] |
| *Vitamin $B_{12}$*: a coenzyme for the reaction that converts homocysteine to methionine; required for normal erythrocyte production and neurological function | *RDA (μg/day)[c]*<br>Males aged 19 to >70 years: 2.4<br>Females aged 19 to >70 years: 2.4 | • Vitamin $B_{12}$ supplementation has not been shown to demonstrate positive effects on physical performance[83,84] |
| *Choline*: a constituent of lecithin; essential in the metabolism of fat; a precursor of the neurotransmitter, acetylcholine | *AI[d] (mg/day)*<br>Males aged 19 to >70 years: 550<br>Females aged 19 to >70 years: 425 | • Strenuous physical activity has been shown to reduce plasma choline concentrations[3]<br>• Choline supplementation appears to lower lipid peroxidation following mild exercise[85]<br>• No effect of choline supplementation during prolonged exercise has been demonstrated on physical performance measures or in delaying fatigue[86,87] |

## TABLE 23.3 (continued)
## Micronutrient Recommendations Based on the DRIs and the Position on Nutrition and Athletic Performance

| Micronutrient/Function | DRI[2,3,5] Recommendations | Nutrient/Exercise Considerations |
|---|---|---|
| **Antioxidants** | | |
| Overall function | Vitamins A, C, E, and selenium may protect cell membranes from oxidative damage. Because exercise can increase oxygen consumption 10- to 15-fold, chronic exercise produces a constant "oxidative stress" on the muscles and other cells. Muscle tissue damage caused by intense exercise can lead to lipid peroxidation of membranes. Increased exercise duration and intensity appear to elevate levels of lipid peroxide by-products[88,89] and may necessitate increases in dietary antioxidants; however, the evidence to date on this topic is conflicting[90,91] and remains uncertain. | |
| Position on Nutrition and Athletic Performance[1] Recommendation | There is no clear consensus on whether supplementation of antioxidant nutrients is necessary. Habitual exercise has been shown to result in an augmented antioxidant system and a reduction of lipid peroxidation. Thus, a well-trained athlete may have a more developed endogenous antioxidant system than a sedentary person. Active individuals at greatest risk for poor antioxidant intakes are those who follow a low-energy, low-fat diet, and have limited dietary intakes of whole grains, fruits, and vegetables. Because antioxidants may be pro-oxidative with potential negative effects, athletes are encouraged not to exceed the UL. | |
| *Vitamin A*: a fat-soluble antioxidant; essential for vision, gene expression, immune function, and growth; beta-carotene, a precursor of vitamin A, also has antioxidant properties | *RDA (as RAE[e] μg/day)*<br>Males aged 19 to >70 years: 900<br>Females aged 19 to >70 years: 700 | • Evidence is lacking to suggest that exercise increases vitamin A needs, since competitive athletes have improved beta-carotene status compared to nonathletes[92]<br>• Supplementation with vitamin A, in combination with vitamins C and E, has been shown to prevent exercise-induced oxidative stress[93] |
| *Vitamin C*: a water-soluble antioxidant; participates in bone formation and scar tissue repair; needed for synthesis of carnitine for fatty acid transport; serves to regenerate vitamin E from its oxidized by-product | *RDA (mg/day)*<br>Males aged 19 to >70 years: 90<br>Females aged 19 to >70 years: 75 | • The requirement for vitamin C may be increased during physical activity due to its roles in immune and antioxidant function and in collagen repair[73]<br>• Vitamin C supplementation does not appear to have a beneficial effect on exercise-induced increases in muscle damage or recovery, or on the hormonal, or immune response after prolonged exercise[94,95] |
| *Vitamin E*: a fat-soluble antioxidant; acts on polyunsaturated fatty acids in cell membranes; essential for maintaining erythrocyte and neurological function | *RDA (mg/day)[f]*<br>Males aged 19 to >70 years: 15<br>Females aged 19 to >70 years: 15 | • Vitamin E deficiency results in oxidative stress and muscle degeneration[73]<br>• Large doses of α-tocopherol supplementation may actually exhibit pro-oxidant effects during high-intensity exercise[96]<br>• Endurance athletes, however, may have a higher need for vitamin E; though future research is warranted |
| *Selenium:* an essential element in the glutathione peroxidase enzyme system; involved in DNA repair, enzyme activation, and immune system function | *RDA (μg/day)*<br>Males aged 19 to >70 years: 55<br>Females aged 19 to >70 years: 55 | • Selenium supplementation, in combination with several other antioxidants, has not been shown to protect against DNA damage or plasma cytokine concentrations following aerobic exercise[97,98]<br>• Selenium supplementation for exercise performance is generally not recommended due to potential toxic effects of overconsumption |
| **Other Micronutrients** | | |
| *Calcium*: needed for growth and repair of bone tissue and the maintenance of blood calcium levels; required for blood clotting, muscle contraction, nerve transmission, and overall bone health | *RDA (mg/day)*<br>Males aged 19–50 years: 1000<br>Females aged 19–50 years: 1000<br>Males aged 51–70 years: 1000<br>Males aged >70 years: 1200<br>Females aged 51 to >70 years: 1200 | • Exercising individuals should strive to meet the recommended intakes for calcium because inadequate dietary calcium increases the risk of osteopenia and stress fractures<br>• Females are at greatest risk for low bone mineral density if energy intakes are low, dairy products are eliminated or restricted in the diet, and menstrual dysfunction is present |
| *Vitamin D*: promotes growth and mineralization of bone by maintaining calcium and phosphorus homeostasis; enhances absorption of calcium; has a role in the modulation of immune cells; regulates the development and homeostasis of skeletal muscle and the nervous system | *RDA (μg/day)[g]*<br>Males aged 19–70 years: 15<br>Females aged 19–70 years: 15<br>Males aged >70 years: 20<br>Females aged >70 years: 20 | • Exercising individuals living at northern latitudes or who train primarily indoors throughout the year (e.g., gymnasts and figure skaters) may be at risk for poor vitamin D status, especially if foods fortified with vitamin D are not consumed; these individuals would benefit from vitamin D supplementation at the level of the DRI[2,8] |

*(continued)*

**TABLE 23.3 (continued)**
**Micronutrient Recommendations Based on the DRIs and the Position on Nutrition and Athletic Performance**

| Micronutrient/Function | DRI[2,3,5] Recommendations | Nutrient/Exercise Considerations |
| --- | --- | --- |
| *Magnesium*: involved in numerous enzymatic reactions such as glycolysis, fat and protein metabolism, adenosine triphosphate hydrolysis, and the second messenger system; regulates neuromuscular, cardiovascular, immune, and hormonal functions | *RDA (mg/day)*<br>Males aged 19–30 years: 400<br>Females aged 19–30 years: 310<br>Males aged 31 to >70 years: 420<br>Females aged 19 to >70 years: 320 | • Magnesium is one of the primary minerals low in the diets of athletes, along with calcium, iron, and zinc; low intakes of these minerals are most often the result of energy restriction or avoidance of animal products<br>• A deficiency in magnesium impairs endurance performance by increasing oxygen requirements to complete submaximal exercise<br>• Among individuals with low-magnesium status, foods high in magnesium should be encouraged, and supplementation at the level of the DRI may be warranted |
| *Iron*: required for the formation of hemoglobin, myoglobin, and cytochromes, and for enzymes involved in energy production | *RDA (mg/day)*<br>Males aged 19–50 years: 8<br>Females aged 19–50 years: 18<br>Females aged 19–50 years who use oral contraceptives:[h] 11<br>Males aged 51 to >70 years: 8<br>Females aged 51 to >70 years: 8 | • Since iron depletion is one of the most prevalent nutrient deficiencies observed in athletic females, there is an increased risk for impaired physical performance associated with symptoms of iron deficiency<br>• Assessment of iron status in physically active females should be done routinely, especially in amenorrheic cases; these individuals may benefit from iron supplementation<br>• Other considerations for iron and athletic performance include blood donation, which adds 0.65 to basal losses, and practicing vegetarianism, which reduces iron absorption from 18% to 10%[5] |
| *Zinc*: important for the growth and repair of muscle and skeletal tissues, maturation and reproduction, wound healing and energy production; functions in a number of metallic enzymes including carbonic anhydrase, alkaline phosphatases, and RNA polymerases; required to maintain the structure of nucleic acid protein | *RDA (mg/day)*<br>Males aged 19 to >70 years: 11<br>Females aged 19 to >70 years: 8 | • Exercising individuals should strive to meet the recommended intakes for zinc, because athletic females, particularly those who are vegetarian, have been shown to have diets low in zinc |

[a]  RDA, Recommended dietary allowances; values are set to meet the needs of almost all (97%–98%) individuals in a group.
[b]  NE, niacin equivalents; 1 mg niacin = 60 mg tryptophan.
[c]  People over the age of 50 are advised to consume vitamin $B_{12}$ from fortified foods and/or supplements.[8]
[d]  AI, Adequate intake; values are set to cover the needs of all individuals in a group, but lack of data or uncertainty in the data prevent being able to specify with confidence the percentage of individuals covered by this intake.
[e]  RAE, Retinol activity equivalents; 1 RAE = 1 μg retinol, 12 μg beta-carotene, 24 μg alpha-carotene, or 24 μg beta-cryptoxanthin.
[f]  As alpha-tocopherol.
[g]  As cholecalciferol; 1 μg cholecalciferol = 40 IU vitamin D; values are in the absence of adequate exposure to sunlight.
[h]  The RDA for iron is reduced for women who use oral contraceptives, because of their lower menstrual iron losses.

The content of this chapter reflects data collected from adults, rather than children, and does not focus on a particular type of athlete or sporting event. Nutrition and hydration guidelines tailored to specific sports, in varying conditions (e.g., altitudes), as well as to child and adolescent athletes, are summarized elsewhere.[9–18] The use of dietary supplements and ergogenic aids by physically active individuals to enhance performance is also beyond the scope of this chapter, but is reviewed both in Poortmans et al.[19] and in Chapter 23. For individualized nutrient assessment, *MyPlate*, developed by the U.S. Department of Agriculture, provides useful dietary and physical activity assessment tools, which are available online at: http://www.choosemy-plate.gov/ (accessed April 1, 2012). Additional information on adopting a healthy lifestyle that includes regular physical activity, fitness, sports participation, and good quality nutrition, has been provided by the President's Council on Fitness, Sports and Nutrition, and can be accessed online at: http://www.fitness.gov/ (accessed April 1, 2012).

## MINIMUM PHYSICAL ACTIVITY RECOMMENDATIONS

In order to achieve the health benefits of an active lifestyle, at least 150–500 min/week of moderately intense or 75–150 min of vigorously intense activities, combined with muscle-strengthening exercises, are currently recommended by national authorities.[8,20,21] According to the most recent (2008) Physical Activity Guidelines for Americans,[20] adults should perform the following:

• Two hours and 30 min/week (150 min) of moderate-intensity, or 1 h and 15 min (75 min)/week of vigorous-intensity aerobic physical activity, or an equivalent combination of moderate- and

**TABLE 23.4**

**Number of Daily Servings in a Food Group Based on Adult Caloric Needs**

| Food Group | 1600 cal | 1800 cal | 2000 cal | 2600 cal | 3100 cal |
|---|---|---|---|---|---|
| Grains[a] | 6 | 6 | 6–8 | 10–11 | 12–13 |
| Vegetables[b] | 3–4 | 4–5 | 4–5 | 5–6 | 6 |
| Fruits[c] | 4 | 4–5 | 4–5 | 5–6 | 6 |
| Low-fat or fat-free dairy foods[d] | 2–3 | 2–3 | 2–3 | 3 | 3–4 |
| Lean meats, poultry, and fish[e] | 3–4 or less | 6 or less | 6 or less | 6 or less | 6–9 |
| Nuts, seeds, and legumes[f] | 3–4/week | 4/week | 4–5/week | 1 | 1 |
| Fats and oils[g] | 2 | 2–3 | 2–3 | 3 | 4 |
| Sweets and added sugars[h] | 3 or less/week | 5 or less/week | 5 or less/week | <2 | <2 |
| Maximum sodium limit[i] | 2300 mg | 2300 mg | 2300 mg | 2300 mg | 2300 mg |

*Source:* Adapted from the 2010 Dietary Guidelines for Americans, Appendix 10: The DASH eating plan at various calorie levels (for adults, 1600–3100 cal). Values are number of servings.

Serving sizes:

[a] One slice bread; 1 oz dry cereal; ½ cup cooked rice, pasta, or cooked cereal.

[b] One cup raw leafy vegetable; ½ cup cut-up raw or cooked vegetable; ½ cup vegetable juice.

[c] One medium fruit; ¼ cup dried fruit; ½ cup fresh, frozen, or canned fruit; ½ cup fruit juice.

[d] One cup milk; 1 cup yogurt; 1 ½ oz cheese.

[e] One oz cooked meats, poultry, or fish; 1 egg.

[f] 1/3 cup or 1 ½ oz nuts; 2 tablespoons peanut butter; 2 tablespoons or ½ oz seeds; ½ cup cooked legumes (dry beans, peas).

[g] One teaspoon soft margarine; 1 teaspoon vegetable oil; 1 tablespoon mayonnaise; 1 tablespoon salad dressing.

[h] One tablespoon sugar, 1 tablespoon jelly or jam; ½ cup sorbet, gelatin dessert; 1 cup lemonade.

[i] Reduce sodium intake to 1500 mg/day among persons who are 51 years of age and older and those of any age who are African American or have hypertension, diabetes, or chronic kidney disease.[8]

vigorous-intensity aerobic physical activity. Aerobic activity should be performed in episodes of at least 10 min, preferably spread throughout the week.

- Additional health benefits are provided by increasing to 5 h (300 min)/week of moderate-intensity aerobic physical activity, or 2 h and 30 min/week of vigorous-intensity physical activity, or an equivalent combination of both.

- Adults should also engage in muscle-strengthening activities that involve all major muscle groups performed on 2 or more days/week.

## ENERGY AVAILABILITY

Meeting energy intake and expenditure requirements is essential for achieving optimal physical performance. Energy balance is defined as an equilibrium between energy intake (from foods, fluids, and supplements) and energy expenditure (from basal metabolic rate, the thermic effect of food, and the thermic effect of activity).[22] Energy availability is defined as the difference between dietary energy intake and exercise energy expenditure normalized to fat-free mass and is the "amount of dietary energy remaining for other body functions after exercise training."[23] In most healthy adults, energy availability occurs between 30 and 45 kcal/kg fat-free mass.[24,25] Both energy intake demands and energy expenditure depend on the type of physical activities performed, the

training regime (duration, frequency, and intensity), as well as the sex and nutritional status of the athlete, and can vary from day to day and by season.[26,27] Participation in strenuous endurance activities (that use predominantly oxidative phosphorylation as the main energy source) produces an increase in overall energy turnover and leads to a loss of body weight and/or a compensatory increase in food intake.

Energy availability is considered optimal when energy intake is sufficient to maintain normal physiological functions in addition to requirements for physical activities. Consistent overconsumption of calories would result in increased energy availability. If energy availability is too high, this can hinder athletic performance due to increases in body weight or undesirable changes in body composition. By contrast, low energy availability (typically, energy intakes less than 1800–2000 kcal/day alone or in combination with excessive exercise) counteracts the benefits of being physically active and can lead to declines in exercise performance (e.g., early fatigue, irritability, loss of strength and endurance, and increased risk of injury), poor macro- and micronutrient intakes, and potentially irreversible health consequences (e.g., increased risk of muscle and bone mass losses, impaired immune, cardiovascular, gastrointestinal, renal, and central nervous system function, and both menstrual and reproductive dysfunction).[1,23,28]

In 1997, the syndrome describing interrelationships among energy availability, menstrual function, and bone health was termed the Female Athlete Triad.[29] This syndrome is often

**TABLE 23.5**

**Timing of Foods and Fluids for Optimal Exercise Performance**

**Timing and Recommendations**

*Pre-exercise*

Goal: to provide sufficient fluid to maintain hydration, be relatively low in fat and fiber to facilitate gastric emptying and minimize gastrointestinal distress, be relatively high in carbohydrates to maximize maintenance of blood glucose, be moderate in protein, be composed of familiar foods, and be well tolerated

The nutrition plan should include

- Sufficient fluid in the 24 h before an exercise session
- 5–7 mL/kg of water or sports drink 4 h before exercise
- 200–300 g carbohydrate in food or fluid consumed 3–4 h before exercise
- Moderate amounts of low glycemic index carbohydrates (may promote the availability of the sustained carbohydrate)
- Limited or no caffeine, alcohol (both increase urine output), or carbonated beverages (may promote stomach fullness)

*During exercise*

Goal: to consume sufficient fluids to replace fluid losses and maintain fluid balance, and carbohydrates (fluid, solid, or gel) to maintain blood glucose levels and muscle glycogen stores that are easily tolerated and are sufficient in calories to prevent hunger during the exercise session; these guidelines are important for endurance events lasting longer than 1 h when the athlete has not consumed adequate food or fluids before exercise, or if an athlete is exercising in an extreme environment (e.g., heat, cold, or high altitude)

The nutrition plan should include

- Carbohydrates (consumed at approximately 30–60 g/h) for maintenance of blood glucose levels, ideally at 15–20 min intervals
- Individualized fluid volume plan, enough to prevent a 2% deficit and avoid exceeding sweat rate (in order to decrease the risk of hyponatremia)
- Fluids containing carbohydrate in concentrations of 6%–8% in addition to water for activities lasting >1 h if both fluid and carbohydrate needs are to be met with beverage only
- Fluids containing carbohydrate in concentrations of 5%–10%, ~20 to 30 mEq/L sodium (chloride as the anion), ~2 to 5 mEq/L potassium when performing prolonged activity in the heat
- Carbohydrates that yield primarily glucose and no more than 2%–3% (2–3 g/100 mL) fructose; or fructose in amounts that do not cause gastrointestinal discomfort/diarrhea
- Caffeine can be considered as an ergogenic aid in some cases of endurance exercise

*Postexercise*

Goal: to provide adequate fluids, electrolytes, energy, and carbohydrates to replace muscle glycogen and ensure rapid recovery; protein consumed after exercise will provide amino acids for building and repair of muscle tissue

The nutrition plan should include

- Carbohydrate intake ~1.0 to 1.5 g/kg body weight during the first 30 min and again every 2 h for 4–6 h to replace glycogen stores after glycogen-depleting exercise and subsequent sessions are within 24 h
- ~16 oz of fluid for every pound of body weight lost during exercise
- 1.5 L of fluid per kg of body weight lost during an exercise session with recovery periods <12 h
- Moderate amounts of high-glycemic index carbohydrates (may promote greater insulin and glucose responses)
- Modest amounts of sodium may be consumed in fluids and/or meals following high-intensity/duration exercise[a]
- Limited or no caffeine or alcohol

Recommendations are targeted toward individuals who perform exercise at a moderate to high intensity and are based on the Position on Nutrition and Athletic Performance[1] and the American College of Sports Medicine Position Stand on Exercise and Fluid Replacement.[9]

[a]   Sodium intake recommendations obtained from the 2010 Dietary Guidelines for Americans report.[8]

evidenced by respective clinical implications such as eating disorders, functional hypothalamic amenorrhea, and osteoporosis, and young female athletes are at particular risk.[28,30] Updated position stands on the Triad were most recently released in 2005 by the International Olympic Committee[31] and in 2007 by the American College of Sports Medicine.[23] The 2007 position stand states that physically active individuals at the greatest risk for low energy availability are those who restrict dietary energy intake, who exercise for prolonged periods, and who limit the types of foods they eat.[23] The overt practice of energy restriction is common among both men and women and both elite and recreational exercisers,

who are driven to achieve a body weight/composition goal believed to be desirable for peak exercise performance. Disordered eating among physically active individuals varies widely but is reported to occur in up to 78% of female athletes.[32,33] Likewise, menstrual dysfunction is common in female athletes (up to 79%),[34] resulting most commonly from low energy availability.[35,36] When energy availability is below 30 kcal/kg fat-free mass/day, luteinizing hormone pulsatility, glucoregulatory hormones, and bone formation are disrupted. In most amenorrheic females, normal menstrual function can return after additional energy is supplied in the diet. However, in prolonged cases of menstrual disturbances where bone resorption exceeds that of bone formation, the rate of bone mass and strength accretion can be slowed (in adolescents) or bone mass and strength loss can occur (in adults).[32,37] Individuals showing any symptoms of the Triad should be referred to a health-care professional, such as a physician, registered dietitian, specialist in sports dietetics, and/or mental health practitioner. However, physically active individuals may not perceive these symptoms as worrisome. These individuals may not seek medical attention until a more obvious symptom, such as a stress fracture, has ensued.[37,38] Though the "first-line strategy" by health-care professionals working with athletes with Triad symptoms is increasing energy availability by increasing dietary energy intake, decreasing energy expenditure, or both, careful selection of nutrient-rich foods and/or dietary supplements to reduce the risk of emergent nutrient deficiencies that impair both health and performance is especially important in cases of caloric restriction, with or without other Triad symptoms.[23,26]

Energy intake recommendations as suggested by the Position on Nutrition and Athletic Performance[1] are included in Table 23.1. These include recommendations from the recently published (2010) Dietary Guidelines for Americans,[8] which are derived from the DRIs.[7] The DRI recommendations for energy (i.e., the estimated energy requirement [EER]) should meet the needs of most active individuals; however, data from competitive elite athletes who participate in high-intensity training for several hours per day (e.g., PAL values >2.5) were not included in establishing the predictive equations for energy needs.[7,39] Therefore, the EER should be modified according to macronutrient recommendations (i.e., the acceptable macronutrient distribution range [AMDR]) addressed in the following text to meet the energy needs of highly trained elite athletes.[39] Accompanied by the recommendations outlined in Table 23.1, the Position on Nutrition and Athletic Performance[1] also directs nutrition professionals to the prediction equations, Cunningham[40] and Harris-Benedict,[41] and/or metabolic equivalents[42] to estimate energy expenditure for the determination of energy intake requirements for physically active individuals.

## MACRONUTRIENTS

Macronutrients supply the energy required by the body as well as important dietary constituents for varying physiological functions. The macronutrient needs of individuals who exercise regularly are influenced by age, sex, total caloric intake, the ratio, timing and quality of macronutrients in the diet, the intensity, duration and type of activity, as well as training history.[43] Table 23.2 summarizes the carbohydrate, protein, and fat intake recommendations based on the Position on Nutrition and Athletic Performance[1] and the current DRI.[7] Included in this DRI report[7] is the AMDR, which represents a range of intakes (as percent of energy) associated with reduced risk of chronic disease within the context of suggested intakes for each macronutrient. The macronutrient needs for physically active individuals should fit within these ranges and should closely resemble specific nutrient

guidelines presented as recommended dietary allowance (RDA) and/or adequate intake (AI) reference standards.[39]

Carbohydrate is the primary energy source used during endurance-type activities and serves as the most efficient fuel for exercise (producing more adenosine triphosphate per unit of oxygen) compared to other macronutrients. Carbohydrates are essential for maintaining blood glucose levels and muscle glycogen stores, and their availability for muscle contraction during exercise is inversely related to the rate of protein catabolism.[43,44] As intensity and duration of exercise increase the source of carbohydrate shifts from muscle glycogen to circulating blood glucose (an ingestion rate of 1 g carbohydrate/min or 0.04 oz/min in beverage form maintains optimal carbohydrate metabolism during endurance exercise).[45,46] About 50%–60% of energy is derived from carbohydrates during 1–4 h of continuous exercise at 70% of maximal oxygen capacity, while the remaining 40%–50% of energy is derived from free fatty acid oxidation.[47] When suboptimal levels of endogenous sources (i.e., muscle and liver glycogen) occur, usually after 60–90 min of exercise, there may be deleterious effects on physical performance. While carbohydrate restriction has been shown to be detrimental to athletic performance,[1] carbohydrate loading to elevate glycogen stores prior to exercise may delay fatigue in activities that are <90 min in duration.[48] Numerous studies support the efficacy of consuming carbohydrates during endurance-type exercise for the purpose of delaying fatigue, improving feelings of perceived exertion, and enhancing overall psychological and physiologic performance.[49,50] Carbohydrate supplementation has also demonstrated glycogen-sparing effects during shorter bouts of intermittent high-intensity exercise and has been shown to suppress the release of cortisol and promote muscle glycogen resynthesis following resistance training exercise.[51–53] Consuming carbohydrate sources (foods and/or fluids) that are easily tolerated is recommended in order to maximize absorption from the gut and minimize gastrointestinal disturbances. For high-intensity activities and activities of long duration, it is important to adequately replace carbohydrate stores during recovery.[26]

Protein serves to repair exercise-induced microdamage to muscle fibers, to aid in the long-term maintenance or gain of muscle and bone, and to improve energy utilization during endurance activities. With an increase in exercise duration, maintenance of blood glucose may occur through gluconeogenesis in the liver.[43,54,55] The consumption of adequate energy, particularly carbohydrates, is important to protein metabolism so that amino acids are spared for protein synthesis and not oxidized to assist in meeting energy needs. While some physically active individuals may need slightly more protein than the current DRI recommendations,[7] depending on the type, frequency, and duration of the exercise(s) performed (Table 23.2), in general, protein should not be consumed in excess of the DRI to enhance exercise performance. Though a varied diet that meets energy requirements will provide sufficient protein for most physically active individuals, there has been evidence that individual amino acids as well as intact, high-quality proteins (e.g., whey, casein, or soy) are effective in the maintenance, repair, and synthesis of skeletal muscle protein in response to training.[56] Increasing dietary protein far beyond the recommended levels is unlikely to result in endurance benefits or additional increases in lean mass because there is a limit to the rate at which protein tissue can be accrued.[54,57,58] Prolonged intakes of excess protein are associated with increased urea production and excretion,[59] and blood urea nitrogen and urine-specific gravity,[60] and may negatively affect hydration status. Therefore, recommendations for supplementation should be conservative and based on individual needs and performance goals.

Dietary fat provides the free fatty acids needed to supply energy for mild- to moderate-intensity endurance exercise. Lipids are transported to the site of oxidation in the exercising muscle where they are used in the oxidative process to supply energy and spare carbohydrate stores.[7] Physically active individuals should consume dietary fat in amounts similar to what is recommended in the DRI report[7] (Table 23.2). Supplementation with free fatty acids is generally not recommended to improve exercise performance. For example, no beneficial effects have been observed with fatty acid supplementation on body composition, muscle strength, exercise fatigue, immune function, or exercise-induced elevation of pro- or anti-inflammatory cytokines.[61,62] The practice of "fat loading" (i.e., consumption of a high-fat diet [65%–70% of total energy]) to increase fat oxidation and spare the use of muscle glycogen during exercise has been shown to either impair or have no effect on high-intensity training efficiency.[63,64]

Consultation with a registered dietitian, particularly among elite athletes who have increased energy requirements, should be encouraged to ensure a balanced macronutrient intake and to assess the need for supplementation on an individual basis.

## MICRONUTRIENTS

Vitamins and minerals facilitate the use of macronutrients for all physiologic processes, including exercise-related energy metabolism, immune response, growth and maintenance of bone mineral, as well as the protection of body tissues from oxidative stress. Table 23.3 outlines the micronutrient intake recommendations, categorized as B-complex vitamins, antioxidants, and other vitamins and minerals, based on the Position on Nutrition and Athletic Performance[1] and the current DRI reports.[2–6] Physical activity was examined as a key factor in approximately one-third of the micronutrients considered for the RDA and AI guidelines (i.e., vitamins $B_6$, C, E, choline, and thiamin, as well as calcium, iron, magnesium, and sodium); however, no specific recommendations within the DRI reports were made with regard to micronutrient needs during exercise.[65] Therefore, the recommendations issued by the DRI panel for micronutrients should be appropriate for most physically active individuals unless otherwise indicated.

The use of nutritional supplements does not compensate for poor food choices and an inadequate diet[26]; however,

during prolonged high-intensity exercise, micronutrient requirements are expected to increase relative to inactive individuals.[65] Since caloric requirements also increase with exercise intensity and duration, micronutrient needs should easily be met with appropriate energy consumption, and supplementation above what is achieved through a well-balanced diet should not be necessary. However, supplementation guidelines unrelated to exercise, such as folic acid recommendations for women of childbearing potential, should be followed.[1] The most common micronutrient concerns in an athlete's diet are calcium, vitamins C, D, E, the B vitamins, iron, zinc, magnesium, beta carotene, and selenium.[1] In cases where energy intake is restricted, food groups omitted, or sun exposure is avoided, there is a greater probability for poor micronutrient status in exercising individuals.[1,26,66] In such cases, consultation with a nutrition professional should be considered to evaluate whether consumption of a multivitamin/mineral supplement is warranted.

Because of their increased energy needs, it may be challenging for highly active individuals (particularly elite athletes) to balance the recommended intakes of vitamins and minerals. That is, there may be a risk for overconsumption of micronutrients, either with food intake alone or with supplement use. The risk may be further exacerbated if one erroneously perceives that consuming "more" of a nutrient marketed to improve exercise performance is actually "better." Most micronutrients in the DRI reports have an assigned tolerable upper intake level (UL), defined as the maximum level of daily nutrient intake that is likely to pose no risk of adverse effects. The UL represents total intake from food, water, and supplements.[67] It would be prudent for exercising individuals to consider the ULs before making decisions about altering their intake of micronutrients. Further discussions concerning the nutrient needs of elite athletes and UL recommendations are available in Chapter 23 and are presented in detail elsewhere.[67,68]

Table 23.4 provides an example from the 2010 Dietary Guidelines for Americans report[8] indicating how the macronutrient- and micronutrient-focused recommendations summarized earlier can be expressed in terms of whole food serving sizes. This example outlines the number of daily servings within each food group to meet recommended nutrient intakes presented across a range of calorie levels. The exact numbers of servings in this eating plan are not intended to be consumed every day, but on average over time. Table 23.1 should serve as a tool to help identify an individual's caloric requirement based on sex, age, and PAL, which can then be applied to the recommendations presented in Table 23.4.

## TIMING OF FOODS AND FLUIDS

The timing of foods and fluids has a considerable impact on athletic performance and is a topic included in reports by national and international consensus authorities.[1,9,26] Before, during, and after exercise are key opportunities for the physically active individual to capitalize on the benefits of energy, nutrient, and fluid intakes for both performance and recovery.

Exercising in a non-fasted state, achieved by consuming foods and/or fluids before and during exercise, has frequently been shown to improve performance and should be integrated into an individual's training plan. Appropriately timed postexercise meals aid in recovery processes and replenishment of nutrients lost during exercise. Table 23.5 highlights recommendations for the timing of foods and fluids, including water and electrolytes, for optimal exercise performance.

Before exercise, the goal should be to consume sufficient fluids and carbohydrates to achieve and maintain a state of euhydration and blood glucose control. In most cases, the timing and size of meals and snacks are inversely related and depend on the intensity of the exercise and an individual's digestive tolerability. For example, smaller meals closer to exercise or competition that allow for gastric emptying are recommended, whereas with a longer duration of exercise, for example, 3–4 h, larger meals can be considered. In general, these meals should be low in fat and fiber, high in carbohydrate, and moderate in protein. Foods consumed prior to activity should also be familiar to the individual, well tolerated, and practiced in preparation for competition or sporting events. During exercise, nutrient composition goals should aim to maximize hydration by replenishing fluid losses and consume carbohydrate to help maintain blood glucose. For events or bouts lasting longer than 1 h, carbohydrates should be consumed at a rate of 30–60 g/h. Intake should ideally begin shortly after the onset of exercise since consuming carbohydrate at 15–20 min intervals for the duration of the activity has been shown to be more effective than the same bolus amount. The duration and intensity of the current, and time between the subsequent, exercise sessions will determine the timing and composition of the postexercise meal or snack. A carbohydrate intake of approximately 1.0–1.5 g/kg body weight within the first 30 min and again at 2 h intervals for 4–6 h should be adequate to replenish glycogen stores, particularly if the next exercise session is within 24 h. Protein in the postexercise meal provides amino acids for muscle protein repair and may promote a more anabolic environment for building new tissue. Individuals who have one or more rest days between intense exercise sessions do not have the same priority on timing as long as adequate carbohydrate is consumed over the course of the first 24 h postexercise.

Optimal exercise performance can occur if the rates of fluid ingestion and absorption are equal to the rate of fluid loss through sweat and urination. However, dehydration occurring from fluid imbalance, when fluid losses exceed fluid intakes, results in impaired exercise performance.[69] Whereas water deficits in excess of 2%–3% of body mass have been shown to decrease exercise performance, dehydration coupled with escalating temperatures increases the risk of potentially life-threatening heat injury. Therefore, fluid intake before, during, and after exercise is an important consideration for both overall health and peak performance. Before exercise, at least 4 h prior, individuals should consume approximately 5–7 mL/kg body weight of water or sports beverage. Depending on the environmental conditions, the activity performed, and the individual, sweat rates can range

from 0.3 to 2.4 L/h. The average sweat sodium concentration is approximately 1 g/L, with sodium being the predominant electrolyte. Potassium, magnesium, and chloride are also lost through sweat, but in smaller amounts. The primary intent of drinking fluids during exercise is to limit total water losses and prevent 2% body weight losses.

Despite the AI recommendation for total water (from foods and fluids), set at 2.7 L/day for females and 3.7 L/day for males,[6] and the idea that drinking according to thirst is adequate to achieve and maintain the hydration status of most Americans,[6,8] these recommendations will likely not compensate for additional fluid losses through the enhanced metabolic demands of exercise. Individualized drinking protocols should be assessed and practiced when possible to achieve adequate hydration throughout exercise sessions. Furthermore, the AI guidelines for water consumption were established for individuals participating in light or moderate activities in relatively mild temperatures (~20°C). For more physically active individuals who may exercise in warmer climates, fluid recommendations must be upwardly adjusted accordingly.[65,70] In higher altitudes (higher than 2500 m), diuresis and respiratory fluid losses increase base fluid recommendations up to 3–4 L/day to maintain kidney function. Since many athletes are not able to keep pace with water losses by consuming enough fluids during exercise, dehydration often occurs. After exercise, 16–24 oz of fluid for every pound of body weight lost during exercise is required for complete recovery from dehydration. Conversely, novice athletes, slow-paced runners, individuals who engage in higher-intensity endurance-type exercises (>4 h in duration) and athletes with relatively low body weight, exercising in extreme hot/cold environments, and/or who have excessive drinking behaviors (e.g., water or sports drinks), are at risk for hyponatremia.[71,72] Individuals at risk for hyponatremia should seek consultation from a qualified nutrition professional to determine their timing and recommendations for fluid intake.

## SUMMARY AND PRACTICAL APPLICATIONS

To enjoy the benefits of a physically active lifestyle, individuals should seek to consume foods and fluids that optimize both psychological and physical performance. Appropriate intakes of energy, macronutrients, micronutrients, and fluids are necessary to ensure optimal performance with exercise. If one or more nutrients associated with the production of energy are limited in the diet, physical functioning during exercise could also be limited. A key strategy to meeting nutrient needs of almost all exercising individuals is to maintain variety in the diet, that is, consume the appropriate number of servings for a given caloric requirement, such as those reported in the 2010 Dietary Guidelines for Americans. If energy intakes are appropriate for energy expenditure, the specific nutrient needs for the exercising individual should not differ considerably from leading recommendations targeted to the general population (e.g., as outlined in the DRI reports). Activities of moderate to vigorous intensity typically require additional energy, predominantly in the form of carbohydrates, and fluids in order to maintain glycogen stores and optimize physical performance. Special considerations related to vigorous activity place several nutrient recommendations for elite and/or endurance athletes above the DRI guidelines, which are most often required in proportion to individual caloric needs.

There is not sufficient scientific evidence to recommend supplementing with individual micronutrients, unless intakes from major food groups, such as fruits and vegetables, are inadequate, or if a specific micronutrient deficiency exists. For individuals on energy-restricted diets, or who are traveling or have other circumstances that interfere with achieving a balanced diet, short-term use of vitamin/mineral supplements may be necessary to improve exercise performance (and at the very least, help achieve DRI recommendations), whereas such supplements may not be as effective in well-nourished individuals. Similarly, the level of training proficiency can impact the metabolic response to nutrients with exercise, where the presence of nutrients (or supplements) in the diet may elicit more pronounced effects on physiological responses in the inexperienced versus the experienced exerciser. As supplementation with certain nutrients above the DRI may actually have a negative impact on exercise performance and overall health, consumption of megadoses of vitamins and minerals is not advised. Furthermore, supplementation with any ergogenic aid is discouraged unless the product has been evaluated for safety, efficacy, potency, and legality. Physically active individuals are encouraged to seek advice from a registered dietitian or sports nutrition specialist to provide advice with regard to food, fluid, and supplement intakes that are based on personalized nutrient needs. In athletes who practice energy restriction or who have disordered eating tendencies, these individuals should be referred to a qualified health professional for evaluation and treatment.

## ACKNOWLEDGMENTS

Sincere appreciation is expressed to Jennifer Ketterly, MS, RD, CCSD, for her clinical practice expertise in reviewing this chapter and for her valuable contribution to the section Timing of Foods and Fluids.

## REFERENCES

1. Rodriguez, NR, DiMarco, NM, Langley, S. *J Am Diet Assoc* 109:509;2009.
2. Institute of Medicine. *Dietary Reference Intakes for Calcium and Vitamin D.* The National Academies Press, Washington, DC; 2011.
3. Institute of Medicine. *Dietary Reference Intakes for Thiamin, Riboflavin, Niacin, Vitamin B6, Folate, Vitamin B12, Pantothenic Acid, Biotin, and Choline.* The National Academies Press, Washington, DC; 1998.
4. Institute of Medicine. *Dietary Reference Intakes for Vitamin C, Vitamin E, Selenium, and Carotenoids.* The National Academies Press, Washington, DC; 2000.
5. Institute of Medicine. *Dietary Reference Intakes for Vitamin A, Vitamin K, Arsenic, Boron, Chromium, Copper, Iodine, Iron, Manganese, Molybdenum, Nickel, Silicon, Vanadium, and Zinc.* The National Academies Press, Washington, DC; 2000.
6. Institute of Medicine. *Dietary Reference Intakes for Water, Potassium, Sodium, Chloride, and Sulfate.* The National Academies Press, Washington, DC; 2004.
7. Institute of Medicine. *Dietary Reference Intakes for Energy, Carbohydrate, Fiber, Fat, Fatty Acids, Cholesterol, Protein, and Amino Acids (Macronutrients).* The National Academies Press, Washington, DC; 2005.
8. U.S. Department of Agriculture and U.S. Department of Health and Human Services. *Dietary Guidelines for Americans;* 2010. http://www.cnpp.usda.gov/dietaryguidelines.htm, Accessed April 1, 2012.
9. Sawka, MN, Burke, LM, Eichner, ER et al. *Med Sci Sports Exerc* 39:377;2007.
10. Maughan, RJ, Shirreffs, SM. *Proc Nutr Soc* 71:112;2012.
11. Jeukendrup, AE. *J Sports Sci* 29:S91;2011.
12. Lundy, B. *Int J Sport Nutr Exerc Metab* 21:436;2011.
13. Stellingwerff, T, Maughan, RJ, Burke, LM. *J Sports Sci* 29:S79;2011.
14. Kechijan, D. *J Spec Oper Med* 11:12;2011.
15. Jeukendrup, A, Cronin, L. *Med Sport Sci* 56:47;2011.
16. Shirreffs, SM. *Scand J Med Sci Sports* 20:90;2010.
17. Mujika, I, Burke, LM. *Ann Nutr Metab* 57:26;2010.
18. Nemet, D, Eliakim, A. *Curr Opin Clin Nutr Metab Care* 12:304;2009.
19. Poortmans, JR, Rawson, ES, Burke, LM et al. *Br J Sports Med* 44:765;2010.
20. U.S. Department of Health & Human Services. *Physical Activity Guidelines for Americans;* 2008. http://www.health.gov/PAGuidelines/guidelines/default.aspx, Accessed April 1, 2012.
21. U.S. Department of Health & Human Services. *Healthy People 2020;* 2010. http://healthypeople.gov/, Accessed April 1, 2012.
22. Donahoo, WT, Levine, JA, Melanson, EL. *Curr Opin Clin Nutr Metab Care* 7:599;2004.
23. Nattiv, A, Loucks, AB, Manore, MM et al. *Med Sci Sports Exerc* 39:1867;2007.
24. Swinburn, B, Ravussin, E. *Am J Clin Nutr* 57:766S;1993.
25. Loucks, AB, Verdun, M, Heath, EM. *J Appl Physiol* 84:37;1998.
26. International Olympic Committee consensus statement on sports nutrition. *J Sports Sci* 29:S3;2010.
27. Melzer, K, Kayser, B, Saris, WH, Pichard, C. *Clin Nutr* 24:885;2005.
28. Beals, KA, Meyer, NL. *Clin Sports Med* 26:69;2007.
29. Otis, CL, Drinkwater, B, Johnson, M et al. *Med Sci Sports Exerc* 29:i;1997.
30. Thein-Nissenbaum, JM, Carr, KE. *Phys Ther Sport* 12:108;2011.
31. Position stand on the female athlete triad. International Olympic Committee Medical Commission Working Group on "Women in Sport;" 2005. http://www.olympic.org/medical-commission?tab=Statements, Accessed April 1, 2012.
32. Loucks, AB, Nattiv, A. *Lancet* 366:S49;2005.
33. Byrne, S, McLean, N. *J Sci Med Sport* 4:145;2001.
34. Warren, MP, Perlroth, NE. *J Endocrinol* 170:3;2001.
35. Dueck, CA, Manore, MM, Matt, KS. *Int J Sport Nutr* 6:165;1996.
36. Harber, VJ. *Exerc Sport Sci Rev* 28(1):19–23;2000.
37. Ducher, G, Turner, AI, Kukuljan, S et al. *Sports Med* 41:587;2011.

38. Zanker, CL, Cooke, CB, Truscott, JG et al. *Med Sci Sports Exerc* 36:137;2004.
39. Zello, GA. *Appl Physiol Nutr Metab* 31:74;2006.
40. Cunningham, JJ. *Am J Clin Nutr* 33:2372;1980.
41. Harris, J, Benedict, F. *A Biometric Study of Basal Metabolism in Man*. Lippincott, Philadelphia, PA; 1919.
42. Ainsworth, BE, Haskell, WL, Whitt, MC et al. *Med Sci Sports Exerc* 32:S498;2000.
43. Lemon, PW. *J Am Coll Nutr* 19:513S;2000.
44. Lemon, PW, Mullin, JP. *J Appl Physiol* 48:624;1980.
45. Coyle, EF. *Am J Clin Nutr* 61:968S;1995.
46. Casa, DJ, Armstrong, LE, Hillman, SK et al. *J Athl Train* 35:212;2000.
47. Coyle, EF, Jeukendrup, AE, Wagenmakers, AJ, Saris, WH. *Am J Physiol* 273:E268;1997.
48. Sedlock, DA. *Curr Sports Med Rep* 7:209;2008.
49. Hargreaves, M. *Nutr Rev* 54:S136;1996.
50. Backhouse, SH, Bishop, NC, Biddle, SJ, Williams, C. *Med Sci Sports Exerc* 37:1768;2005.
51. Bird, SP, Tarpenning, KM, Marino, FE. *Metabolism* 55:570;2006.
52. Roy, BD, Tarnopolsky, MA. *J Appl Physiol* 84:890;1998.
53. Nicholas, CW, Tsintzas, K, Boobis, L, Williams, C. *Med Sci Sports Exerc* 31:1280;1999.
54. Butterfield, GE. *Med Sci Sports Exerc* 19:S157;1987.
55. Lemon, PW. *Int J Sport Nutr* 8:426;1998.
56. Tipton, KD, Elliott, TA, Cree, MG et al. *Am J Physiol Endocrinol Metab* 292:E71;2007.
57. Gaine, PC, Pikosky, MA, Martin, WF et al. *Metabolism* 55:501;2006.
58. Metges, CC, Barth, CA. *J Nutr* 130:886;2000.
59. Young, VR, El-Khoury, AE, Raguso, CA et al. *J Nutr* 130:761;2000.
60. Martin, WF, Cerundolo, LH, Pikosky, MA et al. *J Am Diet Assoc* 106:587;2006.
61. Kreider, RB, Ferreira, MP, Greenwood, M et al. *J Strength Cond Res* 16:325;2002.
62. Huffman, DM, Altena, TS, Mawhinney, TP, Thomas, TR. *Eur J Appl Physiol* 92:584;2004.
63. Havemann, L, West, SJ, Goedecke, JH et al. *J Appl Physiol* 100:194;2006.
64. Burke, LM, Kiens, B. *J Appl Physiol* 100:7;2006.
65. Whiting, SJ, Barabash, WA. *Appl Physiol Nutr Metab* 31:80;2006.
66. Manore, MM. *Sports Med* 32:887;2002.
67. Barr, SI. *Appl Physiol Nutr Metab* 31:61;2006.
68. Barr, SI. *Appl Physiol Nutr Metab* 31:66;2006.
69. Noakes, TD. *Exerc Sport Sci Rev* 21:297;1993.
70. Von Duvillard, SP, Braun, WA, Markofski, M et al. *Nutrition* 20:651;2004.
71. Noakes, TD, Sharwood, K, Speedy, D et al. *Proc Natl Acad Sci U S A* 102:18550;2005.
72. Hew-Butler, T, Almond, C, Ayus, JC et al. *Clin J Sport Med* 15:208;2005.
73. Lukaski, HC. *Nutrition* 20:632;2004.
74. Chen, JD, Wang, JF, Li, KJ et al. *Am J Clin Nutr* 49:1084;1989.
75. Webster, MJ. *Eur J Appl Physiol Occup Physiol* 77:486;1998.
76. Suzuki, M, Itokawa, Y. *Metab Brain Dis* 11:95;1996.
77. Janelle, KC, Barr, SI. *J Am Diet Assoc* 95:180;1995.
78. Heath, EM, Wilcox, AR, Quinn, CM. *Med Sci Sports Exerc* 25:1018;1993.
79. Trost, S, Wilcox, A, Gillis, D. *Int J Sports Med* 18:83;1997.
80. Manore, MM. *Int J Sport Nutr* 4:89;1994.
81. Manore, MN, Leklem, JE, Walter, MC. *Am J Clin Nutr* 46:995;1987.
82. Crozier, PG, Cordain, L, Sampson, DA. *Am J Clin Nutr* 60:552;1994.
83. Montoye, HJ, Spata, PJ, Pinckney, V, Barron, L. *J Appl Physiol* 7:589;1955.
84. Tin May, T, Ma Win, M, Khin Sann, A, Mya-Tu, M. *Br J Nutr* 40:269;1978.
85. Sachan, DS, Hongu, N, Johnsen, M. *J Am Coll Nutr* 24:172;2005.
86. Spector, SA, Jackman, MR, Sabounjian, LA et al. *Med Sci Sports Exerc* 27:668;1995.
87. Deuster, PA, Singh, A, Coll, R et al. *Mil Med* 167:1020;2002.
88. Quindry, JC, Stone, WL, King, J, Broeder, CE. *Med Sci Sports Exerc* 35:1139;2003.
89. Hessel, E, Haberland, A, Muller, M et al. *Clin Chim Acta* 298:145;2000.
90. Schneider, CD, Barp, J, Ribeiro, JL et al. *Can J Appl Physiol* 30:723;2005.
91. Powers, SK, DeRuisseau, KC, Quindry, J, Hamilton, KL. *J Sports Sci* 22:81;2004.
92. Watson, TA, MacDonald-Wicks, LK, Garg, ML. *Int J Sport Nutr Exerc Metab* 15:131;2005.
93. Senturk, UK, Gunduz, F, Kuru, O et al. *J Appl Physiol* 99:1434;2005.
94. Mastaloudis, A, Traber, MG, Carstensen, K, Widrick, J. *J Med Sci Sports Exerc* 38:72;2006.
95. Davison, G, Gleeson, M. *Int J Sport Nutr Exerc Metab* 15:465;2005.
96. McAnulty, SR, McAnulty, LS, Nieman, DC et al. *J Nutr Biochem* 16:530;2005.
97. Davison, GW, Hughes, CM, Bell, RA. *Int J Sport Nutr Exerc Metab* 15:480;2005.
98. Hagobian, TA, Jacobs, KA, Subudhi, AW et al. *Med Sci Sports Exerc* 38:276;2006.

# 24 Nutrient Needs of the Elite Athlete

*Christine Rosenbloom*

## CONTENTS

## INTRODUCTION

The Merriam–Webster dictionary defines "elite" as the best of a class, and that is an apt description for athletes who compete in the professional arena or Olympic games. Athletes at the elite level often work at their sport on a full-time basis, that is, being an athlete is their job and as such they have time to train several times a day, compete with regularity, and often have support from coaches, medical staff, and sports dietitians to help them reach peak performance.

Elite athletes differ from recreational athletes in the time spent in training for sport, usually several hours each day in multiple practice sessions designed to hone their sport skills. Elite athletes usually train at high intensity in addition to long duration. Training usually includes strength and conditioning workouts, sports-specific training, practice sessions, as well as lower level competitions that help an athlete test out his or her training techniques under competitive conditions.

This chapter builds upon the previous chapter (Exercise and Nutrient Needs) by discussing macro- and micronutrient needs for elite level performance, hydration strategies, timing of nutrient intake to support training and competition, and unique needs such as training at altitude, traveling for competition, and dietary supplements purporting to improve performance.

## IMPORTANCE OF NUTRITION FOR TRAINING

In the last several decades, there has been a better understanding of how nutrition can support the adaptations that take place in all tissues in response to the stimulus of training.[1] While providing nutrition support for competition and recovery is still important, nutrition support surrounding training can help maximize changes to cells in the muscle, bone, blood, nervous system, and immune system to enable the athlete to compete under extraordinary conditions.

Carbohydrate intake has long been the nutrient of prime importance for athletes. A newer view of carbohydrate intake is to look at carbohydrate availability to support training and competition. The 2010 International Olympic Committee (IOC) Consensus Statement on Sports Nutrition advises elite athletes to begin competition with adequate stores of carbohydrate to meet their needs.[2] Burke and colleagues propose the term "carbohydrate availability" as the preferable way to discuss carbohydrate intake with athletes.[3] The rationale for this change is that carbohydrate needs for an athlete are not static but rather change based on daily or weekly training, training cycle, injury recovery, and competition. Carbohydrate intake may also need to be adjusted for athletes in skill sports (i.e., baseball) that does not have high energy demand, for smaller athletes who maintain a low body weight (i.e., gymnast), or for an athlete with large body mass who is trying to lose weight (i.e., offensive lineman in American football). Table 24.1 shows carbohydrate intake for a variety of athletes with example of ranges of carbohydrate intake for male and female athletes. As shown in Table 24.1, recommendations for carbohydrate intake are given in absolute ranges in grams per kilogram of body weight. Using percentage of carbohydrate from daily energy intake is an imprecise method for setting carbohydrate goals for elite athletes.

**TABLE 24.1**
**Carbohydrate Intake for Elite Athletes**

| Carbohydrate Intake | Carbohydrate Intake Range (g/kg) | Example for Female Athlete | Example for Male Athlete |
|---|---|---|---|
| Low-intensity or skill-based sports with light training | 3–5 | Female softball player (70 kg): 210–350 g/day | Male golfer (73 kg): 219–365 g/day |
| Athletes with large body mass and moderate training | | | |
| Athletes on energy-restricted diet plans and moderate training | | | |
| Exercise programs of moderate intensity with about 1 h of daily training | 5–7 | Female field event athlete (70 kg): 350–490 g/day | Male field event athlete (75 kg): 375–525 g/day |
| Endurance training Moderate to high intensity for 1–3 h/day | 6–10 | Female marathon runner (55 kg): 330–550 g/day | Male marathon runner (65 kg): 390–650 g/day |
| Ultra-endurance training Moderate- to high-intensity training for more than 4–5 h/day | 8–12 | Female race Across America athlete (60 kg): 480–720 g/day | Male distance cyclist (70 kg): 560–840 g/day |

## PROTEIN INTAKE

Protein intake to support training is important for both power/strength-training athletes as well as endurance athletes but for different reasons. Power and strength athletes need protein to enhance the synthesis of muscle protein while at the same time helping to attenuate muscle protein breakdown to induce muscle hypertrophy. Endurance athletes need protein to help increase mitochondrial protein that will improve oxidative capacity.[4]

The range of protein intake recommended for athletes is 1.2–1.7 g/kg/body weight and depends on several factors including age, training status (well-trained athletes such as elite athletes need less protein than an untrained or novice athlete at the early stages of training), and intensity and durance of activity, but probably the most important is energy intake. Adequate energy consumption is needed to support muscle protein synthesis, so consuming sufficient energy is critical to gaining lean mass.

For the elite athlete trying to alter body composition to increase lean mass while simultaneously decreasing body fat, an intake greater than 1.7 g/kg may be warranted. Mettler and colleagues reported on the effect of protein intake on muscle mass during weight loss in weightlifters.[5] Athletes cut 40% of their usual calorie intake, but the experimental group was given 2.3 g/protein/kg/body weight (35% of energy as protein). Both groups of athletes had the same amount of carbohydrate and calories, but the dietary fat component was manipulated to make up for the difference in protein intake. Both groups lost body fat, but the group with the higher protein intake lost very little lean mass, whereas the control group lost about 1.5 kg of muscle mass.

Perhaps even more important than total protein intake is the timing of protein intake. Resistance training leads to changes in the muscle tissue in the hours (possibly as long as 24 h) after the training stimulus.[1] Research seems to favor the post-workout period as the preferred time to eat protein to supply amino acids for protein synthesis and muscle mass accretion.[6] The amount of protein needed is not very large, about 6 g of essential amino acids or 20 g of high-quality protein (i.e., one that supplies all of the essential amino acids).[7] The IOC Consensus Statement on Sports Nutrition encourages athletes to eat foods or snacks with high-quality protein regularly throughout the day while noting that eating protein-rich foods (15–25 g) after each training session helps to maximize protein synthesis.[2]

Many athletes believe that protein is the most important nutrient for muscle gain and sports performance. However, protein must be pulled into the muscle with exercise training; it cannot be forced into muscle by overconsumption of protein. Very high protein intakes will result in the extra protein being used as a fuel with the excess nitrogen being excreted in the urine. As such, the biggest danger of a very high protein intake in athletes is the risk of dehydration as more urea production leads to more water loss through the kidney.

Fat intake is sometimes overlooked as elite athletes tend to concentrate on carbohydrate and protein intakes. Dietary fats are important to provide essential fatty acids and fat-soluble vitamins, and it is recommended that athletes not consume less than 20% of calories from fat.[8]

## SHOULD ELITE ATHLETES "TRAIN LOW AND COMPETE HIGH"?

In looking to improve training adaptations, some researchers have noticed that in training, when glycogen availability is low, some enhancements are seen including the transcription of some the genes involved in training adaptations.[9] Other effects of training "low" include better utilization of fat during exercise and less reliance on carbohydrate during exercise. Switching to a high carbohydrate intake for competition then allows the athlete to have adequate carbohydrate onboard to fuel sport. This concept has been described as "train low and compete high" and much has been written to both support and discredit the practice. Research on training low is usually conducted in a laboratory setting by having the athlete complete two exercise sessions with the second session under low-carbohydrate availability because there is insufficient time to replenish glycogen lost in the first training session. Other research protocols involve training one leg with two exercise sessions, while the other leg trains less frequently. In these studies, kicking ability of the "train low" leg is improved, but as Burke points out, no medals or awards are given for the muscle that can kick harder due to greater cell-signaling ability or enzyme content.[2] In practice, athletes train under conditions of low glycogen availability (not necessarily adhering to a low-carbohydrate diet as "train low" is frequently described in the lay press, but more likely because of an early morning training session before eating breakfast or when training a second or third time in a day), so muscle adaptation is taking place that might mimic the laboratory findings. The disadvantage of training with low-carbohydrate availability is the inability to work at high intensity for long duration, one of the hallmarks of good training for elite athletes.

## MICRONUTRIENTS AND ELITE ATHLETES

There is a very little research on micronutrient needs in elite athletes. Athletes who eat a nutrient-rich diet are unlikely to have an insufficient intake of vitamins or minerals, with the exception of vegetarian athletes who may have an increased need for nutrients that are typically found in animal foods (iron, calcium, zinc, and vitamins $B_2$, $B_{12}$, and D).[8]

In a recent review of micronutrient needs in athletes, Volpe notes that there are many research limitations in this field of study including a small number of subjects most of whom are male, differences in the type of exercise performed and varying levels of training and fitness,

lack of longitudinal data, differences in research methodology, and varying types and amounts of micronutrient supplementation.[10]

Elite athletes are aware that endurance training increases oxygen delivery to tissues leading to a need for an enhanced antioxidant system to combat free radical production. During exercise, oxygen consumption can be 10–15 times greater than during sedentary periods, leading to increased oxidative stress.[8] Athletes are also interested in the ability of antioxidant nutrients (like Vitamin C) to prevent infections. Athletes involved in contact sports come in close proximity to other athletes (and hence come in contact with their viruses or bacterial infections). A strong immune system can help fight respiratory infections. Endurance athletes complain about increased respiratory infections after a strenuous competition. A simple cold can derail an athlete's training schedule or interfere with an important competition. Do athletes need these nutrients in greater amounts compared to sedentary or recreational athletes? Some research has shown that elite athletes may need more than the recommended dietary allowance (RDA) for both vitamins E and C. Vitamin E may reduce lipid peroxidation in endurance athletes, but research is equivocal, and athletes should not exceed the tolerable upper limit for vitamin E (1000 mg or 1500 IU). Vitamin C intakes of 100–1000 mg/day are suggested for athletes who train and compete in prolonged, strenuous exercise on a regular basis.[8]

Endurance athletes, especially female athletes, need to monitor iron intake to support hemoglobin and myoglobin synthesis. While the true incidence of iron-deficiency anemia in athletes is similar to sedentary individuals (5%–6%), some reports say that as many as 60% of female athletes may have some degree of iron depletion.[11,12] Female athletes should be screened for iron deficiency and iron depletion, and appropriate dietary strategies and/or supplementation regimes should be adopted. Coaches should be cautious about routinely recommending iron supplementation for women without appropriate evaluation. Iron is a pro-oxidant, and supplementing with iron when not needed could have negative health consequences.[13]

Calcium and vitamin D are two bone-building nutrients, and the role of vitamin D in physical activity is gaining increased attention in research. Athletes should consume at least the RDA for calcium (1000–1300 mg/day, depending on age and gender). Bergeron[14] reported that exercising in the heat for long duration results in an increased calcium sweat loss, but it is not known if consuming more than the RDA for calcium is warranted for all elite athletes. Athletes should not exceed the tolerable upper limit of 2500–3000 mg of calcium per day.

Vitamin D is of interest to elite athletes because of its role in muscle function. Elite athletes who live at northern latitudes, who have dark skin pigmentation, or who train indoors are at increased risk for inadequate serum levels of vitamin D.[15,16] While little is known about the vitamin D status of most athletes, some practitioners are recommending that athletes who train or live at latitudes greater than 35° north or south should consider supplementing with vitamin D.[16] The IOC Consensus Statement on Sports Nutrition also notes that supplemental vitamin D may be needed when sun exposure is inadequate.[2]

## HYDRATION BEFORE, DURING, AND AFTER EXERCISE

Proper hydration is critical for both sports performance and good health by preventing heat illness. All athletes should drink enough fluids to minimize dehydration while not overdrinking, increasing the risk for hyponatremia. Recommendations for fluid intake suggest that 2–3 h before exercise an athlete should drink 17–20 oz of water or sport drink containing 6%–8% carbohydrate and 7–10 oz 10–20 min before exercise.[8,17] During exercise, a good hydration plan can help the elite athlete improve performance and reduce the perceived effort of exercise. Athletes are encouraged to know sweat rates and aim to not lose more than 2% of body weight during exercise. Recommendations for fluid intake during exercise should be based on temperature, humidity, sweat rates, and intensity and duration of the activity. Availability of fluids is another consideration for staying well hydrated; some sports limit access to fluids during competition. Sport drinks of 6%–8% carbohydrate are recommended when exercise is longer than 1 h.[8] After exercise, athletes are advised to drink at least 16–20 oz of fluids for every pound lost during exercise to rapidly and completely replace fluid losses. This becomes especially important for elite athletes who compete in multiple events over many days like track and field competitions or swimming heats. Sport drinks are often recommended because the sodium in the beverage encourages fluid consumption and helps the body hold on the fluid by decreasing urine output.[18]

## FOOD INTAKE BEFORE, DURING, AND AFTER EXERCISE

Carbohydrate recommendations before exercise are designed based on the assumption that individuals are eating a diet with sufficient carbohydrate to support exercise by maximizing glycogen stores and replacing glycogen after exercise. This is especially important for the elite athlete who exercises strenuously every day for more than 90 min.[8] Table 24.2 shows the recommended intake of carbohydrate before exercise at 4, 3, 2, and 1 h time frames. Athletes who have more time before an event (i.e., a soccer match played at 4 PM) can eat 4 g/carbohydrate/kg/body weight in a mixed pregame meal about noon and have plenty of time for digestion and absorption of nutrients. Athletes who have early morning competition and have less than an hour before exercise would do better with 30 g of easy to digest carbohydrate foods or fluids. Athletes are

**TABLE 24.2**
**Recommended Intake of Carbohydrate before Exercise**

| Time before Exercise | Recommended Carbohydrate Intake (g/kg) | Example for 70 kg Athlete (g) |
|---|---|---|
| <30 min | 30 | 30 |
| 1 h | 1 | 70 |
| 2 h | 2 | 140 |
| 3 h | 3 | 210 |
| 4 h | 4 | 280 |

encouraged to try fueling strategies in training to know what is tolerated and works best for him or her.

During exercise, 30–60 g of carbohydrate per hour is recommended for endurance events or high-intensity intermittent activities that last longer than an hour. Carbohydrate can be oxidized at a rate of about 1 g/min, hence the recommendation for 30–60 g/h. Consuming carbohydrate during long-duration activities can prevent fatigue, glycogen depletion, and low blood sugar. Researchers have found that carbohydrate oxidation during exercise can be increased to about 1.7 g/min by using multiple sources of carbohydrate. The gut uses different transporters to absorb carbohydrate and mixtures of glucose and fructose or glucose; fructose and sucrose allow athletes to ingest 80–90 g/carbohydrate/h without gastrointestinal upset.[19,20]

After exercise, recovery nutrition should be initiated to restore lost glycogen and provide amino acids for muscle protein synthesis. Replacing muscle and liver glycogen stores is important for recovery for elite athletes who participate in long-duration workouts of high intensity several times a day with a limited amount of time to recover before the next bout of activity. When competing in events where there is less than 6–8 h between activities, an athlete should start consuming carbohydrate immediately after the first exercise session to maximize glycogen resynthesis. One to 1.2 g of carbohydrate/kg/h for the first several hours is recommended after strenuous exercise that depletes muscle glycogen.[8] If the athlete has more time to recover (e.g., one event per day), carbohydrate can be consumed during regular meals and snacks. Many athletes choose to add protein to the recovery feedings, and there is some evidence that when carbohydrate intake is lower than recommended, the addition of protein can help to restore glycogen.[21] Protein also helps provide amino acids for muscle protein synthesis.

## SPECIAL CHALLENGES FOR ELITE ATHLETES

Elite athletes have special challenges to fueling and hydration for sport and maintaining body composition. Among these challenges are travel, competing at altitude, high heat and humidity, and food safety issues surrounding unfamiliar foods.

Elite athletes travel around the world for competition, and the venues can be in developed or developing countries.

Air travel brings with it the stress of jet lag and sleep disturbances. Crossing more than three time zones can affect athletic performance.[22] Air travel can also result in dehydration due to the relatively dry cabin air. Athletes are encouraged to increase fluid intake and minimize alcohol intake during long flights. Athletes should also plan to carry foods onboard as most airlines have limited food availability and some cross-country flights serve only limited foods for purchase. Energy or granola bars, trail mix, dried fruit, nuts, peanut butter sandwiches, and fruit-filled cookies are easy to pack, require no refrigeration, and can supplement the food served onboard the aircraft.

Food safety and water safety are of special concern to elite athletes who travel to developing countries. Athletes should be advised to avoid street food and fresh fruits and vegetables that have been washed with the local water supply. Other high-risk foods include raw or undercooked meat, poultry, fish (including raw fish served in sushi), shellfish, eggs, and unpasteurized dairy foods. Peeling fruits and vegetables can minimize risk of food-borne illness. Bottled or canned drinks are preferable to fountain drinks or tap water served with ice. Elite athletes should work with their governing bodies and a sports dietitian to develop a game plan for safe food and water when traveling.

Elite athletes may have to compete at altitude; certainly alpine skiing events or competitions held in areas of high altitude are included as special concerns for athletes. For example, the 1968 Summer Olympic Games were held in Mexico City with an altitude of 2240 m (7350 ft), considered high altitude. Energy needs are increased at high altitude due to an increase in basal metabolic rate, while at the same time, altitude depresses appetite. Butterfield noted that BMR can be increased as much as 28% at high altitude and can last for about 3 weeks.[23] Carbohydrate oxidation is increased at altitude, and because even highly trained athletes have limited carbohydrate stores in liver, muscle, and blood, carbohydrate intake is crucial for sports performance at altitude. Athletes training and competing at high altitude are encouraged to choose carbohydrate- and calorie-rich foods and fluids to help boost carbohydrate and energy intake when appetite is depressed. Fruit juice, endurance-type sport drinks, and energy-dense granola, cereal, or sport bars are recommended.

Exercising in high heat and humidity is also a challenge for elite athletes. Hydration is always important for peak performance, but in hot environmental conditions, hydration is crucial for staying healthy. Exercising while dehydrated induces physiological changes that compromise health including an increase in heart rate, decrease in stroke volume, and strain on the thermoregulatory system that can lead to an elevated core temperature.[24,25] Athletes who compete when temperatures are high usually acclimate to the conditions by training in environments that mimic heat and humidity of the event several weeks before the event. In the 1996 Centennial Olympic Games, held in the high heat and humidity of summer in Atlanta, Georgia, athletes trained throughout the

southeastern United States in the weeks leading up to the Games. Replacing both fluid and electrolyte losses is critical to performance and safety. Athletes are encouraged to develop a hydration strategy to start competition well hydrated, to drink during events in the heat, and to replace sweat losses after exercise.

## ERGOGENIC AIDS

Ergogenic means to improve the production of energy, and for athletes, that means the ability to be faster or stronger than their opponents. Ergogenic aids can be in the form of equipment (the newest driver in golf promising to give extra distance off the tee), clothing (polyurethane and neoprene speed suits for swimmers), or shoes (athletic shoes made with the lightest materials), but dietary supplements known as ergogenic aids are big business for supplement manufacturers. In the United States, dietary supplements are regulated by Dietary Supplement Health and Education Act of 1994 (DSHEA), which puts supplements in a category with less strict control than over-the-counter drugs or foods. The safety and efficacy of dietary supplements is not a function of the Food and Drug Administration (FDA), so consumers, and especially athletes, use supplements at their own risk.

Few supplements live up to the hype of advertising, and if they do work by enhancing performance, they are likely to be illegal. Elite athletes undergo drug testing, both in training and in competition, so it is imperative that they ingest no ingredient that is on the banned substance list by their governing body and the World Anti-Doping Agency (WADA). WADA publishes a comprehensive list of prohibited substances that is updated yearly in three categories: prohibited at all times, prohibited in competition, and prohibited in particular sports.[26] Unfortunately, some dietary supplements contain prohibited substances, either intentionally or by contamination. Geyer and colleagues conducted an analysis of 54 dietary supplements purchased in the United States for the IOC. They found that 15% of the supplements were contaminated with steroid and/or prohormones that could result in a positive drug test.[27] Supplements labeled as "testosterone boosters" had the highest rate of contamination, followed by "weight loss" and "muscle-building" supplements.

Athletes should ask three critical questions when considering using a supplement: Is it safe, is it effective, and is it contaminated? Unfortunately, it is not that easy to answer those questions without doing extensive investigation and not relying on the marketing and advertising provided by the maker of the supplement.

Table 24.3 shows some of the most popular ergogenic aids with a brief description of the proposed mechanism of action and the pros and cons of using the supplement. In addition to asking if the supplement is safe, effective, and legal, athletes should also consider the ethical aspects to using supplements that might enhance performance.

**TABLE 24.3**
**Popular Ergogenic Aids**

| Ergogenic Aid | Mechanism of Action | Pros | Cons |
|---|---|---|---|
| Beetroot juice | May improve skeletal muscle efficiency by lowering oxygen demand during endurance exercise | Currently used in Australia and Europe by endurance runners; limited research shows it may be effective | Contains a concentrated dose of nitrate; nitrite can be formed from dietary nitrate and combine with dietary amines to form nitrosamines that are carcinogenic; more research is needed to prove safety |
| Beta-alanine | Can increase buffering of muscle pH during high-intensity exercise | Research is equivocal, but several studies show that it can improve performance in high-intensity exercise | More research is needed to prove efficacy and safety |
| Caffeine | Works as a central nervous system stimulant allowing athlete to work harder and decrease perception of effort | Effective ergogenic aid when used in doses of 2–3 mg/kg/body weight | High doses of caffeine have adverse effects on blood pressure, heart rate, and gastrointestinal tract; caffeine in levels >15 µg/L in urine is not allowed by collegiate athletes; use of caffeine in children is not recommended |
| Creatine | Can increase stores of muscle phosphocreatine by 10%–40% in some individuals, allowing for increased training and recovery between training sessions | Safe in recommended doses of 3–5 g/day | Not recommended for children; some athletes are nonresponders to creatine supplementation |

## SUMMARY

Elite athletes have unique nutritional needs to support intense training and top level competition. Nutrition strategies to support elite athletes should be individualized and provide flexibility to cover a wide range of training needs while at the same time providing a nutrient-rich diet. Carbohydrate and protein needs will vary with training demands with the goal of maximizing carbohydrate stores and providing high-quality protein to support muscle protein synthesis and recovery. Elite athletes also have challenges not usually faced by recreational athletes including travel and exercising at extremes in altitude and temperature. Elite athletes also face media pressure and scrutiny that is far greater than is faced by a weekend warrior. Pressure to be perfect and influence from coaches or sponsors can lead to some nutritional recommendations that are not evidence based. Using the services of a registered dietitian who is board certified in sports dietetics (CSSD credential of the Commission on Dietetic Registration of the Academy of Nutrition and Dietetics) can help provide individualized nutrition support using an evidence-based approach. Table 24.4 gives some recommended websites and resources for more information on sports nutrition for elite athletes.

**TABLE 24.4**
**Resources for Nutrient Needs for Elite Athletes**

**Resources**

*Clinical Sports Nutrition*, 4th edn., McGraw Hill, Sydney, Australia, 2009
*Sports Nutrition Care Manual*® (Academy of Nutrition and Dietetics) http://sports.nutritioncaremanual.org/welcome.cfm
*Sports Nutrition: A Practice Manual for Professionals*, 5th edn., Academy of Nutrition and Dietetics, Chicago, IL, 2012

**Websites**

American College of Sports Medicine
http://www.acsm.org/

Australian Institute of Sport
http://www.ausport.gov.au/ais

IOC
http://www.olympic.org/

Professionals in Nutrition for Exercise and Sport
http://www.pinesnutrition.org/i4a/pages/index.cfm?pageid=1

Sports, Cardiovascular, and Wellness Nutrition
http://www.scandpg.org/

Sports Oracle
http://www.sportsoracle.com/

United States Olympic Committee
http://www.teamusa.org/

# REFERENCES

1. Maughan, RJ, Shirreffs, S. *Nutr Soc* 71:105;2012.
2. IOC Consensus Statement on Sports Nutrition 2012. Available at http://www.olympic.org/Documents/Reports/EN/CONSENSUS-FINAL-v8-en.pdf (Accessed March 15, 2012).
3. Burke, LM, Hawley JA, Wong SHS, Jeukendrup AE. *J Sports Sci* 29:S17;2011.
4. Burd, NA, Phillips SM. In: Rosenbloom, CA, Coleman E eds. *Sports Nutrition: A Manual for Professionals*, 5th edn., Chicago, IL, p. 36;2012.
5. Mettler S, Mitchell N, Tipton KD. *Med Sci Sports Exerc* 42:326;2010.
6. Phillips SM, Moore DR, Tang JE. *Int J Sport Nutr Exer Metab* 17:S58;2007.
7. Moore, DR, Robinson MJ, Fry JL et al. *Am J Clin Nutr* 89:161;2009.
8. Rodriguez NR, DiMarco NM, Langley S. *J Am Diet Assoc* 109:509;2009.
9. Hawley, JA, Burke LM. *Exer Sports Sci Rev* 38:152;2010.
10. Volpe SL, Bland R. In: Rosenbloom CA, Coleman E eds. *Sports Nutrition: A Manual for Practitioners*, 5th edn., Chicago, IL, pp. 75;2012.
11. Balaban EP, Cox JV, Snell PV et al. *Med Sci Sports Exerc* 21:643;1989.
12. Cowell BS, Rosenbloom CA, Skinner R, Summers SH. *J Sport Nutr Exerc Metab* 13:277;2003.
13. Rosenbloom CA. *Nutr Today* 43:258;2008.
14. Bergeron MF, Volpe SL, Gelinas Y. *Clin Chem* 44(Suppl.):A167;1998.
15. Ross AC, Manson JE, Abrams SA et al. *J Am Diet Assoc* 11:524;2011.
16. Larson-Meyer DE. *SCAN's Pulse* 29:6;20120.
17. Casa DJ, Armstrong LE, Hillman SK et al. *J Athl Train* 35:212;2000.
18. Shirreffs SM, Taylor AJ, Leiper JB, Maughan RJ. *Med Sci Sports Exerc* 281:1260;1996.
19. Currell K, Jeukendrup AE. *Med Sci Sports Exerc* 40:275;2008.
20. Jeukendrup AE. *Curr Opin Clin Nutr Metab Care* 13:452;2010.
21. Betts JA, Williams C. *Sports Med* 40:941;2010.
22. Young M, Fricker P. In: Burke L, Deakin V. *Clinical Sports Nutrition*, 3rd edn., McGraw-Hill, Sydney, Australia, p.755;2006.
23. Butterfield GE, Gates J, Fleming S et al. *J Appl Physiol* 72;1741;1992.
24. Casa DJ, Stearns RL, Lopez RM et al. *J Athl Train* 45:147;2010.
25. Murray B. In: Rosenbloom CA, Coleman E eds., *Sports Nutrition: A Manual for Practitioners*, 5th edn., Chicago, IL, p. 106;2012.
26. World Anti-Doping Agency. Available at http://www.wada-ama.org/en/ (Accessed March 12, 2012).
27. Geyer H, Parr MK, Mareck U. *Int J Sports Med* 25:124;2004.

# 25 Food and Nutrition for Space Flight

*Helen W. Lane, Sara R. Zwart, Vickie Kloeris, and Scott M. Smith*

## CONTENTS

## INTRODUCTION

The United States has had human space flight programs for over 50 years and now has a continued presence in space on the International Space Station (ISS).[1] Providing nutritious and safe food is imperative for astronauts because space travelers are totally dependent on launched food. The purpose of this chapter is to summarize the state of the United States' space food development and nutrition research and standards, including a historical perspective (Table 25.1). The European and Japanese space agencies collaborate with NASA on research and in providing foods on the U.S. launch platforms including the ISS. The Russian space agency, Roscosmos, has its own nutrition and food research and development programs and provides 50% of all foods for the ISS with 100 different foods and beverages, a significant contribution to the variety of foods available for all crew members.

Over these five decades of U.S. human space flight, the nutritional requirements and food standards have been defined and redefined, and will continuously change with more knowledge. Although much effort has been devoted to defining standards and improving food quality, the major factor limiting our ability to provide nutritious food of good quality to space travelers is the total dependence on processed foods, with no availability of frozen or refrigerated foods and limited availability of fresh foods.

The U.S. astronauts fly on the ISS for 3–6 months, allowing them to participate in months-long nutrition studies while their health is monitored before, during, and after flight. By means of an ever-increasing number of nutritional assessment tools and capabilities, a better understanding of the effect of space flight on astronaut health is achieved. As expected, some of the concerns originally documented in previous human space flight programs still remain, such as the variety of foods, and dietary iron and sodium levels along with concerns about adequate energy and fluid intakes. However, new health concerns appeared because of diligent surveillance and the increasing duration of flights. Thus, the nutrition researchers and food developers are constantly being challenged to meet the health concerns of long-duration flights. As the United States prepares to leave low Earth orbit again for ambitious flights of even longer durations, the health risks increase, and food and nutrition research and development will be the basis of the success of such missions. As part of the effort to meet these needs, NASA uses analogs of space flight to obtain more information. These analogs allow testing of procedures and research methodology on Earth.

## FOOD AND NUTRITION RISKS

NASA's Human Research Program was established in 2005 and sought to identify (1) risks to human health during space flight, (2) gaps in our understanding of the problems and how

**TABLE 25.1**

**Description of the U.S. Space Programs**

| Program Name | Years of Program | Length of Flights[a] | Total Seats per Program[b] | Type of Flight[c] |
|---|---|---|---|---|
| Mercury | 1961–1962 | 15 min–34 h | 6 | Suborbital to low Earth orbit (LEO) |
| Gemini | 1965–1966 | 4 h–4 days | 20 | LEO |
| Apollo | 1968–1972 | Total: 147–301 h; time on the Moon: 22.2–75 h | Total = 51 On the Moon = 12 | Flights to the Moon, 1/6 g for those who worked on the Moon |
| Skylab | 1973 | 28–84 days | 9 | LEO |
| Space shuttle | 1981–2011 | 2–17 days | 852[d] | LEO |
| ISS[4] increments 1–4 | 2000–2001 | 140–102 days | 12 | LEO |
| ISS increments 5–16 | 2002–2007 | 161–215 days | 35 | LEO |
| ISS increments 17–29 | 2008–2011 | 159–198 days | 72 | LEO |

[a] For ISS flights, the longest time for each increment was used. Some crew members flew significantly shorter times. For complete information see websites: http://www.nasa.gov/mission_pages/station/structure/isstodate.html and http://www.nasa.gov/mission_pages/station/expeditions/index.html (May 2012).

[b] Seats are the total number of crew members on each flight. Many crew members were on more than one flight, and on the ISS, some overlapped into the next increment. All seats were counted for this total, which included crew members who were not part of the U.S. astronaut corps.

[c] ISS is International Space Station. Assembly was considered complete in 2011, allowing more scientific studies to be done to learn more about living and working in space and test countermeasures to adverse effects of space flight.

[d] This number includes the astronauts who flew on only one part of the flight, such as to the Mir space station or to ISS, and the astronauts from the two Shuttle tragedies, Challenger (1986) and Columbia (2003).[a]

to counteract them, and (3) tasks to be conducted to help fill these gaps. Risks covered many topic areas, including food system issues and nutrition-related issues. A list of current risks, gaps, and tasks associated with nutrition and space flight can be found at http://humanresearchroadmap.nasa.gov/Risks/?i=76 (May 2012).

In general, nutritional risks increase with the duration of exposure to a closed (or semi-closed) food system and with the use of countermeasures. Understanding nutrient requirements in microgravity or partial-gravity environments and the effect of countermeasures on nutrient requirements is critical to ensure crew health and safety and mission success. Provision of these nutrients in safe amounts (neither high nor low) depends on the provision of appropriate, and palatable foods and the stability of the nutrients for the duration of the mission, actual intake of the nutrients, and the knowledge that countermeasures are not altering requirements.

Inadequate nutrition can compromise crew health, leading to loss of bone and muscle mass and strength; altered immune system function; and impaired cardiovascular performance, gastrointestinal function, endocrine function, oxidative defenses, ophthalmologic health, and psychological health and performance. Food safety is a primary concern for space missions. Beyond understanding nutritional requirements, possibilities exist that food provisions or individual nutrients can be optimized to help mitigate the negative effects of space flight on the human body.

It is critical that crew members be adequately nourished before and during missions. Critical research areas pertaining to the risk of inadequate nutrition include validation of the correct nutritional needs, assessment of the stability of nutrients during long-duration flight, correct packaging and preservation techniques, effects of countermeasures on nutrition, and use of nutrients as countermeasures.

## NUTRITIONAL REQUIREMENTS DURING THE U.S. HUMAN SPACE FLIGHT ERA

The nutritional standards for U.S. space food varied depending on the standards set by the U.S. government through the U.S. Recommended Dietary Allowances (RDAs)[2,3] or the more recent Dietary Reference Intakes (DRIs)[4–6] and the results of space nutrition research. Provided food depended on the capacity of the spacecraft—allowable mass, volume, and power to heat or cool—along with food safety, palatability, and nutritional standards.

Nutritional standards began with the Skylab flights (1973–1974) using the U.S. National Research Council publication, *Recommended Dietary Allowances*.[2] This standard remained until the NASA advisory group commissioned to evaluate the Space Nutritional Standards published a report in 1993.[7] Their recommendations were later updated to keep up with the changes in scientific knowledge, from both ground-based and space flight research, and with agreements with NASA's international partners, primarily Russia, but also including Japan, Canada, and the European Space Agency (ESA).[8,9]

Early Space Shuttle flights (which began in 1981) were short, and thus energy and fluid intakes were the major concerns.[1,10,11] Long-duration stays on the ISS required increased rigor for setting nutritional standards. Also by the time ISS human habitation began in November 2000, nutritional standards were established that reflected the changes resulting from the DRI publications as well as additional space nutrition research.[8,9]

Some notable nutrients of concern were fluid, energy, protein, electrolytes, iron, calcium, and vitamin D. The last Skylab flight and early Space Shuttle experiments confirmed that the energy requirements for astronauts in space were not different from their requirements on the ground.[11] Experiments are currently being conducted with astronauts on the longer-duration flights of the ISS to determine if, over longer periods of time, any differences in energy expenditure develop. Thus the space nutritional standards use the World Health Organization (WHO) formula with a moderate activity factor. This has worked well for food provisions for the ISS. Research on protein turnover suggests that, as on the ground, protein metabolism is related to dietary intake of energy and could be higher in space flight.[12] Yet without strong data, NASA still uses the DRI report for the level of protein for the food provisions.

Studies show that astronauts have normal renal function and endocrine controls, but because of their reduced fluid consumption, lower water turnover, and elevated mineral excretion (calcium), urine may have a high osmotic load. Increased fluid intake ameliorates much of the increase in osmotic load. The U.S. spacecraft maintain cabin temperature and humidity similar to standard room temperature. ISS astronauts may exercise 60 min/day; however, limited research suggests that without convection, there is little evaporative water loss due to sweating.[13] The dietary recommendation is 1–1.5 mL of fluid per kilocalorie of energy consumed, with a minimum of 2 L/day. The recent DRI adequate intake (AI) level is higher at 3.7 L/day from water and beverages.[6] Every effort is made to work with the vehicle engineers and astronauts to accomplish these higher fluid intakes. Fluid intakes impact availability of on-orbit water supplies because for most space vehicles, water has been a limiting resource. Engineering solutions with water recycling were established for the ISS; testing ensures potability of the drinking water. Higher consumption of fluid and other nutrients can also affect the urinary processing system.[14,15]

Beginning with the 1994 space nutritional standards, electrolytes were set at levels below the usual American dietary intakes. At that time, the NASA sodium recommendation was 1.5–3.5 g/day and potassium was 3.5 g/day. The latest U.S. AI recommendation for sodium is 1.5 g/day and for potassium, 4.7 g/day. As shown in Table 25.2, even with the standards set in the early and mid-1990s,[7–9] the space food menus did not meet these standards. Although renal function is not clinically affected, there is concern, especially with the high sodium intakes during long-term space flight, that other physiological adaptations may be harmful, especially the headward shift of fluid and potential changes in intracranial pressure.

Early in the space program, the headward fluid shifts were noted, along with a decreased plasma volume. The decrease

**TABLE 25.2**

**In-Flight Dietary Intake on Apollo, Skylab, Shuttle, and Early, Mid, and Late ISS Missions**

| | Apollo | Skylab | Shuttle | ISS (E[c]1–4) | ISS (E5–16) | ISS (E17–29) |
|---|---|---|---|---|---|---|
| *N* | 33 | 9 | 32 | 6 | 16 | 22 |
| Energy, kcal/day | 1880 ± 415[a] | 2897 ± 447 | 2090 ± 440 | 2011 ± 186 | 2350 ± 547 | 2410 ± 567 |
| Energy,% WHO | 64.2 ± 13.6 | 99.1 ± 8.2 | 74.2 ± 16.0 | 71 ± 11 | 80 ± 20 | 80 ± 18 |
| Protein intake, g/day | 76 ± 19 | 111 ± 18 | 78 ± 19 | 93 ± 19 | 101 ± 26 | 94 ± 31 |
| Protein intake, % of kcal | 16 ± 2 | 16 ± 2 | 15 ± 2 | 19 ± 3 | 17 ± 2 | 16 ± 2 |
| Carbohydrate intake, g/day | 269 ± 49 | 413 ± 59 | 304 ± 67 | | | |
| Carbohydrate intake, % of kcal | 58 ± 7 | 58 ± 9 | 58 ± 5 | | | |
| Fat intake, g/day | 61 ± 21 | 83 ± 14 | 64 ± 18 | | | |
| Fat intake, % of kcal | 29 ± 6 | 27 ± 9 | 27 ± 4 | | | |
| Calcium, mg/day | 774 ± 212 | 894 ± 142 | 826 ± 207 | 955 ± 318 | 949 ± 322 | 1054 ± 308 |
| Phosphorus, mg/day | 1122 ± 325 | 1760 ± 267 | 1216 ± 289 | | | |
| Magnesium, mg/day | | 310 ± 58 | 294 ± 74 | | | |
| Iron, mg/day | | | 15 ± 4 | 19 ± 3 | 23 ± 11 | 19 ± 6 |
| Zinc, mg/day | | | 12 ± 3 | | | |
| Sodium, mg/day | 3666 ± 890 | 5185 ± 948 | 3984 ± 853 | 4252 ± 580 | 4593 ± 1342 | 4415 ± 1461 |
| Potassium, mg/day | 2039 ± 673 | 3854 ± 567 | 2391 ± 565 | | 3164 ± 535 | 3223 ± 877 |
| Water, g/day | 1647 ± 188[b] | 2829 ± 529 | 2223 ± 669 | 1994 ± 391 | 2082 ± 473 | 2085 ± 402 |

*Sources:* Adapted from Alfrey, C.P. et al., *Lancet*, 349, 1389, 1997; Alfrey, C.P. et al., *J. Appl. Physiol.*, 81, 98, 1996; Smith, S.M. et al., *Nutritional Biochemistry of Space Flight*, Nova Science Publishers, Hauppauge, NY, 2009.

[a] All data are mean ± SD. Empty cells show where data were not available.

[b] *n* = 3 for water intake during Apollo missions.

[c] E, Expedition number; ISS data are grouped by early, mid, and more recent missions.

in plasma volume caused the blood to be more concentrated, and experiments on the Space Shuttle[16,17] showed that nascent blood cells were removed from the circulation over the following 10–14 days, until the reduction in blood cells matched the reduction in plasma volume. These events resulted in a reduced circulatory volume, but normal content of most blood constituents. Knowledge of these changes led to research to determine the cause and how these changes affected nutrients such as iron associated with red blood cells. With the first review of space nutritional recommendations in 1991,[8] the recommended dietary iron intake was set at 10 mg/day for men and women astronauts. With additional research on the role of iron and radiation-induced oxidation, this level may be reevaluated, as has happened with the U.S. dietary recommendations. Low iron storage may be an advantage in long-duration space flight.[18]

Skylab researchers completed calcium studies including traditional metabolic balance studies.[19–21] During Space Shuttle flights, calcium balance was determined by subtracting urinary losses from intake along with the use of stable isotopes and markers of bone metabolism.[22,23] Studies on the Russian space station Mir and the ISS provide a better understanding of the effects of long-duration space flight on bone metabolism. In all of these studies, urinary calcium levels increased with microgravity, yet for the Skylab astronauts, the dietary calcium level was about 730 mg/day and most were in calcium balance. For ISS crews,[18] the recommended calcium intake is 1000–1200 mg/day. Although increasing dietary calcium intake alone will not mitigate bone loss, maintaining intake is important nonetheless.

## SPACE FOODS AND SPACE FLIGHT MENUS

Early U.S. space food was very basic.[24,25] The tubes of pureed foods and starch-coated cubes of food are perhaps the best-known items of space food and were engineered to minimize mass and volume. They provided the necessary nutrition but were not very aesthetically pleasing. The food system evolved as the space program evolved (Table 25.3).

The introduction of the spoonbowl package during the Apollo program allowed the addition of utensils to the space dining experience. In addition, thermostabilized foods (cans and pouches) and irradiated foods debuted during Apollo[21,24] (Table 25.4). The Skylab food system in 1973–1974 was the only U.S. space food system to use frozen and refrigerated foods. The Shuttle era, which began in 1981, returned to an all-shelf-stable food system (Table 25.5), an expanded version of which is utilized today on the ISS (Table 25.6). A more detailed

## TABLE 25.3
## Summary of Food and Package Types for U.S. Space Foods

| | Gemini | Late Apollo | Skylab | Shuttle | ISS[a] |
|---|---|---|---|---|---|
| Longest mission duration (days) | 14 | 12 | 84 | 17 | 215 |
| Crew size | 2 | 3 | 3 | Up to 8 | Up to 6 |
| Food warming capabilities (Y/N) | N | N | Y | Y | Y |
| Menu cycle | 4 | 4 | 6 | Up to 16[b] | 8[c] |
| Refrigerator/freezer | | | X | | |
| Food list (number of food and beverage items) | 55 | 90 | 72 | 150 | 206 |
| Food package types | | | | | |
|   Aluminum tubes | X | X | | | |
|   Aluminum cans | X | X | X | X | X |
|   Plastic pouches | X | X | X | X | X |
|   Retort pouches | | X | | X | X |
| Food types | | | | | |
|   Freeze-dried/dehydrated | X | X | X | X | X |
|   Intermediate moisture | X | X | X | X | X |
|   Thermostabilized | | X | X | X | X |
|   Natural form | | X | X | X | X |
|   Irradiated | | X | | X | X |
|   Frozen | | | X | | |
|   Refrigerated or drink chiller[d] | | | X | | X |

[a] International Space Station is still an active program; values recorded here are as of March 2012.

[b] Except on the earliest missions, Shuttle menus were personal preference and thus crew members determined the length of the menu cycle.

[c] This 8 day cycle is for U.S. food only. In instances where the ISS crews share the Russian and U.S. foods, this cycle would be extended for 16 days.

[d] No refrigerated foods have been part of U.S. space food systems with the exception of Skylab. However, a chiller was and is available for chilling beverages for ISS.

**TABLE 25.4**

**Lunar Menu (Apollo Program)**

| Meal | Menu for Day 1 | Food Type | Menu for Day 2 | Food Type |
|------|---------------|-----------|----------------|-----------|
| A | Applesauce | R | Bacon squares | B |
| | Sausage patties | R | Ham and applesauce | R |
| | Apricot cereal cubes | B | Cinnamon-toasted bread cubes | B |
| | Coconut cubes | B | Peanut cubes | B |
| | Cocoa | D | Grapefruit drink (fortified) | D |
| B | Pea soup | R | Potato soup | R |
| | Salmon salad | R | Chicken salad | R |
| | Cheese sandwiches | B | Butterscotch pudding | R |
| | Pineapple fruitcake | B | Sugar-cookie cubes | D |
| | Grapefruit drink (fortified) | D | Pineapple–grapefruit drink | D |
| C | Beef and gravy | R | Corn chowder | R |
| | Potato salad | R | Beef sandwiches | B |
| | Chocolate pudding | R | Cinnamon-toasted bread cubes | B |
| | Brownies | B | Date fruitcake | B |
| | Orange–grapefruit drink | D | Cocoa | D |

[a] B, bite-size; D, beverage powder; R, rehydratable.

discussion of the history of space food is available in the book *Nutritional Biochemistry of Space Flight*.[18]

The current ISS food system uses several types of foods and food-processing technologies to achieve shelf stability. Thermostabilized foods make up about 35% of the U.S. ISS food list, and in all but a very few cases, these products have been processed in retort pouches rather than in cans. The pouches have substantially less weight than cans and are much more efficient to stow in containers, providing two significant advantages for launching food into space. Rehydratable foods represent 24% of the food system. These are foods that require a crew member to add water before consuming them and are packaged in custom packages that facilitate the addition of water on orbit using a rehydration station. Almost all of these are freeze-dried foods, although a few are natural-form cereals packaged with nonfat dry milk. Beverages make up 25% of the food system. All are in powdered form, requiring the addition of hot or cold water, and also having custom packaging to enable the water to be added. Natural-form products (9%) are commercial off-the-shelf foods that fly without further processing, other than repackaging. These include items such as cookies, crackers, nuts, and candies. Irradiated meat products in pouches constitute about 4% of the food list, whereas intermediate-moisture products such as dried fruit are about 2% of the foods. There are currently 206 U.S. space foods and beverages (Table 25.7). Fresh foods, such as apples and citrus fruits, are currently available in very limited quantities after the docking of each Russian-resupply Progress vehicle and crewed Soyuz vehicle.

ISS crew members are involved in the food-selection process to a limited degree. Unlike the Shuttle program, which after the first few flights used 100% personal-preference menus (Table 25.5), the ISS food system has a standard menu that currently repeats every 8 days (Table 25.6). The standard menu was developed when, after several years of ISS expeditions, it became apparent that resupply logistics forced ISS crew members to consume the menu chosen by other crew members during a portion of their stay on the ISS. This was deemed unacceptable by most crew members. The implementation of a generic standard menu that includes all of the U.S. food items provides maximum variety and has been well accepted. Crew members augment the standard menu with a small volume per month of personal-preference foods, called "bonus foods" (Table 25.8). Bonus foods can be additional standard space food items, or they can include commercial food items that have sufficient shelf life and meet microbiological requirements. Table 25.8 gives examples of commercial food types that have been requested by crew members and flown in ISS bonus containers.

## FOOD SAFETY STANDARDS

Food safety has always been the primary focus of the NASA food system. In the 1960s, a joint effort of the Pillsbury Company, NASA, and the U.S. Army Natick Labs (the research lab for military feeding systems) resulted in the development of the Hazard Analysis and Critical Control Point (HACCP) system for food safety. This system emphasizes process control over end product and destructive testing as a means to ensure the safety of the finished food product. HACCP was gradually adopted by the U.S. food industry, with widespread use beginning in the late 1970s, and is mandated by law for certain food facilities such as food plants and restaurants and, in some cases, even school food facilities. HACCP is now internationally recognized as the premier food safety system.

NASA continues to use HACCP as the primary means to ensure food safety for those space foods manufactured in-house at NASA. NASA does augment HACCP with some

**TABLE 25.5**
**Sample Shuttle Menu**

| Breakfast | Lunch | Dinner |
|---|---|---|
| **Day 1** | | |
| Dried apricots (IM) | Mushroom soup (R) | Beef stroganoff w/noodles (R) |
| Oatmeal w/brown sugar (R) | Macaroni and cheese (R) | Rice pilaf (R) |
| Raspberry yogurt (T) | Tuna salad spread (T) | Corn (R) |
| Granola bar (NF) | Tortillas (FF) | Vanilla pudding (T) |
| Orange–grapefruit drink (B) | Pears (T) | Dried pears (IM) |
| Chocolate breakfast drink (B) | Cashews (NF) | Orange–mango drink (B) × 2 |
| | Candy-coated peanuts (NF) | |
| | Orange drink w/A/S (B) × 2 | |
| **Day 2** | | |
| Dried pears (IM) | Mushroom soup (R) | Beef steak (I) |
| Oatmeal w/raisins (R) | Spaghetti w/meat sauce (R) | Macaroni and cheese (R) |
| Sausage pattie (R) | Crackers (NF) × 2 | Asparagus (R) |
| Granola bar (NF) | Cheddar cheese spread (T) | Tapioca pudding (T) |
| Orange–grapefruit drink (B) | Bread pudding (T) | Dried peaches (IM) |
| Cocoa (B) | Cashews (NF) | Orange–pineapple drink (B) × 2 |
| | Lemonade w/A/S (B) × 2 | |
| **Day 3** | | |
| Dried apricots (IM) | Mushroom soup (R) | Beef tips w/mushrooms (I) |
| Oatmeal w/brown sugar (R) | Chicken salad (R) | Mashed potatoes (R) |
| Raspberry yogurt (T) | Macaroni and cheese (R) | Italian vegetables (R) |
| Granola bar (NF) | Tortillas (FF) | Dried pears (IM) |
| Orange–grapefruit drink (B) | Pears (T) | Vanilla pudding (T) |
| Chocolate breakfast drink (B) | Cashews (NF) | Orange–grapefruit drink (B) × 2 |
| | Candy-coated peanuts (NF) | |
| | Orange drink w/A/S (B) × 2 | |
| **Day 4** | | |
| Dried pears (IM) | Mushroom soup (R) | Grilled pork chop (T) |
| Oatmeal w/raisins (R) | Spaghetti w/meat sauce (R) | Macaroni and cheese (R) |
| Sausage pattie (R) | Crackers (NF) × 2 | Candied yams (T) |
| Granola bar (NF) | Cheddar cheese spread (T) | Tapioca pudding (T) |
| Orange–grapefruit drink (B) | Pears (T) | Dried peaches (IM) |
| Cocoa (B) | Cashews (NF) | Orange–pineapple drink (B) × 2 |
| | Lemonade w/A/S (B) × 2 | |
| **Day 5** | | |
| Dried apricots (IM) | Mushroom soup (R) | Beef stroganoff w/noodles (R) |
| Oatmeal w/brown sugar (R) | Macaroni and cheese (R) | Rice pilaf (R) |
| Raspberry yogurt (T) | Tuna salad spread (T) | Corn (R) |
| Granola bar (NF) | Tortillas (FF) | Vanilla pudding (T) |
| Orange–grapefruit drink (B) | Pears (T) | Dried pears (IM) |
| Chocolate breakfast drink (B) | Cashews (NF) | Orange–mango drink (B) × 2 |
| | Candy-coated peanuts (NF) | |
| | Orange drink w/A/S (B) × 2 | |
| **Day 6** | | |
| Dried pears (IM) | Mushroom soup (R) | Beef steak (I) |
| Oatmeal w/raisins (R) | Spaghetti w/meat sauce (R) | Macaroni and cheese (R) |
| Sausage pattie (R) | Crackers (NF) × 2 | Asparagus (R) |
| Granola bar (NF) | Cheddar cheese spread (T) | Tapioca pudding (T) |
| Orange–grapefruit drink (B) | Bread pudding (T) | Dried peaches (IM) |
| Cocoa (B) | Cashews (NF) | Orange–pineapple drink (B) × 2 |
| | Lemonade w/A/S (B) × 2 | |

**TABLE 25.5 (continued)**
**Sample Shuttle Menu**

| Breakfast | Lunch | Dinner |
|---|---|---|
| **Day 7** | | |
| Dried apricots (IM) | Mushroom soup (R) | Beef tips w/mushrooms (I) |
| Oatmeal w/brown sugar (R) | Chicken salad (R) | Mashed potatoes (R) |
| Raspberry yogurt (T) | Macaroni and cheese (R) | Italian vegetables (R) |
| Granola bar (NF) | Tortillas (FF) | Dried pears (IM) |
| Orange–grapefruit drink (B) | Pears (T) | Vanilla pudding (T) |
| Chocolate breakfast | Cashews (NF) | Orange–grapefruit drink (B) × 2 |
| Drink (B) | Candy-coated peanuts (NF) | |
| | Orange drink w/A/S (B) ×2 | |
| **Day 8** | | |
| Dried pears (IM) | Mushroom soup (R) | Grilled pork chop (T) |
| Oatmeal w/raisins (R) | Spaghetti w/meat sauce (R) | Macaroni and cheese (R) |
| Sausage pattie (R) | Crackers (NF) × 2 | Candied yams (T) |
| Granola bar (NF) | Cheddar cheese spread (T) | Tapioca pudding (T) |
| Orange–grapefruit drink (B) | Pears (T) | Dried peaches (IM) |
| Cocoa (B) | Cashews (NF) | Orange–pineapple drink (B) × 2 |
| | Lemonade w/A/S (B) × 2 | |
| **Day 9** | | |
| Dried apricots (IM) | Mushroom soup (R) | Beef stroganoff w/noodles (R) |
| Oatmeal w/brown sugar (R) | Macaroni and cheese (R) | Rice pilaf (R) |
| Raspberry yogurt (T) | Tuna salad spread (T) | Corn (R) |
| Granola bar (NF) | Tortillas (FF) | Vanilla pudding (T) |
| Orange–grapefruit drink (B) | Pears (T) | Dried pears (IM) |
| Chocolate breakfast drink (B) | Cashews (NF) | Orange–mango drink (B) × 2 |
| | Candy-coated peanuts (NF) | |
| | Orange drink w/A/S (B) × 2 | |

A/S, artificial sweetener; B, beverage; FF, fresh food; I, irradiated; IM, intermediate moisture; NF, natural form; R, rehydratable; T, thermostabilized.

endpoint microbiological testing of food products. Some of NASA's microbiological standards are more restrictive than typical U.S. commercial food microbiological standards. Table 25.9 shows the current microbiological standards for U.S. space food.[24]

## FOOD PREPARATION METHODS

Food preparation on orbit is very limited in scope. The earliest space food systems had no food preparation, as tube foods and cubed foods were ready to eat and were squeezed or popped into the mouth after opening. A hand-held rehydration gun was added during Apollo program to allow the addition of water to the rehydratable food items packaged in the spoonbowl. Skylab introduced a dining table (pedestal) that allowed the three crew members to "sit" and dine. The pedestal included the food tray that doubled as the warmer for the foods, including frozen foods. After the first few Shuttle flights, Shuttle orbiters had a galley for food preparation, which consisted of a rehydration station that dispensed hot and chilled water and an oven for warming pouched foods and keeping rehydrated foods warm during the rehydration

process. The ISS now has two food preparation areas or galleys, one in the Russian service module (SM) and one in the U.S. Laboratory module. Unlike in the Shuttle galley, the ISS galley has no chilled water for rehydration, but only for heated and ambient water. A chiller for beverages was added in 2009. The food preparation area in the SM consists of a rehydration station and a table. Built into the table are warmers sized to fit the Russian canned food items. As no method for warming U.S. pouches was available in the SM, NASA modified the suitcase food warmer design that had been used on pre-galley Shuttle flights to make it compatible with ISS power systems. A suitcase food warmer is located in the SM and in the U.S. segment for the warming of U.S. pouched food products. The galley in the U.S. segment was added when the ISS crew size expanded from three to six. This food preparation area has a rehydration station for adding water to foods and beverages, and one of the suitcase food warmers for heating pouched foods. In addition, this galley includes a very small chiller that has the internal volume of a typical home microwave. This chiller allows the crew members to chill beverages before consuming them and has helped to compensate for the lack of chilled water aboard the ISS.

**TABLE 25.6**
**Standard Menu for the ISS**

**Day 1**

Nut and fruit granola bar (NF)/yogurt-
  covered granola bar (NF)

Blueberry–raspberry yogurt (T)

Dried peaches (NF)

Pineapple drink (B)

Minestrone soup (T)

BBQ brisket (I)

Cornbread dressing (R)

Cauliflower w/cheese (R)

Apricot cobbler (T)/lemon curd cake (T)

Chicken w/corn and black beans (T)/chicken
  w/peanut sauce (T)

Potatoes au gratin (R)

Rhubarb applesauce (T)

Butter cookies (NF)

Orange–mango drink (B)

Macadamia nuts (NF)

Butterscotch pudding (T)/banana pudding (T)

Lemonade w/A/S (B)

**Day 3**

Seasoned scrambled eggs (R)

Oatmeal w/brown sugar (R)

Peaches (T)

Orange juice (B)

Vegetarian vegetable soup (T)

Smoked turkey (I)

Baked beans (T)

Macaroni and cheese (R)

Candy-coated peanuts (NF)

Beef steak (I)/meatloaf (T)

Potato medley (T)/pasta w/pesto (T)

Green beans w/mushrooms (R)

Bread pudding (T)

Orange drink w/A/S (B)

Almonds (NF)/cashews (NF)

Dried pears (IM)/dried apricots (IM)

Apple cider (B)

**Day 5**

Granola bar (NF)

Oatmeal w/raisins and spice (R)

Blueberry–raspberry yogurt (T)

Pineapple (T)

Orange–grapefruit drink (B)

Tomato basil soup (T)

BBQ brisket (I)

Teriyaki vegetables (R)

Pasta w/shrimp (R)/shrimp fried rice (R)

Cherry blueberry cobbler (T)

Shrimp cocktail (R)

Tofu w/hoisin (T)/tofu w/hot mustard (T)

Brown rice (T)/rice w/butter (T)

Mixed vegetables (T)

Lemon meringue pudding (T)

Apple cider (B)

Tuna (T)/salmon (T)

Tortillas (NF)

Grape drink (B)

**Day 2**

Breakfast sausage links (I)

Grits w/butter (R)/cheese grits (T)

Waffle (NF)

Vanilla breakfast drink (B)

Hot and sour soup (T)

Grilled chicken (T)/teriyaki chicken (R)

Tomatoes and eggplant (T)

Pears (T)

Chipotle snack bread (NF)

Rice pudding (R)

Chicken strips in salsa (T)

Corn (R)

Strawberries (R)

Vanilla pudding (T)

Tropical punch (B)

Chicken in pouches (T)

Crackers (NF)

Lemonade (B)

**Day 4**

Scrambled eggs (R)

Oat cereal (R)/cornflakes (R)

Apples w/spice (T)

Pineapple drink (B)

Beef stew (T)/beef tips w/mushrooms (I)

Rice pilaf (R)/wild rice salad (R)

Tomatoes and artichokes (R)

Wheat flat bread (NF)

Brownie (NF)

Crawfish etouffee (T)/seafood gumbo (T)

Candied yams (T)/carrot coins (T)

Strawberries (R)

Shortbread cookies (NF)

Cranberry peach drink w/A/S (B)

Cheddar cheese spread (T)

Tortillas (NF)

Mango–peach smoothie (B)

**Day 6**

Mexican scrambled eggs (R)

Granola w/blueberries (R)/granola w/raisins (R)

Chocolate breakfast drink (B)

Orange–pineapple drink (B)

Cream of mushroom soup (R)/Chicken noodle soup (T)

Turkey tetrazzini (R)/Caribbean chicken (R)

Broccoli au gratin (R)

Curry w/vegetables (T)

Applesauce (T)

Lasagna w/meat (T)/fiesta chicken (T)

Italian vegetables (R)/asparagus (R)

Strawberries (R)

Candy-coated chocolates (NF)

Milk (B)

Chicken–pineapple salad (R)

Crackers (NF)

Peach–apricot drink (B)

**TABLE 25.6 (continued)**
**Standard Menu for the ISS**

**Day 7**

Sausage pattie (R)
Homestyle potatoes (T)
Maple top muffin (NF)
Trail mix (IM)
Grapefruit drink (B)
Split pea soup (T)/potato soup (T)
Grilled pork chop (T)
Spicy green beans (R)
Southwestern corn (T)
Chocolate pudding cake (T)
Chicken fajitas (T)/beef fajitas (I)
Red beans and rice (T)/black beans (T)
Tortillas (NF)
Fruit cocktail (T)/citrus fruit salad (T)
Chocolate pudding (T)
Grape drink w/A/S (B)
Peanut butter (T)
Grape jelly (T)/apple jelly (T)
Crackers (NF)
Cocoa (B)

**Day 8**

Vegetable quiche (R)
Granola (R)/multigrain cheerios (R)
Tropical fruit salad (T)
Orange drink (B)
Minestrone soup (T)
Cashew curried chicken (R)
Mashed potatoes (R)
Creamed spinach (R)
Cranapple dessert (T)
Sweet and sour chicken (R)/sweet and sour pork (T)
Teriyaki vegetables (R)
Rice and chicken (R)/noodles and chicken (R)
Candy-coated almonds (NF)
Tropical punch w/A/S (B)
Tuna salad spread (T)
Crackers (NF)
Lemon–lime drink (B)

A/S, artificial sweetener; B, beverage; FF, fresh food; I, irradiated; IM, intermediate moisture; NF, natural form; R, rehydratable; T, thermostabilized.

## IMPACT OF INTERNATIONAL CREW MEMBERS ON FOOD AND NUTRITION

The original food system on the ISS was 50% U.S.-provided foods and 50% Russian-provided foods, as the United States and Russia were the only countries that possessed established space food systems. Today, Russia continues to supply 50% of the food for the six ISS crew members. The remaining 50% is considered the U.S. Operational Segment food system, which can now include food from other International Partners. Foods from other International Partners (Japan, Canada, and the European countries) appeared initially only as bonus foods. As the ISS matured and international crew members from Europe and Japan began to make regular visits to the space station, the ESA and the Japanese Space Agency (JAXA) began to work to establish some of their own space foods.

Currently, ESA has about 20 different space foods produced by commercial food companies and is working with companies to develop more. ESA space foods are shipped to the United States and, upon request, are incorporated into ISS crew member bonus food containers before launch to the ISS. ESA foods are most likely to be on the ISS when an ESA crew member is on board, as that crew member will choose predominately ESA foods for his or her bonus containers.

JAXA has worked with Japanese food companies to establish about 25 space foods. Initially, these JAXA space foods were shipped to the United States as well, but now that JAXA is launching the H II Transfer Vehicle (HTV) from Japan, their space foods are packed in Japan and launched on the HTV. JAXA also packs bonus foods on the HTV; these include a variety of Japanese commercial foods. JAXA foods are available only during ISS increments when a JAXA crew member is on board. Although it has not yet established a Canadian space food system, the Canadian Space Agency (CSA) has identified a variety of commercial Canadian food items that have flown as bonus foods during increments when CSA crew members were on board.

Bonus foods selected by crew members during the 30 ISS increments flown thus far have included commercial foods from additional countries as well. Though foods from countries other than Russia and United States still represent a small percentage of the total ISS food system, the additional variety supplied by these international foods is extremely welcomed by the crew members on board the ISS. Table 25.10 lists the ESA and JAXA standard space foods.

## ADAPTING SPACE FOODS FOR CHANGES IN MISSION REQUIREMENTS

Throughout the history of the U.S. space food system, there have been numerous examples of the food system having to adapt to changing space mission requirements and

**TABLE 25.7**
**Current U.S. Food List for ISS**

**Entrees**

Chicken strips w/salsa (T)
Chicken teriyaki (I)
Chicken w/corn and black beans (T)
Chicken w/peanut sauce (T)
Chicken teriyaki (I)
Chicken w/corn and black beans (T)
Chicken w/peanut sauce (T)
Crawfish etouffee (T)
Curry sauce w/vegetables (T)
Fiesta chicken (T)
Grilled chicken (T)
Grilled pork chop (T)
Lasagna w/meat (T)
Meatloaf (T)
Mexican scrambled eggs (R)
Pasta with shrimp (R)
Salmon (T)
Sausage pattie (R)
Scrambled eggs (R)
Seafood gumbo (T)
Seasoned scrambled eggs (R)
Shrimp cocktail (R)
Shrimp fried rice (R)
Smoked turkey (I)
Spaghetti w/meat sauce (R)
Sweet and sour chicken (R)
Sweet and sour pork (T)
Teriyaki beef steak (I)
Teriyaki chicken (R)
Tofu w/hoisin sauce (T)
Tofu w/hot mustard sauce (T)
Tuna (T)
Tuna noodle casserole (T)
Tuna salad spread (T)
Turkey tetrazzini (R)
Vegetable quiche (R)
Vegetarian chili (R)

**Breads**

Chipotle snack bread (NF)
Tortilla (NF)
Maple top muffin (NF)
Waffle (NF)
Wheat flat bread (NF)

**Cereals**

Oat cereal (R)
Cheese grits (T)
Cornflakes (R)
Granola (R)
Granola w/blueberries (R)
Granola w/raisins (R)
Grits w/butter (R)
Multigrain cheerios (R)
Oatmeal w/brown sugar (R)
Oatmeal w/raisins (R)

**Fruits**

Applesauce (T)
Apples with spice (T)
Berry medley (R)
Citrus fruit salad (T)
Dried apricots (IM)
Dried peaches (IM)
Dried pears (IM)
Fruit cocktail (T)
Peach ambrosia (R)
Peaches (T)
Pears (T)
Pineapple (T)
Rhubarb applesauce (T)
Strawberries (R)
Tropical fruit salad (T)

**Soups**

Beef stew (T)
Chicken noodle (T)
Lentil soup (T)
Minestrone (T)
Cream of mushroom (R)
Potato (T)
Tomato basil (T)
Split pea (T)
Vegetarian vegetable (T)

**Beverages**

Apple cider
Breakfast drink, chocolate
Breakfast drink, strawberry
Breakfast drink, vanilla
Chicken consommé (B)
Cocoa
Cranberry peach drink w/A/S
Decaf coffee, black
Decaf coffee w/A/S
Decaf coffee w/cream
Decaf coffee w/cream and A/S
Decaf coffee w/cream and sugar
Decaf coffee w/sugar
Grape drink
Grape drink w/A/S
Grapefruit drink
Green tea
Green tea w/sugar
Hint of lemon
Hint of lime
Hint of orange
Kona coffee, black
Kona coffee, w/A/S
Kona coffee w/cream
Kona coffee w/cream and A/S
Kona coffee w/cream and sugar
Kona coffee w/sugar
Lemonade

## TABLE 25.7 (continued)
## Current U.S. Food List for ISS

**Starches**

Baked beans (T)
Black beans (T)
Brown rice (T)
Candied yams (T)
Corn (R)
Cornbread dressing (R)
Homestyle potatoes (T)
Macaroni and cheese (R)
Mashed potatoes (R)
Noodles and chicken (R)
Pasta w/pesto sauce (T)
Potatoes au gratin (R)
Potato medley (T)
Red beans and rice (T)
Rice and chicken (R)
Rice pilaf (R)
Rice w/butter (T)
Southwestern corn (T)

**Beverages**

Lemonade w/A/S
Lemon–lime drink
Mango–peach smoothie
Milk
Orange drink
Orange drink w/A/S
Orange–grapefruit drink
Orange juice
Orange–mango drink
Orange–pineapple drink
Peach–apricot drink
Pineapple drink
Raspberry lemonade w/A/S
Strawberry drink
Tea, plain
Tea w/A/S
Tea w/cream
Tea w/cream and sugar

**Vegetables**

Asparagus (R)
Broccoli au gratin (R)
Carrot coins (T)
Cauliflower w/cheese (R)
Creamed spinach (R)
Green beans w/mushrooms (R)
Green beans and potatoes (T)
Italian vegetables (R)
Mixed vegetables (T)
Spicy green beans (R)
Teriyaki vegetables (R)
Tomatoes and artichokes (R)
Tomatoes and eggplant (T)

**Yogurt**

Blueberry–raspberry yogurt (T)
Mocha yogurt (T)

**Snacks and Sweets**

Almonds (NF)
Apple jelly (T)
Apricot cobbler (T)
Banana pudding (T)
Bread pudding (T)
Brownie (NF)
Almonds (NF)
Apple jelly (T)
Apricot cobbler (T)
Banana pudding (T)
Bread pudding (T)
Brownie (NF)
Butter cookies (NF)
Butterscotch pudding (T)
Candy-coated almonds (NF)
Candy-coated chocolates (NF)
Candy-coated peanuts (NF)
Cashews (NF)
Cheddar cheese spread (T)
Cherry blueberry cobbler (T)
Chocolate pudding (T)
Chocolate pudding cake (T)
Crackers (NF)
Cranapple dessert (T)
Dried beef (IM)
Granola bar (NF)
Grape jelly (T)
Lemon curd cake (T)
Lemon meringue pudding (T)
Macadamia nuts (NF)
Nut and fruit granola bar (NF)
Peanut butter (T)
Peanuts (NF)
Rice pudding (R)

*(continued)*

## TABLE 25.7 (continued)
## Current U.S. Food List for ISS

**Snacks and Sweets**
Shortbread cookies (NF)
Trail mix (IM)
Vanilla pudding (T)
Yogurt-covered granola bar (NF)

A/S, artificial sweetener; B, beverage; FF, fresh food; I, irradiated; IM, intermediate moisture; NF, natural form; R, rehydratable; T, thermostabilized.

## TABLE 25.8
## Examples of Commercial Bonus Foods

**Sweets and Snacks**

Almonds
Assorted Russian chocolate candy
Assorted U.S. chocolate candy
Bean dip
Beef jerky
Beef jerky, teriyaki
Chips, commercial in cans/tubes
Cookies, assorted U.S. commercial
Crackers, assorted U.S. commercial
Dark covered espresso beans
Fruit roll-ups and fruit chews
Glazed walnuts
Gummy candy
Hazelnuts
Honey cashews
Honey peanuts
Jelly beans
Licorice
Mixed nuts
Roasted pistachios
Sesame sticks
Sour lemon drops
Variety of trail mix (commercial)
Walnuts
Wasabi green peas

**Beverages (All Packaged in ISS Beverage Package to Allow for Addition of Water on Orbit)**
Cappuccino, instant
Espresso, instant
International coffees, variety of commercial instant
Latte, instant
Powdered beverages, variety of commercial
teas, variety of commercial

**Fruits and Vegetables**

Canned fruit, mixed
Canned fruit, tropical
Dried cranberries
Dried mangoes
Dried mixed berries
Mandarin oranges, canned
Mixed jumbo raisins
Pineapple chunks, canned
Pitted dates
Red grapefruit sections, canned

**Entrees, Sides, and Soups**
Anchovies
Albacore steak, variety of flavors in pouches
Brie cheese
Calabrese sausage
Chicken (pouch)
Chopped clams
Cooked rice, pouch
Crab meat, canned
Dried squid
Flat fillets of anchovies
Indian entrees (pouches)
Italian dry salami
Minced tuna stuffed olives
Mussels in marinade
Oysters
Peanut butter, creamy
Peanut butter, crunchy
Peppered mackerel
Salmon, variety of commercial flavors in pouches
Salted herring
Sardines in tomato sauce
Sardines Mediterranean style
Shrimp, canned
Smoked clams

**Condiments**

Preserves, apricot
Asian mustard
Balsamic vinegar
BBQ sauce plastic bottle
BBQ sauce packets
Cocktail sauce
Dijon mustard
German mustard
Spicy brown mustard
Honey, in squeeze bottles
Honey, packets
Horseradish packets
Hot sauces, variety commercial
Jam, raspberry
Jam, strawberry
Jelly, grape
Mustard with horseradish
Olive oil
Orange marmalade
Paste, garlic
Paste, hot pepper
Paste, pesto
Paste, sun-dried tomato
Paste, wasabi
Picante sauce
Pickles, thermostabilized
Raspberry jelly
Relish packets
Sweet and sour sauce
Tabasco soy sauce

**Breakfast Items**

Granola bars, variety commercial
Food and sports bars, variety commercial

**Et Cetera**

Variety of icing in a tube
Variety of frosting

## TABLE 25.9
## Microbiological Testing for Flight Food Production

| Area/Item | Microorganism Tolerances | |
|---|---|---|
| **Food Product** | **Factor** | **Limits** |
| | Total aerobic count | 20,000 CFU/g for any single sample (or if any 2 of 5 samples from a lot exceed 10,000 CFU/g) |
| | Coliform | 100 CFU/g for any single sample (or if any 2 of 5 samples from a lot exceed 10 CFU/g) |
| Non-thermostabilized[a] | Coagulase-positive *Staphylococci* | 100 CFU/g for any single sample (or if any 2 of 5 samples from a lot exceed 10 CFU/g) |
| | *Salmonella* | 0 CFU/g for any single sample |
| | Yeasts and molds | 1,000 CFU/g for any single sample (or if any 2 of 5 samples from a lot exceed 100 CFU/g or if any 2 of 5 samples from a lot exceed 10 CFU/g *Aspergillus flavus*) |
| Commercially sterile products (thermostabilized and irradiated) | No sample submitted for microbiological analysis | 100% of packages pass package integrity inspection |

[a] Food samples that are considered "finished" products and that require no additional repackaging are tested only for total aerobic counts.
CFU, colony-forming units.

## TABLE 25.10
## International Partners' ISS Baseline Food List

**Breads**

French toast (T) (ESA)

**Cereals**

Muesli (T) (ESA)

**Entrees**

Beef curry (T) (JAXA)
Braised calf's cheeks in balsamic vinegar sauce (T) (ESA)
Chicken curry (T) (JAXA)
Duck breast confit with capers (T) (ESA)
Mackerel w/miso sauce (T) (JAXA)
Mackerel w/teriyaki sauce (T) (JAXA)
Omelet layer cake (T) (ESA)
Pork curry (T) (JAXA)
Ramen noodles, curry flavor (R) (JAXA)
Ramen noodles, seafood flavor (R) (JAXA)
Ramen noodles, soy sauce flavor (R) (JAXA)
Salmon w/candied Menton lemon (T) (ESA)
Sardine w/tomato sauce (T) (JAXA)
Shredded chicken Parmentier (T) (ESA)
Spicy chicken w/Thai vegetables (T) (ESA)
Swordfish Riviera Style (T) (ESA)

**Snacks and Sweets**

Black sugar candy (NF) (JAXA)
Cheese cake (T) (ESA)
Mushroom and truffle legumaise (T) (ESA)
Peppermint candy (NF) (JAXA)
Rich chocolate cake (T) (ESA)
Semolina cake w/dried apricot (T) (ESA)
Sweet red bean paste (T) (JAXA)
Sweet red bean paste 2/chestnut (T) (JAXA)
Tomato, aubergine, and olive dip (T) (ESA)

**Starches**

Cooked rice, plain (R) (JAXA)
Cooked rice w/Japanese red beans (R) (JAXA)
Cooked rice w/vegetables (R) (JAXA)
Puree of white beans (T) (ESA)
Rice ball w/salmon (R) (JAXA)
Rice porridge (T) (JAXA)

**Vegetables**

Carrot tops (T) (ESA)
Celeriac in a fine puree (T) (ESA)

**Condiments**

Mayonnaise (T) (JAXA)
Tomato ketchup (T) (JAXA)
Worchester sauce (T) (JAXA)

A/S, artificial sweetener; B, beverage; FF, fresh food; IM, intermediate moisture; I, irradiated; NF, natural form; R, rehydratable; T, thermostabilized.

NASA's evolving knowledge of crew member medical and nutritional requirements. For example, the original Shuttle food system included a rigid package for the beverages and rehydratable food items. This packaging system worked well for the early Shuttle missions where there were two to five crew members on missions of 5–7 days. As the number of crew members and duration of Shuttle flights increased, the food system had to design flexible packaging to replace these rigid packages to take up less room during launch and less room in the trash, which was returned to Earth on every Shuttle flight.

The most recent example of food system adaptation is a project currently underway to reformulate the U.S. foods used on the ISS to reduce the sodium content. The sodium content in space food systems has always been high due to the abundance of processed foods and the almost complete absence of fresh foods. Several long-duration ISS crew members had a form of vision changes due to increased intracranial pressure. NASA does not consider the high-sodium diet as the cause of the intracranial pressure of long-duration flight, but identified it as a factor that could exacerbate the problem. This led to the current 2 year project to reformulate about 90 foods in the U.S. food system. As crew members are pleased with the current variety of foods on ISS, the strategy was to reformulate existing food items to reduce sodium. Sodium reduction was accomplished in two major ways. First, in many instances, commercial off-the-shelf frozen foods were used as the raw material for our rehydratable food items. These commercial products tend to be very high in sodium, so made-from-scratch formulations of them were developed, and significant sodium reduction was achieved for these in-house formulations. The second major approach used was to reduce sodium content and use more expensive spices and herbs in product formulations to compensate for the reduced sodium levels. Because the quantities of food required per year for space flight are small, use of higher-priced ingredients is a viable option for NASA even though it might not be economically feasible for commercial manufacturers. Although these reduced-sodium products have not yet been consumed on the ISS, ground-based sensory analysis showed that these products had acceptability scores comparable to those of the high-sodium versions. Using the current standard menu on ISS as a basis of comparison, this reformulation project has resulted in a 37% reduction in the average daily sodium content of the ISS menu while actually slightly (1.5%) increasing the average daily caloric content.

## NUTRITIONAL STATUS ASSESSMENT

The impact of long-duration space flight on nutritional status is not well understood and is unknown for several nutrients. In the mid-1990s, as the frequency of extended-duration missions increased, an effort was undertaken to establish a nutritional assessment protocol. This was to ensure that crew members are launched in good nutritional status, their status

was maintained as well as possible during flight, and any deficits identified after flight were addressed by the rehabilitation teams.[10,25] The clinical nutritional status assessment profile includes anthropometric, biochemical, clinical, and dietary intake assessment components. Each component contributes valuable information to the total picture of nutritional status.

Adequate nutrient intake is critical for the maintenance of nutrient status and crew health; however, obtaining precise dietary intake data during space flight is difficult and time-consuming. Methods that have been used for documenting dietary intake during space flight include barcode scanning of food items, logging food intake manually and down-linking files with the information, and food frequency questionnaires (FFQs).[26] Barcode scanning and logging foods takes a great deal of crew time because each food item must be identified and recorded for each meal, and then downlinked, which could add up to many hours over a 6-month period. Currently, a semiquantitative FFQ is used once a week and requires about 5 min of crew time each week. The FFQ was validated in ground-based chamber studies (60 and 91 day studies) at the NASA Johnson Space Center.[25] Intakes of calories, protein, iron, sodium, fluid, and calcium obtained from 1 and 7 day questionnaires were similar to intakes obtained from 3 day weighed food protocols. In addition, in-flight caloric intakes support body mass data obtained during space flight.[27] The FFQ used for space flight has several advantages over typical questionnaires: the food supply in the space food system is limited, and therefore only food items available to a crew member are included on the questionnaire, making a weekly recall of foods more manageable; the menu cycle (about 16 days) is repetitive, making recall easier, especially after the initial weeks of flight; serving sizes are known because the meals are packaged by single servings, and therefore better estimates of intakes can be determined; and lastly, the exact nutrient content of each package is known, based on proximate analysis conducted at the Johnson Space Center's Water and Food Analytical Laboratory.

In addition to dietary intake assessment, a battery of biochemical tests is used to evaluate crew nutritional status before and after space flight. The comprehensive nutritional assessment profile was developed in collaboration with a panel of extramural experts and includes nutrient status indicators for vitamins and minerals, markers of general health and clinical chemistries, antioxidant status, and bone and calcium metabolism. Clinical Nutritional Assessment[10] is a medical requirement for all long-duration (i.e., ISS) crew members and has been since the Expedition 1 crew launched in October 2000. This protocol includes two preflight fasted blood draws and 48 h urine collections (48 h urine was collected at the same time as the blood draw), a landing day blood and urine (48 h) collection, and a blood and 48 h urine collection about 30 days after flight.[25,27] Table 25.11 is a list of the tests included in the Clinical Nutritional Assessment for long-duration crew members.

## TABLE 25.11
## Measurements Included in the Nutritional Status Assessment for Long-Duration Crew Members[a]

**Body Mass and Composition**

**Body weight**
Height
Lean body mass
Bone densitometry

**Protein status**
Retinol-binding protein
Transthyretin
3-Methylhistidine

**Fat-soluble vitamin status**
Retinol
Retinyl palmitate
β-Carotene
Phylloquinone
γ-Carboxyglutamic acid
α-Tocopherol
γ-Tocopherol
Tocopherol:lipid ratio

**Antioxidant status**
Total antioxidant capacity
Superoxide dismutase
Glutathione peroxidase
Malondialdehyde
Lipid peroxides
8-Hydroxy 2′-deoxyguanosine

**General chemistry**
Aspartate aminotransferase
Alanine aminotransferase
Sodium
Potassium
Cholesterol
Triglyceride
Creatinine (serum and urine)

**Iron Status**

Hemoglobin
Hematocrit
Mean corpuscular volume
Transferrin receptors
Transferrin
Ferritin
Ferritin iron

**Mineral status**
Serum/urinary Iron, zinc, selenium, iodine
Ceruloplasmin
Urinary phosphorus, magnesium

**Water-soluble vitamin status**
Erythrocyte transketolase stimulation
Erythrocyte glutathione reductase activity
Erythrocyte nicotinamide adenine dinucleotide
Urinary N-methyl nicotinamide
Urinary 2-pyridone
Erythrocyte transaminase activity
Urinary 4-pyridoxic acid
Red cell folate
Vitamin C

**Bone and calcium status**
25-hydroxyvitamin D
1,25-dihydroxyvitamin D
Intact parathyroid hormone
Osteocalcin (total and undercarboxylated)
Calcium (serum and urine)
Alkaline phosphatase
Bone-specific alkaline phosphatase
Urinary collagen crosslinks
Ionized calcium
Renal stone risk profile

[a] These measurements are conducted twice before and twice after space flight. All measurements are made in serum except those specified as "urinary" or obviously not serum (body weight, etc.).

In 2006, a Nutritional Status Assessment experiment (known as a Supplemental Medical Objective [SMO]) was developed to better understand nutrition during extended-duration space flight. The protocol was designed to expand the nominal medical requirement testing by collecting in-flight blood and urine samples (for postflight analysis), and to expand the number of variables tested beyond those in the medical requirement. The tests included in this experiment are those listed in Table 25.12 in addition to those listed in Table 25.11. As of early 2012, the Nutrition SMO has collected preflight, in-flight, and postflight data on more than 20 crew members, and some of the initial findings have been published.[28–32]

## BODY MASS MEASUREMENT

Body weight, a cornerstone of any nutrition study, cannot be measured in microgravity (often referred to as weightlessness). However, body mass can be measured during space flight and can be used to monitor general health and dietary intake. Measuring body mass requires special hardware, a so-called mass measuring device.[33,34] The Space Linear Acceleration Mass Measurement Device was installed on the ISS during Expedition.[11] Newton's second law of motion (force is equal to mass times acceleration) is used to measure mass from a recorded acceleration and a known force against a crew member. The device can measure mass from 95 to 240 lb. A Russian-built Body

**TABLE 25.12**

**Pre -, In-, and Postflight Tests Added to the Nutrition SMO Experiment Starting in 2006**

| Body Mass and Composition | Iron Status |
|---|---|
| **Antioxidant status** | Hepcidin |
| 8-Iso-prostaglandin F2α | **Mineral status** |
| Protein carbonyls (nitrotyrosine, dityrosine) | Serum magnesium |
| Glutathione (reduced and oxidized) | Serum phosphorus |
| Fibrinogen | **Water-soluble vitamin status** |
| Cytokines (TNFα, IL-1, IL-6, etc.) | Pyridoxal-5′-phosphate |
| Heme | Serum folate |
| C-reactive protein, highly specific | Homocysteine |
| **General chemistry** | Methylmalonic acid |
| High-density lipoprotein (HDL) | 2-methylcitric acid |
| Low-density lipoprotein (LDL) | Cystathionine |
| Uric acid (urine) | **Bone and calcium status** |
| | Osteoprotegerin |
| **Hormones** | Serum receptor activator of nuclear factor kappa B ligand (sRANKL) |
| Free testosterone | C-telopeptide |
| Testosterone, total and bioavailable | **Regulatory factors** |
| Estradiol | Insulin-like growth factor 1 (IGF-1) |
| Cortisol (serum and urine) | Leptin |
| Dehydroepiandrosterone | |
| Dehydroepiandrosterone sulfate | |

a  In addition to those listed in Table 25.11 of this chapter.

Mass Measuring Device is also available on board the ISS. This device measures spring oscillation to calculate mass. Similar devices were also deployed on Skylab and a few Space Shuttle missions.

## NUTRIENT INTAKE

In-flight estimated nutrient intake data are listed in Table 25.2. The ISS data were collected from the weekly FFQ. During Skylab, metabolic experiments required the crew members to consume a eucaloric diet to maintain body weight.[19,35]

## ENERGY BALANCE

The energy requirements for space flight are calculated based on the total energy expenditure as calculated from the 2002 Institute of Medicine DRI reports.[4] Historically, energy intake requirements were defined in 1991[7] and in 1995.[9] These requirements were defined as provision of enough energy to maintain body weight and composition, with continuous monitoring during flight for flights 30–120 days. For missions up to 360 days, energy intake should be sufficient to maintain body weight and composition. For these missions, requirements were calculated for each individual using the WHO equations for men and women.[36] The equations were assumed using a moderate

activity level and an additional 500 cal/day when end-of-mission countermeasures (i.e., intense exercise) or extravehicular activities are being conducted.

A loss of 1%–5% of preflight body weight is a typical finding in the history of space flight, although some crew members have consumed at or above their energy requirements during flight and have maintained body mass.[27] Table 25.13 highlights the changes in body mass during the Shuttle, Skylab, Mir, and ISS programs. ISS Expeditions were divided into early, middle, and more recent missions to illustrate that crew members on recent expeditions have

**TABLE 25.13**

**Changes in Body Weight on the Day of Landing**

| | n | Body Weight (% Change from Preflight) |
|---|---|---|
| Shuttle | 25 | −2.2 ± 2.4 |
| Skylab | 9 | −3.4 ± 1.7 |
| Mir | 19 | −4.5 ± 3.5 |
| ISS expeditions 1–4 | 6 | −4.9 ± 5.7 |
| ISS expeditions 5–16 | 16 | −4.0 ± 2.3 |
| ISS expeditions 17–29 | 22 | −3.4 ± 2.8 |

Data are expressed as percent change from preflight values (average ± SD).

tended to maintain body mass more than crew members on earlier missions.

## BONE, CALCIUM, AND VITAMIN D

Nutrition is integral to maintaining bone and muscle on Earth and during space flight. Too much or too little of a particular nutrient can be detrimental to the musculoskeletal system. For example, although energy deficits in general negatively affect protein synthesis during space flight,[37] providing excess protein above the RDA can have a negative effect on bone as observed in bed rest subjects.[38]

Calcium is indispensable for maintaining bone health, given that it makes up about 40% of the bone mineral hydroxyapatite, and 99% of the body's reserve of calcium is in bone. During space flight, bone resorption increases, leading to an increase in urinary calcium. Skylab studies showed that the loss of bone was not uniform in all parts of the skeleton.[39] Ground-based data have indicated that providing calcium during space flight would likely not protect against bone loss, because calcium absorption has been shown to decrease in space flight and in ground-based models.[22,40]

Other nutrients, including vitamin K, have been proposed as potential countermeasures to bone loss during space flight. Recent data from ISS crew members show no indication of changes in vitamin K status due to space flight.[41] The data represent the first complete picture of a vitamin K status assessment during space flight and support data from ground-based models of space flight, and these data do not support the use of vitamin K supplementation as a countermeasure during space flight to prevent vitamin K deficiency (or mitigate bone loss).

Two nutrition countermeasure studies were conducted on the ISS to investigate the effect of dietary intake patterns on bone resorption. The first, called "SOLO," tests the impact of high sodium intake on acid–base balance and bone resorption. Ground-based bed rest data indicated that high sodium intake during immobilization exacerbates bone resorption.[42] The second study, called "Pro K," investigates the effect of altering the ratio of acidic and basic components of the diet (animal protein:potassium) on bone metabolism. Ground-based studies support the concept that a diet with more acidic than basic components is associated with more bone resorption.[38,43]

NASA is beginning to have a better understanding of vitamin D needs during space flight. Space flight prevents any promotion of vitamin D synthesis by sunlight, and nominal space foods do not contain much vitamin D.[18] The United States provides vitamin D supplements of 20 μg/day (800 IU/day) for men and women, and initial reports show this to be sufficient to maintain vitamin D levels during space flight.[44]

## FLUID AND ELECTROLYTES

Fluid and electrolyte homeostasis is significantly altered during space flight, as reviewed previously.[18,45–47] The hypothesis originally proposed was that upon entering weightlessness, the human body would experience a headward shift of fluids, with subsequent diuresis and dehydration. A series of experiments were conducted to assess fluid and electrolyte homeostasis during space flight, the most comprehensive being flown on the two Spacelab Life Sciences missions of the early 1990s.[23]

Within hours of the onset of weightlessness (the earliest available data point), a reduction in both plasma volume and extracellular fluid volume occurred,[23] accompanied by the typical puffy faces observed early in flight. Initially, the decrement in plasma volume (17%)[23] was larger than the decrement in extracellular fluid volume (10%),[23] suggesting that interstitial fluid volume (the other four-fifths of extracellular fluid) is conserved proportionally more than plasma volume. After this initial adaptation to weightless occurred, extracellular fluid volume decreased between the first days of flight and 8–12 days of flight.[23] After a slight adjustment, plasma volume remained 10%–15% below preflight levels. Plasma volume remains decreased at this level even during flights of extended duration.[48]

It is hypothesized that the extravascular shift of protein and fluid represents an adaptation to weightlessness, and that after several days, some of the extravascular albumin is metabolized, with a loss of oncotic force and a resulting decrease in extracellular fluid volume and increase in plasma volume.[45] This loss of extracellular protein (either intra- or extravascular), and associated decreased oncotic potential, probably plays a role in postflight orthostatic intolerance, which has been considered to result partly from reduced plasma volume at landing.[49] Furthermore, the loss of protein may explain why fluid loading alone does not restore circulatory volume,[50,51] as no additional solute load exists to maintain the fluid volume. In addition, water turnover in flight was directly related to water intake; however, turnover was lower in flight than before launch, probably due to modest reduction in exercise and a 21% decrease in fluid intakes.

The effect of space flight on total body water has been evaluated to assess dehydration. Studies with Shuttle and Skylab astronauts showed about 1% decrease in total body water during flight,[23,52,53] and the percent of body mass represented by water did not change. Thus, the often-proposed weightlessness-induced dehydration does not exist physiologically. However, care must be taken to ensure that astronauts have adequate fluid consumption and avoid prolonged exposure to elevated ambient temperatures.

In-flight sodium intakes during Skylab and Shuttle missions averaged 4–5 g/day and were similar to the astronauts' preflight intakes.[54] The current food system is high in dietary sodium, and typical intakes on the ISS have been in excess of 4.5 g/day (Table 25.2), even with suboptimal food intake.[18,27] Intakes as high as 10–12 g of sodium per day have been observed. Sodium homeostasis and blood sodium levels are maintained during real and simulated space flight.[55] Hypertension is not a primary concern, but there are concerns about other negative health effects of high sodium intake, including effects on bone and renal health.[18,56] In 2009, an effort was initiated to reformulate most of the U.S. space foods to reduce sodium content. With reformulation having been partially implemented (some foods still waiting to be reformulated, some waiting to be flown), sodium intakes have decreased compared to early ISS missions. The next challenge will be for the ISS international partners to reduce sodium content of their foods. The goal is to have intakes of 3–4 g sodium per day, which is still above U.S. recommendations but would be a significant reduction in sodium intake during space flight.

## ANTIOXIDANTS

Space flight increases astronauts' likelihood of having cellular oxidative damage because the space environment contains several sources of oxidative stress. Some of these are high linear energy transfer radiation, hyperoxic (100% oxygen) conditions during extravehicular activities, exercise, and stress, all of which have been associated with initiating reactive oxygen species and oxidative damage in both human and animal studies.[57,58] Currently, not enough data exist to make evidence-based recommendations for antioxidant supplementation during space flight. Some crew members choose to take multivitamin supplements, but there is no evidence for mitigation of oxidative damage in these individuals. Promising results from animal studies show that antioxidants can mitigate oxidative damage from radiation.[59] The next step is to demonstrate the effects with crew members in controlled studies during space flight.

## IRON

Iron is a critical micronutrient involved in many cellular processes. Its functions include oxygen binding, electron transport, and serving as a cofactor for literally hundreds of enzymes. Iron deficiency can have irreversible consequences,[60] and excess iron is toxic. In addition to increasing risks of cardiovascular disease and cancer, iron overload can impair immune function and normal bone metabolism, and cause increased sensitivity to radiation injury,[61] all of which are concerns for space flight. One mechanism for toxicity is related to the ability of superoxide anions to be converted to form highly reactive hydroxyl radicals by iron-mediated Fenton chemistry, which potentiates local oxidative stress. Iron can be liberated from the storage protein ferritin during periods of oxidative stress or exposure to radiation,[62] and thus contribute to oxidative stress. Maintenance of iron homeostasis is therefore extremely important for human health.

During space flight, it is well established that iron homeostasis is altered.[18] Decreased red blood cell mass, increased serum ferritin, decreased transferrin receptors, and increased serum iron document increased iron storage during space flight. Not only is iron availability increased

by neocytolysis of red blood cells,[17] but also iron content of the space food system is very high because many of the commercial food items in the ISS menu are fortified with iron.[18] The mean iron content of the standard 16-day ISS menu is $20 \pm 6$ mg/day. For reference, the defined space flight requirement for iron is 8–10 mg/day for both men and women,[18] which is higher than the current U.S. DRI for males of 8 mg/day.[5]

## VISION

Vision and related ophthalmic changes, including optic disk edema, globe flattening, choroidal folds, and cotton wool spots were identified during and after space flight.[63] Although the etiology of the changes may be related to headward fluid shifts and increased intracranial pressure, data from the Nutrition SMO experiment suggest an underlying mechanism. The data provide evidence that the folate/vitamin $B_6$/vitamin $B_{12}$-dependent one-carbon metabolism pathway may be involved.[30] Homocysteine, 2-methylcitric acid, cystathionine, and methylmalonic acid concentrations were all higher in crew members who had experienced ophthalmic changes than in crew members who did not have changes. The differences were evident before, during, and after flight. Furthermore, in-flight serum folate was lower in crew members with ophthalmic changes than in those with no changes. All of these results are consistent with the presence of polymorphisms of enzymes in the one-carbon pathway in crew members who have ophthalmic changes, but further work is warranted. Throughout the biomedical literature, polymorphisms of enzymes in this one-carbon pathway are reported to be associated with increased risk of vascular events such as stroke and migraine headaches, and even increased risk of decompression sickness.[64-66]

## FLIGHT ANALOGS

Although research and clinical monitoring need to be done during space flight, it is often not possible to conduct research during flight because of many resource limitations, including delayed return from flight and limited crew time, launch mass, on-orbit power or hardware, and perhaps most importantly, a limited number of subjects. Space flight studies are also expensive and time-consuming. Because of these limitations and disadvantages of doing research in space, flight analogs are often used to test countermeasures that are proposed for use during space flight. Ground-based flight analogs are used to test countermeasures for feasibility and side effects. Different flight analogs are used depending on what outcomes are being tested. One example is the Antarctica model. Depending on which Antarctic station is being used, 20–50 subjects can be studied in one winter period. The Antarctica model is good for studying vitamin D during the winter months because ultraviolet light is very low for about half of the year. Other Antarctic

**TABLE 25.14**

**Comparison of Ground-Based Analogs of Space Flight**

| Model | Similarities to Space Flight | Differences from Space Flight | References |
|---|---|---|---|
| **Human** | | | |
| Bed rest | Fluid shifts (if −6° head down tilt), bone loss is ~50% of what is observed in space flight | Mechanism for muscle loss is different from space flight; not as much evidence for an inflammatory/stress response as there is in space flight | 12,67–70 |
| Antarctica | Isolation (months), no fresh food resupply during winter months, little/no ultraviolet light exposure | No bone or muscle loss; no change in gravity | 71,72 |
| NEEMO[a] | Isolation (days/weeks), changes in iron homeostasis and oxidative stress similar to space flight, changes in immune function | No bone or muscle loss | 29,73,74 |
| Dry immersion | Rapid gravitational deconditioning, hypokinesia | | 75 |
| Chambers | Isolation (weeks to months to years), long-duration simulation possible, size of crew quarters similar to space flight | No change in gravity | 25 |
| **Cell culture** | | | |
| HARV[b] | Cells are in a continuous state of free fall | Rotating gravity vector is present | 76,77 |
| Parabolic flight/drop towers | Short duration (up to 30) microgravity (cells, limited human studies), can simulate partial-gravity environments (e.g., moon, Mars) | | |
| **Animals** | | | |
| Hindlimb suspension | Muscle and bone loss, fluid shifts | Animals are restrained and often stressed, body axis differences hinder comparisons | 78,79 |
| Limb immobilization | Muscle atrophy, bone loss | Animals often stressed | |

[a] NEEMO is NASA Extreme Environment Mission (underwater laboratory).

[b] HARV is high-aspect ratio vessel bioreactor.

conditions provide a good model of space flight, including the isolation (and corresponding stress responses) and lack of fresh food supply. Table 25.14 summarizes several ground analogs of space flight and lists similarities with and differences from space flight.

## NEEDED ADVANCES IN FOOD SYSTEM FOR FLIGHT OUTSIDE OF LOW EARTH ORBIT

Advanced food systems are food systems that will be required for NASA's future exploration-class missions that will go beyond low Earth orbit. Such missions could include an extended stay on a lunar or planetary surface and last as long as 2.5 years, which is the estimated time required for a mission to Mars. The spacecraft air and water can be recycled and regenerated, but food cannot, given the limitations of space travel. It is possible that a small quantity of "pick and eat" foods, such as lettuce or cherry tomatoes, could be grown and consumed in transit, but without gravity, more extensive crop growth and processing is implausible. It is generally accepted that there will be no resupply of food during these transits and therein lies the next challenge for space food systems.

The initial mission to Mars would likely require a shelf-stable packaged food system similar to the one in use on the ISS. The chief challenge of providing such a food system

for a trip to Mars is the likelihood that, because a large amount of mass would be involved, most of the food would have to be prepositioned, waiting for the crew when they arrived. This means that these foods would require a shelf life of at least 3 and possibly as much as 5 years.[24] Very few of the current products in the ISS food system have a shelf life long enough to meet this requirement. Although the current ISS foods are safe to eat for that length of time, the quality and nutritional content of these products at the end of that time are likely to be decreased. NASA's Space Food System Laboratory is researching ways to extend the shelf life of shelf-stable foods to meet these extended requirements. Also emerging food processing technologies in the food industry hold promise for extending shelf life by reducing the amount of heat required to achieve shelf stability. Reducing the heat applied to the food during processing has the potential to produce a shelf-stable food with a higher initial sensory quality and higher initial nutritional content, resulting in a longer shelf life.

An extended stay on a lunar or planetary surface in some type of habitat would introduce at least partial gravity to the food system and would likely include the growing of food crops for aid in recycling air and water as well as augmenting the packaged food system or potentially replacing a certain percentage of it. This would introduce a whole new set of requirements for space food systems, as crew members would for the first time actually be harvesting crops, processing them into ingredients, and preparing meals.

To ensure that health is maintained during these advanced missions, continuation of nutrition research is necessary. From the ISS research results, some basic nutrition concerns will be identified. The next step is to ensure that these nutritional concerns or risks can be mitigated with training, crew selection criteria, vehicle health care and food systems, countermeasures, and selection of foods for the space diet.

## REFERENCES

1. Hale, W, Lane, H, Chapline, G, Lulla, K. *Wings in Orbit: Scientific and Engineering Legacies of the Space Station*, 2010, 553pp. http://www.nasa.gov/centers/johnson/wingsinorbit/index.html (May 2012).
2. National Research Council. *Recommended Dietary Allowances. A Report of the Food and Nutrition Board*. National Research Council, 1968, 101pp.
3. National Research Council. *Recommended Dietary Allowances. Report of the Committee on Dietary Allowances and Committee on Interpretation of the Recommended Dietary Allowances*. National Research Council, 1974, 128pp.
4. Institute of Medicine. *Dietary Reference Intakes for Energy, Carbohydrate, Fiber, Fat, Fatty Acids, Cholesterol, Protein, and Amino Acids (Macronutrients)*. The National Academy Press, Washington, DC, 2002, 1045pp.
5. Institute of Medicine. *Dietary Reference Intakes for Vitamin A, Vitamin K, Arsenic, Boron, Chromium, Copper, Iodine, Iron, Manganese, Molybdenum, Nickel, Silicon, Vanadium, and Zinc*. National Academy Press, Washington, DC, 2001, 773pp.
6. Institute of Medicine. *Dietary Reference Intakes for Water, Potassium, Sodium, Chloride, and Sulfate*. The National Academies Press, Washington, DC, 2004, 617pp.
7. National Aeronautics and Space Administration Johnson Space Center. Nutritional requirements for Extended Duration Orbiter missions (30–90 d) and Space Station Freedom (30–120 d). Report No. JSC-32283, National Aeronautics and Space Administration Lyndon B. Johnson Space Center, Houston, TX, 1993.
8. NASA Johnson Space Center. in NASA Conference Publication #3146, Houston, TX, 1991. http://ntrs.nasa.gov/archive/nasa/casi.ntrs.nasa.gov/19920016718_1992016718.pdf (May 2012).
9. National Aeronautics and Space Administration Johnson Space Center. Nutritional requirements for International Space Station (ISS) missions up to 360 days. Report No. JSC-28038, National Aeronautics and Space Administration Lyndon B. Johnson Space Center, Houston, TX, 1996.
10. National Aeronautics and Space Administration Johnson Space Center. Nutritional status assessment for extended-duration space flight. JSC Document #28566, Revision 1, NASA, Washington, DC, 1999.
11. Lane, HW, Gretebeck, RJ, Schoeller, DA et al. *Am. J. Clin. Nutr.* 65, 4;1997.
12. Stein, TP, Blanc, S. *Crit. Rev. Food Sci. Nutr.* 51, 828;2011.
13. Leach, C, Leonard, J, Rambaut, P, Johnson, P. *J. Appl. Physiol.* 45, 430;1978.
14. Marshall Space Flight Center. http://www.nasa.gov/centers/marshall/pdf/104840main_eclss.pdf (May 2012).
15. Carter, DL, Orozco, N. Status of the Regenerative ECLSS Water Recovery System. In: *41st International Conference on Environmental Systems*, AIAA 1021863, July 15–19, 2012, San Diego, CA.
16. Alfrey, CP, Rice, L, Udden, MM, Driscoll, TB. *Lancet* 349, 1389;1997.
17. Alfrey, CP, Udden, MM, Leach-Huntoon, C et al. *J. Appl. Physiol.* 81, 98;1996.
18. Smith, SM, Zwart, SR, Kloeris, V, Heer, M. *Nutritional Biochemistry of Space Flight*. Nova Science Publishers, Hauppauge, NY, 2009.
19. Rambaut, PC, Johnston, RS. *Acta Astronaut.* 6, 1113;1979.
20. Smith, MC, Heidelbaugh, ND, Rambaut, PC et al. Apollo food technology. 437 NASA Scientific and Technical Information, Washington, DC, 1975.
21. Smith, MC, Rapp, RM, Huber, CS et al. Apollo experience report—Food systems. NASA Technical Note TN D-7720, Washington, DC, 1974.
22. Smith, SM, Wastney, ME, Morukov, BV et al. *Am. J. Physiol.* 277, R1;1999.
23. Leach, C, Alfrey, C, Suki, W et al. *J. Appl. Physiol.* 81, 105;1996.
24. Cooper, M, Douglas, G, Perchonok, M. *J. Food Sci.* 76, R40;2011.
25. Smith, SM, Davis-Street, JE, Rice, BL et al. *J. Nutr.* 131, 2053;2001.
26. Soller, BR, Cabrera, M, Smith, SM, Sutton, JP. *Nutrition* 18, 930;2002.
27. Smith, SM, Zwart, SR, Block, G et al. *J. Nutr.* 135, 437;2005.
28. Smith, SM, Heer, M, Wang, Z et al. *J. Clin. Endocrinol. Metab.* 97, 270;2012.
29. Zwart, SR, Jessup, JM, Ji, J, Smith, SM. *PLoS One* 7, e31058;2012.
30. Zwart, SR, Gibson, CR, Mader, TH et al. *J. Nutr.* 142, 427;2012.
31. Zwart, SR, Booth, SL, Peterson, JW et al. *J. Bone Miner. Res.* 26, 948;2011.
32. Zwart, SR, Pierson, D, Mehta, S et al. *J. Bone Miner. Res.* 25, 1049;2010.
33. Pistecky, PV, van Beek, HF, Klinkhamer, JF, Brechignac, F. *Adv. Space Res.* 12, 259;1992.
34. Sarychev, VA, Sazonov, VV, Zlatorunsky, AS et al. *Acta Astronaut.* 7, 719;1980.
35. Leach, CS, Rambaut, PC. In: Johnston, RS, Dietlein, LF eds., *Biomedical Results from Skylab (NASA SP-377)*, National Aeronautics and Space Administration 204;1977. http://lsda.jsc.nasa.gov/books/skylab/Ch01.htm (May 2012).
36. World Health Organization. Energy and protein requirements. Report of a joint FAO/WHO/UNU expert consultation. Technical Report Series 724. WHO, Geneva, Switzerland, 1985.
37. Stein, TP, Leskiw, MJ, Schluter, MD et al. *Am. J. Physiol. Endocrinol. Metab.* 276, E1014;1999.
38. Zwart, SR, Davis-Street, JE, Paddon-Jones, D et al. *J. Appl. Physiol.* 99, 134;2005.
39. Smith, SM, Heer, M. *Nutrition* 18, 849;2002.
40. LeBlanc, A, Schneider, V, Spector, E et al. *Bone* 16(4 Suppl.), 301S;1995.
41. Adlis, D. JSC document 26626A-Extravehicular activity generic design requirements document. NASA/JSC Technical Publication, Johnson Space Center, 1995.
42. Frings-Meuthen, P, Buehlmeier, J, Baecker, N et al. *J. Appl. Physiol.* 111, 537;2011.
43. Zwart, SR, Hargens, AR, Smith, SM. *Am. J. Clin. Nutr.* 80, 1058;2004.

44. Smith, SM, Heer, MA, Shackelford, LC et al. *J. Bone Miner. Res.* 27, 1896;2012.
45. Smith, SM, Krauhs, JM, Leach, CS. *Adv. Space Biol. Med.* 6, 123;1997.
46. Huntoon, CL, Cintrón, NM, Whitson, PA. In: Nicogossian, AE, Huntoon, CL, Pool, SL eds., *Space Physiology and Medicine*, Lea & Febiger, Philadelphia, PA, 1994, p. 334.
47. Leach Huntoon, CS, Grigoriev, AI, Natochin, YV. *Fluid and Electrolyte Regulation in Spaceflight.* American Astronautical Society Science and Technology Series. Vol. 94, Univelt Inc., Escondido, CA, 1998, 219pp.
48. Johnson, P, Driscoll, T, LeBlanc, A. In: Johnston, R, Dietlein, L eds., *Biomedical Results from Skylab (NASA SP-377)*, National Aeronautics and Space Administration, Washington, DC, 1977, p. 235.
49. Bungo, MW, Johnson, PC, Jr. *Aviat. Space Environ. Med.* 54, 1001;1983.
50. Hyatt, KH, West, DA. *Aviat. Space Environ. Med.* 48, 120;1977.
51. Vernikos, J, Convertino, VA. *Acta Astronaut.* 33, 259;1994.
52. Leach, CS, Inners, LD, Charles, JB. In: Bungo, MW, Bagian, TM, Bowman, MA, Levitan, BM eds., *Results of the Life Sciences DSOs Conducted Aboard the Space Shuttle 1981–1986*, Space Biomedical Research Institute, Johnson Space Center, Houston, TX, 1987, p. 49.
53. Thornton, WE, Ord, J. In: Johnston, RS, Dietlein, LF eds., *Biomedical Results from Skylab (NASA SP-377)*, National Aeronautics and Space Administration, Washington, DC, 1977, p. 175.
54. Bourland, C, Kloeris, V, Rice, B, Vodovotz, Y. In: Lane, HW, Schoeller, DA eds., *Nutrition in Spaceflight and Weightlessness Models*, CRC Press, Boca Raton, FL. 2000, p. 19.
55. Lane, HW, Leach, C, Smith, SM. In: Lane, HW, Schoeller, DA eds., *Nutrition in Spaceflight and Weightlessness Models*, CRC Press, Boca Raton, FL, 2000, p. 119.
56. Smith, SM, Zwart, SR. In: Makowsky, G ed., *Adv. Clin. Chem.* Vol. 46, Academic Press, Burlington, VT, 2008, p. 87.
57. Konopacka, M, Rzeszowska-Wolny, J. *Mutat. Res.* 491, 1;2001.
58. Reid, MB. In: Sen, CK, Packer, L, Hänninen, O eds., *Handbook of Oxidants and Antioxidants in Exercise*, Elsevier Science B.V., Amsterdam, the Netherlands, 2000, p. 599.
59. Kennedy, AR, Ware, JH, Carlton, W, Davis, JG. *Radiat. Res.* 176, 62;2011.
60. Beard, J. *J. Nutr.* 133, 1468S,2003.
61. Crichton, RR. *Iron Metabolism from Molecular Mechanisms to Clinical Consequences.* 3rd edn., John Wiley & Sons Ltd., New York, 2009, 461pp.
62. Aubailly, M, Santus, R, Salmon, S. *Photochem. Photobiol.* 54, 769;1991.
63. Mader, TH, Gibson, CR, Pass, AF et al. *Ophthalmology* 118, 2058;2011.
64. Candito, M, Candito, E, Chatel, M et al. *Rev. Neurol.* (Paris) 162, 840;2006.
65. Cronin, S, Furie, KL, Kelly, PJ. *Stroke* 36, 1581;2005.
66. Oterino, A, Toriello, M, Valle, N et al. *Headache* 50, 99;2010.
67. Coker, RH, Wolfe, RR. *Curr. Opin. Clin. Nutr. Metab. Care* 15, 7;2012.
68. Zwart, SR, Crawford, GE, Gillman, PL et al. *J. Appl. Physiol.* 107, 54;2009.
69. Zwart, SR, Oliver, SM, Fesperman, JV et al. *Aviat. Space Environ. Med.* 80, A15;2009.
70. Smith, SM, Nillen, JL, LeBlanc, A et al. *J. Clin. Endocrinol. Metab.* 83, 3584;1998.
71. Smith, SM, Gardner, KK, Locke, J, Zwart, SR. *Am. J. Clin. Nutr.* 89, 1092;2009.
72. Zwart, SR, Mehta, SK, Ploutz-Snyder, RJ et al. *J. Nutr.* 141, 692;2011.
73. Zwart, SR, Kala, G, Smith, SM. *J. Nutr.* 139, 90;2009.
74. Smith, SM, Davis-Street, JE, Fesperman, JV et al. *J. Nutr.* 134, 1765;2004.
75. Navasiolava, NM, Custaud, MA, Tomilovskaya, ES et al. *Eur. J. Appl. Physiol.* 111, 1235;2011.
76. Freed, LE, Vunjak-Novakovic, G. *Adv. Space Biol. Med.* 8, 177;2002.
77. Vunjak-Novakovic, G, Searby, N, De Luis, J, Freed, LE. *Ann. N. Y. Acad. Sci.* 974, 504;2002.
78. Du, F, Wang, J, Gao, Y et al. *Aviat. Space Environ. Med.* 82, 689;2011.
79. Morey-Holton, E, Globus, RK, Kaplansky, A, Durnova, G. *Adv. Space Biol. Med.* 10, 7;2005.

# 26 Vegetarian Diets in Health Promotion and Disease Prevention

*Claudia S. Plaisted Fernandez, Kelly M. Adams, and Martin Kohlmeier*

## CONTENTS

Vegetarianism is rapidly growing in popularity. Technically defined, vegetarians are individuals who do not eat any meat, poultry, or seafood.[1,2] Estimates on the number of vegetarians in the United States vary greatly according to the definition of vegetarianism provided in the survey. True vegetarians who eat no meat, poultry, or fish make up about 3% of the population representing approximately 7 million adults according to a 2009 poll.[2] About one-third of vegetarians follow a vegan eating pattern. Vegetarianism is most common in females ages 18–34 at 5% of the population.[2]

Vegetarian dietary patterns can represent an exceptionally healthy way of eating.[3] One study of Americans, for instance, found that vegan and vegetarians consumed about twice as much fruits and vegetables and several times as much legumes and nuts as nonvegetarians.[4] Another study found that switching to a vegan lifestyle eliminated most saturated fat from the menu and increased intake of dietary fiber and many other protective food constituents.[5] Vegetarian diet patterns are typically rich in vitamins, minerals, phytochemicals, and fiber while often also low in saturated fat and cholesterol.[1] However, each individual diet will need to be assessed for its nutritional adequacy.[3] This chapter provides some guidance in characterizing vegetarian dietary patterns, health benefits, and concerns as well as in identifying sources of various nutrients that may be marginal in many vegetarian diets.

## CHARACTERISTICS OF VEGETARIAN EATING STYLES

When working with someone who follows a vegetarian diet, it is important to ask them a variety of questions about their usual dietary patterns. Many people consider themselves to be vegetarian when they eat nonflesh foods several days a week. Others will claim to be vegetarians when they consume fish or poultry. Table 26.1 lists the types of vegetarian diets and describes what foods fall into or out of those categories.

In popular culture, there are many diets that incorporate principles of vegetarianism and may represent more restrictive ways of eating as described in Table 26.2. For the purposes of this chapter, "vegetarian" will refer to an individual following a lacto and/or an ovo pattern or a vegan dietary pattern. A more restrictive diet makes the individual following it more susceptible to dietary deficiencies and imbalances.[1] Table 26.3 describes the nutrients that may be of concern in many vegetarian diets.

## HEALTH RISKS AND BENEFITS OF VEGETARIANISM

Most health risks associated with a vegetarian diet are found with strict vegetarianism (veganism) only, not with the more liberal forms of intake found in lacto-vegetarians, ovo-vegetarians, or lacto–ovo-vegetarians.[1,6,7] Table 26.4 lists the health risks of vegetarianism, most of which are related to the potential for nutrient deficiencies found with this type of diet. These health risks are not unique to vegetarians, however, as they can be quite common in people following an imbalanced omnivorous diet.

Vegetarian diets are associated with a number of health benefits and can be useful in preventing and treating chronic diseases such as hypertension. Many vegetarians follow a dietary pattern that reduces their risks for common chronic diseases due to many protective factors as noted in Tables 26.5 and 26.6.[8] New vegetarians in particular,

**TABLE 26.1**
**Types of Vegetarian Diets**

| | |
|---|---|
| Vegan | Consumes nuts, fruits, grains, legumes, and vegetables. Does not consume animal-based food products, including eggs, dairy products, red meats, poultry, or seafood. Some vegetarians may avoid foods with animal processing (honey, sugar, vinegar, wine, beer, etc.). |
| Lacto-vegetarian | Consumes milk and other dairy products, nuts, fruits, grains, legumes, and vegetables. Does not consume eggs, red meats, poultry, or seafood. |
| Ovo-vegetarian | Consumes eggs, nuts, fruits, grains, legumes, and vegetables. Does not consume milk or dairy, red meats, poultry, or seafood. |
| Lacto–ovo-vegetarian | Consumes milk and other dairy products, eggs, nuts, fruits, grains, legumes, and vegetables. Does not consume red meats, poultry, or seafood. |
| Pollo vegetarian[a] | Not technically considered a vegetarian type of diet, although often referred to as "vegetarian" in popular culture. Consumes milk and other dairy products, eggs, nuts, fruits, grains, legumes, vegetables, and poultry. |
| Peche vegetarian, also called pesco vegetarian[a] | Not technically considered a vegetarian type of diet, although often referred to as "vegetarian" in popular culture. Consumes milk and other dairy products, eggs, nuts, fruits, grains, legumes, vegetables, and seafood. |
| Omnivore | Consumes from a wide variety of foods, including meats, grains, fruits, vegetables, legumes, and dairy products. Individuals who consume red meats (beef, pork, lamb, etc.), poultry, seafood, or any still or once living nonplant-based matter are not vegetarians. |
| Semi-vegetarian or "flexitarian" | Not technically considered a vegetarian type of diet as it covers a wide range of eating practices. Some individuals may consume meats or animal products as condiments/small amounts, or may only include certain types of these foods in their diet, or may follow meatless eating plans cyclically or periodically. |

[a] This is not technically a vegetarian diet, although it is often referred to as such.

**TABLE 26.2**
**Types of Popular Diets[a] Incorporating Various Principles of Vegetarianism**

| | |
|---|---|
| Fad diets | Popular weight-loss diets often incorporate various principles of vegetarianism, although not generally in nutritious, balanced ways. The cabbage soup diet is an example, which is based on consuming only a vegetable soup based on cabbage as a weight-loss technique. |
| Fruitarian | Consumes botanical fruits (including vegetables such as tomatoes, eggplant, peppers, squash, avocado), nuts and seeds; avoids meats, poultry, seafood, dairy, eggs, and vegetables; may avoid legumes. |
| Macrobiotic | Largely based on grains and in-season foods, including vegetables (except those of the nightshade family), sea vegetables, soups, and beans. Nuts and seeds are not consumed on a daily basis, along with fruits, which are included with the exception of tropical ones. Seafood is sometimes included as well. Processed sweeteners are avoided. Asian foods contribute significantly to food choices. This is an example of a diet following a food-combining philosophy. |
| Natural hygiene or raw foods diet | Generally raw vegetables, fruits, whole grains or sprouted grains (in some cases may be cooked), sprouted or non-sprouted legumes, nuts, and seeds. Some consumers may consume raw dairy products. There is great variation in this diet plan: Many followers do consume cooked foods and some consume meat as well. This is an example of a diet following a food-combining philosophy but has many variations among followers. |

[a] Many variations exist on each of these types of diets. This is not intended as a comprehensive listing.

## TABLE 26.3

## Nutrients Potentially at Risk in Vegetarian Diets, RDA/Adequate Intakes (AIs) from the Dietary Reference Intakes (DRIs), Functions, and Sources

| Vitamin/Mineral | RDA (Unless Otherwise Noted): Adult Value 31–50-Year-Olds, Nonpregnant, per Day | Function | Good Sources in Vegetarian Diet |
|---|---|---|---|
| **Vitamins** | | | |
| Vitamin $B_{12}$ | M: 2.4 μg<br>F: 2.4 μg | Works with folic acid to make red blood cells; important in maintaining healthy nerve fibers; helps the body use fat and protein. | Dairy products, eggs, fortified cereals, fortified soy products/meat substitutes, and fortified nutritional yeast |
| Vitamin D | M: 15 μg<br>F: 15 μg | Promotes absorption of calcium and phosphorus and helps deposit them in bones and teeth. | Fortified milk; made in body when skin is exposed to sunlight |
| Riboflavin ($B_2$) | M: 1.3 mg<br>F: 1.1 mg | Helps the body release energy from protein, fat, and carbohydrates. | Fortified dairy products, fortified breads and cereals, tomatoes, lima beans, raisins, avocado, beans, and legumes |
| **Minerals** | | | |
| Calcium | M: 1000 mg<br>F: 1000 mg | Used to build bones and teeth and keep them strong; important in muscle contraction and blood clotting. | Dairy products, broccoli, mustard, and turnip greens |
| Iron[a] | M: 8 mg<br>F: 18 mg | Carries oxygen in the body, both as a part of hemoglobin (in the blood) and myoglobin (in the muscles). | Whole-grain and enriched cereals, some dried fruits, and soybeans |
| Zinc | M: 11 mg<br>F: 8 mg | Assists in wound healing, blood formation, and general growth and maintenance of all tissues; component of many enzymes. | Plant and animal proteins |
| Manganese[b] | AI:<br>M: 2.3 mg<br>F: 1.8 mg | Found in most of body's organs and tissues, particularly in bones, liver, and kidneys. Serves as a cofactor in many metabolic processes. Deficiency not seen in human populations. | Whole grains, cereal products, tea, some fruits, and vegetables |
| Iodine | M: 150 μg<br>F: 150 μg | Constituent of thyroid hormones (regulation of metabolic rate, body temperature, growth, reproduction, making body cells, muscle function, and nerve growth). | Fortified in salt, found in seaweed, dairy, and plant foods where soil concentration is adequate |
| Copper[c] | M: 900 μg<br>F: 900 μg | Necessary for the formation of hemoglobin; keeps bones, blood vessels, and nerves healthy. | Nuts, legumes, and whole grains |
| Selenium | M: 55 μg<br>F: 55 μg | Antioxidant functions, role in eicosanoid metabolism, regulation of arachidonic acid and lipid peroxidation, and some hormone conversions. | Eggs, whole grains, legumes, and Brazil nuts |
| **Macronutrients and other dietary components** | | | |
| Protein | M: 56 g or 0.8 g/kg<br>F: 46 g or 0.8 g/kg | Building of nearly all body tissues, particularly muscle tissue, energy. | Dairy products, legumes, meat analog products often made from soy; whole grains and vegetables are poorer sources |
| Omega-3 fatty acids | AI:<br>M: 1.6 g<br>F: 1.1 g | Energy source, cell wall structure, may play a role in disease prevention. Fats also play a role in the absorption and transport of fat-soluble vitamins. Linolenic acid cannot be made by the body; omega-3 series fatty acids can be found in grains, seeds, nuts, and soybeans; and the body can manufacture EPA and DHA from these precursors, but conversion is inefficient. | Fats and oils (bean, nut, and grain oils), nuts, and seeds (butternuts, walnuts, and soybean kernels), soybeans, flaxseeds, and flaxseed oil |

*Sources:* Craig, W.J. and Mangels, A.R., *J. Am. Diet. Assoc.*, 109(7), 1266, 2009; Ross, A.C. et al., eds., *Dietary Reference Intakes for Calcium and Vitamin D*, National Academies Press, Washington, DC, 2011; Trumbo, P. et al., *J. Am. Diet. Assoc.*, 102(11), 1621, 2002; Trumbo, P. et al., *J. Am. Diet. Assoc.*, 101(3), 294, 2001; Monsen, E.R., *J. Am. Diet. Assoc.*, 100(6), 637, 2000.

[a]  There is some evidence that vegetarian diets tend to be quite high in iron and that iron deficiency anemia is no more common among vegetarians than in meat eaters.[1]

[b]  Manganese is not usually at risk for deficiency in vegetarians. Most research has found that vegetarians have higher manganese intake than nonvegetarians. However, bioavailability may be a concern.[31,32]

[c]  Copper is not necessarily at risk for deficiency in vegetarians. Some research has indicated that vegetarians have a higher intake of this nutrient; however, bioavailability may be a concern.[8,9]

**TABLE 26.4**
**Health Risks of Vegetarianism**

| Dietary Factor | Risk |
| --- | --- |
| Calcium | Low calcium intake in vegan or macrobiotic diet can lead to low bone-mineral density. |
| Iodine | A strict vegan consuming no iodized salt can develop goiter. |
| Vitamin $B_{12}$ | In strict vegans or in the offspring of vegan mothers only, deficiency can lead to anemia or in far more severe cases, neuropathy. |
| Energy | Impaired growth can result in infants and children with inadequate energy intake or those weaned to "homemade" formulas. |
| DHA | Greatest concern for fetus and young infants. DHA is needed for neural and retinal development. |
| Dairy products | Iron deficiency with excessive consumption of dairy products in young children. Limited evidence exists linking high consumption of dairy products to diabetes (type 1). |

*Source:* Craig, W.J. and Mangels, A.R., *J. Am. Diet. Assoc.*, 109(7), 1266, 2009.

**TABLE 26.5**
**Health Benefits of Vegetarianism**

Lower risk of the following:
    Cancer (particularly colon and lung)
    Obesity
    Heart disease
    Type 2 diabetes
    Hypertension
    Constipation and hemorrhoids
    Kidney stones and kidney disease
    Gallstones
    Hemochromatosis

Potential lower risk for (limited evidence suggesting) the following:
    Rheumatoid arthritis
    Gout
    Dementia and Alzheimer's disease

*Source:* Craig, W.J. and Mangels, A.R., *J. Am. Diet. Assoc.*, 109(7), 1266, 2009.

**TABLE 26.6**
**Protective Factors in the Typical Lacto–Ovo-Vegetarian Diet**

Higher fiber
Lower saturated fat and cholesterol
Higher folate intake
Higher intake of antioxidants
Higher intake of phytochemicals
Higher intake of potassium and magnesium
Lower intake of total and animal protein

*Source:* Craig, W.J. and Mangels, A.R., *J. Am. Diet. Assoc.*, 109(7), 1266, 2009.

**TABLE 26.7**
**Practical Concerns about Vegetarianism**

New vegetarians or those who are vegetarian for philosophical (as opposed to health) reasons may rely heavily on the use of dairy products and eggs.
Whole-milk cheeses, 2% and higher-fat-content milk, eggs, and whole-milk yogurts are rich in saturated fat and cholesterol as well. These can contribute to higher risks for cardiovascular disease in particular and should be evaluated.
For vegetarians who travel extensively, particularly to less urban areas, limited vegetarian options may be available, thus narrowing the field of food choices to higher fat, lower nutrient foods (e.g., macaroni and cheese, bread and cheese), or simply limiting food variety (e.g., only salads on menu meet vegetarian requirements).
Some adolescents with eating disorders may use vegetarianism as a rationalization for avoiding foods or entire food groups.

more critical during specific developmental phases; deficiency of that particular nutrient at that stage of the life cycle can have dramatic consequences.[6,9–11]

## ENERGY AND MACRONUTRIENTS IN THE VEGETARIAN DIET

A common misconception about a vegetarian diet concerns protein. Many new vegetarians are frequently confronted with the question: "So how do you get your protein?" Individuals following a lacto–ovo-vegetarian diet rarely have to worry about protein. Even vegans eating a reasonably balanced diet with adequate calories can easily meet their protein needs.[1] In reality, it is much more likely that the individual is suffering from a dietary deficiency of a micronutrient, such as calcium or zinc, than a protein deficiency. Energy and protein can be of concern with some vegetarian diets, particularly if the individual follows severe and poorly informed dietary restrictions. Inadequate energy and protein intake with such unnecessarily restrictive intake patterns is a concern for infants during the weaning period and for children, particularly during growth spurts.[12] A well-planned

however, may rely heavily on high-fat dairy products, which may actually increase risk for cardiovascular disease. Other practical concerns for new and less experienced vegetarians include risks from unbalanced food patterns (Table 26.7).

Table 26.8 compares the typical dietary intake of vegans and lacto–ovo-vegetarians with omnivores, while the health risks/outcomes associated with specific kinds of vegetarian diets are mentioned in Table 26.9. The nutrients of special concern will vary depending on the type of vegetarian diet followed. As highlighted in Table 26.10, some nutrients are

## TABLE 26.8
## Nutrient Differences between Omnivore, Lacto–Ovo, and Vegan Dietary Patterns

| Dietary Component | Vegan | Lacto–Ovo | Omnivore |
|---|---|---|---|
| Total fat (% of total energy) | 15–30 | 34 | 34 |
| Saturated fat | Lower saturated-fat intake | Slightly lower saturated-fat intake | Generally higher saturated-fat intake |
| P/S ratio (polyunsaturated/saturated fat) | Higher P/S | Mod P/S | Low P/S |
| Fiber (g/day) | 30–60 | 20 | 15 |
| Carbohydrate (% total calories) | 50–65 | 50–55 | <50 |
| Protein (% of total calories) | 10–12 (none from animal sources) | 13.5 (~1/2 from animal sources) | 15 (~2/3 from animal sources) |
| Folate ($\mu$g/day ranges) | 170–385 | 214–455 | 252–471 |
| Cholesterol (mg dietary intake) | 0 | 210 | 300 |

*Sources:* Dewell, A. et al., *J. Am. Diet. Assoc.*, 108(2), 347, 2008; Farmer, B. et al., *J. Am. Diet. Assoc.*, 111(6), 819, 2011.

## TABLE 26.9
## Health Risks of Individuals Following Various Types of Vegetarian Diets

| Type of Vegetarian Diet | Health Risk Profile | Nutrients at Greatest Risk |
|---|---|---|
| Vegan | Lower risk of obesity, heart disease, cancer, hypertension, and diabetes. Vegans may have a lower health risk than lacto–ovo-vegetarians due to the typical lower fat and higher fiber content than either lacto–ovo-vegetarians or nonvegetarians. | Vitamin $B_{12}$<br>Vitamin D<br>Calcium<br>Zinc<br>Energy<br>Potentially iron |
| Lacto-vegetarian | Generally lower risk of obesity, heart disease, cancer, hypertension, and diabetes. Unskilled or new vegetarian may rely heavily on whole-milk-based products, thus consuming high-fat, saturated-fat, and cholesterol intakes, which could increase the risk of cardiovascular-related diseases. | Zinc<br>Potentially iron |
| Ovo-vegetarian | Generally lower risk of obesity, heart disease, cancer, hypertension, and diabetes. Unskilled or new vegetarian may rely heavily on eggs and egg-based products, thus consuming high-fat, saturated-fat, and cholesterol intakes, which could increase the risk of cardiovascular-related diseases. | Vitamin D<br>Calcium<br>Zinc<br>Potentially iron |
| Lacto–ovo-vegetarian | Generally lower risk of obesity, heart disease, cancer, hypertension, and diabetes. Unskilled or new vegetarian may rely heavily on whole-milk- or egg-based products, thus consuming high-fat, saturated-fat, and cholesterol intakes, which could increase the risk of cardiovascular-related diseases. | Zinc<br>Potentially iron |

*Source:* Craig, W.J. and Mangels, A.R., *J. Am. Diet. Assoc.*, 109(7), 1266, 2009.

## TABLE 26.10
## Critical Periods of Importance for Selected Nutrients

| Nutrient | Critical Periods during Life Cycle |
|---|---|
| Vitamin $B_{12}$ | Throughout, particularly critical during pregnancy, infancy, and childhood |
| Riboflavin ($B_2$) | Pregnancy, periods of growth |
| Vitamin D | Childhood and prepuberty, pregnancy, and elderly |
| Calcium | Childhood and prepuberty, elderly |
| Iron | Infancy, childhood, adolescence, pregnancy, and adulthood (women particularly) |
| Zinc | Puberty, pregnancy, and elderly |
| Iodine | Adolescence, pregnancy, and lactation |
| Protein | Infancy, childhood, adolescence, and pregnancy |
| Omega-3 fatty acids (especially DHA) | Pregnancy and infancy |
| Energy | Periods of growth, especially toddlers/preschoolers, due to small stomach capacity |

*Source:* Kohlmeier, M., *Nutrient Metabolism*, Academic Press, London, U.K., 2003.

vegetarian lifestyle, however, is associated with lower obesity risk in childhood and adolescence.[13]

Tables 26.11 through 26.13 provide information about essential and nonessential amino acids and protein complementation. In the 1970s, carefully complementing proteins at each meal was thought to be the only way that vegetarians could avoid protein deficiency. We now know that it is not necessary to combine proteins at each meal,[14] yet it is important to understand the terminology related to the body's protein needs and the principles of complementation.

Table 26.14 compares average protein intakes in the United States, while Tables 26.15 and 26.16 provide information about protein and nutrient-dense/energy-dense food sources. As an arbitrary guideline, foods with 2 g or less of protein were not included. The information about nutrient- and energy-dense foods can be useful for young children who may fill up quickly on a bulky vegetarian diet without meeting their calorie and nutrient needs.[11]

It is relatively easy to get the essential omega-6 fatty acids (linoleic acid, arachidonic acid, and a few others) from

### TABLE 26.11
### Definitions Related to Protein Complementation

| | |
|---|---|
| Complete protein | Contains all essential amino acids in ample amounts to meet biologic needs; amino acid pattern is very similar to humans |
| Incomplete protein | May be low in one or more amino acids; amino acid pattern is very different from humans |
| Limiting amino acid | The essential amino acids that are in the smallest supply in the food |
| Essential amino acid | Cannot be synthesized by the human body. Include histidine, isoleucine, leucine, lysine, methionine, phenylalanine, threonine, tryptophan, and valine |

*Source:* Craig, W.J. and Mangels, A.R., *J. Am. Diet. Assoc.*, 109(7), 1266, 2009.

### TABLE 26.12
### Limiting Essential Amino Acids and Vegan Sources

| Food | Limiting Amino Acids | Vegan Sources of the Limiting Amino Acids |
|---|---|---|
| Legumes | Methionine, cysteine | Grains, nuts, seeds, and soybeans |
| Cereals/grains | Lysine and threonine | Legumes |
| Nuts and seeds | Lysine | Legumes |
| Peanuts | Methionine, lysine, and threonine | Legumes, grains, nuts, seeds, and soybeans |
| Vegetables | Methionine | Grains, nuts, and seeds, and soybeans |
| Corn | Tryptophan, lysine, and threonine | Legumes, sesame and sunflower seeds, and soybeans |

*Source:* Craig, W.J. and Mangels, A.R., *J. Am. Diet. Assoc.*, 109(7), 1266, 2009.

### TABLE 26.13
### Guidelines for Protein Complementation

| Type of Vegetarian Diet | Guidelines for Complementation[a] |
|---|---|
| Lacto–ovo | Dairy products and eggs provide complete protein, as do other animal products. |
| Vegan | A vegan diet that contains a variety of grains, legumes, vegetables, seeds, and nuts over the course of a day in amounts to meet a person's calorie needs will provide adequate amino acids in appropriate amounts. These proteins in combination usually meet human needs for essential amino acids nearly as well as animal foods. |
| Any | It is not necessary to combine proteins in each meal. Young children, however, may need to have the complementary proteins consumed within a few hours of each other. |

*Sources:* Craig, W.J. and Mangels, A.R., *J. Am. Diet. Assoc.*, 109(7), 1266, 2009.

[a] All proteins except gelatin provide all of the amino acids. Some protein sources have relatively low levels of some amino acids, so a large amount of that food would need to be consumed if it were the only source of those "limiting" amino acids.[1]

**TABLE 26.14**

**Protein Intakes in the United States**

| Type of Diet | Percentage of Calories from Protein | Sufficient to Meet RDA? |
|---|---|---|
| Typical U.S. diet | 14–16 | Yes |
| Lacto–ovo-vegetarians | 13–14 | Yes, provided adequate calories are consumed |
| Vegans | 11–13 | Yes, provided adequate calories are consumed |

*Sources:* Haddad, E.H. et al., *Am. J. Clin. Nutr.*, 70(3 Suppl), 586S, 1999; Farmer, B. et al., *J. Am. Diet. Assoc.*, 111(6), 819, 2011.

plant-based foods. Corn oil and soybean oil are pervasive in the modern food supply, and most vegetarians and nonvegetarians get more than enough. It is important to recognize that high intake of these essential omega-6 fatty acids, particularly arachidonic acid from eggs (and meat in omnivores), tends to promote inflammation and other potentially harmful actions.[15]

Omega-3 fatty acids are polyunsaturated fatty acids that are essential in their own right. Omega-6 fatty acids cannot meet omega-3 fatty acid requirements. One type of omega-3 fatty acid, alpha-linolenic acid (ALA), is consumed with many vegetables and flaxseed or linseed oil. Two other types of omega-3 fatty acids are eicosapentaenoic acid (EPA) and docosahexaenoic acid (DHA), which are found mainly in cold-water ocean fish, such as salmon, char, herring, mackerel, and sardine; DHA and EPA are thought to reduce the risk of cardiovascular disease[16] through their effects on triglyceride levels and platelet aggregation.[17] Modest amounts of EPA and DHA can be produced from ALA through a complicated and very inefficient pathway that converts less than 1% of the available precursor ALA.[18] The fetus and the young infant have a dramatically reduced ability to perform this conversion. Growing fetuses and young infants need large amounts of DHA for brain and retinal development. Their mothers have to provide them with these crucial building blocks during pregnancy and breast-feeding. Women have to know that high intake of linoleic acid and other omega-6 fatty acids lower even further their already limited capacity to produce DHA from the ALA precursor. Many convenience foods, such as those with mayonnaise, contain large amounts of omega-6 fatty acids. Women may believe that they follow a particularly healthy diet by using generous amounts of cooking oils rich in linoleic fatty acid, but what counts for their child's and their own health is a high omega-3/omega-6 ratio as well as an adequate amount of omega-3 fatty acids.[15] They should favor foods that are rich in omega-3 fatty acids (flaxseed or linseed oil) and stay away from good sources of omega-6 fatty-rich foods like sunflower seeds and sunflower oil. Vegetarians can boost their long-chain omega-3 fatty acid intake by using DHA-enriched eggs or DHA supplements derived from

microscopic marine algae (phytoplankton). Table 26.17 lists vegetarian dietary sources of the omega-3 fatty acid ALA.

## MICRONUTRIENTS IN THE VEGETARIAN DIET

Although vegetarian dietary patterns can be extremely healthful,[1] certain micronutrients can be challenging to obtain in sufficient quantities depending on the specific dietary restrictions the individual follows. Tables 26.18 through 26.29 provide information about sources of micronutrients that can be of concern for some vegetarian individuals. As a guideline, foods with less than 5%–10% of the recommended amount of that particular nutrient per serving were not included in the table.

A few vitamins, particularly riboflavin (Table 26.18) and vitamin $B_{12}$ (Table 26.19), can be problematic in people who avoid all animal proteins. There is a common misconception that plant foods contain vitamin $B_{12}$. Commercial products from blue-green algae (*Spirulina* species) contain vitamin $B_{12}$–like compounds (cobalamin analogs) along with small amounts[19] of methylcobalamin (authentic vitamin $B_{12}$). However, biological tests indicate that these products cannot meet the vitamin $B_{12}$ requirements of mammals, because intrinsic factor does not mediate absorption well and the small absorbed amounts compete with normal vitamin $B_{12}$.[20] Synthetic vitamin $B_{12}$, free of animal products, is readily available at low cost. Vegetarians should not rely on algal products for their vitamin $B_{12}$ intake.

The issue of vitamin D has shifted in recent years. The Institute of Medicine recommends that younger adults get at least 600 IU/day and people over 70 years of age get 800 IU/day. Practice guidelines of the U.S. Endocrine Society suggest even higher intakes.[21] There is now a consensus that vegetarians and nonvegetarians alike without adequate sun exposure are hard put to get the necessary amounts from foods alone (Table 26.20).

Adolescent females, adult women, and the elderly may need to pay special attention to calcium adequacy. Table 26.21 lists foods and their calcium content. With many foods, the amount of calcium depends upon the brand, particularly in the case of fortified foods.

**TABLE 26.15**
**Protein: Vegetarian Sources and Amounts**

| Food | Portion Size | Protein (g) | kcal |
|---|---|---|---|
| Cereals/Grains | | | |
| Quinoa, cooked | 1 cup | 8.1 | 222 |
| Millet, cooked | 1 cup | 6.1 | 207 |
| Wheat germ, toasted | 0.25 cup | 8.2 | 108 |
| Bagel, plain | 1 medium bagel | 10.5 | 270 |
| Couscous, cooked | 1 cup | 6.0 | 176 |
| Macaroni, enriched, cooked | 1 cup | 8.1 | 221 |
| Pita, whole wheat | 1 large pita | 6.3 | 170 |
| Grape-Nuts, Post™ | 1 cup | 14.5 | 416 |
| Oatmeal crisp, crunchy almond, General Mills™ | 1 cup | 5.4 | 216 |
| Oatmeal, regular and quick | 0.5 cup dry | 5.3 | 154 |
| Oat bran, raw | 0.33 cup | 5.4 | 76 |
| Brown rice, medium grain, cooked | 1 cup | 4.5 | 218 |
| English muffin, plain | 1 muffin | 4.4 | 134 |
| Barley, pearled, cooked | 1 cup | 3.6 | 193 |
| Whole-wheat bread | 1 slice | 3.6 | 69 |
| Corn grits, instant, white, enriched | 1 oz packet dry | 2.2 | 105 |
| Vegetables | | | |
| Peas, green, canned | 0.5 cup | 3.9 | 60 |
| Corn, yellow, boiled | 0.5 cup | 2.5 | 72 |
| Broccoli, boiled | 0.5 cup | 1.9 | 27 |
| Fruits | | | |
| Prunes, dried | 10 prunes | 2.1 | 228 |
| Dairy/Soy Milk | | | |
| Cottage cheese, 1% fat | 1 cup | 28.0 | 163 |
| Yogurt, low fat (1.5% milk fat), plain | 1 cup | 11.9 | 143 |
| Gruyere cheese | 1 oz | 8.5 | 117 |
| Milk, low fat (1%) | 1 cup | 8.2 | 102 |
| Cheddar cheese | 1 oz | 7.1 | 114 |
| Soy milk | 1 cup | 8.0 | 131 |
| American processed cheese | 1 oz | 5.1 | 105 |
| Frozen yogurt, soft serve | 0.5 cup | 2.9 | 114 |
| Ice cream, vanilla, regular (10% fat) | 0.5 cup | 2.3 | 137 |
| Beans/Legumes | | | |
| Soybean nuts, dry, roasted | 0.5 cup | 34.0 | 388 |
| Lentils, boiled | 1 cup | 17.9 | 230 |
| Lima beans, boiled | 1 cup | 11.6 | 209 |
| Kidney beans, canned | 1 cup | 13.4 | 210 |
| Garbanzo beans, canned | 1 cup | 11.8 | 211 |
| Soy Products/Meat Substitutes | | | |
| Tofu, raw, firm | 0.5 cup | 19.9 | 183 |
| Tempeh | 0.5 cup | 15.4 | 160 |
| Griller's original, Morningstar Farms™, frozen | 1 patty | 15.3 | 136 |
| Soybeans, green, boiled | 0.5 cup | 11.1 | 127 |
| Garden veggie patties, Morningstar Farms, frozen | 1 patty | 11.9 | 118 |
| Meatless meatballs | 1 cup | 30.2 | 284 |
| Nuts/Seeds | | | |
| Peanut butter, chunk style/crunchy | 2 T | 7.7 | 188 |
| Sunflower seeds, dried | 1 oz | 5.9 | 165 |
| Almonds, blanched | 1 oz | 6.1 | 167 |
| Sesame butter (tahini) | 2 T | 5.1 | 178 |
| Cashews, dry roasted | 1 oz | 4.3 | 163 |

**TABLE 26.15 (continued)**
**Protein: Vegetarian Sources and Amounts**

| Food | Portion Size | Protein (g) | kcal |
|---|---|---|---|
| Eggs | | | |
|    Egg substitute, frozen | 0.25 cup | 6.0 | 29 |
|    Egg, chicken, whole, fresh/frozen | 1 large | 6.3 | 72 |
|    Egg, chicken, yolk fresh | 1 large | 2.7 | 55 |
| Mixed Foods | | | |
|    Burritos with beans and cheese | 2 burritos | 18.2 | 570 |
|    Biscuit with egg | 1 item | 11.6 | 373 |
|    Potato, baked, with sour cream and chives | 1 potato | 6.7 | 393 |

*Sources:* Trumbo, P. et al., *J. Am. Diet. Assoc.*, 102(11), 1621, 2002; U.S. Department of Agriculture ARS, USDA National Nutrient Database for Standard Reference, Release 24, 2011.

Adult RDA: males 56 g/day, females 46 g/day; taking into account the lower digestibility and amino acid profile, a reasonable RDA for vegans is approximately 10% more protein than omnivores.

One trace element in potentially limited supply in strictly vegetarian foods is iodine. Iodized salt and sea salt are readily available sources. Other sources can be milk (from feed additives and disinfectants) and bread (from iodate conditioners and iodized salt), but the content is unpredictable and has declined in the last few decades.[22] The amounts given in Table 26.23 can only reflect averages and can differ greatly between brands and batches.

Fruits and vegetables contain relatively little iron. Flour and some grains are fortified with iron in the United States and Canada. Legumes contain slightly more iron, but still less than meat. At the same time, much more of the heme iron associated with hemoglobin and myoglobin in meats can be absorbed than of the nonheme iron of plant-based foods. This means that vegetarians have to make sure they get enough iron, particularly young women with their higher iron needs (typically 18 mg/day). Similarly, the zinc content of plant-based foods is very modest compared to meats. Seafood and fish are a very good source of zinc for those who use such foods. Table 26.24 lists nonheme sources of iron, while Table 26.28 shows zinc content of some vegetarian foods.

Some constituents of plant-based foods lower the bioavailability of minerals and decrease the amount that reaches blood and tissues, but other compounds actually improve absorption. Tables 26.25 and 26.29 list factors that may enhance or inhibit the absorption of iron and zinc. Polyphenols (including tannins in tea) and phytates, for example, reduce absorption of nonheme iron, but ascorbic acid and other organic acids in fruits and vegetables are powerful promoters of absorption.[23] Vegetarians should pay close attention, therefore, to food pairings and avoid drinking tea with their main meals. Fruits and fruit juices, on the other hand, help them make the most of their limited trace mineral supplies. Neither inhibitors nor enhancers would significantly affect absorption of heme-iron absorption.

## NONNUTRITIVE AND OTHER IMPORTANT FACTORS IN THE VEGETARIAN DIET

Typical vegetarian diets are rich in many beneficial nonnutritive factors such as dietary fiber and phytochemicals.[24–26] Tables 26.30 and 26.31 provide information about sources of these beneficial but nonnutritive factors.

## EFFECTS OF COOKING, STORAGE, AND PROCESSING ON THE CRITICAL NUTRIENTS

Cooking, storage, and processing methods can influence the amount of a nutrient present in a food. Table 26.32 presents the effects of cooking, storage, and processing on the nutrients that may be of concern in a vegetarian diet.

## GENERAL VITAMIN AND MINERAL DEFICIENCY AND TOXICITY SYMPTOMS

It is important for practitioners to be aware of the symptoms of nutrient deficiencies in any patient. As a group, vegetarians tend to be more health conscious and knowledgeable about nutrition than the general public.[1] Some vegetarians choose megadoses of vitamins or minerals to combat real or perceived threats to their health. Therefore, toxicity may be more of a risk than a nutrient deficiency. Table 26.33 presents deficiency and toxicity symptoms of the nutrients potentially at risk in a vegetarian diet.

## SAMPLE MEAL PLANS

Tables 26.34 through 26.37 present sample meal plans for adults and children following a lacto–ovo or a vegan diet. These menus provide the recommended dietary allowances (RDA) for protein while presenting an appropriate macronutrient breakdown within the estimated energy expenditure.

## TABLE 26.16
## Vegetarian Sources of Energy-Dense, Nutrient-Dense Foods

| Food | Portion Size | kcal |
|---|---|---|
| Cereals/grains | | |
| Granola, low fat, with raisins, Kellogg™'s | 1 cup | 379 |
| Quinoa, cooked | 1 cup | 222 |
| Millet, cooked | 1 cup | 207 |
| Pancakes, blueberry | 3 cakes (4") | 253 |
| Oatmeal Crisp, crunchy almond, General Mills | 1 cup | 216 |
| Grape-Nuts, Post | 0.5 cup | 208 |
| Macaroni, enriched, cooked | 1 cup elbows | 221 |
| Bagel, plain | 1 medium bagel | 270 |
| Raisin Bran, dry | 1 cup | 189 |
| Corn muffin | 1 muffin | 188 |
| Pita, whole wheat | 1 pita (6.5 in diameter) | 170 |
| Blueberry muffin, from recipe | 1 muffin | 162 |
| Oat bran muffin | 1 muffin | 305 |
| Vegetables | | |
| Potatoes, mashed from granules | 1 cup | 227 |
| Fruits | | |
| Avocado, California, raw | 0.5 medium | 114 |
| Raisins, golden, seedless | 0.66 cup | 289 |
| Mixed fruit, dried, diced, Delmonte™ | 0.66 cup | 220 |
| Dairy/soy milk | | |
| Milk shake, thick vanilla | 1 cup | 254 |
| Yogurt, flavored, low fat, 1% milk fat, Breyers™ | 1 cup | 218 |
| Ricotta cheese, part skim | 0.5 cup | 171 |
| Cottage cheese (1% fat) | 1 cup | 163 |
| Pudding, banana, from instant mix, 2% milk | 0.5 cup | 154 |
| Milk, whole | 1 cup | 149 |
| Cheddar cheese | 1 oz | 113 |
| Milk, low fat (1%) | 1 cup | 102 |
| Soy milk, SILK™, plain | 1 cup | 100 |
| Beans/legumes | | |
| Soybean, dried, boiled, mature | 1 cup | 298 |
| Garbanzo beans, canned, solids, and liquids | 1 cup | 211 |
| Lentils, boiled, with salt | 1 cup | 226 |
| Soy products/meat substitutes | | |
| Soybean nuts (dry roasted) | 0.5 cup | 388 |
| Tempeh | 1 cup | 320 |
| Soyburger with cheese | 1 each | 316 |
| Chicken nuggets, meatless | 5 pieces | 238 |
| Frankfurter, meatless | 1 each | 102 |
| Nuts/seeds | | |
| Peanut butter, chunky style | 2 T | 188 |
| Almonds, blanched | 1 oz | 167 |
| Sesame butter (tahini) | 2 T | 178 |
| Sunflower seeds, dry roasted | 1 oz | 165 |
| Mixed foods | | |
| Egg salad | 1 cup | 586 |
| Burritos, with beans | 2 burritos | 447 |
| Potato, baked, with sour cream and chives | 1 potato | 393 |
| Shells and cheese, from mix | 1 cup | 360 |
| Peanut butter and jam sandwich on wheat | 1 each | 344 |
| Cheese enchilada | 1 item | 319 |
| Biscuit with egg | 1 item | 373 |
| Lasagna, no meat, recipe | 1 piece | 298 |
| Chili, meatless, canned | 0.66 cup | 190 |
| Trail mix, regular | 0.25 cup | 173 |

### TABLE 26.16 (continued)
### Vegetarian Sources of Energy-Dense, Nutrient-Dense Foods

| Food | Portion Size | kcal |
| --- | --- | --- |
| Vegetable soup, vegetarian, canned, condensed | 1 cup | 145 |
| Pizza, cheese, fast food chain | 1/8 of 14 in. | 285 |
| Pasta with marinara sauce | 1 cup | 180–450 |

*Sources:* U.S. Department of Agriculture ARS, USDA National Nutrient Database for Standard Reference, Release 24, 2011; Pennington, J., *Bowes & Church's Food Values of Portions Commonly Used*, 17th edn., Lippincott-Raven, Philadelphia, PA, 1998; Hands, E., *Food Finder: Food Sources of Vitamins & Minerals*, ESHA Research, Salem, OR, 1995.

### TABLE 26.17
### Omega-3 Fatty Acids: Vegetarian Sources and Amounts

| Food | Portion Size | ALA(18:3) (mg) | kcal |
| --- | --- | --- | --- |
| Animal products | | | |
| Egg | 1 large | EPA: 2 | 78 |
| Egg from chickens fed flax | 1 egg | DHA: 60–100 | |
| Eggs from chickens fed microalgae | 1 egg | DHA: 100–150 | |
| Cereals/grains | | | |
| Oats, germ | 0.25 cup | 0.4 | 119 |
| Wheat germ | 0.25 cup | 0.2 | 104 |
| Barley, bran | 0.25 cup | 0.1 | 115 |
| Vegetables | | | |
| Soybeans, green, raw | 0.5 cup | 4.1 | 188 |
| Kale, raw, chopped | 1 cup | 0.1 | 34 |
| Broccoli, raw, chopped | 1 cup | 0.1 | 30 |
| Cauliflower, raw | 1 cup | 0.1 | 27 |
| Sea vegetables | | | |
| Nori, dried | 1 sheet | EPA: 0.2 | |
| | | DHA: 0 | |
| Fruits | | | |
| Avocados, California, raw | 1 medium | 0.2 | 306 |
| Dairy/soy milk | | | |
| Cheese, Roquefort™ | 1 oz | 0.2 | 105 |
| Beans/legumes | | | |
| Soybeans, dry roasted | 0.5 cup | 1.5 | 388 |
| Beans, pinto, boiled | 1 cup | 0.2 | 245 |
| Nuts/seeds | | | |
| Butternuts (dried) | 1 oz | 2.4 | 174 |
| Walnuts, dried, English/Persian | 1 oz | 1.9 | 185 |
| Fats/oils/dressings | | | |
| Flaxseed oil | 1 T | 7.5 | 120 |
| Flaxseed, ground | 1 T | 2.2 | 37 |
| Canola oil (rapeseed oil) | 1 T | 1.6 | 124 |
| Walnut oil | 1 T | 1.5 | 120 |
| Salad dressing, comm., mayonnaise, soybean | 2 T | 1.4 | 99 |
| Soybean oil | 1 T | 1.0 | 124 |
| Wheat germ oil | 1 T | 1.0 | 124 |
| Salad dressing, comm., Italian, regular | 2 T | 1.0 | 140 |

*Sources:* Trumbo, P. et al., *J. Am. Diet. Assoc.*, 102(11), 1621, 2002; Pennington, J., *Bowes & Church's Food Values of Portions Commonly Used*, 17th edn., Lippincott-Raven, Philadelphia, PA, 1998; Hands, E., *Food Finder: Food Sources of Vitamins & Minerals*, ESHA Research, Salem, OR, 1995.

Acceptable distribution range: males, 0.6–1.2 g/day; females, 0.6–1.2 g/day; about 10% of this from long-chain omega-3 fatty acids (EPA, DHA, and others).

**TABLE 26.18**
**Riboflavin[a]: Vegetarian Sources and Amounts**

| Food | Portion Size | Riboflavin (mg) | kcal |
|---|---|---|---|
| Cereals[b,c]/grains | | | |
| Raisin Bran, Post | 1 cup (2.1 oz) | 0.43 | 189 |
| Bran flakes | 0.66 cup (1 oz) | 0.38 | 84 |
| Cornflakes, Kellogg's | 1 cup (1 oz) | 0.74 | 102 |
| Bagel, plain | 1 bagel (3.5 in.) | 0.27 | 270 |
| Sesame breadsticks | 2 sticks | 0.22 | 120 |
| Pita, white, enriched | 1 pita (6.5 in. diameter) | 0.20 | 165 |
| Lasagna noodles | 2 oz dry | 0.24 | 219 |
| Corn bread, homemade from 2% milk | 1 slice | 0.19 | 173 |
| English muffin, wheat | 1 muffin | 0.17 | 127 |
| English muffin, plain | 1 muffin | 0.14 | 129 |
| Muffin, blueberry, homemade (2.75 × 2 in.) | 1 muffin | 0.16 | 162 |
| Macaroni, enriched and cooked | 1 cup | 0.19 | 221 |
| Wild rice, cooked | 1 cup | 0.14 | 166 |
| Rye bread | 1 slice | 0.11 | 83 |
| Vegetables | | | |
| Mushrooms, boiled | 0.5 cup | 0.23 | 22 |
| Tomato puree, canned | 1 cup | 0.20 | 95 |
| Sweet potatoes, baked, with skin | 1 medium | 0.12 | 103 |
| Tomato, red, sun dried | 0.5 cup | 0.13 | 70 |
| Garden cress, boiled | 0.5 cup | 0.11 | 16 |
| Fruits | | | |
| Raisins, golden seedless | 0.66 cup | 0.18 | 289 |
| Banana | 1 medium | 0.09 | 64 |
| Raspberries, raw | 1 cup | 0.05 | 60 |
| Avocado, Calif. raw | 0.5 medium | 0.10 | 114 |
| Dairy/soy milk | | | |
| Yogurt, plain, low fat | 1 cup | 0.49 | 143 |
| Milk, whole | 1 cup | 0.41 | 149 |
| Cottage cheese, 1% fat | 1 cup | 0.37 | 163 |
| Milk, nonfat | 1 cup | 0.45 | 83 |
| Feta cheese | 1 oz | 0.24 | 75 |
| Ricotta cheese, part skim | 0.5 cup | 0.23 | 171 |
| Soy milk, plain, SILK | 1 cup | 0.51 | 100 |
| Cheddar cheese, low fat | 1 oz | 0.06 | 49 |
| Cheddar cheese | 1 oz | 0.11 | 114 |
| Goat cheese, soft | 1 oz | 0.11 | 76 |
| Beans/Legumes | | | |
| Soybeans, mature, boiled | 1 cup | 0.49 | 298 |
| Kidney beans, canned, all types | 1 cup | 0.13 | 210 |
| Great northern beans, canned | 1 cup | 0.16 | 299 |
| Pinto beans, canned | 1 cup | 0.04 | 197 |
| Lentils, boiled | 1 cup | 0.14 | 230 |
| Soy products/meat substitutes | | | |
| Chicken nuggets, meatless | 5 pieces | 0.11 | 238 |
| Spicy black-bean burger, Morningstar Farms | 1 patty | 0.20 | 115 |
| Breakfast links, Morningstar Farms | 2 links | 0.27 | 72 |
| Tofu, raw, firm | 0.5 cup | 0.13 | 183 |

**TABLE 26.18 (continued)**
**Riboflavin[a]: Vegetarian Sources and Amounts**

| Food | Portion Size | Riboflavin (mg) | kcal |
|---|---|---|---|
| Nuts/seeds | | | |
| Almonds, dry roasted | 1 oz | 0.27 | 169 |
| Eggs | | | |
| Egg, chicken, hard boiled | 1 large | 0.26 | 78 |
| Egg substitute, frozen | 0.25 cup | 0.23 | 29 |
| Mixed foods | | | |
| Bean burrito | 2 each | 0.61 | 447 |
| Cheese enchilada | 1 each | 0.42 | 319 |
| Egg omelet with onion, pepper, tomato, and mushroom | 1 each | 0.34 | 125 |
| Vegetarian chili, fat-free with black beans, Health Valley™ | 5 oz | 0.26 | 70 |
| Beverages | | | |
| Coffee substitute with milk | 0.75 cup | 0.30 | 120 |
| Miscellaneous | | | |
| Brewer's yeast | 1 T | 0.34 | 23 |

*Sources:* U.S. Department of Agriculture ARS. USDA National Nutrient Database for Standard Reference, Release 24, 2011; Pennington, J., *Bowes & Church's Food Values of Portions Commonly Used*, 17th edn., Lippincott-Raven, Philadelphia, PA, 1998; Yates, A.A. et al., *J. Am. Diet. Assoc.*, 98(6), 699, 1998.

Adult RDA: males 1.3 mg/day, females 1.1 mg/day.

[a] Also called vitamin $B_2$.

[b] Most fortified breakfast cereals contain 0.43–0.51 mg/serving.

[c] Many "100% natural" breakfast cereals are not enriched and contain 0.03–0.12 mg/serving.

**TABLE 26.19**
**Vitamin B₁₂: Vegetarian Sources and Amounts**

| Food | Portion Size | Vitamin B$_{12}$ (µg) | kcal |
|------|-------------|------------------------|------|
| Cereals[a]/grains | | | |
| Total whole grain, General Mills | 1 cup | 8.00 | 133 |
| Complete Oat Bran Flakes, Kellogg's | 1 cup | 8.04 | 140 |
| Cornflakes, Kellogg's | 1 cup | 2.65 | 102 |
| Special K Granola, low fat, Kellogg's | 0.5 cup | 2.08 | 196 |
| Kix, General Mills | 1.5 cup | 2.05 | 132 |
| Eggo low-fat Homestyle waffle, Kellogg's | 2 waffles | 1.10 | 165 |
| Waffle, prepared at home | 1 each | 0.26 | 218 |
| Dairy/soy milk[b] | | | |
| Soy milk, enhanced | 1 cup | 2.62 | 109 |
| Cottage cheese, 1% fat | 1 cup | 1.42 | 163 |
| Milk, skim | 1 cup | 1.22 | 83 |
| Yogurt, flavored, low fat, 1% milk fat, Breyers | 1 cup | 1.20 | 218 |
| Milk, whole | 1 cup | 1.10 | 149 |
| Yogurt, whole, plain | 1 cup | 0.84 | 138 |
| Yogurt, nonfat, vanilla, low-calorie sweetener | 6 oz | 0.73 | 73 |
| Buttermilk, cultured, low fat | 1 cup | 0.54 | 98 |
| Feta cheese | 1 oz | 0.48 | 75 |
| Swiss cheese | 1 oz | 0.95 | 108 |
| Ricotta cheese, part skim | 0.5 cup | 0.36 | 171 |
| American processed cheese food | 1 oz | 0.38 | 94 |
| Cheddar cheese | 1 oz | 0.24 | 114 |
| Soy products/meat substitutes[c] | | | |
| Breakfast links, Morningstar | 2 each | 3.33 | 72 |
| Chik'n Nuggets, Morningstar | 4 pieces | 1.81 | 190 |
| Soy burger with cheese | 1 each | 1.72 | 316 |
| Soy burger | 1 each | 1.14 | 124 |
| Tempeh | 1 cup | 0.13 | 320 |
| Eggs | | | |
| Egg, chicken, hard boiled | 1 large | 0.56 | 78 |
| Mixed foods | | | |
| Spinach soufflé | 1 cup | 0.54 | 230 |
| Cheese pizza | 1 piece (1/8 of a 14 in. pie) | 0.45 | 285 |
| Miscellaneous | | | |
| Fortified nutritional yeast (Red Star T6635) | 1 T | 4.0 | 40 |

*Sources:* U.S. Department of Agriculture ARS, USDA National Nutrient Database for Standard Reference, Release 24, 2011; Pennington, J., *Bowes & Church's Food Values of Portions Commonly Used*, 17th edn., Lippincott-Raven, Philadelphia, PA, 1998; Yates, A.A. et al., *J. Am. Diet. Assoc.*, 98(6), 699, 1998.

Adult RDA: 2.4 µg/day.

[a] Some commercial cereals are not fortified with vitamin B$_{12}$; check labels carefully.
[b] Subject to fortification; unfortified soy milk contains no vitamin B$_{12}$.
[c] Subject of fortification; check labels of individual product carefully.

**TABLE 26.20**

**Vitamin D: Vegetarian Sources and Amounts**

| Food | Portion Size | Vitamin D (IU)[a] | kcal |
|---|---|---|---|
| Cereals/grains | | | |
| Raisin Bran, Post | 1 cup (2.1 oz) | 40 | 189 |
| Corn Pops, Kellogg's | 1 cup | 51 | 124 |
| Lucky Charms, General Mills | 1 cup | 53 | 147 |
| Cornflakes | 1 cup (1 oz) | 36 | 100 |
| Granola, low fat, Kellogg's Special K | 0.33 cup | 26 | 129 |
| Dairy/soy milk | | | |
| Soy milk, plain, SILK | 1 cup | 119 | 100 |
| Milk, nonfat | 1 cup | 115 | 83 |
| Milk, whole | 1 cup | 124 | 149 |
| Pudding, vanilla, instant, with whole milk | 0.5 cup | 49 | 162 |
| Eggs | | | |
| Egg, chicken, hard boiled | 1 large | 44 | 78 |
| Egg yolk, raw | 1 each | 37 | 55 |
| Mixed foods | | | |
| Soup, tomato bisque, with milk | 1 cup | 49 | 198 |
| Egg salad | 0.5 cup | 38 | 293 |
| Egg omelet with mushroom | 1 each (69 g) | 36 | 91 |
| Fats/oils/dressings | | | |
| Margarine, hard, hydrogenated soybean[b] | 1 tsp | 20 | 34 |
| Desserts | | | |
| Egg custard pie, frozen, baked | 1 piece (105 g) | 36 | 220 |
| Chocolate-filled crepe | 1 each (78 g) | 28 | 119 |

*Sources:* Ross, A.C. et al., eds., *Dietary Reference Intakes for Calcium and Vitamin D*, National Academies Press, Washington, DC, 2011; Pennington, J., *Bowes & Church's Food Values of Portions Commonly Used*, 17th edn., Lippincott-Raven, Philadelphia, PA, 1998; Hands, E., *Food Finder: Food Sources of Vitamins & Minerals*, ESHA Research, Salem, OR, 1995.

Adult AI: 15 μg cholecalciferol (600 IU/day).

[a] 1 IU vitamin D = 0.025 μg cholecalciferol.

[b] Subject to fortification; check labels.

**TABLE 26.21**
**Calcium: Vegetarian Sources and Amounts**

| Food | Portion Size | Calcium (mg) | kcal |
|---|---|---|---|
| Cereals/grains | | | |
| Calcium-fortified cereal bars | 1 bar (37 g) | 200 | 120 |
| Vegetables | | | |
| Collards, frozen, boiled | 0.5 cup | 178 | 31 |
| Kale, frozen, boiled | 1 cup | 179 | 39 |
| Turnip greens, canned | 0.5 cup | 138 | 16 |
| Squash, acorn, baked | 1 cup | 90 | 115 |
| Okra, boiled | 0.5 cup | 62 | 18 |
| Squash, butternut, baked | 1 cup | 84 | 82 |
| Broccoli, cooked | 1 cup | 62 | 55 |
| Peas, green, cooked, from frozen | 0.5 cup | 19 | 62 |
| Fruits | | | |
| Calcium-fortified orange juice | 8 oz | 500 | 117 |
| Dairy/soy milk | | | |
| Soy milk, plain, SILK, fortified | 8 oz (1 cup) | 299 | 100 |
| Malted drink mix, chocolate, prepared w/ whole milk | 8 oz | 368 | 231 |
| Evaporated milk, skim | 4 oz | 370 | 100 |
| Evaporated milk, whole | 4 oz | 329 | 169 |
| Goat's milk | 8 oz (1 cup) | 327 | 168 |
| Yogurt, tofu yogurt, frozen | 8 oz | 309 | 254 |
| Cow's milk, skim | 8 oz (1 cup) | 299 | 83 |
| Cow's milk, 1% | 8 oz (1 cup) | 305 | 102 |
| Cow's milk, 2% | 8 oz (1 cup) | 293 | 122 |
| Cow's milk, whole | 8 oz (1 cup) | 276 | 149 |
| Yogurt, fat-free, fruit variety | 8 oz | 345 | 216 |
| Yogurt, low-fat, low-calorie sweetener | 8 oz | 372 | 257 |
| Yogurt, regular | 8 oz | 296 | 149 |
| Swiss cheese | 1 oz | 221 | 106 |
| Cheddar cheese | 1 oz | 202 | 113 |
| American cheese | 1 oz | 293 | 104 |
| Mozzarella cheese, part skim | 1 oz | 222 | 72 |
| Feta cheese | 1 oz | 140 | 75 |
| Soy milk, nonfortified | 8 oz (1 cup) | 61 | 131 |
| Cottage cheese, 1% fat | 0.5 cup | 69 | 81 |
| Beans/legumes | | | |
| Great northern beans, cooked | 0.5 cup | 60 | 104 |
| Soy products/meat substitutes | | | |
| Tofu, raw, firm, prepared w/ calcium sulfate | 0.5 cup | 861 | 183 |
| Tempeh | 1 cup | 184 | 320 |
| Nuts/seeds | | | |
| Almonds, dried | 1 oz (about 24 nuts) | 75 | 163 |
| Desserts | | | |
| Custard, 2% milk | 1 cup | 358 | 274 |
| Sherbet, orange | 1 cup | 80 | 213 |
| Soft-serve ice cream, French vanilla | 1 cup | 225 | 382 |
| Frozen yogurt, soft serve, vanilla | 1 cup | 206 | 229 |
| Ice cream, vanilla, rich | 1 cup | 250 | 533 |

*Sources:* Ross, A.C. et al., eds., *Dietary Reference Intakes for Calcium and Vitamin D*, National Academies Press, Washington, DC, 2011; U.S. Department of Agriculture ARS, USDA National Nutrient Database for Standard Reference, Release 24, 2011.

Adult RDA: males, 1000 mg/day; females, 1000 mg/day.

**TABLE 26.22**
**Copper[a]: Vegetarian Sources[b] and Amounts**

| Food | Portion Size | Copper (mg) | kcal |
|---|---|---|---|
| Cereals/grains | | | |
| Raisin Bran, Kellogg's | 1 cup | 0.255 | 250 |
| Granola, low fat, Quaker™, with raisins | 0.5 cup | 0.133 | 190 |
| Vegetables | | | |
| Vegetable juice cocktail, canned | 1 cup | 0.484 | 61 |
| Potatoes, baked, with skin | 1 each (122 g) | 0.238 | 138 |
| Fruits | | | |
| Avocado, California | 1 each | 0.46 | 227 |
| Prunes, dehydrated, cooked | 0.5 cup | 0.29 | 158 |
| Dairy/soy milk | | | |
| Soy milk | 1 cup | 0.314 | 131 |
| Beans/legumes | | | |
| Beans, adzuki, canned, sweetened | 0.5 cup | 0.38 | 351 |
| Beans, black, cooked, boiled, no salt | 1 cup | 0.359 | 227 |
| Great northern beans | 1 cup | 0.437 | 209 |
| Garbanzo beans, boiled | 0.5 cup | 0.29 | 134 |
| Soy products/meat substitutes | | | |
| Tempeh | 1 cup | 1.11 | 320 |
| Luncheon slice, meatless | 1 piece (67 g) | 0.61 | 127 |
| Soy burger with cheese | 1 each | 0.56 | 316 |
| Tofu, raw, firm, calcium sulfate | 0.5 cup | 0.48 | 183 |
| Miso | 1 cup | 0.289 | 547 |
| Nuts and seeds | | | |
| Cashew, dry roasted | 0.25 cup | 0.76 | 197 |
| Sunflower seeds, toasted | 0.25 cup | 0.61 | 207 |
| Almonds | 1 oz (24 medium nuts) | 0.282 | 169 |
| Hazelnuts/filberts | 1 oz (21 whole nuts) | 0.89 | 178 |
| English walnuts | 1 oz (14 halves) | 0.45 | 175 |

*Sources:* Trumbo, P. et al., *J. Am. Diet. Assoc.*, 101(3), 294, 2001; U.S. Department of Agriculture ARS, USDA National Nutrient Database for Standard Reference, Release 24, 2011; Pennington, J., *Bowes & Church's Food Values of Portions Commonly Used*, 17th edn., Lippincott-Raven, Philadelphia, PA, 1998.

Adult RDA: males, 900 µg/day (0.9 mg); females, 900 µg/day (0.9 mg).

[a] Severe copper deficiency is rare in humans with no dietary deficiency documented. Generally this is only seen with extended supplemental feeding/total nutrition through manufactured nutrition such as total parenteral nutrition or impaired utilization.[32]

[b] High zinc intake (from supplements, denture adhesive, and other sources) can cause copper deficiency.[2]

**TABLE 26.23**
**Iodine: Vegetarian Sources and Amounts**

| Food | Portion Size | Iodine (µg) | kcal |
|---|---|---|---|
| Cereals/grains | | | |
| Rice, white, enriched, cooked, long grain | 0.5 cup (82.5 g) | 52.0 | 81 |
| Bread, corn bread, homemade | 1 piece (65 g) | 44.2 | 176 |
| Fruit flavored, sweetened | 1.1 oz (32 g) | 41.0 | 120 |
| Roll, white | 2 rolls (38 g) | 31.0 | 100 |
| Muffin, blueberry/plain | 1 each (50 g) | 28.5 | 150 |
| Tortilla, flour, 7–8 in. diameter | 1 each (35 g) | 26.3 | 114 |
| Cornflakes | 1 oz (28 g) | 26.0 | 102 |
| Bread, white | 1 slice (28.4 g) | 26.8 | 76.4 |
| Pancakes, from mix, 4" | 1 each (38 g) | 21.0 | 74 |
| Crisped rice | 1 oz (28 g) | 18.5 | 111 |
| Noodles, egg, enriched, boiled | 1 cup (160 g) | 17.6 | 213 |
| Bread, whole wheat | 1 slice (28 g) | 17.6 | 69 |
| Bread, rye, American | 1 slice (32 g) | 15.7 | 83 |
| Vegetables | | | |
| Potato, boiled with peel | 1 each (202 g) | 62.6 | 220 |
| Fruit cocktail, heavy syrup, canned | 0.5 cup (128 g) | 42.2 | 93 |
| Potato, scalloped, homemade | 0.5 cup (122 g) | 37.8 | 105 |
| Navy beans, boiled | 0.5 cup (91 g) | 35.5 | 129 |
| Lima beans, baby, frozen, boiled | 0.5 cup (90 g) | 27.9 | 95 |
| Orange breakfast drink (from dry) | 1 cup | 27.3 | 114 |
| Prunes, heavy syrup | 5 each (86 g) | 26.8 | 90 |
| Cowpeas/black-eyed peas | 0.5 cup (85 g) | 22.1 | 112 |
| Dairy/soy milk | | | |
| Yogurt, low fat, plain | 1 cup | 87.2 | 155 |
| Buttermilk, skim, cultured | 1 cup | 60.0 | 99 |
| 2% fat milk | 1 cup | 56.6 | 137 |
| Cottage cheese 1% fat | 1 cup | 56.5 | 164 |
| Nonfat milk | 1 cup | 56.4 | 85.5 |
| Whole milk, 3.3% | 1 cup | 56.1 | 150 |
| Fruit yogurt, low fat | 1 cup | 45.3 | 250 |
| Eggs | | | |
| Fried in margarine | 1 each (46 g) | 29 | 92 |
| Scrambled, with milk, in margarine | 1 large (61 g) | 26.6 | 101 |
| Soft boiled | 1 each (50 g) | 24 | 78 |
| Mixed foods | | | |
| Grilled cheese on wheat | 1 each (118 g) | 28.9 | 392 |
| Macaroni and cheese, box mix | 0.5 cup | 17.3 | 199 |
| Condiments/seasonings | | | |
| Salt, Morton light salt mixture | 1 tsp | 119 | 0 |

*Sources:* Trumbo, P. et al., *J. Am. Diet. Assoc.*, 101(3), 294, 2001; Pennington, J., *Bowes & Church's Food Values of Portions Commonly Used*, 17th edn., Lippincott-Raven, Philadelphia, PA, 1998; Hands, E., *Food Finder: Food Sources of Vitamins & Minerals*, ESHA Research, Salem, OR, 1995.
Adult RDA 150 µg males and females.

**TABLE 26.24**

**Iron: Nonheme Sources in the Vegetarian Diet**

| Food | Portion Size | Total Iron (mg) | kcal |
|---|---|---|---|
| Cereals/grains | | | |
| Raisin Bran, dry | 0.75 cup (44.25 g) | Range: 5.65–13.5 | 200 |
| Quinoa, cooked | 1 cup (185 g) | 2.76 | 222 |
| Cornflakes, dry | 0.75 cup (15.7–23.28 g) | 3.04–10.13 | 57–83 |
| Oatmeal, instant, fortified, Quaker, regular, organic | 1 packet (41 g) | 1.72 | 150 |
| Special K, regular | 0.75 cup (23.25 g) | 6.51 | 85 |
| Oat bran muffin | 1 med (113 g) | 4.75 | 305 |
| Shredded wheat, dry, plain | 1 oz (46 g) | 1.36 | 155 |
| Bagel, enriched, plain or with seeds | 1, 3.5 in. diameter | 6.35 | 270 |
| Vegetables | | | |
| Potato, baked, flesh and skin | 1 med (173 g) | 1.87 | 161 |
| Asparagus, pieces, frozen, cooked and drained | 1 cup (180 g) | 1.01 | 32 |
| Peas, green, cooked, drained, no salt added | 0.5 cup (80 g) | 1.23 | 67 |
| Spinach, boiled, drained, no salt added | 0.5 cup (90 g) | 3.21 | 21 |
| Fruits | | | |
| Prune juice, canned | 1 cup (256 g) | 3.02 | 182 |
| Figs, dried | 5 each (42 g) | 0.86 | 105 |
| Raisins, seedless | 1 small box (43 g) | 0.81 | 129 |
| Prunes, dried | 5 each (47.5 g) | 0.44 | 114 |
| Soups and beans | | | |
| Split pea soup, canned | 1 cup | 1.95 | 180 |
| Lentil soup, canned | 1 cup | 5.39 | 280 |
| Black bean, canned | 1 cup | 1.85 | 114 |
| Kidney beans, boiled, canned | 0.5 cup (128 g) | 1.50 | 105 |
| Navy beans, canned | 0.5 cup (131 g) | 2.42 | 148 |
| Chickpeas, canned, drained | 0.5 cup (76 g) | 0.81 | 106 |
| Chickpeas, cooked, boiled with salt | 0.5 cup (82 g) | 2.37 | 134 |
| Soybeans, green, boiled | 0.5 cup (90 g) | 2.25 | 127 |
| Pinto beans, frozen, boiled | 3.33 oz (94 g) | 2.55 | 152 |
| Pinto beans, canned | 0.5 cup (1/3 can or 94 g) | 1.33 | 107 |
| Lima beans, cooked | 0.5 cup (94 g) | 2.25 | 108 |
| Soy products/meat substitutes | | | |
| Tofu, raw, regular | 1/2 cup (126 g) | | 183 |
| Garden burger, classic veggie | 1 patty (71 g) | 2.56 | 121 |
| Soy burger, veggie burger | 1 patty (70 g) | 1.69 | 124 |
| Breakfast patties | 1 each (38 g) | 1.33 | 78 |
| Nuts/seeds | | | |
| Pumpkin seed kernel, roasted | 0.25 cup (29.5 g) | 2.38 | 169 |
| Sunflower seeds, kernels, dry | 0.25 cup (35 g) | 1.84 | 204 |
| Cashew, dry roasted | 0.25 cup (34.25 g) | 2.06 | 197 |
| Coconut milk, canned | 0.5 cup (113.5 g) | 3.73 | 223 |
| Almonds, dry roasted | 0.25 cup (34.5 g) | 1.32 | 205 |
| Mixed nuts, dry roasted with peanuts | 0.25 cup (34.25 g) | 1.27 | 203 |
| Miscellaneous | | | |
| Molasses, blackstrap | 1 tbsp (20 g) | 0.94 | 58 |

*Sources:* Trumbo, P. et al., *J. Am. Diet. Assoc.*, 101(3), 294, 2001; U.S. Department of Agriculture ARS. USDA National Nutrient Database for Standard Reference, Release 24, 2011; Pennington, J., *Bowes & Church's Food Values of Portions Commonly Used*, 17th edn, Lippincott-Raven, Philadelphia, PA, 1998; Hands, E., *Food Finder: Food Sources of Vitamins & Minerals*, ESHA Research, Salem, OR, 1995.

Adult RDA: male, 8 mg/day; female, 18 mg/day.

**TABLE 26.25**
**Iron: Absorption Enhancers and Inhibitors**

| Class of Inhibitors | Examples | Found | Effect on Iron Absorption |
|---|---|---|---|
| Polyphenols | Tannic acid, gallic acid, and catechins | Coffee, tea, red wines, certain spices, fruits, and vegetables | Coffee: 35%–40%<br>Tea: 60%<br>Red wine: 50% |
| Phytate | Substance that form insoluble complexes with nonheme iron | Whole grains, bran, soy products | |
| Ethylenediaminetetraacetic acid (EDTA) | Food additive used as sodium EDTA, calcium EDTA (prevents color changes and oxidation in foods) | Used broadly | Possibly up to 50% in some cases |
| Calcium | Calcium chloride (naturally occurring sources of calcium in self-selected diets did not show an inhibitory effect; however, there is a potential effect of other forms of calcium) | Additive to bread products, potential effect of other forms of calcium | Possibly up to 30%–50% in some cases found with calcium chloride fortification |
| Fiber | Insoluble fibers, phytate content may be responsible | Whole grains | Possibly 30%–50% |
| **Class of Enhancers** | | | |
| Organic acids[a] | Malic, ascorbic, citric, and bile acids | Found widely in foods | Enhances absorption |
| Amino acids | Some amino acids such as cysteine | Protein foods, also found widely in vegetables and grains | Enhances absorption |
| Vitamin A and β-carotene | Retinol, retinaldehyde, retinoic acid, β-carotene | Spinach, carrots, squash, sweet potatoes, greens, cantaloupe, and mango | Enhances absorption, possibly by forming a complex with iron |

*Source:* Kohlmeier, M., *Nutrient Metabolism*, Academic Press, London, U.K., 2003.

[a] The presence of these acids with a meal will significantly improve iron absorption and in some cases potentially overcome the inhibitory effects of other components in foods.

## TABLE 26.26
## Manganese: Vegetarian Sources and Amounts

| Food | Portion Size | Manganese (mg) | kcal |
|---|---|---|---|
| Cereals/grains | | | |
| 100% Natural Granola, with raisin, nuts, honey, wheat, Quaker | 1 cup | 1.286 | 213 |
| Raisin Bran, Total | 1 cup | 0.816 | 160 |
| Raisin Bran, Kellogg's | 1 cup | 1.734 | 185 |
| Raisin Bran, Post | 1 cup | 1.73 | 189 |
| Raisin Nut Bran, General Mills | 1 cup | 1.241 | 180 |
| Cheerios, honey nut flavor, General Mills | 1 cup | 0.823 | 110 |
| All Bran, Kellogg's Original | 1 cup | 4.45 | 161 |
| Grape-Nuts | 1 cup | 2.65 | 389 |
| Bran Chex, General Mills | 1 cup | 2.53 | 156 |
| Wheat Chex, General Mills | 1 cup | 1.07 | 160 |
| Wheatena, cooked with water | 1 cup | 2.00 | 136 |
| Noodles, cooked, spinach | 1 cup | 2.10 | 182 |
| Noodles, cooked, macaroni, whole wheat | 1 cup | 1.93 | 174 |
| Rice, brown, cooked | 1 cup | 1.77 | 216 |
| Noodles, cooked, lasagna, whole wheat | 2 each | 1.52 | 136 |
| Vegetables, beans | | | |
| Lima beans, boiled | 0.5 cup | 0.97 | 105 |
| Pinto beans, cooked, boiled | 1 cup | 0.775 | 198 |
| White beans, canned | 1 cup | 1.35 | 299 |
| Fruits | | | |
| Pineapple, chunks | 1 cup | 1.437 | 149 |
| Blackberries | 1 cup | 0.93 | 62 |
| Soy products/meat substitutes | | | |
| Tofu, raw, firm, with nigari | 1 cup | 1.58 | 183 |
| Tempeh | 0.5 cup | 1.19 | 165 |

*Sources:* Trumbo, P. et al., *J. Am. Diet. Assoc.*, 101(3), 294, 2001; U.S. Department of Agriculture ARS, USDA National Nutrient Database for Standard Reference, Release 24, 2011; Pennington, J., *Bowes & Church's Food Values of Portions Commonly Used*, 17th edn., Lippincott-Raven, Philadelphia, PA, 1998.

Manganese is not usually at risk for deficiency in vegetarians. Most research has found that vegetarians have higher manganese intake than nonvegetarians. However, bioavailability may be a concern.[31,32]

AI: males, 2.3 mg/day; female, 1.8 mg/day.

**TABLE 26.27**

**Selenium[a]: Vegetarian Sources and Amounts**

| Food | Portion Size | Selenium (μg) | kcal |
|---|---|---|---|
| Cereals/grains | | | |
| Special K, Kellogg's | 1 cup | 54.9 | 100 |
| Bagel, egg, plain, toasted | 1 each | 27 | 195 |
| Granola, low fat | 1 cup | 22.5 | 422 |
| Pita pocket, 100% whole wheat, toasted | 1 each | 20.2 | 120 |
| Barley, whole, cooked | 0.5 cup | 18.2 | 135 |
| Pita pockct, white | 1 each | 18 | 165 |
| Egg noodles, enriched, cooked | 0.5 cup | 19 | 107 |
| Spaghetti/macaroni, enriched, cooked | 0.5 cup | 19 | 99 |
| Puffed wheat | 1 cup | 14.8 | 44 |
| Whole-wheat bread | 1 slice | 11 | 86 |
| Oatmeal, instant, prepared, raisin, date variety | 0.5 cup | 6 | 159 |
| Buns, hamburger style | 1 each | 12.5 | 129 |
| English muffin, plain | 1 each | 11.5 | 134 |
| Cheerios | 1.25 cup | 10.6 | 111 |
| Matzo, whole wheat | 1 each | 9.89 | 100 |
| Brown rice, long grain, enriched, cooked | 0.5 cup | 10 | 108.5 |
| White rice, long grain, enriched, cooked | 0.5 cup | 6 | 97 |
| Vegetables | | | |
| Brussels sprouts, boiled | 1 cup | 21.1 | 61 |
| Cucumbers, slices with peel | 0.5 cup | 6.19 | 7 |
| Mushrooms, raw | 5 pieces | 14.3 | 32 |
| Fruits | | | |
| Grapes, Thompson seedless | 0.5 cup | 7.70 | 57 |
| Applesauce, canned | 0.5 cup | 6.50 | 53 |
| Dairy/Soy Milk | | | |
| Cottage cheese, 1% | 0.5 cup | 11 | 81 |
| Yogurt, fruit, low fat (12 g protein/8 oz) | 1 cup | 8.09 | 155 |
| Milk, nonfat | 1 cup | 5.15 | 86 |
| Frozen yogurt, chocolate, nonfat | 1 cup | 5.02 | 208 |
| Beans/legumes | | | |
| Black beans, dry, boiled | 1 cup | 13.7 | 227 |
| Lima beans, cooked | 1 cup | 8.19 | 229 |
| Great northern beans, cooked | 1 cup | 7.26 | 209 |
| Chickpeas, boiled | 1 cup | 6.10 | 269 |
| Soy products/meat substitutes | | | |
| Nuts/seeds | | | |
| Brazil nuts, dried | 0.25 cup | 544 | 186 |
| Sunflower seeds, kernels, dry | 0.25 cup | 23 | 165 |
| Cashew, dry roasted, unsalted | 0.25 cup | 8.00 | 197 |
| Eggs | | | |
| Egg, hard cooked | 1 each | 15 | 78 |
| Egg yolk, cooked | 1 each | 7.50 | 59 |
| Egg white, cooked | 1 each | 5.88 | 16.6 |

**TABLE 26.27 (continued)**
**Selenium[a]: Vegetarian Sources and Amounts**

| Food | Portion Size | Selenium (µg) | kcal |
|---|---|---|---|
| Mixed foods | | | |
| Lasagna, no meat, recipe | 1 piece (218 g) | 29.9 | 298 |
| Avocado and cheese sandwich on wheat bread | 1 each | 26.2 | 456 |
| Peanut butter and jam sandwich on wheat | 1 each | 24.3 | 344 |
| Pizza, cheese | 1/8 of 15 in. (120 g) | 20.0 | 268 |
| Bean burrito | 1 each | 14.1 | 224 |
| Cucumber and vinegar salad | 1 cup | 11.1 | 48 |
| Desserts | | | |
| Coffee cake, from mix | 1 piece (72 g) | 11.0 | 229 |
| Carrot, with cream cheese icing, recipe | 1 piece (112 g) | 9.91 | 488 |

*Sources:* Monsen, E.R., *J. Am. Diet. Assoc.*, 100(6), 637, 2000; U.S. Department of Agriculture ARS, USDA National Nutrient Database for Standard Reference, Release 24, 2011; Pennington, J., *Bowes & Church's Food Values of Portions Commonly Used*, 17th edn., Lippincott-Raven, Philadelphia, PA, 1998; Hands, E., *Food Finder: Food Sources of Vitamins & Minerals*, ESHA Research, Salem, OR, 1995.

Adult RDA: males 55 µg/day, females 55 µg/day.

[a] Selenium content of food can vary widely, according to the selenium content of the soil.[35]

**TABLE 26.28**
**Zinc: Vegetarian Sources and Amounts**

| Food | Portion Size | Zinc (mg)[a,b] | kcal |
|---|---|---|---|
| Cereals/grains | | | |
| Total Raisin Bran, General Mills | 1 cup | 15.6 | 160 |
| Product 19, Kellogg's | 1 cup | 15.3 | 100 |
| Bran flakes | 1 cup | 2.0 | 128 |
| Cap'n Crunch, Quaker | 1 cup | 5.82 | 143 |
| Granola, low fat, with raisin, Kellogg's | 0.5 cup | 3.91 | 170 |
| Quinoa | 1 cup | 5.27 | 626 |
| Muffin, oat bran | 1 each (66 g) | 1.21 | 178 |
| Noodle, spaghetti, spinach, cooked | 1 cup | 1.08 | 182 |
| Bagel, plain | 1 medium (105 g) | 2.0 | 270 |
| Pancakes, blueberry, prep from recipe | 3 each (111 g) | 0.62 | 253 |
| Vegetables | | | |
| Hearts of palm, canned | 1 cup (146 g) | 1.68 | 41 |
| Dairy/soy milk | | | |
| Yogurt, frozen, chocolate | 1 cup (146 g) | 2.18 | 208 |
| Yogurt, chocolate, nonfat | 6 oz container | 1.92 | 190 |
| Ricotta cheese, part skim | 0.5 cup (123 g) | 1.65 | 170 |
| Edam cheese | 1 oz (28.35 g) | 1.06 | 101 |
| Buttermilk, cultured, fluid, low fat | 1 cup (245 g) | 1.03 | 98 |
| Soy milk, original and vanilla, unfortified | 1 cup (243 g) | 0.29 | 131 |
| Beans/lLegumes | | | |
| Adzuki, cooked, boiled, without salt | 1 cup (230 g) | 4.07 | 294 |
| Lentils, cooked, boiled, without salt | 1 cup (198 g) | 2.51 | 230 |
| Soybeans, mature, dry roasted | 0.5 cup (86 g) | 4.10 | 388 |
| Soybean, green, boiled without salt | 1 cup (180 g) | 0.91 | 254 |
| Kidney beans, red, cooked, without salt | 1 cup (177 g) | 1.89 | 225 |
| Chickpeas, canned, drained, rinsed | 0.5 cup (76 g) | 0.45 | 105 |
| Soy products/meat substitutes | | | |
| Natto | 1 cup (175 g) | 5.30 | 371 |
| Edamame, frozen, prepared | 1 cup (155 g) | 2.12 | 189 |
| Tempeh, cooked | 100 g | 1.57 | 196 |
| Tofu, raw, firm | 0.5 cup (126 g) | 1.05 | 88 |
| Miso | 1 cup (275 g) | 7.04 | 547 |
| Chili, Worthington Foods™, canned, unprepared | 1 cup (230 g) | 1.84 | 290 |
| Luncheon slice, meatless | 100 g | 1.60 | 189 |
| Nuts/seeds | | | |
| Pumpkin seeds, kernel, dry roasted, salt added | 0.25 cup (29.5 g) | 2.25 | 169 |
| Cashew, dry roasted, no added salt | 0.25 cup (34.25 g) | 1.92 | 197 |
| Almonds, dry roasted, no added salt | 1 oz (34.5 g) | 1.14 | 205 |
| Sunflower seeds, kernels, dry roasted, without salt | 0.25 cup (33.5 g) | 1.78 | 207 |
| Sesame butter/tahini from nonroasted kernels | 1 T (15 g) | 0.69 | 89 |
| Peanuts, dry roasted, with salt | 1 oz (28.35 g) | 0.94 | 166 |
| Peanut butter, smooth, with salt | 2 T (132 g) | 0.94 | 188 |

## TABLE 26.28 (continued)
## Zinc: Vegetarian Sources and Amounts

| Food | Portion Size | Zinc (mg)[a,b] | kcal |
|---|---|---|---|
| **Eggs** | | | |
| Egg substitute, liquid, frozen, fat-free | 0.5 cup (120 g) | 1.18 | 58 |
| **Mixed Foods** | | | |
| Cheese enchilada (fast food) | 1 each (163 g) | 2.51 | 319 |
| Pizza, cheese, frozen | 1/8 of 15 in. (139 g) | 1.83 | 361 |
| **Desserts** | | | |
| Granola bar, fruit filled, nonfat | 1 each/2 oz (56.7 g) | 0.81 | 194 |
| Pecan pie, 1/8 of a 9 in. pie, prepared from recipe | 1 piece (122 g) | 1.24 | 503 |
| Trail mix, regular | 0.25 cup (37.5 g) | 1.21 | 173 |

*Sources:* Monsen, E.R., *J. Am. Diet. Assoc.*, 100(6), 637, 2000; U.S. Department of Agriculture ARS, USDA National Nutrient Database for Standard Reference, Release 24, 2011; Pennington, J., *Bowes & Church's Food Values of Portions Commonly Used*, 17th edn., Lippincott-Raven, Philadelphia, PA, 1998; Hands, E., *Food Finder: Food Sources of Vitamins & Minerals*, ESHA Research, Salem, OR, 1995.

Adult RDA: males 11 mg, females 8 mg.

[a] Zinc content of food is influenced by genetic breeding and fertilizer and soil conditions.

[b] Bioavailability is greater from animal than plant sources.

**TABLE 26.29**

**Zinc: Absorption Enhancers and Inhibitors**

| Possible Absorption Enhancers[a] | Sources | Possible Absorption Inhibitors[b] | Sources |
|---|---|---|---|
| Yeast (acts by breaking down phytates) | Fermented bread dough | Phytates | Whole grains (rye, barley, oatmeal, and wheat), soy products |
| Animal proteins | Animal products | Oxalate | Spinach, Swiss chard, leek, kale, collard greens, okra, rhubarb, raspberries, coffee, chocolate, tea, peanuts, and pecans |
| Histidine | Amino acid widely distributed in foods containing protein | Fiber | Whole grains, fruits, vegetables, and legumes |
| Albumin | Widely distributed in foods containing protein, egg white | | |
| Organic acids | Found widely in foods | Copper | Legumes, whole grains, nuts, seeds, and vegetables |
| | | Calcium | Milk, yogurt, cheese, over-the-counter supplements, multivitamins, some antacids |
| | | Iron supplements | Over-the-counter supplements, multivitamin/mineral |
| | | Casein | Milk |

*Source:* Kohlmeier, M., *Nutrient Metabolism*, Academic Press, London, U.K., 2003.

[a] Yeast and animal proteins are the only noncontroversial zinc absorption enhancers.

[b] Phytate is the only noncontroversial zinc absorption inhibitor.

**TABLE 26.30**

**Fiber: Types, Functions, and Sources**

| Type of Fiber | Fiber Type | Food Sources | Function |
|---|---|---|---|
| Cellulose | Incompletely fermented | Whole-wheat flour, bran, apples, cabbage, peas, green beans, broccoli, cucumbers, peppers, carrots, other vegetables | Increases stool bulk and water absorption, decreases transit time through the GI system |
| Hemicellulose | Incompletely fermented | Bran cereals, whole grains, brussels sprouts, greens, and beetroot | |
| | | | Bacteria in the large intestine produce acetate, propionate, and butyrate, which are partially used for the nourishment of local enterocytes and partially for energy production in the liver |
| Lignin | Incompletely fermented | Breakfast cereals, bran, older vegetables, strawberries, eggplant, pears, green beans, and radishes | |
| Gums | Viscous | Oatmeal, oat products, legumes, oat bran, barley, and guar | Bind bile acids, which tends to lower blood cholesterol levels, are metabolized to short-chain fatty acids in the gut, may slow digestion, glucose absorption and oro-cecal transit time |
| Pectin | Viscous | Squash, apples, citrus fruits, cauliflower, cabbage, dried peas and beans, carrots, and strawberries | |

*Source:* Slavin, J.L., *J. Am. Diet. Assoc.*, 108(10), 1716, 2008.

AI: male, 38 g/day; female, 25 g/day.

## TABLE 26.31
## Common Phytochemicals[a] in Foods

| Chemical Names | Sources | Proposed Mechanism of Action |
|---|---|---|
| Carotenoids | Alpha- and beta-carotenes found in pumpkin, sweet potato; beta-cryptoxanthin found in red pepper, tangerine, papaya; lycopene found in pasta sauce, watermelon; lutein + zeaxanthin found in kale, collard, and turnip greens | |
| Coumestan | Found in pinto beans, mung bean sprouts, and alfalfa sprouts | Weak estrogenic activity |
| Sulforaphane | Isothiocyanates found in broccoli, cauliflower, cress, cabbages, and radishes | Activates phase II enzymes in liver (removes carcinogens from cells) |
| Flavonoids (polyphenols) | Apigenin and luteolin found in celery; kaempferol found in kale, black beans, black and green tea; myricetin found in cranberries, fava beans, green tea; procyanidin found in chocolate, apple; quercetin found in onions, cranberries, vegetable soup | Blocks the cancer-promotion process, weak estrogenic activity; antioxidant activity (anti-peroxyl activity) |
| Isoflavones | Biochanin A found in snow peas, garbanzo, and kidney beans; Daidzein and genistein found in soy foods; Formononetin found in sprouts (clover, alfalfa) | Prevents the formation of capillaries required to nourish tumors |
| Lignins | Matairesinol and secoisolariciresinol found in flaxseed | |
| Phytosterols | Beta-sitosterol found in green and black tea; campesterol found in soybeans and oils (corn, safflower, sunflower), orange; stigmasterol found in soy and kidney beans | |
| Monoterpenes | Perillyl alcohol in cherries<br>Limonene in citrus<br>Ellagic acid in strawberries and blueberries | May inhibit the growth of early cancers |
| Genistein | Soybeans, tofu | Prevents the formation of capillaries required to nourish tumors |
| Indoles | Cruciferous vegetables (broccoli, cauliflower, cress, cabbages, and radishes) | Increase immunity, facilitate excretion of toxins |
| Saponins | Kidney beans, chickpeas, soybeans, and lentils | May prevent cancer cells from multiplying |
| Lycopene | Tomatoes | May fight lung and prostate cancer |

*Source:* Kohlmeier, M., *Nutrient Metabolism*, Academic Press, London, U.K., 2003.

[a] More than 10,000 phytochemicals are thought to exist. This table represents only a partial listing.

## TABLE 26.32
## Effects of Cooking, Storage, and Processing on the Critical Nutrients

| Nutrient | Cooking | Storage | Processing |
|---|---|---|---|
| Riboflavin | Stable to heat; riboflavin in plant sources severely lost to water during boiling process of cooking, destroyed if baking soda is added to soften dried beans or peas | Destroyed by light and irradiation | Half of $B_2$ is lost when grains are milled |
| Vitamin $B_{12}$ | Pasteurization and boiling of milk decreases vitamin $B_{12}$ content; boiling or frying of eggs increases bioavailability | Stable during prolonged storage | |
| Iron | Cooking in cast-iron vessels increases iron content of foods | — | — |
| Omega-3 fatty acids (a polyunsaturated fatty acid) | Stable in baking; unstable if smoking point is reached | May go rancid with prolonged storage | — |

*Sources:* Kohlmeier, M., *Nutrient Metabolism*, Academic Press, London, U.K., 2003; Doscherholmen, A. et al., *Proc. Soc. Exp. Biol. Med.*, 149(4), 987, 1975; Macdonald, L.E. et al., *J. Food Protect.*, 74(11), 1814, 2011; Dong, M.H. et al., *J. Am. Diet. Assoc.*, 76(2), 156, 1980.

**TABLE 26.33**

**General Vitamin and Mineral Deficiency and Toxicity Symptoms**

| Vitamin/Mineral[a] | Deficiency Symptoms[b] | Toxicity Symptoms[c] |
|---|---|---|
| Vitamins | | |
| Vitamin D | Children—rickets<br>Adults—osteomalacia | Excessive bone and soft tissue calcification (lung, kidney, kidney stones, and tympanic membrane)<br>Hyperphosphatemia<br>Hypercalcemia with symptoms of headache, weakness, nausea and vomiting, constipation, polyuria, and polydipsia<br>In infants: retarded growth, gastrointestinal upsets, and mental retardation |
| Vitamin B$_{12}$ | Pernicious (megaloblastic) anemia<br>Smooth red tongue<br>Fatigue<br>Skin hypersensitivity (numbness, tingling and burning of the feet and stiffness and generalized weakness of the legs)<br>Neuropathy, degeneration of peripheral nerves progressing to paralysis<br>Other (glossitis and hypospermia) | Physiological stores substantial (~2000–5000 μg in adults). Stores and enterohepatic recycling may prevent deficiency symptoms for several years (~5) in the absence of intake<br>None known up to 100 μg/day. No known benefit from high doses |
| Riboflavin (vitamin B$_2$) | Anemia (normocytic and normochromic)<br>Neuropathy<br>Purple/magenta tongue<br>Photophobia<br>General B-vitamin deficiency symptoms (soreness and burning of lips, mouth, and tongue)<br>Cheilosis, glossitis, angular stomatitis, seborrheic dermatitis of nasolabial fold, vestibule of the nose, and sometimes the ears and eyelids, scrotum, and vulva | None known, but high intake does not provide greater benefit than adequate intake |
| Minerals | | |
| Calcium | Bone deformities including osteomalacia, osteoporosis, tetany, and hypertension and possibly colon cancer | Hypercalcemia of soft tissues and bone (children and adults)<br>Decreased iron, manganese, and zinc absorption (of particular concern during pregnancy)<br>Increased bone fractures in the elderly<br>Constipation |
| Iron | Hypochromic, microcytic anemia<br>Seen across populations, particularly in women, children, and those from low socioeconomic status<br>Fatigue<br>Spoon-shaped nails | Seen at >45 mg intake<br>Constipation<br>Liver toxicity (due to hemochromatosis)<br>Infections (in hemochromatosis)<br>Potentially increased risk for heart disease and myocardial infarction |
| Zinc | Growth retardation resulting in short stature, mild anemia, low plasma zinc levels, and delayed sexual maturation<br>Possible in diets very rich in fiber and phytate, which chelates the zinc in the intestine, thus preventing absorption<br>Poor taste acuity, poor wound healing, night blindness, baldness, and skin lesions have also been reported<br>Behavioral disturbances<br>Poor immune functioning<br>Impaired appetite | Toxicity is rare (100–300 mg/day)<br>Tolerable upper intake level is 40 mg/day<br>Continuous supplementation with high-dose zinc can interfere with copper absorption<br>Excessive supplementation may decrease HDL and can result in nausea, vomiting, diarrhea, and dizziness<br>Iron and copper losses in urine with doses as low as 25 mg/day and if large doses (10–15 × the RDA) are taken for even short periods of time |

## TABLE 26.33 (continued)
## General Vitamin and Mineral Deficiency and Toxicity Symptoms

| Vitamin/Mineral[a] | Deficiency Symptoms[b] | Toxicity Symptoms[c] |
|---|---|---|
| Copper | Severe copper deficiency: rare in humans | Gastrointestinal distress, liver damage, liver cirrhosis |
| | Adults: neutropenia and microcytic anemia | Seen in genetic diseases such as Wilson's disease (genetic defect of Wilson's disease gene ATP7B) |
| | Children: neutropenia and leukopenia | |
| | Decrease in serum copper and ceruloplasmin levels followed by failure of iron absorption leading to microcytic, hemochromic anemia | Abnormalities in red blood cell formation |
| | Neutropenia, leukopenia, and bone demineralization are later symptoms | Toxicity from food consumption considered impossible |
| | Deficiencies have not been reported in otherwise healthy humans consuming a varied diet | |
| | Subperiosteal hemorrhages | |
| | Hair and skin depigmentation | |
| | Defective elastin formation | |

*Source:* Kohlmeier, M., *Nutrient Metabolism*, Academic Press, London, U.K., 2003.

[a] Absorption of some nutrients is affected by concentration of others; intestinal absorption of some nutrients is competitive.

[b] Deficiency can result from inadequate provision in the diet or via inadequate absorption.

[c] Toxicity is typically from overuse of nutritional supplements, although in some cases can be the cause of improper food fortification procedures (such as milk and vitamin D fortification problems that arose in 1992).

## TABLE 26.34
## Sample Meal Plan for Lacto–Ovo Vegetarian Adult

| Breakfast | Lunch | Dinner | Snack |
|---|---|---|---|
| Raisin Bran (1 cup, 2.15 oz) | Whole-wheat bread, 2 slices | Bean burrito: | Cereal bar, raspberry |
| Milk, 1% fat, 0.75 cup (for cereal) | Griller veg. burger patty, 1 each | Black beans, 1 cup | Dried apricots, 10 halves |
| Milk, 1% fat, 1 cup (beverage) | Mustard | Corn tortilla, 2 each, 6 in. | |
| Orange juice, 1 cup | Tomato, sliced, 1/2 tomato | Rice, brown, 1 cup | |
| Banana, 1 med | Jack cheese, 1 oz | Salsa, 2 tbsp | |
| | Apple, 1 med | Sour cream, 1 tbsp | |
| | | Cheddar cheese, 1 oz | |
| | | Green salad, 2 cups | |
| | | Vinegar and oil dressing (1 tsp olive oil) | |
| | | Broccoli, 1 cup | |
| | | Milk, 1% fat, 1 cup | |

*Sources:* Pennington, J., *Bowes & Church's Food Values of Portions Commonly Used*, 17th edn., Lippincott-Raven, Philadelphia, PA, 1998; Hands, E., *Food Finder: Food Sources of Vitamins & Minerals*, ESHA Research, Salem, OR, 1995.

*Notes:* kcal, 2218; carbohydrate, 374 g (67.35%); protein, 100 g (18.%); fat, 55 g (22.29%).

**TABLE 26.35**

**Sample Meal Plan for Vegan Adult**

| Breakfast | Lunch | Dinner | Snack |
|---|---|---|---|
| Raisin Bran (1 cup, 2.15 oz) | Whole-wheat bread, 2 slices | Bean burrito: | Cereal bar, raspberry |
| Soy milk, 1% fat, 1 cup (for cereal) | Griller veg. burger patty (Morningstar Farms), 1 each, cooked | Black beans, 1 cup | Dried apricots, 10 halves |
| Soy milk, 1% fat, 1 cup (beverage) | Mustard | Corn tortilla, 2 each, 6 in. | |
| Orange juice, 1 cup, Ca fortified | Tomato, sliced, 1/2 tomato | Rice, brown, 1 cup | |
| Banana, 1 med | Almonds, slivered, blanched, 1 oz | Salsa, 2 tbsp | |
| | Apple, 1 med | Walnuts, ground, 0.5 oz | |
| | | Green salad, 2 cups | |
| | | Vinegar and oil dressing (1 tsp olive oil) | |
| | | Broccoli, 1 cup | |
| | | Soy milk, 1 cup | |

*Sources:* Pennington, J., *Bowes & Church's Food Values of Portions Commonly Used*, 17th edn., Lippincott-Raven, Philadelphia, PA, 1998; Hands, E., *Food Finder: Food Sources of Vitamins & Minerals*, ESHA Research, Salem, OR, 1995.

*Notes:* kcal, 2217; carbohydrate, 350g (63%); protein, 90g (16%); fat, 62g (25%).

**TABLE 26.36**

**Sample Meal Plan for Vegan Child Ages 4–6**

| Breakfast | Lunch | Dinner | Snack 1 | Snack 2 |
|---|---|---|---|---|
| 1 packet instant oatmeal | 0.5 cup hummus spread made from chickpeas and sesame butter | Veggie hotdog on bun | 4 oz fortified soy milk | 1.5 oz (~0.25 cup) trail mix |
| 8 oz soy milk fortified with calcium and vitamin B$_{12}$ | 2 slices whole-wheat bread | 0.5 cup mashed potatoes | 4 graham crackers | 4 oz fortified soy milk |
| 1 banana | 6 oz 100% orange pineapple banana juice | 0.5 cup cooked "creamed" spinach | | |
| | Carrot sticks | 0.5 cup applesauce | | |
| | 2 molasses cookies | 8 oz soy milk | | |

*Sources:* Pennington, J., *Bowes & Church's Food Values of Portions Commonly Used*, 17th edn., Lippincott-Raven, Philadelphia, PA, 1998; Hands, E., *Food Finder: Food Sources of Vitamins & Minerals*, ESHA Research, Salem, OR, 1995.

*Notes:* kcal, 1864; carbohydrate, 283 g (60.8%); protein, 68 g (14.5%); fat, 62 g (30%).

**TABLE 26.37**

**Sample Meal Plan for Lacto–Ovo-Vegetarian Child Ages 4–6**

| Breakfast | Lunch | Dinner | Snack 1 | Snack 2 |
|---|---|---|---|---|
| 1 cup Honey Nut Cheerios with 4 oz milk on cereal | 0.5 cup homemade macaroni and cheese | Burrito with salsa and sour cream, made with vegetarian chili | 1.5 oz cheese | Fruit smoothie made with juice, frozen yogurt, and fruit |
| 4 oz 1% milk to drink | celery sticks and 2 tbsp peanut butter | 0.5 cup rice | Five Ritz crackers | |
| Orange slices | Two fruit cookies | 4 oz 1% milk | 4 oz 1% milk | |
| | | 0.5 cup green salad with broccoli | | |
| | | 0.5 cup applesauce | | |

*Sources:* Pennington, J., *Bowes & Church's Food Values of Portions Commonly Used*, 17th edn., Lippincott-Raven, Philadelphia, PA, 1998; Hands, E., *Food Finder: Food Sources of Vitamins & Minerals*, ESHA Research, Salem, OR, 1995.

*Notes:* kcal, 1794; carbohydrate, 255 g (57%); protein, 63 g (14%); fat, 63 g (31.5%).

## SUMMARY

In summary, the term "vegetarianism" may mean different things to different people. Before making or accepting generalizations about vegetarianism, it is important to define the term. A person following a vegetarian lifestyle can have significantly lower risks of many chronic diseases, such as heart disease or cancer, than an omnivore does. However, some nutrients are more difficult to obtain in sufficient quantities and may increase risk of deficiency, especially in children or during other critical life cycle periods.

## DISCLAIMER

The brand names and trademarks appearing in this chapter are mentioned by example only and are not intended to signify endorsement by the author.

## REFERENCES

1. Craig WJ, Mangels AR. Position of the American Dietetic Association: Vegetarian diets. *Journal of the American Dietetic Association* 2009; 109(7): 1266–1282.
2. Stahler C. How many vegetarians are there? *Vegetarian Journal* 2009; (4): 12–13.
3. Mangels R, Messina V, Messina M. *The Dietitian's Guide to Vegetarian Diets. Issues and Applications.* Burlington, MA: Jones & Bartlett Learning; 2011.
4. Haddad EH, Berk LS, Kettering JD, Hubbard RW, Peters WR. Dietary intake and biochemical, hematologic, and immune status of vegans compared with nonvegetarians. *American Journal of Clinical Nutrition* 1999; 70(3 Suppl): 586S–593S.
5. Dewell A, Weidner G, Sumner MD, Chi CS, Ornish D. A very-low-fat vegan diet increases intake of protective dietary factors and decreases intake of pathogenic dietary factors. *Journal of the American Dietetic Association* 2008; 108(2): 347–356.
6. Parsons TJ, van Dusseldorp M, van der Vliet M, van de Werken K, Schaafsma G, van Staveren WA. Reduced bone mass in Dutch adolescents fed a macrobiotic diet in early life. *Journal of Bone and Mineral Research* 1997; 12(9): 1486–1494.
7. Draper A, Lewis J, Malhotra N, Wheeler E. The energy and nutrient intakes of different types of vegetarian: A case for supplements? *British Journal of Nutrition* 1993; 69(1): 3–19.
8. Messina VK, Burke KI. Position of the American Dietetic Association: Vegetarian diets. *Journal of the American Dietetic Association* 1997; 97(11): 1317–1321.
9. Remer T, Neubert A, Manz F. Increased risk of iodine deficiency with vegetarian nutrition. *British Journal of Nutrition* 1999; 81(1): 45–49.
10. Sanders TA. Essential fatty acid requirements of vegetarians in pregnancy, lactation, and infancy. *American Journal of Clinical Nutrition* 1999; 70(3 Suppl): 555S–559S.
11. Sanders TA, Reddy S. Vegetarian diets and children. *American Journal of Clinical Nutrition* 1994; 59(5 Suppl): 1176S–1181S.
12. Van Dusseldorp M, Arts IC, Bergsma JS, De Jong N, Dagnelie PC, Van Staveren WA. Catch-up growth in children fed a macrobiotic diet in early childhood. *Journal of Nutrition* 1996; 126(12): 2977–2983.
13. Van Winckel M, Vande Velde S, De Bruyne R, Van Biervliet S. Clinical practice: Vegetarian infant and child nutrition. *European Journal of Pediatrics* 2011; 170(12): 1489–1494.
14. Young VR, Pellett PL. Plant proteins in relation to human protein and amino acid nutrition. *American Journal of Clinical Nutrition* 1994; 59(5 Suppl): 1203S–1212S.
15. Simopoulos AP. The importance of the omega-6/omega-3 fatty acid ratio in cardiovascular disease and other chronic diseases. *Experimental Biology and Medicine (Maywood)* 2008; 233(6): 674–688.
16. Deckelbaum RJ, Torrejon C. The omega-3 fatty acid nutritional landscape: Health benefits and sources. *Journal of Nutrition* 2012; 142(3): 587S–591S.
17. Guillot N, Caillet E, Laville M, Calzada C, Lagarde M, Vericel E. Increasing intakes of the long-chain omega-3 docosahexaenoic acid: Effects on platelet functions and redox status in healthy men. *FASEB Journal* 2009; 23(9): 2909–2916.
18. Brenna JT, Salem N, Jr., Sinclair AJ, Cunnane SC. alpha-Linolenic acid supplementation and conversion to n-3 long-chain polyunsaturated fatty acids in humans. *Prostaglandins, Leukotrienes, and Essential Fatty Acids* 2009; 80(2–3): 85–91.
19. Kumudha A, Kumar SS, Thakur MS, Ravishankar GA, Sarada R. Purification, identification, and characterization of methylcobalamin from Spirulina platensis. *Journal of Agricultural and Food Chemistry* 2010; 58(18): 9925–9930.
20. Watanabe F, Katsura H, Takenaka S, Fujita T, Abe K, Tamura Y et al. Pseudovitamin B(12) is the predominant cobamide of an algal health food, spirulina tablets. *Journal of Agricultural and Food Chemistry* 1999; 47(11): 4736–4741.
21. Pramyothin P, Holick MF. Vitamin D supplementation: Guidelines and evidence for subclinical deficiency. *Current Opinion in Gastroenterology* 2012; 28(2): 139–150.
22. Pearce EN, Pino S, He X, Bazrafshan HR, Lee SL, Braverman LE. Sources of dietary iodine: Bread, cows' milk, and infant formula in the Boston area. *Journal of Clinical Endocrinology and Metabolism* 2004; 89(7): 3421–3424.
23. Zijp IM, Korver O, Tijburg LB. Effect of tea and other dietary factors on iron absorption. *Critical Reviews in Food Science and Nutrition* 2000; 40(5): 371–398.
24. Baber R. Phytoestrogens and post reproductive health. *Maturitas* 2010; 66(4): 344–349.
25. Peeters PH, Slimani N, van der Schouw YT, Grace PB, Navarro C, Tjonneland A et al. Variations in plasma phytoestrogen concentrations in European adults. *Journal of Nutrition* 2007; 137(5): 1294–1300.
26. Farmer B, Larson BT, Fulgoni VL, III, Rainville AJ, Liepa GU. A vegetarian dietary pattern as a nutrient-dense approach to weight management: An analysis of the national health and nutrition examination survey 1999–2004. *Journal of the American Dietetic Association* 2011; 111(6): 819–827.
27. Ross AC, Taylor CL, Yaktine AL, Del Valle HB, eds. *Dietary Reference Intakes for Calcium and Vitamin D.* Washington, DC: National Academies Press; 2011.
28. Trumbo P, Schlicker S, Yates AA, Poos M. Dietary reference intakes for energy, carbohydrate, fiber, fat, fatty acids, cholesterol, protein and amino acids. *Journal of the American Dietetic Association* 2002; 102(11): 1621–1630.
29. Trumbo P, Yates AA, Schlicker S, Poos M. Dietary reference intakes: Vitamin A, vitamin K, arsenic, boron, chromium, copper, iodine, iron, manganese, molybdenum, nickel, silicon, vanadium, and zinc. *Journal of the American Dietetic Association* 2001; 101(3): 294–301.
30. Monsen ER. Dietary reference intakes for the antioxidant nutrients: Vitamin C, vitamin E, selenium, and carotenoids. *Journal of the American Dietetic Association* 2000; 100(6): 637–640.
31. Gibson RS. Content and bioavailability of trace elements in vegetarian diets. *American Journal of Clinical Nutrition* 1994; 59(5 Suppl): 1223S–1232S.

32. Kadrabova J, Madaric A, Kovacikova Z, Ginter E. Selenium status, plasma zinc, copper, and magnesium in vegetarians. *Biological Trace Element Research* 1995; 50(1): 13–24.

33. Kohlmeier M. *Nutrient Metabolism*. London, U.K.: Academic Press; 2003.

34. U.S. Department of Agriculture ARS. USDA National Nutrient Database for Standard Reference, Release 24, 2011.

35. Pennington J. *Bowes & Church's Food Values of Portions Commonly Used*, 17th edn. Philadelphia, PA: Lippincott-Raven; 1998.

36. Hands E. *Food Finder: Food Sources of Vitamins & Minerals*. Salem, OR: ESHA Research; 1995.

37. Yates AA, Schlicker SA, Suitor CW. Dietary reference intakes: The new basis for recommendations for calcium and related nutrients, B vitamins, and choline. *Journal of the American Dietetic Association* 1998; 98(6): 699–706.

38. Slavin JL. Position of the American Dietetic Association: Health implications of dietary fiber. *Journal of the American Dietetic Association* 2008; 108(10): 1716–1731.

39. Doscherholmen A, McMahon J, Ripley D. Vitamin $B_{12}$ absorption from eggs. *Proceedings of the Society for Experimental Biology and Medicine* 1975; 149(4): 987–990.

40. Macdonald LE, Brett J, Kelton D, Majowicz SE, Snedeker K, Sargeant JM. A systematic review and meta-analysis of the effects of pasteurization on milk vitamins, and evidence for raw milk consumption and other health-related outcomes. *Journal of Food Protection* 2011; 74(11): 1814–1832.

41. Dong MH, McGown EL, Schwenneker BW, Sauberlich HE. Thiamin, riboflavin, and vitamin B6 contents of selected foods as served. *Journal of the American Dietetic Association* 1980; 76(2): 156–160.

# Part IV

## Assessment

# 27 Dietary Guidelines, Food Guidance, and Dietary Quality in the United States

*Eileen Kennedy, Daniel Hatfield, and Jeanne Goldberg*

## CONTENTS

## DIETARY GUIDELINES

The Dietary Guidelines for Americans have served as the cornerstone of nutrition policy in the United States since the first edition was released in 1980. While many factors contributed to the development of that document, two earlier efforts were of particular importance. One was the 1969 White House Conference on Food, Nutrition, and Health,[1] which recommended that the government examine the links between diet and chronic disease. The second was the U.S. Senate Dietary Goals, released in 1977[2]; that document, the product of several years of hearings before the Senate Select Committee on Nutrition and Human Needs, summarized for the first time specific recommendations for diet-related goals for the American public.

The Dietary Guidelines, which came 3 years later, have served as the basis of nutrition standards for all government food programs, including the Supplemental Nutrition Assistance Program (SNAP), formerly known as Food Stamps; National School Lunch and School Breakfast Programs; and the Special Supplemental Nutrition Program for Women, Infants, and Children (WIC). Nutrition education programs at the federal level also must incorporate messages consistent with the Dietary Guidelines. Since approximately one of every five Americans participates in one or more federal nutrition program in a given year,[3] the Dietary Guidelines have a broad impact on the U.S. population.

## HISTORY OF THE DIETARY GUIDELINES FOR AMERICANS

The Dietary Guidelines for Americans aim to address the question, "What should Americans eat to stay healthy?" Specifically, the guidelines provide advice for healthy Americans aged 2 years and over about food choices that promote health and reduce the risk of disease.[4–10] In addition to dietary recommendations, the 2000 Guidelines incorporated recommendations for physical activity, and the 2010 edition increased the focus on maintaining calorie balance to achieve and sustain a healthy weight. This new conceptualization acknowledged the need to address the obesity crisis in the United States.

The basic procedure for revising the Guidelines has been in place since 1985. Every 5 years, the U.S. Department of Agriculture (USDA) and the Department of Health and Human Services (HHS) appoint an external Dietary Guidelines Advisory Committee (DGAC). The committee, composed of highly credentialed nutrition and medical experts, reviews the guidelines and provides recommendations for revisions where indicated by newer evidence. In addition, the committee holds a series of open public meetings to review and discuss the guidelines. Ultimately, it prepares a technical report, which is transmitted to the two secretaries for review within the two departments.

The National Nutrition Monitoring and Related Research Act of 1990 included a statutory mandate from Congress directing the secretary of the Department of Agriculture and the secretary of HHS to jointly publish a report titled Dietary Guidelines for Americans. The act formally required that the report (1) contain nutrition and dietary information and guidelines for the general public, (2) be based on the preponderance of scientific and medical knowledge current at the time of publication, and (3) be promoted by each federal agency in carrying out federal food, nutrition, or health programs. The 1995 edition was the first published under that mandate.

## DIETARY GUIDELINES FOR AMERICANS

### THE 1980, 1985, AND 1990 DIETARY GUIDELINES

The first edition of the Dietary Guidelines for Americans contained seven guidelines, based on a growing body of research linking diet with health outcomes, and particularly with the evidence and recommendations summarized in the 1979 Surgeon General's Report on Health Promotion and Disease Prevention.[11] Some of the seven guidelines focused on goals such as dietary variety and weight maintenance, while three exhorted Americans to "avoid too much" of particular dietary constituents, such as total fat, saturated fat, cholesterol, sugar, and sodium. The guidelines drew controversy from industry and scientific groups, particularly given questions around whether available research was sufficient to demonstrate causal links between dietary components and health.

Such controversy spurred the Senate Committee on Appropriations to direct that a committee be established to review scientific evidence and develop recommendations for future revisions to the guidelines.[12] The first such advisory committee, composed of nine nongovernmental nutrition scientists, issued recommendations that informed the 1985 edition of the Dietary Guidelines. The 1985 report's seven guidelines varied little from those in the 1980 edition but were more widely accepted.

The 1990 Dietary Guidelines maintained the tradition of seven guidelines and represented overall tenets similar to earlier editions. However, this edition incorporated more positive language, as well as a greater focus on the total diet; the 1985 guideline to "Avoid too much fat, saturated fat, and cholesterol," for example, was transformed to "Choose a diet low in fat, saturated fat, and cholesterol." The report also provided more specific numerical recommendations for limiting total dietary fat (<30% of total calories) and saturated fat (<10% of total calories).

### THE 1995 DIETARY GUIDELINES

In the 1995 Dietary Guidelines, emphasis continued to shift toward total diet, with a continued focus on concepts of variety, moderation, and proportionality. The concept of total diet was reflected symbolically through the graphic of the 1995 Dietary Guidelines bulletin, which linked all seven guidelines together. The guidelines were anchored around the recommendation to "Eat a Variety of Food," including each of the five major food groups in the Food Guide Pyramid. Grains, which represented the base of the pyramid, were to form the center of the plate, accompanied by food from the other food groups.

For the first time, the 1995 document recognized that, with careful planning, a vegetarian diet could be consistent with both the Dietary Guidelines and the Recommended Dietary Allowances (RDAs). Weight gain was discouraged for adults, and weight maintenance was encouraged as a first step toward achieving a healthy weight. The benefits of physical activity were also emphasized, and for the first time, the Guidelines included a statement on the benefits of moderate alcohol consumption in reducing the risk of heart disease. On this point, both USDA and HHS were clear that the alcohol guideline was not intended to recommend that people start consuming alcohol. The 1995 Guidelines also directly referred to nutrition education tools, including the Food Guide Pyramid and the Nutrition Facts Label, which consumers could use to build a healthy diet. For the first time, consumer research was conducted to test reactions to specific design and content elements of the 1995 technical report.[13]

### THE 2000 DIETARY GUIDELINES

The Dietary Guidelines 2000, released by President Clinton, broke the tradition of seven guidelines, adding three additional ones. These included a new physical activity guideline: "Be physically active every day." This guideline discussed health benefits of physical activity beyond weight maintenance and offered specific recommendations for the amount of physical activity for adults (30 min or more) and children (60 min or more) per day. There was also a new guideline on food safety, as well as separate guidelines for grains and fruits/vegetables, which were previously grouped together. The 2000 Guidelines not only continued to emphasize a total diet approach, but also stressed a healthy lifestyle. This was reflected clearly in three concepts used as organizing principles: aim for fitness, build a healthy base, and choose sensibly.

Consumer research conducted as part of the Dietary Guidelines 2000 process[14] influenced the development of the recommendations. One clear message from that research was that consumers preferred simple, action-oriented guidelines; therefore, continued emphasis was placed on translating the guidelines into directive recommendations. The 2000 Guidelines were also more consumer-friendly and emphasized practical ways for consumers to put the concepts into practice. For example, the recommendation to choose whole-grain foods was accompanied by a list of examples of whole-grain ingredients, as well as a figure depicting a sample ingredients list for a whole-grain food.

### THE 2005 DIETARY GUIDELINES

The process for developing the Dietary Guidelines 2005 incorporated several adjustments from earlier editions. Since the first edition, it had been clear that the guidelines needed to be based on the preponderance of scientific evidence. For the 2005 edition, it was specified that conclusions from the DGAC must rest on an evidence-based rating system in order to minimize the potential for individual bias to influence decisions. It was further specified that the task of the Advisory Committee would be limited to the preparation of a set of evidence-based recommendations. The committee was not to concern itself with how these recommendations would be communicated to the public. What emerged from the 2005 DGAC was a set of nine key messages. While the general themes remained consistent with earlier editions, the wording for just three guidelines—those for physical activity, food safety, and alcohol—was exactly the same as that in the 2000 Guidelines.

Under the new process for communicating the Dietary Guidelines, an internal group from USDA/DHHS assumed the task of translating the guidelines into a set of recommendations for policymakers, nutrition educators, nutritionists, and health-care providers. These guidelines would then serve as the basis for the development of communications to the public. In essence, this new system divided the process of revising the dietary guidelines into two distinct components, one focusing solely on the science that drives the recommendations and the other on the translation of those recommendations.

The 2005 brochure produced by UDSA/DHHS, "Finding Your Way to a Healthier You," was released on the same day as the guidelines and represented a first attempt at this new approach to consumer communications.[15] In preparing this brochure, the internal USDA/DHHS committee translated the DGAC's messages into a total of 41 key recommendations, including 23 for the general public and 18 for specific population groups. These recommendations were designed to take into account nutrients that were in short supply in the diets of significant numbers of individuals in the population, including vitamin E, calcium, magnesium, potassium, and fiber in children and adults, as well as vitamins A and C in adults. Like previous guidelines, the recommendations emphasized fruits, vegetables, whole grains, and low-fat dairy, along with limits on added sugars, fats, and salt. New recommendations, such as guidance to avoid trans fats, reflected scientific developments since 2000.

## THE 2010 DIETARY GUIDELINES

In developing its report, the 13 members of the 2010 DGAC employed an approach similar to that used in 2005, but modified to further enhance its scientific rigor. The committee developed 180 scientific questions, and 130 of these were answered using the USDA's Nutrition Evidence Library (NEL), founded in 2009. The NEL uses a transparent, systematic evidence-based review process, ensuring that conclusions are informed by the highest quality science and that the DGAC's recommendations align with standards outlined in the Quality of Information Act of 2001. Questions for which the NEL was not used were informed by other analytical methods or reports, such as the 2008 Physical Activity Guidelines for Americans.

While the 2010 DGAC report echoed themes from the 2005 report, several topics received increased emphasis. Most notably, the 2010 report focused largely on the need to reduce the incidence and prevalence of overweight and obesity, with more explicit discussion of the need to reduce caloric intakes and consumption of certain types of foods, like solid fat, alcohol, and added sugars (SoFAAS). The report also added two new chapters: "The Total Diet" and "Translating and Integrating the Evidence," to stress, respectively, the importance of whole dietary patterns as well as the social and environmental dimensions that affect eating behaviors.

The 2010 Dietary Guidelines policy document included 23 recommendations for all Americans, plus six population-specific recommendations, focused largely on the importance of achieving energy balance and consuming nutrient-dense foods (Table 27.1). Like the DGAC report, the guidelines also incorporated a new discussion of social and environmental factors that influence eating and physical activity, calling for "a coordinated system-wide approach … that engages all sectors of society, including individuals and families, educators, communities and organizations, health professionals, small and large businesses, and policymakers" to help Americans engage in healthier behaviors.

## GUIDANCE FOR CHILDREN UNDER 2 YEARS

Since the first Dietary Guidelines were released in 1980, they have applied to individuals aged 2 and older. The United States and most other industrialized countries rely on national pediatric associations to guide the broad policy recommendations for infant feeding and/or feeding practices for the first 2 years of life. In the United States, the American Academy of Pediatrics stresses that human milk is the preferred form of infant feeding.[16] A limited number of other countries do address the needs of children under 2 in their food-based guidelines, and in most cases, the advice relates to a discussion of breast-feeding. Australia, for example, has a guideline to "encourage and support breastfeeding." Similar wording is found in guidelines from the Philippines and Singapore.

## OTHER DIETARY GUIDANCE

The previous section traced the development of the U.S. Dietary Guidelines specifically. In fact, the federal government, and the USDA in particular, has a long, rich history of providing science-based nutrition information and education for the general public that began over 100 years ago, well before the first dietary guidelines were issued. The Organic Act of 1862, which created USDA, mandated that the department "acquire and diffuse among people useful information on subjects connected with agriculture." This mandate led to some of the pioneering work of W.O. Atwater, who in the 1890s began investigating the connections between dietary intakes, food composition, and human health.

**TABLE 27.1**
**2010 Dietary Guidelines for Americans**

Balancing calories to manage weight

- Prevent and/or reduce overweight and obesity through improved eating and physical activity behaviors.
- Control total calorie intake to manage body weight. For people who are overweight or obese, this will mean consuming fewer calories from foods and beverages.
- Increase physical activity and reduce time spent in sedentary behaviors.
- Maintain appropriate calorie balance during each stage of life—childhood, adolescence, adulthood, pregnancy and breast-feeding, and older age.

Foods and food components to reduce

- Reduce daily sodium intake to less than 2300 mg and further reduce intake to 1500 mg among persons who are 51 and older and those of any age who are African American or have hypertension, diabetes, or chronic kidney disease. The 1500 mg recommendation applies to about half of the U.S. population, including children, and the majority of adults.
- Consume less than 10% of calories from saturated fatty acids by replacing them with monounsaturated and polyunsaturated fatty acids.
- Consume less than 300 mg/day of dietary cholesterol.
- Keep *trans* fatty acid consumption as low as possible by limiting foods that contain synthetic sources of *trans* fats, such as partially hydrogenated oils, and by limiting other solid fats.
- Reduce the intake of calories from solid fats and added sugars.
- Limit the consumption of foods that contain refined grains, especially refined grain foods that contain solid fats, added sugars, and sodium.
- If alcohol is consumed, it should be consumed in moderation—up to one drink per day for women and two drinks per day for men—and only by adults of legal drinking age.

Foods and nutrients to increase

- Individuals should meet the following recommendations as part of a healthy eating pattern while staying within their calorie needs.
- Increase vegetable and fruit intake.
- Eat a variety of vegetables, especially dark-green and red and orange vegetables and beans and peas.
- Consume at least half of all grains as whole grains. Increase whole-grain intake by replacing refined grains with whole grains.
- Increase intake of fat-free or low-fat milk and milk products, such as milk, yogurt, cheese, or fortified soy beverages.
- Choose a variety of protein foods, which include seafood, lean meat and poultry, eggs, beans and peas, soy products, and unsalted nuts and seeds.
- Increase the amount and variety of seafood consumed by choosing seafood in place of some meat and poultry.
- Replace protein foods that are higher in solid fats with choices that are lower in solid fats and calories and/or are sources of oils.
- Use oils to replace solid fats where possible.
- Choose foods that provide more potassium, dietary fiber, calcium, and vitamin D, which are nutrients of concern in American diets. These foods include vegetables, fruits, whole grains, and milk and milk products.

*Recommendations for specific population groups*

Women capable of becoming pregnant

- Choose foods that supply heme iron, which is more readily absorbed by the body, additional iron sources, and enhancers of iron absorption such as vitamin C-rich foods.
- Consume 400 μg/day of synthetic folic acid (from fortified foods and/or supplements) in addition to food forms of folate from a varied diet.

Women who are pregnant or breast-feeding

- Consume 8–12 oz of seafood/week from a variety of seafood types.
- Due to their high methyl mercury content, limit white (albacore) tuna to 6 oz/week and do not eat the following four types of fish: tilefish, shark, swordfish, and king mackerel.
- If pregnant, take an iron supplement, as recommended by an obstetrician or other health-care provider.

Individuals ages 50 years and older

- Consume foods fortified with vitamin $B_{12}$, such as fortified cereals, or dietary supplements.

Building healthy eating patterns

- Select an eating pattern that meets nutrient needs over time at an appropriate calorie level.
- Account for all foods and beverages consumed and assess how they fit within a total healthy eating pattern.
- Follow food safety recommendations when preparing and eating foods to reduce the risk of foodborne illnesses.

This seminal science in turn led to the development of a series of USDA food guides. Dissemination of the food guides was facilitated by the 1914 Smith-Lever Act, which created the Cooperative Extension Service and specified that the service provide people with "useful and practical information on subjects relating to agriculture and home economics." "Foods for Young Children," published in 1916, was a five-group system based on what was then known about nutritional needs and food composition. It included milk and meat, cereals, vegetables and fruits, fats and fat foods, and sugars and sugary foods. It was followed a year later by a guide for the general population, entitled "How to Select Foods." This publication was modified slightly over the next several years, providing consumers with information about amounts of food by weight, volume, or count and 100 cal portions to meet the needs of the household.[17]

In the 1930s, to respond to the economic constraints brought about by the depression, the USDA began developing family food plans at four separate cost levels. These food plans have continued to be used, in updated iterations, ever since. The best known of these, the Thrifty Food Plan, served as the nutritional basis for establishing the benefits package of the Food Stamp Program. However, food plans were also developed for higher-income levels, since insufficient understanding of the elements of good nutrition was also common among upper-income Americans; indeed, former Secretary of Agriculture Henry Wallace once commented, "The lack of common-sense knowledge of nutrition even among many well-to-do people in the United States is appalling."[18]

In 1941, the first set of RDAs was released at the National Nutrition Conference for Defense. In that document, USDA scientists noted that consumers spent enough money on food but did not obtain an adequate diet. As a result, the USDA was urged to develop nutrition education and media-type materials to promote good nutrition for the American public. In 1943, USDA released the "National Wartime Nutrition Guide," which included the "Basic Seven" food recommendations. This report communicated a foundational diet thought to meet most of the RDAs for nutrients, while recognizing limited food supplies in the United States. In 1946, the report was revised as the post-war "National Food Guide." While this guide was widely used for the next decade, some considered it overly complex and insufficiently specific in terms of serving sizes. In 1956, a new guide, popularly known as the "Basic Four," was released, providing recommendations for numbers of servings from four food groups: meat, milk, grains, and fruits and vegetables.[17]

This emphasis on nutrition education continued in the 1950s and 1960s. The 1969 White House Conference on Food, Nutrition, and Health was a watershed event in the development of U.S. nutrition policy. In announcing the appointment of Dr. Jean Mayer as the chairman of the Conference, President Richard Nixon underscored the event's importance: "Its conclusions and its goals … will be the basis for action by this administration and the beginning of a national commitment—to put an end to malnutrition and hunger among the poor, to make better use of our agricultural bounty and nutritional knowledge,

and to ensure a healthful diet for all Americans."[19] The conference reinforced the need for aggressive nutrition promotion activities for all Americans, and particularly for low-income populations.

The conference led to a number of developments in the 1970s, as federal agencies increased funding for nutrition programs and nutrition education activities. New programs were created, including School Breakfast and the Special Supplemental Food Program for Women, Infants, and Children, now renamed the Special Supplemental *Nutrition* Program for Women, Infants, and Children. Other programs, such as Food Stamps (now called SNAP) and School Lunch, were expanded nationwide.

The 1977 Food and Agriculture Act named USDA as the lead agency for nutrition research, extension, and teaching. Throughout the 1980s and into the 1990s, USDA placed a renewed emphasis on developing comprehensive, coordinated efforts to promote nutrition for all Americans.

## USDA/DHHS FOOD GUIDE PYRAMID 1992

The release of the 1980 Dietary Guidelines for Americans provided the impetus for the development of a new food guide that would allow consumers to put the Dietary Guidelines into action. Work throughout the 1980s and into the early 1990s culminated in the 1992 USDA Food Guide Pyramid, a graphic that reflected the extensive experience with food guidance systems within the USDA as well as the progression toward providing research-driven materials for consumers. Different visuals were tested with consumers to assess which graphic portrayal most effectively communicated the foundational concepts of variety, balance, and moderation. These tests first targeted adults with at least a high school education and later were expanded to include children and low-literacy and low-income adults. The pyramid shape emerged as the graphic that most effectively communicated the foundational concepts.[20]

The 1992 Food Guide Pyramid communicated a wealth of information with little accompanying text. The Food Guide Pyramid Bulletin explained the complex information provided in the visual, including the differing energy needs of individuals illustrated at 1600, 2200, and 2800 kcal of daily intakes. It also included an in-depth discussion of "How to Make the Pyramid Work for You," covering issues such as serving sizes, different types of fats, and ways to make low-fat selections using the pyramid. The number and amounts of foods recommended in the pyramid were based on three factors:

1. RDAs for age and gender groups
2. Dietary Guidelines for Americans
3. Typical consumption patterns of Americans

The advice provided in the Food Guide Pyramid was designed to provide dietary guidance that ensured nutritional adequacy—defined as meeting the RDAs and Dietary Guidelines—within the framework of typical consumption patterns. Thus, while ostensibly an infinite number of food combinations could be used to ensure nutritional adequacy, the five major food groups emphasized in the USDA Pyramid anchored the food selections to current consumption patterns. In 1999, USDA released a version of the Food Guide Pyramid targeted at children aged 2–6 years. Here again, the concepts of balance, variety, and moderation underpinned the graphic. The icons used in the food groups were based on foods typically consumed by children.

## USDA'S MyPYRAMID, 2005

MyPyramid (Figure 27.1), the first revision to the Food Guide Pyramid, was released just 4 months after the release of the 2005 Dietary Guidelines for Americans to motivate consumers to make healthier choices and to align the USDA's food guidance system with up-to-date nutrition science. Extensive qualitative research was conducted by USDA to guide the development of the new graphic. A series of focus groups in 2002, designed to assess the clarity of messages embedded in the original Food Guide Pyramid, showed that consumers recognized the pyramid but had difficulty understanding the specific messages.[21]

A second series of eight focus groups was completed in 2004 to identify alternative ways to describe the food recommendations so that consumers would understand them. These focus groups also explored consumers' ability to understand nutrition language and messaging about grains, vegetables, types of fats, sugars and added sugars, and physical activity levels. This research showed that consumers did not understand the intended meaning of servings and serving sizes, and more broadly, that their understanding of nutrition terms was limited.[21]

In July 2004, USDA's Center on Nutrition Policy and Promotion (CNPP) solicited public comments on the proposed Food Guidance System and its graphical representation

and educational materials through a notice in the Federal Register. Over 1200 comments were received. CNPP also requested a synthesis of previous research that could inform further revisions to the Food Guidance System. In October 2004, ten 2 h focus groups explored participants' awareness of healthy-eating messages and the information conveyed in those messages. This was the first series that explored different concepts for the new graphic. Two months later, 200 adults participated in a web—TV survey to provide feedback to inform further refinements of the graphic. This phase also included testing of actionable messages.

The MyPyramid graphic ultimately developed not only retained the familiar shape of the Food Guide Pyramid, but also incorporated the physical activity recommendation, represented by a person climbing steps up the side of the pyramid. Unlike the prior pyramid's placement of different food groups at different levels, MyPyramid represented each of the food groups with triangles of varying size, tapering from the base to the top. This representation was designed to show that within each food group, certain foods should be consumed more or less often. That said, the most widely publicized version of the graphic did not include pictures of actual foods; these details were instead communicated through supplementary materials like the MyPyramid website, which provided interactive tools for personalizing the recommendations.

Publicity on the day that MyPyramid was released was extensive; its website received 48 million hits in the 24 h following the release.[22] As reported in the media, many members of the academic community reacted negatively, pointing out that the new materials did not provide sufficiently specific messages about which foods to eat more of and which to eat in lesser quantities. Some contended that the new materials catered to the food industry.[23]

## MyPLATE, 2010

Launched following the release of the 2010 Dietary Guidelines, MyPlate (Figure 27.2) represented a significant shift from previous food guidance graphics, motivated in part by a 2010 report by the White House Task Force on Childhood Obesity, which noted that, "Despite its popularity and prominence, the Food Pyramid has been subject to significant criticism for failing to communicate effective, actionable messages to consumers, which many observers have suggested are critical in changing behavior."[24]

In an effort to develop a new, more actionable food guidance icon that reflected the 2010 Dietary Guidelines, the USDA launched an iterative research process, which included interviews with Federal nutrition education staff, assessment of news coverage of the 2005 Dietary Guidelines, a literature review, and analysis of six other successful health communication programs. The USDA also held 14 focus groups in four U.S. cities, with an equal distribution of individuals who perceived themselves as "Strugglers" or "Succeeders" in terms of implementing healthy eating behaviors. Finally, two

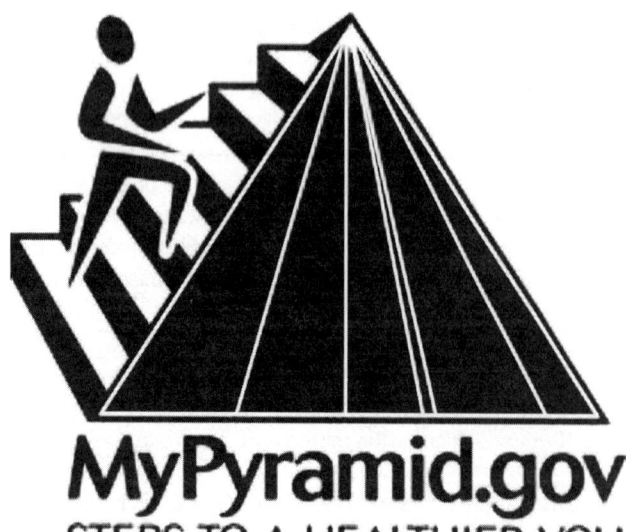

**FIGURE 27.1** MyPyramid.

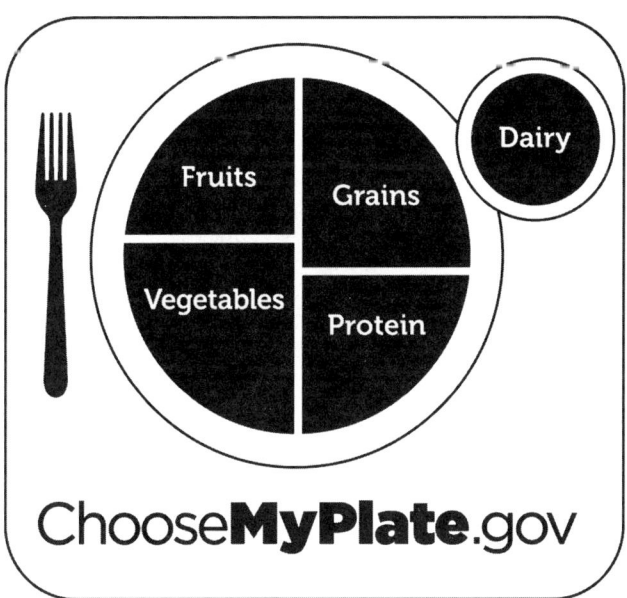

**FIGURE 27.2** MyPlate.

quantitative surveys of children and adults, with oversampling of low-education and low-income segments, further tested images and language for the new icon.[25]

The USDA research suggested that consumers generally understood the basic components of a healthy diet, but struggled with concepts around weight management, particularly with regard to portion sizes and calorie control. In addition, consumer focus groups revealed a preference for messages that were not only directive, but also realistic; messages such as "Enjoy what you eat, just eat less of it" and "Save half your plate for fruits and vegetables," for example, had high consumer appeal. Ultimately, three different icons were tested with consumers: an updated pyramid graphic, a plate icon, and a thought-bubble graphic depicting different food groups. While no one graphic had universal appeal or comprehensively captured all messages in the Dietary Guidelines, the plate was ultimately selected as the most effective option, particularly given its simplicity and familiarity.[25] The icon was fine-tuned based on findings from the quantitative consumer survey, and the final image, a simple plate-and-cup icon showing the recommended distribution of food groups, was launched by First Lady Michelle Obama in June 2011.

## DIET QUALITY MEASURES

Since the early 1900s, the major areas of concern in public health nutrition have shifted from problems of nutritional deficiency to problems of excesses and imbalances. In the United States, problems of relative overconsumption are, on average, more prevalent today than are problems of underconsumption. Until the 1990s, most measures of Americans' dietary quality were somewhat selective in the components included and did not fully align with the U.S. Dietary Guidelines' growing focus on total diet.[26,27] In an effort to measure how well American diets conform to recommended healthy eating patterns, USDA developed the

Healthy Eating Index (HEI), which was originally created in 1995 and later revised in 2005.

## HEALTHY EATING INDEX—1995

The HEI was designed originally to measure various aspects of a healthful diet.[28] As shown in Table 27.2, the HEI-1995 is a 10-component index. Components 1–5 measure the degree to which a person's diet conforms to age- and gender-specific serving recommendations for the five major food groups in the Food Guide Pyramid: grains, vegetables, fruits, milk, and meat. The index used food groups rather than nutrients to provide consumers with an easier standard against which to judge their dietary patterns, as well as to incorporate components in foods that would not be picked up by measuring nutrients alone. Components 6–9 measure various recommendations of the Dietary Guidelines, including total fat, saturated fat, cholesterol, and sodium, respectively. Component 10 provides a measure of dietary variety. Each of the 10 components has a score ranging from 0 to 10; thus, the total HEI-1995 score can vary from 1 to 100.

The HEI-1995 was applied to nationally representative data derived from the Continuing Survey of Food Intake by Individuals (CSFII) for three time periods: 1989–1990, 1994–1996, and 1999–2000. For each of these periods, the combined score for the U.S. population fell between 63.5 (1995) and 63.9 (1989–1990),[29–31] suggesting that there was little variation in overall U.S. dietary quality across this 11 year period. The distribution of the average HEI scores likewise did not vary dramatically over the period of 1989–2000. Throughout this time period, the majority of individual scores fell in the 51–80 range, the "needs improvement" category, and no more than 12% of individuals fell in the "good diet" category at any point in time.

## HEALTHY EATING INDEX—2005

Following the release of the 2005 Dietary Guidelines for Americans, the HEI was revised to be more consistent with new recommendations, including those for whole grains, specific categories of fruits and vegetables, and discretionary calories.[32] The new, 12-component index included each of the food groups in the 2005 MyPyramid (e.g., Total Fruit and Total Vegetables); these were generally the same as components in the original HEI, though the Oils category was new. The HEI-2005 eliminated the prior category of "Variety" and instead added three specific categories of foods recommended in the Dietary Guidelines: Whole Fruit, Dark Green and Orange Vegetables and Legumes, and Whole Grains. Cholesterol was also removed as a component in the Index, and Solid Fat, Alcohol, and Added Sugars was added. In total, nine of the categories were designated "adequacy components," representing sufficient nutrient intakes; the remaining three components were "moderation categories."

The scoring of each of the categories was also adapted. Each food group in MyPyramid maintained a total maximum score of 10; in some cases, this total was split between

**TABLE 27.2**

**Original HEI and HEI-2005 Components and Standards for Scoring**

| Component | 0 | 5 | 8 | 10 | 20 |
|---|---|---|---|---|---|
| | | | | Points | |
| **Original HEI** | | | | | |
| Total fruit | 0 ←——————→ | | | 2–4 servings (approx. 1–2 cups[a]) | |
| Total vegetables | 0 ←——————→ | | | 3–5 servings (approx. 1.5–2.5 cups[a]) | |
| Total grains | 0 ←——————→ | | | 6–11 servings (approx. 6–11 oz eq[a]) | |
| Milk | 0 ←——————→ | | | 2–3 servings (2–3 cups[b]) | |
| Meat (and beans) | 0 ←——————→ | | | 2–3 servings (approx. 5.5–7.0 oz eq[a]) | |
| Sodium | ≥4.8 ←——————→ | | | ≤2.4 g | |
| Saturated fat | ≥15 ←——————→ | | | ≤10% energy | |
| Total fat | ≥45 ←——————→ | | | ≤30% energy | |
| Cholesterol | ≥450 ←——————→ | | | ≤300 mg | |
| Variety | ≤6 ←——————→ | | | ≥16 different foods in 3 days[c] | |
| **HEI-2005[d]** | | | | | |
| Total fruit | 0 ←——→ ≥0.8 cup eq/1000 kcal | | | | |
| Whole fruit | 0 ←——→ ≥0.4 cup eq/1000 kcal | | | | |
| Total vegetables | 0 ←——→ ≥1.1 cup eq/1000 kcal | | | | |
| Dark green and orange vegetables and legumes | 0 ←——→ ≥0.4 cup eq/1000 kcal | | | | |
| Total grains | 0 ←——→ ≥3.0 oz eq/1000 kcal | | | | |
| Whole grains | 0 ←——→ ≥1.5 oz eq/1000 kcal | | | | |
| Milk | 0 ←——————→ | | | ≥1.3 cup eq/1000 kcal | |
| Meat and beans | 0 ←——————→ | | | ≥2.5 oz eq/1000 kcal | |
| Oils | 0 ←——————→ | | | ≥12 g/1000 kcal | |
| Saturated fat | ≥15 ←——→ | | 10 ←→ ≤7% of energy | | |
| Sodium | ≥2.0 ←——→ | | 1.1 ←→ ≤0.7 g/1000 kcal | | |
| Calories from SoFAAS[e] | ≥50 ←————————————————→ | | | | ≤20% of energy |

[a] According to gender and age.

[b] According to age.

[c] In 1994–1996 and 1999–2000, 8 or more different foods in 1 day.

[d] See appendix 1: foods included in components of the healthy eating index-2005.

[e] Solid fat, alcohol, and added sugar.

two subcategories. For example, five points were allocated for each Total Grains and Whole Grains, in keeping with the Dietary Guidelines' recommendation that Americans make at least half their grains whole. Saturated fat and sodium were each scored on a 0–10 scale and SoFAAS on a 0–20 scale. Whereas the original HEI scoring was based primarily on daily servings from each group, the HEI-2005 was reconfigured to represent food and nutrient intakes based on density (i.e., amounts per 1000 kcal). SoFAAS were evaluated based on the proportion of total energy intakes.

The HEI-2005 was tested for several psychometric properties, including content validity, construct validity, and reliability. For example, each of the components of the HEI-2005 was checked against the Dietary Guidelines for Americans 2005. In addition, 10 NHANES 24 h dietary recalls were scored against the HEI to test for face validity. Diet scores against HEI-2005 were also compared with scores against the original HEI. Diets with high scores in HEI-2005 generally also had high scores in the original HEI. However, the inverse was not always true, particularly because of the HEI-2005's incorporation of Whole Fruit, Whole Grains, and Dark Green and Orange Vegetables and Legumes.[32]

In addition to other tests of content validity, HEI scores were computed for several dietary plans recommended by nutrition experts, including MyPyramid, Harvard's Healthy Eating Pyramid, the DASH Eating Plan, and the American Heart Association's No-Fad Diet. Each plan scored over 90 on the HEI-2005.

The HEI-2005 was applied to dietary intake data from the 1994 to 1996 CSFII and from NHANES 2001 to 2002. No change in dietary quality was observed, as both assessments yielded average overall scores of 58.2 out of 100. The highest component scores relative to the maximum were for Total Grains and Meat and Beans, while the lowest scores were for Whole Grains, Dark Green and Orange Vegetables and Legumes, Sodium, and SoFAAS.[33]

Another analysis using 2003–2004 NHANES data suggested that overall dietary scores were not statistically different for low-income Americans (56.5) and higher-income Americans (57.8), though lower-income Americans did score significantly lower in several component areas, including Total Vegetables, Dark Green and Orange Vegetables and Legumes, and Whole Grains.[34] HEI-2005 scores for older Americans were generally higher than the national average, though no significant change was observed in this subgroup from 1994–1996 (65.4) to 2001–2002 (67.6),[35] Analysis of NHANES 2004–2005 dietary intake data yielded an overall score of 55.9 among American children aged 2–17 years and suggested a particular need to increase intakes of whole fruit, whole grains, and dark green and orange vegetables and legumes and to decrease intakes of solid fats and added sugars.[36]

These HEI scores provide an understanding of the degree to which the overall population and subpopulations meet the recommendations in the Dietary Guidelines for Americans. This insight should provide a roadmap for future guidelines as well as for tailoring food and nutrition programs to meet Americans' needs.

## SUMMARY

Since 1980, U.S. dietary guidance has evolved to reflect a growing understanding of the relationship between diet and health. While many foundational precepts underlying dietary guidance have largely remained unchanged (e.g., benefits of fruits and vegetables and the importance of limiting sodium and sugars), the emergence of new science-based evidence has led to greater specificity in much of the guidance. Americans' changing needs have led to further adaptations to the recommendations. In particular, the obesity epidemic has largely shifted the principal focus from nutrient adequacy toward eating and physical activity behaviors that support calorie balance. Today, the gap between the Dietary Guidelines 2010 and the eating behavior of most Americans remains wide. For nutrition professionals, understanding how to close that gap will be a key challenge.

## REFERENCES

1. *Proceedings of the White House Conference on Food, Nutrition and Health.* White House, Washington, DC, 1970, 16p. http://www.nns.nih.gov/1969/full_report/White_House_Report2_S1a.pdf. Accessed January 10, 2012.
2. U.S. Senate Select Committee on Nutrition and Human Needs. *Dietary Goals for the United States.* U.S. Government Printing Office, Washington, DC, 1977, 79p.
3. Oliveira V. Informing food and nutrition assistance policy: 10 Years of research at ERS, p. 4, 2007. http://www.ers.usda.gov/Publications/MP1598/MP1598.pdf. Accessed January 10, 2012.
4. U.S.D.A. and U.S. D.H.H.S. *Nutrition and Your Health: Dietary Guidelines for Americans.* Home and Garden Bulletin 232. U.S. Government Printing Office, Washington, DC, 1980, 11p.
5. U.S.D.A. and U.S.D.H. H.S. *Nutrition and Your Health: Dietary Guidelines for Americans.* Home and Garden Bulletin 232. U.S. Government Printing Office, Washington, DC, 1985, 24p.
6. U.S.D.A. and U.S.D.H.H.S. *Nutrition and Your Health: Dietary Guidelines for Americans.* Home and Garden Bulletin 232. U.S. Government Printing Office, Washington, DC, 1990, 29p.
7. U.S.D.A. and U.S.D.H.H.S. *Nutrition and Your Health: Dietary Guidelines for Americans.* Home and Garden Bulletin 232. U.S. Government Printing Office, Washington, DC, 1995, 48p.
8. U.S.D.A. and U.S. D.H.H.S. *Nutrition and Your Health: Dietary Guidelines for Americans.* Home and Garden Bulletin. U.S. Government Printing Office, Washington, DC, 2000, 42p.
9. U.S.D.A. and U.S.H.H.S. *Dietary Guidelines for Americans.* U.S. Government Printing Office, Washington, DC, 2005, 80p.
10. U.S.D.A. and U.S.D.H.H.S. *Dietary Guidelines for Americans.* U.S. Government Printing Office, Washington, DC, 2010, 97p.
11. Office of the Surgeon General. *Healthy People: The Surgeon General's Report on Health Promotion and Disease Prevention.* U.S. Government Printing Office, Washington, DC, 1979,179p.
12. U.S. Senate Agricultural Appropriations Committee. Senate Report 1030, 96th Congress, 1st session, 1980.
13. Prospect Associates. *Dietary Guidelines Focus Group Report.* USDA Center for Nutrition Policy and Promotion, Washington, DC, 1995.
14. Systems Assessment & Research, Inc. Final Report: Focus Groups on Nutrition and Your Health: Dietary Guidelines for Americans, 4th edn., Lanham, MD, 1999.
15. U.S.D.A. and U.S.D.H.H.S. *Finding Your Way to a Healthier You.* U.S. Government Printing Office, Washington, DC, 2005, 12p.
16. Gartner LM, Morton J, Lawrence RA et al. Breastfeeding and the use of human milk. *Pediatrics* 115: 496, 2005.
17. Davis C, Saltos E. Dietary recommendations and how they have changed over time. In: Frazao E, ed. *America's Eating Habits: Changes and Consequences.* Agriculture Information Bulletin No. 750, Economic Research Service, U.S. Department of Agriculture, Washington, DC, 1999, p. 33.
18. Wallace H. *Foreword. Yearbook of Agriculture.* U.S. Government Printing Office, Washington, DC, 1939, p. 5. http://naldc.nal.usda.gov/download/IND50000141/PDF. Accessed January 11, 2012.
19. Nixon R. *Statement on the White House Conference on Food, Nutrition, and Health.* Washington, DC. http://www.presidency.ucsb.edu/ws/index.php?pid=2093#axzz1jB30uSCk. Accessed January 11, 2012.
20. Welsh S, Davis C, Shaw A. Development of the food guide pyramid. *Nutrition Today* 26: 12, 1992.
21. Britten P, Haven J, Davis C. Consumer research for development of educational messages for the mypyramid food guidance system. *Journal of Nutrition Education & Behavior* 38: S108, 2006.
22. Johnston CS. Uncle sam's diet sensation: MyPyramid—An overview and commentary. *Medscape General Medicine* 7: 78, 2005.
23. Nestle M. *What to Eat.* North Point Press, New York, 2006, p. 149.
24. Barnes M. Solving the problem of childhood obesity within a generation: White House Task Force on Childhood Obesity Report to the President, Washington, DC, p. 15, 2010. http://www.letsmove.gov/sites/letsmove.gov/files/TaskForce_on_Childhood_Obesity_May2010_FullReport.pdf. Accessed January 11, 2012.
25. U.S.D.A. Development of 2010 dietary guidelines for Americans consumer messages and new food icon: Executive summary of formative research. 2011. http://www.choosemyplate.gov/food-groups/downloads/MyPlate/ExecutiveSummaryOfFormativeResearch.pdf. Accessed January 11, 2012.
26. Kant A, Schatzkin A, Harris T et al. Dietary diversity and subsequent mortality in the first national health and nutrition examination survey epidemiologic follow-up study. *American Journal of Clinical Nutrition* 57: 434, 1993.

27. Patterson RE, Haines PS, Popkin BM. Diet quality index: Capturing a multidimensional behavior. *JADA* 94: 57, 1994.

28. Kennedy ET, Ohls J, Carlson S, Fleming K. The healthy eating index: Design and applications. *JADA* 95: 1103, 1995.

29. Center for Nutrition Policy and Promotion. *The Healthy Eating Index.* U.S. Department of Agriculture, Washington, DC, 1995. http://www.cnpp.usda.gov/publications/hei/HEI89-90report.pdf. Accessed January 11, 2012.

30. Bowman SA, Lino M, Gerrior SA, Basiotis PP. *The Healthy Eating Index: 1994–1996.* Center for Nutrition Policy and Promotion, U.S. Department of Agriculture, Washington, DC, 1998. http://www.cnpp.usda.gov/publications/hei/hei94-96report.PDF. Accessed January 11, 2012.

31. Basiotis PP. *The Healthy Eating Index: 1999–2000.* Center for Nutrition Policy and Promotion, U.S. Department of Agriculture, Washington, DC, 2002. http://www.cnpp.usda.gov/publications/HEI/HEI99-00report.pdf. Accessed January 11, 2012.

32. Guenther P, Reedy J, Krebs-Smith S et al. *Development and Evaluation of the Healthy Eating Index-2005: Technical Report.* Center for Nutrition Policy and Promotion, U.S. Department of Agriculture, Washington, DC, 2007. http://www.cnpp.usda.gov/Publications/HEI/HEI-2005/HEI-2005TechnicalReport.pdf. Accessed January 11, 2012.

33. Guenther PM, Juan WY, Reedy J et al. *Diet Quality of Americans in 1994–96 and 2001–02 as Measured by the Healthy Eating Index-2005.* Center for Nutrition Policy and Promotion, U.S. Department of Agriculture, Washington, DC, 2007. http://www.cnpp.usda.gov/Publications/NutritionInsights/Insight37.pdf. Accessed January 11, 2012.

34. Guenther PM, Juan WY, Lino M et al. *Diet Quality of Low-Income and Higher Income Americans in 2003–2004 as Measured by the Healthy Eating Index-2005.* Center for Nutrition Policy and Promotion, U.S. Department of Agriculture, Washington, DC, 2008. http://www.cnpp.usda.gov/Publications/NutritionInsights/Insight42.pdf. Accessed January 11, 2012.

35. Juan WY, Guenther PM, Kott PS. *Diet Quality of Older Americans in 1994–1996 and 2001–2002 as Measured by the Healthy Eating Index-2005.* Center for Nutrition Policy and Promotion, U.S. Department of Agriculture, Washington, DC, 2008. http://www.cnpp.usda.gov/Publications/NutritionInsights/Insight41.pdf. Accessed January 11, 2012.

36. Fungwe T, Guenther P, Juan W et al. *The Quality of Children's Diets in 2003–04 as Measured by the Healthy Eating Index-2005.* Center for Nutrition Policy and Promotion, U.S. Department of Agriculture, Washington, DC, 2009. http://www.cnpp.usda.gov/Publications/NutritionInsights/Insight43.pdf. Accessed January 11, 2012.

# 28 Dietary Guidelines around the World
## *Regional Similarities and Differences and New Innovations*

*Odilia I. Bermudez, Johanna T. Dwyer, and Erin Bury*

## CONTENTS

## INTRODUCTION AND OVERVIEW

Dietary guidelines are "recommendations for achieving appropriate diets, and healthy lifestyles."[1] In this chapter, we examine the similarities, differences, strengths, and weaknesses of some representative examples of dietary guidelines from various regions of the world. The chapter concludes with a review of some innovations and new resources that are now available as adjuncts to the guidelines in many countries.

The regions we have chosen represent different health and economic realities, as well as different foodways, culinary traditions, and eating habits. For example, the European, American, Canadian, some of the Asian (Japan), and Australian/New Zealand guidelines are examples of highly industrialized, affluent populations. The Indian, Latin American, and African guidelines represent populations that are in the midst of the "nutrition transition." The term "nutrition transition" refers to the shift from a pattern of high fertility and high mortality, to a pattern of low fertility and low mortality.[2] It also refers to the shift from prevalent infectious diseases associated with malnutrition, famine, and poor environmental sanitation to a pattern chronic and degenerative diseases associated with affluent urban-industrial.[2–5] Both highly affluent and very poor populations that differ in their degree of urbanization and standards of living all live within each of these countries. Dietary guidelines from many other countries are also available at a Food and Agricultural Organization's website.[6]

## CHARACTERISTICS OF EFFECTIVE GUIDELINES

Effective dietary guidelines have several elements in common. Good ones are designed to address and mitigate the major diet-related nutrition problems of the population to which they are addressed. They are also timely; since health problems change over time, the recommendations cannot be static but must also be updated periodically, as is done with the Dietary Guidelines for Americans.[1,7]

Effective guidelines also are evidence-based, with strong supportive scientific evidence underlying them. Eating habits, cultural beliefs, and food supplies available are also considered in effective guidelines.[6] The dietary guideline messages conveyed are reviewed and tested prior to their finalization to ensure that the guidelines are communicated effectively. Successful guidelines are also integrated with other nutritional guidance of a public health nature, since they are but one of groups of essential components of effective food and nutrition policies.

Other factors present in effective guidelines include mention of a variety of safe and affordable foods that are easily accessible with available economic and environmental resources, with attention to sustainability. Ideally, once successful guidelines are promulgated, they are followed up by studies to evaluate their effectiveness.

## DIETARY GUIDELINES IN ENGLISH-SPEAKING NORTH AMERICA AND AUSTRALIA/NEW ZEALAND

### Overview

In English-speaking North America, Europe, Australia, New Zealand, and parts of Asia such as Japan and Singapore, guidelines and other health education have addressed excessive as well as inadequate dietary patterns, weight, and physical activity since they were first formulated in the late 1970s and early 1980s. All of these affluent countries share similar nutrition-related problems, including dietary patterns that are frequently excessive in calories, fat, salt, sugars, and alcohol, and too low in fruits, vegetables, and whole grains.

Today, diet-related diseases formerly considered as affecting only affluent countries and populations (such as obesity, type 2 diabetes, heart disease, and certain cancers) are common among all socioeconomic groups. Therefore, these issues are a major focus of the dietary guidelines of these countries, and they are also being incorporated in the guidelines in countries undergoing the nutrition transition.

### Formulation

Table 28.1 shows the approaches used in the development of the dietary guidelines in these affluent countries and their key characteristics. In dietary guideline development, all of these countries used nutrition experts and scientists, and all of the guidelines were endorsed by a relevant government agency. All four of these well-off countries address their guidelines to both the general population and health professionals or other policy makers.

### United States

The United States' 2010 Dietary Guidelines for Americans (DGA), presented in Table 28.2, is a combination of food-based and ingredient-based recommendations.[8] They are for individuals 2 years and older and are not segregated by age.

The 2010 DGA usually follows the precedents established in earlier versions. Compared to earlier editions, in the 2010 Dietary Guidelines for Americans, some changes simply involve a change in wording. For example, the American guideline regarding sugar has evolved from "Avoid too much sugar" in 1980[9] to "Use sugars only in moderation" in 1990[10] and "Choose a diet moderate in sugars" in 1995[11] to the 2000 "Choose beverages and foods that limit your intake of sugars,[12] in 2005 "Choose and prepare foods and beverages with little added sugars or caloric sweeteners,"[13] and in 2010 "Limit the consumption of foods that contain refined grains, especially refined grain foods that contain solid fats, added sugars, and sodium."[8] Other changes are more innovative.

The United States added new guidelines on food safety in 2000 and expanded them in 2005.[13,14] The 2010 guidelines also included recommendations for specific population groups at high nutritional risk.[8] Since the report of the 2005 Dietary Guidelines for Americans Scientific Committee,[13] American guidelines have been increasingly oriented toward policy makers and health professionals, rather than to the general public. Their intent is to summarize current knowledge regarding individual nutrients and food components into recommendations for a pattern of eating that can guide federal food programs and that can be adapted for use by consumers. Simplified consumer-friendly messages with key images for consumers have been also prepared to help people to choose diets like those recommended in the DGA, including the *MyPyramid* icon in earlier DGA[15] and more recently *MyPlate*.[8]

In the United States, the National Nutrition Monitoring and Related Research Act of 1990 required that the Dietary Guidelines for Americans be updated every 5 years and be

**TABLE 28.1**
**Development of Dietary Guidelines in the United States, Canada, Australia, and New Zealand**

| Country | United States | Canada | Australia | New Zealand |
|---|---|---|---|---|
| Title of guidelines | Dietary Guidelines for Americans | Eating well with Canada's food guide | Dietary Guidelines for All Australians | Food and Nutrition Guidelines |
| Year | 2010 | 2007 | 2003 | 2003 |
| Endorsing unit | U.S. Department of Agriculture and Department of Health and Human Services | Department of National Health and Welfare | National Health and Medical Research Council | Nutrition Task Force at the Ministry of Health |
| Approaches[a] | 1–5, 7 | 1–5, 7 | 1–5 | 1–5 |
| Number of guidelines | 27 | 11 | 13 | 6 |
| Target audiences[b] | G, H, P, N | G, H, P, N | G, H, P | G, H, P |
| Major nutrition problems addressed in guidelines[c] | C,E,I,O | C,E,I,O | C,E,I,O | C,E,I,O |
| Graphic representation | MyPlate | Rainbow | Pyramid | None |
| Other dietary guidelines | National Cancer Institute American Institute for Cancer Research American Heart Association | Dietary guidelines for: • Children • Women of childbearing age • Men and women over 50 | National physical activity guidelines | Dietary guidelines for: • Healthy infants and toddlers • Healthy children • Healthy adolescents • Healthy breast-feeding women • Healthy pregnant women • Healthy older people |

[a] 1, Nutrition experts, nutrition scientists views; 2, review of former guidelines; 3, from food groups; 4, from consumption/nutrition survey; 5, definition of nutritional objectives; 6, economic data; 7, consumer focus groups.
[b] G, general population; H, health professionals; P, policy makers; N, nutrition education of school children.
[c] C, diet-related chronic degenerative diseases; I, dietary inadequacy; E, dietary excess (other nutrients); O, overnutrition (energy); PEM, protein–energy malnutrition.

**TABLE 28.2**

**Dietary Guidelines for the United States**

**United States 2010**

**Key Recommendations**

1. Prevent and/or reduce overweight and obesity through improved eating and physical activity behaviors
2. Control total calorie intake to manage body weight. For people who are overweight or obese, this will mean consuming fewer calories from food or beverages
3. Increase physical activity and reduce time spent in sedentary behaviors
4. Maintain appropriate calorie balance each stage of life—childhood, adolescence, adulthood, pregnancy and breast-feeding, and older age
5. Reduce daily sodium intake to less than 2300 mg and further reduce intake to 1500 mg among persons who are 51 and older and those of any age who are African American or have hypertension, diabetes, or chronic kidney disease
6. Consume less than 10% of calories from saturated fatty acids by replacing them with monounsaturated and polyunsaturated fatty acids
7. Consume less than 300 mg/day of dietary cholesterol
8. Keep *trans*-fatty acid consumption as low as possible by limiting foods that contain synthetic sources of *trans* fats, such as partially hydrogenated oils, and by limiting other solid fats
9. Reduce the intake of calories from solid fats and added sugars
10. Limit the consumption of foods that contain refined grains, especially refined grain foods that contain solid fats, added sugars, and sodium
11. If alcohol is consumed, it should be consumed in moderation—up to one drink per day for women and two drinks per day for men—and only by adults of legal drinking age
12. Increase vegetable and fruit intake
13. Eat a variety of vegetables, especially dark-green and red and orange vegetables and beans and peas
14. Consume at least half of all grains as whole grains. Increase whole-grain intake by replacing refined grains with whole grains
15. Increase intake of fat-free or low-fat milk and milk products, such as milk, yogurt, cheese, or fortified soy beverages
16. Choose a variety of protein foods, which include seafood, lean meat and poultry, eggs, beans and peas, soy products, and unsalted nuts and seeds
17. Increase the amount and variety of seafood consumed by choosing seafood in place of some meat and poultry
18. Replace protein foods that are higher in solid fats with choices that are lower in solid fats and calories and/or are sources of oils
19. Use oils to replace solid fats where possible
20. Choose foods that provide more potassium, dietary fiber, calcium, and vitamin D, which are nutrients of concern in American diets. These foods include vegetables, fruits, whole grains, and milk and milk products

reviewed by the Departments of Health and Human Services and Agriculture. The latest Dietary Guidelines for Americans were issued in 2010 and are summarized in Table 28.2.[8] The traditional pyramid (MyPyramid) was replaced in 2011 with MyPlate as a graphic tool consistent with the new dietary guidelines.[8]

## CANADA

Table 28.3 presents Canada's dietary guidelines. They were first developed in 1942 and have been updated many times since. After reviewing the 1992 dietary guidelines, some challenges were identified in understanding and using the dietary information presented in the guidelines. The 2007 "Eating well with Canada's food guide"[16] reflects current nutritional recommendations, that is, the Dietary Reference Intakes (produced jointly by the Institute of Medicine, National Academy of Sciences, and Health Canada), as well as changes in the Canadian food supply, changes in the patterns of food use, and special emphasis on a central message: *Eat well and be active today and every day!*

## AUSTRALIA AND NEW ZEALAND

Since 2003 Australia has had a hybrid of food-based and nutrient-based recommendations.[17] After a recent review and update of the Australian Guidelines, the National Health

and Medical Research Council (NHMRC) released the draft Australian Dietary Guidelines and Australian Guide to Healthy Eating for public consultation, and new guidelines should be issued later in 2012.[18]

As reflected in Table 28.3, each current guideline deals with a specific health issue, for example, "maintain a healthy body weight by balancing physical activity and food intake," (New Zealand 2003) and describes the increasing prevalence of overweight and obesity within the population. In the past, the dietary guidelines were numbered, but this practice has since been discontinued. The National Health and Medical Research Council felt that numbering the guidelines gives the wrong impression that one is more important than the other. The dietary guidelines work together and act much like individual pieces to a "good puzzle."[17]

In 1991, the New Zealand Nutrition Task Force recommended the development of population-based food and nutrition guidelines. These dietary guidelines are based on a series of population-specific food and nutrition guideline background papers started in 2003 for healthy adults.[19] Those addressing specific age groups were developed in the succeeding years after the task force's recommendation. Each guideline background paper is accompanied by an educational resource for use by the general public. These papers include information for infants 0–2 years of age, children ages 2–12, adolescents, children and young people

**TABLE 28.3**

**Dietary Guidelines for Selected North American and Oceanic Countries**

| Canada 2007 | Australia 2003 | New Zealand 2003 |
|---|---|---|
| 1. Make each serving count (7–8 servings)<br>2. Make at least half of your grain products whole grains (7 servings)<br>3. Drink skim, 1%, or 2% milk each day (2 servings)<br>4. Select lean meat and alternatives prepared with little or no added fat or salt (2 servings)<br>5. Consume 2–3 Tbsp of unsaturated fat each day<br>6. For children: don't restrict nutritious foods due to fat content; give small nutritious meals and snacks<br>7. Women of childbearing age: take an MVI; pregnant women need iron, and pregnant and breast-feeding women need extra calories<br>8. Adults over 50 need vitamin D<br>9. Physical activity for 30–60 min each day for adults, 90 min for children/youth<br>10. Limit foods and beverages high in calories, fat, sugar, or salt<br>11. Read and compare food labels | 1. Prevent excess weight gain<br>2. Enjoy a variety of nutritious foods<br>3. Eat plenty of vegetables, legumes, and fruits<br>4. Eat plenty of cereals, preferably whole grain<br>5. Include lean meats, fish, poultry, or alternatives<br>6. Include milk, yogurt, cheese, or alternatives<br>7. Drink plenty of water<br>8. Limit saturated fats and moderate total fat intake<br>9. Choose foods low in salt<br>10. Limit your alcohol intake if you choose to drink<br>11. Consume only moderate amounts of sugars and foods containing added sugars<br>12. Care for your food; prepare and store it safely<br>13. Encourage and support breast-feeding | 1. Eat a variety of foods from each of the four major food groups each day<br>2. Prepare meals with minimal added fat (especially saturated fat), salt, and sugar<br>3. Choose prepared foods, drinks, and snacks that are low in fat (especially saturated fat), salt, and sugar<br>4. Maintain a healthy body weight by regular physical activity and by healthy eating<br>5. Drink plenty of liquids each day<br>6. If drinking alcohol, do each day so in moderation |

2–18 years, pregnant and breast-feeding women, adults, and older people. Subsequent revisions have been made since the original dietary guidelines and continue to be made with the findings of new research, including the nutrient reference values.[19]

The United States, Canada, and Australia have graphical representations for their dietary recommendations. The United States now uses a plate (MyPlate), to promote healthy eating along with the dietary guidelines. Canada uses a rainbow graphic to depict the components of a healthy diet. Australia has two graphics: a pyramid and a circular plate, which was used in the past. Although New Zealand did not use a graphic representation of its dietary guidelines, authorities there have produced educational pieces with several illustrations of those guidelines that reflect their emphasis in the education of its population.

## SIMILARITIES

Food-based guidelines are thought to be easier for consumers to implement than nutrient-based guidelines since human beings eat foods and not specific nutrients. All of these affluent countries have guidelines that include recommendations for certain nutrients or ingredients like sugar or salt and also for groups of foods, such as fruits/vegetables, grains, dairy, and meats.

The problems addressed by the guidelines also are similar in all of these countries since heart disease, hypertension, diabetes with its complications and certain cancers are the leading causes of death in each of them.[8,20,21] Obesity, which is also prevalent, increases the severity and adverse outcomes from many of these diseases.[8,16,22]

The core messages in all of these dietary guidelines are also similar: eat a variety of foods and include physical activity to achieve and/or maintain a healthy weight. The

U.S. dietary guidelines have recently adopted a particularly strong emphasis on weight control through diet and physical activity, and now state that that major causes of illness and death are related to both a poor diet and to a sedentary lifestyle.

The background and supporting information accompanying the dietary guidelines of these countries provides the rationale for quantitative suggestions for intakes of specific nutrients.[8,17,23] All of these countries have guidelines that suggest that 50%–55% of total calories should come from carbohydrates. They vary in the amount of total fat from 30% to 35% of calories.

Moderation in the consumption of saturated fat is also addressed, with recommendations for consumption of less saturated fat (Australia and New Zealand) consumption of less than 10% of calories from saturated fat in the U.S. guidelines and Canadian guidelines that advise the population to "consume 2–3 Tbsp of unsaturated fat each day".

All of these affluent countries have recommendations on limiting fat, salt, and alcohol and increasing fruits, vegetables, and whole grains. The United States, Canada, and New Zealand all suggest limiting alcoholic beverages to less than two drinks/day for men and one for women. Australia has a higher limit: less than four drinks for men and two for women/day.

The United States, Canada, Australia, and New Zealand all are affluent, but each of them has sizeable minority populations. According to the U.S. 2010 census data, the diversity of the American population is widening with over 16% being of Hispanic origin and 13% African Americans.[24] Therefore, guidelines need to be easily adaptable to the eating patterns of these and other ethnic groups, such as American Indian and Alaska Natives, Native Hawaiian and other Pacific Islanders, and Asian Americans.

In addition to race/ethnic minority populations, in the United States there is growing attention to the problems of the chronically ill, which themselves constitute a minority of sorts. In the United States, several professional associations have also promulgated dietary guidelines for those at risk or already suffering from chronic degenerative diseases such as cancer and heart disease.[25,26] These are usually based on the dietary guidelines but are more disease specific. As example, the 2006 recommendations from the American Heart Association (AHA) address more strict reduction of dietary saturated and *trans*-fatty acids for people affected by a cardiovascular disease than those for the general U.S. population.[26] AHA also addresses the importance of minimizing consumption of food and beverages with added sugars; eating a diet rich in vegetables, fruits, and whole-grain foods; and avoiding use of and exposure to tobacco products, while emphasizing in physical activity and weight control.[26]

The American Cancer Society (ACS) promulgated the latest version (2012) of its nutrition guidelines on nutrition and physical activity for cancer prevention, which include recommendations for individual choices and recommendations for community action.[25] The ACS guidelines for individual action include recommendations related to healthy weight, physical activity, and moderation in alcohol consumption. ACS dietary guidelines include an overall recommendation for healthy eating based on giving emphasis to plant foods instead of animal products, plus four specific guidelines: daily consumption of at least 2.5 cups of vegetables and fruits, limiting consumption of processed meat and red meat, choosing whole grains instead of refined grain products, and choosing foods and beverages in amounts that help achieve and maintain a healthy weight.[25]

Canada has a sizeable aboriginal population. This group includes the Indian, Inuit, and Métis peoples of Canada.[27] In 2007, food-based dietary guidelines (FBDG) were developed to reflect the cultural differences and recommendations for this population group. These dietary guidelines also emphasize the spiritual and physical importance of traditional aboriginal foods and include the role of nontraditional foods in contemporary diets.[23]

In Australia, the Aboriginal and Torres Strait Islander people comprise only about 2.5% of the entire population,[20] but they often live under impoverished, overcrowded conditions that put them at nutritional risk.[20] They also have a high prevalence of android (apple) pattern obesity, which is associated with many health problems.[20] In New Zealand 13% of the population belongs to the rapidly growing Maori minority, and another 5% of the population is Pacific Islanders.[28] Some of these minority groups have increased risks of chronic degenerative diseases that are developing rapidly as they move away from traditional customs to modern diets and lifestyles. The information accompanying the Australian and New Zealand dietary guidelines deals with these special problems of minority populations, although the dietary guidelines are targeted to the general population.

## DIFFERENCES

There are some differences in the issues the guidelines of these highly industrialized countries cover. In the 2000 edition of the U.S. guidelines, food safety was first addressed and it has continued to be included. Elderly people and pregnant women are especially vulnerable to risks associated with food-borne illnesses. Australia's food safety guidelines specifically address food safety in the elderly (care for your food: prepare and store it correctly) and the New Zealand guidelines discuss risks from *Listeria monocytogenes* in the information specifically directed to pregnant women.[68] Canada does not discuss food safety in its guidelines.

The guidelines for the United States and Canada are for all healthy individuals over age 2 years,[8,16] except for the fat guideline in Canada, which does not apply to children under 5 years of age. Australia and New Zealand both have specific guidelines for infants, toddlers, school-age children, adolescents, and the elderly that also include other health recommendations related to nutrition, such as breast-feeding of infants and physical activity for everyone.[18,19] New Zealand also has dietary guidelines for pregnant and breast-feeding women. Both countries also focus some specific guidelines on poor and disadvantaged populations. Another health recommendation that is included in New Zealand's guidelines is nonsmoking, especially for adolescents and pregnant and breast-feeding women. Also, the elderly, who may suffer from isolation and therefore poor nutrition, are encouraged to "make mealtime a social time." Australia encourages its elderly to eat at least 3 meals/day.

## CONCLUSIONS

The guidelines for these well-off English-speaking countries in different parts of the world are very similar, reflecting the affluent lifestyles, climates, and common foodways that they share.

# LATIN AMERICA

Dietary guidelines were first formulated in Latin America in the late 1980s.[29] Guidelines from Argentina, Chile, Guatemala, Ecuador, Mexico, Panama, Venezuela, and Uruguay are provided as examples of dietary guidelines in the region.

Latin America is a region with great inequalities in the distribution of wealth and also large variations in the nutritional health of its population groups. There has been a shift from dietary deficiency disease to problems of dietary excess in many countries of the region over the past two decades as incomes have risen and the nutritional transition progresses in all of them.[30–34]

In Chile, the prevalence of protein–calorie malnutrition in children has declined rapidly, but the prevalence of chronic degenerative diseases associated with excesses and imbalances in food intake and sedentary lifestyles is rising[35–37] as incomes have increased. In contrast, in Guatemala,[38,39] Ecuador,[40] and Mexico,[41] poverty-related undernutrition

## TABLE 20.4
## Development of Dietary Guidelines in Latin American Countries

|  | Chile | Guatemala | Mexico | Panama | Venezuela |
|---|---|---|---|---|---|
| Title of guidelines | Food guidelines for Chile | Food guidelines for Guatemala | Food guidelines—Mexico | Food guidelines for Panama | Food guidelines for Venezuela |
| Year | 2005 | 1998 | 1993 | 1995 | 2003 |
| Endorsing unit | Ministry of Health, Food Technology and Nutrition Institute, and University of Chile | Food guidelines national committee | National nutrition institute | Ministry of Health | CAVENDES Foundation, National Institute of Nutrition, several universities |
| Approaches[a] | 1, 3, 4 | 1, 3, 6 | 1, 3, 4, 5, 6 | 1, 3, 4, 5 | 1, 2, 5, 6 |
| Target audiences[b] | G, P, N | G | G | G, P | G, P, N |
| Graphic representation | Pyramid | Family pot | Pyramid | Pyramid | None |
| Other guidelines | For school-age children and for the elderly | Food safety | None | For the first year of age | For the preschooler, school-age children, and for the elderly |

[a] 1, Nutrition experts, nutrition scientists views; 2, review of former guidelines; 3, from food groups; 4, from consumption/nutrition survey; 5, definition of nutritional objectives; 6, economic data.

[b] G, general population; H, health professionals; P, policy makers; N, nutrition education of school children.

and dietary deficiency diseases are still prevalent especially among children and women of reproductive age in rural areas. At the same time, the prevalence of diet-related chronic diseases is rising, especially among the affluent in cities. Venezuela is an oil-exporting country, but it still has large economic inequalities and grapples with poverty-related malnutrition as well as dietary excess. Argentina faces similar problems among its diverse population. Children are at particular risk for health-related problems due to lack of clean water and environmental pollutants in that country.

In most Latin American countries, food consumption patterns are influenced to some extent by the same factors that are also evident in the United States. Changing cultural and economic influences, rural–urban migration, greater availability of processed foods, and advertising are all also affecting food consumption.[42] Both over- and undernutrition may result.[41,43,44] Residence in poor ghettos in and around metropolitan areas, short lactation periods, low wages, and low maternal educational levels are associated with undernutrition in young children. The interactions of urbanization, sedentary lifestyles, lack of nutrition education, and excessive consumption of cheap foods low in nutritional value make diseases of overconsumption, such as obesity, diabetes, and cardiovascular disease common.[31,32,45]

### FORMULATION

Out of the 33 countries from Latin America and the Caribbean, 18 have listed their national dietary guidelines in the webpage of the Food and Agriculture Organization of the United Nations (FAO).[6] However, there are other countries that, although not listed in the FAO site, have already established their dietary guidelines; this is the case for Costa Rica and Honduras.[46,47] The dietary guidelines for the Mexican

population have been issued for many years by the Mexican Institute of Nutrition.[6,48] Venezuela issued dietary guidelines in the late 1980s that were later revised and updated.[6,49] The dietary guidelines have been implemented in many ways in that country. For example, they have been incorporated into Venezuelan kindergarten, elementary, and secondary school curricula.[50,51]

Table 28.4 provides details about the dietary guidelines development process in the Latin American countries of Chile,[52] Guatemala,[53] Mexico,[49] Panama,[54] and Venezuela.[49] All have dietary guidelines for the general population. Some also have guidelines for specific population groups (Chile, Panama, and Venezuela) or target certain groups because of specific concerns (e.g., Guatemala focusing on food safety among the poor). Governmental or quasi-governmental organizations develop and promulgate the guidelines based on the views and opinions of experts and scientists in these countries. Some guidelines also use background data from food consumption surveys (Chile, Mexico, and Panama) and economic data (Venezuela, Mexico) to supplement expert opinion in constructing their guidelines. Most of the countries also refer to food groups rather than nutrients in their dietary guidelines.

Four of the countries, Chile, Panama, Mexico, and Guatemala, also use graphic representations of food groups to visualize the advice in the guidelines and provide supporting messages. Chile and Panama adopted the food guide pyramid used in the United States until 2011. Mexico uses a plate rather than the pyramid it formerly employed. Guatemala summarizes its food groups and dietary guidelines in a family pot resembling a jar or "crock-pot" graphic. Venezuela has no graphic, but the government has produced an extensive set of educational materials directed at different target groups.[50,51]

Tables 28.5 through 28.7 summarize the dietary guidelines for selected Latin American countries. The number of guidelines varies a great deal, ranging from 4 in Ecuador to 17 in Mexico; Venezuela has issued 9 guidelines and also 40 educational messages to facilitate the implementation of the guidelines.

## SIMILARITIES

Guatemala is categorized by the World Bank as a lower-middle-income nation, as its population gross national income (GNI) felt in the bracket of $1026 to $4035 per capita.[55]

Guatemala emphasizes getting adequate amounts of grains, fruits, and vegetables per day for its population. Ecuador, Chile, Panama, Venezuela, Mexico, and Argentina have more affluent economic environments, classified by the World Bank as upper-middle-income economies (GNI per capita between $4,036–$12,475).[55] With more of the population economically secure, these countries can focus more on educating their citizens more on specific nutrients, rather than on simply getting enough to eat. All of the dietary guidelines provide recommendations for specific nutrients, fat, salt, and sugar, and address concerns for chronic diseases. The guidelines also suggest variety in the

---

## TABLE 28.5
### Dietary Guidelines for Selected Lower-Middle-Income Latin American Countries

| Bolivia 2000 | El Salvador 2009 | Guatemala 1998 |
|---|---|---|
| 1. Eat every day balanced meals increasing cereals, grains, fruits, and vegetables | 1. Eat a varied diet | 1. Include, at each meal, grains, cereals, or potatoes, because they are nutritious, tasty, and have low cost |
| 2. At least three times per week eat liver, meat, fish, or dried meat | 2. Include in all meals grains, root crops, and plantains | 2. Eat every day vegetables and greens to benefit your body |
| 3. Increase your consumption of eggs and low-fat dairy products | 3. Eat tortillas and beans every day | 3. Every day, eat some types of fruit, because they are healthy, easy to digest, and nutritious |
| 4. Always use iodized salt with your meals without excesses | 4. Eat vegetables and leafy greens every day | 4. If you can eat tortilla and beans every day, eat one spoonful of beans with each tortilla to make more nutritious |
| 5. Prefer vegetable oil and avoid reheated fats and oils | 5. Include fruits in season as part of your daily eating | 5. At least twice a week, eat one egg, or one piece of cheese, or drink one glass of milk, to complement your diet |
| 6. Wash your hands after using the bathroom and before cooking or eating | 6. Eat eggs, milk, and milk products at least 3 times a week | 6. At least once per week, eat a serving of liver (beef) or meat to strengthen your body |
| 7. Reduce your consumption of tea and coffee and replace them with porridges ("mazamorras") made with native products | 7. Eat meats, liver, or other entrails at least once a week | 7. To stay healthy, eat a variety of foods as indicate in the household pot |
| 8. Avoid elevated consumption of sugar, sweets, and drinks | 8. Make sure the salt you consume is fortified with iodine | |
| 9. Practice frequently some sports and physical activity | 9. Make sure the sugar you consume is fortified with vitamin A | |
| | 10. Drink plenty of water every day | |

---

## TABLE 28.6
### Dietary Guidelines for Selected Upper-Middle-Income Latin American Countries

| Chile 2005 | Ecuador 1999 | Panama 1997 | Venezuela 2003 |
|---|---|---|---|
| 1. Consume dairy products such as milk, yogurt, cheese or fresh cheese, 3 times a day | 1. Two servings of grain legume + 1 vegetable + oil = nutrient mixture | 1. Eat a variety of foods | 1. Eat foods from all food groups |
| 2. Eat three fruits of different colors and at least two dishes of vegetables every day | 2. It is very important to eat foods from each of the groups | 2. Eat sufficient grains, roots, vegetables, and fruits | 2. Daily, do 30 min of physical activity |
| 3. Eat beans, chickpeas, lentils, or peas at least two times per week, in place of meat | 3. Iron: prevents anemia of pregnant women and helps the formation of fetal blood | 3. Select a diet low in saturated fat, cholesterol, and oil | 3. Practice hygienic habits in your food preparation |
| 4. Eat fish, boiled, baked, steamed, or grilled, a minimum of 2 times a week | 4. Common problems during pregnancy: For dizziness and morning sickness, eat easily digested foods—crackers, toast, rice, noodles—before getting up in the morning and during periods of nausea; for cramps, increase foods rich in calcium and potassium, like salsa, Guinea, or spinach | 4. Eat sugar and sweets in moderation | 4. Use your money wisely in your food selection and expenditures |
| 5. Choose foods that are lower in saturated fat and cholesterol | | 5. Eat salt and sodium and moderation | 5. Breast milk is the only food without substitute for infants below 6 months of age |
| 6. Reduce consumption of sugar and salt | | 6. Maintain a healthy weight | 6. Increase your consumption of fruit, vegetables, legumes, and cereals |
| 7. Drink six to eight glasses of water per day | | | 7. Use moderation in consumption of sugar, salt, and alcoholic beverages |
| | | | 8. Consume animal products in moderate amounts |
| | | | 9. Water is indispensable for life, and its consumption helps to maintain health |

## TABLE 20.7
## Dietary Guidelines for Selected Upper-Middle-Income Latin American Countries

| Argentina 2000 | Mexico 2006 | Uruguay 2004 |
|---|---|---|
| 1. Eat a variety of foods. Eat with moderation and include a variety of foods for nutrients in all your meals. | 1. Make meal times enjoyable with family and friends. | 1. To maintain health, consume a varied diet that includes foods from different groups. |
| 2. Eat regular meals/eat breakfast. If possible, eat 4 times a day. | 2. Consume fruits and raw vegetables that are in season. | 2. Eat in moderation the necessary portions of each food group to maintain weight. |
| 3. Enjoy eating/read food labels as social part of eating. Take advantage of mealtimes to meet and talk with others. | 3. Consume moderate amounts of fat (margarine, vegetable oil, and mayonnaise among others), sugar (soft drinks, honey, jam, sweets, and table sugar), and salt. | 3. Begin each day with a breakfast that includes milk and fruit bread. |
| 4. Eat moderate amounts of food and sufficient energy and to meet the body's requirements. Eat with moderation. | 4. Eat according to your needs and conditions, neither more nor less. | 4. Eat at least a pint of milk per day. You can substitute with yogurt or cheese. This food group is required for all ages. |
| 5. Consume adequate fluids. Drink abundant clean and safe water throughout the day. | 5. Eat moderate amounts of food of animal origin, and prefer legumes. | 5. Increase your daily intake of fruits and vegetables in season including them in every meal. |
| 6. Eat complex carbohydrates and whole grains. Consume a variety of breads, cereals, pastas, flours, starch, and legumes. | 6. Combine (tortilla, bread, or pasta) cereals with legumes such as beans, chickpeas, or lentils. | 6. Control the consumption of meat, deli meat, butter, cheese, cream, mayonnaise, and fried foods for their high fat content. |
| 7. Eat more vegetables and fruits. Consume fruits and vegetables every day of all types and colors. | 7. Try to choose whole grains such as corn tortilla chips, whole-grain bread, oatmeal, and amaranth, rather than refined grains. | 7. Eat fewer sweets, sweetened beverages, sugar, desserts, candies, and pastries. |
| 8. Drink enough milk and consume calcium-rich foods. Consume milk, yogurt, or cheese every day; they are necessary at all ages. | 8. Try to eat fish and skinless chicken twice a week, rather than red meat. | 8. Reduce salt intake. Broth cubes, concentrated soups, sauces, sausages, cold cuts, hamburgers, and canned and snack bar products have very high salt content. |
| 9. Consume fish, poultry, eggs, lean meat, legumes, and pulses. Eat a wide variety of red and white meats, removing the visible fat. (Legumes are promoted in the group of cereals.). | 9. If you eat eggs, do so in moderation. | 9. More expensive foods are not necessarily more nutritious. Choose from each food group best suited to your budget. |
| 10. Moderate fat intake. Prepare your foods preferably with raw oils and avoid cooking with grease. | 10. Avoid alcoholic drinks, or drink them only sporadically because, among other factors, they are high in calories (7 kcal/g). | 10. Take care of food hygiene when buying, storing, preserving, preparing, and serving. Improperly handled food can cause serious illness. |
| 11. Moderate salt intake. Decrease intake of salt. | | |
| 12. Moderate sugar intake. Decrease intake of sugar. | | |
| 13. Moderate alcohol consumption. Decrease consumption of alcoholic beverages; avoid with children, teenagers, and pregnant or lactating women. | | |
| 14. Achieve and maintain a healthy body weight and exercise regularly. Enjoy physical activity various times during the week that helps in overall well-being. | | |
| 15. Exclusive breast-feeding is recommended from birth to at least 4–6 months. Exclusive breast-feeding is recommended until 6 months. | | |
| 16. Complementary feeding can be started between 4–6 months. Weaning should start at 6 months. | | |

daily diet, maintenance of a healthy weight, and tackling overconsumption patterns.

## DIFFERENCES

Recommendations on alcohol intake are included in the Venezuelan and Argentinean guidelines. Breast-feeding recommendations are included with Mexican, Venezuelan, and Argentinean recommendations. Panama has special dietary guidelines for infants that recommend exclusive breast-feeding during the first 6 months of life and for complementary feeding thereafter. Venezuelan guidelines also encourage hygiene when preparing food and food safety. Prudence in the management of financial resources is also encouraged.

The Ecuadorian guidelines provide recommendations for the makeup of a healthy plate: two servings of grain, legume, vegetable, and some oil. It also includes information for dealing with common problems during pregnancy, including nausea and cramps.

Guatemala, a country with low literacy rates, also emphasizes nutrients but in simple, short messages; it singles out energy, protein (both animal and vegetable), vitamins A and C, calcium, iron, zinc, and fiber.[53] This emphasis reflects Guatemala's goals of preventing both dietary deficiencies and excesses. It is recommended that those with limited resources eat meats, eggs, and dairy products at least once or twice a week. Since dairy products can be costly, and much of the population does not prefer milk, the guidelines recommend consuming milk once or twice a week. They also recommend consuming fruit and vegetables every day to improve health. Finally, there is considerable emphasis on the importance of hand washing, and keeping food and water well covered and free from vermin is displayed in its graphic.

## CONCLUSIONS

Dietary guidelines for the Latin American countries we reviewed reflect the diversity in socioeconomic situations and nutritional problems in the region and each country's unique perspectives. They offer the general public, service providers, and policy makers actionable recommendations for improving nutrition and health status. Some countries, like Mexico, still need to evaluate the applicability of their guidelines to the eating practices of the ethnically and economically diverse Mexican population. Dietary guidelines in Guatemala were directed to the poor; however, problems associated with overconsumption of foods and sedentary lifestyles still need to be addressed.

## ASIA

Asia's diversity is reflected in many cuisines and cultural practices. However, the countries all present similarities in their nutritional problems related to under- and overconsumption that are present in most other developing countries described in this chapter: China,[56] India,[57] Indonesia,[58] Japan,[59] Korea,[60] Malaysia,[61] Philippines,[62] Singapore,[63] and Thailand.[64]

Until the mid-1950s, poverty-related malnutrition was the major problem in Asia. The primary concern was to ensure adequate energy intakes and prevention or control of prevalent dietary deficiency diseases.[58,62,65] Today, nutrition problems in Asia cover the entire spectrum from deficiency disease to excess.[56,62,65] Most countries in this region are experiencing new affluence, and increasingly, issues of chronic degenerative disease are also becoming common.[56]

Most of the Asian dietary guidelines focus on reducing or preventing both chronic deficiencies and chronic degenerative diseases since both problems are often prevalent.[59,60,66,67] Presently, India still has high rates of protein–energy malnutrition among some groups, but it also has very affluent population groups, which suffer from chronic degenerative disease and obesity.[57,65] The Indian national guidelines address both groups. In countries such as Korea, Japan, and Singapore, deficiency diseases have declined dramatically in the past four decades.[59,60,63] Countries such as Thailand and China have low rates of protein–energy malnutrition, but micronutrient deficiencies (iron, Iodine, vitamin A, and riboflavin) are still common.[56,68] Indonesia and the Philippines face both persistent problems of undernutrition and deficiency disease among the poor, coupled with emerging problems of overnutrition and increased chronic degenerative disease rates, particularly among the affluent.[58,62] Filipino guidelines for the more affluent members of the population focus on chronic degenerative diseases and avoiding excess, whereas a different set of Filipino guidelines that exist for the poor emphasize achieving sufficiency of nutrient intakes.[62]

### FORMULATION

Table 28.8 shows the various approaches used in developing dietary guidelines in these countries in Asia. The guidelines are all intended to provide nutrition education and dietary

## TABLE 28.8
## Development of Dietary Guidelines in Asian Countries

| Country | China | India | Indonesia | Japan | Korea |
|---|---|---|---|---|---|
| Title of guidelines | FBDGs in China | Dietary guideline for Indians | 13 Core messages for a balanced diet | Guidelines for health promotion: dietary guidelines | National dietary guidelines |
| Year | 2007 | 2010 | 1995 | 1985 | 1990 |
| Endorsing unit | Chinese Nutrition Society | National Institute of Nutrition | National Development and Planning Coordinating Board | Ministry of Health and Welfare | Korean Nutrition Society/Ministry of Health and Welfare |
| Approaches[a] | 1–5 | 1–6 | 1 | 1, 2, 3, 5 | 1, 2, 4 |
| Target audiences[b] | G, H | G, H, N | G | G, H | G |
| Graphic representation | Pagoda | Stairs | None | Numeral 6 | Pagoda |
| Title of guidelines | Proposed dietary guidelines for Malaysia | Nutritional guidelines for Filipinos | Guidelines for a healthy diet | Dietary guidelines for the population | The Thai dietary guidelines for better health |
| Year | 1996 | 1990 | 1993 | 1995 | 1995 |
| Endorsing unit | Ministry of Health | Department of Science and Technology (National Guidelines Committee) | National Advisory Committee on Food and Nutrition, Ministry of Health | Department of Health | Division of Nutrition, Department of Health, and Ministry of Public Health |
| Approaches[a] | 1, 2, 3 | 1–5 | 1 | 1 | 1 |
| Target audiences[b] | G, H | G, H | G | G | G |
| Graphic representation | Pyramid | Pyramid, 6-sided star | Pyramid | Plum flower | None |

[a] 1, Nutrition experts, nutrition scientists views; 2, review of former guidelines; 3, from food groups; 4, from consumption/nutrition survey; 5, definition of nutritional objectives; 6, economic data.

[b] G, general population; H, health professionals; P, policy makers; N, nutrition education of school children.

guidance to the general public in terms that are understand-able to most consumers. They are also used to help officials in the health, agricultural, and educational sectors in program planning. All of the countries surveyed rely on government agencies and/or professional societies to develop and endorse their official guidelines. Some countries (such as the Philippines, Korea, and Japan) formulate guidelines based on findings from national nutrition or food consumption surveys. Others develop their dietary guidelines based on what experts deem to be appropriate.

Graphics or icons have been adopted by many of the Asian countries to help the public visualize these dietary guidelines and food guides. These include the "Healthy Food Pyramid" in Singapore,[69] the Malaysian food guide pyramid,[70] the "Food Guide Spinning Top" for Japan,[71] a new version of the traditional "food pagoda" in China,[56] and a "nutrition flag" in Thailand.[68]

Table 28.10 provides dietary recommendations for China, Malaysia, and Thailand. The World Bank categorizes these countries as upper-middle income. Table 28.11 summarizes the guidelines for India, Indonesia, and the Philippines, three Asian lower-income countries. All of these countries have guidelines focused on reducing obesity, salt intake, food safety, and food variety. The Indian and Thai guidelines also warn against overconsumption of sugar. Indonesia, Thailand, China, and the Philippines ask the public to avoid alcoholic beverages. Fat intake is found in all of the guidelines with the exception of the Filipino recommendations.

Tables 28.9 through 28.11 present additional information on representative dietary guidelines from the Asian region. Table 28.9 shows Japan, Singapore, and Korea; Table 28.10

represents China, Malaysia, and Thailand; Table 28.11 depicts India, Indonesia, and Philippines.

## SIMILARITIES

Most of the guidelines are general and are food rather than nutrient-based. The exception is Singapore, which has guidelines that are quantitative and nutrient-specific.[63] There is a common core of food-based messages in all the guidelines, they include: choose a diet composed of a wide variety of foods; eat enough food to meet bodily needs and maintain or improve body weight; select foods that are safe to eat; and enjoy your food. Other dietary guidelines are also common to all Asian countries. One of these is to eat clean and safe foods; such recommendations are especially important in areas such as those where the climate is very hot and foods are easily spoiled. The hygienic messages range from "consume food that is hygienically prepared" in Malaysia,[61] to "eat clean and safe food to prevent food-borne disease in the family" in the Philippines.[62] There is also a similar guideline for China population: "Choose fresh and sanitary foods."[56]

The majority of these guidelines also stress common nonfood-related healthy behaviors such as not smoking, dental hygiene, stress management, weight control, and physical activity. Asian dietary guidelines also specify the settings (places or environments) or other circumstances surrounding food and eating. Most countries in this region also acknowledge the impacts of lifestyle changes on health and emphasize attaining a healthy body weight to prevent diet-related disease. India, for example, addressed their growing

## TABLE 28.9

## Dietary Guidelines for Selected High-Income Asian Countries: Japan, Republic of Korea, and Singapore

| Japan 1985 | Republic of Korea 2003 | Singapore 1993 |
|---|---|---|
| 1. Obtain well-balanced nutrition with a variety of foods (30 foods a day); take staple food, main dish, and side dishes together | 1. Ensure to have adequate intakes of energy and protein based on the RDAs | 1. Eat a variety of foods |
| 2. Match daily energy intake with daily physical activity | 2. Increase the intakes of calcium, iron, vitamin A, and riboflavin | 2. Maintain a desirable body weight |
| 3. Be aware that both the quality and quantity of fats consumed are important; avoid too much fat; use vegetable oils rather than animal fats | 3. Try to limit fat intake not to exceed 20% of total calories | 3. Restrict total fat intake to 20%–30% of total energy intake |
| 4. Avoid eating too much salt; aim for a salt intake of less than 10 g/day; resourceful cooking cuts down on excessive salt intake | 4. Keep salt intake less than 10 g/day. (This is the first step to lower salt intake down to 6 g/day, eventually.) | 4. Modify composition of fat in diet to one-third polyunsaturated, one-third monounsaturated, and one-third saturated |
| 5. Make all activities pertaining to food and eating pleasurable activities; use the mealtime as an occasion for family communication; appreciate home cooking | 5. Decrease alcohol consumption. | 5. Reduce cholesterol intake to less than 300 mg/day |
| | 6. Maintain healthy weight ($18.5 \leq BMI < 25$) | 6. Maintain intakes of complex carbohydrates at about 50% total energy intake |
| | 7. Keep a desirable dietary habit | 7. Reduce salt intake to less than 5 g a day (2000 mg Na) |
| | 8. Promote our traditional dietary culture | 8. Reduce intake of salt-cured, preserved, and smoked foods |
| | 9. Keep and prepare food safely | 9. Reduce intake of refined and processed sugar to less than 10% of energy |
| | 10. Reduce food waste | 10. Increase intake of fruit and vegetables and whole-grain cereal products thereby increasing vitamin A, vitamin C, and fiber intakes |
| | | 11. For those who drink, have not more than 2 standard drinks (about 30 g alcohol)/day |
| | | 12. Encourage breast-feeding in infants until at least 6 months of age |
| | | 13. Lose weight if obesity is a problem |

## TABLE 28.10
### Dietary Guidelines for Selected Asian Upper-Middle-Income Countries: China, Malaysia, and Thailand

**China 2007**

1. Eat a variety of foods, mainly cereals including appropriate amount of coarse grains
2. Consume plenty of vegetables, fruits, and tubers
3. Consume milk, soybean, or dairy or soybean products every day
4. Consume appropriate amounts of fish, poultry, eggs, and lean meat
5. Use less cooking oil; choose a light diet that is also low in salt
6. Do not overeat, exercise every day, and maintain a healthy body weight
7. Rationally distribute the daily food intake among three meals; correctly chose snacks
8. Drink sufficient amount of water every day; rationally select beverages
9. If you drink alcoholic beverages, do so in limited amounts
10. Choose fresh and sanitary foods

**Malaysia 2010**

1. Eat a variety of foods within your recommended intake
2. Maintain body weight in a healthy range
3. Be physically active every day
4. Eat adequate amount of rice, other cereal products (preferably whole grain), and tubers
5. Eat plenty of fruits and vegetables every day
6. Consume moderate amounts of fish, meat, poultry, egg, legumes, and nuts
7. Consume adequate amounts of milk and milk products
8. Limit intake of foods high in fats, and minimize fats and oils in food preparation
9. Choose and prepare foods with less salt and sauces
10. Consume foods and beverages low in sugar
11. Drink plenty of water daily
12. Practice exclusive breast-feeding from birth until 6 months and continue to breast-feed until two years of age
13. Consume safe and clean foods and beverages
14. Make effective use of nutrition information on food

**Thailand 1998**

1. Eat a variety of foods from each of the five food groups and maintain proper weight
2. Eat adequate amount of rice or alternative carbohydrate sources
3. Eat plenty of vegetables and fruits regularly
4. Eat fish, lean meat, eggs, legumes, and pulses regularly
5. Drink milk in appropriate quality and quantity for one's age
6. Eat a diet containing appropriate amounts of fat
7. Avoid sweet and salty foods
8. Eat clean and safe food
9. Avoid or reduce the consumption of alcoholic beverages

## TABLE 28.11
### Dietary Guidelines for Selected Lower-Middle-Income Asian Countries

**India 2010**

1. Eat variety of foods to ensure a balanced diet
2. Ensure provision of extra food and healthcare to pregnant and lactating women
3. Promote exclusive breast-feeding for 6 months, and encourage breast-feeding till 2 years
4. Feed home-based semisolid foods to the infant after 6 months
5. Ensure adequate and appropriate diets for children and adolescents both in health and sickness
6. Ensure moderate use of edible oils and animal foods and very less use of ghee/butter/vanaspati
7. Overeating should be avoided to prevent overweight and obesity
8. Use salt in moderation/restrict salt intake to minimum
9. Ensure the use of safe and clean foods
10. Practice right cooking methods and healthy eating habits
11. Drink plenty of water and take beverages in moderation
12. Minimize the use of processed foods rich in salt, sugar, and fats
13. Include micronutrient-rich foods in the diets of elderly people to enable them to be fit and active
14. Eat plenty of vegetables and fruits
15. Exercise regularly and be physically active to maintain ideal body

**Indonesia 1994**

1. Eat a wide variety of foods
2. Consume foods that provide sufficient energy
3. Obtain about half of total energy requirements from complex CHO-rich foods
4. Obtain not more than a quarter of total energy intake from fats or oils
5. Use only iodized salt
6. Consume iron-rich foods
7. Breast-feed your baby exclusively for 4 months
8. Have breakfast every day
9. Drink adequate quantities of fluids that are free from contaminants
10. Take adequate exercise
11. Avoid drinking alcoholic beverages
12. Consume foods hygienically
13. Read the labels of packaged foods

**Philippines 2000**

1. Eat a variety of foods every day
2. Breast-feed infants exclusively from birth to 4–6 months, and then, give appropriate foods while continuing breast-feeding
3. Maintain children's normal growth through proper diet, and monitor their growth regularly
4. Consume fish, lean meat, poultry, or dried beans
5. Eat more vegetables, fruits, and root crops
6. Eat foods cooked in edible/cooking oil daily
7. Consume milk, milk products, and other calcium-rich foods such as small fish and dark-green leafy vegetables every day
8. Use iodized salt, but avoid excessive intake of salty foods
9. Eat clean and safe food
10. For a healthy lifestyle and good nutrition, exercise regularly, do not smoke, and avoid drinking alcoholic beverages

concerns about overweight and obesity in their recently promulgated dietary guidelines.[57,65]

Filipino and Indian guidelines recommend increasing consumption of green leafy vegetables, and the Filipino and Thailand guidelines also stress the importance of milk and milk products in the diet to increase calcium consumption. In India, a special guideline for the elderly suggests eating nutrient-rich food and remaining fit and active.

The Filipino and Chinese guidelines focus on achieving dietary adequacy, emphasizing food rather than nutrient-based interventions. Most of the countries in this region include guidelines to address deficiency. In Indonesia, people are advised to "use iodized salt."[58] The Filipino guidelines include a recommendation to consume calcium-rich foods such as small fish and dark-green leafy vegetables.[62]

The World Bank lists Malaysia with other upper-middle-income countries. Dietary recommendations for the Malaysian population include obesity and physical activity; fat and salt intake; food variety; and breast-feeding. Malaysia recommends choosing foods from each of the food groups daily.[61] Guidelines for nutrients are more general: minimizing fat in food preparation and using or choosing foods with only a small amount of salt in food preparation. Increasing consumption of rice, cereal products, legumes, and fruits and vegetables is also recommended for the Malaysian population. The even more affluent countries classified as high income by the World Bank, such as Singapore, Korea, and Japan emphasize moderation in fat, saturated fat, and/or simple sugars.

## Differences

The major difference between the various guidelines in Asian countries is in the amounts and the relative balance suggested between dietary constituents. The Asian guidelines on moderation in fat and salt intake vary greatly. Some simply say to avoid excess or limit/restrict the use of fat (see guidelines for India, Malaysia, and China), and others specify the type of fat to be consumed. For example, the Japanese guidelines recommend use of vegetable oil instead of animal fat.[59] Japan and Korea recommend a specific guideline for salt as well, aiming to keep daily consumption of salt <10 g/day, with Korea's ultimate goal to keep salt intake <6 g/day. Singapore is more specific still, recommending eating less than 5 g of salt or 2000 mg of sodium/day.[63]

Singapore is listed as high income by the World Bank. Its dietary guidelines are the most specific when it comes to nutrient intake. They recommend restricting fat intake to 20%–30% of energy intake; modification of dietary fat consumption to evenly distributing fat intake between poly-unsaturated, monounsaturated, and saturated fat; reducing cholesterol intake to less than 300 mg/day; maintaining intake of complex carbohydrates to 50% of total energy intake; and keeping intake of processed and refined sugar to less than 10% of daily energy intake.[63]

Japan and Korea are two other affluent Asian countries with different cuisines. The Japanese guidelines recommend eating 30 or more different kinds of food daily to assure a well-balanced diet.[59] Korea mentions achieving and maintaining energy balance by balancing intakes and expenditure.[60] Korean guidelines also address dietary deficiency diseases. They include guidelines for increasing intakes of calcium, iron, vitamin A, and riboflavin.

Asian guidelines recognize that eating is more than just "refueling" from the physiological standpoint. They recognize that food provides pleasure and has strong links to family, tradition, and culture. Therefore, enjoyment of meals is a concern in all countries, but it is especially evident in the Japanese and Korean guidelines. In Japan, dietary guidelines that promote family values are included; citizens are advised to "make all activities pertaining to food pleasurable ones." Another Japanese guideline also advices to enjoy cooking and use mealtimes as occasions for family communication."[59] In Korea, eating is viewed as a way to keep harmony between diet and other aspects of daily life, and this is stated in the guidelines.[60]

The guidelines of these countries differ with respect to the number and relative emphasis given to balance, adequacy, moderation, and restriction. Although all of the Asian dietary guidelines recommend eating a variety of foods, they differ in suggestions on achieving such a varied pattern. Some include recommendations for frequency of consumption of specific foods or meals. Eating breakfast daily is recommended in the Indonesian guidelines, and having regular meals is recommended in the Korean guidelines.[60] Other guidelines recommend specific amounts of different kinds of foods as the ways to achieve a varied pattern.

## Conclusions

Dietary guidelines for the Asian countries are all directed to the general population. Many countries, including Malaysia, Indonesia, China, and Japan, also have specific guidelines and recommendations for food intakes focusing on those of different ages, sexes, and physiological conditions, such as infants and pregnant and lactating women.[56,58,59,61] For example, breast-feeding in early infancy is a common recommendation in the dietary guidelines of many Asian countries. Breast milk is recognized as the best food for infants. Encouragement of breast-feeding and recognition of breast milk's unique properties are included in the guidelines. The duration of exclusive breast-feeding ranges from 4 months (Indonesia) to 4–6 months (Philippines) and to 6 months in Singapore. Another difference is age of weaning, introduction of other foods in addition to breast milk. For example, it is at 4–6 months in the Philippines, but in the Malaysian guidelines weaning is recommended at no earlier than 5–6 months, with breast-feeding continuing for up to 2 years.

## AFRICA

Africa consists of more than 50 nations, most of which are developing countries. Food insecurity is a prominent phenomenon in most of this continent. Protein–energy malnutrition, nutrient deficiencies, infectious diseases such as HIV AIDS, tuberculosis, and malaria are prevalent, especially in Central Africa,

**TABLE 28.12**

**Development of Dietary Guidelines in African Countries**

| Country | South Africa | Republic of Namibia | Nigeria |
|---|---|---|---|
| Title of guidelines | South African guidelines for healthy eating | Food and nutrition guidelines for Namibia food choices for a healthy life | Food guidelines for Nigeria |
| Year | 2001 | 2000 | 2001 |
| Endorsing unit | Department of Health, Association for Dietetics in South Africa, Nutrition Society of South Africa | National Food Security and Nutrition Council | Ministries of Health and Agriculture and Rural Development and other organizations |
| Approaches[a] | 1, 2, 3, 4, 5 | 1, 2, 4 | 1, 2, 4 |
| Number of guidelines | 11 | 10 | |
| Target audiences[b] | G, H, P | G, H, P | G, H, P |
| Major nutrition problems addressed in guidelines[c] | O, C, PEM, I | O, C, PEM, I | O, C, PEM, I |
| Graphic representation | | | |
| Other guidelines | | | |

[a] 1, Nutrition experts, nutrition scientists views; 2, review of former guidelines; 3, from food groups; 4, from consumption/nutrition survey; 5, definition of nutritional objectives.

[b] G, general population; H, health professionals; P, policy makers.

[c] C, diet-related chronic degenerative diseases; I, dietary inadequacy; O, overnutrition (energy); PEM, protein–energy malnutrition.

**TABLE 28.13**

**Dietary Guidelines for Selected Upper-Middle-Income African Countries**

| South Africa 2004 | Republic of Namibia 2000 |
|---|---|
| 1. Enjoy a variety of foods | 1. Eat a variety of foods |
| 2. Be active | 2. Eat vegetables and fruit every day |
| 3. Make starchy foods the basis of most meals | 3. Eat more fish |
| 4. Eat dry beans, split peas, lentils, and soy regularly | 4. Eat beans and meat regularly |
| 5. Chicken, fish, milk, meat, or eggs can be eaten daily | 5. Use whole-grain products |
| 6. Drink lots of clean, safe water | 6. Use only iodized salt, but use less salt |
| 7. Eat plenty of vegetables and fruits every day | 7. Eat at least three meals a day |
| 8. Eat fats sparingly | 8. Avoid drinking alcohol |
| 9. Use salt sparingly | 9. Consume clean and safe water and food |
| 10. Use food and drinks containing sugar sparingly and not between meals | 10. Achieve and maintain a healthy body weight |
| 11. If you drink alcohol, drink sensibly | |

while diseases of affluence raise concerns in more wealthy and developed Southern African countries. Guideline development details of the dietary guidelines for South Africa,[72] Nigeria,[73] and the Republic of Namibia[74] are presented in Table 28.12. And the specific dietary guidelines for those African countries are summarized in Tables 28.13 and 28.14.

### FORMULATION

South Africa's Guidelines for Healthy Eating were promulgated in the year 2000.[72] Subsequently, they were revised and adopted at the Ministry of Health, Directorate of Nutrition in 2004[75] (see Table 28.12). The guidelines aim to improve health as well as to relieve chronic diseases, overweight, nutrient deficiencies, and malnutrition. In the process of dietary guidelines formulation, scientific findings, dietary recommendations from other countries, World Health Organization (WHO) guidelines, and health status surveys were reviewed.

Dietary guidelines for Nigeria, published in four languages spoken in the country, were established collaboratively by several ministries, WHO, and other professional organizations and were updated in 2003, as detailed in Table 28.12.[73]

The Food and Nutrition Guidelines for Namibia were prepared by the National Food Security and Nutrition Council in 2000.[74] However, there is only limited information related to the development process that was involved in the Nigerian and Namibian guidelines.

South Africa published its dietary guidelines in a brochure with detailed illustration and suggested applications on each guideline in 2004.[75] This upper-middle-income country

## TABLE 28.14
## Dietary Guidelines for Nigeria, a Lower-Middle-Income African Nation

**Nigeria 2003**

1   Good nutrition
  - No single food by itself (except breast milk) provides all the nutrients in the right amounts that will promote growth and maintain life
  - To achieve good nutrition, therefore, it is necessary to consume as wide a variety of foods as possible from the age of 6 months

1.1   Infants (0–6 months)
  - Start exclusive breast-feeding immediately after birth and continue for 6 months
  - There should be no bottle-feeding

1.2   Infants (6–12 months)
  - Continue breast-feeding
  - Introduce complementary feeds made from a variety of cereals, tubers, legumes, fruits, and animal foods, and give with cup and spoon

1.3   Toddlers (12–24 months)
  - Continue to breast-feed until child is 2 years
  - Give enriched pap or mashed foods twice daily
  - Give family diet made soft with less pepper and spices
  - Give fruits and vegetables in season

1.4   Children (25–60 months)
  - Give diet that contains a variety of foods in adequate amounts
  - Add palm oil or vegetable oil to raise the energy level of complementary foods
  - Gradually increase food intake to four to five times daily as baby gets older
  - Provide dark-green leafy vegetables, yellow-/orange-colored fruits, citrus fruits, cereals, legumes, tubers, and foods of animal origin
  - Limit the consumption of sugary food
  - Continue feeding even when child is ill

1.5   School-age children (6–11 years)
  - Give diet that contains a variety of foods in adequate amounts
  - Encourage consumption of good quality snacks, but limit the consumption of sugary snacks

1.6   Adolescents (12–18 years)
  - Consume diet containing a variety of foods
  - Most of the energy should be delivered from roots/tubers, legumes, cereals, and vegetables and less from animal foods
  - An increase in total food intake is very important at this stage, so is the need to enjoy family meals
  - Snacks especially pastry and carbonate drinks should not replace main meals. If you must eat out, make wise food choices
  - Liberal consumption of whatever fruit is in season should be encouraged
  - Females need to eat more iron-containing foods like meat, fish, poultry, legumes, cereals, as well as citrus fruits to enhance body's use of iron

1.7   Adults (male and female)
  - Total food intake should take into consideration the level of physical activity
  - Individuals who do manual work need to consume more food than those who do sedentary work
  - Limit fat intake from animal foods
  - Diet should consist of as wide a variety of foods as possible, e.g., cereals, legumes, roots/tubers, fruits, vegetables, fish, lean meat, and local cheese (wara)
  - Limit intake of salt, bouillon cubes, and sugar
  - Liberal consumption of whatever fruit is in season is encouraged

1.8   Pregnant women
  - Eat a diet that contains a variety of foods in adequate amounts
  - Consume enough food to ensure adequate weight gain
  - Eat more cereals, legumes, fruits, vegetables, dairy products, and animal foods
  - Take iron and folic acid supplements as prescribed
  - Avoid alcohol, addictive substances, and smoking

1.9   Breast-feeding mothers
  - Eat a diet that contains a variety of available food items like cereals, tubers, legumes, meat, fish, milk, fruits, and vegetables
  - Consume more foods rich in iron such as liver, fish, and beef
  - Eat fruits in season at every meal
  - Consume fluids as needed to quench thirst
  - Avoid alcohol, addictive substances, and smoking

(*continued*)

**TABLE 28.14 (continued)**

**Dietary Guidelines for Nigeria, a Lower-Middle-Income African Nation**

1.10   The elderly
- Eat diets that are prepared from a variety of available foods, e.g., cereals, tubers, fruits, and vegetables
- Increase consumption of fish and fish-based diets
- Eat more of fruits and vegetables
- Eat more frequently

2     Physical activity/exercise: Physical activity both as short periods of intense exercise or prolonged periods of modest activity on a daily basis generally has beneficial effects
- Children and adolescents should engage in leisure time exercise
- Adults should undertake some form of exercise as recommended by their doctors

3     Healthy lifestyles: Some habits and lifestyles, e.g., tobacco use and excessive alcohol consumption have been found to be bad for health. Prolonged indulgence in these lifestyles predisposes to noncommunicable diseases like cancer, diabetes, heart problems, and hypertension

3.1   Alcohol: Too much alcohol consumption can lead to risk of hypertension, liver damage, malnutrition, and various cancers. There is also the problem of alcohol abuse
- If you must drink, take alcohol in moderation
- Avoid drinking alcohol when driving a vehicle or operating any machinery

3.2   Tobacco: Tobacco use is associated with lung cancer and other chronic disorders. Smoking during pregnancy can harm the developing baby and can result in low-birth-weight babies
- Avoid the use of tobacco in any form

recommends specific numbers of servings on each food group, but similar features in the Namibia and Nigeria guidelines are not present. No graphic representations of dietary guidelines were found for the African countries.

While the South African guidelines were targeted to all adults and children older than 7 years of age, Nigerian guidelines were presented in 10 age categories. The Namibian guidelines were not age-specific.

Dietary guidelines for South Africa and Namibia are summarized in Table 28.13 and Nigeria in Table 28.14. Dietary guidelines from all four African countries are food-based instead of nutrient-based. While South Africa has 11 dietary guidelines and Namibia has 9, Nigeria presents over 40 recommendations in 3 general sections—Good Nutrition, Physical Activity, and Healthy Lifestyle.

### SIMILARITIES

All the African dietary guidelines are similar in several ways. All three sets of guidelines recommend choosing a variety of foods and at the same time emphasize vegetable and fruit intake. All of the African guidelines suggest consuming beans, meat, and fish regularly or daily. Also, advice on reducing salt intakes as well as avoiding or limiting alcohol intake is found in most guidelines. Furthermore, South Africa and Nigeria recommend limitations on sugar and fat intake. Only Namibia advocates consuming whole-grain products. Only South Africa alone suggests daily milk intake.

All African guidelines recognize the importance of maintaining a healthy body weight with physical activities. South Africa, but not Nigeria and Namibia, further defines healthy body weight in terms of body mass index (BMI) and provides specific guidelines on the duration and ways to be physically active (see Tables 28.13 and 28.14).

South Africa and Namibia include food safety guidelines and suggest drinking clean and safe water only. Both South Africa and Nigeria emphasize enjoyment of meals.

### DIFFERENCES

Nigeria has developed different guidelines on food intake along the life cycle, categorizing the lifespan into infants of 0–6 months, infants of 7–12 months, toddlers, preschool children, school-age children, adolescents, adults, and elderly. Guidelines for pregnant and lactating women are also available. Breast-feeding is suggested as the sole nutrition for infants under 6 months of age and to be continued until 2 years of age with other foods. Such age-specific division is not observed in South African and Namibian dietary guidelines.

### CONCLUSIONS

Dietary guidelines for Africa reflect the large economic differences among African countries. South Africa, a more wealthy country, emphasizes on promotion of balanced diet and prevention of diseases of affluence. In contrast, others, such as Namibia and Nigeria, aim to advocate food safety and adequacy of nutrition intake. Education and literacy level also affect the content and complexity of dietary guidelines in these countries. Although many other African countries may already have their own dietary guidelines, there is lack of publications containing details of dietary guidelines to guide proper and healthy eating among their population groups.

## EUROPE

With a rich and varied history, Europe has a variety of economic, political, and healthcare conditions. European countries have numerous differences in culture and dietary

**TABLE 28.15**

**WHO FBDG and Number of European Countries, by Region, That Incorporated Them into Their National Dietary Guidelines**

| | Southeastern Europe and Central Asia 11 | Central and Eastern Europe 6 | Western Europe 9 | Southern Europe 10 | Nordic Countries 5 | Other European Countries[a] 10 |
|---|---|---|---|---|---|---|
| **Total Number of Countries in Region** | **Number of Countries that Adopted the WHO FBDG** | | | | | |
| 1. A varied diet, consisting mainly of plant foods | 4 | 5 | 7 | 7 | 5 | 5 |
| 2. Daily intake of bread, grains, rice, potatoes, and pasta | 4 | 4 | 5 | 6 | 5 | 6 |
| 3. Daily intake of fresh and local vegetables and fruits | 6 | 4 | 6 | 6 | 5 | 3 |
| 4a. Healthy BMI range | 3 | 3 | 5 | 5 | 4 | 5 |
| 4b. Physical activity | 2 | 3 | 4 | 3 | 4 | 3 |
| 5a. Low fat intake (total fat) | 3 | 6 | 7 | 7 | 5 | 6 |
| 5b. Low fat intake (saturated fat) | 3 | 6 | 5 | 6 | 5 | 6 |
| 6. Intake of lean meat, poultry, fish, and legumes | 3 | 5 | 6 | 7 | 4 | 6 |
| 7. Intake of low-fat milk and low-fat dairy products | 2 | 5 | 6 | 5 | 5 | 6 |
| 8. Low sugar intake | 3 | 4 | 5 | 7 | 5 | 6 |
| 9. Low salt intake | 3 | 5 | 7 | 6 | 5 | 6 |
| 10. Limited alcohol intake | 3 | 5 | 6 | 4 | 4 | 5 |
| 11. Hygienic preparation of food[b] | 3 | 0 | 4 | 0 | 1 | 4 |
| 12. Exclusive breast-feeding[b] | 3 | 4 | 2 | 3 | 5 | 5 |

[a]  Include Baltic countries and Commonwealth of Independent States.

[b]  Many countries include guidelines on these areas in separate guidelines.

habits. In 2000, the WHO Regional Office for Europe developed a Countrywide Integrated Noncommunicable Disease Intervention (CINDI) dietary guide that included a section on "Twelve Steps to Healthy Eating" as seen in Table 28.15,[76] which served as the basis for formulating country-specific dietary guidelines in European countries. Most countries in the Nordic, western, southern, and central eastern regions of Europe have their national dietary guidelines in various stages of development and have incorporated some of the 12 steps to healthy eating in their own national guidelines. The heterogeneous nature of European populations makes the review of these guidelines both interesting and complex.

Beginning in the late 1990s the European countries started a regional process of development and implementation of FBDG,[77] following the recommendations issued by the WHO in 1996.[78] The evolution of the process is a regional enterprise coordinated by regional groups who work closely with the national sectors involved in the establishment of their FBDG. The efforts in developing FBDG are continuing and are changing rapidly because the European countries are at different stages in guidelines development, as reported in the workshop about FBDG held in Budapest, Hungary in 2009.[79] The European Food Information Council (EUFIC) summarized in a 2009 report[79] the steps followed by the European countries for the promulgation of their FBDG, which included: (1) the

identification of diet–health relationships; (2) identification of country-specific diet-related problems; (3) identification of nutrients of public health importance; (4) identification of foods relevant for FBDG; (5) identification of food consumption patterns; (6) testing and optimizing FBDG; and (7) graphical representation of FBDG. With respect to graphical representations of FBDG, most European countries opted for the pyramid-based pictorial design formerly used in the United States and many other world countries.

## FORMULATION

To illustrate this section, we arbitrarily selected a group of European countries—United Kingdom,[80] Spain,[81] Ireland,[82] Greece,[83] Italy,[84] the Netherlands,[85] France,[86] Germany,[87] and Portugal,[88] which all had enough literature in English, Spanish, or Portuguese to be easily comprehensible—and analyzed their process for the establishment and implementation of their FBDG. All of these dietary guidelines are based on scientific reviews and what was in the former guidelines of the countries. All of the countries chosen as examples also use national government bodies for defining and formulating them (Tables 28.16 through 28.21). The European countries represented in here are designated by the World Bank as high-income nations and will be compared together.[55]

## TABLE 28.16

### Development of Dietary Guidelines in Selected European Countries

|  | United Kingdom | Germany | Spain | Greece | Finland | Portugal |
|---|---|---|---|---|---|---|
| Title of guidelines | Guidelines for a healthier diet | 10 Guidelines of the German nutrition society for a wholesome diet | The Bilbao declaration | Dietary guidelines for adults in Greece | Finnish nutrition recommendations |  |
| Year |  |  | 2000 | 1999 | 1999 | 1997 |
| Number of guidelines | 9 | 10 | 10 | (Not listed in bullets) | (not listed in bullets) | 9 and 11 |
| Endorsing unit | Institute of Food Research | German Nutrition Society | Spanish Society of Community Nutrition | Ministry of Health and Welfare, Supreme Scientific Health Council | National Nutrition Council | National Council of Food and Nutrition |
| Other guidelines | Vegetarian diet guidelines |  |  |  |  |  |
| Graphic representation | Food plate | Food plate | Pyramid | Pyramid | Food pyramid, food plate, and food circle | Food wheel |

## TABLE 28.17

### Dietary Guidelines for Selected High-Income European Countries: United Kingdom, Ireland, and Greece

| United Kingdom | Ireland 2005 | Greece 1999 |
|---|---|---|
| 1. Enjoy your food | 1. Choose at least 6 or more breads, cereals, and potatoes each day. If physical activity is high, may need up to 12 servings | 1. Do not exceed the optimal body weight for your height |
| 2. Enjoy a variety of different foods | 2. Choose at least 5 or more fruits and vegetables per day | 2. Eat slowly, preferably at regular times during the day and in a pleasant environment |
| 3. Eat the right amount to be a healthy weight | 3. Choose 3 milk, yogurt, and dairy products each day | 3. Prefer fruits and nuts as snacks, instead of sweets or candy bars |
| 4. Eat plenty of food rich in starch and fiber | 4. Choose 2 meat, fish, and meat alternatives per day. Choose 3 servings during pregnancy | 4. Prefer whole-grain bread or pasta |
| 5. Eat plenty of fruits and vegetables | 5. Use about 1oz low-fat spread/low-fat butter or ½ oz margarine or butter each day. Use oils sparingly | 5. Always prefer water over soft drinks |
| 6. Don't eat too many foods that contain a lot of fat | 6. If you drink or eat snacks containing sugar, limit the number of times you take them throughout the day. Eat high-fat snacks in only small amounts and not too frequently. Choose lower-fat, sugar-free alternatives | 6. Healthy adults, with the exception of pregnant women, do not need dietary supplements when they follow a balanced diet |
| 7. Don't have sugary foods and drinks too often | 7. Drink alcohol in moderation, preferably with meals and have some alcohol-free days | 7. Light foods are not a substitute for physical activity when it comes to controlling excess body weight; furthermore, their consumption in large quantities has been shown to promote obesity |
| 8. If you drink alcohol, drink sensibly |  | 8. Although the indicated diet is the ultimate goal, gradual adoption may be more realistic for some people |

## SIMILARITIES

WHO advocates the use of FBDG for better comprehension and application by the general public. All of the European dietary guidelines examined present their key recommendations in terms of food, following the framework established by the working group 2 of Eurodiet,[89] and summarized in the report published by EUFIC.[79] Among the European dietary guidelines reviewed, Portugal offered the most detailed nutrient-based recommendations, which it presents in addition to the food-based guidelines. Portugal has one set of 9 nutrient-based guidelines and a separate set of 11 food-based dietary recommendations, which are available for different purposes (planning for nutrients and communications to the public for the food-based guidelines).

Virtually all of the European guidelines categorize foods into different food groups, but the food groups are slightly different from country to country. For example, most countries consider potatoes in the starch group, but Greece discusses potatoes separately and classifies them in neither the vegetable nor the starch groups.

Nearly all of the European countries include a variety guideline and emphasize fruit, vegetables, and whole grains, and all have some guideline for the amount of alcohol and fat in the diet. All countries except Spain have a guideline on limiting salt, and all have guidelines about limiting sugar.

## TABLE 20.10
## Dietary Guidelines for Selected High-Income European Countries: Italy, Netherlands, and Germany

| Italy | Netherlands 1993 | Germany |
|---|---|---|
| 1. Watch your weight and be active | 1. Eat a variety of foods | 1. Choose from among many different foods |
| 2. More cereals, vegetables, tubers, and fruit | 2. Be moderate with fat | 2. Cereal products several times per day and plenty of potatoes |
| 3. Fat—choose quality and limit the amount | 3. Eat plenty of carbohydrates and fiber | 3. Fruit and vegetables—take "5 a day" |
| 4. Sugars, sweets, sweet drinks—just the right amount | 4. Eat three meals a day and do not snack more than four times in between meals | 4. Milk and dairy products daily; fish once a week; meat, sausages, and eggs in moderation |
| 5. Drink plenty of water every day | 5. Be careful with salt | 5. Low-fat diet |
| 6. Salt? Better if little | 6. Drink at least daily 1.5 L fluid. Be moderate with alcohol | 6. Sugar and salt in moderation |
| 7. Alcoholic drinks—only if in limited amounts | 7. Keep your body weight at its correct level | 7. Plenty of liquid |
| 8. Make varied choices | 8. Prevent food-borne infections with good hygiene | 8. Make sure your dishes are prepared gently and taste well |
| 9. Special advice for special people | 9. Keep in mind the presence of harmful substances in food | 9. Take your time and enjoy eating |
| 10. The safety of your food depends also on you | 10. Read the information on the label | 10. Watch your weight and be active |

Countries differ to the extent they are nutrient-based and which nutrients they concentrate upon; for example, Portugal is more quantitative in terms of nutrient recommendations, whereas Spain and Greece are more food-based. Portugal recommends keeping total fat intake less than or equal to 30% per day, while Spain's guideline is more general, "achieve a healthier lipid profile in the diet by enhancing a relevant contribution of monounsaturated fatty acids (MUFAs)…".

European guidelines are consistent in that variety in food choices is encouraged, but the message is conveyed in various ways. Germany promotes the idea that there is no "forbidden food" and that people should pay attention to the quantity of food intake.

European guidelines also agree in promoting fruit and vegetable intakes. Although most countries do not specify the appropriate amounts of fruits and vegetables, Spain recommends consumption of at least 250 g of vegetables and 400 g of fruits daily, and Germany advocates "5 a day" for 5 portions of fruits and vegetables on each day. The majority of European countries suggest daily consumption of dairy products and an increase in fish intake, but there is no consensus concerning the optimal amount of intake.

All countries suggest moderation in eggs, meats, and poultry, reflecting the fact that these protein-rich foods are abundant in current diets in these countries. All European dietary guidelines also urge limiting sugar and consumption of sweets, but the recommended numbers of servings from these guidelines vary. Greece suggests half a serving of sweets per day, while Spanish recommends having sweets on no more than "four occasions" per day. United Kingdom and Spain relate sugar intake to dental problems and/or obesity.

All countries except for Greece, which does not specify a fat amount, recommend limiting fat intake to 30%–35% of total food energy. In Mediterranean countries such as Greece, Portugal, and Spain, use of olive oil is encouraged over other types of lipids.

## DIFFERENCES

Body weight is mentioned in most of the European guidelines. Although some guidelines simply advise for a "healthy" or "desirable" weight, the Portuguese and Spanish guidelines discuss energy balance. Spain and France offer specific recommendations for a healthy BMI; France also recommends to the public to increase their physical activity by 25% daily or engage in at least 30 min of brisk walking 5 days a week. Virtually all of the countries with the exception of the United Kingdom have physical activity guidelines. All countries address weight control.

Interestingly, only Germany encourages the leisurely enjoyment of meals and avoiding stress and haste in eating. The German guidelines also mention that food should be appetizing and processed as little as possible.

In addition to written documents, graphic presentations of dietary guidelines are available in most of the European countries. The icons used to represent the guideline are usually a pyramid (Spain, Greece, Ireland), a wheel with spokes representing the amounts of recommended foods (Portugal), a tabulated list (France), or a food plate (United Kingdom, Germany).

France takes a different approach and has health-specific guidelines. These include recommendations for reducing blood pressure, reducing the prevalence of obesity, and the percentage by which one should increase his physical activity daily. French guidelines also have recommendations for reducing iron deficiency during pregnancy, improving folate status in women of childbearing age, and improving calcium, iron, and vitamin D status is children and adolescents.

## CONCLUSIONS

In contrast to many parts of the world, most of the European countries have developed dietary guidelines.[79] Many of these guidelines were developed using the WHO CINDI dietary guidelines as a template.[76] The dietary guidelines

**TABLE 28.19**

**Dietary Guidelines for Selected High-Income European Countries, Continued**

| France 2009 | Portugal 1997 | Spain 2000 |
|---|---|---|
| 1. Increase consumption of fruits and vegetables at least 25%<br><br>2. Increase the consumption of calcium to reduce by 25% those with calcium intakes below the recommended values while reducing the prevalence of vitamin D deficiency by 25%<br><br>3. Reduce total dietary fat intake to less than 35% of daily energy intake with a reduction of 25% of the consumption of saturated fatty acids<br><br>4. Increase the consumption of carbohydrates so that they contribute to more than 50% of daily energy intake by promoting the consumption of food, reducing current consumption of simple sugars to 25%; increase fiber consumption by 50%<br><br>5. Reduce yearly alcohol consumption (as much as possible) until you reach the suggested levels (8.5 L/year/person)<br><br>6. Reduce cholesterol intake by 5%<br><br>7. Reduce systolic blood pressure by an average of 2–3 mm Hg in adults<br><br>8. Reduce by 20% the prevalence of overweight and obesity (BMI > 25 kg/m²) in adults, and stop the increasing prevalence of obesity among children<br><br>9. Increase your daily physical activity by 25%, the equivalent of at least 30 min of brisk walking 5 days a week<br><br>10. Reduce the average intake of sodium to 8 g /person/day<br><br>11. Reduce iron deficiency during pregnancy<br><br>12. Improve folate status in women of childbearing age, especially if they desire to become pregnant<br><br>13. Promote breast-feeding<br><br>14. Improve iron, calcium, and vitamin D status for children and adolescents<br><br>15. Prevent, detect, and reduce malnutrition of older people, and improve their calcium and vitamin D status<br><br>16. Reduce the frequency of iodine deficiency to 8.5% in males and 10.8% females<br><br>17. Improve feeding of disadvantaged persons including reducing their vitamin and mineral deficiencies<br><br>18. Don't follow restrictive diets as they lead to vitamin and mineral deficiencies<br><br>19. Take food allergies into account when planning your diet | *Nutrition-based guidelines*<br>1. Total carbohydrates should contribute a total daily energy value of 50%–70%<br><br>2. Fiber intake should vary between 27–40 g/day<br><br>3. Total lipids consumption ≤30% daily energy intake<br><br>4. Consumption of saturated fatty acids <10% of total daily energy<br><br>5. Cholesterol consumption <300 mg/day<br><br>6. Total saccharose <20–30 g/day<br><br>7. Salt <6 g/day<br><br>8. Reduce cholesterol consumption<br><br>9. Calcium—total daily intake of 800 mg<br>*Food-based guidelines*<br>1. Breast-feeding in the first months of a baby's life, especially during the first 6 months<br><br>2. Adequate consumption of cereals and cereal products<br><br>3. Increase of the consumption of vegetable products and fresh fruit<br><br>4. Reduction of the consumption of fats, especially solid and overheated fats, preference given to olive-oil consumption<br><br>5. Increase of fish consumption<br><br>6. Reduction of sugar and sugar-like productions consumption<br><br>7. Reduction of salt consumption<br><br>8. Moderate consumption of alcoholic drinks. Pregnant women, children, and those younger than 17 should not drink alcohol<br><br>9. Adequate consumption of milk and dairy products<br><br>10. Weight control kept through a balanced diet and physical activity<br><br>11. A balanced meal first thing in the morning | 1. To adjust intake to energy output in order to achieve an energy balance conductive to maintain BMI within the desirable range<br><br>2. To harmonize the percentage contribution of macronutrients to energy intake<br><br>3. To achieve a healthier lipid profile in the diet by enhancing a relevant contribution of monounsaturated fatty acids (MUFAs), mostly from olive oil<br><br>4. To stimulate changes in the carbohydrate profile, through a higher proportion of complex carbohydrates<br><br>5. To adjust daily frequency of consumption +gary foods to less than four occasions per day<br><br>6. A daily consumption of vegetables equal to or greater than 250 g is recommended, including at least one portion as fresh raw vegetables in a salad. A consumption of 400 g or more of fruit/person/day is also recommended<br><br>7. Moderation in the consumption of alcoholic beverages is advised, within the Mediterranean consumption pattern, i.e., small amounts of wine with meals<br><br>8. Introducing moderate physical exercise for at least 30 min within daily practices is highly recommended<br><br>9. It would be advisable that public administrations and institutions stimulate, support, and implement programs at developing individual skills contributing to food choices and preparations conductive to a healthy food pattern. Actions targeted to socially deprived environments should be a priority<br><br>10. The need to draw global strategies to protect and recover traditional cooking styles is also noticed (gastronomic heritage) as a source of cultural and health wellness |

from different European countries are quite similar in their main ideas. Key common recommendations are food-based, and they encourage the public to increase fruit and vegetable intake; to decrease fat and sugar usage; to moderate meat, dairy, and egg consumption; and to increase physical activities. Despite the similarity among European dietary guidelines, there are variations between each of the country to cater the unique cultural and health concerns of each country.

Some European countries offer additional guidelines for children and elderly. Countries like Greece referred to other publications like the "European Union Project on Promotion of Breastfeeding in Europe" for specific breast-feeding guidelines.

## INNOVATIONS

Many of the countries discussed in this chapter have taken to technology and especially the Internet, to engage their populations. The United States, for example, offers electronically the interactive website Choose *MyPlate*.gov, where interested members of the population can find the

**TABLE 28.20**

**Commonalities among National Food-Based Guidelines in Various Countries**

| Country | Overweight/ Obesity/PA | Fat Intake | Salt Intake | Sugar Intake | Alcohol | Food Safety | Food Variety | Breast-Feeding |
|---|---|---|---|---|---|---|---|---|
| United States | × | × | × | × | × | | × | |
| Canada | × | × | × | × | | | | |
| Australia | × | × | × | × | × | × | × | × |
| New Zealand | × | × | × | × | × | | × | |
| Chile | × | × | × | × | | | × | |
| Guatemala | | | | | | | × | |
| Mexico | × | × | × | × | | × | × | × |
| Panama | × | × | × | × | | | × | |
| Venezuela | × | × | × | × | × | × | × | × |
| China | × | × | × | | × | × | × | |
| India | × | × | × | × | | × | × | × |
| Indonesia | × | × | × | | × | × | × | × |
| Japan | × | × | × | | | | | × |
| Korea | × | × | × | | × | × | | |
| Malaysia | × | × | × | | | | × | × |
| Philippines | × | | × | | × | × | × | × |
| Singapore | × | × | × | × | × | | × | × |
| Thailand | × | × | × | × | × | × | × | |
| South Africa | × | × | × | × | × | × | × | |
| Republic of Namibia | × | | × | | × | | × | |
| Nigeria | | × | | × | | | × | |
| United Kingdom | × | × | | × | × | | × | |
| Germany | × | × | × | × | | | × | |
| Spain | × | × | | × | × | | | |
| Ireland | | × | | × | × | | | |
| France | × | × | × | × | × | | × | × |
| Greece | × | × | | × | | | | |
| Portugal | × | × | × | × | × | | | × |
| Italy | × | × | × | × | × | × | × | |
| the Netherlands | × | × | × | | × | × | × | |
| Argentina | × | × | × | × | × | | × | × |
| Uruguay | | × | × | × | | × | × | |
| Ecuador | | | | | | × | × | |
| Malaysia | × | × | × | | | | × | × |

dietary guidelines, keep track of their food intake, and get the latest news related to nutrition.[90] Canada has a similar website that provides information on the guidelines, tips for planning meals, smart snacking ideas, and how to make healthy choices when eating out.[16] The website also helps visitors learn how to read food labels and become familiar with serving sizes. The United Kingdom's interactive website provides information for specific age groups, provides nutrition news, and includes healthy-eating tools such as those to assess a diet and plan meals.[80] Spain's Society for Community Nutrition provides the population with nutrition resources and information about specific nutrients, including salt, fats, carbohydrates, protein, sugars, and proper hydration.[81]

## CONCLUSION

In this chapter we examined and reviewed the dietary guidelines of different countries throughout the world. Dietary guidelines should change and adapt to meet the needs of the population they are designed to influence. Each region represented included countries of different affluence. The dietary guidelines differed depending on economic and social status of the country in question, but the countries in each region also had many similarities. Most of the world's countries have recommendations on limiting salt and sugar, controlling calories, and eating a balanced diet. Each of these guidelines continues to evolve as science discovers new ways to keep the world healthy.

**TABLE 28.21**

**Countries Classified by Income Group[a]**

| High Income | Upper-Middle Income | Lower-Middle Income |
|---|---|---|
| United States | Argentina | Bolivia |
| Canada | Chile | El Salvador |
| Australia | Ecuador | Guatemala |
| New Zealand | Mexico | India |
| Japan | Panama | Indonesia |
| Republic of Korea | Venezuela | Philippines |
| Singapore | Uruguay | Nigeria |
| United Kingdom | China | |
| Germany | Malaysia | |
| Spain | Thailand | |
| Ireland | South Africa | |
| Greece | Republic of Namibia | |
| Portugal | | |
| Italy | | |
| the Netherlands | | |
| France | | |

[a] Income group: According to estimates from the World Bank for the year 2011, world economies are divided according to 2011 GNI per capita, calculated using the World Bank Atlas method. The groups are as follows: high income, $12,476 or more; upper-middle income, $4,036–$12,475; lower-middle income, $1,026–$4,035; and low income, $1,025 or less (URL: http://data.worldbank.org/about/country-classifications).

## ACKNOWLEDGMENTS AND SUPPORT

This work was supported in part by the U.S. Department of Agriculture, Agricultural Research Service, under agreement No. 58-1950-7-707. Any opinions, findings, conclusions, or recommendations expressed here are those of the authors and do not necessarily reflect the view of the U.S. Department of Agriculture.

We thank the following individuals who assisted in the preparation of earlier editions of this chapter: Winifred Yu, BS, RD; Linda G. Tolstoi, BA, BS, MS, MEd; Lei Chi Chang, PhD; Karen Koehn, MS; and Chin Ling Chan, MS.

## REFERENCES

1. Miraglia ML, Dwyer JT. Dietary recommendations for primary prevention: An update. *Am J Lifestyle Med* 2011, 5: 144–155.
2. Popkin BM, Lu B, Zhai F. Understanding the nutrition transition: Measuring rapid dietary changes in transitional countries. *Public Health Nutr* 2002, 5: 947–953.
3. Popkin BM. Nutrition in transition: The changing global nutrition challenge. *Asia Pac J Clin Nutr* 2001, 10 (Suppl): S13–S18.
4. Popkin BM, Adair LS, Ng SW. Global nutrition transition and the pandemic of obesity in developing countries. *Nutr Rev* 2012, 70: 3–21.
5. Popkin BM, Gordon-Larsen P. The nutrition transition: Worldwide obesity dynamics and their determinants. *Int J Obes Relat Metab Disord* 2004, 28 (Suppl 3): S2–S9.
6. Food and Agriculture Organization of the United Nations. 2009. Food-based dietary guidelines: Food guidelines by country. URL: http://www.fao.org/ag/humannutrition/nutritioneducation/fbdg/en/ (Accessed September 2010).
7. Dwyer JT. Dietary guidelines for cancer prevention. In *Nutritional Oncology*, Chapter 47. Ed. Heber D. New York: Elsevier, 2006, pp. 757–778.
8. U.S. Department of Agriculture, Center for Nutrition Policy and Promotion. *Dietary guidelines for Americans, 2010.* URL: http://www.cnpp.usda.gov/DGAs2010-PolicyDocument.htm (Accessed March 26, 2012).
9. U.S. Department of Agriculture, U.S. Department of Health, Dietary Guidelines Advisory Committee. *Report of the Dietary Guidelines Advisory Committee on the Dietary Guidelines for Americans.* Springfield, IL: National Technical Information Service, 1980.
10. U.S. Department of Agriculture, U.S. Department of Health, Dietary Guidelines Advisory Committee. *Report of the Dietary Guidelines Advisory Committee on the Dietary Guidelines for Americans.* Springfield, IL: National Technical Information Service, 1990.
11. U.S. Department of Agriculture, U.S. Department of Human Health. *Nutrition and Your Health: Dietary Guidelines for Americans*, Home and Garden Bulletin No. 232, 4th edn., Washington, DC: US Government Printing Office, 1995.
12. U.S. Department of Agriculture, U.S. Department of Health. *A Dietary Guidelines Advisory Committee: Report of the Dietary Guidelines Advisory Committee on Dietary Guidelines for American, 2000*, to the secretary of health and human services and the secretary of agriculture. Springfield, IL: National Technical Information Service, 2000.

13. U.S. Department of Health and Human Services, U.S. Department of Agriculture. *Dietary Guidelines for Americans, 2005*, 6th edn., Washington, DC: US Government Printing Office, 2005.

14. U.S. Department of Agriculture, Dietary Guidelines Advisory Committee. *Report of the dietary Guidelines Advisory Committee on Dietary Guidelines for American.* Springfield, IL: National Technical Information Service, 2000.

15. U.S. Department of Health and Human Services, U.S. Department of Agriculture. *Finding Your Way to a Healthier You: Based on the Dietary Guidelines for Americans*, 2005. URL: www.healthierus. gov/dietaryguidelines (Accessed February 15, 2006).

16. Health Canada. *Eating Well with Canada's Food Guide.* URL: www.healthcanada.gc.ca/foodguide (Accessed March 26, 2012).

17. Australian Government, National Health and Medical Research Council. *Dietary Guidelines for Australians, 2003.* Canberra, Australia: Population Health Publications Officer, Commonwealth Department of Health and Ageing. Reprinted in May 2005.

18. Australian Government, National Health and Medical Research Council. dietary guidelines for Australians. Draft for public consultation (Closed in February 2012). NHMRC, Canberra, Australia, 2011.

19. New Zealand Ministry of Health: Food and nutrition guidelines for healthy adults. A background paper, 2003. URL: http://www.moh.govt.nz/moh.nsf/0/fe468ceed06b0771cc256 cd600709490?OpenDocument (Accessed August 20, 2010).

20. Australian Bureau of Statistics. The health and welfare of Australia's Aboriginal and Torres Strait Islander peoples, 2010. URL: http://www.abs.gov.au/AUSSTATS/abs@.nsf/lookup/4704.0Chapter2302010 (Accessed April 5, 2012).

21. Centers for Disease Control and Prevention. Cancer prevention and control. URL: http://www.cdc.gov/cancer/nper/register.htm.CDC, Washington, DC (Accessed March 22, 2000).

22. Mokdad AH, Serdula MK, Dietz WH, Bowman BA, Marks JS, Koplan JP. The spread of the obesity epidemic in the United States, 1991–1998. *JAMA* 1999, 282: 1519–1522.

23. Health Canada on-line. Nature and dimensions of nutrition related problems. URL: http://www.hc-sc.gc.ca. Minister of Public Works and Government Services Canada. (Accessed March 15, 2010).

24. U.S. Census Bureau. Overview of race and Hispanic origin. 2010 census briefs. URL: http://www.census.gov/prod/cen2010/briefs/c2010br-02.pdf (Accessed March 26, 2012).

25. Kushi LH, Doyle C, McCullough M, Rock CL, Demark-Wahnefried W, Bandera EV, Gapstur S, Patel AV, Andrews K, Gansler T, and the American Cancer Society. 2010. Nutrition and physical activity guidelines advisory committee: American cancer society guidelines on nutrition and physical activity for cancer prevention. *CA Cancer J Clin* 2012, 62: 30–67.

26. Lichtenstein AH, Appel LJ, Brands M, Carnethon M, Daniels S, Franch HA, Franklin B, Kris-Etherton P, Harris WS, Howard B et al. Diet and lifestyle recommendations revision 2006. A scientific statement from the American Heart Association nutrition committee. *Circulation* 2006, 114: 82–96.

27. Health Canada on-line. A statistical profile on the health of first nations in Canada. URL: http://www.hc-sc.gc.ca/fniah-spnia/intro-eng.php. Minister of Public Works and Government Services Canada. (Accessed April 5, 2012).

28. Statistics New Zealand. Māori population estimates 1990–2011. URL: http://www.stats.govt.nz/browse_for_stats/population/estimates_and_projections/maori-population-estimates.aspx (Accessed April 5, 2012).

29. Bengoa J, Torun B, Behar M, Scrimshaw N. Nutritional goals and food guides in Latin America. Basis for their development (Spanish). *Arch Latinoam Nutr* 1988, 38: 373–426.

30. Albala C, Vio F, Kain J, Uauy R. Nutrition transition in Latin America: The case of Chile. *Nutr Rev* 2001, 59: 170–176.

31. Albala C, Vio F, Kain J, Uauy R. Nutrition transition in Chile: Determinants and consequences. *Public Health Nutr* 2002, 5: 123–128.

32. Barria RM, Amigo H. Nutrition transition: A review of Latin American profile. *Arch Latinoam Nutr* 2006, 56: 3–11.

33. Monteiro CA, Conde WL, Popkin BM. Independent effects of income and education on the risk of obesity in the Brazilian adult population. *J Nutr* 2001, 131: 881S–886S.

34. Vio F, Albala C, Kain J. Nutrition transition in Chile revisited: Mid-term evaluation of obesity goals for the period 2000–2010. *Public Health Nutr* 2008, 11: 405–412.

35. Stanojevic S, Kain J, Uauy R. The association between changes in height and obesity in Chilean preschool children: 1996–2004. *Obesity (Silver Spring)* 2007, 15: 1012–1022.

36. Stanojevic S, Kain J, Uauy R. Secular and seasonal trends in obesity in Chilean preschool children, 1996–2004. *J Pediatr Gastroenterol Nutr* 2008, 47: 339–343.

37. Uauy R, Kain J, Mericq V, Rojas J, Corvalan C. Nutrition, child growth, and chronic disease prevention. *Ann Med* 2008, 40: 11–20.

38. Lee J, Houser RF, Must A, de Fulladolsa PP, Bermudez OI. Socioeconomic disparities and the familial coexistence of child stunting and maternal overweight in Guatemala. *Econ Hum Biol* 2012, 10: 232–241.

39. Lee J, Houser RF, Must A, deFulladolsa PP, Bermudez OI. Disentangling nutritional factors and household characteristics related to child stunting and maternal overweight in Guatemala. *Econ Hum Biol* 2010, 8: 188–196. Epub 2010 May 2027.

40. Buitron D, Hurtig AK, San Sebastian M. Nutritional status of Naporuna children under five in the Amazon region of Ecuador (Spanish). *Rev Panam Salud Publica* 2004, 15: 151–159.

41. Barquera S, Peterson KE, Must A, Rogers BL, Flores M, Houser R, Monterrubio E, Rivera-Dommarco JA. Coexistence of maternal central adiposity and child stunting in Mexico. *Int J Obes (London)* 2007, 31: 601–607.

42. Bermudez OI, Tucker KL. Trends in dietary patterns of Latin American populations. *Cad Saude Publica* 2003, 19 (Suppl 1): S87–S99.

43. Garrett JL, Ruel MT. Stunted child-overweight mother pairs: An emerging policy concern? Discussion paper No.148. Washington, DC: International Food Policy Research Institute, 2003.

44. Garrett JL, Ruel MT. Stunted child-overweight mother pairs: Prevalence and association with economic development and urbanization. *Food Nutr Bull* 2005, 26: 209–221.

45. Altimir O. United Nations Development Programme, Occasional Paper No. 29, 1996. URL: http://www.undp.org/hdro/oc29.htm (Accessed February 25, 2000).

46. Molina V. *Guías Alimentarias y Promoción de la Salud en América Latina.* Guatemala, GT: Nutrition Institute for Central America and Panama, 2000, p. 6.

47. Peña M, Molina V. *Food Based Dietary Guidelines and Health Promotion in Latin America.* Washington, DC: Pan American Health Organization and Institute of Nutrition of Central America and Panama, 1999.

48. Chavez MM, Chavez A, Rios E, Madrigal H. *Guias de Alimentacion: Consejos Practicos para Alcanzar y Mantener un buen Estado de Nutricion y Salud*. Mexico, DF: Salvador Zubiran National Institute of Nutrition, 1993.

49. Instituto Nacional de Nutrición, Fundación Cavendes. *Guías de Alimentación para Venezuela*. Caracas, Venezuela: Fundación Cavendes, 1991, p. 88.

50. Ministerio de la Familia, Fundación Cavendes. *Guías de Alimentación para Venezuela del Niño menor de seis Años. Manual para Hogares y Multihogares de Cuidado Diario*. Caracas, Venezuela: Fundación Cavendes, 1996, p. 131.

51. Ministerio de la Familia, Fundación Cavendes. *Guías de Alimentación en el Niño menor de 6 Años. Orientacion Normativa*. Caracas, Venezuela: Fundación Cavendes, 1997, p. 44.

52. Chilean Ministry of Health, Institute of Nutrition and Food Technology, Nutrition Center at the University of Chile. *Dietary Guidelines for the Chilean Population*. Santiago, Chile: Ministry of Health, 1997.

53. Comisión Nacional de Guías Alimentarias de Guatemala. *Guías alimentarias para Guatemala: Los siete Pasos para una Alimentación Sana*. Guatemala, GT: Comisión Nacional de Guías Alimentarias, 1998, pp. 44.

54. Ministry of Health of Panama. *Dietary Guidelines for Panama (Spanish)*. Panama City, Panama: Ministry of Health, 1995, p. 40.

55. The World Bank. How we Classify Countries. URL: http://data.worldbank.org/about/country-classifications (Accessed May 21, 2012).

56. Ge K. The transition of Chinese dietary guidelines and food guide pagoda. *Asia Pac J Clin Nutr* 2011, 20: 439–446.

57. Indian Council of Medical Research and National Institute of Nutrition. Dietary Guidelines for Indians, Revision 2010. URL: http://www.indg.in/health/nutrition/dietary-guidelines-for-indians (Accessed April 10, 2012).

58. Usfar AA, Fahmida U. Do Indonesians follow its dietary guidelines?—Evidence related to food consumption, healthy lifestyle, and nutritional status within the period 2000–2010. *Asia Pac J Clin Nutr* 2011, 20: 484–494.

59. Nakamura T. Nutritional policies and dietary guidelines in Japan. *Asia Pac J Clin Nutr* 2011, 20: 452–454.

60. Jang YA, Lee HS, Kim BH, Lee Y, Lee HJ, Moon JJ, Kim CI. Revised dietary guidelines for Koreans. *Asia Pac J Clin Nutr* 2008, 17 (Suppl 1): 55–58.

61. Tee ES: Development and promotion of Malaysian dietary guidelines. *Asia Pac J Clin Nutr* 2011, 20: 455–461.

62. Tanchoco CC. Food- based dietary guidelines for Filipinos: Retrospects and prospects. *Asia Pac J Clin Nutr* 2011, 20: 462–471.

63. Lee B. Dietary guidelines in Singapore. *Asia Pac J Clin Nutr* 2011, 20: 472–476.

64. Sirichakwal PP, Sranacharoenpong K, Tontisirin K: Food based dietary guidelines (FBDGs) development and promotion in Thailand. *Asia Pac J Clin Nutr* 2011, 20: 477–483.

65. Krishnaswamy K. Developing and implementing dietary guidelines in India. *Asia Pac J Clin Nutr* 2008, 17 (Suppl 1): 66–69.

66. Chiang CE, Wang TD, Li YH, Lin TH, Chien KL, Yeh HI, Shyu KG, Tsai WC, Chao TH, Hwang JJ et al. 2010 Guidelines of the Taiwan Society of Cardiology for the Management of Hypertension. *J Formos Med Assoc* 2010, 109: 740–773.

67. Kusharto CM, Hardinsyah, Rimbawan. Nutritional guidelines for Indonesia. In *Dietary guidelines in Asia-Pacific*. Florencio CA (Ed.). Quezon City, Philippines: ASEAN-New Zealand IILP Project 5, 1997, p. 52.

68. Sirichakwal PP, Sranacharoenpong K. Practical experience in development and promotion of food-based dietary guidelines in Thailand. *Asia Pac J Clin Nutr* 2008, 17: 63–65.

69. Singapore Government, Health Promotion Board. Healthy food pyramid. URL: http://www.hpb.gov.sg/foodforhealth/article.aspx?id=2638 (Accessed April 18, 2012).

70. Nutrition Society of Malaysia. Eat right with the new Malaysian food pyramid. URL: http://thestar.com.my/health/story.asp?file=/2010/11/6/health/7342546&sec=health (Accessed April 18, 2012).

71. Yoshiike N, Hayashi F, Takemi Y, Mizoguchi K, Seino F. A new food guide in Japan: The Japanese food guide spinning top. *Nutr Rev* 2007, 65: 149–154.

72. Vorster HH, Love P, Browne C: Development of food-based dietary guidelines for South Africa—The process. *South African J Clin Nutr* 2001, 14 (Suppl): S3–S6.

73. FAO. Food Guidelines by Country. Dietary Guidelines for Nigeria. URL: http://www.fao.org/ag/agn/nutrition/education_guidelines_nga_en.stm (Accessed February 13, 2006).

74. FAO. Food Guidelines by Country. Dietary Guidelines for Namibia. URL: http://www.fao.org/ag/agn/nutrition/education_guidelines_nam_en.stm (Accessed February 13, 2006).

75. South African Department of Health, Directorate of Nutrition. South African guidelines for healthy eating, 2004. URL: ftp://ftp.fao.org/es/esn/nutrition/dietary_guidelines/zaf_eating.pdf. (Accessed on May 21, 2012).

76. WHO Regional Office for Europe. The CINDI dietary guide for Europe. Countrywide integrated noncommunicable disease intervention (CINDI) programme, 2000. URL: http://www.euro.who.int/__data/assets/pdf_file/0010/119926/E70041.pdf (Accessed May 21, 2012).

77. International Life Sciences Institute. National food-based dietary guidelines: Experiences, implications and future directions. In Summary Report of a *Workshop on National Food-Based Dietary Guidelines*, ILSI Europe, Budapest, Hungary, 2004.

78. World Health Organization, Food and Agriculture Organization. Preparation and use of food-based dietary guidelines. In *Report of a joint FAO/WHO consultation Nicosia, Cyprus* (WHO/NUT/96.6 ed.). Nutrition Programme. Geneva, Switzerland: WHO, 1996.

79. European Food Information Council, FAO. In Summary Report of a *Workshop on Food Based Dietary Guidelines*, Budapest, Hungary. URL: http://www.fao.org/ag/humannutrition/18893-0f5791b5218038c61824252703117b8b4.pdf (Accessed May 21, 2012).

80. The United Kingdom National Health Service. Healthy Eating. URL: http://www.eatwell.gov.uk/ (Accessed February 2011).

81. Spanish Society of Community Nutrition. Guide for Healthy Eating (Spanish). URL: http://www.nutricioncomunitaria.org/generica.jsp?tipo=docu&id=3 (Accessed May 21, 2012).

82. FAO. Food-based dietary guidelines. Dietary guidelines for Ireland. URL: http://www.fao.org/ag/humannutrition/nutritioneducation/fbdg/49851/en//irl/ (Accessed May 21, 2012).

83. Greek Ministry of Health and Welfare. Dietary guidelines for adults in Greece, 1999. URL: http://www.mednet.gr/archives/1999-5/pdf/516.pdf (Accessed December 2010).

84. Italian National Research Institute for Food and Nutrition. Guidelines for Healthy Eating (Italian). URL: http://sapermangiare.mobi/linee_guida.html (Accessed May 21, 2012).

85. The Netherlands Bureau for Food and Nutrition Education. The Food Guide. Explanation and Background. The Hague. URL: http://www.fao.org/ag/humannutrition/nutritioneducation/fbdg/49851/en/nld/ (Accessed May 21, 2012).

86. French Ministry of Health. Food eating guide for all (French). URL: http://www.sante.gouv.fr (Accessed May 21, 2012).

87. Federal Ministry of Food, Agriculture and Consumer Protection of Germany. Healthy diet. URL: http://www.bmelv.de/EN/Food/Healthy-Diet/healthy-diet_node.html (Accessed May 21, 2012).

88. Porto University, School of Food and Nutrition Sciences. The new wheel of foods. A guide for selecting daily foods (Portuguese). URL: http://www.fao.org/ag/humannutrition/17282-0ffdf74091278ac33097e975219536e08.pdf (Accessed May 21, 2012).

89. Euro Diet, Nutrition and Health for Healthy Living in Europe. A framework for food-based dietary guidelines in the European union, 2000. Eurodiet reports from working group 2. Chair Michael Gibney, Institute of European Food Studies, Trinity College, Dublin, Ireland. URL: http://eurodiet.med.uoc.gr/ (Accessed May 21, 2012).

90. U.S. Department of Agriculture. Choose MyPlate. Gov. URL: http://www.choosemyplate.gov/ (Accessed May 21, 2012).

# 29 Nutrition Monitoring in the United States

*Margaret A. McDowell*

## CONTENTS

## INTRODUCTION

Nutrition monitoring and related research, defined by the U.S. Congress as "the set of activities necessary to provide timely information about the role and status of factors that bear on the contribution that nutrition makes to the health of the people of the United States,"[1] plays a vital role in formulating the U.S. nutrition research, programs, and policies. Traditionally, the scope of nutrition monitoring in the United States has included federal and state-sponsored survey and surveillance systems, policy initiatives, and research to assess and improve the health and nutritional status of the general population and population subgroups that may be at increased risk of disease. Nutrition and public health professionals have worked together for more than three decades to build and strengthen the U.S. nutrition monitoring system.

The national nutrition monitoring efforts undertaken by many federal, state, and local partners grew from the National Nutrition Monitoring System (NNMS) formed in 1978 to a comprehensive National Nutrition Monitoring and Related Research Program (NNMRRP) with the passage of the National Nutrition Monitoring and Related Research Act of 1990. When the Act expired in 2002, nutrition monitoring program activities continued. Today, a comprehensive, albeit decentralized network of federal, state, and nongovernment activities collect and report comprehensive information in the five key NNMRRP measurement areas: nutrition and related health measurements; food and nutrient consumption; knowledge, attitudes, and behavior assessments; food composition and nutrient databases; and food-supply and expenditure patterns.

Previous editions of this handbook described the establishment of a NNMS to support federal nutrition research and policy. The first half of this chapter includes a brief review of NNMRRP history, an updated list of major nutrition monitoring surveys and surveillance programs, and the descriptions of several new nutrition monitoring initiatives and resources that have been added since the second edition of this handbook was published in 2005. The second half of the chapter describes nutrition monitoring program, research, and policy activities. The chapter concludes with personal reflections on the factors that have shaped recent national nutrition monitoring activities and future challenges for the NNMS.

## HISTORY OF NUTRITION MONITORING IN THE UNITED STATES

Jean Mayer remarked during a ceremony for the founding of the Tufts Nutrition Institute in 1977, "*Nutrition is not simply a science, it is an agenda.*"[2] Perhaps this analogy can also be used for nutrition monitoring considering that the nation's nutrition monitoring system reflects an ever-changing public health and nutrition agenda. In the United States, the national nutrition monitoring agenda evolved from public health programs that were rooted in state health departments, voluntary health agencies, and federal–state partnerships formed to improve maternal and child health and eliminate undernutrition and deficiency disorders to a comprehensive population-based system that considers under- and overnutrition and its effects on health status.[3] Today, nutrition and health status are now viewed within a broader context of diet and health systems, both of which are impacted by global, domestic, and regional food policies, programs, and resources.

### EARLY YEARS: NATIONAL NUTRITION MONITORING IN THE UNITED STATES (1977–1989)

The Food and Agriculture Act of 1977 required the U.S. Department of Agriculture (USDA) and the U.S. Department of Health Education and Welfare (now the Department of Health and Human Services [DHHS]) to develop a plan to coordinate the DHHS National Health and Nutrition Examination Survey (NHANES) and USDA Nationwide Food Consumption Survey (NFCS).[4] The Act mandated the development of a reporting system and the delivery of periodic reports to Congress based on survey results and related nutrition monitoring activities. A proposal for a comprehensive nutrition monitoring system was submitted to Congress in 1978 with NHANES and NCFS as the cornerstones of the first NNMS.

The Joint DHHS/USDA Nutrition Monitoring Evaluation Committee was formed in 1983, and one of its deliverables

was the Committee's first report entitled, *First Progress Report on Nutrition Monitoring in the United States.*[5] The report provided a comprehensive summary of the dietary and nutritional status of the U.S. population. The Committee made several recommendations for future survey data collection and nutrition monitoring. The nation's leading nutrition policymakers, researchers, and academicians responded to the report with a flurry of papers, many of which articulated expanded roles and opportunities for nutrition monitoring programs, policies, and research.[6–8] Slow, steady progress was made in the years that followed, and a formal operational plan for the NNMS was released in 1987.[9] In 1988, the Interagency Committee on Nutrition Monitoring was formed to enhance planning, coordination, and communication on nutrition monitoring activities within federal government.[10] A second comprehensive report entitled *Second Progress Report on Nutrition Monitoring in the United States* was prepared by the Life Sciences Research Office (LSRO) of the Federation of American Societies for Experimental Biology (FASEB) and delivered to Congress in 1989.[11] Later that year, the first *Directory of Federal Nutrition Monitoring Activities*, a comprehensive reference for all nutrition monitoring surveys and related activities, was published.[12]

### NATIONAL NUTRITION MONITORING AND RELATED RESEARCH ACT OF 1990: NUTRITION MONITORING (1990–2002)

The enactment of the National Nutrition Monitoring and Related Research Act of 1990, establishing the NNMRRP, was the culmination of efforts to establish a coordinated, comprehensive collaboration between federal, state, and local government groups that were engaged in nutrition monitoring activities.[13] The Act provided a mandate for a wide range of activities, though no funds were appropriated by the Congress to carry them out. The Act also stipulated that NNMRRP implementation and reporting were to be undertaken jointly by the secretaries of the co-lead agencies, USDA and DHHS. The Interagency Committee on Nutrition Monitoring was replaced by the Interagency Board for Nutrition Monitoring and Related Research (IBNMRR) in 1991. The IBNMRR was composed of representatives from the 22 federal agencies that contributed or used national nutrition monitoring data. The Assistant Secretary for Health, DHHS, and the Assistant Secretary for Food and Consumer Services, USDA, cochaired the board.

The IBNMRR provided leadership and oversight for the federal nutrition monitoring budget and NNMRRP reporting activities until the Act expired in 2002. During its tenure, the IBNMRR directed the development and implementation of the DHHS/USDA Ten-Year Comprehensive Plan, a blueprint for nutrition monitoring and research activities.[14] The primary goals of the plan were to (1) collect continuous, comprehensive, and reliable data in a timely coordinated manner; (2) develop and implement comparable methods to collect and report federal survey data; (3) conduct nutrition research; and (4) efficiently and effectively disseminate and exchange information with data users. The board coordinated the production biennial progress reports to the President and the Congress, the nutrition policy updates, and the scientific research reports describing the nutritional and health status of the U.S. population.

The Act also included provisions for the formation of an external advisory group. In 1992, the National Nutrition Monitoring Advisory Council was appointed to provide guidance and scientific and technical oversight to the IBNMRR. The Advisory Council was comprised of nine appointees— five presidential and four congressional appointees who had expertise in public health, human nutrition, food production and distribution, and nutrition policy. During the time period from 1991 to 1993, the *Directory of Federal Nutrition Monitoring Activities* was updated and expanded with information about state-based surveillance activities.[15] A user-friendly data chartbook was produced with input from IBNMRR agencies to highlight major activities in the five major NNMRRP measurement areas.[16]

Communication and coordination among the IBNMRR member agencies were enhanced through the efforts of several work groups. The survey comparability group, co-led by DHHS National Center for Health Statistics (NCHS) and the USDA Agricultural Research Service (ARS), assisted the IBNMRR in its efforts to improve federal survey and surveillance system coordination and communication and work toward the development of a common automated dietary intake assessment methodology and database system for national surveys. The Federal–State Relations and Information Dissemination and Exchange Group was formed to improve the capacity of states and local groups to engage in nutrition monitoring activities. The food composition group, led by USDA/ARS, was charged with maintaining existing databases and identifying future food composition data needs. Following the enactment of welfare reform legislation in 1996, a Welfare Reform, Nutrition, and Data Needs Working Group comprised of federal and non-federal members was formed to foster collaborative research on nutrition and welfare reform and to coordinate efforts to assess the impact of welfare reform legislation on nutrition, hunger, and health status.

In 1995, the LSRO under contract with USDA, and under the joint leadership of DHHS and USDA, prepared the *Third Report on Nutrition Monitoring in the United States.*[17] In addition to providing a profile of the nutrition-related health status of the U.S. population and the nutritional quality of the U.S. diet, the report documented rising rates of overweight and chronic diet-related health conditions in the U.S. population including coronary heart disease, stroke, and bone fracture. With respect to eating patterns and diet quality, a gap was noted between public health recommendations and consumers' practices. Less than one-third of U.S. adults reported consuming five or more servings of fruits and vegetables per day, and intakes of total fat, saturated fatty acids, and cholesterol were higher than recommended for a large proportion of the U.S. population. Furthermore, despite the fact that per capita food and nutrient availability was adequate overall to prevent undernutrition and nutritional

deficiencies, approximately 9%–13% of Americans residing in low income households experienced food insufficiency.[17]

The integration of the DHHS, NHANES, and USDA Continuing Survey of Food Intakes of Individuals (CSFII) was a major initiative undertaken between 1997 and 2002. The Act provided the impetus for coordinating national dietary survey data collection. Survey integration was formally initiated in 1998 with the signing of a memorandum of understanding between the NHANES lead agency, the NCHS, and the CSFII lead, the USDA ARS, and an expert panel on survey integration was formed later that year; a formal plan to integrate NHANES and CSFII was developed by the lead agencies in 2000. The third and the final *Directory of Federal and State National Nutrition Monitoring and Related Research Activities* produced when the Act was still in effect was published in 2000.[18]

The goal of an integrated national nutrition survey program was achieved in January 2002 with the launch of *What We Eat in America* (WWEIA), the dietary component of NHANES.[19,20] Survey integration and concomitant advances in information technology have increased efficiencies in data collection, data release, and statistical reporting. The USDA/ARS automated multiple pass (AMPM) dietary interview and processing system has been used to collect NHANES in-person baseline (day 1) dietary recalls and telephone-mode (day 2) dietary recalls since 2002, thus achieving the NNMRRP goal of a single unified dietary data collection and processing system for national dietary surveys.[19,20]

## NATIONAL NUTRITION MONITORING ACTIVITIES: 2003–PRESENT

The National Nutrition Monitoring and Related Research Act of 1990 and the NNMRRP Ten-Year Plan guided federal nutrition monitoring nutrition surveillance, research, policy, and program activities from 1992 to 2002. Numerous attempts were made by nutrition monitoring stakeholders to garner support for reauthorization of 1990 legislation. Prior to the expiration of the Act and shortly thereafter, several public meetings and professional society reports were issued:

- The National Academy of Sciences (NAS) sponsored a public symposium in 1999 entitled "Nutrition Monitoring in the US: Preparing for the Next Millennium" as a means of engaging nutrition monitoring stakeholders in federal, research, industry, and consumer arenas on the important uses of NNMRRP data and future opportunities to optimize data systems and reporting activities.
- The Council of American Society for Nutritional Sciences Nutritional Sciences formed a working group to review the current status and future plans of the NNMRRP. The working group issued a formal statement urging reauthorization and expansion of national nutrition monitoring activities.[21]

- DHHS and USDA cosponsored a workshop entitled "Future Directions for the Integrated CSFII-NHANES: What We Eat in America-NHANES" in 2002 to discuss current and future nutrition monitoring activities and research needs.[22]
- The NAS National Research Council (NRC) Committee on National Statistics (CNSTAT) issued a report on food and nutrition data needs in 2004.[23]
- In 2005, the NRC Panel on Enhancing the Data Infrastructure in Support of Food and Nutrition Programs, Research, and Decision Making issued a report entitled Improving Data to Analyze Food and Nutrition Policies.[24] The expert group considered future nutrition monitoring data needs and made recommendations to enhance the survey data collection systems and thus improve the utility of federal nutrition monitoring data.

Nutrition monitoring advocacy groups have made at least two unsuccessful attempts to garner Congressional support for reauthorization of the Act:

- Formal legislation to reauthorize and extend the 1990 Act for 10 years was introduced in Congress in 2005. House of Representatives (HR) 2844, known as *The National Health, Nutrition, and Physical Activity Monitoring Act of 2005*, was introduced into the 109th Congress (2005–2006), but the bill never left committee.[25]
- In 2008, the U.S. Farm Bill (also known as the *Food, Conservation, and Energy Act of 2008*) included a section on joint nutrition monitoring and related research activities supporting and reaffirming joint nutrition monitoring activities through fiscal year 2012.[26] Section 4403 of the 2008 Act states that that the Secretaries of DHHS and USDA shall "*continue to provide jointly for continuous collection of dietary, health, physical activity, and diet and health knowledge data on a nationally representative sample, periodically collect data on special at-risk populations; distribute information on health, nutrition, the environment, and physical activity to the public in a timely fashion; continuously update food composition tables; and engage in research and development of data collection methods and standards.*"

Accordingly, today, DHHS, USDA, and numerous other federal and state partners are engaged in nutrition monitoring activities, albeit under a decentralized system. Additionally, many new interagency and public–private partnerships have emerged in recent years to augment federal, state, and local government efforts. Previous editions of this handbook authored by Bialostosky et al.[27] and Pennington,[28] and elsewhere (Briefel[29] PKN 2005 and Briefel and McDowell[30]), provided comprehensive updates on national nutrition monitoring surveys and surveillance

program activities. The next section includes updated information on the national nutrition monitoring surveys and surveillance activities featured in earlier editions of this handbook and descriptions of several new initiatives (Table 29.1).

## MAJOR FEDERAL NUTRITION MONITORING SURVEYS, SURVEILLANCE ACTIVITIES, DATABASES, AND NUTRITION ASSISTANCE PROGRAMS BY NUTRITION MONITORING COMPONENT

### NUTRITION AND RELATED HEALTH MEASUREMENTS

New and expanded data collection efforts are supporting efforts to monitor health and nutritional status of the U.S. population and targeted subpopulations. National efforts to reverse the increasing rates of child and adult overweight and obesity have taken center stage. Comprehensive data are collected as part of national initiatives to improve the food security and nutritional status of low-income populations, the nutritional quality of foods served in schools and other congregate settings, and the health of risk groups such as older adults, pregnant women, infants, and children. Surveys and evaluation studies are described in the next section. Findings from many of these studies are reported in annual meetings sponsored by federal partners and public health and professional associations.

*Administration on Aging (AOA) Initiatives and Evaluation Studies*[31]: The Older Americans Act (OAA) nutrition program was established to reduce hunger and food insecurity, promote socialization among older adults, and promote health and well-being of older individuals and delay the onset of adverse health conditions through access to comprehensive preventive health and nutrition programs. Congregate Nutrition Services, Home-Delivered Nutrition Services, and the Nutrition Services Incentive Program are administered under the OAA. Grants for Congregate Nutrition Services and Home-Delivered Nutrition Services are allocated to states and territories by a formula based on their share of the population aged 60 and over. Nutrition Services Incentive Program grants are additional grants for food only to states, territories, and Indian tribal organizations based on their proportional share of the total number of meals served in the prior federal fiscal year. Completed and ongoing evaluation activities are listed on the AOA website.

*NHANES*[32]: CDC/NCHS has conducted a program of studies to assess the health and nutritional status of adults and children in the United States since the 1960s. Periodic NHANES were conducted between 1971 and 1994. NHANES became a continuous annual survey program in 1999. The NHANES is unique that it uses household interview and physical examination methods. Initially, health interviews are completed in respondents' homes; health examinations including the first of two dietary recall

**TABLE 29.1**

**National Nutrition Monitoring Surveys, Programs, and Technical Files by NNMRRP Measurement Area**

| Department/Agency(IES) | Surveys and Programs |
|---|---|
| Measure—nutrition and health status | |
| DHHS/AOA | Evaluation studies of nutrition programs for older Americans |
| DHHS/CDC | NHANES |
| DHHS/CDC | NHCS |
| DHHS/CDC | NHIS |
| DHHS/CDC | NIS |
| DHHS/CDC | NSFG |
| DHHS/CDC | National Survey of mPINC |
| DHHS/CDC | NVSS |
| DHHS/CDC | NCHS linked mortality data files (multiple surveys) |
| DHHS/CDC | PedNSS |
| DHHS/CDC | PNSS |
| DHHS/CDC | SLAITS |
| DHHS/HRSA | NSCH |
| DHHS/NIH | FAB survey |
| DHHS/NIH | HINTS |
| DHHS/NIH | Add Health |
| DOL/BLS | NLSY79 |
| USDA/FNS | Studies of CACFP |
| USDA/FNS | SNDA |
| USDA/FNS | PC |
| Measure—food and nutrient intake | |
| DHHS/CDC | SHPPS |
| DHHS/CDC | NHANES—WWEIA component |
| DHHS/FDA | TDS |
| DoEd | ECLS |
| DOL/BLS; USDA/ERS | CPS-FSS |
| USDA/FNS | WIC studies |
| Measure—health and nutrition knowledge, attitudes, and behavior | |
| DHHS/CDC | BRFSS |
| DHHS/CDC | YRBSS |
| DHHS/CDC | PRAMS |
| DHHS/CDC | NHANES 2005–2010 Flexible Consumer Behavior module |
| DHHS/CDC, FDA; others | IFPS |
| DHHS/FDA | HDS |
| DHHS/FDA; USDA/FSIS | FSSs |
| DHHS/NIH; DOL/BLS; USDA/ERS | ATUS EH module of the CPS |
| Measure—food and dietary supplement composition | |
| DHHS/FDA | FLAPS |
| DHHS/NIH | Dietary Supplements Labels Database |
| USDA/ARS | DSID |
| USDA/ARS | NNDSR |
| USDA/ARS | FNDDS |
| USDA/ARS | FPED (formerly MPED) |
| Measure—food-supply determinations | |
| Commercial | AC Nielsen ScanTrack and Homescan (NCP) services |
| DOC | Fisheries of the U.S. survey |
| DOL/BLS | CES |
| USDA/ERS | U.S. Food and Nutrient Supply Series |
| USDA/ERS, FNS | National Household FoodAPS |

*Abbreviations*: AOA, Administration on Aging; ARS, Agricultural Research Service; BLS, Bureau of Labor Statistics; CDC, Centers for Disease Control and Prevention; DHHS, Department of Health and Human Services; DOC, Department of Commerce; DoEd, Department of Education; DOL, Department of Labor; ERS, Economic Research Service; FDA, Food and Drug Administration; FNS, Food and Nutrition Service; FSIS, Food Safety Inspection Service; HRSA, Health Resources and Services Administration; NIH, National Institutes of Health; USDA, U.S. Department of Agriculture.

interviews are completed in mobile examination centers (MECs). The MECs are staffed by health interviewers and examiners. The NHANES teams travel to 15 geographic locations/year. Approximately 5000 individuals, all ages, are interviewed and examined annually. Selected population subgroups such as Hispanics, blacks, and older adults are oversampled to improve the statistical reliability of the subgroup estimates. Asians will be among the subgroups oversampled in NHANES 2011–2014. Each NHANES survey has unique components, and these are described in the website materials for each survey period. NHANES data remain the cornerstone of national nutrition monitoring in the United States and are used to assess nutritional status, estimate the prevalence of major diseases and risk factors for diseases, and evaluate progress toward achieving long-term national health promotion and disease prevention objectives.

*National Health Care Surveys (NHCS)*[33]: CDC/NCHS surveys health-care providers and health-care facilities. The NHCS surveys are designed to answer key questions of interest to health-care policy makers, public health professionals, and researchers such as the factors that influence the use of health-care resources; the quality of health care, including safety; and the disparities in health-care services provided to population subgroups in the United States.

*National Health Interview Survey (NHIS)*[34]: NHIS conducted by CDC/NCHS has been used to monitor the health of the nation since 1957. NHIS data are obtained through personal household interviews. Interviewers visit 35,000–40,000 households across the country annually and collect data on about 75,000–100,000 individuals. The NHIS core content covers a broad range of health topics. Supplemental questions that change from year to year may be included in the NHIS to address emerging health issues and topics.

*National Immunization Survey (NIS)*[35]: The CDC NIS is an annual survey conducted jointly by CDC/NCIRD and CDC/NCHS to monitor immunizations of the U.S. children nationwide. Breastfeeding questions have been included in the survey since 2001. NIS consists of a list-assisted random-digit-dialing (RDD) telephone survey followed by a mailed survey to children's immunization providers. NIS began data collection in April 1994 to monitor childhood immunization coverage. The target population for the NIS is children between the ages of 19 and 35 months living in the United States at the time of the interview. More than 24,000 children were included in the 2010 NIS.

*National Survey of Family Growth (NSFG)*[36]: Periodic data collection occurred from 1973 to 2002; continuous, annual surveys have been conducted since 2006. Men and women 15–44 years are interviewed (4400–5000 persons annually). The survey content topics include family life, marriage and divorce, pregnancy, infertility, use of contraception, breastfeeding, and men's and women's health.

*National Survey of Maternity Practices in Infant Nutrition and Care (mPINC)*[37]: CDC has conducted a biennial national survey of maternity care practices and policies every 2 years since 2007 because evidence has shown that specific practices in medical care settings affect the rates of breastfeeding initiation and duration. The survey is mailed to all facilities with registered maternity beds in the United States and the U.S. territories. CDC produces benchmark and state reports and calculates scores for every participating facility and state to indicate their performance on the mPINC survey.

*National Vital Statistics System (NVSS)*[38]: CDC/NCHS collects and disseminates the nation's official vital statistics data. Vital statistics data are provided through contracts between NCHS and vital registration systems operated in the jurisdictions that are legally responsible for registering vital events such as births, deaths, marriages, divorces, and fetal deaths. In the United States, legal authority for the registration of these events resides individually with the 50 states, 2 cities (Washington, DC, and New York City), and 5 territories (Puerto Rico, the Virgin Islands, Guam, American Samoa, and the Commonwealth of the Northern Mariana Islands). Standard forms for the collection of the data and model procedures for the uniform registration of the vital events have been developed and are recommended for nationwide use through the cooperative activities of the jurisdictions and NCHS.

*NHANES Linked Mortality Follow-Up Studies (Multiple Surveys)*[39]: NCHS currently links several NCHS surveys with death certificate records from the National Death Index (NDI). The NDI linkage provides the opportunity to conduct an extensive array of outcome studies designed to investigate the association of a wide variety of health factors with mortality. Linked mortality data are available for the following NCHS surveys: NHIS; NHANES I Epidemiologic Follow-up Study; NHANES II, 1976–1980; NHANES III, 1988–1994; the Second Longitudinal Study of Aging; and the National Nursing Home Surveys.

*Pediatric Nutrition Surveillance System (PedNSS)*[40]: CDC's PedNSS* is a child-based public health surveillance system that began in the 1970s to provide data to describe the nutritional status of low-income U.S. children who attend federally funded maternal and child health and nutrition programs. CDC has partnered with USDA/FNS and other public health programs across the country to operate the PedNSS. The program uses existing data from the Special Supplemental Nutrition Program for Women, Infants, and Children (WIC); the Early and Periodic Screening, Diagnosis, and Treatment (EPSDT) Program; and the Title V Maternal and Child Health Program (MCH) for nutrition surveillance activities. Information on birth weight, short stature, underweight, overweight, anemia, and breastfeeding is obtained on infants, children, and adolescents from birth to 20 years who receive routine care, nutrition education, and supplemental foods at public health clinics.

*Pregnancy Nutrition Surveillance System (PNSS)*[41]: CDC's PNSS* is a program-based public health surveillance system that began in the 1970s to monitor risk factors associated with infant mortality and poor birth outcomes among low-income pregnant women who participate in federally funded public health programs. PNSS uses existing data from the WIC and Title V MCH for nutrition surveillance. PNSS tracks maternal health indicators such as prepregnancy weight status, maternal weight gain, parity, inter-pregnancy intervals, anemia, diabetes, and hypertension during pregnancy. Data on maternal behavioral indicators include medical care, WIC enrollment, multivitamin dietary supplement use, and tobacco and alcohol use.

*PedNSS and PNSS Program Note*: Extensive data are available from population surveys such as NHANES, NHIS, NIS, and PRAMS, BRFSS, and YRBS and the USDA/FNS WIC Participant Characteristics (PC) study, which provides comparable statistics across all of the states on many PedNSS and PNSS indicators. Therefore, CDC will discontinue both systems in 2012 after the 2011 PedNSS and PNSS data and reports are released.

*State and Local Area Integrated Telephone Survey (SLAITS)*[42]: SLAITS collects health-care data at the state and local levels as a means of supplementing national data collection efforts. SLAITS uses the same RDD telephone design approach and sampling frame as the ongoing NIS program. SLAITS is funded through sponsorship of specific questionnaire modules. Sponsors include both government agencies and nonprofit organizations. Data are obtained on a variety of health topics to meet varied program and policy needs. The National Survey of Children's Health (NSCH) and the National Survey of Children with Special Health Care Needs (2009–2010) were conducted as SLAITS modules.

*NSCH*[43]: NSCH is sponsored by the Maternal and Child Health Bureau of HRSA, conducted as a module of the SLAITS. NSCH data are used to produce national- and state-specific prevalence estimates for physical, emotional, and behavioral health indicators and measures of children's experiences with the health-care system. NSCH includes questions about the family (e.g., parents' health status, stress and coping behaviors, family activities) and respondents' perceptions of the neighborhoods where their children live. Surveys were completed in 2003, 2007, and 2011 with telephone samples of households with children less than 18 years residing in each of the 50 states and the District of Columbia.

*Food Attitudes and Behaviors (FAB) Survey*[44]: The National Institutes of Health (NIH)/NCI conducted a one-time panel survey of approximate 3400 U.S. adults 18 and older in 2007. Interview questionnaires included attitudes and behaviors related to fruit and vegetable intake, dietary behaviors, leisure-time physical activity, and self-reported height and weight information.

*Health Information National Trends Survey (HINTS)*[45]: HINTS is a biennial survey of the U.S. adults in all 50 states, conducted by NIH/NCI since 2002. HINTS data are used to understand how the U.S. adults access and use cancer and general health information.

*National Longitudinal Study of Adolescent Health (Add Health)*[46]: The NIH National Institute of Child Health and Development in collaboration with other NIH institutes and other groups. Data collection began in 1994 and occurred most recently in 2008 (wave IV). Data collection is performed by the University of North Carolina at Chapel Hill. Add Health targets the U.S. adolescents in grades 7 through 12. Data collection includes an in-school questionnaire. Add Health data are used to explore the social, the behavioral, and the biological linkages in the health trajectories of the U.S. adolescents.

*National Longitudinal Survey of Youth 1979 (NLSY79)*[47]: The objective of the study is to collect data about demographics, health, and life/work trajectories of individuals who were between the ages of 14 and 22 years and residing in the United States in 1979. It began in 1979 and conducted annually through 1994 and biennially thereafter. The most recent year available is 2008; data for 2010 will be available in the spring of 2012. Food security, eating away from home, self-reported height and weight, and frequency, type, and intensity of physical activity are among the interview topics. The DOL (Department of Labor)/BLS (Bureau of Labor Statistics) website has information about other longitudinal surveys conducted by the agency.

*School Nutrition Dietary Assessment Surveys (SNDA)*[48,49]: SNDA consists of a series of USDA/Food and Nutrition Service (FNS)-funded studies. Information is obtained on the nutritional quality of meals and snacks served in public schools that participate in the National School Lunch Program (NSLP) and the School Breakfast Program (SBP). SNDA-I (1991–1992) assessed the content of school meals offered to students and meals consumed by students; study findings showed that overall, school lunches were not consistent with *Dietary Guidelines for Americans* recommendations for total-fat and saturated-fat intake. At the time, school food service programs were not required to offer meals that were consistent with the *Dietary Guidelines*. USDA launched the School Meals Initiative (SMI) for Healthy Children in 1995. Data from the SNDA-II (1998–1999) provided data to evaluate progress on achieving the SMI standards. SNDA-III (2004–2005) provided information on the school meal programs, the school environment that affects the programs, the nutrient content of school meals, and the contributions of school meals to students' diets. Estimations of usual nutrient intakes were produced using a statistical method recommended by the Institute of Medicine (IOM). SNDA-IV (January to June 2010) examined school food environments and meal service operations, including policies and availability of competitive foods (foods offered outside the school meal programs), school wellness policies, food safety, the nutrient content of school meals, and the contributions of school meals to students' diets.

*Studies of the Child and Adult Care Food Program (CACFP)*[50]: CACFP is a nutrition assistance program that is administered by the USDA FNS through grants to states—typically to state educational agencies. CACFP serves infants, preschool children, and children younger than 12 years in child care centers and homes; older children in at-risk after-school programs and emergency shelters; and disabled and older adults in adult day care centers. The IOM reviewed and assessed the nutritional needs of the populations served by CACFP and provided recommendations to revise the meal requirements for CACFP.[51]

*WIC Participant Characteristics (PC) Study*[52]: FNS has produced biennial reports on participant and program characteristics in the WIC program since 1998. This information is used for general program monitoring as well as for managing the information needs of the program. The biennial reports include information on the income and nutritional risk characteristics of WIC participants, breastfeeding initiation rates and durations by the state, data on WIC program participation for migrant farm worker families, and information on WIC participation that is deemed appropriate by the Secretary of Agriculture.

## FOOD AND NUTRIENT CONSUMPTION

Efforts to characterize the food and nutrient intakes of the U.S. food supply are challenged by the sheer size and diversity of the U.S. food supply. For example, the typical U.S. supermarket contains more than 38,000 food items.[53] Additionally, many of the foods consumed by the United States are imported—from more than 175 different countries, thus adding to the challenge of reporting representative food intake and nutrient composition values for the U.S. food supply.[54] Among the notable accomplishments in food and nutrient intake assessment are improved methods to estimate usual intakes of foods and nutrients from foods and total nutrient intakes from foods and dietary supplements. Research findings using the new estimation methods have been presented at national and international professional society meetings, at conferences convened by the NAS/IOM, and at federal agency meetings and workshops. The next section describes federal food and nutrient consumption data collection activities.

*School Health Policies and Practices Study (SHPPS)*[55]: SHPPS is a national survey conducted periodically to assess school health policies and practices at the state, district, school, and classroom levels. SHPPS was conducted in 1994, 2000, and 2006 and will be fielded again in 2012.

*NHANES*[32,56]: NHANES has always included a comprehensive nutritional status assessment component consisting of anthropometry, nutritional biochemistry and hematology tests, clinical tests, a 24 h dietary recall interview, and extensive health and nutrition questionnaire data. Detailed questionnaire information is obtained on dietary supplement use, food security, food and nutrition program participation, dietary habits, breastfeeding, healthcare utilization, access to health care, and health status. DHHS–USDA survey integration in 2002 resulted in the introduction of WWEIA, as the new dietary component of NHANES. Comprehensive dietary intake data collection is conducted jointly by CDC/NCHS and USDA/ARS staff

using the USDA/ARS AMPM system described earlier. The continuous NHANES dietary and nutrition assessment components are modified periodically to meet emerging data needs. Extensive information is collected on diet and health behavior, consumer knowledge and practices, food security status, and dietary supplement use.

NHANES collected accelerometry data on children and adults 6 years and over in NHANES 2003–2006 and accelerometry returned to the survey for NHANES 2011–2012. Additionally, a special 1-year NHANES Physical Activity and Fitness Survey to assess physical activity and fitness of youth was launched in 2012. The youth study includes accelerometry assessments with youth 3 years and older. Cardiorespiratory fitness, muscular strength, muscular endurance, and flexibility will be assessed in school-aged youngsters, and motor skill development will be assessed in preschool-aged children.

*Total Diet Study (TDS)*[57]: The TDS is an ongoing FDA program that determines the levels of selected contaminants and nutrients in foods consumed by the U.S. population. The TDS began in 1961 as a means of monitoring radioactive contamination of foods and now includes pesticide residues, industrial chemicals, and toxic and nutrient elements. The foods that are sampled for the TDS program are prepared as they would be consumed (i.e., table ready) prior to chemical analysis. Thus, the analytical results provide the basis for realistic estimates of dietary intake of the analytes by the U.S. population. National food consumption survey data are used to compile dietary intake estimates for 14 sex–age groups. The number of foods sampled in the TDS has increased from 82 food items in the early 1960s to about 280 foods in the current program. The TDS food list is updated periodically to reflect changing U.S. food consumption patterns. Beginning with the 2006 TDS, the TDS data will be summarized in 5-year increments.

*Early Childhood Longitudinal Study (ECLS) Program*[58]: The ECLS program consists of nationally representative studies of early childhood development and educational experiences. Detailed information on children's health, early care, and early school experiences is collected including cognitive, social, emotional, and physical development; home environment; home educational practices; school and classroom environment; classroom curriculum; and teacher qualifications. The nutrition topics in the studies pertain to WIC and USDA food assistance program participation, infant feeding practices, children's household food security, and children's height and weight. The three ECLS cohorts are the following: (1) Birth cohort of the ECLS-B is a sample of children born in 2001 and followed from birth through kindergarten entry; (2) kindergarten class of 1998–1999 cohort is a sample of children followed from kindergarten through the eighth grade; (3) kindergarten class of 2010–2011 cohort will follow a sample of children from kindergarten through the fifth grade.

*Current Population Survey (CPS) Food Security Supplement (FSS)*[59]: The CPS is a monthly labor force survey of about 50,000 households conducted by the Census Bureau for the DOL/BLS. In December of each year, after completing the labor force interview, the sampled households (nationally representative) also respond to the FSS module consisting of food security questions and questions about food spending and the use of federal and community food assistance programs. The CPS-FSS is the source of national- and state-level statistics on food insecurity used in USDA/ERS's annual reports on household food insecurity.

*WIC Program*[60]: WIC is administered by USDA FNS. The program is designed to safeguard the health of low-income pregnant, postpartum, and breastfeeding women, infants, and children up to age 5 years. WIC provides nutritious foods to supplement diets, information on healthy eating including breastfeeding promotion and support, and referrals to health care.

## KNOWLEDGE, ATTITUDES, AND BEHAVIOR ASSESSMENTS

Consumer knowledge, attitudes, and behavior are among the factors that shape diet quality and health outcomes. DHHS, USDA, and other federal partners collect and monitor information on the food and health habits, attitudes, and behaviors of the U.S. consumers. The next section provides updated information on continuing programs and information about several new initiatives.

*American Time Use Survey (ATUS) Eating and Health (EH) Module of the CPS*[61]: Time-use surveys measure the amount of time people spend doing everyday activities, such as work, child care, housework, watching television, eating and drinking, volunteering, and socializing. The Census Bureau has conducted time-use surveys for the DOL/BLS since 2003. The Eating and Health (EH) Module of the ATUS, co-funded by USDA/ERS and the NIH, National Cancer Institute (NCI), collects additional data to analyze relationships among time-use patterns and eating patterns, nutrition, and obesity; food and nutrition assistance programs; and grocery shopping and meal preparation. Yearly EH Module results for the time period 2006–2008 are available on the Internet.

*Behavioral Risk Factor Surveillance System (BRFSS)*[62]: BRFSS, the world's largest ongoing health survey system, has tracked health conditions and risk behaviors in the United States annually since 1984. Currently, BRFSS data are collected in all 50 states, the District of Columbia, Puerto Rico, the U.S. Virgin Islands, and Guam. BRFSS uses a cross-sectional, telephone interview mode design. Surveys are conducted by state health departments with technical and methodological assistance provided by the CDC. Every year, states conduct monthly telephone surveillance using a standardized questionnaire to determine the distribution of risk behaviors and health practices among noninstitutionalized adults 18 years or older. In 2010, 451,075 adults surveyed as part of BRFSS.

The states forward their survey responses to the CDC; monthly data are aggregated for each state. The data are returned to the states and subsequently published on the BRFSS website. The BRFSS questionnaire consists of core questions and optional modules. All states administer the core questions. State-specific BMI results have been reported widely based on self-reported height and weight data collected in the core component of BRFSS. The optional modules are standardized questions that are supported by CDC that cover additional health topics or more detailed questions on core health topics. States select the optional modules they want to use based on the particular needs of their state.

*Consumer Expenditure Survey (CES)*[63]: This DOL/BLS survey provides information on the buying habits of American consumers, including data on their expenditures, income, and consumer unit (families and single consumers) characteristics. Since 1960, USDA has used CES data to produce annual reports with estimates of expenditures on children from birth through age 17. Food expenditures are one of the major budgetary components included in the CES.

*FDA/CFSAN Food Safety Surveys (FSSs)*[64]: FDA conducted RDD telephone surveys in 2006 and 2010 with English- or Spanish-speaking adults 18 years and older in the 50 states and the District of Columbia to track consumer knowledge, behavior, and perceptions on several food-safety-related topics.

*Health and Diet Surveys (HDS)*[65]: Since 1982, FDA/CFSAN has conducted telephone surveys of noninstitutionalized adults 18 and older residing in the 50 states and the District of Columbia to assess self-reported behaviors, knowledge, attitudes and beliefs about health and diet. A *Dietary Guidelines* Supplement was fielded in 2004 and 2005; the most recent survey was conducted in 2008.

*Infant Feeding Practices Survey (IFPS)*[66]: FDA conducted the first IFPS in 1993–1994. FDA collaborated with CDC and others to support IFPS II, 2004–2005, a longitudinal study designed to examine infant feeding practices and diets of women from their third trimester to 12 months postpartum. Infant feeding behaviors included breastfeeding patterns, formula feeding, and solid food intake. Monthly mail questionnaires were sent to a sample drawn from a national mail panel, with an over sampling of African-American and Hispanic women.

*NHANES 2005–2010 Flexible Consumer Behavior Module*[67]: ERS established the Consumer Data and Information Program (CDIP) in 2005 as a means of collecting data to understand how consumer behavior and market dynamics shape diet quality and health outcomes. As part of the CDIP initiative, ERS partnered with CDC/NCHS to gather and track information on changing food habits, attitudes, and dietary behaviors of the U.S. consumers through a consumer behavior module in the NHANES. The ERS-sponsored module known as the Flexible Consumer Behavior Survey (FCBS) was added to the 2007–2008 NHANES; a second round of FCBS was fielded in the 2009–2010 NHANES.

The FCBS modules will help shed light on diet–health connections, especially in relation to nutrition assistance and education programs, food security monitoring, and obesity prevention.

*Pregnancy Risk Assessment Monitoring System (PRAMS)*[68]: PRAMS is a surveillance project of the CDC and state health departments. Since 1987, state-specific, population-based data on maternal attitudes and experiences before, during, and shortly after pregnancy have been collected. The goal of the project is to improve the health of mothers and infants by reducing adverse outcomes such as low birth weight, infant mortality and morbidity, and maternal morbidity. PRAMS provides state-specific data for planning and assessing health programs and for describing maternal experiences that may contribute to maternal and infant health. The PRAMS sample consists of women who have had a recent live birth and is drawn from the state's birth certificate file. Each participating state samples between 1300 and 3400 women per year. Women from some population subgroups are sampled at a higher rate to ensure adequate data are available in smaller but higher risk populations. Data collection procedures and instruments are standardized to allow comparisons between states. The PRAMS questionnaire has two parts: Core questions are asked by all states. The core portion of the questionnaire includes questions about the attitudes and feelings about the most recent pregnancy, content and source of prenatal care, maternal alcohol and tobacco consumption, physical abuse before and during pregnancy, pregnancy-related morbidity, infant health care, contraceptive use, and mother's knowledge of pregnancy-related health issues, such as adverse effects of tobacco and alcohol, benefits of folic acid, and risks of HIV. The remaining questions on the questionnaire are chosen from a pretested list of standard questions developed by CDC or developed by states on their own. As a result, each state's PRAMS questionnaire is unique.

*Youth Risk Behavior Surveillance System (YRBSS)*[69,70]: CDC developed the YRBSS program in 1990 to monitor priority youth risk behaviors that contribute to the leading causes of death, disability, and social problems among U.S. youth. The behaviors include those that contribute to unintentional injuries and violence, tobacco use, alcohol and other drug use, sexual risk behaviors, unhealthy dietary behaviors, and physical inactivity. YRBSS also monitors the prevalence of obesity and asthma. YRBSS has reported national, state, and local estimates of body mass index (BMI) calculated from self-reported height and weight data since 1999. National-, state-, territorial-, tribal-, and local school–based YRBS surveys of representative samples of students in grades 9 through 12 are conducted every 2 years, usually during the spring semester. The national survey, conducted by CDC, provides data representative of 9th through 12th grade students in public and private schools in the United States. The state, territorial, tribal, and local surveys, conducted by departments of health and education, provide data representative of public high school students in each jurisdiction. YRBSS data are used to determine the prevalence of health risk behaviors, monitor progress toward achieving *Healthy People* objectives and other health and nutrition program indicators, and provide comparable data to compare national, state, territorial, tribal, and local data.

## FOOD AND DIETARY SUPPLEMENT PRODUCT COMPOSITION DATA AND DATABASES

Interest in food composition and dietary supplement product databases and research has fostered new research and significant database development and exchange. Food and dietary supplement composition data are used to report national health and nutrition survey results, examine the association of diet and health, and assess the impact of food fortification policy and monitoring programs. In the United States, the annual *National Nutrient Databank Conference* meetings have provided an active forum for scientists, nutrient database developers, and users to engage with one another, share information, and identify future research and database priorities.[71]

The *International Network of Food Data Systems (INFOODS)* established in 1984 has helped stimulate and coordinate the availability of high-quality food composition data among international partners.[72] The Food and Agriculture Organization has coordinated INFOODS activities since 1999, providing leadership and an administrative framework to support the development of standards and guidelines for the collection, compilation, and reporting of food component data. INFOODS established and coordinates a global network of regional food composition data centers and serves as the generator and repository of special international databases.[73]

Since 1997, federal food and dietary supplement product database activities have been coordinated through the *National Food and Nutrient Analysis Program (NFNAP)* initiative.[74] NFNAP is directed by the USDA/ARS Nutrient Data Laboratory (NDL) in collaboration with NIH/NCI and other supporting NIH offices and institutes and other agencies. The five specific aims of NFNAP are to (1) establish a monitoring program for key foods and critical nutrients (key foods are frequently consumed foods and ingredients, which contributed, collectively, more than 75% of the intake of any specific nutrient for the U.S. population), (2) conduct comprehensive analyses of selected key foods, (3) develop databases for high-priority foods consumed by U.S. ethnic subpopulations, (4) develop databases for new bioactive components, and (5) develop a validated database for ingredients in dietary supplements. For each specific aim, the process includes the identification of foods for analysis, the development of unique statistically based sampling plans, and the application of validated analytical chemistry. The primary outcome of the Program is to develop comprehensive nutrient composition databases having unprecedented analytical quality.

Dietary supplements database activities have developed from the NFNAP initiative. The NIH *National Library of Medicine Dietary Supplements Labels Database*[75] contains information on more than 6000 brands of dietary supplement products. Another initiative, *the Dietary Supplements Ingredients Database (DSID)*,[75] provides analytical data on dietary supplement product ingredients. The DSID is led by the USDA/ARS NDL in collaboration with the NIH Office of Dietary Supplements (ODS) and other federal agencies. The goals of the DSID project are to develop reliable baseline estimates of nutrients and other bioactive components in dietary supplement products, compare analyzed levels of ingredients to labeled values, support efforts to improve total dietary intake assessments in research and release, and maintain a publicly available dietary supplement database. The first data release, DSID-1, provides information on chemically analyzed levels of nutrients found in a nationally representative set of adult multivitamin/mineral (MVM) products used in the United States.[76] The release of DSID-2, a database containing updated analytical data on adult's and children's MVM products, is planned in 2012.

*FDA/CFSAN Food Label and Package Survey (FLAPS)*[77]: The FLAPS, an FDA study of processed and packaged food labels in the U.S. food supply, provides comprehensive label information on current U.S. food products. The 2006–2007 FLAPS is the 13th survey to be conducted since the project began in 1976–1978.

*Food and Nutrient Database System for Dietary Studies (FNDDS)*[78]: The FNDDS is a multi-file database system. FNDDS includes a database of foods, nutrient values, gram weights for typical food portions, and extensive file documentation. The foods data are used to analyze dietary recall data from WWEIA, the dietary intake component of NHANES. The underlying food composition data are from the USDA National Nutrient Database for Standard Reference (NNDSR).

*Food Patterns Equivalents Database (FPED)*[79]: The FPED is the future successor to the MyPyramid Equivalents Database (MPED).The FPED translates the amounts of food eaten in WWEIA into numbers of food groupings that are related to the USDA Food Patterns found in the *Dietary Guidelines for Americans* (2010). Future postings on the USDA/ARS website will provide updates on the FPED.

*NNDSR*[80]: NNDSR (abbreviated SR in reports) is the major source of food composition data in the United States. Over the years, the SR series has been the foundation for most of the food composition databases developed by the public and private sectors. The SR series is updated as new information becomes available. SR Release 24 or "SR24" was released in September 2011 and contains data on 7906 food items and up to 146 food components. The USDA/NDL also produces special food composition data files. An updated USDA database containing data on five subclasses of flavonoids measured in 500 food items was released in 2011.[81]

## FOOD-SUPPLY DETERMINATIONS

The U.S. food supply today can be characterized as being both plentiful and diverse. Two recent trends in our food supply with respect to food production and marketing are noteworthy. The United States has been a net exporter of agricultural products since 1959. This trend could soon be reversed if current trends in important food continue.[82] Increased consumer demand is driving the growth of the imported foods market in the United States. Currently, imported foods account for approximately 11% of the food consumed in the United States.[83] The diverse and increasingly global U.S. food supply has an impact on efforts to monitor the safety of the U.S. food supply, determine representative food composition values of foods consumed, and ultimately, characterize the food consumption patterns of the U.S. population.

In addition to the growing imported food component of the food supply, there is a movement in the United States to adopt more ecological food production systems and to conserve natural resources and improve ecological balance.[84] One example in the United States is the expanding market for organic foods. Sales of organic products have increased at a higher rate compared to the general food supply and now account for $24.8 billion in sales (OTC).[85] The USDA/AMS National Organic Program was created to facilitate trade and ensure the integrity of organic foods, establish organic foods standards, and enforce compliance with the Organic Food Production Act of 1990.[86,87] The implications for programs that track chemical exposures in foods, report nutrient intakes, and study consumer purchasing behavior and attitudes are great.

*AC Nielsen ScanTrack and National Consumer Panel (Formerly Homescan) Data*[88]: USDA/ERS, FNS, and CNPP purchase monthly and annual proprietary sales data from the AC Nielsen Company. ScanTrack scanner data include records of weekly dollar sales and units sold for all Universal Product Code (UPC) transactions at participating grocery stores. ScanTrack does not track sales of foods random-weight items without UPC codes (e.g., some fresh fruits and vegetables, baked goods, and deli items), foods obtained from restaurants or food outlets, or foods sold at discount and warehouse centers. The National Consumer Panel (NCP) panel began in 1989. The 2008 NCP panel included more than 60,000 U.S. households; households reported all UPC and random-weight transactions from all outlet channels, including grocery, drug, mass-merchandise, club, supercenter, and convenience stores. USDA/CNPP created a food price dataset using NCP data to evaluate the nutritional adequacy of the Thrifty Food Plan.

*Fisheries of the U.S. Survey*[89]: The National Marine Fisheries Service (NMFS) calculation of per capita consumption is based on a "disappearance" model. The total U.S. supply of imports and domestic landings is converted to edible weight and decreases in supply such as exports are subtracted out. The remaining total is divided by a population value to estimate per capita consumption. Data on per capita edible weight (pounds) have been reported annually since 1910.

*Food Availability (per capita) Data System*[90]: This USDA/ERS data system includes three distinct but related data series on food and nutrient availability for consumption: (1) The food availability data series that reports estimates of per capita availability for hundreds of food commodities are useful for time-series data presentations; (2) loss-adjusted food availability, used to obtain estimates of per capita availability of daily calories and daily food patterns equivalents (formerly MyPyramid Equivalents), also provides per capita availability estimates after adjusting for losses); and (3) nutrient availability data series are useful to obtain estimates of calories and 27 nutrients and dietary components available per capita per day.

*National Household Food Acquisition and Purchase Survey (FoodAPS)*[91]: FoodAPS, also called the National Food Study, is cosponsored by USDA's ERS and FNS. The objectives of the study are to determine if households have access to healthy foods at affordable prices. A nationally representative sample of approximately 5000 low- and higher-income households will be selected. Information about foods people obtain during a 1-week period will be collected. Additionally, information about food expenditures and food sources, distance traveled to obtain food, and access to healthy food will be ascertained. Participating households will receive a scanner to scan barcodes on foods brought into their home. Booklets will be provided to attach receipts and record all the places where food was obtained. A field test was conducted in early 2011. Updated information is posted on The National Food Study website.

## NUTRITION MONITORING RESOURCES FOR NUTRITION SURVEILLANCE, RESEARCH, PUBLIC HEALTH PRACTICE, AND EDUCATION

In addition to national survey data sources and technical files, numerous nutrition and health surveillance activities, technical reports, and resources for public health practice, research, and education are available. The next section includes a list of resources grouped by major topic area (Table 29.2) and brief descriptions of their relevance to national nutrition monitoring.

**TABLE 29.2**

**Nutrition Monitoring Resources for Nutrition Surveillance, Research, Public Health Practice, and Education**

| Agency | Name (References) |
| --- | --- |
| Surveillance tools and reports | |
| DHHS/CDC | Breastfeeding Report Card |
| DHHS/CDC | Interactive Database Systems |
| DHHS/CDC | National Reports on Human Exposure to Environmental Chemicals |
| DHHS/CDC | Norovirus outbreak surveillance network (CaliciNet) |
| DHHS/CDC | Water (drinking and recreational) data and statistics |
| DHHS/CDC, FDA; USDA/FSIS | Foodborne Diseases Active Surveillance Network (FoodNet) |
| USDA/ARS, ERS | FICRD |
| USDA/ERS | Food Desert Locator |
| USDA/ERS | Your Food Environment Atlas |
| USDA/FNS | SNAP data system |
| USDA/NIFA | KYF |
| Resources for nutrition research and public health practice | |
| DHHS/CDC | CDC growth charts |
| DHHS/CDC | Physical activity resources for health professionals |
| DHHS/CDC | NHANES web tutorials |
| DHHS/NIH | HNRIM |
| DHHS/NIH | Dietary supplement research and literature: CARDS and PubMed® subset |
| DHHS/ODPHP | Health communication tools |
| NAS/IOM | DRIs reports and updates |
| DHHS/NIH | Resources for diet and health research |
| USDA/CNPP | USDA NEL |
| Partnership | Health data tools and statistics |
| Nutrition education resources | |
| DHHS/CDC | Nutrition topics for consumers |
| DHHS/NIH | DHHS and USDA nutrition education materials for general and clinical populations |
| DHHS/ODPHP | Health.gov website |
| NIH/NIH | Dietary supplements information for consumers and health professionals |
| USDA/CNPP | ChooseMyPlate.gov website |
| USDA/NAL | Food and nutrition resources for consumers: Nutrition.gov website |

## SURVEILLANCE TOOLS AND REPORTS

*CDC Breastfeeding Report Card*[92]: Data collection for this annual reporting system began in 2007. The Report Card combines state-specific information on breastfeeding practices in individual states. The system is used to track state and national trends in breastfeeding initiation, duration, as well as progress in achieving *Healthy People 2020* breast-feeding goals.

*CDC Interactive Database Systems*[93]: CDC maintains a list of interactive database systems that provide continuous data and reports on major public health topics.

*CDC National Reports on Human Exposure to Environmental Chemicals*[94]: CDC produces comprehensive assessments of environmental chemical exposure in the U.S. population. CDC has measured 219 chemicals in blood or urine using NHANES specimens for children and adults. The first report was released in 1999, and the fourth report was produced in 2009; updated tables were released in 2011.

*Norovirus Outbreak Surveillance Network (CaliciNet)*[95]: Caliciviruses, which include the noroviruses, are responsible for the majority of foodborne outbreaks of viral gastroenteritis in the United States. CDC developed and implemented this electronic surveillance system in collaboration with state and local public health laboratories to improve national norovirus surveillance. CaliciNet compares norovirus gene sequences to expedite the identification of common food sources during outbreaks and to identify emerging norovirus strains. Currently, 17 states are certified for participation in the Network.

*CDC Drinking Water Information*[96]: The CDC website features a compilation of information on numerous drinking water topics including the nutritional aspects related to water consumption and health, water fluoridation, and health and safety issues related to the U.S. drinking water supply.

*CDC Foodborne Diseases Active Surveillance Network (FoodNet)*[97]: This is a collaborative program established in 1995 with CDC, 10 state health departments, USDA/FSIS, and FDA. The objectives of the program are to determine the burden of foodborne illness in the United States, monitor trends in the burden of specific foodborne illness overtime, identify foods and settings that contribute to foodborne illnesses, and disseminate information to improve public health practice and prevent foodborne illness.

*USDA Food Intakes Converted to Retail Commodities Databases (FICRCD)*[98]: The databases that were developed jointly by USDA/ARS and ERS convert food intakes reported in national dietary intake surveys to retail commodity-level groupings. Foods reported in the surveys are converted into 65 retail-level commodities. The commodities were regrouped into eight major food categories: dairy products; fats and oils; fruits; grains; meat, poultry, fish, and eggs; nuts; caloric sweeteners; and vegetables, dry beans, and

legumes. Databases were developed for CSFII 1994–1996 and 1998, NHANES 1999–2000, and NHANES–WWEIA 2001–2002.

*USDA/ERS Food Desert Locator*[99]: Healthy Food Financing Initiative (HFFI), a partnership between the U.S. Treasury Department, DHHS and USDA, and a working group composed of agency representatives defined the term "food desert" to mean a low-income census tract where a substantial number or share of residents has low access to a supermarket or a large grocery store. The Food Desert Locator tool was developed as a means of creating maps showing food-desert census tracts, viewing statistics on selected population characteristics in food-desert census tracts, and accessing census-level information about food-desert areas.

*USDA/ERS Food Environment Atlas*[100]: The Atlas provides statistics on food choices, health and well-being, and community characteristics for all communities in the United States. The smallest geographic level of data in the Atlas is the county.

*USDA/ERS Supplemental Nutrition Assistance Program (SNAP) Data System*[101]: The USDA/ERS Food Economics Division studies and evaluates SNAP and other USDA nutrition programs. USDA/FNS information is used for the SNAP Data System. The data system provides time-series data on state- and county-level estimates of SNAP participation and benefit levels, combined with the area estimates of total population and the number of persons in poverty.

*USDA/NIFA Know Your Farmer, Know Your Food (KYF) Compass*[102]: This USDA/NIFA electronic resource provides information about USDA-supported projects and programs related to local and regional food systems. An interactive KYF map feature shows the location and focus of many USDA-supported local and regional food projects.

## RESOURCES FOR RESEARCH AND PUBLIC HEALTH PRACTICE

*CDC Growth Charts*[103]: CDC maintains an information site on the development, clinical use, and interpretation of CDC and World Health Organization growth chart data for infants and children birth to 20 years.

*CDC Physical Activity Resources for Health Professionals*[104]: These are resources and tools for health departments, educators, community coalitions, public health program planners, health-care planners, and others who are engaged in physical activity program planning.

*DHHS Office of Disease Prevention and Health Promotion (ODPHP) Health Communications Resources*[105]: Health communication tools, research and reports, and resources for public health and health communication professionals are available.

*NIH/DRNC Human Nutrition Research and Information Management (HNRIM)*[106]: The HNRIM is a searchable database of nutrition research and research training activities supported by the federal government. HNRIM is maintained by the NIH Division of Nutrition Research Coordination (DNRC). HNRIM data are useful to examine trends in nutrition research funding, institutions and investigators involved in nutrition research, and topic areas of federal agency support. Annual updates are completed by the DNRC with information provided by participating federal agencies.

*Computer Access to Research on Dietary Supplements (CARDS) Database and PubMed® Bibliographic Retrieval Tools on Dietary Supplements*[107,108]: CARDS is a database of federally funded research on dietary supplement products. The database dates from 1988 and includes projects funded by USDA, DOD, and NIH. Projects funded by other federal agencies will be added to CARDS as they become available.

Bibliographic retrieval of citations and abstracts from the vast dietary supplement literature can be accomplished more efficiently by using a new PubMed® subset, "Dietary Supplements." The subset was created by the ODS and the National Library of Medicine (NLM) to succeed the International Bibliographic Information on Dietary Supplements (IBIDS) database.

*NIH/NCI Diet and Health Assessment and Resources*[109]: The NCI Division of Cancer Control and Population Sciences conducts and supports a comprehensive research program in genetic, epidemiologic, behavioral, social, and surveillance research. Among the NCI resources are dietary assessment tools such as the Diet History Questionnaire, the NCI Automated Self-Administered 24-Hour Dietary Recall System (ASA24™), resources for analyzing national health survey datasets on dietary intake and physical activity, questionnaire design resources, health research collaborations, and scientific publications.

*NHANES Web Tutorials*[110]: CDC/NCHS and others collaborated to develop a series of web-based tutorials. Tutorials are available for periodic and continuous NHANES. The tutorial modules provide descriptive information about surveys, instructions for accessing and reviewing data, recommended statistical analysis methods, and statistical analysis programs. A special tutorial section is devoted to dietary data analysis, featuring information provided by NIH/NCI and USDA/ARS researchers.

*USDA Nutrition Evidence Library (NEL)*[111]: The USDA NEL was created to inform federal nutrition policies and programs and to provide an accessible resource on food and nutrition research to the broader health and nutrition community. NEL provides a mechanism to conduct systematic reviews on nutrition topics using a consistent and objective methodology. The scientific evidence is reviewed, synthesized, and graded by trained abstractors. The NEL website provides a detailed evidence portfolio for each of the 2010 Dietary Guidelines Advisory Committee (DGAC) systematic reviews.

*Comprehensive Health Data Tools and Statistics Resource List*[112]: A collaborative effort undertaken by the U.S. government agencies, public health organizations, and health sciences libraries led to the development of a timely, comprehensive website containing links to major public health resources that are available on the Internet.

## NUTRITION EDUCATION

Title III of the National Nutrition Monitoring and Related Research Act of 1990 (PL 101–445) mandates that all dietary guidance materials that are developed by federal agencies for the general population or identified subpopulations undergo joint review by DHHS and USDA (Act REF). The DHHS Nutrition Policy Board Committee on Dietary Guidance and the USDA Dietary Guidance Working Group work together to complete the review process.[113]

*CDC Nutrition Topics for Consumers and Public Health Practice*[114]: CDC compiled timely information on federal and state nutrition and health programs. Program planning, professional training and development, and reports and recommendations for public health professionals are available.

*USDA/Center for Nutrition Policy Promotion (CNPP) MyPlate*[115]: Information and education materials and interactive web tools developed by CNPP to disseminate the *Dietary Guidelines for Americans* (2010).

*USDA/National Agricultural Library (NAL) Nutrition. gov*[116]: The USDA NAL maintains a website listing government resources on food and nutrition for consumers.

*DHHS/NIH*[117]: The NIH/DNRC compiles nutrition education resources for child and adult target groups. Most of the materials were developed by federal agencies. Materials that are intended for the general population have been reviewed for consistency with the *Dietary Guidelines for Americans*.

*NIH/ODS Dietary Supplements Information for Consumers and Health Professionals*[118]: The NIH/ODS website features timely information on dietary supplement products. Information is provided on dietary supplement research, product ingredients and labeling, and health and safety related to dietary supplement product use. The information materials target general consumer and health professional audiences.

# USES OF NATIONAL NUTRITION MONITORING DATA IN FEDERAL NUTRITION POLICIES AND PROGRAMS

Nutrition monitoring data are used to formulate evidence-based federal nutrition and public health policies and programs and to evaluate their impact on population health and nutritional status. This section provides information about major U.S. nutrition and public health programs and policy initiatives.

## FEDERAL DIETARY AND PHYSICAL ACTIVITY GUIDELINES

The *Dietary Guidelines for Americans* are the federal government's evidence-informed nutritional guidance.[119]

The recommendations are used to promote health and to reduce risk for major chronic diseases through diet and physical activity. By law, the *Dietary Guidelines for Americans* are reviewed, updated if necessary, and published every 5 years.[120] USDA and DHHS jointly produce each edition of the *Dietary Guidelines*. The *Dietary Guidelines for Americans (2010)* is based on the *Report of the DGAC on the Dietary Guidelines for Americans* (2010) and consideration of federal agency and public comments.[119] Traditionally the *Dietary Guidelines for Americans* have been intended for healthy Americans ages 2 years and older. The 2010 *Dietary Guidelines* reflect rising concerns about the health of the U.S. population with their focus on balancing calories with physical activity. The *Dietary Guidelines* also encourage Americans to consume vegetables, fruits, whole grains, fat-free and low-fat dairy products, and seafood and less sodium, saturated and *trans* fats, added sugars, and refined grains.[119] Consumer-friendly dietary guidance messages and consumer education materials, including ChooseMyPlate.gov and Health.gov, will be used to disseminate the Dietary Guidelines recommendations to the general public.[115,121]

## 2008 DHHS Physical Activity Guidelines

The DHHS *2008 Physical Activity Guidelines for Americans* provides science-based guidance to help Americans aged 6 and older improve their health through appropriate physical activity.[122] The *Physical Activity Guidelines* complement the *Dietary Guidelines for Americans* as a means of promoting good health and reducing the risk of chronic diseases. The *Physical Activity Guidelines for Americans* describe the major research findings on the health benefits of physical activity and provide guidelines for children and adolescents, adults, and selected subpopulation groups. The data on recent trends in physical activity in the United States were based on national nutrition monitoring survey data, principally BRFSS, NHANES, NHIS, and YRBSS.[122] Plans are under way to develop a plan to conduct full reviews of the physical activity literature every 10 years. In the interim, a midcourse review of the Guidelines has been proposed as a means of identifying strategies that have been shown to be effective in increasing levels of physical activity levels of children, youth, and young adults. The midcourse review will also identify new evidence that has emerged since the 2008 Guidelines were published and support ongoing efforts to strengthen the communication component of the federal physical activity initiative.

## National Health Agenda: Healthy People 2020

*Healthy People 2020* is the fifth in a series of national health initiatives and provides a science-based, 10-year national health agenda to improve the health of the U.S. population.[123,124] Broad input was solicited from groups and individuals, including consumers, during the planning process. Webinar meetings, nationwide public meetings, and a public online comment website were used to gather input for the initiative. A Federal Interagency Workgroup coordinated the review of the comments and made final

recommendations for the objectives. A reliable data source, baseline measures, and targets for specific improvements to be achieved by 2020 were specified for each objective. As with previous *Healthy People* initiatives, nutrition monitoring survey and surveillance program data products will be used extensively to monitor national progress toward efforts to achieve a healthier nation. Twenty-two Nutrition and Weight Status objectives are included in *Healthy People 2020*. The *Healthy People 2020* website includes program planning tools, webinar announcements, and information updates to keep the public health community engaged.[123,124]

## ASSESSING THE HEALTH AND NUTRITIONAL STATUS OF THE U.S. POPULATION

At the national level, the continuous NHANES remains the cornerstone of national nutrition monitoring efforts in terms of providing the most comprehensive national data on body weight and health status, food and nutrient intakes, health conditions, and nutritional biomarkers.[32] Additionally, NHIS, CPS-FSS, BRFSS, NIS, surveillance programs, and food and nutrition program evaluation studies are all integral to describing population health and nutritional status. In recent years, the use of automated data collection and processing systems has expedited survey data releases, thus improving the timeliness and the efficiency of data collection, processing, and reporting. A majority of national survey data files, documentation, and reports are available on the Internet.

*Assessing the Food Security Status of Children and Adults in the United States*: USDA-sponsored CPS-FSS data collection and reporting activities have been conducted annually since 1995 to monitor domestic food insecurity.[59] USDA also engages in research to evaluate the FSS questionnaires and food insecurity terminology and methodology. In 2006, an independent expert panel was convened by the CNSTAT of the National Academies at USDA's request to consider the use of the word "hunger" in connection with food insecurity. The panel concluded that in official statistics, resource-constrained hunger (i.e., physiological hunger resulting from food insecurity) "...should refer to a potential consequence of food insecurity that, because of prolonged, involuntary lack of food, results in discomfort, illness, weakness, or pain that goes beyond the usual uneasy sensation."[125] The new food insecurity terminology was adopted after the report was released. The methods used to assess households' food security did not change, however. Therefore, the food security statistics for 2005 and later years are directly comparable with those for earlier years for the corresponding categories. Food security is also assessed in NHANES and in the 1998–1999 and 2001 ECLS.

## PARTNERSHIPS AND COLLABORATIONS

Collaborative and partnership initiatives have expanded the scope and impact of many traditionally federal initiatives by engaging diverse partners from nongovernment sectors. Several examples of collaborative efforts that are designed to improve nutritional and health status include the following:

- First Lady Michelle Obama's *Let's Move* campaign, a nationwide campaign, was launched in 2010 to address the challenge of childhood obesity within a generation.[126]
- The *National Collaborative on Childhood Obesity Research* (NCCOR) was launched in 2009. The CDC, the NIH, the USDA, and the Robert Wood Johnson Foundation (RWJF) are working to identify intervention needs, improve child obesity surveillance, improve research and evaluation methodologies, and provide national leadership to implement evidence-based practice and policy. NCCOR also works with many non-health partners to develop sustainable environmental design and food systems strategies to reach high-risk populations and communities.[127]
- USDA/CNPP *Nutrition Communicators Network* and *Community Partners* Initiatives: The Nutrition Communicators Network and the Community Partners initiatives were organized by CNPP to engage national companies and organizations (Network) and community dietitians, educators, doctors, and others (Partners) to disseminate the *Dietary Guidelines for Americans* and promote nutrition.[128]
- NIH/National Institute of Diabetes and Digestive and Kidney Diseases (NIDDK) *Weight-control Information Network (WIN)*: WIN provides the general public, health professionals, and community partners with evidence-based nutrition education curricula, consumer information, and up-to-date science-based information on weight control, obesity, physical activity, and related nutritional issues.[129]
- NIH *Ways to Enhance Children's Activity and Nutrition (We Can!)*[130]: Four institutes of the NIH: the National Heart, Lung, and Blood Institute (NHLBI), the NIDDK, the Eunice Kennedy Shriver National Institute of Child Health and Human Development (NICHD), and the NCI developed the program. *We Can!* is designed to engage community partners in a national effort to promote healthy weight status for children 8–13 years. The program provides evidence-based tools, and education resources are available for parents, health professionals, and community partners.

## Assessments of Nutrient Adequacy

*Revised Dietary Reference Intakes (DRIs) for Calcium and Vitamin D*: DRIs consist of four nutrient-based reference values that serve as a guide for good nutrition and provide the scientific basis for the development of national nutrition policy and food guidelines in the United States and Canada.[131] In 2009, the IOM convened an ad hoc expert panel to review the 1997 DRI recommendations for calcium and vitamin D.[132] NHANES biomarker and dietary intake estimates were a key component of the IOM panel's review. An expanded, updated, and improved USDA food composition database of vitamin D values for U.S. foods was used to produce dietary vitamin D intake estimates for the U.S. population.[133-135] NHANES serum 25-hydroxyvitamin D [25(OH)D] data were used to assess vitamin D status of the U.S. children and adults. The panel's final report, released in 2011, included estimated average requirements, recommended dietary allowances, and tolerable upper intake levels for calcium and vitamin D.[136]

## Regulatory and Policy Initiatives

Significant legislative and policy activities in recent years lead to the passage of health reform legislation, child nutrition program and food safety regulations, and proposals for food and menu labeling and initiatives to reduce dietary sodium intakes of the U.S. population and reduce the sodium content of the U.S. food supply.

*Health Reform Legislation*: The *Patient Protection and Affordable Care Act* became law on March 23, 2010.[137] The legislation aims to improve access to health care, control health-care costs, expand access to preventive health-care services, and reduce health-care fraud. The Act established a National Prevention Council chaired by the U.S. Surgeon General and a Prevention and Public Health Fund to support community-level efforts such as Communities Putting Prevention to Work. Section 4205 of the Act requires restaurants and similar retail food establishments with 20 or more locations to list calorie content information for standard menu items on restaurant menus and menu boards. The Act also requires vending machine operators who own or operate 20 or more vending machines to disclose calorie content for certain items.

*Healthy Hunger-Free Kids Act of 2010*[138]: This legislation authorizes funding and sets policy for USDA's core child nutrition programs—the NLSP, the SBP, and the WIC; the Summer Food Service Program, and the CACFP. The Act allows USDA to make major reforms to the programs and thus improve child nutritional status.[139]

*Food Front-of-Package Labeling*: A wide variety of nutrition rating systems are currently used by food manufacturers. Congress directed the CDC to undertake a study with the IOM. Accordingly, a two-phase effort was undertaken by the CDC with support from FDA and USDA/CNPP. The first phase, completed in 2010, provided an in-depth analysis of the current nutrition rating systems and the scientific research that underlies them.[140] The second phase of the project, completed in 2011, examined consumer use and understanding of front-of-package label systems.[141] Both reports will inform future food labeling regulatory activities and policies.

*Food Safety Modernization Act*[142]: The legislation is designed to prevent outbreaks of foodborne illness by strengthening collaborations between federal, state, local, territorial, tribal, and foreign food safety agencies. Among the provisions, FDA will have a well-delineated regulatory framework and mandatory recall authority for all food products.[143]

*National Salt Reduction Initiative (NSRI)*[144]: A voluntary framework and partnership was launched in 2008 to engage federal, state, and local health groups and commercial food producers in a joint effort with two overarching goals. The first goal is to reduce the U.S. population sodium intakes by 20% within 5 years and, second, to reduce the sodium content in the U.S. food supply by 25% in 5 years. The partnership is committed to assessing population sodium intakes with dietary intake and biomarker data, maintaining a comprehensive food composition database to track sodium reduction in the food supply, and establishing voluntary sodium-reduction targets for packaged and restaurant foods. To date, more than two dozen companies have committed to the Initiative.[144]

## CHALLENGES AND FUTURE NEEDS FACING THE U.S. NATIONAL NUTRITION MONITORING SYSTEM

The U.S. NNMS has continued to evolve in the decade following the expiration of the NMRRP Act in 2002, thus giving pause for thought. Often, when a legislative mandate ends, activities and interest in a topic cease. One could surmise that several factors have contributed to the continued growth of the system. First, there has always been a core group of committed leaders to advocate for nutrition research, food and nutrition assistance programs, and public health, thus providing a strong support and a steady vision for nutrition monitoring. In recent years, new alliances have formed, bringing diverse groups with shared vision and purpose. Whereas in years past, federal, state, and local governments were the major drivers for change, today federal, state, and nonfederal nutrition and public health partners are working together to solve problems, address needs, and pool their expertise and resources.

Second, ecological and systems approaches are being utilized to address the underlying causes of nutrition and health disparities in the United States. Ecological frameworks utilize expertise from diverse disciplines to solve complex problems related to food supplies, nutritional status, and health. For example, by improving access to healthy food; supporting local food producers; creating safe, pedestrian-friendly communities; and promoting healthy school and worksite designs and food service operations, there is greater opportunity to influence population and individual-level behaviors to improve health and prevent disease.[145,146] Ecological perspectives provide the conceptual framework for the *2008 Physical Activity Guidelines for Americans*, the *Dietary Guidelines for Americans (2010)*, and the *Healthy People 2020*.[119,122,123]

Third, innovations in information technology have broadened the reach of the nutrition monitoring community and changed the way we collect, process, and disseminate nutrition research findings. Communication resources and tools that are widely available on the Internet and interactive tools, mobile applications, and social media have revolutionized the way we communicate and disseminate information to colleagues and stakeholders around the world. From a survey perspective, information technology has improved the efficiency of research and survey data collection and reporting. Automated processes are now used to collect, process, and report research and survey results. Activities that once took years to complete can be accomplished in a matter of weeks or months.

From a research and data user perspective, the information technology innovations have made it possible to access a majority of national nutrition survey data files, methodology manuals, protocols, questionnaires, and data reports free of charge via the Internet. Additionally, researchers have free, online access to the latest journal articles, reports, web tutorials, and statistical analysis resources. Computer programming and data analysis tasks that once required complex computer hardware systems can now be accomplished using mobile and portable devices. Electronic media have largely replaced printed reports and hard copy data files, thus expanding dissemination capability while saving staff time and production costs.

## FUTURE CHALLENGES FOR NATIONAL NUTRITION MONITORING

The last 5 years have been marked by truly remarkable accomplishments in nutrition programs, policy, and research. If the past provides lessons for the future, the nutrition monitoring community must continue to innovate, collaborate, and advocate for nutrition and public health programs, policy, and research. This will be a formidable challenge because government, industry, and academia are constrained by budget shortfalls and limited staff resources to support complex research and program activities. As such, now might be an opportune time to consider adopting a formal, comprehensive national strategy and long-term plan to frame future national nutrition monitoring research and activities. This undertaking could provide a central coordination focus with input from public and private partners, many of whom are already working together. An action plan specifying specific activities, commitments, and plans for future reporting would serve to formalize this process, demonstrate commitment, and provide a long-term vision for the nutrition community. Furthermore, a formal plan would reaffirm the foundation of the U.S. nutrition monitoring system that is evidence-based policy and research. Evidence-based initiatives have advanced the national nutrition monitoring agenda for more than 30 years. Thus, a renewed commitment to the science base for future nutrition monitoring programs and policies is essential to advance the nation's national nutrition monitoring agenda in the twenty-first century.

## ACRONYMS

| Acronym | Name |
|---|---|
| AOA | Administration on Aging |
| ARS | Agricultural Research Service |
| ATUS | American Time Use Survey |
| BLS | Bureau of Labor Statistics |
| BMI | Body mass index |
| BRFSS | Behavioral Risk Factor Surveillance System |
| CACFP | Child and Adult Care Food Program |
| CARDS | Computer Access to Research on Dietary Supplements |
| CDC | Centers for Disease Control and Prevention |
| CES | Consumer Expenditure Survey |
| CNPP | Center for Nutrition Policy Promotion |
| CPS | Current Population Survey |
| CSFII | Continuing Survey of Food Intake by Individuals |
| DHHS | Department of Health and Human Services |
| DNRC | Division of Nutrition Research Coordination |
| DOC | Department of Commerce |
| DoEd | Department of Education |
| DOL | Department of Labor |
| DRI | Dietary Reference Intake |
| DSID | Dietary Supplements Ingredients Database |
| ECLS | Early Childhood Longitudinal Studies |
| ERS | Economic Research Service |
| FDA | Food and Drug Administration |
| FLAPS | Food Label and Package Survey |
| FNDDS | Food and Nutrient Database System for Dietary Studies |
| FNS | Food and Nutrition Service |
| FoodAPS | Food Acquisition and Purchase Survey |
| FSIS | Food Safety Inspection Service |
| FSS | Food Security Supplement |
| HDS | Health and Diet Survey |
| IBIDS | International Bibliographic Information on Dietary Supplements |
| IBNMRR | Interagency Board on Nutrition Monitoring and Related Research |
| IFPS | Infant Feeding Practices Survey |
| IOM | Institute of Medicine |
| LSRO | Life Sciences Research Office |
| mPINC | Maternity and Nutrition Practices in Infant Care |
| NAS | National Academy of Sciences |
| NCHS | National Center for Health Statistics |
| NCI | National Cancer Institute |
| NFNAP | National Food and Nutrient Analysis Program |
| NHANES | National Health and Nutrition Examination Survey |
| NHIS | National Health Interview Survey |
| NIFA | National Institute of Food and Agriculture |
| NIH | National Institutes of Health |
| NIS | National Immunization Survey |
| NLM | National Library of Medicine |
| NNDB | National Nutrient Databank |
| NNDSR | National Nutrient Database for Standard Reference |
| NNMRRP | National Nutrition Monitoring and Related Research Program |
| NSCH | National Survey of Children's Health |
| NSFG | National Survey of Family Growth |
| OAA | Older Americans Act |
| ODPHP | Office of Disease Prevention and Health Promotion |
| ODS | Office of Dietary Supplements |
| PC | Participant Characteristics |
| PedNSS | Pediatric Nutrition Surveillance System |
| PNSS | Pregnancy Nutrition Surveillance System |
| PRAMS | Pregnancy Risk Assessment Monitoring System |
| SHPPS | School Health Policies and Practices Study |
| SLAITS | State and Local Area Integrated Telephone Survey |
| SNDA | School Nutrition and Dietary Assessment Surveys |
| TDS | Total Diet Study |
| USDA | U.S. Department of Agriculture |
| WIC | Special Supplemental Nutrition Program for Women, Infants, and Children |
| WWEIA | What We Eat in America |
| YRBSS | Youth Risk Behavior Surveillance System |

## DISCLAIMER STATEMENT REQUESTED BY NIH ETHICS OFFICE

Dr. McDowell's work as an editor and author was performed outside the scope of her federal employment. This work represents her personal and professional views and not necessarily those of the U.S. government.

## REFERENCES

1. U.S. Code-Title 7; Chapter 84, Section 5302 Definitions. National nutrition monitoring and related research. Available at http://uscode.house.gov/download/pls/07C84.txt. Accessed March 12, 2012.
2. Kennedy, E et al. *Food Nutr Bull* 32: 60; 2011.
3. Egan, MC. *JADA* 94: 298; 1994.
4. U.S. Congress, Publication L. 95–113. *Food and Agriculture Act of 1977*, 95th Congress, Washington, DC, September 29, 1977.
5. U.S. Department of Health and Human Services (HHS) and U.S. Department of Agriculture (USDA). *Nutrition Monitoring in the United States: A Progress Report from the Joint Nutrition Monitoring Evaluation Committee*. DHHS Publication No. (PHS) 86–1255. U.S. Government Printing Office, Washington, DC, 1986 (1st report).
6. Calloway, W. *JADA* 84: 1179; 1984.
7. Ostenso, GL. *JADA* 84: 1181; 1984.
8. Brown Jr, GE. *JADA* 84: 1185; 1984.
9. USDHHS and USDA. *Operational Plan for the National Nutrition Monitoring System*. U.S. Department of Health and Human Services, Public Health Service and U.S. Department of Agriculture, Food and Consumer Services, Washington, DC, p. 47, 1987.

10. U.S. Department of Health and Human Services, Interagency Committee on Nutrition Monitoring. *Fed Reg* 134. 53–26505; 1988.

11. Life Sciences Research Office, Federation of American Societies for Experimental Biology. *Nutrition Monitoring in the United States: An Update Report on Nutrition Monitoring*. DHHS Publication No. (PHS)89-1255. U.S. Government Printing Office, Washington, DC, 1987.

12. Interagency Committee on Nutrition Monitoring. *Nutrition Monitoring in the United States: The Directory of Federal Nutrition Activities*. DHHS Publication No (PHS) 89-1255-1. Public Health Service, Washington, DC, 1989.

13. U.S. Congress, Publication L. 101–445. *National Nutrition Monitoring and Related Research Act of 1990*, 101st Congress, Washington, DC, October 22, 1990.

14. U.S. Department of Health and Human Services (HHS) and U.S. Department of Agriculture (USDA). *Fed Reg* 58: 32752–32806; 1993.

15. Interagency Board for Nutrition Monitoring and Related Research. *Nutrition Monitoring in the United States: The Directory of Federal and State Nutrition Monitoring Activities*, DHHS Publication No (PHS) 92-1225-1. Hyattsville, MD, 1992.

16. Interagency Board for Nutrition Monitoring and Related Research. *Nutrition Monitoring in the United States: Chartbook I: Selected Findings from the National Nutrition Monitoring and Related Research Program*. Hyattsville, MD, 1993.

17. Life Sciences Research Office (LSRO). Federation of American Societies for Experimental Biology. Third Report on Nutrition Monitoring in the United States, Vol. 1 and 2, U.S. Government Printing Office, Washington, DC, 1995.

18. U.S. Department of Health and Human Services, NCHS. Nutrition monitoring in the United States: The directory of federal and state nutrition monitoring and related research activities. Hyattsville, MD, 2000. Available at: http://www.cdc.gov/nchs/data/misc/direc-99.pdf. Accessed March 12, 2012.

19. U.S. Department of Agriculture. What we eat in America-an integrated federal food survey. Available at: http://www.ars.usda.gov/Services/docs.htm?docid=13793. Accessed March 12, 2012.

20. U.S. Department of Agriculture, What we eat in America. USDA automated multiple-pass methodology. Available at: http://www.ars.usda.gov/Services/docs.htm?docid=7710. Accessed March 12, 2012.

21. Woteki, CE et al. *J Nutr* 132: 3782; 2002.

22. Dwyer, J, Picciano, MF, and Raiten, DJ. *J Nutr* 133: 576S; 2003.

23. National Research Council, Institute of Medicine, Committee on National Statistics. *Summary of Workshop on Food and Nutrition Data Needs*. National Academies Press, Washington, DC, 2004.

24. National Research Council. *Improving Data to Analyze Food and Nutrition Policies*. The National Academies Press, Washington, DC, 2005.

25. U.S. Congress, *National Health, Nutrition, and Physical Activity Monitoring Act of 2005 (H.R. 2844)*, 109th Congress. June 9, 2005. Available at: http://www.gpo.gov/fdsys/pkg/BILLS-109hr2844ih/pdf/BILLS-109hr2844ih.pdf. Accessed March 12, 2012.

26. U.S. Congress, Pub.L.110–234. *Food, Conservation, and Energy Act of 2008*, Section 4403, 110th Congress. *Cong Rec* 154, May 22, 2008.

27. Bialostosky, K, Briefel, RR, and Pennington, J. In *Handbook of Nutrition and Food*, Berdanier, CD, ed., CRC Press, Washington, DC, 2002, p. 407.

28. Pennington, J. In *Handbook of Nutrition and Food*, 2nd edn., Berdanier, CD, ed., CRC Press, Washington, DC, 2002, p. 451.

29. Briefel, RR. Nutrition monitoring in the United States. In B. Bowman and R. Russell (eds.), *Present Knowledge in Nutrition*, 9th edn., Vol. II. ILSI Press, Washington, DC, pp. 838–858, 2006.

30. Briefel, RR, McDowell, MA. Nutrition Monitoring in the United States. In JW Erdman, Jr., IA MacDonald, and SH Zeisel (eds.), *Present Knowledge in Nutrition*, 10th edn., Chapter 65, Wiley-Blackwell, Hoboken, NJ, September 2012.

31. U.S. Department of Health and Human Services, AOA. Evaluation studies of nutrition programs for older Americans. Available at: http://www.aoa.gov/aoaroot/aoa_programs/hcltc/nutrition_services/index.aspx#purpose and http://www.aoa.gov/AoARoot/Program_results/Program_Evaluation.aspx. Accessed March 12, 2012.

32. U.S. Department of Health and Human Services, CDC, NCHS. National health and nutrition examination survey (NHANES). Available at: http://www.cdc.gov/nchs/nhanes.htm. Accessed March 12, 2012.

33. U.S. Department of Health and Human Services, CDC, NCHS. National health care surveys (NHCS) (multiple surveys). Available at: http://www.cdc.gov/nchs/dhcs.htm. Accessed March 12, 2012.

34. U.S. Department of Health and Human Services, CDC, NCHS. National health interview survey (NHIS). Available at: http://www.cdc.gov/nchs/nhis/about_nhis.htm. Accessed March 12, 2012.

35. U.S. Department of Health and Human Services, CDC. National immunization survey (NIS). Available at: http://www.cdc.gov/breastfeeding/data/NIS_data/index.htm. Accessed March 12, 2012.

36. U.S. Department of Health and Human Services, CDC, NCHS. National survey of family growth (NSFG). Available at: http://www.cdc.gov/nchs/nsfg.htm. Accessed March 12, 2012.

37. U.S. Department of Health and Human Services, CDC. National survey of maternity and nutrition practices in infant care (mPINC). Available at: http://www.cdc.gov/breastfeeding/data/mpinc/index.htm. Accessed March 12, 2012.

38. U.S. Department of Health and Human Services, CDC, NCHS. National vital statistics system (NVSS). Available at: http://www.cdc.gov/nchs/nvss/about_nvss.htm. Accessed March 12, 2012.

39. U.S. Department of Health and Human Services, CDC, NCHS. NCHS linked mortality data files (multiple surveys). Available at: http://www.cdc.gov/nchs/data_access/data_linkage/mortality.htm. Accessed March 12, 2012.

40. U.S. Department of Health and Human Services, CDC. Pediatric nutrition surveillance system (PedNSS). Available at: http://www.cdc.gov/pednss/what_is/pednss/index.htm. Accessed March 12, 2012.

41. U.S. Department of Health and Human Services, CDC. Pregnancy nutrition surveillance system (PNSS). Available at: http://www.cdc.gov/pednss/what_is/pnss/. Accessed March 12, 2012.

42. U.S. Department of Health and Human Services, CDC, NCHS. State and local area integrated telephone survey (SLAITS). Available at: http://www.cdc.gov/nchs/slaits.htm. Accessed March 12, 2012.

43. U.S. Department of Health and Human Services, HRSA. National survey of children's health (NSCH). Available at: http://www.cdc.gov/nchs/slaits/nsch.htm. Accessed March 12, 2012.

44. U.S. Department of Health and Human Services, NIH. Food attitudes and behaviors survey (FAB). Available at: http://cancercontrol.cancer.gov/brp/fab/index.html. Accessed February 21, 2013.

45. U.S. Department of Health and Human Services, NIH. Health information national trends survey (HINTS). Available at: http://hints.cancer.gov/. Accessed February 21, 2013.

46. U.S. Department of Health and Human Services, NIH. National longitudinal survey of adolescent health (AddHealth). Available at: http://www.nichd.nih.gov/health/topics/add_health_study.cfm. Accessed March 12, 2012.

47. U.S. Department of Labor. National longitudinal surveys of youth. Available at http://www.bls.gov/nls/. Accessed March 12, 2012.

48. U.S. Department of Agriculture, FNS. School nutrition dietary assessment survey (SNDA)-SNDA-III. Available at: http://www.fns.usda.gov/ora/menu/Published/CNP/FILES/SNDAIII-Vol1ExecSum.pdf. Accessed March 12, 2012.

49. U.S. Department of Agriculture, FNS. School nutrition dietary assessment survey (SNDA)-SNDA IV. Available at: http://www.mathematica-mpr.com/nutrition/snda_IV.asp. Accessed March 12, 2012.

50. U.S. Department of Agriculture, FNS. Studies of child and adult care food program (CACFP). Available at: http://www.fns.usda.gov/cnd/care/default.htm. Accessed March 12, 2012.

51. National Research Council. *Child and Adult Care Food Program (CACFP): Aligning Dietary Guidance for All*. The National Academies Press, Washington, DC, 2011.

52. U.S. Department of Agriculture, FNS, WIC Program and Participant Characteristics Study (PC). WIC Studies information. Available at: http://www.fns.usda.gov/ora/menu/Published/WIC/WIC.htm. Accessed March 12, 2012.

53. Food Market Institute. Supermarket facts. Industry overview. 2010. Available at http://www.fmi.org/facts_figs/?fuseaction=superfact. Accessed March 12, 2012.

54. Harkness J. U.S. food system deeply at risk. The Institute for America's Future, Washington, DC, 2007. Available at http://www.tompaine.com/articles/2007/05/31/us_food_system_deeply_at_risk.php. Accessed March 12, 2012.

55. U.S. Department of Health and Human Services, CDC. School health policies and practices study (SHPPS). Available at: http://www.cdc.gov/HealthyYouth/shpps/index.htm. Accessed March 12, 2012.

56. U.S. Department of Agriculture, ARS. NHANES-What we eat in America (WWEIA) Component. Available at: http://www.ars.usda.gov/Services/docs.htm?docid=13793. Accessed March 12, 2012.

57. U.S. Department of Health and Human Services, FDA. Total diet study (TDS). Available at: http://www.fda.gov/Food/FoodSafety/FoodContaminantsAdulteration/TotalDietStudy/default.htm. Accessed March 12, 2012.

58. U.S. Department of Education. Early childhood longitudinal study program (ECLS). Available at: http://nces.ed.gov/ecls/. Accessed March 12, 2012.

59. U.S. Department of Agriculture. ERS. Current population survey (CPS) food security supplement (FSS). Available at: http://www.ers.usda.gov/Data/foodsecurity/cps/. Accessed March 12, 2012.

60. U.S. Department of Agriculture, FNS. Supplemental nutrition program for women, infants, and children (WIC) studies. Available at http://www.fns.usda.gov/ora/menu/Published/WIC/WIC.htm. Accessed March 12, 2012.

61. U.S. Department of Agriculture, ERS. American time use survey (ATUS)-eating and health (EH) module of the CPS. Available at: http://www.ers.usda.gov/Data/ATUS/. Accessed March 12, 2012.

62. U.S. Department of Health and Human Services, CDC. Behavioral risk factor surveillance system (BRFSS). Available at: http://www.cdc.gov/brfss/technical_infodata/surveydata/2009.htm. Accessed March 12, 2012.

63. U.S. Department of Labor, BLS. Consumer expenditure survey (CES). Available at http://www.bls.gov/cex/. Accessed March 12, 2012.

64. U.S. Department of Health and Human Services, FDA. Food safety surveys (FSS). Available at: http://www.fda.gov/Food/ScienceResearch/ResearchAreas/ConsumerResearch/default.htm. Accessed March 12, 2012.

65. U.S. Department of Health and Human Services, FDA. Health and diet survey (HDS). Available at: http://www.fda.gov/Food/ScienceResearch/ResearchAreas/ConsumerResearch/default.htm. Accessed March 12, 2012.

66. U.S. Department of Health and Human Services, CDC. Infant feeding practices survey (IFPS). Available at: http://www.cdc.gov/ifps/. Accessed March 12, 2012.

67. U.S. Department of Agriculture, ERS. Flexible consumer behavior survey (FCB). Available at http://www.ers.usda.gov/briefing/dietquality/flexible.htm. Accessed March 12, 2012.

68. U.S. Department of Health and Human Services, CDC. Pregnancy risk assessment monitoring system (PRAMS). Available at: http://www.cdc.gov/PRAMS/. Accessed February 21, 2013.

69. U.S. Department of Health and Human Services, CDC. Youth risk behavior surveillance system (YRBSS). Available at: http://www.cdc.gov/HealthyYouth/yrbs/index.htm. Accessed March 12, 2012.

70. U.S. Department of Health and Human Services, CDC. Methodology of the youth risk behavior surveillance system. MMWR 53:1;2004. Available at: http://www.cdc.gov/mmwr/preview/mmwrhtml/rr5312a1.htm. Accessed February 21, 2013.

71. National Nutrient Databank Conference. Home page. Available at http://nutrientdataconf.org/. Accessed March 12, 2012.

72. International Network of Food Data Systems (INFOODS). http://www.fao.org/infoods/index_en.stm

73. International Nutrient Databank Directory. Available at http://www.nutrientdataconf.org/indd/. Accessed March 12, 2012.

74. U.S. Department of Agriculture, NDL: National Food and Nutrient Analysis Program. NFNAP fact sheet. Available at: http://www.ars.usda.gov/Research/docs.htm?docid=9446. Accessed March 12, 2012.

75. U.S. Department of Health and Human Services, NIH, NLM. Dietary supplements labels database. Available at: http://dietarysupplements.nlm.nih.gov/dietary/. Accessed March 12, 2012.

76. U.S. Department of Agriculture, ARS. Dietary supplements ingredients database (DSID). Available at: http://www.ars.usda.gov/Aboutus/docs.htm?docid=6255. Accessed March 12, 2012.

77. U.S. Department of Health and Human Services, FDA. Food label and package survey (FLAPS). Available at: http://www.fda.gov/Food/LabelingNutrition/ReportsResearch/ucm275404.htm. Accessed March 12, 2012.

78. U.S. Department of Agriculture, ARS. Food and nutrient database system for dietary studies (FNDDS). Available at: http://www.ars.usda.gov/Services/docs.htm?docid=12089. Accessed March 12, 2012.

79	U.S. Department of Agriculture, Food Patterns Equivalents Database (formerly MyPyramid Equivalents Database-MPED). Food patterns database is under development. Updated information is available at: http://www.ars.usda.gov/Services/docs.htm?docid=17558. Accessed March 12, 2012.

80.	U.S. Department of Agriculture, ARS. National nutrient database for standard reference (NNDSR). Available at: http://www.ars.usda.gov/Services/docs.htm?docid=8964. Accessed March 12, 2012.

81.	U.S. Department of Agriculture, NDL. USDA database for the flavonoid content of selected foods, Release 3. 2011. Available at http://www.ars.usda.gov/Services/docs.htm?docid=6231. Accessed February 21, 2013.

82.	U.S. Department of Agriculture, ERS. Amber waves-the economics of food, farming, natural resources, and rural America. February 2004. Available at http://www.ers.usda.gov/AmberWaves/February04/Features/USTradeBalance.htm. Accessed March 12, 2012.

83.	U.S. Department of Agriculture, ERS. Electronic outlook report from the economics research service. Import share of U.S. food consumption stable at 11 Percent. FAU-79–01. July 2003. Available at http://www.ers.usda.gov/publications/fau/july03/fau7901/fau7901.pdf. Accessed March 12, 2012.

84.	Underwood TJ et al. *Hunger Environ Nutr* 6: 398–423; 2011.

85.	Organic Trade Association. Organic foods facts. 2010. Available at http://www.ota.com/organic/mt/food.html. Accessed March 12, 2012.

86.	Title 21 of P.L. 101–624, *The Food, Agriculture, Conservation, and Trade Act of 1990*. November 28, 1990 Available at http://www.ams.usda.gov/AMSv1.0/getfile?dDocName=STELPRDC5060370&acct=nopgeninfo. Accessed March 12, 2012.

87.	Electronic Code of Federal Regulations website (e-CFR). Title 7, Part 205, *National Organic Program* (current as of January 12, 2012). Available at http://ecfr.gpoaccess.gov/cgi/t/text/text-idx?c=ecfr&sid=3f34f4c22f9aa8e6d9864cc2683cea02&tpl=/ecfrbrowse/Title07/7cfr205_main_02.tpl. Accessed March 12, 2012.

88.	AC Nielsen SCANTRACK and National Consumer Panel Services. Available at: http://www.nielsen.com/us/en.html. Accessed February 21, 2013.

89.	U.S. Department of Commerce, NMFS. Fisheries of the U.S. survey. Available at: http://www.st.nmfs.noaa.gov/st1/fus/fus10/index.html. Accessed February 21, 2013.

90.	U.S. Department of Agriculture, ERS. U.S. food and nutrient supply series. Available at: http://www.ers.usda.gov/data/foodconsumption/. Accessed February 21, 2013.

91.	U.S. Department of Agriculture, ERS. National household food acquisition and purchase survey (FoodAPS). Available at: http://www.ers.usda.gov/Briefing/DietQuality/food_aps.htm. Accessed March 12, 2012.

92.	U.S. Department of Health and Human Services, CDC. CDC breastfeeding report card. Available at: http://www.cdc.gov/breastfeeding/data/reportcard.htm#Background. Accessed March 12, 2012.

93.	U.S. Department of Health and Human Services, CDC. Interactive database systems. Available at: http://www.cdc.gov/surveillancepractice/data.html. Accessed March 12, 2012.

94.	U.S. Department of Health and Human Services, CDC. National reports on human exposure to environmental chemicals. Available at: http://www.cdc.gov/exposurereport/. Accessed February 21, 2013.

95.	U.S. Department of Health and Human Services, CDC. Norovirus outbreak surveillance network (CaliciNet). Available at: http://www.cdc.gov/foodsafety/resources.html. Accessed February 21, 2013.

96.	U.S. Department of Health and Human Services, CDC. CDC drinking water information website. Available at: http://www.cdc.gov/healthywater/drinking/index.html. Accessed February 21, 2013.

97.	U.S. Department of Health and Human Services, CDC. Foodborne diseases active surveillance network (FoodNET). Available at: http://www.cdc.gov/foodnet/. Accessed February 21, 2013.

98.	U.S. Department of Agriculture, ARS. Food intakes converted to retail commodities databases (FICRCD). Available at: http://www.ars.usda.gov/Services/docs.htm?docid=21993. Accessed February 21, 2013.

99.	U.S. Department of Agriculture, ERS. Food desert locator. Available at: http://www.ers.usda.gov/Data/FoodDesert/. Accessed February 21, 2013.

100.	U.S. Department of Agriculture, ERS. Food environment atlas. Available at: http://www.ers.usda.gov/FoodAtlas/. Accessed February 21, 2013.

101.	U.S. Department of Agriculture, ERS. Supplemental nutrition assistance program (SNAP) data system. Available at: http://www.ers.usda.gov/Data/SNAP/. Accessed February 21, 2013.

102.	U.S. Department of Agriculture, NIFA. Know your farmer, know your food (KYF) compass. Available at: http://www.usda.gov/wps/portal/usda/usdahome?navid=KYF_COMPASS. Accessed March 12, 2012.

103.	U.S. Department of Health and Human Services, CDC. CDC growth charts website. Available at: http://www.cdc.gov/growthcharts/

104.	U.S. Department of Health and Human Services, CDC. Physical activity resources for health professionals. Available at: http://www.cdc.gov/physicalactivity/professionals/index.html. Accessed March 12, 2012.

105.	U.S. Department of Health and Human Services, ODPHP. Health communications and health literacy resources. Available at: http://www.health.gov/communication/Default.asp. Accessed February 21, 2013.

106.	U.S. Department of Health and Human Services, NIH, DRNC. Human nutrition research and information system (HNRIM). Available at: http://hnrim.nih.gov/. Accessed February 21, 2013.

107.	U.S. Department of Health and Human Services, NIH, ODS. Computer access to research on dietary supplements database (CARDS). Available at: http://ods.od.nih.gov/Research/CARDS_Database.aspx. Accessed February 21, 2013.

108.	U.S. Department of Health and Human Services, NIH, ODS. PubMed® bibliographic retrieval tools on dietary supplements. Available at: http://ods.od.nih.gov/Health_Information/IBIDS.aspx. Accessed March 12, 2012.

109.	U.S. Department of Health and Human Services, NIH, NCI. Diet and health assessment and resources. Available at: http://cancercontrol.cancer.gov/. Accessed February 21, 2013.

110.	U.S. Department of Health and Human Services, CDC, NCHS. NHANES web tutorials. Available at: http://www.cdc.gov/nchs/tutorials/Nhanes/index.htm. Accessed February 21, 2013.

111.	U.S. Department of Agriculture. Nutrition evidence library (NEL). Available at: http://www.nutritionevidencelibrary.com/default.cfm. Accessed February 21, 2013.

112. Partners in Information Access for the Public Health Workforce. Home page is available at: http://phpartners.org/index.html. Accessed March 12, 2012.

113. Pennington, JAT and Hubbard, VS. *J Nutr Ed Behavior* 34: 53; 2002.

114. U.S. Department of Health and Human Services, CDC. Nutrition topics for consumers and public health practice. Available at: http://www.cdc.gov/nutrition. Accessed March 12, 2012.

115. U.S. Department of Agriculture, CNPP. ChooseMyPlate. Available at: http://www.choosemyplate.gov/. Accessed February 21, 2013.

116. U.S. Department of Agriculture, National Agricultural Library (NAL): Food and nutrition resources for consumers. Available at: www.nutrition.gov. Accessed March 12, 2012.

117. U.S. Department of Health and Human Services, NIH. Educational resource list compiled by the NIH/DNRC. Available at: http://dnrc.nih.gov/. Accessed March 12, 2012.

118. U.S. Department of Health and Human Services, NIH. Dietary supplements information for consumers and health professionals. Available at: http://ods.od.nih.gov/. Accessed March 12, 2012.

119. U.S. Department of Agriculture and U.S. Department of Health and Human Services. *Dietary Guidelines for Americans, 2010*, 7th edn., U.S. Government Printing Office, Washington, DC, December 2010. Available at: http://www.cnpp.usda.gov/dietaryguidelines.htm. Accessed March 12, 2012.

120. U.S. Congress. National Nutrition Monitoring and Related Research Act of 1990, Pub. L. 101–445, Title III, 7 U.S.C. 5301 et seq.

121. U.S. Department of Health and Human Services, ODPHP. Health.gov portal. Available at: http://health.gov/. Accessed March 12, 2012.

122. U.S. Department of Health and Human Services. *2008 Physical Activity Guidelines for Americans*. Office of Disease Prevention and Health Promotion Publication No. U0036. Washington, DC. Available at: http://www.health.gov/paguidelines/pdf/paguide.pdf. Accessed March 12, 2012.

123. U.S. Department of Health and Human Services. Healthy people 2020 website. Available at: http://www.healthypeople.gov/2020/default.aspx. Accessed February 21, 2013.

124. U.S. Department of Health and Human Services. Healthy people 2020. Website home page and resources. Available at: http://www.healthypeople.gov/2020/implementing/default.aspx. Accessed March 12, 2012.

125. National Research Council. *Food Insecurity and Hunger in the United States: An Assessment of the Measure*. The National Academies Press, Washington, DC, 2006.

126. Let's Move. A campaign against childhood obesity. http://www.letsmove.gov/. Accessed March 12, 2012.

127. National Collaborative on Childhood Obesity Research (NCCOR). http://nccor.org/. Accessed March 12, 2012.

128. U.S. Department of Agriculture, CNPP. Partnership initiatives. Available at: http://www.choosemyplate.gov/Partnerships/index.aspx. Accessed March 12, 2012.

129. U.S. Department of Health and Human Services, NIH. Weight-control Information Network (WIN). Available at: http://win.niddk.nih.gov/. Accessed February 21, 2013.

130. U.S. Department of Health and Human Services, NIH. Ways to enhance children's activity and nutrition *(We Can!)*. Available at: http://www.nhlbi.nih.gov/health/public/heart/obesity/wecan/index.htm. Accessed March 12, 2012.

131. Institute of Medicine. *Dietary Reference Intakes. The Essential Guide to Nutrient Requirements*. The National Academies Press, Washington, DC, 2006, p. 543.

132. Institute of Medicine. *Dietary Reference Intakes for Calcium, Phosphorus, Magnesium, Vitamin D, and Fluoride*. The National Academies Press, Washington, DC, 1997, p. 448.

133. Yetley, EA et al. *J Nutr* 140: 2030S; 2010.

134. U.S. Department of Agriculture, ARS. *Vitamin D Addendum to USDA Food and Nutrient Database for Dietary Studies 3.0*. Beltsville, MD, 2009. Available at: http://www.ars.usda.gov/Services/docs.htm?docid=18807. Accessed March 12, 2012.

135. U.S. Department of Agriculture, ARS. Nutrient intake tabulations from NHANES WWEIA 2001–2008. Available at: http://www.ars.usda.gov/Services/docs.htm?docid=18349. Accessed March 12, 2012.

136. National Research Council. *Dietary Reference Intakes for Calcium and Vitamin*. The National Academies Press, Washington, DC, 2011, p. 1115. Report Link: http://www.nap.edu/catalog.php?record_id=13050. Accessed March 12, 2012.

137. U.S. Congress, P.L. 111–148. *The Patient Protection and Affordable Care Act*, 111th Congress, Washington, DC, March 23, 2010. Available at http://www.gpo.gov/fdsys/pkg/PLAW-111publ148/pdf/PLAW-111publ148.pdf. Accessed March 12, 2012.

138. U.S. Congress, P.L. 111–296. *Healthy Hunger-Free Kids Act of 2010*, 111th Congress, Washington, DC, December 13, 2010. Available at: http://www.gpo.gov/fdsys/pkg/PLAW-111publ296/pdf/PLAW-111publ296.pdf. Accessed February 21, 2013.

139. U.S. Department of Agriculture, FNS. *Healthy Hunger-Free Kids Act of 2010* Information Website. Available at: http://www.fns.usda.gov/cnd/governance/legislation/CNR_2010.htm. Accessed March 12, 2012.

140. National Research Council. *Examination of Front-of-Package Nutrition Rating Systems and Symbols: Phase I Report*. The National Academies Press, Washington, DC, 2010.

141. National Research Council. *Front-of-Package Nutrition Rating Systems and Symbols: Promoting Healthier Choices*. The National Academies Press, Washington, DC, 2011.

142. U.S. Congress, P.L. 111–353. The *Food Safety Modernization Act of 2011*, 111th Congress, Washington, DC, January 4, 2011. Available at http://www.fda.gov/Food/FoodSafety/FSMA/ucm247548.htm. Accessed March 12, 2012.

143. U.S. Department of Health and Human Services, FDA. *Food Safety Modernization Act of 2011. FDA* information website. Available at http://www.fda.gov/Food/FoodSafety/FSMA/ucm238000.htm. Accessed March 12, 2012.

144. U.S. Department of Health and Human Services, CDC. Sodium reduction initiative website. Available at http://www.cdc.gov/about/grand-rounds/archives/2011/April2011.htm?source=govdelivery. Accessed March 12, 2012.

145. Gordon-Larsen, P and Popkin, B. *J Am Diet Assoc* 111: 1816; 2011.

146. Mabry, PL, Olster, DH, Morgan, GD, Abrams, DB. *Am J Prev Med* 35: S211; 2008.

# 30 Nutrition Monitoring and Research Studies
## *Observational Studies*

*Katherine H. Ingram and Gary R. Cutter*

## CONTENTS

## INTRODUCTION

The purpose of this chapter is to provide an overview and to give current examples of observational studies. Specifically we focus on cohort observational studies that incorporate nutritional assessment in this chapter. After a brief review of the types and purposes of observational studies, a detailed description of the characteristics, advantages, and disadvantages of a cohort study is provided. Next, several cohort studies that have utilized nutritional assessments are discussed to demonstrate the use of the cohort design in nutrition research. This chapter is not meant as an all-inclusive summary but a sampling of work with this focus in mind. Finally, selected nutrition-related publications from these cohort studies are referenced along with the corresponding measured nutritional variables.

## OBSERVATIONAL STUDIES

Epidemiology is classically known as the study of the distribution of disease in human populations; however, the definition expands and often overlaps with other areas of research. Observational studies in epidemiology include natural history studies, case–control studies, prevalence (cross-sectional

or population) studies, and cohort (incidence) studies. The research question of interest dictates which type of observational study (OS) is used (see Table 30.1). For example, the diagnosis or frequency of a disease would be facilitated by using the prevalence study design. Cohort studies provide an opportunity to observe populations prospectively, thereby enabling the observation of incidence rates, as well as prevalence rates, and further provide the ability to calculate relative risks. Risk factors and prognosis of a disease can be identified through several different types of observational studies.

### OBSERVATIONAL STUDIES AND CLINICAL TRIALS

In this section, we are primarily concerned with observational studies, but will briefly discuss the relationship between observational studies and randomized clinical trials (CTs). The primary difference between these two types of research is the randomization of subjects into study groups facilitating an experimental maneuver, be it a treatment or an intervention. In CTs, subjects are randomized into various treatment or control groups. Conversely, in observational studies, the subjects are examined according to their natural selection or evolution into groups.[1] In many instances, the results from randomized CTs and cohort studies do not agree.

**TABLE 30.1**

**Question and Appropriate Design**

| Question | Observational Studies |
|----------|----------------------|
| Diagnosis | Prevalence |
| Prevalence | Prevalence |
| Incidence | Cohort |
| Risk factors | Cohort, case/control, nested case–control, prevalence |
| Prognosis | Cohort, natural history |

**TABLE 30.2**

**Characteristics of a Cohort or Incidence Study**

1. Selection of a study cohort WITHOUT disease
2. Follow study cohort over time (prospective)
3. Measurement of incidence and/or absolute risk (new cases developed in a time period)
4. Comparison of incidence in those with and without the risk factor (relative risk and attributable risk)

For example, observational studies have consistently found an association between low β-carotene levels and elevated risk of lung cancer in smokers; however, CTs have failed to find beneficial effects of supplementary β-carotene and have even provided evidence of harm.[2–4] Similarly, observational studies have shown hormone-replacement therapy (HRT) to have a protective effect against myocardial infarction, but randomized trials have shown a slight increase in risk.[5–8] These two examples have raised many questions regarding the validity of observational studies compared to randomized trials.

A major reason for the discrepancy in results between randomized trials and cohort studies pertains to measurement error of the exposure variable of interest, otherwise known as selection bias or residual confounding. This measurement error can result from confounding either from unmeasured variables, often in a form called confounding by indication, or from error in the measurement of variables. In the smoking and β-carotene studies mentioned earlier, it has been suggested that residual confounding occurred in the observational studies due to imprecise measurement of smoking status.[9] If smoking exposure is imprecisely measured and β-carotene is related to true smoking exposure, but β-carotene is found to be unrelated to decreased risk of lung cancer, then there will still be an apparent protective effect of β-carotene on lung cancer even after controlling for smoking exposure. Confounding by indication can occur when participants are observed on certain treatments; however, the reason they are on those treatments is that they failed on other treatments or were switched based on characteristics associated with their condition.

A number of statistical methods exist to address this potential confounding after the fact, but may not be able to sufficiently adjust for all the biases. However, taking preventive measures to reduce the problem in the design of the cohort study may be a better, and ultimately a more convincing, strategy. Restricting the research topics, designs, and analyses may help observational research to attain some of the desired benefits of randomization.[10]

## COHORT STUDIES

As noted in Table 30.1, the purpose of a cohort study is to identify the risk factors associated with a disease of interest, to obtain the incidence of disease, or to determine the prognosis of disease.[11] Cohort studies allow the development of a disease to be described and, as such, are often considered to be the preferred type of OS.[12]

Some of the defining characteristics of a cohort study are given in Table 30.2. The first characteristic is the identification of a study cohort that currently does not have the disease of interest. Any group of individuals who have either been exposed to the same occurrence, live in a defined geographic area, or have the same risk factors may be identified as a cohort.[1,12,13] When similar risk factors identify a cohort, a second similar cohort without the identified risk factors and the disease of interest must also be obtained for comparison purposes.[12] Both groups may be identified within the same cohort, but must be defined in advance by the design.

A second characteristic is that the study cohort(s) is followed over time. Because the study cohort(s) is disease free, the cohort(s) is followed over time to identify which individuals develop the disease of interest.[1,12,13] The new cases of a particular disease that developed within a specified time period are then assessed to define the incidence and absolute risk of that particular disease. Finally, the incidence in individuals with specific risk factors can be compared to the incidence in those without the risk factors to assess relative risk and attributable risk of these factors on the development of the disease.

Some consider placebo groups of CTs to be well-suited for use as cohort studies. This may or may not be true and depends on the entrance criteria used for the trial. For example, a prevention study within the general population may provide useful data as a cohort study; however, a trial on prostate cancer prevention would likely introduce bias from the all-male gender requirement and the likelihood of self-selection for participation by "healthy" at-risk participants.

### Advantages and Disadvantages of Cohort Studies

There are several advantages and disadvantages associated with the use of cohort studies, as compared to other types of observational studies (see Table 30.3). With respect to the advantages, cohort studies make it easier to distinguish cause from simply an association. Because the risk factors are measured prior to the development of the disease of interest, temporal order is established. Temporal order is one of eight factors classically associated with causality (see Table 30.4)[14] and strengthens a causal conclusion instead

## TABLE 30.3
### Advantages and Disadvantages of a Cohort Study

| Advantages | Disadvantages |
| --- | --- |
| Easier to distinguish cause from association | Large N may be needed |
| Incidence can be obtained | Results are delayed for low incidence or long incubation |
| Multiple outcomes can be studied | Expensive in resources |
| Standard questions and measurements can be used | Methods, criteria, and exposure status may change over time |
| May lead to identification of variables that can be experimentally examined | Losses may bias results |

## TABLE 30.4
### Factors Associated with Causality

1. The magnitude of the association's strength
2. The ability to show the association's consistency through replication
3. The association's identification of one risk factor to one outcome
4. The risk factor must precede the outcome
5. The outcome is sensitive to different levels of the risk factor
6. The association's logical adherence to current theory
7. The association's consistency with other information about the outcome
8. The association's correspondence to other causal associations

of simply describing the relationship between risk factors and outcome.[1,11,14] A comparison of cohorts based on differences in risk factors carries the assumption that both cohorts are similar in all other factors. Because this assumption can rarely be completely supported, causal implications are restricted.[11]

Another important advantage of cohort studies is that the incidence of an observed disease can provide estimates of the impact of preventive programs. This information can then be used to identify programmatic needs and to support budgetary plans needed to achieve specific reductions over a given time period.[14] Moreover, cohort studies make it possible to examine multiple outcomes, and standard measures allow for the comparison of cohorts from one study to the another. For example, the Framingham Heart Study (FHS) has provided important information on blood pressure, cholesterol, diet, eye disease, and a number of other risk factors and outcome measures.[15–21] Other studies, such as the Coronary Artery Risk Development in Young Adults (CARDIA) study, were designed with many similarities to FHS. In CARDIA, 22 variables were included in the baseline examination because of their known or suspected relationships to cardiovascular disease and can be compared to FHS results. The availability of multiple and often-related endpoints within the same population further enables researchers to study the temporal development of these endpoints as they relate to disease progression and also to study

their interrelatedness. Finally, cohort studies may permit the study of relationships between other variables and the outcome measures, which may then be selected for further experimental examination.[13]

One of the most obvious disadvantages of cohort studies is that the duration of the study has to be adequate for the development of the disease or surrogate of interest.[11,14] For example, consider blood pressure and cardiovascular disease. Cardiovascular disease is the ultimate outcome of interest, but the development of the surrogate measure blood pressure may be sufficiently linked to the outcome to make it a reasonable outcome in its own right. For diseases or surrogates with low incidence or long incubation periods, the results are delayed. With low disease incidence rates, the sample size for each study cohort may need to be extremely large in order to make the necessary comparisons.[11,14] From a statistical perspective, power is often directly related to the number of events and not just the sample size. The lengthy process and large sample size needed to conduct the study can result in hefty research expenses or unacceptably long durations of study.[4]

Another disadvantage of a cohort study is that participant loss may lead to biased results. The ability to recapture the study participants at the end of the study is influenced by study duration and ultimately depends on their geographic mobility, interest in continuing the study, and their mortality rates.[14] An inability to capture study participants and take account of their experience may result in bias[11,12] by so-called informative censoring. Even when these biases are not present, low follow-up rates may cause a suspicion of bias that is difficult to overcome.

A final disadvantage of cohort studies is that methods, criteria, and exposure status may change over the course of the study. For example, environmental, cultural, or technological changes may influence the risk factors identified and the measurement of the variables under study, and this is especially true of biological risk factors such as weight.[12,14]

A nested case–control study design can be used to reduce the costs of a cohort study. This type of study is a modification of the basic cohort study design and is created by inserting a case–control study into a retrospective or prospective cohort study.[1] In a nested case–control design, the baseline risk factor data are collected for the entire cohort and all of the participants are followed for development of the disease. Once a predetermined number of positive cases have been identified, the specific risk factor is then evaluated in only these cases and a comparison group of controls. This type of study design can be conducted at a fraction of the cost of conducting a typical cohort study. While nested case–control studies cannot estimate the relative risk of occurrence, they are able to offer more information than a stand-alone case–control study because of the specific cohort used for study. These studies estimate the odds ratio associated with the risk factor, which provides an excellent estimate of the relative risk when the incidence is relatively low (10% or less). However, when the incidence exceeds 10%, the odds ratio always is greater than the relative risk.

## SUMMARY OF OBSERVATIONAL STUDIES

Observational studies play an important role in epidemiological research. They allow diseases to be studied in their natural environment. Among the types of observational studies, cohort studies provide the most valuable approach for identifying temporal relationships between risk factors and outcomes. The primary characteristic of a cohort study is that it enables the cohort (or subgroup) to be identified as disease-free at the onset of the study, thereby making it possible for researchers to study the incidence of disease. The development of the disease of interest can then be measured and compared across cohorts. Like all observational studies, cohort studies have both advantages and disadvantages. The primary advantage of using a cohort study design is the ability to distinguish cause from association. The primary disadvantage is the considerable expense in time, money, sample size, and potential loss of subjects, which can lead to substantive bias in the inferences.

### EXAMPLES OF COHORT STUDIES UTILIZING NUTRITION ASSESSMENT

The remainder of this chapter focuses on eight selected examples of cohort studies that utilized some form of nutritional assessment (see Table 30.5). Although there are many

cohort studies available and additional cohort studies that include nutritional assessments, the following examples were selected to include a range of nationally and internationally recognized studies, unique uses of the cohort design, and different methods of collecting dietary intake information.

The selected examples include the following studies:

1. FHS
2. Nurses' Health Study
3. Health Professionals Follow-up Study
4. Coronary Artery Risk Development in Young Adults (CARDIA)
5. Atherosclerosis Risk in Communities (ARIC)
6. Women's Health Initiative (WHI) Observational Study
7. Reasons for Geographic and Racial Differences in Stroke (REGARDS)
8. European Prospective Investigation into Cancer and Nutrition (EPIC)

### Framingham Heart Study

The FHS was initiated to provide a population-based prospective examination of the development of cardiovascular disease and its risk factors.[22] The original sample

## TABLE 30.5
## Examples of Cohort Studies Utilizing Nutrition Assessments

| Cohort Study | Years Conducted | Sample Studied | Primary Outcomes | Dietary Intake Measurement |
| --- | --- | --- | --- | --- |
| Framingham Heart Study | 1949–ongoing | 5,209 men and women, primarily whites, 30–62 years old | Cardiovascular risk factors | Semi-Quantitative Food Frequency Questionnaire (Willet) |
| The Nurses' Health Study | 1976–ongoing | 121,700 female registered nurses, primarily whites, 30–55 years old | Cancer risk factors | Semi-Quantitative Food Frequency Questionnaire (Willet) |
| The Health Professionals Follow-Up Study | 1986–ongoing | 51,529 male health professionals, primarily whites, 40–75 years old | Heart disease and cancer risk factors | Semi-Quantitative Food Frequency Questionnaire (Willet) |
| Coronary Artery Risk Development in Young Adults (CARDIA) | 1985–ongoing | 5,116 men and women, blacks and whites, 18–30 years old | CHD risk factors | Baseline: Diet History Questionnaire (Interview Administered) Year 2: NCI (Block) Food Frequency Questionnaire |
| Atherosclerosis Risk in Communities (ARIC) | 1987–ongoing | 15,792 men and women | CHD risk factors and atherosclerosis and CHD events | Semi-Quantitative Food Frequency Questionnaire (Willet) |
| Women's Health Initiative Observational Study | 1993–2006 | 93,721 women, primarily whites 50–79 years old | Causes of morbidity and mortality in postmenopausal women | WHI Food Frequency Questionnaire |
| Reasons for Geographic and Racial Differences in Stroke (REGARDS) | 2003–ongoing | 30,239 men and women, equal number of whites and African Americans, aged 45 years and older with in-home interview | Underlying causes for the geographic and racial differences in stroke mortality | NCI (Block 98) self-administered food-frequency questionnaire completed after in-home interview |
| European Prospective Investigation into Cancer and Nutrition (EPIC) | 1992–ongoing | 520,000 men and women residing in 10 European countries | Relationships between nutrition and cancer | 1. Semiquantitative food-frequency questionnaire, both self- and interviewer-administered 2. 7-day food record 3. 14-day food record |

consisted of 5209 primarily non-Hispanic white men and women between the ages of 30 and 62 years who lived in Framingham, Massachusetts.[22,23] Measurements have been taken biennially since 1949, representing one of the first prospective observational studies of its kind. Exam 31, conducted between 2008 and 2011, had 91 attendees with a mean age of 92 years. Measurements include blood analyses, extensive medical history questionnaires, anthropometric measurements, and comprehensive physical examinations.[22] Additional assessments related to psychological conditions, dietary intake, and physical activity have been added to the study over the years. In 1971, the FHS Offspring Cohort was initiated with 5124 participants and, in 2002, the FHS Generation 3 Cohort examinations of 4095 volunteers began, providing researchers with a wealth of information on genetic contributors to cardiovascular disease.[24] FHS Omni Cohorts 1 and 2 were added to the Framingham studies in 1994 and 2003, respectively, to include ethnically diverse samples of 916 men and women of African American, Hispanic, Asian, Indian, Pacific Islander, and Native American origins who resided in or near Framingham at the time of enrollment. The information collected from the FHS has led to over 2300 publications between 1950 and 2011.[24] The expanded Willet Semi-Quantitative Food Frequency Questionnaire[23] was used as part of the examination protocol for the Original Cohort from Exam 20 (1986–1990) through Exam 22 (1990–1994), in the Offspring Cohort from Exam 3 (1983–1987) through Exam 8 (2005–2008), and in the Generation 3 Cohort Exam 1 (2002–2005). This questionnaire asks about the frequency of eating specific food items during the previous year. It includes 126 specific food items, 20 vitamin and mineral supplements, and 10 questions regarding fats and sugars used during food preparation.[24]

## Nurses' Health Study

Initially, the purpose of the Nurses' Health Study was to examine the long-term consequences of oral contraceptive use.[25] The study has since been expanded to examine the influence of other lifestyle factors, such as diet, exercise, and quality-of-life on the development of chronic disease.[26] The sample consisted of 121,700 registered female nurses from 11 states in the United States who were 30–55 years of age. Nurses were chosen because they were expected to be more accurate when reporting the incidence of diseases and lifestyle factors and, additionally, were expected to have higher participation and retention rates.[25,28]

Questionnaires have been requested biennially since 1976, and blood and toenail samples have been requested only occasionally. Unique to this study, researchers did not have personal contact with the nurse participants; instead, all contact was maintained through the mail. That is, study participants were required to mail in their bodily samples, anthropometric information, and the various questionnaires.[25–30] Only when a participant was nonresponsive to mailing in the measurements were telephone interviews conducted. Measurements included basic demographics,

medical history including the use of medications, blood and toenail samples, anthropometrics, lifestyle factors such as diet, exercise, and cigarette smoking, quality of life, and social support questionnaires.[25,27] In order to confirm the presence of a specified outcome (e.g., cancer, myocardial infarction, diabetes, or fractures), medical chart reviews were conducted when participants indicated an outcome's existence.[25,28,30] In 1989, the Nurses' Health Study II was initiated and enrolled 116,686 women between the ages of 25 and 42 years. The study is ongoing, and the cohort members continue to receive questionnaires every 2 years. The first food-frequency questionnaire was administered to this cohort in 1991. Nutrition intake is measured with Willett's semiquantitative food-frequency questionnaire, which assessed the consumption frequency of specified portions of food within the last year.[25,28–30] In 1980, the food-frequency questionnaire identified only 61 common foods,[25] while the 1984, 1986, 1990, and 1994 measures were expanded to include 120 common foods and both vitamin and mineral supplementations.[26] Recently, results from the Nurses' Health Study revealed that a higher milk and vitamin D intake during pregnancy was associated with a reduced risk of developing MS in the offspring.[31]

## Health Professionals Follow-up Study

The Health Professionals Follow-Up Study is an all-male OS designed to complement the all-female Nurse's Health Study. This study examines the relationship between diet and chronic illness, particularly heart disease and cancer.[32] The original sample consisted of 51,529 primarily white male health professionals who were 40–75 years of age.[30,32,33] The health professions included dentists, optometrists, osteopaths, pharmacists, podiatrists, and veterinarians.

Questionnaires have been administered biennially since 1986.[30,32,33] Similar to the Nurses' Health Study, the measures were all self-administered, mailed, and the outcome identifications were verified through medical chart reviews.[30,33–35] The measurements included demographics, medical history, anthropometrics (height, weight, and body mass index [BMI]), chronic disease risk factors (heart disease and cancer in particular), and lifestyle factors such as diet, physical activity, cigarette smoking, and alcohol use.[32–36]

Dietary intake was assessed with Willett's 131-item semiquantitative food-frequency questionnaire used as the expanded version in the Nurse's Health Study.[30,34] As in the Nurse's Health Study, the food-frequency questionnaire assessed the consumption frequency of specified portions of food within the last year.[30,34,36] Dietary intake was first assessed in 1986 and continues to be assessed every 4 years; however, vitamin use is assessed biannually.[37]

## Coronary Artery Risk Development in Young Adults

The purpose of the CARDIA study was to identify risk factors that either contributed to or protected young adults from coronary heart disease (CHD).[39] The sample consisted of 5116 black and white men and women from four cities, who were 18–30 years of age at enrollment.[38,39] Measurements were taken at baseline (1985 through 1986) and at years 2, 5, 7, 10, and every 5 years thereafter.[38–42] Baseline measurements included a sociodemographic questionnaire, medical (family history, current medical history, and use of medications), anthropometrics (weight, height, skinfolds, and various circumferences), lab work (lipids, apolipoprotein, insulin, and cotinine), blood pressure, lifestyle (treadmill test, questions on tobacco and marijuana use, and nutrition intake), and psychosocial questionnaires (type A/B personality, life satisfaction, hostility, social support, and job demand or latitude).[39] Subsequent examinations have varied with continually evolving specific aims related to cardiovascular disease and have included echocardiography, obesity-related questionnaires, chest and abdominal CT scans, carotid ultrasound, and brain MRI.[43]

Dietary intake was assessed with an interview-administered Diet History Questionnaire at baseline, year 7, and year 20, as well as the NCI (Block) Food Frequency Questionnaire at year 2.[38,41] Reliability and validity of the Diet History Questionnaire were assessed in a preliminary study prior to its use in the main study. Reliability was measured through the simple correlation between a 1-month test and retest methods of the Diet History Questionnaire.[40,43] Validity was assessed through comparisons with seven 24 h recalls. The nutrient intakes and mean caloric intakes of the Diet History Questionnaire were compared to the same variables derived from 24 h recalls,[40,43] NCI (Block) Food Frequency Questionnaire,[41] NHANES II,[40] and RDA's Body Mass Index[40] as an assessment of concurrent validity. For both reliability and validity, the Diet History Questionnaire appears to be more applicable for whites than for blacks, which has become an increasingly important consideration in research focusing on health disparities.[43]

### Atherosclerosis Risk in Communities Study

ARIC is a complementary study to CARDIA and was designed to examine the associations of established and suspected CHD risk factors with both atherosclerosis and new CHD events in an adjacent older age group. Participants include 15,792 men and women from four geographically diverse communities.[44] The study consists of two components: a community surveillance of morbidity and mortality and a cohort component with repeated examinations. The community surveillance component is an ongoing observational investigation of cardiovascular events (hospitalized myocardial infarction, inpatient heart failure, and CHD deaths) in the four defined communities. The cohort component is an examination of randomly selected samples of 4000 individuals aged 45–64 from a defined population in each of the four communities. In this cohort study, participants received an extensive examination at which time medical, social, and demographic data

were collected. Atherosclerosis was measured by carotid ultrasonography. The collected risk factor data include blood lipids and lipoproteins, plasma hemostatic factors, blood chemistries and hematology, blood pressure, anthropometry, fasting blood glucose and insulin, electrocardiography, physical activity levels, dietary intake, cigarette and alcohol use, and family history.[44] Dietary intake was assessed using a semiquantitative food-frequency questionnaire adapted from the questionnaire developed by Willett.[45–47] The questionnaire was administered at baseline and then at each of 3-year follow-up visits. All cohort participants were examined four times at 3-year intervals (baseline occurring in 1987–1989, the second in 1990–1992, the third in 1993–1995, and the final exam in 1996–1998). Since the final exam, the participants have been contacted annually to update their medical histories with any major medical events.[48]

### Women's Health Initiative Observational Study

The WHI was an extremely large and complex clinical investigation designed to explore the prevention and control of the common causes of morbidity and mortality, particularly cancer, cardiovascular disease, and osteoporosis, in postmenopausal women and to identify new risk factors for these diseases. Women aged 50–90 were enrolled in either a CT including 64,500 women or an OS of 93,676 women.[49] Forty clinical centers throughout the United States enrolled the participants between October 1, 1993, and December 31, 1998. The OS group included those who were ineligible for the randomized trial components of the WHI (including not wanting to be randomized), but were willing to be followed. The OS women were followed for 8 years on average.[50] All OS women had a physical examination at baseline and 3 years. Additional data regarding risk exposures, health behaviors, and other less common diseases were obtained with annual mailed questionnaires. Demographic, family, and medical history data, as well as risk exposure, were collected by self-report through standardized questionnaires. Physical measurements including blood pressure, height and weight, as well as blood samples were collected at the clinic visits. Dietary intake was assessed using the WHI Food Frequency Questionnaire,[49] which was derived from survey instruments used in previous studies.[51–54] The WHI food-frequency questionnaire comprised three sections including 19 adjustment questions used to calculate nutrient content of specific food items, 122 foods or food groups with questions on portion size and usual frequency of intake, and several summary questions on usual intake of fruits, vegetables, and fat during the previous 3 months.[55] Key findings from this study have had enormous impact on the understanding of women's health in the United States. One of the most rapid translations of CT results occurred in response to findings from the WHI-OS, leading to the rapid withdrawal of millions of women from postmenopausal HRT due to excess breast cancer risks.

## TABLE 30.6
## Selected Nutrition-Related Publications from the Six Cohort Examples

| Reference | Nutrition Variables and Primary Outcome |
|---|---|
| Framingham Heart Study[61] | Analyzed protein intake (total, animal, and plant) of 807 men and women as a continuous variable and by tertile of intake in relation to the number of falls reported by participants. Protein intake was associated with reduced risk of falls in older participants. |
| Framingham Heart Study[62] | Examined associations between atrial fibrillation (AF) and consumption of alcohol, caffeine, fiber, and fish-derived PUFAs in 4,526 participants with Cox proportional hazards regression. Dark fish was significantly and negatively associated with AF risk. None of the other variables were found to be related to AF risk. |
| Nurses' Health Study[63] | Assessed the association of maternal milk intake, maternal dietary vitamin D intake, and predicted maternal serum 25-hydroxyvitamin D (25(OH)D) during pregnancy in 35,794 participants and the risk of MS in the offspring. The multivariate adjusted rate ratio revealed an association between offspring MS and maternal intake of milk and vitamin D during pregnancy. |
| Nurses' Health Study[64] | Studied dairy product consumption from food-frequency questionnaire pertaining to high school diet in 37,038 women. Higher dairy product intake during adolescence is associated with a lower risk of T2D in adulthood. |
| Health Professionals Follow-up Study[65] | Examined the impact of sugar-sweetened (e.g., sodas) and artificially sweetened (e.g., diet sodas) beverages on incident fatal and nonfatal CHD (myocardial infarction) using proportional hazard models. Consumption of sugar-sweetened, but not artificially sweetened, beverages was associated with increased risk of CHD and associated biomarkers. |
| Health Professionals Follow-up Study[66] | Calculated three low-carbohydrate diet scores (high total protein and fat, high animal protein and fat, and high vegetable protein and fat) and compared them with incident T2D using Cox models. A low-carbohydrate diet high in animal protein and fat was positively associated with the risk of T2D in men. |
| Health Professionals Follow-up Study[67] | Assessed whole-grain intake and compared to incident hypertension in 31,684 men. An inverse association was found. |
| Health Professionals Follow-up Study/Nurses' Health Study[68] | Assessed potential protein substitutions for red meat, including fish, poultry, nuts, legumes, low-fat dairy, and whole grains. A substitution of 1 serving/day in place of red meat was associated with a 7%–19% lower mortality risk. |
| Coronary Artery Risk Development in Young Adults[69] | Evaluated relations of dietary meat, dairy, and plant foods (whole grains, refined grains, fruit, vegetables, nuts, or legumes) at years 0 and 7 with the 15-year incidence of elevated blood pressure (EBP) in 4,304 participants with proportional hazards regression. Plant food intake had a beneficial effect on blood pressure risk, while meat intake had an adverse effect. |
| Coronary Artery Risk Development in Young Adults[70] | Assessed associations between food price, dietary intake, overall energy intake, weight, and homeostatic model assessment insulin resistance (HOMA-IR) scores in 5,115 participants using conditional log–log and linear regression models. As the cost of soda or pizza increased, improvements were seen in body weight, energy intake, and HOMA-IR. |
| Coronary Artery Risk Development in Young Adults[71] | Calculated the 100-point Diet Quality Index (2005 DQI) in 4,913 black and white men and women to compare diet quality to 20-year weight gain. Longitudinal models adjusted for physical activity, smoking, energy intake, age, education, sex, and initial BMI showed that higher-quality diets were associated with less weight gain with in each race/gender group. |
| Atherosclerosis Risk in Communities[72] | Examined association between glycemic index (GI) or glycemic load (GL) of diets calculated from food-frequency questionnaires of 13,051 patients and risk of developing CHD. Proportional hazards regression showed a positive relationship between both GI and GL and the risk for CHD. |

(continued)

**TABLE 30.6 (continued)**
**Selected Nutrition-Related Publications from the Six Cohort Examples**

| Reference | Nutrition Variables and Primary Outcome |
| --- | --- |
| Atherosclerosis Risk in Communities[73] | Assessed whether shellfish consumption is associated with an increased risk of CHD in 13,355 participants using proportional hazards regression. An adjusted model found no increased risk of experiencing a coronary event in moderate- or high-intake groups compared to a low-intake group. |
| Women's Health Initiative Observational Study[74] | Nested case–control study tested whether dietary patterns predicted CHD events among 1,224 women with centrally confirmed CHD, fatal, or nonfatal myocardial infarct compared to matched controls. Diets rich in energy, total fat, and trans fatty acids were associated with higher CHD risk, while diets rich in carbohydrate, vegetable protein, fiber, dietary vitamin K, folate, carotenoids, α-linolenic acid, linoleic acid, and supplemental calcium and vitamin D were associated with lower risk. |
| Women's Health Initiative Observational Study[75] | Assessed whether dairy products were associated with risk for type 2 diabetes. Results indicated that a diet high in low-fat, but not high-fat, dairy products is associated with lower diabetes risk in postmenopausal women, and particularly in those who are obese. |
| Women's Health Initiative Observational Study[76] | Examined the association between dietary fat and cognitive decline in 482 women aged 60 and older. Results showed that high intakes of saturated fats, trans fats, and cholesterol were not associated with cognitive decline, while high monounsaturated fat intake was associated with less cognitive decline. |
| Reasons for Geographic and Racial Differences in Stroke[77] | Investigated the relationships between both race and region with intakes of fiber, saturated fat, trans fat, sodium, potassium, magnesium, calcium, and cholesterol among 9,229 American men. Multivariable linear regression revealed that race and region were significant predictors of most nutrient intakes. |
| European Prospective Investigation into Cancer and Nutrition[78] | Assessed the association between olive oil intake and breast cancer risk in 62,284 postmenopausal women. Cox proportional hazards regression results showed no association between olive oil and breast cancer. |
| European Prospective Investigation into Cancer and Nutrition[79] | Investigated the association between caffeinated and decaffeinated coffee consumption and the risk of chronic diseases, including type 2 diabetes, myocardial infarction, stroke, and cancer, in 42,659 participants. Multivariate Cox regression models indicated that coffee consumption does not increase the risk of chronic disease, but it may be associated with a lower risk of type 2 diabetes. |
| European Prospective Investigation into Cancer and Nutrition[80] | Examined the association between vegetable and fruit consumption and breast cancer risk in over 31,000 women. Adjusted Cox proportional hazard models revealed an inverse association between consumption of all vegetables and breast cancer risk. Leafy vegetables, fruiting vegetables, and raw tomatoes were particularly protective. |

## Reasons for Geographic and Racial Differences in Stroke

The purpose of the REGARDS study is to understand the underlying causes for the geographic and racial differences in stroke mortality.[56] REGARDS is an ongoing population-based longitudinal cohort study. Participants include 30,239 men and women over the age of 45 who enrolled in the program between January 2003 and October 2007. This cohort consists of an equal representation of whites and African Americans who were randomly selected by computer from a commercially available mailing list. Approximately one-half of the participants were selected from the Southern United States (Stoke Belt and Stroke Buckle regions), while the others were from other regions of the United States. Participants were recruited by mail and then by telephone.[56] Data on stroke risk factors, sociodemographic, lifestyle, and psychosocial characteristics were collected at the initial telephone interview. Physical measures, including an echocardiogram and fasting blood samples, were collected during a subsequent in-home visit.[56,57] The NCI (Block 98) semiquantitative food-frequency questionnaire[58] is used to collect dietary information. Participants were given this questionnaire at their in-home visit and were asked to return it by mail. Patients are followed via telephone at 6-month intervals to collect information about stroke-like symptoms and events. This is an ongoing study, and the participants will be followed for many years.[57]

## European Prospective Investigation into Cancer and Nutrition

EPIC is an ongoing cohort study designed to explore the relationship between cancer and nutrition and is currently the largest single resource for prospective investigations on nutrition, lifestyle, and cancer. Participants include 366,521 women and 153,457 men who were enrolled between 1992 and 2000 at 23 centers in 10 European countries. At enrollment, anthropometric measures (weight, height, and hip and waist circumferences) and blood samples were collected, and questionnaires regarding lifestyle were administered.[59] Data were collected on diet, physical activity, sexual maturation and reproductive history, alcohol and tobacco use, previous illnesses, and medication.[60] Blood samples were analyzed for various biomarkers including circulating levels of vitamins and provitamins, hormones, and growth factors, among others. Participants are contacted every 3–4 years to collect updated information regarding tobacco exposure, alcohol consumption, physical activity, weight, pregnancies, menopause, and other variables.[59]

While only one physical activity questionnaire was administered, three different dietary assessment methods were used for this study depending on the testing center location. In Italy, The Netherlands, Germany, Spain, France, and Greece, the questionnaires were extensive, containing up to 260 food items and estimated the individual portion sizes systematically or by structured meals. These were self-administered, except for Greece, Spain, and the Ragusa region of Italy, where the questionnaires were administered by interviewers in order to increase compliance. In Denmark, Norway, and the cities of Naples, Italy, and Umea, Sweden, semiquantitative food-frequency questionnaires were used, with standard portions assumed for all participants. In the United Kingdom, both a semiquantitative food-frequency questionnaire and a 7 day record were used, while participants in Malmo, Sweden, were given a short nonquantitative food-frequency questionnaire and a 14 day record on hot meals. Since the study had a multicenter design, a software program EPIC-SOFT was designed to standardize the questionnaire responses. EPIC-SOFT was adapted for each participating country and translated into nine languages.[60] The study is designed to follow the participants for life.[60]

Selected nutrition-related publications from the aforementioned studies and their respective measured nutrient variables and primary outcomes are displayed in Table 30.6.

## SUMMARY

In summary, this chapter briefly describes the use of observational studies indicating their use for nutrition monitoring and particularly focuses on the cohort study. Cohort studies make it possible for researchers to study the incidence of disease in the natural environment and, importantly, distinguish cause from association. On the other hand, cohort studies require a large commitment of time, money, number of subjects, and potential subject loss. In this chapter, eight large cohort studies using nutritional monitoring were described.

## REFERENCES

1. Hennekens, CH, Burning, JE. *Epidemiology in Medicine* Boston, MA: Little, Brown and Company, 1987.
2. Hirvonen, T, Virtamo, J, Korhonen, P et al. *Cancer Causes Control* 12: 789; 2001.
3. Holick, CN, Michaud, DS, Stolzenberg-Solomon, R et al. *Am J Epidemiol* 156: 536; 2002.
4. Woodson, K, Tangrea, JA, Barrett, MJ et al. *J Natl Cancer Inst* 91: 1738; 1999.
5. Beral, V, Banks, E, Reeves, G. *Lancet* 360: 942; 2002.
6. Hu, FB, Grodstein, F. *Am J Cardiol* 90: 26F; 2002.
7. Lawlor, DA, Davey, SG, Ebrahim, S. *Int J Epidemiol* 33: 464; 2004.
8. Vandenbroucke, JP. *Int J Epidemiol* 33: 456; 2004.
9. Stram, DO, Huberman, M, Wu, AH. *Am J Epidemiol* 155: 622; 2002.
10. Vandenbroucke, JP. *Lancet* 363: 1728; 2004.
11. Monsen, ER, Cheney, CL. *JADA* 88: 1047; 1988.
12. Friedman, GD. *Primer of Epidemiology*. New York: McGraw-Hill Book Company, 1987.
13. Zolman, JF. *Biostatistics: Experimental Design and Statistical Inference*. New York: Oxford University Press, 1993.
14. Slome, T. *Basic Epidemiological Methods and Biostatistics: A Workbook*. Monterey, CA: Wadsworth Health Sciences Division, 1982.
15. Atwood, LD, Wolf, PA, Heard-Costa, NL et al. *Stroke* 35: 1609; 2004.
16. Dhingra, R, Pencina, MJ, Benjamin, EJ et al. *Am J Hypertens* 17: 891; 2004.
17. Fox, CS, Coady, S, Sorlie, PD et al. *JAMA* 292: 2495; 2004.
18. Fox, CS, Cupples, LA, Chazaro, I et al. *Am J Hum Genet* 74: 253; 2004.
19. Massaro, JM, D'Agostino, RB, Sr., Sullivan, LM et al. *Stat Med* 23: 351; 2004.
20. Peeters, A, Bonneux, L, Nusselder, WJ et al. *Obes Res* 12: 1145; 2004.
21. Weiner, DE, Tighiouart, H, Stark, PC et al. *Am J Kidney Dis* 44: 198; 2004.
22. Dawber, TR. *The Framingham Study: The Epidemiology of Atherosclerotic Disease*. Cambridge, MA: Harvard University Press, 1980.
23. Tucker, KL, Selhub, J, Wilson, PW, Rosenberg, IH. *J Nutr* 126: 3025; 1996.
24. Framingham Heart Study. http://www.framinghamheartstudy.org/about, Retrieved March 15, 2012.
25. Colditz, GA. *J Am Med Womens Assoc* 50: 40; 1995.
26. The Nurses' Health Study. http://www.channing.harvard.edu/nhs/, Retrieved March 10, 2012.
27. Colditz, GA, Coakley, E. *Int J Sports Med* 18 Suppl 3: 162S; 1997.
28. Hu, FB, Stampfer, MJ, Manson, JE et al. *Am J Clin Nutr* 70: 1001; 1999.
29. Liu, S, Manson, JE, Stampfer, MJ et al. *Am J Public Health* 90: 1409; 2000.
30. Michels, KB, Edward, G, Joshipura, KJ et al. *J Natl Cancer Inst* 92: 1740; 2000.
31. Mirzaei, F, Michels, KB, Munger, K et al. *Ann Neurol* 70: 30; 2011.
32. Rimm, EB, Giovannucci, EL, Willett, WC et al. *Lancet* 338: 464; 1991.
33. van Dam, RM, Huang, Z, Giovannucci, E et al. *Am J Clin Nutr* 71: 135; 2000.

34. Giovannucci, E, Rimm, EB, Colditz, GA et al. *J Natl Cancer Inst* 85: 1571; 1993.

35. Platz, EA, Willett, WC, Colditz, GA et al. *Cancer Causes Control* 11: 579; 2000.

36. Giovannucci, E, Rimm, EB, Wolk, A et al. *Cancer Res* 58: 442; 1998.

37. Harvard School of Public Health, Health Professionals Follow Up Study. http://www.hsph.harvard.edu/hpfs/hpfs_qx.htm, Retrieved March 20, 2012.

38. Bild, DE, Sholinsky, P, Smith, DE et al. *Int J Obes Relat Metab Disord* 20: 47; 1996.

39. Friedman, GD, Cutter, GR, Donahue, RP et al. *J Clin Epidemiol* 41: 1105; 1988.

40. McDonald, A, Van Horn, L, Slattery, M et al. *J Am Diet Assoc* 91: 1104; 1991.

41. Slattery, ML, Dyer, A, Jacobs, DR, Jr. et al. *J Clin Epidemiol* 47: 701; 1994.

42. CARDIA. Coronary Artery Risk Development in Young Adults. http://www.cardia.dopm.uab.edu/overview.htm, Retrieved March 26, 2012.

43. Liu, K, Slattery, M, Jacobs, D, Jr. et al. *Ethn Dis* 4: 15; 1994.

44. Atherosclerosis Risk in Communities (ARIC). http://www.cscc.unc.edu/aric/2006, Retrieved March 25, 2012.

45. Diez-Roux, AV, Nieto, FJ, Caulfield, L et al. *J Epidemiol Community Health* 53: 55; 1999.

46. Houston, DK, Stevens, J, Cai, J, Haines, PS. *Am J Clin Nutr* 81: 515; 2005.

47. Steffen, LM, Jacobs, DR, Jr., Stevens, J et al. *Am J Clin Nutr* 78: 383; 2003.

48. Atherosclerosis Risk in Communities (ARIC). http://www.cscc.unc.edu/aric/, Retrieved April 5, 2012.

49. Langer, RD, White, E, Lewis, CE et al. *Ann Epidemiol* 13: 107S; 2003.

50. The Women's Health Initiative Study Group. *Control Clin Trials* 19: 1; 1998.

51. Henderson, MM, Kushi, LH, Thompson, DJ et al. *Prev Med* 19: 115; 1990.

52. Kristal, AR, Patterson, RE, Glanz, K et al. *Prev Med* 24: 221; 1995.

53. Kristal, AR, Feng, Z, Coates, RJ et al. *Am J Epidemiol* 146: 856; 1997.

54. White, E, Shattuck, AL, Kristal, AR et al. *Cancer Epidemiol Biomarkers Prev* 1: 315; 1992.

55. Hsia, J, Rodabough, R, Rosal, MC et al. *Am J Med* 113: 384; 2002.

56. Howard, VJ, Cushman, M, Pulley, L et al. *Neuroepidemiology* 25: 135; 2005.

57. Reasons for Geographic and Racial Differences in Stroke (REGARDS). http://www.regardsstudy.org/about, Retrieved March 29, 2012.

58. Benedict, JA, Block, G. In: St. Jeor S, ed. *Obesity Assessment: Tools, Methods, Interpretations*. New York: Chapman and Hall, 1997.

59. Riboli, E, Hunt, KJ, Slimani, N et al. *Public Health Nutr* 5: 6B; 2002.

60. Riboli, E, Kaaks, R. *Int J Epidemiol* 26: 1S; 1997.

61. Zoltick, ES, Sahni, S, McLean, RR, Quach, L, Casey, VA, Hannan, MT. *J Nutr Health Aging* 15(2): 147–152; 2011.

62. Shen, J, Johnson, VM, Sullivan, LM, Jacques, PF, Magnani, JW, Lubitz, SA, Pandey, S et al. *Am J Clin Nutr* 93(2): 261–266; 2011.

63. Mirzaei, F, Michels, KB, Munger, K, O'Reilly, E, Chitnis, T, Forman, MR, Giovannucci, E, Rosner, B, Ascherio, A. *Ann Neurol* 70: 30–40; 2011.

64. Malik, VS, Sun, Q, van Dam, RM, Rimm, EB, Willett, WC, Rosner, B, Hu, FB. *Am J Clin Nutr* 94(3): 854–861; 2011.

65. de Koning, L, Malik, VS, Kellogg, MD, Rimm, EB, Willett, WC, Hu, FB. *Circulation* 125(14): 1735–1741; 2012.

66. de Koning, L, Fung, TT, Liao, X, Chiuve, SE, Rimm, EB, Willett, WC, Spiegelman, D, Hu, FB. *Am J Clin Nutr* 93(4): 844–850; 2011.

67. Flint, AJ, Hu, FB, Glynn, RJ, Jensen, MK, Franz, M, Sampson, L, Rimm, EB. *Am J Clin Nutr* 90(3): 493–498; 2009.

68. Pan, A, Sun, Q, Bernstein, AM, Schulze, MB, Manson, JE, Stampfer, MJ, Willett, WC, Hu, FB. *Arch Intern Med* 172(7): 555–563; 2012.

69. Steffen, L, Kroenke, C, Jacobs, D, VanHorn, L, Pereira, M, Gross, M, Slattery, M, Yu, X. *Am J Clin Nutr* 82: 1169–1177; 2005.

70. Duffey, KJ, Gordon-Larsen, P, Shikany, JM, Guilkey, D, Jacobs, DR, Jr., Popkin, BM. *Arch Intern Med* 170(5): 420–426; 2010.

71. Zamora, D, Gordon-Larsen, P, Jacobs, DR, Jr., Popkin, BM. *Am J Clin Nutr* 92(4): 784–793; 2010.

72. Hardy, DS, Hoelscher, DM, Aragaki, C, Stevens, J, Steffen, LM, Pankow, JS, Boerwinkle, E. *Ann Epidemiol* 20(8): 610–616; 2010.

73. Matheson, EM, Mainous, AG III, Hill, EG, Carnemolla, MA. *J Am Diet Assoc* 109(8): 1422–1426; 2009.

74. Horn, LV, Tian, L, Neuhouser, ML, Howard, BV, Eaton, CB, Snetselaar, L, Matthan, NR, Lichtenstein, AH. *J Nutr* 142(2): 284–291; 2012.

75. Margolis, KL, Wei, F, de Boer, IH, Howard, BV, Liu, S, Manson, JE, Mossavar-Rahmani, Y, Phillips, LS, Shikany, JM, Tinker, LF. *J Nutr* 141(11): 1969–1974; 2011.

76. Naqvi, AZ, Harty, B, Mukamal, KJ, Stoddard, AM, Vitolins, M, Dunn JE. *J Am Geriatr Soc* 59(5): 837–843; 2011.

77. Newby, PK, Noel, SE, Grant, R, Judd, S, Shikany, JM, Ard J. *J Nutr* 141(2): 296–303; 2011.

78. Buckland, G, Travier, N, Agudo, A, Fonseca-Nunes, A, Navarro, C, Lagiou, P, Demetriou, C et al. *Int J Cancer* 131(10): 2465–2469; 2012.

79. Floegel, A, Pischon, T, Bergmann, MM, Teucher, B, Kaaks, R, Boeing, H. *Am J Clin Nutr* 95(4): 901–908; 2012.

80. Masala, G, Assedi, M, Bendinelli, B, Ermini, I, Sieri, S, Grioni, S, Sacerdote, C et al. *Breast Cancer Res Treat* 132(3): 1127–1136; 2012.

# 31 Nutritional Screen Monitoring Tools

*Ronni Chernoff*

## CONTENTS

## INTRODUCTION

Malnutrition is not a condition that occurs rapidly; it is a chronic condition that develops slowly over time. It is widely accepted that malnutrition from any etiology is not a positive factor in health status and may have a negative impact on other health conditions. There have been many reports of the health consequences of malnutrition, particularly in hospitalized individuals where poor nutritional status has been associated with increased lengths of hospital stay, poor wound healing, other comorbidities, complications, incomplete rehabilitation, readmissions, and mortality.[1–6] This is particularly important because it has been estimated that 85% of noninstitutionalized older adults have one or more chronic conditions, many of which are related to nutritional status.[7] If it is possible to identify indicators of risk for the development of malnutrition, and these factors are reversible conditions, then interventions that will alleviate risk can be instituted before malnutrition becomes overt and worsens chronic conditions.[8]

## SCREENING FOR MALNUTRITION

Nutritional screening is of value if it (1) reliably identifies the existence of risk factors for malnutrition, (2) recognizes the existence of poor nutritional status, (3) contributes to the avoidance of malnutrition, (4) minimizes suffering, and (5) the condition causing the malnutrition can be reversed.[7,9] Reuben et al.[7] describe criteria necessary to define the potential effectiveness of interventions; these criteria are whether or not identification of malnutrition can be achieved more accurately with screening than without it and whether or not individuals who have malnutrition detected early have a better outcome than those who have malnutrition detected later in the course of their illness. Rush[10] defines the role of nutrition screening in older adults in different terms. He describes another criteria set for screening including specificity, sensitivity, inexpensive screening devices, and interventions in which health benefit is not sacrificed by not treating those who are at moderate or low risk. He indicates that screening is appropriate where there is a relatively small but important proportion of the population that is affected, where those who are affected can be identified by an easily applied tool, and where there is an effective intervention.

There is no doubt that screening for poor nutritional status in older adults is more difficult than screening in children or young adults due to the increasing heterogeneity among people as they age. There are very few established norms for measurement parameters in older people, and the existence of chronic conditions, multiple medications, variable hydration status, and changes in body composition and habitus contributes to the challenge of objective assessment.[11] The selection of a screening tool raises several issues that need to be considered, including reliability, validity, sensitivity, and specificity and, in the case of older adults, the appropriateness of the reference values.

Despite these challenges, a proliferation of screening tools have been developed to try to discriminate between individuals who are at risk and those who are not at risk for malnutrition. Some tools focus on risk factors, others on the need for interventions; some tools are designed for use in a defined population group and others for general use or application in a specific care delivery setting.[12] Examining the efficacy and applicability of these screening tools has been the focus of analysis in the international literature.[12–14]

### Subjective Global Assessment

One of the first tools developed for screening was the Subjective Global Assessment (SGA). Devised by a group of clinicians in Canada, the SGA uses a brief set of history and physical assessment items to make an evaluation of nutritional status.[15] The SGA includes an analysis of weight changes, dietary change, gastrointestinal symptoms, functional capacity, medical status, and physical assessment (Figure 31.1). This tool relies on a subjective rating by using clinical judgment on weight loss, dietary intake, loss of subcutaneous tissue, functional capacity, fluid retention, and apparent muscle wasting.[8,15] This tool has been successfully adopted and used by physicians and nurses in clinical settings. The SGA has been tested in the clinical setting with different assessors with a high degree of inter-rater reliability (0.91).[16,17] Most of the validity reports of the SGA were conducted on hospitalized subjects with a mean age of 50 years or older, which may contribute to some questions about its general applicability. In a report by a group of German investigators, the SGA was able to identify malnutrition-related muscle dysfunction, validated by using a measure of grip strength.[18] However, the addition of laboratory values to the SGA did not improve its validity.[16]

Nursal et al.[19,20] explored different approaches to increasing the reliability of the SGA in predicting malnutrition in hospitalized patients. In a series of 2211 patients, they examined two approaches for evaluating malnutrition and found that the issue of unintended weight loss and loss of subcutaneous fat on the SGA predicted malnutrition with 93% accuracy. In a subsequent study,[20] these investigators found that weighting several items on the SGA (MQ-SGA) outperformed the usual SGA in predictive value. The most important factor was loss of subcutaneous fat, whereas the least effective item on the SGA was weight loss during the previous 6 months. The sensitivity and specificity were derived from statistical tests conducted on their data from a sample of 2167 patients and those among them who had a score of 18 on the MQ-SGA, which is highly predictive of malnutrition. The most heavily weighted items were the loss of subcutaneous fat (10 points), sacral edema (6 points), and ascites (3 points).

Although the SGA is a short tool that can be used successfully by health practitioners, there are limitations as to its use as a screening tool. It requires a trained clinician to administer it because there is some clinical judgment involved, which would not be expected in someone who is not a health professional. It requires that the individual being assessed is undressed, which does not lend itself to community-based assessment programs, and able to be turned, which may not be possible for extremely ill patients.

A. History
1. Weight change
Overall loss in past 6 months: amount = # ________ kg; % loss = # ________
Change in past 2 weeks: ________ increase
________ no change
________ decrease
2. Dietary intake change (relative to normal
________ No change
________ Change Duration = # ________ weeks
Type: ________ suboptimal solid diet ________ full liquid diet
________ hypocaloric liquids ________ anorexia
3. Gastrointestinal symptoms (that persisted for >2 weeks)
________ none ________ nausea ________ vomiting ________ diarrhea ________ anorexia
4. Functional capacity
________ No dysfunction (e.g., full capacity)
________ Dysfunction Duration = # ________ weeks
Type: ________ working suboptimally
________ ambulatory
________ bedridden
5. Disease and its relation to nutritional requirements ________
Primary diagnosis (specify) ________
Metabolic demand (stress): ________ no stress ________ low stress
________ moderate stress ________ high stress
B. Physical (for each trait specify: 0 = normal, 1 + = mild, 2+ = moderate, 3 + = severe)
# ________ loss of subcutaneous fat (triceps, chest)
# ________ muscle wasting (quadriceps, deltoids)
# ________ ankle edema
# ________ sacral edema
# ________ ascites

C. SGA rating (select one)
________ A = Well nourished
________ B = Moderately (or suspected of being) malnourished
________ C = Severely malnourished

**FIGURE 31.1** Components of the SGA.

## NUTRITION SCREENING INITIATIVE

Keeping these criteria in mind, and looking for a way to make both professional and volunteer care providers more attentive to the malnutrition risks encountered by older adults, the Nutrition Screening Initiative (NSI) was established as a public awareness initiative with tools that could easily be used by community and health-care workers who have regular contact with older adults. The tools include a checklist to identify risk factors, and level I and level II nutrition assessment instruments. These tools were developed as a joint venture project, begun in 1990, of the American Dietetic Association, the American Academy of Family Physicians, and the National Council on the Aging. The premise of the NSI is that, if factors associated with malnutrition risk are identified early, interventions can be instituted that may delay or avoid the progression of the risk factors toward overt malnutrition.[21,22]

The NSI was developed as a nested set of tools that serve to identify risk factors for poor nutrition status and then to diagnose malnutrition. The items on the tools were developed by reviewing the literature and achieving consensus among a technical advisory committee of experts. The checklist was tested using a follow-up sample from a previous study of nutritional status in older people.[23]

### Checklist

The checklist was created as a public awareness screening tool for use by health-care and social services personnel and other providers who work in community-based programs in which older adults participate. The checklist was conceived and designed to bring awareness to nutritional issues that may impact on the health status of elderly clients. It is widely available for reproduction and information collection.

The checklist was titled "DETERMINE Your Nutritional Health" based on a mnemonic that contains the risk factors for malnutrition listed on the reverse side of the checklist (Figure 31.2a and b). The checklist is a one-page questionnaire that can be used in community, long-term care, or acute health settings by volunteers, health aides, or health professionals. The objective of awareness of potential nutritional problems in older people was easily achieved; those who have been critical have built their criticisms on the basis of assumptions that have gone further than the original intent of the tool or the Nutritional Screening Initiative campaign.[24]

The items on the checklist were developed using the reference literature, expert opinion, existing databases, and pilot testing.[21–23] Using biochemical or laboratory parameters to define nutritional status may be misleading because the most commonly used measures, such as serum proteins, are affected by so many different factors that are independent of diet or nutritional status.[25]

### Implementation Strategies

Screening can be conducted in many settings and by health professionals as well as health-care workers or lay volunteers. Involving interested participants (nurses, aides, admission clerks, etc.) will increase the likelihood that data collection (weights, heights, completion of screening instruments) is more complete.

Modifications that allow the screening tools to be used in different settings, and for unique purposes, make this approach and instrument user friendly, applicable, and relevant. A tool that is flexible, valid, and reliable and allows different applications in diverse settings is very valuable. The easier and less time consuming it is to collect data that give insights into an individual's nutrition and health status, the more valuable the information. One example is the slight modifications made to the NSI Checklist for use in a dental office (Figure 31.3).[26,27] Dental professionals are in a unique position to monitor their patients' nutritional status as many of the consequences of poor nutrition manifest themselves in the oral cavity (bleeding or swollen gums; pain in mouth, teeth, and gums; angular cheilosis; alterations in the surface of the tongue). Additionally, oral health problems may contribute to the development of inadequate nutritional status because of lesions, loose or missing teeth, poorly fitting dentures, dry mouth, tooth decay or disease, and difficulty in chewing or swallowing.

The checklist can also be modified for use in specialized community or clinical settings. One example is the use of the checklist in a rural community setting as reported by Jensen et al.[28] They found that the checklist items indicating poor appetite, eating problems, low income, eating alone, and depression were associated with functional limitation.

### Implementation Partners

The NSI was designed to be a project that included many health professionals working in partnership to identify nutritional problems in older adults. It is important to include any professional who has direct patient contact. Therefore, nurses are essential partners and participants in nutrition screening. They are the best individuals to gather anthropometric data and health history information; they are well-positioned to evaluate individuals' functional status by assessing ability to engage in activities of daily living (ADL) (self-care) and instrumental activities of daily living (IADL) (managing independence). Clinical nurse specialists are uniquely positioned to conduct health and nutrition screenings in clinic settings, particularly to identify risk factors that are modifiable before nutritional status begins a slippery slope downward. The advantage of implementing health promotion programs before or concurrently with the emergence of risk-associated conditions should be apparent.[29]

Other health practitioners (dentists, social workers, physical therapists, speech pathologists, etc.) may also use the screening tool for clients who may have risk factors for the development of malnutrition. Community workers who run senior centers, senior meal programs, home health agencies, and so on, can also use the checklist to help identify those clients who may require more attention to their dietary intake, social circumstance, and chronic disease management.

The NSI contributed a unique approach to addressing the issues of malnutrition in older adults. It also opened the creativity of others to develop and test new tools in nutrition screening and assessment.

## MINI-NUTRITIONAL ASSESSMENT

The Mini-Nutritional Assessment (MNA) is a tool that was developed to be used easily to evaluate the nutritional status of frail elderly individuals.[30,31] This instrument was developed to meet a perceived need to go beyond the DETERMINE checklist developed by the NSI, which was designed to raise the awareness of potential malnutrition risks, and the SGA, which was designed for use with hospitalized individuals. The MNA, therefore, was created to complement the screening tools already described.

The objectives for the MNA were to meet the criteria of (1) a reliable instrument, (2) defined thresholds, (3) ability to be used with minimal training, (4) ability to be free of rater bias, (5) ability to be minimally intrusive to patients, and (6) ability to be inexpensive. The tool was designed to collect 18 items that combine objective and subjective data. These data include simple anthropometric measures (height, weight, arm and calf circumferences, and weight loss), general geriatric assessment items, a brief general dietary assessment, and self-assessment of health and nutrition perception (Figure 31.4).

### *The warning signs of poor nutritional health are often overlooked. Use this checklist to find out if you or someone you know is at risk.*

# Determine Your Nutritional Health

Read the statements below. Circle the number in the yes column for those that apply to you or someone you know. For each yes answer, score the number in the box. Total your nutritional score.

|  | YES |
|---|---|
| I have an illness or condition that made me change the kind and/or amount of food I eat. | 2 |
| I eat fewer than 2 meals per day. | 3 |
| I eat few fruits or vegetables, or milk products. | 2 |
| I have 3 or more drinks of beer, liquor, or wine almost every day. | 2 |
| I have tooth or mouth problems that make it hard for me to eat. | 2 |
| I don't always have enough money to buy the food I need. | 4 |
| I eat alone most of the time. | 1 |
| I take 3 or more different prescribed or over-the-counter drugs a day. | 1 |
| Without wanting to, I have lost or gained 10 pounds in the last 6 months. | 2 |
| I am not always physically able to shop, cook, and/or feed myself. | 2 |
| **TOTAL** |  |

## Total Your Nutritional Score. If it's -

**0-2  Good!** Recheck your nutritional score in 6 months.

### 3-5  You are at moderate nutritional risk.
See what can be done to improve your eating habits and lifestyle. Your office on aging, senior nutrition program, senior citizens counter, or health department can help. Recheck your nutritional score in 3 months.

### 6   You are at high nutritional risk.
**or more** Bring this checklist the next time you see your doctor, dietitian, or other qualified health or social service professional. Talk with them about any problem you may have. Ask for help to improve your nutrition health.

(a)

*These materials developed and distributed by the Nutrition Screening Initiative, a project of:*

 AMERICAN ACADEMY OF FAMILY PHYSICIANS

 THE AMERICAN DIETETIC ASSOCIATION

 NATIONAL COUNCIL ON THE AGING

**Remember that warning signs suggest risk, but do not represent diagnosis of any condition. Turn this page to learn more about the warning signs of poor nutritional health.**

**FIGURE 31.2** DETERMINE your nutritional health. (a) The DETERMINE Your Health Checklist.

**The Nutrition Checklist is based on the Warning Signs described below.**
**Use the word DETERMINE to remind you of the Warning Signs.**

**DISEASE**

Any disease, illness, or chronic condition which causes you to change the way you eat, or makes it hard for you to eat, puts your nutritional health at risk. Four out of five adults have chronic diseases that are affected by diet. Confusion or memory loss that keep getting worse is estimated to affect one out of five or more older adults. This can make it hard to remember what, when, or if you've eaten. Feeling sad or depressed which happens to about one in eight older adults, can cause big changes in appetite, digestion, energy level, weight, and well-being.

**EATING POORLY**

Eating too little and eating too much both lead to poor health. Eating the same foods day after day or not eating fruit, vegetables, and milk products daily will also cause poor nutritional health. One in five adults skips meals daily. Only 13% of adults eat the minimum amount of fruit and vegetables needed. One in four older adults drinks too much alcohol. Many health problems become worse if you drink more than one or two alcoholic beverages per day.

**TOOTH LOSS/MOUTH PAIN**

A healthy mouth, teeth, and gums are needed to eat. Missing, loose, or rotten teeth, or dentures which don't fit well or cause mouth sores make it hard to eat.

**ECONOMIC HARDSHIP**

As many as 40% of older Americans have incomes of less than $6000 per year. Having less - or choosing to spend less - than $25 to 30 per week for food makes it very hard to get the foods you need to stay healthy.

**REDUCED SOCIAL CONTACT**

One-third of all older people live alone. Being with people daily has a positive effect on morale, well-being, and eating.

**MULTIPLE MEDICINES**

Many older Americans must take medicines for health problems. Almost half of older Americans take multiple medicines daily. Growing old may change the way we respond to drugs. The more medicines you take, the greater the chance for side effects such as increased or decreased appetite, change in taste, constipation, weakness, drowsiness, diarrhea, nausea, and others. Vitamins or minerals when taken in large doses act like drugs and can cause harm. Alert your doctor to everything you take.

**INVOLUNTARY WEIGHT LOSS/GAIN**

Losing or gaining a lot of weight when you are not trying to is an important warning sign that must not be ignored. Being overweight or underweight also increases your chance of poor health.

**NEEDS ASSISTANCE IN SELF CARE**

Although most older people are able to eat, one of every five has trouble with walking, shopping, and buying and cooking food, especially as they get older.

**ELDER YEARS ABOVE AGE 80**

Most older people lead full and productive lives, but as age increases, risk of frailty and health problems increase. Checking your nutritional health regularly makes good sense.

The Nutrition Screening Initiative, 1010 Wisconsin Avenue, NW, Suite 800, Washington, D.C. 20007
The Nutrition Screening Initiative is funded in part by a grant from Ross Laboratories, a division of Abbott Laboratories.

(b)

**FIGURE 31.2 (continued)** DETERMINE your nutritional health. (b) Definitions of the mnemonic for DETERMINE.

This tool has been validated in many clinical studies by comparing the scores with the judgments of trained nutrition clinicians, the NSI instruments, and a comprehensive nutritional assessment that collected in-depth data about the nutritional status of the subjects.[32] The MNA has also been tested in a variety of populations including cognitively impaired elderly[33] linked to other conditions common in older adults, such as osteoporosis,[34] long-term care residents, and elderly individuals in different populations throughout the world.[32–43] These studies found that the threshold for the well-nourished on this instrument with a 30-point scale was 22–24 points; the threshold for malnutrition was 16–18 points on this scale. A short form with only six items[44] has been used with some success as a quick screening tool.[45]

The MNA meets its objectives of being a practical non-invasive tool that contributes to the rapid evaluation of an elderly subject's nutritional status, contributing early intervention to correct nutritional deficits. This tool is easily used in a variety of settings including hospital, nursing home, home care settings, or physician offices or clinics.

## UNIQUE NUTRITIONAL SCREENING TOOLS

Investigators from around the world have developed tools, using validated nutrition screening instruments such as the MNA as a starting point but modified for their unique populations. One example is the Chinese nutrition screen that uses the MNA as a base and adjusts for Chinese eating

The warning signs of poor nutritional health are often overlooked. A checklist can help determine
if someone is a nutritional risk:

Read the statements below. Circle the number in the yes column for those that apply to you.
For each yes answer, score the number in the box. Total your nutritional score.

|  | Yes |
|---|---|
| An illness or condition makes me change the kind and/or amount of food I eat. | 2 |
| I avoid eating a food group, i.e., meat, dairy, vegetables, and/or fruit. | 2 |
| I have two or more drinks of beer, liquor, or wine almost every day | 2 |
| I have tooth pain or mouth sores that make it hard to eat or make me avoid certain foods. | 2 |
| I snack or drink sweetened beverages two or more times per day between meals. | 2 |
| I had three or more new cavities at a recent dental check-up | 2 |
| I don't always have enough money to buy the food I need. | 4 |
| I eat alone most of the time. | 1 |
| I have a dry mouth, which makes me drink or use gum, hard candy, cough drops, or mints to moisten my mouth two or more times per day. | 1 |
| I take three or more different prescription or over-the-counter drugs daily. | 1 |
| Without wanting to, I have lost or gained 10 lb in the last six months. | 2 |
| I am not always physically able to shop, cook, and/or feed myself. | 2 |
| Total | |

Totally your nutritional score, if it is:

0–2        Good! recheck your nutritional score in 6 months.
3–5        You are at moderate nutritional risk. Try to improve your
             eating habits and lifestyle.
6 or more  You are at high nutritional risk. take with your doctor,
             dental hygienist, or dietitian about any problems you may have.
             Ask for help to improve your nutritional health.

**FIGURE 31.3**   Nutritional assessment form modified for use in dental office.

patterns, health-care system, and culture. Using physicians' physical examinations as a method of validation, this tool had a 60% chance of correctly identifying people at nutrition risk.[46,47]

Another instrument using the MNA as a base was tested for use with elderly South Africans and validated using measures of ADL and IADL. The investigators[48] reported a sensitivity of 87.5% and a specificity of 95%.

Another group in Iceland, using the MNA as a base along with a screening sheet for malnutrition and a full nutrition assessment as validation, identified four items predictive of malnutrition (body mass index [BMI], unintended weight loss, recent surgery, and loss of appetite). The investigators suggest validation of this screening tool in other populations.[49]

The British Association for Parenteral and Enteral Nutrition (BASPEN) developed a nutrition screening tool (NST) based on four parameters (weight, height, recent unintentional weight loss, and appetite).[50] This tool, malnutrition universal screening tool (MUST), is strongly supported by the British Dietetic Association, the Royal College of Nursing, and the Registered Nursing Homes Association, as well as the Malnutrition Advisory Group of BASPEN.[51] Another screening tool was developed and validated using interrater reliability between dietitians and nurses for the South Manchester University Hospitals Trust; this instrument used BMI, mid-upper-arm circumference, percentage of weight loss, and energy intake using the patients' first full hospital day intake.[52]

Investigators in the Netherlands developed and validated a short nutritional assessment questionnaire for early detection and screening for malnutrition in hospital patients.[53] The questions most predictive of malnutrition focused on unintentional weight loss, a decrease in appetite, and use of supplemental drinks or tube feedings. Another group in the Netherlands focused on community interventions for elderly people in a randomized controlled trial[54] of an EASYcare instrument that includes IADLs, cognition evaluation, mood, and a goal-setting item, which were assessed in follow-up visits at 3 and 6 months after inclusion in this validation study.

A Danish meta-analysis of randomized controlled clinical trials examining the predictability of screening instruments leads to a new method of nutrition risk screening. The review, working with the European Society of Parenteral and Enteral Support Education Committee, reexamined 75 studies. The authors assumed that indications for nutritional interventions relied on two criteria: severity of undernutrition and an increase in nutritional needs associated with disease severity. Although not a universally available data set, dietary history was included as a variable in the analysis. The resulting tool for use in hospital patients is the Nutritional Risk Screening (NRS-2002); the authors recommend that this new tool and its associated

# MINI NUTRITIONAL ASSESSMENT
## MNA™
ID# _____

Last Name: _____  First Name: _____ M.I. _____  Sex: ____  Date: _____

Age: _____  Weight,kg: _____  Height, cm: _____  Knee Height, cm: _____

*Complete the form by writing the numbers in the boxes. Add the numbers in the boxes and compare the total assessment to the Malnutrition Indicator Score.*

### ANTHROPOMETRIC ASSESSMENT

| | Points |
|---|---|
| 1. Body Mass Index (BMI) (weight in kg) / (height in m)² <br> a. BMI < 19 = 0 points <br> b. BMI 19 to < 21 = 1 points <br> c. BMI 21 to < 23 = 2 points <br> d. BMI ≥ 23 = 3 points | ☐ |
| 2. Mid-arm circumference (MAC) in cm <br> a. MAC < 21 = 0.0 points <br> b. MAC 21 ≤ 22 = 0.5 points <br> c. MAC > 22 = 1.0 points | ☐.☐ |
| 3. Calf circumference (CC) in cm <br> a. CC < 31 = 0 points  b. CC ≥ 31 = 1 point | ☐ |
| 4. Weight loss during last 3 months <br> a. weight loss greater than 3kg (6.6 lbs) = 0 points <br> b. does not know = 1 point <br> c. weight loss between 1and 3 kg <br> (2.2 and 6.6 lbs) = 2 points <br> d. no weight loss = 3 points | ☐ |

### GENERAL ASSESSMENT

| | Points |
|---|---|
| 5. Lives independently (not in a nursing home or hospital) <br> a. no = 0 points  b. yes = 1 point | ☐ |
| 6. Takes more than 3 prescription drugs per day <br> a. yes = 0 points  b. no = 1 point | ☐ |
| 7. Has suffered psychological stress or acute disease in the past 3 months <br> a. yes = 0 points  b. no = 2 points | ☐ |
| 8. Mobility <br> a. bed or chair bound = 0 points <br> b. able to get out of bed/chair but does <br> not go out = 1 point <br> c. goes out = 2 points | ☐ |
| 9. Neuropsychological problems <br> a. severe dementia or depression = 0 points <br> b. mild dementia = 1 point <br> c. no psychological problems = 2 points | ☐ |
| 10. Pressure sores or skin ulcers <br> a. yes = 0 points  b. no = 1 point | ☐ |

### DIETARY ASSESSMENT

| | Points |
|---|---|
| 11. How many full meals does the patient eat daily? <br> a. 1 meal = 0 points <br> b. 2 meals = 1 point <br> c. 3 meals = 2 points | ☐ |

| | Points |
|---|---|
| 12. Selected consumption markers for protein intake <br> • At least one serving of dairy products (milk, cheese, yogurt) per day? yes ☐ no ☐ <br> • Two or more servings of legumes or eggs per week? yes ☐ no ☐ <br> • Meat, fish, or poultry every day? yes ☐ no ☐ <br> a. if 0 or 1 yes = 0.0 points <br> b. if 2 yes = 0.5 points <br> c. if 3 yes = 1.0 points | ☐.☐ |
| 13. Consumes two or more servings of fruits or vegetables per day? <br> a. no = 0 points  b. yes = 1 point | ☐ |
| 14. Has food intake declined over the past three months due to loss of appetite, digestive problems, chewing or swallowing difficulties? <br> a. severe loss of appetite = 0 points <br> b. moderate loss of appetite = 1 point <br> c. no loss of appetite = 2 points | ☐ |
| 15. How much fluid (water, juice, coffee, tea, milk,...) is consumed per day? (1 cup = 8 oz.) <br> a. less than 3 cups = 0.0 points <br> b. 3 to 5 cups = 0.5 points <br> c. more than 5 cups = 1.0 points | ☐.☐ |
| 16. Mode of feeding <br> a. Unable to eat without assistance = 0 points <br> b. self-fed with some difficulty = 1 point <br> c. self-fed without any problem = 2 points | ☐ |

### SELF ASSESSMENT

| | Points |
|---|---|
| 17. Do they view themselves as having nutritional problems? <br> a. major malnutrition = 0 points <br> b. does not know or moderate malnutrition = 1 point <br> c. no nutritional problem = 2 points | ☐ |
| 18. In comparison with other people of the same age. how do they consider their health status? <br> a. not as good = 0.0 points <br> b. does not know = 0.5 points <br> c. as good = 1.0 points <br> d. better = 2.0 points | ☐.☐ |

**ASSESSMENT TOTAL** (max.30 points): ☐☐.☐

| MALNUTRITION INDICATOR SCORE | | |
|---|---|---|
| ≥ 24 points | well-nourished | ☐ |
| 17 to 23.5 points | at risk of malnutrition | ☐ |
| < 17 points | malnourished | ☐ |

**FIGURE 31.4**  MNA form.

algorithm be used in hospital and be added to the existing armamentarium of the MUST tool for use in the community and the MNA used in institutionalized elderly.[55]

In Canada, another screening tool was designed and tested for validity in community-living older adults. Based on four factors (food intake, adaptation, physiologic, and functional domains), a self-report tool, SCREEN I (Seniors in the Community: Risk Evaluation for Eating and Nutrition) consists of 15 items. A factor analysis linked the four domains to nutrition risk indices. This was found to

be a reliable tool although the author recommends further refinement of the instrument for use in community-dwelling older adults.[56]

The Geriatric Nutritional Risk Index is another screening tool specifically designed for older patients; it focuses on albumin as an indicator of nutritional status and weight changes as evaluated by comparing actual weight to desirable weight. This instrument seems to be less reliable in detecting differences among nutrition parameters commonly used but seems to have a higher prognostic value; the recommendation is that this tool be used in conjunction with the MNA for a more reliable and valid assessment of nutrition risk.[57]

Locally developed NSTs are proliferating. One example is the Glasgow NST. This screening tool was validated using the MUST as its comparison. The Glasgow NST proved to be at least as sensitive in identifying nutrition risk as MUST; it identified a greater number of patients with nutrition risk but that may be attributed to a lack of specificity. The local tool had been used in the study setting, and the users were comfortable with it; the study demonstrated that the local tool identified patients at risk, and its specificity and sensitivity were not of concern to the assessors.[58]

One criticism of NSTs is that they are not often adequately specific for certain diseases. While these tools are designed for general use in health care settings, disease specific tools would be useful. A nutrition screen that is applicable for cancer patients, specifically one that can identify risk for cancer cachexia. A study was undertaken to validate a new screening tool for cancer patients. This nutrition screen, a malnutrition screening tool (MST) for hospitalized cancer patients (MSTC), was evaluated through comparison with a short version of the SGA. Compared to the SGA, the MSTC had a sensitivity of 94% and a specificity of 84.2%. This screening tool was recommended for use in hospitalized cancer patients.[59]

In another trial, three screening tools were compared to determine which had a better malnutrition screening value in oncology patients. This study, conducted in a Portuguese cancer clinic, compared an MST with MUST and with NRS-2002. MUST identified the highest proportion of nutritionally at-risk patients (43.8%) when compared with the NRS-2002 (28.5%) and the MST (17.7%). The investigators concluded that the MUST tool better identified patients most at risk for nutritional complications that lead to a longer hospital stay.[60]

Yet another screening tool, the Imperial Nutritional Screening System (INSYST), was developed to overcome the challenge of obtaining reliable and valid measures to determine the BMI. When compared to MUST and the MNA, INSYST had a high sensitivity (95%–100%) but a lower specificity (65%–83%). Based on the results obtained when comparing these three instruments, the authors recommend the INSYST tool particularly when height and weight cannot be determined or accurately measured.[61]

Having a wide selection of NSTs to select from has lead to a variety of comparison studies.[62–65] Different study groups have come to different conclusions, often linked to the uniqueness of the population studied and the setting in which the study was undertaken. It is evident that adjustments and refinements will continue to be made to NSTs so that the available validated reliable instruments can meet the needs of unique populations. Although there are screening instruments that are widely used, adapting these tools to make them more useful in different settings with different racial or ethnic groups is important. The underlining outcome, which more care providers are focusing on nutritional status of their patients, is most important regardless of the screening tool used.

## NUTRITIONAL ASSESSMENT IN OLDER ADULTS

The descriptions of the screening tools used to define nutritional status among elderly people highlight the fact that one of the more difficult determinations in elderly people is the accurate assessment of their nutritional status. This evaluation is more challenging in older adults because of the physiologic changes that occur with normal aging. Many of the commonly used assessment standards are not reliable in this population for a variety of reasons, one being the lack of validated standards.[66]

### ANTHROPOMETRIC MEASURES

Anthropometric measures, including height, weight, and skinfold measures, are usually important components of a nutritional assessment. These parameters are the ones most affected by the aging process.[66–70] The most apparent age-related change occurs in height. Height decreases as people get older because of changes in skeletal integrity, most noticeably affecting the spinal column. Loss of height may be due to thinning of the vertebrae, compression of the vertebral disks, development of kyphosis, and the effects of osteomalacia and osteoporosis.[71] Loss of height occurs in both males and females, although it may occur more rapidly in elderly women with osteoporosis. Therefore, stature changes and body appearance may be altered.

Height is difficult to measure in individuals who are unable to stand erect, cannot stand unaided, cannot stand at all owing to neuromuscular disorders, paralysis, or loss of lower limbs, or are bed-bound due to other medical problems. One estimate of stature in these individuals is to measure their recumbent height or the bone lengths of extremities.[72] This estimate of stature may not be very reliable, but it provides some estimate of height to help determine whether body weight is appropriate for height.

Weight is another important anthropometric measure that is altered with advancing age. Weight changes occur at different rates among elderly people. Use of most standard height and weight tables is not valid in older people as most reference tables do not include elderly people in their subject pool, and most are not age-adjusted.

BMI is a commonly used measure to evaluate relative weight for height using a mathematical ratio of weight (in kilograms) divided by height (meters squared).

$$\frac{\text{Weight (kg)}}{\text{Height (m}^2)}$$

This formula yields a whole number that should be greater than 21 and less than approximately 30–35.[21] (*Note*: The upper healthy limit in older people is a matter of current dispute, but most experts consider that the limit is somewhat higher than that in younger persons.) Nomograms and tables are available that minimize the need for calculation. Use of the BMI depends on accurate height and weight measures. It is used frequently to evaluate weight for height but standards are not available for an elderly population.[73]

In recent years, waist circumference has become a widely used anthropometric measure. In a recent meta-analysis of 29 studies across the globe, waist circumference has been shown to be a better predictor of mortality risk than is BMI. It appears to be a reasonable alternative that is easy to measure.[74]

Skin-fold measurements (triceps, biceps, subscapular, suprailiac, and thigh) are often included in a thorough nutritional assessment. However, loss of muscle mass, shifts in body fat compartments, changes in skin compressibility and elasticity, and lack of age-adjusted references serve to decrease the reliability of skin-fold measures in the assessment of nutritional status in elderly people.[66]

## BIOCHEMICAL MEASURES

Biochemical assessment parameters are also affected by advancing age.[75] Laboratory measures may reflect an age-related decline in renal function, fluid imbalances or hydration status, or the effects of long-term chronic illnesses. Among the commonly used biochemical markers of nutritional status, serum transferrin is one that is markedly affected by advancing age. As tissue iron stores increase with age, circulating serum transferrin levels are reduced. A lower-than-normal serum transferrin should be evaluated in relation to other biochemical measures and serum iron levels, if obtainable.[76]

The most commonly used predictor of nutritional status in elderly people is serum albumin. Serum albumin below 4.0 g/dL (depending on local laboratory normal ranges) is not usual in an older person unless the subject is overhydrated, has cancer, renal or hepatic disease, or is taking medications that may interfere with hepatic function. Recent evidence suggests that serum albumin is also altered when there is an inflammatory response, common with the presence of chronic disease, infection, or injury.[25] A depressed serum albumin level seems to be a primary prognostic indicator of rehospitalization, extended lengths of stay, and other complications associated with protein energy malnutrition in elderly people.[77,78] However, this malnutrition may be secondary to other causes and not correctable by increasing food intake.[79,80] Unless there are medical reasons, most biochemical measures should remain within normal limits.

Serum cholesterol has been considered a risk factor for coronary heart disease, but a depressed serum cholesterol level is also associated with poor health status in older people.[81,82] It may be predictive of impending mortality[83] and should be evaluated carefully within the context of other health measures.

## IMMUNOLOGIC ASSESSMENT

Tests for immunocompetence are often included as part of a nutritional assessment because malnutrition results in compromised host-defense mechanisms. However, the incidence of anergy is reported to increase with advanced age and the response to skin test antigens appears to peak after longer intervals in older people.[84] The value of these tests is limited in elderly people.

## SOCIOECONOMIC STATUS

Social history, economic status, drug history, oral health condition, family and living situations, and alcohol use should be evaluated along with the physical and physiologic measures usually assessed.[66] It is also useful to assess elderly individuals using instruments that evaluate how well elderly people perform the ADL. Available tools assess the capability of an individual in managing the activities necessary for independence; these tools add another valuable dimension to the assessment of elderly people (Tables 31.1 and 31.2).[85,86]

**TABLE 31.1**
**Activities of Daily Living**

Toileting
    Cares for self; no incontinence
    Needs to be reminded or needs help with cleanliness; accidents rare
    Soiling or wetting at least once a week
    No control of bladder or bowels
Feeding
    Eats without assistance
    Eats with minor assistance or with help with cleanliness
    Feeds with assistance or is messy
    Requires extensive assistance with feeding
    Relies on being fed
Dressing
    Independent in dressing and selecting clothing
    Dresses and undresses with minor assistance
    Requires moderate assistance with dressing and undressing
    Needs major assistance with dressing but is helpful
    Completely unable to dress and undress oneself
Grooming
    Always neatly dressed and well groomed
    Grooming adequate; may need minor assistance
    Requires assistance in grooming
    Needs grooming care but is able to maintain groomed state
    Resists grooming
Ambulation
    Totally independent
    Ambulates in limited geographical area
    Ambulates with assistance (cane, wheelchair, walker, railing)
    Sits unsupported in chair or wheelchair but needs help with motion
    Bedridden
Bathing
    Bathes independently
    Bathes self with help getting into bath or shower
    Washes hands and face but needs help with bathing
    Can be bathed with cooperation
    Does not bathe and is combative with those trying to help

*Source:* Adapted from Lawton, M.P., *J. Am. Geriatr. Soc.*, 19, 4465, 1971.

**TABLE 31.2**
**Instrumental Activities of Daily Living**

Ability to use telephone
Shopping
Food preparation
Housekeeping
Laundry
Mode of transportation
Responsibility for own medications
Ability to handle finances

*Source:* Adapted from Lawton, M.P., *J. Am. Geriatr. Soc.*, 19, 4465, 1971.

## SUMMARY

Nutrition monitoring, screening, and assessment in the older adult population pose challenges to health-care professionals because of the heterogeneity of this group and the wide range of their health status. The difficulty in using the tools discussed here is that people age at different rates and in different ways related to their health status, their lifestyle, and their genetic inheritance. In particular in long-term care, the available instruments, particularly the Minimum Data Set (MDS 2.0), are not sensitive or specific for malnutrition risk.[88] Although there are a variety of reasonable approaches to nutrition assessment and monitoring in the older population, it is wise for the clinician to understand that the definitive tool or definition of malnutrition in older people has yet to be reported and that there are vast opportunities for research in this area.

## REFERENCES

1. Bauer, J.M., Kaiser, M.J., Sieber, C.C. *Curr Opin Clin Nutr Metab*, 13: 8–13; 2010.
2. Herrmann, F.R., Safran, C., Levkoff, S.E. et al. *Arch Intern Med*, 152: 125; 1992.
3. Galanos, A.N., Pieper, C.F., Cornoni-Hunt, J.C. et al. *J Am Geriatr Soc*, 42: 368; 1994.
4. Harris, C.L., Fraser, C. *Ostomy Wound Manage*, 50: 10; 2004.
5. Donini, L.M., De Bernardini, L., De Felice, M.R. et al. *Aging Clin Exp Res*, 16: 132; 2004.
6. O'Flynn, J., Peake, H., Hickson, M. et al. *Clin Nutr*, 24: 1078; 2005.
7. Reuben, D.B., Greendale, G.A., Harrison, G.G. *J Am Geriatr Soc*, 43: 415; 1995.
8. Chernoff, R. In Chernoff, R. (ed.). *Geriatric Nutrition: A Health Professional's Handbook*, 4th edn. Boston, MA: Jones & Barlett Publishers, in press.
9. MacLellan, D.L., Van Til, L.D. *Can J Public Health*, 89: 342; 1998.
10. Rush, D. *Ann Rev Nutr*, 17: 101; 1997.
11. Green, S.M., Watson, R. *J Adv Nurs*, 54(4): 477–490; 2006.
12. Elia, M., Stratten, R.J. *Curr Opin Clin Nutr Metab Care*, 14: 425–433; 2011.
13. Skipper, A., Ferguson, M., Thompson, K. et al. *J Parenter Enteral Nutr*, 36(3): 292–298; 2012.
14. Elia, M., Stratton, R.J. *Nutrition*, 28: 477–494; 2012.
15. Detsky, A.S., McLaughlin, J.R., Baker, J.P. et al. *J Parenter Enteral Nutr*, 11: 8; 1987.
16. Detsky, A.S., Baker, J.P., Mendelson, R.A. et al. *J Parenter Enteral Nutr*, 8: 153; 1984.
17. Baker, J.P., Detsky, A.S., Wesson, D. et al. *N Eng J Med*, 306: 969; 1982.
18. Norman, K., Schütz, T., Kemps, M. et al. *Clin Nutr*, 24: 143; 2005.
19. Nursal, T.Z., Noyan, T., Atalay, B.G. et al. *Nutrition*, 21: 659; 2005.
20. Nursal, T.Z., Noyan, T., Tarim, A. et al. *Nutrition*, 21: 666; 2005.
21. Lipschitz, D.A., Ham, R.J., White, J.V. *Am Fam Phys*, 45: 601; 1992.
22. Wellman, N.S. *Nutr Today*, II: 44S; 1994.
23. Posner, B.M., Jette, A.M., Smith, K.W., Miller, D.R. *Am J Public Health*, 83: 972; 1993.
24. Rush, D. *Am J Public Health*, 83: 944; 1993.
25. Sullivan, D.H. *J Gerontol*, 56A: M71; 2001.
26. Boyd, L.D., Dwyer, J.T. *J Dent Hyg*, 72: 31; 1998.
27. Saunders, M.J. *Spec Care Dent*, 15: 26; 1995.
28. Jensen, G.L., Kita, K., Fish, J. et al. *Am J Clin Nutr*, 66: 819; 1997.
29. Curl, P.E., Warren, J.J. *Clin Nurse Spec*, 11: 153; 1997.
30. Guigoz, Y., Vellas, B., Garry, P.J. *Nutr Rev*, 54: 59S; 1996.
31. Guigoz, Y., Vellas, B., Garry, P.J. *Facts Res Gerontol*, 4(Suppl 2): 15; 1994.
32. Vellas, B., Guigoz, Y., Baumgartner, M. et al. *J Am Geriatr Soc*, 48: 1300; 2000.
33. Arellano, M., Garcia-Caselles, M.P., Pi-Figueras, M. et al. *Arch Gerontol Geriatr Suppl*, 9: 27; 2004.
34. Gerber, V., Krieg, M.A., Cornuz, J. et al. *J Nutr Health Aging*, 7: 140; 2003.
35. Saletti, A., Lindgren, E.Y., Johansson, L. et al. *Gerontology*, 46: 139; 2000.
36. Cohendy, R., Gros, T., Arnaud-Battandier, F. et al. *Clin Nutr*, 18: 345; 1999.
37. de Rezende, C.H.A., Cunha, T.M., Júnior, V.A. et al. *Gerontol*, 51: 316; 2005.
38. Kuzuya, M., Kanda, S., Koike, T. et al. *Nutrition*, 21: 498; 2005.
39. Kucukerdonmez, O., Koksal, E., Rakicioglu, N. et al. *Saudi Med J*, 26: 1611; 2005.
40. Soini, H., Routasalo, P., Lagstrom, H. *Eur J Clin Nutr*, 58: 64; 2004.
41. Ruiz-Lopez, M.D., Artacho, R., Olivia, P. et al. *Nutrition*, 19: 767; 2003.
42. Chubb, P.E. *Asia Pac J Clin Nutr*, 14: 70S; 2005.
43. de la Montana, J., Miguez, M. *J Nutr Health Aging* 15(3): 187–191; 2011.
44. Guigoz, Y., Lauque, S., Vellas, B.J. *Clin Geriatr Med*, 18: 737; 2002.
45. Ranhoff, A.H., Gjoen, A.U., Mowe, M. *J Nutr Health Aging*, 9: 221; 2005.
46. Woo, J., Chumlea, W.C., Sun, S.S. et al. *J Nutr Health Aging*, 9: 203; 2005.
47. Lok, K., Woo, J., Hui, E. et al. *J Nutr Health Aging*, 13(2); 96; 2009.
48. Charlton, K.E., Kolbe-Alexander, T.L., Nel, J.H. *Public Health Nutr*, 8: 468; 2005.
49. Thorsdottir, I., Jonsson, P.V., Asgeirsdottir, A.E. et al. *J Hum Nutr Diet*, 18: 53; 2005.
50. Weekes, C.E., Elia, M., Emery, P.W. *Clin Nutr*, 23: 1104; 2004.

51. Stratton, R.J., Hackston, A., Longmore, D. et al. *Br J Nutr*, 92: 799–808; 2004.

52. Burden, S.T., Bodey, S., Bradburn, Y.J. et al. *J Hum Nutr Diet*, 14: 269; 2001.

53. Kruizenga, H.M., Seidell, J.C., de Vet, H.C.W. et al. *Clin Nutr*, 24: 75; 2005.

54. Melis, R.J.F., van Eijken, M.I.J., Borm, G.F. et al. *BMC Health Serv Res*, 5: 65; 2005.

55. Kondrup, J., Rasmussen, H.H., Hamberg, O. et al. *Clin Nutr*, 22(3): 321–336; 2003.

56. Keller, H. *J Clin Epidemiol*, 59: 836–841; 2006.

57. Cereda, E., Pedrolli, C. *Curr Opin Clin Nutr Metab Care*, 12: 1–7; 2009.

58. Gerasimidis, K., Drongitis, P., Murray, L. et al. *Eur J Clin Nutr*, 61: 916–921; 2007.

59. Kim, J.-Y., Wie, G.-A., Cho, Y.-A. et al. *Clin Nutr*, 30: 724–729; 2011.

60. Amaral, T.F., Antunes, A., Cabral, S. et al. *J Hum Nutr Dietet*, 21: 575–583; 2008.

61. Tammam, J.D., Gardner, L., Hickson, M. *J Hum Nutr Dietet*, 22: 536–544; 2009.

62. Tsai, A.C., Chang, T.-L., Chen, J.T. et al. *Int J Nurs Stud*, 46: 1431–1438; 2009.

63. Raslan, M., Gonzalez, M.C., Torrinhas, R.S. et al. *Clin Nutr*, 30: 49–53; 2011.

64. Kyle, U.G., Kossovsky, M.P., Karsegard, V.L. et al. *Clin Nutr*, 25: 409–417; 2006.

65. Putwatana, P., Reodecha, P., Sirapo-ngam, Y. et al. *Nutrition*, 21: 691–697; 2005.

66. Mitchell, C.O. Chernoff, R. (ed.). *Geriatric Nutrition: The Health Professional's Handbook*, 4th edn. Boston, MA: Jones & Bartlett Publishers, in press.

67. Mitchell, C.O., Lipschitz, D.A. *Am J Clin Nutr*, 35: 398; 1982.

68. Roberts, S.B., Rosenberg, I. *Physiol Rev*, 86: 651–667; 2006.

69. Solemdal, K., Sandvik, L., Møinichen-Berstad. et al. *Gerodontology*, 29(2): e1038–e1044; 2012.

70. McDowell, M.A., Fryar, C.D., Ogden, C.L. *Vital Health Stat 11*, 249: 1–68; 2009.

71. Chumlea, W.C., Garry, P.J., Hunt, W.C. et al. *Hum Biol*, 60: 918; 1988.

72. Martin, A.D., Carter, J.E.L., Hendy, K.C. et al. In Lohman, T.G., Roche, A.F., Martorell, R. (eds.). *Anthropometric Standardization Reference Manual*. Champaign, IL: Human Kinetics Publishers, Inc., 1988.

73. Cook, Z., Kirk, S., Lawrenson, S. et al. *Proc Nutr Soc*, 64: 313; 2005.

74. de Hollander, E.L., Bemelmans, W.J., Boshuizen, H.C. et al. *Int J Epidemiol*, 41(3): 805–817; 2012.

75. Fleming, D.J., Jacques, P.F., Dallal, G.E. et al. *Am J Clin Nutr*, 67: 722; 1998.

76. Ferguson, R.P., O'Connor, P., Crabtree, B. et al. *J Am Geriatr Soc*, 41: 545; 1993.

77. Sullivan, D.H., Walls, R.C., Lipschitz, D.A. *Am J Clin Nutr*, 53: 599; 1991.

78. Wilson, P.W.F., Anderson, K.M., Harris, T. et al. *J Gerontol Med Sci*, 49: M252; 1994.

79. Dennis, R.A., Johnson, L.E., Roberson, P.K. et al. *J Am Geriatr Soc*, 56(7): 1270–1275; 2008.

80. Sullivan, D.H., Johnson, L.E., Dennis, R.A. et al. *J Nutr Health Aging*, 15(4): 311–315; 2011.

81. Alsheikh-Ali, A.A., Trikalinos, T.A., Kent, D.M. et al. *J Am Coll Cardiol*, 52(14): 1141–1147; 2008.

82. Williams, P.T. *J Am Geriatr Soc*, 60: 430–436; 2012.

83. Rudman, D., Mattson, D.E., Nagraj, H.S. et al. *J Parenter Enteral Nutr*, 12: 155; 1988.

84. Pawelec, G., Koch, S., Gouttefangeas, C. et al. *Rejuvenation Res*, 9(1): 111–116; 2006.

85. Katz, S. *J Am Geriatr Soc*, 31: 721; 1983.

86. Spector, W.D. In Spilker, B. (ed.). *Quality of Life Assessments in Clinical Trials*. New York: Raven Press Ltd., 1990.

87. Lawton, M.P. *J Am Geriatr Soc*, 19: 4465; 1971.

88. Bowman, J.J., Keller, H.H. *Can J Diet Pract Res*, 66: 155; 2005.

# 32 Dietary Intake Assessment
## *Methods for Adults*

*Helen Smiciklas-Wright, Diane C. Mitchell, and Dara Wheeler*

## CONTENTS

## INTRODUCTION

Dietary assessment is a challenging undertaking. Individuals may consume many different foods at several eating occasions on any given day and do so both at home and away from home. Social, environmental, and cognitive events can affect the ability and/or willingness to report what is consumed. Expanding food market places and an increasing number of health-related dietary components require consistent updates of food composition databases. Despite assessment challenges, dietary data are widely used to provide dietary guidance for individuals and institutions, to interpret clinical and laboratory data, to evaluate intervention outcomes, and to establish dietary guidelines and intake recommendations.

This chapter is organized to review dietary methodology at three stages: dietary intake methods, data processing/analysis, and dietary quality assessments. The use of technology continues to increase. Where appropriate, information will be presented on recent technological advances in dietary assessment methods.

## DIETARY INTAKE METHODS

The most common methods for assessing intake by adults are prospective methods, daily food records/diaries, and retrospective daily food recalls and food frequency methods. Many advances in assessing food intake/exposure including computer-assisted techniques have become widely used in recent years. Applicability of methods, sources of error, and improvements in assessment procedures have been considered in review papers.[1–6] There is no single optimal assessment method. Some 40 years ago, Christakis advised that the assessment methods selected should be no more detailed, no more cumbersome, and no more expensive than necessary.[7] This advice is still sound. Assessment protocols may need to provide highly quantitative and detailed data on food consumption as would be the case for research studies such as clinical trials. More qualitative data are likely to be appropriate when food intake information is used for dietary guidance and counseling.

## DAILY INTAKE METHODS

### Records

Food records/diaries provide a prospective account of foods and beverages consumed. Records have been used to identify diet and disease associations,[8,9] and to calibrate other dietary methods.[10–12] The use of records for self-monitoring is related to more successful achievement of dietary goals[13] and greater weight loss and weight maintenance.[14,15]

Records are usually kept for brief periods of 1–7 days, but have been kept for a month[16] and up to a year[17] in methodological studies. Multiple days are recommended for assessing usual intake. The demands of record keeping, however, can lead to fatigue, with one study reporting significant dropouts after no more than three consecutive days.[18]

Respondents are asked to identify and describe foods and indicate amounts consumed. Food portions may be either weighed or estimated. While weighing foods will increase the accuracy of recorded portions, it can also increase respondent burden. Scales that do not disclose food weights to respondents are available[19] but at increasing cost.

When circumstances preclude self-reporting, food records may be kept by observers. Observed intakes are usually reported in institutions, primarily extended care facilities. The Omnibus Budget Reconciliation Act[20] requires that all Medicare- and Medicaid-certified facilities implement a standardized comprehensive assessment, including a measure of dietary intake for all residents. Designated staff estimate the portion of each served item consumed (e.g., from

"all" to "none").[21] More detailed estimates of intake require well-trained observers.[22] Digital photography has also been proposed for measuring food intake in settings that allow direct observation.[23]

When using food records, instruction should be clear as to how and when the form is to be filled out, guiding respondents about maintaining usual eating patterns. Comprehensive instruction is essential for improving record keeping, reducing error rates and costs of administration and analyses.[24,25] Table 32.1 provides instructions for a food record when detailed information is needed for food group and nutrient analysis.

After records have been completed, they should be reviewed (i.e., documented) to ensure that all necessary information has been provided. When reviewed with respondents, probing questions may be used to clear any ambiguities and to provide missing information. When records are to be further analyzed, they need to be processed using standard methods.

Subject burden can be high when intakes are recorded. Participant's willingness and ability are critical to the success of record data. The need for literacy may be a limiting factor for their use. Record keeping can introduce biases.[26] Respondents may make dietary changes that alter typical intakes.[27] Respondent characteristics may affect record keeping with consequential response bias. In a mailed study, women with higher weight status returned fewer records,[28] and in another study, those with higher weights presented records with more missing portion sizes and records with less sufficient food descriptors.[29]

Much of the foregoing discussion pertains to traditional written paper records. Technological advance have led to explorations of alternative record-keeping modes. Camera phones,[30] automated imaging with camera phones,[31] and personal digital assistant-based food diaries[32,33] are among instruments undergoing testing. Much of the work is in developmental stages

---

## TABLE 32.1

### Sample Instructions for the Administration of a Food Record

To help us do the best analysis of your food intake, please follow these instructions.

1. *Maintain your usual eating pattern*: Try not to modify your food intake because you are keeping a record.
2. *Record everything you eat or drink*: Be sure to include all snacks and drinks. Also include any vitamin or mineral supplements and the dosage for each day.
3. *Write foods down as soon as you eat them*: Daily record pages are provided. Please write clearly.

*Details are important!*

Completing the food record form

1. *Date*. Please record the date at the top of each form.
2. *Name*. Please write your name in the space at the top of the form.
3. *Time of day*. Record the time of the day you ate each meal, including AM or PM.
4. *Meal/where prepared?* Record the name of the meal eaten (i.e., breakfast, lunch, dinner, supper, or snack) and where the meal was prepared (i.e., at home, at a restaurant).
5. *Food item*. Write the name of each food item eaten.
6. *Description/preparation*. Include information on how each food was prepared.
7. *Amount*. Record the amount of each food either by using the poster provided or common household measures.

with testing often on small samples and respondents with some technical skills. Availability and cost of alternative modes and their feasibility for diverse populations must be explored. While there is much work to be done, the new technologies hold promise for improving record quality.

## Recalls

Recalls are used to assess diet and disease parameter associations,[34,35] clinical trial outcomes,[36,37] for validation of other instruments,[38] and for monitoring in nationwide surveys.[39]

Recalls provide a retrospective record of intake over a defined time period. While dietary recall may be for any length of time, this method is almost always administered to cover a 24 h time period and is generally termed the 24-hour recall (24 HR). To estimate the usual intake of individuals, multiple recalls are needed, preferably on random, nonconsecutive days, including weekends and weekdays.[3,17] Intake from one-day recalls available in large surveys can be estimated from analyses applied to multiple days in a population subsample.[40,41]

The 24 HR recall has become a favored way of collecting dietary data[42] as recalls can be administered easily and quickly with low respondent burden. Depending on the objectives of the recall, the amount and depth of information collected will vary. The 24 HR method is becoming the gold standard particularly as methodological improvements[42–45] and technological capabilities[46] increase validity. With the emergence of technological aids in dietary assessment, it is becoming more common for interviewers to collect intake data using interactive software, entering intake data directly into a computer as it is collected.

Recalls have traditionally and continue to be conducted as in-person interviews. In the 1980s, telephone interviews became more widely used in survey research. Technology enabled interview data entry into a computer system file, increased efficiency, and decreased costs of recalls.[46] Recalls by telephone interview have been shown to be practical, valid, and cost-effective.[46,47] They are becoming an increasingly popular mode of data collection, especially for research and population-monitoring purposes.[39] Initial concerns about telephone surveys were biases of noncoverage and nonresponse. Dramatic changes in telecommunication since the 1980s need to be reviewed to address potential for similar biases in telephone surveys.

Trained interviewers are essential for administering 24 HR whether face-to-face or by telephone. The costs of data collection have prompted the development of automated self-administered recalls.[48–50] Arab et al. reported high rates of return when the Internet was used to obtain eight self-administered recalls from African American and White adults.[50] The National Cancer Institute and its contractor, Westat, have made available a self-administered tool, the Automated Self-Administered 24-Hour Dietary Recall (ASA24™) for use by researchers, clinicians, and educators.[51]

A 24 HR requires a respondent's memory of food eaten. The development of a multiple-pass technique with

structured probes into a standardized interview protocol can reduce reporting errors. A multiple-pass technique provides respondents several opportunities (i.e., passes) to recall foods eaten using both free recall and cued (probed recall) strategies.[43–45,52] Historically, the strategy involves three passes: an introductory opening sequence in which a respondent is asked to recall all items eaten; an interactive, structural probe sequence to elicit detailed food descriptions and amounts; and a final review of the recall. The multiple-pass technique is theoretically sound and, when incorporated into a well-structured interactive interview process, may decrease reporting errors for groups of individuals. More recently, Conway et al. have developed and tested newer multiple-pass methodologies that include five passes: (1) a quick list or uninterrupted listing of all foods and beverages; (2) a forgotten foods list or questions about nine food categories that are often forgotten; (3) time of day foods were consumed and the eating occasion; (4) detailed questions about each food including preparation and amounts consumed; and (5) a final review and probe of all foods consumed.[52] Research using these newer methods has demonstrated in an experimental setting that individuals are able to accurately report intakes within 10% of actual intake for obese and normal-weight men and women.[52] While these studies are encouraging for the presentation of group data, there is room for improvement in assessing individuals' intakes.[43]

Prior to conducting recalls, training of interviewers is important. This is particularly relevant when more quantitative data are required, increasing the need to use multiple-pass and probing techniques. Figure 32.1 provides a sample probing sequence to elicit detailed information regarding one specific food (i.e., macaroni and cheese). The complexity of this probing sequence exemplifies the potentially complex nature of probing questions and need for good interviewer training. More qualitative food intake data can be achieved with more limited questions.

A multiple-pass technique can be facilitated by the use of interactive software.[53] This allows for a greater level of detail and facilitates data collection, but the technology is generally expensive and is not used commonly in clinical settings. However, written tools, such as probing guides, may be used to mimic this process when quantitative analysis is critical.

## FOOD FREQUENCY METHODS

Food frequency methods are designed to obtain information about usual long-term food consumption patterns. The methods evolved from the dietary history method originally developed by Burke.[54] The dietary history interview included a 24 HR, a 3-day food record, and a checklist of foods with questions about likes, dislikes, and consumption over the previous month. It was time consuming to administer and process the dietary information. However, the checklist with its list of foods and consumption options was the basis of

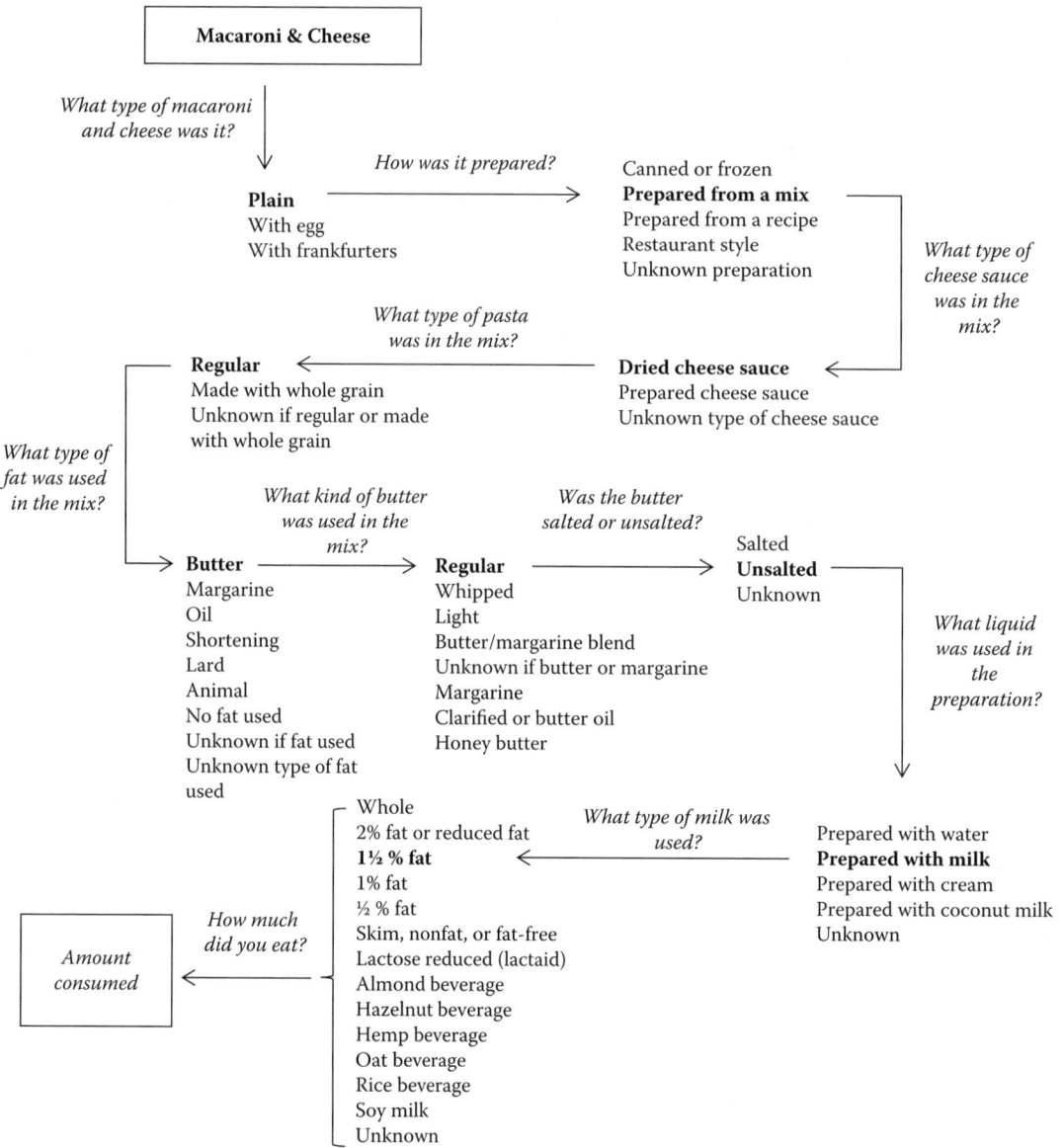

**FIGURE 32.1** A sample probing scheme. This scheme could be used with recalls to elicit more information from a respondent that consumed macaroni and cheese. Bold font indicates respondent's reply. Probing questions, which are specific for each response, are italicized. (Adapted from Nutrition Data System for Research software, developed by the Nutrition Coordinating Center, University of Minnesota, Minneapolis, MN.)

food frequency questionnaires (FFQs). FFQs are widely used in epidemiologic studies primarily because of their low cost to administer and analyze relative to dietary recall and food record methodology.

FFQs consist of a list of foods and frequency-of-use response categories and may also include portion size response categories. A comprehensive list of foods that represents the diet of a target population is necessary to provide reasonable estimates of total intake. Careful consideration is needed when deciding on whether to group similar foods together or to list them individually. Grouping foods together can lead to underestimation of intake; however, listing too many foods individually can overestimate intake. Generally,

it is easier to aggregate if needed for analysis, but difficult to separate groupings once data are collected. Asking participants to determine the frequency of a food that is sometimes eaten alone or in combination is cognitively difficult.

Commonly used FFQs are the Nurses' Health Study Dietary Questionnaire[4] and the NCI FFQ developed by Block et al.[55] Many of the food frequencies used are modifications of these questionnaires. Modifying existing questionnaires is more cost effective than developing a new one; however, careful consideration should be given to the existing questionnaires' intended purpose. In a review of nearly 200 food frequency validation studies, less than half had a clearly stated purpose, and in some cases, a FFQ would not be recommended.[56] FFQs are not as useful in studies involving small numbers of participants, short-term interventions, for monitoring nutrient intakes, or when absolute nutrient intakes are required.

Subar has provided a succinct but thorough summary of considerations in selecting an FFQ.[57] A basic question is whether to select or adapt a commonly used questionnaire or to develop and validate a new instrument. Willett[4] and others[58,59] have described the very intensive processes involved with the development of new FFQs. An example of the development process and the use of cognitive interviewing is described for the National Cancer Institute Diet History Questionnaire (NCI DHQ).[60] The original Block FFQ and the NCI DHQ were developed from a nationally representative sample of the U.S. population. For this reason, these instruments were used for many research studies but may not be as appropriate for population subgroups where intakes could be dramatically different than those of the general population.

Validating a new instrument or administration of a standard instrument on a specific population is also challenging. FFQs are commonly validated by calibrations with other dietary assessment methods.[12,60,61] Both dietary recalls or food records conducted over longer period of time and are representative of the time frame of the FFQ are recommended.[56] Kipnis et al. used biomarkers for energy and protein validation in the Observing Protein and Energy Nutrition (OPEN) study.[62] Correlation between the reference method and the food frequency is the most common statistics used to determine validation. However, correlation analyses in combination with other methods such as Bland–Altman plots are recommended. Bland–Altman plots show the agreement between both the test and the reference method across a range of intake. For example, a Bland–Altman plot determines whether the test method (or FFQ) is less valid or more valid at higher or lower intakes compared to the reference method. If the purpose of the FFQ is to identify those at risk of low intakes, the instruments' inability to accurately assess high intakes may be irrelevant. Other useful validation methods include sensitivity or specificity analysis and classification of intakes into percentiles of intakes. Both methods will provide information on how well individuals are classified or ranked by their nutrient intakes.

FFQs without portion size information generally provide qualitative data. If portion size information is included, nutrient intakes may be estimated to enable relative ranking of intakes. Several investigators have studied the use of standard versus reported portion intakes. Laus et al.[63] found little difference in nutrient estimates when a standard (medium size) portion was substituted for reported sizes. In a meta-analysis conducted by Molag et al.,[64] the use of standard portion sizes resulted in higher correlations for some nutrients than specific portion sizes. However, others have indicated that the use of standard portion size data may attenuate relationships between diet and disease.[65]

FFQs are commonly self-administered mostly because of the higher cost and time involved in interviewer-administered questionnaires. Self-administered questionnaires should include a review process that includes some follow-up by telephone or face-to-face to complete missed or incomplete items. Most self-administered instruments are computer scanned eliminating the time-consuming, error-prone data entry. FFQs can also be collected by telephone, which can result in higher response rates[46] than mailed self-administered methods and are more cost effective than interviewer administered. For the longer FFQs, telephone-administered methods may still be too time consuming and cost prohibitive especially for large studies. As technology has progressed, Internet-based methods are gaining in popularity.[66] These methods eliminate the need for a review process since respondents are prompted when items are skipped or incomplete and provide an automated analysis that does not require computer scanning or data entry. Internet-based methods can also provide better portion size estimation tools that may improve accuracy.

## DIETARY SCREENERS

Dietary screeners are abbreviated questionnaires designed to provide rapid cost-effective estimates of usual intake. Screeners are usually presented in the form of food frequency type questionnaires. Screeners may be used to assess overall intake.[67] More typically, screeners are designed to assess intakes and adherence to recommendations of nutrients (e.g., fat[68,69] calcium[70]), and foods or food groups (e.g., fruits and vegetables[71]). Screeners can help to identify individuals at nutritional risk who may require more in-depth evaluation and dietary intervention.[67,72] Programs have been developed for computerized dietary screeners. Toobert et al. reported that computerized as well as paper-and-pencil screeners were significantly correlated with 24 HR in assessing fruit, vegetable, and fat intakes.[73]

The brevity of screeners poses challenges for validity assessment.[74] Many screeners have not shown adequate reliability or validity. Those demonstrating validity have been based on subpopulation studies.[67,75–78]

## DIETARY SUPPLEMENTS

Approximately one-third of children and adolescents and one-half of adults in the U.S. report use of dietary supplements.[79,80] Supplement intake of special populations such as those individuals with cancer diagnosis can be much higher, as high as 80% in some studies.[81] Many types of supplements are available as shown in Table 32.2.

Knowledge of dietary supplements as well as an understanding of assessment methods is critical to the overall assessment of nutrient and other dietary components. Supplement intake data can be assessed in a variety of ways and is usually collected by questionnaire, including FFQs, or as part of intake data collected by 24 HR or by food records. When collected by "daily" methods, it is important to recognize that the intake of supplements for the day of data collection may not reflect the pattern of intake over an extended period of time.[82] Detailed questionnaires, which are better

**TABLE 32.2**
**Categories of Supplements**

| Category | Examples |
|---|---|
| Vitamins (single or multiple formulations) | Vitamin C, E, D, B$_6$ |
| Minerals (single or multiple formulations) | Iron, calcium, chromium, zinc |
| Vitamin(s) with mineral (s) | Calcium with vitamin D; vitamin E with selenium |
| Herbs and other botanicals | St. John's Wort, ginkgo biloba, ginseng, saw palmetto |
| Flavonoids | Quercetin, rutin, hesperidin, diadzin |
| Carotenoids | Lycopene, zeaxanthin, lutein, dried carrot extract, other vegetable extracts |
| Fatty acids/fish oils, other oils | Linoleic acid, omega 3 fatty acids, DHA EPA |
| Amino acids/nucleic acids/proteins including coenzymes, enzymes, and hormones | L-Glutamine, coenzyme Q-10, bromelain, tryptophan |
| Microbial preparations/probiotics | *Lactobacillus acidophilus*, *Bifidobacterium bifidus*, *Lactobacillus bulgaricus* |
| Glandular and other organ preparations | Desiccated glands such thyroid and adrenal |
| Miscellaneous | Shark cartilage, pycnogenol, chrondoitin sulfate |

for capturing long-term intake and frequency of intake, are used frequently in research studies, clinical practice, and nutrition monitoring and surveys.[83]

Quantifying supplement intake can be complicated.[82] When collecting supplement information, it is important to identify what level of detail is needed to describe or quantify total nutrient intakes. Strategies may include having individuals bring in their supplement labels or photocopy the labels. Other strategies include having the participants respond to questionnaires that provide lists of single vitamins and minerals as well as common brand names for multiple formulations. For herbal and botanical ingredients and other components not typically found in common formulations, it might be necessary to identify the active components and, above all else, to obtain brand name and label information. Bailey et al., however, noted that estimating mineral intake in their study was limited by depending on label and not analytic values.[82]

## ISSUES AFFECTING VALIDITY

In his address at the First International Conference on Dietary Assessment Methods, Beaton stated, "There has been a great deal published about the errors in dietary data...

this is understandable, but unfortunate because it can easily leave the impression that dietary data are worthless."[84] He reminded his audience that, while dietary intake data cannot and never will be estimated without error, a serious limitation is not the errors themselves, but failure to understand the nature of the errors and the consequent impact on data analysis and interpretation. Several reviews have delineated potential sources of error for different assessment methods,[3-5] a discussion of which follows. Benefits to minimizing errors are outlined in Table 32.3.

## MEMORY

Daily recalls and FFQs require that respondents remember intakes, albeit for different time frames. Food records intended for completion at the times of meals may be delayed thus requiring recalls of foods eaten.

Our understanding of memory for diet assessment has been developed from advances in cognitive psychology as described by Dwyer et al.[85] Critical memory processes include encoding information, transmission to long-term memory, and retrieval.[86,87] Early studies described strategies for encoding information as well as strategies for retrieving memories, such as free recall, recognition, and cued recall.

**TABLE 32.3**
**Benefits Derived from Minimizing Assessment Errors**

Clinical setting
    Improve ability to detect inadequate, imbalanced, or excessive dietary intake
    Provide a better basis for nutrition counseling and interventions
    Improve ability to monitor dietary changes
Research setting
    Improve accuracy of nutrient intake estimations
    Decrease attenuation between intake data and biomarkers
    Provide a better basis for nutrition education program
    Provide a better basis for elucidation of diet–disease relationships

The memory model of cognitive psychology is applicable to dietary recall.[88] To accurately report intake, people must be able to remember what foods were consumed, how the foods were prepared, and the quantities of foods eaten. This requires the acquisition of specific food memories and the ability to retrieve the memories. Individuals that pay little attention to foods consumed as well as people that have difficulty storing information in memory and those that lack the cognitive ability to retrieve food memories may have difficulty in recalling dietary intake.

Several techniques have been developed to reduce memory-related error in dietary data. For the 24 HR, techniques such as probing (see Figure 31.1), encoding strategies,[88] and multiple-pass memory retrieval cues[43–46] have been employed to improve memory. Campbell and Dodd's[89] classic paper showed that probing elicited additional information with significant impact on total caloric intake. Ervin and Smiciklas-Wright found that older adults were able to remember more foods when a deeper processing strategy was used during encoding and a recognition task was used for memory retrieval.[88] Record-assisted recalls may be used to help reduce memory-related error in food records.[90,91]

## FOOD DESCRIPTION

Identifying and describing foods can be a challenge when detailed information is required. As more foods are eaten away from home, it is difficult to describe the components of mixed dishes and the methods of preparation. Databases that include detailed restaurant data may provide some of the information for analysis. Food frequency methods and dietary screeners may provide limited response options in food names and amounts that may influence data accuracy. In describing the limitations of a brief screener to estimate fast-food and beverage consumption among adolescents, Nelson and Lytle[75] argued that population-specific rather than common instruments may better enable subpopulations to relate to food descriptions.

## RESPONSE BIAS

Various response biases can affect who responds and how accurately people provide dietary data. Response bias can be induced by methods with a high participant burden. For example, the burden of keeping food records may lead subjects to submit incomplete records[18,29] or fail to return instruments.[28]

Social desirability (the tendency to respond in ways consistent with societal beliefs) and social approval (tendency to seek praise) can lead to biased intake data.[92] Some individuals selectively omit foods that may be regarded as unacceptable (e.g., alcohol and high-fat foods),[5] while others may report eating a healthier diet than was actually consumed. Hebert et al. have studied the influence of social desirability among diverse study participants finding difference by gender, education level, food group studied, pre- and post-intervention assessment, and type of instrument used.[92,93] They argue that

the magnitude of bias may distort estimates of diet and health effects and may require models adjusting for biases in data analyses.

For both interviewer-assisted and self-completed assessments, questions should be reviewed for face validity to help ensure that the participant's comprehension of the questions is appropriate. Quality control procedures and monitoring of interviewers can avoid leading questions and verbal and non-verbal cues that may appear to be judgmental.

## CONSUMPTION FREQUENCY

Accurate estimation of how often foods are consumed is important for assessments by FFQ. The cognitive demands required to estimate consumption frequency contribute to the error involved with these methods. For FFQs, frequency of consumption estimates may contribute more error than portion size estimates, and frequency of consumption is a better predictor of contribution to diet than typical serving size.[94,95] Incorporation of portion size and frequency of consumption questions continue to be debated.[95] Willett[4] considers the challenges to selecting proper response format. Options include multiple-choice versus open-ended responses. It has been suggested that the precision of FFQs can be increased by not using predefined consumption frequency categories (i.e., multiple choice), instead allowing participants to simply enter a number to reflect intake (i.e., open-ended).[91] However, multiple-choice categories may lead to fewer errors than open-ended categories. Decisions about the number of response options may also affect ease of recall and precision of responses. Not surprisingly, Willett alludes to FFQ formats as appearing simple but providing opportunities for pitfalls.[22]

## VARIABILITY OF INTAKE

Day-to-day variation of food intake has been well documented in the literature.[17,96–98] Accordingly, assessment of an individual's total dietary intake, particularly by quantitative daily methods, may not yield an accurate measure of usual intake. Basiotis et al.[98] found that over 100 days of dietary data may be needed to accurately estimate an individual's typical intake for certain nutrients, such as vitamin A. Errors associated with variability are seen in 24 HRs, which may not adequately capture day-to-day variation and are also subject to random errors in reporting.[99] To lessen the effect of day-to-day dietary variation when using 24 HRs, assessment should be done on multiple, random, nonconsecutive days[17,100] that include both weekends and weekdays. For food records and 24 HRs, increasing the number of assessment days will decrease error related to variation in food intake; however, this must be balanced with subject tolerability and assessment objectives.

Several statistical approaches have been developed for estimating usual dietary intake distributions at the population level when intake data are collected by 24 HRs. A method developed at Iowa State University, the ISU method, based its estimates from distributions available for two independent days from a subsample of individuals.[40,41] A recent paper by Bailey et al.[83] illustrates the use of the NCI method[101] in estimates of minimum requirements. The National Research Council (NRC) method functions similarly to the ISU method.[102] While these two methods adjust for within-person variability, they do not adequately adjust for underreporting. Freedman et al.[102] adjusted 24 HR energy intake estimates in the OPEN study using doubly labeled water (DLW) as the reference biomarker, allowing for adjustment of underreporting. In doing so, they created the National Research Council Biomarkers (NRC-B), which allows for adjustment of within-person variability as well as underreporting.[99]

## PORTION SIZES

Many individuals have difficulty estimating amounts of foods and beverages. Subar et al.[103] reviewed three factors affecting portion size estimation: perception, conceptualization, and memory (Table 32.4).

Another factor that may affect estimates is unfamiliarity with portion size estimate units. The properties of foods and amounts eaten can contribute to estimating errors. Amorphous foods are more difficult to estimate.[104] Smaller portions tend to be overestimated and larger portions to be underestimated. This is a challenge as larger portions are more widely consumed.[105] Harnack et al. reported that typically used models resulted in underreporting of several foods served in a restaurant. With larger-sized models, reported amounts more closely matched amounts actually consumed.[106] This is consistent with cognitive studies that support respondents' preferences for aids more similar to portions eaten.[104] Cognitive psychologists have recommended aids such as moldable objects or modifiable computer images to assist in portion estimation.[104] Various portion size estimation aids are available (Table 32.5). Aids vary in sophistication and cost. Choice of tools is dictated partially by feasibility. In a clinical setting, aids such as measuring utensils,[39] food replicas,[107] real foods, graduated food models,[108] and food picture books[109] may be more appropriate. For interviews conducted by phone, tools that are compact for mailing, such as a chart with two-dimensional portions,[110] would be more appropriate. Digital photography and computerized portion size estimates are more recent approaches to reducing estimation errors.

## TABLE 32.4
### Factors Affecting Portion Estimations

| | |
|---|---|
| Perception | The ability to relate a food actually present to a portion size aid |
| Conceptualization | The ability to develop a mental picture of a food not present to an aid |
| Memory | The ability to recall an amount of food eaten |

*Source:* Adapted from Subar, A.F. et al., *J. Am. Diet Assoc.*, 134, 1836, 2004.

## TABLE 32.5
### Tools for Portion Size Estimation

| Type | Examples |
|---|---|
| Household measures | • Measuring cups and spoons |
| | • Rulers |
| Food models | • Food replicas |
| | • Graduated food models |
| | • Thickness sticks |
| Pictures | • 2-Dimensional portion shape drawings |
| | • Portion photos of popular foods |
| | • Portion drawings of popular foods |
| | • Computer-based food photography |
| Food labels | • Nutrition facts label |
| | • Food package weights |

Williamson et al.[23] found that estimate by distal photography correlated highly with weighed foods in a study of test meals. Turconi et al. reported that a food photography atlas with foods presented in three portion sizes was valid at the group level for quantifying food portions.[111] Computer-based photographs have been developed for use with self-administered 24 HR.[103] In a 1997 review of the validity of portion estimation aids, the authors concluded that they could not draw conclusive conclusions about guidelines for use given an insufficient research base.[112] The challenge remains given the many types of aids and cognitive factors as well as characteristics of foods.

## SUMMARY

Valid assessment of dietary intake is critical for understanding associations between food, beverage, and supplement intake and health and disease. Inaccurate information can obscure true relationships. Unquestionably, providing valid information is a challenge. Individuals may under- or over-report intakes for reasons already discussed. Considerable attention has focused on energy intakes underreported from 10% to 40%[43,113–115] with consequences for assessment of dietary components.[115] A number of prediction equations have been developed for estimating minimum energy requirements and establishing cutoffs for plausible, under-, and overreporters.[116,117] Plausible reporting, but not underreporting, has been shown to be a significant predictor of body mass index in young girls.[118] Reporting inaccuracies occur with all methods. Reviews of methods and comparisons of methods continue. In their study of dietary misreporting in the OPEN Study, using DLW as reference, Subar et al.[119] found more underreporting with an FFQ than 24 HRs. They also indicated that accuracy declines the more respondents consume, suggesting that more foods and larger portion sizes present a challenge to accurate reporting. Recently, Carroll et al. examined issues of bias, power, and sample when discussing the use of 24 HR and FFQ in cohort studies. With the development of Internet-based 24 HR and FFQ, the authors proposed circumstances in which multiple 24 HR alone or 24 HR and an FFQ could be appropriate.[120] Given the importance of dietary data, it is not surprising that it is a dynamic field of study with new methods such as computer-assisted techniques undergoing development and testing. Much work is needed to reduce both systematic and random errors. Development of new, innovative techniques and rigorous assessment of methodological validity will strengthen confidence in dietary data assessments.

## DATA ANALYSIS

Data analysis is the second phase in deriving information about foods/beverages and dietary components consumed. While data entry and database are critical components, there is a synergy as more interactive software programs are available.

### DATA ENTRY

Data entry is the link between the information provided by the respondent and the database used to analyze reported intakes. Data entry requires decisions to adapt intake information to meet the demands of a selected data analysis system.[121] Data entry staff must decide on reasonable substitutions if respondents provide insufficient information about food descriptions and portion sizes or the database lacks information about specific foods consumed. The use of interactive software programs with detailed probing guides and automatic coding has facilitated the data entry process. Nevertheless strict coding and data entry rules and documentation of decisions are essential in research studies.

### DATABASES

Complete and accurate food and nutrient databases are essential for the assessment of dietary intakes and are an integral part of most software used to collect, process, and analyze dietary data (see Chapters 1 and 6). The core nutrient and food values in most U.S. databases or dietary analysis software programs are based on the U.S. Department of Agriculture National Nutrient Database for Standard Reference (SR).[122] Food composition data have been made available by USDA's Nutrient Data Laboratory (NDL) for over 115 years providing analytical data when possible on most foods. Today the SR database contains values for nearly 8000 foods and 146 nutrients and is a publicly available database that can be used by anyone. In addition to common nutrient values, the NDL provides special interest data tables for other food components such choline and choline metabolites and phytonutrients such as flavonoids, isoflavone, and oxalic acid.

The SR database is used to develop the Food and Nutrient Database for Dietary Studies (FNDDS), which is the database that is used to analyze national survey data or What We Eat in America, the dietary intake portion of the National Health and Nutrition Examination Survey (NHANES).[123] The FNDDS is developed and maintained by USDA's Food Surveys Research Group and uses the SR database for its nutrient values used to assess and monitor dietary behaviors of the American population.

In addition, there are many other commercially available databases. These databases and software programs also rely heavily on USDA's SR database for the development of their databases. Databases such as the University of Minnesota's Nutrition Database for Research (NDSR)[124] uses the SR database for core foods but have greatly expanded on the nutrient and other food components as well as a large database of brand-specific and ethnic foods. The primary differences in databases are in the number of foods, the details about foods including preparation and ingredients, brand specificity, number of nutrients, completeness of nutrients values or number of missing values, and the accuracy of the nutrient values. No database is 100% complete, and many nutrients and other food component values may be imputed from other similar foods rather than based on analytical data. It is important to explore the documentation provided by software companies about their databases. Among the concerns that should be explored are the source of the data for nutrients and foods of interest, missing data and completeness of the data, appropriateness of foods available in the database including how often is it updated, and how reflective of the marketplace are the data for the time period of data collection.

## DIETARY QUALITY INDICATORS

Assessing dietary quality can be challenging given the many dietary factors that can affect health. An ever-growing variety of foods, many dietary components, food preparation methods, and eating behaviors may function in ways that are antagonistic or synergistic to good health. The following are some of the strategies developed to capture dietary quality.

### INDEXES

Many dietary quality indexes have been developed to assess relationships between diet, health, and disease. Kant described the following three major types of indexes: indexes derived from nutrients only; indexes derived from foods/food groups only; and those based on combination of nutrients and foods.[125] To Kant's three categories can be added indexes that include eating behaviors such as eating motivation and dietary restraint.[126] Some indexes are developed for general population use, others for specific groups (e.g., children,[127] older adults[128]).

Indexes based only on nutrients frequently estimated intakes to recommended nutrient intakes such as the Dietary Reference Intakes.[129] The Nutrient Adequacy Ratio (NAR) is calculated by dividing estimated intake by recommended intake.[130] A Mean Adequacy Ratio (MAR) is derived as a multiple nutrient index from individuals NARs.[131] Drewnowski proposed a "naturally nutrient rich" score based on a nutrient-to-energy intake ratio.[132] de Koning et al. have used a similar approach to calculate carbohydrate scores based on percentages of energy from carbohydrates, fats, and proteins.[133]

Food-only indexes are estimates of the number of servings or cup/ounce equivalents of selected items such as coffee[134] or grains.[135] Estimated intakes can be compared with national guidelines such as those developed by the U.S. Department of Agriculture[136] or other groups.[137]

Increasingly, global nutrition indexes have been proposed in total diet quality assessment. The Healthy Eating Index,[138] the Alternative Healthy Eating Index,[139] the Diet Quality Index,[140] and the Diet Quality Index Revised[141] are only a few of the many indexes developed in the United States and internationally, and which may include nutrients and foods, as well as eating behaviors and dietary variety. Some indexes are developed primarily to assess population intakes against national guidelines,[138] and others may be more focused on disease risk assessment[139] or clinical trial outcomes.[141] Differences in food group schemes, on placement of foods into groups, on definitions of serving sizes, and on scoring algorithms present methodological challenges in comparing indexes.

## Dietary Patterns

Dietary pattern analysis is used increasingly to reflect the complexity and interrelatedness of dietary intakes. Anderson et al. described dietary pattern analysis as follows:

> Dietary pattern analysis can capture the complexity of the diet because it accounts for the high correlation among intakes of specific foods and nutrients as well as interactive effects of foods and nutrients, which are often interdependent in their bioavailability. (p. 84)[142]

Dietary patterns have been derived from FFQs,[142,143] daily intake methods,[144] and dietary screeners.[131] A number of statistical techniques including factor, cluster, and principle component analyses have been used to examine dietary patterns. With these methods, foods are combined into composite variables or patterns that are reasonably homogeneous. As with indexes, many food grouping schemes are used in the numerous dietary pattern studies. Across many studies, however, patterns that are identified as "prudent," "healthy," and "nutrient dense" are characterized by higher intakes of fruits, vegetables, low-fat dairy, fish and poultry, and whole grains. Dietary patterns with higher levels of red meats, sugar-sweetened beverages, high-fat dairy products, and desserts are associated with increased risk of many chronic diseases and mortality.[142,145]

## Energy Density

Energy density is another way that dietary quality can be addressed. Energy density refers to the amount of energy in a particular weight of food. It is generally presented as the number of calories in a gram. Foods with a low-energy density provide less energy relative to their weight than foods with a high-energy density. Energy density values, which are influenced by the moisture content and macronutrient composition of foods, range from 0 to 9 kcal/g. The component of food with the greatest impact on energy density is water.[146] Water has an energy density of 0 kcal/g as it contributes weight but not energy to foods. Foods with high water content, such as fruits and vegetables, have a relatively low energy density. Fiber also has a relatively low energy density, providing 1.5–2.5 kcal/g and can lower the energy density of foods. However, the influence of fiber on energy density is more modest than that of water since only a limited amount can be added to foods. On the opposite end of the energy density spectrum, fat is the most energy-dense component of food. Fat increases the energy content of foods, providing 9 kcal/g, more than twice as many as carbohydrates or protein, which provide 4 kcal/g.

Energy density values reported in the literature have been calculated by a variety of different methods that include only food, as well as food and various combinations of beverages, such as all beverages, all beverages excluding water, energy-containing beverages, milk, juice, and so forth, with no current standard method of calculation.[147] Though commonly studies exclude all beverages since energy density values vary widely depending on the beverage inclusion method, studies investigating energy density should clearly define the treatment of beverages.[147] Although insufficient data are available to state definitively which beverage calculation method is superior, calculations based on food, excluding all beverages, are becoming increasingly common. This method lacks some of the controversies associated with other methods. For example, values based on food and all beverages (including water) are rarely reported in the literature, as water intake is not commonly collected in research studies. Calculations based on food and all beverages excluding water may not provide meaningful measures of dietary energy density because noncaloric beverages such as diet cola, coffee, and tea are not excluded. Additionally, values based on food- and energy-containing beverages may lead to increased within-person variance values, which may diminish associations with outcome variables.[148]

While calculating dietary energy density can be challenging due to the data coding and manipulations necessary to appropriately deal with beverages, evidence indicates that there exists a positive association between energy density and body weight.[147] Though some mixed results do exist,[147,149–153] clinical trials have evidenced that reduced dietary ED is associated with successful weight loss and maintenance.[154,155] Furthermore, given that low-energy-dense diets have been associated with high intakes of fruits and vegetables, high intakes of fiber, high intakes of a variety of vitamins and minerals, and good overall diet quality,[156] the dietary energy density values appear to be a marker for a healthy diet pattern.

## Glycemic Index/Glycemic Load

Because of the considerable attention given to low-carbohydrate diet approaches and the new Dietary Guidelines emphasis on whole grains, interest in carbohydrate quality as assessed by glycemic index and glycemic load is increasing.[157] International tables of glycemic index values[158] are quickly becoming integrated into nutrient databases used to enter, collect, and analyze dietary data.

Glycemic index is the scale used to classify the quality of carbohydrate by its potential to increase blood glucose independent of its carbohydrate content, whereas the glycemic load of the diet reflects the total glycemic effect of the diet and is the product of the carbohydrate content of each food and its glycemic index value.[158] Carbohydrate-containing foods vary widely with respect to their glycemic response. Many dietary factors such as grain size and structure, fiber content, cooking methods, amylose content, previous meal, and satiety all play a role in the total glycemic effect of the diet.[159] Glycemic index is measured in vivo by comparing the glucose responses of a test food with an amount of carbohydrate equivalent to a reference food (usually 25 or 50 g of glucose or starch). Because of the differences in methodology and the wide variety of factors affecting glycemic response, the glycemic values of foods vary considerably, and for this reason, assessing glycemic is still somewhat controversial. Databases are still somewhat incomplete, and not unlike nutrient databases and other food component databases, they are subject to errors in measurement and interpolation.

A lower dietary glycemic index and glycemic load of the diet has, nevertheless, been shown to have beneficial health effects by altering metabolic endpoints such as improved blood glucose, insulin, and lipid levels; improved glycemic control in diabetes; decreased fat mass; and reduced colon cancer risk.[160–165] Recently, Davis et al. studied the glycemic load of older adults, finding that a healthier dietary pattern was associated with a lower glycemic index and glycemic load.[157]

Any method of assessing an individual's dietary intake is dependent on the methods of interpretation. More comprehensive methods of interpretation may facilitate the identification of more specific patterns of intake and their relationship to disease.

## Summary

The importance of dietary data as well as the challenges in collecting, analyzing, and interpreting what people eat and drink has been presented in this report. Advances at all three levels (i.e., collection, analysis, and interpretation) have been considered.[6] Most notably, technological innovations have impacted collection and processing of dietary data. Innovative methods continue to be developed and validated. Devices that can allow participants to record food as it is eaten, can capture photographic records of foods, and can transmit to software may help reduce respondent burden and facilitate data processing.[166] The expertise of nutritionists and other health professionals will remain paramount in applying dietary data to improving health of individuals and communities.

## REFERENCES

1. Bingham, S, *Nutr Abstr Rev (Series A)* 57:705;1987.
2. Life Sciences Research Office, Guidelines for use of dietary intake data, Federation of American Societies for Experimental Biology, Bethesda, MD, 1996.
3. Gibson, RS, *Principles of Nutrition Assessment*, 2nd edn., Oxford University Press, New York, 2005.
4. Willett, W, *Nutritional Epidemiology*, 2nd edn., Oxford University Press, New York, 1998.
5. Dwyer, J, In: Shils, ME, Olson, JA, Shike, M, Ross, AC, eds., *Modern Nutrition in Health and Disease*, 9th edn., Williams & Wilkins, Philadelphia, PA, 1999, p. 937.
6. Millen, BE, *J Am Diet Assoc* 110:1166;2010.
7. Christakis, G, *Am J Public Health* 63:1S;1973.
8. Bingham, S, Luben, R, Welch, A et al., *Int J Epidemiol* 37:978;2008.
9. Key, TJ, Abbleby, PN, Cairns, BJ, *Am J Clin Nutr* 201:1043;2011.
10. Feskanich, D, Rimm, EB, Giovannuci, EL et al., *J Am Diet Assoc* 93:790;1993.
11. Kristal, AR, Feng, Z, Coates, RJ et al., *Am J Epidemiol* 146:856;1997.
12. Kumanyika, S, Mauger, D, Mitchell, DC et al., *Ann Epidemiol* 13:111;2003.
13. Sushama, DA, Elci, OU, Sereika, SM, *J Am Diet Assoc* 111:583;2011.
14. Baker, RC, Kirschenbaum, DS, *Behav Ther* 24:377;1993.
15. Helsel, DL, Jakicic, JM, Otto, AD, *J Am Diet Assoc* 107:1807;2007.
16. St. Jeor, ST, Guthrie, HA, Jones, MB, *J Am Diet Assoc* 83:155 1983.
17. Tarasuk, V, Beaton, GH, *Am J Clin Nutr* 54:464;1991.
18. Gersovitz, M, Madden, JP, Smiciklas-Wright, H, *J Am Diet Assoc* 73:48;1978.
19. Bingham, SA, *Ann Nutr Metab* 35:117;1991.
20. Omnibus Budget Reconciliation Act of 1990, Public Law 101-508;1990.
21. Andrews, YN, Castellanos, VH, *J Am Diet Assoc* 103:873;2003.
22. Gittelsohn, J, Shankar, AV, Pokhrel, RP, West, KP, Jr., *J Am Diet Assoc* 94:1273;1994.
23. Williamson, DA, Allen, HR, Martin, PD et al., *J Am Diet Assoc* 103:1139;2003.
24. Kolar, AS, Patterson, RE, White, E et al., *Epidemiology* 16:579;2005.
25. Kwan, ML, Kushi, LH, Song, J et al., *Am J Epidemiol* 172:1315;2010.
26. Craig, ML, Kristal, AR, Cheney, CL, Shattuck, AL, *J Am Diet Assoc* 100:421;2000.
27. Rebro, SM, Patterson, RE, Kristal, AR, Cheney, CL, *J Am Diet Assoc* 98, 1163;1998.
28. Lancaster, KJ, Smiciklas-Wright, H, Kumanyika, SK et al., *J Am Diet Assoc* 100:1532;2000.
29. Sudo, N, Perry, C, Reicks, M, *J Am Diet Assoc* 110:95;2010.
30. Six, BL, Schap, TE, Zhu, FM et al., *J Am Diet Assoc* 110:74;2010.
31. Arab, L, Winter, A, *J Am Diet Assoc* 110:1238;2010.
32. McClung, HL, Sigrist, LD, Smith, TJ et al., *J Am Diet Assoc* 109:1241;2009.

33. Mathiessen, TB, Steinberg, FM, Kaiser, LL, *J Am Diet Assoc* 111:750;2011.

34. Austin, GL, Ogden, LG, Hill, JO, *Am J Clin Nutr* 93:836;2011.

35. Arab, L, Cambou, MC, Craft, N et al., *Am J Clin Nutr* 93:1102;2011.

36. Copeland, T, Grosvenor, M, Mitchell, DC et al., *J Am Diet Assoc* 100:1186;2000.

37. Hendrie, GA, Golley, GK, *Am J Clin Nutr* 93:1117;2011.

38. Satia, JA, Watters, JL, Galanko, JA, *J Am Diet Assoc* 109:502;2009.

39. Centers for Disease Control and Prevention, National Health and Nutrition Examination Survey, http://www.cdc.gov/nchs/nhanes.htm, accessed March 26, 2012.

40. Nusser, SM, Carriquiry, AL, Dodd, KW, Fuller, WA, *J Am Stat Assoc* 91:1440;1996.

41. Guenther, PM, Kott, PS, Carriquiry, AL, *J Nutr* 127:1106;1996.

42. Buzzard, IM, Faucett, CL, Jeffery, RW et al., *J Am Diet Assoc* 96:574;1996.

43. Jonnalagadda, SS, Mitchell, DC, Smiciklas-Wright, H et al., *J Am Diet Assoc* 100:303;2000.

44. Johnson, RK, Driscoll, P, Goran, MI, *J Am Diet Assoc* 96:1140;1996.

45. Conway, JM, Ingerwersen, LA, Vinyard, BT, Moshfegh, AJ, *Am J Clin Nutr* 77:1171;2003.

46. Fox, TA, Heimendinger, J, Block, G, *J Am Diet Assoc* 92:729;1992.

47. Derr, JA, Mitchell, DC, Brannon, D et al., *Am J Epidemiol*, 136:1386;1992.

48. Baranowski, T, Islam, N, Baranowski, J et al., *J Am Diet Assoc* 102:380;2002.

49. Subar, AF, Thompson, FE, Potischman, N et al., *J Am Diet Assoc* 107:1002;2007.

50. Arab, L, Wesseling-Perry, K, Jardack, P et al., *J Am Diet Assoc* 110:857;2010.

51. http://riskfactor.cancer.gov/tools/instruments/asa24/, accessed March 26, 2012.

52. Conway, JM, Ingwersen, LA, Mushfegh, AJ, *J Am Diet Assoc* 104:95;2004.

53. Nutrition Coordinating Center, Nutrient Data Systems for Research (NDS-R) software, University of Minnesota, Minneapolis, MN.

54. Burke, BS, *J Am Diet Assoc* 23:1041;1947.

55. Block, G, Hartman, AM, Naughton, D, *Epidemiology* 1:58;1990.

56. Cade, J, Thompson, R, Burley, V et al., *Pub Health Nutr* 5(4):567;2002.

57. Subar, AF, *J Am Diet Assoc* 104:769;2004.

58. Subar, AF, Dodd, KW, Guenther, PM et al. *J Am Diet Assoc* 106:1556;2006.

59. Subar, AF, Thompson, FE, Smith, AF et al., *J Am Diet Assoc* 95:781;1995.

60. Potischman, N, Carroll, RJ, Iturria, SJ et al., *Nutr Cancer* 34:70;1999.

61. Lund, SM, Brown, J, Harnack, L, *Eur J Clin Nutr* 52:S53;1998.

62. Kipnis, V, Subar, AF, Midthune, D et al., *Am J Epidemiol* 158:14;2003.

63. Laus, MJ, Cohen, NL, Smickilas-Wright, HA et al., *J Nutr Elder* 18:1;1999.

64. Molag, ML, de Vries, JHM, Ocke, MC et al., *Am J Epidemiol* 166(12):1468;2007.

65. Clapp, JA, McPherson, RS, Reed, DB et al., *J Am Diet Assoc* 91(3):316;1991.

66. NutritionQuest, Berkeley, CA, NutrtionQuest Home Page, http://www.nutritionquest.com/, accessed March 15, 2012.

67. Bailey, RL, Miller, PE, Mitchell, DC et al., *Am J Clin Nutr* 90:177;2009.

68. Mochari, H, Gao, Q, Mosca, L, *J Am Diet Assoc* 108:817;2008.

69. Williams, GC, Hurley, TG, Thompson, FE et al., *J Nutr* 138:212S;2008.

70. Hacker-Thompson, A, Robertson, TP, Sellmeyer, DE, *J Am Diet Assoc* 109:1237;2009.

71. Peterson, KE, Hebert, JR, Hurley, TG, *J Nutr* 138:218S;2008.

72. McNaughton, SA, Ball, K, Crawford, D et al., *J Nutr* 138:86;2008.

73. Toobert, DJ, Strycker, LA, Hampson, SE et al., *J Am Diet Assoc* 111:1578;2011.

74. Nelson, MC, Lytle, LA, *J Am Diet Assoc* 109:730;2009.

75. Ceni, H, Rossi, C, Turconi, G, *Eur J Nutr* 47:1;2008.

76. Thompson, FE, Midthune, D, Subar, AF et al., *J Am Diet Assoc* 107(S):760;2007.

77. Wiens, L, Schulzer, M, Chen, C, Parinas, K, *J Am Diet Assoc* 110:101;2010.

78. Phillips, MB, Foley, AL, Barnard, R et al., *Asia Pac J Clin Nutr* 19:440;2010.

79. Picciano, MF, Dwyer, JT, Radimer, KL et al., *Arch Pediatr Adolesc Med* 161:978;2007.

80. Bailey, RL, Gahche, JJ, Lentino, CV et al., *J Nutr* 141:261;2011.

81. Winters, BL, Mitchell, DC, Grosvenor, M et al., *FASEB J* 13:A253;1999.

82. Dwyer, J, Picciano, MF, Raiten, DJ, *J Nutr* 133:590S;2003.

83. Bailey, RL, Fulgoni, VL 3rd, Keast, DR, Dwyer, JT, *Am J Clin Nutr* 94:1376;2011.

84. Beaton, GH, *Am J Clin Nutr* 59:253S 1994.

85. Dwyer, JT, Krall, EA, Coleman, KA, *J Am Diet Assoc* 87:1509;1987.

86. Wessells, MG, *Cognitive Psychology*, Harper & Row Publishers, New York, 1982.

87. Craik, FIM, *Philos Trans R Soc Lond B Biol Sci* 302:341;1993.

88. Ervin, RB, Smiciklas-Wright, H, *J Am Diet Assoc* 98:984;1998.

89. Campbell, VA, Dodds, ML, *J Am Diet Assoc* 51:29;1967.

90. Lytle, LA, Nichaman, MZ, Obarzanek, E et al., *J Am Diet Assoc* 93:1431;1993.

91. Eldridge, AL, Smith-Warner, SA, Lytle, LA, Murray, DM, *J Am Diet Assoc* 98:777;1998.

92. Hebert, JR, Peterson, KE, Hurley, TG et al., *Ann Epidemiol* 11:417;2001.

93. Hebert, JR, Hurley, TG, Peterson, KE et al., *J Nutr* 138:2265; 2008.

94. Flegal, KM, Larkin, FA, Metzner, HL et al., *Am J Epidemiol* 128:749;1988.

95. Thompson, FE, Subar, AF, In: Coulson, AM, Rock, CL, Monsen, ER, eds., *Nutrition in the Prevention and Treatment of Disease*, Academic Press, San Diego, CA, p. 3, 2001.

96. Guthrie, HA, Crocetti, AF, *J Am Diet Assoc* 85:325;1985.

97. McAvay, G, Rodin, *J Appetite* 11:97;1988.

98. Basiotis, PP, Welsh, SO, Cronin, FJ et al., *J Nutr* 117:1638;1987.

99. Yaneetz, R, Carroll, RJ, Dodd, KW, *J Am Diet Assoc* 108:455;2008.

100. Hartman, AM, Brown, CC, Palmgren, J et al., *Am J Epidemiol* 132:999;1990.

101. National Cancer Institute, Usual dietary intakes: The NCI method, 2009, http://riskfactor.cancer.gov/diet/usualintakes/method.html, accessed March 26, 2012.

102. Freedman, LS, Midthune, D, Carroll, RJ et al., *J Nutr* 134:1836;2004.

103. Subar, AF, Crafts, J, Zimmerman, TP et al., *J Am Diet Assoc* 134:1836;2004.

104. Chambers, E IV, Godwin, SL, Vecchio, FA, *J Am Diet Assoc* 100:891;2000.

105. Smiciklas-Wright, H, Mitchell, DC, Mickle, SJ et al., *J Am Diet Assoc* 103:41;2003.

106. Harnack, L, Steffen, L, Arnett, DK et al., *J Am Diet Assoc* 104:804;2004.

107. NASCO, *Nasco Nutrition Teaching Aids*, 1990–2000 Catalog, Number 437, NASCO, Fort Atkinson, WI, 1999.

108. National Center for Health Statistics, Dietary intake source data: United States, 1976–1980 (DHHS publication no. PHS 83-1681), Series 11, No. 231, U.S. Department of Health and Human Services, Washington, DC, 1983.

109. Hess, MA, *Portion Photos of Popular Foods*, Ed. American Dietetic Association Center for Nutrition Education, University of Wisconsin, Stout, WI, 1997.

110. Nutrition Consulting Enterprises, *Food Portion Visual*, Nutrition Consulting Enterprises, Framingham, MA, 1981.

111. Turconi, G, Guarcello, M, Berzolari, FG et al., *Eur J Clin Nutr* 59:923;2005.

112. Cypel, YS, Guenther, PM, Petot, GJ, *J Am Diet Assoc* 97:289;1997.

113. Schoeller, DA, *Metabolism* 44:18;1995.

114. Seale, JL, Klein, G, Friedmann, J et al., *Nutrition* 18:568;2002.

115. Millen, AA, Tooze, JA, Subar, AF et al., *J Am Diet Assoc* 109:1194;2009.

116. McCrory, MA, Hajduk, CL, Roberts, SB, *Public Health Nutr* 5:873;2002.

117. Huang, TT, Howarth, NC, Lin, BH et al., *Obes Res* 12:1875;2004.

118. Savage, JS, Mitchell, DC, Smiciklas-Wright, H et al., *J Am Diet Assoc* 108:131;2008.

119. Subar, AF, Kipnis, V, Troiano, RP et al., *Am J Epidemiol* 158:1;2003.

120. Carroll, RJ, Midthune, D, Subar, AF et al., *Am J Epidemiol* 175:340;2012.

121. Lacy, JM. Coder variability in computerized dietary analysis, Research Bulletin Number 729, Massachusetts Agricultural Experiment Station, MA, 1990.

122. U.S. Department of Agriculture, Agricultural Research Service, USDA National Nutrient Database for Standard Reference, Release 24, Nutrient Data Laboratory Home Page, 2011, http://www.ars.usda.gov/nutrientdata

123. Ahuja, JKA, Montville, JB, Omolewa-Tomobi, G, Heendeniya, KY, Martin, CL, Steinfeldt, LC, Anand, J, Adler, ME, LaComb, RP, and Moshfegh, AJ, USDA Food and Nutrient Database for Dietary Studies, 5.0. U.S. Department of Agriculture, Agricultural Research Service, Food Surveys Research Group, Beltsville, MD, 2012.

124. Nutrition Data System for Research (NDSR), University of Minnesota, Nutrition Coordinating Center Nutrition Coordinating Center Home Page, http://www.ncc.umn.edu/index.html, accessed March 5, 2012.

125. Kant, AK, *J Am Diet Assoc* 96:785;1996.

126. Cahill, JM, Freeland-Graves, JH, Shah, BS et al., *J Am Diet Assoc* 109:1593;2009.

127. Kranz, S, Hartman, T, Siega-Riz, AM, Herring, AH, *J Am Diet Assoc* 106:1594;2006.

128. Kourlaba, G, Polychronopoulos, E, Zampelas, A et al., *J Am Diet Assoc* 109:1022;2009.

129. Food and Nutrition Board, *Dietary Reference Intakes for Calcium and Vitamin D*, National Academy Press, Washington, DC, 2011.

130. Guthrie, HA, Scheer, JC, *J Am Diet Assoc* 78:240;1981.

131. Bailey, RI., Mitchell, DC, Miller, CK et al., *J Nutr* 137:1;2007.

132. Drewnowski, A, *Am J Clin Nutr* 82:721;2005.

133. de Koning, L, Fung, TT, Liao, X et al., *Am J Clin Nutr* 93:844;2011.

134. Kempf, K, Herder, C, Erlund, I et al., *Am J Clin Nutr* 91:950;2010.

135. Newby, PK, Maras, J, Bakun, P et al., *Am J Clin Nutr* 85:1745;2007.

136. ChooseMyPlate.gov-USDA, accessed March 15, 2012.

137. Appel, LJ, Champagne, CM, Harsha, DW et al., *JAMA* 289:2083;2003.

138. Guenter, PM, Reedy, J, Krebs-Smith, SM, *J Am Diet Assoc* 108:1896;2008.

139. McCullough, ML, Feskanich, D, Stampfer, MJ et al., *Am J Clin Nutr* 76:1261;2002.

140. Patterson, RE, Haines, PS, Popkin, BM, *J Am Diet Assoc* 94:57;1994.

141. Snyder, DL, Sloane, R, Haines, PS et al., *J Am Diet Assoc* 107:1519;2009.

142. Anderson, AL, Harris, TB, Tylavsky, FA et al., *J Am Diet Assoc* 111:84;2011.

143. Tucker, KL, Dallal, GE, Rush, D, *J Am Diet Assoc* 92:1487;1992.

144. Ledikwe, JH, Smiciklas-Wright, H, Mitchell, DC et al., *J Am Geriatr Soc* 52:589;2004.

145. Mitrou, PN, Kipnis, V, Thiebaut, AC et al., *Arch Int Med* 167:2461;2007.

146. Rolls, BJ, Bell, EA, In *Medical Clinics of North America*, Jensen, MD, ed., W.B. Saunders Company, Philadelphia, PA, p. 84, 401, 2000.

147. Vernarelli, JA, Mitchell, DC, Hartman, TJ, Rolls, BJ, *J Nutr* 141:12;2011.

148. Cox, DN, Mela, DJ, *Int J Obes* 29:49;2000.

149. Ledikwe, JH, Blanck, HM, Kettel Khan, L et al., *Am J Clin Nutr* 83:6;2006.

150. Kant, AK, Graubard, BI, *Int J Obes* 29:8;2005.

151. Stookey, JD, *Eur J Clin Nutr* 55:5;2001.

152. Howarth, NC, Murphy, SP, Wilkens, LR et al., *J Nutr* 136:8;2006.

153. de Castro, JM, *J Nutr* 132:2;2004.

154. Ledikwe, JH, Rolls, BJ, Smiciklas-Wright, H et al., *Am J Clin Nutr* 85:5;2007.

155. Ello-Martin, JA, Roe, LS, Ledikwe, JH et al., *Am J Clin Nutr* 85:6;2007.

156. Ledikwe, JH, Blanck, HM, Kettel-Khan, L et al., *J Am Diet Assoc* 106:8;2006.

157. Davis, MS, Miller, CK, Mitchell DM, *J Am Diet Assoc* 104:1828;2004.

158. Foster-Powell, K, Holt, SH, Brand-Miller, JC, *Am J Clin Nutr* 76 (1):51;2002.

159. Venn, BJ, Mann JI, *Eur J Clin Nutr* 58:1443;2004.

160. Giacco, R, Parillo, M, Rivellese, AA et al., *Diabetes Care* 23:1461;2000.

161. Jarvi, AE, Karlstrom, BE, Granfeldt, YE et al., *Diabetes Care* 23:10;1999.

162. Jenkins, DJ, Kendall, CW, Augustin, LS et al., *Am J Clin Nutr* 76 (Suppl): 266S;2002.

163. Chiu, C-J, Liu, S, Willett, WC et al., *Nutr Rev* 69(4):231;2011.

164. Salmeron, J, Manson, JE, Stampfer, MJ et al., *J Am Med Assoc* 277:472;1997.

165. Bouche, C, Rizkalla, SW, Luo, J et al., *Diabetes Care* 25:822;2002.

166. Thompson, FE, Subar, AF, Loria, CM et al., *J Am Diet Assoc* 110:48;2010.

# 33 Use of Food Frequency Questionnaires in Minority Populations

*Rebecca S. Reeves*

## CONTENTS

Food frequency questionnaires (FFQs) are selected by investigators to assess the usual food or nutrient intakes of groups or individuals because they are relatively easy to administer, are less expensive than other dietary assessment methods, and can be adapted to all racial and ethnic populations in the United States.[1] Investigators can also modify these dietary instruments for telephone interviews or a self-administered mailed survey. FFQs are commonly used in epidemiological studies on diet and disease but are also chosen by investigators as the dietary assessment instrument in clinical intervention studies. The use of these questionnaires in minority populations in the United States is increasing for several reasons: The country is becoming more racially and ethnically diverse,[2] government agencies have placed emphasis on including minority populations in health-related research,[3] and variations in disease incidence and dietary practices within and across ethnic minorities offer important opportunities for examining the role of diet in relation to risk of chronic disease.[4]

This chapter reviews 23 published studies evaluating the validity and/or reliability of FFQs used in measuring dietary intakes in adult minority populations in the United States over the last 23 years. Also included in this chapter are selected samples of FFQs and information on obtaining copies of them. Recommendations on the use of these FFQs are discussed.

A search of the National Library of Medicine's (Bethesda, MD) MEDLINE system was conducted using various terms such as *validity, reliability, reproducibility, diet,* FFQ, *minority, Hispanic, Black, Asian, Pacific islander, and Native America* to identify articles published between 1980 and 2005. These searches were supplemented by cross-referencing from author reference lists.

Articles were selected that described the evaluation of any FFQ that assessed the usual daily diet and provided data on the validity and/or reliability of the instrument in a specific U.S. ethnic minority population or a diverse population representing at least 40% minority persons. The degree of reliability or validity of the instrument reported was not considered an inclusion factor. Validity and reliability studies that were reported in the same article were considered separately and are referenced in different tables. The measures of performance that were chosen were reliability, comparison of means (when available), and validity because these are usually reported to describe the results of the evaluation of the FFQ. Correlation coefficients were selected as indicators of reliability and validity because they are commonly used and are more easily summarized. Factors that can influence correlation coefficients are the number of days between the times the questionnaire is administered (reliability coefficients) and the number of days of food records or 24 h recalls used for the referent period (validity coefficients). Adjusted and unadjusted correlation coefficients are reported in the tables. The methods for adjusting the coefficients are discussed in each article.

The terms used to describe FFQs in the tables are as follows:

*Quantitative*—quantity of food consumed was estimated using weights, measures, or food models. Responses were open-ended.

*Semiquantitative*—quantity of food consumed was estimated using a standard portion size, serving, or a predetermined amount and the respondent was asked about the number of portions consumed.

*Nonquantitative*—quantity of food was not assessed.

*Self-administered*—an adult completed the dietary assessment without assistance.

*Interviewer administered*—a trained interviewer collected the dietary information from the adult in a one-on-one setting.

The 23 studies reviewed for this chapter included adult groups representing ethnic minorities, African-American, Hispanic, Asian, or a combination of an ethnic minority and a Caucasian group. Eight[5–12] studies represent only ethnic minorities and 15[13–27] are a combination of an ethnic minority and white participants.

The review of the validation studies on FFQs was not conclusive. Pearson's correlations (Table 33.1) between questionnaire-based estimates of nutrient intakes and estimates derived from 24 h recalls or records were not consistent for ethnic groups, but trends were suggested. Pearson correlations for black males and females across validation studies were in the range of 0.27–0.70 for Hispanic females, 0.32–0.49 except for two studies, one conducted in Starr County, Texas, which reported a correlation of 0.75,[9] and one conducted with low-income Hispanic males and females living in San Francisco Bay area, which reported a correlation of 0.68,[10] and for white males and females, 0.53, and Asian males and females, 0.53. If one considers a measure of ≥0.05 as satisfactory or good, 0.30–0.49 as fair, and <0.30 as poor,[22] then these correlations suggest that black and Hispanic groups do not perform well on FFQs unless special efforts are made to administer the questionnaires.

The validation correlations for total energy, total fat, and vitamin A were inconsistent across studies. In Table 33.2, the correlation coefficients for total fat ranged from 0.18 to 0.65 with the higher correlations usually found in the Asian or white populations. A similar trend was found for energy among the various groups. The correlation coefficients for Hispanic and black populations were commonly in the range of 0.24–0.43, but in the white and Asian groups, the coefficients ranged from 0.41 to 0.61. Values for vitamin A were more inconsistent ranging from 0.15 to 0.67 across all groups. The number of days of food records and recalls that are compared against FFQs can explain some of these low correlations especially for vitamin A. Many days are required to provide a precise estimate of vitamin A intake, and in these studies, the greatest number of daily recalls or records collected over 1 year was 28. Even in this study certain subgroup correlations for vitamin A were still 0.23 and 0.29.

Four studies report serum nutrient concentrations of carotenoids, vitamin E, lycopene, and lutein as a referent.[7,12,25,27] One of these studies reported correlations that were much lower for smokers <0.02 than for non-smokers <0.40.[5] In the study by Satia et al.,[25] the authors examined the validity of a 92 item antioxidant nutrient questionnaire. For most nutrients, there were linear trends of increasing plasma concentrations with higher questionnaire-derived intakes. The investigators of these studies summarized that using nutrient biomarkers demonstrated

their FFQs are reasonably valid for use in southern, urban, low-income black populations except for the analysis of lutein and lycopene. Another study comparing adipose tissue fatty acids and dietary fat intake collected from eight different 24 h recalls and a 200 item FFQ confirmed previous findings that 24 h recalls are valid for assessing dietary intake of different types of fat.[14] The correlation of FFQ values for fat intake to adipose tissue fatty acids resulted in correlations in the order of 0.4–0.6.[14]

In most of the studies reviewed, the FFQ overestimated the mean of the referent recall or records and in some cases by nontrivial amounts. One explanation for this difference was again the number of days of recalls or records collected for comparison to the FFQ. Depending on which nutrient is of interest in the study and the time period the participant is asked to recall on the FFQ, more than 4–7 days may be required to capture the actual intake of the individual.

The reliability coefficients across all diverse and minority studies were much higher than the validity coefficients (Table 33.3). The median correlations for black males and females across studies were in the range of 0.51–0.88; for Hispanic females, 0.51–0.58, except for one study conducted in Starr County, Texas, which reported a median correlation of 0.85[9]; and for white males and females, 0.64–0.71. These coefficients would suggest that within minority and diverse populations, the FFQ can usually describe with some consistently, the food or nutrient intakes of individuals when administered at two points in time.

In most of the studies reviewed, the investigators made suggestions and recommendations for improving the performance of the FFQ in minority populations. It was repeatedly mentioned that a "gold standard" referent method was not available so collecting valid dietary intake data remains challenging. The need to identify a complete food list on the FFQ that captures all of the foods in the usual diet of the study population was highly recommended. Depending on the study, the food list should include foods that will contribute substantially to the nutrients under investigation. This importance of a food list capturing the usual intake of study participants was demonstrated in the study conducted in Starr County, Texas.[9] Because of the limited number of overall foods that the participants consumed, the food list of the FFQ was able to reflect the major sources of food and nutrient intake of these individuals. Because of this unique situation, the nutrient values from the FFQ were more likely to agree with the values from the food records.

Several suggestions were made regarding the administration of the dietary assessment forms in minority populations. It is recommended that any staff person who is responsible for interviewing a subject for any dietary assessment measure whether the conversation takes place in person or over the phone should be of the same ethnic background of the subject. In several of the studies, investigators found that interviewer-administered FFQs produced much better nutrient estimates compared to 24 h recalls than self-administered FFQs.

**TABLE 33.1**

**Median and Reported Range of Correlation Coefficients**

| Study | Validity Coefficients | Reliability Coefficients |
|---|---|---|
| *Diverse Groups* | | |
| Baumgartner et al.[21] | 0.50 (0.21–0.57) HF + WF (adjusted value) | 0.62 (0.40–0.71) unadjusted |
| Hankin et al.[22] | 0.63 (0.58–0.67) Chinese females | |
| | 0.46 (0.38–0.64) white females | |
| | 0.56 (0.49–0.60) Filipino females | |
| | 0.38 (0.29–0.41) Hawaiian females | |
| | 0.60 (0.23–0.68) Japanese females | |
| | 0.58 (0.38–0.68) Chinese males | |
| | 0.45 (0.34–0.64) white males | |
| | 0.57 (0.21–0.84) Filipino males | |
| | 0.36 (0.26–0.62) Hawaiian males | |
| | 0.55 (0.46–0.77) Japanese males | |
| Knutsen et al.[17] | 0.41 (0.51–0.13) SFA black M and F | |
| | 0.435 (0.68–0.34) MonoFA black M and F | |
| | 0.61 (0.77–0.23) PolyFA black M and F | |
| | 0.31 (0.57–0.08) SFA white M and F | |
| | 0.27 (0.48–0.13) MonoFA white M and F | |
| | 0.31 (71–0.05) PolyFA white M and F | |
| Kristal et al.[18] | Baseline | |
| | 0.31 (0.26–0.46) black females | 0.51 (0.37–0.60) black females |
| | 0.35 (0.25–0.48) Hispanic females | 0.51 (0.19–0.75) Hispanic females |
| | 6 months (control group) | |
| | 0.40 (0.29–0.49) black females | |
| | 0.37 (−0.01–0.48) Hispanic females | |
| Larkin et al.[14] | 0.43 (0.26–62) white males | 0.70 (0.60–0.91) white males and females |
| | 0.23 (0.09–0.41) black males | |
| | 0.44 (0.27–0.57) white females | |
| | 0.32 (0.24–0.43) black females | |
| Liu et al.[15] | 0.64 (0.50–0.86) white males | |
| | 0.53 (0.13–0.68) white females | 0.58 (0.45–0.85) black males and females |
| | 0.42 (0.23–0.67) black males | |
| | 0.27 (0.04–0.53) black females | |
| Mayer-Davis et al.[19] | 0.58 (0.30–0.77) white females, urban | 0.71 (0.43–0.82) white females |
| | 0.38 (0.22–0.62) black females, urban | 0.62 (0.26–0.69) black females |
| | 0.57 (0.24–0.68) white females, rural | 0.64 (0.25–0.88) white females, rural |
| | 0.32 (0.21–0.44) Hispanic females, rural | 0.58 (0.33–0.66) Hispanic females, rural |
| Morris et al.[16] | 0.47 (0.67–0.31) black + white males and females | 0.60 (0.70–0.50) black + white males and females |
| Stram et al.[23] | Average correlation for amount | |
| | 0.30 (0.16–0.41) black males and females | |
| | 0.43 (0.27–0.62) Hispanic males and females | |
| | 0.57 (0.48–0.64) white males and females | |
| | 0.48 (0.31–0.67) Japanese males and females | |
| Forsythe et al.[13] | | 0.88 (0.69–0.98) females |
| Suitor et al.[20] | 0.32 (0.12–0.52) all females combined | 0.88 (0.80–0.94) all females |
| *Minority Groups* | | |
| Coates et al.[5] | 0.34 (−0.02–0.45) nonsmokers | |
| | 0.08 (−0.02–0.20) smokers | |
| Kumanyika et al.[6] | 0.33 (0.51–0.15) black females | |
| Lee et al.[8] | 0.46 (0.21–0.66) Chinese females | |
| McPherson et al.[9] | 0.75 (0.53–0.77) Hispanic males and females | 0.85 (0.84–0.90) Hispanic males and females |
| Resnicow et al.[7] | 0.31 (0.35–0.02) black males M + F | |

**TABLE 33.2**
**FFQ Validity Studies among Adult Populations in the United States**

| Reference | Sample | Instrument | Response Categories | Validation Standard | Design | Results |
|---|---|---|---|---|---|---|
| Baumgartner et al.[21] | 43 HF (Hispanic) 89 NHF | 140 items; interviewer administered; open-ended; referent period was previous 4 weeks | Included per month, week, or day | 4-day food records | Compared subject's report of past month's food intake against four randomly selected nonconsecutive day food records; third FFQ taken 6 months after 1st FFQ to recall original month then compared against subject's 4-day FR | Pearson correlation coefficients (log transformed and energy adjusted); nutrients that differed significantly by ethnicity between FFQ2 + FFQ3 and food records<br>Protein (g)<br>HF: 0.40<br>NHF: 0.35<br>Vitamin A<br>HF: 0.67<br>NHF: 0.38<br>Vitamin C<br>HF: 0.34<br>NHF: 0.64<br>Calcium<br>HF: 0.49<br>NHF: 0.58 |
| Block et al.[10] | 89 HMF | 112 items: interviewer administered after the first 24 h recall | Included maximum of every day, twice per day, or 5 times/day | Three 24 h dietary recalls over 2 months | Compared subject's FFQ of past 12-month food intake against mean and median nutrient intakes of three 24 h recalls | Pearson correlation coefficients (deattenuated, energy adjusted) between FFQ and mean of three 24 h recalls<br>Protein<br>HMF: 0.61<br>Carbohydrate<br>HMF: 0.61<br>Fat<br>HMF: 0.78<br>Saturated fat<br>HMF: 0.68<br>Dietary fiber<br>HMF: 0.68 |
| Carithers et al.[11] | Jackson Heart Study 273 BF (black) 163 BM (black) | 158 item (short) FFQ derived from the 283 (long) FFQ both interviewer administered. Short FFQ administered initial clinic visit, long | 10 included never to 2 or more/day | Four 24 h dietary recalls scheduled about 1 month apart | Both short and long FFQs were compared to the mean of four 24 h recalls | Pearson correlation coefficients (energy adjusted and deattenuated) between nutrient intakes of each of the FFQs and the mean of the 24 h recalls (only 6 nutrients shown) |

administered 4 months later 1 week after last 24 h recall

Protein: short
BM: 0.39
BF: 0.37
Carbohydrate: short
BM: 0.70
BF: 0.44
Fat: short
BM: 0.49
BF: 0.39
Saturated fat: short
BM: 0.54
BF: 0.36
Sodium: short
BM: 0.20
BF: 0.23
Calcium: short
BM: 0.48
BF: 0.49
Protein: long
BM: 0.45
BF: 0.50
Carbohydrate: long
BM: 0.67
BF: 0.53
Fat: long
BM: 0.46
BF: 0.44
Saturated fat: long
BM: 0.50
BF: 0.57
Sodium: long
BM: 0.33
BF: 0.27
Calcium: long
BM: 0.57
BF: 0.56

Coates et al.[5]

91 BF

HHHQ—original 98 item FFQ revised to include 19 ethnic/regional foods resulting in 117 item FFQ; past year

4 (times/day, week, month, or year)

Serum carotenoids, alpha-tocopherol, lycopene, cryptoxanthin, lutein/zeaxanthin

Compared female's FFQ responses to 15 mL nonfasting venous blood sample

Pearson correlations (log transformed, unadjusted) between FFQ and serum for nonsmokers:
alpha-tocopherol (food only)—0.19
Provitamin A
Carotenoids: 0.37
Beta-carotene: 0.34
Cryptoxanthin: 0.37

(continued)

**TABLE 33.2 (continued)**
**FFQ Validity Studies among Adult Populations in the United States**

| Reference | Sample | Instrument | Response Categories | Validation Standard | Design | Results |
|---|---|---|---|---|---|---|
| | | | | | | Lycopene: (−0.02) |
| | | | | | | Lutein: 0.12 |
| | | | | | | Pearson correlations (log transformed, unadjusted) for smokers were as follows: |
| | | | | | | Alpha-tocopherol: −0.12 |
| | | | | | | Provitamin A |
| | | | | | | Carotenoids: 0.07 |
| | | | | | | Beta-carotene: 0.11 |
| | | | | | | Cryptoxanthin: 0.18 |
| | | | | | | Lycopene: (−0.02) |
| | | | | | | Lutein: 0.11 |
| | | | | | | Results suggest that FFQ was reasonably valid for black females. Analysis of lycopene and lutein may not reflect validity of the assessment of these nutrients. |
| Forsythe et al.[13] | 80 BF ethnic mix of African blacks, Asian Indians, Caribbean whites, Guyanese Amerindians, and Caribbean Chinese | FFQ 82 items compiled from Caribbean food tables, Willett FFQ, Stower prenatal food guide, and regional recipes | Unknown (weekly intake patterns) | 3, 24 h recalls | Compared female's report of intake against 3, 24 h recalls, one recall at prenatal visit and two others by phone during next 7 days. Second FFQ administered 3 weeks later | Paired t-tests examined differences between the food recall means and the means of the FFQ at time. (1) Most of the 14 nutrients were significantly different using the two instruments, with the exception of saturated fat, vitamin A, and caffeine. The percentage of energy from protein, CHO, and fat showed no significant differences on either method of assessment. Mean difference scores were computed between food recalls and time. (2) FFQ responses in the subsample. Significant differences were found for energy, CHO, and vitamin C and the percentage of energy from CHO. The 24 h recalls did not fully support the responses provided on the FFQs. |

| Reference | Population | FFQ | Response categories | Reference method | Comparison | Results |
|---|---|---|---|---|---|---|
| Hankin et al.[22] | Japanese 29M + 29F, Chinese 29M + 26 F, Filipino 22 M + 25 F, Hawaiian 19M + 28F, Caucasian 29 M + 26 F | Hawaiian Cancer Research Center 47 items, semiquantitative; administered; covers past 12 months; color photographs showing S, M, and L portion sizes were used by subjects to estimate intake on FFQ and FR. | 8 (never or hardly ever to 2 or more times/day) | 4, 1 week food records at approximately 3-month intervals | Compared subject's report of nutrient intake (FFQ) against average of 4, 1 week FR collected at 3-month intervals during a 1-year period. FFQ collected at end of 12-month period | Intraclass correlations (log transformed) between the subjects' reports on FFQs and average 7-day FR<br>Total fat: JapM: 0.55, WM: 0.34, ChinM: 0.39, FilM: 0.60, HawM: 0.26, JapF: 0.65, WF: 0.44, ChinF: 0.61, FilF: 0.55, HawF: 0.40<br>Vitamin A: JapM: 0.74, WM: 0.38, ChinM: 0.65, FilM: 0.53, HawM: 0.35, JapF: 0.23, WF: 0.40, ChinF: 0.64, FilF: 0.53, HawF: 0.29. Intraclass correlation for total fat for all males was 0.48 and for all females 0.60. FFQ overestimated means of FR by large amounts, but results on the agreement of the FFQ with FR were generally satisfactory. |
| Kristal et al.[18] | 555 white F, 271 black F, 159 Hispanic F recruited at three clinical centers. Because Hispanics recruited at Miami clinic only, their data were compared with WF from same clinic; data for WF and BF at two other centers were collapsed and compared. | 100 items, self-administered, semiquantitative; covering last 3 months; portion sizes were S, M, and L. FFQ collected at screening, baseline, and 6 months. Printed in both English and Spanish | 9 (never or < once/month to 2 or more times/day for foods and 6+/day for beverages) | 4-day food records collected at baseline and 6 months | Compared subject's recall of baseline FFQs with the baseline food records and at 6 months, and the 6-month FFQ with the 6-month food records | FFQ overestimated % of energy from fat compared with FR. Pearson correlations (log transformed) between FFQ and 4-day FR<br>Baseline<br>Fat (% energy adjusted)<br>BF: 0.26<br>WF: 0.49<br>HF: 0.35 (Miami clinic)<br>WF: 0.35<br>Saturated fat (% energy adjusted)<br>BF: 0.32<br>WF: 0.50<br>HF: 0.37<br>WF: 0.56 |

(continued)

**TABLE 33.2 (continued)**
**FFQ Validity Studies among Adult Populations in the United States**

| Reference | Sample | Instrument | Response Categories | Validation Standard | Design | Results |
|---|---|---|---|---|---|---|
| | | | | | | Beta-carotene (unadjusted) |
| | | | | | | BF: 0.42 |
| | | | | | | WF: 0.32 |
| | | | | | | HF: 0.26 |
| | | | | | | WF: 0.30 |
| | | | | | | Correlations at baseline were significantly larger among whites than blacks and tended to be larger for whites than Hispanics. |
| | | | | | | Six months—control group |
| | | | | | | Fat (% energy) |
| | | | | | | BF: 0.49 |
| | | | | | | WF: 0.52 |
| | | | | | | HF: 0.48 (Miami) |
| | | | | | | WF: 0.61 |
| | | | | | | Saturated fat (% energy) |
| | | | | | | BF: 0.47 |
| | | | | | | WF: 0.53 |
| | | | | | | HF: 0.48 (Miami) |
| | | | | | | WF: 0.68 |
| | | | | | | Beta-carotene (unadjusted) |
| | | | | | | BF: 0.34 |
| | | | | | | WF: 0.23 |
| | | | | | | HF: 0.27 (Miami) |
| | | | | | | WF: 0.57 |
| | | | | | | Educational level associated with poor validity of FFQ and/or FR measures |
| Kumanyika et al.[6] | 408 BF | NCI FFQ (short form) 11 items added to short resulting in food list of 68 items; semiquantitative; collected at baseline | 9 (never or <1/month through 2 + times/day) | 3 telephone, 24 h. recalls obtained during a different season; 1 written 3-day food record; all data collected over a 1-year period | Compared dietary data over a 1-year period to baseline FFQ data for 12 dietary constituents with relevance to chronic disease including fat, sat fat, protein, carbohydrate, fiber, calcium, iron, B-carotene, folate, and vitamin E | Pearson correlation coefficients (energy adjusted) between FFQ and mean of combined recall and diary data |
| | | | | | | Fat: 0.32 |
| | | | | | | Saturated fat: 0.37 |
| | | | | | | Protein: 0.31 |
| | | | | | | Carbohydrate: 0.30 |
| | | | | | | Dietary fiber: 0.51 |
| | | | | | | Calcium: 0.28 |
| | | | | | | Iron: 0.33 |
| | | | | | | Vitamin C: 0.43 |

| Study | Sample | FFQ | Frequency categories | Reference method | Comparison | Results |
|---|---|---|---|---|---|---|
| | | | | | | Folate: 0.47<br>Beta-carotene: 0.40<br>Vitamin E: 0.15 |
| Larkin et al.[14] | 43 BM<br>48 BF<br>64 WM<br>73 WF<br>(40% subjects black) | University of Michigan FFQ: 113 food items based on data from NFCS 77–78; semiquantitative; collected food intake over past 12 months | 9 (not in past year to more than once a day) | 1, 24 h recall + 3-day food record collected 4 times/year about 3 months apart. FRs administered and reviewed in subject's home. FFQ administered in subject's home about 3 months after fourth set of records had been completed | Compared by sex and ethnic group (BM, BF, WM, WF) report of food intake (four sets of food record) against the FFQ | Pearson correlation (nonadjusted) values between FFQ and 16 days of FR<br>Energy<br>BM: 0.23<br>BF: 0.26<br>WM: 0.41<br>WF: 0.43<br>Protein (g)<br>BM: 0.23<br>BF: 0.40<br>WM: 0.41<br>WF: 0.36<br>Total fat (g)<br>BM: 0.23<br>BF: 0.35<br>WM: 0.44<br>WF: 0.39<br>Vitamin A(IU)<br>BM: 0.15<br>BF: 0.28<br>WM: 0.26<br>WF: 0.27<br>FFQ showed larger mean nutrient intakes compared to FR.<br>Black M + F had lower coefficients between FFQ and FR than white M + F. |
| Lee et al.[8] | 74 Chin W | 84 items; interviewer administered; past year; portion size asked for foods eaten >1/week; 3D actual size food models used; type of fat used in cooking asked | 5 (day, week, month, year, or not at all) | One 24 h recall (typical day during past month) | Compared female's report of frequency of intake against the one 24 recall | Pearson correlations between the FFQ and the food recall<br>Total kcal: 0.05<br>Total fat: 0.21<br>Protein: 0.56<br>Vitamin A: 0.46<br>Nutrient intakes by FFQ that were significantly higher than 24 h recall were total kcal, total fat, vitamin A, saturated fat, cholesterol, and beta-carotene. Use of only one 24 h recall could explain the modest correlations. |

(continued)

**TABLE 33.2 (continued)**
**FFQ Validity Studies among Adult Populations in the United States**

| Reference | Sample | Response Categories | Instrument | Validation Standard | Design | Results |
|---|---|---|---|---|---|---|
| Liu et al.[15] | 33 BM<br>32 BF<br>30 WM<br>33 WF | Open-ended | About 300 items in 20 categories; interviewer-administered quantitative FF based on the Western Electric dietary history; referent period is past month. | Seven 24 h food recalls collected by phone | Compared subject's recall of last 30 days against seven 24 h food recalls | Mean nutrient values for WM are similar between two methods; for WF, values from FFQ are generally higher than recalls (vitamin A significantly different); for BM + BF, values from history are much higher than recalls (vitamin A + kcal significantly different).<br>Pearson correlations (log transformed)<br>Total calories<br>  WM: 0.64<br>  WF: 0.47<br>  BM: 0.43<br>  BF: 0.21<br>Total fat<br>  WM: 0.65<br>  WF: 0.37<br>  BM: 0.36<br>  BF: 0.23<br>Vitamin A<br>  WM: 0.67<br>  WF: 0.62<br>  BM: 0.62<br>  BF: 0.32 |
| Mayer-Davis et al.[19] | 32 WF (urban)<br>63 BF (urban)<br>30 WF (rural)<br>61 HF (rural) | 9 (never or <1/month to 2 or more times/day) | 114 item, interviewer-administered FFQ; modified from NCI-HHHQ to include regional and ethnic food choices; past year | Eight 24 h recalls over course of 1 year (randomly selected days, about every 6 weeks) | Compared subject's report of frequency of intake from FFQ2 to average of eight 24 h recalls | Pearson correlations (log transformed) between FFQ2/FR<br>Energy<br>  WF (urban): 0.61<br>  BF (urban): 0.37<br>  WF (rural): 0.56<br>  HF (rural): 0.27<br>Total fat<br>  WF (urban): 0.66<br>  BF (urban): 0.59<br>  WF (rural): 0.58<br>  HF (rural): 0.40 |

| Study | Sample | FFQ description | Reliability | Reference measure | Method of comparison | Results |
|---|---|---|---|---|---|---|
| | | | | | | Vitamin A<br>WF (urban): 0.38<br>BF (urban): 0.28<br>WF (rural): 0.62<br>HF (rural): 0.43<br>Correlations by educational status:<br>Total fat<br>&lt;12 grade: 0.05<br>12 grade: 0.59<br>Total CHO<br>&lt;12 grade: 0.19<br>12 grade: 0.53<br>Saturated fat<br>&lt;12 grade: 0.07<br>12 grade: 0.63<br>Vitamin A<br>&lt;12 grade: 0.31<br>12 grade: 0.21 |
| McPherson et al.[9] | 33 HM + F | 38 mutually exclusive food types; interviewer administered; referent period last 4 weeks | Unknown | 3 random nonconsecutive food records | Compared subject's report of past month's food intake against three 24 h food records | Pearson correlation coefficients (unadjusted) between FFQ and records<br>Energy: 0.77<br>Total fat: 0.76<br>Cholesterol: 0.61<br>None of the differences between nutrients on FFQ1 and FR were significant. |
| Morris et al.[16] | 60 BF<br>58 BM<br>65 WF<br>49 WM | Modified, semiquantitative Harvard FFQ, measured food intake over 1 year; 139 food items and vitamin and mineral supplements; self-administered | NA | Six 24 h dietary recall interviews conducted at 2-month intervals over 1 year (Average no. RC/person was 3.6) | Compared analysis of 15 nutrients from the 3.6 average FR/person with 1 FFQ covering food intake over 1 year | Pearson's correlation between a 12-month SFFQ and avg. 24 h dietary recalls for total sample of 232 participants<br>Protein: 0.31<br>Carbohydrate: 0.42<br>Saturated fat: 0.47<br>Poly fat: 0.36<br>Mono fat: 0.40<br>Cholesterol: 0.39<br>Vitamin E: 0.67<br>Vitamin C: 0.60<br>Vitamin D: 0.51<br>Calcium: 0.56<br>Folate: 0.50<br>Vitamin B6: 0.51<br>Vitamin B12: 0.38 |

*(continued)*

**TABLE 33.2 (continued)**
**FFQ Validity Studies among Adult Populations in the United States**

| Reference | Sample | Instrument | Response Categories | Validation Standard | Design | Results |
|---|---|---|---|---|---|---|
| Quandt et al.[24] | African-American 18M + 23F Native Americans 23M + 21F White 17M + 20F All participants: >65 years old, <12 years education, low income | Modified NCI-HHHQ 94 item semiquantitative; administered; covers past 6 months; a second FFQ same food and beverage line items, but color picture of food was presented to subject. | 9 (never or less than once/month to 2 or more/day) | Six 24 h recalls collected in homes at 1-month intervals | Compared average of six 24 h and the FFQ and the picture-sort FFQ. First 6 FR collected monthly followed by FFQ and picture-sort FFQ collected last 3 weeks | Pearson correlation coefficients adjusted for energy intake calculated between 24 h, FFQ, and picture-sort FFQ. Ethnicity not distinguished (only six nutrients shown) FFQ energy F: 0.22 M: 0.53 FFQ protein F: 0.34 M: 0.34 FFQ carbohydrate F: 0.19 M: 0.13 FFQ fat F: 0.11 M: 0.18 FFQ dietary fiber F: 0.54 M: 0.38 FFQ sodium F: 0.34 M: 0.35 PSFFQ energy F: 0.27 M: 0.43 PSFFQ protein F: −0.06 M: −0.30 PSFFQ fat F: 0.17 M: 0.18 PSFFQ CHO F: 0.02 M: 0.03 PSFFQ diet fiber F: 0.45 M: 0.42 |

| Reference | Population | Instrument | Frequency | Validation method | Results |
|---|---|---|---|---|---|
| | | | | | PSFFQ sodium<br>F: 0.23<br>M: 0.39<br>M: 0.43 |
| Resnicow et al.[7] | African-American M and F recruited from 14 churches | 1. 7 item fruit and vegetable (F and V) FFQ based on intake of last month;<br>2. item F and V measure asking servings consumed each day;<br>3. 36 item FFQ of F and V intake based on HHHQ, version 2.1. Asked consumption of F and V in last week. Portion size was fixed at medium;<br>4. one 24 h recall by telephone; 5. three 24 h recalls by telephone | Varied by instrument | Serum carotenoid levels (lycopene, lutein, cryptoxanthin, alpha-carotene, and beta-carotene). Comparison of four methods of assessing F and V intake with serum carotenoid levels | Validity correlations based on transformed values for the 36 item FFQ that proved generally as strong as both 1 and 3 days of dietary recalls are provided:<br>Lycopene: 0.02<br>Lutein: 0.21<br>Cryptoxanthin: 0.26<br>Alpha-carotene: 0.34<br>Beta-carotene: 0.31<br>Total carotenoids: 0.32<br>Carotenoids without lycopene: 0.3 |
| Satia et al.[25] | African-American 83 (53% female) White 81 (52% female) | 92 item self-administered FFQ designed to capture usual dietary and supplemental intakes of carotenoids, vitamin C, vitamin E. Responses collected from past month | Eight less than once/month to 2/day | Four unannounced telephone-administered 24 h recalls (2 weekdays and 2 weekend days) Semifasting blood sample analyzed for carotenoids, retinols, tocopherols, cholesterol, and vitamin C. Compared mean of four 24 h with FFQ and nutrient biomarkers | Pearson correlation coefficients (adjusted and deattenuated) compared to antioxidant FFQ (data not presented by sex)<br>Beta-carotene<br>Whites: 0.56<br>African A: 0.44<br>Beta-cryptoxanthin<br>Whites: 0.27<br>African A: 0.34<br>Lutein + zeaxanthin<br>Whites: 0.49<br>African: 0.51<br>Lycopene<br>Whites: 0.17<br>African A: 0.11<br>Retinols<br>Whites: 0.17<br>African A: 0.12<br>Vitamin C<br>Whites: 0.45<br>African A: 0.37 |

(continued)

**TABLE 33.2 (continued)**
**FFQ Validity Studies among Adult Populations in the United States**

| Reference | Sample | Instrument | Response Categories | Validation Standard | Design | Results |
|---|---|---|---|---|---|---|
| | | | | | | Pearson correlation coefficients and nutrient biomarkers<br>Beta-carotene<br>Whites: 0.33<br>African A: 0.27<br>Beta-zeaxanthin<br>Whites: 0.28<br>African A: 0.33<br>Lutein + zeaxanthin<br>Whites: 0.24<br>African A: 0.32<br>Lycopene<br>Whites: 0.12<br>African A: 0.11<br>Retinols<br>Whites: 0.12<br>African A: 0.23<br>Vitamin C<br>Whites: 0.15<br>African A: 0.10 |
| Jaceldo-Siegl et al.[26] | Adventist church members<br>Whites: 550<br>M: 35.5%<br>F: 64.5%<br>Blacks: 461<br>M: 30.7%<br>F: 69.3% | Adventist Health Study-2 FFQ, quantitative instrument consisting of 204 foods, 54 questions about food preparation, and 46 fields for open-ended questions. Mailed to home and returned by mail during the 6-month study period and covered foods and beverages consumed in past year | Frequency categories varied with food type to allow response with greater specificity (never or rarely to 2, 4, or 6 times/day depending on food) | Two sets of three unannounced dietary recalls collected by phone interview | Average deattenuated energy-adjusted validity correlations calculated and compared to mean daily nutrient estimate | Deattenuated energy-adjusted correlations between the FFQ and 24 h recalls<br>Fat<br>Whites: 0.57<br>Blacks: 0.43<br>Saturated fat<br>Whites: 0.71<br>Blacks: 0.45<br>Animal protein<br>Whites: 0.85<br>Blacks: 0.68<br>Vegetable protein<br>Whites: 0.68<br>Blacks: 0.57<br>Total carbohydrate<br>Whites: 0.58<br>Blacks: 0.31 |

| | | | | | | |
|---|---|---|---|---|---|---|
| Signorello et al.[27] | Members of the Southern Community Cohort Study African-Americans F: 63 M: 62 F: 64 M: 66 | 89 item FFQ administered through a computer-assisted in-person interview. Represents major foods and sources of energy for AA and non-AA in the South and does not list portion sizes but assigns sex/race average portion size estimates | 9 never, rarely to 2+/day | 20 mL nonfasting venous blood sample. Plasma alpha-carotene, beta-carotene, beta-cryptoxanthin, lutein + zeaxanthin, lycopene, and alpha-tocopherol were measured | From FFQ calculated estimates of average daily intakes for five major carotenoids to compare with biochemical indicators | Partial correlation coefficients between FFQ and biochemical measurements of selected nutrients Adjusted correlation coefficients Alpha-carotene African A: 0.44 White: 0.23 Beta-carotene African A: 0.35 White: 0.23 Beta-cryptoxanthin African A: 0.41 White: 0.29 Lutein/zeaxanthin African A: 0.23 White: 0.32 Lycopene African A: 0.06 White: 0.31 |
| Stram et al.[23] | African-American 151 BM, 186 BF Japanese 224 JM, 222 JF Hispanics 136 HM, 123 HF Caucasians 264 WM, 264 WF | Based on Hawaiian Cancer Research Center FFQ; quantitative by placing serving size photos beside the amount category; eight frequency categories for food and nine for beverages | Unknown; highest response for food is >2 times/day; for beverages, 4 times/day | Three random, 24 h recalls conducted by phone | An initial FFQ was mailed to random sample of prospective subjects; three 24 h recalls were collected by phone after the initial contact; a second FFQ was sent 4–6 weeks after the recalls were completed; the subjects' responses on the second FFQ were compared against the 24 h recall values | Corrected correlations for the regression of mean 24 h recalls on the second FFQ by ethnic/sex group for following nutrients: Total kcal BM: 0.16, BF: 0.17 JM: 0.34, JF: 0.19 HM: 0.33, HF: 0.40 WM: 0.48, WF: 0.28 Total protein BM: 0.17, BF: 0.22 JM: 0.31, JF: 0.25 HM: 0.27, HF: 0.35 WM: 0.51, WF: 0.38 |

(continued)

**TABLE 33.2 (continued)**
**FFQ Validity Studies among Adult Populations in the United States**

| Reference | Sample | Instrument | Response Categories | Validation Standard | Design | Results |
|---|---|---|---|---|---|---|
| | | | | | | Total fat<br>BM: 0.29, BF: 0.24<br>JM: 0.41, JF: 0.32<br>HM: 0.33, HF: 0.57<br>WM: 0.57, WF: 0.39<br>Vitamin A<br>BM: 0.30, BF: 0.22<br>JM: 0.45, JF: 0.49<br>HM: 0.62, HF: 0.52<br>WM: 0.59, WF: 0.58 |
| Suitor et al.[20] | Initially who provided three diet recalls: WF: 54; BF: 20; HF: 18 Subjects who provided FFQ2 and FR = 62 but no ethnic breakdown | Willett (Harvard University) 111 items, self-administered (edited foods, portion size information deleted); developed as a prenatal FFQ | Unknown (recall of past 2 weeks) | Three 24 h recalls conducted by phone | Compared female's report of food intake between food recalls and FFQ2 that were mailed | Pearson correlation (unadjusted, log-transformed values) between FFQ2s and recalls<br>Energy: 0.41<br>Protein: 0.33<br>Vitamin A: 0.12<br>Calcium: 0.52 |

| Talegawkar et al.[12] | Jackson Heart Study 247 BF 155 BM | 158 item (short) FFQ derived from the 283 (long) FFQ both interviewer administered. Short FFQ administered initial clinic visit, long administered 4 months later 1 week after last 24 h recall. FFQ listed typical foods and beverages of the region | 10 never to 2 or more/day | Four 24 h dietary recalls scheduled about 1 month apart. Fasting sample of blood collected in vacutainer | Estimates of carotenoid intake from both short and long FFQs and mean of four 24 h recall were compared to biochemical values of carotenoids | Adjusted Pearson correlation coefficients between serum carotenoid nutrient biomarkers and carotenoid intakes from long and short FFQs, and 24 h. |
|---|---|---|---|---|---|---|

24 h recalls

Alpha-carotene
  All participants: 0.37
Beta-carotene
  All participants: 0.35
Beta-cryptoxanthin
  All participants: 0.42
Lutein + zeaxanthin
  All participants: 0.33
Lycopene
  All participants: 0.37

Short FFQ

Alpha-carotene
  All participants: 0.35
Beta-carotene
  All participants: 0.26
Beta-cryptoxanthin
  All participants: 0.34
Lutein/zeaxanthin
  All participants: 0.15
Lycopene
  All participants: 0.19

Long FFQ

Alpha-carotene
  All participants: 0.21
Beta-carotene
  All participants: 0.28
Beta-cryptoxanthin
  All participants: 0.26
Lutein/zeaxanthin
  All participants: 0.17
Lycopene
  All participants: 0.14

**TABLE 33.3**
**FFQ Reliability Studies among Adult Minority Populations in the United States**

| References | Sample | Instrument | Response Categories (Range) | Design | Results |
|---|---|---|---|---|---|
| Baumgartner et al.[21] | 43 HF (Hispanic) 89 WF | 140 items; interviewer administered; semiquantitative; referent period was previous 4 weeks | Included per month, week, or day | Compared 6-month test–retest reproducibility of nutrient estimates from FFQ2 and FFQ3. Reproducibility coefficients were not reported by ethnic group except for two nutrients | Pearson coefficients (log transformed, adjusted) by ethnic group between the 2 FFQs for two nutrients<br>Saturated fat<br>HF: 0.57<br>WF: 0.77<br>Retinol<br>HF: 0.50<br>WF: 0.80 |
| Forsythe et al.[13] | 80 BF ethnic mix of African blacks, Asian Indians, Caribbean whites, Guyanese Amerindians, and Caribbean Chinese | FFQ 82 items compiled from Caribbean food tables, Willett FFQ, Stower prenatal food guide, and regional recipes | Unknown (weekly intake patterns) | Compared 3-week test–retest reproducibility of nutrient estimates from FFQs and food recalls | Paired t-tests examined differences between the food recall means and the means of the FFQ at time. 1. Most of the 14 nutrients were significantly different using the two instruments, with the exception of saturated fat, vitamin A, and caffeine. The percentage of energy from protein, CHO, and fat showed no significant differences on either method of assessment. Mean difference scores were computed between food recalls and time 2 FFQ responses in the subsample. Significant differences were found for energy, CHO, and vitamin C and the percentage of energy from CHO.<br>Pearson correlations between the 2 FFQs were<br>Energy: 0.91<br>Protein: 0.97<br>Total fat: 0.89<br>Vitamin A: 0.73 |
| Kristal et al.[18] | 555 WF, 271 BF, 159 HF recruited at three clinical centers. Because Hispanics recruited at Miami clinic only, their data were compared with WF from same clinic; data for WF and BF at two other centers were collapsed and compared | 100 items, self-administered, semiquantitative; last 3 months; portion sizes were S, M, and L. FFQ collected at screening, baseline, and 6 months | 9 (never or <once/month to 2 or more times/day) | Compared 6-month test–retest reproducibility of selected nutrient estimates from baseline and 6-month FFQs in the control group only. Analyses were also stratified on level of education | Pearson coefficients (log transformed) between the 2 FFQs were<br>Fat (% energy)<br>BF: 0.37<br>WF: 0.51<br>HF: 0.45 (Miami Center)<br>WF: 0.34<br>Vitamin C (unadjusted)<br>BF: 0.60<br>WF: 0.67<br>HF: 0.75 (Miami Center)<br>WF: 0.44 |

| Source | Sample | Questionnaire | Comparison | Results |
|---|---|---|---|---|
| | | | | Beta-carotene (unadjusted)<br>BF: 0.54<br>WF: 0.61<br>HF: 0.62 (Miami Center)<br>WF: 0.46<br>Little evidence that reliability was affected by poor education |
| Liu et al.[15] | 33 black M<br>32 black F<br>30 white M<br>33 white F | About 300 items in 20 categories; interviewer-administered quantitative history based on the Western Electric dietary history; referent period is past month | Open-ended | Compared subject's history of last 30 days against baseline history<br>Sex-adjusted partial correlation coefficients (log transformed, not calorie adjusted) between the first and last histories Energy<br>WM + F: 0.76<br>BM + F: 0.50<br>Total fat<br>WM + F: 0.73<br>BM + F: 0.56<br>Protein<br>WM + F: 0.70<br>BM + F: 0.57<br>Vitamin A<br>WM + F: 0.77<br>BM + F: 0.74 |
| Morris et al.[16] | 97 black adults<br>95 white adults | Modified, semiquantitative Harvard FFQ; self-administered; referent period is past 12 months | NA | Comparison of 15 nutrients between 2 self-administered FFQs at the beginning and end of a 12-month period<br>Intraclass correlations between 2 SFFQs 12 months apart for total sample for the following nutrients:<br>Protein: 0.57<br>Carbohydrate: 0.65<br>Saturated fat: 0.60<br>Poly fat: 0.54<br>Mono fat: 0.61<br>Cholesterol: 0.57<br>Vitamin E: 0.67<br>Vitamin C: 0.62<br>Vitamin D: 0.60<br>Calcium: 0.51<br>Folate: 0.70<br>Vitamin B6: 0.58<br>Vitamin B12: 0.50 |
| McPherson et al.[9] | 20 HM + F | 38 mutually exclusive food types; interviewer administered; referent period last 4 weeks | Unknown | Compared 1-month test–retest reproducibility of nutrient estimates between FFQ2 and 3 and FFQ2 and 4<br>Absolute nutrient intake from FFQ2 was greater than those of FFQ3 and FFQ4.<br>Pearson coefficients (unadjusted) between FFQ2 and FFQ3:<br>Energy: 0.90 |

(continued)

**TABLE 33.3 (continued)**
**FFQ Reliability Studies among Adult Minority Populations in the United States**

| References | Sample | Instrument | Response Categories (Range) | Design | Results |
|---|---|---|---|---|---|
| | | | | | Total fat: 0.85 |
| | | | | | Cholesterol: 0.85 |
| | | | | | Coefficients (unadjusted) between FFQ2 and FFQ4 were |
| | | | | | Energy: 0.84 |
| | | | | | Total fat: 0.70 |
| | | | | | Cholesterol: 0.79 |
| Mayer-Davis et al.[19] | 32 WF (urban) 63 BF (urban) 30 WF (rural) 61 HF (rural) | 114 item, first FFQ was interviewer administered and second was conducted over phone; modified from NCI-HHHQ to include regional and ethnic food choices; past year | 9 (never or <1/month to 2 or more times/day) | Compared 2–4-year test–retest reproducibility of baseline FFQ1 with FFQ2 | Pearson coefficients (log transformed, unadjusted) between 2FFQs were Energy WF (urban): 0.81 BF (urban): 0.64 HF (rural): 0.83 WF (rural): 0.61 Total fat (g) WF (urban): 0.81 BF (urban): 0.69 HF (rural): 0.87 WF (rural): 0.63 Vitamin A (IU) WF (urban): 0.67 BF (urban): 0.26 HF (rural): 0.63 WF (rural): 0.53 Reproducibility of FFQs was similar across all subgroups evaluated including educational attainment. |
| Suitor et al.[20] | Initially who provided three diet recalls: WF: 54; BF: 20; HF: 18 Subjects who provided FFQ1 and FFQ2 = 43 but no ethnic breakdown | Willett (Harvard University) 111 items, self-administered (edited foods, portion size information deleted); developed as a prenatal FFQ | Unknown (recall of past 2 weeks) | Compared female's report of food intake between baseline FFQ1 that was completed in the clinic and FFQ2 that was mailed. Those returning FFQ2 were unrepresentative of the original sample | Pearson correlation (unadjusted, log-transformed values) between FFQ1 and FFQ2 Energy: 0.92; protein: 0.87; vitamin A: 0.89; calcium: 0.80 |

Educational attainment of participants appeared to be a major determinant of the validity of the dietary assessment measures in several studies. Agreement between the food frequency and the criterion measure of 24 h dietary recalls was substantially compromised among individuals with less than a high school education. This was particularly true within two Hispanic group studies. In another study, it was found that increasing validity with increased education suggested that poor education is a barrier to accurate completion of the FFQ, the food record, or both. In this same study, low educational levels did not affect reliability measures. These findings would suggest that special efforts are needed when using dietary assessment tools with participants of low educational status or culturally diverse dietary habits. Small group instruction and practice in using the dietary tools could improve the dietary information collected. Instructing participants by videotape on completing dietary forms is another method to help improve the accuracy of information. If possible, incorporating interviewer-administered FFQs using graphic portion size models could improve collection of dietary information.

This section includes examples of the FFQs that have been used or adapted for studies of minority populations. This is not intended to be a complete list of all the questionnaires that were used in the 23 studies reviewed nor is inclusion in this set of examples an implied endorsement of one instrument. The FFQs included are those that are widely available. The FFQs in this set were originally selected by an investigator for modification to his/her population, or the FFQ is the actual instrument used to assess dietary intake. Readers who are interested in using or adapting these dietary assessment tools should contact the resource people listed with each tool.

In selecting an FFQ, the reader should consider several points:

1. What is the primary purpose of the project or study you are planning to conduct and how does the food intake data relate to the outcome?
2. What length of time are you interested in assessing food intake? 12 months, 3 months?
3. How current is the food list? Does it reflect the current food supply?
4. Does the food list contain foods that contribute significantly to the nutrients you are interested in assessing?
5. Does the food list reflect the traditional or cultural foods eaten by your population?
6. Is the portion size listed on the FFQ easy to interpret by the participant? Consider expressing the portion size in some graphic manner such as 2- or 3D portion size models.
7. Is the nutrient software analysis program updated on a regular basis to reflect the changing composition of our food supply?
8. Can you individualize the food list of the FFQ to your specific population? How much latitude do you

have to modify the existing questionnaire? Can the existing software be modified to reflect the changes you wish to make?
9. Request a list of the validity and reliability studies that investigators have conducted using the FFQ you are considering. Were these studies conducted with populations similar to the groups of persons you wish to recruit into your study?

## BLOCK FOOD FREQUENCY QUESTIONNAIRES

NutritionQuest was founded by Dr. Gladys Block in 1993, initially to provide services to health researchers. All of the Block questionnaires are derived from and based on Dr. Block's landmark research into the development of valid, user-friendly assessment methods.

The full-length dietary questionnaire was originally developed by Dr. Gladys Block at the National Cancer Institute (NCI), for research into the role of diet in health and disease, and since that time, it has been continually updated and improved. The questionnaire was developed in a scientific- and data-based fashion and has been extensively studied and validated. It is in use by over 700 research and public health groups, in university and public health settings all around the country. Eleven different FFQs developed by Dr. Block and associates including two specifically designed for children can be found at http://www.nutritionquest.com/company/

## DIET HISTORY QUESTIONNAIRE

Investigators at the NCI have developed a new self-administered, scannable FFQ, the Diet History Questionnaire (DHQ). The instrument was designed with particular attention to cognitive ease and has been updated with respect to the food list and nutrient database using national dietary data (USDA's 1994–1996 Continuing Survey of Food II). This instrument is available on the Internet and can be downloaded from the site http://appliedresearch.cancer.gov. The data analysis program that accompanies this questionnaire became available for downloading from this site in November 2005. Validity studies have been completed but not within minority populations.

## HARVARD UNIVERSITY FOOD FREQUENCY QUESTIONNAIRE ("WILLETT QUESTIONNAIRE")

Several FFQs are available from the Harvard School of Public Health including this current version designed for use in African-American populations. This is a scannable, self-administered FFQ and is referred to as the "green version." This questionnaire contains a section on the assessment of vitamin and mineral intake that is followed by approximately 174 food items. The assessment period of the FFQ is the past 12 months and respondents are asked to average seasonal use of foods over the entire year. This tool is designed to enhance an individual's ability to respond more appropriately to the food items. For example, the response categories are individualized for each item ranging from "never" to "6 or more times per day," and probing questions are asked regarding specific characteristics of foods consumed. Information can be found at https://regepi.bwh.harvard.edu/health

*Resource:*
Laura Sampson, MS, RD
HSPH—Nutrition
Bldg. #2, Room 335
665 Huntington Avenue
Boston, MA 02115
nhlas@channing.harvard.com

## FRED HUTCHINSON CANCER RESEARCH CENTER FOOD FREQUENCY QUESTIONNAIRE ("KRISTAL QUESTIONNAIRE")

This questionnaire links answers from an extensive list of food questions to specific food frequency items to derive more precise nutrient estimates for those items. The FFQ is machine readable and is accompanied by a software system to process the questionnaire. The format has nine frequency categories and a small, medium, and large portion size. The food list is composed of 122 foods and is preceded by 19 behavioral questions related to preparation techniques and types of food selected. Answers to these questions are used directly in the program to choose more appropriate nutrient composition values for certain foods in the food list. This questionnaire is available in Spanish.

*Resource:*
Alan R. Kristal, DrPH
Fred Hutchinson Cancer Research Center
Cancer Prevention Research Program
1100 Fairview Avenue N
MP-702
Seattle, WA 98109-1024
Phone: 206 667 4686
Fax: 206 667 5977
akristal@fhcrc.org

## CANCER RESEARCH CENTER OF HAWAII'S DIETARY QUESTIONNAIRE (THE HAWAII CANCER RESEARCH SURVEY)

The Cancer Research Center of Hawaii, part of the University of Hawaii, has developed a variety of quantitative FFQs for use with the multiethnic population of Hawaii. Recently, a questionnaire was developed to assess the diets of the five main ethnic groups in the Hawaii–Los Angeles Multiethnic Cohort Study: Hispanics, African-Americans, Japanese, Hawaiians, and Caucasians. Unlike previous questionnaires, the cohort questionnaire was designed to be

self-administered. Three day measured food records were collected from all ethnic groups in advance and were used to identify food items for inclusion in the questionnaire. To ensure more accurate specifications of amounts usually consumed, photographs showing three portion sizes were printed on the questionnaire. A customized, and in part ethnic-specific, food composition table was developed for the cohort questionnaire. A calibration study, comparing questionnaire responses to three 24 h recalls for the same subjects, showed highly satisfactory correlations, particularly after energy adjustment.

*Resource:*
Donna Au, MPH, RD
Research Dietitian Supervisor
Cancer Research Center of Hawaii
University of Hawaii
1236 Lauhala St.
Honolulu, HI 96813
Phone: 808 564 5950
Fax: 808 586 2982
Email: dtakemor@crch.hawaii.edu

## NEW MEXICO WOMEN'S HEALTH STUDY, EPIDEMIOLOGY, AND CANCER CONTROL PROGRAM, UNIVERSITY OF NEW MEXICO HEALTH SCIENCES CENTER

This FFQ was developed for an adjunct trial to the New Mexico Women's Health Study, a population-based case–control study of breast cancer in non-Hispanic and Hispanic women. The 140 item FFQ was a modified version of a questionnaire developed by the Human Nutrition Center, University of Texas School of Public Health, Houston, for a Texas Hispanic population. The FFQ was revised to include important food sources of energy, macronutrients, and vitamins that were identified following an analysis of food intake recalls. Emphasis was placed on specific, rather than grouped, food items because recall is considered better for specific items. Usual portion size, based on 2D food models, included data on number of servings, the type of food model, and thickness of food. Common serving descriptions were included for each food item and were based either on food models or a defined portion size. This FFQ was translated into Spanish.

*Resource:*
R. Sue Day, Ph.D.
Director Human Nutrition Center
Associate Professor of Epidemiology and Nutrition
University of Texas-Houston School of Public Health
1200 Herman Pressler
Houston, TX 77030
Phone: 713 500 9317
Fax: 713 500 9329
Email: rena.s.day@uth.tmc.edu

## INSULIN RESISTANCE ATHEROSCLEROSIS STUDY FOOD FREQUENCY QUESTIONNAIRE, SCHOOL OF PUBLIC HEALTH, UNIVERSITY OF SOUTH CAROLINA

The Insulin Resistance Atherosclerosis Study (IRAS) provided the opportunity to evaluate the comparative validity and reproducibility of an FFQ within and across subgroups of non-Hispanic white, Hispanic, and African-American individuals. The 114 item questionnaire was modified from the NCI–Health Habits and History Questionnaire (HHHQ) that was originally created by Gladys Block, PhD. This interviewer-administered FFQ was modified to include regional and ethnic food choices that were commonly consumed by the participants of the study. The FFQ contains nine categories of possible responses ranging from "never or less than once per month" to "two or more times per day." Portion sizes are determined as "small, medium, or large compared to other men/women about your age." At the end of the FFQ, an open-ended question is asked to describe foods that are usually eaten "at least once per week" that were not asked on the FFQ. Also nine additional questions probe for information regarding common food preparation methods, specific fats used in cooking, and frequency of consumption of fruits and vegetables.

*Resource:*

Mara Z. Vitolins, DrPH, RD, LDN, Associate Professor
Wake Forest University School of Medicine
Department of Public Health Sciences
Medical Center Blvd.
Piedmont Plaza 2, Suite 512
Winston-Salem, NC 27157-1063
Phone: 336 716 2886
Fax: 336 716 4300
Email: mvitolin@wfubmc.edu

## REFERENCES

1. Coates, RJ, Monteilh, CP. *Am J Clin Nutr* 65(Suppl 4): 1108S; 1997.
2. Spencer, G. US Department of Commerce, Bureau of Census (Series P-25), Washington, DC, 1989.
3. National Institutes of Health. *Fed Reg* 59: 14508; 1994.
4. Hankin, JH, Wilkens, LR. *Am J Clin Nutr* 59(Suppl 1): 198S; 1994.
5. Coates, RJ, Eley, JW, Block, G et al. *Am J Epidemiol* 5: 658, 1991.
6. Kumanyika, SK, Manager, D, Mitchell, DC. *Ann Epidemiol* 13: 111; 2003.
7. Resnicow, K, Odom, E, Wang, T et al. *Am J Epidemiol* 152: 1072; 2000.
8. Lee, MM, Lee, F, Ladenla, SW, Miike, R. *Ann Epidemiol* 4: 188; 1994.
9. McPherson, RS, Kohl, HW, Garcia, G et al. *Ann Epidemiol* 5: 378; 1995.
10. Block, G, Wakimoto, P, Jensen, C et al. *Prev Chronic Dis* 3: A77, July 2006, http://www.cdc.gov/pcd/issues/2006/jul/05/_0219.htm
11. Carithers, TC, Talegawkar, SA, Rowser, ML et al. *J Am Diet Assoc* 109: 1184; 2009.
12. Talegawkar, SA, Johnson, EJ, Carithers, TC et al. *Public Health Nutr* 11: 989; 2008.
13. Forsythe, HE, Gage, B. *Am J Clin Nutr* 59(Suppl 1): 203; 1994.
14. Larkin, FA, Metzner, HL, Thompson, FE et al. *JADA* 89: 215; 1989.
15. Liu, K, Slattery, M, Jacobs, D et al. *Ethn Dis* 4: 15; 1994.
16. Morris, MC, Tangney, CC, Bienias, JL et al. *Am J Epdemiol* 158: 1213; 2003.
17. Knutsen, SF, Fraser, GE, Beeson, WL et al. *Ann Epidemiol* 13: 119; 2003.
18. Kristal, AR, Feng, Z, Coates, RJ et al. *Am J Epidemiol* 146: 856; 1997.
19. Mayer-Davis, JE, Vitolins, MZ, Carmichael, SL et al. *Ann Epidemiol* 9: 314; 1999.
20. Suitor, C, Gardner, J, Willett, WC. *J Am Diet Assoc* 89: 1786; 1989.
21. Baumgartner, KB, Gilliland, FD, Nicholson, CS et al. *Ethn Dis* 8: 81; 1998.
22. Hankin, JH, Wilkens, LR, Kolonel, LN, Yoshizawa, CN. *Am J Epidemiol* 15: 616; 1991.
23. Stram, DO, Hankin, JH, Wilkens, LR et al. *Am J Epidemiol* 15: 358; 2000.
24. Quandt, SA, Vitolins, MZ, Smith, SL et al. *Public Health Nutr* 10: 524; 2006.
25. Satia, JA, Watters, JL, Galanko, JA. *J Am Diet Assoc* 109: 502; 2009.
26. Jaceldo-Siegl, K, Knutsen, SF, Sabate, J et al. *Public Health Nutr* 13: 812; 2009.
27. Signorello, LB, Buchowski, MS, Cai, Q et al. *Am J Epidemiol* 171: 488; 2010.

# 34 Methodologies and Tools for Dietary Intake Assessment

*Marian L. Neuhouser*

## CONTENTS

## INTRODUCTION

Dietary intake is one of the most important modifiable determinants of health and longevity. Comprehensive reviews of the literature have consistently concluded that there are clear causal links between food intake and major causes of morbidity and mortality, such as coronary heart disease, certain forms of cancer, diabetes, and obesity.[1–4] In addition, undernutrition contributes to substantial health problems, particularly in resource-poor countries.[5–7]

Given the importance of diet in human health, assessment of dietary intake plays a pivotal role in efforts to improve the health of individuals and populations throughout the world. Dietary intake data are used for three major purposes:

1. At the individual level, assessment of dietary intake is necessary for determining a person's dietary adequacy or risk, assessing adherence to recommended dietary patterns, and tailoring education and counseling efforts.

2. Dietary intake assessment is an integral part of research studies investigating how diet determines the health of individuals and populations. Etiologic studies assess dietary intake as an exposure for association with disease outcomes. Behavioral research assesses dietary intake (or change in intake) as an outcome in studies designed to develop and test strategies to encourage adoption of healthful eating patterns.

3. Finally, at the population level, assessment of dietary intake is necessary to identify national health priorities and develop public health dietary recommendations. These data are used to determine the success of public health interventions to improve dietary patterns and for identification of population subgroups at risk or in need of special assistance. Nutrition monitoring also serves a key role in food assistance programs, fortification initiatives, food safety evaluations, and food labeling programs.

It is clear that dietary assessment is a cornerstone of efforts to improve the health of individuals and groups. However, concerns have arisen in recent years about the accuracy and usefulness of self-reported dietary data.[8–10] The challenges associated with assessing dietary intake are well known and related to day-to-day variation in intake, respondent reporting errors and biases, limitations of the assessment instruments, and limitations in food composition databases.[9,11,12] Several different assessment methods and tools have been developed to address these difficulties, and each method has different strengths and weaknesses with regard to the type and quality of data produced. In addition, there are substantial differences between these assessment methods in practical matters of respondent burden and overall cost of administration. Therefore, it is necessary to carefully consider the specific objectives of each specific dietary assessment as a precursor to choosing the best or most appropriate method. Perhaps the first and most important question is whether the data will be used for assessing intake in individuals or groups.

Here, we describe the three major types of dietary assessment methods: (1) food records and 24 h dietary recalls, (2) food frequency questionnaires (FFQs), and (3) brief assessment instruments. We summarize both the scientific and practical advantages and disadvantages of each of these methods. Then, we consider the use of these three dietary assessment methods for assessing diet in individuals versus groups. More specifically, we discuss these three assessment methods when used for (1) determination of an individual's dietary adequacy for purposes of counseling, (2) research studies of dietary intake and disease risk, and (3) nutrition monitoring of populations.

## DESCRIPTION OF THE THREE MAJOR DIETARY ASSESSMENT METHODS

### FOOD RECORDS AND DIETARY RECALLS (RECORDS/RECALLS)

For many years, food records were considered the "gold standard" of dietary assessment methods. Briefly, food records or diaries require individuals to record everything consumed over a specified period of time, usually 1–7 days, with 3–4 days being the most common. Participants are typically asked to carry the record with them and to record foods as eaten in real time. Intensive protocols require participants to weigh or measure foods before eating, while less stringent protocols use food models, measuring cups, rulers,

photographs, and other aids to instruct respondents on estimating serving sizes. While most protocols specify that the food record be reviewed by a dietitian to confirm portion sizes of foods, fats, and salt added in cooking and at the table and other food details, one study showed that when detailed instructions about completion of the food record are given to participants, the review and documentation by a dietitian may not be necessary.[13] Regardless of the data collection protocol, ultimately the food consumption information from records/diaries is entered into a specialized software program for calculation of nutrient intakes. This data-entry step is a time-consuming task and requires trained data technicians or nutritionists.

Food records can be somewhat burdensome for clients or study participants to complete. In addition, they are costly to administer since staff are required to code and data-enter the recorded foods into a food and nutrient database. For this reason, much recent research has evolved around the use of digital cameras, mobile telephones, and other electronic devices both to record and transmit food intake data.[14–17] In one recent study, an application for mobile telephones was developed where participants captured digital photographs of foods instead of using paper and pencil photographs. Refinement of portion size and direct coding into a nutrient database were also part of the study.[16] Results suggest that using digital devices and other technologies will become more common and will be a critical piece of future dietary assessment methods.[18]

A dietary recall is a 20–30 min interview in which the respondent is asked to recall all foods and beverages consumed over the previous 24 h. Use of dietary supplements can and should be used in this assessment as they contribute substantially to total nutrient intake for many people.[19,20] Dietary recall interviews can be conducted in person or by telephone; when the latter is used, it is typically using a computer-assisted telephone interview (CATI) system. In some settings, dietary recall data are captured on paper forms and subsequently entered into a software program for nutrient analysis. However, ideally the interview will be conducted simultaneously with direct data entry into the software program. It is very important that the interviewer be well trained; tone of voice, body posture (when in person), and reactions to participant descriptions of foods consumed can influence the quality of the data.

The use of portion size estimate aids increases the reliability of the recall data. Recalls conducted in person utilize 3D food models, while those conducted over the telephone often use 2D booklets or photographs. For the latter approach, the portion size aids should be sent to clients or study participants in advance of the recall. Before the recall begins, the interviewer should ask the participant to retrieve the portion size aid to use during the course of the interview. In some special population groups, in-person training in the proper use of the portion size estimators may improve the quality of the data. Among older adults with poor memory, additional memory cues such as recall of the previous day's activities may be needed to stimulate recollection of food intake.

One of the most widely used approaches to collect standardized dietary recall data is the United States Department of Agriculture (USDA) Automated Multiple-Pass Method that is currently in use in the national survey, "What We Eat in America," which is part of the National Health and Nutrition Examination Surveys (NHANES).[21,22] This five-step method includes the following sequence of queries:

1. *Quick list*: Trained interviewers first ask participants to list all foods and beverages consumed during the previous 24 h.
2. *Forgotten food list*: Interviewers probe for details about foods or additions to foods that are frequently forgotten. Examples of foods that are often added to this list are milk on cereal, sugar in coffee, and between meal snacks and beverages.
3. *Time and place*: The interviewer asks the participant to recall the time of day and the location (e.g., home, school, restaurant) of the food consumption. This time and place memory probe frequently helps participants to better recall the foods consumed.
4. *Detail cycle*: The interviewer probes for details about each food named in the quick list and forgotten list, including cooking methods, portion size, brand names, type, and amount of fat added during cooking and at the table. These details include the collection of information on mixed dishes and recipes. The questions in the detail cycle are highly standardized with computerized prompts to ensure uniform data collection.
5. *Final review*: The interviewer does a final review of the foods and beverages consumed and queries participants about any additional items that may have been omitted.

In addition to the standard telephone or in-person 24 h recalls, the United States National Cancer Institute has developed an automatic recall called the automated self-administered 24 h recall (ASA24). Details of this web-based system may be found at http://riskfactor.cancer.gov/tools/instruments/asa24/. There is no charge for use of the ASA24. As noted earlier, other technologies, such as use of mobile telephone cameras to capture and transmit food intake data to a coding database, are also under development or emerging.[15,16]

## Advantages and Disadvantages of Records/Recalls

Both records and recalls provide the same type of data: detailed information on all foods and beverages consumed on specified days. In theory, a food record provides a "perfect" snapshot of intake since the intent is that all foods will be recorded in real time and thus items should not be forgotten. In reality, however, there are significant limitations associated with this method for assessing food intake. The principal problems are the large respondent burden of recording food intake and the impact on usual food consumption caused by record keeping. Respondents may alter their normal food choices merely to simplify record keeping because they are sensitized to food choices. For example, participants may choose to avoid complicated foods with multiple ingredients due to the recording burden, or they may skip desserts or sugar-sweetened beverages if these foods are perceived as less socially desirable. These recording biases appear to be more common among women, restrained eaters, obese respondents, or participants in a dietary intervention.[9,23,24] Other sources of error by respondents include mistakes or omissions in describing foods and assessing portion sizes.

Unannounced, interviewer-administered 24 h dietary recalls are often recommended because respondents cannot change what they ate retrospectively. One major disadvantage of dietary recalls is that they rely on the respondent's memory and ability to estimate portion sizes, although the latter limitation can be alleviated by the use of portion size aids. In addition, it cannot be verified that social desirability does not influence self-report of the previous day's intake.[25] A noteworthy benefit of recalls is that they are appropriate for low-literacy populations and children.[26–29]

Both records and recalls are expensive and time-consuming methods of assessing dietary intake. However, the major scientific issue with records/recalls concerns the issue of day-to-day variability in intake, which means that several days of records/recalls are required to characterize usual intake. This is particularly true in the United States where a great deal of food diversity is available and an increasing number of meals are consumed away from home. Other important, yet often overlooked, limitation of records and recalls is the difficulty that can be encountered in capturing episodically consumed foods that may contribute in meaningful ways to overall dietary intake but may not be captured in these methods that assess only a few days at a time. For example, fatty fish, such as tuna and salmon, are some of the most important sources of long-chain omega-3 fatty acids. Yet, these would be considered episodic foods. Even if a person consumed these foods once or twice a month, the probability of capturing the days of fish intake using standard methods may be quite low.

Using data on variability in intake from food records completed by 194 participants in the Nurses' Health Study,[30] the number of days needed to estimate the mean intakes for individuals within 10% of "true" means would be 57 days for fat, 117 days for vitamin C, and 67 days for calcium. For estimating food consumption for individuals, variability can be even greater. For example, the number of days needed to estimate the following foods within 10% of "true" means would be 55 days for white fish and 217 days for carrots. Unfortunately, research has shown that reported energy intake, nutrient intake, and recorded numbers of foods decrease with as few as 4 days of recording dietary intake.[31] These changes may reflect reduced accuracy and completeness of recording intake or actual changes in dietary intake to reduce the burden of recording intake. In either case, there are considerable limitations on the usefulness of this methodology for characterizing usual intake in individuals.

## Food Frequency Questionnaires

FFQs were developed for conducting research on dietary intake and chronic diseases, such as heart disease and cancer.[30] Because these diseases develop over 10 or more years, the biologically relevant exposure is long-term diet consumed many years prior to disease diagnosis. Therefore, instruments that only capture data on short-term or current intake (i.e., food records or recalls) may be less useful for chronic disease research.

FFQs are designed to capture standardized, semiquantitative data on current or past, long-term diet. Although these questionnaires vary, they usually include three sections: (1) adjustment questions, (2) the food list, and (3) summary questions. Adjustment questions assess the nutrient content of specific food items. For example, participants are asked what type of milk they usually drink and are given several options (e.g., whole, skim, and soy), which saves space and reduces participant burden compared to asking for the frequency of consumption and usual portion sizes of many different types of milk. Adjustment questions also permit more refined analyses of fat intake by asking about food preparation practices (e.g., removing skin from chicken) and types of added fats (e.g., use of butter or margarine on bread or vegetables).

The main section of an FFQ consists of a food or food group list, with questions on usual frequency of intake and portion size. To allow for machine scanning of these forms, frequency responses are typically categorized from "never or less than once per month" to "2+/day" for foods and "6+/day" for beverages. Portion sizes are often assessed by asking respondents to mark "small," "medium," or "large" in comparison to a given medium portion size, often conveyed with a cartoon picture or a photograph. However, some questionnaires only ask about the frequency of intake of a "usual" portion size (e.g., 3 oz meat).

The food list in an FFQ is chosen to capture data on (1) major sources of energy and nutrients in the population of interest, (2) between-person variability in food intake, and (3) specific scientific hypotheses. The choice of a food list is part data-driven and part scientific judgment. One data-based approach uses record/recall data to determine the foods that are the major nutrient sources in the diet (i.e., the contribution of specific foods to the total population intake of nutrients). Information on food sources of nutrients in the American population has been an important part of the NHANES/"What we Eat in America" surveys.[21] Details about nutrients are limited, though, for foods consumed in specific population groups that may not be included on the food list (e.g., immigrants who retain their food habits), and there are very limited data on bioactive constituents of foods that are not considered nutrients but nonetheless have biologic actions (e.g., isothiocyanates).

However, a food is only informative if intake varies from person to person such that it discriminates between respondents. Therefore, another data-based approach to choosing the food list is to start with an extensive list of foods that is completed by a representative sample of the larger population. Stepwise regression analysis is performed where the dependent variable is the nutrient and the independent variable is frequency of consumption of foods.[30] In this process, the computer algorithm ranks foods by the degree to which they explain the most between-person variance in nutrient intake, which is reflected in change in cumulative $R^2$. In addition to these two data-driven methods, items are often added to a questionnaire because of specific hypotheses (e.g., does consumption of soy foods reduce breast cancer or prostate cancer risk?).

A particularly challenging issue in FFQ food lists has to do with assessing intake of mixed dishes. For example, many FFQs ask about frequency of pizza consumption. However, from a nutrient perspective, there is no accurate way to define "pizza." Depending on whether it is meat or vegetarian, thick or thin crust, tomato or pesto sauce (and so forth), pizza may be either low fat and high carbohydrate or extremely high fat and high protein. However, it is unreasonable to ask individuals to disaggregate their pizza into servings of (1) breads, (2) vegetables, (3) meats, (4) cheese, and (5) added fats. Therefore, FFQs typically strike an uneasy compromise between asking about some mixed dishes (e.g., pizza, hamburgers, and tacos) while also asking the respondent to provide information on foods contained in their mixed dishes: "cheese, including cheese added to foods and in cooking." Unfortunately, asking about both "lasagna" and "cheese in cooking" presents the peril of double counting. There are little or no data to guide an investigator in making these judgments.

Finally, to save space and reduce respondent burden, similar foods are often grouped into a single line item (e.g., white bread, bagels, and pita bread). When grouping foods, important considerations include whether they are nutritionally similar enough to be grouped and whether the group will make cognitive sense to the respondent. For example, a food group composed of rice, macaroni, and cooked breakfast cereal may be nutritionally sensible. However, this question could be difficult to answer, because it requires summing food consumption events across different meal occasions.

Finally, FFQ summary questions that ask about usual intake of fruits and vegetables are often included in the questionnaire, because the long lists of these foods needed to capture micronutrient intake can lead to overreporting of intake.[32] Algorithms using the summary question are typically applied to the sum of the line items all fruits and vegetables consumed to give a more conservative estimate of fruit and vegetable consumption.

In recent years, FFQs have come under a great deal of scrutiny and criticism.[33,34] Several studies have shown that FFQs are more prone to measurement error compared to other assessment methods.[8,9] In particular, data suggest that misreporting of dietary intake on FFQs (particularly for energy) may vary by personal characteristics; for example, those who are overweight or obese have a greater tendency to underreport energy intake compared to normal-weight people.[9] Fortunately, statistical techniques are emerging to correct for some of this measurement error.[12] Such correction for the measurement error biases may ultimately render the FFQ and other measures of dietary self-report useful tools to measure diet in large population-based studies.[35]

## Assessing the Reliability and Validity of FFQs

Because records and recalls are open-ended, they can (in theory) be applied in a standardized manner across populations with markedly different eating patterns. However, as noted earlier, FFQs are close-ended forms with limited food lists. Because the food list varies from questionnaire to questionnaire, every FFQ will have different measurement characteristics. In addition, a questionnaire with appropriate foods and portion sizes for one population group (e.g., older non-Hispanic white men) may be wholly inappropriate for another subgroup (e.g., adolescent African American females). Finally, given the changes in the food supply over time, such as the introduction of specially manufactured low-fat or low-carbohydrate foods/those with added vitamins, minerals, etc., questionnaires can become obsolete. Therefore, the measurement characteristics (i.e., reliability and validity) of an FFQ ideally need to be assessed for each new questionnaire and each new population group being assessed. However, scarce resources may dictate that validation studies may not always be possible.

Reliability generally refers to reproducibility or whether an instrument will measure an exposure (e.g., nutrient intake) in the same way twice on the same respondents. Validity, which is a higher standard, refers to the accuracy of an instrument. Generally, a validity study compares a practical, epidemiologic instrument (e.g., an FFQ) with a more accurate but more burdensome and expensive method (e.g., dietary recalls).

Reliability and validity of an FFQ are typically investigated using measures of bias and precision. Bias is the degree to which the FFQ accurately assesses mean intakes in a group. Lack of bias is especially important when the goal is to measure absolute intakes for comparison to dietary recommendations or some other objective criteria.[36] For example, when the aim is to estimate how close Americans are to meeting the dietary recommendation to eat at least five servings of fruits and vegetables per day, it is critical to know whether the assessment instrument being used under- or overestimates fruit and/or vegetable intake. Precision concerns whether an FFQ accurately ranks individuals from low to high nutrient intakes, which is typically the information needed to assess associations of dietary intake with risk of disease. It is important to remember that an instrument can be reliable without being accurate (valid or precise). That is, it can yield the same nutrient estimates two times and be wrong (e.g., biased upward) both times.[36] Alternatively, an instrument can be reliable and consistently yield an accurate group mean (e.g., unbiased) but have poor precision such that

it does not accurately rank individuals in the group from low to high in nutrient intake.

A reliability study compares intake estimates from two administrations of the FFQ in the same group of respondents. If an instrument is reliable, the mean intake estimates should not vary substantially between the two administrations. In addition, correlation coefficients between nutrient intakes estimated from two administrations of the FFQ in the same group of respondents should be high and are generally in the range of 0.6–0.7. Reliability is easy to measure and gives an upper bound as to the accuracy of an instrument.[36] While a high reliability coefficient does not imply a high validity coefficient, a low reliability coefficient clearly means poor validity. That is, if an instrument cannot measure a stable phenomenon (such as usual nutrient intake) the same way twice, it clearly cannot be accurate.

In a validity study, bias is assessed by comparing the mean estimates from an FFQ to those from multiple days of records/recalls in the same respondents. This comparison allows us to determine whether nutrient intake estimates from an FFQ appear to be under- or overreported in comparison to the criterion measure. Precision is measured as the correlation coefficients between nutrient intake estimates from the FFQ in comparison to a criterion measure and typically ranges from 0.4 to 0.6. However, lower correlation coefficients (<0.4) are not unusual for nutrients that are poorly estimated with an FFQ, such as energy.[37] In addition, inclusion of dietary supplement use will often markedly improve correlation coefficients (>0.8), because supplement use may be more accurately assessed and its doses can be extraordinarily high compared to dietary intake and thereby markedly increase the variability in intake for a nutrient. Some studies also assess precision by ranking nutrient intake estimates, dividing them into categories (e.g., quartiles) and comparing these to similar categories calculated from another instrument. However, classifying a continuous exposure into a small number of categories does not reduce the effects of measurement error, and, therefore, this analysis does not provide additional information above correlation coefficients.[36]

The early theory behind these (so-called) validity studies is that the major sources of error associated with FFQs are independent of those associated with records and recalls, which avoids spuriously high estimates of validity resulting from correlated errors.[38] The errors associated with FFQs are the limitations imposed by a fixed list of foods and the respondents' ability to report usual frequency of food consumption (and usual portion sizes) over a broad time frame. Since recent studies have documented the increase in typical food and meal portion sizes of American meals over the past 30 years, the fixed portion sizes on FFQs may quickly become obsolete.[39,40] For example, most FFQs list a 12 oz soft drink as a medium portion, when it is more likely "small" using today's portion standards. In contrast, diet records are open-ended, do not depend on memory, and permit measurement of portion sizes. Errors in food records result from coding errors and changes in eating habits while keeping the records. Errors in recalls result from estimation of portion sizes, participant memory, and coding errors. All dietary assessment methods are limited by the food composition databases used to derive nutrient estimates. Despite the early assumptions that different methods of self-reported dietary assessment did not have correlated errors, recent studies suggest that in fact there are correlated errors between FFQs and records or recalls.[12,35,38] Social desirability could influence how participants record or recall food intake across all types of dietary assessment instruments.[41] Participant errors in estimating portion sizes could bias recall and FFQ estimates of intake in similar ways. There are also correlated errors in nutrient databases. Finally, research using doubly labeled water to estimate total energy expenditure and 24 h urine samples to estimate protein consumption has demonstrated significant underreporting of energy and protein intakes from records, recalls, and FFQs.[8,9] This underreporting varies by participant characteristics such as age, sex, body mass index, and various psychosocial characteristics.[9,35,41] Taken together, current data suggest that it is important to be aware of the limitations of records and recalls as criterion measures of dietary intake and cautiously interpret results using these assessment tools. Additional methodological work is still needed in this area to improve measures of self-reported dietary intake that minimizes measurement error.[12]

A final note is that an FFQ cannot, in and of itself, be validated. Only individual nutrient intake estimates can be validated by comparison of a nutrient estimate from the FFQ to a more accurate measure.

### Advantages and Disadvantages of FFQs

The major advantage of FFQs is that they attempt to assess usual long-term diet, either current or in the past. In addition, they have relatively low respondent burden and are simple and inexpensive to analyze, because they can be self-administered and are machine scannable. A disadvantage of these questionnaires is that respondents must estimate usual frequency of consumption of more than 100 foods and the associated usual portion sizes. These types of questions (i.e., this cognitive task) can be exceedingly difficult for many respondents, as evidenced by the prevalence of energy estimates from FFQs that are well outside of the realm of plausibility.[30,42] For example, it is not unusual for respondents to report usual energy intakes that are less than 500 kcal/day or greater than 5000 kcal/day. In addition, the format of the questionnaire itself is not user-friendly. Because FFQs are machine scannable, respondents need to indicate their responses by filling in circles in a food-by-frequency matrix, similar to that used in standardized testing. Some population groups may be unfamiliar or uncomfortable with such data collection methods. As might be hypothesized, validity studies of FFQs suggest that these forms may be less valid in less-educated respondents and among those for whom English is a second language.[43] Elderly participants with poor eyesight may have difficulty completing the questionnaire.

Another major disadvantage of these questionnaires is related to the close-ended nature of the form. The limited food list and fixed portion size will not be appropriate for all individuals in a population, and different forms have different measurement characteristics across various populations. For example, the use of an FFQ with a typical American food list is not likely to be useful in some special populations or in places outside the United States. There is continued need to develop FFQs that can be used outside the United States as well as among various ethnic groups within the United States.[44–46] Therefore, data from different FFQs are not directly comparable, nor are data from the same FFQ used in different populations, nor are data from the same FFQ used at different points in time (because of changes in the food supply). Finally, dependent upon the food list chosen by an investigator, the validity of nutrient intake estimates will vary from nutrient to nutrient.

### BRIEF DIETARY ASSESSMENT INSTRUMENTS

Comprehensive dietary assessments (records/recalls and FFQs) are not always necessary or practical, which has led to the development of a diverse collection of brief assessment instruments. These brief methods include three general types: (1) ecologic-level measures such as food disappearance data or household food inventories, (2) short instruments that target a limited number of foods and nutrients, and (3) questionnaires that assess dietary behaviors.

### Ecologic-Level Measures

One well-known ecologic assessment of dietary intake is per capita food consumption estimated using national data on the total food supply. Publications from the Food and Agricultural Organization (FAO) of the United Nations and other international organizations provide data on a country's total food supply from which nonconsumption uses (such as exports, livestock feed, and industrial uses) are subtracted, after which the total remaining food available can be divided by the population to obtain the per capita estimate of intake. These population intakes have been correlated with disease incidence across countries in provocative hypothesis generating studies.[4,47] One caution about the use of these data is that it is not always clear how the nonhuman uses are tallied and subtracted due to fluctuating market demand for the agricultural goods. For example, soybean farmers may sell their crop in 1 year to an oil manufacturer for human use, but in the process of oil purification, some of the by-product may be drawn off and sold for industrial use. Another limitation is that total food supplies usually do not include foods produced at home and not sold commercially. Thus, the best use of food supply data is to give an overall snapshot of food availability.

Other ecologic measures, such as supermarket and restaurant sales receipts,[48] have been developed and evaluated.

Household food inventories are another example of ecologic measures of diet. In one study, the presence (in the house) of 15 high-fat foods was found to correlate with household members dietary fat intake at 0.42 ($p < 0.001$).[49] Individuals with ≤4 high-fat foods in their house had a mean of 32% energy from fat compared to 37% for those with ≥8 high-fat foods. However, other household inventories may be less precise in their ability to assess food intake, particularly among certain ethnic groups.[50] Poor household food availability has also been shown to be significantly associated with greater individual-level measures of food insecurity. Household inventories may be especially good assessment tools to use with new immigrants where language or cultural barriers may preclude use of records, recalls, or FFQs.[44]

## Targeted Instruments

Dietary assessment instruments that measure a limited number of foods or nutrients are most useful when the target food/nutrient is not widely distributed throughout the food supply. For example, dietary fat is widely distributed in dairy foods, meats, added fats, desserts, and prepared foods. Therefore, short instruments that attempt to estimate fat intake tend to be biased and imprecise.[51] Alternatively, intake of the isoflavones genistein and daidzein, which are largely limited to soy foods, can be captured with relatively short instrument (15 foods).[52,53] Similarly, a focused recall that can be completed in 5–7 min has been shown to give carotenoid estimates that are comparable to those obtained from a full 30 min, 24 h recall.[54] A questionnaire designed to assess sweetened beverage and snack (both salty and sweet snacks) was just as effective using a 16 item questionnaire as using a comprehensive multiple-day food record.[55] Other novel, targeted instruments include food propensity questionnaires and short fruit and vegetable questionnaires.[56,57] In many situations, the lower participant or patient burden, cost, and staff time associated with targeted instruments may be strong motivations for their use particularly if the research question at hand is in regard to a specific food (e.g., sweetened beverages).[55]

## Food Checklists

Food checklists and food preference lists have been developed primarily for use as screening tools. In format, they are similar to a short FFQ but include no portion size information and may be limited to a certain class of foods, such as sweets or fruits and vegetables.[57,58] These instruments may be appropriate to use when monitoring adherence to a dietary intervention, to determine eligibility for an intervention study, or to use as a counseling tool.[59]

## Behavioral Instruments

The development of diet behavioral instruments was motivated by problems with assessing dietary intervention effectiveness, particularly low-fat interventions. Traditional comprehensive instruments, such as records and FFQs, yield fairly imprecise estimates of fat intake that may not be sensitive to an intervention focused on changing participants' dietary behavior. One of the best-known instruments of this type is the fat-related diet habit questionnaire.[60] This instrument was based on an anthropologic model that described low-fat dietary change as four types: (1) avoiding high-fat foods (exclusion), (2) altering available foods to make them lower in fat (modification), (3) using new, specially formulated or processed, lower-fat foods instead of their higher-fat forms (substitution), and (4) using preparation techniques or food ingredients that replace the common higher-fat alternative (replacement).[61] Although originally developed for intervention assessment, the diet habit questionnaire has since been used as a short assessment instrument in other research settings. A new behavioral instrument designed to assess "mindful eating" may be particularly useful in behavioral and/or weight loss interventions.[62]

## Advantages and Disadvantage of Brief Assessment Instruments

The principal advantage of ecologic measures is that they are simple, inexpensive, nonintrusive, and objective measures of nutritional status. However, these environmental indicators do not provide precise measures of individual intake, and it can be difficult to disentangle human consumption from livestock and industrial use.

Targeted questionnaires also tend to yield rather imprecise food or nutrient estimates. For example, short questionnaires for assessing fruit and vegetable intake have been extensively used in surveillance and intervention research. The typical approach uses two summary questions to capture consumption of most fruits and vegetables ("How often did you eat a serving of fruit [not including juices]?" and "How often did you eat a serving of vegetables [not including salad and potatoes]?"), to which are added usual consumption of juice, salad, and potatoes.[32] Comparison of this brief measure with food records, food frequency estimates, and serum carotenoids indicates that this method yields particularly biased (underestimated) and imprecise measures of vegetable intake, likely because vegetables in mixed foods such as casseroles or sandwiches may be forgotten and unreported.[32] However, more detailed, but short, targeted questionnaires are an improvement to the more global questions mentioned earlier.

The major advantage of the behavioral questionnaires is that they are short and simple (i.e., low respondent burden) and can be easily data-entered and scored. The disadvantage of these tools is that the diet "score" derived from these measures can be difficult to interpret, because it is not comparable to nutrient or food intake measures. In addition, because these questionnaires have typically been "validated" in relation to records or recalls, which have many sources of error and bias, the degree to which these questionnaires accurately reflect dietary intake is unknown.

## USE OF DIETARY ASSESSMENT METHODS IN INDIVIDUALS VERSUS GROUPS

### DETERMINATION OF AN INDIVIDUAL'S DIETARY ADEQUACY FOR PURPOSES OF COUNSELING

#### Records/Recalls

Records and recalls are used in clinical and counseling settings to assess dietary intake and are often used in a qualitative fashion. That is, respondents are asked to describe a usual day's intake and the nutritionist simply "eyeballs" the eating pattern for estimating dietary adequacy or risk, adherence to a prescribed diet, or areas for improving eating habits. The individualized nature of the interview can allow for probing and personalization of the feedback.

Whether these methods are used in a quantitative or qualitative manner, records and recalls can provide useful and understandable information to a respondent. The respondent can observe that the dietary recommendations are based directly on the food intake information provided and can use the advice to alter future food choices, food preparation techniques, or portion sizes. Therefore, on an individual level, records and recalls can serve an important teaching function. In addition, there is a considerable literature indicating the act of keeping records (i.e., self-monitoring) is a significant predictor of success in achieving weight loss or making other dietary changes.[63–65]

#### Food Frequency Questionnaires

FFQs tend to produce imprecise dietary intake estimates because of respondent error and inappropriate food lists and fixed portion sizes that may have little relationship to portions actually consumed. In addition, the data input (usual frequency of intake and portion sizes) and nutrient calculation algorithms are a "black box" to the respondent. Therefore, the respondent cannot easily use this information to make more healthful food choices. For these reasons, FFQs are not generally useful for assessing an individual's nutrient intake for purposes of counseling.

However, data on food consumption from FFQs have been used for individual feedback. For example, Kristal et al. developed computer programs for tailored feedback to participants in a self-help dietary intervention that used FFQ data to provide food-specific recommendations to reach nutritional goals (e.g., "if you use low-fat mayonnaise instead of regular mayonnaise, you will cut your fat by 28 g/week").[66] Because the feedback being provided to the participants is food based and taken directly from their responses (e.g., type of mayonnaise used and frequency consumed), this approach avoids the black box problems associated with using FFQs to estimate nutrient intake.

#### Brief Assessment Instruments

These instruments are diverse, and therefore it is difficult to generalize regarding their use. Ecologic measures are intended to be environmental indicators and, therefore, are generally not appropriate for individuals. However, it is clear that some simple targeted instruments can be very useful for individual counseling. For example, a rather short set of questions can likely assess usual fruit and vegetable consumption or sweetened beverage intake sufficiently well for purposes of advising a respondent whether their intake appears to be adequate, inadequate, or excessive in the case of foods that should be consumed in moderation. These types of questionnaires may also be useful for nutritionists who need to assess an individual or family's food scarcity.

### RESEARCH STUDIES OF DIETARY INTAKE AND DISEASE RISK

#### Records/Recalls

Historically, records and recalls have not generally been used in large-scale studies of diet and disease risk for scientific and practical reasons. Scientifically, records/recalls only assess current, short-term diet, and in most etiologic studies of chronic disease risk, usual long-term (and often past) diet is the exposure of biologic significance. Practically, records and recalls are infeasible because of costs and respondent burden. However, records and recalls are often used in subsamples of the parent study for the following purposes:

1. FFQ reliability and validity substudies
2. Evaluating dietary interventions where the goal is to compare mean intakes in the intervention versus the control group
3. As a check of the main study assessment instrument (such as an FFQ)
4. As a substudy conducted among certain participants to address specific hypothesis, for example, a nested case–control or case–cohort study

#### Food Frequency Questionnaires

As noted earlier, the major advantage of an FFQ is that it attempts to assess the exposure of interest in most applications: usual dietary intake in an individual. The main use of these instruments is to rank study participants from low to high intake of many foods and nutrients for comparison (on the individual level) with disease risk. However, these questionnaires produce food and nutrient estimates containing considerable random error resulting from inadvertently marking the wrong frequency column, skipping questions, and failures in judgment. These errors introduce "noise" into nutrient estimates such that our ability to find the "signal," such as an association of dietary fat and breast cancer, is masked or attenuated (i.e., biased toward no association).

However, a more important concern in research studies is systematic error. Systematic error refers to under- or overreporting of intake across the population and person-specific sources of bias. For example, studies indicate that obese people are more likely to underestimate dietary intake than normal-weight people.[9,24] Systematic error may result in either null associations or spurious associations.

Prentice used data from FFQs collected in a low-fat dietary intervention trial to simulate the effects of random and systematic error on an association of dietary fat and breast cancer, where the true relative risk (RR) was assumed to be 4.0.[69] Assuming only random error exists in the estimate of fat intake, the projected (i.e., observed) RR for fat and breast cancer would be 1.4. Assuming both random error and systematic error exist, the projected RR would be 1.1, similar to that reported in a recent meta-analysis on dietary fat and breast cancer.[70] The data on systematic error from biomarker studies, combined with these types of statistical simulations, clearly suggest that measures of self-reported dietary intake may not be adequate to detect many associations of diet with disease, even when a strong relationship exists. It is important to note that records/recalls are not exempt from these biases.

Finally, FFQs cannot provide detailed information on specific foods (e.g., brand names), restaurant type (e.g., fast food), or eating patterns (e.g., meals and snacks per day or consumption of breakfast) that may be important in some research studies.

### Brief Assessment Instruments

Most brief instruments were developed for very specific research applications. The biggest concern when using a brief instrument is that it is often impossible to anticipate all the questions regarding diet that may become important by the end of a study. Therefore, the choice of a brief instrument limits the future questions that can be addressed. Nonetheless, data collection for research purposes is a compromise between what is ideal and what is practical, and a comprehensive dietary assessment may not always be possible either from the standpoint of study budget or participant burden.

## NUTRITION MONITORING OF POPULATIONS

### Records/Recalls

Records and recalls have proven very useful for nutrition monitoring. Recalls are the primary assessment tool used in NHANES/"What we eat in America."[21] This important survey provides the primary data used to make important policy decisions about the nutritional status of Americans. In these large surveys, a single day's recall intake can provide estimates of the average intake of large groups that are comparable to those obtained with more burdensome techniques. Because these methods are open-ended, they are especially useful for assessing mean intake across population groups with markedly different eating patterns.[21]

However, a single day's intake cannot be used to study distributions of dietary intake, because on any one day, an individual's diet can be unusually high (e.g., a celebratory meal) or low (e.g., a sick day). These days are not representative of an individual's intake even though they may be perfectly recorded. This day-to-day variation in intake is random and does not bias the mean intake for a group,

although this variability does result in an increased distribution of observed intake (i.e., a wide standard deviation).[30] However, if multiple measures (per person) are collected on a subsample of the population, it is possible to obtain an estimate of the within- versus between-person variance and calculate the "true" standard deviation around the mean for the population. This procedure allows the investigator to determine the percent of individuals above (or below) a specified cut point.[30]

Although the use of records/recalls in nutrition monitoring appears straightforward, there is actually considerable subtlety about the data needed to address public health dietary objectives. For example, assume that a public health objective is to reduce total fat intake to less than or equal to 30% energy from fat. A critical clarification of this objective is whether

1. The population mean intake should be 30% energy from fat, in which case approximately half of the group will have intakes exceeding that level.
2. The entire population should have intakes less than or equal to 30% energy from fat, in which case the group mean will be several percentage points below 30%.

If the public health objective is the first goal listed, then nutrition monitoring can be appropriately performed with a single 24 h record/recall for determination of mean intake in the population. Alternatively, if the public health objective is the second one listed earlier, then multiple records/recalls (per person) will need to be collected for assessment of the distribution of intakes in the population to determine the proportion of individuals consuming more than 30% energy from fat. These issues have important implications for food labeling and policy decisions.[71]

### Food Frequency Questionnaires

FFQs have proven most useful in nutritional epidemiologic studies when the objective is to rank individuals from low to high intake for a food or nutrient. However, as described earlier, FFQs are close-ended forms with a limited food list and the accuracy of FFQs will vary considerably across groups with different eating patterns. Therefore, when the goal is to assess mean intakes in population subgroups with markedly different dietary patterns or to track changes in intake over time, the FFQ is not the instrument of choice.

### Brief Assessment Instruments

The accuracy of several of these instruments is particularly sensitive to differences in dietary patterns across population groups. For example, the validity of a fat-related behavioral questionnaire depends entirely on knowledge of those dietary behaviors that influence fat intake. In populations with different dietary patterns, the instrument would be useless for assessment of fat intake. Overall, it is helpful to remember

## TABLE 34.1
## Summary of the Major Advantages and Disadvantages of Dietary Assessment Methods

| Characteristics | Single Record/Recall | Multiple Record/Recalls per Person | Food Frequency Questionnaire | Brief Assessment Instruments |
|---|---|---|---|---|
| Brief description | Detailed recording of everything consumed in 1 day | Multiple days (per person) of recording of everything consumed | Measure of usual intake determined from frequencies of consumption of about 100 foods (or food groups) | Diverse group of short tools developed to target a limited number of foods, nutrients, and/or dietary behavior |
| **Scientific Features** | | | | |
| Advantages | Open-ended format appropriate for all types of eating patterns | (Same as single records/recalls) | Captures data on usual, long-term intake | Ideal for studies where comprehensive assessment is not needed |
| | Provides detailed information on foods consumed | 3–4 days of records/recalls have been used to characterize usual intake in individuals | Can be used retrospectively | Some are nonintrusive and therefore relatively objective. |
| | Provide data that are comparable across populations and time | | | Behavioral assessments may be more sensitive to dietary interventions than nutrient estimates |
| | Recalls cannot affect (past) food choices | | | |
| Disadvantages[a] | Can only capture information on current intake, and 1 day's intake does not characterize usual intake. | (Same as single records/recalls) | Accurate reporting of usual intake of foods is very difficult for some respondents | Typically provide fairly imprecise estimates of nutrient intakes |
| | Records can change eating behavior | Because of day-to-day variability in intake, even 3–4 days of intake only roughly approximate usual intake | Limited food list will not be appropriate for all respondents | Because of targeted nature of these instruments, future scientific questions on other foods or nutrients cannot be addressed |
| | Recalls depend on respondent memory | | Different questionnaires are needed for different populations and therefore do not produce comparable nutrient estimates | |
| **Practical Features** | | | | |
| Advantages | Recalls do not require literate respondents. | (Same as single records/recalls) | Fairly low respondent burden | Low respondent burden |
| | Because recalls are interviewer administered, data can be collected in a standardized way | | Once developed, scannable FFQs are inexpensive and easy to analyze | Usually simple and inexpensive to code and analyze |
| Disadvantages | Expensive to collect, code, and analyze | (Same as single records/recalls) | FFQ development costs are extremely high | |
| | | Multiple records or recalls are extremely burdensome for participants | | |

[a] All types of dietary self-report are subjective and are subject to underreporting and person-specific biases associated with sex, obesity, social desirability, etc.

**TABLE 34.2**

**Summary of the Issues Regarding Use of Data from Dietary Intake Assessment Methods**

| Data | Single Record/Recall | Multiple Record/Recalls per Person | Food Frequency Questionnaire | Brief Assessment Instruments |
|---|---|---|---|---|
| Appropriate use of data | To estimate absolute mean values for intakes of foods and nutrients<br>Group means and standard deviations for comparison to other groups | As an approximation of usual intake in an individual if used with caution and recognition that there will be considerable attenuation of associations with other variables | Ranking individuals from low to high intakes for foods or nutrients | Ranking individuals from low to high intakes for the specific food or nutrient being targeted |
| Inappropriate use of data[a] | Ranking respondents from low to high intakes<br>For determination of the percent of population above (or below) some cut point | | Estimation of absolute nutrient intakes for comparison to other questionnaires or populations<br>Just because an FFQ has been "validated" does not mean that it assesses all nutrients with good, or equal, accuracy. | Estimation of absolute intakes for nutrients |
| Data not available | These methods cannot be used to assess dietary intake in the past | (Same as single record/recall) | Eating pattern information (e.g., meals per day)<br>Detailed information on foods consumed, such as brand names | (Same as FFQ) |

[a] Because of considerable random and systematic error, no forms of dietary self-report data should be regarded as "truth."

that brief dietary assessment instruments are developed for very specific objectives and caution needs to be taken when applying them to other populations or using them for other purposes.

## SUMMARY

Much of what has been presented here is summarized in Tables 34.1 through 34.3. Specifically, Table 34.1 summarizes the major scientific and practical advantages and disadvantages of the major dietary assessment methods. Table 34.2 provides an overview of the issues regarding use of data from dietary intake assessment methods. Table 34.3 gives a summary of consideration regarding use of dietary intake assessment in individuals versus groups.

The use of sophisticated computerized technologies and Internet accessibility has the potential to address many of the practical and logistic limitations of the major dietary intake assessment methods. For example, a computer screen could provide life-size pictures of foods to help respondents more accurately estimate serving sizes. A user-friendly, computer-administered dietary recall, such as the ASA24, could eliminate the costs associated

with this method of collecting data. A touch-screen FFQ program, with algorithms for limiting questions to foods eaten with some minimal frequency, could eliminate the unfriendly format of the questionnaire and tailor the food list. Nonetheless, these practical advances will not eliminate the scientific problems inherent in dietary self-report. In particular, the issues of systematic and person-specific biases in self-report can likely only be addressed by use of objective biomarkers for identification, quantification, and correction of random and systematic error.[9,12,35]

It is clear that from this brief overview, choosing the appropriate dietary assessment method is a complex decision based on the specific objective, with an eye toward the competing demands of accuracy and practicality. There is no right or wrong approach but only the best possible measure given the specific objectives of the assessment. In many cases, multiple measures of dietary assessment may be preferable to a single measure, although this approach certainly has implications for cost and participant or client burden. Despite all the challenges and limitations of dietary assessment methods, these data will continue to serve an essential role in efforts to improve the health and longevity of individuals and groups.

**TABLE 34.3**

**Summary of Consideration Regarding Use of Dietary Intake Assessment in Individuals versus Groups**

| | Single Record/Recall | Multiple Record/Recalls per Person | Food Frequency Questionnaire | Brief Assessment Instruments |
|---|---|---|---|---|
| **Individual Assessment** | | | | |
| Appropriate use | Qualitative use in clinical setting<br>Teaching tool regarding food composition<br>For self-monitoring | (Same as single record/recall) 3–4 days can be used as an approximation of usual intake | To provide feedback regarding respondent consumption of a food versus recommended intake | Targeted instrument may be appropriate for individual counseling for the food or nutrient being assessed |
| Inappropriate use | As estimate of usual intake | | Nutrient intake estimates too imprecise for individual counseling | Reliable estimate of absolute intakes |
| **Research Studies** | | | | |
| Appropriate use | For comparing mean intakes in control versus intervention group<br>As a check of FFQ mean intake estimates for a group | (Same as single record/recall) Validity substudies for comparison of nutrient intake estimates to FFQ | For ranking individuals from low to high intakes for determination of associations with disease risk | Where costs or logistic realities prohibit use of a comprehensive assessment instrument |
| Inappropriate use | When characterization of usual, long-term diet is the exposure of interest | (Same as single record/recall) In study population where respondent burden will result in poor-quality data | For estimation of absolute intakes<br>When comparable data needed across markedly different populations | In cases where there is the potential for important, new research questions to emerge |
| **Nutrition Monitoring of Populations** | | | | |
| Appropriate use | Nutrition monitoring of group means, including trend analyses<br>Descriptive data on population eating patterns<br>For international comparisons of food and nutrient intake | (Same as single record/recall) 3–4 days can approximate usual intake in individuals. | | |
| Inappropriate use | To determine percentage of population meeting a dietary recommendation or at risk | | For estimation of absolute intakes<br>For time trend analyses because changing food supply can make questionnaires obsolete | To estimate absolute intakes |

# REFERENCES

1. Villareal, D. T., Miller, B. V., Banks, M. et al., *Am J Clin Nutr*, 84: 1317; 2006.
2. Mozaffarian, D., Appel, L. J., van Horn, L., *Circulation*, 123: 2870; 2011.
3. Lichtenstein, A. H., Appel, L. J., Brands, M. et al., *Circulation*, 114: 82; 2006.
4. World Cancer Research Fund/AICR, *Food, Nutrition, Physical Activity, and the Prevention of Cancer: A Global Perspective.* AICR, Washington, DC, 2007.
5. Pi-Sunyer, F. X., *Am J Clin Nutr*, 72: 533S; 2000.
6. Bhaskaram, P., *Nutr Rev*, 60: 40; 2002.
7. Enwonwu, C. O., *Nigerian J Clin Biomed Res*, 1: 6; 2006.
8. Subar, A., Kipnis, V., Troiano, R. P. et al., *Am J Epidemiol*, 158: 1; 2003.
9. Neuhouser, M. L., Tinker, L., Shaw, P. A. et al., *Am J Epidemiol*, 167: 1247; 2008.
10. Freedman, L. S., Potischman, N. A., Kipnis, V. et al., *Int J Epidemiol*, 35: 1011; 2006.
11. Prentice, R. L., *J Natl Cancer Inst*, 88: 1738; 1996.
12. Prentice, R. L., Huang, Y., *Can J Stat*, 39: 498; 2011.
13. Kolar, A. S., Patterson, R. E., White, E. et al., *Epidemiology*, 16: 579; 2005.
14. Beasley, J., Riley, W. T., Jean-Mary, J., *Nutrition*, 21: 672; 2005.
15. Hughes, D., Andrew, A., Denning, T. et al., *J Diabetes Sci Technol*, 4: 429; 2010.
16. Six, B. L., Schap, T. R. E., Zhu, F. M. et al., *J Am Diet Assoc*, 110: 74; 2010.
17. Williamson, D. A., Martin, P. D., Alfonso, A. et al., *Eat Weight Disord*, 9: 24; 2004.

18. Williamson, D. A., Allen, H. R., Martin, P. D. et al., *J Am Diet Assoc*, 103: 1139; 2003.
19. Dwyer, J. T., Holden, J., Andrews, K. et al., *Anal Bioanal Chem*, 389: 37; 2007.
20. Neuhouser, M. L., *J Nutr*, 133: 1992S; 2003.
21. Dwyer, J., Picciano, M. F., Raiten, D. J., *J Nutr*, 133: 590; 2003.
22. Dwyer, J., Picciano, M. F., Raiten, D. J., *J Nutr*, 133: 624S; 2003.
23. Kristal, A. R., Andrilla, C. H., Koepsell, T. D. et al., *J Am Diet Assoc*, 98: 40; 1998.
24. Johnson, R. K., Soultanakis, R. P., Matthers, D. E., *J Am Diet Assoc*, 98: 1136; 1998.
25. Klesges, L. M., Baranowski, T., Beech, B. et al., *Prev Med*, 38: S78; 2004.
26. Baranowski, T., Domel, S. B., *Am J Clin Nutr*, 59: 212S; 1994.
27. Lindquist, C. H., Cummings, T., Goran, M. I., *Obese Res*, 8: 2; 2000.
28. Moore, G. F., Tapper, K., Murphy, S. et al., *Eur J Clin Nutr*, 61: 420; 2007.
29. Sobo, E. J., Rock, C. L., Neuhouser, M. L. et al., *J Am Diet Assoc*, 100: 428; 2000.
30. Willett, W., *Nutritional Epidemiology*. Oxford University Press, New York, 1998.
31. Rebro, S., Patterson, R. E., Kristal, A. R. et al., *J Am Diet Assoc*, 98: 1163; 1998.
32. Kristal, A. R., Vizenor, N. C., Patterson, R. E. et al., *Cancer Epidemiol Biomarkers Prev*, 9: 939; 2000.
33. Kristal, A. R., Peters, U., Potter, J. D., *Cancer Epidemiol Biomarkers Prev*, 14: 2826; 2005.
34. Willett, W. C., Hu, F. B., *Cancer Epidemiol Biomarkers Prev*, 15: 1757; 2006.
35. Prentice, R. L., Mossavar-Rahmani, Y., Huang, Y. S. et al., *Am J Epidemiol*, 174: 591; 2011.
36. White, E., Armstrong, B. K., Saracci, R., *Principles of Exposure Measurement in Epidemiology*. Oxford University Press, New York, 2008.
37. Patterson, R. E., Kristal, A. R., Tinker, L. F. et al., *Ann Epidemiol*, 9: 178; 1999.
38. Kipnis, V., Midthune, D., Freedman, L. S. et al., *Am J Epidemiol*, 153: 394; 2001.
39. Kant, A. K., Graubard, B. I., *Am J Clin Nutr*, 84: 1215; 2006.
40. Nielsen, S. J., Popkin, B. M., *JAMA*, 289: 450; 2003.
41. Tooze, J. A., Subar, A. F., Thompson, F. E. et al., *Am J Clin Nutr*, 79: 795; 2004.
42. Bingham, S., Luben, R., Welch, A. et al., *Lancet*, 362: 212; 2003.
43. Kristal, A. R., Feng, Z., Coates, R. J. et al., *Am J Epidemiol*, 146: 856; 1997.
44. Satia, J. A., Patterson, R. E., Kristal, A. R. et al., *Public Health Nutr*, 4: 241; 2001.
45. Satia, J. A., Patterson, R. E., Taylor, V. M. et al., *J Am Diet Assoc*, 100; 934; 2000.
46. Makhoul, Z., Kristal, A. R., Gulati, R. et al., *Am J Clin Nutr*, 91: 777; 2010.
47. Prentice, R., Sheppard, L., *Cancer Causes Control*, 1: 81; 1990.
48. Ayala, G. X., Mueller, K., Lopez-Madurga, E. et al., *J Am Diet Assoc*, 105: 38; 2005.
49. Patterson, R. E., Kristal, A. R., Shannon, J. et al., *Am J Public Health*, 87: 272; 1997.
50. Neuhouser, M. L., Thompson, B., Coronado, G. et al., *J Am Diet Assoc*, 107: 672; 2007.
51. Neuhouser, M. L., Kristal, A. R., Mclerran, D. et al., *Cancer Epidemiol Biomarkers Prev*, 8: 721; 1999.
52. Kirk, P., Patterson, R. E., Lampe, J., *J Am Diet Assoc*, 99: 558; 1999.
53. Frankenfeld, C. L., Patterson, R. E., Horner, N. K. et al., *Am J Clin Nutr*, 77: 674; 2003.
54. Neuhouser, M. L., Patterson, R. E., Kristal, A. R. et al., *Public Health Nutr*, 4: 73; 2001.
55. Neuhouser, M. L., Lilly, S., Lund, A. et al., *J Am Diet Assoc*, 109: 1587; 2009.
56. Subar, A. F., Dodd, K. W., Guenther, P. M. et al., *J Am Diet Assoc*, 106: 1556; 2006.
57. Thompson, F. E., Subar, A. F., Smith, A. F. et al., *J Am Diet Assoc*, 102: 1764; 2002.
58. Kristal, A. R., Abrams, B. F., Thornquist, M. D. et al., *Am J Public Health*, 80: 1318; 1990.
59. Kristal, A. R., Shattuck, A. L., Henry, H. J. et al., *Am J Health Promotion*, 4: 288; 1990.
60. Kristal, A. R., Shattuck, A. L., Henry, H. J., *J Am Diet Assoc*, 90: 214; 1990.
61. Shannon, J., Kristal, A. R., Curry, S. J. et al., *Cancer Epidemiol Biomarkers Prev*, 6: 355; 1997.
62. Framson, C., Kristal, A. R., Schenk, J. M. et al., *J Am Diet Assoc*, 109: 1439; 2009.
63. Tinker, L. F., Patterson, R. E., Kristal, A. R. et al., *J Am Diet Assoc*, 101: 1031; 2001.
64. Yon, B. A., Johnson, R. K., Harvey-Berino, J. et al., *J Am Diet Assoc*, 106: 1256; 2006.
65. Burke, L. E., Warziski, M., Starrett, T. et al., *J Renal Nutr*, 15: 281; 2005.
66. Kristal, A. R., Curry, S. J., Shattuck, A. L. et al., *Prev Med*, 31: 380; 2000.
67. Bingham, S. A., Luben, R., Weich, A. et al., *Lancet*, 362(9379): 212–214; 2003.
68. Prentice, R. L., *Lancet*, 362(9379): 182–183; 2003.
69. Prentice, R. L., *J Natl Cancer Inst*, 88: 1738; 1996.
70. Hunter, D. J., Speigelman, D., Adami, H. O. et al., *N Engl J Med* 334: 356; 1996.
71. Murphy, S. P., Barr, S. I., *Nutr Rev* 63: 267–271; 2005.
72. Prentice, R. L., Sugar, E., Wang, C. Y. et al., *Public Health Nutr* 5: 977–984; 2002.

# 35 Validity and Reliability of Dietary Assessment in School-Age Children

R. Sue McPherson Day, Deanna M. Hoelscher,
Courtney Byrd-Williams, and Michelle L. Wilkinson

## CONTENTS

## INTRODUCTION

Unique methodological challenges plague researchers' ability to validly and reliably assess school-age children's dietary intake. These challenges have inspired creative study designs to determine the efficacy of dietary assessment methodologies applicable to school-age children. Lessons learned from the last 42 years of research exploring the validity and reliability of 24 h recalls, food records, food frequency questionnaires (FFQs), checklists, screeners, and observations among school-age children are summarized in this report. This review of 195 validity and reliability studies of dietary assessment methods for school-age children combines recent published reports with the authors' three previous reviews on this topic.[1–3] Highlights of this review include the addition of two new categories: a food record reliability and an observation validity category. The most active area of dietary assessment methods research among school-age children has been in studies of FFQs, checklists, and screeners with a 124% increase in the number of reports since our last review.[3] At the close of this review are recommendations, comments on emerging diet assessment approaches, and suggestions for future research.

## REVIEW METHODOLOGY

The validity and reliability (reproducibility) of dietary assessment methods for use with school-age children is the review focus. The methodologies include either in-person-, telephone-, or computer-technology-assisted versions of 24 h recalls (full and partial day); food records; FFQs, food checklists, and screener-type questionnaires; diet histories; and observations. A total of 136 validity and 59 reliability studies used at least one of these methodologies and met the following review criteria: (1) publication in a peer-reviewed English journal between January 1970 and March 2012, (2) inclusion of school children ages 5–18 years living in an industrialized country with an advanced economy, (3) inclusion of validity or reliability assessment measures of nutrient or food variables, and (4) reporting specific reliability and/or validity tests from a minimum sample of 30 children in either the main study sample or a subsample (denoted by age, gender, or ethnicity), after the publishing author's exclusions for analyses. Studies were identified by Ovid Medline and PubMed searches using the following keywords: diet, nutrition, adolescent, child, adolescent nutrition, child nutrition, nutrition assessment, nutrition index, diet, eating, food, nutrition survey, questionnaires, reproducibility, repeatability, reliability, validity, sensitivity, and specificity. Studies not specifically using the word validity, reliability, reproducibility, or repeatability in the results or discussion may not have been identified. Additional articles were identified by cross-referencing from author reference lists and published review papers during the eligible period. The degree of validity or reliability of the reported diet assessment method was not considered an inclusion factor. However, the referent period for validity studies had to reasonably coincide with that of the stated validation standard for inclusion. Multiple validity or reliability studies included within a single published article were evaluated and presented separately in the tables and the reference repeated accordingly.

## TABLE 35.1
### Table Entry Format

*General*

Study entries are listed in ascending order by age except in Table 35.8

*Definitions*

*Adults required*—adults provided all of the intake information or were required to supplement and assist the child's report

*Quantitative*—quantity of food consumed was estimated using weights, measures, or food models. Responses were open-ended

*Semiquantitative*—quantity of food consumed was estimated using a standard portion size, a serving, or a predetermined amount, and respondent was asked about the number of portions consumed

*Nonquantitative*—quantity of food consumed was not assessed

*Self-administered*—child completed the dietary assessment without assistance

*Group administered*—child completed the dietary assessment with help from a proctor, teacher, or caregiver in a group setting

*Interviewer administered*—a trained interviewer elicited the dietary assessment information from the child in a one-on-one setting

*Phantom foods or intrusions*—foods reported eaten that were known to have not been eaten

*Omissions*—foods not reported eaten that were known to have been eaten

*Match*—foods reported eaten that were known to have been eaten

MPR—questioning for a recall that includes a quick list of foods and drinks consumed, a detailed description of each food, and a review for missed foods

*Results section*

Omission of any of the following components indicates the item was not included in the article or it was not provided from a sample of at least 30 children. Statistical significance of measures is noted with clarifications as to whether significance testing was shown in the article or only reported via a statement from the publishing authors. The results are ordered as follows:

Correlations for energy, protein, and total fat between methodologies or administrations

Range of correlations, kappa statistics, intraclass correlation (ICC), Cronbach's alpha, or Wilcoxon scores between methodologies or administrations for the nutrients or foods assessed

For validity studies: the absolute values and percent difference in energy intake between the validation standard and the instrument ([instrument-validation standard]/validation standard × 100)

For reliability studies: the absolute values and percent difference in energy intake between first and follow-up assessment ([follow-up instrument-first instrument]/follow-up instrument × 100)

Percent agreement between categories

Comparison of mean intake of nutrients assessed

Comparison of foods or food groups consumed with low to high range of select food items

Comparison of portion size

Results by age, gender, or ethnicity

## DIETARY ASSESSMENT METHODOLOGIES

Each of the following sections defines a dietary assessment method and refers to the corresponding validity and reliability tables. The format of table entries is described in Table 35.1. Table entries are ordered by chronologic age or grade of the children to facilitate identification of age-specific methodological results.

## 24 H RECALL

The 24 h recall consists of a structured interview in which a trained nutritionist or other professional asks the child and/or adult caregiver to list everything the child ate or drank during a specified time period, typically the previous day (Tables 35.2 and 35.3). The 24 h recall is an estimate of actual intake usually incorporating a detailed description of foods, including brand names, ingredients of mixed dishes, food preparation methods, and portion sizes consumed. Prompts for quantification of portion size such as 2D or 3D food models or detailed food pictures are typically employed. Nutrient intake can be calculated for the designated day or portion of the day with this level of detail. When conducted with a randomly sampled population, a single 24 h recall is appropriate for estimating group means, but it is not a tool to describe usual individual intake or to predict individual-level health outcomes such as serum cholesterol levels. Because of intra-individual variation in intake, multiple recalls are needed to accurately estimate usual food and nutrient intake. Nelson and colleagues have addressed how to calculate the number of days of recalls or records required to estimate intakes of individual nutrients for children ages 2–17 years.[4]

Researchers have creatively modified basic delivery techniques for the 24 h recall to include self-administered recalls using computer-prompted recalls,[31,32,34,37] recalls using a structured list of foods as prompts,[35] recalls using food records as a prompt,[14,16,39] recalls of specific foods,[33] recalls using a multiple-pass approach (MPR),[7,8,23,27,32,34] and recalls of foods eaten without obtaining portion-size information.[9,12,13,35]

The majority (69%) of recall validity studies used a portion of the day or selected meals/foods as the basis of the validity evaluation. MPRs have been tested with school-age children, and for young children, minimization of the prompts may increase accuracy.[10] The MPR review and reinterview on foods

## TABLE 35.2
### Recall Validity Studies among School-Age Children

| References[a] | Sample | Age/Grade | Instrument | Validation Standard | Design | Results |
|---|---|---|---|---|---|---|
| Basch et al.[5] | 18 m[b] 28 f[b] Hisp[d] | 4–7 years Adults required[c] | Evening meal recall; quantitative | Observation | Compared mothers' recall of what child ate against observation of the meal. Excerpted evening meal from 24 h recall | Pearson correlations (energy adjusted) between recalled and observed evening meals were 0.71 for energy, 0.50 for protein, and 0.52 for total fat. The range of correlations for 18 nutrients assessed was −0.10 for phosphorus to 0.82 for iron. Recalled energy intake was 9% higher than observed intake (507 vs. 465 kcal/meal). Seven nutrients were significantly overestimated by recalled intake of the meal (significance testing not shown). 15.5% of reported portion sizes were smaller and 33.5% of portions were greater than those observed (significance testing not shown). |
| Eck et al.[6] | 33 m and f | 4–9.5 years Adults required | Lunch recall; quantitative | Observation | Compared mother's, father's, or both parents plus child's (consensus) recall of lunch against observation of lunch. Excerpted lunch meal from 24 h recall | Pearson correlations between consensus recall of lunch and observed lunch were 0.87 for energy, 0.91 for protein (% kcal), and 0.85 for total fat (% kcal). The range of correlations for nine nutrients assessed was 0.75 for carbohydrate (% kcal) to 0.91 for protein (% kcal). Pearson correlations between observed intake and fathers' recall were 0.83 for energy, 0.79 for protein (% kcal), and 0.72 for total fat (% kcal). Pearson correlations between observed intake and mother's recall were 0.64 for energy, 0.56 for protein (% kcal), and 0.65 for total fat (% kcal). Recalled energy intake from the consensus, fathers', and mothers' recalls was 2% (558 kcal/meal), 5% (545 kcal/meal), and 4% (550 kcal/meal) lower than observed intake (572 kcal/meal), respectively. Only mothers' recall of energy from dairy foods/beverages and snacks/desserts was significantly different from observed intake. There were no significant differences in mean nutrient intake between any pairs compared. |
| Fisher et al.[7] | 76 m 73 f 99 m and f White 50 m and f AA[g] | 4.4–11.5 years Adults required | Two to three 24 h MPR[e]; semiquantitative | TEE[f] by doubly labeled water | Compared average of child's parent-assisted recalls against 14-day TEE | Correlation between average recalled intake and TEE was 0.27 for energy. Average recalled energy intake was 10% higher than TEE (1881 vs.1704 kcal/day). No associations were found between reporting accuracy and age, gender, and ethnicity. |
| Montgomery et al.[8] | 32 m 31 f | 4.5–6.9 years Adults required | Three 24 h MPR; semiquantitative | TEE by doubly labeled water | Compared mother's recall of child's intake against 10 day TEE | Recalled energy intake was 0.58% higher than TEE (6910 vs. 6870 kJ/day) for males. Recalled intake was 4.67% higher than TEE (6280 vs. 6000 kJ/day) for females. |
| Warren et al.[9] | 103 m 100 f | 5–7 years | Lunch recall; nonquantitative | Observation | Compared child's recall of packed lunch or school lunch 2 h after consumption against observation of lunch with school lunch discards noted and packed lunch checked before and after meal | Correlation between the number of recalled and observed lunch foods was 0.22 for children eating packed lunch and 0.16 for children eating school lunch. Percent of accurate recall of the number of foods was significantly higher for packed lunch (70%) than for school lunch (58%). Percent report of phantom foods was 22% for packed lunch and 11% for school lunch. Main dishes and drinks were items best recalled by packed lunch children, while fried accompaniments and main dishes were best recalled by school lunch children. Vegetables were not well recalled by either group. |

(continued)

**TABLE 35.2 (continued)**
**Recall Validity Studies among School-Age Children**

| References[a] | Sample | Age/Grade | Instrument | Validation Standard | Design | Results |
|---|---|---|---|---|---|---|
| Baxter et al.[10] | 12 m White<br>12 m AA<br>12 f White<br>12 f AAs<br>12 m White<br>12 m AA<br>12 f White<br>12 f AAs | First grade<br>First grade<br>First grade<br>First grade<br>Fourth grade<br>Fourth grade<br>Fourth grade<br>Fourth grade | Lunch recall; semiquantitative | Observation | Compared child's recall of lunch intake using three prompting methods (preferences, food category, or visual) against observation of school lunch | Average recall inaccuracy after specific prompting for all three groups was increased by 0.5 servings for first graders and decreased by 0.1 servings for fourth graders. |
| Lindquist et al.[11] | 17 m<br>13 f<br>17 White<br>13 AA | 6.5–11.6 years<br>Adults required | Three 24 h recalls, one phone, two interview; quantitative | TEE by doubly labeled water | Compared average of three child's parent-assisted recalls against 14-day TEE | Pearson correlation between average recalled intake and TEE was 0.32 for energy. Recalled energy intake was 0.5% higher than TEE from doubly labeled water (7.90 vs. 7.86 mJ/day). Inaccuracy in energy reporting was not predicted by age, gender, ethnicity, social class, or adiposity. |
| Reynolds et al.[12] | 18 m and f<br>25 m and f<br>31 m and f | 7–8 years<br>9–10 years<br>11–12 years | Three daytime recalls; nonquantitative | Observation | Compared average of three child's recalls of daytime meals against observation of daytime meals. Exchange units of foods were developed from the recalls for analyses. | Recalled energy intake was 34% lower for 7- to 8-year-olds (1818 vs. 2751 kcal/daytime meals), 21% lower for 9- to 10-year-olds (2291 vs. 2887 kcal/daytime meals), and 17% lower for 11- to 12-year-olds (2643 vs. 3185 kcal/daytime meals) than observed intake. Children significantly underestimated their energy, carbohydrate, and fat consumption as compared to observers, with younger children having larger differences. Exact agreement for the nine exchange groups ranged from 94% for lean fat meat to 17% for the fat group. Females were significantly more accurate in reporting medium fat meat exchange units than males, 62% vs. 50%, respectively (significance testing not shown). |
| Edmunds et al.[13] | 204 m and f | 7–9 years | 24 h recall, Day in the Life Questionnaire (DILQ); group administered; nonquantitative | Observation | Compared child's recall of fruit and vegetables on school-day meals against observation of school morning break and lunch. Excerpted intake of fruits and vegetables from school-day meals from 24 h recall | Kappas for the two assessment periods were 68.5 and 74.0 for count of fruit and vegetables. There were no significant gender differences (significance testing not shown). |
| Lytle et al.[14] | 49 m and f | Third grade | 24 h recall assisted by food record; quantitative | Observation | Compared child's food record-assisted recalls against observation of school lunch and breakfast by trained personnel and other meals at home by parents | Pearson correlations between recalled and observed intakes were 0.59 for energy, 0.62 for protein (% kcal), and 0.64 for total fat (% kcal). The range of correlations for the 8 nutrients assessed was 0.41 for polyunsaturated fat (% kcal) to 0.79 for saturated fat (% kcal). Recalled energy intake was 10% higher than observed intake (1823 vs. 1650 kcal/day). There was an overall 77.9% agreement in the types of food items recalled and observed. Food portions were recalled within 10% of observed portions 35% of the time; overestimation occurred 42% and underestimation occurred 23% of the time. |

| Study | Sample | Age | Method | Validation | Description | Results |
|---|---|---|---|---|---|---|
| Van Horn et al.[15] | 18 m / 14 f | 8–10 years | 24 h recall by phone; quantitative | Observation | Compared child's recall of intake against parent's observation | Pearson correlations between recalled intake and observation of intake were 0.76 for energy, 0.74 for protein (% kcal), and 0.73 for total fat (% kcal). The range of correlations for the 10 nutrients assessed was 0.64 for saturated fat (% kcal) to 0.93 for iron. Recalled energy intake was 2% lower than recorded intake (1799 vs. 1836 kcal/day). There were no significant differences between child and parent reports of nutrient intake (significance testing not shown). |
| Weber et al.[16] | 54 m and f / NA[b] | 8–10 years | Breakfast and lunch recall assisted by food record; quantitative | Observation | Compared child's food record-assisted recalls of school breakfast and lunch against observation of school meals. Excerpted breakfast and lunch meals from 24 h recall | Pearson correlations between recalled breakfast and lunch combined and observed breakfast and lunch were 0.52 for energy, 0.68 for protein, and 0.57 for total fat. The range of correlations for the seven nutrient measures assessed was 0.52 for energy to 0.86 for both carbohydrate (% kcal) and protein (% kcal). Recalled energy intake was 13% higher than observed intake (862 vs. 761 kcal/daytime meals). There was an overall 75% agreement in the types of food items recalled and observed. Food portions were recalled within 10% of observed portions 57% of the time; overestimation occurred 30% of the time and underestimation occurred 13% of the time. |
| Todd et al.[17] | 30 m and f Chinese / 31 m and f Hisp | 8–11 years | Breakfast and lunch recall; quantitative | Observation | Compared child's recall of school breakfast and lunch against observation of school meals with plate waste subtracted. Excerpted breakfast and lunch meals from 24 h recall | Pearson correlations between recalled lunch and observed lunch for Chinese were 0.49 for energy, 0.62 for protein, and 0.25 for total fat and for Hisps were 0.53 for energy, 0.51 for protein, and 0.46 for total fat. The range of correlations for the 15 nutrients assessed for Chinese was −0.10 for sodium to 0.63 for thiamin and for Hisps was 0.34 for niacin to 0.81 for vitamin C. Chinese children's recalled energy intake was 10% lower than observed intake (686 vs. 765 kcal/two meals). Chinese children recalled consistently less food than consumed that was significantly lower for 4 of the 15 nutrients. Hisp children's recalled energy intake was 6% higher than observed intake (665 vs. 630 kcal/two meals). Hisp children's recalled intake vs. consumed intake was inconsistent and was significantly higher for two nutrients and lower for 1 of the 15 nutrients assessed. For Chinese, food item omissions ranged from 4% for milk to 35% for vegetables. For Hisps, food item omissions ranged from 0% for juice and milk to 35% for vegetables. |
| Samuelson[18] | 56 m and f / 43 m and f | 8 years / 13 years | Lunch recall; quantitative | Chemical analysis of food | Compared child's recall of lunch against weighed chemical analyses of a double portion of lunch, with plate waste subtracted. Excerpted lunch meal from 24 h recall | Spearman correlations between recalled lunch and chemical analyses of lunch for 8- and 13-year-olds for energy were 0.68 for 8-year-olds and 0.71 for 13-year-olds. Correlations for protein of 8- and 13-year-olds were 0.55 and 0.45, respectively. Correlations for total fat of 8- and 13-year-olds were 0.61 and 0.69, respectively. The range of correlations for the four nutrients assessed for 8-year-olds was 0.55 for protein to 0.68 for energy. The range of correlations for 13-year-olds was 0.45 for protein to 0.71 for energy. Among 8-year-olds, recalled energy intake was 18% higher than chemical analyses (472 vs. 399 kcal/meal). Among 13-year-olds, recalled energy intake was 1% higher than chemical analyses (494 vs. 491 kcal/meal). Median portion size estimated by child compared to weighing was not significantly different for 8-year-olds and was 14% lower among 13-year-olds (significance testing not shown). |

(continued)

**TABLE 35.2 (continued)**
**Recall Validity Studies among School-Age Children**

| References[a] | Sample | Age/Grade | Instrument | Validation Standard | Design | Results |
|---|---|---|---|---|---|---|
| Baxter et al.[19] | 374 m and f 96% AA | Fourth grade | 24 h recall in person and by phone; quantitative | Observation | Compared child's breakfast and lunch recall at morning, afternoon, and evening for prior 24 h and previous day against observation of breakfast and lunch | Pearson correlations between recalled breakfast and lunch and observation for the prior 24 h were 0.36 for energy, 0.33 for protein, 0.39 for carbohydrate, and 0.46 for fat. Pearson correlations between recalled breakfast and lunch and observation for the previous day were 0.36 for energy, 0.34 for protein, 0.38 for carbohydrate, and 0.35 for fat. |
| Baxter et al.[20] | 374 m and f 96% AA | Fourth grade | 24 h recall in person and by phone; quantitative | Observation | Compared child's breakfast and lunch recall at morning, afternoon, and evening for prior 24 h and previous day against observation of breakfast and lunch | Average recall inaccuracy was 5.41 servings for the prior 24 h and 7.53 for the previous day. Omission rates and intrusion rates were 46% and 28% for the prior 24 h and 65% and 55% for the previous day, respectively. For the prior 24 h, omission rates for morning, afternoon, and evening interviews were 55%, 42%, and 41% and 59%, 69%, and 68% for the previous day, respectively. For the prior 24 h, intrusion rates for morning, afternoon, and evening interviews were 34%, 22%, and 28% and 41%, 59%, and 62% for the previous day, respectively. |
| Baxter et al.[21] | 374 m and f 96% AA | Fourth grade | 24 h recall in person and by phone; quantitative | Observation | Compared child's breakfast and lunch recall at morning, afternoon, and evening for prior 24 h and previous day against observation of breakfast and lunch | Mean recalled energy intake for breakfast for prior 24 h morning, afternoon, and evening and previous-day morning, afternoon, and evening were 289, 309, and 282 kcal and 281, 315, and 337 kcal, respectively, compared with mean observed intake of 282, 315, and 267 kcal and 260, 262, and 266 kcal. Mean recalled energy intake for lunch for prior 24 h morning, afternoon, and evening and previous-day morning, afternoon, and evening were 410, 444, and 444 kcal and 495, 370, and 430 kcal, respectively, compared with mean observed intake of 467, 566, and 520 kcal and 603, 500, and 496 kcal. |
| Harrington et al.[22] | 379 m and f 50.4% m 49.6% f 57.3% White 39.6% AA 3.2% others | Fourth grade | Lunch recall; interviewer administered; semiquantitative | Observation | Compared child's recall of previous day's school lunch with lunch observation | Recalled fruits were overestimated by 22.8% and underestimated by 22.8%, and vegetables were over reported by 37.0% and underestimated by 22.6% as compared to the observation. Match, omission, and intrusion rates between food item recall and observation were for fruits, 78%, 12.7%, and 15%, respectively, and for vegetables, 73%, 20.3%, and 32%, respectively. Rates for portion matching were 54% for fruits and 40% for vegetables. |

| Study | Sample | Grade | Method | Standard | Comparison | Results |
|---|---|---|---|---|---|---|
| Baxter et al.[23] Baxter et al.[24] Baxter et al.[25] Baxter et al.[26] | 25 m White 24 m AA 28 f White 27 f AA | Fourth grade | One to three 24 h MPR; quantitative | Observation | Compared child's report of food items from 1–3 recall interviews for school breakfast and lunch against observation of school meals. Compared child's breakfast and lunch recall in forward and reverse order against observed breakfast and lunch. Excerpted breakfast and lunch food from 24 h recall | Mean omission rate of foods on the recalls compared to observation was 51% and mean intrusion rate was 39%. Correspondence rates for breakfast for interviews 1–3 were 36%, 41%, and 44% and for lunch were 46%, 50%, and 57%, respectively, for energy. Total inaccurate servings for breakfast for interviews 1–3 were 3.3, 3.2, and 3.2 and for lunch were 4.3, 3.9, and 3.5, respectively. Inaccuracy of reports significantly decreased from the first to third recall. Pearson correlations between forward-ordered interviews for girls and boys, respectively, for energy were 0.51 and 0.25, for protein were 0.57 and 0.32, for carbohydrate were 0.21 and 0.21, and for fat were 0.50 and 0.42. Pearson correlations between reverse-ordered interviews for girls and boys, respectively, for energy were 0.28 and 0.28, for protein were 0.41 and 0.19, for carbohydrate were 0.37 and 0.28, and for fat were 0.17 and 0.40. Total inaccurate servings for boys for breakfast in forward and reverse were 3.4 and 2.8 and for lunch were 4.1 and 3.6, respectively. Total inaccurate servings for girls for breakfast in forward and reverse were 2.5 and 2.4 and for lunch were 3.7 and 4.0, respectively. |
| Baxter et al.[27] | 10 m AA 8 m White 8 f AA 7 f White | Fourth grade | 24 h MPR in person; semiquantitative | Observation | Compared child's recall of school breakfast and lunch from in-person interview against observation of school meals. Excerpted breakfast and lunch meals from same-day recall | Mean omission rate of foods on the recalls compared to observation was 34% and mean intrusion rate was 19%. Accuracy of reporting was not significantly different whether obtained in person or by telephone. |
| Baxter et al.[27] | 8 m AA 8 m White 11 f AA 9 f White | Fourth grade | 24 h MPR by phone; semiquantitative | Observation | Compared child's recall of school breakfast and lunch from telephone interview against observation of school meals. Excerpted breakfast and lunch meals from same-day recall | Mean omission rate of foods on the recalls compared to observation was 32% and mean intrusion rate was 16%. Accuracy of reporting was not significantly different whether obtained in person or by telephone. |
| Baxter et al.[28] | 120 m 117 f 58 White 179 AA | Fourth grade | Lunch recall; quantitative | Observation | Compared child's recall of food items from school lunch either the same day or the following day against observation of that lunch | Average matched food rates from recall of lunch and observation of lunch were 84% and 68% for same-day and next-day intervals, respectively. Rates for omitted and added (phantom) foods were significantly lower for the same-day recalls (16% vs. 5%) than next-day recalls (32% vs. 13%). Children were least likely to omit beverages and main dishes and most likely to omit condiments and miscellaneous foods. There were no significant gender, ethnic, or time interval differences in the accuracy of recalling the amount of food consumed (significance testing not shown). |

(continued)

**TABLE 35.2 (continued)**
**Recall Validity Studies among School-Age Children**

| References[a] | Sample | Age/Grade | Instrument | Validation Standard | Design | Results |
|---|---|---|---|---|---|---|
| Lytle et al.[29] | 238 m 248 f 253 White 146 Asian 73 AA 14 others | Fourth grade | Lunch recall; quantitative | Observation | Compared child's recall of school lunch against observation of lunch. Excerpted lunch meal from 24 h recall | Pearson correlation between recalled and observed intakes for energy was 0.44. The range of correlations for the five nutrients assessed was 0.39 for beta-carotene to 0.61 for vitamin C. Recalled energy intake was 14% higher than observed intake (600 vs. 526 kcal/meal). There were significant differences between recalled and observed nutrient intakes for all nutrients except beta-carotene (borderline significant). Correlations ranged from 0.42 for vegetables to 0.65 for fruit. |
| Moore et al.[30] | 374 m and f 157 m 215 f 2 unknown | 9–11 years | Diet recall questionnaire (RQ); self-administered; previous-day intake and same-day breakfast; semiquantitative | One 24 h diet recall interview | Compared diet RQ with 24 h diet recall interview for two breakfasts (same day and previous day) and rest of day reported foods | Comparisons of consumers and nonconsumers for same-day and previous-day breakfasts were made for 10 food and beverage items: fruit, bread, cereal, milk, milk adjusted, sweet items, crisps, water, drink, and others. Kappa coefficients ranged from 0.31 to 0.71 for same day and 0.03 to 0.46 for previous day. For seven out of nine categories, females had greater agreement of kappa statistics than boys for both same-day and previous-day breakfasts. |
| Moore et al.[31] | 72 m and f | 9–11 years Adults required | Computerized 24 h recall (checklist); three food types (fruit, sweets/chocolate/biscuit (SCB), crisps); self-administered; semiquantitative | One 24 h recall interview | Compared child's computerized 24 h recall with 24 h recall interview. Computerized 24 h recall was preceded by a 24 h food diary; child's parent-assisted diary was not available during computerized 24 h recall but was available during 24 h recall interview | Mean intake from computerized 24 h recall overestimated fruit by 59% (0.35 vs. 0.22 servings) and crisps by 33% (0.81 vs. 0.61 servings) and underestimated SCB by 22% (1.06 vs. 1.36 servings) compared to 24 h recall interview, during periods 2–3. During periods 1–6, mean intake was overestimated for fruit by 136.6% (2.13 vs. 0.90 servings) and crisps by 67% (1.67 vs. 1.00 servings) and underestimated for SCB by 4% (4.28 vs. 4.46 servings). Kappa statistics indicated higher agreement during the periods 2–3 (0.29 fruit, 0.25 SCB, 0.22 crisps) as opposed to periods 1–6 (0.06 fruit, 0.00 SCB, 0.03 crisps). Match rates for consumption were highest for fruit during periods 2–3, 81%, and ranged from 60% for fruit periods 1–6 to 75% for crisps periods 1–6. |
| Baranowski et al.[32] | 91 m and f White, AA, Hisp, others | Fourth grade, 9–11 years | 24 h MPR by Food Intake Recording Software System (FIRSSt); self-administered; quantitative | Observation | Compared child's recall of food items from school lunch by FIRSSt against observation of lunch. Excerpted lunch foods from 24 h FIRSSt recall | To control for game exploration using FIRSSt by some children, two sets of data were analyzed: restricted (first n foods reported within each meal or snack: n = 5 for breakfast, three for morning snack, six for lunch, three for afternoon snack, five for dinner, three for evening snack) and unrestricted (all foods reported). For restricted data, there was a mean food match rate of 46%, omission rate of 30%, and intrusion rate of 24%. For unrestricted data, there was a mean food match rate of 40%, omission rate of 36%, and intrusion rate of 23%. |

| Source | Sample | Age | Instrument | Reference method | Comparison | Results |
|---|---|---|---|---|---|---|
| Baranowski et al.[32] | 91 m and f; White, AA, Hisp, others | Fourth grade, 9–11 years | 24 h MPR; quantitative | Observation | Compared child's recall of lunch foods by 24 h MPR against observation of the lunch. Excerpted lunch meal from 24 h MPR | To control for game exploration using FIRSSt by some children, two sets of data were analyzed: restricted (foods reported within each meal or snack: n = 5 for breakfast, three for morning snack, six for lunch, three for afternoon snack, five for dinner, three for evening snack) and unrestricted (all foods reported). For restricted data, there was a mean food match rate of 59%, omission rate of 24%, and intrusion rate of 17%. For unrestricted data, there was a mean food match rate of 53%, omission rate of 26%, and intrusion rate of 20%. |
| Baranowski et al.[32] | 137 m and f; White, AA, Hisp, others | Fourth grade, 9–11 years | 24 h recall by FIRSSt; self-administered; quantitative | 24 h MPR | Compared child's recall of food items from school lunch by FIRSSt against child's recall of foods by 24 h MPR. Excerpted lunch foods from FIRSSt recall and 24 h recall | To control for game exploration using FIRSSt by some children, two sets of data were analyzed: restricted (first n foods reported within each meal or snack: n = 5 for breakfast, three for morning snack, six for lunch, three for afternoon snack, five for dinner, three for evening snack) and unrestricted (all foods reported). For restricted data, there was a mean food match rate of 60%, omission rate of 24%, and intrusion rate of 15%. For unrestricted data, there was a mean match rate of 56%, omission rate of 24%, and intrusion rate of 20%. Hisp children reported more problems with using FIRSSt than other ethnic groups. |
| Andersen et al.[33] | 36 m 49 f | Sixth grade | 24 h recall of fruit, fruit juice and vegetables; group administered; semiquantitative | One 7-day food record with precoded list of foods; semiquantitative | Compared child's recall of fruit, fruit juice, vegetable, and potato intake against child's report of intake on 7-day food records. Excerpted fruit and vegetable intake from 7-day food record with precoded list of foods | Reported intake from the 24 h recall was significantly higher than from the 7-day precoded food records for fruit, fruit juice, and potato; fruit and vegetable without fruit juice and potato; and fruit, fruit juice, vegetable, and potato, but not for vegetable. The same results were found by gender except for potato that was not significant (significance testing not shown). Recalled fruit and vegetable (including fruit juice and potato) intake from the 24 h recall was 159% (4.4 vs. 1.7 portions/day) higher than food record intake. |
| Hanning et al.[34] | 201 m and f 82 m 119 f | Sixth to eighth grade | 24 h MPR recall, web-based Food Behavior Questionnaire (FBQ); quantitative | 24 h MPR recall | Compared child's recall of intake using the web-based FBQ against child's report of intake from dietitian-led recall | ICCs between FBQ recall and dietitian-led recall were 0.56 for energy, 0.58 for protein, and 0.52 for total fat. The range of correlations for the 22 nutrients assessed 0.35 for vitamin B6 to 0.92 for vitamin B12. Recalled energy was 10.5% lower on the web-based FBQ than in the dietitian-led recall (1975 vs. 2274 kcal/day). Underreporting was predominantly from carbohydrate foods. |
| Johnson et al.[35] | 41 m 55 f | 11–13 years | 24 h recall of 41 items (10 fatty, 13 sugary, 10 fibrous, and 3 low-sugar foods and 5 alternative fats), Food Intake Questionnaire (FIQ); self-administered; past 3 months; nonquantitative | One 3-day food record with interview | Compared child's recall of foods from previous day on FIQ against nutrient intake from child's 3-day food diary 2 weeks later | Pearson correlation between the 24 h recall scores and 3-day food diary for energy and the fatty group score was 0.20 and for fat (% kcal) and the fatty group was 0.36. The range of correlations for the four nutrients and three food groups assessed was −0.057 (not significant) for fiber and the fatty group to 0.36 for fat (% kcal) and the fatty group. |

(continued)

**TABLE 35.2 (continued)**
**Recall Validity Studies among School-Age Children**

| References[a] | Sample | Age/Grade | Instrument | Validation Standard | Design | Results |
|---|---|---|---|---|---|---|
| Mullenbach et al.[36] | 22 m<br>18 f | Sixth to ninth grade<br>Adults required | 24 h recall by phone; quantitative | One 3-day food record | Compared child's parent-assisted recall against child's parent-assisted 3-day food records completed 2–4 weeks prior to recalls | Pearson correlations between recall and food records were 0.42 for energy, 0.42 for protein, and 0.33 for total fat. The range of correlations for the 19 nutrients assessed was 0.09 for cholesterol to 0.57 for riboflavin. Recalled energy intake was 12% lower than recorded energy intake (1835 vs. 2097 kcal/day). There were no significant differences between recalled and recorded average nutrient intakes, although the 24 h recall estimates were all lower than those from the food record. |
| Vereecken et al.[37] | 55 m<br>46 f | 11–14 years | 24 h recall computer-assisted Young Adolescent's Nutrition Assessment on Computer (YANA-C); self-administered; quantitative | 24 h recall | Compared child's recall of intake by the YANA-C against child's 24 h recall | Spearman correlations between YANA-C and interview were 0.66 for energy, 0.67 for protein, and 0.59 for fat. The range of correlations for the eight nutrients assessed was 0.44 for iron and 0.86 for calcium. Recalled energy intake from the YANA-C recall was 5% higher than recalled intake (8240 vs. 7812 kJ). Spearman correlations for amount/portion agreement ranged from −0.02 for fish to 0.90 for milk. Percent agreement of food matches ranged from 67% for sauces and butter to 97% for bread. |
| Vereecken et al.[37] | 44 m<br>92 f | 12–14 years | 24 h recall computer-assisted YANA-C; self-administered; quantitative | 1-day food record | Compared child's recall of intake by the YANA-C against child's 1-day food record | Spearman correlations between YANA-C and food record were 0.64 for energy, 0.44 for protein, and 0.58 for fat. The range of correlations for the eight nutrients assessed was 0.44 for protein and 0.79 for vitamin C. Recalled energy intake from the YANA-C recall was 13% higher than food record intake (9336 vs. 8236 kJ). Spearman correlations for amount/portion agreement ranged from 0.15 for cereals to 0.97 for eggs. Percent agreement of food matches ranged from 76% for pastry and cookies to 97% each for bread, cereals, and fish. |
| Rankin et al.[38] | 44 m<br>81 f | 13–18 years | 24 h recall; interviewer administered; quantitative | TEE by basal metabolic rate (BMR) and physical activity levels (PALs) | Compared reported energy intake from seven 24 h recalls with TEE by BMR and PALs | Pearson correlation between 24 h recall and TEE at baseline was 0.20 for girls and 0.04 for boys. Mean energy intake was underestimated by 14% for girls and 11% for boys in the 24 h recall at baseline. |

[a] Results of all subgroups not reported due to samples below the N = 30 criterion.
[b] Males (m), females (f).
[c] Adult assistance required for instrument administration.
[d] Hisp, includes Hispanic, Latino(a), Hispanic/Latino(a), Hispanic White, and Hispanic Black; see author definitions.
[e] MPR, multiple-pass recall.
[f] TEE, total energy expenditure.
[g] AA, African American.
[h] NA, includes Native American, American Indian, and Alaskan Native; see author definitions.

**TABLE 35.3**
**Recall Reliability Studies among School-Age Children**

| References[a] | Sample | Age/Grade | Instrument | Design | Results |
|---|---|---|---|---|---|
| Edmunds et al.[13] | 204 m and f[b] | 7–9 years | 24 h recall, DILQ; group administered; nonquantitative | Compared 2-week test–retest of fruit and vegetable intake from DILQ | Wilcoxon test for difference in total number of fruits and vegetables consumed at time 1 vs. 2 was significant for only 1 school that had documented no servings of vegetable on the lunch menu for the day of the second visit. There were no differences by gender (significance testing not shown). |
| Moore et al.[30] | 1024 m and f | 9–11 years | 24 h diet RQ; self-administered; previous-day intake and same-day breakfast; semiquantitative | Compared 4-month test–retest of mean intakes of "healthy" and "unhealthy" breakfast and food items | Spearman correlations between baseline and 4-month follow-up for "healthy" and "unhealthy" items were 0.60 and 0.56 for same day and 0.48 and 0.47 for previous day, respectively. Correlations for food items consumed during the rest of the day ranged from 0.33 for fruit to 0.75 for crisps. |
| Moore et al.[31] | 178 m and f 91 m 87 f | 9–11 years Adults required[c] | Computerized 24 h recall (checklist); three food types (fruit, sweets/chocolate/biscuit (SCB), crisps); self-administered; semiquantitative | Compared 8-day test–retest for fruit, SCB, and crisps intake from 24 h recall checklists. The first administration was preceded by a 24 h food diary reporting assisted by parents. | Mean reported intake for periods 1–6 of fruit, SCB, and crisps was lower for the second administration than for the first, −58%, −15%, and −26%, respectively. Mean reported intake for periods 2–3 of fruit, SCB, and crisps was 0, 5%, and −4%, respectively, between the two measurements. |
| Andersen et al.[33] | 54 m 60 f | Sixth grade | 24 h recall of fruit and vegetables; group administered; semiquantitative | Compared 2-week test–retest of fruit and vegetable intake from 24 h recalls | Reported intakes from the two 24 h recalls were not significantly different for fruit, fruit juice, potato, and vegetable. There were significant differences for the combined groups, fruit and vegetable without fruit juice and potato, and fruit, fruit juice, vegetable, and potato. No differences were seen between times 1 and 2 for combined genders (significance testing not shown) except for between times 1 and 2 for girls for combined fruits and vegetables without juice and potato, but not for boys. |
| Vereecken et al.[37] | 37 m and f | 11–14 years | 24 h recall computer-assisted YANA-C; self-administered; quantitative | Compared 1-week test–retest of food and nutrient intake from YANA-C 24 h recall | Mean recalled energy intake from the first assessment was 0.25% (8791 vs. 8813 <J) lower than the second assessment. |
| Johnson et al.[35] | 45 m 53 f | 13–14 years | 24 h recall of 41 items (10 fatty, 13 sugary, 10 fibrous, and 3 low-sugar foods and 5 alternative fats), FIQ; self- administered; past 3 months; nonquantitative | Compared 3-month test–retest of food intake from child's recall on FIQ | Spearman correlations between times 1 and 2 were 0.58 for sugary foods, 0.45 for fiber, and 0.59 for fatty foods; correlations between times 1 and 3 were 0.62 for sugary foods, 0.42 for fiber, and 0.55 for fatty foods; correlations between times 2 and 3 were 0.69 for sugary foods, 0.44 for fiber, and 0.59 for fatty foods. |

[a] Results of all subgroups not reported due to samples below the N = 30 criterion.
[b] Males (m), females (f).
[c] Adult assistance required for instrument administration.

may cause phantom foods to appear. Substantive progress has been made to understand the role of phantom and missing foods (intrusions and exclusions) associated with children's recalls.[19–21,23–28] Understanding the origin and negative effects of intrusions and exclusions on recall validity has substantively advanced the field. This research also indicates repeated recalls over time do not increase these types of reporting errors.

Child observations were used as the validity standard in 60% of the recall validity studies and another 14% used total energy expenditure (TEE) or food chemical analyses. Eight- to 10-year-olds are the youngest age group reporting a complete 24 h recall without adult assistance.[15] Energy intake was assessed in 16 of the recall validity study groups and was overestimated in 10 and underestimated in 6, as compared to the standard.

Five of the six recall reproducibility studies are a partial-day recall and one a full-day recall. The partial-day studies include those focused on selected foods such as fruits and vegetables. Foods were excerpted from a recall for the evaluation. Children ages 7–14 years have participated in studies. The study designs include a 1 week and up to a 4-month reproducibility assessment. The heterogeneity of the designs and populations does not allow for further summarization.

## FOOD RECORD

Food records are written accounts of actual intake of the food and beverages consumed during a specified time period, usually 3, 5, or 7 days (Table 35.4).[39] A single food record is a measure of actual intake and, like the 24 h recall, is appropriate for estimating group means and is not a tool to predict individual-level health outcomes. The work of Nelson and colleagues can be used to calculate the number of days of records necessary to determine nutrient intake with precision.[4] Respondents record detailed information about their dietary intake, such as brand names, ingredients of mixed dishes, food preparation methods, and estimates of amounts consumed. By collecting the information at the time of consumption, error due to memory loss is reduced, and thus, food records often serve as a validation standard. Prompts for quantification of food portions, such as 2D or 3D food models, are frequently used to aid respondents.

The food records evaluated for validity ranged from 1 to 8 days in length and 63% required parental assistance for completion. Two of the studies used computer approaches[32,43] to collect the food record and two study groups used only a portion of a day for the validation.[43] Seven studies used TEE, five used observation, one used 24 h urine, and one used serum folate as the validation standard.

Audiotaping food records and photography of food consumed has been explored as an alternative to pen and paper records.[11,15] A precoded-style food record has been described in two studies for children as young as fourth grade.[46,50] Energy intake was assessed in 10 of the record validity study groups and was overestimated in 4 and underestimated in 6, as compared to the standard.

Accurate completion of food records is greatly dependent on the ability of the child to read and write. Caution is suggested when interpreting studies using child-completed food records as the validation standard because young children less than 9 years have not been shown to accurately complete food records independently. The validity of food records for measuring long-term or usual food intake improves with more days of recording,[32] which indicates that multiple records may be needed. Multiple food records/recalls can introduce compliance issues for children because of the high respondent burden. Since a high degree of cooperation is required from children for food records, it is essential that children be motivated to participate and be cognitively able to complete the records or be provided assistance.

## FOOD FREQUENCY QUESTIONNAIRES AND CHECKLISTS

FFQs determine usual food intake and are often utilized in epidemiologic studies because they are relatively easy to administer, less expensive than other assessment methods, and easily adapted for population studies (Tables 35.5 and 35.6). A measure of usual intake can be used to rank respondents by intake levels and is useful for predicting health outcomes at both group and individual levels. Respondents typically report their usual intake over a defined period of time in the past year, month, or week, although frequency of intake on the previous day has also been assessed. The FFQ can be self-administered, interviewer administered, parent completed, or group administered and is well suited for computerized applications. The burden of work for the researcher is on the front end developing the food list for the FFQ. The appropriateness of the FFQ food list for the population is key to the accuracy of usual intake estimates. Respondents are typically asked to report frequency of consumption and sometimes the portion size for a defined list of foods. FFQs can be classified as quantitative, semiquantitative, or nonquantitative. Data from nonquantitative FFQs are generally used to assess frequency of consumption of food; however, these frequencies may also be associated with standard portions to estimate nutrient amounts. Semiquantitative FFQs have standard portions, servings, or predetermined amount (a description or a picture) to guide the respondent. Studies do not generally use standard portion sizes adjusted for children's level of intake. In 2006, our review[3] found 12% of the studies adjusted portion sizes for children, and in this review, 16.6% adjusted portions for children. This may enhance the lack of agreement between the FFQ and validation standard if the validation-standard-defined standard portions differ from those of the FFQ.

Researchers developed short food frequency-type questionnaires, called checklists or screeners, to assess intake of a specific list of foods or food groups. Some of these are developed from longer FFQs and assess a particular food group (fruits or vegetables) or intake of a nutrient. These short FFQs typically did not assess portion size and ranged

**TABLE 35.4**
**Food Record Validity and Reliability Studies among School-Age Children**

| Validity References[a] | Sample | Age/Grade | Instrument | Validation Standard | Design | Results |
|---|---|---|---|---|---|---|
| O'Connor et al.[40] | 22 m[b] 25 f[b] | 6–9 years Adults required[c] | 3-day food record; quantitative | TEE[d] by doubly labeled water | Compared average of child's parent-assisted food record against 10-day TEE. | Mean recorded energy intake was 4% greater than TEE from doubly labeled water (7.51 vs. 7.4 mJ/day). |
| Lindquist et al.[11] | 17 m 13 f 17 White 13 AA[e] | 6.5–11.6 years Adults required | 3-day audiotaped food record; quantitative | TEE by doubly labeled water | Compared average of child's parent-assisted reports of intake from audiotaped food records against 14-day TEE. | Mean recorded energy intake from 3-day records was 14% lower than TEE from doubly labeled water (6.73 vs.7.86 mJ/day). Age was significantly related to reporting accuracy with underestimation of energy intake from audiotaped food records increasing with age. |
| Bokhof et al.[41] | 137 m and f 102 m and f | 7–8 years 11–13 years Adults required | 1-day weighed dietary record; quantitative | 24 h urine samples | Compared 1-day weighed dietary record with simultaneously collected 24 h urine samples. | Pearson correlations between weighed record and 24 h urine for protein intake and energy-adjusted protein intake were 0.56 and 0.50 for 7–8 years and 0.59 and 0.56 for 11–13 years, respectively. |
| Lambert et al.[42] | 65 m | 7–11 years | Two 5-day smart card food records; semiquantitative | Observation | Compared food items recorded on smart card (adjusted for portion-size error and weighed tray waste) with observed items selected. | Percent agreement between smart card selected and smart card observed was 95.9%. |
| Knuiman et al.[43] | 30 m | 8–9 years Adults required | 3-day lunch food record; quantitative | Observation | Compared average of child's parent-assisted record of lunch intake against observation of lunch with weighed duplicate portions. Excerpted lunch meal from 7-day nonconsecutive food records collected over 15 days. | Correlations between mean values from recorded lunch intake and observed lunch intake were 0.71 for energy, 0.66 for protein, and 0.63 for total fat. The range of correlations for 14 nutrients (i.e., both absolute and density values) assessed was 0.62 for saturated fatty acids (% kcal) to 0.92 for polyunsaturated fat (% kcal). Recorded energy intake was 25% higher than observed intake (456 vs. 365 kcal/meal). Ten nutrients were significantly overestimated by recorded intake of lunch as compared to observation. |
| Knuiman et al.[43] | 68 m | 8–9 years Adults required | 7-day dinner food record; quantitative | Chemical analysis of food | Compared average of mothers' record of dinner intake against chemical analyses of duplicate portions of dinner. Excerpted dinner from 7-day nonconsecutive food records collected over 15 days. | Correlations between mean values from recorded dinner intake and chemical analyses of dinner were 0.52 for energy, 0.56 for protein, and 0.58 for total fat. The range of correlations for the 14 nutrients (i.e., both absolute and density values) assessed was 0.45 for polyunsaturated fat (% kcal) to 0.85 for cholesterol. Recorded energy intake was 31% higher than chemical analysis of food (647 vs. 495 kcal/meal). Nine nutrients were significantly overestimated by mother's record of dinner as compared to chemical analysis of dinner. |
| Van Horn et al.[15] | 33 m and f | 8–10 years | 1-day audiotaped food record; quantitative | Observation | Compared child's report of intake from audiotaped food record against parent's observation recorded as a food record. | Pearson correlations between child's record and parent's record were 0.68 for energy, 0.82 for protein (% kcal), and 0.82 for total fat (% kcal). The range of correlations for the 10 nutrients assessed was 0.68 for energy to 0.96 for iron. Child's recorded energy intake was 2% lower than parents' recorded energy intake (1882 vs. 1913 kcal/day). There were no significant differences between child and parent reports of nutrient intake (significance testing not shown). |

(continued)

**TABLE 35.4 (continued)**

**Food Record Validity and Reliability Studies among School-Age Children**

| Validity References[a] | Sample | Age/Grade | Instrument | Validation Standard | Design | Results |
|---|---|---|---|---|---|---|
| Bandini et al.[44] | 109 f; White, AA, Hisp[f], others | 8–12 years; Adults required | 7-day food record; quantitative | TEE by doubly labeled water | Compared average of child's adult-assisted food record against 14-day TEE. | Mean recorded energy intake was 13% lower than TEE from doubly labeled water (7.00 vs. 8.03 mJ/day). Age was significantly related to reporting accuracy with underestimation of energy intake from food records increasing with age. There were no significant differences by ethnicity. |
| Lillegaard et al.[45] | 109 m and f; 55 m; 45 f | Fourth grade; 9 years; Adults required | 4-day precoded food diary (PFD); parent's child-assisted record; semiquantitative | Weighed records | Compared average of 4-day PFD intake against intake from 4-day weighed record started 3 days late. | Spearman correlation coefficients for energy, protein, and fat were 0.43, 0.47, and 0.41 for girls and 0.41, 0.48, and 0.37 for boys, respectively. Correlations of 13 nutrients ranged from 0.37 for added sugar (g) to 0.61 for fiber (g) for girls and 0.32 for iron (mg) to 0.62 for retinol (µg) for boys. Mean energy intake was overreported by 8% (8.0 vs. 7.4 mJ) for girls and underreported by −4.7% for boys (8.0 vs. 8.4 mJ). For all 13 nutrients, girls overestimated intake on PFD; boys overestimated for 7 out of 13 nutrients. |
| Lillegaard et al.[46] | 51 m and f; 24 m; 27 f | Fourth grade; 9 years; Adults required | 4-day PFD; semiquantitative | TEE by position-and-movement monitor | Compared energy intake from PFD with TEE during simultaneous 4-day period. | Pearson's correlation between energy intake and TEE was 0.28. Classification into the same quartile with both PFD and TEE by position-and-movement monitor was 37%, classification into the correct or adjacent quartiles was 75%, and gross misclassification was 10%. Correlations by gender between energy intake and TEE were 0.23 for girls (excluding overreporters of energy intake) and 0.46 for boys. |
| Baranowski et al.[32] | 138 m and f; 45% m; 55% f; 34% White; 30% AA; 15% Hisp; 21% others | Fourth grade; 9–11 years | 1-day software-recorded food record; quantitative; self-administered | Observation; 24 h recall | Compared average of food recall entered into FIRSSt with school lunch observations and 24 h recall. | Correlation between portion-size estimates for FIRSSt against 24 h recall was 0.75 and against observation was 0.73. Compared against observation, FIRSSt attained lower match (46%) and higher intrusion (24%) and omission (30%) rates than 24 h recall (59%, 17%, 24%, respectively). |
| Champagne et al.[47] | 118 m and f; 60 m; 58 f; 62 White; 56 AA | 9–12 years; Adults required | 8-day food record; quantitative | TEE by doubly labeled water | Compared average of child's parent-assisted food record against 8-day TEE. | Mean recorded energy intake was 24% lower than TEE from doubly labeled water for males (1953 vs. 2555 kcal/day) and 27% lower for females (1633 vs. 2232 kcal/day). Mean recorded energy intake was 28% lower than TEE from doubly labeled water for AAs (1678 vs. 2346 kcal/day) and 22% lower for Whites (1909 vs. 2441 kcal/day). |
| DiNoia et al.[48] | 89 m and f; 48% m; 52% f AA | 11–14 years | 3-day CD-ROM-mediated food record; quantitative; self-administered | Observation | Compared Healthy Eating Self-Monitoring Test (HEST) CD-ROM-mediated food record with observation of breakfast, lunch, and dinner for three consecutive days at summer camps. | The range of correlations for HEST-recorded and HEST-observed fruit and vegetable intake was 0.38–0.52. Spearman correlations for 3-day intake of fruits, vegetables, and juices were 0.39, 0.58, and 0.28, respectively. |

| References | Sample | Age/Grade | Instrument | Design | Results |
|---|---|---|---|---|---|
| Livingstone et al.[49] | 34 m and f; 50% m; 50% f; 35% 12 years; 35% 15 years; 29% 18 years | 12–18 years; Adults required | 7-day weighed food record; quantitative | TEE by doubly labeled water. Compared average of child's parent-assisted food record against 10–14-day TEE. | Energy intake from weighed food records was less than TEE in 29 of 34 children. |
| Andersen et al.[50] | 41 m and f; 31 m and f | 13 years | 4-day precoded energy intake food diary; semiquantitative | TEE by position-and-movement monitor. Compared PFD with TEE. Study 1 participants completed 4-day food diary on weekdays and recorded TEE during same time period. Study 2 participants completed 4-day food diary on 3 weekdays and 1 weekend day and recorded TEE for 7 days starting 3 days before beginning the food diary. | Pearson correlations between energy intake and TEE were 0.47 in study 1 and 0.74 in study 2. Mean energy intake from PFD was 34% lower in study 1 (7.8 vs. 11.9 mJ/day) and was 22% lower in study 2 (8.0 vs. 10.3 mJ/day) compared to TEE. |
| Green et al.[51] | 14 f; 19 f; 29 f; 43 f | 16 years; 17 years; 18 years; 19 years | 3-day food record; quantitative | Serum folate, red blood cell (RBC) folate, and serum vitamin B-12. Compared average of child's food record against serum micronutrient levels collected 1 week before food records. | Pearson correlations between recorded folate intake and serum folate were 0.65, between recorded folate intake and RBC folate were 0.50, and between recorded vitamin B-12 intake and serum B-12 were 0.32. |
| **Reliability** | **Sample** | **Age/Grade** | **Instrument** | **Design** | **Results** |
| Martin et al.[52] | 23 m; 20 f | Sixth grade | 5-day digital photography lunch record; quantitative | Compared 5-day food record reproducibility of food selection, plate waste, and food intake by two dietitians. | Correlation coefficients between the two dietitians were 0.93 for energy, 0.93 for fat (kcal), 0.89 for protein, and 0.94 for carbohydrate. |

[a] Results of subgroups not reported due to samples below the N = 30 criterion.
[b] Males (m), females (f).
[c] Adult assistance required for instrument administration.
[d] TEE, total energy expenditure.
[e] AA, African American.
[f] Hisp, includes Hispanic, Latino(a), Hispanic/Latino(a), Hispanic White, and Hispanic Black; see author definitions.

**TABLE 35.5**
**FFQ[a] and Checklist Validity Studies among School-Age Children**

| References[b] | Sample | Age/Grade | Instrument | Response Categories (Range) | Validation Standard | Design | Results |
|---|---|---|---|---|---|---|---|
| Blom et al.[53] | 13 m[c] 17 f | 2–16 years Adults required[d] | 36 items (sucrose, protein, fat, fiber, nitrite, vitamin C); self-administered; referent period not specified; nonquantitative | Unknown (<1/week to ≥4 times/ day) | 7-day food record | Compared child's parent-assisted report of intake on FFQ of foods with high content of sucrose, protein, fat, fiber, nitrite, and vitamin C against child's parent- and other adult-assisted report of intake on 7-day consecutive food record completed 6–8 weeks before the FFQ. | Spearman correlations between FFQ and food records for frequency of food groups with high content of protein and fat were 0.69 and 0.69, respectively. The range of correlations for six food groups assessed was 0.52 for sucrose to 0.76 for vitamin C. Compared to the food record, two food groups were significantly overestimated and three were significantly underestimated by the FFQ. Of 34 food items, 5 were significantly overestimated and 8 were significantly underestimated by the FFQ. |
| Taylor et al.[54] | 26 m 41 f | 3–6 years Adults required | 35 items (calcium); self-administered; past year; semiquantitative | Open-ended (never to number of times/month) | 4-day food record | Compared parent's frequency of intake of calcium foods on FFQ against parent's report of child's 4-day food record. | FFQ significantly overestimated mean calcium intake by 18% compared to the food record (942 vs. 798 mg/day). |
| Cade et al.[55] | 180 m and f 100 m 80 f | 3–7 years Adults required | <92-item (12 fruits, 10 vegetables, 4 beans/seeds, 7 drinks) Child and Diet Evaluation Tool (CADET); group administered; past 24 h; nonquantitative | 2 (yes/no) | 1-day semiweighed food record | Compared child's parent- and other adult-assisted FFQs of intake of foods with 1-day semiweighed food record completed by parent and researcher. FFQ and food record were completed on the same day. | Correlations between the FFQ and food record were 0.41 for energy, 0.41 for protein, and 0.46 for fat and ranged from 0.32 for polyunsaturated fat to 0.68 for carotene for 10 nutrients. Correlations for fruit and vegetable intake were 0.52 (fruit), 0.56 (vegetable), and 0.40 (fruit and vegetable). FFQ overestimated mean energy by 15% (1800 vs. 1563 kcal) compared to the food record. Classification in the same tertile ranged from 57% for fiber to 43% for energy; extreme misclassification ranged from 12% for protein to 7% for calcium. Correlations between FFQ and food record for girls were higher for energy, carbohydrate, calcium, iron, and fat and lower for protein, fiber, and vitamin C than boys. |

| Reference | Sample | Instrument | Items/frequency | Reference method | Comparison | Results |
|---|---|---|---|---|---|---|
| Kobayashi et al.[56] | 48 m and f 41 m and f Adults required | 75-item Children's FFQ (CFFQ); self-administered; previous month; semiquantitative; child portions | Dependent on food type | 4-day weighed food record | Compared parent's report of child's frequency of intake of foods on FFQ against parent's report on 4-day weighed food record collected once a week for the 4 weeks prior to completing the FFQ. | For 3- to 11-year-olds, Pearson correlations between the CFFQ and food records were 0.66 for energy, 0.66 for protein, and 0.51 for fat and ranged from 0.37 (alpha-linolenic acid) to 0.73 (manganese) for 12 fatty acids and 24 additional nutrients. CFFQ underestimated energy intake by 1% compared to food records (1533 vs. 1547 kcal/day). For 12- to 16-year-olds, Pearson correlations between the CFFQ and food records were 0.33 for energy, 0.37 for protein, and 0.14 for fat and ranged from 0.04 (linoleic acid) to 0.42 (niacin and arachidonic acid) for 12 fatty acids and 24 additional nutrients. CFFQ underestimated energy intake by 14% compared to food records (1781 vs. 2078 kcal/day). |
| Kobayashi et al.[56] | 48 m and f 41 m and f Adults required | 76-item Adult's FFQ (AFFQ): self-administered; previous month; semiquantitative; adult portions | Dependent on food type | 4-day weighed food record | Compared parent's report of child's frequency of intake of foods on FFQ against parent's report on 4-day weighed food record collected once a week for the 4 weeks prior to completing the FFQ. | For 3- to 1-year-olds, Pearson correlations between AFFQ and food records were 0.57 for energy, 0.55 for protein, and 0.41 for fat and ranged from 0.09 (cholesterol) to 0.71 (manganese) for 12 fatty acids and 24 additional nutrients. AFFQ overestimated energy intake by 14% compared to food records (1757 vs. 1547 kcal/day). For 12- to 16-year-olds Pearson correlations between AFFQ and food records were 0.31 for energy, 0.25 for protein, and −0.07 for fat and ranged from 0.01 (alpha-tocopherol) to 0.40 (copper) for 12 fatty acids and 24 additional nutrients. AFFQ overestimated energy intake by 9% compared to food records (2257 vs. 2078 kcal/day). |
| Kaskoun et al.[57] | 22 m 23 f White, NA[e] 4–6 years Adults required | <111 items; self-administered; past year; semiquantitative; adult portions | 9 (<1/month to ≥6 times/day) | TEE[f] by doubly labeled water | Compared parent's report of child's frequency of intake of foods on FFQ against 14-day TEE completed after or at the same time as the FFQ. | FFQ significantly overestimated total energy intake by 59% compared to TEE (9.12 vs. 5.74 mJ/day). |
| Persson et al.[58] | 477 m and f 4 and 8 years Adults required | 27 items; interviewer administered; referent period not specified; nonquantitative | 8 (none to ≥4 times/day) | 7-day food record | Compared parent's report of child's frequency of intake of foods on FFQ against parent's report of child's intake on 7-day food records. Foods from the records were translated into food categories of the FFQ. | FFQ significantly overestimated intake of 15 food items and underestimated intake of 9 items as compared to the food record. |
| Wilson et al.[59] | 61 f 50 White 10 AA[g] 1 Asian 4–9 years Adults required | 109 items; (Block 98 FFQ) interviewer administered; past year; quantitative | 9 (none or <1/month to 2+ times/ day; three portion sizes) | 3-day food record | Compared parent's child-assisted report of frequency of intake of foods on FFQ against parent's report of child's intake from 3-day food record. | Correlations between Block98 FFQ and food records ranged from 0.40 for energy to 0.55 for three macronutrients. Block98 FFQ energy intake was 25% higher than the diet record (2180 vs. 1749 kcal/day). |

(continued)

**TABLE 35.5 (continued)**
**FFQ[a] and Checklist Validity Studies among School-Age Children**

| References[b] | Sample | Age/Grade | Instrument | Response Categories (Range) | Validation Standard | Design | Results |
|---|---|---|---|---|---|---|---|
| Hammond et al.[60] | 150 m and f | 5–11 years Adults required | 35 items (fat, energy, fiber); self-administered; past month; nonquantitative | 10 (none to 7 days/week) | 14-day food checklist | Compared child's parent-assisted report of frequency of intake of foods on FFQ against child's parent-assisted report of intake on 14-day food checklists. Food checklists consisted of two sets of 7-day consecutive food records 1 and 2 months after the FFQ and contained the same food categories as the FFQ. | Median difference in days/week consumption between the FFQs and food checklists was equal to 0 for 17 foods, >0 for 5 foods, and <0 for 13 foods (significance testing not shown). Differences ranged from −1 (cakes, chips) to 1 (green vegetables). Percentage of responders classified to within ± 1 day/week of frequencies reported on checklists ranged from 46.8% for low-fiber cereal to 99.3% for lamb, other fish, and liver. |
| Burrows et al.[61] | 93 m and f | 5–12 years Adults required | 137 items (21 vegetables, 11 fruits); self-administered; past 6 months; semiquantitative; "natural" or child portions | Unknown | Plasma carotenoids | Compared parent's report of child's frequency of intake of foods on FFQ against child's fasting plasma carotenoid concentration. | Pearson correlations between FFQ and plasma concentration of carotenoids after adjusting for BMI were 0.56 for β-carotene, 0.51 for α-carotene, 0.32 for cryptoxanthin, and 0.42 for lycopene. |
| Byers et al.[62] | 43 m 54 f White, AA | 6–10 years Adults required | 35 items (15 fruits, 20 vegetables); self-administered; past 3 months; semiquantitative; adult portions | 9 (none or <1 time/month to ≥6 times/day) | Serum carotenoids vitamins A, C, and E | Compared parent's report of child's frequency of intake on FFQ of fruit and vegetables against child's serum micronutrient levels. | Spearman correlations between FFQ and serum nutrients were 0.16 for carotene, 0.39 for vitamin C, 0.14 for vitamin A, and 0.32 for vitamin E. Correlations between frequencies of intake of total fruits and vegetables and serum levels of carotene, vitamin C, vitamin A, and vitamin E were 0.24, 0.29, 0.14, and 0.17, respectively. There were no differences by gender or ethnicity (significance testing not shown). |
| Marcotte et al.[63] | 18 m 24 f 28 White 8 AA 6 others | 7–8 years Adults required | 19 items (15 calcium foods and 4 dummy foods); interviewer administered; past 24 h; child portions | Open-ended | One 24 h recall | Compared child's report of frequency of food intake on checklist against child's parent-assisted report of intake on 24 h recall. Checklist and recall were administered in randomly determined order, 1.5 h apart. | Spearman correlations between the checklist and 24 h recall were 0.28 for total calcium (from all foods) and 0.51 for dairy calcium (from dairy foods). Total calcium intake from the checklist and 24 h recall was similar (935 vs. 1053 mg). Calcium intake from calcium foods on checklist and 24 h recall was similar (766 vs. 698 mg). |

| Muckelbauer et al.[64] | 35 m and f<br>15 m<br>20 f | 7–9 years<br>Adults required | 24 h RQ (7 beverage categories); self-administered; past 24 h; semiquantitative | 2 (yes/no; full, half-full, and empty glass) | One 24 h weighed diet record | Compared child's report of beverage volume and consumption with parent's report of 24 h weighed record. | Spearman correlations for beverage volume between RQ and weighed record ranged from 0.86 for soft drinks to 0.91 for juices. Correlation for total 24 h volume between RQ and weighed record was 0.72. Classification of participants into the correct tertile was 49% for total 24 h volume, 80% for mineral/tap water, 71% for milk, and 22% for juices/soft drinks. Gross misclassification ranged from 0% for milk to 3% for total 24 h volume, mineral/tap water, and juices/soft drinks. Correct classification of children into consumers vs. nonconsumers for each beverage category for match rates ranged from 91% for tap water to 97% for juices, tea, and others; omission rates ranged from 0% for juices and other to 3% for mineral water, tap water, milk, soft drinks, and tea; intrusion rates ranged from 0% for tea to 6% for tap water. |
| Zemel et al.[65] | 104 m and f<br>61 f<br>43 m<br>34 7–8 years<br>70 9–10 years<br>22 AA<br>82 non-AA | 7–10 years<br>Adults required | 41-item Calcium Counts! FFQ (CCFFQ); administered to parent/child by RD; previous 4 weeks; semiquantitative; typical serving sizes | Number of servings per day, week, or month (or never) | 7-day parent-completed food record | Compared child's parent-assisted CCFFQ report against 7-day parent-completed food record completed the week following the visit. | Pearson correlations between CCFFQ and 7-day record were 0.61 for calcium. CCFFQ calcium intake was significantly higher (300 mg/day) vs. 7-day record. Differences were larger for younger children (367 mg/day) vs. older children (268 mg/day), females (318 mg/day) vs. males (275 mg/day), and lower for AA (164 mg/day) vs. non-AA (337 mg/day). When quintiles between FFQ and 7-day record were compared, 74% of items were correctly classified (same or adjacent quintile). Correlations for calcium intake between FFQ and 7-day record were 0.43 for ages 7–8, 0.67 for ages 9–10, 0.59 for females, 0.54 for males, 0.35 for AA, and 0.66 for non-AA. |
| Arnold et al.[66] | 77 f | 7–12 years<br>Adults required | 160 items; self-administered; past year (inferred); semiquantitative; adult portions | Open-ended (none to number of months/year) | Two sets of 7-day food record | Compared child's parent-assisted report of frequency of intake from two FFQ administrations against child's parent-assisted report of intake on two sets of consecutive 7-day food records. Records were completed 1 month after each FFQ and the two FFQs were 6 months apart. | Pearson correlations (log transformed, energy adjusted) between the first FFQ and the first 7-day food record and the second FFQ and second 7-day food record were 0.29 and 0.22 for energy, 0.17 and 0.25 for protein, and 0.05–0.38 for fat, respectively. The range of correlations for 16 nutrients assessed at the first assessment was 0.00 for unsaturated fat to 0.51 for vitamin B2 and at the second assessment was 0.?3 for starch to 0.60 for fiber. For the first FFQ, energy intake was 24% higher than the first food record (2319 vs. 1867 kcal/day). For the second FFQ, energy intake was 16% higher than the second food record (2205 vs. 1902 kcal/day). Both FFQs overestimated intake for all 16 nutrients compared to food records (significance testing not shown). |

(continued)

**TABLE 35.5 (continued)**
**FFQ[a] and Checklist Validity Studies among School-Age Children**

| References[b] | Sample | Age/Grade | Instrument | Response Categories (Range) | Validation Standard | Design | Results |
|---|---|---|---|---|---|---|---|
| Marshall et al.[67] | 63 m 66 f | 8 years Adults required | 75-item Block Kids' Food Questionnaire; self-administered; past week; semiquantitative | Unknown | 3-day food record | Compared parent's child-assisted report of child's frequency of intake on FFQ against parent's child-assisted report of child's intake on food record. Block Kids' Food Questionnaire was completed within 4 months of food records. | Spearman correlations between FFQ and food records were 0.26 for energy, 0.31 for protein, and 0.27 for fat. Spearman correlations for five additional nutrients ranged from 0.20 for carbohydrates to 0.56 for energy-adjusted calcium. FFQ energy intake was 2.2% lower (1701 vs. 1740 kcal) than from the food record. Spearman correlations for beverages ranged from 0.22 for juice drinks to 0.57 for milk. Percent agreement of quartile placements for 5 beverages ranged from 32.6% for juice drinks to 46.0% for milk. |
| Marshall et al.[67] | 106 m 117 f | 8–9 years Adults required | 22-item (bone nutrients, e.g., calcium, vitamin D, fluoride) targeted nutrient questionnaire; self-administered; past week; semiquantitative | Unknown | 3-day food record | Compared parent's child-assisted report of child's frequency of intake of foods on targeted nutrient questionnaire against parent's child-assisted report of child's intake on food record. Targeted nutrient questionnaires were completed 4–9 months after food records. | Spearman correlations between the nutrient questionnaire and the food records were 0.46 for calcium, 0.49 for vitamin D, and 0.53 for fluoride. Spearman correlations for beverages ranged from 0.25 for soda pop to 0.57 for milk. The questionnaire significantly underestimated calcium, vitamin D, and fluoride; underestimated milk; and overestimated 100% juice. Percent agreement on classification of quartile placements for beverages ranged from 34.1% for soda pop and water to 47.5% for 100% juice. |
| Baranowski et al.[68] | 1530–1570 m and f White, AA | Third grade | Seven items (three fruits, four vegetables); group administered; past month; semiquantitative; "serving" portions | 10 (none to ≥5 times/day) | 7-day food record | Compared child's report of servings of fruits and vegetables against child's report of intake on 7-day food records. Foods from the records were abstracted into the FFQ categories by a dietitian. | Pearson correlations between the FFQ and food records for fruits and vegetables, fruits and juices, and vegetables were 0.20, 0.24, and 0.15, respectively. Mean total serving of fruits and vegetables per week as measured by the FFQ was 50.9 and by the food record was 15.9. The FFQ significantly overestimated intake of food items in all seven food categories, both aggregate and individual items (significance testing not shown). |
| Bellu et al.[69] | 165 m 158 f | 8–10 years Adults required | 116 items; self-administered; past 6 months; semiquantitative; "average" portions | Unknown | One 24 h recall | Compared parent's report of child's frequency of intake on FFQ of foods against mother's report of child's intake on 24 h recall. | Mean energy estimates from the 24 h recall for females were 27% higher than the 24 h recall for females (2156 vs. 1703 kcal/day) and 25% higher for males (2281 vs. 1821 kcal/day). Intake was overestimated by the FFQ as compared to the recall for one nutrient and underestimated for two among females. Among males, the FFQ overestimated three nutrients and underestimated one. |

| Reference | Sample | Age | Instrument | Response | Comparison method | Description | Results |
|---|---|---|---|---|---|---|---|
| Mariscal-Arcas et al.[70] | 241 m and f; Adults required | 8–15 years | Unknown number of items; interviewer administered; previous day, week, and year; semiquantitative | Open-ended (consumed or not, times consumed per day, week, or month during previous year) | Three 24 h recalls | Compared child's report of frequency of food intake on FFQ against child's report of intake on three 24 h recalls completed the 3 days before the FFQ. | Median intakes were similar between FFQ and 24 h recalls for energy (8.2 vs. 8.1 MJ), protein (71.7 vs. 70.8 g), fat (88.5 vs. 85.6 g), and carbohydrates (215.5 vs. 224.4 g). Mean intake from 24 h recalls minus mean intake from FFQ was −0.01 mJ for energy, 0.64 g for protein, −2.85 g for fat, and 0.70 g for carbohydrate. Wilcoxon tests comparing FFQ and 24 h recalls were not significant for energy, protein, fat, or carbohydrates. |
| Perks et al.[71] | 23 m; 27 f | 8–16 years | 131-item Youth/Adolescent Questionnaire (YAQ); self-administered; past year; semiquantitative; child portions | Dependent on food type | TEE by doubly labeled water | Compared child's report of frequency of intake of foods on YAQ against TEE. Child completed YAQ within 1 year of TEE measurement. | Mean energy intake from YAQ was 1.93% higher, yet not significant, than TEE from doubly labeled water (10.03 vs. 9.84 mJ/day). Body weight and percentage body fat were significantly correlated to the discrepancy in energy intake (YAQ-TEE). |
| Stiegler et al.[72] | 101 m and f; 52 m; 49 f | 9–11 years; Adults required | 82-item FFQ; parent-assisted; past year; semiquantitative; pictures of food portion sizes with options to choose parts of a portion | 9 (never and once/month to 2–3 times/day and 4 times/day or more) | One parent-assisted telephone 24 h recall | Compared child's parent-assisted FFQ with one parent-assisted 24 h telephone recall completed 2–3 weeks after the FFQ. The 24 h recall was conducted using only weekday data. Food items and nutrients from the FFQ and 24 h recall were compared. | Mean energy intake from the FFQ was 7.9% higher than from the 24 h recall (8554 vs. 7926 kJ/day). The percentage of nutrient intakes correctly classified by tertiles using the two methods was about 40%, with about 10%–15% classified into adjacent tertiles. Classification in the same tertile ranged from 31.7% for vitamin E to 45.5% for total fat intake; extreme misclassification ranged from 8.9% for SFA to 23.8% for MUFA. CHO. FFQ overestimated food group intakes by more than 10% for 13 food groups and underestimated nine food groups more than 10% as compared to the recall. |
| Thiagarajah et al.[73] | 110 m and f; 47% m; 53% f | 9–11 years | 54-item School Physical Activity and Nutrition (SPAN) questionnaire; group administered; yesterday; nonquantitative | Unknown | One 24 hour recall | Compared child's responses on the SPAN survey with similar items on the child's 24 hour recall. | Spearman correlations between SPAN and recall for 20 food groups ranged from 0.25 (bread and bread products) to 0.67 (gravy). The percent agreement ranged from 26% for bread and related products to 90% for gravy. Kappa statistics ranged from 0.06 for chocolate candy to 0.60 for beans. |
| Wallen et al.[74] | 125 m and f; 51% m; 49% f | Fourth grade; 9–11 years | DILQ-Colorado (DILQ-CO); group administered; "yesterday to today" or "today to yesterday"; semiquantitative with symbols | 4 (all, more than half, less than half, none) | Observation and weighed plate waste | Compared child's DILQ-CO of school meals to observation and weighed plate waste estimates. Trained staff observed and recorded students' food selections and measured plate waste after the children left the lunchroom. | Spearman correlations between DILQ-CO responses and plate waste range from 0.31 for turkey wrap to 0.72 for flavored milk. Correlations between DILQ-CO and plate waste were significant for 5 of 10 lunch items. Percent matches between DILQ-CO responses and plate waste ranged from 61% for dessert to 99% for sandwiches, with kappa statistics ranging from 0.23 for dessert to 0.97 for sandwiches. |

*(continued)*

**TABLE 35.5 (continued)**
**FFQ[a] and Checklist Validity Studies among School-Age Children**

| References[b] | Sample | Age/Grade | Instrument | Response Categories (Range) | Validation Standard | Design | Results |
|---|---|---|---|---|---|---|---|
| Domel et al.[75] | 160–165 m and f White, AA | Fourth to fifth grade | 45 items (15 fruits, 30 vegetables); group administered; past month; semiquantitative; "serving" portions | 7 (none or <1/ month to several per day) | 22-day food record | Compared child's report of frequency of fruit and vegetable intake (mean of 2 administrations) against child's report of intake on 22 consecutive days of food records. Records were collected between FFQ administrations; foods from the records were abstracted by a dietitian into servings of fruit and vegetables. | Spearman correlations between month 1 FFQ and food records and month 2 FFQ and food records were 0.12 and 0.17 for total fruit, −0.04 and 0.02 for total vegetables, and −0.05 and 0.01 for total fruit and vegetable. The range of correlations for eight fruit/vegetable groupings assessed was −0.05 for total fruit and vegetables to 0.32 for fruit and vegetable juice. Mean daily servings of total fruit and vegetables were 409% higher for the month 1 FFQ compared to the corresponding food records (11.7 vs. 2.3) and 135% higher for the month 2 FFQ compared to the food records (5.4 vs. 2.3). Both administrations of the monthly FFQ significantly overestimated mean daily servings for all eight fruit/vegetable groupings compared to the corresponding food records. |
| Domel et al.[75] | 154–156 m and f White, AA | Fourth to fifth grade | 45 items (15 fruits, 30 vegetables); group administered; past week; semiquantitative; "serving" portions | 5 (none or <1/ week to several per day) | 7-day food record | Compared child's report of frequency of fruit and vegetable intake (mean of 2 administrations) against child's report of intake on 7-day food records. Records were collected between FFQ administrations; foods from the records were abstracted by a dietitian into servings of fruit and vegetables. | Spearman correlations between week 1 FFQ and food records and week 2 FFQ and food records were 0.18 and 0.18 for total fruit, −0.01 and 0.11 for total vegetable, and 0.00 and 0.05 for total fruit and vegetable. The range of correlations for eight fruit/vegetable groupings assessed was −0.01 for total vegetable to 0.25 for total legumes and fruit. Mean daily servings of total fruits and vegetables were 295% higher for week 1 FFQs compared to the corresponding food record (8.3 vs. 2.1) and 306% higher for week 2 FFQ (7.3 vs. 1.8). Both administrations of the FFQ significantly overestimated mean daily servings for all eight fruit and vegetable groupings compared to the food records. |
| Moore et al.[76] | 107 m | 9–12 years | 41-item calcium focus rapid assessment method (RAM); interviewer administered; typical day; semiquantitative visual aids to approximate serving sizes | Open-ended (number of servings/day) | One 24 h recall | Compared child's report of daily calcium intake on interviewer-administered RAM against child's calcium intake from 24 h recall (typical day). The 24 h recall covered the day prior to the interview. Both instruments were administered at the same time. | ICC between RAM and 24 h recall for daily calcium intake was 0.46. RAM calcium intake was 57% higher than from the 24 h recall (1576 vs. 1003 mg). |

(continued)

| Study | Sample | Age | FFQ | Frequency | Reference method | Comparison | Results |
|---|---|---|---|---|---|---|---|
| Bellu et al.[77] | 39 m 49 f | 9–12 years Adults required | 116 items; self-administered; past 6 months; semiquantitative; "average" portions | Unknown | 14-day weighed food record | Compared parent's report of child's frequency of intake of foods on FFQ against parent's report of child's intake on 14-day weighed food records. Records consisted of two sets of 7-day consecutive food records at the beginning of the study and 6 months later, before and after the FFQ. | Pearson correlations between FFQ and food records were 0.46 for energy, 0.34 for protein, and 0.39 for fat. The range of correlations for 18 nutrients assessed was 0.07 for vitamin A to 0.52 for carbohydrates. FFQ energy intake was 40% higher than the diet record (2620 vs. 1865 kcal/day). The FFQ significantly overestimated six nutrients and significantly underestimated five nutrients compared to the food records. |
| Field et al.[78] | 51 m and f 58 m and f 84% AA | Fourth to fifth grade Sixth to seventh grade | 97 items (11 fruits and fruit juices, 14 vegetables); group administered to fourth to fifth grade; self-administered to sixth to seventh grade; past year; semiquantitative; child portions | Dependent on food type | Four 24 h recalls | Compared child's report of frequency of intake of foods on FFQ against child's report of intake from four, nonconsecutive 24 h recalls administered 3 months apart and within 1 year of FFQ. Recalls were not conducted during the summer or on Saturdays. | Pearson correlations (unadjusted log-transformed values) between FFQ and mean of recalls among fourth to fifth graders were 0.26 for energy, 0.20 for protein, and 0.26 for fat. Correlations among sixth to seventh graders were 0.34 for energy, 0.23 for protein, and 0.24 for fat. The range of correlations among fourth to fifth graders for the 10 nutrients assessed was 0.01 for fat (% kcal) to 0.31 for saturated fat. The range among sixth to seventh graders was from 0.04 for fat (% kcal) to 0.50 for vitamin C. Spearman correlations (unadjusted) between FFQ and recalls among fourth to fifth graders ranged from −0.01 for servings of fruits and juice to 0.16 for vegetables. Among sixth to seventh graders, the range was from 0.13 for vegetables to 0.30 for fruit juice. Median FFQ energy intake was 87% higher than recalls (3136 vs. 1677 kcal/day) among fourth to fifth graders. Median FFQ energy intake was 15% higher than recalls (2297 vs. 1992 kcal/day) among sixth to seventh graders. |
| Watson et al.[79] | 113 m and f | 9–16 years | 120-item Australian Child and Adolescent Eating Survey (ACAES); self-administered; previous 6 months; semiquantitative; natural serving sizes for ages 9–16 years | Varied by food type (ranged from "never" to " or more times per day") | Four 1-day interviewer-assisted food records or recalls | Compared child's ACAES administered at the beginning (FFQ1) and end (FFQ2) of a 5-month period against four 1-day interviewer-assisted FRs collected between the two FFQs. If child had a missing food record, the interviewer did a 24 h recall instead. The average of food records was used to compare with FFQ2 and the mean of FFQs 1 and 2. | Spearman correlations (deattenuated, transformed) between FFQ2 and FRs were 0.22 for energy, 0.18 for protein, and 0.31 for total fat. The range of correlations for 21 nutrients assessed was 0.03 for retinol to 0.56 for magnesium. FFQ median energy intake was 7.9% higher than food records (10.0 vs. 9.3 mJ/day). The strength of agreement was slight for 9 nutrients (K ≤ 0.2) and fair for 13 nutrients (0.2 < K ≤ 0.4). |

**TABLE 35.5 (continued)**
**FFQ[a] and Checklist Validity Studies among School-Age Children**

| References[b] | Sample | Age/Grade | Instrument | Response Categories (Range) | Validation Standard | Design | Results |
|---|---|---|---|---|---|---|---|
| Watson et al.[79] | 101 m and f | 9–16 years | 120-item ACAES; self-administered; previous 6 months; semiquantitative; natural serving sizes for ages 9–16 years | Varied by food type (ranged from "never" to "four or more times per day") | Four 1-day interviewer-assisted food records or recalls | Compared child's ACAES administered at the beginning (FFQ1) and end (FFQ2) of a 5-month period against child's interviewer-assisted four 1-day food records collected between the two FFQ administrations. If child had a missing food record, the interviewer did a 24 h recall instead. The average of food records was used to compare with the FFQ2 and the mean of FFQs 1 and 2. | Spearman correlations (deattenuated, transformed) between FFQ2 and FRs were 0.32 for energy, 0.32 for protein, and 0.39 for total fat. The range of correlations for 21 nutrients assessed was 0.03 for retinol to 0.56 for calcium. FFQ median energy intake was 13.1% higher than food records (10.5 vs. 9.3 mJ/day). The strength of agreement was slight for two nutrients ($K \leq 0.2$), fair for 18 nutrients ($0.2 < K \leq 0.4$), and moderate ($K > 0.4$) for 2 nutrients. |
| Rockett et al.[80] | 261 m and f | 9–18 years | 126-item FFQ YAQ; self-administered; semiquantitative; portion sizes for ages 9–18 years and "natural" serving size | 8 (ranged from never to 4 or more/day) | Three 24 h recalls | Compared child's responses to YAQ against child's three 24 hour recalls. Two YAQs 1 year apart; recalls collected every 4 months during year. | Pearson correlations between YAQ and recalls were 0.35 for energy, 0.37 for protein, and 0.49 for total fat. The range of correlations for 29 nutrients assessed was 0.21 for sodium to 0.58 for folate. YAQ energy intake was 1.2% higher than recalls (2196 vs. 2169 kcal/day). Mean corrected correlation for all nutrients was 0.46. |
| Rockett et al.[80] | 261 m and f | 9–18 years | 26-item FFQ derived from 126-item FFQ; self-administered; past year; semiquantitative; portion sizes for ages 9–18 year and "natural" serving size | 8 (ranged from never to 4 or more/day) | Three 24 h recalls | Compared child's responses to the short YAQ against child's three 24 h recalls conducted about every 4 months over 1 year. Two YAQs 1 year apart; recalls collected each 4 months during year. | Pearson correlations between the 26-item YAQ and the recalls were 0.34 for energy, 0.30 for protein, and 0.41 for total fat. The range of correlations for 29 nutrients assessed was 0.05 for sodium to 0.58 for folate. The short list YAQ energy intake was 40.2% lower than recalls (1296 vs. 2169 kcal/day). Mean corrected correlation for all nutrients was 0.42. |
| Rockett et al.[81] | 122 m 139 f 96% White | 9–18 years | 131-item YAQ; self-administered; past year; semiquantitative; child portions | Dependent on food type | Three 24 h recalls | Compared child's report of frequency of intake of foods (mean of 2 administrations 1 year apart) on YAQ against child's report of intake on three 24 h recalls. Recalls were collected by telephone in the year between YAQ administrations. | Pearson correlations (unadjusted log-transformed values) between YAQ and recalls were 0.35 for energy, 0.30 for protein, and 0.41 for fat. The range of correlations for 28 nutrients assessed was 0.09 for copper to 0.46 for vitamin C. YAQ energy intake was 1% higher than the recalls (2196 vs. 2169 kcal/day). Of the 31 nutrients assessed, 16 were overestimated by the YAQ and 8 were underestimated (significance testing not shown). Correlations did not show a consistent pattern by gender or age (significance testing not shown). |

| | Sample | Age | Instrument | Frequency | Reference method | Results |
|---|---|---|---|---|---|---|
| Preston et al.[82] | 94 m and f 40 m 54 f | Fifth grade | 97-item FFQ including supplements; interviewer administered; past month; semiquantitative | Unknown | 3-day parent-assisted food records | Compared child's report of intake on second FFQ against the mean of child's 3-day food records. Food records were completed beginning on the day after completion of the first FFQ. The second FFQ was completed 2 weeks after the first FFQ. | Spearman correlations between the second FFQ and the food record means were 0.23 for energy, 0.05 for protein, and 0.15 for total fat. The range of correlations for 12 nutrients assessed was 0.05 for vitamin C, vitamin B6, and vitamin D to 0.23 for energy. FFQ energy intake was 2.9% lower than diet records (2136 vs. 2200 kcal/day). The FFQ significantly overestimated 4 of the 12 nutrients. Gross misclassifications of nutrients (>2 quartiles) ranged from 7.3% for energy and calcium to 14.6% for vitamin C. The range of correlations for 18 nutrients assessed for girls was 0.02 for vitamin B6 and vitamin D to 0.37 for energy; for boys, the range was 0.00 for carbohydrates to 0.12 for calcium. |
| Roumelioti et al.[83] | 200 m and f 47% m 53% f | Fourth to sixth grade 10–12 years | 65-item FFQ interviewer administered; forthcoming 7 days (week); semiquantitative with photographs of two differently sized portions for 40 typical Greek foods | 3 (1–7 days/ week, 1–2 days/month, or never) | 65-item FFQ; parent completed for child's intake | Compared child's interviewer-completed FFQ against child's parent-completed FFQ over the same time period. | Spearman correlations for food groups ranged from 0.58 for cornflakes to 0.90 for milk. Kappa statistics ranged from 0.36 for potatoes to 0.81 for milk. Using kappa statistics criteria, 1 food group was classified as very good agreement, 7 food groups were classified as good agreement, 14 food groups and breakfast consumption were classified as fair agreement, and 4 food groups were classified as poor agreement. |
| Wilson et al.[84] | 117 m and f | 10–12 years | 14-item questionnaire with six food scores and one score related to healthy food behaviors; usual or recent (previous/ current day) group administered; nonquantitative | Dependent on food type (5-point Likert scales and ranged from none to five times a day and never consumed to one to three times per week to more than five serves/day) | 7-day food record | Compared child's modified food scores from the questionnaire against child's scores from the 7-day food records completed 8–36 days after the questionnaire. | Spearman correlations between the FFQ and the 7-day record ranged from 0.34 for sweetened beverages to 0.48 for fruit. Mean bias (differences in scores from questionnaire and the 7-day records) ranged from −1.2 for sweetened beverages to 0.6 for noncore (e.g., chocolate, cookies, pizza) foods. |

(continued)

**TABLE 35.5 (continued)**
**FFQ[a] and Checklist Validity Studies among School-Age Children**

| References[b] | Sample | Age/Grade | Instrument | Response Categories (Range) | Validation Standard | Design | Results |
|---|---|---|---|---|---|---|---|
| Vereecken et al.[85] | 101 m and f 52% m 48% f | Fifth to sixth grade | 15-item (fiber, calcium foods, and foods relevant to youth food culture) Health Behavior in School-Aged Children (HBSC) FFQ: group administered; yesterday; nonquantitative | 7 (never to more than once a day) | 7-day food record structured on meal segments | Compared child's report of frequency of intake of foods on HBSC against child's report of frequency of food items abstracted from food record. To identify misclassification and percent agreement, HBSC and records were translated into three comparable categories of frequency of consumption. | Spearman correlations between the HBSC and the food record ranged from 0.10 for crisps to 0.65 for semiskimmed milk. The Wilcoxon test used to compare mean consumption indicates the HBSC significantly overestimated intake for all items except two: cheese and soft drinks. Percent agreement ranged from 34% for vegetables (excluding composite dishes) to 66% for crisps. The percentage gross misclassification ranged from 1% for chips to 21% for diet soft drinks. |
| DiNoia et al.[86] | 64 m and f 92 m and f 55% f AA | 10–11 years 12–14 years | 7-item (fruit, vegetable, and juice) five-a-day FFQ (FADFFQ); self-administered; past month; nonquantitative | Dependent on food type | 3-day plate waste by direct observation | Compared child's report of frequency of fruit and vegetable intake on FFQ against child's plate waste estimated by direct observation. FADFFQ was completed after three consecutive days of direct observation. Responses were transformed to servings per day to allow for comparison. | Pearson correlation between FADFFQ and observation was 0.39, and intake was significantly overestimated using the FADFFQ by 19.7% (5.41 vs. 6.74 servings/day). Pearson correlations for fruit, vegetable, and juice intake ranged from 0.15 (juice) to 0.28 (vegetable) and were significant for fruit and vegetable intake but not for juices. Intake of vegetables by FADFFQ was higher than vegetable intake by observation (2.32 vs. 1.26, p < 0.01). Pearson correlations for total intake were 0.36 for 10- to 11-year-olds and 0.43 for 12- to 14-year-olds. Correlations did not differ by age or gender (significance not shown). |
| Koehler et al.[87] | 66 m 54 f White, Hisp,[h] NA | Fifth to eighth grade | 33-item Yesterday's Food Choices- (YFC); self-administered; past day; nonquantitative | 3 (yes, not sure, and no) | One 24 h recall | Compared child's report of frequency of food intake on YFC against child's 24 h recall, both completed on same day. | Spearman correlations between scores on the YFC and 24 h recall were 0.71 for low-fat foods, 0.35 for high-fiber foods, 0.29 for fruits and vegetables, and 0.40 for high-fat foods. |
| Magkos et al.[88] | 162 m 189 f | 10–15 years | 30-item calcium; self-administered; previous year; semiquantitative | Open-ended (never or rarely or times per month or per week or per day) | One 24 h recall | Compared child's report of frequency of food intake on FFQ against child's report on 24 h recall. | Pearson correlations for calcium intake between FFQ and 24 h recall were 0.64 for boys and 0.63 for girls. FFQ underestimated calcium intake by 8.9% for boys (906 vs. 995 mg/day) and 6.4% for girls (885 vs. 946 mg/day). Cross classification showed that 85% of boys and 87% of girls were classified into the same or adjacent quartile of calcium intake. |

| Study | Sample | Age | Instrument | Response | Reference method | Comparison | Results |
|---|---|---|---|---|---|---|---|
| Cullen et al.[89] | 83 m and f 53% f 57% Hisp 23% White 21% AA | 10–17 years | 72-item Block Kids Questionnaire; interviewer administered; past 7 days; semiquantitative | 6 (from none to everyday) | Two 24 h recalls | Compared child's report of frequency of intake of foods on FFQ against child's report on 24 h recalls. Two 24 h recalls were completed within a 7-day period, and FFQ was completed at the end of the week. | ICCs between the FFQ and the 24 h recalls were 0.63 for energy, 0.35 for percent energy from fat, and 0.21 for percent energy from protein. ICCs for 10 other foods and nutrients ranged from −0.17 for fruit (servings) to 0.68 for sodium (mg). FFQ significantly underestimated the energy intake by 22% compared to the recall (1560 vs. 1991 kcal). Pearson correlations for energy were 0.38 for children (≤12 years) and 0.58 for adolescents (>12 years). More than twice as many Pearson correlations for food and nutrients were weak (<0.30) for children as compared to adolescents (4 vs. 9). Among children, FFQ significantly underestimated the energy intake by 38% compared to recall (1245 vs. 2017 kcal). Among adolescents, FFQ underestimated energy intake by 8.6%, though not significantly (1801 vs. 1971 kcal). |
| Yang et al.[90] | 745 f (baseline) | Sixth grade | 15-item Brief Calcium Assessment Tool (BCAT); self-administered; past month; semiquantitative | Unknown (weighted to frequency/day) | Bone mineral content (BMC) determined by dual-energy x-ray absorptiometry (DEXA) | Compared child's BCAT calcium score against child's BMC at baseline and 12-month data. BMC for total body, spine, total hip, and femoral neck was determined at baseline and at 12 months for a subset (n = 265) of the original sample. BCAT was administered at these same time points. | Correlations between BCAT and BMC at baseline ranged from 0.748 for femoral neck to 0.853 for total body. Significant positive associations were seen for BCAT with BMC at total hip and femoral neck. Prospective associations using 12-month cata ranged from 0.931 for femoral neck to 0.954 for total body; significant positive associations were seen for total-body BMC with BCAT score. |
| Haraldsdottir et al.[91] | 93 m 112 f | 11–12 years | 6 items (5 fruits and vegetables, and 1 potato); self-administered; "usual intake"; semiquantitative | 8 (never to >2 times/day) | 7-day weighed food record | Compared child's report of frequency of fruit and vegetable intake on FFQ against child's report on 7-day food record completed 1–8 days later. The FFQ and the food records were translated into quartiles of intake (g/day) to identify misclassification and percent agreement. | Spearman correlations between FFQ and 7-day food records for total fruit and vegetable intake in ranged from 0.40 (Portugal) to 0.53 (Iceland). Spearman correlations ranged from 0.43 (Portugal) to 0.5 (Iceland) for fruit, from 0.38 (Denmark and Norway) to 0.53 (Iceland) for vegetables, and from 0.13 (Portugal) to 0.55 (Iceland) for orange juice. Cross classification showed that 25%–50% of participants were classified into the same quartile for fruit, vegetable, total fruit and vegetable, and orange juice. Between 70% and 88% were classified into the same or adjacent quartile. Between 0% and 12% were classified into the opposite quartile. |

(continued)

**TABLE 35.5 (continued)**
**FFQ[a] and Checklist Validity Studies among School-Age Children**

| References[b] | Sample | Age/Grade | Instrument | Response Categories (Range) | Validation Standard | Design | Results |
|---|---|---|---|---|---|---|---|
| Andersen et al.[33] | 36 m 49 f | Sixth grade | 16 items (7 fruits and vegetables); self-administered; past 3 months; nonquantitative | 10 (never to several times per day) | 7-day food record with precoded list of 277 foods | Compared child's report of fruit and vegetable intake on FFQ against child's report of intake on 7-day food records. Excerpted fruit and vegetable intake from 7-day food record with precoded list of foods. | Spearman correlations between FFQ and food record were 0.21 for fruit; 0.21 for potato; 0.23 for fruit, fruit juice, vegetable, and potato; 0.28 for vegetable; 0.28 for fruit juice; and 0.32 for fruit and vegetable without fruit juice and potato. The percentage correctly classified by tertiles for six food groups ranged from 35% for fruit to 47% for fruit, fruit juice, vegetable, and potato. Spearman correlation coefficients were higher among girls than boys (significance testing not shown). |
| Jenner et al.[92] | 61 m 57 f | 11–12 years | 175 items; group administered; past week; nonquantitative | 6 (none to every day) | 14-day food record | Compared child's report of frequency of food intake on FFQ against child's report of intake on 14-day food records. Seven sets of two consecutive day records were collected in the 3 months following administration of the FFQ. Nutrient estimates from FFQ completed by parents were also compared to the 14-day diet records. | Pearson correlations (log transformed) between the child's FFQ and diet records were 0.25 for energy, 0.18 for protein, and 0.19 for total fat. The range of correlations for 13 nutrients assessed was 0.11 for monounsaturated fat to 0.42 for complex carbohydrates. Correlations between the parents' FFQs and diet records were 0.38 for energy, 0.26 forprotein, and 0.30 for total fat. The range of correlations was 0.26 for protein to 0.47 for complex carbohydrates. Children's FFQ energy intakes were 36% higher than diet records (10.9 vs. 8.0 mJ/day). Parents' FFQ estimates of children's energy intake were 21% higher than children's diet records (9.7 vs. 8.0 mJ/day). All 13 nutrients were overestimated by both the child and the parent FFQs (significance testing not shown). |
| Johnson et al.[93] | 96 m and f 41 m 55 f | 11–13 years | 56-item (inferred) FIQ categorized in sugary, fatty, fiber, and negative and positive markers; previous day; self-administered; nonquantitative | 2 (yes/no) | 3-day interviewer-assisted food record | Compared child's FIQ with child's 3-day food record completed two weeks after FIQ. On the fourth day, the child was interviewed about portion size and to clarify dietary information of their food record. FIQ was completed 3 times all on weekdays at roughly equal intervals over a 3-month period. | Pearson correlations between FIQ and 3-day food record energy intake were 0.20 for fatty, 0.28 for sugary, 0.03 for fiber, 0.23 for negative markers, and 0.01 for positive markers. Pearson correlations between FIQ and 3-day food record fat were 0.36 for fatty, 0.27 for sugary, −0.17 for fiber, 0.34 for negative markers, and −0.06 for positive markers. |

| Author | Sample | Age | Instrument | Categories | Reference method | Comparison | Results |
|---|---|---|---|---|---|---|---|
| Lietz et al.[94] | 37 m and f | 11–13 years | Unknown number of items; European Prospective Investigation of Cancer (EPIC) FFQ; interviewer administered; past year; semiquantitative | 9 (<1 time/month to >6 times/day) | 7-day weighed food record | Compared child's report of intake from frequency of intake of foods on EPIC against child's 7-day weighed food record completed 1 day after the EPIC interview. | Spearman correlations (unadjusted) between EPIC and food records were 0.33 for energy, 0.30 for protein, and 0.52 for total fat. The range of correlations for 13 nutrients assessed was 0.27 for potassium and 0.61 for total fat (% kcal). Energy-adjusted correlations were 0.31 for protein and 0.66 for fat and ranged from 0.26 for sodium to 0.66 for total fat. FFQ energy intake was 30% higher than the diet record (10.4 vs. 8.0 mJ/day). The percentage correctly classified into tertiles by the two methods ranged from 29.7% for total fat (% kcal) to 48.6% for potassium and total carbohydrate. The percentage misclassified in opposite thirds ranged from 8.1% each for calcium, potassium, carbohydrate (% kcal), and sugar (% kcal) to 16.2% for Englyst fiber (median 10.8%). |
| Harnack et al.[95] | 92 m and f 156 m and f 60.5% f 68.5% White 19.4% AA 6.5% others 6.0% Somali American 5.6% Hisp 3.6% NA | 11–12 years 13–14 years | 10-item calcium FFQ; self-administered; past month; semiquantitative | Unknown (never or less than 1 time/month to 3 or more times/day) | Three 24 h recalls | Compared child's report of frequency of intake on FFQ against child's parent-assisted report of three 24 h recalls that were collected after the second administration of the FFQ. | ICCs between the calcium (mg/day) estimates from FFQ and 24 h recalls were 0.43 for the total sample, 0.59 for 11- to 12-year-olds, 0.33 for 13- to 14-year-olds, 0.45 for girls, and 0.40 for boys. Calcium intakes from FFQ were lower than 24 h recall calcium intake estimates: 856.0 vs. 993.3 mg/day for total sample, 855.8 vs. 1008.0 for 11- to 12-year-olds, 856.1 vs. 984.6 for 12- to 13-year-olds, 825.6 vs. 907.3 for girls, and 902.5 vs. 1125.0 for boys. Calcium intake was significantly underestimated by the FFQ compared to the recalls in the total sample, in 11- to 12-year-olds and 13- to 14-year-olds, and in girls and boys. |
| Harnack et al.[95] | 92 m and f 156 m and f 60.5% f 68.5% White 19.4% AA 6.5% others 6.0% Somali American 5.6% Hisp 3.6% NA | 11–12 years 13–14 years | 1-item YRBS (calcium question); self-administered; past week; semiquantitative | Unknown | Three 24 h recalls | Compared child's report of frequency of intake of milk against child's parent-assisted report of three 24 h recalls. | ICCs between the calcium intake (mg/day) estimates from 24 h recalls and YRBS question were 0.37 for total sample, 0.40 for 11- to 12-year-olds, 0.35 for 13- to 14-year-olds, 0.46 for girls, and 0.29 for boys. Calcium intakes from YRBS question were lower than 24 h recall calcium intake estimates: 422.7 vs. 993.3 mg/day for total sample, 408.7 vs. 1008.0 for 11- to 12-year-olds, 430.9 vs. 984.6 for 13- to 14-year-olds, 415.4 vs. 907.3 for girls, and 433.8 vs. 1125.0 for boys. Calcium intake was significantly underestimated by the YRBS compared to recalls in the total sample and 11–12- and 13- to 14-year-olds. |

(continued)

**TABLE 35.5 (continued)**
**FFQ[a] and Checklist Validity Studies among School-Age Children**

| References[b] | Sample | Age/Grade | Instrument | Response Categories (Range) | Validation Standard | Design | Results |
|---|---|---|---|---|---|---|---|
| Yaroch et al.[96] | 57 f AA | 11–17 years | 18 items; (13 related to low-fat or high-fat eating behaviors) qualitative dietary fat index questionnaire (QFQ); usual; interviewer administered; nonquantitative | 4 (never to always) | Three 24 h recalls | Compared child's report of food intake on QFQ against the mean of child's three 24 h recalls administered within 2 weeks after QFQ. The 18 low-fat and high-fat items were summed to create a total QFQ score with a higher score indicating lower-fat intake behaviors. | Pearson correlations (log transformed) between QFQ score and mean of recalls were −0.23 for energy, −0.31 for total fat, and 0.23 for fat (% kcal). |
| Wong et al.[97] | 161 m and f 81 m 80 f 86 11–14 years 75 15–18 years 56 White 58 Hisp 47 Asian | 11–18 years | 80-item computerized FFQ; self-administered; moderators; past month; semiquantitative photos and visual portion sizes | 4–7 (ranging from "never or less than once/month" to "4 or more servings/day") | Two in-person, interviewer-assisted 24 h recalls | Compared child's FFQ2 against the child's 24 h recalls. | Spearman correlations between the FFQ2 and the mean 24 h recall intake were 0.51 for calcium. FFQ calcium intake was 11% lower than the 24 h recalls (1045 vs. 1172 mg/day). Correlations were 0.48 for males and 0.47 for females, 0.47 for ages 11–14 and 0.54 for ages 15–18, and 0.57 for Asian, 0.50 for Hisps, and 0.45 for Whites. |
| Nelson et al.[98] | 59 m and f 26 m | 11–18 years | 22-item screener FFQ (9 beverages and 13 fast-food items); self-administered; time frame varied by question, from usually to past month; some questions were semiquantified, others were not; usual portion sizes | Dependent on food type (ranged from yes/no to 9 response categories) | Three telephone 24 h recalls | Compared child's screener with child's three 24 h recalls administered on 2 weekdays and 1 weekend day within a 15-day period. | Kappa statistics between screener and recalls for beverage amount ranged from 0.19 (regular soda) to 0.20 (water) and for beverage frequency from 0.11 (other sweetened beverages) to 0.38 (regular soda). Kappa statistics between screener and recalls for overall fast-food frequency was 0.03. No significant differential misclassification in tertiles for soda, other sweetened beverages, milk, or fast food. The screener overestimated sports drink intake compared to the recalls in 32% of participants. |
| Vereecken et al.[85] | 7072 m and f 47.4% m 52.6% f | 11–18 years | 15-item (fiber, calcium, and foods relevant to youth culture) HBSC FFQ; group administered; yesterday; nonquantitative | 7 (never to more than once a day) | One 24 h food behavior checklist (FBC) | Compared child's report of frequency of intake of foods on HBSC against child's report of intake of foods on FBC adjusted for weekly time period. | The percent agreement of foods with responses "never" or "once a day, every day" and "everyday, more than once" on HBSC with the FBC foods ranged from 89% for other milk products to 99.3% for alcohol, with a mean agreement for all food items of 95.3% (data not shown). No differences were found between genders or between students aged 11–12, 13–14, 15–16, and 17–18 (significance testing not shown). |

| Study | Sample | Age/grade | Instrument | Scale | Reference method | Comparison | Results |
|---|---|---|---|---|---|---|---|
| Prochaska et al.[99] | 61 m and f | 12 years (mean age) | Two-item fruits and vegetables; self-administered; typical day; semiquantitative | 4 (none to 4 or more/day) | 3-day food record; 2 weekdays and 1 weekend | Compared child's fruit and vegetable brief questionnaire to child's 3-day food record. Food recording occurred prior to fruit and vegetable brief questionnaire administration. | Spearman's correlation between the fruit and vegetable brief and the 3-day food record was 0.23 for fruits and vegetables. Among boys, the correlation was 0.25 and for girls 0.20. |
| Watanabe et al.[100] | 63 f | 12–13 years | 82-item FFQ (FFQW82) with pictures; self-administered; past 1 month; semiquantitative; small, medium, and large portion sizes | 6 ("absolutely do not eat" to "always eat at breakfast or lunch or dinner") | 7-day weighed food record and photos of food consumed | Compared child's FFQW82 against child's 7-day weighed food record (using photos to reconstruct foods). | Spearman correlations between FFQ2 and 7-day weighed food records were 0.28 for energy, 0.33 for protein, and 0.32 for total fat. The range of correlations for the entire day's consumption for 10 nutrients was 0.19 for salt to 0.55 for calcium. The range of correlations for 11 food groups for entire day was 0.12 for grains to 0.74 for milk, with a correlation of 0.28 for all food groups. Median difference between FFQ energy intake and 7-day food records was 0.769 mJ (769 kJ), with FFQ reporting higher intake. Spearman correlations for food groups were higher for breakfast (0.49) compared to lunch (0.37) and dinner (0.25). |
| Neuhouser et al.[101] | 46 m and f 18 m 28 f 56.5% White 13.0% AA 6.5% Hisp 6.5% Asian 15.22% others | Seventh grade | 19-item Beverage and Snack Questionnaire (BSQ); self-administered; past week; nonquantitative | 7 (never or less than once/week to 4+ times/day) | 4-day food record (3 school days and 1 weekend day) | Compared child's mean frequency/week of items on BSQ with mean frequency/week of foods on child's food records, using binary coding rules for intake of food categories (e.g., milk) and location (at school vs. outside of school). | Pearson correlations between BSQ and food records were 0.71, 0.70, and 0.69 for beverages, snacks and sweets, and fruit and vegetables, respectively. Pearson correlations for food items ranged from 0.48 for cookies, brownies, pies, and cakes not consumed at school to 0.87 for fruit drinks consumed at school. Estimates for food categories consumed at and away from school were similar. |
| Smith et al.[102] | 243 m and f | Seventh grade | 40 items; (foods high in total fat, saturated fat, and sodium) Child and Adolescent Trial for Cardiovascular Health (CATCH) Food Checklist (CFC); group administered; yesterday; nonquantitative | 2 (yes/no) | One 24 h recall | Compared child's reported frequency of intake of foods on CFC against child's 24 h recall. The children were in two groups: the first group completed the recall at least 2 h after the CFC and the second group completed the recall at least 2 h before the CFC. For each of the 40 foods, a score of 0 (low intake) to 5 (high intake) was assigned and a total score summed for each nutrient—total fat, saturated fat, and sodium. | Pearson correlations between the CFC nutrient scores and the 24 h recall using equal weights were 0.22 for percent total fat, 0.23 for percent saturated fat, and 0.24 for sodium. Kappa statistics between the CFC food items and foods on recall ranged from 0.21 for butter to 0.84 for pizza and lasagna. The mean kappa value was higher for students who completed the CFC after the recall (kappa = 0.60) than for those who completed the CFC first (kappa = 0.45). Male students reported greater intake of all three nutrients on the CFC than females; however, CFC scores were only significantly different for sodium. |

(continued)

**TABLE 35.5 (continued)**

**FFQ[a] and Checklist Validity Studies among School-Age Children**

| References[b] | Sample | Age/Grade | Instrument | Response Categories (Range) | Validation Standard | Design | Results |
|---|---|---|---|---|---|---|---|
| Cullen et al.[103] | 89 m and f 41% m 59% f 54% AA 46% Hisp | Seventh to eighth grade | 152-item YAQ; group administered; past year; semiquantitative; child portions | Dependent on food type | 6-day food record | Compared nutrient intake from child's report of frequency of food intake on YAQ against child's report of intake from 6-day food record. | Spearman correlations between YAQ and mean of food records were 0.19 for energy and 0.09 for fat (% kcal). Spearman correlations for the four fruit and vegetable groupings ranged from 0.02 for high-fat vegetables to 0.23 for regular vegetables. Among AAs, the Spearman correlations ranged from 0.02 for fruit to 0.25 for juice and among Hisps ranged from −0.06 for high-fat vegetables to 0.38 for regular vegetables. |
| Truthmann et al.[104] | 1213 m and f 582 m 631 f 416 12–13 years 427 14–15 years 370 16–17 years | 12–17 years | 45-item FFQ "what do you eat"; self-administered; "during the last few weeks"; semiquantitative; usual portion size (five-item-specific categories) | 10 (never, once a month, 2–3 times a month, 1–2 times/week, 3–4 times/week, 5–6 times/week, once a day, 2–3 times/day, 4–5 times/day, >5 times/day) | Diet history interview (DISHES) | Compared child's FFQ responses against child's diet history interview. FFQ was completed 3–4 weeks after diet history, so both methods covered the same time period. DISHES uses methods similar to 24 h recalls. | Spearman correlations ranged from 0.22 for pasta/rice to 0.69 for margarine. Participants classified in the same and adjacent quartiles ranged from 70.1% for pasta/rice to 90.8% for coffee, while misclassifications ranged from 1.9% for soda/mineral water to 9.7% for tap water. Cohen's weighted kappa statistics ranged from 0.21 to 0.60 for food items. Mean food group intake differences/day between the two methods ranged from 1.4% for milk to 100.3% for pasta/rice. Correlations for vegetables and sports energy drinks were lower in girls compared to boys, and the correlation for poultry was higher than boys (CI did not overlap). Correlations for 16–17 years were higher for fish and white bread compared to younger adolescents; correlations were higher in 16–17 years for coffee and breakfast cereals than in 12–13 years and higher in fast food than 14–15 years. |
| Taylor et al.[105] | 107 f 62 White 2 AA 2 Asian 9 others | 12–18 years | 40-item (calcium and vitamin D) FFQ; administered by a research dietitian; semiquantitative | Open-ended (servings/day or servings/ week) | 4-day food records (3 weekdays and 1 weekend) | Compared child's FFQ responses against mean of child's 4-day record; nutrient intakes were adjusted per 1000 kcal. | Spearman's rank correlation between FFQ and food record was 0.60 for calcium and 0.75 for vitamin D. Correlations overall were weaker for adjusted food records and FFQ for calcium (0.32) but stronger for adjusted vitamin D (0.62). For calcium intake, there were 0% gross misclassifications (>2 quartiles apart); only one subject was grossly misclassified for vitamin D intake. |

| Source | Sample | Age | Instrument | Response categories | Comparison | Method | Results |
|---|---|---|---|---|---|---|---|
| Matthys et al.[106] | 104 m and f | 12–18 years | 69 items; web based; self-administered; past month; quantitative; portions based on adolescent serving sizes | 6 (<1 day/month to every day) | 3-day food record (2 weekdays and 1 weekend day) | Compared child's web-based FFQ to mean of child's 3-day food record intake of 15 food groups. | Spearman correlation between the FFQ and the food records for foods was 0.30. The average Spearman correlation for individual items was 0.38 and ranged from 0.20 for pasta to 0.64 for breakfast cereals. The web-based FFQ underestimated some food groups (soft drinks, sweet and savory snacks/fillings, sauces, and fat spreads, cheese, pasta/rice, and vegetables), and overestimated others (milk and milk products). |
| Prochaska et al.[107] | 59 m and f 37% m 63% f 37% White 25% Asian 12% Hisp 3% AA | Seventh to 12th grade | 21-item (high-fat foods) PACE+; self-administered; past 7 days; nonquantitative | 6 (did not eat it this week to more than twice each day) | 3-day food record | Compared child's report of frequency of food intake on PACE+ and fat measure against child's report of intake on 3-day food record. | Pearson correlation between PACE+ and fat score and food records was 0.36 for total fat (% kcal), P < 0.01. |
| Prochaska et al.[107] | 59 m and f 37% m 63% f 37% White 25% Asian 12% Hisp 3% AA | Seventh to 12th grade | Four categories (four high-fat food groups); self-administered; past 7 days; nonquantitative | 6 (did not eat it this week to more than twice each day) | 3-day food record | Compared fat measure scores from child's report of frequency of food intake against child's report of intake on 3-day food records. | Pearson correlation between 4-category fat measure and food records was 0.12 for total fat (% kcal), P < 0.31. |
| van Assema et al.[108] | 50 m and f | 12–18 years | 35-item (19 foods high in total fat and saturated fat) fat list; self-administered; past 6 months; semiquantitative | Open ended | 7-day food record | Compared child's total fat score from fat list against child's report of intake on 7-day food record kept consecutively after the fat list was completed. For each of the 19 foods, a fat score of 0 (low-fat intake) to 5 (high-fat intake) was assigned and a total score summed for all foods. | Pearson correlations between fat list score and food records were 0.56 for energy and 0.61 for fat. The range of correlations for five nutrients assessed was 0.14 for saturated fat (% kcal) to 0.61 for fat. |
| Hoelscher et al.[109] | 103 m 106 f 79 White 36 AA 85 Hisp 9 others | Eighth grade | 63-item (17 items tested for validity) School-Based Nutrition Monitoring (SBNM) Questionnaire; group administered; yesterday; nonquantitative | 4 (0 times/day to 3+ times/day) | One 24 h recall | Compared child's report of frequency of intake of foods on SBNM against child's report of intake on 24 h recall. Using two groups, the first group completed the recall at least 2 h after the SBNM and the second group completed the recall at least 2 h before the SBNM. Excerpted foods from recall to match the 17 SBNM food items. | Spearman correlations between SBNM items and 24 h recall ranged from 0.32 for any type of bread, bun, bagel, tortilla, and roll to 0.68 for milk and for beans. Kappa statistics ranged from 0.12 for any type of bread, bun, bagel, tortilla, and roll to 0.59 for beans. Percent agreement ranged from 38% for any type of bread, bun, bagel, tortilla, and roll to 89% for gravy. |

(continued)

**TABLE 35.5 (continued)**
**FFQ[a] and Checklist Validity Studies among School-Age Children**

| References[b] | Sample | Age/Grade | Instrument | Response Categories (Range) | Validation Standard | Design | Results |
|---|---|---|---|---|---|---|---|
| Johnson et al.[35] | 1822 m and f 32% m 68% f 1666 White 144 non-White 36 unknown | 13–16 years | 23-item Adolescent Food Habits Checklist (AFHC); self-administered; usual intake; nonquantitative | True/false (10 items, also have a non-applicable option) | Number of portions of fruits and vegetables; Dietary Instrument for Nutrition Education (DINE) FFQ | Compared child's score from AFHC against child's report of fruit and vegetables portions and frequency of intake using DINE FFQ. AFHC score was the number of "healthy" responses (23/number of items completed). | Pearson correlations between AFHC score and DINE FFQ were −0.46 for dietary fat, 0.16 for dietary fiber, and 0.45 for portions of fruit and vegetable intake. Among females, the correlations were 0.44 for fruit and vegetable intake and −0.41 for dietary fat and 0.18 for dietary fiber. Among males, the correlations were 0.45 for fruit and vegetable intake and −0.46 for dietary fat and 0.24 for dietary fiber. |
| Vereecken et al.[110] | 48 m and f 46% f | 13–17 years | 137-item HELENA FFQ; online; self-administered; past 30 days; semiquantitative; "standard" portion sizes | Dependent on food type ("units per day," "units per week," "units during the last 30 days") includes consumption frequency and average amount per occasion | Four nonconsecutive computer-based 24 h recalls (Young Adolescents' Nutrition Assessment on Computer (YANA-C); 1 weekend and 3 weekdays | Compared HELENA FFQ with data from the four nonconsecutive 24 h recalls (YANA-C). | Spearman correlation between HELENA FFQ and YANA-C was 0.70 for energy. Spearman correlations between FFQ and YANA-C for nutrients ranged from 0.32 for fiber to 0.64 for fat. FFQ energy intake was 23% higher than YANA-C (2629 vs. 2131 kcal). Correlations between FFQ and YANA-C for food groups ranged from −0.08 for other snacks to 0.80 for milk. FFQ/YANA-C ratios ranged from 0.68 for cheese to 3.37 for other snacks. |
| Kinlay et al.[111] | 57 m 48 f | 13–17 years Adults required | 12 items (fat, saturated fat); Fat-Habits Score Questionnaire; self-administered; past week; semiquantitative | Dependent on food type | 180-item CSIRO-FFQ | Compared child's parent-assisted report of frequency of intake on Fat-Habits Score Questionnaire against child's parent-assisted report of food intake on a CSIRO-FFQ. | Spearman correlations between the Fat-Habits Score Questionnaire and the CSIRO-FFQ were 0.40 for total fat as% of kcal and 0.54 for saturated fat as% of kcal. |
| Li et al.[112] | 16 m 30 f 11 White 33 Asian 2 others | Eighth to 12th grade | Unknown number of items; self-administered; previous week; semiquantitative | Unknown | 24 h food record | Compared child's report of fruit and vegetable intake on FFQ against child's report on 24 h dietary record. | Pearson correlation for fruit and vegetable intake between the FFQ and the 24 h record was 0.52. Mean servings of vegetable and fruit intake on the FFQ significantly overestimated daily servings by 27.5% compared with the 24 h record (6.9 vs. 5.0 servings). |

| Reference | Sample | Age | Instrument | Response | Comparison instrument | Description of analysis | Results |
|---|---|---|---|---|---|---|---|
| Ambrosini et al.[113] | 403 m 380 f | 14 years Adults required | 212 items; self-administered; past year; semiquantitative; "standard" portions | 5 (never to number of times/month, week, or day) | 3-day parent-assisted food record and plasma biomarkers | Compared dietary pattern scores derived from parent's child-assisted report of frequency of intake of foods on FFQ against dietary pattern scores derived from child's parent-assisted 3-day food record. Dietary pattern scores were compared to nutrient intakes and serum biomarkers (glucose, lipids, erythrocyte n – 3, and erythrocyte VLC n – 3). | Two major dietary patterns, "healthy" and "western," were identified in the FFQ and food record (factor loadings were generally weaker in food record). Spearman energy-adjusted correlations between FFQ and food record "healthy" pattern scores were 0.42 for girls and 0.47 for boys and for "western" pattern scores were 0.34 for boys and 0.38 for girls. Correlations for the 3 reported biomarkers ranged from –0.10 to 0.17 for FFQ dietary pattern scores. |
| Ambrosini et al.[114] | 403 m 382 f | 14 years Adults required | 212 items; self-administered; past year; semiquantitative; "standard" portions | 5 (never to number of times/month, week, or day) | 3-day parent-assisted food record | Compared parent's child-assisted report of frequency of intake of foods on FFQ against child's parent-assisted 3-day food record. | Pearson correlations between FFQ and food records for energy were 0.24 (girls) and 0.29 (boys), for protein were 0.20 (girls) and 0.28 (boys), and for fat were 0.20 (girls) and 0.25 (boys). Pearson correlations for 19 other nutrients ranged from 0.11 (polyunsaturated fat, girls) to 0.51 (thiamin, boys). FFQ energy intake was 7.5% higher than food record for girls (8,882 vs. 8,266 kJ) and 1.4% lower for boys (10,412 vs. 10,559 kJ). The limits of agreement ranged from 27% (retinol) to 976% (carotene), with most nutrients being overestimated by the FFQ. The FFQ classified 80%–90% of subject's intake into the same or adjacent tertile as the food record. |
| Moore et al.[76] | 55 m | 14–16 years | 41-item calcium focus RAM; interviewer administered; typical day; semiquantitative visual aids to approximate serving sizes | Open ended (number of servings/day) | One 24 h recall | Compared child's report of daily calcium intake on interviewer-administered RAM against child's calcium intake from 24 h recall (typical day). The 24 h recall covered the day prior to the interview. Both instruments were administered at the same time. | ICC between RAM and 24 h recall for daily calcium intake was 0.43. RAM calcium intake was 62% higher than from the 24 h recall (1873 vs. 1155 mg). |
| Davis et al.[115] | 35 f Hisp | 14–17 years | 22 items (9 beverages, 13 fast-food consumptions); self-administered; past month; semiquantitative | Dependent on food type | 3-day food records | Compared child's report of frequency of beverage and fast-food intake on screener against child's report of food intake on 3-day food records done 7 days prior to the screener. Tertiles of beverage and fast-food frequencies and amounts were computed. | The agreement of classification between the screener and the diet records for overall fast-food frequency using kappa was 0.08. Kappa estimates of the frequency or amount of beverage and fast food ranged from 0.01 (regular soda) to 0.18 (milk). Percent agreement on classification of tertile rankings ranged from 37% (soda) to 49% (milk). |

(continued)

**TABLE 35.5 (continued)**
**FFQ[a] and Checklist Validity Studies among School-Age Children**

| References[b] | Sample | Age/Grade | Instrument | Response Categories (Range) | Validation Standard | Design | Results |
|---|---|---|---|---|---|---|---|
| Field et al.[116] | 102 m and f<br>50% m<br>50% f<br>35% White<br>24% AA<br>15% Hisp | Ninth to 12th grade | 27-item (12 fruits, 15 vegetables) YAQ; self-administered; past year; semiquantitative | Unknown (<1/month to ≥2 times/day) | Three nonconsecutive 24 h recalls | Compared child's report of frequency of fruit and vegetable intake on YAQ against child's report of intake on three nonconsecutive 24 h recalls completed 2 weeks apart. YAQ was administered 2–4 weeks after the third recall. | Spearman correlations between the YAQ and the mean of three 24 h recalls were 0.33 for fruit only, 0.29 for fruit juice, 0.33 for fruit and juice, 0.32 for vegetables, and 0.41 for fruit (including juice) and vegetables. |
| Field et al.[116] | 102 m and f<br>50% m<br>50% f<br>35% White<br>24% AA<br>15% Hisp | Ninth to 12th grade | Four-item (two fruits, two vegetables) Youth Risk Behavior Surveillance System Questionnaire (YRBSS); self-administered; previous day; semiquantitative | 4 (none to ≥3 times/day) | Three nonconsecutive 24 h recalls | Compared child's report of frequency of fruit and vegetable intake on YRBSS against child's report of intake on three nonconsecutive 24 h recalls completed 2 weeks apart. YRBSS was administered 2–4 weeks after third recall. | Spearman correlations between YRBSS items and mean of 24 h recalls were 0.17 for fruit only, 0.07 for fruit juice, 0.21 for fruit and juice, 0.24 for vegetables, and 0.28 for fruit (including juice) and vegetables. |
| Field et al.[116] | 102 m and f<br>50% m<br>50% f<br>35% White<br>24% AA<br>15% Hisp | Ninth to 12th grade | Six-item (two fruits, four vegetables) Behavioral Risk Factor Surveillance System Questionnaire (BRFSS); self-administered; previous day; semiquantitative | 4 (none to ≥3 times/day) | Three nonconsecutive 24 h recalls | Compared child's report of frequency of fruit and vegetable intake on BFRSS against child's report of intake on three nonconsecutive 24 h recalls completed 2 weeks apart. BFRSS was administered halfway between the two recalls. | Spearman correlations between previous-day BRFSS and mean of 24 h recalls were 0.33 for fruit only, 0.30 for fruit juice, 0.34 for fruit and juice, 0.14 for vegetables, and 0.30 for fruit (including juice) and vegetables. |
| Field et al.[116] | 100 m and f<br>50% m<br>50% f<br>35% White<br>24% AA<br>15% Hisp | Ninth to 12th grade | Six-item (two fruits, four vegetables) BRFSS; self-administered; past year; semiquantitative | 6 (none to ≥5 times/day) | Three nonconsecutive 24 h recalls | Compared child's report of frequency of fruit and vegetable intake on BRFSS child's report of intake on three nonconsecutive 24 h recalls completed 2 weeks apart. BRFSS was administered preceding the third recall. | Spearman correlations between past-year BRFSS and mean of 24 h recalls were 0.36 for fruit only, 0.36 for fruit juice, 0.35 for fruit and juice, 0.33 for vegetables, and 0.43 for fruit (including juice) and vegetables. |

| Author | Sample | Age | FFQ description | Frequency | Reference method | Comparison | Results |
|---|---|---|---|---|---|---|---|
| Papadopoulou et al.[117] | 250 m and f<br>120 m<br>130 f | 15.3 years (mean age) | 108-item Greek Adolescent FFQ (GAFFQ); self-administered; semiquantitative; serving portion | 8 (1–7 times/week or >7 times/week) | 3-day weighed food recall; 2 weekdays and 1 weekend | Compared child's GAFFQ against mean of 3-day weighed food recall. Food recall occurred 1-week before completion of GAFFQ. | Pearson correlations between GAFFQ and recall were 0.83 for energy, 0.77 for protein, and 0.78 for fat. Correlations ranged from 0.34 for folate to 0.77 for phosphorus. GAFFQ overestimated energy intake by 5.7% compared to food recall (2661.93 vs. 2516.36 kcal). |
| Preston et al.[82] | 89 m and f<br>42 m<br>47 f | 11th grade | 97-item FFQ including supplements; interviewer administered; past month; semiquantitative | Unknown | 3-day parent-assisted food records | Compared child's report of intake on second FFQ against the mean of child's 3-day food records. Food records were completed beginning on the day after completion of the first FFQ. The second FFQ was completed 2 weeks after the first FFQ. | Spearman correlations between the second FFQ and the food record means were 0.23 for energy, 0.15 for protein, and 0.15 for total fat. The range of correlations for 12 nutrients assessed was 0.10 for carbohydrate to 0.53 for vitamin B6. FFQ energy intake was 13.6% higher than diet records (2476 vs. 2179 kcal/day). FFQ significantly overestimated 8 of the 12 nutrients compared to diet records. Misclassifications of nutrients (>2 quartiles) ranged from 3.1% for 6 nutrients to 10.4% for 3 nutrients. The range of correlations for 12 nutrients assessed for girls was 0.01 for protein to 0.57 for vitamin B6; for boys, the range was 0.08 for energy to 0.53 for magnesium and folate. |
| Andersen et al.[118] | 13 m<br>36 f | 11th grade Adults required | 190 items; group administered; past year; semiquantitative | Dependent on food type | 7-day weighed food record | Compared child's parent-assisted report of frequency of food intake on FFQ against child's report of intake on 7-day weighed food records completed 2–3 months after FFQ administration. Records consisted of four consecutive days, a 1-week interval, and three consecutive days. | Spearman correlations between FFQ and food records were 0.51 for energy, 0.48 for protein, and 0.57 for total fat. The range of correlations for 18 nutrients was 0.14 for vitamin D to 0.66 for monounsaturated fat. FFQ energy intake was 24% higher than diet records (10.7 vs. 8.6 mJ/day). FFQ significantly overestimated 16 of the 18 nutrients and 8 of 13 food items compared to food records. |
| Green et al.[51] | 14 f<br>19 f<br>29 f<br>43 f | 16 years<br>17 years<br>18 years<br>19 years | 116 items; self-administered; past year; semiquantitative | Unknown | Serum folate, RBC folate, and serum vitamin B-12 | Compared child's report of frequency of intake of foods on FFQ against serum micronutrient levels. | Pearson correlations were 0.48 between folate from the FFQ and serum folate, 0.42 between folate from the FFQ and RBC folate, and 0.25 between vitamin B-12 intake from the FFQ and serum B-12. |

a FFQ, food frequency questionnaire.
b Results of all subgroups not reported due to samples below the N = 30 criterion.
c Males (m), females (f).
d Adult assistance required for instrument administration.
e NA, includes Native American, American Indian, and Alaskan Native; see author definitions.
f TEE, total energy expenditure.
g AA, African American.
h Hisp, includes Hispanic, Latino(a), Hispanic/Latino(a), Hispanic White, and Hispanic Black; see author definitions.

**TABLE 35.6**
**FFQ and Checklist Reliability Studies among School-Age Children**

| References[a] | Sample | Age/Grade | Instrument | Response Categories (Range) | Design | Results |
|---|---|---|---|---|---|---|
| Lanfer et al.[119] | 113 m[b] 145 f[b] | 2–9 years Adults required[c] | 43 items; Children's Eating Habits Questionnaire (CEHQ)-FFQ[c]; past 4 weeks; nonquantitative | 8 (never to 4 or more times/day) | Compared test–retest of frequency of food intake from CEHQ-FFQ completed by the parents up to 354 days apart. | Kappa coefficients between 2 CEHQ-FFQs ranged from 0.23 (soft drink, diet) to 0.68 (milk, sugar added) for 43 foods assessed. Spearman correlations ranged from 0.32 (soft drink, diet) to 0.76 (milk, sugar added). Longer time between FFQ administrations (>128 days) resulted in lower reproducibility for 38 foods. Spearman correlation coefficients were significantly different for 10 foods in North European countries (Sweden, Estonia, Belgium) compared to South European countries (Hungary, Italy, Cyprus). |
| Kobayashi et al.[56] | 89 m and f | 3–16 years Adults required | 75 items; Children's FFQ (CFFQ); self-administered; previous month; semiquantitative; child portions | Dependent on food type | Compared 1-month test–retest of food intake from FFQs completed by the children and parents. | Pearson correlations between the two CFFQs were 0.73 for energy, 0.77 for protein, and 0.76 for total fat and ranged from 0.54 (linoleic acid) to 0.84 (pantothenic acid) for 12 fatty acids and 25 additional nutrients. Median Pearson correlation coefficient was 0.76. Pearson correlations were positive and significant for energy, 26 nutrients, and 12 fatty acids assessed. |
| Kobayashi et al.[56] | 89 m and f | 3–16 years Adults required | 76 items; AFFQ; self-administered; previous month; semiquantitative; adult portions | Dependent on food type | Compared 1-month test–retest of food intake from FFQs completed by the children and parents. | Pearson correlations between the two AFFQs were 0.80 for energy, 0.73 for protein, and 0.71 for total fat and ranged from 0.39 (manganese) to 0.83 (carbohydrate) for 12 fatty acids and 25 additional nutrients. Median Pearson correlation coefficient was 0.73. Pearson correlations were positive and significant for energy, 26 nutrients, and 12 fatty acids assessed. |
| Basch et al.[120] | 166 m and f Hisp[g] | 4–7 years Adults required | ~116 items; interviewer administered; past 6 months; semiquantitative; child portions | 9 (none or <1/month to ≥6/day) | Compared both 3-month and 1-year tests–retests of nutrient estimates from FFQs completed by the parent. | Pearson correlations (log transformed) between the two FFQs at 3 months were 0.53 for energy, 0.49 for protein, and 0.56 for total fat. The range of correlations for 12 nutrients assessed at 3 months was −0.06 for sucrose to 0.61 for crude fiber. At 1 year, correlations were 0.46 for energy, 0.40 for protein, and 0.47 for total fat. The range of correlations for 12 nutrients assessed at 1 year was 0.06 for sucrose to 0.57 for polyunsaturated fat. |
| Metcalf et al.[121] | 90 m and f | 5–14 years Adults required | 117 items; Children's Nutrition Survey FFQ; self-administered; past 4 weeks; semiquantitative | 7 (never or less than once per month to 2 or more times per day) | Compared 2-week test–retest of FFQs completed by parent/caregiver or parent/caregiver and child. | Pearson correlations (log transformed) between the two FFQs for the 17 food groups ranged from 0.35 for bread (slices) to 0.86 for rice among 5- to 9-year-olds and from 0.49 for spreads to 0.91 for red meats among 10- to 14-year-olds. Spearman correlations (log transformed) between the two FFQs for the 17 food groups ranged from 0.38 for bread (slices) to 0.85 for rice among 5- to 9-year-olds and from 0.54 for mixed meat dishes to 0.89 for convenience meals among 10- to 14-year-olds. Standardized Cronbach's alpha between the two FFQs ranged from 0.52 for bread (slices) to 0.92 for rice among 5- to 9-year-olds and from 0.64 for spreads to 0.95 for red meats among 10- to 14-year-olds. Pearson and Spearman correlations and Cronbach's alpha were generally lower among 5- to 9-year-olds compared to 10- to 14-year-olds. |

| Reference | Sample | Age/Grade | Instrument | Response | Comparison | Results |
|---|---|---|---|---|---|---|
| Marcotte et al.[63] | 28 m, 21 f, White, AA[f], others | 6–8 years; Adults required | 19 items (15 calcium foods and 4 dummy foods); interviewer administered; past 24 hours; child portions | Open ended | Compared 1 h test–retest of calcium intake from checklists completed by the child. | Spearman correlations between the two checklists for calcium intake were 0.58 for total calcium (calcium from all foods) and 0.57 for dairy calcium (calcium from dairy foods). Percent agreement between the two checklists for individual food consumption was >80% for most foods. |
| Zemel et al.[65] | 61 m and f, 62% f, 30% AA | 7–10 years; Adults required | 41 items; Calcium Counts! FFQ; administered to parent/child by RD; previous 4 weeks; semiquantitative; typical serving sizes | Number of servings per day, week, month (or never) | Compared 3.6-month test–retest (median time interval was 32 days, range of 7–111 days) of calcium from child's parent-assisted FFQ. | Pearson correlations between the two FFQs for calcium were 0.74 (0.77, deattenuated). Correlations were 0.69 (deattenuated r = 0.73) for 9–10 years and 0.89 (deattenuated r = 0.90) for 7–8 years. Correlations (deattenuated) were 0.74 for females, 0.86 for males, 0.72 for AA, and 0.82 for non-AA. |
| de Assis et al.[122] | 227 m and f | 7–10 years; Adults required | 21-item Previous-Day Food Questionnaire (PDFQ); group administered; previous day; nonquantitative | 2 (yes/no) | Compared a same-day test–retest of food intake from PDFQs completed by child. Excerpted midmorning meal, lunch, and afternoon snack. | Kappa coefficients ranged for midmorning meal from 0.68 for bread/pasta to 0.74 for sweets, for lunch from 0.54 for fruits to 0.77 for rice and dried beans, and for afternoon snack from 0.59 for bread/pasta to 0.81 for fruits. |
| Arnold et al.[66] | 77 f | 7–12 years; Adults required | 160 items; self-administered; past year; semiquantitative; adult portions | 5 (open-ended, none to number of months/year) | Compared 6-month test–retest of nutrient estimates from FFQs completed by the parent and child. | Pearson correlations (log transformed, energy adjusted) between the two FFQs were 0.60 for energy, 0.51 for protein, and 0.14 for total fat. The range of correlations for 16 nutrients assessed was 0.14 for total fat to 0.71 for fiber. Mean energy intake was 5% higher in the first FFQ compared to the second (2319 vs. 2205 kcal/day). Mean intake of 15 nutrients was higher in the first FFQ compared to the second; 1 nutrient was lower (significance testing not shown). |
| Garcia-Dominic et al.[123] | 138 m and f | Third grade | 73 items; Block Kids FFQ; self-administered; 7 days; semiquantitative; "usual" portion | 6 (none to 5 or more times a day) | Compared 2-week test–retest of food intake from FFQs completed by the child. | Spearman correlation between the two FFQs was 0.81. |
| Garcia-Dominic et al.[123] | 138 m and f | Third grade | 41 items; Block Kid Screener; self-administered; semiquantitative | 6 (none to 5 or more times a day) | Compared 2-week test–retest of food intake from screeners completed by the child. | Spearman correlation between the 2 screeners was 0.73. |
| Tak et al.[124] | 302–372 m and f | 9–10 years; Adults required | Unknown number of items (fruit and vegetables); group administered; semiquantitative: usual intake | Varied dependent on food (weighted to frequencies/day) | Compared 1-year test–retest of child's teacher-assisted FFQ report of fruit and vegetable intake at baseline and year 1 and parents report of intake of child at baseline and year 1. | Mean fruit and vegetable intake was overreported by children a baseline as compared to 1 year, 1.72 vs. 1.04 pieces/day and 102.5 vs. 93.2 g/day, respectively. Mean fruit and vegetable intake of children as reported by parents was underreported at baseline as compared to 1 year 1.08 vs. 1.11 g/day and 67.1 vs. 72.2 g/day, respectively. |

(continued)

**TABLE 35.6 (continued)**

**FFQ and Checklist Reliability Studies among School-Age Children**

| References[a] | Sample | Age/Grade | Instrument | Response Categories (Range) | Design | Results |
|---|---|---|---|---|---|---|
| Lee et al.[125] | 153 m and f Korean | 9–11 years | 7 items; self-administered; last week; nonquantitative | 7 (almost never to ≥3 times/day) | Compared 1-month test–retest of frequency of intake of food typical by Korean school children completed by the children. | Spearman correlations between the intake frequencies of seven items from two FFQs were 0.22 (spaghetti), 0.32 (ddeokbokki), 0.51 (kimchi), 0.33 (ham roast), 0.31 (pork cutlet), 0.43 (dairy products and ices), and 0.47 (fruits). |
| Domel et al.[75] | 146 m and f White, AA | Fourth to fifth grade | 45 items (15 fruits, 30 vegetables); group administered; past week; semiquantitative; "serving" portions | 5 (none or <1/week to several times/day) | Compared 1-week test–retest of fruit and vegetable intake from FFQs completed by the child. The order of fruit (15 items) and vegetables (30 items) was reversed between the first and second administrations. | Spearman correlations between the two FFQs were 0.50 for total fruit, 0.48 for total vegetable, and 0.54 for total fruit and vegetable intake. The range of correlations for eight fruit and vegetable groupings assessed was 0.39 for fruit and vegetable juice to 0.54 for total fruit and vegetables. Mean daily servings of total fruits and vegetables were 12% higher for week 1 FFQ compared to week 2 FFQ (8.3 vs. 7.3). Mean daily servings of 6 fruit and vegetable groupings of eight assessed were higher for week 1 FFQ compared to week 2 FFQ (significance testing not shown). |
| Domel et al.[75] | 156 m and f White, AA | Fourth to fifth grade | 45 items (15 fruits, 30 vegetables); group administered; past month; semiquantitative; "serving" portions | 7 (none or <1/month to several times/day) | Compared 1-month (3.5-week) test–retest of fruit and vegetable intake from FFQs completed by the child. The order of fruit (15 items) and vegetables (30 items) was reversed between the first and second administrations. | Spearman correlations between the two FFQs were 0.43 for total fruit, 0.37 for total vegetable, and 0.47 for total fruit and vegetable intake. The range of correlations for eight fruit and vegetable groupings assessed was 0.28 for fruit and vegetable juice to 0.47 for both legumes and total fruit and vegetable intake. Mean daily servings of total fruits and vegetables were 54% higher for month 1 FFQ compared to month 2 FFQ (11.7 vs. 5.4). Mean daily servings of 8 fruit and vegetable groupings were higher for month 1 FFQ compared to month 2 FFQ (significance testing not shown). |
| Penkilo et al.[126] | 322 m and f 48% m 52% f 73% White 14% AA 13% Hisp | 9–12 years | 54 items (21 food intake–related items); SBNM; group administered; yesterday; nonquantitative | 4 (0 times/day to ≥3 times/day) | Compared a >2 h test–retest of "yesterday" questions. The SBNM was administered Tuesday to Friday. | Spearman correlations between the 2 SBNMs for 21 food and meal choice behaviors ranged from 0.64 for eating snacks to 0.88 for both meats and peanuts. Kappa statistics ranged from 0.51 for breads to 0.87 for vitamin pills. The percent agreement ranged from 66.6% for breads to 94.0% for gravy. |
| Field et al.[78] | 35 m and f 34 m and f | Fourth fifth grade Sixth to seventh grade | 97 items (11 fruits and fruit juices, 14 vegetables; group administered to fourth to fifth grade; self-administered to sixth to seventh grade; past year; semiquantitative; child portions | Dependent on food type | Compared a 1-year test–retest of FFQs completed by child. | Spearman correlations between the 2 FFQs among fourth to fifth graders were 0.24 for energy, 0.25 for protein, and 0.15 for total fat. Correlations between the 2 FFQs among sixth to seventh graders were 0.21 for energy, 0.23 for protein, and 0.18 for total fat. The range of correlations for the 11 nutrients assessed was from 0.03 for phosphorous to 0.30 for carbohydrates among fourth to fifth graders. Among sixth to seventh graders, correlations ranged from 0.18 for total fat to 0.47 for iron. Spearman correlations between the 2 FFQs among fourth to fifth graders were −0.26 for vegetables, 0.07 for fruit and vegetables, 0.36 for fruit, and 0.40 for fruit juice. Among sixth to seventh graders, correlations were 0.18 for fruit juice, 0.28 for vegetables, 0.29 for fruit and vegetables, and 0.33 for fruit. |

| Study | Subjects | Age | Instrument | Response options | Comparison | Results |
|---|---|---|---|---|---|---|
| Watson et al.[79] | 101 m and f | 9–16 years | 120 items; ACAES; self-administered; previous 6 months; semiquantitative; natural serving sizes for data from children aged 9–16 | Varied, depending on food (ranged from never to ≥4 times/day) | Compared a 5-month test–retest of the ACAES completed by the children. | Pearson correlations log transformed and energy adjusted between the 2 FFQs were 0.44 for energy, 0.36 for protein, and 0.31 for total fat. The range of correlations for 22 nutrients assessed was 0.18 for vitamin A to 0.50 for calcium. Mean energy intake was 4.8% higher in first FFQ compared to the second (10.5 mJ vs. 10.0 mJ/day). Weighted kappa statistics for 22 nutrients ranged from 0.36 for sugars to 0.54 for niacin. The proportion of individuals correctly classified into the same quintile ranged from 39% for niacin equivalent to 23% for sugars. Gross misclassifications ranged from none for vitamin C to 5% for fiber. |
| Yang et al.[90] | 41 m and f 42% m 59% f 76% 9–14 years 24% 15–20 years 68% Asian 29% White 2% mixed | 9–20 years | 15 items; BCAT; self-administered; past month; semiquantitative | Unknown (weighted to frequencies/day) | Compared a 1-week test–retest of the BCAT. | Pearson correlation between the 2 FFQs for calcium was 0.76. No significant differences in scores between the first and second administrations. |
| Rockett et al.[127] | 75 m 101 f 3 N/A[d] multiethnic | 9–18 years | 151 items; YAQ; self-administered; past year; semiquantitative; adult portions | 9 (none or <1/month to ≥6/day) | Compared 1-year test–retest of nutrient estimates from YAQ completed by the child. | Pearson correlations (log transformed, energy adjusted) between the 2 YAQs were 0.49 for energy, 0.26 for protein, and 0.41 for total fat. The range of correlations for seven nutrients assessed was 0.26 for protein and iron to 0.58 for calcium. Mean energy intake was 10% higher in the first YAQ compared to the second (2477 vs. 2222 kcal/day). Mean intake of six nutrients assessed was significantly higher in the first YAQ compared to the second. The range of correlations for eight food groups assessed was 0.39 for meats to 0.57 for soda. Pearson correlations (log transformed) for servings/day were 0.49 for fruits, 0.48 for vegetables, and 0.48 for fruits and vegetables. Of the eight food groups, mean serving frequencies of five were significantly higher in the first YAQ compared to the second. Reproducibility of nutrient intake was significantly higher for females than males' mean correlation for all nutrients and was 0.44 and 0.34, respectively. There were no significant differences by age or ethnicity. |
| Preston et al.[82] | 94 m and f 40 m 54 f | Fifth grade | 97 items; FFQ including supplements; interviewer administered; past month; semiquantitative | Unknown | Compared 2-week test–retest of the FFQ administered by interviewers. | Spearman correlations between the two FFQs were 0.30 for energy, 0.11 for protein, and 0.26 for total fat. The range of correlations for 12 nutrients assessed was 0.11 for protein to 0.33 for vitamin B12. Mean energy intake was 34% higher in the first FFQ compared to the second (2856 vs. 2136 kcal/day). Correlation coefficients for all nutrients averaged 0.21. Spearman correlations between FFQ1 and FFQ2 ranged from 0.12 for protein to 0.40 for vitamin B12 for girls and from 0.05 for calcium to 0.48 for total fat for boys. |

(continued)

**TABLE 35.6 (continued)**
**FFQ and Checklist Reliability Studies among School-Age Children**

| References[a] | Sample | Age/Grade | Instrument | Response Categories (Range) | Design | Results |
|---|---|---|---|---|---|---|
| Wilson et al.[84] | 134 m and f<br>62% f<br>36% fifth grade<br>33% sixth grade<br>31% seventh grade | 10–14 years | 14 items; questionnaire with six food scores and one score for healthy food behaviors; group administered; usual, recent/current, or previous day; nonquantitative | Unknown (none to 5 times/day, never to 1–3 times/week, and more than 5 serves/day) | Compared 8–36 day (mean = 24 days) test–retest of questionnaire. Developed 12 scores divided into 5 categories. Questionnaires were administered on Tuesday to Friday. | ICCs between intake scores of the two questionnaires were 0.47 for noncore foods to 0.66 for fruits and vegetables. Cronbach's alpha identified four items in three scores as unnecessary, including breakfast frequency, fast food, and number of fruits and vegetables, never consumed, or not known. After modification, Cronbach's alpha values were 0.50 for healthy behavior and fruit and vegetable environment scores. |
| Haraldsdottir et al.[91] | 93 m<br>112 f | 11–12 years | Six items (five fruits and vegetables, one potato); self-administered; "usual intake"; semiquantitative | 8 (never to >2 times/day) | Compared 7–12-day test–retest of fruit and vegetable intake from FFQs completed by the child in six countries (Denmark, Norway, Iceland, Belgium, Portugal, Spain). | Spearman correlations between the two FFQs averaged across six countries were 0.65 for fruit, 0.67 for vegetables, 0.69 for total intake of fruit and vegetables, and 0.72 for orange juice. Cross classification showed that between 39% and 72% of participants were classified in the same quartile fruit, vegetable, total fruit and vegetable, and orange juice. Between 85% and 98% were placed in the same or adjacent quartile. Only 0%–8% were misclassified into the opposite quartile. |
| Andersen et al.[33] | 54 m<br>60 f | Sixth grade | 16 items (7 fruits and vegetables); self-administered; past 3 months; nonquantitative | 10 (never to several times/day) | Compared a 2-week test–retest of fruit and vegetable intake from FFQs completed by the child. | Spearman correlations between the 2 FFQs were 0.62 for fruit; 0.70 for vegetable; 0.75 for fruit and vegetable without fruit juice and potato; 0.77 for fruit juice; 0.78 for fruit, fruit juice, vegetable, and potato; and 0.83 for potato. |
| Vereecken et al.[85] | 207 m and f<br>43% m<br>57% f | 11–12 years | 15 items (fiber, calcium foods, and foods relevant to youth food culture); HBSC FFQ; group administered; yesterday; nonquantitative | 7 (never to more than once a day) | Compared a 7–15-day test–retest of HBSC completed by the child. | Spearman correlations between the two HBSCs for the 15 foods ranged from 0.52 for chips to 0.82 for semiskimmed milk. Mean weighted kappa value between the two HBSCs was 0.58. The range of kappa values for the 15 foods was 0.44 for other milk products to 0.70 for semiskimmed milk. The percent agreement between the two HBSCs ranged from 39% for other milk products to 87% for alcoholic beverage with an overall mean agreement of 55%. |
| Harnack et al.[95] | 92 m and f<br>156 m and f<br>60.5% f<br>68.5% White<br>19.4% AA<br>6.5% others<br>6.0% Somali American<br>5.6% Hisp<br>3.6% NA[b] | 11–12 years<br>13–14 years | 10 items; calcium FFQ; self-administered; past month; semiquantitative | Unknown (never or less than 1 time/ month to ≥3 times/ day) | Compared 7-day test–retest of calcium intake from FFQs completed by the child. | ICCs of calcium intake between the two FFQs were 0.74 for total sample, 0.74 for 11- to 12-year-olds, 0.75 for 12- to 13-year-olds, 0.79 for girls, and 0.66 for boys. |

| Study | Sample | Age | Instrument | Response categories | Comparison | Results |
|---|---|---|---|---|---|---|
| Buzzard et al.[128] | 415 m and f; 46% m; 54% f; 56% White; 32% AA; 12% Asian, Hisp, Indian | Sixth grade 11–14 years | 35 items (25 measuring fat, fiber, and fruit and vegetable intake); goals for health; self-administered; usual intake; nonquantitative | 7 (Never to ≥3 times/day) | Compared a 4-month test–retest of nutrient scores from FFQs completed by the child. | Pearson correlations (log transformed) between nutrient scores from the two FFQs were 0.58 for total fat, 0.49 for fiber, and 0.51 for fruit and vegetables. Correlations of the 25 frequency items ranged from 0.24 for donuts, sweet rolls, and muffins to 0.59 for mayonnaise on sandwiches. The mean correlation was 0.41. |
| Speck et al.[129] | 31 m and f; 42% m; 58% f; 56% White; 44% AA | Sixth to eighth grade | 140 items (14 food habit questions, 83 food frequency questions past week, and 43 quantity of foods eaten/day questions); EHQ: group administered; past week; quantitative | 5 (never to almost every day); 6 for beverage items (never to ≥3 times/day); 4 for quantity items (0 to ≥5 servings) | Compared a 48 h test–retest of FFQs completed by the child. | Pearson correlations between the two FFQs for the 10 food groupings ranged from 0.46 for dairy to 0.85 for meats/fish/casseroles. |
| Speck et al.[129] | 31 m and f; 55% m; 45% f; 57% White; 43% AA | Sixth to eighth grade | 140 items (14 food habit questions, 83 food frequency questions past week, and 43 quantity of foods eaten/day questions); EHQ: group administered; past week; quantitative | Five for food items (never to almost every day); six for beverage items (never to ≥3 times/day); four for quantity items (0 to ≥5 servings) | Compared a 2-week test–retest of FFQs completed by the child. | Correlations between the initial and the 2-week FFQs ranged from 0.08 for dairy to 0.76 for sweet snacks. |
| Nelson et al.[98] | 33 m and f 15 m | 11–18 years | 22-item screener FFQ (9 beverages, 13 fast-food items); self-administered; usually to past month; semiquantified, others were not; usual portion sizes | Varied by depending on question (ranged from yes/no to 9 response categories) | Compared a 2–21-day test–retest of screener completed by child. | Spearman correlations ranged from 0.63 for frequency of diet soda consumption to 0.84 for frequency of milk consumption; overall fast-food consumption was 0.67. Kappa statistics ranged from 0.10 for consumption at bakery/donut shop to 0.80 for consumption of fried chicken. |
| Wong et al.[97] | 161 m and f; 50% m; 50% f; 53% 11–14 years; 47% 15–18 years; 36% Hisp; 35% White; 29% Asian | 11–18 years | 80 items; computerized FFQ with photos and visual portion sizes and audio script; self-administered with moderators; past month; semiquantitative | 4–7 frequency responses, (ranged from never or <once/month to ≥4 servings/day) | Compared 1 and 4-week test–retest of FFQ completed by the children. | Daily calcium intakes were 16% higher in the first FFQ compared to the second (1210 vs. 1045 mg). Pearson transformed correlations were 0.72 for calcium intake for the total sample. Correlations for boys were 0.59 vs. 0.81 for girls. Correlations by age were 0.65 for 11–14 years and 0.82 for 15–18 years. By race/ethnicity, correlations were 0.73 for Asians, 0.76 for Hisps, and 0.61 for Whites. |
| Prochaska et al.[99] | 218 m and f | 12 years (mean age) | Two-item fruit and vegetable brief; self-administered; typical day; semiquantitative | 4 (none to 4 or more/day) | Compared same-day to 1-month test–retest of the fruit and vegetable brief questionnaire completed by the child. | ICC between the two brief questionnaires for fruits and vegetables was 0.68; ranging from 0.80 for same-day retest to 0.47 for a retest up to 1 month. The overall kappa was 56% and ranged from 53% for same-day retest to 44% for up to 1-month retest. |

*(continued)*

**TABLE 35.6 (continued)**
**FFQ and Checklist Reliability Studies among School-Age Children**

| References[a] | Sample | Age/Grade | Instrument | Response Categories (Range) | Design | Results |
|---|---|---|---|---|---|---|
| Watanabe et al.[100] | 63 f | 12–13 years | 82-item FFQ (FFQW82) with pictures; self-administered; past 1 month; semiquantitative; small, medium, and large portion sizes | 6 ("absolutely do not eat" to "always eat at breakfast (or lunch or dinner)") | Compared a 1-month test–retest of the FFQW82. | Spearman correlations between the two FFQs were were 0.58 for energy, 0.56 for protein, and 0.34 for total fat. The range of correlations for 10 nutrients assessed was 0.34 for fat to 0.70 for carbohydrate. Pearson correlations between the two FFQs were similar but slightly higher. Spearman correlations between 11 food groups ranged from 0.13 for total fats to 0.86 for fruits, with an average of 0.58. |
| Neuhouser et al.[101] | 46 m and f 18 m 28 f 56.5% White 13.0% AA 6.5% Hisp 6.5% Asian 15.2% others | Seventh grade | 19 items (beverages and snacks); Beverage and Snack Questionnaire (BSQ); self-administered; past week; nonquantitative | 7 (never or <once/week to ≥4 times/day) | Compared a 4–6-week test–retest of the BSQ completed by the child during class time in school. | Pearson correlations for 19 individual food items ranged from 0.61 for low-fat and nonfat frozen desserts consumed at school and at home to 0.89 for 100% juices not consumed at school. Pearson correlations for food categories (n = 6) ranged from 0.72 for snacks and sweets consumed at school to 0.85 for fruits and vegetables consumed at school. Reliability was similar for foods consumed at school (0.70) or away from school (0.67). |
| Smith et al.[102] | 122 m and f | Seventh grade | 40 items; (foods high in total fat, saturated fat, and sodium); CATCH CFC; group administered; yesterday; nonquantitative | Yes/no | Compared a morning and afternoon test–retest of CFCs completed by the child. The second administration occurred at least 2 h after the first administration. | Pearson correlations between scores from the two CFCs were 0.89 for total fat, 0.85 for saturated fat, and 0.86 for sodium. Kappa statistics for individual items between the two CFC food items ranged from 0.66 for pork to 0.94 for pickles/olives and for pretzels (median = 0.85). |
| Cullen et al.[103] | 89 m and f 41% m 59% f 54% AA 46% Hisp | Seventh to eighth grade | 152 items; YAQ; group administered; past year; semiquantitative; child portions | Dependent on food type | Compared a 3-week test–retest of YAQs completed by the child. | Spearman correlations between the two YAQs were 0.72 for energy and 0.19 for total fat (% kcal). Correlations for the five fruit and vegetable groupings ranged from 0.37 for fruit juice to 0.67 for total fruit, juice, and vegetables. Mean daily nutrient intakes were higher in the first YAQ than the second YAQ for all items except total fat (% kcal). Correlations between the two YAQs among Hisps were 0.61 for energy and 0.11 for total fat (% kcal) and for the five fruit and vegetable groupings ranged from 0.30 for high-fat vegetables to 0.68 for total fruit, juice, and vegetables. Among AA children, correlations between the two YAQs were 0.80 for energy and 0.31 for total fat (% kcal) and for the five fruit and vegetable groupings ranged from 0.44 for juice to 0.66 for total fruit, juice, and vegetables and also for high-fat vegetables. The reliability coefficients were generally lower for the Hisp children compared to the AA children. |
| Frank et al.[130] | 189 m and f White, AA | 12–17 years | 64 items; group administered; past week; semiquantitative; adult portions | 6 (none to >3 times/day) | Compared 2-week test–retest of food intake from FFQs completed by the child. | Two-thirds of the children reported similar responses for the frequency of consumption of low-fat milk, diet carbonated soft drinks, and shellfish. Twelve food groups had percent agreement of 50% or better (significance testing not shown). |

| Study | Sample | Age/Grade | Instrument | Categories | Comparison | Results |
|---|---|---|---|---|---|---|
| Matthys et al.[106] | 66 m and f | 12–18 years | 69 items; self-administered; past month; quantitative; web based; portions based on adolescent serving sizes | 6 (<1 day/month to every day) | Compared at least 1-month test–retest of median food group intakes from FFQ completed by the child. | Spearman correlation for all foods collectively was 0.62; correlations ranged from 0.27 for fish/eggs/meat to 0.87 for alcoholic beverages. |
| Prochaska et al.[107] | 40 m<br>26 f<br>57 m<br>104 f<br>41% White<br>26% AA<br>16% Asian<br>4% Hisp | Seventh to eighth<br>Seventh to eighth<br>9–12th<br>9–12th grade | 21 items (21 high-fat foods); PACE+; self-administered; past 7 days; nonquantitative | 6 (did not eat it this week to more than twice each day) | Compared a 1–2-week test–retest of high-fat food intake from FFQs completed by the child. | ICC of the fat intake measures between the two FFQs was 0.64 for the full sample of males and females grades 7–12, 0.62 for males grades 7–8, 0.55 for males grades 9–12, and 0.68 for females grades 9–12. Internal consistency, as calculated by coefficient α, was 0.88 at time 1 and 0.87 at time 2. |
| Prochaska et al.[107] | 40 m<br>26 f<br>57 m<br>104 f<br>41% White<br>26% AA<br>16% Asian<br>4% Hisp | Seventh to eighth<br>Seventh to eighth<br>9–12th<br>9–12th grade | Four categories (four high-fat food groups); self-administered; past 7 days; nonquantitative | 6 (did not eat it this week to more than twice each day) | Compared a 1–2-week test–retest of high-fat food intake from FFQs completed by the child. | ICCs of the fat intake measures between the two FFQs were 0.65 for the full sample of males and females grades 7–12, 0.50 for males grades 7–8, 0.71 for males grades 9–12, and 0.65 for females grades 9–12. Internal consistency, as calculated by coefficient α, was 0.74 at time 1 and 0.76 at time 2. |
| Hoelscher et al.[109] | 254 m and f<br>48% m<br>52% f<br>74% White<br>6% AA<br>16% Hisp<br>5% others/missing | Eighth grade | 63 items (19 food items tested for reproducibility); SBNM; group administered; yesterday; nonquantitative | 4 (0 times/day to ≥3 times/day) | Compared a morning and afternoon test–retest of SBNM completed by the child. The second administration of SBNM occurred after lunch and at least 2 h after first administration from Tuesday to Friday. | Spearman correlations between the two SBNMs for the 19 food groupings ranged from 0.66 for French fries or chips to 0.97 for gravy. Kappa statistics ranged from 0.54 for French fries or chips to 0.93 (adjusted) for gravy. Percent agreement ranged from 70% for any type of bread, bun, bagel, tortilla, and roll to 70% for French fries or chips to 98% for gravy. No significant gender differences were detected. |
| Hoelscher et al.[109] | 259 m and f<br>49% m<br>51% f<br>75% White<br>6% AA<br>14% Hisp<br>5% others/missing | Eighth grade | 63 items (11 food habit items tested for reproducibility); SBNM; group administered; usual intake; nonquantitative | 4 (0 times/day to >3 times/day) | Compared a 9–14-day test–retest of SBNM completed by the child. The SBNM was administered Tuesday to Friday. | Spearman correlations between the two SBNMs for 11 food and meal choice behaviors ranged from 0.43 for eating dinner to 0.87 for type of milk (fat content). Kappa statistics ranged from 0.41 for eating dinner to 0.79 for type of milk (fat content). Percent agreement ranged from 62% for type of sweet roll, doughnuts cookies, brownies, and pies cakes (fat content) to 96% for vegetarian status. No significant gender differences were detected. |
| Vereecken et al.[85] | 560 m and f<br>60% m<br>40% f | 13–14 years | 15 items (fiber, calcium foods, and foods relevant to youth food culture); HBSC FFQ; group administered; yesterday; nonquantified | 7 (never to more than once/day) | Compared a 6–10-day test–retest of traditional paper FFQ and a computerized version of FFQ completed by the child. | Spearman correlations between the two FFQs for the 15 foods ranged from 0.57 for chips and other milk products to 0.78 for brown bread. The mean weighted kappa value between the two FFQs was 0.55. The range of kappa values for the 15 foods was 0.43 for other milk products to 0.66 for white bread and brown bread. Percent agreement between the two FFQs ranged from 37% for other milk products to 68% for chips with an overall mean percent agreement of 52%. |

*(continued)*

**TABLE 35.6 (continued)**
**FFQ and Checklist Reliability Studies among School-Age Children**

| References[a] | Sample | Age/Grade | Instrument | Response Categories (Range) | Design | Results |
|---|---|---|---|---|---|---|
| Johnson et al.[93] | 98 m and f 45 m 53 f | 13–14 years | 56-item (inferred) FIQ five food groups: sugary, fatty, fiber, and negative and positive markers; previous day; self-administered; nonquantitative | Yes/no | Compared food groups in three FFQs completed over 3 months time at regular intervals by children. | Pearson correlations for food groups between FFQ1 and FFQ2 ranged from 0.45 for fiber to 0.68 for negative markers, between FFQ1 and FFQ3 ranged from 0.42 for fiber to 0.76 for negative markers, and between FFQ2 and FFQ3 ranged from 0.44 for fiber to 0.71 for negative markers. |
| Vereecken et al.[110] | 48 m and f 46% f | 13–17 years | 137 items; HELENA FFQ; online self-administered; past 30 days; semiquantitative; standard portion sizes | Based on "units per day," "units per week," "units during the last 30 days"; varied from 10 units to 30 units; for some frequency and average amount per occasion | Compared a 1–2-week test–retest of the online HELENA FFQ completed by the adolescent. | Spearman correlations between the two FFQs were 0.65 for energy and 0.65 for total fat. The range of correlations for 11 nutrients assessed was 0.46 for calcium to 0.65 for energy, total fat, and iron, with an average of 0.58. Mean energy intake was 5% higher in the first FFQ compared to the second (2629 vs. 2509 kcal/day). Spearman correlations between 22 food groups ranged from 0.46 for water to 0.90 for alcoholic beverages, with an average of 0.64. |
| Li et al.[112] | 43 m and f White, Asian | Eighth to 12th grade | Unknown, modified NCI Vegetable Fruit By Meal Questionnaire; number of items; self-administered; previous week; semiquantitative | Unknown | Compared 2-month test–retest of fruit and vegetable intake from FFQs completed by the child. | Pearson correlation for the 2 FFQs was 0.46. Mean fruit and vegetable intake did not differ significantly between 2 FFQs (8.7 and 9.1 servings on the 1st and 2nd FFQs, respectively). |
| Davis et al.[115] | 35 f Hisp | 14–17 years | 22 items (9 beverages, 13 fast-food consumptions); self-administered; past month; semiquantitative | Dependent on food type | Compared 7-day test–retest of fast-food and beverage intake from screeners completed by the child. | Spearman correlation between the two screeners for overall fast-food frequency was 0.49 and for beverage frequency ranged from 0.37 (sweetened beverages) to 0.71 (coffee drinks). Kappa statistics for beverage amount ranged from 0.44 (regular soda) to 0.61 (water) and for fast-food type ranged from 0.08 (coffee shop) to 0.73 (bakery/donut shop). |

| Turconi et al.[131] | 68 m and f | 106 items (28 food frequencies and 14 food habit/portion questions); self-administered; usual day or weekly intake; semiquantitative | Dependent on question | Compared a 1-week test–retest of FFQs completed by the child. | Pearson correlations for 28 items in the food frequency section ranged from 0.45 for pasta/rice/bread/potatoes and sweets to 0.90 for milk/milk and coffee/cappuccino/yogurt and beer. Pearson correlation for food habit scores between FFQs was 0.88, with a Cronbach's alpha of 0.75. |
| Preston et al.[82] | 89 m and f<br>42 m<br>47 f | 97-item FFQ including supplements; interviewer administered; past month; semiquantitative | Unknown | Compared a 2-week test–retest of the FFQ, administered by interviewers. | Spearman correlations between the two FFQs were 0.30 for energy, 0.42 for protein, and 0.45 for total fat. The range of correlations for 12 nutrients assessed was 0.30 for energy to 0.51 for folate. Mean energy intake was 27% higher in the first FFQ compared to the second (3150 vs. 2476 kcal/day). Correlation coefficients for all nutrients averaged 0.43. Spearman correlations between FFQ1 and FFQ2 ranged from 0.23 for iron to 0.66 for folate for girls and from 0.26 for both vitamin C and vitamin B6 to 0.57 for magnesium for boys. |
| Andersen et al.[118] | 53 m<br>50 f | 190 items; FFQ group administered; past year; semiquantitative | Dependent on food type | Compared 6-week test–retest of nutrient estimates from FFQs completed by the child and parent. | Spearman correlations (energy adjusted) between the two FFQs were 0.87 for energy, 0.86 for protein, and 0.86 for total fat. The range of correlations for 18 nutrients assessed was 0.72 for vitamin C to 0.91 for alcohol. Median energy intake was 11% higher in the first FFQ compared to the second (12.3 vs. 10.9 mJ/day). Median intake of 15 nutrients was significantly higher in the first FFQ compared to the second FFQ. Differences in median correlations for nutrient intake were not significant between females and males (0.78 vs. 0.74, respectively). |

<sup>a</sup> Results of all subgroups not reported due to samples below the N = 30 criterion.

<sup>b</sup> Males (m), females (f).

<sup>c</sup> Adult assistance required for instrument administration.

<sup>d</sup> N/A, not applicable.

<sup>e</sup> FFQ, food frequency questionnaire.

<sup>f</sup> AA, African American.

<sup>g</sup> Hisp, includes Hispanic, Latino(a), Hispanic/Latino(a), Hispanic White, and Hispanic Black; see author definitions.

<sup>h</sup> NA, includes Native American, American Indian, and Alaskan Native; see author definitions.

between 1 and 40 items. The majority of the FFQ validity studies (78%) included an instrument with less than 97 items, and the range of FFQ items was 1–212 items from all studies. Seventy-two percent of the FFQs were semiquantitative and 23% nonquantitative. Adults were needed to assist children in 30% of all studies and for almost all studies of children under 9 years and some over the age of 9. Multiple food records and/or 24 h recalls were used 83% of the time as the validation standard for the FFQs. Seventy-six percent of the FFQs overestimated children's intake using nutrients or food measures.

Although the number of FFQ reliability studies has more than doubled since the last review in 2008, the conclusions do not change appreciably. Results indicate the FFQ has an acceptable reproducibility for select nutrients and foods. The studies indicate older youth had more reliable FFQ reports than younger youth. Shorter intervals between administrations of the FFQ typically resulted in higher agreement between foods or nutrients. Test–retest periods ranged from a few hours up to 1 year, with most periods just a few weeks or months.

## DIET HISTORY

Diet histories assess the past diet of an individual in the form of usual meal patterns, food intake, and food preparation practices through an extensive interview or questionnaire (Table 35.7).[39] The diet history provides a measure of usual intake appropriate for ranking individuals and predicting health outcomes. In contrast to other methods of dietary assessment, a diet history is usually more qualitative than quantitative, allowing detailed information about food preparation, eating habits, and food consumption to be collected by a highly trained interviewer. This method requires children and/or parents to recall dietary intake from the past, understand spatial relationships, be able to apply math skills, and have the stamina to complete the typical 1–2 h interview. Because of the respondent burden, diet histories are not often used to assess children's diets. This review identified two diet history validity studies and one reliability study. One validity study underestimated energy intake and the other overestimated intake. One diet history was compared to TEE and the other to a 7-day food record as the standard. More studies are needed before broad conclusions can be made about the utility of this method among children.

## OBSERVATION

Observation is useful for assessing children who are preliterate (third grade or younger), either in a lunchroom setting with school meals or in controlled school or group activities (Table 35.7). Intensively trained observers unobtrusively watch the children, sometimes many at a time, to ascertain foods, brand names, and portion sizes consumed. A single observation provides a measure of actual intake appropriate for estimating group means and cannot be used to predict health outcomes. Multiple observations can provide a measure of usual intake. Observer recordings are interpreted

after the collection process and coded to a nutrient database to calculate nutrient intake for each child. Adult observations of children have frequently been used as the standard for comparison for recalls, records, and FFQs, yet this review identified the first validity study on observation among children.[132] It has been generally accepted that observing what a child ate would be the best measure of what a child really ate. This validity study compared observer's ability to assess intake of a child using a prepared checklist as compared to a weighed food record. Observation had similar energy estimates as the standard and percent agreement of 60%. The one reliability study of paired adult observations of children eating lunch indicates high agreement of nutrient amounts.

## SUMMARY

There has been a 91% increase in the number of studies on dietary assessment methods in children in the four years since our previous review (Table 35.8). Particular emphasis is seen with validating new FFQs, checklists, and screeners and new techniques for administering 24 h recalls. There was an increase in new styles of food frequency-type questionnaires referred to as checklists and screeners. This heightened attention to dietary assessment methods resulted in the appearance of several 24 h recall validity and reliability studies, one observation, and one diet history validity study.

This review allows comparison of dietary methods to determine the most effective dietary data collection instruments to use with particular research questions.[137,138] The reader may, for example, scan each table for age-appropriate instruments with higher or lower nutrient correlations with a particular validity standard, or look for instruments that children can complete with or without adult assistance, or look for methods with no portion-size estimation, or identify instruments specific to assessing intake of food groups. Highlights of each dietary assessment method and its validity, advantages, and disadvantages for using the methods are summarized in Table 35.8.

The FFQ both under- and overestimates energy intake more than any other methodology. The addition of new studies to this review has widened the range of nutrient correlations for every dietary assessment measure. Overall, results indicate food records tend to underestimate children's energy intake less and overestimate intake more than recalls. FFQs consistently overestimate usual energy and macronutrient intake at a higher percentage than other methods. FFQs are best used for ranking children's intake. Younger children underestimate intakes more frequently than older children, and as age increases, overestimation increases.

In the 4 years since our previous literature review on dietary assessment methods for school-age children, the literature has almost doubled, but the summary results are telling us the same thing as the older studies: the current assessment methods and the standards of comparison need to be altered to increase their accuracy and repeatability. The ranges of the validity nutrient correlations and energy intake

**TABLE 35.7**
**Diet History and Observation Validity and Reliability Studies among School-Age Children**

| Validity References[a] | Sample | Age/Grade | Instrument | Response Categories (Range) | Validation Standard | Design | Results |
|---|---|---|---|---|---|---|---|
| Kremer et al.[132] | 106 m[b] and f[b] 41 m 65 f | 5–12 years Adults required[c] | Observation; 20 food and beverage categories School Food Checklist (SFC); lunch only; semiquantitative | 2 (yes/no; open-ended) | Weighed record | Compared same-day observer recorded energy intake from SFC with staff-administered WR of lunch. | Pearson correlation for energy intake between SFC and weighed record was 0.77. Mean energy intake was similar between SFC and record (2992 vs. 3008 kJ). The percentage of children classified in the same tertiles for energy was 60% and misclassification into opposite tertiles was 4%. |
| Waling et al.[133] | 85 m and f 52% m 48% f | 8.3–12.4 years | Diet history; general meal pattern and previous 2 weeks detailed; quantitative; group administered | Open-ended | Doubly labeled water; SenseWear armband | Compared energy intake from a 2-week diet history interview with TEE[a] from SenseWear armband and doubly labeled water. | Mean reported energy intake from diet history was 14% lower than TEE from SenseWear armband (9.20 vs. 10.9 mJ/day) and from doubly labeled water (9.12 vs. 10.8 mJ/day). Mean reported energy intake was 16% lower for boys and 12% lower for girls than TEE from SenseWear armband. Mean reported energy intake was 17% lower for boys and 11% lower for girls than TEE from doubly labeled water. |
| Sjöberg et al.[134] | 51 f | 15–16 years | Diet history; habitual intake; interviewer-assisted group administration and interview; quantitative | Fixed categories of frequency and amount of foods | 7-day diet record | Compared child's report of diet history of foods, nutrients, and meals against child's 7-day food record. | Spearman correlations between diet history and records were 0.63 for energy, 0.67 for protein, and 0.63 for total fat. The range of correlations for 11 nutrients assessed were 0.25 for alcohol to 0.71 for fiber. Mean daily energy intake was 3% higher in the diet history as compared to the 7-day records (8.1 vs. 7.5 mJ). Spearman correlations for 20 food groups ranged from 0.30 for buns, pastry, and biscuits to ice cream to 0.71 for sweets. |

(continued)

**TABLE 35.7 (continued)**
**Diet History and Observation Validity and Reliability Studies among School-Age Children**

| Reliability References | Sample | Age/Grade | Instrument | Design | Results |
|---|---|---|---|---|---|
| Rasane[135] | 47 m and f<br>50 m and f<br>37 m and f | 5 years<br>9 years<br>13 years<br>Adults required | Diet history; past year; interviewer administered; quantitative | Compared 7-month test–retest of nutrient intake from diet histories completed by child and parent. | Pearson correlations between the first and second interviews were 0.59 for energy, 0.60 for protein, and 0.57 for total fat. The range of correlations for 11 nutrients assessed was 0.41 for ascorbic acid to 0.60 for protein. Mean daily energy intake was 27% higher in the first diet history interview as compared to the second interview (3256 vs. 2573 kcal/day). |
| Simons-Morton et al.[136] | 45 m and f | Three to fifth grade<br>Adults required | Observation; lunch only; quantitative | Compared two simultaneously collected adult observers' estimates of nutrient intake and food items from observations of lunch. | ICCs between paired observers ranged from 0.81 to 0.90 for energy and from 0.74 to 0.88 for fat. Of the six nutrients assessed, ICCs were lowest for total fat (0.74–0.88) and highest for vitamin A (0.96–0.98). Interobserver percent differences in mean energy intake ranged from 0.1% to 6.8%. Overall agreement on food items between observers was 84%; percent agreement was highest for chips and condiments and lowest for desserts. Differences in portion-size estimates accounted for most of the energy and nutrient differences between observers. |

a   Results of subgroups not reported due to samples below the N = 30 criterion.
b   Males (m), females (f).
c   Adult assistance required for instrument administration.
d   TEE, total energy expenditure.

**TABLE 35.8**

**Summary of Dietary Assessment Methods for School-Age Children**

| Method and Number of Studies Reviewed | Ages Evaluated | Energy Validity[a] | Protein Validity[a] | Total-Fat Validity[a] | Energy Intake Compared with Standard[b] | Advantages of Method | Disadvantages of Method |
|---|---|---|---|---|---|---|---|
| *Food recall* Validity—35 Reliability—6 | 4–14 years Adult assistance needed for <16 years | 0.04–0.87 | 0.19–0.91 | 0.17–0.85 | −34% to 18% | Short administration time Defined recall time Intake can be quantified. Procedure does not alter habitual dietary patterns. Low respondent burden Can be telephone administered Procedure can be automated. | Recall depends on memory. Portion size difficult to estimate Trained interviewer required Expensive to collect and code |
| *Food record* Validity—16 Reliability—1 | 3–23 years Adult assistance needed for <12 years | 0.28–0.74 | 0.47–0.82 | 0.37–0.82 | −34% to 31% | Record not rely on memory Defined record time Intake can be quantified. Training can be group administered. Procedure can be automated. | Recorder must be literate. High respondent burden Food eaten away from home less accurately recalled Procedure alters habitual dietary patterns. Validity may decrease as recording days increase. Expensive to collect and code |
| *Food frequency* Validity—82 Reliability—50 | 2–19 years Adult assistance needed for <17 years | 0.13–0.83 | 0.05–0.77 | −0.07–0.78 | −38% to 87% | Trained interviewers not needed Interviewer or self-administered Relatively inexpensive to collect Procedure does not alter habitual dietary habits. Low respondent burden Total diet or selected foods or nutrients can be assessed. Can be used to rank according to nutrient intake Procedure can be automated. | Recall depends on memory. Period of recall imprecise Quantification of intake imprecise because of poor recall or use of standard portion sizes Specific food descriptions not obtained Food list may not represent the population's diet and lead to misclassification. |
| *Diet history* Validity—2 Reliability—1 | 8.3–16 years Adult assistance needed for all ages | 0.63 | 0.67 | 0.63 | −17% to 8% | Literacy not required Procedure does not alter habitual dietary habits. Can obtain highly detailed descriptions of foods and preparation methods | Recall depends on memory. Highly trained interviewers required Period of recall imprecise Very high respondent burden Requires long interview time Quantification of intake imprecise because of poor recall or use of standard portion sizes Expensive to administer |
| *Observation* Validity—1 Reliability—1 | 5–12 years Adult assistance needed for all ages | 0.77 | None | None | −0.53% | Literacy not required Procedure does not alter habitual dietary habits. Procedure does not rely on memory. Defined observation time Intake can be quantified. Multiple days give measure of individual or group intake. | Highly trained observers required Requires long observation period Expensive to administer |

a  Pearson and Spearman correlations of nutrients both unadjusted and adjusted for % kcal.

b  Calculation of percentage = ([instrument-validation standard]/validation standard).

comparisons to a standard are not improving from repeating the same approaches. Many of the same challenges noted in the earlier review still exist and have not been overcome. Generally, comparisons across studies were limited by differences in instruments, research design, validation standards, and populations. The paucity of data in some areas also made it difficult to draw generalized conclusions.

It is evident that many of the validation standards used in the reviewed articles are imperfect, especially for children. In this review, food records or recalls were the most common choice for validation standards, and information on the validity of these methods for children noted in the review is mixed. Observations were the most common validity standard for recall validity studies and there is only one study regarding the validity of this measure for assessing children's intake. Thus, the validation standards used may have inconsistent validity or use a referent period differing from that used for the instrument. Heterogeneity of the studies also makes it difficult to draw conclusions; the differences in study administrations and study populations often make comparisons uncertain both within a type of assessment method and between methods. For the field to advance, we must understand the validity of our standard measures among children.

In evaluating validation studies, the effect of correlated errors between the method being evaluated and the validation standard should be considered. All dietary assessment methods have inherent errors; for validation studies, it is important these errors be as independent as possible.[139] For example, if errors between the methods are similar (e.g., both methods rely on dietary information from a respondent such as FFQ and recalls), correlations between the two methods will be artificially inflated. In contrast, errors inherent in physiologic measures (e.g., doubly labeled water measurements or serum micronutrients) or observational data do not rely on information provided by respondents and would be a more independent comparison to a respondent-based measure.[140] Comparisons of physiologic endpoints, such as blood nutrient levels, to dietary assessment methods have not been widely used with school-age children and offer other problems since food intake may not be directly correlated with physiologic endpoints.

Selecting a validation standard can be a difficult task because often there is not an assessment tool available for validation with the same referent period as the dietary assessment tool. Thus, a compromise may need to be made in the study design. For example, an FFQ measures usual food consumption over a period of 6 months to a year, while a food record generally is used to measure food consumption on a day-to-day basis. In order to validate an FFQ, it would be necessary to complete several sets of food records over the referent period for the FFQ. Clearly, validation studies using a week of continuous consecutive food records may not capture seasonal variation in diet. Similarly, a food recall, which is generally used to measure one complete day of consumption, should be validated by a method assessing an entire day, not just a portion of the day.

Selection of the measure of truth for validation studies is also challenging because there is not always a good choice when the referent periods differ so markedly between instruments and the potential effect of correlated errors is considered. Physiologically based measures, such as doubly labeled water, chemical analyses of food, or serum micronutrient concentrations, represent a type of standard with considerable appeal and merit further study, since these measures are not affected by respondent error. In addition, studies that compare multiple validation standards for a particular assessment method would allow comparisons of the validation standards best suited for particular situations. Future studies need to address the timing of the referent period that best suits the assessment instrument in the design phase.

The problem of referent periods also influences the experimental design for reliability studies. Because there is much day-to-day variation in diet, readministration should be close enough in time to reflect the same referent period. Since some methods reflect diet over a short span of time (e.g., 1-day records and 24 h recalls), theoretically the reliability testing should be completed on the same day as the assessment tool, which may allow memory effects from the first assessment to bias the readministration. Studies examining reliability should alternate administrations in order to eliminate bias as much as possible. Because FFQs usually include a longer referent period, it is easier to develop reproducibility studies for this method.

The studies reviewed adapted adult dietary assessment methods for administration to a pediatric population. Specific adaptations included incorporating parental or adult assistance, adjusting portion-size information, using shorter referent times, using food pictures, using computer programs designed for children, and administering the instrument in the school setting. Children younger than 8–9 years of age need adult assistance to provide accurate dietary information for all the methods because they usually have limited reading skills and adults control most of the food offered, including the timing and frequency of eating occasions.[141,142] This review found that almost all of the validity and reliability studies among children less than 8–9 years of age, with the exception of a few of the recall and FFQ studies, included adult participation. The addition of studies from the last 4 years has not found any different results. Thus, to obtain valid reliable data, researchers need to develop approaches to assess children's diet incorporating parents into the process.

Children generally have difficulty estimating portion sizes.[57,143,144] A recent review of portion-size aids was unable to make guidelines for portion-size estimation for children or even adults.[145] Both 2D and 3D models have been used to enhance children's portion-size estimation.[5,6,14,15,36,43,120,135,136,146–148] Pictures of food and portions have been incorporated in assessments to enhance children's understanding; however, the addition of pictures did not increase accuracy among third graders.[149] Among the newer tools for dietary assessment are reference books with life-size photographs of portion sizes that have been credited as being both easy and accurate.[150–153] Training to improve portion-size estimation among children has been attempted with significant improvements in estimation; however, even with training, some errors were reported to be as high as 100%.[154] Until portion-size issues are adequately addressed, children's intakes will continue to be biased.

The dietary habits of children, especially young children who are preliterate, are inherently difficult to study. Special consideration must be given to the age and cognitive ability of the child as well as methodological issues associated with nutrient analyses, food coding, and portion sizes. Both age and cognitive ability relate to the child's understanding of the method used and the thought processes that contribute to self-reporting of food choices. Unfortunately, assessment techniques that work reasonably well among adult men and women may not be useful for youth, especially those less than 8–9 years of age, who may need assistance from a proxy or special prompting techniques to estimate portion size. Because parents/adults are often the respondents for young children, the methods used to interview them may resemble those used best with adults, while methods for the child need to be age appropriate. Creative portion-size tools must be developed to estimate children's portion sizes to enhance the quality of nutrient estimates. Systematic evaluations of children's ability to estimate portion size utilizing various approaches by age, gender, ethnicity, and body size are needed.

This review found little research on the effects of age, gender, or ethnicity. Given the multiplicity of minority groups in the United States and the rising obesity epidemic among children, it is essential to determine the accuracy of these dietary assessment tools within major subgroups. Other areas, such as the effect of body size on reporting of dietary intake, need further study. For example, a recent study suggested that children with central fat distribution had higher rates of underreporting of energy intake than lean or obese children or those with peripheral fat distribution.[43] Another study reported energy intake was significantly lower in obese children than nonobese children when compared to doubly labeled water as a percentage of energy expenditure.[155] Underreporting of dietary intake by obese adolescents is consistent with recent findings that obese adults underreport their dietary intake.[155] With the increasing prevalence of obesity among children and adolescents, it is essential to determine whether body size differences significantly affect accuracy of dietary assessment instruments.[156] Methodological studies will need to plan for adequate sample size for the weight categories for subgroup analyses.

The field of nutritional epidemiology needs to shape definitions for the checklists and screener-type questionnaires to allow a clear demarcation from the definition of an FFQ. Currently, there are short FFQs with the same number of items and frequency options as another tool that may be called a checklist or a screener. There are other FFQ-type tools with no name. To allow comparisons and consistent reporting, these definitions are essential.

In summary, it appears the work in dietary assessment methods for children has plateaued. It is time to take a step back and look carefully at what should be accomplished through future research. We are not generating new insights from the continuing validity studies of FFQ-type questionnaires. The extensive evaluation of 24 h recalls to understand the role of intrusions and exclusions is an excellent example of formative methodological research that is advancing how recalls can be used with children. Similar research is needed for every method discussed in this review.

This 42-year review serves as a guide to the status of dietary assessment methods for school-age children. The key to advancing the field is to build on our current base of methods, refine those techniques that are useful, and develop new approaches to overcome obstacles identified in their methodology for use with children of all ages. Dietary assessment is rapidly expanding into the preschool population; thus, parents must be embraced as a vital part of diet assessment in children. We must be able to accurately assess the dietary intake of children to monitor dietary intake trends, make accurate research and policy decisions, and develop and effectively evaluate nutrition interventions.

## ACKNOWLEDGMENT

The authors would like to thank Cerissa Roman, RD, MPH, and Sam Weiss for assisting with the review process.

## REFERENCES

1. McPherson, RS, Hoelscher, DM, Alexander, M et al. In: Berdanier, C eds. *Handbook of Nutrition and Food*, CRC Press, Boca Raton, FL, 2002.
2. McPherson, RS, Hoelscher, DM, Alexander, M et al. *Prev Med* 31:S11;2000.
3. Day, RS, Hoelscher, DM, Eastham, CA, Koers, EM In: Berdanier, C eds. *Handbook of Nutrition and Food*, 2nd edn., CRC Press, Boca Raton, FL, pp. 543, 2008.
4. Nelson, M, Black, AE, Morris, JA, Cole, TJ. *Am J Clin Nutr* 50:155;1989.
5. Basch, CE, Shea, S, Arliss, R et al. *Am J Public Health* 80:1314;1990.
6. Eck, LH, Klesges, RC, Hanson, CL. *J Am Diet Assoc* 89:784;1989.
7. Fisher, JO, Johnson, RK, Lindquist, C et al. *Obes Res* 8:597;2000.
8. Montgomery, C, Reilly, JJ, Jackson, DM et al. *Am J Clin Nutr* 80:591;2004.
9. Warren, JM, Henry, CJ, Livingstone, MB et al. *Public Health Nutr* 6:41;2003.
10. Baxter, SD, Thompson, WO, Davis, HC. *J Am Diet Assoc* 100:911;2000.
11. Lindquist, CH, Cummings, T, Goran, MI. *Obes Res* 8:2;2000.
12. Reynolds, LA, Johnson, SB, Silverstein, J. *J Pediatr Psychol* 15:493;1990.
13. Edmunds, LD, Ziebland, S. *Health Educ Res* 17:211;2002.
14. Lytle, LA, Nichaman, MZ, Obarzanek, E et al. *J Am Diet Assoc* 93:1431;1993.
15. Van Horn, LV, Gernhofer, N, Moag-Stahlberg, A et al. *J Am Diet Assoc* 90:412;1990.
16. Weber, JL, Lytle, L, Gittelsohn, J et al. *J Am Diet Assoc* 104:746;2004.

17. Todd, KS, Kretsch, MJ. *Nutr Res* 6:1031;1986.
18. Samuelson, G. *Nutr Metab* 12:321;1970.
19. Baxter, SD, Guinn, CH, Royer, JA et al. *J Am Diet Assoc* 110:1178;2010.
20. Baxter, SD, Hardin, JW, Guinn, CH et al. *J Am Diet Assoc* 109:846;2009.
21. Baxter, SD, Guinn, CH, Royer, JA et al. *Eur J Clin Nutr* 63:1394;2009.
22. Harrington, KF, Kohler, CL, McClure, LA, Franklin, FA. *J Am Diet Assoc* 109:36;2009.
23. Baxter, SD, Thompson, WO, Litaker, MS et al. *J Am Diet Assoc* 102:386;2002.
24. Baxter, SD, Royer, JA, Hardin, JW et al. *J Nutr Educ Behav* 39:126;2007.
25. Baxter, SD, Smith, AF, Hardin, JW, Nichols, MD. *Prev Med* 44:34;2007.
26. Baxter, SD, Smith, AF, Hardin, JW, Nichols, MD. *J Am Diet Assoc* 107:595;2007.
27. Baxter, SD, Thompson, WO, Litaker, MS et al. *J Nutr Educ Behav* 35:124;2003.
28. Baxter, SD, Thompson, WO, Davis, HC, Johnson, MH. *J Am Diet Assoc* 97:1293;1997.
29. Lytle, LA, Murray, DM, Perry, CL, Eldridge, AL. *J Am Diet Assoc* 98:570;1998.
30. Moore, GF, Tapper, K, Murphy, S et al. *Eur J Clin Nutr* 61:420;2007.
31. Moore, L, Tapper, K, Dennehy, A, Cooper, A. *Eur J Clin Nutr* 59:809;2005.
32. Baranowski, T, Islam, N, Baranowski, J et al. *J Am Diet Assoc* 102:380;2002.
33. Andersen, LF, Lande, B, Trygg, K, Hay, G. *Public Health Nutr* 7:757;2004.
34. Hanning, RM, Royall, D, Toews, JE et al. *Can J Diet Pract Res* 70:172;2009.
35. Johnson, B, Hackett, A, Roundfield, M, Coufopoulos, A. *J Hum Nutr Diet* 14:457;2001.
36. Mullenbach, V, Kushi, LH, Jacobson, C et al. *J Am Diet Assoc* 92:743;1992.
37. Vereecken, CA, Covents, M, Matthys, C, Maes, L. *Eur J Clin Nutr* 59:658;2005.
38. Rankin, D, Ellis, SM, Macintyre, UE et al. *Eur J Clin Nutr* 65:910;2011.
39. Thompson, FE, Byers, T. *J Nutr* 124:2245S;1994.
40. O'Connor, J, Ball, EJ, Steinbeck, KS et al. *Am J Clin Nutr* 74:643;2001.
41. Bokhof, B, Gunther, AL, Berg-Beckhoff, G et al. *Public Health Nutr* 13:826;2010.
42. Lambert, N, Plumb, J, Looise, B et al. *J Hum Nutr Diet* 18:243;2005.
43. Knuiman, JT, Rasanen, L, Ahola, M et al. *J Am Diet Assoc* 87:303;1987.
44. Bandini, LG, Cyr, H, Must, A, Dietz, WH. *Am J Clin Nutr* 65:1138S;1997.
45. Lillegaard, IT, Loken, EB, Andersen, LF. *Eur J Clin Nutr* 61:61;2007.
46. Lillegaard, IT, Andersen, LF. *Br J Nutr* 94:998;2005.
47. Champagne, CM, Baker, NB, DeLany, JP et al. *J Am Diet Assoc* 98:426;1998.
48. Di Noia, J, Contento, IR. *Public Health Nutr* 12:3;2009.
49. Livingstone, MB, Prentice, AM, Coward, WA et al. *Am J Clin Nutr* 56:29;1992.
50. Andersen, LF, Pollestad, ML, Jacobs, DR, Jr. et al. *Public Health Nutr* 8:1315;2005.
51. Green, TJ, Allen, OB, O'Connor, DL. *J Nutr* 128:1665;1998.
52. Martin, CK, Newton, RL, Jr, Anton, SD et al. *Eat Behav* 8:148;2007.
53. Blom, L, Lundmark, K, Dahlquist, G, Persson, LA. *Acta Paediatr Scand* 78:858;1989.
54. Taylor, RW, Goulding, A. *Eur J Clin Nutr* 52:464;1998.
55. Cade, JE, Frear, L, Greenwood, DC. *Public Health Nutr* 9:501;2006.
56. Kobayashi, T, Kamimura, M, Imai, S et al. *Nutr J* 10:27;2011.
57. Kaskoun, MC, Johnson, RK, Goran, MI. *Am J Clin Nutr* 60:43;1994.
58. Persson, LA, Carlgren, G. *Int J Epidemiol* 13:506;1984.
59. Wilson, AM, Lewis, RD. *J Am Diet Assoc* 104:373;2004.
60. Hammond, J, Nelson, M, Chinn, S, Rona, RJ. *Eur J Clin Nutr* 47:242;1993.
61. Burrows, TL, Warren, JM, Colyvas, K et al. *Obesity* 17:162;2009.
62. Byers, T, Trieber, F, Gunter, E et al. *Epidemiology* 4:350;1993.
63. Marcotte, L, Hennessy, E, Dwyer, J et al. *Public Health Nutr* 11:57;2008.
64. Muckelbauer, R, Libuda, L, Kersting, M. *Public Health Nutr* 13:187;2010.
65. Zemel, BS, Carey, LB, Paulhamus, DR et al. *Am J Hum Biol* 22:180;2010.
66. Arnold, JE, Rohan, T, Howe, G, Leblanc, M. *Ann Epidemiol* 5:369;1995.
67. Marshall, TA, Eichenberger Gilmore, JM, Broffitt, B et al. *J Am Diet Assoc* 108:465;2008.
68. Baranowski, T, Smith, M, Baranowski, J et al. *J Am Diet Assoc* 97:66;1997.
69. Bellu, R, Riva, E, Ortisi, MT et al. *Nutr Res* 16:197;1996.
70. Mariscal-Arcas, M, Velasco, J, Monteagudo, C et al. *Nutr Hosp* 25:1006;2010.
71. Perks, SM, Roemmich, JN, Sandow-Pajewski, M et al. *Am J Clin Nutr* 72:1455;2000.
72. Stiegler, P, Sausenthaler, S, Buyken, AE et al. *Public Health Nutr* 13:38;2010.
73. Thiagarajah, K, Fly, AD, Hoelscher, DM et al. *J Nutr Educ Behav* 40:305;2008.
74. Wallen, V, Cunningham-Sabo, L, Auld, G, Romaniello, C. *J Nutr Educ Behav* 43:50;2011.
75. Domel, SB, Baranowski, T, Davis, H et al. *J Am Coll Nutr* 13:33;1994.
76. Moore, M, Braid, S, Falk, B, Klentrou, P. *Nutr J* 6:24;2007.
77. Bellu, R, Ortisi, MT, Riva, E et al. *Nutr Res* 15:1121;1995.
78. Field, AE, Peterson, KE, Gortmaker, SL et al. *Public Health Nutr* 2:293;1999.
79. Watson, JF, Collins, CE, Sibbritt, DW et al. *Int J Behav Nutr Phys Act* 6:62;2009.
80. Rockett, HR, Berkey, CS, Colditz, GA. *Int J Pediatr Obesity* 2:31;2007.
81. Rockett, HR, Breitenbach, M, Frazier, AL et al. *Prev Med* 26:808;1997.
82. Preston, AM, Palacios, C, Rodriguez, CA, Velez-Rodriguez, RM. *P R Health Sci J* 30:58;2011.
83. Roumelioti, M, Leotsinidis, M. *Nutr J* 8:8;2009.
84. Wilson, AM, Magarey, AM, Mastersson, N. *Int J Behav Nutr Phys Act* 5:5;2008.
85. Vereecken, CA, Maes, L. *Public Health Nutr* 6:581;2003.
86. Di Noia, J, Contento, IR. *J Am Diet Assoc* 109:1785;2009.
87. Koehler, KM, Cunningham-Sabo, L, Lambert, LC et al. *J Am Diet Assoc* 100:205;2000.
88. Magkos, F, Manios, Y, Babaroutsi, E, Sidossis, LS. *J Hum Nutr Diet* 19:331;2006.

89. Cullen, KW, Watson, K, Zakeri, I. *J Am Diet Assoc* 108:862;2008.
90. Yang, YJ, Martin, BR, Boushey, CJ. *J Am Diet Assoc* 110:111;2010.
91. Haraldsdottir, J, Thorsdottir, I, de Almeida, MD et al. *Ann Nutr Metab* 49:221;2005.
92. Jenner, DA, Neylon, K, Croft, S et al. *Eur J Clin Nutr* 43:663;1989.
93. Johnson, F, Wardle, J, Griffith, J. *Eur J Clin Nutr* 56:644;2002.
94. Lietz, G, Barton, KL, Longbottom, PJ, Anderson, AS. *Public Health Nutr* 5:783;2002.
95. Harnack, LJ, Lytle, LA, Story, M et al. *J Am Diet Assoc* 106:1790;2006.
96. Yaroch, AL, Resnicow, K, Petty, AD, Khan, LK. *J Am Diet Assoc* 100:1525;2000.
97. Wong, SS, Boushey, CJ, Novotny, R, Gustafson, DR. *J Am Diet Assoc* 108:539;2008.
98. Nelson, MC, Lytle, LA. *J Am Diet Assoc* 109:730;2009.
99. Prochaska, JJ, Sallis, JF. *J Adoles Health* 34:163;2004.
100. Watanabe, M, Yamaoka, K, Yokotsuka, M et al. *Public Health Nutr* 14:297;2011.
101. Neuhouser, ML, Lilley, S, Lund, A, Johnson, DB. *J Am Diet Assoc* 109:1587;2009.
102. Smith, KW, Hoelscher, DM, Lytle, LA et al. *J Am Diet Assoc* 101:635;2001.
103. Cullen, KW, Zakeri, I. *J Am Diet Assoc* 104:1415;2004.
104. Truthmann, J, Mensink, GB, Richter, A. *Nutr J* 10:133;2011.
105. Taylor, C, Lamparello, B, Kruczek, K et al. *J Am Diet Assoc* 109:479;2009.
106. Matthys, C, Pynaert, I, De Keyzer, W, De Henauw, S. *J Am Diet Assoc* 107:605;2007.
107. Prochaska, JJ, Sallis, JF, Rupp, J. *Prev Med* 33:699;2001.
108. Van Assema, P, Brug, J, Ronda, G et al. *Nutr Health* 16:85;2002.
109. Hoelscher, DM, Day, RS, Kelder, SH, Ward, JL. *J Am Diet Assoc* 103:186;2003.
110. Vereecken, CA, De Bourdeaudhuij, I, Maes, L. *Eur J Clin Nutr* 64:541;2010.
111. Kinlay, S, Heller, RF, Halliday, JA. *Prev Med* 20:378;1991.
112. Li, L, Levy-Milne, R. *Can J Diet Pract Res* 69:213;2008.
113. Ambrosini, GL, O'Sullivan, TA, de Klerk, NH et al. *Br J Nutr* 105:625;2011.
114. Ambrosini, GL, de Klerk, NH, O'Sullivan, TA et al. *Eur J Clin Nutr* 63:1251;2009.
115. Davis, JN, Nelson, MC, Ventura, EE et al. *J Am Diet Assoc* 109:725;2009.
116. Field, AE, Colditz, GA, Fox, MK et al. *Am J Public Health* 88:1216;1998.
117. Papadopoulou, SK, Barboukis, V, Dalkiranis, A et al. *Int J Food Sci Nutr* 59:148;2008.
118. Andersen, LF, Nes, M, Lillegaard, IT et al. *Eur J Clin Nutr* 49:543;1995.
119. Lanfer, A, Hebestreit, A, Ahrens, W et al. *Int J Obes* 35:S61;2011.
120. Basch, CE, Shea, S, Zybert, P. *Am J Public Health* 84:861;1994.
121. Metcalf, PA, Scragg, RK, Sharpe, S et al. *Eur J Clin Nutr* 57:1498;2003.
122. de Assis, MA, Kupek, E, Guimaraes, D et al. *Appetite* 51:187;2008.
123. Garcia-Dominic, O, Trevino, RP, Echon, RM et al. *Health Promot Pract* 2011,
124. Tak, NI, te Velde, SJ, de Vries, JH, Brug, J. *J Hum Nutr Diet* 19:275;2006.
125. Lee, S, Ahn, HS. *Nutr Res Pract* 1:313;2007.
126. Penkilo, M, George, GC, Hoelscher, DM. *J Nutr Educ Behav* 40:20;2008.
127. Rockett, HR, Wolf, AM, Colditz, GA. *J Am Diet Assoc* 95:336;1995.
128. Buzzard, IM, Stanton, CA, Figueiredo, M et al. *J Am Diet Assoc* 101:1438;2001.
129. Speck, BJ, Bradley, CB, Harrell, JS, Belyea, MJ. *J Adolesc Health* 28:16;2001.
130. Frank, GC, Nicklas, TA, Webber, LS et al. *J Am Diet Assoc* 92:313;1992.
131. Turconi, G, Celsa, M, Rezzani, C et al. *Eur J Clin Nutr* 57:753;2003.
132. Kremer, PJ, Bell, AC, Swinburn, BA. *Asia Pac J Clin Nutr* 15:465;2006.
133. Waling, MU, Larsson, CL. *J Nutr* 139:522;2009.
134. Sjoberg, A, Hulthen, L. *Eur J Clin Nutr* 58:1181;2004.
135. Rasanen, L. *Am J Clin Nutr* 32:2560;1979.
136. Simons-Morton, BG, Forthofer, R, Huang, IW et al. *J Am Diet Assoc* 92:219;1992.
137. Cullen, KW, Baranowski, T, Baranowski, J et al. *J Am Diet Assoc* 99:849;1999.
138. Eldridge, AL, Smith-Warner, SA, Lytle, LA, Murray, DM. *J Am Diet Assoc* 98:777;1998.
139. Willett W. 2nd edn. *Nutritional Epidemiology*, Oxford University Press, New York, 1998.
140. Bingham, SA. *Am J Clin Nutr* 59:227S;1994.
141. Frank, GC. *Am J Clin Nutr* 59:207S;1994.
142. Baranowski, T, Hearn, MD. In: Gochman, DS eds. *Handbook of Health Behavior Research I: Personal and Social Determinants*, 1st edn. Plenum Press, New York, pp. 303, 1997.
143. Buzzard, IM, Sievert, YA. *Am J Clin Nutr* 59:275S;1994.
144. Contento, IR, Balch, GI, Bronner, YL et al. *J Nutr Educ* 27:279;1995.
145. Cypel, YS, Guenther, PM. *J Am Diet Assoc* 97:289;1997.
146. Crawford, PB, Obarzanek, E, Morrison, J, Sabry, ZI. *J Am Diet Assoc* 94:626;1994.
147. Frank, GC, Berenson, GS, Schilling, PE, Moore, MC. *J Am Diet Assoc* 71:26;1977.
148. McPherson, RS, Nichaman, MZ, Kohl, HW et al. *Pediatrics* 86:520;1990.
149. Baranowski, T, Dworkin, R, Henske, JC et al. *J Am Diet Assoc* 86:1381;1986.
150. Nelson, M, Atkinson, M, Darbyshire, S. *Br J Nutr* 72:649;1994.
151. Nelson, M, Atkinson, M, Darbyshire, S. *Br J Nutr* 76:31;1996.
152. Faggiano, F, Vineis, P, Cravanzola, D et al. *Epidemiology* 3:379;1992.
153. Hess, MA. *Portion Photos of Popular Foods*, The American Dietetic Association, Chicago, IL, 1997.
154. Weber, JL, Cunningham-Sabo, L, Skipper, B et al. *Am J Clin Nutr* 69:782S;1999.
155. Bandini, LG, Schoeller, DA, Cyr, HN, Dietz, WH. *Am J Clin Nutr* 52:421;1990.
156. Goran, MI. *Pediatrics* 101:505;1998.

# 36 Anthropometric Assessment
## Stature, Weight, and Body Mass Index (Adults)

*Stefan A. Czerwinski, Wm. Cameron Chumlea, and Michael J. LaMonte*

## CONTENTS

## INTRODUCTION

Direct anthropometric measurements and derived indices describe body size, shape, and composition. They infer information about the body at the tissue level, and they are affected by and reflect changes due to aging and disease. Weight is a limited indicator, because it is related to stature, for example, on average, tall people are heavier than short people. This limitation is reduced in weight divided by stature indices, such as the body mass index or BMI. Stature and weight are covariates in statistical models of body composition[1] and BMI values are associated with morbidity and mortality.[2] Standardized anthropometric techniques are required to compare clinical and research data, and text and video media describing these techniques are available.[3,4] Individuals needing to use anthropometric methods and equipment should consult these available resources for additional information.

## KEY MEASUREMENTS

### STATURE

Stature describes general body size and length, and variation in stature from the normal range can be associated with disease. Measuring stature is useful in screening for osteoporosis, among the elderly experiencing bone loss, and in interpreting body weight. Stature is easily measured with a variety of fixed or portable commercially available stadiometers. There are also methods of predicting stature when it cannot be measured, such as in disabled persons or in those with mobility impairments.[5,6] In some instances, recumbent length can be substituted, but an adjustment of 1.5 cm is subtracted to account for the systematic differences between it and stature. Reference data for stature are available from the Centers for Disease Control and Prevention, National Center for Health Statistics (CDC/NCHS) (http://www.cdc.gov/nchs), and from the World Health Organization (WHO) (http://www.who.int/research/en).

### Measurement Technique

Measurement of stature requires a vertical surface with an attached metric rule, and a horizontal headboard attached to the vertical surface, that is brought into contact with the most superior point on the head. The subject is barefoot or wears thin socks, and little clothing, so that the position of the body is clear. The subject stands upright without assistance, with heels close together, legs straight, arms at the sides, and shoulders relaxed. The subject stands erect facing away from the vertical portion of the stadiometer. The buttocks, shoulders, and head are positioned in contact with the vertical portion of the stadiometer, and the heels are placed together, so that the subject stands straight when viewed from the side. It may not be possible for some subjects to place their buttocks, shoulders and head against the stadiometer due to adipose tissue on the buttocks. These subjects are positioned with only the buttocks in contact with the vertical portion of the stadiometer, and the body is positioned vertically above and below the waist, so that the subject stands straight when viewed from the side. The head is positioned vertically from left to right with the subject looking straight ahead, and the head is positioned horizontally, so that a line from the lower margin of the bony socket containing the eye and the opening of the external ear is parallel to the floor. The subject inhales deeply and stands fully erect, and the horizontal measuring piece is lowered to make contact with the top of the head. Hair ornaments, buns, braids, etc., are removed as necessary to obtain an accurate measurement. The measurer's eyes should be level with the headpiece to avoid reading errors due to parallax. The subject's stature is recorded to the nearest 0.1 cm. Mean inter-measurer differences range from 1.4 (SD = 1.5 mm) to 2.1 mm (SD = 2.1 mm) for adults between 20 and 85 years of age.[3]

## WEIGHT

Weight is an overall composite measure of total body size and composition, and changes in weight reflect corresponding changes in body water, and fat and lean tissues. A weight change with or without the presence of chronic disease is a possible indicator of potential health problems. Weight tends to increase through middle age due to increased fatness; thus, it is the obvious measure of overweight and obesity, as most adults with high body weights tend to have high amounts of body fat. However, this is not always true, as in the case of athletes who can have high body weights due to increased bone and skeletal muscle mass, rather than high amounts of fat, or in elderly persons with sarcopenic obesity in which stable or even low body weights occur with increased percent body fatness.[7] Reference data for weight are available from CDC/NCHS (http://www.cdc.gov/nchs) and from the WHO (http://www.who.int/research/en/).

### Measurement Technique

Weight is the most commonly recorded anthropometric variable, and generally it is measured accurately. Weight is measured using a beam scale or a calibrated digital scale that must be level and resting on a hard or firm surface. The subject stands in the middle of the scale platform with head and eyes looking straight ahead. Light indoor clothing can be worn, excluding shoes, dresses, long trousers, and sweaters, but it is best to standardize the clothing, for example, with a disposable paper gown. It is not necessary to subtract the weight of the paper gown from the observed weight. In studies to assess short-term changes, weights must be recorded at standardized times, but this is not necessary for a single measurement. Weight is recorded to the nearest 100 g, and mean inter-measurer differences are 1.5 g (SD = 3.6 g) and

inter-measurer and intra-measurer technical errors are about 1.2 kg, for pairs of measurements made 2 weeks apart.[3]

Handicapped subjects, those with amputations and mobility impairments, can be weighed using a chair scale or bed scale. Scales that can be moved from one location to another are useful, but they should be calibrated each time they are moved.

## BMI

Weight is related to stature, in that a weight of 100 kg has a completely different meaning if it is associated with a stature of 150 cm compared to 190 cm, as are the corresponding associations with body fatness. An index of weight, independent of stature, provides a better descriptor of body fatness than weight alone. The BMI is weight (kg) divided by stature (m) squared, and Lambert Adolf Jacques Quetelet developed this concept in 1835.[8] In the middle of the twentieth century, several indices were proposed that attempted to reduce the association of weight with stature, by calculating weight divided by stature raised to a power of one-third or greater. The BMI has been compared against several of these indices by Keys et al., Benn, and many others.[9–13] The current consensus is that there is little if any significant improvement or utility of these other weight-for-stature indices over that of BMI in describing associations with body fatness. Additional advantages of BMI over other indices are the availability of extensive national reference data worldwide for it, its established relationships with levels of body composition, and its strong association with the risk of developing chronic diseases and with premature mortality.[14] Reference data for BMI are available from the CDC/NCHS (http://www.cdc.gov/nchs) and from the WHO (http://www.who.int/en).

### Measurement Technique

BMI includes measures of stature and weight that are recorded accurately in metric units or converted from English values to kilograms and meters or centimeters. BMI is calculated easily with a calculator or from one of many websites that perform this task, using either English or metric measurement values.

### BMI, Race, and Ethnicity

Race and ethnic variations in BMI and body composition are associated with differences in socioeconomic status, diet, health-care utilization, and degrees of genetic admixture within and between countries.[12,15] For example, African-American and Hispanic women tend to have higher mean levels of BMI and body fatness than non-Hispanic white women. Compared with African-American and non-Hispanic white men, Hispanic men tend to have higher mean levels of body fat, but not BMI.[16] Race and age-specific reference data for BMI in the U.S. population are available from the CDC/NCHS (http://www.cdc.gov/nchs).

### BMI, Weight, and Obesity

Weight and BMI are used to screen for and monitor the effectiveness of treatment of overweight and obesity, but both

## TABLE 36.1
## BMI Value Ranges, Health Classifications, and Comorbidity Risk

| BMI Ranges | Health Classification | Risk of Comorbidity |
|---|---|---|
| ≤18.5 | Possible wasting | Increased |
| 18.5–24.9 | Normal | Average |
| 25–29.9 | Overweight | Increased |
| 30.0–34.9 | Obese class I | Moderate |
| 35–39.9 | Obese class II | Severe |
| ≥40 | Obese class III | Very severe |

measurements are imperfect tools for evaluating fatness. A weight change of 3.5 kg is necessary to produce a one unit change in BMI. Body builders, wrestlers, and athletes can have high weight and BMI values due to high levels of muscularity, rather than high body fatness. Conversely, in the elderly, BMI and weight may be normal or even low, in spite of a high level of relative body fatness due to declines in stature, bone mass, and fat-free mass with age.[17] Correlations between BMI values and standardized measures of body fat range from <0.1 to >0.8 depending on the initial percentage of body fatness, levels of physical activity, and fitness, gender, race, and age, that is, a BMI of 28 does not have the same meaning in relation to body fatness in all adults, but must be used in context with other related factors.[18] On an individual basis, weight and BMI can be of limited value, but for the "average" adult, they are both useful and important screening tools.

The WHO categorizes grades of BMI values in relation to health risk, primarily its association with obesity (Table 36.1). Adults with BMI levels below 18 and above 25 have higher risks for health problems than adults with BMI levels from 18 to 25. A BMI of 30 or greater defines obesity. Obesity is further categorized into three classes of severity (Table 36.1). Based upon these criteria, the prevalence of obesity is 20%–30% for non-Hispanic white, non-Hispanic black, and Mexican-American men; 25%–40% for non-Hispanic white and Mexican-American women; and as high as 46%–53% for non-Hispanic black women. The prevalence of BMI-defined overweight in each of these groups is even higher.[2] Similar health associations and prevalence of overweight and obesity exists for adult populations in Europe and among urban areas of Mexico, the Middle East, India, and China.[19–22]

### BMI and Central Obesity

Obese adults typically also have increased amounts of intra-abdominal fat, which is not directly assessed by BMI. A measure of abdominal circumference is a valuable addition in assessing weight-related health risk. The ratio of abdominal circumference (sometimes incorrectly referred to as "waist" circumference) to the hip circumference has also been used to describe central adipose tissue distribution or fat patterning,[23,24] but is only moderately correlated with intra-abdominal adipose tissue. Thus, abdominal circumference is now the reference measure used to screen for

and assess health risks due to intra-abdominal fatness.[25–29] Abdominal circumference thresholds are used to define components of the metabolic syndrome, a cluster of interrelated risk factors that when present, significantly increase the risk of CVD events and type 2 diabetes.[30,31] The relationship of abdominal circumference with total body fatness and mortality risk is affected by age, sex, and fitness levels.[32–34] Cut points for abdominal circumference associated with BMI have been established, according to the risk for developing chronic diseases, particularly type 2 diabetes and mortality.[19,35] Abdominal circumference cut points are reported to be independent of BMI.[36–38] Thus, their recommended clinical application is to refine BMI-defined assessment of health risk.[39,40] Abdominal circumference is potentially of greater clinical utility than BMI in describing obesity by providing additional information regarding central adiposity,[41] but its utility is not universally recommended.[42] Because a large abdomen can also be a thick abdomen, measurements such as the sagittal diameter or trunk depth may provide a better indicator of abdominal obesity.[43] Unfortunately, attempts at standardizing this measurement have been inconsistent, and little reference data are available.[25]

### BMI, Morbidity, and Mortality

As a result of the WHO classification of BMI values and their relation to increasing risk of developing chronic diseases and premature mortality, BMI is commonly used in epidemiological studies of adults.[22,44] BMI values of 18 and less are potential indicators of possible wasting conditions, such as malnutrition, tuberculosis, depression, chronic obstructive pulmonary disease, and lung and stomach cancer. The morbidities associated with BMI values of 30 and higher include impaired mobility, compromised cardiovascular and pulmonary function, sleep apnea, increased prevalence and incidence of cerebrovascular and cardiovascular disease (CVD), diabetes, a number of specific cancers, and a high prevalence of chronic disease risk factors, including impaired glucose intolerance, dyslipidemia, and hypertension, and a high risk for continued obesity, chronic disease, and hospitalization.[19,39,45] Further, risks for many clinical outcomes rapidly increase at BMI values greater than 35. The descriptive utility of BMI depends, in part, on its positive association with overall levels of body fatness,[9,46,47] but this association and BMI's correlation with risk of disease deteriorates with age, sex, and ethnicity.[18,36,48–50]

The relationship between BMI and total and cause-specific mortality in adults is characterized as linear in some studies but curvilinear in others.[2,22,39,51,52] The patterns of association between BMI and mortality also vary by age, sex, race–ethnicity, smoking status, and cause of death.[18,36,39,48–50] The association between BMI and mortality varies within population subgroups in the United States.[53] When adjusted for poverty, smoking, and elevated blood pressure, a high BMI is associated with a slightly increased mortality risk in white men, but not in white women. By contrast, in the Framingham Heart Study, the relationship of BMI with mortality was positive in nonsmoking men and women over

65 years of age.[54] However, adults with BMI levels above the 70th percentile (28.5 for men; 28.7 for women) had lower survival than those with moderate BMI levels. Underlying these population differences in the BMI–mortality relationship are, in part, the previously mentioned differences in the relationship between BMI and levels of body fat among population subgroups.[9,46,47,55] There are major challenges to disentangling the complex multifactorial etiology of obesity and health outcomes, and limited epidemiological information is available regarding the concurrent links among BMI, body fatness, central fat distribution, and subsequent mortality.[32,56,57]

In many, but not all, studies, the strength of association between mortality and BMI and body composition is reduced when physical activity or cardiorespiratory fitness is a covariate.[32,58–62] These relationships are illustrated in Figures 36.1 and 36.2 in data on 21,925 men aged 30–83 years whose percent body fat and cardiorespiratory fitness were measured at baseline and who were followed for an average of 8 years for total and CVD mortality.[32] In Figure 36.1, a curvilinear J-shaped association is seen between increments of body fat and all-cause mortality, much like that noted with BMI, but a linear relationship occurred between body fat and CVD mortality. Next, the men were grouped into categories of fit (upper 80% of exercise duration) and unfit based on duration of a symptom-limited maximal treadmill exercise test, and mortality rates were cross-tabulated on body fat and fitness levels. In each incremental category, fit men had a lower rate of total and CVD mortality than unfit men (Figure 36.2). In fact, men in the highest category of fatness who were fit had lower death rates than their unfit lean counterparts. As the U.S. population ages, and as the prevalence of BMI-defined obesity and of abdominal obesity continues to increase, the role of physical activity and fitness in ameliorating some of the adverse health risk associated with excessive adiposity is of high public health significance. Recent national surveillance reports from NHANES (1999–2010) indicate that among U.S. adults ≥60 years in all race–ethnic groups combined, the prevalence of overall obesity (BMI ≥ 30) is 36% in men and 42% in women,[63]

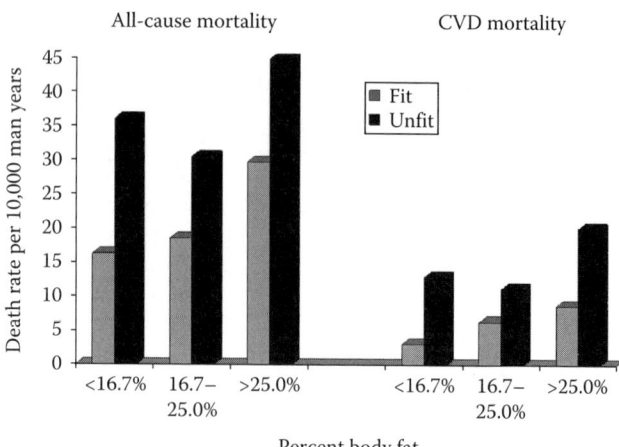

FIGURE 36.2 Rates of all-cause and CVD mortality according to levels of cardiorespiratory fitness and percent body fat in 21,925 men in the Aerobics Center Longitudinal Study—1971–1989. The number of deaths for each bar from left to right was 68, 14, 127, 60, 65, and 94 for all-cause mortality, and was 13, 5, 43, 22, 19, and 42 for CVD mortality.

whereas the prevalence of abdominal obesity (abdominal circumference: >88 cm women, >102 cm men) was 60% in men and 73% in women.[64] The mortality benefit of higher fitness among older adults with obesity has recently been shown in a follow-up on 2603 adults 60 years and older who completed symptom-limited treadmill exercise testing and extensive assessment of body size and adiposity.[65] When fitness and abdominal circumference were considered simultaneously and adjusting for age and sex, rates (per 1000 person years) of all-cause mortality were significantly lower in fit adults compared to their unfit peers in those with abdominal obesity (death rates: fit, 6.2; unfit, 13.5) and without abdominal obesity (death rates: fit, 5.1; unfit, 14.5). In fact, the death rate in older adults with abdominal obesity who were fit was lower than the death rate among those without abdominal obesity who were unfit. Similar patterns were seen when BMI and percent body fat from hydrodensitometry or skinfolds were analyzed. Another particularly intriguing observation pertaining to the importance of skeletal muscle fitness to longevity in older adults comes from the Health ABC Study in which 2292 adults 70–79 years were followed for mortality after having completed assessments on physical activity habits, muscular strength, and body size and composition.[66] The multivariable-adjusted relative risk of mortality was 32% (p < 0.05) lower with each 1 SD unit higher quadriceps muscle strength (assessed by isokinetic dynamometry), even after adjustment for chronic disease status, systemic inflammation, aerobic physical activity habits, and both body composition (by DXA) and quadriceps cross-sectional area. These findings suggest two important implications among older adults prone to sarcopenic obesity. First, muscle quality may be more influential than muscle size on healthy aging. Second, skeletal muscle function may confer important metabolic and prognostic benefit, especially in older adults, through pathways that are related to, but separate from, aerobic activity and fitness.[67]

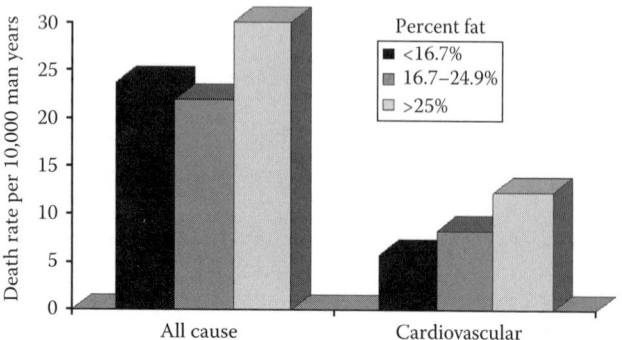

FIGURE 36.1 All-cause and CVD death rates by levels of percent body fat in 21,925 men in the Aerobics Center Longitudinal Study—1971–1989. The number of deaths in each incremental level of body fat was 82, 187, and 159 for all-cause mortality, and was 18, 65, and 61 for CVD mortality.

Physical inactivity can be an antecedent or a consequence of obesity,[68,69] but it is difficult to know how much of the increased morbidity and mortality associated with high BMI results from excessive body fat, from physical inactivity, or from both. Data from exercise intervention studies have shown that increases in physical activity result in weight loss and changes in body composition and fat distribution.[70–72] Higher levels of physical activity and fitness are also associated with favorable chronic disease risk factor profiles in men and women,[73–76] and several studies report an inverse association between physical activity or fitness exposures and the occurrence of nonfatal diseases such as hypertension,[77–82] type II diabetes,[82–90] metabolic syndrome,[82,91] myocardial infarction,[92,93] stroke,[93,94] and certain cancers.[95–97] Several studies have also demonstrated a strong, graded, and inverse association between physical activity or fitness exposures and mortality.[94,98–100] This pattern of association is generally consistent in all adults and is independent of conventional risk factors including body weight and BMI.[99,101] Three expert panels concluded that low levels of physical activity and fitness are likely to be causal factors in the development of overweight and obesity and that improvements in physical activity and fitness levels will result in favorable changes in chronic disease risk factors and lower risk of morbidity and mortality in the normal weight and overweight alike.[102–104] This position on obtaining broad health benefits through moderate amounts and intensities of regular aerobic physical activity and resistance exercises (e.g., 30 min of brisk walking daily), in adults across a wide range in body weight and BMI, is emphasized in the seminal 2008 federal guidelines on physical activity for Americans.[105]

## BMI Paradox

Several studies have shown a U-shaped relationship of BMI with all-cause mortality, characterized by increased risk among adults with a BMI < 18.5, little or no risk observed across BMI levels between 18.5 and 30, and increasingly pronounced mortality risk beyond a BMI of 30.[19,22,39] This U-shaped relationship is associated with an age-related paradox. Between about 40 and 60 years of age, both low and high BMI are associated with increased mortality risk. However, after about 70 years of age, only low BMI is associated with a higher mortality, whereas little if any excess mortality is seen at high BMI levels,[106] although high levels of BMI are reported to be related to increased risk of hospitalization and all-cause mortality by others.[45] This has been interpreted to indicate that a moderate weight gain in later years might be beneficial to health.[2,107] However, there is no clear description of a favorable association between changes in weight or BMI status and the occurrence or severity of disease across the middle and later years of life. A key to clarifying this paradox requires a more thorough evaluation of the purported link between changes in weight from middle to old age and subsequent health status. Age-related weight loss associated with worsening health conditions typically occurs in those persons who have the greatest weight between 40 and 60 years of age, but if health is maintained during aging, then a low body weight often is not an important risk factor.[106] Some important issues must be considered in regard to existing information on this paradox. Most analyses associated with the BMI–mortality paradox are limited to individuals less than 70 years of age, and little is known about this issue among persons of more advanced ages.[106] Unfortunately, data on body weight are often self-reported, which can lead to misclassification of initial weight status as well as erroneous tracking of weight changes.[108] Thus, the underlying changes in body composition (e.g., fat and lean mass) that are associated with the patterns of change in weight from middle to old age cannot be quantified. Therefore, the interaction of changes in weight and body composition with health conditions remains largely unknown. However, a recent follow-up study of women and men in the NHANES I and II cohorts found a U-shaped relationship between baseline BMI and all-cause mortality, fat-free mass had a monotonically inverse relationship with mortality, and fat mass had a monotonically positive relationship with mortality.[109] This study demonstrates that because BMI is not able to discriminate fat mass from lean tissue, it might obscure important underlying mechanisms linking body composition with disease that could be detected with additional measures of fat distribution, such as waist circumference. Leanness might have beneficial effects on longevity that in some degree counter the negative effects of excessive adiposity. Most studies do not have longitudinal data with serial measures of body weight and composition, and fat distribution in women and men over a large age range to track relationships with health status during the middle to later years of life. In addition, the effects of smoking, diet, levels of physical activity, and genetics may further confound many of these associations.

## SUMMARY

Stature, weight, and BMI are useful measures of body size and indices of body composition in adults. There are extensive reference data available in many countries that describe the current status of the distributions of these indicators in their respective populations. Given the increased prevalence of overweight and obesity worldwide among adults, weight and weight-for-stature indices, such as BMI, have significant health importance in characterizing health risk relationships and as a screening tool for determining chronic disease risk and the risk of early mortality.

## ACKNOWLEDGMENTS

This work was supported by the following National Institutes of Health (Bethesda, MD) grants: HD012252, DK064870, DK064391, and AR052147.

## REFERENCES

1. Sun, SS, Chumlea, WC. In: Heymsfield, SSB, Lohman, TTG, Wang, Z (eds.), *Human Body Composition*, Human Kinetics, Champaign, IL, p. 151; 2005.
2. Flegal, KM, Graubard, BI, Williamson, DF. *J Am Med Assoc* 15: 1861; 2005.

3. Lohman, TG, Roche, AF, Martorell, R. *Anthropometric Standardization Reference Manual*. Human Kinetics, Champaign, IL, 177p., 1988.

4. Kuczmarski, RJ, Chumlea, WC. Third National Health and Nutrition Examination Survey (NHANESIII) anthropometric procedures video. 1997.

5. Chumlea, WC, Guo, SS, Steinbaugh, ML. *J Am Diet Assoc* 12: 1385; 1994.

6. Chumlea, WC, Guo, SS, Wholihan, K. *J Am Diet Assoc* 2: 137; 1998.

7. Gallagher, D, Ruts, E, Visser, M. *Am J Physiol Endocrinol Metab* 2: E266; 2000.

8. Quetelet, LA. *Sur L'homme et le Developpement de ses Facultes, ou essai de Physique Sociale*. Bachelier, Paris, France, 327p., 1835.

9. Keys, A, Fidanza, F, Karvonen, MJ. *J Chronic Dis* 6: 329; 1972.

10. Garn, SM, Pesick, SD. *Am J Clin Nutr* 4: 573; 1982.

11. Benn, RT. *Br J Prev Soc Med* 1: 42; 1971.

12. Gallagher, D, Visser, M, Sepulveda, D. *Am J Epidemiol* 3: 228; 1996.

13. Abdel-Malek, AK, Mukherjee, D, Roche, AF. *Hum Biol* 3: 415; 1985.

14. French, SA, Folsom, AR, Jeffery, RW. *Am J Epidemiol* 6: 504; 1999.

15. Wildman, RP, Gu, D, Reynolds, K. *Am J Clin Nutr* 5: 1129; 2004.

16. Chumlea, WC, Guo, SS, Kuczmarski, RJ. *Int J Obes Relat Metab Disord* 12: 1596; 2002.

17. Donini, LM, Chumlea, WC, Vellas, B. *J Nutr Health Aging* 52; 2006.

18. Gallagher, D, Heymsfield, SB, Heo, M. *Am J Clin Nutr* 3: 694; 2000.

19. WHO. *Obesity: Preventing and Managing the Global Epidemic*. WHO, Geneva, Switzerland, 276p., 1998.

20. James, PT, Leach, R, Kalamara, E. *Obes Res* 9(4): 228S; 2001.

21. Deitel, M. *Obes Surg* 3: 329; 2003.

22. Gu, D, He, J, Duan, X. *J Am Med Assoc* 7: 776; 2006.

23. Seidell, JC, Oosterlee, A, Thijssen, MA. *Am J Clin Nutr* 1: 7; 1987.

24. Fujimoto, WY, Newell-Morris, LL, Grote, M. *Int J Obes* 15(2): 41; 1991.

25. Pouliot, MC, Despres, JP, Lemieux, S. *Am J Cardiol* 7: 460; 1994.

26. Despres, JP, Prud'homme, D, Pouliot, MC. *Am J Clin Nutr* 3: 471; 1991.

27. Bray, GA. Obesity, In: Ziegler, EE and Filer, LJ (eds.), *Present Knowledge in Nutrition*, 7th edn. International Life Sciences Institute, Washington, DC, pp. 19–32, 1994.

28. Nicklas, BJ, Penninx, BW, Cesari, M. *Am J Epidemiol* 8: 741; 2004.

29. Okosun, IS, Chandra, KM, Boev, A. *Prev Med* 1: 197; 2004.

30. Grundy, SM. *Endocrinol Metab Clin North Am* 2: 267; 2004.

31. Katzmarzyk, PT, Janssen, I, Ross, R. *Diabetes Care* 2: 404; 2006.

32. Lee, CD, Blair, SN, Jackson, AS. *Am J Clin Nutr* 3: 373; 1999.

33. Kuk, JL, Lee, S, Heymsfield, SB. *Am J Clin Nutr* 6: 1330; 2005.

34. Janssen, I, Katzmarzyk, PT, Ross, R. *Obes Res* 3: 525; 2004.

35. Yarnell, JW, Patterson, CC, Thomas, HF. *J Epidemiol Commun Health* 5: 344; 2000.

36. Van Pelt, RE, Evans, EM, Schechtman, KB. *Int J Obes Relat Metab Disord* 8: 1183; 2001.

37. Iwao, S, Iwao, N, Muller, DC. *Obes Res* 11: 685; 2001.

38. Bigaard, J, Frederiksen, K, Tjonneland, A. *Int J Obes (Lond)* 7: 778; 2005.

39. NHLBI. Clinical guidelines on the identification, evaluation, and treatment of overweight and obesity in adults: The evidence report. Rockville, MD, 228p., 1998.

40. Zhu, S, Heymsfield, SB, Toyoshima, H. *Am J Clin Nutr* 2: 409; 2005.

41. Wang, Y, Rimm, EB, Stampfer, MJ. *Am J Clin Nutr* 3: 555; 2005.

42. Rexrode, KM, Buring, JE, Manson, JE. *Int J Obes Relat Metab Disord* 7: 1047; 2001.

43. Bouchard, C. *Int J Obes (Lond)* 10: 1552; 2007.

44. Lamon-Fava, S, Wilson, PW, Schaefer, EJ. *Arterioscler Thromb Vasc Biol* 16(12): 1509; 1996.

45. Yan, LL, Daviglus, ML, Liu, K. *J Am Med Assoc* 2: 190; 2006.

46. Garrow, JS, Webster, J. *Int J Obes* 2: 147; 1985.

47. Kuczmarski, RJ, Flegal, KM. *Am J Clin Nutr* 5: 1074; 2000.

48. Rimm, EB, Stampfer, MJ, Giovannucci, E. *Am J Epidemiol* 12: 1117; 1995.

49. Stevens, J, Plankey, MW, Williamson, DF. *Obes Res* 4: 268; 1998.

50. Fernandez, JR, Heo, M, Heymsfield, SB. *Am J Clin Nutr* 1: 71; 2003.

51. Van Itallie, TB. *Ann Intern Med* 6(Pt 2): 983; 1985.

52. McGee, DL. *Ann Epidemiol* 2: 87; 2005.

53. Tayback, M, Kumanyika, S, Chee, E. *Arch Intern Med* 5: 1065; 1990.

54. Harris, T, Cook, EF, Garrison, R. *J Am Med Assoc* 10: 1520; 1988.

55. Jackson, AS, Stanforth, PR, Gagnon, J. *Int J Obes Relat Metab Disord* 6: 789; 2002.

56. Hubbard, VS. *Am J Clin Nutr* 5: 1067; 2000.

57. Katzmarzyk, PT, Craig, CL, Bouchard, C. *Int J Obes Relat Metab Disord* 8: 1054; 2002.

58. Church, TS, LaMonte, MJ, Barlow, CE. *Arch Intern Med* 18: 2114; 2005.

59. Wei, M, Kampert, JB, Barlow, CE. *J Am Med Assoc* 16: 1547; 1999.

60. Barlow, CE, Kohl, HW, III, Gibbons, LW. *Int J Obes Relat Metab Disord* 19(4): S41; 1995.

61. Katzmarzyk, PT, Church, TS, Janssen, I. *Diabetes Care* 2: 391; 2005.

62. Wei, M, Gibbons, LW, Kampert, JB. *Ann Intern Med* 8: 605; 2000.

63. Flegal, KM, Carroll, MD, Kit, BK. *JAMA* 307(5): 483; 2012.

64. Ford, ES, Li, C, Zhao, G. *Int J Obes (Lond)* 35(5): 736; 2011.

65. Sui, X, LaMonte, MJ, Laditka, JN. *JAMA* 298(21): 2507; 2007.

66. Newman, AB, Kupelian, V, Visser, M. *J Gerontol A Biol Sci Med Sci* 1: 72; 2006.

67. LaMonte, MJ, Kozlowski, KF, Cerny, F. In: Maughan, RJ (ed.), *The Olympic Textbook of Science in Sport*. Blackwell Publishing, Boston, MA, p. 401, 2009.

68. Di Pietro, L, Dziura, J, Blair, SN. *Int J Obes Relat Metab Disord* 12: 1541; 2004.

69. Petersen, L, Schnohr, P, Sorensen, TI. *Int J Obes Relat Metab Disord* 1: 105; 2004.

70. Stefanick, ML. *Exerc Sport Sci Rev* 21: 363; 1993.

71. Ross, R, Katzmarzyk, PT. *Int J Obes Relat Metab Disord* 2: 204; 2003.

72. Ross, R. *Sports Med* 1: 55; 1997.

73. Cooper, KH, Pollock, ML, Martin, RP. *J Am Med Assoc* 2: 166; 1976.

74. Gibbons, LW, Blair, SN, Cooper, KH. *Circulation* 5: 977; 1983.

75. LaMonte, MJ, Eisenman, PA, Adams, TD. *Circulation* 14: 1623; 2000.

76. Dannenberg, AL, Keller, JB, Wilson, PW. *Am J Epidemiol* 1: 76; 1989.

77. Paffenbarger, RS, Jr., Wing, AL, Hyde, RT. *Am J Epidemiol* 3: 245; 1983.

78. Hayashi, T, Tsumura, K, Suematsu, C. *Ann Intern Med* 1: 21; 1999.

79. Hu, G, Barengo, NC, Tuomilehto, J. *Hypertension* 1: 25; 2004.

80. Blair, SN, Goodyear, NN, Gibbons, LW. *J Am Med Assoc* 4: 487; 1984.

81. Sawada, S, Tanaka, H, Funakoshi, M. *Clin Exp Pharmacol Physiol* 20(7–8): 483; 1993.

82. Carnethon, MR, Gidding, SS, Nehgme, R. *J Am Med Assoc* 23: 3092; 2003.

83. Helmrich, SP, Ragland, DR, Leung, RW. *N Engl J Med* 3: 147; 1991.

84. Hu, FB, Sigal, RJ, Rich-Edwards, JW. *J Am Med Assoc* 15: 1433; 1999.

85. Wannamethee, SG, Shaper, AG, Alberti, KG. *Arch Intern Med* 14: 2108; 2000.

86. Wei, M, Gibbons, LW, Mitchell, TL. *Ann Intern Med* 2: 89; 1999.

87. Sawada, SS, Lee, IM, Muto, T. *Diabetes Care* 10: 2918; 2003.

88. Manson, JE, Nathan, DM, Krolewski, AS. *J Am Med Assoc* 1: 63; 1992.

89. Manson, JE, Rimm, EB, Stampfer, MJ. *Lancet* 8770: 774; 1991.

90. Hu, G, Lindstrom, J, Valle, TT. *Arch Intern Med* 8: 892; 2004.

91. Laaksonen, DE, Lakka, HM, Salonen, JT. *Diabetes Care* 9: 1612; 2002.

92. O'Connor, GT, Hennekens, CH, Willett, WC. *Am J Epidemiol* 11: 1147; 1995.

93. Salonen, JT, Slater, JS, Tuomilehto, J. *Am J Epidemiol* 1: 87; 1988.

94. Lee, IM, Skerrett, PJ. *Med Sci Sports Exerc* 33(Suppl 6): S459; 2001.

95. Slattery, ML, Edwards, S, Curtin, K. *Am J Epidemiol* 3: 214; 2003.

96. Oliveria, SA, Kohl, HW, III, Trichopoulos, D. *Med Sci Sports Exerc* 1: 97; 1996.

97. McTiernan, A, Kooperberg, C, White, E. *J Am Med Assoc* 10: 1331; 2003.

98. DHHS CDC. *Physical Activity and Health: A Report of the Surgeon General.* NCCDPHP, Atlanta, GA, 278p., 1996.

99. Blair, SN, Cheng, Y, Holder, JS. *Med Sci Sports Exerc* 33(Suppl 6): S379; 2001.

100. Kohl, HW, III. *Med Sci Sports Exerc* 33(Suppl 6): S472; 2001.

101. Blair, SN, Brodney, S. *Med Sci Sports Exerc* 31(Suppl 11): S646; 1999.

102. Grundy, SM, Blackburn, G, Higgins, M. *Med Sci Sports Exerc* 31(Suppl 11): S502; 1999.

103. Jakicic, JM, Clark, K, Coleman, E. *Med Sci Sports Exerc* 12: 2145; 2001.

104. Saris, WH, Blair, SN, van Baak, MA. *Obes Rev* 2: 101; 2003.

105. DHHS. *2008 Physical Activity Guidelines for Americans: Be Active, Helathy, and Happy!* Washington, DC, 2008.

106. Losonczy, KG, Harris, TB, Cornoni-Huntley, J. *Am J Epidemiol* 4: 312; 1995.

107. Andres, R, Muller, DC, Sorkin, JD. *Ann Intern Med* 7(Pt 2): 737; 1993.

108. McAdams, MA, Van Dam, RM, Hu, FB. *Obesity (Silver Spring)* 1: 188; 2007.

109. Allison, DB, Zhu, SK, Plankey, M. *Int J Obes Relat Metab Disord* 3: 410; 2002.

# 37 The "How" and "Why" of Body Composition Assessment (Adults)

*Stefan A. Czerwinski and Wm. Cameron Chumlea*

## CONTENTS

## INTRODUCTION

A variety of direct and indirect methods are available to quantify human body composition at the following levels: (1) the atomic level for the elements of carbon, calcium, potassium, and hydrogen; (2) the molecular level for amounts of water, protein, and fat; (3) the cellular level for extracellular fluid and the body cell mass and; (4) the tissue level for amounts and distributions of adipose, skeletal, and muscle tissues. These methods are based upon assumptions regarding the concentrations of elements, water, and electrolytes, the density of body tissues, the biological interrelationships between body components and body tissues, and their distributions among groups of normal-weight adults. Detailed aspects of body composition methodology, its theories, general applications, equipment, and analytical techniques are found in several references,[1–3] and readers interested in a specific method and its details should consult these references.

In most instances, body composition assessments quantify amounts of lean or fat-free mass (FFM) and fat mass (FM). Other reasons for a body composition assessment may include, but are not limited to, the determination of (1) bone mineral content (BMC) and bone mineral density (BMD) to screen for and diagnose osteoporosis, (2) total body water (TBW) and extracellular water (ECW) in adults with end-stage renal disease or other disorders affecting body fluids, or (3) monitoring changes in body composition during clinical treatment. Direct assessments, like neutron activation and total body counting, quantify chemical elements in the body

from the atomic level up to the tissue level, while indirect methods estimate body composition from the molecular level through the tissue level, via data collected from and validated against another method and a reference sample. Indirect methods view the body as a compartmental system consisting of TBW, ECW, BMC, FFM, and FM. These compartments are quantified from models using the hydration level, density, chemical composition, and BMC of FFM; the density of FM; and the reference samples used to validate them; they are not "gold standards" for in vivo body composition assessment.

Indirect methods quantify body components by measuring a body property such as its volume (total and molecular), density, and conductivity or describe amounts and distributions of muscle and adipose tissues via x-ray or magnetic imaging techniques. Some indirect methods can quantify only total body composition, while others quantify both total and regional body composition. All indirect methods depend on biological interrelationships between directly measured body components and tissues and their distributions among normal adults. Indirect methods include hydrometry (isotope dilution), densitometry, bioelectrical impedance analysis (BIA), dual-energy x-ray absorptiometry (DXA), computed x-ray tomography (CT), and magnetic resonance imaging (MRI). Large errors can occur when using indirect methods, and the results are affected by individual and sample specificity, as well as the presence of disease. Some indirect methods rely on prediction equations to estimate body composition that are developed from direct and other indirect methods, and their reference samples. Prediction equations using anthropometry are also available to estimate body composition values. However, prediction equations lose accuracy when applied to individuals or groups differing from the validation group, and the predicted results will vary and can require interpretation. In this chapter, current indirect body composition assessments are reviewed and evaluated regarding their methodologies, applications, and limitations in adults.

## INDIRECT BODY COMPOSITION METHODS

### HYDROMETRY

TBW is quantified by isotope dilution using deuterium or tritium in urine, saliva, or plasma with mass spectrometry, infrared spectrometry, or nuclear magnetic resonance spectroscopy.[4,5] There are good levels of agreement in TBW estimates among subjects, isotopes, specimens, and laboratory methods, but some differences for individuals are as much as 2–3 L. These differences are within the range expected in comparisons between body composition methods. The accepted equilibration time for isotope dilution is about 2–3 h, but this time is not well documented and the variation in equilibration times with body size is poorly documented. TBW measures need to be corrected for natural abundance and isotope exchange,[3] especially for deuterium, which is a naturally occurring isotope. ECW is also quantified by dilution using bromide as NaBr or other chemical elements similar to chloride[6,7] that estimate the volume of chloride space, which is all extracellular. Bromide concentration in plasma is measured by high-pressure liquid chromatography. It is not necessary to measure the natural abundance of bromide in the body, but this increases accuracy.

Body water is easy to measure in an adult because it does not require undressing or any real physical participation, but this methodology is limited in the obese. Hydrometry presupposes FFM can be calculated from TBW based upon an assumed average proportion of TBW in FFM of 73%, but this proportion ranges from 67% to 80%.[8,9] In addition, about 15%–30% of TBW is present in adipose tissue as ECW, and this proportion increases with the degree of adiposity, but available reference values are out of date. These proportions are higher in women than men, are higher in the obese, and can produce underestimates of FFM and overestimates of FM. Variation in the distribution of TBW due to diseases associated with obesity, such as diabetes and renal failure, further affects estimates of FFM and FM.

### DENSITOMETRY

Densitometry estimates body composition using measures of body weight and body volume corrected for residual lung volume. Densitometry uses an adult's body weight to displace a volume of either air or water as in the Archimedes principle of underwater weighing. Underwater weighing requires a large tank of water sufficient for an adult to completely submerge and have his or her weight recorded at full expiration.

Air displacement measures the change in the volume of air created by the presence of the body within a closed container of known volume, but it is hampered by potentially faulty assumptions.[10] Accurate and reliable measures by both water and air displacement are compromised for overweight or obese adults. It is difficult for an overweight or obese adult to submerge underwater, and weight belts can help correct the difficulty with submersion but not all other aspects of performance. Air displacement devices[10–12] are limited to adults who are "moderately" obese at best. Regardless, most overweight and obese adults are reluctant to put on a bathing suit and participate in body density measurements.

Historically, body density has been converted to the percentage of body weight as fat using the two-compartment models of Siri[9] or Brozek et al.,[13] but more recently, a multicompartment model is used.[14] Two-compartment models divide the body into FM and FFM based on densities of 0.9 and 1.10 g/mL, respectively. The density of FM has little interindividual variation across age, but the density of FFM varies depending upon the relative proportions of water, protein, and osseous and non-osseous mineral, as well as the sex, race, and age.[15] Two-compartment models are not sex- and race-specific, and thus, a variation of only 0.02 g/mL in the density of FFM can produce an error of 5% body fat. Multi-compartment models combine body density with measures of bone density from DXA and TBW volume to calculate body fatness.[16] Multi-compartment models estimate body composition more accurately than two-compartment models because they include measures of bone mineral and water that better reflect between-individual variance in body composition estimates across age, race, and sex.

### BIOELECTRIC IMPEDANCE ANALYSIS

Bioelectric impedance at a frequency of 50 kHz is used to estimate TBW or FFM and subsequently FM by measuring the resistance of the body as a conductor to a very small amperage-alternating electric current,[17,18] and bioelectric impedance at multiple frequencies from 1 to 1000 kHz can also differentiate the proportions of intra and extracellular fluid volumes.[19] Body composition estimates from single and multifrequency bioelectrical impedance in healthy individuals are well established, but all bioelectrical impedance methods employ some form of predictive modeling to estimate outcomes.[19] Bioelectrical impedance is useful in describing body composition for groups, but large errors for an individual limit its clinical use, especially in the presence of disease or with repeated assessments. The predictive errors for an individual are large, so that repeated estimates are insensitive to small responses to treatment.

The tetrapolar method was the common way to measure single and multifrequency BIA. Early measures of impedance were taken with the subject supine and the electrodes were connected to the right hand–wrist and right ankle–foot, but BIA measurements now depend on the model and manufacturer of the BIA analyzer. For most commercially available BIA instruments, an adult stands barefoot on them, much like using a bathroom scale.

The conductor of the body is its water content, and all BIA machines measure the impedance of this fluid conductor. Impedance is the vector relationship between resistance and reactance measured at a current frequency. Resistance is the opposition of the conductor to the alternating current, as in nonbiological conductors, and reactance is from the capacitant effect of cell membranes, tissue interfaces, and nonionic tissues.[19] From Ohm's law, a conductor's volume is proportional to its length squared divided by its resistance, and BIA utilizes this same relationship in the body where stature (S) is squared and divided by resistance (R) as an index of body volume; thus, $S^2/R$, is directly related to the volume of TBW. The impedance index is used to estimate FFM and FM, but this is based upon the fraction of 73% of TBW in FFM. Since the hydration fraction of FFM is not constant, $S^2/R$ is combined with anthropometric data to predict body composition based upon results from other methods.

The theory behind multifrequency BIA is the same as that of single-frequency BIA, except that multifrequency BIA uses at least two different frequencies. At low frequency, the current cannot pass through the cell membrane due to its capacitance, so that low-frequency currents are conducted only through ECW of the body. High-frequency currents penetrate cell membranes and thus are used to estimate TBW.

When predicting body fluid volumes with multifrequency BIA, the analysis is adjusted for the effects of the fluid containing materials of differing conductive capacity. This is done using mixture theory,[20,21] which adjusts for the nonlinear relationship between R and water volume in a mixed medium system. The mixture effects are greatest at low frequency because the conductive volume, presumably ECW, is a smaller proportion of the total volume. Hanai[20] developed an equation to describe the effect on the conductivity of a conducting material having nonconductivity entities in suspension and hypothesized that the theory could be applied to tissues with nonconductivity materials ranging from 10% to 90%. This approach has been used successfully by a number of investigators to monitor changes in ECW, TBW, and FFM under a variety of conditions.[22–25]

Numerous BIA prediction equations for estimating body composition have been published that describe statistical associations based on biological relationships for a specific population. As such, the equations are useful only for adults that closely match the reference population in body size and shape. BIA has been applied to overweight or obese samples[26,27] in a few studies, but the majority of BIA prediction equations are not applicable to overweight or obese adults. The ability of BIA to predict fatness in obese adults is further limited, because there is a large proportion of body mass and body water accounted for by the trunk, the hydration of FFM is lower, and the ratio of ECW to TBW is increased. There are also prediction equations resident in commercial single-frequency impedance analyzers, and these equations are usually not provided and therefore not recommended unless additional information is provided by the manufacturer regarding the predictive accuracy, errors, and the samples used to develop them. While BIA is used most often to determine whole body composition, it can be used for segmental assessments also.

## DUAL-ENERGY X-RAY ABSORPTIOMETRY

DXA is the most popular method for quantifying amounts of total body and regional fat and lean and skeletal tissues. The primary use of DXA in the clinical setting is measuring BMC and BMD of the hip and spine for diagnosing osteoporosis. The two low-radiation energy levels used in DXA and their differential attenuation throughout the body and subsequent computer calculations allow discrimination and quantification of total body adipose, lean mass, and bone mass. DXA is an easy and convenient method for measuring body composition in the majority of the population, and it is currently included in the ongoing National Health and Nutrition Examination Survey.[28] DXA software has inherent assumptions regarding levels of hydration, potassium content, and density in estimating fat and lean tissue, and these assumptions vary by manufacturer.[29,30] DXA estimates of body composition are also affected by differences among manufacturers in the technology, machine models and software utilized, methodological problems, and intra- and inter-machine differences.[29,31–33]

A computer printout provides the DXA body composition analysis for body segments and the whole body. Adipose or fat tissue weight is given on the printout, and total body FFM is calculated as the sum of the weights of soft tissue and BMC. The sum of the total body weights of FFM, BMC, and FM should approximate measured body weight within 2.0 kg; otherwise, concern should be raised for measurement and machine accuracy. Inter-machine and inter-method comparisons of DXA body composition estimates should be made cautiously. DXA accurately measures BMC compared to neutron activation, and several studies have shown that DXA soft tissue estimates of FFM and FM are equivalent to results obtained from other methods in weight-stable individuals. Regular maintenance and calibration are needed to preserve the accuracy of DXA machines.

The DXA methodology is limited by restrictions on body weight, length, thickness, and width as a function of the available table scan area with each manufacturer and type of DXA machine, i.e., pencil or fan beam. Although some innovative adaptations have been proposed, many overweight and obese adults are too wide and too thick for a whole body DXA scan that requires lying supine with current machines.[34] Jebb et al.[35,36] reported that estimates of BMD were affected by tissue depth or thickness, with an increasing error when measuring BMD in tissue greater than 20 cm in depth. In weight-stable adults, measurement of soft tissue composition is similar to reference techniques, but concern about BMD in large adults is warranted.[31]

# IMAGING METHODS

Imaging systems, such as CT and MRI, are frequently limited to clinical situations and are often not practical for obese adults. CT accommodates large body sizes but has high radiation exposures and is inappropriate for whole body assessments, but it has been used to measure intra-abdominal fat. MRI is not able to accommodate large body sizes in many instances but can be used for whole body assessments and poses no known health risks. Both of these methods require time and software to provide whole body and regional quantities of FM and FFM.

## COMPUTED TOMOGRAPHY

CT is an x-ray device for specific medical diagnoses with an unacceptable radiation dose except for clinical examinations and studies.[37] Rossner et al.[37] compared adipose tissue depths measured directly from cadavers to CT images from 21 cross-sectional abdominal images and found a significant relationship between the two methods for total adipose tissue (r = 0.94) and intra-abdominal adipose tissue (r = 0.83). Work by Ross et al. on rats demonstrated a relationship between CT images and chemical analysis of lipids (r = 0.98).[38] Validation and checking the accuracy of this technique are constrained by the need for human cadaver analysis or chemical analysis of animals.

## MAGNETIC RESONANCE IMAGING

MRI involves an interaction between a very strong magnetic field and the nucleus of the hydrogen atom. Hydrogen is the most abundant element in the body, and the proton in the hydrogen nucleus acts like a tiny magnet. The very strong magnetic field of the MRI instruments aligns the hydrogen protons in a known direction, at which time a pulsed radio frequency is applied to the body part within the magnetic field. The hydrogen protons absorb the radio energy and change alignment or directional orientation like a spinning gyroscope falling out of position. When the radio frequency is turned off, the protons release the absorbed energy and return to their normal position or orientation within the magnetic field. The released energy is detected and converted into images by computer software.

Foster et al.[39] first reported MRI measures of adipose tissue and adjacent muscle tissue, and this work continued with carcass and cadaver. Work by Abate et al.[40] demonstrated that MRI measurements of adipose tissue in humans were similar to direct measurement of visceral and subcutaneous adipose tissue on cadavers. Supporting documentation for the accuracy of MRI has compared MRI to CT scan results,[41] and in general, the relationship between CT and MRI for the assessment of adipose tissue is good, with correlations ranging from 0.79 for subcutaneous to 0.98 for visceral and 0.99 for total adipose tissue. MRI is now used regularly to measure intra-abdominal amounts of visceral adipose tissue

in epidemiological studies related to risk of cardiovascular disease and the metabolic syndrome.

MRI images involve no radiation, making them a low-risk method for body composition assessment. MRI, like CT imaging, requires multiple scans in order to obtain adipose tissue distribution information. Two different research teams used multiple MRI images over the entire body. Fowler et al.[42] acquired 28 images from head to foot, while Ross et al.[38] obtained 40+ images from head to foot to determine adipose tissue and lean tissue distribution in both males and females. Fowler demonstrated that as few as four MR images could be used, while Ross showed that one image at the level of the L4-L5 lumbar vertebrae could be used to predict total adipose tissue volume. While as few as a single measure can provide an estimate of fat and lean components, there is some recent information that suggests that abdominal adipose tissue patterning differs by age, sex, and ethnicity. This work suggests that a single image may not be fully informative and that multiple image approaches may provide additional useful information regarding fat patterning for health studies.[43,44]

# STATISTICAL MODELS OF BODY COMPOSITION

Statistical modeling can predict body composition for groups or individuals[45] using regression equations. For example, one such model might use age and sex to predict the amount of central adiposity as measured by MRI. The selection of predictor variables depends on their biological and statistical relationships to the outcome variable of interest, because the strength of these relationships affects the accuracy or precision of the prediction equation. Several regression methods are available, such as forward selection, stepwise, and backward elimination regression. These are used if the predictor variables are not very interrelated. Predictor variables such as S and weight are interrelated and if used together in the same equation can reduce the precision and accuracy of the predictions. In such cases, a maximum $R^2$ or all-possible subsets of regression procedure are appropriate analytical choices.

Regression analysis assumes bivariate relationships between an outcome and its predictor variables are linear; otherwise, the prediction equations have large errors and poor performance. It is assumed that the dependent variable is normally distributed in order to allow statistical inferences about the significance of the regression parameters. A large sample results in more precise and accurate prediction equations than a small sample, but the necessary sample size is a function of the correlations between the outcome and predictor variables. The sample size required to achieve accuracy on cross-validation depends on the number of predictor variables, the bivariate relationships among the dependent variable and the predictor variables, and the variance of the dependent variable in the cross-validation sample.

Numerous prediction equations for TBW, FFM, FM, and %FM from anthropometry and for TBW and FFM from bioelectrical impedance for non-Hispanic white, non-Hispanic black, and Mexican-American adults have been published.[10] Unless specified, these equations are not recommended for obese adults or groups. Many of these equations are for whites only, but there are a limited number for Native-American, Hispanic-American, and non-Hispanic black American samples.[46,47] Using a multicomponent body composition validation model, BIA prediction equations for TBW and FFM are available for non-Hispanic white, non-Hispanic black, and Mexican-American adults.[16] These anthropometric and BIA equations provide reasonable prediction for individuals except at the extremes of the body composition distribution.

## AVAILABLE REFERENCE DATA

Body composition references are available from national survey data collected by the National Center for Health Statistics, Centers for Disease Control and Prevention. These surveys use multiple methods of data collection including interviews, physical examinations, physiological testing, and biochemical assessments from large representative samples of the U.S. population to monitor the nation's health and nutritional status. Plots of estimated means from single-frequency BIA for TBW, FFM, FM, and %FM of non-Hispanic white, non-Hispanic black, and Mexican-American adults from the third National Health and Nutrition Examination Survey are presented in Figures 37.1 through 37.4.[48] The data in these figures represent estimates for these groups of American adults between 1988 and 1994. More recent data based upon

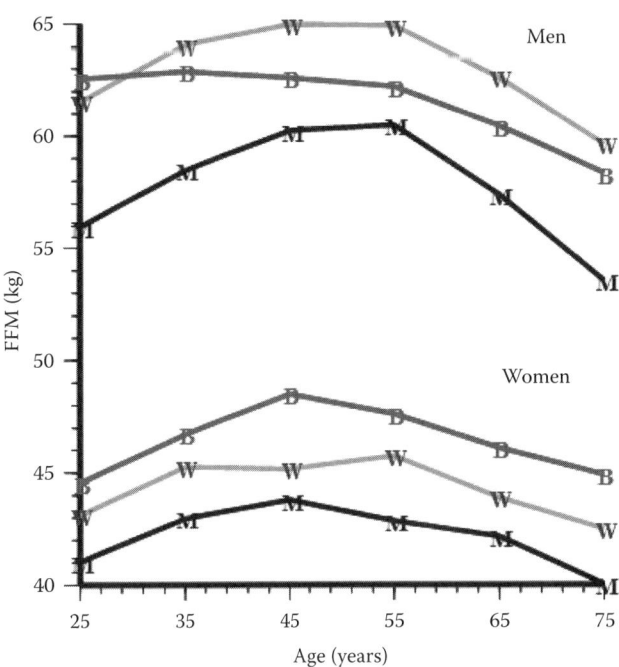

FIGURE 37.2 Estimated means for FFM by 10-year age groups from 20 to 80 years for non-Hispanic white (W), non-Hispanic black (B), and Mexican-American (M) men and women.

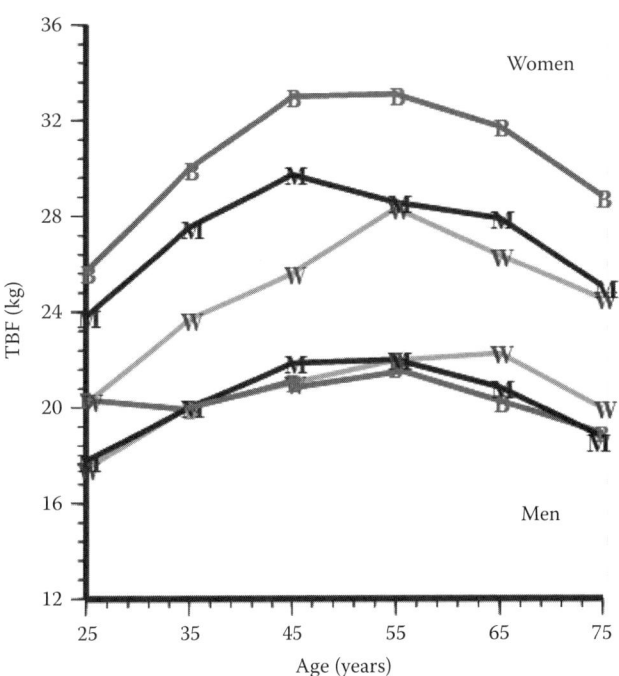

FIGURE 37.3 Estimated means for TBF by 10-year age groups from 20 to 80 years for non-Hispanic white (W), non-Hispanic black (B), and Mexican-American (M) men and women.

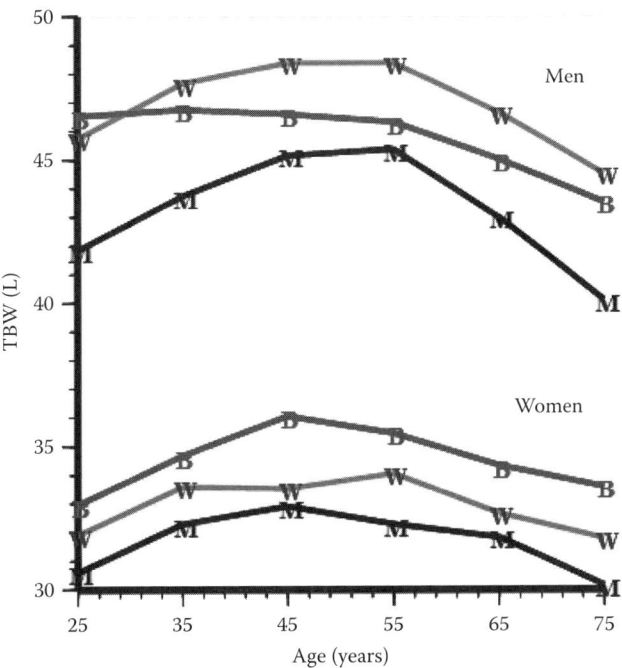

FIGURE 37.1 Estimated means for TBW from NHANES III by 10-year age groups from 20 to 80 years for non-Hispanic white (W), non-Hispanic black (B), and Mexican-American (M) men and women.

the body mass index or BMI have been published for data collected since 1998, and these body composition estimates are being augmented by body composition values measured by DXA in more recent National Health and Nutrition Examination Surveys.[28]

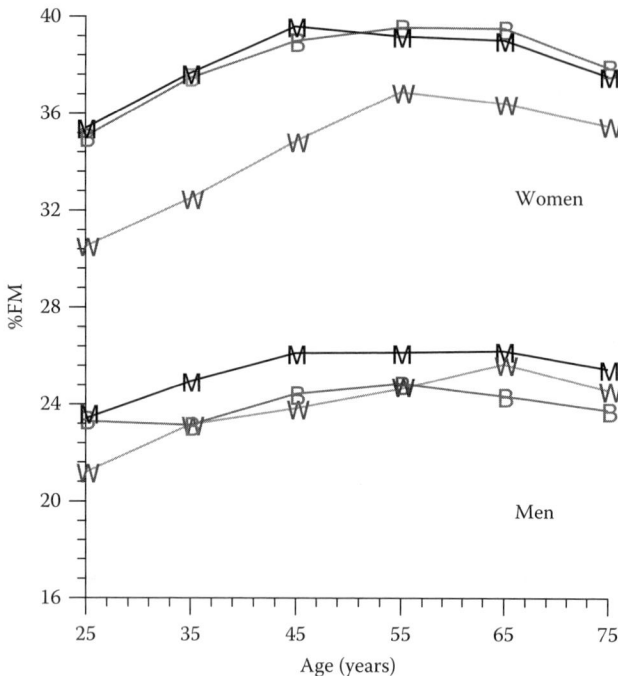

**FIGURE 37.4** Estimated means for %FM by 10-year age groups from 20 to 80 years for non-Hispanic white (W), non-Hispanic black (B), and Mexican-American (M) men and women.

## SPECIAL POPULATIONS AND METHODOLOGICAL ISSUES

Direct and indirect assessment methods and their reference data are applicable to adults but exclude most of the obese and many of the elderly. Obese (and wasted) adults have metabolic and hormonal profiles accompanied by comorbid conditions that alter assumptions underlying the validity of body composition methods applicable to normal-weight individuals.[49] Body composition assessments are of limited use among most obese adults, because their bodies are too large for the available equipment. Because of the challenges of collecting such data from sufficient numbers of obese individuals, epidemiological and national obesity prevalence data are not based completely on actual measures of body fatness. It is also difficult to monitor and treat obesity without a commonly accepted assessment method or index and a reference population. There is no universally accepted method of clearly measuring body fatness or quantifying overweight and obesity. Current body composition analysis is hampered by problems of nonuniversal assumptions, limited by application of methodology, or affected by chronic disease or subject size and performance, and these are special problems for the obese patient.

It is important in interpreting results from any body composition assessment to recognize its limitations. Direct assessments have an error of about 2%–3% body fat at best when compared with corresponding results from other direct methods. With indirect methods, an error of about 5% body fat is expected, and an error of 5%–10% is more realistic for predicted body composition. In addition, many assessments use technology and software that are proprietary to

a manufacturer. Basic understanding of this technology is important as is an understanding of the accuracy and reliability of the equipment; these equipment details are frequently available only from the manufacturer and should be evaluated critically.

## CONCLUSION

Researchers and clinicians currently have the ability to assess body composition in a variety of ways. Direct and some indirect methods are impractical for most clinical examinations or community studies because of the scarcity of equipment and testing centers and due to high costs. CT and MRI are used to image the total body or specific body parts for the presence of pathology, disease, or injury. These methods can also be used to quantify body fat and lean tissue amounts with specific software. However, this use is frequently limited due to scheduling issues, with clinical needs being prioritized over research study access. DXA machines are commonly utilized for both clinical diagnosis and in large community-based studies. Although DXA examinations are conducted clinically, the methodology is practical for both the patient and the testing center. Estimating body composition through prediction equations is the easiest for the patient or study participant and works fairly well for population trends, but is not always the best estimate for an individual. When choosing the most appropriate body composition assessment method for a particular study, the characteristics of the patient population should be balanced with equipment needs and availability and appropriate interpretations of the results.

## ACKNOWLEDGMENTS

This work was supported by the following National Institutes of Health (Bethesda, MD) grants: HD012252, DK064870, DK064391, and AR052147.

## REFERENCES

1. Heymsfield, S. *Human Body Composition*. Human Kinetics, Champaign, IL, 2005; 523pp.
2. Lohman, TG. *Advances in Body Composition Assessment*. Human Kinetics Publishers, Champaign, IL, 1992; 150pp.
3. Roche, AF, Heymsfield, S, Lohman, TG. *Human Body Composition*. Human Kinetics, Champaign, IL, 1996; 366pp.
4. Khaled, MA, Lukaski, HC, Watkins, CL, *Am J Clin Nutr* 1:1;1987.
5. Rebouche, CJ, Pearson, GA, Serfass, RE, *Am J Clin Nutr* 2:373;1987.
6. Cheek, DB, *J Pediatr* 58:103;1961.
7. Vaisman, N, Pencharz, PB, Koren, G, *Am J Clin Nutr* 1:1;1987.
8. Chumlea, WC, Guo, SS, Zeller, CM, *Kidney Int* 6:2250;2001.
9. Siri, W, *Techniques for Measuring Body Composition*. National Academy Press, Washington, DC, 1961; 223pp.
10. Demerath, EW, Guo, SS, Chumlea, WC, *Int J Obes Relat Metab Disord* 3:389;2002.
11. Dempster, P, Aitkens, S, *Med Sci Sports Exerc* 12:1692;1995.

12. McCrory, MA, Gomez, TD, Bernauer, EM, *Med Sci Sports Exerc* 12:1686;1995.

13. Brozek, J, Grande, F, Anderson, JT, *Ann N Y Acad Sci* 113;1963.

14. Guo, SS, Chumlea, WC, Roche, AF, *Int J Obes Relat Metab Disord* 12:1167;1997.

15. Lohman, TG, *Exerc Sport Sci Rev* 325;1986.

16. Sun, SS, Chumlea, WC, Heymsfield, SB, *Am J Clin Nutr* 2:331;2003.

17. Chumlea, WC, Guo, SS, *Nutr Rev* 4:123;1994.

18. Lukaski, HC, Johnson, PE, Bolonchuk, WW, *Am J Clin Nutr* 4:810;1985.

19. Chumlea, WC, Sun, SS. *Human Body Composition*. Human Kinetics, Champaign, IL, 2005; 523pp.

20. Hanai, T. *Emulsion Science*. Academic Press, London, U.K., 1968; 496pp.

21. Macdonald, JR. *Impedance Spectroscopy: Emphasizing Solid Materials and Systems*. Wiley, New York, 1987; 346pp.

22. De Lorenzo, A, Andreoli, A, Matthie, J, *J Appl Physiol* 5:1542;1997.

23. Van Loan, M, Withers, P, Mattie, J. *Human Body Composition: In Vivo Methods, Models, and Assessment*. Plenum Press, New York, 1993; 400pp.

24. Van Loan, MD, Kopp, LE, King, JC, *J Appl Physiol* 3:1037;1995.

25. Van Loan, MD, Strawford, A, Jacob, M, *AIDS* 2:241;1999.

26. Gray, DS, Bray, GA, Gemayel, N, *Am J Clin Nutr* 2:255;1989.

27. Kushner, RF, Kunigk, A, Alspaugh, M, *Am J Clin Nutr* 2:219;1990.

28. Binkley, N, Kiebzak, GM, Lewiecki, EM, *J Bone Miner Res* 2:195;2005.

29. Roubenoff, R, Kehayias, JJ, Dawson-Hughes, B, *Am J Clin Nutr* 5:589;1993.

30. Kohrt, WM, *Med Sci Sports Exerc* 10:1349;1995.

31. Schoeller, DA, Tylavsky, FA, Baer, DJ, *Am J Clin Nutr* 5:1018;2005.

32. Guo, SS, Wisemandle, WA, Tyleshevski, F, *J Health Nutr Aging* 1:29;1997.

33. Hangartner, TN, *Osteoporos Int* 4:513;2007.

34. Tataranni, PA, Ravussin, E, *Am J Clin Nutr* 4:730;1995.

35. Jebb, SA, Goldberg, GR, Jennings, G. *Human Body Composition: In Vivo Methods, Models, and Assessment*. Plenum Press, New York, 1993; 400pp.

36. Jebb, SA, Goldberg, GR, Jennings, G, *Clin Sci (Lond)* 3:319;1995.

37. Rossner, S, Bo, WJ, Hiltbrandt, E, *Int J Obes* 10:893;1990.

38. Ross, R, Leger, L, Morris, D, *J Appl Physiol* 2:787;1992.

39. Foster, MA, Hutchison, JM, Mallard, JR, *Magn Reson Imaging* 3:187;1984.

40. Abate, N, Burns, D, Peshock, RM, *J Lipid Res* 8:1490;1994.

41. Seidell, JC, Bakker, CJ, van der Kooy, K, *Am J Clin Nutr* 6:953;1990.

42. Fowler, PA, Fuller, MF, Glasbey, CA, *Am J Clin Nutr* 1:18;1991.

43. Demerath, E, Sun, SS, Lee, M, *Circulation* 8:e221;2007.

44. Demerath, E, Sun, SS, Rogers, NL, *Obesity* 12:2984;2007.

45. Sun, SS, Chumlea, WC. *Human Body Composition*. Human Kinetics, Champaign, IL, 2005; 523pp.

46. Lohman, TG, Caballero, B, Himes, JH, *Int J Obes Relat Metab Disord* 8:982;2000.

47. Wagner, DR, Heyward, VH, Kocina, PS, *Med Sci Sports Exerc* 7:969;1997.

48. Chumlea, WC, Guo, SS, Kuczmarski, RJ, *Int J Obes Relat Metab Disord* 12:1596;2002.

49. Moore, FD, Oelsen, KH, McMurrey, JD. *The Body Cell Mass and Its Supporting Environment: Body Composition in Health and Disease*. W.B. Saunders Company, Philadelphia, PA, 1963; 535pp.

# 38 Height, Weight, and Body Mass Index in Childhood

*Ellen W. Demerath, Stefan A. Czerwinski, and Wm. Cameron Chumlea*

## CONTENTS

## INTRODUCTION

In childhood, height (stature) and weight are the two most frequently used measures of growth and nutritional status. In addition, indices of weight for height, especially BMI, are used as a proxy for body fatness or obesity. As growth is the most sensitive indicator of overall health in childhood, it is essential that accurate measurements be made on a regular basis during routine health supervision of children and adolescents to identify and address significant deviations in a timely manner.

Pediatric health professionals take two basic anthropometric measurements on each child: *recumbent length* (for children *under* 2 years of age) or *standing height* (for children *over* 2 years of age) and *weight*. From these two measurements, *body mass index (BMI)* can be derived from a reference chart or calculated by formula. This chapter will focus on these measures: height (or length), weight, and BMI. For each measurement, the following aspects will be discussed: definition, normal patterns of change, measurement techniques, and interpretation of values using reference growth charts. As most practicing pediatricians in the United States, as well as other health professionals who care for children, record their measurements in inches and pounds, these units will be used in the discussion.

## HEIGHT

### DESCRIPTION

Height, or stature, is a linear measure from the base on which the child is standing to the firm top of the child's head. Height is measured in children over 2 years of age. It is measured with the child standing with erect posture and without shoes. From birth to 2 years of age, the infant or toddler's stature is measured as recumbent length. This is the total length of the child—from the bottom of the feet (positioned at a 90° angle) to the top of the head. Recumbent length is slightly greater than standing height measured in the same individual.

### NORMAL PATTERNS OF LINEAR GROWTH IN CHILDHOOD

There is a wide range of normal variation in human linear growth during childhood: During the first year of life, babies increase in recumbent length about 10 in. on average, from about 20 in. at birth to 30 in. by their first birthday. During the second year of life, their length increases by 4–5 in., or about $1/_3$ in. per month, on average. After age 2 years, height is measured in the standing position. Growth continues at a slower but steady rate of about 2½ in. per year until about the age of 11 in girls and 13 in boys, when the growth spurt associated with puberty usually begins. Puberty is characterized by a greater rate of growth, culminating in a peak height velocity (inches grown per year) comparable to the rate of growth during the second year of life. The peak height velocity for girls is about 2½–4 ½ in. per year, and for boys is about 3–5 in. per year. For both boys and girls, however, puberty and the pubertal "growth spurt" may occur several years earlier or later than average and still be within a normal range. Linear growth is complete when the epiphyses (ends) of the long bones fuse with the shaft, which usually occurs between 14 and 16 years of age for girls and between 16 and 18 years of age for boys.

## Measuring Length

The stature of subjects less than 2 years of age is measured as recumbent length. This is done most accurately with a measuring board with an inflexible headpiece against which the top of the head is positioned and a moveable footboard against which the feet are placed at a 90° angle. The child should be relaxed, wearing only a diaper, with legs fully extended, and the child should be looking directly upward, with the head positioned so that a line connecting the outer margin of the eyes with the ears is at a 90° angle with the bottom of the measuring board (i.e., in the "Frankfurt plane"). Recumbent length is measured from the top of the head to the bottom of the feet. It should be measured to the nearest 0.1 cm or 1/8 in. and recorded in the child's chart. Measurement of recumbent length on an examining table without a board should also be from the top of the head to the bottom of the feet, which are positioned at a 90° angle. It is recommended that the same examiner measure the child at each visit to minimize interexaminer variability. It is also recommended that the individual measuring is assisted by another to maintain the infant in the proper position. Measuring between two pencil marks on an exam table does not provide an accurate measurement. Using such inappropriate equipment for recumbent length measurement has a tendency to measure "short." Length should be measured twice, and the two measurements should agree within ¼ in. If the difference exceeds the tolerance limit of ¼ in., the infant should be remeasured a third time.

Because recumbent length is slightly greater than standing height, it is recommended that measurements of both length and height be obtained for two visits between 2 and 3 years of age. With these simultaneous recumbent length and standing height values, measurement discrepancy can be distinguished from actual change in growth rate.

## Measuring Height

The height of subjects older than 2 years of age is measured, without shoes, with a stadiometer. A stadiometer consists of a measuring tape affixed to a vertical surface, such as a wall or a rigid freestanding measuring device, and a movable block, attached to the vertical surface at a right angle, which can be brought down to the crown of the head. If possible, height should not be measured on a platform scale, because the

moveable measuring rod is too narrow and unsteady and can be easily bent. The subject should stand with heels together and back as straight as possible; the heels, buttocks, shoulders, and head should touch the wall or the vertical surface of the measuring device. The weight of the subject is distributed evenly on both feet and the head is positioned in the horizontal plane. The arms hang freely by the sides with the palms facing the thighs. The subject should be asked to inhale deeply and maintain a fully erect position. The examiner positions the movable block until it touches the head, applying sufficient pressure to compress the hair. The height marker is read while pressing firmly on the headpiece. The number on the height bar immediately behind the indicator line of the height marker is read. The examiner's eyes should look directly at the indicator line at about the same height in order to avoid parallax error in reading the measurement. The height is measured to the nearest 0.1 cm or 1/8 in. As is the case for recumbent length, the child should be repositioned for a second measurement, and the two measurements should agree within 1 cm or ¼ in. If the difference exceeds this tolerance limit, a third measure should be obtained. Record the average of the two heights that match most closely on the child's chart.

Height has diurnal variation. Children are tallest in the morning and shrink as much as a centimeter during the course of a day as the fibrous intervertebral cartilaginous disks are compressed. Diurnal variation in height is completely due to changes in the height of the vertebral column, and full height is regained when the child lies supine for about 30 min.

## Reference Charts for Length and Height

Growth charts are simple grids that are used to plot a child's height according to age and sex. Pediatric health professionals should measure and plot height on a growth chart at every visit, at least every 6 months before school age and annually thereafter. Growth charts are derived from the heights of large numbers of healthy children of all ages, separating the wide ranges of normal heights into percentiles by statistical techniques. The spaces between the percentile lines are called channels. Age in years is plotted along the horizontal axis at the bottom of the chart and length or height in inches (or centimeters) is plotted along the vertical axis on the left of the chart. Growth charts' percentile curves are commonly provided percentiles between the 5th and 95th percentiles, 3rd and 97th percentiles, or 2nd and 98th percentiles of the population distribution values. The 50th percentile curve represents the median height at each age for the reference population. As growth charts are generally cross-sectional in nature, it does not represent the expected growth pattern of an individual child.

For children aged 2–20 years, the United States Centers for Disease Control and Prevention (CDC) recommends using the stature-for-age growth reference charts for boys and girls that it published in 2000 (Figure 38.1 for boys and Figure 38.2 for girls), which was a revision of the 1977 National Center for Health Statistics (NCHS) growth charts for ages from birth to 17 years, using new national survey data and improved statistical smoothing procedures.

CDC Growth Charts: United States

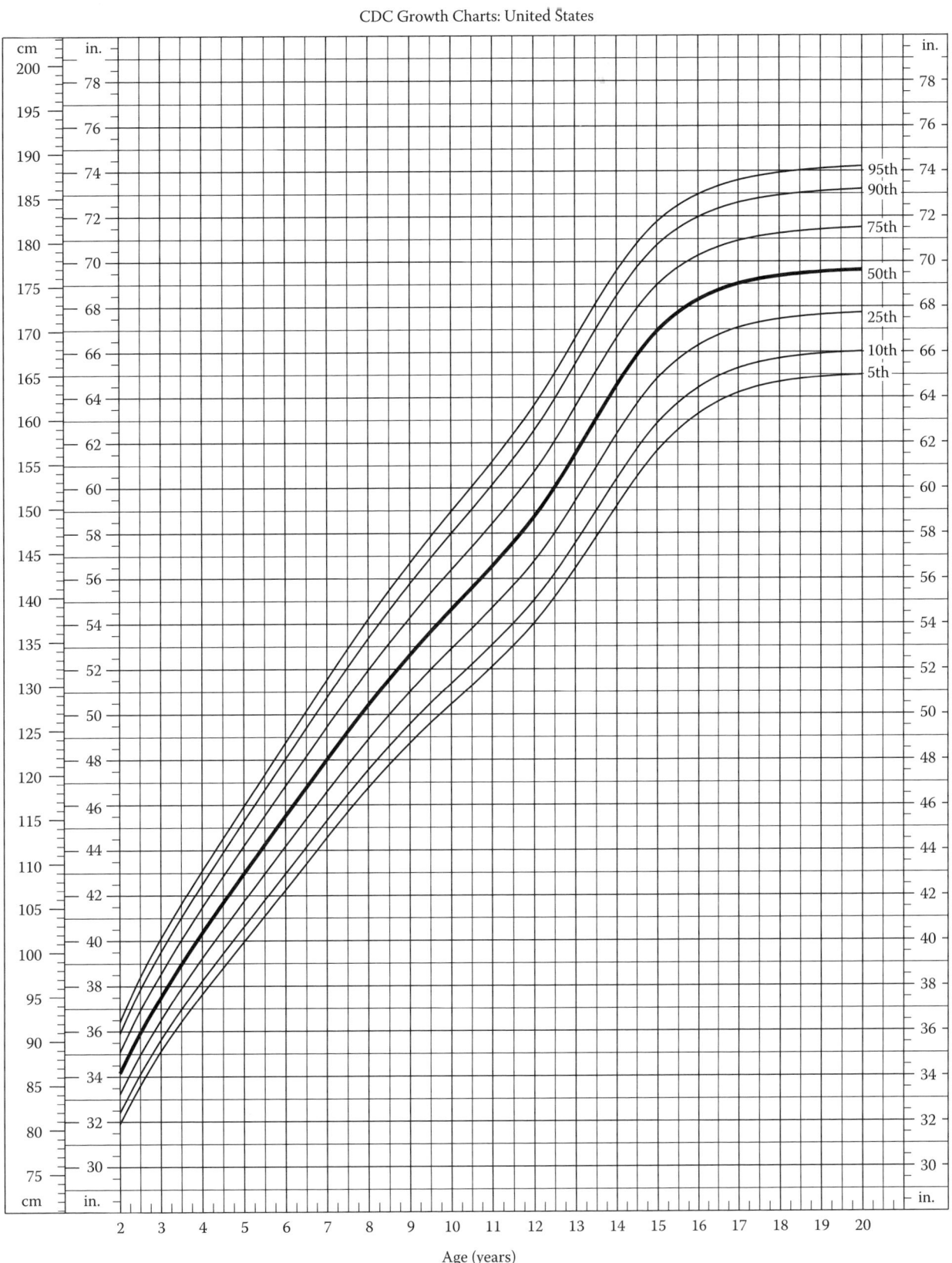

Age (years)

**FIGURE 38.1** Stature-for-age percentiles: Boys, 2 to 20 years. (Developed by the National Center for Health Statistics in collaboration with the National Center for Chronic Disease Prevention and Health Promotion, Hyattsville, MD. May 30, 2000, and publicly available at http://www.cdc.gov/growthcharts/clinical_charts.htm).

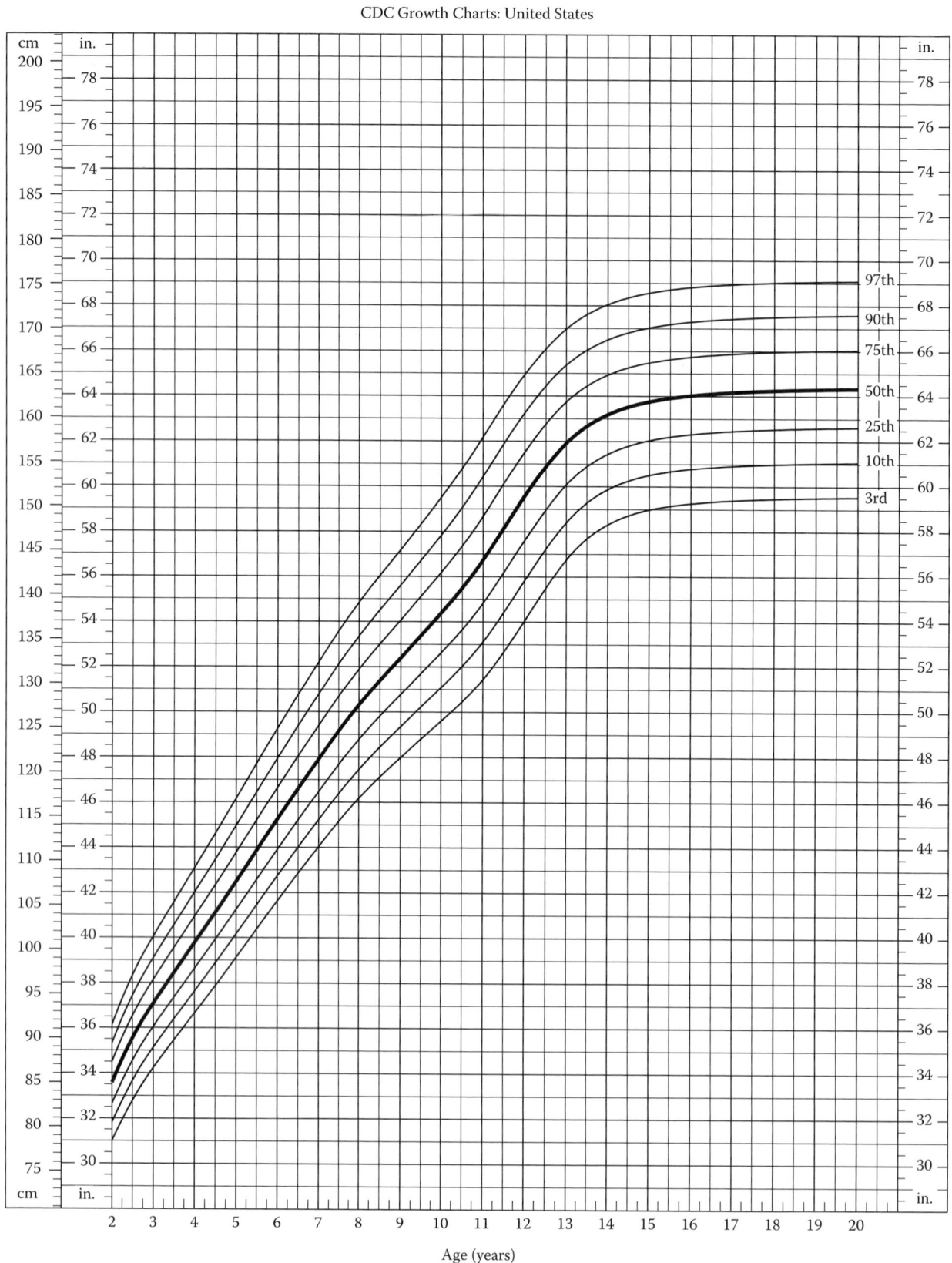

**FIGURE 38.2**  Stature-for-age percentiles: Girls, 2 to 20 years. (Developed by the National Center for Health Statistics in collaboration with the National Center for Chronic Disease Prevention and Health Promotion, Hyattsville, MD. May 30, 2000, and publicly available at http://www.cdc.gov/growthcharts/clinical_charts.htm).

For children aged 0–2 years (including very low birth weight and premature infants after discharge), the CDC recommends use of the World Health Organization international growth charts (Figure 38.3 for boys and Figure 38.4 for girls). The 2006 WHO charts are growth standards, describing how we think infants should grow. These charts are derived from an international sample of exclusively breast-feeding, non-smoking mothers of moderate to high socioeconomic status, who had optimal prenatal care. The CDC 2000 charts are growth references, describing the length and height of U.S. children from a series of health and nutrition surveys, without extensive exclusions; for instance, infants in the sample included both breast milk- and formula-fed children. It is a description of how children did grow at a certain period of time. The reason the CDC now recommends use of an international growth standard for infant growth monitoring is because it brings the growth chart into alignment with current infant-feeding guidelines, including exclusive breast-feeding for 6 months and continued breast milk feeding for 12 months. Differences in length growth between the two sets of charts are of minimal clinical significance. The 2000 CDC and 2006 WHO/CDC charts may be downloaded from the CDC website: http://ww.cdc.gov/growthcharts.

### INTERPRETATION OF LENGTH AND HEIGHT MEASUREMENTS

Depending on the genetic endowment that a child inherits from their parents, children after birth tend to gravitate toward a specific percentile or channel of the reference length (or height) charts and this process of "canalization" results in frequent percentile crossing during the first 2 years of life, particularly in the first 6 months. After 2 years of age, most children track close to that percentile or channel, maintaining a stable position relative to their peers.

Children who track consistently along the lowest height percentiles may have *familial short stature,* in which the parents are short and the child has inherited the same genetic variants influencing stature. Other short children may have *constitutionally delayed growth* characterized by a slower rate of growth in the first 2–3 years of life, followed by normal growth velocity that tracks along a height percentile or channel lower than expected for the family. These children often have delayed skeletal development (bone age younger than chronological age), later onset of puberty and its accompanying growth spurt, as well as a parent who followed a similar pattern of growth as a child. Final adult height is generally appropriate for parental height expectations.

Children who decelerate in linear growth and shift downward, crossing 1–2 percentile lines, deserve medical evaluation and continued growth monitoring. Poor linear growth may reflect inadequate nutrition, an underlying disease affecting a major organ system, or a genetic abnormality. Children in whom linear growth accelerates and shifts upward to a higher percentile also deserve medical evaluation. Increased rate of linear growth may reflect overnutrition, early or precocious onset of puberty, or another endocrine or genetic abnormality. Definitions of low length for age, low weight for age, underweight, overweight, and obesity are found in Table 38.1.

# WEIGHT

## DESCRIPTION

Body *weight* is a measure of body mass, which is a composite of each contributing tissue (e.g., adipose tissue, muscle, and bone). Although weight should ideally be measured without clothing, this is often impractical. Weight should be measured without shoes and with the child either in underwear only or in light indoor clothing.

## AVERAGE PATTERNS OF WEIGHT GAIN IN CHILDHOOD

As with height, there is a wide variation in normal patterns of weight gain in childhood. On average, infants double their birth weight by 6 months of age and triple it by their first birthday. From 1 to 2 years of age, toddlers who are tracking along the 50th percentile for weight gain about 5–6 lb, or about ½ lb per month, and during the third year of life weight gain averages about 4 lb. Children tracking along higher percentiles gain more, and those tracking on the lower percentiles gain proportionately less.

## MEASUREMENT TECHNIQUES

Weight should be measured using a standard beam balance scale with moveable weights or with an electronic scale of equivalent accuracy. It is recommended that the scale be calibrated at least monthly using standard weights. For infants, the child should be wearing a diaper only. For older children, the child should be weighed in underwear only if possible, or in light indoor clothing, without shoes. Belts and items carried in pockets should be removed. The beam of the platform scale must be graduated so that it can be read from both sides. The subject stands still over the center of the platform with body weight evenly distributed between both feet. The weight is measured to the nearest 0.01 kg or 1/2 oz. Two measurements are obtained, and if they do not agree within 0.01 kg (1/2 oz) for infants or 0.1 kg (1/4 lb) for children and adolescents, a third measurement should be obtained and the mean of the two closest measurements recorded.

Weight, like height, has diurnal variation. In contrast to height, however, weight is lowest in the morning after emptying the bladder and increases gradually through the day, depending on diet and physical activity.

## REFERENCE CHARTS FOR WEIGHT

Weight charts are available to plot a child's weight according to age and sex. Weight charts are also constructed from the weights of large numbers of healthy children of all ages, separating the wide range of weights into percentiles by statistical techniques. As for the height charts, the spaces between percentile lines are called channels. Age in years is plotted along the horizontal axis at the bottom of the chart and weight in pounds (or kilograms) is plotted along the vertical axis on the left of the chart. Most weight charts may provide percentile curves between the 5th and 95th percentiles, between the 3rd and 97th percentiles, or between the 2nd and 98th percentiles.

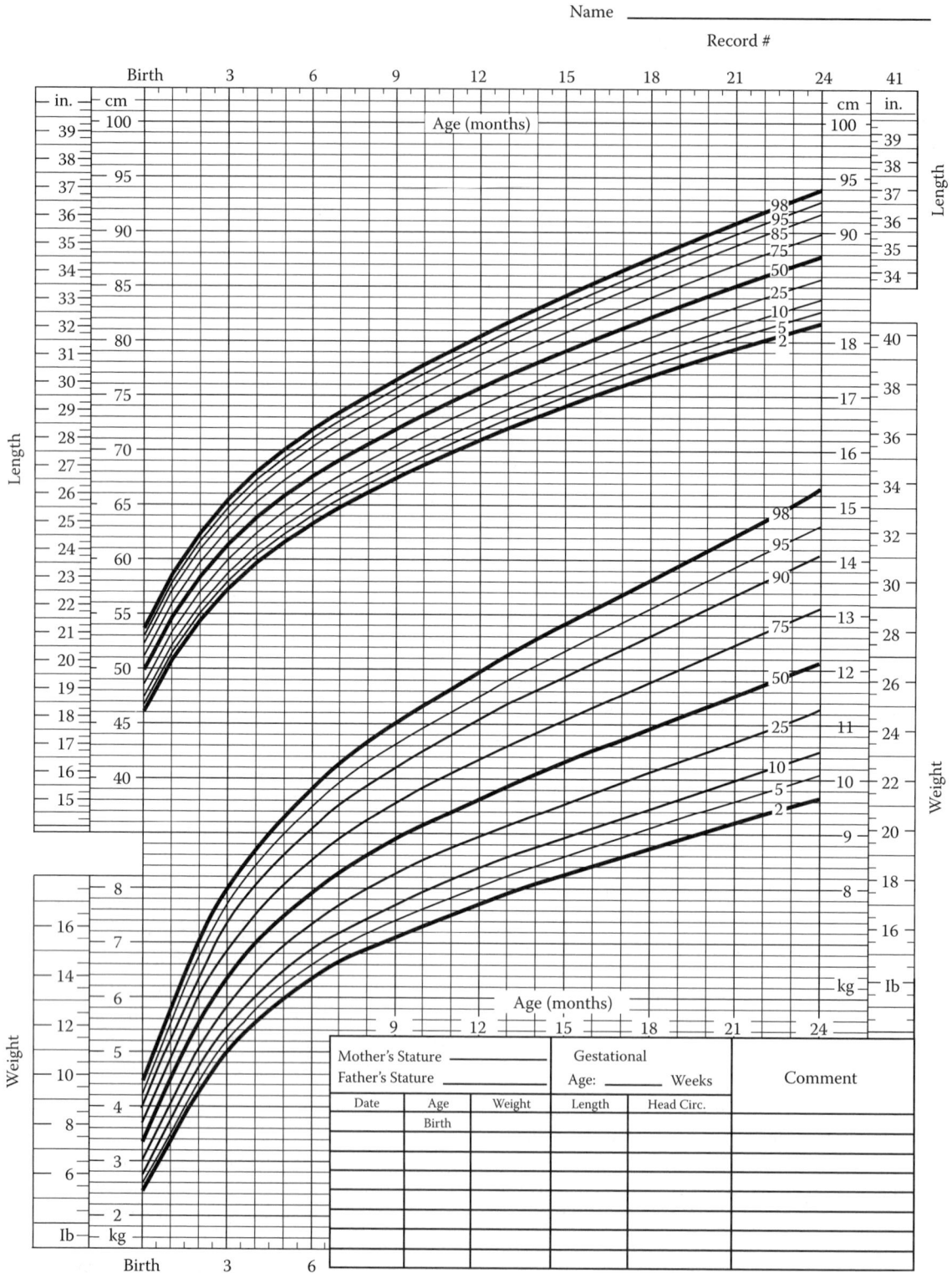

**FIGURE 38.3** Length-for-age and weight-for-age percentiles: Boys, birth to 24 months. (Published by the Centers for Disease Control and Prevention, November 1, 2009, and publicly available at http://www.cdc.gov/growthcharts/who_charts.htm; WHO Child Growth Standards, Geneva, Switzerland, http://www.who.int/childgrowth/en).

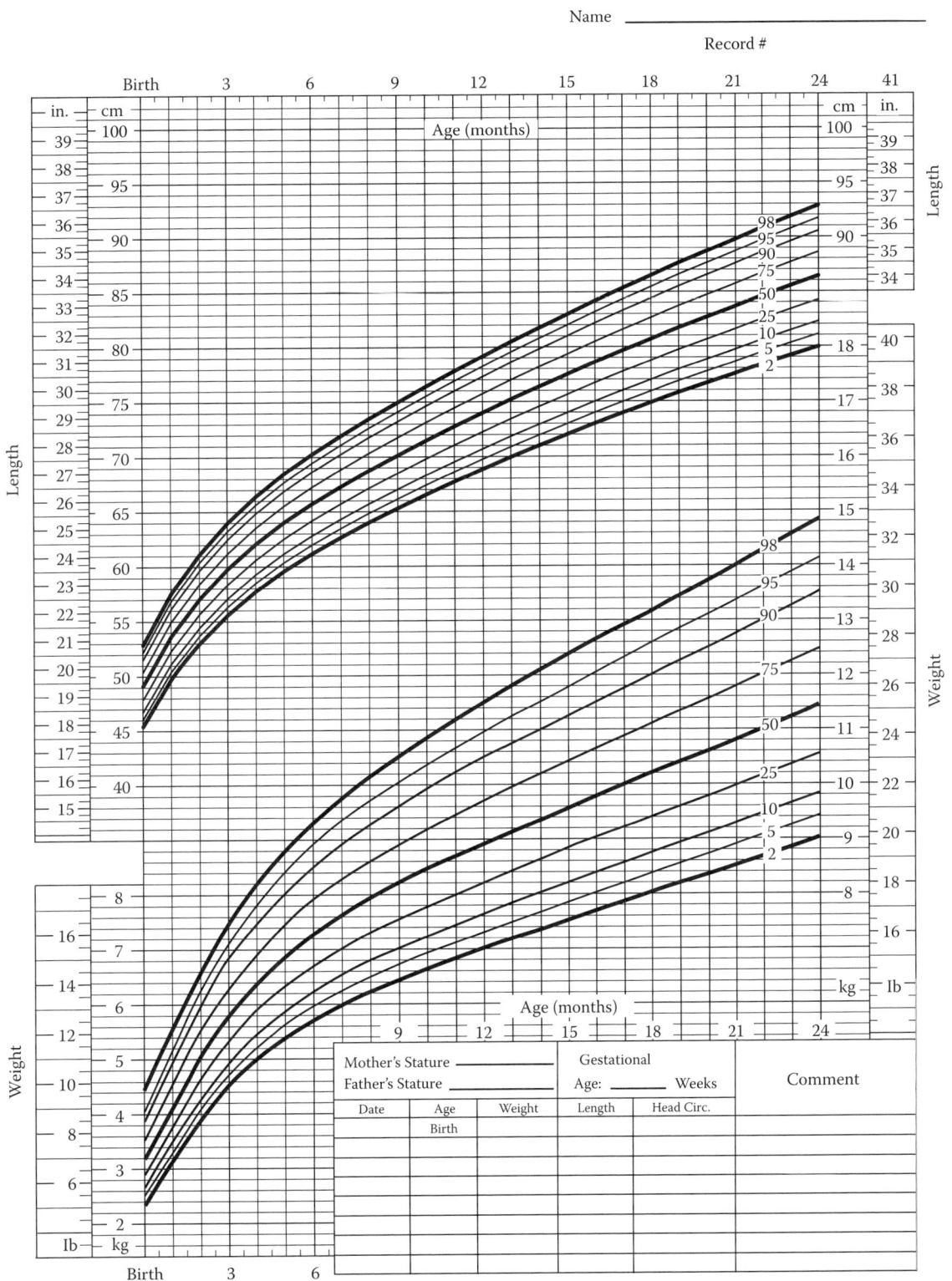

**FIGURE 38.4** Length-for-age and weight-for-age percentiles: Girls, birth to 24 months. (Published by the Centers for Disease Control and Prevention, November 1, 2009, and publicly available at http://www.cdc.gov/growthcharts/who_charts.htm; WHO Child Growth Standards, Geneva, Switzerland, http://www.who.int/childgrowth/en).

**TABLE 38.1**

**Growth Indicator Thresholds Used during Child Growth Monitoring**

| Nutritional Status Indicator | Age < 2 Years | | Age ≥ 2 Years | |
| --- | --- | --- | --- | --- |
| | Growth Indicator | Definition | Growth Indicator | Definition |
| Short stature | 2006 WHO/CDC length-for-age percentile | <2nd percentile | 2000 CDC height-for-age percentile | <5th percentile |
| Underweight | 2006 WHO/CDC weight-for-length percentile | <2nd percentile | 2000 CDC BMI-for-age percentile | <5th percentile |
| Overweight | NA | NA | 2000 CDC BMI-for-age percentile | ≥85th to <95th percentile |
| Obese | 2006 WHO/CDC weight-for-length percentile | >98th percentile | 2000 CDC BMI-for-age percentile | ≥95th percentile |

To evaluate weight in children 2–20 years of age, the CDC recommends use of the CDC 2000 growth charts for boys and girls (Figure 38.3 for boys and Figure 38.4 for girls). These charts, although essentially descriptive as in the case of the stature charts, did remove weight data from children aged 6 years and older who were seen in the NHANES III survey (conducted 1988–1994) so that the increase in child obesity prevalence seen at that time did not lead to inappropriately high weight-for-age, weight-for-length, and BMI-for-age percentile values. This means the prevalence of high weight-for-age overweight should be correctly estimated using the CDC 2000 charts.

To evaluate weight in infants 0–2 years of age, the CDC recommends use of the 2006 WHO weight-for-age percentiles, which are presented on the same charts as the 2006 WHO length-for-age percentiles discussed previously (Figure 38.5 for boys and Figure 38.6 for girls). Due to the differences in weight gain of breast milk- and formula-fed infants, clinicians should be aware that there are differences in the rate of low weight for age and high weight for length obtained using the two growth charts. A comparison is provided in Figure 38.7.

## Interpretation of Weight Measurements

As with length, body weight and patterns of weight gain and adiposity in childhood are the result of gene–environment interactions. A child's genotype reflects the genetic variants inherited from his or her parents. Expressed growth phenotypes are both heavily influenced by genotype and by environmental factors such as diet and physical activity. Most children gravitate toward a specific percentile curve of the standard weight charts during the first few years of life. However, in the present situation of increasing prevalence of childhood obesity in the United States, it is not uncommon for children's weights to gradually cross upward across percentiles, rather than maintaining a consistent percentile position relative to their peers. It is recommended that body weight, height, and calculated BMI values all be monitored carefully during routine health supervision so that children and adolescents who begin to deviate from normal growth patterns may receive further evaluation and treatment.

Children's weight percentile may be similar to their height percentile, or may be somewhat above or below and still be "normal" or healthy if their BMI is below the 85th percentile for age, which indicates overweight status (see as follows). It is important to recognize that at the upper height percentiles, just because weight percentile is similar to the height percentile does not mean that BMI will necessarily be within the normal range.

Healthy children who consistently track along the lower weight percentiles throughout childhood are considered normal if their weight is proportional to their height (close to the same percentile) and consistent with parental heights and weights. Thus, the most important indicator of adequate growth is that the child is following a consistent growth pattern in weight and height, similar to their previous growth centile curves.

Significant deviation from their previous pattern of weight gain requires additional monitoring and nutritional and medical assessment. Children whose weight percentile declines across 1–2 percentile lines and children who lose weight or do not gain any weight between scheduled growth assessments (except in the case of overweight children on medically supervised treatment) should be medically evaluated to determine the cause. Poor weight gain or unexplained weight loss may reflect inadequate nutrition, an eating disorder, an underlying disease affecting a major organ system, depression, or the presence of other conditions.

Overweight children who are placed on medically supervised treatment to either slow the rate of weight gain or lose weight should be carefully monitored to ensure adequate intake of (1) essential nutrients through a balanced calorie-controlled diet and (2) calories to maintain linear growth throughout treatment.

## BODY MASS INDEX

BMI (weight/height$^2$) provides a guideline based on weight and height to determine underweight or overweight status. BMI is not an exact measure of fatness because levels of fatness vary among children at a given BMI. This is so because BMI reflects (1) frame size, (2) leg length, and (3) the amount of lean and fat tissue, all of which are affected by maturational status. Although BMI correlates less well with the percent of body weight that is fat than more direct measures of fat such as triceps skinfold thickness or other body composition techniques, the readily available weight and height data make BMI a more useful tool for clinical assessment of overweight or underweight.

BMI in children and adolescents compares well with laboratory measurements of body fat, particularly at higher

CDC Growth Charts: United States

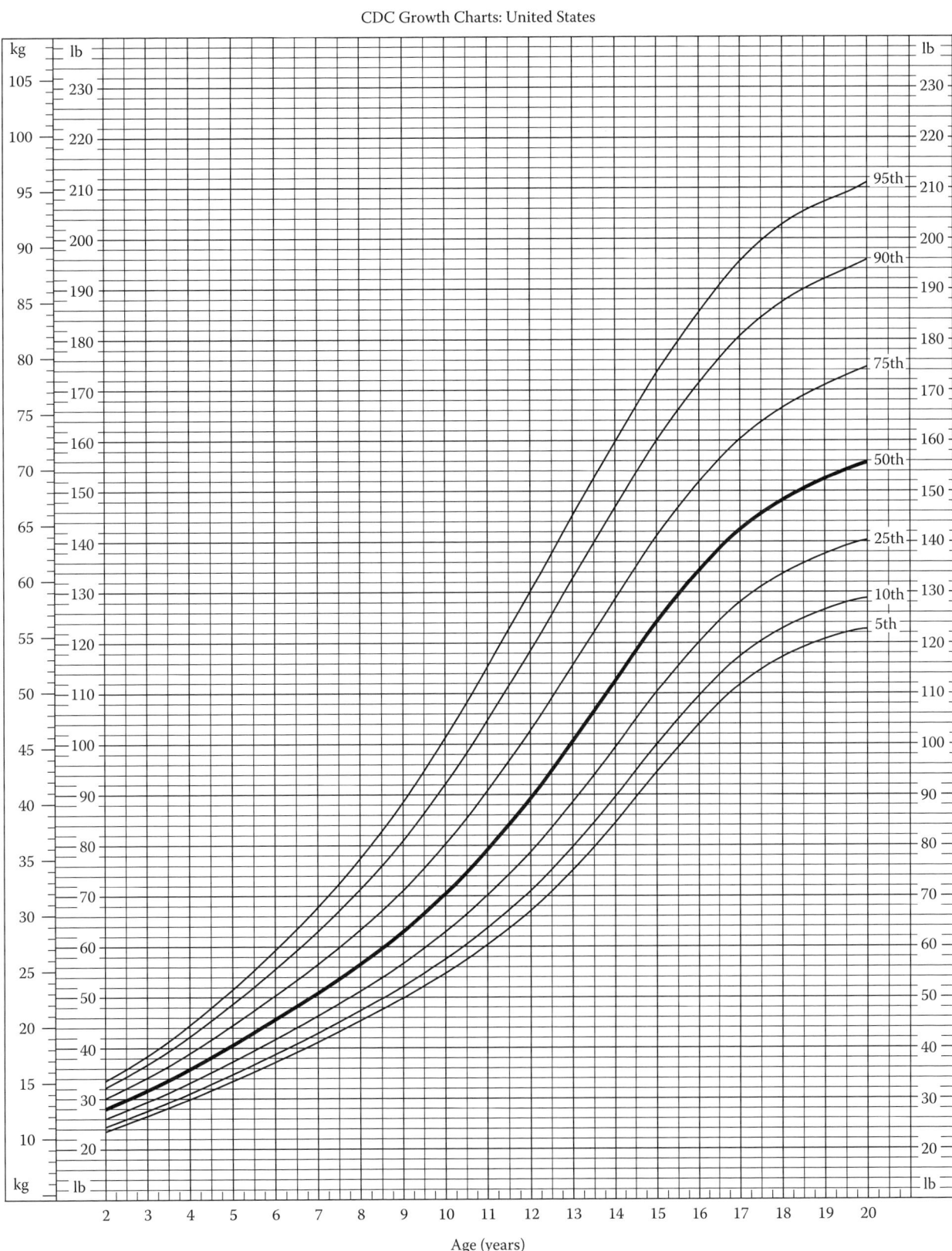

**FIGURE 38.5** Weight-for-age percentiles: Boys, 2 to 20 years. (Developed by the National Center for Health Statistics in collaboration with the National Center for Chronic Disease Prevention and Health Promotion, Hyattsville, MD. May 30, 2000, and publicly available at http://www.cdc.gov/growthcharts/clinical_charts.htm).

CDC Growth Charts: United States

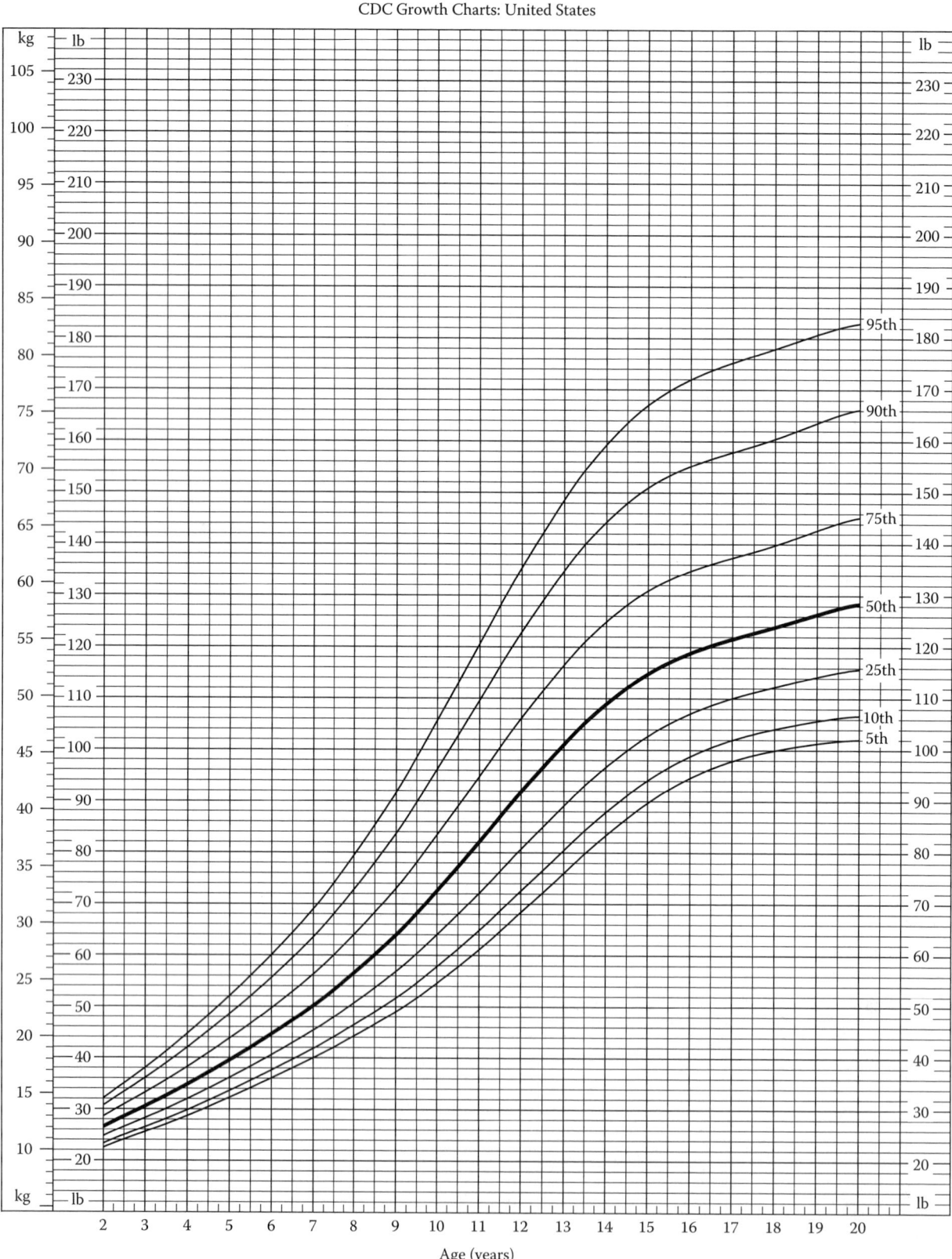

Age (years)

**FIGURE 38.6**  Weight-for-age percentiles: Girls, 2 to 20 years. (Developed by the National Center for Health Statistics in collaboration with the National Center for Chronic Disease Prevention and Health Promotion, Hyattsville, MD. May 30, 2000, and publicly available at http://www.cdc.gov/growthcharts/clinical_charts.htm).

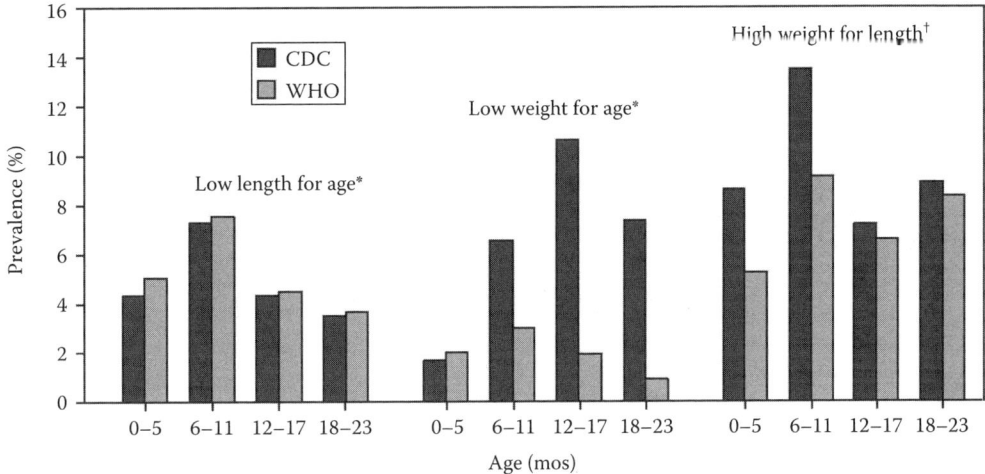

**FIGURE 38.7** Comparison of WHO and CDC growth chart prevalences of low length for age, low weight for age, and high weight for length among children aged <24 months—United States, 1999–2004. * ≤5th percentile shown on the CDC charts; ≤2nd percentile shown on the WHO charts. † ≥95th percentile shown on the CDC charts; ≥98th percentile shown on the WHO charts. (Data from National Health and Nutrition Examination Survey, 1999–2004; Center for Disease Control and Prevention, Use of the World Health Organization and CDC growth charts for children aged 0–59 months in the United States, *MMWR*, 59(No. RR-9), 1, 2010.)

percentile values. Children and adolescents with a BMI for age above the 95th percentile are classified as obese. This threshold is used because BMI above the 95th percentile (1) reflects increased adiposity, (2) is consistent across age groups, and (3) is predictive of morbidity.

The percentage of children and adolescents who are obese in the United States has more than tripled since the 1960s, and the sharpest increase has occurred since the late 1980s. In the United States in 2009–2010, 12.1% of 2–5-year-old children, 18.0% of 6–11-year-old children, and 18.4% of youth 12–19 years of age were obese, and an additional 17% or more of children 2–19 years were overweight. Rates vary by ethnicity, with African American girls and Hispanic American boys at particularly high risk.

The rationale for using pediatric BMI classification is based on studies indicating that BMI is related to health risks. Overweight children are likely to become overweight adults, with risk increasing with severity and duration of the problem. Sixty percent of youth with a BMI for age above the 95th percentile have at least one risk factor for cardiovascular disease, while 20% have two or more risk factors. High blood pressure, abnormal blood lipid levels (elevated total cholesterol, low-density lipoprotein [LDL] cholesterol, and/or triglycerides and low levels high-density lipoprotein [HDL] cholesterol), insulin resistance, and type II diabetes mellitus are some of the risk factors observed in obese children and adolescents. Overweight and obese children are at increased risk of a wide range of other medical and psychological problems. Obese girls are also more likely to have earlier onset of menarche (first menses).

## AVERAGE PATTERNS OF BMI DURING CHILDHOOD AND ADOLESCENCE

BMI increases rapidly during the first year of life, reaching a maximum around 9 months of age, and then decreases to its lowest value on average between 4 and 6 years of age.

After reaching this nadir, BMI again begins a slow increase throughout the rest of childhood and adolescence. The upward shift of the BMI curve, after reaching the lowest point, has been termed "adiposity rebound." Studies suggest that children who begin their adiposity rebound earlier than average are at greater risk for later obesity.

## MEASUREMENT OF BMI

BMI, also known as the weight–height index or Quetelet index, is calculated as the quotient of weight divided by height squared: The *English formula* (in inches and pounds) is as follows:

$$BMI = Weight\,(lb) \div Stature\,(in.) \div Stature\,(in.) \times 703$$

The *metric formula* (in centimeters and kilograms) is as follows:

$$BMI = Weight\,(kg) \div Stature\,(cm) \times Stature\,(cm) \times 10,000$$

To use the English formula, it is necessary to convert ounces (for weight) and fractional inches (for height) to decimal values, using Table 38.2.

## TABLE 38.2
### Conversion of Fractional Inches and Ounces to Decimal Values to Allow Calculation of BMI

| Fraction (Height) | Ounces (Weight) | Decimal Value |
|---|---|---|
| 1/8 | 2 | 0.125 |
| 1/4 | 4 | 0.25 |
| 3/8 | 6 | 0.375 |
| 1/2 | 8 | 0.5 |
| 5/8 | 10 | 0.625 |
| 3/4 | 12 | 0.75 |
| 7/8 | 14 | 0.875 |

CDC Growth Charts: United States

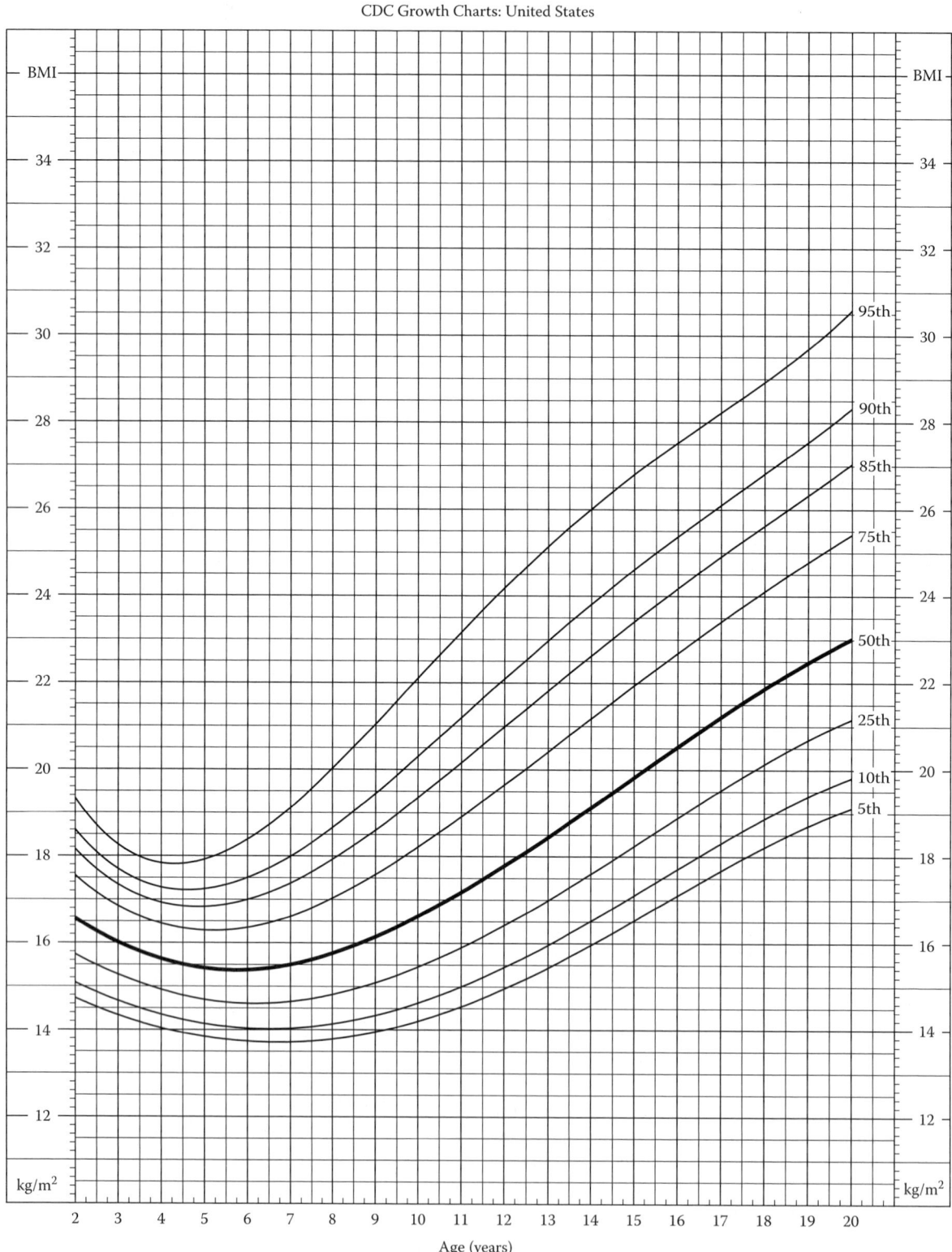

**FIGURE 38.8** Body mass index-for-age percentiles: Boys, 2 to 20 years. (Developed by the National Center for Health Statistics in collaboration with the National Center for Chronic Disease Prevention and Health Promotion, Hyattsville, MD. May 30, 2000, and publicly available at http://www.cdc.gov/growthcharts/clinical_charts.htm).

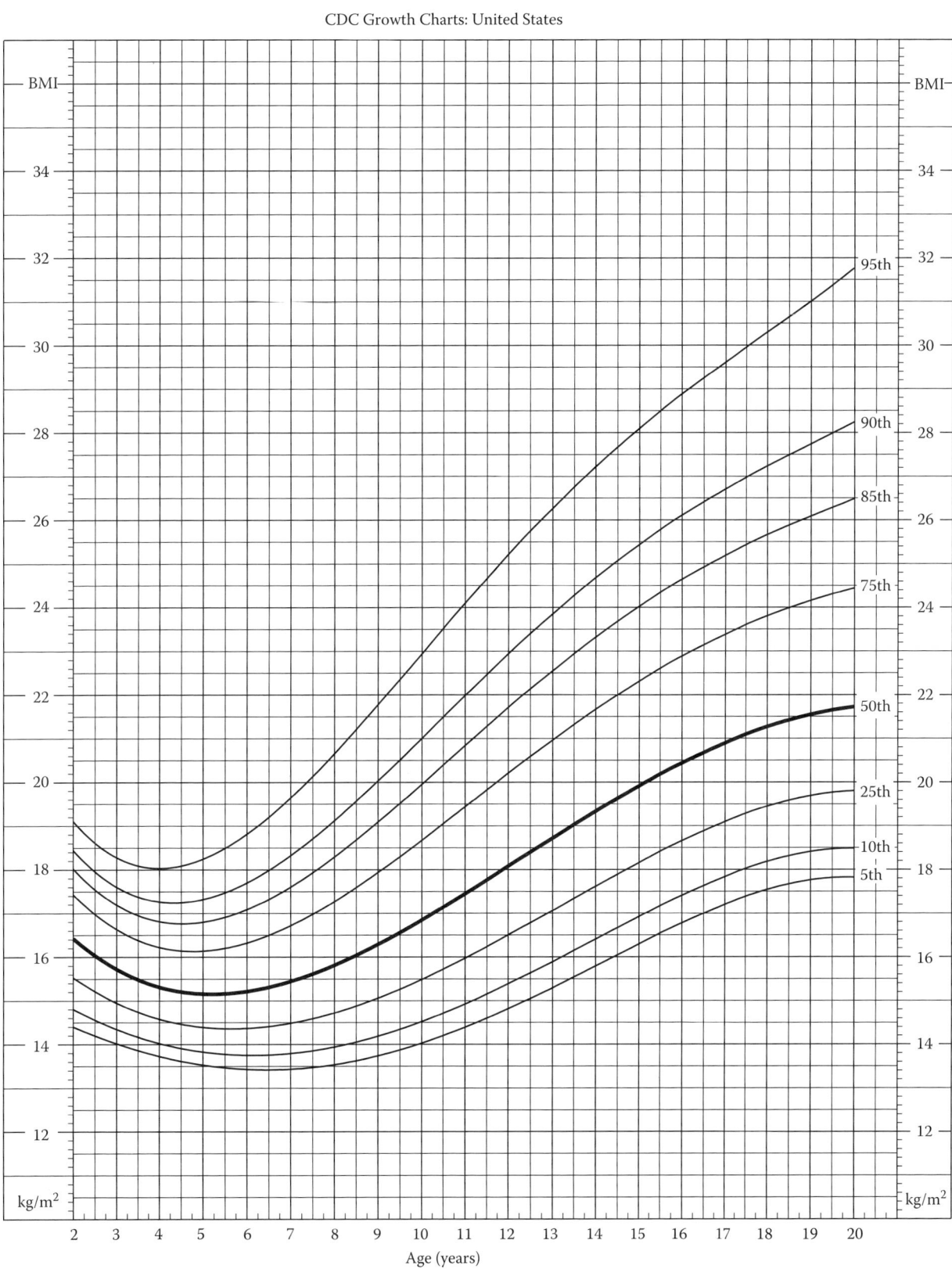

CDC Growth Charts: United States

**FIGURE 38.9** Body mass index-for-age percentiles: Girls, 2 to 20 years. (Developed by the National Center for Health Statistics in collaboration with the National Center for Chronic Disease Prevention and Health Promotion, Hyattsville, MD. May 30, 2000, and publicly available at http://www.cdc.gov/growthcharts/clinical_charts.htm).

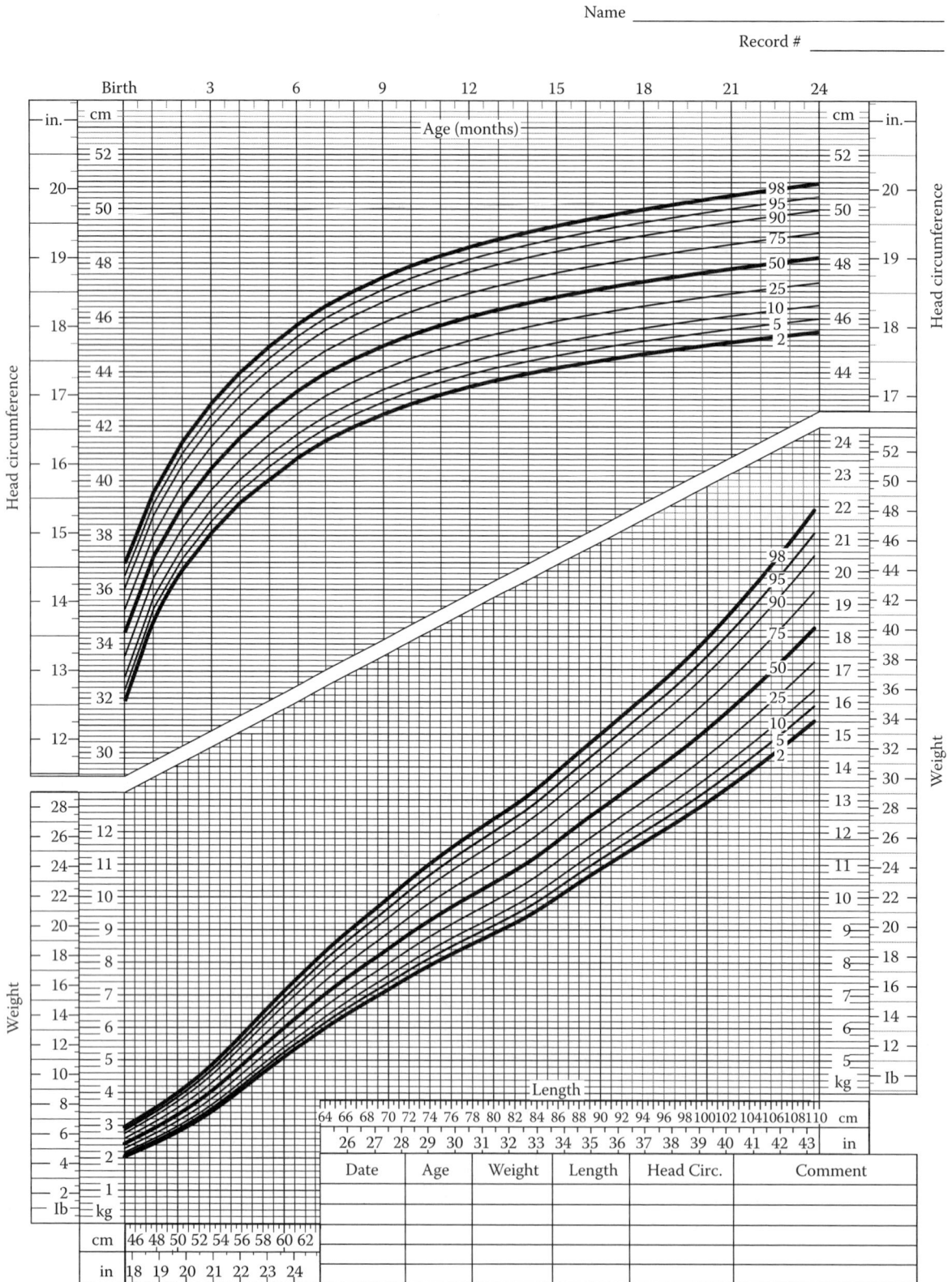

**FIGURE 38.10** Head circumference-for-age and weight-for-length percentiles: Boys, birth to 24 months. (Published by the Centers for Disease Control and Prevention, November 1, 2009 and publicly available at http://www.cdc.gov/growthcharts/who_charts.htm; WHO Child Growth Standards, Geneva, Switzerland, http://www.who.int/childgrowth/en).

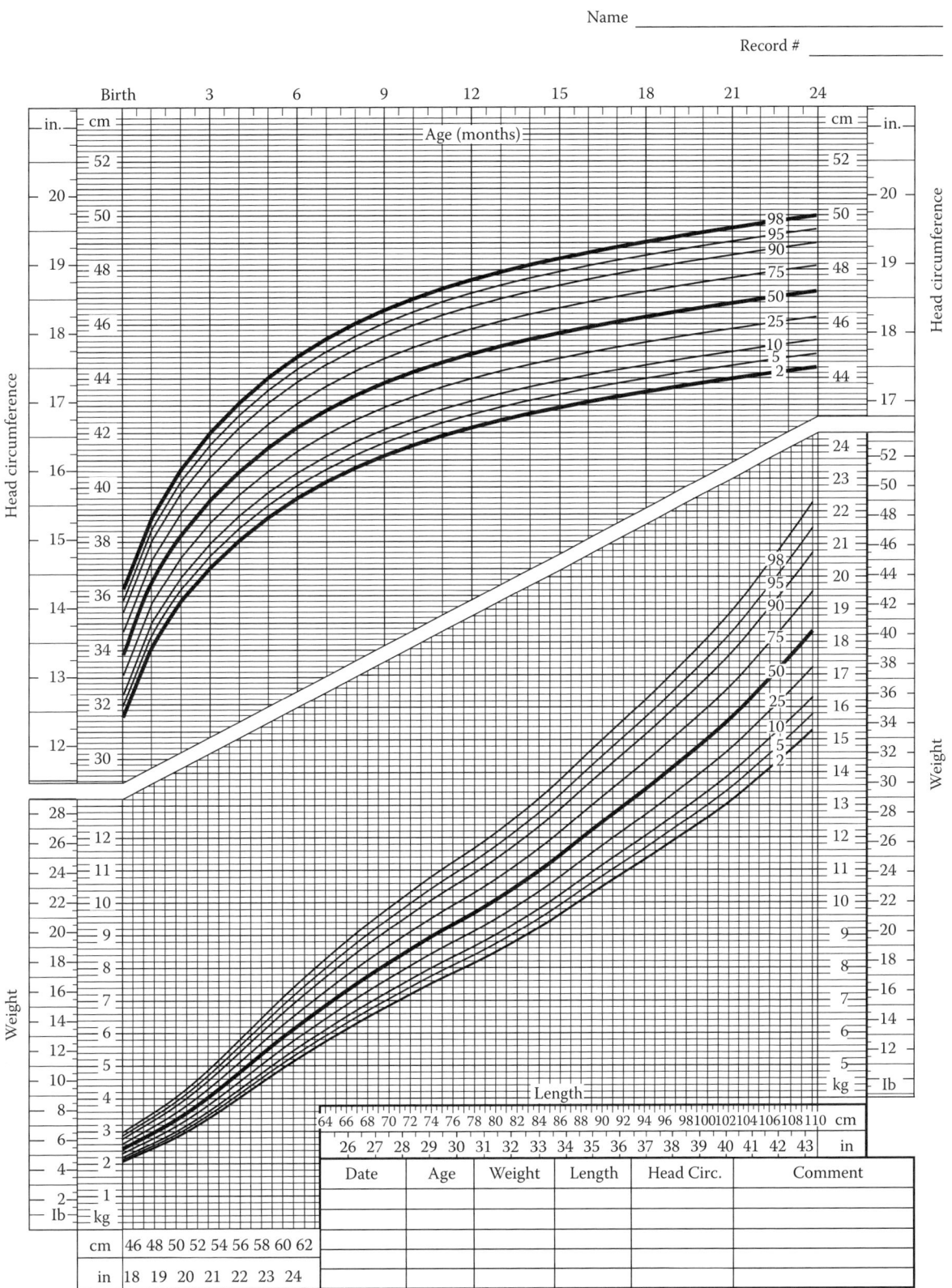

**FIGURE 38.11** Head circumference-for-age and weight-for-length percentiles: Girls, birth to 24 months. (Published by the Centers for Disease Control and Prevention, November 1, 2009, and publicly available at http://www.cdc.gov/growthcharts/who_charts.htm; WHO Child Growth Standards, Geneva, Switzerland, http://www.who.int/childgrowth/en).

## REFERENCE CHARTS FOR BMI AND WEIGHT FOR LENGTH

The CDC has published BMI-for-age charts: one for boys, ages 2–20 years, and another for girls, 2–20 years of age (Figure 38.8 for boys and Figure 38.9 for girls). These charts may be downloaded from the CDC website: http://www. cdc.gov/growthcharts. In addition, numerous BMI calculation tools and educational resources may also be downloaded at http://www.cdc.gov/nccdphp/dnpao/growthcharts/ resources/index.htm. Clinicians can avoid having to calculate BMI values by using an extensive set of tables covering heights from 29 to 78 in. and weights from 18 to 250 lb at this site as well.

With the earlier onset of obesity in children today, there is increasing interest in the timing of infant peak BMI, which may presage early adiposity rebound. Although WHO 2006 charts did produce BMI charts from birth, the CDC does not currently recommend using BMI during infancy to assess relative weight or adiposity. For infants 0–2 years old, the WHO 2006 weight-for-length percentile charts should be used (Figures 38.10 and 38.11).

## INTERPRETATION OF BMI VALUES

Unlike adult BMI, BMI during childhood changes rapidly during growth and development, and for this reason, there is no one particular BMI value defining overweight and obese. Interpretation of BMI depends on the sex and age of the child, as boys and girls differ in their body fatness as they mature. Therefore, BMI is plotted on age- and sex-specific charts. Established cutoff points are used to identify infants and children who are underweight or overweight as indicated in Table 38.1.

## SUMMARY

Monitoring child growth in height, weight, and BMI using appropriate growth charts is a central part of preventive medicine. Growth charts are not intended to be the sole diagnostic instrument for the assessment of nutritional status but are important tools that contribute to forming an overall clinical impression of child health.

## FURTHER READING

Argyle J. Approaches to detecting growth faltering in infancy and childhood. *Ann Hum Biol* 2003; 30(5): 499–519.

Barlow SE and the Expert Committee. Expert committee recommendations regarding the prevention, assessment, and treatment of child and adolescent overweight and obesity: Summary report. *Pediatrics* 2007; 120(Supplement December 2007): S164–S192.

Center for Disease Control and Prevention, Use of the World Health Organization and CDC growth charts for children aged 0–59 months in the United States, *MMWR* 2010; 59(No. RR-9): 1.

Cole TJ. The LMS method for constructing normalized growth standards. *Eur J Clin Nutr* 1990 January; 44(1): 45–60.

de Onis M, Garza C, Victora CG, Onyango AW, Frongillo EA, Martines J. For the WHO multicentre growth reference study group. The WHO multicentre growth reference study: Planning, study design, and methodology. *Food Nutr Bull* 2004; 25(Suppl 1): S15–S26.

Dewey KG. Growth characteristics of breast-fed compared to formula-fed infants. *Biol Neonate* 1998; 74(2): 94–105.

Dietz WH. Health consequences of obesity in youth: Childhood predictors of adult disease. *Pediatrics* 1998; 101: 518–525.

Dietz WH, Bellizzi MC. Introduction: The use of BMI to assess obesity in children. *Am J Clin Nutr* 1999; 70(Suppl): 123s–125s.

Freedman DS, Mei Z, Srinivasan SR, Berenson GS, Dietz WH. Cardiovascular risk factors and excess adiposity among overweight children and adolescents: The Bogalusa Heart Study. *J Pediatr* 2007; 150(1): 12.e2–17.e2.

Guo SS, Chumlea WC. Tracking of BMI In children in relation to overweight in adulthood. *Am J Clin Nutr* 1999; 70(Suppl): 145s–148s.

Guo SS, Chumlea WC, Roche AF et al. The predictive value of childhood BMI values for overweight at age 35 years. *Am J Clin Nutr* 1994; 59: 810–819.

Guo SS, Khoury PR, Sprecker B. Prediction of fat-free mass in black and white preadolescent girls from anthropometry and impedance. *Am J Human Biol* 1993; 5: 735–745.

Gutin B, Basch C, Shea S et al. Blood pressure, fitness, and fatness in 5- and 6-year-old children. *JAMA* 1990; 264: 1123–1127.

Himes JH, Deitz WH. Guidelines for overweight in adolescent preventive services: Recommendations from an expert committee. *Am J Clin Nutr* 1994; 59: 307–316.

Kuczmarski RJ, Ogden CL, Grummer-Strawn LM et al. *CDC Growth Charts: United States. Advance Data from Vital Statistics; No. 314.* National Center for Health Statistics, Hyattsville, MD, 2000.

Kuczmarski RJ, Ogden CL, Guo SS et al. 2000 CDC growth charts for the United States: Methods and development. *Vital Health Stat* 2002; 11(246): 1–190.

Lazarus R, Baur L, Webb K et al. BMI in screening for adiposity in children and adolescents: Systematic evaluation using receiver operator curves. *Am J Clin Nutr* 1996; 63: 500–506.

Mei Z, Grummer-Strawn LM, Thompson D, Dietz WH. Shifts in percentiles of growth during early childhood: Analysis of longitudinal data from the California Child Health and Development Study. *Pediatrics* 2004 June; 113(6): e617–e27.

Mei Z, Ogden CL, Flegal KM, Grummer-Strawn LM. Comparison of the prevalence of shortness, underweight, and overweight among US children aged 0 to 59 months by using the CDC 2000 and the WHO 2006 growth charts. *J Pediatr* 2008; 153(5): 622–628.

Morrison JA, Payne G, Barton BA, Khoury PR, Crawford P. Mother-daughter correlations of obesity and cardiovascular disease risk factors in black and white households: the NHLBI Growth and Health Study. *AJPH* 1994; 84: 1761–1767.

Ogden CL, Carroll MD, Kit BK, Flegal KM. *Prevalence of Obesity in the United States, 2009–2010. NCHS Data Brief, No. 82.* National Center for Health Statistics, Hyattsville, MD, 2012.

Ogden CL, Kuczmarski RJ, Flegal KM et al. Centers for disease control and prevention 2000 growth charts for the United States: Improvements to the 1977 national center for health statistics version. *Pediatrics* 2002; 109: 45–60.

Pietrobelli A, Faith M, Allison DB, Gallagher D, Chiumello G, Heymsfeld SB. Body mass index as a measure of adiposity among children and adolescents: A validation study. *J Pediatr* 1998; 132: 204–210.

Rames LK, Clark WR, Connor WE et al. Normal blood pressures and the evaluation of sustained blood pressure elevation in childhood: The Muscatine study. *Pediatrics* 1978; 61: 245–251.

Rosenbloom ST, Qi X, Riddle WR, Russell WE, DonLevy SC, Giuse D, Sedman AB, Spooner SA. Implementing pediatric growth charts into an electronic health record system. *J Am Med Inform Assoc* 2006 May–June; 13 (3): 302–308. Epub 2006 February 24.

Serdula MK, Ivery D, Coates RJ, Freedman DS. Williamson DF. Byers T. Do obese children become obese adults? A review of the literature. *Prev Med* 1993; 22: 167–177.

Sutherland ER. Obesity and asthma. *Immunol Allergy Clin North Am* 2008, 28 (3). 589–602, ix.

Taylor ED, Theim KR, Mirch MC et al. Orthopedic complications of overweight in children and adolescents. *Pediatrics* June 2006; 117(6): 2167–2174.

Whitaker RC, Pepe MS, Wright JA, Seidel KD, Dietz WH. Early adiposity rebound and the risk of adult obesity. *Pediatrics* 1998; 101(3): E5. http://www.pediatrics.org/cgi/content,/full/101-3/e5

Whitlock EP, Williams SB, Gold R, Smith PR, Shipman SA. Screening and interventions for childhood overweight: A summary of evidence for the US Preventive Services Task Force. *Pediatrics* 2005; 116(1): e125–e144.

WHO Multicentre Growth Reference Study Group. WHO child growth standards based on length/height, weight and age. *Acta Paediatr Suppl* 2006 April; 450: 76–85.

# 39 Frame Size, Circumferences, and Skinfolds

*Barbara J. Scott*

## CONTENTS

## INTRODUCTION

Numerous studies conducted over the past 85+ years provide a large body of evidence that simple methods of quantifying body size and proportions can be used with different populations to estimate and evaluate weight, body composition, and regional fat distribution. Applications for these measurements include monitoring of normal growth and development, evaluating response to treatment, and assessing disease risk. This chapter will discuss the strengths and weaknesses and potential best applications of three field anthropometric methods: frame size (FS), skinfolds (SFs), and circumferences. These methods have been widely studied and yield valid and reliable results when applied correctly. They are noninvasive, inexpensive, portable, and relatively simple to perform.

### APPLICATIONS TO PRACTICE

Applications for measurement and analysis of body composition and body dimensions using these methods include the following:

- *Surveillance*: evaluating how individuals or groups are faring in general or in response to public health efforts and changing economic or political situations (e.g., new leadership, prolonged drought or famine, war, changes in expenditures for health services, increase in number of individuals or families living in poverty, and increased cost of food)
- *Treatment efficacy*: monitoring individual response to specific therapeutic interventions (changes in diet and activity, surgery, medication, chemotherapy)

- *Assessment*: making comparisons of actual weight and body composition with "ideal"
- *Diet and lifestyle prescription*: formulating exercise or dietary programs/regimens
- *Treatment risk assessment*: providing prognostic indicators in certain disease states linked to body composition (diabetes, certain types of cancer, osteoporosis, cystic fibrosis, HIV/AIDS)
- *Outcomes evaluation*: providing periodic feedback regarding achievement of goals resulting from lifestyle modifications (diet, exercise, smoking cessation)
- *Disease risk assessment*: for chronic disease (cardiovascular, cancer, diabetes, osteoporosis) and monitoring relative risk over time

Precise methods for measuring body composition, such as computed tomography (CT), magnetic resonance imaging (MRI), and dual-energy x-ray absorptiometry (DEXA), are becoming more widely available in many clinical and research settings. The purpose of this chapter is to discuss indirect field methods that use circumferences and SFs. While these measures tend to be less precise, they will still be needed and used when other methods are too expensive or impractical. In reality, decisions regarding which measures to use are based most often on what is practical given the considerations of cost, availability of equipment, staff (number of personnel and expertise), and portability. The degree of precision needed will also guide selection of methods to be used. While field methods tend to be less precise, they may be acceptable if the focus is on generalized risk assessment or documenting change in a diet or exercise program. More precise methods will be desired if the information is needed for establishing health policy or making clinical decisions about disease treatment or prognosis. Ongoing research to develop more accurate reference methods to validate or refine equations for SF, FS, and circumference measurements with different populations will provide clinicians with the necessary information and tools to continue using these practical methods with confidence.

There appears to be greater standardization of methodology in many of the body composition validation studies done over the past decade with greater adherence to and more detailed documentation of use of commonly accepted measurement protocols, inclusion of both a test and a validation sample in the study design, and use of similar statistical methods to examine results. With regard to the analysis of results, more studies are using what has become known as the Bland–Altman method, whereby agreement between measurements is examined using a plot of the difference between methods against their mean.[1] This standardization of analytical design should be helpful to clinicians and field researchers as they make decisions as to selection of the best methods to use in practice. Similarly, reporting of precision and accuracy of measurements using the technical error of measurement will enhance this body of research.[2]

## APPLICATION TO DIFFERENT POPULATIONS

Many variables have been found to affect the validity of measurements of body composition including age, gender, ethnicity, measurement site selection, weight status, and health status.[3] Therefore, it is imperative that methods selected are those that are best suited to the persons or population being measured or studied. Depending on the setting and application, it may be necessary to use different methods and different anatomical sites or to apply different equations to the same methods. This is particularly critical because the population in the United States and other countries has become more overweight and more ethnically diverse and more people are living to be very old. Indeed, because so many of the long-standing prediction equations were developed on very homogenous samples, the preponderance of recent studies has been done to examine the validity of these existing prediction equations on specific population groups of interest (children, elderly, pregnant, overweight or obese persons, dialysis patients, Hispanic adults, etc.). Studies have been selected for summarization in this chapter to represent these diverse populations.

## VALIDATION OF FIELD METHODS
## AGAINST "GOLD STANDARDS"

Many different methods have been employed over the past decades to measure the composition of the human body,[4] and new technologic developments and findings from validation studies both inform and complicate decisions about which method(s) to select for a given purpose. A primary consideration in the selection of a method is whether it can provide valid information for the specific application and population of interest. Many different statistical tests have been employed to compare body composition derived from

experimental or indirect methods (predictor variables) with those from a direct method or a reference standard method (dependent or outcome variables). These include analysis of variance (examining differences), correlation coefficients (examining similarities), standard error, coefficient of variation (examining the size of the standard deviation relative to the mean [focusing on variability]), level of bias (difference between the "gold standard" and experimental measure), regression analyses (examining the unique and additive contributions of different measures in improving the predictive power of body composition equations), intra- and interobserver variance, and the Bland–Altman method mentioned earlier. Development of greater consensus and understanding by researchers regarding statistical methods for comparing clinical measurement methods and reporting results is adding clarity to this body of knowledge.

From a practical standpoint, there is no one perfect method to use to measure and find the true value for body composition in living humans. However, the more body compartments that can be directly measured, the greater is the accuracy. Conversely, the fewer compartments that are measured and the more assumptions that have to be made, the less is the accuracy because the assumptions are often violated due to wide variations in hydration and bone mineral content (BMC) between people who differ by age, gender, ethnicity, or health status.

There appears to be consensus that a four-compartment model (body density, total body water, bone mineral mass, and residual nonbone mineral and protein) for body composition is an excellent standard against which to compare and validate other methods. However, because the four-compartment model uses a variety of methods to independently estimate body fat (BF) (hydrostatic weighing, deuterium oxide dilution, and DEXA), it is not practical to perform on a large number of subjects. Therefore, use of the DEXA (that employs a three-compartment body composition model that directly measures fat mass, lean mass, and bone[5]) is gaining acceptance as a practical reference model. It has essentially replaced hydrostatic weighing (employing a two-compartment model that divides body composition into fat and fat-free components and assumes constant densities for these tissues that are not universally applicable[4]) as the measurement against which the majority of field measures of FS, circumferences, and SFs are now being evaluated. DEXA measures are currently included in the periodic National Health and Nutrition Examination Survey (NHANES) studies, providing current information for comparison of field methods with population norms. However, while the DEXA technology is easier and more convenient for the operator and subject, it has a number of limitations[6]: The software used to interpret results relies on and uses assumptions about levels of hydration, potassium content, and tissue density, and these assumptions may vary by manufacturer. The machines must be routinely calibrated, they utilize different scan types (pencil or fan), and they impose physical limitations on the size (weight, length, thickness) of individuals to be scanned. Therefore, ideally it is wise not to rely on a single method but rather to use multiple methods whenever possible to simultaneously measure the different body compartments to establish and/or validate field methods on diverse populations.[7]

Direct methods used in recent studies to examine amount and location (subcutaneous vs. intra-abdominal) of central BF as a risk factor for cardiovascular disease (CVD) include CT (CAT scan) and MRI. Additional methods of body composition analysis that have been used in recent studies to validate or compare results from field methods include bioelectrical impedance analysis (BIA) and air displacement plethysmography (ADP) (the "BOD POD").

## MEASUREMENT ERROR

Once a field method has been selected as appropriate to the application at hand, adherence to guidelines for achieving acceptable levels of measurement error[8,9] is needed to ensure the quality of data collected (see Table 39.1).

Guidelines for training and certification of measurement staff direct a repeated-measures protocol where the trainee and trainer measure the same subjects until the difference between them is very small. However, the definition or description of "small difference" is constrained to some extent by the technique (how precise it can be), by the equipment (how exactly it can be calibrated, how fine the scale is),

## TABLE 39.1
### Data Quality and Anthropometric Measurement Error

| Goal of Quality Measurement | Terminology, Definitions, and Causes or Contributing Factors |
|---|---|
| Repeated measures give the same value | *Reliability*: Differences between measures on a single subject (within-subject variability) are not caused by errors in measurement (site or technique) or physiologic variation. |
| | *Imprecision*: Different results are obtained for a single subject when measurements are done either by one person (intraobserver differences) or two or more persons (interobserver differences) and reflect measurement errors. |
| | *Undependability*: Different results are due to physiologic factors (such as differences over the course of a day in weight [due to weight of food eaten or fullness of the bladder] or height [due to compression of the spine]). |
| | *Unreliability*: The sum of errors due to imprecision and undependability. |
| Measurement represents a "true" value | *Inaccuracy*: A systematic bias is present due to instrument errors or errors of measurement technique. |
| | *Validity*: Measurement is as close to the true value as it is possible to determine. |

*Sources:* Ulijaszek, S.J. and Kerr, D.A., *Br. J. Nutr.*, 82, 165, 1999; Nordhamm, K. et al., *Int. J. Obes.*, 24, 652, 2000.

## TABLE 39.2
### Recommendations for Evaluating Measurement Differences between Trainer and Trainee

| Measurement | Difference between Trainer and Trainee | | | |
|---|---|---|---|---|
| | Good | Fair | Poor | Gross Error |
| Height (length) (cm) | 0–0.5 | 0.6–0.9 | 1.0–1.9 | 2.0 or > |
| Weight (kg) | 0–0.1 | 0.2 | 0.3–0.4 | 0.5 or > |
| Arm circumference (cm) | 0–0.5 | 0.6–0.9 | 1.0–1.9 | 2.0 or > |
| SFs (any) (mm) | 0–0.9 | 1.0–1.9 | 2.0–4.9 | 5.0 or > |

and by the magnitude of the potential size of the measurement itself (measured in many centimeters such as height vs. in few millimeters such as some SFs).

Some targets for difference to be achieved that are acceptably small to certify competency have been proposed (Table 39.2).[10] Given the limits of what level of accuracy is possible, investigators must also be aware of the proportion of the total measurement that is represented by the acceptable difference.[11]

## METHODS

Even though literally hundreds of anthropometric studies have been done comparing methods and developing predictive equations,[12] there is neither clear evidence nor scientific consensus as to which methods, sites, or equations should be used. Thus, best practice is to select a method with a preponderance of supporting evidence for the specific setting, population, and application, use good equipment, train staff well, understand the limitations, and be able to interpret the results within these limitations. Specific instructions for taking measurements or locating anatomical sites will not be covered in this chapter because excellent detailed anthropometric manuals are available.[13–15]

Once a method and site(s) of measurement have been selected as appropriate to the purpose for which the information is needed, then the next steps include the "logistics" of selecting, calibrating, and using equipment and training and certifying staff in the actual measurement procedures.

## FRAME SIZE

It seems intuitive that it is fat weight that is unhealthy and that persons with larger frames (relatively more bone and more muscle and less fat) can weigh more and still be healthy. While there is general agreement that frame is a valid consideration in the assessment of weight for height, identifying an exact method for classifying FS has been problematic.[16] The literature includes a variety of different concepts of FS: body type and body proportions (length of trunk relative to total height), bone and skeletal size and thickness, and muscularity. There are two general "schools of thought" about frame: one that frame is primarily a skeletal concept and the other that it also encompasses the fat-free mass (FFM, everything that is not fat, including bone and muscle). Most researchers agree that a valid measure of frame must be independent of body fatness, while others believe that it must also be somewhat independent of height to be of value in the assessment of weight. However, studies have shown varying degrees of correlation of different measures of skeletal size and dimension with height (the linear dimension of the skeleton) and correlation of measures of both bone and muscle with body weight and fatness. Therefore, additional criteria for validity of FS measures have been proposed: (1) The correlation of the measure with FFM should be greater than the correlation of height alone with FFM and (2) the measure should have little or no association with BF beyond that accounted for by the association of FFM with fat.[17]

Others have proposed more generalized methods or observations for classifying frame according to body type or morphology. The categories of somatotypes (ectomorph, mesomorph, or endomorph) use the conceptualization of the human body as like a cylinder with its mass determined by height, breadth, and depth.

The main purpose for assessing FS is to evaluate weight and recommend an optimal weight that would be associated with the best state of health and longest life expectancy. One of the first proposed common uses of FS was with weight tables published by the Metropolitan Life Insurance Company in 1954 that were based on mortality rates of insured adults in the United States and Canada.[18] These early tables suggested "ideal" weights by gender and by ranges of height and FS

(small, medium, and large) but provided no method or instructions for assessing frame.[19] The tables were updated in 1983 and provided instructions for measuring elbow breadth (EB) and applying cutoffs for classifying FS using data from the U.S. NHANES (1971–1975) that were to result in approximately 50% of persons falling in medium frame and 25% in small and large frame categories, respectively (see Table 39.3).[20] When these cutoffs were subsequently tested on a large Canadian sample (n = 12,348 males and 6,957 females), they were found to classify only a small percent of the sample as having large frames thereby increasing the probability of misclassification into incorrect FS categories and consequent unrealistic weight recommendations.[21]

Practical evaluation of measures of FS is complicated by several factors including a lack of national reference standards for any measure except EB (see Table 39.4). Because FS cannot be directly measured by any single parameter, there is no "gold standard" by which to judge proposed surrogate measures. Neither is there consensus on how to assign cut points for categorizing small, medium, or large frames nor a standard upon which to base expectations of how FS is (or should be) distributed in a normal population. Different conceptualizations include the following:

- Distribution by percentiles
- Terciles (equal numbers in each of three frame categories)

**TABLE 39.3**
**Approximation of FS by 1983 Metropolitan Height and Weight Tables**

| Women | | Men | |
| --- | --- | --- | --- |
| Height (in.) in 1 in. Heels | EB (in.) | Height (in.) in 1 in. Heels | EB (in.) |
| 58–59 (4 ft 10 in.–4 ft 11 in.) | 2 1/4–2 1/2 | 62–63 (5 ft 2 in.–5 ft 3 in.) | 2 1/2–2 7/8 |
| 60–63 (5 ft 0 in.–5 ft 3 in.) | 2 1/4–2 1/2 | 64–67 (5 ft 4 in.–5 ft 7 in.) | 2 5/8–2 7/8 |
| 64–67 (5 ft 4 in.–5 ft 7 in.) | 2 3/8–2 5/8 | 68–71 (5 ft 8 in.–5 ft 11 in.) | 2 3/4–3 |
| 68–71 (5 ft 8 in.–5 ft 11 in.) | 2 3/8–2 5/8 | 72–75 (6 ft–6 ft 3 in.) | 2 3/4–3 1/8 |
| 72 (6 ft 0 in.) | 2 1/2–2 3/4 | 76 (6 ft 4 in.) | 2 7/8–3 1/4 |

**TABLE 39.4**
**FS by EB by Gender and Age**

| Age (Years) | Males | | | Females | | |
| --- | --- | --- | --- | --- | --- | --- |
| | Small Frame | Medium Frame | Large Frame | Small Frame | Medium Frame | Large Frame |
| 18–24 | ≤6.6 | >6.6 and <7.7 | ≥7.7 | ≤5.6 | >5.6 and <6.5 | ≥6.5 |
| 25–34 | ≤6.7 | >6.7 and <7.9 | ≥7.9 | ≤5.7 | >5.7 and <6.8 | ≥6.8 |
| 35–44 | ≤6.7 | >6.7 and <8.0 | ≥8.0 | ≤5.7 | >5.7 and <7.1 | ≥7.1 |
| 45–54 | ≤6.7 | >6.7 and <8.1 | ≥8.1 | ≤5.7 | >5.7 and <7.2 | ≥7.2 |
| 55–64 | ≤6.7 | >6.7 and <8.1 | ≥8.1 | ≤5.8 | >5.8 and <7.2 | ≥7.2 |
| 65–74 | ≤6.7 | >6.7 and <8.1 | ≥8.1 | ≤5.8 | >5.8 and <7.2 | ≥7.2 |

*Source:* Frisancho, A.R., *Am. J. Clin. Nutr.*, 40, 808, 1984.

- Distribution by quartiles where the lowest and highest quartiles constitute the small and large frame categories, respectively, with the middle two quartiles combined to indicate medium frame
- Distribution by varying "border values" defined at the 15th, 20th, or 25th and 75th, 80th, or 85th percentiles for small and large frames
- Defining cut points by standard deviations with medium frame falling within plus or minus one standard deviation of the mean and those with small and large frames falling below or above these values

Many different skeletal measurements, including segmental lengths, breadths, circumferences, and radiographs, have been examined for assessing FS (see Table 39.5). These include the following:

- Wrist and arm circumference
- Elbow, knee, shoulder, chest, hip, wrist, and ankle breadths
- Combination measurements
- Ratio of wrist circumference to height
- Frame index ([EB (mm)/height (cm)] × 100)
- Regression of the sum of bitrochanteric and biacromial breadths (large calipers) on height
- Ratio of sitting to standing height

## CIRCUMFERENCES

Circumference measurements have been widely examined because of advantages of being relatively easy to perform, inexpensive, and noninvasive and requiring only a tape measure and minimal training of personnel. Primary applications include the following:

- Monitoring brain growth in children
- Monitoring effectiveness of treatments (including physical exercise) to measure reduction or increase in selected body areas
- As a marker of protein–energy malnutrition
- Estimation of the relative proportion of body weight from fat vs. lean both as an independent measure and as a measure of FS
- Description of body shape or the relative distribution of body weight using single measures or ratios of two circumference measures such as waist and hip

Techniques for taking circumference measures are relatively simple. However, significant errors can result from improper positioning or placement of the tape and from differences in tension applied. In general, the tape is placed perpendicular to the long axis of the body, but exceptions include head and neck where the measurement is made at the widest and narrowest point, respectively. In almost all cases except the head, the tension on the tape is just enough to place it snug against the skin without causing an indentation. However, if the purpose of the circumference is to estimate FS (or skeletal size), it is not entirely clear whether the tape should be pulled more tightly to get as close to the bone as possible. "Equipment" includes a flexible but non-stretchable tape measure that is relatively narrow (0.7 cm). Special anthropometric tapes are available such as those that are already interlocked to slip over the arm or head with arrows to make reading the measurement or finding the midpoint of the back of the arm easier. Detailed instructions for technique for measurement of the head, neck, chest, waist, abdomen, hips or buttocks, thigh, calf, ankle, forearm, and wrist are described by Callaway et al. who recommend intra- and intermeasurer limits of agreement of 0.2 cm for relatively small sites (calf, ankle, wrist, head, arm, forearm) and 1.0 for the larger sites (waist, abdomen, buttocks, chest).[22]

One of the most commonly measured and clinically practical anthropometric indices is the arm muscle area that was originally developed for use in the field for the evaluation of undernourished children.[23] Arm circumference and triceps SF measurement can be used to compare an individual to a reference population[24] and to estimate the relative proportion of fat and muscle[25] or to estimate the severity of undernutrition in seriously ill hospitalized patients.[26] The use of arm circumference has importance when either undernutrition or overnutrition is of concern, and it can be easily used in the field, hospital, or community setting. Similarly, head circumference is a common measurement for infants in the first 2–3 years of life that can be plotted on standard growth charts to be compared with population norms.

Because of some of the difficulties of applying traditional height–weight tables to individuals who are either very lean or very fat and because of the practicality of doing circumference measurements, various researchers have evaluated the validity of using circumferences to estimate body composition and physical fitness. Using underwater weighing as the "gold standard," tables such as Table 39.6 have been developed to estimate percent body fat (% BF) within 2.5%–4% for women and men using the following circumferences[27]:

The U.S. Navy requires personnel to pass certain physical fitness screening tests including having an appropriate weight for height. In this setting, it is quite important to use a method that provides more specific information than traditional height–weight indices in differentiating individuals who have excess lean weight from those individuals with excess fat. Because of the large numbers of potential recruits and enlisted personnel being measured, practicality is also very important. Equations using circumference measures have been used to estimate % BF and body density since the early 1980s (see Table 39.7 for selected studies of circumference measures).

**TABLE 39.5**
**Selected Validation Studies of Determinants of FS**

| FS Measure | Subjects[a] | Methods and Criterion[b,c] | Results |
|---|---|---|---|
| Bony chest breadth[59] | n = 2201, men, Scotland | Bony chest breadth measured by x-ray. Criterion tested: 1, 3, and sig > in wt with > in FS. | a. Correlation of bony chest breadth to wt > correlation of ht to wt.<br>b. Wt > about 3.7 kg/each cm > in bony chest breadth.<br>c. Wt > about 12 kg/FS (S→M→L)<br>d. Wt to bony chest breadth ratio correlated with FFM. |
| Ratio of height (cm) to wrist circumference (cm)[60] | 100% and & adult patients at a university medical center, United States | Wrist measured distal to styloid process at wrist crease on right arm. FS (S, M, L) assigned using this ratio by gender. | a. Method for assigning FS not stated. It appears that some sort or "normal" distribution was applied, but no other criteria of validity were tested.<br>b. FS assigned by ht to wrist ratio<br>% S, >10.4; M, 9.6–10.4; L, <9.6<br>% S, >11.0; M, 10.1–11.0; L, <10.1. |
| Elbow and bitrochanteric breadths[61] | n = 16,494; age range, 18–74; M and F; black and white; U.S. NHANES 1971–1974 | Criterion tested: 1, 3, and 4. BF determined by sum of triceps and SFs. | a. Correlation coefficients of weight, elbow, and bitrochanteric breadth to log-transformed sum of SF values done by gender, by three age groups, by race demonstrate lowest correlation with EB.<br>b. Categories of SML FS established for EB with cut points at the 15th and 85th percentiles (values given by gender, race, and age group) demonstrate significant gender differences and some racial differences.<br>c. Greater differences were observed for mean weights of subjects when they were categorized by FS (S, M, L) vs. height (short, medium, tall), demonstrating that FS is more effective in weight discrimination. |
| EB[44] | n = 21,752; "adults" age range 25–54; "elderly" age 55–74; M and F; multiracial; U.S. NHANES I and II | Based on this large data set, percentiles of weight, SFs (triceps and subscapular), and bone-free upper arm muscle were developed by height, gender, and FS (using EB) for two age groups. | a. Values of EB for S, M, L FS are given for males and females by age (see Table 39.4).<br>b. These standards can be used to identify persons who are at risk of being undernourished or overfat. |
| Height (H) and sum of biacromial (A) & bitrochanteric (T) (HAT method) Body fatness estimated by hydrostatic weighing[62] | Mean age = 22; n = 113 M, 182F; Υ; university students; ht & wt representative of U.S. population for this age group; Caucasian, United States | Criterion: 3, 5 Bivariate model developed based on height (H) and sum of biacromial (A) & bitrochanteric (T) breadths. Boundaries for FS (S, L) set by gender using mean ht + 1 sd. | a. Criterion satisfied.<br>b. For % differences in wt between FS primarily due to differences in FFM.<br>c. For & there was small but sig increase in FM per FS but no increase in FFM per FS.<br>d. FS equations: % ht (8.239) + (A + T); & ht (10.357) + (A + T).<br>e. HAT FS boundaries: % S <1459.3; M 1459.4–1591.9; L >1592.0; & S <1661.9; M 1662.0–1850.7; L >1850.8. |
| Wrist, biacromial, elbow, hip, knee, and ankle breadths Body fatness estimated by hydrostatic weighing[15] | n = 225 M and 215 F; age range = 18–59 Canada, Quebec City, French descent. Tended to be leaner than either Canadian or U.S. reference populations | Criterion: 5–6 Differences in lean weight between FS categories (assigned by terciles) > differences in % BF. | a. All bone breadth measures were shown to be associated with FFM.<br>b. Biacromial, elbow, hip, and knee did not meet criterion 6.<br>c. Both criteria satisfied for wrist and ankle breadths. (Data not shown for FS cut points.) |
| Actual FS (AFS)[d] Body composition determined by JP, Br[63] | n = 17; 0 age = 20.9 ± 1.4; Υ; M; Caucasian; United Kingdom | Criterion: 1–5 and correlation with proposed measure AFS. | a. Lack of agreement in assigning FS between methods 2–5.<br>b. Criterion satisfied: ankle breadth & EB 1–5; AFS and hand length 1–3 & 5; HAT 1–3; chest breadth 1–4; wrist breadth 2 and 3; height/wrist 3.<br>c. Additional correlations: ht→wt r = 0.68 (s); ht→FFM r = 0.70 (s); FFM→FM r = 0.20 (ns). |

## TABLE 39.5 (continued)
## Selected Validation Studies of Determinants of FS

| FS Measure | Subjects[a] | Methods and Criterion[b,c] | Results |
|---|---|---|---|
| Frame index 5[64] | n = 21,648 M; 21,391 F (sample size planned for 96% statistical confidence); age range = 18–70; Germany | Developed percentile curves for weight, height, and BMI by gender and age. Three categories of frame index using 20th and 80th percentiles as border values. Median values for BMI and %BF by gender and age for each FS. | a. Graph of median curves for frame-specific BMI by age (18–64) demonstrates important differences with age and gender and consistently higher BMI with larger frame.<br>b. Graph of median curves for frame-specific % BF by age (18–64) also demonstrates age and gender differences and consistently higher BF with larger FS.<br>c. Values used for cut points for frame index (at the 20th and 80th percentiles by gender and age) are not given for this sample. However, those published by Frisancho (derived from U.S. NHANES data) could be used for other studies. |
| Biacromial, bi-iliocristal, wrist, and knee diameters and sitting height<br>Body composition: DW[65] | n = 2512 men; age range = 45–59; South Wales | Criterion of effectiveness, improvement in correlation of BMI with body fatness when BMI is adjusted for FS. | a. All 4 breadth frame measures were positively associated with BF (range of r = 0.16 [wrist]–0.45) and with height (range of r = 0.32–0.43). (Correlation of sitting height with BF or total ht not reported.)<br>b. Adjusting BMI for FS did not improve the association of BMI with BF.<br>c. Correlations of the BMI adjusted for FS by wrist and sitting height (both r = 0.74) were essentially the same as for BMI alone (r = 0.76).<br>d. Correlations of the BMI adjusted for FS by biacromial, bi-iliocristal, and knee diameters (range of r = 0.60–0.66) were lower than for BMI alone (r = 0.76), indicating a possible inflating effect of subcutaneous fat on these diameter measures. |
| EB and height to wrist ratio<br>Body composition: BIA-Lu[66] | n = 42 &; 38 men; age range = 18–55; United States | Criterion tested: 3<br>Measures result in normal distribution of FS and produce the same FS in an individual. | a. Criterion 3 met for % but not &<br>b. Both measures resulted in an FS distribution highly skewed to small frame (53%–73% of subjects) with 0%–3% in large frame.<br>c. These two FS measures produced the same FS in 69% of the subjects. |
| Arm and wrist circumferences; ankle, elbow, and wrist breadths; SSFs; frame index 2; ht and wt; visual assessment[67] | n = 300 (71 M and 229 F); mean age = 72.6 ± 5.1; &; Caucasian; Midwest, United States | Criterion tested: 3 and agreement across methods in classifying FS. | a. Distribution of FS designation varied by determinant but was not influenced by age.<br>b. Visual assessment and EB 19 classified about 75% of subjects as medium frame. EB 21 and frame index 2.5 resulted in more even distribution of FS.<br>c. Association with "fatness" (SSF) was noted for women with EB and for men with height/wrist.<br>d. Ankle and wrist breadth had lowest correlations with SSF, but lack of population-based standards limits their application. |
| Wrist and knee width used as FS measures Ht and wt; sitting ht Slenderness index (ht/wrist + knee width) %BF measured by UWW and BIA.[68] | n = 120, matched for age, gender, and BMI. China (Singapore and Beijing: Chinese; Netherlands: Caucasian) | Measured %BF compared by matched BMI between ethnic groups. %BF calculated from BMI compared to measured. Skeletal mass calculated from ht, wrist, and knee width. | a. %BF differences observed between groups for the same BMI, with %BF > with > FS.<br>b. %BF calculated vs. measured not different for Beijing Chinese and Dutch.<br>c. %BF calculated underpredicted true value by 4% in Singapore Chinese.<br>d. Differences in FS are at least partially responsible for differences in relationship of BMI→%BF among different ethnic groups. |

*(continued)*

**TABLE 39.5 (continued)**
**Selected Validation Studies of Determinants of FS**

| FS Measure | Subjects[a] | Methods and Criterion[b,c] | Results |
|---|---|---|---|
| Wrist circumference (WC) and EB[69] | n = 224; (127 M; 117 F); adults; ϒ; Venezuela | Distribution of FS[e] (S, M, L) determined by two methods—WC (Grant, 1980) and EB (Frisancho, 1989)—and used to compare weight for height classification. | Distribution of FS: <br> a. WC: S = 57%; M = 38%; L = 6% <br> b. EB: S = 16%; M = 60%; L = 25%. <br> Significant differences are observed in weight for height classification within the same group of persons depending on the FS method used. EB achieved more "normal" distribution. |
| Height, weight, skeletal dimensions (shoulder width, hip width, chest width and depth, limb lengths), circumferences (head, trunk, limbs), SFs (triceps, subscapular, abdominal)[70] | n = 1260 (middle-class adult women); ϒ; mean age = 49 years (range = 18–100); Australia | Criterion tested: 3 & 6. Survey organized by a garment industry company aimed at improvement in apparel sizing standards. More than 60 dimensions measured. FS calculated as bi-iliocristal hip width times sitting height and weight to trunk ratio. | Vertical dimensions weak correlations with fatness. Body frame circumferences and transverse dimensions correlated with fatness (each explaining from 3% to 44% of variation in SF thickness). Skeletal dimensions explained up to 50% of variation in SF, especially for chest width and depth and hop width. Body frame dimensions reflect trunk volume and trunk/limb proportions (larger lean trunk size associated with greater fatness). |

[a] Subjects (all information provided in the original reference is given): n, number of subjects; age in years; health status: ϒ, healthy; gender: M, male; F, female.

[b] Criterion applied: 1, highly correlated with weight; 2, highly correlated with FFM; 3, minimally correlated with body fatness; 4, minimally correlated with height; 5, correlation with FFM is greater than the correlation of height alone with FFM; 6, little or no association with BF beyond that accounted for by the association of FFM with fat.

[c] Methods for determining body composition: UWW, underwater weighing; BIA, bioelectrical impedance analysis; JP, regression equations of Jackson and Pollack[71,72]; Br, formula of Brozek et al.[73]; DW, regression equation of Durnin and Wormersley[74]; BIA-Lu, bioelectrical impedance analysis using the equations of Lukaski et al.[75]

[d] In this study, the authors propose a reference measure "AFS" comprised of the sum of a battery of 22 different skeletal measures (11 breadths, 9 lengths, and 2 depths) as described in text of Lohman et al.[12]

[e] *Abbreviations*: WC, wrist circumference; EB, elbow breadth; FS, frame size; S, M, L, small, medium, large; ht, height; wt, weight; FFM, fat-free mass; FM, fat mass; %BF, percent body fat; r, correlation coefficient; sig, statistically significant; ns, not statistically significant; sd, standard deviation.

**TABLE 39.6**
**Circumferences Used to Estimate % BF**

| Young Women (Ages 17–26) | Older Women (Ages 27–50) | Young Men (Ages 17–26) | Older Men (Ages 27–50) |
|---|---|---|---|
| Abdomen | Abdomen | Right upper arm | Buttocks |
| Right thigh | Right thigh | Abdomen | Abdomen |
| Right forearm | Right calf | Right forearm | Right forearm |

## SKINFOLD MEASUREMENTS

The SF (sometimes referred to as fatfold) technique is performed by pinching the skin and underlying fat at a given location between the thumb and forefinger, pulling the fold slightly away from the body, placing the calipers on the fold, and measuring its thickness. Some SF sites are relatively easy to locate and measure, while others are not.

There are many individual factors that affect the accuracy of SF measurements:

- Degree of leanness or fatness
- Muscle tone (including presence of muscle wasting)
- Changes with growth
- Younger or older age (as they affect accuracy of assumptions about tissue composition, muscle tone, SF compressibility, and elasticity)
- Subject cooperation (small children may be frightened or uncooperative)
- Ethnicity
- Health status (bedridden vs. ambulatory)
- Hydration status

Use of this method relies on two main assumptions: (1) SFs provide good measures of subcutaneous fat and (2) there is a good relationship between subcutaneous fat and total BF. The ability to predict total BF varies by site, with some sites

**TABLE 39.7**

**Selected Studies of Circumference Measures**

| Circumference Site(s) | Subjects[a] | Methods | Results |
|---|---|---|---|
| Neck, abdomen, thigh[77] | n = 5,710 M and 477 F, Navy personnel, United States | 1. %BF estimated from standardized Navy equations for men: %BF = (0.740 × abdomen)–(1.249 × neck) + 0.528[76] <br> 2. Men: Body Density = [0.19077 × Log 10 (abdomen – neck)] + [0.15456 × Log 10 (height)] + 1.0324; %BF = [(4.95/ body density) – 4.5] × 100; Women: %BF = (1.051 × biceps) – (1.522 × forearm) – (0.879 × neck) + (0.326 × abdomen) + (0.597 × thigh) + 0.707 <br> %BF estimates correlated with three measures of physical fitness | Estimates of %BF derived from these circumference measurements and equations correlated better with performance on the Navy's physical fitness tests than did commonly used weight–height indices. |
| Waist, hip[80] | n = 32,978; age range = 25–64; participants in 19 male and 18 female groups participating in a WHO MONICA project | Identification of obesity compared by cut points for waist circumference at two levels (1. % ≥94 cm; & ≥80 cm; 2. % ≥102 cm; & ≥88 cm) vs. cut points for BMI (≥25 kg/m²) and WHR (% ≥0.95; & ≥0.80). | Sensitivity was lowest in populations with fewer overweight individuals and highest in populations with more overweight. Use of waist cut points vs. BMI or WHR cut points would correctly identify most people without obesity but miss some with obesity. Optimal screening cutoff points for waist circumference may be population specific. |
| Waist, hip umbilical[81] | n = 91, women; age range = 20–54; BMI = 18–34 kg/m² | %BF by DEXA compared with %BF from predictive equations | Comparability and precision of %BF estimates from predictive equations can be improved by adjusting for umbilical circumference and BMI. |
| Waist, hip[82] | n = 385 (140 M and 245 F); mean age = 80 (range = 65–96); United States | %BF by DEXA and BIA. BF distribution by SFs | %BF < % vs. &, upper body obesity > % vs. & even in older age; strong age-adjusted correlations among obesity measures (BMI, %BF [DEXA & BIA], SFs) were observed for both % and &; weak associations among measures of upper body obesity differed by gender. |
| Neck[83] | n = 979 (460 M and 519 F); mean age = 51 + 17 years); visiting Family Medicine clinic for any reason; Israel | Examined correlation between neck circumference (NC) and measures of obesity (BMI, weight, waist and hip circumference and ratio) | NC simple and time-saving measure can be used to identify potentially overweight patients. Men with NC < 37 cm and women with NC < 34 cm are not considered overweight. Men with NC > 37 and women with NC > 34 require additional evaluation of overweight or obesity status. |
| Waist, hip, WHR[82] | n = 385 (140 M; 245 F); age range = 65–96; United States | %BF by DEXA | For both men and women, waist circumference is more strongly correlated with BMI and %BF by DEXA than WHR. <br> For subjects >80 years, <br> a. W:H not correlated with any measure of obesity or fat distribution for % and only with SSF in & <br> b. Waist correlated significantly with almost all measures of central obesity. |

[a] Subjects (all information provided in the original reference is given): n, number of subjects; health status: ϒ, healthy; gender: M, male; F, female.

[b] Method for determining intra-abdominal fat (IAF): MRI, magnetic resonance imaging.

[c] Methods for determining body composition: UWW, underwater weighing; DEXA, dual-energy x-ray absorptiometry; DD, deuterium dilution; TBK, total body potassium; BIA, bioelectrical impedance analysis; SKF, JP, regression equation of Jackson and Pollack[55,56]; Br, formula of Brozek et al.[57]; DW, regression equation of Durnin and Wormersley[58]; BIA-Lu, bioelectrical impedance analysis using the equations of Lukaski et al.[59].

[d] *Abbreviations*: SFs, skinfolds; IAF, intra-abdominal fat; WHR, waist-to-hip ratio; ht, height; wt, weight; BMI, body mass index; FFM, fat-free mass; FM, fat mass; %BF, percent body fat; r, correlation coefficient; sig, statistically significant; ns, not statistically significant; sd, standard deviation.

**TABLE 39.8**
**Reliability of Selected SF Measurement Sites**

| Site | Intermeasurer Error | Intrameasurer Error |
|---|---|---|
| Subscapular | SEM: 0.88–1.53 mm | SEM: 0.88–1.16 mm |
| Midaxillary | SEM: ±0.36; 1.47 mm (children); ±0.64 mm (adults) | SEM: children: ±0.95 mm Adults: ±1.0, 1.22, 2.08 mm |
| Pectoral (chest) | R: 9, 93, 97; SEM: 2.1 mm | R: 91–97 mm; SEM: ±1–2 mm |
| Abdominal | | R: 979; SEM: 0.89 mm |
| Suprailiac | SEM: 1.53 mm (children); 1.7 mm (adults) | R: 97; SEM: 0.3–1.0 mm |
| Thigh | R: >0.9, 97, 975; SEM: ±2.1, ±2.4, 3–4 mm | R: 91, 98, 985; SEM: 0.5–0.7, 1–2 mm |
| Medial calf | | R: 94, 98, 99; SEM: 1.0–1.5 mm |
| Tricep | SEM: 0.8–1.89 mm | SEM: 0.4–0.8 mm |
| Bicep | SEM: ±1.9 mm | SEM: 0.2–0.6, ±1.9 mm |
| Children ages 6–9: (measurements investigated in five different countries)[84] SFs Circumferences | Agreement >88% same | 0.12–0.47 mm 0.09–1.24 cm |
| Neonatal (within 24 h of delivery) multiethnic birth cohort study[85] SFs: subscapular (SSF) Triceps (TSF) Circumferences: head, mid-upper arm (MUAC), and abdomen | 0.17–0.63 mm (SSF) 0.15–0.54 mm (TSF) 0.2–0.36 cm (head); 0.19–0.39 cm (MUAC); 0.39–0.77 cm (abdomen) | 0.14–0.25 mm (SSF) 0.22–0.35 mm (TSF) All <0.4 cm |

*Source:* Unless otherwise referenced, the information in this table is summarized from Harrison, G.G. et al., Skinfold thickness and measurement technique, in: Lohman, T.G., Roche, A.F., and Martorell, R. (eds.), *Anthropometric Standardization Reference Manual*, Human Kinetics, Champaign, IL, pp. 55–80, 1988. This chapter includes the specific citations for the reliability studies.

*Abbreviations:* SEM, standard error of measurement; R, reliability coefficient.

*Note:* Multiple error estimates represent differing results from different studies.

highly correlated with total fat and others relatively independent of total fat. Studies show that the relationship between subcutaneous and total BF (ranging from 20% to 70%) is affected by age, gender, degree of fatness, and race.[28–30] Thus, as has been mentioned previously, it is important to review the literature carefully and select sites and predictive equations that have been validated for the population being measured and provide sufficient precision for the desired application.

Guidelines for SF measurement technique, location of measurement sites, and information on reliability of measurement at the various sites have been published.[31] Considerable supervised practice is required before an individual can take accurate SF measurements. Training by an experienced person should be conducted and measures practiced until consistency is achieved between the expert and trainee and by the trainee on within-subject repeated measures. Experts agree on the importance of using standardized techniques in both locating the site and using calipers to take the measurement, yet some argue that in light of the many biologic variables affecting body composition, technical errors in SF measurement are of comparatively little importance.[32] Nonetheless, given a standard level of training and care in measurement, high levels of reliability can be achieved (see Table 39.8).

Many different models of SF calipers are available, but only those that are designed to maintain a constant tension (10 g/mm) between the jaws should be used. However, even with the higher-quality calipers, there is a difference in the pressure exerted by the jaws and therefore in the degree of compression of the SF.[33] Differences in compression have also been attributed to differences in caliper jaw surface area such that calipers with smaller surface area and lighter spring tension (such as the Lange) give larger values than calipers with larger surface area and tighter spring tension (Holtain and Harpenden).[34] Because of these differences attributable to the calipers themselves, it is important to calibrate often[35] and consistently use the same equipment in order to compare data within or across subjects.

The greater availability of DEXA equipment in the past decade and recognition of the four-compartment model as the best reference standard have allowed for the reexamination of some of the most widely used equations using SF measures to predict percent body fat in different populations. The results of some of these studies are summarized in Table 39.9.

## TABLE 39.9

## Selected Update and Validation Studies Examining the Utility of Field Methods in Predicting or Estimating Body Composition in Different Populations

| Subjects | Methods | Results |
|---|---|---|
| Healthy young to middle-age adults: n = 681 (360 M; 321 F); mean age ~35. Primarily Caucasian (FELS study), United States[86] | %BF measured by the four-compartment model (4 cm) compared with %BF estimated using common SF equations (Durnin & Wormersley (DW), Jackson and Pollack) | %BF from SF thickness equations < %BF from 4 cm. Results from new predictive equations developed from SF yielded results close to 4 cm: %: 22.7% (sf) vs. 22.8% (4 cm) &: 32.6% (sf) vs. 32.8% (4 cm) |
| Fit and healthy young adults: n = 52 (21 M; 31 F); mean age ~22. United Kingdom[87] | %BF measured by DEXA and the 4 cm model (& only) compared with %BF estimated from upper body SFs (UBSF) vs. lower body (LBSF) | Thigh SF had highest correlation with %BF by DEXA % and & and also with %BF by the four-compartment model for &. Sum of the LBSF explained more of variance in %BF by DEXA than did sum of the UBSF Authors conclude: important to include lower body SF when assessing %BF in young adults |
| Healthy young to middle-age men: n = 160; age range = 18–62; primarily Caucasian; United States[88] | %BF measured by DEXA compared with %BF estimated using three of the most common and professionally recommended equations (Jackson and Pollack: seven-site equation and two different three-site equations) | %BF from SF equations underestimated by ~3% compared to DEXA New predictive equation developed using sum of 7 SFs (chest, midaxillary, triceps, subscapular, abdomen, thigh) and age. |
| Healthy adults: n = 117 (46 M; 71 F); Normal weight and obese (BMI =19–39); mean age validation group ~48 years; cross-validation group ~58 years; age range = 26–67 years; Caucasian; Germany[89] | %BF by DEXA compared with %BF by SF (equations by DW and Peterson). Additional measures collected [SF (chin, biceps, triceps, subscapular, chest, abdomen, hip, thigh, knee, calf), circumferences (waist, hip, thigh, calf), breadths (chest, elbow, knee, wrist, ankle, and chest depth)] | New predictive equations developed combining SF, circumferences, and breadths: a. Men: waist circumference and SF (log triceps, subscapular, abdomen) b. Women: hip circumference, SF (log chin, triceps, subscapular), and knee breadth %BF estimates from new equations showed excellent correspondence to DEXA and had negligible tendency to underestimate %BF in subjects with higher BMI. |
| Asian (n = 242) and white (n = 445) adults: age 18–94; United States[90] | Correlations examined between BMI and %BF by DEXA and 6 circumferences and 8 SF compared for Asians vs. whites | Asians had lower BMI but higher %BF. SF revealed greater subcutaneous fat in Asians and different fat distribution (> upper body) than whites. Magnitude of difference between races > in women vs. men New predictive equations developed for each race and gender based on BMI, age, and SF. |
| African American Women: n = 134; age range = 18–40, premenopausal, United States[91] | %BF estimated from five different SF equations: Jackson and Pollack (three and seven sites), DW (generalized and age-specific equations), and Wang compared with DEXA | Comparison of predictive accuracy of the five equations found Jackson–Pollack seven sites to be most valid, explaining 75% of variance in reference body density and no significant difference from %BF by DEXA. |
| Pregnant women: n = 200. United States[92] | %BF measured by the four-compartment model (DEXA done 2–4 weeks postpartum) | Estimates of %BF measured at gestation weeks 14 and 37 (early and late pregnancy) using four widely used predictive equations yielded significantly higher values than the four-compartment model. New predictive equations developed that were found to be valid for pregnant women with different prepregnancy BMI, different pregnancy weight gains, and different ethnicity and SES. Field methods used in these equations include a. Change in FM: thigh SF b. Fat at term: biceps SF, thigh SF, wrist circumference |
| Young children: n = 98 (49 M; 49F); mean age = 6.6; Caucasian, United States[93] | %BF by SF (using Slaughter equation based on triceps and calf SF) and BIA with DEXA | %BF by DEXA significantly < than %BF by SF or BIA New predictive equations developed for this age and ethnic group |

*(continued)*

**TABLE 39.9 (continued)**

**Selected Update and Validation Studies Examining the Utility of Field Methods in Predicting or Estimating Body Composition in Different Populations**

| Subjects | Methods | Results |
|---|---|---|
| Children:<br>n = 86 (34 M; 52F); mean age = 11; range = 7–18; African American (~30% of sample) and Caucasian, United States[96] | %BF estimated from triceps SF (Dezenberg equation[94]) compared with %BF from DXA and ADP[95] | Triceps SF accounted for only 13% of the variance in %BF change<br>Authors conclude<br>a. There appears to be no noninvasive, simple method to measure changes in children's %BF change accurately and precisely.<br>b. ADP could prove useful for measuring change %BF in children. |
| Children in adiposity rebound period:<br>n = 75 (34 M; 41F); mean age ~6; range = 3–8); Hispanic (~16% of sample) and Caucasian, United States[99] | %BF estimated from SF (using equations of Slaughter [method 1 and 2],[97] Deurenberg (D),[98] and Dezenberg) compared with BIA and DEXA | All methods except D significantly underestimated %BF as determined by DEXA.<br>BMI underestimated more than SF or BMI<br>Correlations with %BF by DEXA<br>a. Slaughter method 2: high (r = 0.82)<br>b. BMI: moderate (r = 0.61–0.75)<br>c. BIA: low (r = 0.30) |
| Latino children:<br>n = 96; mean age ~11; range = 7–13; Hispanic, United States[100] | %BF estimated using equations of Dezenberg (weight, triceps, gender) compared with DEXA | %BF by method of Dezenberg et al. significantly different (−3.43 ± 4.32 kg) than DEXA<br>New predictive equations developed<br>Authors conclude weight (as single most significant predictor) can be used alone to estimate %BF. Adding age and gender increases precision. |
| African American (AA) and White (W) Adolescent Girls: n = 112 (40 AA; 72 W), mean age = 13; United States[101] | %BF from 4 cm compared with %BF estimated from SF using eight equations (three logarithmic, two quadratic, three linear)<br>Bland–Altman plot method used to determine bias and limits of agreement | %BF estimated using quadratic equations agreed most closely with 4 cm.<br>The quadratic equation of Slaughter et al. recommended for population studies in adolescent females because of accuracy and simplicity (uses triceps and calf sites vs. "invasive" subscapular, suprailiac, or thigh SFs or buttocks circumference)<br>%BF can be over- or underestimated in an individual by ~10% when this equation is used. (Hence, recommended for use in population studies.) |
| Black African children:<br>n = 214 (118 M; 96F); prepubescent; mean age = 9.5 years; Tanner stage 1; South Africa[102] | %BF estimated using equations of Slaughter and Dezenberg compared with DEXA.<br>Validation and cross-validation samples.<br>Bland–Altman plot method used to determine bias and limits of agreement | %BF significantly underestimated by Slaughter and Dezenberg equations compared with DEXA<br>New predictive equations developed:<br>Boys: triceps, biceps, subscapular, suprailiac, thigh<br>Girls: biceps, subscapular, suprailiac, thigh calf |
| Adolescent girls:<br>n = 59; age 14–17 year; eumenorrheic; ballet dancers; Israel[103] | %BF estimated from sum of four SF (triceps, biceps, subscapular, suprailiac) and compared to DEXA and BIA | Correlation of SF with DEXA (r = 0.8) > BIA with DEXA<br>Authors conclude SF measures can be successfully used to estimate %BF in homogeneous group of female ballet dances and can be used to determine minimal healthy body weight. |
| Men:<br>n = 67; age = 20–95; Italy[104] | %BF estimated from age-specific equations using SF and BMI compared with BIA and DEXA. Results for subjects >80 years examined separately | Equations based on BMI and BIA systematically overestimated %BF as compared to DEXA in all ages.<br>%BF difference SF vs. DEXA < differences BMI or BIA vs. DEXA, but in subjects >80 years, %BF by SF significantly underestimated.<br>Authors conclude age-related differences in total body bone mineral mass and FFM mineralization in elderly >80 require further research to develop and validate practical field methods for estimating %BF. |

## TABLE 39.9 (continued)
## Selected Update and Validation Studies Examining the Utility of Field Methods in Predicting or Estimating Body Composition in Different Populations

| Subjects | Methods | Results |
|---|---|---|
| Elderly: n = 204 (76 M; 128F); age range = 60–87; healthy; Netherlands.[105] | %BF by SF (triceps, biceps, subscapular, suprailiac [all subjects] and umbilicus, quadriceps, fibula [subset of subjects]) compared with %BF by hydrostatic weight (UW) | %BF predicted from SF using existing published equations generally underestimated %BF from UW. Three new predictive equations developed found to be valid for elderly based on gender and a. Sum of 2 SF (biceps, triceps) (SEE %BF = 5.6%) b. Sum of 4 SF (biceps, triceps, suprailiac, subscapular) (SEE %BF = 5.4%) c. BMI (SEE %BF = 4.8%) |
| Elderly: n = 286 (125 M; 161F); age = 75; Sweden[106] | %BF by 4 CM compared with %BF estimated from SF using three equations: DW, D, and Visser (V) Bland–Altman plot method used to assess limits of agreement | Difference %BF by 4 cm vs. SF equation: a. DW: overestimate in % by 3.12% and underestimate in & by 1.06% b. D: overestimate % by 3.26% and & by 9.56% c. V: overestimate % by 3.63% and & by 9.23% New predictive equation developed using $\log_{10}$ sum of biceps, triceps, subscapular, suprailiac SF, gender, weight, and height (r = 0.86; mean difference %BF 4 cm %BF new equation = 0). Authors conclude population-based prediction equations are preferable in the elderly. |
| Obese women: n = 16 nonobese (BMI ~22; mean age = 28.6) and 21 obese (BMI ~34.5; mean age 39.3); Turkey[107] | %BF by DEXA compared with BIA and SF (biceps, triceps, subscapular, suprailiac) using equation of DW | Preliminary analysis using correlation coefficients: Nonobese: DEXA-BIA $r^2$ = 0.93; DEXA-SF $r^2$ = 0.89 Obese: DEXA-BIA $r^2$ = 0.84; DEXA-SF $r^2$ = 0.75 Reanalysis of data by the Bland–Altman method a. Lack of agreement between DEXA-BIA and DEXA-SF methods in obese subjects b. %BF underestimated by BIA and SF as compared to DEXA in both groups Authors conclude DEXA should be considered method of choice in obese patients. |
| Dialysis patients: n = 30 (15 M; 15 F); mean age = 47; clinically stable; Brazil[108] | %BF by DEXA compared with BIA and SF (biceps, triceps, subscapular, suprailiac) using equation of DW | For all patients, %BF estimates not significantly different between methods. Bland–Altman plot revealed agreement between DEXA and SF (0.47 ± 2.8 kg) and DEXA and BIA (−0.39 ± 3.3 kg). When results examined by gender, BIA had greater variability and mean prediction error. |
| Adolescents followed to adulthood (1976–2000); n = 335 (168 M; 182 F); healthy; Amsterdam[109] | Prospective measurements of 8 BMI and SF analyzed in relation to adult body fatness measured at mean age of 37 years with DEXA | Adolescent SF (sum of 4) more strongly associated with adult body fatness than BMI. Authors conclude SF thickness during adolescence is better predictor of high body fatness during adulthood than is BMI. |
| Representative cross-sectional sample of U.S. adults enrolled in the NHANES[110] n = 12,901 | Examination of the relationships between waist circumference (waist circ.), waist–stature ratio (WSR), and BMI and % BF (as measured by DEXA) | The three measures were more closely related to each other than they were to %BF and performed similarly as indicators of %BF. Men: %BF more correlated with WC than BMI. Women: %BF more correlated with WC. Percentile values of all three measures correspond to percentiles of %BF. More than 90% of the sample was categorized within one category of %BF by each measure. Authors conclude these measures would not be accurate to determine % BF for an individual, but they are useful in distinguishing categories of %BF. |

## IMPORTANCE OF FRAME SIZE, SKINFOLDS, AND CIRCUMFERENCES TO DISEASE RISK

A variety of approaches have been employed to better understand the validity of using these field measurements for the assessment of risk for the most prevalent and serious diseases: heart disease, diabetes, cancer, and osteoporosis. Major interest has been in evaluating these measures for their ability to measure, estimate, or predict:

- Total fat or % BF
- Fat or weight patterning or distribution
- Skeletal size or density
- Biochemical markers such as lipids and insulin sensitivity/resistance
- Prevalence of childhood allergic disease and asthma[36,37]
- Lipodystrophy in HIV-infected persons[38]
- Health outcomes such as elevated blood pressure, morbidity, or mortality (cancer, diabetes, coronary artery disease, myocardial infarction)

The preponderance of studies relating anthropometric measures to disease has been in the area of CVD in an attempt to identify potentially modifiable body factors and to understand potential markers for and predictors of disease. An extensive summary of studies done in men illustrates the methodological and statistical difficulties that are encountered when assessing the relationship between CVD and various body measurements.[39] In general, studies have not shown a consistent relationship between obesity using a variety of measures (weight for height, relative weight, total BF, etc.) and CVD. The strength of association between central fat distribution and CVD is stronger than that of BF alone, yet a large percent (30%–50%) of the variation remains unexplained. Potential sources of difficulty in conducting these studies include inability to identify adequate surrogates for obesity, confounding effects of cigarette smoking or subclinical disease, short follow-up periods, and inadequate methodology for identifying subgroups of obese persons who are at risk.

In light of the rise in pediatric overweight and obesity, more research has been initiated to determine the utility of using field measures of SFs and waist circumference in addition to the BMI percentiles to assess and prevent obesity in children and its advancement to obesity in adulthood, to minimize overdiagnosis or misclassification, and to identify those at highest risk for associated comorbidities. There is agreement in principle that body fatness and likely central obesity add to disease risk, but findings have been somewhat mixed relative to the utility of using waist circumference or SFs along with BMI percentiles to assess this additional disease risk in children. The general opinion at this time seems to be that high BMI for age percentiles based on national reference data remain the

optimal criteria for defining obesity in children and that neither SFs nor waist circumferences provide significant additional information.[40-44] However, it appears that there is broad global interest in improving our early detection and prevention efforts and in establishing more accurate methods to identify children at highest risk for associated disease.[45] Recently published reference curves for triceps and subscapular skinfold thicknesses in children and adolescents in the United States (based on 32,783 children and adolescents who also had complete data for BMI) suggest an interesting degree of independence between BMI and SF thicknesses at the upper percentiles of the BMI distribution.[46] An Italian study of 986 children (ages 8–12 years) found BMI percentiles to have high specificity but low sensitivity in detecting excess adiposity with sensitivity being improved with the addition of information from SFs.[47] Another study provides evidence that the measurement of SF thicknesses does increase the ability to accurately predict adiposity, but the authors conclude that improvements over using BMI alone in overweight children are relatively small.[48] Therefore, while there currently are no strong supporting data for using any measures besides BMI percentile to detect obesity in children, the growing body of literature in this area may provide sufficient evidence and data to establish reference standards that may eventually change practice.

There is general agreement that adults who have a greater central distribution of BF have higher risk for CVD, diabetes, hypertension, and possibly some cancers, and several studies suggest that those who develop this pattern early in life may have even greater disease risk.[49,50] While one study of three distinct populations found a consistent direct association between abdominal obesity as measured by waist circumference and waist-to-hip ratio (WHR) and dyslipidemia,[51] others have found the sagittal abdominal diameter (SAD) (distance from surface to top of abdomen measured at the level of iliac crest with subject supine on firm surface; also referred to as abdominal height) to be a better marker of intra-abdominal adiposity and predictor of risk than BMI, waist circumference, or WHR.[52,53] One group of Swedish investigators have developed cutoffs for SAD of 22 cm for men and 20 cm for women based on measurements from a population-based study of 4032 men and women.[54] Recent studies have been conducted using MRI or CT scans and/or DEXA as reference standards against which to compare the utility of more practical field methods in estimating total central fat and partitioning it into intra-abdominal vs. subcutaneous fat. Results of selected studies conducted with samples of varying age and ethnicity are summarized in Table 39.10. An excellent review of methods used for measuring waist and hip circumferences; impact of variations attributable to gender, age, and ethnicity; and recommendations for cutoff points and a review of the relationships of these measurements to disease risk and mortality have been published by the World Health Organization (WHO).[55]

**TABLE 39.10**

**Selected Studies Examining the Utility of Field Methods in Predicting or Estimating Central BF**

| Anthropometric Measures | Subjects | Methods | Results |
|---|---|---|---|
| Weight, BMI, waist circumference, WHR, SSF[111] | n = 157 (97 M; 60 F); age range = 48–68; predominantly Caucasian; United States | Field methods compared to results from reference standard: MRI. IAF and subcutaneous abdominal fat area (SAF) measured | Gender differences identified<br>a. Women had more > SAF and = IAF than men and tended to deposit IAF at a constant rate as weight >.<br>b. Men have more IAF at relatively lower weight than women, and fat is more uniformly deposited at higher body weights.<br>After correction for age, IAF associated with BMI, waist, weight, and SSF.<br>Men: quadratically<br>Women: linear relationship<br>Anthropometric measures tended to predict less of total variance in IAF for % than for &.<br>Anthropometric indices linearly associated with SAF and predicted more of variance in SAF than IAF. |
| Waist circumference, sagittal diameter[112] | n = 150 (75 M; 75 F); age range = 70–79; African American and Caucasian; Netherlands | Visceral fat (VF) and total abdominal fat (TAF) by reference standard CT compared to TAF by DEXA with and without field methods | TAF: good correlation between DEXA and CT but DEXA underestimated TAF by ~10%<br>VF: association of VF by CT with DEXA comparable to association of CT with sagittal diameter. Combination of information from DEXA + anthropometrics gave only limited improvement in predicting VF. |
| Abdominal SF and waist circumference[113] | n = 113; prepubertal children age range = 4–10 years; African American and Caucasian; United States | IAF and SAF measured by CT. Total fat and trunk fat measured by DEXA | IAF by CT most strongly and similarly correlated with abdominal SF and trunk fat by DEXA.<br>SAT most strongly correlated with trunk fat and total fat by DEXA and waist circumference.<br>Authors' conclusion: IAF and SAF can be accurately estimated in this population from anthropometry with or without DEXA data. |
| Waist (waist circ.) and hip circumference, WHR; abdominal sagittal diameter (ASD)[114] | n = 76; age range = 20–80; Caucasian; United States | TAF and VF measured by CT | For both M and F, waist circ. and ASD but not W:H strongly associated with TAF (r = 0.87–0.93) and VF (r = 0.84–0.93) from CT. |
| Waist, WHR[115] | n = 40 (18 M and 22 F); age range = 26–57; BMI: ≥30. Scotland | Observational, cross-sectional study<br>Reference methods: IAF measured by MRI and central abdominal fat (CAF) measured by DEXA | Obese &: waist, WHR and CAF by DEXA equally well correlated with IAF by MRI<br>Obese M: waist, WHR not sig correlated with IAF; CAF by DEXA moderately correlated with IAF by MRI |
| Waist, hip, wrist, and arm circumferences; WHR; sagittal diameter[116] | n = 692 (black: 91 M; 137 F; white: 227 M; 237 F); age range = 17–65; United States | VF and SAF measured by CT. %BF determined by hydrostatic weighing | VF of white M and F > than black M and F (independent of BMI, W:H, wrist circumference, and age.) VF of M > F<br>Using VF from CT as reference: combination of sagittal diameter, SAF, age, and race accounted for 84% of variance in % and 75% in &.<br>Two valid generalized field equations developed for predicting VF using the following: (1) BMI, W:H, age, and race ($r^2$ = 0.78%; 0.73 &) and (2) BMI (& only), wrist, age, and race ($r^2$ = 0.78%; 0.72 &). Accuracy of predictive ability decreases as VF increases. |

*(continued)*

**TABLE 39.10 (continued)**

**Selected Studies Examining the Utility of Field Methods in Predicting or Estimating Central BF**

| Anthropometric Measures | Subjects | Methods | Results |
|---|---|---|---|
| SF (bicep, tricep, subscapular, suprailiac, midaxillary, abdominal) and circumferences (midarm, abdomen, hip, midthigh, calf)[117] | n = 129 (54 M; 75 F); mean age 60.4 at baseline (followed 9.4 years); United States | VF and TAF measured by CT. %BF determined by hydrostatic weighing | Waist and hip circumference changes were best anthropometric predictors of total fat change. Thigh circumference change more strongly associated with FFM change than with FM change in women. Authors conclude SF cannot be used to assess changes in BF because of age-related fat redistribution. Waist and thigh girths should be considered for use in longitudinal studies in the elderly to capture information about increased abdominal adiposity and sarcopenia. |
| SAD, waist circumference (waist circ.), WHR[118] | Healthy adult women: 107 immigrants from the Middle East living in Sweden; 50 native Swedes | Anthropometric measures all measured in supine position and compared to cardiovascular risk factors (C-reactive protein [CRP], insulin, glucose, insulin resistance, blood pressure, serum lipids) using linear regression analysis | SAD showed slightly higher correlation with CVD risk factors: insulin resistance, insulin, CRP, apolipoprotein B, and triglycerides. BMI was better predictor of HDL cholesterol. Authors conclude SAD identifies insulin resistance, subclinical inflammation in this population; larger studies are need with larger population to confirm usefulness of SAD as CVD risk marker. |
| SAD, waist circumference (waist circ.), WHR, BMI[119] | High-risk group of moderately obese men: n = 59; ages 35–65 years; BMI 32.6 ± 2.3 | Anthropometric measures compared to insulin sensitivity, plasma concentrations of proinsulin, specific insulin, C-peptide, glucose, serum IGF binding protein-1 using univariate and multiple regression analyses | SAD showed stronger correlations to all metabolic variables than any of the other anthropometric measures. SAD explained largest degree of variation in insulin sensitivity and was only independent predictor of insulin resistance and hyperproinsulinemia. Authors conclude SAD is better indicator of CVD risk in obese men that other anthropometric measures and could represent a simple, inexpensive, noninvasive tool. Results need confirmation in larger studies that also include women. |

*Abbreviations*: M, male; F, female

*Other Abbreviations*: Central fat measures: SAF, subcutaneous abdominal fat; IAF, intra-abdominal fat; VF, visceral fat; TAF, total abdominal fat; CAF, central abdominal fat. Comparison ("gold standard") measures: DEXA, dual-energy x-ray absorptiometry; CT, computed tomography; MRI, magnetic resonance imaging; BMI, body mass index; CVD, cardiovascular disease; waist circ., waist circumference; BF, body fat.

## TABLE 39.11
## Selected Studies Examining the Relationships between Anthropometric Measures and Bone Mass or BMD

| Anthropometric Measures | Subjects | Methods | Results |
|---|---|---|---|
| Frame: biacromial, bi-iliac, bicofemoral, bicohumeral, and wrist breadths<br>SF: triceps, biceps, forearm, subscapula, suprailium, calf, abdomen, thigh<br>Circumferences: calf, waist, upper arm, abdomen<br>Height and weight[121] | n = 342; mean age = 44.1 (range = 25–79); &; United States | Correlation of anthropometric measures to<br>a. Measured (photon absorptiometry) BMD (g/cm$^2$) at the radius, femoral neck, Ward's triangle, trochanter, lumbar spine<br>b. Constructed summary of bone density score (radius, spine, femoral neck)<br>Muscle mass (termed "muscularity") estimated from circumferences and SFs[120]<br>Multiple regression models constructed to test the usefulness of measures in predicting bone mass | a. For all skeletal sites, one frame measure (biacromial width [BW]), one SF (SSF), and one circumference (calf [CC]) provided the strongest correlations.<br>b. The greater trochanter was more strongly correlated with all anthropometric measures than any other skeletal site.<br>c. After inclusion of age, BW, SSF, and muscularity in the multiple regression model, BW was a significant predictor for all sites except the radius, and SSF and muscularity were significant for all sites.<br>d. Neither height nor weight contributed significantly to the model after BW, SSF, and CC or muscularity were included.<br>e. Despite the strength of the associations, none of the models accounted for more than 40%–45% of the variability in bone mass at any site and therefore are not adequate to predict bone mass for individuals.<br>f. No measures of distribution of BF were significantly associated with bone mass.<br>g. Cross-sectional data not adequate to address questions of rates of bone loss |
| EB<br>Height, weight, and BMI<br>WHR[122] | n = 6,705; & mean age = 71.2 ± 5, Nonblack, United States | BMD measured by single photon (proximal and distal radius and calcaneus) and DEXA (lumbar spine and proximal femur)<br>Adiposity measured by bioelectrical impedance | a. Weight was the major determinant of BMD at all sites, explaining 6%–20% of the variability. (Weight explained more of the variability at direct weight-bearing sites—proximal femur and os calcis.) Effect of weight on BMD did not seem to vary with age. (Age had independent significant effect on BMD decline.)<br>b. Although the measures of BMI, EB, height, and WHR resulted in statistically significant (P < 0.001) improvements in fit of the model, they added very little explanatory power over weight alone.<br>c. A modest proportion of the weight effect was explained by adiposity (36%–63% at weight-bearing sites and 8%–12% at forearm sites).<br>d. These data suggest that both mechanical loading and metabolic mechanisms affect BMD. |

**TABLE 39.11 (continued)**

**Selected Studies Examining the Relationships between Anthropometric Measures and Bone Mass or BMD**

| Anthropometric Measures | Subjects | Methods | Results |
|---|---|---|---|
| WHR, wt, BMI, arm muscle, and fat area[123] | n = 1873 & (97% postmenopausal), Italy | BMC and BMD evaluated by DEXA as normal (N), osteopenic (OPN), or osteoporotic (OPR) | Body wt., BMI, arm muscle, and fat sig > in N than either OPN or OPR groups. WHR not different between groups Wt and age sig predictors of BMC and BMD, but high levels of variation in BMC for the same level of wt (under, normal, over) negate its usefulness as a predictive indicator. |
| SFs at four sites, waist, hip, WHR, BMI[124] | n = 100; postmenopausal &, mean age = 55; Turkey | BMC, BMD, and whole body composition (lean and fat) determined by DEXA | Lean mass (but not fat mass) correlated with BMD at all sites measured (range r = 0.312–0.636; all p < 0.01). |
| Waist circumference, SSF, sum of SF measures[125] | n = 41 4-year-old children; 28 boys; 28 normal weight; 13 obese | Anthropometric measures compared with BMC and density from heel DEXA | Significant positive correlations were found between BMC and BMD and waist circumference, subscapular SF, and sum of SF measures. |

*Abbreviations*: M, male; F, female

*Other Abbreviations*: Central fat measures: SAF, subcutaneous abdominal fat; IAF, intra-abdominal fat; VF, visceral fat; TAF, total abdominal fat; CAF, central abdominal fat. Comparison ("gold standard") measures: DEXA, dual-energy x-ray absorptiometry; CT, computed tomography; MRI, magnetic resonance imaging; BMI, body mass index; CVD, cardiovascular disease; waist circ., waist circumference; BF, body fat.

Several studies evaluating the ability of simple anthropometric measures to identify those at risk for low bone mass and fractures have found a strong association between weight and bone mineral density (BMD), while others have not (see Table 39.11). Possible factors affecting the relationship between body weight and/or size and BMD include simple mechanical loading (because a larger and heavier body will need a stronger skeletal support), the influence of endogenous sex steroids, and possibly muscularity (either directly by its contribution to total body weight or indirectly by its association with increased activity). For these reasons, anthropometric measures related to gender-related weight distribution (central vs. lower body), FS, and measures of muscularity/adiposity have been investigated for their value in estimating BMD.

## CONCLUSION

Findings from recent studies using more precise reference methods have added important information to the already extensive body of literature in this area, thus improving our ability to use field methods of FS, circumferences, or SFs to estimate body composition, predict disease risk, or evaluate treatment outcomes. In particular, more data are available from well-designed studies of specific subgroups identified by age or life-stage, gender, ethnicity, and health condition. These data provide a more solid evidence base from which clinicians and researchers can select and apply these practical, inexpensive, and portable techniques when evaluating individuals and populations.

## REFERENCES

1. Bland JM, Altman DG. *Lancet* 1: 307; 1986.
2. Perini TA, de Oliveira GL, Ornellas JS, de Oliveira FP. *Rev Bras Med Esporte* 11: 86; 2005.
3. Wang J, Thornton JC, Kolesnik S, Pierson RN Jr. *Ann NY Acad Sci* 904: 317; 2000.
4. Sutcliffe JF. *Phys Med Biol* 41: 791; 1996.
5. Wagner DR, Heyward VH. *Res Q Exerc Sport* 70: 135; 1999.
6. Chumlea WC, Guo SS. *Endocrine* 13: 135; 2000.
7. Heyward VH, *Sports Med* 22: 146; 1996.
8. Frisancho AR. *Anthropometric Standards for the Assessment of Growth and Nutritional Status.* University of Michigan Press, Ann Arbor, MI, 1990.
9. Ulijaszek SJ, Mascie-Taylor CGN (eds.). *Anthropometry: The Individual and the Population.* Cambridge University Press, Cambridge, U.K., 1994.
10. Zerfas AJ. *Checking Continuous Measures: Manual for Anthropometry.* Division of Epidemiology, School of Public Health, University of California, Los Angeles, CA, 1985.
11. Ulijaszek SJ, Lourie JA. *Coll Antropol* 21: 429; 1997.
12. Fuller NJ, Sawyer MB, Elia M. *Int J Obes* 18: 503; 1994.
13. Lohman TG, Roche AF, Martorell R. *Anthropometric Standardization Reference Manual.* Human Kinetics, Champaign, IL, 1998.
14. Heyward VH, Stolarczyk LM. *Applied Body Composition Assessment.* Human Kinetics, Champaign, IL, 1996.
15. US Department of Health and Human Services: CDC 2005. http://www.cdc.gov/nchs/data/nhanes/nhanes_05_06/BM.pdf (accessed April 8, 2012).
16. Van Itallie TB. *Am J Public Health* 75: 1054; 1985.
17. Himes JH, Bouchard C. *Am J Public Health* 75: 1076; 1985.
18. Metropolitan Life Insurance Co. *Stat Bull* 40: 1; 1959.
19. Weigley ES. *JADA* 84: 417; 1984.

20. Metropolitan Life Insurance Co. Metropolitan height and weight tables. *Stat Bull* 64. 2–9, 1983.
21. Faulkner RA, Dailey DA. *Can J Public Health* 80: 369; 1989.
22. Callaway CW, Chumlea WC, Bouchard C et al. Circumferences. In: Lohman TG, Roche AF, Martorell R (eds.), *Anthropometric Standardization Reference Manual*. Human Kinetics Books, Champaign, IL, pp. 39–55, 1988.
23. Jelliffe EFP, Jelliffe DB. *J Trop Pediatr* 15: 179; 1969.
24. Frisancho AR. *Am J Clin Nutr* 34: 2540; 1981.
25. Gurney JM, Delliffe DB. *Am J Clin Nutr* 26: 912; 1973.
26. Heymsfield SB, McManus C, Smith J et al. *Am J Clin Nutr* 36: 680; 1982.
27. Katch FI, McArdle WD. *Nutrition, Weight Control, and Exercise*. Lea & Febiger, Philadelphia, PA, 1988.
28. Vickery SR, Cureton KJ, Collins MA. *Hum Biol* 60: 135; 1988.
29. Behnke AR. New concepts in height-weight relationships. In: Wilson NL (ed.), *Obesity*. FA Davis Company, Philadelphia, PA, pp. 25–54, 1988.
30. Lohman TG. *Hum Biol* 53: 181; 1981.
31. Harrison GG, Buskirk ER, Carter JEL et al. Skinfold thickness and measurement technique. In: Lohman TG, Roche AF, Martorell R (eds.), *Anthropometric Standardization Reference Manual*. Human Kinetics, Champaign, IL, p. 55; 1988.
32. Durnin JVGA, DeBruin H, Feunekes GIJ. *Br J Nutr* 77: 3; 1997.
33. Schmidt PK, Carter JEL. *Hum Biol* 62: 369; 1990.
34. Gruber JJ, Pollack ML et al. *Res Q* 61: 184; 1990.
35. Gore CJ, Woolford SM, Carlyon RG. *J Sports Sci* 13: 355; 1995.
36. Usaad SM, Patterson T, Ericksen J et al. *J Allergy Clin Immunol* 123: 1321; 2009.
37. Yao TC, Ou LS, Yeh KW et al. *J Asthma* 48: 503; 2011.
38. Padilla S, Gallego JA, Ardoy F et al. *Curr HIV Res* 5: 459; 2007.
39. Williams SRP, Jones E, Bell W, Cavies B, Bourne MW. *Eur Heart J* 18: 376; 1997.
40. Reilly JJ. *J Hum Nutr Diet* 23: 205; 2010.
41. Reilly JJ, Kelly J, Wilson DC. *Obesity* 11: 645; 2010.
42. Freedman DS, Katzmarzyk PT, Dietz WH et al. *Am J Clin Nutr* 90: 210; 2009.
43. Mei Z, Grummer-Strawn LM, Wang J et al. *Pediatrics* 119: e13067; 2007.
44. Reilly JJ, Dorosty AR, Ghomizadeh NM et al. *Int J Pediatr Obes* 5: 151; 2010.
45. Schwandt P. *Int J Prev Med* 2: 1; 2011.
46. Addo OY, Himes JH. *Am J Clin Nutr* 91: 635; 2010.
47. Bedogni G. Iughetti L, Ferrari M et al. *Ann Hum Biol* 30: 132; 2003.
48. Freedman DS, Wang J, Ogden CL et al. *Ann Hum Biol* 34: 183; 2007.
49. Freedman DS. *Am J Med Sci* 310: S72; 1995.
50. Van Lenthe FJ, Kemper HCG, Van Mechelen W, Twist JWR. *Int J Epidemiol* 25: 1162; 1996.
51. Paccaud F, Schluter-Fasmeyer V, Wietlisbach V, Bovet P. *J Clin Epidemiol* 53: 393; 2000.
52. Ohrvall M, Berglund L, Vessby B. *Int J Obes* 24: 497; 2000.
53. Gustat J. Elkasabany A, Srinivasan S, Berenson GS. *Am J Epidemiol* 151: 885; 2000.
54. Riserus U, de Faire U, Berglund L, Hellenius ML. *J Obes* 2010: 757939; 2010.
55. World Health Organization. http://whqlibdoc.who.int/publications/2011/9789241501491_eng.pdf (accessed April 3, 2012).
56. Ulijaszek SJ, Kerr DA. *Br J Nutr* 82: 165; 1999.
57. Nordhamm K, Sodergren E et al. *Int J Obes* 24: 652; 2000.
58. Frisancho AR. *Am J Clin Nutr* 40: 808; 1984.
59. Garn SM, Pesick SD, Hawthorne VM. *Am J Clin Nutr* 37: 315; 1983.
60. Grant JP. *Handbook of Total Parenteral Nutrition*. WB Saunders, Philadelphia, PA, 1980.
61. Frisancho AR, Flegel PN. *Am J Clin Nutr* 11: 418; 1983.
62. Katch VL, Freedson PS. *Am J Clin Nutr* 36: 669; 1982.
63. Peters DM, Eston R. *J Sports Sci* 11: 9; 1993.
64. Greil H, Trippo U. *Coll Antropol* 2: 345; 1998.
65. Fehily AM, Butland BK, Yarnell JWG. *Eur J Clin Nutr* 44: 107; 1990.
66. Nowak RK, Olmstead SL. *J Am Diet Assoc* 87: 339; 1987.
67. Mitchell MC. *J Am Diet Assoc* 93: 53; 1993.
68. Deurenberg P, Deurenberg YM, Wang J, Lin FP, Schmidt G. *Int J Obes Relat Metab Disord* 23: 537; 1999.
69. Hernandez RA, Hernandez deValera Y. *Arch Latinoam Nutr* 48: 13; 1998.
70. Henneberg M, Ulijaszek SJ. *Am J Hum Biol* 22: 83; 2010.
71. Jackson AS, Pollock ML. *Br J Nutr* 40: 497; 1978.
72. Jackson AS, Pollock ML, Ward A. *Med Sci Sports Exerc* 12: 175; 1980.
73. Brozek J, Grande F, Anderson JT et al. *Ann NY Acad Sci* 110: 113; 1963.
74. Durnin JVGA, Womersley J. *Br J Nutr* 32: 77; 1974.
75. Lukaski HC, Johnson PE, Bolonchuk WW, Lykken GI. *Am J Clin Nutr* 41: 1985; 1984.
76. Wright HF, Dotson CO, Davis PO. *US Navy Med* 72: 23; 1981.
77. Conway TL, Cronan TA, Peterson KA. *Aviat Space Environ Med* 60: 433; 1989.
78. Hodgdon JA, Beckett MB. Prediction of percent body fat for US Navy men from body circumferences and height. Technical Report No. 84-29, Naval Health Research Center, San Diego, CA, 1984.
79. Wright HF, Dotson CO, Davis PO. *US Navy Med* 71: 15; 1980.
80. Molarius A, Seidell JC, Sans S et al. *J Clin Epidemiol* 52: 1213; 1999.
81. Rutishauser IHE, Pasco JA, Wheeler CE. *Eur J Clin Nutr* 49: 248; 1995.
82. Goodman-Gruen D, Barrett-Connor E. *Am J Epidemiol* 143: 898; 1996.
83. Ben-Noun L, Sohar E, Laor A. *Obes Res* 9: 470; 2001.
84. Stomfai S, Ahrens W, Gammann K et al. *Int J Obes* 35: S45; 2011.
85. West J, Manchester B, Wright J et al. *Paediatr Perinat Epidemiol* 25: 164; 2011.
86. Peterson MJ, Czerwinski SA, Siervogel RM. *Am J Clin Nutr* 7: 1186; 2003.
87. Eston RG, Rowlands AV, Charlesworth S et al. *Eur J Clin Nutr* 59: 695; 2005.
88. Ball SD, Altena TS, Swan PD. *Eur J Clin Nutr* 58: 1525; 2004.
89. Garcia AL, Wagner K, Hothorn T et al. *Obes Res* 13: 626; 2005.
90. Wang J, Thornton JC, Russell M et al. *Am J Clin Nutr* 60: 23; 1994.
91. Irwin ML, Ainsworth BE, Stolarczyk LM, Heyward VH. *Med Sci Sports Exerc* 30: 1654; 1998.
92. Paxton A, Lederman SA, Heymsfield SB et al. *Am J Clin Nutr* 67: 104; 1998.
93. Goran MI, Driscoll P, Johnson R, Nagy TR, Hunter G. *Am J Clin Nutr* 63: 299; 1996.
94. Dezenberg CV, Nagy TR, Gower BA et al. *Int J Obes Relat Metab Disord* 23: 253; 1999.

95. Dempster P, Aitkens S. *Med Sci Sports Exerc* 27: 1692; 1995.
96. Elberg J, McDuffie JR, Sebring NG et al. *Am J Clin Nutr* 80: 64; 2004.
97. Slaughter MH, Lohman TG, Boileau RA et al. *Hum Biol* 60: 709; 1998.
98. Deurenberg P, Pieters JJ, Hautvast JG. *Br J Nutr* 63: 293; 1990.
99. Eisenmann JC, Heelan KA, Welk GJ. *Obes Res* 12: 1633; 2004.
100. Huang TTK, Watkins MP, Goran MI. *Obes Res* 11: 1192; 2003.
101. Wong WW, Stuff JE, Butte NF et al. *Am J Clin Nutr* 72: 348; 2000.
102. Cameron N, Griffiths PL, Wright MM et al. *Am J Clin Nutr* 80: 70; 2004.
103. Eliakim A, Ish-Shalom S, Giladi A et al. *Int J Sports Med* 21: 598; 2000.
104. Ravaglia G, Forti P, Mailoi F et al. *J Gerontol A Biol Sci Med Sci* 54: M70; 1999.
105. Visser M, Van Den Heuvel E, Deurenberg P. *Br J Nutr* 71: 823; 1994.
106. Gause-Nilsson I, Deay DK. *J Nutr* 9: 19; 2005.
107. Erselcan T, Candan F, Saruhan S, Ayca T. *Ann Nutr Metab* 44: 243; 2000.
108. Kamimura MA, Avesani CM, Cendoroglo M et al. *Nephrol Dial Transplant* 18: 101; 2003.
109. Nooyens ACJ, Koppes LJ, Visscher TLS et al. *Am J Clin Nutr* 85: 1533; 2007.
110. Flegel KM, Sheperd JA, Looker AC et al. *Am J Clin Nutr* 89: 500; 2009.
111. Schreiner PJ, Terry JG, Evans GW et al. *Am J Epidemiol* 15: 335; 1996.
112. Snijder MB, Visser M, Dekker JM et al. *Int J Obes Relat Metab Disord* 26: 984; 2002.
113. Goran MI, Gower BA, Treuth M, Nagy TR. *Int J Obes Relat Metab Disord* 22: 549; 1998.
114. Clasey JL, Bouchard C, Teates CD et al. *Obes Res* 7: 256; 1999.
115. Kamel EG, McNeill G, Van Wijk MC. *Obes Res* 8: 36; 2000.
116. Stanforth PR, Jackson AS, Green JS et al. *Int J Obes Relat Metab Disord* 28: 925; 2004.
117. Hughes VA, Roubenoof R, Wood M et al. *Am J Clin Nutr* 80:47; 2004.
118. Petersson H, Daryani A, Riserus U. *Cardiovasc Diabetol* 6: 10; 2007.
119. Riserus U, Arnlov J, Brismar K et al. *Diabetes Care* 27: 8; 2004.
120. Ross WD, Crawford SM, Kerr DS et al. *Am J Phys Anthropol* 77: 169; 1998.
121. Slemenda CW, Hui SL, Williams CJ et al. *Bone Miner* 11: 101; 1990.
122. Glauber HS, Vollmer WM, Nevitt MC et al. *J Clin Endocrinol Metab* 80: 1118; 1995.
123. Bedogni G, Simonini G, Viaggi S et al. *Ann Hum Biol* 26: 561; 1999.
124. Sahin G, Polat G, Baethis S et al. *Rheumatol Int* 23: 87; 2003.
125. Tubic B, Magnusson P, Swolin-Eide D, Marild S. *Int J Obes* 35: S119; 2011.

# 40 Psychological Assessment for Adults and Children

*Craig A. Johnston, Jennette P. Moreno, and John P. Foreyt*

## CONTENTS

## PSYCHOLOGICAL TESTS

Psychological factors play a significant role in many nutritional abnormalities. These factors include mood (e.g., depression, anger, and anxiety), emotional eating, distorted body image, low self-esteem, poor self-efficacy and quality of life, dietary restraint, stress, susceptibility to external cues to eat, and locus of control. They contribute to a number of nutritional abnormalities including obesity, and eating disorders such as anorexia nervosa (AN), bulimia nervosa (BN), and binge eating disorder (BED). The assessment of obesity and eating disorders requires not only a medical evaluation but also assessment of the contributing psychological factors. In this chapter we discuss instruments that assess psychological factors relevant to nutritional goals and concerns.

## OBESITY

Obesity is epidemic in our modern society.[1,2] Currently, 31.8% of children are considered to be overweight and obese.[2] The problem is only compounded in adulthood, with 74.1% of adult males and 64.5% of adult females having a BMI in the overweight or obese range.[1] While there appears to be a slowing in the increasing rates of obesity overall, the prevalence rates among male youths and adults continue to increase.[1,2] The abundance of palatable, energy-dense food is a significant factor fueling these high rates of obesity. Aromas, advertisements, and social gatherings are some of the environmental cues that trigger eating behavior. An individual's susceptibility to external cues to eat, perceptions of ability to control behavior, and feelings of self-efficacy and self-esteem are factors that interact with the environment to determine behavioral responses.

Despite awareness of the seriousness of obesity in the United States and the chronic and debilitating conditions related to it, many people do not attempt to change behaviors that contribute to the problem. Though a number of reasons for this failure to act have been given (e.g., lack of self-confidence, perception that change is too difficult, and lack of knowledge), to date research has not shown exactly why people maintain unhealthy habits. Of those who attempt change, the majority fail to maintain their weight loss goals.[3,4]

The ability to measure psychological states and traits may facilitate the planning of the treatment for disordered eating. Many of the instruments do not provide norms for obese populations; however, in light of the evidence indicating no significant differences in levels of psychopathology between obese and non-obese individuals, the lack of obesity-specific norms may not be a major problem.[5,6]

## EATING DISORDERS

AN, BN, and BED are eating disorders described in the *Diagnostic and Statistical Manual*, Fourth edition, Text Revised (DSM-IV-TR) published by the American Psychiatric Association.[7] AN is marked by a failure to maintain a minimal healthy body weight and a fear of gaining weight. BN is characterized by the uncontrollable eating of unusually large amounts of food (binge eating) followed by compensatory behavior such as vomiting. BED was proposed as an eating disorder for inclusion in the DSM-IV-TR. Although it was not accepted as a formal disorder, the DSM-IV-TR included research criteria to encourage further investigation of the condition.[7] BED is characterized by recurrent episodes of eating unusually large amounts of food within discrete periods of time, which are associated with feelings of being out of control. Three of the following features must also be present to meet the DSM-IV-TR criteria for BED: rapid eating; eating until uncomfortably full; eating when not physically hungry; and feelings of embarrassment, disgust, depression, and/or guilt. Additionally, the behavior must occur at least 2 days/week for a period of 6 months.[7]

These eating disorders are often comorbid with other psychological abnormalities. For example, the cardinal features of AN include fear of being out of control and distorted body image.[8] Comorbid major depression or dysthymia has been reported in 50%–75% of AN patients.[9] According to Maxmen and Ward,[8] 75% of BN patients develop major depression. Increased rates of anxiety were reported in 43% of individuals with AN.[9] Restrained eating and emotional eating due to stress are believed to be related to BED.[10] Large and unplanned changes in body weight are oftentimes symptoms of depression.[7]

We have identified instruments that measure psychological characteristics related to obesity and eating disorders in adults and children (Tables 40.1 and 40.2) and describe them in this chapter. Each description explains what the instrument measures, how it measures it, why it is important, administration and scoring procedures, norms, psychometrics, and availability.

## BROAD BASED MEASURES OF PSYCHOPATHOLOGY

### Symptom Checklist 90-R (SCL90-R)

The Symptom Checklist 90-R (SCL90-R)[11] is a 90-item self-report instrument designed to assess psychopathology in individuals 13 and older along 9 dimensions: somatization, obsessive–compulsive, interpersonal sensitivity, depression, anxiety, hostility, phobic anxiety, paranoid ideation,

**TABLE 40.1**

**Adult Psychological Instruments and What They Measure**

| | General Measure of Psychopathology | Eating Disorders | Symptoms of Eating Disorders | Binge Eating | Body Image | Mood | QOL | Self-Efficacy | Locus of Control | Stages of Change |
|---|---|---|---|---|---|---|---|---|---|---|
| SCL-90-R | x | | | | | x | | | | |
| EDI3 | | x | | | x | | | | | |
| EDE | | x | | | x | | | | | |
| SCOFF | | x | | | x | | | | | |
| EI | | | x | | | | | | | |
| DEBQ | | | x | | | | | | | |
| BULIT-R | | | x | x | x | | | | | |
| BEDT | | | x | x | x | | | | | |
| BES | | | x | x | | | | | | |
| FRS | | | | | x | | | | | |
| BIA | | | | | x | | | | | |
| BIA-O | | | | | x | | | | | |
| BDI-II | | | | | | x | | | | |
| CES-D | | | | | | x | | | | |
| SF-36 | | | | | | | x | | | |
| GWB | | | | | | x | x | | | |
| HeRQoLEDv2 | | | | | | | x | | | |
| ESES | | | | | | | | x | x | |
| DBS | | | | | | | | | x | |
| SOCA | | | | | | | | | | x |
| URICA | | | | | | | | | | x |
| ANSOCQ | | | | | | | | | | x |

**TABLE 40.2**

**Child Psychological Instruments and What They Measure**

| | General Measure of Psychopathology | Eating Disorders | Symptoms of Eating Disorders | Body Image | Family Health Environment | Mood | QOL |
|---|---|---|---|---|---|---|---|
| SCL-90-R | x | | | | | x | |
| BASC-2 | x | | | | | x | |
| EDI3 | | x | | x | | | |
| ChEDE | | x | | x | | | |
| KEDS | | x | | x | | | |
| DEBQ | | | x | | | | |
| DEPQ-P, -C | | | x | | | | |
| FHBS | | | | | x | | |
| FEAHQ | | | | | x | | |
| FNPA | | | | | x | | |
| PEAS | | | | | x | | |
| CDI 2 | | | | | | x | |
| PEDS-QL | | | | | | | x |

and psychosis. The scales of particular interest to clinicians are anxiety, hostility, and depression because they measure characteristics that may be related to abnormal eating behaviors.[8] The items describe physical and psychological conditions, and respondents are asked to assess the degree to which the conditions have affected them over the past 7 days. Responses are selected from a 5-point Likert scale that ranges from "not at all" (0) to "extremely" (4). The subscale scores are determined by averaging the scores of the items comprising each subscale.

The SCL-90-R has extensive normative data for psychiatric and non-psychiatric populations, white and non-white populations, men, women, and adolescents.[11] The subscales have good internal consistency with Cronbach alpha coefficients

($\alpha$) ranging from 0.77 to 0.90, as well as good test–retest reliability with Pearson Product Moment Coefficients (r) ranging from 0.78 to 0.90.[12] The SCL-90-R has also been evaluated in a bariatric surgery-seeking population and has shown to have excellent internal consistency ($\alpha$ = 0.76–0.97) and to discriminate between patients who have a history of inpatient psychiatric treatment.[13]

A weakness of the SCL90-R is a lack of evidence supporting the discriminant validity of the subscales.[14] The test appears to have the ability to measure general distress; however, its ability to discriminate between types of distress is not supported. The SCL-90-R is available from Pearson Assessments. The web address for this instrument is http://www.pearsonassessments.com/tests/scl90r.htm

## BEHAVIOR ASSESSMENT SYSTEM FOR CHILDREN, SECOND EDITION (BASC-2)

A similar instrument to the SCL90-R that can be used with children as young as 2 years of age is the BASC-2.[15] The BASC-2 provides a multidimensional approach to evaluating behavior and personality in children. It includes Teacher Rating Scales (TRS), Parent Rating Scales (PRS), and a Self-Report of Personality (SRP). The BASC-2 contains clinical scales (i.e., Aggression, Anxiety, Attention Problems, Atypicality, Conduct Problems, Depression, Hyperactivity, Learning Problems, Somatization, and Withdrawal) and adaptive scales (i.e., Activities of Daily Living, Adaptability, Functional Communication, Leadership, Study Skills and Social Skills). This instrument produces four composite scores including Externalizing Problems, Internalizing Problems, Behavioral Symptom Index, and Adaptive Skills. The TRS also contains an additional Learning Problems clinical scale, Study Skills adaptive scale, and a School Problems composite score.

Adequate reliability and validity have been shown for this measure.[15] Specifically, internal consistency ranges from 0.65 to 0.90 for all subscales and 0.85–0.95 for all composite scores. Test–retest reliability ranges from 0.65 to 0.89. The BASC-2 is available from Pearson Assessments. The web address for this instrument is http://www.pearsonassessments.com/HAIWEB/Cultures/en-us/Productdetail.htm?Pid=PAa30000.

## ASSESSMENT OF EATING DISORDERS

### EATING DISORDER INVENTORY

The Eating Disorder Inventory (EDI)[16] is a popular 91-item self-report instrument used to assess eating attitudes and behaviors along three subscales: drive for thinness, bulimia, and body dissatisfaction. Measurement of these factors is important because of their relation to serious nutrition-related conditions such as anorexia and bulimia.

The drive for thinness and the bulimia subscales assess attitudes and behaviors toward weight and eating. The body dissatisfaction scale is most related to body image. It assesses attitudes and behaviors toward the shapes of nine different body parts. Individuals indicate the degree to which they relate to statements by choosing from six possible answers ranging from "never" to "always." The three most pathological responses are scored 3, 2, and 1 in order of descending severity. The three least pathological responses are not scored. Scores are computed by summing all responses for each subscale. Normative data are available for male and female college-age eating-disordered and non-eating-disordered respondents[17] as well as for adolescents.[18] The body dissatisfaction subscale has been found to be reliable with children as young as 8 years old.[18]

In reports on internal consistency, reliability estimates of the eight scales ranged from 0.82 to 0.93. One year test–retest reliability in a non-disordered sample ranged from 0.41 to 0.75.[17] Test–retest reliability after a 3-week span was above 0.80 on all scales in a similar sample.[19]

Both the Eating Disorder Symptom Checklist (EDI-3SC) and the Eating Disorder Referral Form (EDI-3RF) are based on the EDI-3. The EDI-3SC is a self-report form that provides information on the frequency of eating-disordered symptoms. The EDI-3RF is an abbreviated form that is intended to identify individuals who have or are at high risk for having an eating disorder. The most current version is the EDI-3 and is available from Psychological Assessment Resources, Odessa, FL. The web address for this instrument is http://www4.parinc.com/Products/Product.aspx?ProductID=EDI-3

### EATING DISORDERS EXAMINATION

The Eating Disorders Examination (EDE)[20] is a 62-item semi-structured interview that measures the presence of disorders along four subscales: shape concern, weight concern, eating concern, and dietary restraint. Shape concern consists of general feelings of dissatisfaction and preoccupation with issues related to body image. Weight concern refers to the desire to lose weight and the importance given to it. The eating concern subscale measures fear and guilt about eating as well as any preoccupation with food. The dietary restraint scale attempts to quantify the degree to which individuals are guided by strict rules concerning type and quantity of food.

In addition to subscale items, the examination also has items used in making a clinical diagnosis of eating disorders. The EDE was originally developed with individuals suffering from BN and AN. Hence, the examination is useful in determining specific areas of concern as well as in making formal clinical diagnoses of eating disorders. It is a mature instrument that underwent many revisions before publication.

The items used in calculating the four subscales are scored using a severity indicator expressed by a Likert scale that ranges from 0 to 6. These items are organized within a set of 23 higher-order categories such as pattern of eating, restraint, and fear of losing control. The 4 subscales comprised the 23 higher-order items, with the restraint scale consisting of 5 items, the eating concern scale 5, the weight concern scale 5, and the shape concern scale 8. Subscale values are computed by summing the severity indicators of the related items and then dividing by the number of valid items. A global score, defined as the sum of the individual subscale scores divided by the number of valid subscales, may also be computed. The diagnostic items are scored in terms of frequency (e.g., frequency of binge days over the preceding 2 months).

The EDE is a preferred method for assessing binge eating. It is designed to be administered and scored by trained interviewers familiar with eating disorders. It measures eating behavior using a 28-day recall method, although some questions extend out to the previous 3 and 6 months. Even when administered by trained interviewers, requiring a recall of eating over the past 14 days prior is problematic. Administration may take 1 h or more when properly given. The authors of the instrument recommend that the interviewer first seek to develop a rapport with the respondent. The belief is that good rapport and a feeling of trust facilitates disclosure and contributes in a positive way to the validity of the process.

The EDE appears to have satisfactory internal consistency. With a sample of 100 eating-disordered patients and 42 controls, Cooper et al.[21] reported α coefficients ranging from 0.68 to 0.82 for the four subscales. Another study measuring internal consistency in a sample of 116 eating-disordered people reported α coefficients ranging from 0.68 to 0.78.[22] In studies of inter-rater reliability, very good correlations were reported across all items.[23,24] The EDE appears in an article by Fairburn and Cooper.[20]

The EDE Questionnaire (EDE-Q) is adapted from the EDE for a pencil and paper format.[25] It consists of 33 items with the same 4 subscales as the EDE. It has excellent internal consistency and test–retest reliability.[26] Overall, the EDE and the EDE-Q are similar in the assessment of behavioral symptoms.[25] There may be greater variability between the EDE and EDE-Q when assessing binge eating, and caution should be taken in using and interpreting individual subscales in nonclinical populations of young adolescents.[27] The full version of this questionnaire can be found in a chapter by Fairburn and Beglin.[28]

In order to better address developmental differences, the EDE is also adapted for use with children.[29] The Child Eating Disorder Examination (ChEDE) is a semistructured clinical interview very similar to the adult version, but modified to assess intent rather than actual behavior. The language of the EDE was also modified to be appropriate for children ages 8–14. The ChEDE is reported to have sufficient inter-rater reliability (r = 0.91–1.0), internal consistency (α = 0.80–0.91) and discriminant validity.[30] In addition to having been used to assess eating disorders, the ChEDE has been used to examine overeating and loss of control in a severely obese child population.[31] The primary source for this measure is an article by Bryant-Waugh et al.[29]

### KIDS EATING DISORDER SURVEY

The Kids Eating Disorder Survey (KEDS)[32] is a 12-item self-report questionnaire used to assess symptoms of eating disorders in children.[33] It has two subscales: purging/restriction

and weight dissatisfaction, which have been shown to discriminate between children with and without eating disorders.[33] Scores of 16 or more are considered to be elevated on either scale. A KEDS total score is also provided. Two administered items are not accounted for on either of the subscales, but are included in the total score.[33]

The questionnaire has been found to be reliable and valid in children between 10 and 13 years of age.[32] However, an interview format has been used to assist younger children interpret questions.[34] Results have indicated that the KEDS has adequate internal consistency (α = 0.73) and good test–retest reliability (r = 0.83).[32] Overall, the KEDS was found to be useful in identifying children with eating disorders as determined by a clinical interview.[33] The KEDS appears in an article by Childress et al.[33]

### SCOFF

The SCOFF questionnaire is a brief and easy-to-use screener for AN and BN.[35] Each letter represents one of the five questions, targeting one of the core features of eating disorders. Purging (make yourself **S**ick), disinhibition (lost **C**ontrol), rapid weight loss (lost **O**ne stone or 15 lb), body image disturbance (view yourself as **F**at when others say you are thin), and preoccupation with food (**F**ood dominates your life). This measure was designed for use by non mental health specialists such as primary care doctors.[36] The short and easy-to-remember format allows for quick administration during a medical visit, but can also be completed in a paper and pencil format. This questionnaire is not intended to be used for diagnostic purposes, but will identify whether further evaluation by a specialist is needed. If a respondent answers in the affirmative to two of the five questions, further evaluation is recommended.

The SCOFF has demonstrated high sensitivity, correctly identifying 84.6% of eating disorder patients and high specificity, correctly identifying 89.6% who do not have an eating disorder.[36] Reliability between written and oral formats is high (κ = 0.82). Additionally, the SCOFF has demonstrated strong convergent validity with other measures of eating disorders. There is some evidence that the EDE-Q may out perform the SCOFF; however, this should be considered in combination with the brevity of the SCOFF which may make it preferable for use as a screening tool.[27] The SCOFF has been published in the *British Medical Journal*.[35]

## MEASURES OF SPECIFIC SYMPTOMS OF EATING DISORDERS

### EATING INVENTORY, ALSO KNOWN AS THE THREE-FACTOR EATING QUESTIONNAIRE

The Three-Factor Eating Questionnaire (TFEQ-R)[37] is a 51-item self-report instrument that was developed as a measure of behavioral restraint in eating in adults. Measuring restraint is important in the nutritional context of obesity because severe caloric restriction may lead to binge eating and increased metabolic efficiency, promoting weight gain.[38,39]

Restriction also has nutritional sequelae such as vitamin deficiency and related morbidity.

The instrument is divided into two parts. The first part consists of 36 true/false questions. The second part has 14 questions presented in a four-level Likert format with choices ranging from *rarely* to *always*, plus an additional question that is a six-point rating of perceived self-restraint. Questions ask about cues to eat, ability to control eating, and willingness to diet. Respondents are asked to indicate how often each statement applies to their personal behavior patterns. The questionnaire contains three subscales: Cognitive Control of Eating, and Disinhibition, Susceptibility to Hunger. The Cognitive Control subscale is related to one's awareness of and ability to cognitively control or restrain eating behavior. Disinhibition assesses the tendency to periodically lose control of eating, and the Susceptibility to Hunger subscale refers to one's ability to resist cues to eat.

Scoring is described in the Eating Inventory (EI) Manual.[40] The control subscale has 21 questions, the disinhibition subscale has 16, and the hunger subscale has 14. Each question has a value of zero or one. Individual subscale scores are calculated by summing the scores of the related questions. Scores above 13, 11, and 10 are considered to be in the clinical range for the control, disinhibition, and hunger subscales, respectively.

The TFEQ-R appears to have good construct validity. Food diaries and doubly labeled water techniques have been used to assess the construct validity of the subscales. These studies have shown that high scores on the restraint scale are correlated in the hypothesized direction with low levels of caloric intake.[41,42] The test also has good internal consistency ($\alpha = 0.80$–$0.93$)[37] and test–retest reliability of 0.80–91 over 2 weeks.[43] The inventory appears in an article by Stunkard and Messick.[37] The inventory and related scoring materials are available from the Psychological Corporation, San Antonio, Texas. The web address for this instrument is http://www.pearsonassessments.com/HAIWEB/Cultures/en-us/Productdetail.htm?Pid=015-8102-258.

An 18-item version of the TFEQ-R has been developed (TFEQ-R18V2).[44] Questions are rated on a 4-point Likert format. The short form has demonstrated adequate internal consistency ($\alpha = 0.70$–$0.92$). Additionally, there is strong evidence for the factor structure within both obese and nonobese populations. The TFEQ-R18V2 and its scoring instructions are provided in an article by Cappelleri et al.[44]

## Dutch Eating Behavior Questionnaire

The Dutch Eating Behavior Questionnaire (DEBQ)[45] is a 33-item self-report instrument that measures eating behavior along three subscales: restrained eating, emotional eating, and eating in response to external cues. The diagnostic capabilities of this instrument are useful for identifying overeating triggers when designing effective behavioral interventions, as well as for the identification of individuals with restrained eating patterns. The reading level of this instrument is between the fifth and eighth grade.[46] In research, it has been used with children as a measure of dieting behavior, though it is designed for use in adults.[47,48]

The instrument consists of questions related to eating behavior. Each item is presented in a 5-point Likert response format with possible answers being: *never, seldom, sometimes, often,* and *very often.* Some of the items have an additional *not relevant* category. Subscale scores are computed by summing the scores of the related items and dividing by the number of items. Items scored as not relevant are omitted from the subscale score.

The restraint scale has received most of the research attention, and some norms are available for this scale.[49] In general, they indicate that women have higher restraint scores than men, and that obese people have higher restraint scores than non-obese. Internal consistency of the scales was reported in the range from 0.80 to 0.95.[49] Two-week test–retest reliability of the restraint scale was 0.92.[42] The DEBQ is published in an article by Van Strien et al.[45]

The DEBQ-P is a parent report measure of emotional, external, and restrained eating in children ages 11–14.[50] The DEBQ-P was developed to address inadequacy of self-report measures to address overeating in children. The DEBQ-P has also been shown to have good internal consistency ($\alpha = 0.81$–$0.87$). The construct validity of the scale has been established through factor analysis. The restrained eating subscale of the DEBQ-P has been shown to discriminate between normal weight and overweight and obese children. One limitation of the parent report of this measure is that it has not been validated in an English speaking sample. The primary source for this questionnaire is an article by Caccialanza et al.[50]

A child self-report version of the DEBQ has been developed for children 7–12 years old.[51] The DEBQ-C contains fewer items (20 items) in order to better complement the shorter attention spans of younger children and has simplified language. The three subscales of the DEBQ-C (i.e., emotional, external, and restrained eating) demonstrated adequate internal consistency ($\alpha = 0.73$–$0.82$), and there is evidence for the construct and concurrent validity of the scale. Interestingly, researchers have found children to more commonly report engaging in restrained eating which is often thought to lead to subsequent overeating. However, in boys, the frequency of restrained eating is linked with the amount of time spent engaged in sports. In girls, dietary restraint was related to skipping breakfast and body dissatisfaction, suggesting that dietary restraint in girls is not likely to be healthy. This questionnaire has been adapted for children in an article by Van Strien et al.[51]

# ASSESSMENT OF BINGE EATING

## Bulimia Test–Revised and Binge Eating Disorder Test

The Bulimia Test–Revised (BULIT-R) is a 36-item self-report measure of binge eating, compensatory behavior, and weight and shape concerns.[52] It was originally developed in 1984 based in the DSM-III criteria for bulimia.[53] The revised version was published in 1991.[52] A total of 28 of the 36 items are used to compute a total score. Items are scored on a 5-point Likert scale and a cutoff score of 104 is recommended for optimal sensitivity and specificity, though others have recommended alternative cutoff values.[54,55] The BULIT-R has demonstrated high internal consistency ($\alpha = 0.97$) and test–retest reliability ($r = 0.95$). There is also strong evidence of the concurrent and discriminant validity for assessing BN in adolescent and adult samples.[55,56] The BULIT-R has also been used as a screener for BED, which is likely to be added as a new diagnosis in the DSM-V.[57] The primary source for this measure is an article by Thelen et al.[52]

The Binge Eating Disorder Test (BEDT)[57] contains 23 of the items from the BULIT-R which assess binge eating, loss of control, and body image factors, and excludes items related to compensatory behaviors. The BEDT has demonstrated strong internal consistency ($\alpha = 0.96$). The BEDT has been shown to correctly classify whether a person meets criteria for BED for 100% of respondents using a cutoff score of 75. The BEDT is considered to be superior to the BULIT-R as a screener for BED, though the BULIT-R allows for assessment of potential compensatory behaviors.[57] Items used in this measure are available in an article by Thelen et al.[52]

## BINGE EATING SCALE

The Binge Eating Scale (BES)[58] is a 16-item scale designed to assess binge eating in individuals who are obese. It has also been used with non-obese populations. Eight items of the BES measure binge eating behavior and the other eight measure associated feelings and thoughts. Each item consists of a cluster of self-statements. Respondents are asked to select the statement that most closely resembles their feelings. Responses are given different weights. The scale score is computed by summing weighted scores of the 16 items. The BES does not assess all of the information necessary to make a clinical diagnosis, but does measure behavioral features and cognitions associated with binge eating. The scale score has been interpreted as an indication of severity of binge eating.[64] The range of potential scores is 0–46, with higher scores indicating higher levels of binge eating. A score above 27 suggests severe binge eating.

The original work by Gormally et al.[58] demonstrates that the BES has adequate internal consistency. The scale discriminates well between individuals with BN (non-purging) and normal controls.[59] The BES has good test–retest reliability.[60] The BES, along with norms and instructions for scoring, appears in an article by Gormally et al.[58]

## WEIGHT DISSATISFACTION

### FIGURE RATING SCALE

The figure rating scale (FRS)[61] is a popular instrument used to assess an individual's level of dissatisfaction with their physical appearance. Dissatisfaction with physical appearance is a core feature of eating disorders and is included in the diagnostic criteria for AN and BN.[7] The instrument consists of a set of nine figures of increasingly larger size. Administration is done in two parts. First, respondents select the figure that most closely resembles their current size. Next, the figure that most closely resembles their ideal size is selected. The difference (discrepancy score) between selections represents their level of body dissatisfaction.

The FRS has been shown to have good test–retest reliability as well as strong evidence of validity.[62,63] Two-week test–retest reliability was 0.82 for ideal size and 0.92 for current size in a sample of 34 men, and 0.71 for ideal size and 0.89 for current size in a sample of 58 women.[62] In a sample of 146 women, correlations between discrepancy scores and other measures of self-image were moderate to strong.[62] Furthermore, the FRS has been shown to be highly correlated with actual BMI.[63] The scale appears in chapter by Stunkard et al.[61] A similar scale has been developed for use in African American populations and has demonstrated strong cultural relevance.[64]

The use of figure scales for children has been discouraged for several reasons. First, most of the instruments are age-specific. This is problematic because the shape of children's bodies change so rapidly, and images from one age group to another do not generalize. Second, reliability coefficients for most of the scales fall well below 0.70.[65] Finally, most of the stimuli were made using obvious Caucasian characteristics.[66] For a measure of body dissatisfaction in children, the reader is directed to the previous descriptions of the EDI-3 and the KEDS.

## BODY IMAGE ASSESSMENT AND THE BODY IMAGE ASSESSMENT FOR OBESITY

Similar to the FRS, the Body Image Assessment (BIA) is a figure stimulus method of assessing body images.[67] The original version of the scale contains nine female and male figures ranging in size from very thin to overweight. Raters are asked to select their actual or current body size and their ideal body size. The discrepancy between current body size and ideal body size is an approximation of dissatisfaction with body size. The BIA is available in an article by Williamson et al.[67]

The Body Image Assessment for Obesity (BIA-O) added an additional nine figures ranging in size from overweight to severely obese.[68] The figures are presented on separate cards and presented one at a time in a random order. As with the original BIA, raters are asked to select their current and ideal body size, but also a body size that they believe is reasonable to maintain for a long period of time. The BIA-O yields five measures: current body size, ideal body size, reasonable body size, the discrepancy between current body size and ideal body size, and the discrepancy between current body size and reasonable body size. The two discrepancy scores are considered measures of body size dissatisfaction.

The BIA-O has demonstrated good test–retest reliability for both the male ($r = 0.65$–81) and female ($r = 0.77$–0.93) versions of the scale. Additionally, both the discrepancy scores were highly correlated with other measures of body size dissatisfaction demonstrating evidence of good concurrent validity. The BIA-O is published in the *International Journal of Obesity.*[68]

## ASSESSMENT OF FAMILY HEALTH ENVIRONMENT

### FAMILY HEALTH BEHAVIORS SCALE

Due to the increasing rates of childhood obesity, greater attention is being paid to factors in the family environment which may be contributing to obesity. These factors are often referred to as obesogenic behaviors. Several measures have been developed to assess the presence of healthy and obesogenic behaviors in the family environment. These measures often assess both parent and child behaviors.

The Family Health Behaviors Scale (FHBS) is a 27-item parent-report measure of family and child behaviors related to obesity in children between 5 and 12 years old.[69] Caregivers rate the frequency of healthy and obesogenic behaviors using a 5-point Likert scale ranging from 0 "almost never" to 4 "nearly always." Obesogenic items are reverse scored. Higher scores on the FHBS and its subscales indicate a greater frequency of health-promoting behaviors. The scale yields a total score and four subscales measuring Parent Behaviors (10 items), Physical Activity (6 items), Mealtime Routines (5 items), and Child Behaviors (6 items).

The FHBS has demonstrated good internal consistency with coefficient α's ranging from 0.66 to 0.86 as well as test–retest reliability with correlation coefficients ranging from 0.56 to 0.85. Additionally, higher scores on the FHBS predicted a decreased likelihood of being overweight or obese. The construct validity of the FHBS has been established through factor analysis in an ethnically and economically diverse sample. The FHBS is available in an article by Moreno et al.[69]

### FAMILY EATING AND ACTIVITY HABITS QUESTIONNAIRE

The Family Eating and Activity Habits Questionnaire (FEAHQ) is a 21-item parent-report measure of family behaviors and environmental factors related to weight gain or weight loss.[70] It comprised four variables: activity level, stimulus exposure, eating related to hunger, and eating style. Subscale scores are calculated for each member of the family (mother, father, and child). The measure has shown acceptable levels of test–retest reliability (r = 0.78–0.90) and internal consistency (α = 0.83). The FEAHQ appears to be sensitive to behavior changes during treatment. The FEAHQ has demonstrated concurrent validity with obese children having significantly higher scores on the FEAHQ than healthy weight children. Additionally, the content validity of the measure has been evaluated by an expert panel, though additional research is needed to support the concurrent and discriminant validity of the measure.

The FEAHQ seeks to measure several important factors such as parenting behaviors, environmental factors, and

eating and physical activity behaviors. The FEAHQ may have potentially useful clinical applications such as identifying target behaviors for treatment and monitoring treatment progress. The FEAHQ has been published in the *European Journal of Clinical Nutrition.*[70]

### FAMILY NUTRITION AND PHYSICAL ACTIVITY SCREENING TOOL

The Family Nutrition and Physical Activity (FNPA) is a 21-item questionnaire of behaviors related to children's risk for being overweight.[71] The questionnaire measures 10 constructs: breakfast and family meals, modeling of nutrition, nutrient-dense foods, high-calorie beverages, restriction and reward, parent modeling of physical activity, child's physical activity, screen time, TV in bedroom, and sleep routines.[72] Higher scores on this measure indicate more health-promoting behaviors and lower scores indicated greater risk for obesity.

Support for the validity and reliability of the FNPA was established in a large urban school district. The FNPA has been shown to discriminate between overweight and healthy weight children[71] and to explain the unique variance in follow-up child BMI even when controlling for baseline BMI, parent BMI, gender, and ethnicity.[72] The reliability of the FNPA has not been evaluated. The FNPA is available through the American Dietetic Association using the following website: http://adaf.eatright-fnpa.org/public/partner.cfm.

### PARENTING STRATEGIES FOR EATING AND ACTIVITY SCALE

The Parenting Strategies for Eating and Activity Scale (PEAS) is a 26-item measure of parenting behaviors related to children's eating and physical activity behaviors.[73] It is available in both English and Spanish and was developed and validated in a Latino sample. The PEAS measures five constructs: limit setting, monitoring, discipline, control, and reinforcement related to eating and physical activity behaviors in children. High internal consistency has been established for all five subscales (α = 0.81–0.82), and there is strong evidence of concurrent validity with other measures which measure behavioral strategies. There is less evidence for the ability of the PEAS to predict standardized BMI (zBMI). Only the control scale was correlated with zBMI, indicating that parents with fewer controlling behaviors were more likely to have children with higher BMIs. The PEAS has been published in the journal *Appetite.*[73]

## MOOD

### BECK DEPRESSION INVENTORY–SECOND EDITION

The comorbidity of depression and eating disorders is well documented.[74,75] Depressive symptoms are more severe among obese individuals who also binge eat than among non-bingers.[76] The assessment of mood in people receiving treatment for obesity and eating disorders is important because disorders such as depression may have a negative impact on program adherence,[77] and intervention outcomes.[70,79] Specifically, treatment outcomes for individuals with eating-related disorders and comorbid depression may be improved by treating the depression first.

The Beck Depression Inventory—Second Edition (BDI-II)[80] is a 21-item instrument commonly used to measure depression. The items explore changes in mood, activity level, self-concept, and feelings of self-worth. The BDI-II has been used with a broad array of people ranging from young adolescents through adults. It is easy to understand and takes only about 10 min to complete.

Each item offers a choice of four self-descriptive statements that range in severity from 0 to 3. The instrument is scored by summing the values of the individual items. The range of possible scores is 0–63. Cutoff scores for interpretation of the instrument are 0–13, minimal; 14–19, mild; 20–28, moderate; and 29–63, severe depression.[80]

The BDI-II has demonstrated high internal consistency ($\alpha = 0.92$), good retest reliability ($r = 0.93$), and strong construct and convergent validity.[80,81] The BDI-II is available from Pearson Assessment. The web address for this instrument is http://psychcorp.pearsonassessments.com/HAIWEB/Cultures/en-us/Productdetail.htm?Pid=015-8018-370&Mode=summary.

## CHILDREN'S DEPRESSION INVENTORY SECOND EDITION

Similar to the BDI-II, the Children's Depression Inventory Second Edition (CDI 2) is a multi-rater (i.e., parent, self, and teacher) measure of depression in youth ages 7–17.[82] The CDI 2 self-report measure yields a total score, two scale scores (i.e., Emotional Problems and Functional Problems), and four subscale scores (i.e., Negative Mood/Physical Symptoms, Negative Self-Esteem, Interpersonal Problems, and Ineffectiveness). For quick screening purposes, a short form of 12 items is also available. The reading level of the CDI is at the first grade, which is the lowest reading level for any measure of depression in children.[83]

Each item offers a choice of three possible answers that range in severity from 0 (absence of symptoms) to 2 (definite symptom). The range of possible scores is 0–56. Reliability and validity have been found to be good.[82] The CDI 2 is available in paper and pencil, software, and online formats from MHS. The web address for this instrument is http://www.mhs.com/product.aspx?gr=edu&prod=cdi2&id=overview.

## CENTER FOR EPIDEMIOLOGIC STUDIES DEPRESSION SCALE

The Center for Epidemiologic Studies Depression Scale (CES-D)[84] is another self-report instrument used to screen for recent symptoms of depression. The CES-D is a 20-item measure, with each item offering four possible response choices which range in severity from 0 to 3. The range of possible scores is 0–60, with higher scores indicative of greater distress. Scores greater than or equal to 16 are reflective of significant distress.[84]

The CES-D is a widely used screening instrument for adults of various ages and ethnicities[85] and has been found to be a reliable instrument with high internal consistency and good test–retest reliability.[84,86] The CES-D has also been demonstrated to have good factorial and discriminant validity.[86] The CES-D is available online at no cost, and can be found on several websites, including: http://www.chcr.brown.edu/pcoc/cesdscale.pdf.

## QUALITY OF LIFE

### MEDICAL OUTCOMES STUDY SHORT-FORM 36 HEALTH STATUS SURVEY (SF-36)

Quality of life is a global construct that incorporates emotional, social, and physical functioning. It provides a comprehensive assessment of both physical and psychosocial factors that may impact a patient. Quality of life may be used as an outcome to determine if an intervention has improved multiple areas of a patient's life. Health-related quality of life has been shown to be significantly impaired in people who are overweight, and as weight increases, quality of life decreases.[87] The quality of life of obese children has also been shown to be lower than that of healthy children and more similar to that of children with cancer.[88]

The SF-36[89] was developed to provide a general assessment of health status. The measure has 36 items, representing 8 domains: physical functioning, pain, social functioning, vitality, general health, emotional well-being, role limitations caused by physical problems as well as those caused by emotional problems. Participants self-report their responses, and domains are scored separately with scores ranging from 0 (low) to 100 (high). Thus, the SF-36 is useful as an indicator of the extent to which weight presents problems in various aspects of health. The use of the SF-36 has been supported in diverse groups of participants, and the measure is available in numerous languages. This instrument is widely accepted as a valid measure of health-related quality of life with reliability coefficients for the domains ranging from 0.65 to 0.94.[90] There is an updated second version of the SF-36 which is the SF-36v2. The web address for this instrument is www.sf-36.org.

### GENERAL WELL BEING SCHEDULE

The General Well Being Schedule (GWB)[91] is comprised of 18 items indicating subjective feelings of psychological well-being and distress. GWB total scores are computed by summing across all 18 items and subtracting 14, since the items are on both 6-point and 11-point Likert scales. Scores range from 0 to 110, with low scores representing greater distress.[91] Proposed cutoffs representing three levels of distress are 0–60 (severe distress), 61–72 (moderate distress), and 73–110 (positive well-being). In addition, this measure assesses six hypothesized dimensions including anxiety, depression, general health, positive well-being, self-control, and vitality.[92]

Adequate test–retest reliability has been reported for the GWB Total, with reliability coefficients ranging from

0.68 to 0.85.[93,94] High internal consistency has been demonstrated for the GWB, with all correlations reported to be over 0.90.[94] Previous studies have also consistently demonstrated concurrent validity between the GWB and depression scales[95] and with use of psychiatric services.[93] The GWB is available in a book by McDowell and Newell.[96] It is also available online: http://www.mhhe.com/socscience/hhp/fahey7e/wellness_worksheets/wellness_worksheet_023.html.

### PEDIATRIC QUALITY OF LIFE SCALE

The Pediatric Quality of Life Scale (PedsQL) 4.0[97] is a 23-item self-report measure that assesses health-related quality of life in children and adolescents. Each item is answered using a 5-point scale that ranges from "Never" to "Almost Always." The measure yields 4 generic core scales of functioning (physical, 8 items; emotional, 5 items; social, 5 items; and school, 5 items) and 3 summary scales (total scale, 23 items; physical health, 8 items; and psychosocial health, 15 items).

The scale has demonstrated reliability with a Cronbach α reliability coefficient of 0.90 for the total scale score and with all subscale scores exceeding Cronbach α of 0.70.[98] Validity of the scale is supported based on its ability to distinguish between healthy and physically ill children. In addition, the scale has been shown to respond to clinical change over time and has been normed and used in a variety of ethnic minority groups.[98] The web address for this instrument is www.pedsql.org/conditions.html.

### HEALTH-RELATED QUALITY OF LIFE FOR EATING DISORDERS

The Health-Related Quality of Life for Eating Disorder (HeRQoLED)[99] is a 55-item self-report measure used to assess an individual's health-related quality of life as related to eating disorders. The scale assesses nine domains of functioning: symptoms, restrictive behaviors, binge eating, body image, mental health, emotional role, physical role, personality traits, and social relations. The scores in each domain are converted into a range from 0 to 100, with higher scores indicative of worse functioning.[100] The HeRQoLED is appropriate for ages 16–60.[101]

Patients with AN have been found to have higher scores on the HeRQoLED when compared to the general population, though their scores have been shown to increase post-treatment.[102] The most recent version of the HeRQoLED is the second version (HeRQoLEDv2).[100] The initial version has been published in the *Journal of Clinical Epidemiology*.[99]

## SELF-EFFICACY

### EATING SELF-EFFICACY SCALE

For many people, today's environment is filled with opportunities and encouragement to consume large quantities of food. This is especially challenging for those who eat in response to stress. Understanding a person's behavioral response in the presence of gastronomical opportunities and stress is important in the design of programs to normalize eating.

The Eating Self-Efficacy Scale (ESES)[103] is a self-report instrument designed to measure perceived ability to control eating behavior in 25 challenging situations. Perceived ability to control eating is evaluated along two subscales: control in socially acceptable situations and control when experiencing negative effect. Items are rated on a Likert scale that presents answers in a 7-point format. Ten of the items make up the social acceptability subscale and the other 15 make up the negative effect subscale. Subscale scores are computed by summing the scores of the associated items. The instrument appears to have good internal consistency across subscales. Alpha coefficients for a sample of 484 female undergraduates were 0.85 for the negative effect subscale and 0.85 for the social acceptability subscale.[103] Seven-week test–retest reliability using a sample of 85 female undergraduates was 0.70.[103] The ESES appears in an article by Glynn and Ruderman.[103]

## LOCUS OF CONTROL

### DIETING BELIEFS SCALE

The Dieting Beliefs Scale (DBS)[104] is a 16-item scale that measures weight-specific locus of control. Weight locus of control is a method for categorizing beliefs about factors influencing weight. Individuals with an internal locus of control have the expectancy that they can control, to some extent, their own weight. An external locus of control implies a more fatalistic orientation marked by beliefs that weight is determined by factors outside of personal control (e.g., genetics, environment, and/or social context).

The utility of this instrument is in the planning of treatment of obese and overweight individuals. Theoretically, individuals who believe that they have control over factors determining their weight would be expected to have greater success in weight management programs. Identifying individuals with an external locus of control might be valuable in the process of treatment planning because it would cue the counselor to be particularly mindful to avoid interventions that might inadvertently reinforce pre-existing negative expectations. For example, very modest and frequently measured short-term goals may be set for individuals with external loci of control in an effort to encourage them toward more positive expectations.

The 16 items are statements expressing either internal or external locus of control viewpoints: eight are internal and eight are external. The items are presented in a 6-point Likert format ranging from *not at all descriptive of my beliefs* (1) to *very descriptive of my beliefs* (6). Eight of the items are reverse scored. The instrument is scored in the internal direction so that high scores indicate more of an internal locus of control.

The DBS has three subscales: internal control, uncontrolled factors, and environmental factors. The internal control subscale is related to the belief that individuals can control their weights through internal means such as willpower and effort. The uncontrolled factors subscale is associated with belief in the importance of factors such as genetics and fate. The environmental factors subscale is related to beliefs in the importance of context and social setting. The subscales are scored by summing the individual items that make up the scale.

The scale demonstrates moderate internal consistency (Chronbach's α = 0.69) and good stability in a sample of undergraduate students.[104] The DBS is published in an article by Stotland and Zuroff.[104]

## STAGE OF CHANGE

### STAGES OF CHANGE ALGORITHM

The Stages of Change Algorithm (SOCA)[105] is a self-report instrument that assesses weight loss activities and intentions. The instrument is based on the transtheoretical model,[106] which conceptualizes change as a six-stage process. The stages are precontemplation, contemplation, preparation, action, maintenance, and termination. The purpose of the model is to maximize successful behavior change. The model posits that optimal intervention strategies vary according to a person's position in the change process. The purpose of the SOCA is to facilitate treatment planning by identifying the individual's position in the process. Persons in the precontemplation stage may not at all be concerned with their condition. These individuals might benefit from efforts to raise their awareness and to personalize their risk factors. People in the contemplation stage may be concerned but not yet decided on taking action. Such people might benefit from information regarding possible treatment alternatives. The preparation stage is characterized by having decided to do something about the condition and have taken some steps aimed at changing. Encouragement to take action and to make a commitment to their health may help people move to the action stage. Individuals in the action stage have recently shown behavior change and may benefit most from behavioral interventions such as goal setting and self-monitoring. Moral support and recognition might be best for people in the maintenance stage as they have implemented changes over a period of time. The SOCA uses only four of the stages: precontemplation, contemplation, action, and maintenance. The model is of particular interest in the context of nutrition because of the refractory nature of dysfunctional eating behavior.

The SOCA consists of four yes/no items. The scoring is simple and the determination of the person's stage of change is quickly determined.[105] Data describing the reliability of the SOCA for weight loss are not available. The SOCA was found to be reliable when applied to similar problems. For example, in their investigation of the processes of change in smoking-related behavior, Prochaska et al.[107] observed α coefficients ranging from 0.69 to 0.92, with the majority being above 0.80. The SOCA is published in an article by Rossi et al.[105]

### UNIVERSITY OF RHODE ISLAND CHANGE ASSESSMENT SCALE

The University of Rhode Island Change Assessment Scale (URICA)[108,109] is a 32-item Likert scale designed to measure a person's position in the four-stage change process: precontemplation, contemplation, action, and maintenance. It is similar in concept to the SOCA. It is different in that it has 28 more items, and each stage of change is implemented as a scale. The URICA produces a score for each scale. When viewed together, the scale scores can be interpreted as a profile. This approach is richer than the SOCA because it provides a framework that allows attitudes and behaviors characteristic of different stages of change to coexist in a single individual. Thus, the URICA may be able to detect gradual shifts from one stage to another. The URICA is general in format and not specific to any particular problem area. It has been widely used across an array of problem areas.

Items are presented in a 5-point format. Scale scores are computed by summing the responses to the scale items. Good internal consistency is indicated by numerous studies reporting α coefficients ranging from 0.69 to 0.89 across all scales.[108–110] The general version of the URICA is published in an article by McConnaughy et al.[108] A version designed for use in a weight control context is available in an article by Rossi et al.[105]

### ANOREXIA NERVOSA STAGES OF CHANGE QUESTIONNAIRE

The Anorexia Nervosa Stages of Change Questionnaire (ANSOCQ) is a self-report instrument used to assess patients' readiness to recover from AN. The questionnaire was developed based on the stages of change model[111] and contains 20 items which are rated on a scale from 1 to 5, with higher scores being more indicative of a patient's readiness to change.[112] The instrument has been found to be a psychometrically sound instrument regarding both measures of reliability and validity.[112,113] The questionnaire can be found in an article by Rieger et al.[112]

## STAGE OF CHANGE FOR CHILDREN

Although no specific algorithm for stages of change is readily available for children, several researchers have provided direction in this area. Kristal et al.[114] were the first to specifically propose using parental stage of change to determine the appropriateness of intervening with a child. Based on this suggestion, Rhee et al.[115] examined this with parents of overweight children between the ages of 2 and 12. More specifically, questions regarding increasing fruit and vegetable intake, decreasing juice consumption, and changing to lower fat food items were included. A flow chart of questions to be asked is included in an article by Rhee et al.[115]

## SUMMARY

Having a better understanding of a person's psychological state should facilitate planning of nutritional interventions for both adults and children. The instruments presented in this chapter are used for such purposes. Brief explanations of the psychological factor to be measured as well as the importance of the factor have been presented. Additionally, instrument-specific information has been included to assist the health care professional in determining the usefulness of the measure for a particular patient. Though not exhaustive, these measures represent factors relevant to nutrition-related treatment.

## ACKNOWLEDGMENTS

Thanks to Chermaine Tyler and Victor Pendleton for their contributions to an earlier version of this chapter. Preparation of this paper was supported, in part, by USDA ARS 2533759358.

## REFERENCES

1. Flegal KM, Carroll MD, Kit BK, Ogden CL, *JAMA* 307:491; 2012.
2. Ogden CL, Carroll MD, Kit BK, Flegal KM, *JAMA* 307:483; 2012.
3. de Zwaan M, Hilbert A, Herpertz S et al., *Obesity* 16:2535; 2008.
4. McGuire MT, Wing RR, Hill JO, *Int J Obes Relat Metob Disord* 23:1314; 1999.
5. Perri MG, Nezu AM, Viegener BJ. *Improving the Long-term Management of Obesity: Theory, Research, and Clinical Guidelines*. John Wiley & Sons, New York, 1992.
6. Zeller MH, Saelens BE, Roehrig H et al., *Obes Res* 12:1576; 2004.
7. American Psychiatric Association. *Diagnostic and Statistical Manual of Mental Disorders*, 4th edn. Text Revision. American Psychiatric Association, Washington, DC, 2000.
8. Maxmen JS, Ward NG. *Essential Psychopathology and Its Treatment*, 2nd edn. W.W. Norton & Company, New York, 1995.
9. Halmi KA, Eckert E, Marchi P et al., *Arch Gen Psychiatry* 48:712; 1991.
10. Polivy J, Herman CP. In: Fairburn CG, Wilson G, eds. *Binge Eating: Nature, Assessment, and Treatment*. Guilford Press, New York, 1993, p. 173.
11. Derogatis LR. *Symptom Checklist-90-R (SCL-90-R) Administration, Scoring and Procedures Manual*, 3rd edn. National Computer Systems, Minneapolis, MN, 1994.
12. Derogatis LR, Cleary PA, *J Clin Psychol* 33:981; 1977.
13. Ransom D, Ashton K, Windover A, Heinberg L, *Surg Obes Relat Dis* 6:622; 2010.
14. Paap MC, Meijer RR, Van Bebber J et al., *Int J Methods Psychiatr Res* 20(3): e39; 2011: doi: 10.1002/mpr.347.
15. Reynolds CR, Kamphaus RW. *Behavior Assessment System for Children*, 2nd edn. AGS Publishing, Circle Pines, MN, 2004.
16. Garner DM, Olmstead MP, Polivy J, *Int J Eat Disord* 2:15; 1982.
17. Espelage DL, Mazzeo SE, Aggen SH et al., *Psychol Assess* 15:71; 2003.
18. Garner D. *Manual for the Eating Disorder Inventory-2 (EDI-2)*. Psychological Assessment Resources, Odessa, FL, 1991.
19. Wear RW, Pratz O, *Int J Eat Disord* 6:767; 1987.
20. Fairburn CG, Cooper Z. In: Fairburn CG, Wilson GT, eds. *Binge Eating: Nature, Assessment, and Treatment*, 12th edn. Guilford Press, New York, 1993, p. 317.
21. Cooper Z, Cooper PJ, Fairburn CG, *Br J Psychiatry* 154:807; 1989.
22. Beumont P, Kopec-Schrader E, Talbot P, Touyz S, *Aust NZ J Psychiatry* 27:506; 1993.
23. Cooper Z, Fairburn C, *Int J Eat Disord* 6:1; 1986.
24. Wilson G, Smith D, *Int J Eat Disord* 8:173; 1989.
25. Fairburn CG, Beglin SJ, *Int J Eat Disord* 16:363; 1994.
26. Luce KH, Crowther JH, *Int J Eat Disord* 25:349; 1999.
27. Túry F, Güleç H, Kohls E, *J Psychosom Res* 69:601; 2009.
28. Fairburn CG, Beglin SJ. In: Fairburn CG, ed., *Cognitive Behavior Therapy and Eating Disorders*. Guilford, New York, 2008, p. 311.
29. Bryant-Waugh RJ, Cooper PJ, Taylor CL, Lask BD, *Int J Eat Disord* 19:391; 1996.
30. Watkins B, Frampton I, Lask B, Bryant-Waugh R, *Int J Eat Disord* 38:183; 2005.
31. Levine MD, Ringham RM, Kalarchian MA et al., *Int J Eat Disord* 39:135; 2006.
32. Childress AC, Jarrell MP, Brewerton TD, *Eat Disord J Treat Prev* 1:123; 1993.
33. Childress AC, Brewerton TD, Hodges EL, Jarrell MP, *J Am Acad Child Adolesc Psychiatry* 32:843; 1993.
34. Epstein LH, Paluch RA, Saelens BE et al., *J Pediatr* 139:58; 2001.
35. Morgan JF, Reid FJ, Lacey H, *BMJ* 319:1467; 1999.
36. Hill LS, Reid F, Morgan JF, Lacey JH, *Int J Eat Disord* 4:344; 2010.
37. Stunkard AJ, Messick S, *J Psychosom Res* 29:71; 1985.
38. Klesges RC, Isbell TR, Klesges LM, *J Abnorm Psychol* 101:668; 1992.
39. Polivy J, Herman C, *Am Psychol* 40:193; 1985.
40. Stunkard AJ, Messick S. *Eating Inventory Manual*. Harcourt Brace Jovanovich, San Antonio, TX, 1988.
41. Laessle RG, Tuschl RJ, Kotthaus BC, Prike KM, *J Abnorm Psychol* 98:504; 1989.
42. Tuschl RJ, Laessle RG, Platte P, Pirke KM, *Appetite* 14:9; 1990.
43. Allison DB, Kalinsky LB, Gorman BS, *Psychol Assess* 4:391; 1992.
44. Cappelleri JC, Bushmakin AG, Gerber RA et al., *Int J Obesity* 33:611; 2009.
45. Van Strien T, Frijters JE, Van Staveren WA et al., *Int J Eat Disord* 5:747; 1986.
46. Allison DB, Franklin RD, *Psychother Priv Pract* 12:53; 1993.
47. Hill AJ, Oliver S, Rogers PJ, *Br J Clin Psychol* 31:95; 1992.
48. Wardle J, Marsland L, *J Psychosom Res* 34:377; 1990.
49. Gorman BS, Allison DB. In: Allison DB, ed. *Handbook of Assessment Methods for Eating Behaviors and Weight-related Problems: Measures, Theory, and Research*. Sage Publications, Inc., Thousand Oaks, CA, 1995, p. 149.
50. Caccialanza R, Nicholls D, Cena H et al., *Eur J Clin Nutr* 58:1217; 2004.
51. Van Strien T, Oosterveld P, *Int J Eat Disord* 41:72; 2008.
52. Thelen, MH, Farmer J, Wonderlick S, Smith M, *Psychol Assess* 3:119; 1991.
53. Smith MC, Thelen MH, *J Consult Clin Psychol* 52:863; 1984.
54. Thelen MH, Mintz LB, Vander Wal JS, *Psychol Assess* 8:219; 1996.
55. Welch G, Thompson L, Hall A, *Int J Eat Disord* 14:95; 1993.
56. Vincent MA, McCabe MP, Ricciardelli LA, *Behav Res Ther* 37:1129; 1999.
57. Vander Wal JS, Stein RI, Blashill AJ, *Eat Behav* 12:267; 2001.
58. Gormally J, Black S, Daston S, Rardin D, *Addict Behav* 7:47; 1982.

59. Marcus MD, Wing RR, Hopkins J, *J Consult Clin Psychol* 56:433; 1988.
60. Wilson G. In: Fairburn CG, Wilson GT, eds. *Binge Eating: Nature, Assessment, and Treatment*. Guilford Press, New York, 1993, p. 227.
61. Stunkard A, Sorenson T, Schlusinger F. In: Kety S, Rowland LP, Sidman RL, Matthysse SW, eds. *The Genetics of Neurological and Psychiatric Disorders*. Raven Press, New York, 1983, p. 115.
62. Thompson J, Altabe MN, *Int J Eat Disord* 10:615; 1991.
63. Stunkard A, *Percept Mot Skills* 90:930; 2000.
64. Pulvers KM, Lee RE, Kaur H et al., *Obes Res* 12:1641; 2004.
65. Thompson JK. In: Thompson JK, ed. *Body Image, Eating Disorders, and Obesity*. American Psychological Association, Washington, DC, 1996, p. 49.
66. Altabe M. In: Thompson JK, ed. *Body Image, Eating Disorders, and Obesity*. American Psychological Association, Washington, DC, 1996, p. 129.
67. Williamson DA, Davis CJ, Bennett SM et al., *Behav Assess* 11:433; 1989.
68. Williamson DA, Womble LG, Zucker NL et al., *Int J Obes Relat Metab Disord* 24:1326; 2000.
69. Moreno JP, Kelley ML, Landry DN et al., *Int J Pediatr Obes* 6:e480; 2011.
70. Golan M, Weizman A, *Eur J Clin Nutr* 52:771; 1998.
71. Ihmels MA, Welk GJ, Eisenmann JC, Nusser SM, *Int J Behav Nutr Phys Act* 6:1; 2009.
72. Ihmels MA, Welk GJ, Eisenmann JC et al., *Ann Behav Med* 38:60; 2009.
73. Larios SA, Ayala GX, Arredondo EM et al., *Appetite* 52:166; 2008.
74. Garner DM, Olmsted MP, Davis R et al., *Int J Eat Disord* 9:1; 1990.
75. Strober M, Katz JL, *Int J Eat Disord* 6:171; 1987.
76. Marcus MD. In: Fairburn CG, Wilson G, eds. *Binge Eating: Nature, Assessment and Treatment*. Guilford Press, New York, 1993, pp. 77–96.
77. Webber EM, *J Psychol* 128:339; 1994.
78. Clark MM, Niaura R, King TK, Pera V, *Addict Behav* 21:509; 1996.
79. Tanco S, Linden W, Earle T, *Int J Eat Disord* 23:325; 1998.
80. Beck AT, Steer RA, Brown G. *Manual for the Beck Depression Inventory*, 2nd edn. Psychological Corporation, San Antonio, TX, 1996.
81. Whisman MA, Perez JE, Ramel W, *J Clin Psychol* 56:545; 2000.
82. Kovacs M. *Children's Depression Inventory*, 2nd edn. Technical Manual. Multi-Health Systems, North Tonawanda, NY, 2010.
83. Kovacs M. *Manual for the Children's Depression Inventory*. Multi-Health Systems, North Tonawanda, NY, 1992.
84. Radloff LS, *Appl Psychol Meas* 1:385; 1977.
85. Ros L, Latorre JM, Aguilar MJ, *Int J Aging Hum Dev* 72(2):83; 2011.
86. Orme JG, Reis J, Herz EJ, *J Clin Psychol* 42(1):28; 1986.
87. Hassan MK, Joshi AV, Madhavan SS, Amonkar MM, *Int J Obes Relat Metab Disord* 27:1227; 2003.
88. Schwimmer JB, Burwinkle TM, Varni JW, *JAMA* 289:1813; 2003.
89. Ware JE, Sherbourne CD, *Med Care* 30:473; 1992.
90. McHorney C, Ware JE, Lu J, Sherbourne CD, *Med Care* 32:40; 1994.
91. Dupay HJ. *Proceedings of the American Public Health Association Meeting*, Los Angeles, CA, October 17, 1978.
92. Brook RH, Ware JE, Davies-Avery A et al., *Med Care* 17:1; 1979.
93. Edwards DW, Yarvis RM, Mueller DP et al., *Eval Q* 2:275; 1978.
94. Monk M, *Clin Invest Med* 4:183; 1981.
95. Simpkins C, Burke FF. Comparative analyses of the NCHS General Well-Being Schedule: Response distributions, community vs. patient status discriminations, and content relationships (Contract No. HRA 106-74-13). Center for Community Studies, George Peabody College, Nashville, TN, 1974.
96. McDowell I, Newell C. *Measuring Health: A Guide to Rating Scales and Questionnaires*. Oxford University Press, New York, 1987.
97. Varni JW, Seid M, Rode CA, *Med Care* 37:126; 1999.
98. Varni JW, Seid M, Kurtin PS, *Med Care* 39:800; 2001.
99. Las Hayas C, Quintana JM, Padierna JA et al., *J Clin Epidemiol* 60(8): 825; 2006.
100. Las Hayas C, Quintana JM, Padierna JA et al., *Health Qual Life Outcomes* 8:29; 2010.
101. Tirico PP, Stefano SC, Blay SL, *J Nerv Ment Dis* 198(12):854; 2010.
102. Munoz P, Quintana JM, Las Hayas C et al., *Qual Life Res* 18(9):1137; 2009.
103. Glynn SM, Ruderman AJ, *Cognit Ther Res* 10:403; 1986.
104. Stotland S, Zuroff DC, *J Pers Assess* 54:191; 1990.
105. Rossi JS, Rossi SR, Velicer WF, Prochaska JO. In: Allison DB, ed. *Handbook of Assessment Methods for Eating Behaviors and Weight-related Problems: Measures, Theory, and Research*. Sage Publications, Inc., Thousand Oaks, CA, 1995, p. 387.
106. Prochaska JO, DiClemente CC, Norcross JC, *Am Psychol* 47:1102; 1992.
107. Prochaska JO, Velicer WF, DiClemente CC, Fava J, *J Consult Clin Psychol* 56:520; 1988.
108. McConnaughy EA, DiClemente CC, Prochaska JO, Velicer WF, *Psychotherapy* 26:494; 1989.
109. McConnaughy EA, Prochaska JO, Velicer WF, *Psychotherapy* 20:368; 1983.
110. DiClemente CC, Hughes SO, *J Subst Abuse* 2:217; 1990.
111. DiClemente CC, Prochaska JO, *Addict Behav* 7:133; 1982.
112. Rieger E, Touyz SW, Beumont PJ, *Int J Eat Disord* 32(1):24; 2002.
113. Rieger E, Touyz S, Schotte D et al., *Int J Eat Disord* 28:387; 2000.
114. Kristal AR, Glanz K, Curry SJ, *J Am Diet Assoc* 99:679; 1999.
115. Rhee KE, De Lago CW, Arscott-Mills T et al., *Pediatrics* 116:e94; 2005.

# 41 Energy Assessment
## *Physical Activity*

*Nancy L. Keim and Lisa Jahns*

## CONTENTS

## INTRODUCTION

Physical activity is an important contributor to total energy expenditure (TEE). Physical activity can vary greatly within an individual from day-to-day, or between individuals because preferred physical activities, practices, and routines differ from one person to the next. These variations impact total daily energy expenditure (EE) and could potentially change energy balance. Accurately measuring the physical activity levels (PALs) of individuals is challenging due to the multi-faceted nature of movement, the limitations of measurement devices and/or self-report, and the potentially high respondent burden it imposes on those who are being measured.

The purpose of this chapter is to provide an overview of physical activity assessment, describe important assessment issues, discuss relevant aspects to be considered when selecting a method for assessing physical activity, and review the different methods available. Although recent advancements in technology have yielded new and improved devices for activity monitoring, there is still no single measure able to accurately assess physical activity in all individuals or groups of the population, in all settings, and for all aspects and types of physical activity.[1] Some methods that are deemed more accurate for measuring EE of individuals may not be feasible for use in large population studies because subject or investigator burden may be too high, or costs may be prohibitive. Careful consideration of the accuracy, validity, and

feasibility of available methods to assess physical activity is necessary to best meet objectives.

## CONCEPTS AND DEFINITIONS

Physical activity is defined as bodily movement produced by contraction of skeletal muscle resulting in increased EE over resting levels.[2] Exercise is a more vigorous form of physical activity that is "planned, structured, repetitive, and purposive" in that it can result in improved physical fitness.[3] Components of TEE include sleeping metabolic rate (SMR), basal metabolic rate (BMR), resting energy expenditure (REE), thermic effect of food (TEF), and physical activity energy expenditure (PAEE). The classic definition of BMR is the amount of heat produced by an individual while in a state of complete muscular repose, 12–14 h after ingestion of the last meal.[4] BMR represents the energy needed to sustain the metabolic activity of cells, tissues, and organs at rest. REE also represents the energy expended under restful conditions, but generally is about 10% higher than BMR due to less stringent measurement conditions such as shorter period of time since eating or being active. REE typically accounts for about 60%–70% of TEE; within-subject variability is small and can be predicted from body size and age with reasonable accuracy for the majority of individuals.[5] TEF, or diet-induced thermogenesis, represents the energy needed for eating, digesting, absorbing, transporting, metabolizing, and storing usable forms of energy derived from food. Generally, this represents about 10% of TEE. PAEE represents the energy used for bodily movement, and because persons choose to be inactive, moderately active, or very active, the contribution of PAEE to TEE can be negligible, small, or significant.

Qualitative descriptions of physical activity include activities of daily living, non-volitional movement such as fidgeting and toe-tapping, occupational and household tasks, recreation, structured exercise, complex sports, and hard physical labor. These types of activities fall in the general domains of occupational, household-related, transport, and leisure; energy expended in activities that are not considered purposeful exercise is referred to as non-exercise activity thermogenesis.[6,7] Quantitative dimensions of physical activity include frequency, intensity, and duration. Depending on the type of activity, its associated EE may vary on an individual basis with body weight, body composition, and efficiency of performance,[8] contributing to differences in amount of energy expended.

The unit of measurement for activity-related EE is total kilocalories (or kilojoules), and it can be expressed per unit of time (minutes) or per unit of body mass (kilogram) or both. The intensity of activity can be defined in qualitative terms (light, moderate, or vigorous) or in quantitative terms related to actual EE. The energy expended in physical activity or exercise is often expressed in metabolic equivalents (METs). An MET is a numerical value that represents a multiple of REE for a given activity. MET values can be converted to rates of oxygen consumption or EE using the equation $1\ \text{MET} = 3.5\ \text{mL} \cdot \text{kg}^{-1} \cdot \text{min}^{-1}$ or $1\ \text{kcal} \cdot \text{kg}^{-1} \cdot \text{h}^{-1}$, but this approach should be used cautiously since it is derived from measurements taken on one 70 kg, 40-year-old man.[9] Nonetheless, based on this approach, the *Compendium of Physical Activities*[10] provides MET values for a large selection of physical activities for adults. MET values are also available for activities performed by children and adolescents[11] and for disabled persons with spinal cord injuries.[12] MET values between 1.0 and 1.5 are considered *sedentary*, and values ranging between 2.0 and 12.0 represent the typical physical activity spectrum from light to intense. In general, activities with MET values ranging from 3.0 to 5.9 are of moderate intensity and are associated with health benefits.[2] Vigorous intensity activities are defined as those with MET values of 6 and higher.[2] For aerobic endurance-type exercises, it is also common to see intensity described in terms of oxygen uptake values relative to maximal oxygen uptake ($VO_2$max). When performing exercise against resistance, such as weight-lifting, pedaling against a load, or running up a flight of stairs, power output can be measured. These power tests measure work accomplished per unit time, and the results are expressed in Watts, Joules, Newton-meters, or kilogram-meters.

An individual's PAL is a quantitative summary of the different types of physical activity engaged in for various amounts of time during a specified time period, usually 24 h. PAL is defined as the ratio of TEE to REE and can be determined by measuring TEE using the doubly labeled water method and REE using indirect calorimetry. In the absence of these measures, PAL can be estimated as a weighted average of MET values assigned to all activities constituting the 24 h period, including sleep and rest. The Dietary Reference Intakes for Macronutrients[13] define PAL values for *sedentary* ≥1.0 to <1.4; *low active* ≥1.4 to <1.6; *active* ≥1.6 to <1.9; *very active* ≥ 1.9 to <2.5.

## WHY IT IS IMPORTANT TO ASSESS PHYSICAL ACTIVITY

Strong scientific evidence exists to support the idea that regular participation in physical activity is linked to better health status in children, adolescents, adults, and the elderly, across the racial and ethnic groups studied to date.[2] The majority of evidence describing the relationship between physical activity and health-related outcome measures was established using self-reported physical activity. Physical activity is also assessed for surveillance purposes to determine whether individuals of all ages are meeting public health physical activity recommendations and whether or not patterns are changing over time. In the United States, the Behavioral Risk Factor Surveillance System (BRFSS) has been operational since 1984, tracking health and risk behaviors, including physical activity and exercise, by a telephone survey.[14] Since self-report of physical activity is subject to bias (toward overestimation),[15] surveillance and intervention research would be improved by including objective measures since the costs of certain monitoring devices are declining. In fact, physical activity assessment for the National Health and Nutrition Examination Survey (NHANES) included physical activity monitoring with an accelerometer for the 2003–2006 and 2011–2012 cycles.[16] Concern has been expressed by experts that the use and interpretation of the NHANES physical activity data need better standardization.[17] Certainly, use of standardized methods that are valid, reliable, non-reactive, and precise will provide greater understanding about the specific type and amount of habitual physical activity necessary to gain protective effects against degenerative diseases, to maintain a healthy body weight, and to improve metabolic fitness. A standardized toolkit for assessing physical activity, physical fitness, and associated mediators and moderators is now available to researchers for use in epidemiological studies and intervention studies.[18] Use of these tools will facilitate comparisons of data across studies. Important advancements such as this one will deepen our understanding of critical activity–disease relationships and provide valuable information to public health professionals, teachers, researchers, policymakers, and others responsible for physical activity interventions.

## IMPORTANT ASPECTS TO CONSIDER IN CHOOSING THE MOST APPROPRIATE MEASURE

Whether evaluating a physical activity intervention program, determining the prevalence of activity in a population, establishing the associations between physical activity and health outcomes, or determining whether activity guidelines are being met, it is necessary to choose an appropriate physical activity assessment method. Ideally, the method chosen should be accurate, valid, simple, not time-consuming, inexpensive, and suitable for use in a wide range of individuals under a wide range of conditions. A multitude of methods are available, and the market is expanding rapidly. Choosing the most appropriate method or combination of methods depends on a variety of factors.

## PURPOSE OF THE ASSESSMENT

The purpose and objectives of a research study or an intervention program are the primary factors to consider when selecting the physical activity assessment method. If the purpose is population surveillance of physical activity, it may be sufficient to classify individuals into broad activity categories such as sedentary, moderately active, or highly active. This can be accomplished by relatively simple and inexpensive methods such as completion of a short questionnaire on general activity patterns. Physical inactivity has been identified as an important public health concern for adults and children[19]; therefore, assessing sedentary activities may be equally as important as measuring physical activity in observational or intervention studies.

Another factor to consider in selecting a physical activity assessment method in an intervention study is the content of the intervention. If the study will emphasize fitting more walking into daily routines, a detailed questionnaire on walking times, amounts, intensity, frequency, and duration would be appropriate, and the use of a pedometer as an assessment tool would provide a low-cost objective measure. In clinical counseling situations, it is often important to assess an individual's activity level for the purposes of self-monitoring, goal setting, and evaluating progress. In this case, it is necessary to have data that accurately reflect the person's activity. Thus, a combination of self-assessment and objective monitoring would be ideal.

## CHARACTERISTICS OF PHYSICAL ACTIVITY

Specific dimensions of physical activity may have different effects on various health outcomes. Thus, it is important to characterize physical activity using both quantitative and qualitative methods. Quantitatively, the energy expended in physical activity is a key measurement needed to predict daily energy intake needs to maintain energy balance. Indirect calorimetry is a valid measure of EE based on measuring the rates of oxygen consumption ($VO_2$) and carbon dioxide production ($VCO_2$); it is commonly used in a laboratory setting to measure PAEE of specific activity and exercise protocols. The use of a stable isotope tracer technique using doubly labeled water as the tracer is also a validated measure of EE that is appropriately applied to free-living individuals. However, this method can only provide an estimate of PAEE averaged over a number of days, and one must assume that REE and TEF remain constant over that time. Also there are qualitative and quantitative aspects of physical activity that cannot be measured such as type, duration, and frequency of physical activity, which may also be important in the regulation of energy balance and health.

## PHYSICAL ACTIVITY PATTERNS

It is important to know how regularly an individual engages in physical activity and also how patterns of activity vary at different times. The majority of health benefits are acquired as chronic adaptations to exercise, and this requires that habitual

patterns of physical activity be assessed. Generally, adults have relatively regular daily patterns that may only change for different seasons or during holidays, whereas children have more erratic patterns of activity. Significant differences have been found between weekdays and weekends in type and amount of activity.[20] The level of an individual's physical activity may be higher in some seasons and lower in others, in most age and sex groups.[21–28] Seasonal differences occur because of weather,[21,23,29] length of daylight hours, and presence of holidays.[24,28] Among children and adolescents, school schedules also contribute to patterns of activity. For people who choose to actively commute to work, weather conditions such as precipitation, temperature, and wind represent significant barriers.[30] In industrialized countries, in northern climates, people tend to be more active outdoors during summer than winter months.

Adults who are habitually active may increase activity in clement months by adding additional outdoor activities to their regimen.[27] In southern climes, extreme summer conditions invert the seasonal relationship; more activity is reported in the temperate winter months.[31] The association of physical activity and season is measured by perception of seasonal change, by self-report,[32] or by objective means such as accelerometers or pedometers.[23,25,33] Therefore, a careful consideration of the effects of seasonality is suggested when attempting to measure habitual physical activity.[28,32]

Walking is the form of physical activity that contributes to PAEE in people capable of ambulation, regardless of whether they are mostly sedentary or very active. According to the American Time Use Survey conducted in 2003–2005, adults walk for many utilitarian purposes; most frequently reported were shopping, transportation, and walking the dog.[34] Only 5% of respondents walked for exercise, despite the fact that walking is consistently reported as a preferred form of exercise.[35] Pedometers (discussed later) are the most sensitive devices for capturing walking behaviors[36] and their use has been shown to actually increase PALs.[37]

## NATURE OF THE STUDY POPULATION

The nature of the population to be examined is an important consideration for choosing an assessment method. Methods developed for adults may not be appropriate for children. Since children appear to have more variation than adults in patterns of activity, and they perform activities over shorter time periods, their intermittent and frequently changing pattern of activity often requires a different strategy than that used for adults.[38] Physical activity has been assessed in children and adolescents by various methods including self-report by questionnaire or interview, which is of limited value in younger children, and report by proxies such as parents or teachers. Objective measures such as heart rate monitors, motion sensors, stable isotope tracers, and indirect calorimetry have been used frequently in small-scale studies. A comprehensive approach to measurement issues in assessing children's physical activity has been presented by Welk et al.[38] Points to be considered when selecting a physical activity measurement for children and adolescents are that 7 days of monitoring are required to obtain stable estimates of overall activity patterns,[39] both weekend and weekdays need to be included in the assessment,[40] and motion sensors need to be worn for the entire day or at least for multiple times over the course of the day.[39]

In adults, other considerations include age, gender, and possibly socioeconomic factors also may often be important. Information is available on specific activity assessment methods for specific racial or ethnic groups.[41] Physical activity varies with age, with general population data showing a gradual decline and the highest prevalence of sedentary behavior observed in elderly persons, especially women.[42] However, there may be substantial differences in activity patterns in retired individuals. For some, most of the activity might be housework and yard work, for others it might be walking, and perhaps for those living in retirement centers the major activities might be recreational activities such as golf or dancing. It is not possible to select a single activity assessment method for use with older individuals, but it is important to consider the type of older population that will be included in the project.

In summary, the nature of the population to be monitored is important to consider when selecting a physical activity assessment method. In general, younger persons are more active than older individuals, men are more active than women, and members of minority groups tend to be less active than non-Hispanic whites. Nonetheless, it is not possible to simply select a method based on age, gender, or racial/ethnic group status. Many other factors such as educational level, health status, geography, climate, and occupational group must be considered. Ideally, it would be useful to collect some pilot data, perhaps by open-ended questionnaires and conducting focus groups, to obtain information on types of activity most often reported by the target population.

## SAMPLE/POPULATION SIZE

The characteristics or the size of a sample must be taken into account before selecting the activity measure. A national survey or a large population study is not likely to use labor-intensive or high-cost techniques. A validation study or clinical trial with a relatively small sample means that the cost, time, logistical complexity, and other resources per person can be increased, allowing the use of more sophisticated, time-consuming, and accurate techniques.

## PERIOD OF MEASUREMENT

For instruments that measure activity over periods of time, an important question is the appropriate length of the monitoring period. This may differ for adults as compared with children and adolescents. According to Janz et al.,[43] four or more days of activity monitoring are needed to achieve satisfactory reliability, although Gretebeck and Montoye[44] suggested that at least 5 or 6 days of monitoring are needed to minimize intra-individual variance. More recently, Trost et al.[39] concluded that a 7-day monitoring period was required for accelerometers to assess usual activity in children and adolescents and account for apparent differences between weekday and weekend activity behaviors in the same way as within daily differences. Similarly, Matthews et al.[45]

found that reliable accelerometer measures of activity in adults require at least 7 days of monitoring.

In addition to considering the length of the monitoring period, it is also necessary to consider whether multiple periods need to be monitored over the course of a year. It is obvious that seasonal or climatic effects could have an influence on physical activity, but this has not been studied adequately. Most epidemiological studies on physical activity and health have obtained activity measurements at one time point. However, some of these approaches have asked about activity over periods of various lengths—past week, past month, past 3 months, past year, or usual activity. There is insufficient evidence to determine whether any single approach is better than any other, so at this time investigators should simply select the recall period that seems logical for their specific population.

## COST AND FEASIBILITY

Although objective measures are a useful adjunct to self-reports for assessing physical activity, the higher cost of some of these methods does not allow for them to be used in some studies. For example, the stable isotope tracer method would not be considered feasible for use in large-scale population studies because of cost and participant burden. Motion sensors (reviewed in more detail later) may be good choice, but technical support may be required, which would add additional costs. Other factors that must be considered with the use of objective monitoring devices include participant cooperation that might include multiple visits to the study laboratory, and participant compliance that would involve proper body placement and continuous use of the device as specified by the research protocol.

## SUMMARY

It is not possible to give a few simple guidelines for selecting a physical activity assessment method, and we have presented several factors that need to be considered when making a decision. The purpose of the study, type of physical activity that is of interest, nature of the study group, size and complexity of the study, and the available resources are all essential elements to be evaluated in order to select the most appropriate method for measuring physical activity. It is important to spend sufficient time in planning and selecting an assessment method to avoid later problems.

# PHYSICAL ACTIVITY ASSESSMENT METHODS

Physical activity assessment methodology is a rapidly growing field, stimulated by the surge in obesity-prevention research, public interest in personal health, and advancements in technology. An extensive variety of methods exists for obtaining qualitative and quantitative measures of physical activity. Matching one's study objectives, participant population, and resources with the appropriate physical activity measurement tool(s) requires knowledge of the uses, strengths, and limitations of different approaches. A summary of methods, divided into subjective and objective categories, is provided below and in Table 41.1.

**TABLE 41.1**
**Methods of Physical Activity Assessment**

| Instrument | Unit of Measurement | Period of Measurement | Activity Parameters Assessed | | | | | | Cost | Subject Burden | Sample Size |
|---|---|---|---|---|---|---|---|---|---|---|---|
| | | | Field Measure | Total Volume | Duration | Intensity | Type | Frequency | | | |
| Subjective measures | | | | | | | | | | | |
| I. Questionnaires[57] Retrospective quantitative history[108,109] Global[110,111] Recall[56,112] | | Days to year | X | X | X | X | X | X | $ | Light | Large |
| II. PA records/diary[81,113] | kcal/day[a] | Days | X | X | X | X | X | X | $–$$ | Heavy | Small |
| Objective measures | | | | | | | | | | | |
| I. Direct observation[61,62] | Activity minutes | Hours | X | | X | X | X | X | $$ | None | Small |
| II. Indirect calorimetry | | | | | | | | | | | |
| Whole-room calorimetry[66] | TEE, PAEE | 1–3 days | | X | X | X | X | X | $$$ | Heavy | Small |
| Metabolic cart[63] | PAEE, REE | <1 h | | | X | X | | | $$$ | Heavy | Small |
| Portable gas analyzer[65] | PAEE | Hours | X | | X | X | | | $$ | Heavy | Small |
| III. Doubly labeled water[67,68] | TEE (PAEE derived) | 7–14 days | X | X | | | | | $$$ | Light | Small–med um |
| IV. Pedometers[114–116] | Steps; EE[a] | Days, weeks | X | X | X | | | X | $ | Light | Medium–large |
| V. Accelerometers[73,74,116] | Counts, PAEE; TEE[a] | 1–2 weeks | X | X | X | X | | X | $$ | Light | Medium–large |
| VI. Inclinometers[76–78] | PAEE | Days | X | X | X | X | | X | $$ | Light | Medium–large |
| VII. Heart rate monitors[84] | HR, PAEE; TEE[a] | Days | X | X | X | X | | X | $$ | Light–moderate | Medium |
| VIII. Recent developments | | | | | | | | | | | |
| IDEEA[85,86] | PAEE, TEE, qualitative measures | Days | X | X | X | X | X | X | $$$ | Heavy | Small |
| Tracmor[87] | Counts, PAEE | Days | X | X | X | X | | X | $$ | Light | Small–medium |
| SenseCam[88] | Qualitative measures | Hours | X | | | | X | | $$ | Light | Small–medium |
| Actiheart[90–92] | HR, PAEE, TEE | Days | X | X | X | X | | X | $$ | Light | Small–medium |
| SenseWear Armband[93–95] | HR, PAEE, TEE | Days | X | X | X | X | | X | $$ | Light–moderate | Small–medium |
| GPS loggers | PAEE, qualitative measures | Days, weeks | X | X | X | X | X | X | $$ | Light–moderate | Small–medium |

*Cost:*   $, $$, $$$ = low, moderate, high.

[a] Estimated.

## SUBJECTIVE METHODS

Subjective measures of physical activity rely on study participant or proxy self-report. Information is obtained by questionnaire or diary/log through manual or computer-assisted means. Time and material costs vary across methods, as does the degree of detail in data collected. The benefits of flexibility in mode of administration (e.g., telephone, internet, or in-person; self-administered or interviewer-assisted) and relatively simple scoring for subjective assessment methods must be weighed against their susceptibility to participant misreporting.[46] Also important to consider is the influence of questionnaire administration mode on response bias.[47,48] Self-report methods are not recommended for use in children younger than 10 years of age due to the diverse range and sporadic nature of children's activities and their inability to accurately recall and record multiple aspects of physical activity.[49,50] Recently, Ainsworth et al. provided a framework to reduce errors in self-reported estimates of physical activity.[51]

*Questionnaires*: Questionnaires are self-completed by the subject or proxy, or administered by research staff. Large-scale epidemiological studies frequently use questionnaires to evaluate the relationship between physical activity and health outcomes. Three general types of physical activity questionnaires, listed in increasing length and degree of detail, are global self-report, recall, and quantitative history. Questionnaires should address the occupation, household, transportation, and leisure domains of physical activity and establish frequency, intensity, and duration of the activities with the goal of classifying general activity levels or specific values of EE. Guidelines have been published for using information derived from questionnaires to select an appropriate PAL factor in calculating TEE.[52] The accuracy, repeatability, and utility of self-report physical activity measures have been reviewed.[1,53–56] A compilation of physical activity questionnaires can be found in Pereira.[57]

*Records/diaries and logs*: The terms physical activity records, diaries, and logs are used variously in the literature but generally refer to a detailed, ongoing account of physical activity performed over a defined period of time.[58] At regular time intervals, subjects record the duration of time spent performing specified types of physical activity. The listing of physical activity categories can be customized for evaluating a particular population (e.g., the elderly) or outcome measure (e.g., exercise intensity). EE scores are calculated by multiplying the summed time spent in each physical activity category by the rate of EE (or MET) for that category. Important to note, methods using average MET values listed in the Compendium of Physical Activity[10] to estimate PAEE may not produce accurate results for individuals. This limitation has been discussed by the Compendium authors and was investigated by Bryne et al.[9] Another factor to consider is the substantial effort required of subjects and staff to keep and score, respectively, physical activity records. Electronic logging of physical activities has become increasingly popular as

availability of mobile phones or PDAs become widespread. Ecologic Momentary Assessment (EMA), which captures information on the context of a behavior in real time, has been applied successfully to physical activity assessment by means of electronic diary.[59]

## OBJECTIVE METHODS

Objective approaches to physical activity assessment utilize an external measure of activity, such as electronic activity monitors or direct observation. Objective methods carry generally higher costs for purchase, maintenance, and operation than do subjective methods, yet they avoid inaccuracies associated with subject misreporting and are appropriate for use across most populations, including children.

*Direct observation*: In direct observation, the subject's physical activity is coded according to type, intensity, duration, etc. by a trained observer. Direct observation is used as a criterion measure and is frequently employed to assess physical activity in children.[60–62] Coding can be performed in real time or during review of a camera recording. Care must be taken to assure reliability between coders. Direct observation allows multiple dimensions of physical activity, such as social and physical context, to be reliably and objectively assessed, but the number of subjects observed and the time period and location of observation are limited.

*Indirect calorimetry*: Indirect calorimetry determines EE from rates of oxygen consumption and carbon dioxide production. As an established method, it is often used as a criterion measure to validate other physical activity assessment methods. Respiratory gas exchange is commonly measured over short time intervals by means of an automated metabolic gas analyzer.[63] Recent advances in instrumentation have produced small, portable gas analyzers that can be used in field settings otherwise inaccessible to stationary metabolic carts.[64,65] While these newer compact devices enable measurement PAEE outside of the laboratory, they are cumbersome to wear, relatively expensive, and best applied to measuring EE of specific structured exercise or sporting activities. Indirect calorimetry is also used to measure EE over longer time periods, typically 24 h, within a whole-room calorimeter.[66] The calorimeter is ideal for measuring sleeping EE and TEE under predominantly sedentary conditions. However, the space limitation and generally slower response time of calorimeter gas exchange limit its usefulness for measuring EE of discrete bouts of activity or exercise.

*Doubly labeled water*: Doubly labeled water (DLW) method is considered the gold standard for measuring TEE.[67,68] In this method, stable isotopes of water (deuterium and oxygen-18) are orally administered to the subject, and carbon dioxide production is estimated from analysis of the isotopes remaining in urine samples collected over time (usually 7–14 days). From this, average 24 h TEE is calculated using regression analysis.[69] PAEE is derived by subtracting REE and TEF from TEE. The DLW method imposes minimal burden on free-living subjects; however, it is a technically complex and expensive technique that provides no descriptive physical activity information (e.g., type, duration, frequency).

*Activity monitors*: Activity monitors comprise a variety of electronic and mechanical devices that include pedometers (step counters) and accelerometers (acceleration detectors). Pedometers record the number of steps accumulated over a period of time. Their light-weight, low cost (for most models), and ability to provide feedback to the wearer are ideal for use in large-scale walking intervention studies. A major limitation of pedometers is that the output cannot be converted to EE.[70] Pedometers capture movement of the lower body, and do not measure the added work associated with walking on an incline or carrying extra weight.[71] Many health promotion programs, including the Physical Activity Guidelines for Americans,[2] recommend 30 min of moderate intensity physical activity on most days of the week. Although a simple pedometer does not automatically gauge intensity of locomotion, research has shown that moving at a pace of at least 100 steps/min roughly translates to moderate intensity activity.[71]

More detailed physical activity assessment requires the greater sophistication of an accelerometer. Most accelerometers contain a piezoelectric sensor that generates a voltage in response to movement in one or more planes of motion. The voltage is translated by a microprocessor to create a digital count value that can be further processed to yield EE. Typical accelerometer output displays the duration and energy cost of physical activity by intensity category for each recording hour. Accelerometers are easy to wear on the waist, wrist, or ankle, yet their operation and data management are significantly more complicated than that for pedometers. Reviews of accelerometry, including validation and reliability studies, are available.[72–74]

*Inclinometers*: Inclinometers are used to assess sedentary activities. Reclining, sitting, standing and short bouts of activity may all be classified as sedentary.[75] Inclinometers are typically worn on the thigh and are used to identify posture, sitting, standing and brief bouts of stepping. Inclinometer devices often are combined with accelerometers, and vice versa.[76–78] As many people spend large amounts of time working in offices, accurate identification of low levels of activity is important.[79]

*Heart rate monitors*: Heart rate monitoring is a common method used to describe the intensity and duration of physical activity. The basis of this method is the linear relationship between heart rate and oxygen uptake across a range of moderate to vigorous aerobic activities. Most monitors have software for converting heart rate data into an estimate of EE. However, when a higher level of data accuracy is desired, a graded exercise test is required in order to calibrate the individual's heart rate to simultaneous oxygen consumption. From this, a calibration curve can be constructed for estimating EE at moderate to strenuous levels of exercise. A limitation of employing heart rate as a surrogate for EE is that the relationship between heart rate and oxygen

consumption is weak at low activity levels, which are the levels characteristic of most sedentary individuals. Another important consideration in utilizing heart rate monitors for physical activity assessment is usability. Depending on model design, heart rate monitor chest transmitters are uncomfortable for some subjects to wear, resulting in poor compliance,[80,81] but new non-woven fabric sensors built into functional clothing may provide greater comfort.[82] Reviews of heart rate monitoring as a marker for physical activity are available.[55,83,84]

*Recent developments*: Devices that render novel applications to or combine traditional physical activity assessment methods have been introduced in recent years. One is a sophisticated system for recording posture and movement, called the IDEEA (Intelligent Device for Energy Expenditure and Activity). It is composed of a microcomputer worn on the hip with flexible wire extensions that attach to the feet, legs, and chest. Data output describes physical activity by type, intensity, duration, and energy cost. Validity and reliability studies have been conducted with encouraging results.[85,86]

Another promising device is the Directlife triaxial accelerometer (Tracmor), which is a miniaturized device worn against the lower back. Tracmor is well tolerated for long wear periods and has been validated for determining TEE, PAEE, and PAL.[87]

The SenseCam is a small, wearable camera that takes approximately 3600 time-stamped photos daily and is useful for capturing activities directly, without relying upon self-report or inferences from activity monitors.[88]

Mobile phone technology provides a major advancement for measuring physical activity and transmitting data. Although the burgeoning market of smart phone "apps" are geared toward the health-conscious consumer to provide motivation and feedback, the technology can be useful in research settings for real-time data collection and monitoring compliance to a physical activity intervention.[89]

Two examples of combination methods are the Actiheart (heart rate monitor + accelerometer) and the SenseWear™ armband (accelerometer + multiple temperature sensors). The Actiheart has shown reliability and validity (against indirect calorimetry) in estimating PAEE[90,91] and has demonstrated superior accuracy compared to accelerometry alone.[92] The SenseWear armband is a portable device worn on the upper arm that contains an accelerometer and sensors for temperature and galvanic skin response. Recent studies evaluating the armband conclude that it provides a reasonably accurate measure of daily EE under free-living conditions,[93] but EE is underestimated during high-intensity endurance exercise[94] and during resistance exercise with circuit weight training protocols,[95] suggesting that at this stage of development of the armband exercise-specific algorithms are necessary to accurately estimate PAEE.

Global Positioning System (GPS) technology has been applied to physical activity assessment methodology, particularly as a complement to accelerometry.[96] GPS contributes spatial data on locomotion, such as position, speed, incline, and stride length and frequency, all of which influence the energy cost of movement.[97,98]

In combination with accelerometry (measures movement) and heart rate monitors (indicates intensity), GPS systems can add the context of the activity being performed by providing where, how far, and how fast. For example, a hip-worn activity monitor may not detect a person cycling as moving. Heart rate would be elevated, but this would still not identify the activity. Adding GPS would show that person moving from one location to another at a moderate speed, allowing an accurate characterization of the trip.[99–101] GPS systems are a powerful tool for assessing the relationship between the activity and the environment, particularly active transport.[102,103]

GPS loggers are small and unlike heart rate monitors and accelerometers, wear position does not affect accuracy. Units are most often worn on the hip; in studies of children, wrist or chest-worn monitors improve compliance.[101,104] Current devices have fairly short battery life, and nightly charging is burdensome for participants. Satellite communication can be lost in areas with dense tree cover or in urban canyons. The use of GPS devices in health research is increasing rapidly, and technologies for collecting and interpreting data are improving rapidly.[105]

## SUMMARY

The scope of physical activity assessment methodology has expanded in response to the need for comprehensive, accurate approaches to quantifying and qualifying physical activity. Exciting advances in electronic and computer technologies have resulted in increasingly small, portable devices capable of measuring multiple aspects of free-living physical activity. Changing demographics, including increased cultural diversity and a growing elderly population, in the United States and other nations has led to the development of population-specific physical activity questionnaires (e.g., for Spanish-speaking[106] and older individuals[107]). Such methodological advancements have not only improved the accuracy and descriptiveness of physical activity assessment but also increased the accessibility of physical activity measurement tools to a wide range of health care and research professionals. The unique perspectives contributed by these investigators in the context of a global effort to promote physical activity will continue to spur the progress of physical activity assessment methodology.

## REFERENCES

1. Sallis JF, Saelens BE. *Res Q Exerc Sport* 71: S1; 2000.
2. US Department of Health and Human Services. *Physical Activity Guidelines for Americans.* Washington, DC: U.S. Department of Health and Human Services, 2008.
3. Casperson CJ, Powell KE, Chrisstenson GM. *Public Health Rep* 100: 126; 1985.
4. Harris JA, Benedict FG. *Proc Natl Acad Sci U S A* 4: 370; 1918.
5. Frankenfield D, Roth-Yousey L, Compher C. *J Am Diet Assoc* 105: 775; 2005.
6. Levine JA. *Nutr Rev* 62: S82; 2004.
7. Levine JA, Vander Weg MW, Hill JO et al. *Arterioscler Thromb Vasc Biol* 26: 729; 2006.
8. Goran MI, Sun M. *Am J Clin Nutr* 68: 944S; 1998.
9. Byrne NM, Hills AP, Hunter GR et al. *J Appl Physiol* 99: 1112; 2005.
10. Ainsworth BE, Haskell WL, Hermann SD et al. *Med Sci Sports Exerc* 43: 1575; 2011.
11. Ridley K, Ainsworth BE, Olds TS. *Int J Behav Nutr Phys Act* 5: 45; 2008.
12. Collins EG, Gater D, Kiratli J et al. *Med Sci Sports Exerc* 42: 691; 2010.
13. Institute of Medicine, Food and Nutrition Board. *Dietary Reference Intakes for Energy, Carbohydrate, Fiber, Fat, Fatty Acids, Cholesterol, Protein, and Amino Acids (Macronutrients).* Institute of Medicine, Food and Nutrition Board; The National Academies Press, Washington, DC, 2004.
14. Center for Disease Control and Prevention, Office of Surveillance, Epidemiology and Laboratory Services. The Behavioral and Risk Factor Surveillance System. Available at http://www.cdc.gov/brfss/ (accessed August 4, 2012).
15. Hagstromer M, Ainsworth BE, Oja P et al. *J Phys Act Health* 7: 541; 2010.
16. Center for Disease Control and Prevention, National Center for Health Statistics, Office of Information Services. Available at http://www.cdc.gov/nchs/nhanes/htm/accessed (accessed August 4, 2012).
17. Tudor-Locke C, Camhi SM, Troiano RP. *Prev Chronic Dis* 9: E113; 2012.
18. Haskell WL, Troiana RP, Hammond JA et al. *Am J Prev Med* 42: 486; 2012.
19. Matthews CE, Chen KY, Freedson PS et al. *Am J Epidemiol* 167: 875; 2008.
20. Racette SB, Weiss EP, Schechtman KB et al. *Obesity* 16: 1826; 2008.
21. Tucker P, Gilliland J. *Public Health* 121: 909; 2007.
22. Carson V, Spence JC. *Pediatr Exerc Sci* 22: 81; 2010.
23. Chan CB, Ryan DA. *Int J Environ Res Public Health* 6: 2639; 2009.
24. Shephard RJ, Aoyagi Y. *Eur J Appl Physiol* 107: 251; 2009.
25. Buchowski MS, Choi L, Majchrzak KM et al. *J Phys Act Health* 6: 252; 2009.
26. Kolle E, Steene-Johannessen J, Andersen LB et al. *Int J Behav Nutr Phys Act* 6: 36; 2009.
27. Pivarnik JM, Reeves MJ, Rafferty AP. *Med Sci Sports Exerc* 35: 1004; 2003.
28. Matthews CE, Freedson PS, Hebert JR et al. *Am J Epidemiol* 153: 172; 2001.
29. Belanger M, Gray-Donald K, O'Loughlin J et al. *Ann Epidemiol* 19: 180; 2009.
30. Flynn BS, Dana GS, Sears J et al. *Prev Med* 54: 122; 2012.
31. Baranowski T, Thompson WO, DuRant RH et al. *Res Q Exerc Sport* 64: 127; 1993.
32. Rifas-Shiman SL, Gillman MW, Field AE et al. *Am J Prev Med* 20: 282; 2001.
33. Plasqui G, Westerterp KR. *Obes Res* 12: 688; 2004.
34. Tudor-Locke C, Ham SA. *J Phys Act Health* 5: 633; 2008.
35. Tudor-Locke C. *Prev Med*; 55: 540–541 doi:10.1016/j.ypmed. 2012.07.009; 2012.

36. Bassett DR, Mahar MT, Rowe DA et al. *Med Sci Sports Exerc* 40: S529; 2008.

37. Bravata DM, Spangler CS, Sundaram V et al. *JAMA* 298: 2296; 2007.

38. Welk GJ, Corbin CB, Dale D. *Res Q Exerc Sport* 71: S59; 2000.

39. Trost SG, Pate RR, Freedson PS et al. *Med Sci Sports Exerc* 32: 426; 2000.

40. Sallis JF. *J Sch Health* 61: 215; 1991.

41. Masse LC, Fulton JE, Watson KL et al. *Res Q Exerc Sport* 70: 212; 1999.

42. US Department of Health and Human Services. *Physical Activity and Health: A Report of the Surgeon General.* Center for Disease Control and Prevention, Atlanta, GA 1996.

43. Janz KF, Witt J, Mahoney LT. *Med Sci Sports Exerc* 27: 1326; 1995.

44. Gretebeck RJ, Montoye HJ. *Med Sci Sports Exerc* 24: 1167; 1992.

45. Matthews CE, Ainsworth BE, Thompson RW et al. *Med Sci Sports Exerc* 34: 1376; 2002.

46. Troiano RP, Macera CA, Ballard-Barbash R. *J Nutr* 131: 451S; 2001.

47. Pridemore WA, Damphousse KR, Moore RK. *Soc Sci Med* 61: 976; 2005.

48. Perlis TE, Des Jarlais DC, Friedman SR et al. *Addiction* 99: 885; 2004.

49. Sallis JF, Buono MJ, Roby JJ et al. *Med Sci Sports Exerc* 22: 698; 1990.

50. Sallis JF, Buono MJ, Roby JJ et al. *Med Sci Sports Exerc* 25: 99; 1993.

51. Ainsworth BE, Caspersen CJ, Matthews CE et al. *J Phys Act Health* 9(Suppl 1): S76; 2012.

52. Black AE. *Int J Obes Relat Metab Disord* 24: 1119; 2000.

53. Shephard RJ. *Br J Sports Med* 37: 197; 2003.

54. Lamonte MJ, Ainsworth BE. *Med Sci Sports Exerc* 33: S370; 2001.

55. Haskell WL, Kiernan M. *Am J Clin Nutr* 72: 541S; 2000.

56. Matthews CE. In: Welk GJ, ed. *Physical Activity Assessments for Health-Related Research.* Champaign, IL: Human Kinetics, 2002.

57. Pereira MA, Fitzer Gerald SJ, Gregg EW et al. *Med Sci Sports Exerc* 29: S1; 1997.

58. Conway JM, Seale JL, Jacobs DR, Jr. et al. *Am J Clin Nutr* 75: 519; 2002.

59. Dunton GF, Whalen CK, Jamner LD et al. *Am J Prev Med* 29: 281; 2005.

60. Reilly JJ, Coyle J, Kelly L et al. *Obes Res* 11: 1155; 2003.

61. Robertson RJ, Goss FL, Aaron DJ et al. *Med Sci Sports Exerc* 38: 158; 2006.

62. Trost SG, Sirard JR, Dowda M et al. *Int J Obes Relat Metab Disord* 27: 834; 2003.

63. Macfarlane DJ. *Sports Med* 31: 841; 2001.

64. Duffield R, Dawson B, Pinnington HC et al. *J Sci Med Sport* 7: 11; 2004.

65. Mc Naughton LR, Sherman R, Roberts S et al. *J Sports Med Phys Fitness* 45: 315; 2005.

66. Levine JA. *Public Health Nutr* 8: 1123; 2005.

67. Schoeller DA, Ravussin E, Schutz Y et al. *Am J Physiol* 250: R823; 1986.

68. Schoeller DA. *J Nutr* 118: 1278; 1988.

69. Racette SB, Schoeller DA, Luke AH et al. *Am J Physiol* 267: E585; 1994.

70. Schneider PL, Crouter SE, Lukajic O et al. *Med Sci Sports Exerc* 35: 1779; 2003.

71. Marshall SJ, Levy SS, Tudor-Locke CE et al. *Am J Prev Med* 36: 410; 2009.

72. Chen KY, Bassett DR, Jr. *Med Sci Sports Exerc* 37: S490; 2005.

73. Butte NF, Ekelund U, Westerterp KR. *Med Sci Sports Exerc* 44: S5; 2012.

74. Plasqui G, Westerterp KR. *Obesity* 15: 2371; 2007.

75. Pate RR, O'Neill JR, Lobelo F. *Exerc Sport Sci Rev* 36: 173; 2008.

76. Grant PM, Ryan CG, Tigbe WW et al. *Br J Sports Med* 40: 992; 2006.

77. Kozey-Keadle S, Libertine A, Lyden K et al. *Med Sci Sports Exerc* 43: 1561; 2011.

78. Carr LJ, Mahar MT. *J Obes*; 2012. DOI: 10.1155/2012/460271.

79. Kozey-Keadle S, Libertine A, Staudenmayer J et al. *J Obes*; 2012. DOI: 10.155/2012/2823303.

80. Lof M, Hannestad U, Forsum E. *Br J Nutr* 90: 961; 2003.

81. Forrest A, Gustafson-Storms M, Gale B et al. *FASEB J* 18: A112; 2004.

82. Kang TH, Merritt CR, Grant E et al. *IEEE Trans Biomed Eng* 55: 188; 2008.

83. Ainslie P, Reilly T, Westerterp K. *Sports Med* 33: 683; 2003.

84. Janz KF. In: Welk GJ, ed. *Physical Activity Assessments for Health-Related Research.* Champaign, IL: Human Kinetics, 2002.

85. Zhang K, Pi-Sunyer FX, Boozer CN. *Med Sci Sports Exerc* 36: 883; 2004.

86. Zhang K, Werner P, Sun M et al. *Obes Res* 11: 33; 2003.

87. Bonomi AG, Plasqui G, Goris AHC et al. *Obesity* 18: 1845; 2010.

88. Kelly P, Doherty A, Berry E et al. *Int J Behav Nutr Phys Act* 8: 44; 2011.

89. Freedson P, Bowles HR, Troiano R et al. *Med Sci Sports Exerc* 44: S1; 2012.

90. Brage S, Brage N, Franks PW et al. *Eur J Clin Nutr* 59: 561; 2005.

91. Crouter SE, Churilla JR, Bassett DR. *Eur J Clin Nutr* 62: 704; 2008.

92. Corder K, Brage S, Wareham NJ et al. *Med Sci Sports Exerc* 37: 1761; 2005.

93. Johannsen DL, Calabro MA, Stewart J et al. *Med Sci Sports Exerc* 42: 2134; 2010.

94. Drenowatz C, Eisenmann JC. *Eur J Appl Physiol* 111: 883; 2011.

95. Benito PJ, Neiva C, Gonzalez-Quijano PS et al. *Eur J Appl Physiol* 112: 3155; 2012.

96. Rodriguez DA, Brown AL, Troped PJ. *Med Sci Sports Exerc* 37: S572; 2005.

97. Schutz Y, Herren R. *Med Sci Sports Exerc* 32: 642; 2000.

98. Terrier P, Ladetto Q, Merminod B et al. *Med Sci Sports Exerc* 33: 1912; 2001.

99. Maddison R, Mhurchu CN. *Int J Behav Nutr Phys Act* 6: 73; 2009.

100. Rodriguez DA, Brown AL, Troped PJ. *Med Sci Sports Exerc* 37: S572; 2005.

101. Duncan JS, Badland HM, Schofield G. *J Sci Med Sport*; 12: 583–585; 2009.

102. Krenn PJ, Mag D, Titze S et al. *Am J Prev Med* 41: 508; 2011.

103. Duncan MJ, Badland HM, Mummery WK. *J Sci Med Sport* 12(5): 549; 2009.

104. Cooper AR, Page AS, Wheeler BW et al. *Am J Prev Med* 38: 178; 2010.

105. Kerr J, Duncan S, Schipperjin J. *Am J Prev Med* 41: 532; 2011.

106. Elosua R, Garcia M, Aguilar A et al. *Med Sci Sports Exerc* 32: 1431; 2000.

107. Stewart AL, Mills KM, King AC et al. *Med Sci Sports Exerc* 33: 1126; 2001.

108. Reiff GG, Montoye HJ, Remington RD et al. *J Sports Med Phys Fitness* 7: 135; 1967.

109. Taylor HL, Jacobs DR, Jr., Schucker B et al. *J Chronic Dis* 31: 741; 1978.

110. Schechtman KB, Barzilai B, Rost K et al. *Am J Public Health* 81: 771; 1991.

111. Weiss TW, Slater CH, Green LW et al. *J Clin Epidemiol* 43: 1123; 1990.

112. Sallis JF, Haskell WL, Wood PD et al. *Am J Epidemiol* 121: 91; 1985.

113. Irwin ML, Ainsworth BE, Conway JM. *Obes Res* 9: 517; 2001.

114. Schneider PL, Crouter SE, Bassett DR. *Med Sci Sports Exerc* 36: 331; 2004.

115. Tudor-Locke C, Ainsworth BE, Thompson RW et al. *Med Sci Sports Exerc* 34: 2045; 2002.

116. Bassett DR, Jr., Ainsworth BE, Swartz AM et al. *Med Sci Sports Exerc* 32: S471; 2000.

# 42  Environmental Challenges and Assessment

*Suzanne Phelan and Gary D. Foster*

## CONTENTS

## INTRODUCTION

The prevalence of obesity in the United States has increased dramatically since the 1970s. Data from the 2007–2010 National Health and Nutrition Examination Survey (NHANES) show that 69% of the adult population in the United States is currently overweight, which is defined as having a body mass index (BMI) greater than 25 kg/m$^2$, compared with 46% in NHANES I, conducted between 1971 and 1974 (Figure 42.1).[1–4] The prevalence of obesity, defined as BMI greater than 30 kg/m$^2$, has also increased dramatically, from 14% in 1971–1974 to 36% in 2007–2010 (Figure 42.1).[3,5,6] Since 2003, obesity prevalence appears to have more or less plateaued,[7] while severe obesity rates have increased with no evidence of slowing.[8] Based on prevalence data over the past few decades, Finkelstein et al.[9] predicted that over the next two decades obesity prevalence would increase by 33% and severe obesity by 130%. Children are also affected, with the prevalence of obesity in children and adolescents near tripling since the early 1970s (from 6% to 17%) (Figure 42.2). The World Health Organization has declared obesity as one of the top 10 risk conditions in the world and one of the top 5 in developed nations.[10]

In this chapter, the major environmental factors that have contributed to the rise in obesity will be examined. In addition, methods of assessing environmental influences at the population and clinical levels will be reviewed.

## ETIOLOGY OF OBESITY

Obesity is the result of an energy imbalance in which intake exceeds expenditure. Clearly, genetic, biological, and behavioral factors play a role in the etiology of obesity[11–13]; however, environmental factors appear to be the driving force behind the increasing prevalence of obesity.[14,15] The environment of industrialized countries has been viewed as so severely promoting obesity that it has been labeled "toxic."[16] In order to better understand the environmental influences on obesity, both energy intake and expenditure must be examined.

## ENVIRONMENTAL FACTORS

### ENERGY INTAKE

Food consumption in industrialized and western nations has increased significantly over the past few decades, particularly in women. U.S. data from NHANES indicate

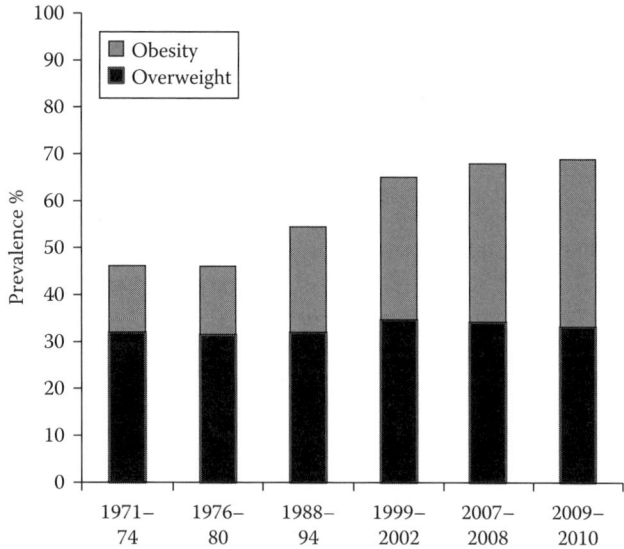

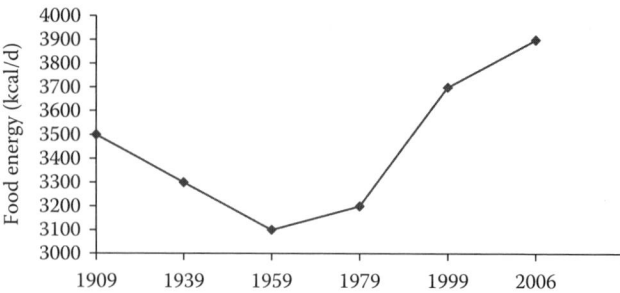

**FIGURE 42.3** Food energy per capita per day in the United States. (From Center for Urban Transportation Research, *Public Transit in America: Results from the 2001 National Household Travel Survey,* National Center for Transit Research, Tampa, FL, 2005; U.S. Department of Transportation, Nationwide personal transportation survey, 2009, www-cta.ornl.gov/npts.)

**FIGURE 42.1** Prevalence of overweight (BMI ≥ 25–29.9 kg/m²) and obesity (BMI ≥ 30 kg/m²) in the United States from 1960 to 2010. Based on data from the National Health and Nutrition Examination Surveys. (From Flegal, K.M. et al., *Int. J. Obes.,* 22, 39, 1998; Hedley, A.A. et al., *JAMA.,* 291, 2847, 2004; Gerrior, S. et al., *Nutrient Content of the U.S. Food Supply, 1909–2000,* U.S. Department of Agriculture, Center for Nutrition Policy and Promotion, Washington, DC, 2004; Centers For Disease Control and Prevention, *MMWR Morb. Mortal. Wkly. Rep.,* 52, 764, 2003.)

representing an 11% increase.[2,18] Other indicators, including increases in portion sizes and the widespread availability of highly palatable and energy-dense foods, further suggest that increases in energy intake account, in part, for the rising prevalence of obesity.[19]

**Larger Portions and Decreased Costs**

Several lines of research have shown that when portion sizes are increased, individuals consume more food and calories.[20,21] Unfortunately, during the past 20 years, the "supersizing" of America has been ubiquitous. Portion sizes of virtually all foods and beverages have increased[22,23]—from individually packaged, ready-to-eat foods to foods served at fast food, chain, and privately owned restaurants.[22,24] A study comparing servings sizes of food available in the 1950s vs. 2002 found enormous increases in portion sizes available for French fries, burgers, drinks, muffins, and chocolate bars (Table 42.1). Packaged cereal portions (intended to be eaten at one time) are two to three times larger today than the single unit size sold previously.[22,24]

As portion sizes in the marketplace have grown, so have individuals' perceptions of appropriate and reasonable

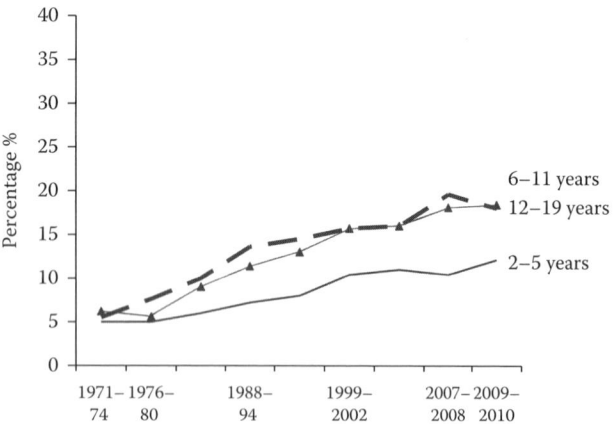

**FIGURE 42.2** Prevalence of overweight and obesity (BMI ≥ 95th percentile) in children and adolescents in the United States, 1963–2010.

that between 1971 and 2008, the average energy intake increased from 1542 and 1771 kcal/day to 2450 and 2504 kcal/day for men and women, respectively.[17] Data from the U.S. Department of Agriculture (USDA) also indicate a significant increase in the amount of food available for consumption per capita per day over the past few decades (Figure 42.3). Specifically, the amount of food available has increased from 3500 kcal per capita per day in 1909 to an average of 3900 kcal per capita per day in 2006,

**TABLE 42.1**
**Maximal Portion Sizes of Foods and Beverages Available in the 1950s and 2002**

| Food or Beverage | 1950s (oz) | 2002 (oz) |
|---|---|---|
| French fries | 2.4 | 7.1 |
| Fountain soda | 7.0 | 64 |
| Hamburger patty | 1.6 | 8.0 |
| Hamburger sandwich | 3.9 | 12.6 |
| Muffin | 3.0 | 6.5 |
| Chocolate bar | 0.6ᵃ | 8 |

*Source:* Adapted from Young, L.R. and Nestle, M., *J. Am. Diet. Assoc.,* 103, 231, 2003.
ᵃ Serving size in 1908.

portion sizes.[25] One study assessed the quantity of food young adults selected as a typical portion of breakfast and lunch foods during the 1980s and then again in 2003.[26] Results indicated that participants served themselves typical portion sizes of cereal, juice, and even fruit salad that were more than 50% larger in 2003 than in 1984.

Consumption of larger portions is further enhanced by attractive size/quantity discounts. "Value meals" offering larger portions of energy-dense food and drinks for only a small increase in cost have continued to gain in popularity both among consumers and vendors. Similarly, supermarkets "add value" by offering larger sizes that cost progressively less per ounce; for example, huge boxes of cereal and even double packs are often found in warehouse club or box stores. Marketing data suggest that supersizing and multiple unit-pricing (i.e., "2 for $1.00" instead of "50 cents each") translate into greater food consumption.[27] This applies both to unhealthy, energy-dense foods and to lower calorie, healthy foods. Thus, research suggests that when the price per ounce of low-fat foods is reduced, sales increase; when price per unit of unhealthy foods, such as soft drinks, is increased, sales decline.[28,29] This line of research has led to suggestions that policymakers alter the cost of unhealthy, energy-dense foods through fiscal pricing (tax or subsidy),[30,31] but further research is clearly needed in this area.

### Energy-Dense and Convenience Foods

Based on surveys of individual intake, calorie intake in the U.S. population has increased over the past few decades due, in large part, to an increase in percentage of energy intake from carbohydrates. NHANES data indicate that between 1971 and 2008, the percentage of calories from carbohydrates increased from 44% to 49%, resulting in a decline in the percentage of energy from fat (from 37% to 34%).[32,33]

The rise in carbohydrate consumption is thought due, in large part, to an influx in amount of sugar and sweets available and consumed in the food supply. Since 1909, the per capita availability of sugar and sweets in the U.S. food supply has increased by 40% (Figure 42.4).[34] Moreover, availability

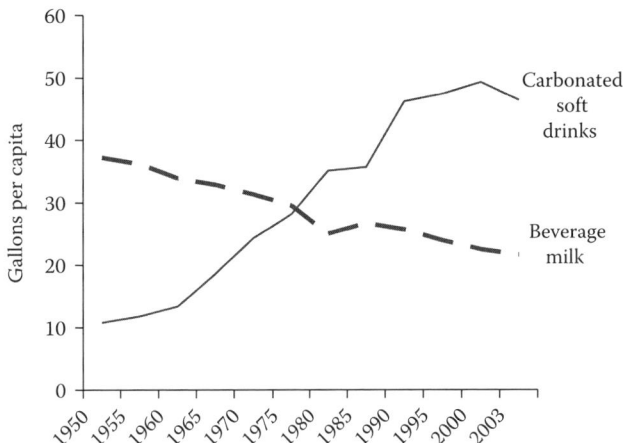

**FIGURE 42.5** Per capita availability of milk and carbonated soft drinks in the United States, 1950–2003. (From USDA, Food availability data system. 2011; http://www.ers.usda.gov/Data/FoodConsumption/FoodAvailSpreadsheets.htm#fruitcan)

of soft drinks has increased fourfold (Figure 42.5) and consumption increased by 131% since 1977.[35] Intake of sugars from beverages now comprises 16% of total energy intake in the American diet and is even higher among adolescents, comprising 20% of total energy intake.[36] Several studies indicate that greater intake of sugar-sweetened beverages is related to greater risk of weight gain, and a recent review concluded that sugar-sweetened drinks accounted for at least 20% of the increase in weight in the United States between 1977 and 2007.[37] However, additional research is needed in this area, as the magnitude of the effect of sugar-sweetened beverages on body weight remains under dispute.[38]

Clearly, access to highly palatable, energy-dense, convenience foods has increased substantially since the 1970s. Fast food franchises and inexpensive convenient dining options have proliferated, and food and drinks are now quickly available from a multitude of different places, including vending, drug stores, book stores, hardware stores, and big box stores. Money spent on food away from home has correspondingly

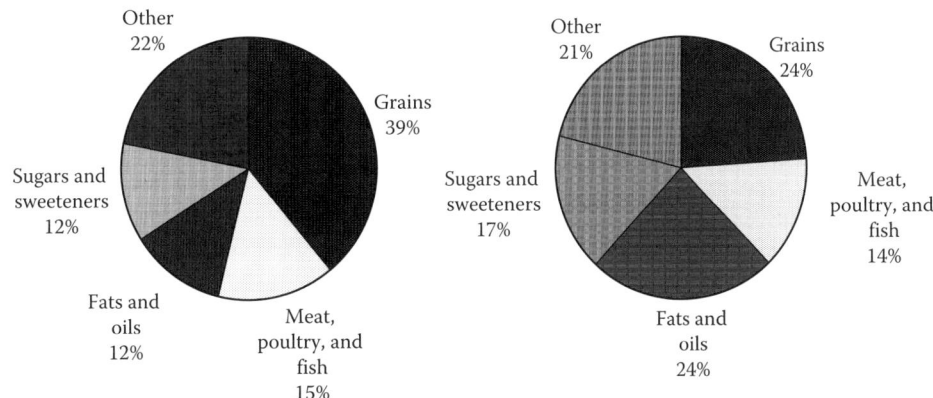

**FIGURE 42.4** Sources of food energy in the U.S. food supply 1909, 2006. USDA Center for Nutrition Policy and Promotion. (From Gerrior, S. et al., *Nutrient Content of the U.S. Food Supply, 1909–2000: A Summary Report*, U.S. Department of Agriculture, Center for Nutrition Policy and Promotion, 2004.)

continued to grow, and the proportion of money spent at restaurants rose from 9% in 1929 to 37.5% in 2010.[39] Estimates suggest that 37% of adults and 42% of children eat in a fast food restaurant on any given day.[40] Continued fast food consumption has been shown to predict increased BMI in both children and adults.[41–44] Moreover, adults and children who report eating fast food have higher intakes of sugar-sweetened soft drinks as well as total energy and fat.[40,44] Nonetheless, more research is needed to determine the degree to which increasing access to fast food restaurants is responsible for the rise in obesity prevalence.[45,46]

## Summary

The available research, based principally on self-report, reveals significant increases in energy intake over the past few decades. The principal factors that appear to be responsible are increasing portion sizes and greater accessibility to highly palatable, energy-dense foods at affordable prices.

## ENERGY EXPENDITURE

Although nearly one-third of U.S. adults do not engage in any physical activity during their leisure time, there is little evidence that physical activity levels have changed significantly over the past decade (Figure 42.6).[47,48] Nonetheless, it is generally accepted that with the modernization of society, energy expenditure has decreased and is at least partly responsible for the increasing prevalence of obesity.[13,49,50] The decrease in energy expenditure is most likely due to changes in activities of daily living.[50]

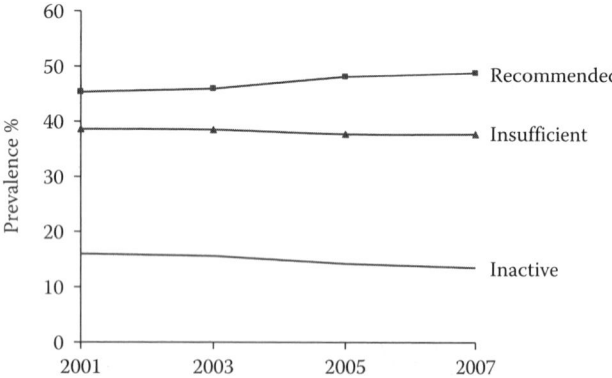

**FIGURE 42.6**  Trends in leisure-time physical activity of adults aged 18+ years, Behavioral Risk Factor Surveillance System, United States, 2001–2007. Recommended level = moderate intensity activity ≥5 times/week for ≥30 min each time/day or vigorous intensity ≥3 times/week for ≥200 min each time, or both; Insufficient = some activity but not enough to be classified as moderate or vigorous; Inactive = no leisure time physical activity during the preceding month. (From Centers for Disease Control and Prevention, *MMWR. Morb. Mortal. Wkly. Rep.*, 50(9), 166, 2001; Pickrell, D. and Schimek, P., *Transportation*, 1998; Flegal, K.M. et al., *JAMA*, 307(5), 491, 2012; Division of Nutrition Physical Activity, and Obesity, National Center for Chronic Disease Prevention and Health Promotion, Summary of physical activity, 2010, http://apps.nccd.cdc.gov/PASurveillance/StateSumResultV.asp?CI=&Year=2001&State=0#data)

**TABLE 42.2**
**Energy Savers**

Personal computers
Tele-commuting
Cellular phones
E-mail/Internet
Personal digital assistants (PDAs)
Shopping by phone
Food delivery services
Phone extensions
Dishwashers
Escalators/elevators
Cable movies
Drive-thru windows
Computer games
Intercoms
Moving sidewalks
Remote controls
Garage door openers
Snow blowers
Riding-lawnmowers

Table 42.2 lists some of the ways time (and energy) is saved each day. In particular, computers have clearly changed the American workplace, as their number has increased exponentially in the past two decades. It has been suggested that the impact that sending an email rather than walking to the office next door to communicate information in the workplace may decrease energy expenditure by half.[14] Computer use in the home has also increased dramatically, from 8% in 1984 to 61.8% in 2003.[51] Estimates suggest that adults spend an average of 28 h/week watching television, and children and adolescents watch an average of 25 h a week.[52] Television viewing is strongly related to increasing prevalence of obesity among children[53–55] and to the level of obesity in adults.[56,57] Children spend more time watching television than any other activity with the exception of sleeping, and by the age 18 the average teenager has spent more time watching television than learning in the classroom.[19,58] The number of screens in the home has also been directly related to increasing weight and amount of sedentary behavior in both adults and children.[59,60] Conversely, children and adults participate in more activity when a greater amount of space and physical activity cues (e.g., treadmills, active toys for children) are present in the home.[61–63] The proliferation of televisions and other energy-saving devices has also been linked with shorter sleep durations, which is an independent predictor of weight gain.[64]

Automobiles are clearly the preferred mode of travel over walking in both the United States (Figure 42.7)[65] and the United Kingdom,[66] and people are less likely to walk or bike for transportation than in previous years. The environmental barriers to use of bicycling and walking for transportation include lack of bike trail access, safety concerns (e.g., crime), lighting, and traffic, lack of changing facilities at work, lack of employer support, and inconvenience.[67] More research is needed on trends in other labor-saving

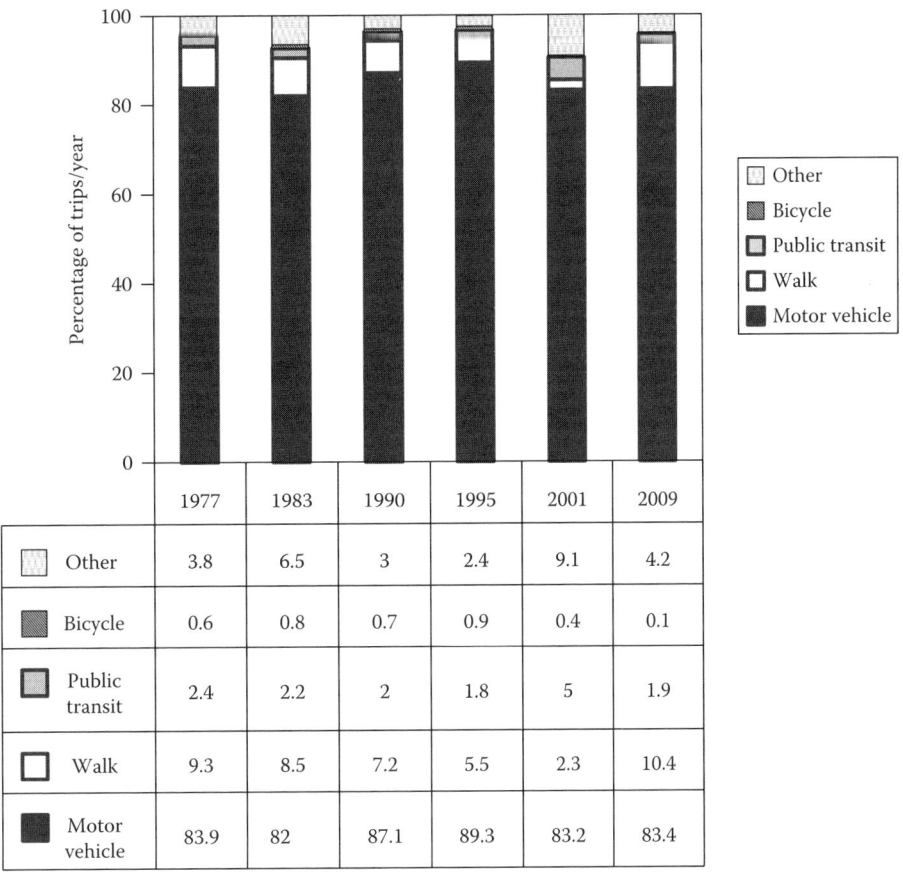

**FIGURE 42.7** Mode of travel in the United States from 1977 to 2009. Nationwide Personal Transportation Surveys, 1998, 2001, 2009. (From Center for Urban Transportation Research, *Public Transit in America: Results from the 2001 National Household Travel Survey*, National Center for Transit Research, Tampa, FL, 2005.)

devices or on their potential impact on physical activity levels, including use of such labor-saving devices as escalators and leaf blowers.

## CULTURAL AND SOCIAL FACTORS

The increasing prevalence of overweight is also associated with cultural and social factors. Obesity affects every group and income level but some racial or ethnic groups are disproportionately obese. Specifically, the prevalence of obesity in the United States is greatest among non-Hispanic blacks and Mexican-American women (Figure 42.8).[1,4] This may reflect cultural values and beliefs that limit the motivation for weight control and effectiveness of weight control programs or specific behaviors such as lower levels of physical activity.[68,69] Metabolic factors may also play a role, including decreased energy expenditure among obese African-American women relative to Caucasian women.[70]

Obesity is also more common among low-income populations.[71] Low-income populations often experience differential access to health care services[72,73] due to cost barriers, unavailability of health insurance, and discrimination in health care.[74,75] Economic status may also impact families' nutritional patterns, level of concern about nutrition, and knowledge of foods to purchase and consume.[76,77]

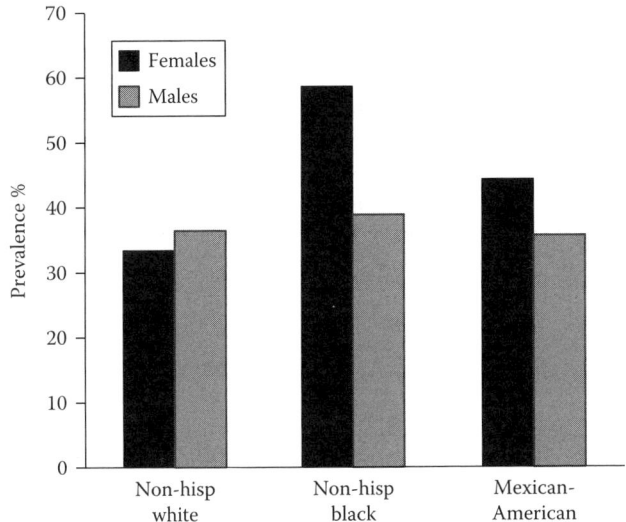

**FIGURE 42.8** Prevalence of obesity (BMI $\geq$ 30 kg/m$^2$) in the United States by race-ethnic group for men and women aged 20 years and older, 2009–2010. (From Flegal, K.M. et al., *JAMA*, 307(5), 491, 2012.)

## ASSESSMENT OF ENVIRONMENTAL CHALLENGES

A detailed review of measures of food intake and physical activity can be found in Chapters 31 and 41 of this book and other comprehensive texts (e.g., Allison[78]). Therefore, only a brief review of assessment tools will be provided here.

### EPIDEMIOLOGIC ASSESSMENT

#### Physical Activity

Although physical activity tends to be over-reported,[48,79] questionnaires are frequently used in epidemiologic studies to classify levels of physical activity.[80,81] Although several physical activity measures exist (e.g., diaries, retrospective histories), recall surveys appear to be the least likely to influence behavior and generally require the least amount of effort by respondents.[48,80] Among the most frequently used measures are the Physical Activity Recall (PAR)[82] and the Paffenbarger.[83] The PAR is available in interviewer- and self-administered versions[82] and categorizes activities by their intensity; the Paffenbarger is a one-page questionnaire that evaluates habitual daily and weekly activity. Measures of sedentary promoting behaviors, such as television viewing and computer use, are only beginning to be utilized and validated. However, sedentary behavior can be simply assessed by the number of reported minutes per day spent in sedentary behaviors (e.g., watching television, using the computer, video-games, and driving). Questionnaire measures may be used to document the amount and type of exercise equipment and media available in the home for both adults[26] and children,[62,84,85] but more validation studies are needed, particularly in measures for children.[86] While not possible in large numbers, accelerometry remains the most objective assessment of levels of physical activity in children and adults.

#### Food Intake

As noted earlier, food intake tends to be underreported, particularly in obese individuals.[87] Nonetheless, several methods of assessment exist to measure nutrient intake. The 24 h recall has been used in many large-scale studies (e.g., the National Health and Nutrition Examination Surveys) to assess nutrient intake. The 24 h recall takes about 20 min to complete, requires no record keeping on the part of respondents, and, unlike other measures (e.g., food diaries), does not cause subjects to alter their intake.[88] The 24 h recall is typically administered by trained interviewers, but can also be completed in a self-administered online format through the National Cancer Institute (ASA-24; http://riskfactor.cancer.gov/tools/instruments/asa24.html).

Alternatively, if assessment of subjects' average, long-term intake is needed (rather than a more precise measurement of short-term consumption), food frequency questionnaires (FFQ) are an appropriate alternative, although potentially more reliable in adults[89] than in

children.[90] FFQ (e.g., the Block[89]) assesses the frequency and quantity of habitual consumption of food items listed in a questionnaire in reference to the past week or month. These are easy to administer and do not require trained interviewers. Checklists are available to assess availability and accessibility of high-fat and low-fat foods in the home of adults,[52,76,91] and children,[62,84,85] but more validation studies are needed, particularly for children and for racial/ethnic minority populations.[86]

#### Neighborhood/Community Environment

Given the role of the wider "macro" environment in the development of obesity, there has been a consistent call for assessing community-level food and activity environments. A common methodology used to assess the community environment is Geographic Information Systems (GIS) technology. In this method, global position technologies are used to assess spatial distributions of community food environments (e.g., fast food outlets, supermarkets, other restaurants) and physical activity–related parameters (e.g., street connectivity, presence of green open space, access to public transportation, density of public transition stations, etc.).[92–94] Buildings are evaluated for the presence of vending machines, snack shops, recreational space, office layouts that encourage walking, and recreational facilities. Schools are assessed for vending, cafeterias, classroom space for movement versus sitting, access via walking, and the presence of safe playgrounds.

Other methods have also been developed to assess consumer food environments, including observational surveys,[95,96] intercept surveys,[97] questionnaires,[98] sales analyses,[99] menu analyses,[100] and nutrient analyses[101] that assess the quality of fresh produce in stores, types of food offered through lunches, vending and a la carte option at schools, menu options in restaurants, and food sales in worksites. However, relatively little work has been done that evaluates psychometric properties of these instruments.[102]

Research is in its infancy on ways to assess the impact of governmental policies, laws, and regulations on the obesogenic environment. An "obesity impact assessment" has been proposed that assesses the effects on obesity of legislation pertaining to public liability, urban planning, transport, food safety, marketing, school food rules, taxes/levies, agriculture, and trade.[103] Assessment of governance and governing systems, the way policy debate is framed, and the interactions between stakeholders in the policy process are additional avenues of future investigation on impacts of policy on obesity.[104]

### CLINICAL ASSESSMENT

#### Physical Activity

The questionnaires reviewed earlier (i.e., PAR[82] and the Paffenbarger[83]) may also be useful in assessing physical activity in the clinical setting. Alternatively, a few simple questions may provide practical and efficient means of assessing physical activity. These include, "How many minutes do you spend each week in planned physical activity?" "Approximately how many city blocks do you walk each day?" and "How many flights of stairs do you climb each day?" Television viewing, computer and videogame use, and driving time may also be evaluated in the clinical setting by weekly number of minutes for each activity. Pedometers, which provide a count of the total number of steps taken each day, can be very useful in monitoring changes in physical activity. Finally, for a brief assessment of the home physical activity environment, number of screens in the home, presence of home exercise equipment and a yard can also be assessed.

## Food Intake

The most commonly used means to assess energy and nutrient intake in the clinical setting is the food record. Food records are patients' daily notations of the type, quantity, and calories of food and liquid consumed. Patients are instructed to record all meals, drinks, and snacks immediately after eating. Patients may also record the number of fat grams consumed, place of consumption, and minutes of television viewing per day. It should also be noted that food records are also commonly used as an intervention tool.[105]

If a less reactive and more immediate assessment of intake is required, FFQ or 24 h recalls may be used. Fast food eating can be assessed at the time of the clinic assessment with the question, "How many times per week, on average, do you eat at fast food restaurants?" Measures of food availability in the home tend to be quite lengthy but may be useful in some clinical encounters.[52,62,76,84,85,91]

## Assessment Model

The ultimate challenge of environmental assessment is to integrate the multiple factors that influence obesity. As Figure 42.9 illustrates, food intake and physical activity may result from a combination of influences (e.g., large portion sizes, use of labor-saving devices) that interact with cultural and social factors to promote obesity. In this model, excess food intake may be due to larger portion sizes at restaurants, but other factors must also be considered. For example, cultural taste preferences and economic status may also influence restaurant selection. Although distinguishing among the several overlapping environmental influences can be difficult, an awareness of such interrelationships is critical for designing public health and clinical interventions aimed to decrease the rising prevalence of obesity.

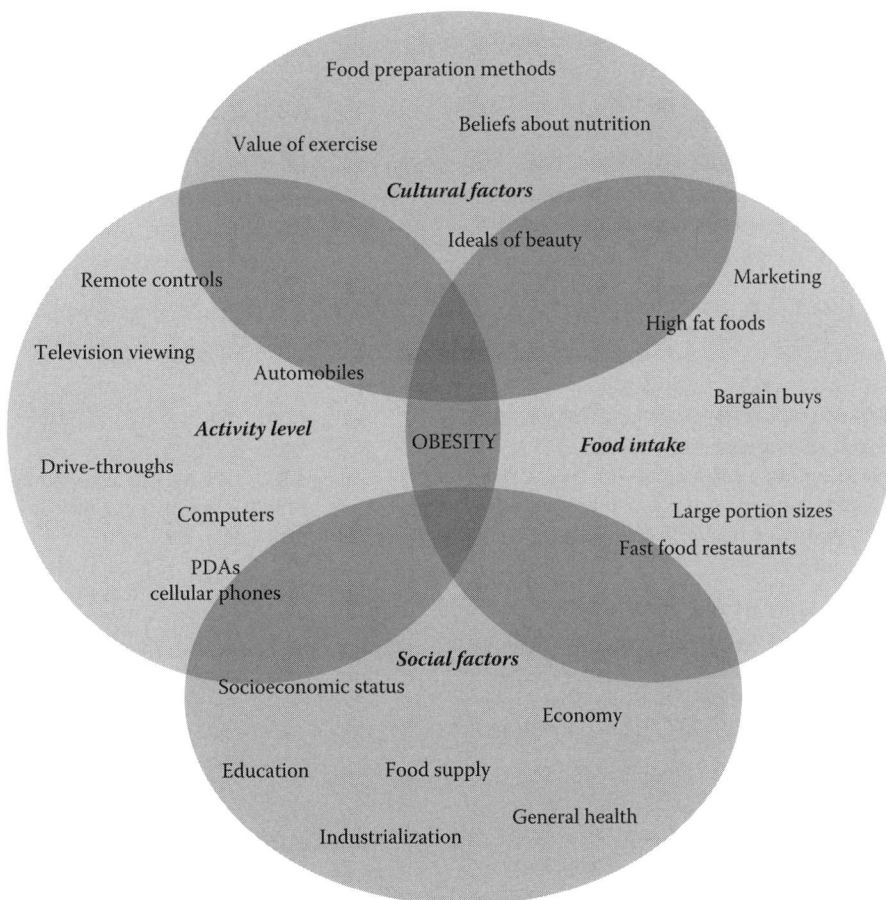

**FIGURE 42.9** Environmental influences on obesity.

## SUMMARY AND CONCLUSION

In summary, obesity is due to an imbalance of energy intake and expenditure. Both biological and behavioral factors are implicated. Several environmental changes have occurred over the past few decades that appear to contribute to the increase in obesity in industrialized nations. In particular, portion sizes have increased and highly palatable, energy-dense foods are heavily marketed and readily available at a low cost. In addition, the amount of energy expended in activities of daily living appears to have declined.

Given the complexity of the relationship between the environment, individual behaviors, and obesity, a multilevel approach is likely needed to curb current obesity rates. Policy and industry level measures have been initiated, including The Walt Disney Company restricting the advertising and sale in its theme parks of energy-dense foods,[106] the First Lady Michelle Obama's "Let's Move" program (www. Letsmove.gov) to increase activity and make healthy foods available, the Patient Protection and Affordable Care Act of 2010 mandating that calorie labels be added to menus of chain restaurants,[107] and New York's proposal to restrict the serving sizes of soda offered for sale.[108] As these and other policies move forward, it is critically important that rigorous evaluation of these environmental changes be undertaken to inform future policy decisions.[109] Ultimately, promoting healthy nutrition will require targeting multiple environmental components and a partnership among various sectors of society, including the government, food industry, the media, and the scientific community.

## REFERENCES

1. Hedley AA, Ogden CL, Johnson CL, Carroll MD, Curtin LR, Flegal KM. Prevalence of overweight and obesity among US children, adolescents, and adults, 1999–2002. *JAMA* 2004; 291(23): 2847–2850.
2. Gerrior S, Bente L, Hiza H. *Nutrient Content of the US Food Supply, Development Between 2000–2006*. Washington, DC: USDA, 2011.
3. National Center for Health Statistics/Division of Data Services. www.cdc.gov/nchs/data/hus/hus05.pdf#chartbookontrends2005 (accessed July 30, 2012).
4. Ogden CL, Carroll MD, Curtin LR, Lamb MM, Flegal KM. Prevalence of high body mass index in US children and adolescents, 2007–2008. *JAMA* 2010; 303(3): 242–249.
5. Ogden CL, Lamb MM, Carroll MD, Flegal KM. Obesity and socioeconomic status in adults: United States, 2005–2008. *NCHS Data Brief* 2010; 50: 1–8.
6. Ogden CL. *Obesity and Socioeconomic Status in Children and Adolescents: United States, 2005–2008*. Hyattsville, MD: U.S. Department of Health and Human Services, Centers for Disease Control and Prevention, National Center for Health Statistics, 2010.
7. Flegal KM, Carroll MD, Ogden CL, Curtin LR. Prevalence and trends in obesity among US adults, 1999–2008. *JAMA* 2010; 303(3): 235–241.
8. Ogden CL, Carroll MD, McDowell MA, Flegal KM. Obesity among adults in the United States—No statistically significant chance since 2003–2004. *NCHS Data Brief* 2007; 1: 1–8.
9. Finkelstein EA, Khavjou OA, Thompson H, Trogdon JG, Pan L, Sherry B, Dietz W. Obesity and severe obesity forecasts through 2030. *Am J Prev Med* 2012; 42(6): 563–570.
10. Obesity and Overweight. Media Centre. World Health Organization; Fact sheet Number 311. May 2012. http://www.who.int/mediacentre/factsheets/fs311/en/ (accessed July 30, 2012).
11. Centers For Disease Control and Prevention (CDC). Prevalence of physical activity, including lifestyle activities among adults—United States, 2000–2001. *MMWR Morb Mortal Wkly Rep* 2003; 52(32): 764–769.
12. USDA. Food availability data system. 2011; http://www.ers.usda.gov/Data/FoodConsumption/FoodAvailSpreadsheets.htm#fruitcan (accessed July 30, 2012).
13. Weinsier RL, Hunter GR, Heine AF, Goran MIS, Sell SM. The etiology of obesity: Relative contribution of metabolic factors, diet, and physical activity. *Am J Med* 1998; 105: 145–150.
14. French SA, Story M, Jeffery RW. Environmental influences on eating and physical activity. *Ann Rev Pub Health* 2001; 22: 309–335.
15. Hill JO, Wyatt HR, Reed GW, Peters JC. Obesity and the environment: Where do we go from here? *Science* 2003; 299(7): 853–855.
16. Brownell K. Toward optimal health: Dr. Kelly Brownell discusses [corrected] the influence of the environment on obesity. Interview by Jodi R. Godfrey. *J Womens Health (Larchmt)* 2008; 17(3): 325–330.
17. Wright JD, Wang CY. Trends in intake of energy and macronutrients in adults from 1999–2000 through 2007–2008. *NCHS Data Brief* 2010; 49: 1–8.
18. Gerrior S, Bente L, Hiza H. *Nutrient Content of the U.S. Food Supply, 1909–2000: A Summary Report*. U.S. Department of Agriculture, Center for Nutrition Policy and Promotion, Washington, DC, 2004.
19. Brantley PJ, Myers VH, Roy HJ. Environmental and lifestyle influences on obesity. *J Louis St Med Soc* 2005; 156: S19–S27.
20. Wansink B. Can package size accelerate usage volume? *J Marketing* 1996; 60: 1–14.
21. Rolls BJ, Roe LS, Meengs JS, Wall DE. Increasing the portion size of a sandwich increases energy intake. *J Am Diet Assoc* 2004; 104(3): 367–372.
22. Young LR, Nestle M. Expanding portion sizes in the US marketplace: Implications for nutrition counseling. *J Am Diet Assoc* 2003; 103(2): 231–234.
23. Penisten MB, Litchfield RE. Nutrition education delivered at the state fair: Are your portions in proportion? *J Nutr Educ Behav* 2004; 36(5): 275–277.
24. Young LR, Nestle M. The contribution of expanding portion sizes to the US obesity epidemic. *Am J Public Health* 2002; 92(2): 246–249.
25. Geier AB, Rozin P, Doros G. Unit bias. A new heuristic that helps explain the effect of portion size on food intake. *Psychol Sci* 2006; 17(6): 521–525.
26. Schwartz J, Byrd-Bredbenner C. Portion distortion: Typical portion sizes selected by young adults. *J Am Diet Assoc* 2006; 106(9): 1412–1418.
27. Center for Science in the Public Interest. The pressure to eat. *Nutr Action Health Lett* 1998; 25: 3–6.
28. French S, Jeffery R, Story M, Hannan P, Snyder M. A pricing strategy to promote low-fat snack choices through vending machines. *Am J Public Health* 1997; 87(5): 849–851.
29. Jeffery RW, French SA, Raether C, Baxter JE. An environmental intervention to increase fruit and salad purchases in a cafeteria. *Prev Med* 1994; 23: 788–792.

30. Powell LM, Chaloupka FJ. Food prices and obesity: Evidence and policy implications for taxes and subsidies. *Milbank Q* 2009; 87(1): 229–257.

31. Cotti C, Tefft N. Fast food prices, obesity, and the minimum wage. *Econ Hum Biol* 2012 (accessed July 30, 2012).

32. Centers for Disease Control and Prevention. Trends in intake of energy and macronutrients—United States, 1971–2000. *Morb Mortal Wkly Rep* 2004; 53(4): 80–82.

33. Austin GL, Ogden LG, Hill JO. Trends in carbohydrate, fat, and protein intakes and association with energy intake in normal-weight, overweight, and obese individuals: 1971–2006. *Am J Clin Nutr* 2011; 93(4): 836–843.

34. Putnam JJ, Gerrior S. Trends in the US food supply, 1970–1997. In: Frazao E (ed.), *America's Eating Habits: Changes and Consequences*. Washington, DC: USDA Economic Research Service, 1999.

35. Subar AF, Heimendinger J, Patterson BH, Krebs-Smith SM, Pivonka E. Fruit and vegetable intake in the United States: The baseline survey of the five a day for better health program. *Am J Health Promot* 1995; 9: 352–360.

36. Guthrie JF, Morton JF. Food sources of added sweeteners in the diets of Americans. *JADA* 2000; 100: 43–51.

37. Institute of Medicine (U.S.). Committee on Accelerating Progress in Obesity Prevention. In: Glickman D (ed.), *Accelerating Progress in Obesity Prevention*. Washington, DC: National Academic Press; 2012.

38. Mattes RD, Shikany JM, Kaiser KA, Allison DB. Nutritively sweetened beverage consumption and body weight: A systematic review and meta-analysis of randomized experiments. *Obes Rev* 2011; 12(5): 346–365.

39. USDA Economic Research Service. Food CPI and expenditures: Table 15. 2010; http://www.ers.usda.gov/briefing/cpifoodandexpenditures/Data/Expenditures_tables/table15.htm, 2012 (accessed July 30, 2012).

40. Paeratakul S, Ferdinand DP, Champagne CM, Ryan DH, Bray GA. Fast-food consumption among US adults and children: Dietary and nutrient intake profile. *JADA* 2003; 103(10): 1332–1338.

41. Jeffery RW, French S. Epidemic obesity in the United States: Are fast foods and television viewing contributing? *Am J Public Health* 1998; 88(2): 277–280.

42. Pereira MA, Kartashov AI, Ebbeling CB, Van Horn L, Slattery ML, Jacobs DR, Ludwig DS. Fast-food habits, weight gain, and insulin resistance (the CARDIA study): 15-year prospective analysis. *Lancet* 2005; 367(9453): 36–42.

43. French S, Story M, Neumark-Sztainer D. Fast food restaurant use among adolescents: Associations with nutrient intake, food choices, and behavioral and psychosocial variables. *Int J Obes Relat Metab Disord* 2001; 25: 1823–1833.

44. Bowman SA, Vinyard BT. Fast food consumption of US adults: Impact on energy and nutrient intakes and overweight status. *J Am Coll Nutr* 2004; 23(2): 163–168.

45. Fleischhacker SE, Evenson KR, Rodriguez DA, Ammerman AS. A systematic review of fast food access studies. *Obes Rev* 2011; 12(5): e460–e471.

46. Fraser LK, Edwards KL, Cade J, Clarke GP. The geography of fast food outlets: A review. *Int J Environ Res Public Health* 2010; 7(5): 2290–2308.

47. Division of Nutrition Physical Activity, and Obesity, National Center for Chronic Disease Prevention and Health Promotion. Summary of physical activity. 2010; http://apps.nccd.cdc.gov/PASurveillance/StateSumResultV.asp?CI=&Year=2001&State=0#data (accessed July 30, 2012).

48. U.S. Department of Health and Human Services. The surgeon general's report on nutrition and health. In Neatle M (ed.), *The Reports of the Surgeon General*. Department of Health and Human Services, Washington, DC: Government Printing Office; 1996, pp. 88–50210.

49. Prentice AM, Jebb SA. Obesity in Britain: Gluttony or sloth? *Br Med J* 1995; 311: 437–439.

50. Hill JO, Wyatt HR, Melanson EL. Genetic and environmental contributions to obesity. *Med Clin N Am* 2000; 84: 333–346.

51. U.S. Bureau Census; Web-Site Database. 2005; http://www.census.gov (accessed July 30, 2012).

52. Nielsen Media Research. *2000 Report on Television: The First 50 Years*. New York: AC Nielsen Co.; 2000.

53. Dietz WH, Gortmaker SL. Do we fatten our children at the television set? *Pediatrics* 1985; 75: 807–812.

54. Gortmaker SL, Must A, Sobol AM, Peterson K, Colditz GA, Dietz WH. Television viewing as a cause of increasing obesity among children in the United States, 1986–1990. *Arch Pediatr Adolesc Med* 1996; 150(Title): 356–362.

55. Andersen RE, Crespo CJ, Bartlett SJ, Cheskin LJ, Pratt M. Relationship of physical activity and television watching with body weight and level of fatness among children. *JAMA* 1998; 279(12): 938–942.

56. Tucker LA, Friedman GM. Television viewing and obesity in adult males. *Am J Public Health* 1989; 79(4): 516–518.

57. Tucker LA, Bagwell M. Television viewing and obesity in adult females. *Am J Public Health* 1991; 81: 908–911.

58. Kotz K, Story M. Good advertisements during children's Saturday morning television programming: Are they consistent with dietary recommendations? *JADA* 1994; 94: 1296–1300.

59. Saelens BE, Sallis JF, Nader PR, Broyles SL, Berry CC, Taras HL. Home environmental influences on children's television watching from early to middle childhood. *J Dev Behav Pediatr* 2002; 23(3): 127–132.

60. Phelan S, Liu T, Gorin A, Lowe M, Hogan J, Fava J, Wing RR. What distinguishes weight-loss maintainers from the treatment-seeking obese? Analysis of environmental, behavioral, and psychosocial variables in diverse populations. *Ann Behav Med* 2009; 38(2): 94–104.

61. Fees B, Trost S, Bopp M, Dzewaltowski DA. Physical activity programming in family child care homes: Providers' perceptions of practices and barriers. *J Nutr Educ Behav* 2009; 41(4): 268–273.

62. Spurrier NJ, Magarey AA, Golley R, Curnow F, Sawyer MG. Relationships between the home environment and physical activity and dietary patterns of preschool children: A cross-sectional study. *Int J Behav Nutr Phys Act* 2008; 5: 31.

63. Jakicic JM, Wing RR, Butler BA, Jeffery RW. The relationship between presence of exercise equipment in the home and physical activity level. *Am J Health Promot* 1997; 11(5): 363–365.

64. Cappuccio FP, Taggart FM, Kandala NB, Currie A, Peile E, Stranges S, Miller MA. Meta-analysis of short sleep duration and obesity in children and adults. *Sleep* 2008; 31(5): 619–626.

65. Pickrell D, Schimek P. Trends in personal motor vehicle ownership and use: Evidence from the nationwide personal transportation survey. Boston: US Department of Transportation Volpe Center, 1998.

66. DiGuiseppi C, Roberts I, Li L. Influence of changing travel patterns on child death rates from injury: Trend analysis. *Br Med J* 1997; 314: 710–713.

67. U.S. Department of Transportation. *Final Report: The National Bicycling and Walking Study: Transportation Choices for a Changing America*. Washington, DC: U.S. Department of Transportation; 1994. FHWA-PD-023.

68. Kumanyika S, Wilson JF, Guilford-Davenport M. Weight-related attitudes and behaviors in black women. *JADA* 1993; 93: 416–422.

69. Kumanyika S, Morssink C, Agurs T. Models for dietary and weight change in African American women. *Ethn Dis* 1992; 2: 166–175.

70. Foster GD, Wadden TA, Swain RM, Anderson DA, Vogt RE. Changes in resting energy expenditure after weight loss in obese African American and white women. *Am J Clin Nutr* 1999; 69: 13–17.

71. Sobal J, Stunkard AJ. Socioeconomic status and obesity: A review of the literature. *Psychol Bull* 1989; 105(Title): 260–275.

72. Ginzberg E. Access to health care for Hispanics. *JAMA* 1991; 262: 238–241.

73. Finucane TE, Carrese JA. Racial bias in presentation of cases. *J Gen Int Med* 1990; 5: 120–121.

74. Wenneker MB, Epstein AM. Racial inequalities in the use of procedures for patients with ischemic heart disease in Massachusetts. *JAMA* 1987; 261: 253–257.

75. Carlisle DM, Leake BD, Shapiro MF. Racial and ethnic differences in the use of invasive cardiac procedures among cardiac patients in Los Angeles County. *Am J Public Health* 1995; 85: 352–356.

76. U.S. Department of Health Education and Welfare, Center for Disease Control, Ten-State nutrition survey, 1968–1970; 1975 Publication Number (HSM) 72-8132.

77. Hulshof KF, Lowik MR, Kik FJ, Wedel M, Brants HA, Hermus RJ, Hoor F. Diet and other life-style factors in high and low socio-economic groups. *Eur J Clin Nutr* 1991; 45: 441–450.

78. Allison DB, Baskin ML. *Handbook of Assessment Methods for Eating Behaviors and Weight-Related Problems: Measures, Theory, and Research*, 2nd edn. Los Angeles, CA: Sage Publications; 2009.

79. Lichtman SW, Pisarska K, Berman ER, Pestone M, Dowling H, Offenbacher E, Weisel H, Heshka S, Matthews DE, Heymsfield SB. Discrepancy between self-reported and actual caloric intake and exercise in obese subjects. *N Engl J Med* 1992; 327(Title): 1893–1898.

80. LaPorte RE, Montoye HJ, Caspersen CJ. Assessment of physical activity in epidemiologic research: Problems and prospects. *Public Health Rep* 1985; 100: 131–146.

81. Caspersen CJ. Physical activity epidemiology: Concepts, methods, and applications to exercise science. *Exerc Sport Sci Rev* 1989; 17: 423–473.

82. Blair SN. How to assess exercise habits and physical fitness. In: Matarazzo JD, Weiss SM, Herd JA, Miller NE (eds.), *Behavioral Health: A Handbook of Health Enhancement and Disease Prevention*. New York: Wiley, 1984, pp. 424–427.

83. Blair SN, Haskell PH, Paffenbarger RS, Vranizan KM, Farquhar JW, Wood PD. Assessment of habitual physical activity by a seven-day recall in a community survey and controlled experiments. *Am J Epidemiol* 1985; 122(Title): 794–804.

84. Gattshall ML, Shoup JA, Marshall JA, Crane LA, Estabrooks PA. Validation of a survey instrument to assess home environments for physical activity and healthy eating in overweight children. *Int J Behav Nutr Phys Act* 2008; 5: 3.

85. Larios SE, Ayala GX, Arredondo EM, Baquero B, Elder JP. Development and validation of a scale to measure Latino parenting strategies related to children's obesigenic behaviors. The parenting strategies for eating and activity scale (PEAS). *Appetite* 2009; 52(1): 166–172.

86. Pinard CA, Yaroch AL, Hart MH, Serrano EL, McFerren MM, Estabrooks PA. Measures of the home environment related to childhood obesity: A systematic review. *Public Health Nutr* 2011; 7: 1–13.

87. Schoeller DA. Limitations in the assessment of dietary energy intake by self-report. *Metabolism* 1995; 44(2 Title): 18–22.

88. Wolper C, Heshka S, Heymsfield SB. Measuring food intake: An overview. In: Allison DB (ed.), *Handbook of Assessment Methods for Eating Behaviors and Weight Related Problems. Measures, Theory and Research*. Thousand Oaks: Sage, 1995, pp. 215–240.

89. Block G, Woods M, Potosky A, Clifford C. Validation of a self-administered diet history questionnaire using multiple diet records. *J Clin Epidemiol* 1990; 43(12): 1327–1335.

90. Borradaile KE, Foster GD, May H, Karpyn A, Sherman S, Grundy K, Nachmani J, Vander Veur S, Boruch RF. Associations between the Youth/Adolescent Questionnaire, the Youth/Adolescent Activity Questionnaire, and body mass index z score in low-income inner-city fourth through sixth grade children. *Am J Clin Nutr* 2008; 87(6): 1650–1655.

91. Bryant M, Stevens J. Measurement of food availability in the home. *Nutr Rev* 2006; 64(2 Pt 1): 67–76.

92. Pearce J, Witten K, Bartie P. Neighbourhoods and health: A GIS approach to measuring community resource accessibility. *J Epidemiol Commun Health* 2006; 60(5): 389–395.

93. Austin SB, Melly SJ, Sanchez BN, Patel A, Buka S, Gortmaker SL. Clustering of fast-food restaurants around schools: A novel application of spatial statistics to the study of food environments. *Am J Public Health* 2005; 95(9): 1575–1581.

94. Handy SL, Boarnet MG, Ewing R, Killingsworth RE. How the built environment affects physical activity: Views from urban planning. *Am J Prev Med* 2002; 23(2 Suppl): 64–73.

95. Glanz K, Sallis JF, Saelens BE, Frank LD. Nutrition environment measures survey in stores (NEMS-S): Development and evaluation. *Am J Prev Med* 2007; 32(4): 282–289.

96. Voss C, Klein S, Glanz K, Clawson M. Nutrition environment measures survey-vending: Development, dissemination, and reliability. *Health Promot Pract* 2012; 13(4): 425–430.

97. Borradaile KE, Sherman S, Vander Veur SS, McCoy T, Sandoval B, Nachmani J, Karpyn A, Foster GD. Snacking in children: The role of urban corner stores. *Pediatrics* 2009; 124(5): 1293–1298.

98. Mujahid MS, Diez Roux AV, Morenoff JD, Raghunathan T. Assessing the measurement properties of neighborhood scales: From psychometrics to ecometrics. *Am J Epidemiol* 2007; 165(8): 858–867.

99. Abarca J, Ramachandran S. Using community indicators to assess nutrition in Arizona-Mexico border communities. *Prev Chronic Dis* 2005; 2(1): A06.

100. Cassady D, Housemann R, Dagher C. Measuring cues for healthy choices on restaurant menus: Development and testing of a measurement instrument. *Am J Health Promot* 2004; 18(6): 444–449.

101. Cullen KW, Watson K, Zakeri I, Ralston K. Exploring changes in middle-school student lunch consumption after local school food service policy modifications. *Public Health Nutr* 2006; 9(6): 814–820.

102. McKinnon RA, Reedy J, Morrissette MA, Lytle LA, Yaroch AL. Measures of the food environment: A compilation of the literature, 1990–2007. *Am J Prev Med* 2009; 36(4 Suppl): S124–S133.

103. Swinburn BA. Obesity prevention: The role of policies, laws and regulations. *Aust N Z Health Policy* 2008; 5: 12.

104. Shill J, Mavoa H, Allender S, Lawrence M, Sacks G, Peeters A, Crammond B, Swinburn B. Government regulation to promote healthy food environments—A view from inside state governments. *Obes Rev* 2012; 13(2): 162–173.

105. Wadden TA, Foster GD. Behavioral treatment of obesity. *Med Clin N Am* 2000; 84: 441–462.

106. Battle against diabetes and obesity moves to Disneyland. *The New York Times*. June 11, 2012; The Times in Plain English.

107. Swartz JJ, Braxton D, Viera AJ. Calorie menu labeling on quick-service restaurant menus: An updated systematic review of the literature. *Int J Behav Nutr Phys Act* 2011; 8: 135.

108. Grynbaum MM. New York plans to ban sale of big sizes of sugary drinks. *The New York Times*. May 30, 2012; N.Y./Region.

109. Whitacre P, Tsai P, Mulligan J, Institute of Medicine (U.S.). Board on Population Health and Public Health Practice. National Research Council (U.S.). Food and Nutrition Board. Board on Agriculture and Natural Resources. *The Public Health Effects of Food Deserts: Workshop Summary*. Washington, DC: National Academies Press, 2009.

110. Flegal KM, Carroll MD, Kuczmarski RJ, Johnson CL. Overweight and obesity in the United States: Prevalence and trends. *Int J Obes* 1998; 22(Title): 39–47.

111. Gerrior S, Bente L, Hiza H. *Nutrient Content of the U.S. Food Supply, 1909–2000*. Washington, DC: U.S. Department of Agriculture, Center for Nutrition Policy and Promotion; 2004.

112. Center for Urban Transportation Research. *Public Transit in America: Results from the 2001 National Household Travel Survey*. Tampa, FL: National Center for Transit Research; 2005.

113. U.S. Department of Transportation. Nationwide personal transportation survey. 2009; www-cta.ornl.gov/npts (accessed July 30, 2012).

114. Ogden CL, Carroll MD, Kit BK, Flegal KM. Prevalence of obesity and trends in body mass index among US children and adolescents, 1999–2010. *JAMA* 2012; 307(5): 483–490.

115. Centers for Disease Control and Prevention (CDC). Physical activity trends—United States, 1990–1998. *MMWR Morb Mortal Wkly Rep* 2001; 50(9): 166–169.

116. Flegal KM, Carroll MD, Kit BK, Ogden CL. Prevalence of obesity and trends in the distribution of body mass index among US adults, 1999–2010. *JAMA* 2012; 307(5): 491–497.

# 43 Oral Health Screening and Assessment for Nutrition Professionals

*Melissa Page, Johanna T. Dwyer, and Carole A. Palmer*

## CONTENTS

## INTRODUCTION: WHY NUTRITION SCREENING FOR ORAL HEALTH?

Why should nutritionists and other non-dental professionals screen for oral health? It is because, unfortunately, many individuals with serious dental problems rarely or never see a dentist. Unless others in the health professions whom they are more likely to interact with identify these problems, they will go unrecognized and untreated, often with severe consequences to both oral and overall health. This is why screening and assessment tools for non-dental professionals are necessary to provide baseline evaluation of oral and nutrition status. Conducting oral health nutrition screenings can prevent the development of oral health and nutrition issues. This chapter will discuss how nutrition professionals can help to identify major oral health issues in order to promote optimal health.

## MALNUTRITION AND ORAL HEALTH

Today's nutrition professionals should be aware of the significant effects nutrition can have on the oral health status of their patients. The consequences of decreased nutritional status can be profound on the oral cavity.[1] It is important to be aware of the connections between nutrition status and oral health to use this information to assess patient's nutritional status, and to be able to recognize oral health issues at different stages of life and in patients who have complicated and extensive medical histories.

Health care is undergoing a rapid transformation. Until 50 years ago, medical care was traditionally centered in the hospital or primary care provider's office, but now venues for delivery of care include additional settings such as nutrition clinics, sports clubs, urgent care centers, and pharmacies. There is also a broader array of stakeholders and practitioners, including nurse practitioners, physician assistants, and nutrition professionals. Health care providers are being required to broaden their knowledge of physiological systems and to assume new responsibilities to better manage their patients. Screening and assessment, to help identify health problems, including oral health issues, are now essential parts of clinical practice for nutritionists and other allied health professionals. In order to provide the most comprehensive and accurate care, clinicians other than dental professionals need to recognize oral health issues and/or diseases that could be related to them. Although dietitians and clinical nutritionists are not experts in dental medicine, they can screen for oral health problems and refer problems to dental health experts. More extensive oral health assessment and treatment will require collaboration and consultation between dental, medical, and nutrition professionals.

The connections between oral and systemic health and their reciprocal relationships highlight the importance of multidisciplinary teamwork among clinicians. The mouth is a primary indicator of general health. Clinically evident signs of disease, including nutritional disorders, are often evident first in the oral cavity. This is due, in part, to the more rapid soft tissue turnover in the oral cavity as compared to other tissues of the body.[2] Conversely, nutrition can affect tooth development prior to eruption (which is irreversible), and oral tissue turnover (soft tissue, oral bone, salivary glands, etc., some of which are reversible) throughout life. Dietary habits are the primary etiologic factors in dental caries. This new understanding of the mouth as a health indicator has led to changes in the treatment and prevention of disease and how health professionals view risk factors for oral health. The bidirectional impact of oral health and general health further supports the use of oral health screening and assessment as an effective tool in nutrition practice. Several diseases including diabetes, autoimmune disorders, cardiovascular disease, cancers of the head and neck, and some developmental disorders have a bidirectional impact on oral and systemic health, and the presence of these conditions should prompt appropriate collaboration between dentist, primary physician and/or nurse practitioner, and registered dietitian.

The type of multidisciplinary and integrative work that is being called for today requires the development of easy-to-use screening tools that will allow all clinicians to screen for oral health problems and provide anticipatory guidance for addressing these issues. This chapter provides a review of common oral conditions and their nutritional implications, and provides guidelines for oral health/nutrition screening for nutrition professionals.

## NUTRITION SCREENING

Table 43.1 provides definitions of nutrition screening and assessment.[3] Nutrition screening is the process of identifying the characteristics known to be associated with dietary or

## TABLE 43.1
## Definitions of Nutrition Screening and Assessment

| | |
|---|---|
| Nutrition screening | The process of identifying characteristics known to be associated with dietary or nutritional problems. Its purpose is to differentiate individuals who are at high risk of nutritional problems or who have poor nutritional status. |
| Nutrition assessment | The measurement of indicators of dietary or nutrition-related factors to identify the presence, nature, and extent of impaired nutritional status of any type, and to obtain the information needed for intervention, planning, and improvement of nutritional care. |

nutritional problems.[3] Nutrition screening for oral health is required in order to prevent later oral health issues that have nutritional implications from arising. It is also designed to screen and diagnose problems in the mouth early on so that interventions can be tailored accordingly.

### DENTAL PROFESSIONALS AND ORAL HEALTH ASSESSMENT

Dentists, dental hygienists, dental assistants, laboratory technicians, and other dental professional staff provide dental care in the United States. Enhancements in dental treatment and the development of new technologies have broadened the scope of practice for dental professionals, requiring the use of more preventive versus treatment strategies. Although dental treatment procedures such as extractions have decreased since the 1980s, the nation's growing aging population requires more crown placements and periodontal treatment.[4]

How do nutrition professionals address dental health issues in their practice and what criteria do they need to refer to other specialties? The registered dietitian and other health professionals are key players in the screening of patients with chronic conditions such as diabetes, therefore oral health

screening can easily be accomplished by incorporating questions addressing oral health during routine clinic visits. These simple questions include biting, chewing, and swallowing difficulties, and conducting a brief oral exam.[5,6] The Academy of Nutrition and Dietetics Position Paper on Oral Health[5] calls for Registered Dietitians to "... include oral health screening as a component of nutrition care process tasks, including nutrition screening, nutrition assessment (e.g., cranial nerve function, occlusion, soft tissue, edentulism, masticatory ability, swallowing, salivary adequacy, intervention, and monitoring)." The goal of the oral health screening is to identify any potential abnormal finding, to determine what impact this has on diet intake and nutrition status, and to refer the patient to the appropriate professionals or specialists when needed.[7]

Nutrition professionals are responsible for identifying nutritional risk factors that will affect their patient's overall health. In the dental arena, compromised dietary intake and nutritional status may have many causes, including pain from dental caries or root caries, missing teeth, and dentures, or periodontal disease.[5] Nutritionists should use oral health screening and assessment tools in their practice in order to identify and address nutrition issues or refer those beyond their expertise to the appropriate health professional.

## ORAL PROBLEMS WITH NUTRITIONAL IMPLICATIONS

Figure 43.1 shows the anatomy of the oral cavity and the nomenclature of the teeth, and Figure 43.2 describes the different parts of the tooth. The major oral disorders with nutrition implications are periodontal disease, dental caries, mucosal disease, and dysphagia. Each is described briefly later, with some steps non-dental professionals can take to help in their prevention and treatment.

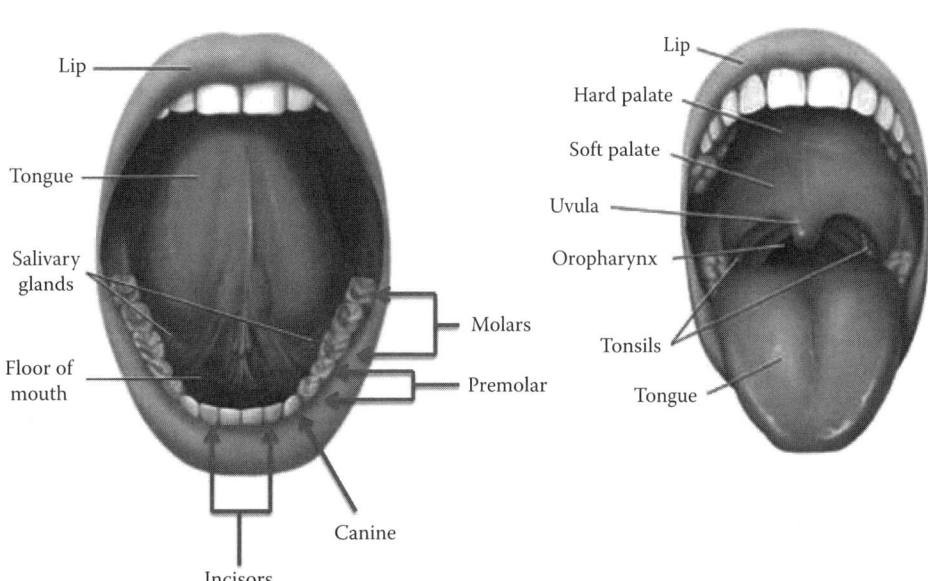

**FIGURE 43.1** Parts of the mouth.

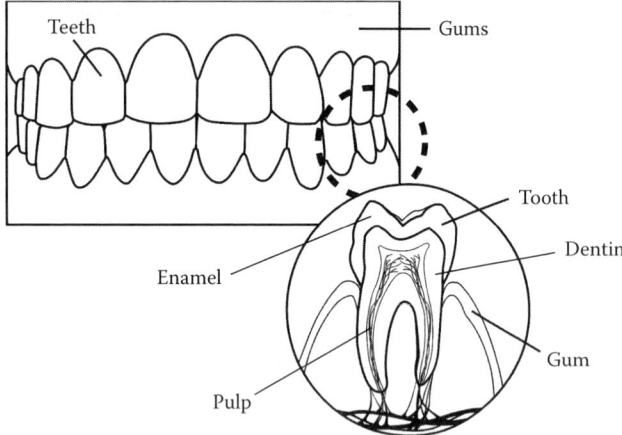

**FIGURE 43.2**  Tooth anatomy.

## PERIODONTAL DISEASE

### ETIOLOGY

Periodontal disease is a progressive disease that can cause major nutritional and overall health problems. Periodontal diseases impact the supporting structures (gingiva) of the teeth and are characterized by an infiltration of dental plaque bacteria into the gingiva (soft tissue) surrounding the tooth. The gums become swollen, inflamed, and bleed, eventually leading to deterioration of the alveolar bone supporting the teeth, and tooth loss. Systemic diseases, such as diabetes, can have a major impact on the progression of periodontal disease.[8]

### NUTRITIONAL IMPLICATIONS

Malnutrition does not cause periodontal disease; however, patients who are malnourished do have an increased risk of developing disease.[9] Malnutrition, including underweight and vitamin/mineral deficiencies, can exacerbate the condition through a compromised immune system, which is less able than normal to combat the periodontopathic bacteria. Saliva contains antibacterial properties that can be compromised in malnutrition.[10] This can lead to proliferation of oral bacteria and increased risk of periodontal disease.

Antioxidant nutrients have also been studied for their potential for preventing periodontal disease. In the presence of periodontal pathogens, which cause an inflammatory response, neutrophils release oxidants that damage the oral cavity.[11] Certain antioxidants found in the diet, including vitamin C, vitamin E, and beta-carotene, protect against these destructive oxidants. One study found that patients with reduced levels of antioxidants present in salivary secretions had higher rates of periodontal disease than patients with normal levels of antioxidant activity.[12] However, data are still not secure enough, and current recommendations do not suggest that supplementing patients with antioxidants in large amounts above the Recommended Dietary Allowances

**TABLE 43.2**
**Risk Factors for Periodontal Disease**

Age—The risk of developing periodontal disease increases with age
Tobacco use
Diabetes mellitus
Lack of oral hygiene/build-up of plaque

(RDA) is useful.[1] Periodontal disease can lead to edentulism if not addressed appropriately by a dental professional. This can have significant effects on dietary intake and lead to malnutrition. Masticatory function is reduced in patients who have lost teeth, which can lead to decreased intake of tough, crunchy foods, which contain essential vitamins and minerals.[13,14]

Although these associations between deficiencies and periodontal disease are interesting, the findings do not mean that most Americans need to take dietary supplements, because their diets are generally adequate without them. Until there is more conclusive evidence, patients should aim to meet the RDA for vitamins and minerals for optimal gum health.[15] Following the MyPlate[16] eating plan will help to accomplish this. If supplements are desired, a multivitamin mineral supplement not exceeding 100% of the Daily Values (DV) should suffice.

### PERIODONTAL DISEASE PREVENTION/TREATMENT

The first step is to assess the patient's risk of developing periodontal disease. The risk factors for periodontal disease are outlined in Table 43.2. After estimating the patient's risk, if it is high, he or she should be referred to a dentist. It is also important to educate the patient on preventive measures, including adequate intake of vitamins and minerals and proper oral hygiene practices, such as brushing, flossing, and frequent visits to a dental health professional. Patients should also be urged to follow the MyPlate[16] and the Dietary Guidelines for Americans recommendations and consume at least the RDA/Adequate Intake (AI) levels of nutrients.

## DENTAL CARIES

### ETIOLOGY

Dental caries is a microbial disease that results from the dissolution and destruction of calcified tooth structure.[8] The oral flora in the mouth contains millions of bacteria that form a film on the tooth, called plaque. These bacteria ferment sugars to form acids. The acids erode the tooth enamel and expose the dentin, which is then invaded by oral bacteria. If left untreated, the bacterial infection can move into the blood stream and cause systemic infection as well.[17]

The risk factors for dental caries development include: lack of good oral care (tooth brushing and flossing, lack of topical fluoride (from water and dentifrice) on a consistent basis, and dietary factors. Any type of disease or medication

TABLE 43.3

## Oral Medications That Can Decrease Salivary Flow

| Antihypertensive | Antihistamines | Antipsychotic Agents | Anti-Parkinsonian Agents |
|---|---|---|---|
| Captopril | Bendadryl | Thorazine | Benztropine |
| Lisinopril | Hydrocodone | Clozaril | Ansemet |
| Cozaar | Cystagon | Prolixin | Akineton |
| Lopressor | Sudafed | Haldol | Parlodel |
| Timolol | Claritin | Loxapine | Dopar |
| Norvasc | Guaifenex | Moban | Levsin SL |
| Cardizem | | Compazine | Permax |
| | **Antidepressants** | | Kemadrin |
| **Benzodiazepines** | Nardil | **Diuretics** | Eldepryl |
| Xanax | Parnate | Hydrochlorothiazide | Artane |
| Buspar | Prozac | Methylclothiazide | |
| Klonopin | Marplan | Bumex | |
| Tranzene | Serzone | Lasix | |
| Diastat | Paxil | Aldactone | |
| Ativan | Zoloft | Dyrenium | |
| Vistaril | Effexor | | |
| | Elavil | | |
| | Amoxapine | | |

that reduces salivary flow can increase the risk of developing dental caries. Several medications, particularly certain antihypertensive and antidepressant medications, are antisialogogues and can impair the secretions of the salivary gland, increasing the risk of dental caries in these individuals.[18,19] Table 43.3 lists typical medications that patients may use, which decrease salivary function. Other conditions that can significantly decrease salivary secretions include Sjogren's syndrome (an autoimmune disease) and radiation therapy for head and neck cancers. These conditions can have significant impacts on the development of dental caries and should be addressed during routine dental assessments by the dentist.[20] Children with developmental disorders that affect activities of daily living, such as tooth brushing, are at a higher risk of developing dental caries. Individuals who have a previous history of dental caries are also at a higher risk of caries development in the future and they should be evaluated for significant underlying causes of this disorder, especially the diet-related causes such as those listed earlier.[8]

## EFFECTS OF SYSTEMIC NUTRITION ON DENTAL CARIES AND TOOTH DEVELOPMENT

Malnutrition can affect the developing dentition, leading to increased vulnerability and risk for dental caries due to alterations in tooth structure. Enamel hypoplasia is evident in very severely malnourished children in developing countries and also in patients in the United States on anti-seizure drugs for long periods of time.[1] Linear enamel hypoplasia (the presence of surface defects, including pits, fissures, or areas of missing enamel)[21] is a diet-related defect, which can

be caused by protein-energy malnutrition in early childhood or severe maternal malnutrition. It results in an increased risk of dental caries in children.[1] Undernutrition can also cause delayed eruption of the dentition, putting these patients at an increased risk of developing dental caries as well.[11] However, it is the direct effects of diet on teeth, and not the systemic effects, that play the essential roles in caries risk.

## DIRECT TOPICAL EFFECTS OF DIET

Factors such as the frequency and form of dietary carbohydrates have a direct adverse impact on the development of dental caries. Several studies have concluded that consumption of dietary sugars is a major risk factor for the development of dental caries. Sreenby[22] and Ruxton et al.[23] conducted epidemiological studies looking at sugar consumption in different countries and the rates of dental caries and concluded that 52% and 28% (respectively) of the variation in dental caries prevalence was related to the amount of sugar available in those countries. However, human intervention studies have found that the amount of sugar consumption is not as significant as the high frequency of fermentable carbohydrates on caries development.[24] The type of fermentable carbohydrate consumption has been studied as well, with little difference found between the different types of mono- and disaccharides.[25]

Fermentable carbohydrates include sugars, honey, syrups, as well as starchy foods. Starches are long chains of glucose and have two forms, amylose and amylopectin. Starches can be found in many different types of foods including wheat, oats, potatoes, corn, rice, squash, peas, barley, etc. When starches enter the oral cavity, salivary amylase hydrolyzes the amylose and amylopectin into maltose, maltriose, and dextrins, which cariogenic bacteria can feed on to form acids and initiate dental caries.[26] Recent innovations have introduced foods to the consumer market that contain many different kinds of sugars and starches with varying degrees of processing, and varying degrees of bioavailability for bacteria to ferment in the oral cavity.[27] Frequency and retention of starches in the mouth are important factors in cariogenicity. Kashket et al.[28] found that starch particles (broken down into maltose and maltriose) were retained in the mouth longer than food particles that contained smaller amounts of starch, but higher levels of sucrose and other fermentable sugars. This is important because the longer maltose and maltriose sugars are in contact with plaque bacteria, the more acid is formed, and the greater the caries risk. Thus, starches (when hydrolyzed to sugars and when serving as vehicles for sugar retention in the mouth) contribute to the dangers of the cariogenic diet.[27]

Adequate saliva production is also essential to the health of the oral cavity. Saliva has a pH of 7, which is a high enough pH to deter the colonization of bacteria. Saliva also contains calcium and phosphate, which promote remineralization of tooth structures that have been damaged by aciduric bacteria.[29] Conditions in which saliva production is limited include Sjogren's syndrome, diseases or treatments that cause damage to salivary secretions, and certain antisialogogic drugs. These drugs are listed in Table 43.3.

## EARLY CHILDHOOD NUTRITION AND ORAL HEALTH ISSUES

From birth to 36 months, even though the child's teeth have not fully erupted, the oral cavity is undergoing growth and development of the jawbone and primary teeth. It is of utmost importance for the infant to be well nourished to provide adequate nutrients for the teeth and bones. Mothers are encouraged not to provide fluoride to their children under 6 months of age due to the risk of fluorosis in the developing teeth.[30] Infants can obtain virtually all of their nutritional requirements from breast milk or from infant formula for the first 4–6 months of life. However, mothers should be encouraged not to allow their children to sleep with their bottles to reduce the risk of developing early childhood caries (ECC). Caries development in children is still a major health problem, although much progress has been made in recent years. According to the Surgeon General's Report on Oral Health, childhood caries is the single most common chronic childhood disease.[4] ECC is defined as one or more teeth with evidence of decay (noncavitated or cavitated lesions), filled tooth surfaces in any primary teeth, or missing teeth (from decay) in any child aged 71 months or younger. In children under 3 years of age, any sign of smooth-surface caries is a sign of severe early childhood caries (S-ECC).[31] Dental caries in young children usually look like brown, rough breaks on usually smooth surfaces of the enamel.[32] If left untreated, childhood caries can cause major nutrition and overall health problems. Pain, failure to thrive, premature tooth loss, and compromised chewing abilities are all signs and symptoms of dental caries that can have an effect on the dietary intake of children.

Long-term use of baby bottles filled with fermentable sugars (such as cow's milk, breast milk, infant formula, fruit juice, soda), for example, while sleeping, is a major risk factor for the development of dental caries in infants.[33] When a baby is fed from a bottle, if the infant is lying down, the liquid pools around the infant's teeth and provides the environment favorable for oral bacterial fermentation of the sugars.[34] To prevent the development of ECC, parents should be encouraged to avoid allowing infants to sleep or nap with a bottle containing fermentable sugars, and to replace the milk or juice with water if the child is resistant. It is also helpful to establish a breastfeeding schedule that does not include frequent night feedings. Infants should be consuming several ounces every few hours and avoid ad libitum breast-feeding, especially if the infant is consuming other carbohydrate-containing foods. Caretakers should avoid continuous feedings, introduce solid foods after 6 months and encourage consumption of non-cariogenic foods.[34] Some examples of non-cariogenic foods for infants are pureed vegetables like green beans, carrots, and squash, dairy foods like yogurt, and protein foods such as turkey or chicken.

To prevent childhood caries, caretakers should provide a balanced diet emphasizing non-cariogenic foods and discourage eating between meals and continuously sipping on bottles or cups filled with fermentable sugars like juice, soda, or milk. Some cariogenic foods, such as starches, cannot and should not be eliminated from the diet completely. However, these foods should be consumed at meals rather than between meals. Children should also brush their teeth after every meal and (when old enough) chew sugar-free gum, preferably with xylitol, to prevent dental caries.[34] These habits should be sustained through later childhood, adolescence, and into adulthood.

Dental caries can increase the risk of developing growth and eating problems that, if extreme, can lead to malnutrition and failure to thrive. Failure to thrive is defined as a decrease in weight-for-age on the National Center for Health Statistics (NCHS) standardized growth curve,[35] growth that falls below the fifth percentile, or growth that drops two major percentiles during the first 3 years of life. Undernutrition during this key time of development and growth can cause major health and behavioral implications for these children. Developmental delays and nutrient deficiencies are often associated with failure to thrive.

Childhood obesity is on the rise in the United States. Currently, 17% (or approximately 12.5 million) children in the United States aged 2–19 years are obese, and since 1980 obesity prevalence among children and adolescents has tripled.[36] Research on associations between dental caries and childhood obesity is interesting if equivocal.[37,38] Macek and Mitola[39] concluded that there was no statistically significant association between body mass index (BMI), BMI-for-age, and dental caries in children with primary or permanent teeth. Also, overweight children with a past history of dental caries had fewer decayed, missing, or filled teeth compared to normal weight children. Marshall et al.[40] hypothesized that low socioeconomic status (SES) was a common risk factor for obesity and dental caries that could explain the association, since low SES increased the risk of both dental caries and obesity.

When screening for patients with oral health issues, it is important to consider their SES. Low SES patients may have difficulties purchasing enough food to maintain their nutritional status. Providing education to the patient about food assistance programs, such as the Supplemental Nutrition Assistance Program (SNAP) and the National School Lunch Program, can help the patient in purchasing the adequate amount of food.

## ADULT DENTAL CARIES

Root caries are dental caries (primarily in adults) that develop when the receding gingiva exposes the cementum of the tooth, which is less highly mineralized than enamel, and thus more susceptible to caries.[41] The prevalence of root caries increases with age: 9% among persons aged 20–39 years, 18% among those aged 40–59 years, and 32% among those aged ≥60 years.[42] The xerostomia, which accompanies cancer therapy and is a side effect of many medications used by adults and elders, significantly increases the risk of developing root caries.[18] The amount and frequency of consumption of fermentable carbohydrates are associated with root caries as well as crown caries.[43] An added factor is that people with xerostomia may use hard candies to help overcome the dryness, thus increasing sugar retentiveness in the oral cavity. The role of the nutrition professional is to identify these patients at risk and provide nutrition education on a low cariogenic diet. Also, brushing with a fluoride toothpaste and flossing regularly will help to decrease the risk of root caries.

## DENTAL CARIES PREVENTION/TREATMENT

Caries prevention and intervention strategies have been developed on several fronts, including public health approaches, recommendations from dental professionals, and on a personal hygiene level. Nutrition professionals should be key players in the prevention and treatment of dental caries and dental erosion.

### Oral Hygiene: Brush, Swish, and Floss

Dental hygiene is key in the prevention of dental caries. Brushing after each meal and flossing daily removes the bacterial colonization on the surface of the tooth. Flossing is essential for dental hygiene practices because it reaches areas of the teeth that the toothbrush cannot clean. Flossing keeps the tooth root clean and free of plaque and bacteria so that root caries will not form. Dental professionals may also recommend using electric toothbrushes to effectively clean the surface of the teeth and stimulate the gums.

### Fluoride

Currently, fluoridation of the water supply is as an important public health intervention strategy used for the prevention of dental caries both in the United States and in many other industrialized countries. Fluoride functions to increase the resistance of dental enamel, inhibit enamel demineralization, enhance remineralization, and inhibit the activity of bacterial organisms in the dental plaque.[4] The greatest benefit from fluoride is through topical sources (fluoridated water, dentifrices, and rinses) after tooth eruption throughout life.

Fluoride supplementation is not recommended in patients younger than 6 months because of the risk for developing fluorosis, which is the ingestion of too much fluoride during tooth formation. However, children 6 months and older should be receiving sufficient fluoride either through the public water system or through supplements. Parents are encouraged to find out about the fluoride level of their water to determine the fluoride concentration and to supplement their children accordingly if necessary to meet the recommendations of 1.0 ppm/day for optimal caries prevention.[44] Adults also benefit from the fluoride present in the public water system and in fluoride toothpastes. Fluoride rinses are also being used to address dental caries in children. They have been shown to reduce the prevalence of dental caries from 20% to 50% in these types of interventions.[4]

Currently, about 95% of commercial toothpaste products contain fluoride. Fluoride toothpastes have been shown to be effective and preventative against dental caries in children. A systematic review by Twetman et al.[45] concluded that daily use of fluoride toothpaste had a significant caries-reducing effect in young permanent teeth.[45]

### Sugarless Gum/Xylitol

Chewing sugarless gum helps to decrease the risk of dental caries by stimulating the secretion of saliva, which buffers the acidic effects of carbohydrate foods and promotes remineralization of the tooth enamel.[46–50] Sugarless gum should be chewed for at least 20 min after each meal or snack to prevent dental caries and promote remineralization. Xylitol, a non-cariogenic sugar alcohol, actually interferes with the bacteria that cause dental caries, such as *Streptococcus mutans*. Xylitol interferes with plaque's ability to colonize and stick to oral tissues, and stimulates salivary flow.

### Non-Cariogenic Dietary Patterns

Diet is a major contributor to the development of dental caries. It is up to the nutrition professional to educate the patient on a non-cariogenic diet in order to prevent dental caries. Much research has been related to the consumption of sugar, sugar-sweetened beverages, and starchy sugary retentive foods in the diet and the increased risk of dental caries. Table 43.4 lists potentially cariogenic and non-cariogenic foods that people commonly eat.

Cariogenic foods promote the development of dental caries. They are the simple mono- and disaccharide carbohydrates. The length of time that any of these carbohydrates are

**TABLE 43.4**
**Potentially Cariogenic Foods**

| Highly Cariogenic | Low Cariogenicity |
|---|---|
| Dried fruits | Raw vegetables |
| Candy, hard candy | Raw fruits |
| Cake, cookies, pie | Milk |
| Crackers | |
| Chips | **Non-cariogenic** |
| | Meat, fish, poultry |
| **Moderately Cariogenic** | Fats and oils |
| Fruit juice | |
| | **Cariostatic** |
| **Sweetened, Canned fruit** | Cheeses |
| Soft drinks | Nuts |
| Breads | Xylitol |

**TABLE 43.5**
**Cariogenic Dietary Patterns**

| Factors Increasing Risk | Factors Decreasing Risk |
|---|---|
| Eaten or sipped often | Consumed infrequently |
| Eaten or sipped for prolonged periods | Consumed fast |
| Highly retentive in mouth | Liquid or fast removal from mouth |
| No rinsing or brushing after | Oral hygiene after |
| Xerostomia | No xerostomia |

in contact with dental plaque is the most important risk factor for caries. Therefore, minimizing the number of eating/drinking periods and having less orally retentive foods are strategies which will reduce caries risk. Since between-meal snacks/beverages seem to be the most damaging, it seems prudent to recommend having sweets at meal times, rather than between meals. See Table 43.5 for examples of beneficial and risky eating patterns and Table 43.4 for examples of potential cariogenicity of foods. Over the past 20 years, there has been a decrease in milk consumption and an increase in sugar-sweetened beverage (soda and juice) consumption.[51] Milk or milk-based products contain lactose and in some cases added fermentable sugars; however, milk also contains calcium, phosphorous, and fat, which can be caries protective. Snacking frequency and consumption of sugary, starchy foods is also on the rise. This increases the risk for dental caries, both from the cariogenicity and the frequency of consumption of these foods, which is coupled with lack of oral hygiene following snacking.

## Sealants

Sealants, in combination with the use of fluoride treatments, are virtually 100% effective at preventing dental caries on the chewing surfaces of newly erupted children's teeth (as long as the sealant stays in place). Dental sealants are clear plastic resinous materials that protect the rough pits and fissures that are hard to reach with a toothbrush. Once sealants have been bonded to the enamel adjacent to pits and fissures, these areas are sealed-off from decay-causing bacteria in the mouth for as long as the sealant remains in place on the tooth. In addition, sealing a tooth kills most of the bacteria colonizing the pit or fissure, and essentially all the remaining microorganisms soon become nonviable from lack of food and air.[52]

## Sialogogues

Saliva has a host of benefits in caries prevention. It helps cleanse the mouth of food debris, has antibacterial effects, and contains calcium and phosphorus that can help remineralize dental enamel. Certain conditions, such as Sjogren's syndrome and radiation treatment to the head and neck that exposes the salivary glands to excessive radiation, cause a decrease in salivary secretion, resulting in rampant caries development in the dental cavity.[53] Sialogogues are medications that stimulate the salivary glands to secrete more saliva.[54] Pilocarpine is one sialogogue that is effective in increasing salivary flow in patients with xerostomia. Another option is to recommend artificial saliva, such as Saliva Orthana™, to keep the mouth moist and to prevent tooth decay and promote remineralization. Nutrition professionals should screen for patients with xerostomia, as these patients will be at a higher risk for dental caries.

## Mouthwashes and Rinses

Mouth rinses containing fluoride are effective at preventing dental caries in children and adults. They are solutions of sodium fluoride used to prevent dental caries and promote remineralization against plaque.[55] Patients with a high risk of dental caries (previous dental caries, cariogenic diet, xerostomia, etc.) should rinse with mouthwash daily to protect against dental caries. Mouth rinses can be bought over-the-counter in brand names such as Listerine™ and Act™. Patients suffering from dry mouth can also use products such as Biotene that contain enzymes to help fight dental caries and relieve the symptoms of dry mouth.

## TOOTH LOSS

### ETIOLOGY

Most tooth loss results from periodontal disease or dental caries.[56,57] The rate of edentulism (toothlessness) for adults 18 and older is around 10%, but the rate actually jumps to 33% in adults over 65 years old. Periodontal disease and dental caries can lead to tooth loss if not treated quickly and appropriately. The infection or damage to the tooth can destroy the tissues and bone surrounding the tooth and cause the tooth to loosen. This can necessitate tooth extraction in order to protect the oral cavity from further infection.[4]

### NUTRITION IMPLICATIONS

Masticatory function is significantly reduced in patients who have lost teeth.[13,14,58,59] The logical assumption would be to conclude that decreased masticatory function would be related to a decreased intake of nutritious foods, like meat, poultry, and fibrous fruits and vegetables, because these foods are usually difficult to chew. However, the research associating edentulism with nutrition status is not at all clear. Many studies are cross-sectional or longitudinal and have limited power to make any definitive conclusions. Also, nutrition status itself can affect tooth loss and so it is hard to eliminate this risk factor in older persons with dentures.[60] Several large studies have shown decreased nutrient intakes in older persons with dentures. Sheiham et al.[61] concluded that nutrient intake was associated with nutritional status in older people. Protein, energy, fiber, calcium, non-heme iron, niacin, and vitamin C intake were all decreased in patients with dentures.[61] Nowjack-Raymer and Sheiham[62] concluded that patients with dentures had lower intakes of some nutrient-rich foods, and beta-carotene, folate, and vitamin C serum levels were significantly lower.[62] Furthermore, Papas et al.[63] studied 691 subjects in the New England area and found that denture wearers had lower intakes of calories, protein, and folate than subjects without dentures. This evidence shows the possible nutritional problems of edentulous patients and the importance of nutrition professionals in screening and assessing patients for tooth loss and edentulism.

### EDENTULISM PREVENTION/TREATMENT

When screening and assessing patients with tooth loss or edentulism, subjective information from the patient is key. Asking questions such as "Do you have any difficulty biting, chewing, swallowing? If yes, please specify," are simple ways to gather more information about issues potentially affecting oral health and/or nutrition status. It is also important to ask patients who wear their dentures if they keep their dentures in while eating and during the day. The jaw can change and cause ill-fitting dentures if they are worn only occasionally. If patients do not use their dentures, they also may have trouble chewing and swallowing, and eventually the dentures will not fit and become painful. Fit of the dentures is also important to evaluate because ill-fitting dentures can cause decreased dietary intake.[64] If the patient's dentures do not fit well, it is appropriate to refer to a dental professional to adjust the dentures, so as not to impede dietary intake. Nutrition professionals should also monitor the patient's weight. Frequently, 24 h recalls can also give the nutritionist a good idea of dietary intake and indicate if the patient is missing any important food groups in their diet.

## AUTOIMMUNE DISORDER: SJOGREN'S SYNDROME

### ETIOLOGY

Sjogren's syndrome is the second most common autoimmune disease, following rheumatoid arthritis.[65] Patients with this disorder have similar symptoms to patients with fibromyalgia, including xerostomia and generalized muscle pain. Sjogren's attacks the exocrine and salivary glands, resulting in

xerostomia and dry eyes. Xerostomia can have major impacts on the development of dental caries, due to the decreased production of saliva, which protects against dental caries. Patients with significant xerostomia often suffer from pooling of saliva in the mouth, and dry oral mucosa. They also have increased incidence of surface caries, dental erosion, and candidiasis.[66]

### DENTAL AND NUTRITIONAL IMPLICATIONS

Xerostomia has the most notable nutritional implications for Sjogren's syndrome. Dry mouth leads to rampant dental caries and can decrease dietary intake and increase risk of undernutrition due to problems lubricating, masticating, tolerating, tasting, and swallowing food. Rhodus[67] found that elderly patients with Sjogren's syndrome, both institutionalized and free-living, consumed less calories, protein, fiber, vitamins A, C, thiamin, riboflavin, iron, vitamin B-6, calcium, potassium, and zinc than patients without Sjogren's syndrome. The Sjogren's patients also experienced significant dysgeusia (taste changes) and/or hypogeusia (decreased taste) due to their dry mouths.

### SJOGREN'S SYNDROME TREATMENT/ NUTRITIONAL MANAGEMENT

Currently there is no cure for Sjogren's. The primary treatment methods involve minimizing the symptoms, such as dry mouth and dry eyes. Nutrition professionals should screen for xerostomia routinely to identify patients who are at risk of dental caries, periodontal disease, and decreased dietary intake. If a patient is experiencing dry mouth and has not seen a dentist to address the issue, a referral to a dental professional is appropriate to evaluate for oral health problems. Artificial saliva may also be helpful for these patients. For the nutrition professional, it is appropriate to recommend certain dietary modifications to help with the signs and symptoms from dry mouth and to increase dietary intake. Table 43.6 provides some dietary tips for patients with xerostomia. Patients should stay hydrated and increase their fluid intakes to help keep the oral cavity moist so that patients can tolerate dietary intake.

---

**TABLE 43.6**

**Common Side Effects of Cancer Treatment and Ways to Address Them**

Decreased appetite
    Recommend small, frequent meals with high protein and calorie intake.
    Offer a variety of foods and flavors to adjust for taste changes.
    Decrease food odors.

Xerostomia
    Puree foods to liquid consistency to reduce friction in the oral cavity.
    Use dairy products, such as Greek yogurt, cottage cheese, or bean soups as protein sources.
    Use lip balm to keep the lips moist.
    Always carry water or artificial saliva with you to stay hydrated and to moisten the mouth.

---

## HIV-AIDS

### ETIOLOGY

Human immunodeficiency virus (HIV) is a condition in which the body's immunological defense system deteriorates and develops opportunistic infections and many complications, including oral health conditions.[68] Patients with HIV often have mouth pain due to lesions in the oral cavity that can inhibit them from eating or drinking enough. Also, these patients are required to take a large amount of medications, some of which cause xerostomia and increase dental caries risk.[69] One of the major signs of HIV in the mouth is an increased prevalence of oral lesions and ulcerations in the oral cavity. Patients with HIV may also have signs and symptoms of xerostomia due to decreased salivary function.[70] Decreased salivary flow further increases the risk for oral infections and dental caries.

### NUTRITIONAL IMPLICATIONS/TREATMENT

Patients with HIV often find it challenging to achieve optimal nutrition status. Economic insecurity is prevalent among them, as are hunger and food insecurity. Low SES, living situation, ability to cook and purchase food, and possible substance use should always be considered when treating and recommending nutrition interventions to these patients.[71] HIV can affect nutrition status, independent of SES, and results in compromised nutritional status due to micro- and macronutrient deficiency. HIV-AIDS patients also exhibit significant wasting of fat and lean body mass.[72,73] Having an adequate dietary intake is an important part of maintaining lean body mass and fighting infection. Through managing the patient's symptoms of xerostomia and pain from oral lesions, the nutrition professional can help patients maintain adequate nutritional status.

Nutritional status has an impact on the body's ability to fight HIV infections. When weight decreases by 54%, patients are at an increased risk of death, even without the presence of an infectious complication.[74] Patients with HIV are at an increased risk of protein energy malnutrition due to the pain and difficulty eating associated with oral lesions. Oropharyngeal infections can cause burning sensations and result in dysphagia. Painful ulcerations associated with stomatitis and periodontitis can impede oral intake as well. It is up to the nutrition professional to recognize oral lesions or oral health conditions, such as dental caries or candidiasis that affect the ability to eat adequate amount of nutrients and to refer the patient to a physician or dentist. The following tips are helpful for patients with xerostomia. Patients should use moist foods without added spices or strong flavors; suck on sugar-free hard candy, ice chips, frozen grapes, sugar-free gum or sugar-free ice pops. Patients should also remember to use xylitol gums to prevent dental caries that arise from dry mouth. Try to carry a bottle of water around to keep the mouth moist. Opt for mashed or soft foods instead of hard, chewy foods such as steak or crackers. Try canned vegetables or fruit instead of raw, because the texture is smoother. HIV patients will also need to see a dental professional if they have not within the past 6 months in order for them to monitor for dental caries and oral infections.

## ORAL HEALTH/SYSTEMIC DISEASE RELATIONSHIPS

There is a significant bidirectional connection between oral health and nutritional status.[75–79] Research on associations between oral health and systemic disease has increased in recent years, so it is important for nutrition professionals to understand these associations and their nutritional implications. They need to screen for oral health issues affecting patients with these disorders.

### PERIODONTAL DISEASE AND CARDIOVASCULAR DISEASE

The development of periodontal disease is characterized by the loss of connective tissue surrounding the tooth and alveolar bone loss, which can eventually result in tooth loss.[80] There are several theories on the pathogenesis of periodontal disease and its effect on cardiovascular disease and stroke incidence. Systemic inflammation and development of inflammatory markers are thought to be the primary causes. Some theories identify the bacterial infiltration of periodontal disease as the cause of the inflammatory cell proliferation and eventual hepatic synthesis of clotting factors, platelet aggregation, and direct damage to cell walls of arteries and veins in the development of cardiovascular events.[81–84]

Research showing the connection between periodontal disease and cardiovascular disease has strengthened over the past two decades.[82,85–87] The first reports of connections between these two conditions were epidemiological studies that found that patients with a past history of myocardial infarctions also had a higher incidence of periodontal infections.[88] This led to further research on the association and cause of cerebrovascular disease and periodontal disease. After two decades of research, the association is now viewed as primarily rooted in the development of inflammation in both of these disease states. Chronic inflammation of the vessels of the heart plays a critical role in the pathogenesis of atherosclerosis, and conditions such as periodontal disease can contribute to this chronic state of inflammation.[89] This is evident in the increased blood levels of C-reactive protein (a biomarker of inflammation, in patients with atherosclerosis).[89,90]

Currently, dietary modification has been the primary treatment for cardiovascular disease, including a reduction of LDL cholesterol through decreased intake of dietary saturated and trans-fat,[91,92] and decreased hypertension through weight control and decreased sodium and alcohol intake. There are no specific guidelines for nutrition in periodontal disease other than the recommendation to follow a sound, nutritious diet.

### PERIODONTAL DISEASE AND DIABETES MELLITUS

Diabetes mellitus also can have significant impact on the oral cavity. Diabetes is the third leading cause of mortality and morbidity in the United States with prevalence rates doubling from 6 million in 1980 to 12 million in 2000. Type 1 diabetes is caused by an autoimmune response that damages the insulin-secreting beta cells in the pancreas. Conversely,

Type 2 diabetes is a result of decreased sensitivity to otherwise adequate amounts of insulin. Both of these conditions result in hyperglycemia, causing polydipsia, polyphagia, and polyuria. These and other pathologic changes cause other complications including, in severe cases, end-stage renal disease, limb amputation, blindness, hypertension, neuropathy, impaired immunity, and myocardial infarction.[93] Along with its systemic complications, diabetes can also cause significant oral complications as a result of poorly controlled blood glucose levels, including periodontitis, xerostomia, candidiasis, dental caries, and mucosal disease.[94] The pathogenesis of periodontitis and diabetes has been researched extensively within the past decade. Several theories suggest that the relationship is directly causal, with the hyperglycemic environment causing the expression of periodontal disease.[78,79,95] One common supposition is that there is production of pro-inflammatory cytokines (interleukin [IL]-1, IL-6, and tumor necrosis factor-$\alpha$) in the presence of hyperglycemia and hyperlipidemia. This results in changes of the cellular and connective tissue, increasing the susceptibility to infection and vascular changes present in periodontal disease. The complexity of this relationship is evident in the research looking at the bidirectional as well as unidirectional relationship of these two conditions.[79,80] The theory is that both periodontitis and diabetes are modulated by the same gene sets (HLA on chromosome 6) that could result in a host who is susceptible to both conditions, therefore making the development of these diseases not strictly unidirectional.[96]

## ORAL AND PHARYNGEAL CANCER

Oral and pharyngeal cancers involve the lip, oral cavity, pharynx, and/or salivary glands. Oral cancer accounts for roughly 2% of all cancers diagnosed annually in the United States. Approximately 35,000 people will be diagnosed with oral cancer each year and about 7,600 will die from the disease. A diagnosis of cancer in the oral cavity can have major implications for both nutritional and overall health status. More than half of the patients with head and neck cancer are malnourished when they present for medical care.[97,98] Patients with oral and/or pharyngeal cancer can suffer from facial disfigurement, swallowing difficulties, chewing and/or speech impairment, emotional stress, decreased quality of life, and reduced survival.[99] These factors can affect nutrition status and should be taken into consideration when evaluating patients for nutrition risk. Although most cases of oral cancer are linked to cigarette smoking and/or heavy alcohol use, diet and nutrition can increase risk or be potential preventive and therapeutic factors.

Oral complications of cancer treatment depend on the various forms and degrees of severity of the cancer and also on the individual and the cancer treatment chosen. Chemotherapy may impair the function of bone marrow, suppressing the formation of white blood cells, red blood cells, and platelets. Some cancer treatments are described as stomatotoxic because they have toxic effects on the oral tissues. Table 43.7 lists some of the signs and symptoms common to

---

## TABLE 43.7

## Oral Complications Common to Both Chemotherapy and Radiation

Complications common in patients undergoing chemotherapy and radiation

  Oral mucositis: inflammation and ulceration of the mucous membranes; can increase the risk for pain, oral and systemic infection, and nutritional compromise.

  Infection: viral, bacterial, and fungal; results from myelosuppression, xerostomia, and/or damage to the mucosa from chemotherapy or radiotherapy.

  Xerostomia/salivary gland dysfunction: dryness of the mouth due to thickened, reduced, or absent salivary flow; increases the risk of infection and compromises speaking, chewing, and swallowing. Medications other than chemotherapy can also cause salivary gland dysfunction. Persistent dry mouth increases the risk for dental caries.

  Functional disabilities: impaired ability to eat, taste, swallow, and speak because of mucositis, dry mouth, trismus, and infection.

  Taste alterations: changes in taste perception of foods, ranging from unpleasant to tasteless.

  Nutritional compromise: poor nutrition from eating difficulties caused by mucositis, dry mouth, dysphagia, and loss of taste.

  Abnormal dental development: altered tooth development, craniofacial growth, or skeletal development in children secondary to radiotherapy and/or high doses of chemotherapy before age 9.

Other complications of chemotherapy

  Neurotoxicity: persistent, deep aching and burning pain that mimics a toothache, but for which no dental or mucosal source can be found. This complication is a side effect of certain classes of drugs, such as the vinca alkaloids.

  Bleeding: oral bleeding from the decreased platelets and clotting factors associated with the effects of therapy on bone marrow.

Other complications of radiation therapy

  Radiation caries: lifelong risk of rampant dental decay that may begin within 3 months of completing radiation treatment if changes in either the quality or the quantity of saliva persist.

  Trismus/tissue fibrosis: loss of elasticity of masticatory muscles that restricts normal ability to open the mouth.

  Osteonecrosis: blood vessel compromise and necrosis of bone exposed to high-dose radiation therapy; results in decreased ability to heal if traumatized.

*Source:* National Institute of Dental and Craniofacial Research, National Institutes of Health, Bethesda, MD.

both chemotherapy and radiation therapy, and complications specific to each type of treatment. Nutrition professionals must consider the possibility of these complications when they evaluate cancer patients.

## PREVENTION/TREATMENT OF ORAL HEALTH PROBLEMS FOR PATIENTS WITH ORAL AND PHARYNGEAL CANCER

The nutrition professional is integral in the management of patients with oral and pharyngeal cancer. Because these patients are at a higher risk of malnutrition, their nutrition status and eating behaviors should be monitored before, during, and after treatment to help improve patient prognosis and decrease the chance of secondary malnutrition.[100] The nutrition professional's key objective is to provide strategies for overcoming side effects of cancer treatment to improve nutrition and oral health status. Table 43.6 lists some treatment methods for managing patients suffering from head and neck cancer. Smoking cessation should be encouraged immediately. This will help with the dry mouth symptoms and help increase dietary intake. The practitioner should also encourage eating a variety of foods consistent with the MyPlate[16] guidelines and aim for the RDA/DV of vitamins and minerals. Nutrition professionals should monitor their patient's weight to ensure maintenance of lean body mass and urge patients to limit consumption of alcoholic beverages. To prevent dental caries, the patient should brush their teeth after every meal and chew sugar-free or xylitol gum to promote remineralization. If the patient suffers from dry mouth, foods should be recommended that will not irritate or cause pain when eating, such as mashed potatoes, creamy soups, Greek yogurt, pudding, oral nutrition supplements, etc.

## EATING DISORDERS AND ORAL HEALTH

The oral cavity is one of the first places in the body that the signs of bulimia and anorexia nervosa become evident. Approximately 80% of bulimic patients show signs of tooth decay from the reflux of destructive acids of the stomach, which are regurgitated into the mouth. These gastric acids can cause erosion of the dental enamel on the tongue side and biting surfaces of teeth. The telltale signs of bulimia nervosa are sore throat, hoarseness, redness of the throat and palate, dry mouth, and dry lips.[101] Nutrition professionals should be aware of the damaging effects of eating disorders on the oral cavity in order to screen for both oral health issues and for patients suffering from eating disorders. Table 43.8 lists the warning signs of eating disorders. Other oral health issues associated with eating disorders are tooth erosion, dental caries, periodontal disease, decreased saliva production, and oral mucosal lesions secondary to nutrient deficiencies.[102] Dental erosion is the most dramatic manifestation of chronic regurgitation that is found in patients with bulimia nervosa.[103,104] Patients who suffered from anorexia nervosa, but did not

---

**TABLE 43.8**
**Warning Signs of Eating Disorders**

Marked weight loss
Abnormal preoccupation with weight, food, calories, and diet
Denial of hunger
Avoidance of meal times
Evidence of purging behavior
Lack of sleep
Hormonal changes
Depression
Stomach pain
Withdrawal from one's usual group of friends and activities

---

vomit, had more dental erosion than control subjects, but less dental erosion than patients suffering from bulimia nervosa.[105] The damage to the oral mucosa is a generally recognized indicator of eating disorders and malnutrition in these patients as well. Many oral mucosal lesions may develop from severe deficiencies such as iron, B vitamins, and folate. These deficiencies impede the rapid turnover of cells in the oral mucosa and result in painful lesions such as angular cheilitis and glossitis.[103] Angular cheilitis is well established as a sign related to both nutritional deficiency and manifestation of an oral infection, otherwise known as *Candida albicans*. Another key complication of eating disorders is xerostomia, the decreased production of saliva, due to sialadenosis, or the swelling of the salivary gland. Sialadenosis (enlargement of the parotid and salivary glands) is a common feature in patients with eating disorders, and the xerostomia creates an environment in the oral cavity that is susceptible to dental caries and oral infections.[102]

## PREVENTION/TREATMENT OF DENTAL PROBLEMS FOR EATING DISORDERS

Nutrition professionals should use the warning signs found in Table 43.8 to screen for patients with potential eating disorders. These patients are at risk for dental caries and dental erosion due to decreased saliva production and damage from stomach acids present in the oral cavity. If a patient presents with signs and risk factors for an eating disorder, a referral to the appropriate physician and/or psychologist should be considered to address the underlying eating issues. A referral to a dental professional will also be necessary to address the many oral health problems listed earlier that are often involved.

## DYSPHAGIA

Several disorders can lead to swallowing difficulty, or dysphagia, including stroke, head and neck cancer, and multiple sclerosis.[77] The characteristics of dysphagia include dysphonia (unable to produce voice sounds), dysarthria (motor speech disorder), abnormal gag reflex, cough, abnormal lip closure, disordered tongue movement, oral discoordination, delayed oral and pharyngeal transit, and regurgitation.[106] Swallowing difficulties may limit dietary intake and have dramatic consequences for nutritional status and oral health. Decreased energy and protein intake may lead to weight loss and protein energy malnutrition, which can impede recovery and cause oral health issues, such as ill-fitting dentures.[107] Dysphagic patients are also at very high risk for aspiration pneumonia.[108] Brody et al.[109] studied the involvement of registered dietitians in the screening process and found that they were key players in the identification of patients with dysphagia. This multidisciplinary collaboration with speech pathologists and primary care providers leads to quicker referrals for swallowing evaluations and better outcomes in patients at risk for dysphagia. The *Oral Health Risk Evaluation* presented later in this chapter provides some questions to assess patients with potential problems with dysphagia.

The National Dysphagia Diet,[110] developed by the Academy of Nutrition and Dietetics, is a four-stage diet therapy used to address the swallowing and chewing difficulties associated with dysphagia. The key objective of this dietary advice is to provide safe oral nutrition and hydration, meeting the dysphagic patient's recommended needs for maintaining optimal lean body mass and preventing weight loss.[109] The four stages of the diet provide a sequence in the thickness and texture of foods in each of the stages, and examples of foods that fit into these categories of diet therapy.[110] The stages of the diet are as follows:

- Stage 1 is *dysphagia pureed*, which includes uniform, pureed consistency. Examples of foods include smooth hot cereals, cooked to a "pudding consistency," mashed potatoes, applesauce, etc.
- Stage 2 is *mechanically altered* and includes soft-textured, moist foods. Examples of foods include soft pancakes, cooked cereals, moist ground meat, scrambled eggs, etc.
- Stage 3 is *dysphagia advanced* and includes regular foods with exception of very hard, sticky, or crunchy foods. Examples of foods include moist breads, tender, thin-slided meats, eggs, rice, baked potato, etc.
- Stage 4 is a *regular diet*, which allows all foods.

The difficulties in finding foods appropriate and safe for patients on dysphagia diets can be challenging. Many patients do not care for the taste of pureed or moistened foods and will find it difficult to meet their needs for energy and protein with these foods. Hospitals have developed techniques to make pureed or softened foods that look like meat, carrots, or other tough-textured foods not allowed on the dysphagia diet. Products are also available commercially, however they can be expensive. It is up to the nutrition professional and the food service team to decide if the cost of these resources will result in better outcomes in

**TABLE 43.9**
**Modified Foods for Dysphagia Patients**

| Product, Brand Name | Use in Clinical Practice |
| --- | --- |
| Thick-It® | Thick-It is a product that can be added to liquids to make them thicker and therefore easier for patients with dysphagia to swallow. There are several different recipes that can be used to modify foods to the appropriate thickness, based on the diet appropriate for the patient. |
| Thick & Easy® | Instant food thickener that can be added to liquids, including nutritional supplements to make them easier for patients with dysphagia to swallow. There are several different recipes that can be used to modify foods to the appropriate thickness, based on the diet appropriate for the patient. |
| Puree Food Molds® | Commercial tray molds; food service operations can puree food into molds that look like foods not allowed on dysphagia diet. For example, a pork chop mold is available for pureed protein products. |

their patients.[111] Some sources of food products for patients with dysphagia are listed in Table 43.9.

## PREVENTION/TREATMENT FOR PATIENTS WITH DYSPHAGIA

The primary role of the nutrition professional in the treatment of dysphagia is to ensure safe and adequate dietary intake for the patient. Because this condition has several subdiagnoses depending on swallowing ability, the nutritional management of these patients will differ greatly. During the nutrition evaluation, the first step is to simply interview the patient on his or her swallowing and chewing ability. If the patient reveals difficulties swallowing or chewing, then the nutrition professional should consider a referral to a speech pathologist for a full swallowing evaluation. Swallowing evaluations include observation of a range of foods with different textures and the patient's ability to safely swallow these foods. The speech pathologist diagnoses the patient's specific degree of dysfunction and aspiration risk and educates the patient about their diagnosis.[106]

When the patient and health care providers are already aware of his or her swallowing and/or chewing difficulties, then the next step is to evaluate nutrition status and determine what specific issues are present that affect dietary intake. Factors such as food or liquid consistency and/or elimination of certain foods can be modified to ensure safety of the patient, while also providing adequate protein and energy. For patients with mechanical disorders that cause dysphagia, liquid or pureed diets might be the only foods that they can tolerate. However, these foods are not appropriate for patients with oropharyngeal dysphagia, who often better tolerate semisolid foods that are easy to chew.[111]

## DEVELOPMENTAL DISABILITIES

Several developmental disabilities have a significant impact on oral health. Patients with autism, cerebral palsy, Down syndrome, and intellectual disabilities have problems that begin at birth or shortly thereafter, and last an entire lifetime. These patients often struggle with self-care activities such as showering, dressing, eating, and cleaning their teeth. People with disabilities often need extra help to perform these activities and maintain good oral health status. However, some patients that do not have access to these resources will suffer from periodontal disease, dental caries, and other issues related to oral health hygiene. People with serious intellectual disabilities have more untreated caries and a higher prevalence of gingivitis and other periodontal diseases than the general population. Some of the common pharmaceuticals used for people with special needs can also cause oral problems such as xerostomia or Dilantin hyperplasia (overgrowth of gum tissue). Nutrition professionals must recognize that these patients are at a higher risk for oral health problems and to screen and refer these patients to a dental professional when it is necessary.

## PREVENTION/TREATMENT FOR PATIENTS WITH DEVELOPMENTAL DISABILITIES

During an oral health screen, patients with severe intellectual and behavioral disabilities should be screened for potential issues with feeding abilities or oral health issues. Some of these patients are fed by their caregivers and they cannot articulate pain or other sensations that other patients could express, so it is important to identify symptoms of subjective discomfort and of malnutrition or oral health problems through physical signs and symptoms. For example, patients with swallowing difficulties could show signs of dysphagia by coughing, choking, wet breathing, etc.[112] If a patient is showing these types of signs, a speech pathologist will need to evaluate the patient for dysphagia.

Other potential issues that arise for patients with disabilities can be overweight and underweight. According to Rimmer et al.,[113] patients with developmental disabilities and Down syndrome have a higher incidence of overweight and obesity. Monitoring the patient's weight frequently (and tracking along standardized growth charts for children/adolescents with developmental disabilities) will help determine if growth is appropriate. Table 43.10 shows the common oral health issues related to patients with intellectual disabilities and strategies for care.

## QUALITY OF LIFE

Not only does oral health status have an impact on other systems in the body, but oral health status also can have a potent impact on patients' quality of life.[114] Several investigators have developed different modalities for measuring quality of life related to health, such as oral health status.[115] Oral health problems can indeed affect activities of daily living

associated with these conditions.[116–119] By measuring activities that oral health can affect, such as eating and communicating, conclusions can be made about the broader overall connection between oral health and psychosocial well-being as well as life satisfaction.[120] Strauss and Hunt[121] found that older adults felt that the presence of teeth enhanced their appearance, ability to eat, and enjoyment of food. They also found a positive effect on enjoyment, confidence, comfort, speech, and longevity.

Several quality of life measures have been developed to screen patients for oral health issues. The Surgeon General's Report on Oral Health in America[4] provides a complete review of these tools and their effectiveness at assessing the quality of life. All of the measures identified included questions regarding oral health issues and the effect on dietary intake. Specifically, the review found that oral and craniofacial diseases contributed to compromised ability to chew, bite, and swallow foods, creating limitations on food selection and lead to malnutrition.[4] Incorporating quality of life measures in nutrition screening can provide more information about the health and nutrition status in patients experiencing significant oral health problems.

## SCREENING AND ASSESSMENT TOOLS

Nutrition professionals are responsible for identifying nutritional risk factors that will affect their patient's overall health. In the dental arena, compromised dietary intake and nutritional status may have many causes, including pain from dental caries or root caries, missing teeth, and dentures, or periodontal disease.[5] Nutritionists should use oral health screening and assessment tools in their practice in order to identify and address nutrition issues or refer those beyond their expertise to the appropriate health professional. The following section identifies tools for screening and assessment that are useful for determining oral health risk in children and adults. Table 43.11 lists the different screening and assessment tools provided and the advantages of each of these tools.

## NUTRITION SCREENING INITIATIVE

The Nutrition Screening Initiative (NSI) was a national volunteer effort supported by 25 national health care organizations to "make nutrition a vital sign" in the delivery of health care in the United States. They developed materials to identify older Americans who were at risk of nutrition problems, to assess the problems, and to provide interventions to address them. The NSI developed tools to quickly screen the nutritional status of older Americans. The DETERMINE Checklist (Figure 43.3), the primary screening and educational tool developed by the NSI, is a brief generic health risk-appraisal questionnaire that older persons, their family members, or practitioners can use to assess the nutritional risk associated with chronic disease and oral problems.[3] The Checklist is effective in

**TABLE 43.10**

**Oral Health Problems in Intellectual Disability and Strategies for Care**

| Problem | Periodontal Disease | Dental Caries | Malocclusion, Missing Permanent Teeth, Delayed Eruption, and Enamel Hypoplasia |
|---|---|---|---|
| Causes | Medications, malocclusion, multiple disabilities, and poor oral hygiene combine to increase the risk of periodontal disease. | People with intellectual disability develop caries at the same rate as the general population. The prevalence of untreated dental caries, however, is higher among people with intellectual disability, particularly those living in non-institutional settings. | The prevalence of malocclusion in people with intellectual disability is similar to that found in the general population, except for those with coexisting conditions such as cerebral palsy or Down syndrome. The ability of the patient or caregiver to maintain good daily oral hygiene is critical to the feasibility and success of treatment. |
| Steps for patients and for caregivers | Encourage independence in daily oral hygiene.<br>Ask patients to show you how they brush, and follow up with specific recommendations on brushing methods or toothbrush adaptations.<br>Involve your patients in hands-on demonstrations of brushing and flossing.<br>Talk to caregivers about daily oral hygiene. | Emphasize noncariogenic foods and beverages as snacks. Advise caregivers to avoid using sweets as incentives or rewards.<br>Advise patients taking medicines that cause xerostomia to drink water often. | Examine a child by his or her first birthday and regularly thereafter to help identify unusual tooth formation and patterns of eruption. |
| Steps for patients and caregivers | Emphasize that a consistency in location and method.<br>Mouth rinses, such as Chlorhexidine, can be used but consider the patient's limits. Rinsing, for example, may not work for a patient who has swallowing difficulties or one who cannot expectorate.<br>Chlorhexidine applied using a spray bottle or toothbrush is equally efficacious.<br>If use of particular medications has led to gingival hyperplasia, emphasize the importance of daily oral hygiene and frequent professional cleanings. | Recommend preventive measure such as fluorides and sealants. | Take appropriate steps to reduce sensitivity and risk of caries in your patients with enamel hypoplasia. |

*Source:* National Institute of Dental and Craniofacial Research, National Institutes of Health, Bethesda, MD.

**TABLE 43.11**

**Nutrition Screening and Assessment Tools**

| Screening Tools | Target Population | Advantages |
|---|---|---|
| Nutrition Screening Initiative: DETERMINE Checklist | Older Americans | Focuses on health issues pertinent to older Americans.<br>Can be used by the patient or family members for self-assessment. |
| Oral Health Risk Evaluation Tool | Adults over 18 years of age | Practitioner can identify problems through the screening tool and provide recommendations accordingly. |
| Tufts University School of Dental Medicine's Food, Oral Health and You Tool | Adults over 18 years of age | Provides recommendations for altering diet according to dietary recall. |
| Nutrition Risk Assessment for Children | Children >1 year of age | Caregiver answers questions related to child's diet. Assesses diet cariogenicity. |

increasing awareness of these nutrition-related problems in older adults.[122] If problems related to teeth and oral health are identified, further exploration is necessary with a second checklist.

The Determine Checklist for Oral Health (Figure 43.4), which was also developed by the NSI, provides a rapid way for nutritionists and other non-dental professionals to assess oral health status and further identify these oral health issues. Table 43.12 describes each item on the DETERMINE Checklist for Oral Health, why it is important, and what the next steps are for the patient. Taken together, these screening and counseling tools are helpful in identifying individuals with potential nutritional and/or oral health problems, and can provide a starting point for nutrition professionals to assess health status in older persons.

*The warning signs of poor nutritional health are often overlooked. Use this checklist to find out if you or someone you know is at nutritional risk.*

Read the statements below. Circle the number in the yes column for those that apply to you or someone you know. For each yes answer, score the number in the box. Total your nutritional score.

# Determine Your Nutritional Health

|  | YES |
|---|---|
| I have an illness or condition that made me change the kind and/or amount of food I eat. |  |
| I eat fewer than 2 meals per day. |  |
| I eat few fruits or vegetables, or milk products. |  |
| I have 3 or more drinks of beer, liquor, or wine almost every day. |  |
| I have tooth or mouth problems that make it hard for me to eat. |  |
| I don't always have enough money to buy the food I need. |  |
| I eat alone most of the time. |  |
| I take 3 or more different prescribed or over-the-counter drugs a day. |  |
| Without wanting to, I have lost or gained 10 pounds in the last 6 months. |  |
| I am not always physically able to shop, cook, and/or feed myself. |  |
| Total |  |

## Total Your Nutritional Score. If it's -

**0–2**  **Good!** Recheck your nutritional score in 6 months.

**3–5**  **You are at moderate nutritional risk.** See what can be done to improve your eating habits and lifestyle. Your office on aging, senior nutrition program, senior citizens center or health department can help. Recheck your nutrition score in 3 months.

**6 or more**  **You are at high nutritional risk.** Bring this checklist the next time you see your doctor, dietitian, or other qualified health or social service professional. Talk with them about any problems you may have. Ask for help to improve your nutritional health.

*These materials developed and distributed by the Nutrition Screening Initiative, a project of:*

AMERICAN ACADEMY OF FAMILY PHYSICIANS

THE AMERICAN DIETETIC ASSOCIATION

NATIONAL COUNCIL ON THE AGING

**Remember that warning signs suggest risk, but do not represent diagnosis of any condition. Turn this page to learn more about the warning signs of poor nutritional health.**

**FIGURE 43.3**  DETERMINE Checklist. (From Nutrition Screening Initiative, *Report of Nutrition Screening I: Toward a Common View*, Nutrition Screening Initiative, Washington, DC, 1991.)

The Nutrition Checklist is based on the warning signs described below. Use the word DETERMINE to remind you of the warning signs.

**Disease:** Any disease, illness or chronic condition which causes you to change the way you eat, or makes it hard for you to eat, puts your nutritional health at risk. Four out of five adults have chronic diseases that are affected by diet. Confusion or memory loss that keeps getting worse is estimated to affect one out of five or more of older adults. This can make it hard to remember what, when or if you've eaten. Feeling sad or depressed, which happens to about one in eight older adults, can cause big changes in appetite, digestion, energy level, weight and well being.

**Eating Poorly:** Eating too little and eating too much both lead to poor health. Eating the same foods day after day or eating fruit, vegetables, and milk products daily will also cause poor nutritional health. One in five adults skip meals daily. Only 13% of adults eat the minimum amount of fruit and vegetables needed. One in four older adults drink too much alcohol. Many health problems become worse if you drink more than one or two alcoholic beverages per day.

**Tooth Loss/Mouth Pain:** A health mouth, teeth and gums are needed to eat. Missing, loose or rotten teeth or dentures, which don't fit well or cause mouth sores make it hard to eat.

**Economic Hardship:** As many as 40% of older Americans have incomes of less than $6,000 per year. Having less— or choosing to spend less— than $25-30 per week for food makes it very hard to get the foods you need to stay healthy.

**Reduced Social Contact:** One-third of all older people live alone. Being with people daily has a positive effect on morale, well-being and eating.

**Multiple Medicines:** Many older Americans must take medicines for health problems. Almost half of older Americans take multiple medicines daily. Growing old may change the way we respond to drugs. The more medicines you take, the greater the chance for side effects such as increased or decreased appetite, change in taste, constipation, weakness, drowsiness, diarrhea, nausea, and others. Vitamins or minerals when taken in large doses act like drugs and can cause harm. Alert your doctor to everything you take.

**Involuntary Weight Loss/Gain:** Losing or gaining a lot of weight when you are not trying to do so is an important warning sign that must not be ignored. Being overweight or underweight also increases your chance of poor health.

**Needs Assistance and Self Care:** Although most older people are able to eat, one of every five have trouble walking, shopping, buying and cooking food, especially as they get older.

**Elder Years Above Age 80:** Most older people lead full and productive lives. But as age increases, risk of frailty and health problems increase. Checking your nutritional health regularly makes good sense.

**FIGURE 43.3 (continued)** DETERMINE Checklist. (From Nutrition Screening Initiative, *Report of Nutrition Screening I: Toward a Common View*, Nutrition Screening Initiative, Washington, DC, 1991.)

Once the patient has been screened for oral health problems, a more comprehensive health assessment is necessary. This includes an evaluation of an individual's overall health status, including any risk factors and personal needs that can affect health and treatment options.[4] A dietitian or other nutrition professional can manage the risk of dental caries or risk of demineralization from diet, as well as oral pain or xerostomia. For other risk indicators revealed by the screening, such as dysphagia, the patient can be referred to the appropriate health professional (such as a speech therapist), who can further assess or treat the patient's problem. The remainder of this section focuses on several common problems and their management.

## ORAL HEALTH RISK EVALUATION TOOLS
### FOR NUTRITION PROFESSIONALS

A variety of different types of information are necessary in order to evaluate a patient's risk of oral health issues. The nutrition professional should collect subjective information, such as current and recent diet, feeding abilities, and weight change. Asking the right questions is key to obtaining the most relevant information. Objective information can also be an excellent indicator of oral health risk. Different settings in which health professionals work have different capabilities to assess objective information regarding oral health risk. Objective information includes height, weight, and pertinent lab values. The Oral Health Risk Evaluation Tool does assess both subjective and objective information.

## ORAL HEALTH RISK EVALUATION TOOL

The *Oral Health Risk Evaluation Tool* (Figure 43.5) was developed for nutrition professionals who do not have access to laboratory data at the time of evaluation. In the *Oral Health Risk Evaluation* the subjective portion of the assessment includes questions that can identify major oral health risks, including xerostomia, dental caries, protein energy malnutrition, low SES, use of multiple medications, etc. Each section is presented separately to isolate these various risks. If a patient checks the box next to any question within a section, it will indicate to the nutrition professional that there is a need to evaluate the patient for an oral health problem and provide the appropriate recommendations for it.

The nutrition professional can interview the patient and visually observe the patient's mouth to determine if the patient has any carious lesions or missing teeth. The patient's weight and height are helpful in determining if the patient is malnourished or overweight. Weight history may reveal undernutrition and poverty that have a likely impact on oral and nutrition status. Unintentional weight loss can indicate undernutrition and should be addressed immediately.

*Oral health can affect your nutritional health. A healthy mouth, teeth and gums are needed to eat.*

# Determine Your Oral Health

If you answered "yes" to "I have tooth or mouth problems that make it hard for me to eat," on the determine your nutrition health checklist, answer the questions below.

**Check all that apply:**

**Do you have tooth or mouth problems that make it hard for you to eat, such as loose teeth, ill-fitting dentures, etc.?**

**Is your mouth dry?**

**Do you have problems with:**

**Lips (soreness or cracks in the corners of your mouth)?** ........................ ————

**Tongue (pain/soreness)?** ............................................. ————

**Sores that do not heal?** ............................................. ————

**Bleeding or swollen gums?** ........................................... ————

**Toothaches or sensitivity to hot or cold?** .............................. ————

**Pain or clicking your jaw?** ........................................... ————

**Have you visited a dentist:**

**Within the past 12 months?** .......................................... ————

**In the last 2 years?** ................................................ ————

**Never been to a dentist?** ............................................ ————

**If you have visited a dentist, was the main reason for your visit:**

**Regular checkup.** .................................................. ————

**To have denture made.** ............................................. ————

**To have teeth cleaned.** ............................................. ————

**Bleeding or score gums.** ............................................ ————

**To have tooth filled.** ............................................... ————

**Loose teeth/loose tooth.** ........................................... ————

**To have tooth pulled or other surgery.** ................................ ————

**Oral or facial pain.** ................................................ ————

**To have a root canal** ............................................... ————

**Adjustments or repair of denture** .................................... ————

**Other** ........................................................... ————

Discuss with your care provide what can be done to correct the problems you have indicated. Also, bring this checklist to your dentist the next time you visit. Remember that warning signs suggest risk, but do not represent diagnosis of any condition

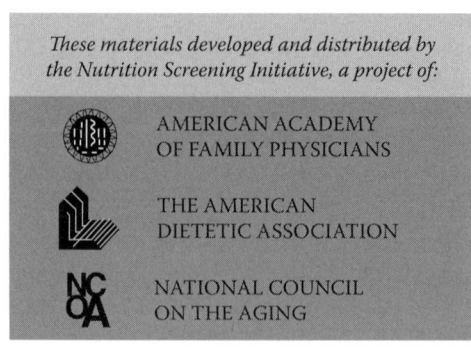

*These materials developed and distributed by the Nutrition Screening Initiative, a project of:*

AMERICAN ACADEMY OF FAMILY PHYSICIANS

THE AMERICAN DIETETIC ASSOCIATION

NATIONAL COUNCIL ON THE AGING

**FIGURE 43.4** DETERMINE Checklist for oral health. (From Nutrition Screening Initiative, *Report of Nutrition Screening I: Toward a Common View*, Nutrition Screening Initiative, Washington, DC, 1991.)

A 24 h diet recall can help the nutrition professional determine what kinds of foods and the amount the patient is eating. Further questioning helps to identify patients that are not eating enough, eliminating a whole food group, or eating cariogenic foods frequently throughout the day.

All of these factors pose risks to oral and nutritional health. The assessment and planning portion of the evaluation is where the practitioner decides the oral health risk and the caries risk. The 24 h recall and the responses on the first page determine what steps to take next. According to

**TABLE 43.12**
**DETERMINE Oral Health Checklist and Interventions**

| Oral Health Issue on Checklist | Next Steps for Nutrition Professionals |
|---|---|
| Mouth Pain | Identify location of pain and, if possible, source |
| | Note additional symptoms and relationship to eating |
| | Contact dentist with all relevant information |
| | If appropriate, ask for permission to contact dentist, regarding mouth pain |
| | Recommend ways for older patients to modify diet-soft/liquid diet recommendations |
| | Screen for chronic disease and anatomic anomalies |
| Caries | Modify diet to eat fewer sugary (especially sticky) foods and drinks |
| | Avoid frequent snacking |
| | Practice proper oral hygiene (brushing, flossing) |
| | Contact dentist |
| | Give older adults visual materials on proper oral hygiene |
| | Assist older adults with proper food selection and eating habits |
| | Administer food frequency form with Palmer Classification of Cariogenicity and make dietary recommendations |
| Loose teeth, bleeding gums | Improve oral hygiene (brushing, flossing) |
| | Modify diet to eat more foods with fiber and fewer soft foods that stick to teeth and gums |
| | Contact dentist |
| | Give older adults visual materials on proper oral hygiene |
| | Assist older adults with proper food selection |
| | Screen for nutrient deficiency—recommend dietary changes |
| | Oral hygiene instruction |
| | Screen for chronic disease |
| Dry mouth | Eat foods that require a lot of chewing (such as sugarless chewing gum), snack on hard sugarless candies |
| | Drink plenty of water and other fluids |
| | Contact dentist and/or doctor |
| | Encourage older adults to participate in social dining |
| | Assist older adults with proper food selection and adequate hydration |
| | Prepare special snacks |
| | Offer mouth rinses |
| | Review older patient's diet and eating habit and make appropriate recommendations |
| | Screen for drug–nutrient interactions |
| | Screen for chronic disease |
| Soft tissue sores, lesions in moth, inflammation (tongue, lips, gums) | Stop alcohol and/or tobacco use |
| | Contact dentist and/or doctor |
| | Assist older adults with proper food selection and preparation |
| | Refer to dietitian |
| | All prior interventions |
| | Soft/liquid diet recommendations |
| | Screen for allergies, chronic and infectious disease, nutrient deficiencies (especially vitamin B, C) |
| Pain or clicking jaw | Nizel et al. suggests the use of an acrylic night guard followed by construction of fixed bridgework or a partial denture relief of TMJ pain. |

*Source:* Nutrition Screening Initiative, *Incorporating Nutrition Screening and Interventions Into Medical Practice: A Monograph for Physicians,* Nutrition Screening Initiative, Washington, DC, 1991.

the recommendations in Step 4, if the patient responds with a check mark in the "dental caries" section, then the patient should be provided with nutrition education on the proper diet for reducing the risk of dental caries and also referred to a dentist, if the patient has not seen the dentist in more than 6 months. The criteria for scoring the dietary assessment are based on the amount and frequency of cariogenic foods that contribute significantly to the risk of developing dental caries. If the patient has a high dental caries risk score (e.g., consuming five or more cariogenic foods per day), then that patient will benefit from dietary education on non-cariogenic dietary practices.

## Tufts University School of Dental Medicine's Food, Oral Health, and You Tool

This tool (see Figure 43.6) is a caries risk assessment tool developed for dentists to identify patients who need further evaluation for possible nutrition-related issues. This form is used in a dental professional's practice and includes questions on eating habits, functional eating issues, food access, and diet quality. It also provides a small amount of nutrition education after the patient is scored and the risk of caries related to nutrition has been determined. This tool is helpful in that it combines self-assessment and education into one form. Patients are presented with nutrition education tips while they assess their own oral nutrition status. After patients complete the 24 h diet recall, they are instructed to assess their intake and determine if they are eating adequate and balanced amounts of each food group. This recall also alerts the practitioner if a patient is missing a key food group,

**Oral Health Risk Evaluation**

Directions: For each "yes" answer, please give 1 point. For each "no", please give zero point. For each section that has at least 1 point, please evaluate for further oral problems and/or refer to dental health professional. Also, nutrition recommendations are provided at the end of the evaluation.

**Step 1: Subjective Assessment:** Please answer the questions below to the best of your ability.

A — Total = ______

1. Do you have any tooth or mouth pain that interface with your ability to eat 2 or more meals per day? ☐
2. Have you been diagnosed with any one of these conditions within the past year? ☐
   - Head and/or Neck Cancer ☐
   - Diabetes Mellitus (Type 1 or Type 2) ☐
   - Osteoporosis ☐
   - Autoimmune disorders, such as Sjogren's syndrome, Pernicious Anemia, Pemphigus Vulgaris, Benign Musous Membrane Pemphigoid, Systemic Lupus Erythematosus, or Rheumatoid Arthritis ☐
   - HIV/AIDS ☐
   - Eating disorder
3. Do you have a developmental disorder that inhibits you from performing basic ☐ activities of daily living? ☐

B — Total = ______

4. Do you have difficulty shopping for, or preparing foods? ☐
5. Do you ever run of money for food during the month? ☐
6. Have you visited the dentist:
   - Within the past 12 months? ☐
   - In the last 2 years? ☐
   - Never been to a dentist. ☐

Questions 4 and 5 would require a referral to social services.

7. Do you take any vitamins, minerals, or other dietary supplements? ☐
   - If yes, please list type and dosage: ______

C — Total = ______

8. Do you have pain or difficulty chewing or swallowing food? ☐
9. Can you eat meal or snack without needing liquids? ☐
10. Have there been any changes in your medications? ☐
    - If yes, please list them here ______

D — Total = ______

Caries risk evaluation:

1. Do you eat or drink more than five times per day? ☐
2. Do you chew sugar-free/xylitol-containing gum after eating? ☐
3. Do you suffer from dry mouth (xerostomia)? ☐
4. If you snack between meals, do you eat candies, chips, crackers, pastries, etc.? ☐
5. Do you drink sweetened beverages, such as coffee, tea, soda, or juice more than 1 time per day? ☐
6. Do you drink milk, cheese, yogurt, or calcium-fortified non-dairy drinks at least once per day? ☐

E — Total = ______

Dysphagia risk evaluation:

1. Do you experience drooling of liquids or solids while eating? ☐
2. Do you experience coughing dring or after swallowing, or feeling like you are choking? ☐
3. Do you find it difficult to complete at least half of your meals? ☐

(a)

**FIGURE 43.5** Oral health risk evaluation.

**Step 2: Objective Assessement**

1. Does the patient have carious lesions currently? If yes, how many? _____
2. Is the patient missing any teeth due to carious lesions? If yes, how many? _____
3. What is the patient's weight? _____
   - Has the patient lost more than 10 Ibs. in 6 months?        _____
4. What is the patient's height? _____

---

**Diet Intake (24-hour Recall)**

| Time of Day | Foods Eaten | Amount |
|---|---|---|
| | | |

---

**Step 3: Dietary Assessment:** It is the responsibility of the nutrition professional to rate the diet for risk of cariogenicity. Here are some questions that will help to identify risk for dental caries.

- How many times did the patient eat (meals and snacks)?
- Did the patient use any sugar-free gum or xylitol gum after a meal or snack?
- How many snacks contained cariogenic foods?
- Did the patient eat immediately before bed?

**Step 4: Recommendations/Plan:** After you have determined the risk level of the patient's oral health it is time to develop and intervention strategy. According to the subjective assessement from step 1, provide recommendations below corresponding to the lettered section.

| | |
|---|---|
| Section A: Protein energy Malnutrition | Recommend nutritional supplements, such as ensure or boost, to increase oral intake and maintain lean body mass stores. |
| Section B: Socioeconomic Status | Referral to social services for evaluation of food assistance programs and discount dental insurance programs |
| Section C: Xerostomia | Suggest foods without added spices or strong flavors. Opt for mashed or soft foods instead of hard, chewy foods such as steak or crackers. Such on sugar-free hard candy or ice chips. Use xylitol gums to prevent dental caries that arise from dry mouth. Carry a bottle of water around to keep the mouth moist. Try canned vegetables or fruit instead of raw. Try to buy canned vegetables with "no salt added." |
| Section D: Dental Caries | Emphasize the importance of oral hygiene: brushing after every meal and flossing regularly. Use fluoride toothpaste to promote remineralization after meals. Chew sugar-free or xylitol gum to prevent dental caries Visit the dentist regularly to have your teeth cleaned. (every 6 months) |
| Section E: Dysphagia | Referral to speech pathologist for swallowing evaluation. Once swallowing ability is assessed, modify diet based on the *National Dysphagia Diet.* |

(b)

**FIGURE 43.5 (continued)**    Oral health risk evaluation.

---

What you eat can have helpful or harmful effects on your mouth and teeth.

Good nutrition keeps oral tissues healthy, aids in wound healing, helps keep your immune system strong to fight gum disease, and helps prevent tooth decay.

This tool will help you see how your nutrition and oral health shape up.

**Part 1 –Promoting good nutrition**

Please begin by answering the following:

Are you being treated for any other condition involving nutrition?

Do you have any dental problems which affect your eating?
Have you changed your eating habits in the past 6 months?
If yes, gained or lost?

Do you drink more than 3 alcoholic beverages daily?

Do you take vitamins or nutritional supplements?

If you answered YES to any of the above, please explain:

---

**Diet Recall: What do you eat in a typical day?**

Please list all of the foods, including snacks and beverages, that you eat in a typical day (for example, yesterday.)

Give your best estimate of amounts and times consumed

| Time of Day | Foods Eaten | Amount |
|---|---|---|
| | | |

Now move to the next page and see how your diet compares to what is recommended

---

(a)

**FIGURE 43.6**    Tufts University School of Dental Medicine: Food, Oral Health and You. (From Division of Nutrition and Preventive Dentistry, Tufts University School of Dental Medicine, Boston, MA.)

*(continued)*

**How does your diet rate?**
For each food you listed on the previous page, put
a check in the appropriate food pyramid box below
for each serving you had.

**Results**
If you were below the lowest recommended servings
in any of the food groups in the Food Guide Pyramid,
you may be at nutritional risk. Plot your risk below

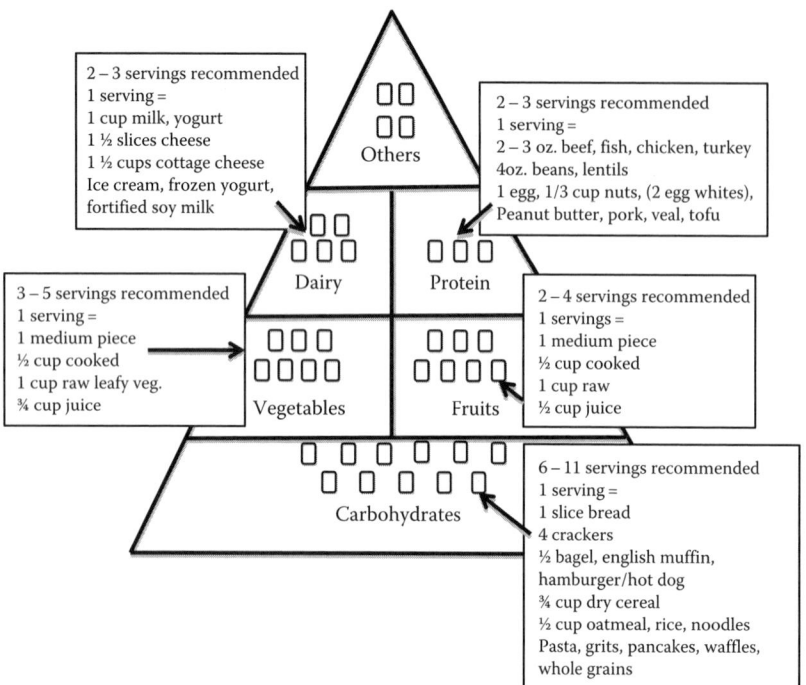

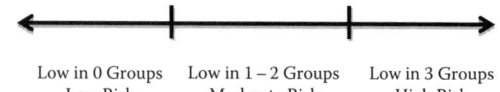

Low in 0 Groups   Low in 1 – 2 Groups   Low in 3 Groups
Low Risk          Moderate Risk         High Risk

Here are some suggestions for how to add more
nutritious foods to your everyday diet.

| Food Group | Diet Benefits | Suggestions |
|---|---|---|
| Dairy | Calcium, protein, vitamin D | Have a yogurt or cheese for a snack. add milk to coffee or tea. |
| Protein | Protein, zinc, iron, B-vitamins | Put peanut butter on crackers. Use tofu as a filler. Use more beans. |
| Vegetable | Vitamins A & C, antioxidants, potassium, folate | Have more salads. Use raw vegetables as snacks. Add to sandwiches, stir fry. |
| Fruit | Vitamins A & C, antioxidants, fiber, potassium | Have on cereal. Eat as snack or dessert. |
| Grains | B-vitamins, fiber, complex carbohydrates | Snack on pretzels, popcorn, crackers. Have whole grain rice or pasta with meals. |

(b)

## Part II
### Diet and Your Teeth
Frequent eating or drinking of sugar-containing foods is a
major risk factor for developing dental caries (tooth decay).

| Do you have a dry mouth | Yes | No |
|---|---|---|
| Do you chew gum? If yes, what type? | Yes | No |
| Do you often such on hard candy, cough drops etc.? | Yes | No |

| A<br>Circle any foods you eat regularly (at least once a week) | B<br>How many of the circled foods do you normally eat each day | C<br>Multiply the number from column "B" by the number in the box next to it. Record the total at the bottom. |
|---|---|---|
| LIQUID<br>Soft drinks, fruit drinks, cocoa, sugar and honey in beverages, non-dairy creamers, flavored yogurt, pudding, custard, ice cream, frozen yogurt, sherbert, popsicles, jello | | × 1 = |
| SOLID AND STICKY<br>Bananas, canned fruit in syrup, crackers, potato chips, pretzels, cake, cupcakes, donuts, sweet rolls, pastry, cookies, chocolate candy, caramel, toffee, jelly beans, other chew candy, chewing gum, dried fruit, jelly jam, marshmallows | | × 2 = |
| SLOWLY DISSOLVING<br>Hard candies, breath mints, antacid tablets, cough drops | | × 3 = |

**Total** _____ ➡

## Oral Health Results
### Your Risk for Dental Caries
Using your total from the previous page, plot your risk for
dental caries below.

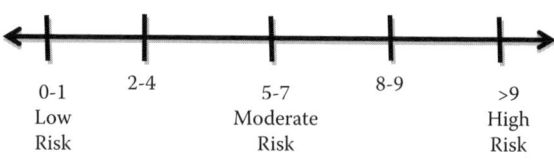

0-1          2-4          5-7          8-9          >9
Low                       Moderate                  High
Risk                      Risk                      Risk

Points to keep in mind to lower your risk for caries:

- Cut down on the frequency of between-meals sweets
- Don't sip constantly on sweetened beverages
- Avoid using slowly dissolving items like hard candy, cough drops, or breath mints
- Eat more non-decay promoting foods such as low-fat cheese, raw vegetables, crunchy fruits, popcorn, nuts, artificially sweetened beverages and natural spring waters

To promote general oral health, eat adequate
amounts from each of the Pyramid food groups.

**A good diet, adequate fluoride, and effective
oral hygiene are the keys to oral health.**

(c)

**FIGURE 43.6 (continued)**   Tufts University School of Dental Medicine: Food, Oral Health and You. (From Division of Nutrition and
Preventive Dentistry, Tufts University School of Dental Medicine, Boston, MA.)

**Dental Nutrition Risk Assessment** (questions for parent or caregiver)

- Does your child take any sugar-containing medications or vitamins on a regular basis? Yes (enter 1) _____
  No (enter 0) _____

- How many snacks does your child eat per day?
  0, 1, or 2 snacks (enter 0) _____
  3 snacks (enter 1) _____
  more than 3 snacks (enter 2) _____
  constant snacking (enter 3) _____

- Which best describes when your child eats sweets (candy, cookies, cake other desserts)?
  never (enter 0) _____
  with meals (enter 0) _____
  at the end of meals (enter 1) _____
  with or as snacks (enter 2) _____

- How often does your child snack before bedtime?
  Never (enter 0) _____
  Occasionally (enter 1) _____
  Often ( enter 2) _____

- How often does your child use slowly dissolving candies and/or lozenges?
  Never/rarely (enter 0) _____
  Often (enter 1) _____
  Once a day (enter 2) _____
  More than once a day (enter 3) _____

- How often does your child drink fruit juice, soda, or other carbonated beverages?
  Never/rarely (enter 0) _____
  Often, but not every day (enter 1) _____
  Daily, one (enter 2) _____
  Daily, more than one (enter 3) _____
  If sipped slowly (enter 3) _____

- Does your child chew sugar-free gum?
  Yes (enter 0) _____
  No (enter 1) _____

**RESULTS:**

**If end score was:**
3+ = High risk Needs nutrition counseling.
1-2 = Moderate risk. Needs caries prevention guidelines and methods.
0–1 = Low risk. Will benefit from review of caries prevention guidelines and methods.

**FIGURE 43.7** Dental nutrition risk assessment. (From Carole A. Palmer, EdD, RD, LDN, Tufts University Dental School, Boston, MA.)

which could be a risk factor for malnutrition. Nutritionists can also use this tool to determine if a patient is at risk of a diet-related issue that can be addressed by in the nutrition as well as the dental setting.

## NUTRITION RISK ASSESSMENT FOR CHILDREN

Figure 43.7 provides a nutrition and oral health screening tool developed for parents to assess dietary factors that are related to the risk of developing dental caries in their children. It asks parents questions about cariogenic dietary intake and the frequency of meals throughout the day. This tool is helpful for parents to fill out to determine if their child needs further education on a healthy diet for caries risk reduction.

## CONCLUSIONS

Nutrition professionals can have a significant impact on the oral health of their patients. By identifying high-risk patients, assessing nutritional and oral health issues, educating the patients and referring those who need dental experts, nutritionists can make a real difference. They can provide not only referrals but also recommendations for care to other health professionals (dentists, dental hygienists, physicians, etc.) and provide related nutritional care, if it is needed, for individuals of all ages. In the future, oral health assessment protocols will need to be developed for other health care practitioners who will have clients with oral health problems. The new settings will include physical and occupational therapy centers as well as speech and language therapy centers. This will require further collaborations between specialists and dental professionals and continue the trend toward more effective multidisciplinary care.

## REFERENCES

1. Moynihan, PJ, Lingström, P. In: Touger-Decker, R, Sirois, DA, Mobley, CC, eds. *Nutrition and Oral Medicine*. Humana Press, Totowa, NJ, 2005, p. 107.
2. Squier, CA, Kremer, MJ. *JNCI Monographs* 2001:7;2001.
3. Dwyer, JT, Campbell, D. Nutrition Screening Initiative, Washington, DC, 1991.
4. National Institute of Dental and Craniofacial Research. Surgeon general's report on oral health. National Institutes of Health, Bethesda, MD, 2000.
5. Touger-Decker, R, Mobley, C, *J Am Diet Assoc* 107: 1418–1428;2007.
6. Touger-Decker, R, Sirois, DA. In: Powers, MA, ed. *Handbook of Diabetes Medical Nutrition Therapy*. Aspen Publishers, Gaithersburg, MD, 1996.
7. Rigassio, D, Touger-Decker, R. *Today's Dietitian* 9:24;2000.
8. Touger-Decker, R, Sirois, D, Mobley, CC. *Nutrition and Oral Medicine*. Humana Press, Totowa, NJ, 2005, p. 63.
9. Enwonwu, C. *Am J Clin Nutr* 61:430S;1995.
10. Johnson, DA. *The Salivary System*. CRC Press, Boca Raton, FL, 1987, p. 136.
11. Enwonwu, C. *Arch Oral Biol* 18:95;1973.
12. Sculley, DV, Langley-Evans, SC. *Proc Nutr Soc* 61:137;2002.
13. Wayler, AH, Chauncey, HH. *J Prosthet Dent* 49:427;1983.

14. Chauncey, H, Muench, M, Kapur, K et al. *Int Dent J* 34:98;1984.
15. Oliver, W, Leaver, A, Scott, P. *J Periodont Res* 7:29;1972.
16. United States Department of Agriculture. Available at http://www.choosemyplate.gov. Accessed May 2, 2012.
17. Selwitz, RH, Ismail, AI, Pitts, NB. *Lancet* 369:51;2007.
18. Guggenheimer, J, Moore, PA. *J Am Dent Assoc* 134:61;2003.
19. Tenovuo, J. *Commun Dent Oral Epidemiol* 25:82;1997.
20. D'Hondt, E, Eisbruch, A, Ship, JA. *Spec Care Dentist* 18:102;1998.
21. Infante, P, Gillespie, G. *Arch Oral Biol* 19:1055;1974.
22. Sreebny, LM. *Commun Dent Oral Epidemiol* 10:1;1982.
23. Ruxton, C, Garceau, F, Cottrell, R. *Eur J Clin Nutr* 53: 503;1999.
24. Gustafsson, BE, Quensel, CE, Lanke, LS et al. *Acta Odontol* 11:232;1953.
25. Moynihan, P, Petersen, PE. *Public Health Nutr* 7:201;2004.
26. Mörmann, J, Mühlemann, H. *Caries Res* 15:166;1981.
27. Lingstrom, P, Van Houte, J, Kashket, S. *Crit Rev Oral Biol Med* 11:366;2000.
28. Kashket, S, Zhang, J, Van Houte, J. *J Dent Res* 75:1885;1996.
29. Arends, J, Ten Bosch, J, Leach, S et al. In: Leach, SA. *Factors Relating to Demineralization and Remineralization of the Teeth*. IRL Press Limited, Oxford, U.K., 1985, 11p.
30. Burt, B. *J Dent Res* 71:1228;1992.
31. American Academy of Pediatric Dentistry. Available at http://www.aapd.org/media/Policies_Guidelines/D_ECC.pdf. Accessed May 3, 2012.
32. Kagihara, LE, Niederhauser, VP, Stark, M. *J Am Acad Nurse Pract* 21:1;2009.
33. Kaste, LM, Gift, HC. *Arch Pediatr Adolesc Med* 149:786;1995.
34. Fitzsimmons, D, Dwyer, JT, Palmer, C et al. *J Am Diet Assoc* 98:182;1998.
35. Centers for Disease Control and Prevention. Available at http://www.cdc.gov/growthcharts/clinical_charts.htm. Accessed May 3, 2012.
36. Centers for Disease Control and Prevention. Available at http://www.cdc.gov/obesity/data/childhood.html. Accessed May 3, 2012.
37. Reifsnider, E, Mobley, C, Mendez, D. *J Multicult Nurs Health* 10:24;2004.
38. Tuomi, T. *Commun Dent Oral Epidemiol* 17:289;1989.
39. Macek, MD, Mitola, DJ. *Pediatr Dent* 28:375;2006.
40. Marshall, TA, Eichenberger-Gilmore, JM, Broffitt, BA et al. *Commun Dent Oral Epidemiol* 35:449;2007.
41. Albandar, J, Brunelle, J, Kingman, A. *J Periodontol* 70: 13;1999.
42. Beltrán-Aguilar, ED, Barker, LK, Canto, MT et al. *MMWR Surveill Summ* 54:1;2005.
43. Papas, AS, Joshi, A, Palmer, CA et al. *Am J Clin Nutr* 61:423S;1995.
44. Palmer, C, Wolfe, SH, *J Am Diet Assoc* 105:1620;2005.
45. Twetman, S, Axelsson, S, Dahlgren, H et al. *Acta Odontol* 61:347;2003.
46. Edgar, W. *Br Dent J* 169:96;1990.
47. Jensen, M, Wefel, J. *Br Dent J* 167:204;1989.
48. Yankell, SL, Emling, RC. *J Clin Dent* 1:51;1988.
49. Jensen, ME. *J Clin Dent* 1:6;1988.
50. Wennerholm, K, Emilson, CG. *Eur J Oral Sci* 97:257;1989.
51. Guenther, PM. *J Am Diet Assoc* 86:493;1986.
52. Siegal, MD, Farquhar, CL, Bouchard, JM. *Public Health Rep* 112:98;1997.
53. Atkinson, J, Fox, P. *Clin Geriatr Med* 8:499;1992.
54. Wiseman, LR, Faulds, D. *Drugs* 49:143;1995.

55. Reich, E, Petersson, L, Netuschil, L et al. *Int Dent J* 52: 337;2002.
56. Phipps, KR, Stevens, VJ. *J Public Health Dent* 55:250;1995.
57. Niessen, LC, Weyant, RJ. *J Public Health Dent* 49:19;1989.
58. Joshipura, KJ, Kent, RL, DePaola, PF. *J Periodontol* 65: 864;1994.
59. Johan, HS. *Acta Odontol* 43:139;1985.
60. Kerr, R, Touger-Decker, R. *Nutrition and Oral Medicine.* Humana Press, Inc., Totowa, NJ, 2005, p. 129.
61. Sheiham, A, Steele, J, Marcenes, W et al. *J Dent Res* 80:408;2001.
62. Nowjack-Raymer, R, Sheiham, A. *J Dent Res* 82:123;2003.
63. Papas, AS, Palmer, CA, Rounds, MC et al. *Spec Care Dentist* 18:17;1998.
64. Sahyoun, NR, Krall, E, *J Am Diet Assoc* 103:1494;2003.
65. Thomas, E, Hay, E, Hajeer, A et al. *Rheumatology* 37:1069;1998.
66. Sirois, DA, Touger-Decker, R. In: Touger-Decker, R, Sirois, DA, Mobley, C, eds. *Nutrition and Oral Medicine.* Humana Press, Inc., Totowa, NJ; 2005, p. 241.
67. Rhodus, NL, DMD M. *J Nutr Elder* 10:1;1991.
68. Castro, KG, Ward, J, Slutsker, L et al. *MMWR Recomm Rep* 41:1;1992.
69. Patel, A, Glick, M. In: Touger-Decker, R, Sirois, DA, Mobley, C, eds. *Nutrition and Oral Medicine.* Humana Press, Totowa, NJ; 2005, p. 223.
70. Lin, A, Johnson, D, Stephan, K et al. *J Dent Res* 82:719;2003.
71. Fields-Gardner, C, Fergusson, P et al. *J Am Diet Assoc* 104:1425;2004.
72. Strawford, A, Hellerstein, M. *Semin Oncol* 25(2 Suppl 6):76;1998.
73. Mulligan, K, Tai, VW, Schambelan, M. *J Acquir Immun Defic Syndr* 15:43;1997.
74. Kotler, DP, Tierney, AR, Wang, J et al. *Am J Clin Nutr* 50:444;1989.
75. Demmer, RT, Desvarieux, M. *J Am Dent Assoc* 137:14S;2006.
76. Genco, R, Offenbacher, S, Beck, J. *J Am Dent Assoc* 133:14S;2002.
77. Elmståhl, S, Bülow, M, Ekberg, O et al. *Dysphagia* 14:61;1999.
78. Grossi, SG, Genco, RJ. *Ann Periodontol* 3:51;1998.
79. Löe, H. *Diabetes Care* 16:329;1993.
80. Nagasawa, T, Noda, M, Katagiri, S et al. *Intern Med* 49:881;2010.
81. Nieto, FJ. Am J Epidemiol 148:937;1998.
82. Beck, J, Garcia, R, Heiss, G et al. *J Periodontol* 67: 1123;1996.
83. Lopes-Virella, MF, Virella, G. *Clin Immunol Immunopathol* 37:377;1985.
84. Rivers, R, Hathaway, W, Weston, W. *Br J Haematol* 30: 311;1975.
85. Persson, GR, Persson, RE. *J Clin Periodontol* 35:362;2008.
86. Joshipura, KJ, Rimm, E, Douglass, C et al. *J Dent Res* 75:1631;1996.
87. Meurman, JH, Sanz, M, Janket, SJ. *Crit Rev Oral Biol Med* 15:403;2004.
88. Simonka, M, Skaleric, U, Hojs, D. *Zobozdrav Vestn* 43:81;1988.
89. Danesh, J, Wheeler, JG, Hirschfield, GM et al. *N Engl J Med* 350.1387,2004.
90. Shah, SH, Newby, LK. *Cardiol Rev* 11:169;2003.
91. Chobanian, AV, Bakris, GL, Black, HR et al. *Hypertension* 42:1206;2003.
92. Ockene, IS, Miller, NH. *Circulation* 96:3243;1997.
93. Touger-Decker, R, Sirois, D, Vernillo, A. *Nutrition and Oral Medicine.* Humana Press, Totowa, NJ, 2005, p. 185.
94. Little, JW, Faace, D, Miller, C et al. *Dental Management of the Medically Compromised Patient.* Mosby, St. Louis, MO; 1997, 664p.
95. Yalda, B, Offenbacher, S, Collins, JG. *J Periodontol* 2000 6:37;1994.
96. Hart, TC, Kornman, KS. *J Periodontol* 2000 14:202;1997.
97. Goodwin Jr, WJ, Torres, J. *Head Neck Surg* 6:932;1984.
98. Laviano, A, Meguid, MM. *Nutrition* 12:358;1996.
99. Morse, DE. In: Touger-Decker, R, Sirois, DA, Mobley, CC, eds. *Nutrition and Oral Medicine.* Humana Press, Inc., Totowa, NJ, 2005, p. 205.
100. Minasian, A, Dwyer, JT. *Oncology (Williston Park)* 12:1155;1998.
101. Ritter, D, André, V. *J Esthet Restor Dent* 18:114;2006.
102. Frydrych, A, Davies, G, McDermott, B. *Aust Dent J* 50:6;2005.
103. Ruff, J, Koch, MO, Perkins, S. *Gen Dent* 40:22;1992.
104. Steinberg, B. *J Dent Educ* 63:271;1999.
105. Robb, N, Smith, B, Geidrys-Leeper, E. *Br Dent J* 178:171;1995.
106. Perry, L, Love, CP. *Dysphagia* 16:7;2001.
107. Bending, A. *Commun Nurse* 7:13;2001.
108. Finestone, HM, Greene-Finestone, LS. *Can Med Assoc J* 169:1041;2003.
109. Brody, RA, Touger-Decker, R, VonHagen, S et al. *J Am Diet Assoc* 100:1029;2000.
110. National Dysphagia Diet Task Force, American Dietetic Association. *National Dysphagia Diet: Standardization for Optimal Care.* American Dietetic Association, Chicago, IL, 2002.
111. Kamer, AR, Sirois, DA, Huhmann, M. In: Tougher-Decker, R, Sirois, DA, Mobley, CC, eds. *Nutrition and Oral Medicine.* Humana Press, Totowa, NJ, 2005, p. 63.
112. Van Riper, C. *J Am Diet Assoc* 110:296;2010.
113. Rimmer, JH, Rowland, JL, Yamaki, K. *J Adolesc Health* 41:224;2007.
114. Needleman, I, McGrath, C, Floyd, P et al. *J Clin Periodontol* 31:454;2004.
115. Slade, GD. *Measuring Oral Health and Quality of Life.* University of North Carolina, Chapel Hill, NC, 1996.
116. Reisine, S. *Commun Dent Health* 5:63;1988.
117. Atchison, KA, Dolan, TA. *J Dent Educ* 54:680;1990.
118. Locker, D, Slade, G. *Gerodontology* 11:108;1994.
119. Palmer, C. In: Touger-Decker, R, Sirois, DA, Mobley, CC, eds. *Nutrition and Oral Medicine.* Humana Press, Totowa, NJ, 2005, p. 63.
120. Locker, D, Clarke, M, Payne, B. *J Dent Res* 79:970;2000.
121. Strauss, R, Hunt, R. *J Am Dent Assoc* 124:105;1993.
122. Sahyoun, NR, Jacques, PF, Dallal, GE et al. *J Am Diet Assoc* 97:760;1997.

# 44 Herbal Supplements in the Prevention and Treatment of Cancer

*Donato F. Romagnolo and Ornella I. Selmin*

## CONTENTS

## INTRODUCTION

Although problems persist with the interpretation of cancer data from non-randomized studies of herbal treatment, ~48% of cancer patients are estimated to use complementary and alternative medicine (CAM). The lack of universal success and side effects associated with chemotherapy are two main reasons for cancer patients to seek therapy from dietary supplements including herbals. Cancer patients who use CAM are usually younger females with a higher level of education than non-users [1,2]. The use of herbal supplements was estimated to be one of the most popular practices (~60%) during or after chemotherapy [3], and among cancer patients (~20%) [4] with less advanced disease, i.e., patients receiving potentially curative treatment compared to the general population [5,6].

A survey of dietary supplements used in the United States reported about 18% of American adults used natural products in the past 12 months [7,8] including herbals such as green tea, garlic, Echinacea, chamomile, ginseng, and gingko biloba [5]. American Indians, Alaskan natives, and white adults are more likely to use CAM including natural products, than Asians or black adults. Examples of traditional medical systems based on botanicals include Ayurvedic and Traditional Chinese Medicine (TCM) [9]. Herbal supplements used in Ayurvedic and TCM were suggested to be useful in cancer prevention and treatment [10,11]. For example, preclinical studies in vitro and animal models reported Triphala, a traditional Ayurvedic herbal supplement composed of pericarps from *Emblica officinalis*, *Terminalia belerics*, and *Terminalia chebula* fruits, exerted anticarcinogenic effects in various models of breast, skin, stomach, and pancreatic cancer [12]. *E. officinalis*, a component of Triphala, is widely used in Ayurvedic medicine. It contains various anticancer compounds such as ellagic acid, kaempferol, and gallic acid.

Studies that investigated the use of CAM in a cancer survivor population residing in Australia revealed herbal supplements were used by 8%–15% of subjects compared to 23% for nutritional supplements and vitamins [13,14]. Interestingly, ~83% of cancer patients residing in Turkey reported using herbals as a form of complementary therapy [15]. Across a number of European countries, the use of herbal products increased from ~5% to ~14% after cancer diagnosis [16]. Type of herbs used varied by country and included green tea (Scotland), mistletoe (Switzerland), ginseng (Czech Republic, Sweden), and olive leaves (Greece). Since 2011, herbal medicine in European countries has been regulated by Good Manufacturing Practice regulations [17]. Examples of herbal supplements used in cancer therapy are summarized in Table 44.1.

Information is lacking about the adverse effects of bioactive compounds present in herbal supplements in cancer patients undergoing treatment [2]. Interactions with prescription drugs and other dietary supplements have been suspected to induce secondary and undesirable effects [7,18]. Therefore, caution should be exercised when considering complementing chemotherapies with herbal supplements. For example, herbal supplement–drug interactions have been reported for bioactive compounds present in garlic and gingko that influence metabolism of drugs by P450 enzymes [6,19]. The following paragraphs summarize results of preclinical and clinical cancer studies with selected herbals.

**TABLE 44.1**

**Preclinical Studies of Herbal Supplements and Cancer**

| Cancer | Reference | Herbal Supplement | Model | Outcome of Study |
|---|---|---|---|---|
| Multiple | Baliga [12] | Triphala[a] | MCF-7, T47D PC-3, nu/nu mice | Reduced proliferation, skin and liver tumor incidence; induced apoptosis |
| | Ngamkitidechakul et al. [98] | E. officinalis | A549, HepG2, Hela, MDA-OV3, SW620 | Inhibited proliferation, DMBA-induced skin tumors; induced apoptosis |
| | Wang et al. [53] | Spatholobus suberectus | MCF-7, HT-29 | Inhibited cell growth,; induced G2/M arrest, reduced growth of tumor xenografts |
| | Yadav et al. [99] | Withania somnifera | PC-3, DU-145, HCT-15, A549, IMR-32 | Induced cytotoxicity |
| Prostate | Yang et al. [30] | Saw Palmetto | LNCaP | Induced apoptosis, p21, p53; reduced growth of tumor xenografts |
| | Du et al. [27] | PC-SPES II | PC-3 | Induced apoptosis, Bax; reduced Bcl-2 |
| | Ye et al. [32] | S. baicalensis | LNCaP, PC-3 | Reduced PGE2, COX-2 activity; PSA and cyclin D1 in LNCaP; reduced cdk1 and induced G2/M in PC-3 |
| | Ikezoe et al. [28] | PC-SPES | LNCaP | Reduced activation of AR and PSA expression |
| | Ikezoe et al. [29] | Oridonin (Rabdosia r.) | LNCaP | Induced G0/G1 arrest and apoptosis |
| | Chung et al. [34] | PC-SPES | PC-3 | P. notoginseng exerted antagonistic effects against other PC-SPES herbs |
| | Adams et al. [33] | PC-SPES | 22Rv1 | S. baicalensis and G. uralensis inhibited each other |
| | Bonham et al. [35] | PC-SPES | LNCaP | Reduced expression of α-tubulin and growth of CWR22R AR-independent tumor xenografts |
| | Bonham et al. [31] | S. baicalensis | LNCaP, PC-3 | Baicalein, wogonin, neobaicalein reduced expression of AR-regulated PSA gene and induced G1 arrest. Wogonin, neobaicalein, and skullcapflavone induced G2 arrest in PC-3 cells |
| Lung | Ikezoe et al. [39] | PC-SPES | NSCLC | Reduced COX-2 expression, NFκB, C/EBPβ |
| | Hegde et al. [42] | Viscum album | A549 | Inhibition of COX-2 expression and PGE2 secretion |
| | Liu et al. [40] | PC-SPES | A549, GLC-82 | Ponicidin (R. rubescens) induced apoptosis |
| Colon | Huerta et al. [51] | PC-SPES | SW620 | Induced G2/M arrest, apoptosis; reduced β-tubulin |
| | | | APCMin | Reduced tumor number (58%) and load (56%) |

| | Reference | Supplement | Model | Effect |
|---|---|---|---|---|
| | Encalada et al. [52] | *M. officinalis* | HCT-116 | Reduced proliferation by extract and rosmarinic acid fraction |
| | Wang et al. [53] | PHY906 | BDF-1 mice | Enhanced antitumor effects of irinotecan |
| | Kummar et al. [55] | PHY906 | Colon 39 | Improved antitumor activity of irinotecan in Phase I |
| | Volate et al. [57] | Ginseng powder, quercetin, curcumin, rutin, silymarin | Male F344 | Decreased the number of ACF and induced apoptosis |
| | Ryu et al. [100] | Bojanggunbi-tang | ICR mice | Reduced colon inflammation |
| | Lam et al. [54] | PHY906 | BFD1 38 | Restored Wnt signaling and expression of stem cell markers |
| | Brandin et al. [56] | Ginger supplement | LS180 | Induced CYP1A2, CYP3A4, MDR1 |
| | Yi and Wetzstein [101] | Thyme, rosemary, sage, spearmint, peppermint | SW-480 | Inhibited cell growth |
| | Sze et al. [102] | Tian Xian[b] | HT-29 | Induced p21; reduced cyclin D1, PCNA |
| | Lee et al. [103] | *Gleditsia sinensis* | HCT-116 | Induced G2/M arrest, p53, ERK, JNK, p38 |
| | | | | Reduced cyclin B1, cdc25c, tumor growth xenografts |
| | Yusup et al. [104] | Savda Munziq | Caco-2 | Induced G0/G1 arrest, apoptosis, Bax; reduced Bcl-2 |
| | Xu et al. [105] | Rosmarinic acid (*Prunella vulgaris*) | Ls174-T | Reduced MMP-2, MMP9, growth tumor xenografts |
| | Chia et al. [106] | Tien-Hsien | CT-26 | Reduced pulmonary metastasis, MMP-2, MMP-9 |
| | Tang et al. [107] | *Houttunya cordata* | HT-29 | Induced apoptosis, cytochrome c, procaspase-9 and -3 |
| | Wang et al. [108] | American ginseng | SW-480 | Induced apoptosis |
| Blood | Battle et al. [109] | Honokiol (*Magnolia* sp.) | B-CLL | Induced caspase-3, -8, and 9, apoptosis |
| Brain | Jeong et al. [110] | *Moris fructus* | A172 | Induced apoptosis, Bax, cytochrome c, caspase; reduced growth and PCNA in tumor xenografts |

a *E. officinalis, T. belerics,* and *T. chebula.*

b Tian Xian: *Cordyceps sinensis, Astragulus membranaceus, Ganoderma lucidum, Panax ginseng, Atractylodes macrocephalae, Dioscorea batatas, Codnopsis pilosula, Pogostemon cablin, Lycium barbarum, Pteria margaritifera, Ligustrum lucidum, Radix glycyrrhizae.*

## CANCER STUDIES

### PROSTATE CANCER

A herbal supplement that has been investigated for the treatment of hormone refractory prostate cancer (HRPC) is PC-SPES, which contains extracts from eight herbs based on TCM (Table 44.1). According to the National Cancer Institute, "PC-SPES is a patented mixture of eight herbs that was sold as a dietary supplement to support and promote healthy prostate function. Each herb used in PC-SPES has been reported to have anti-inflammatory, antioxidant, or anticarcinogenic properties. However, PC-SPES was recalled and withdrawn from the market because certain batches were contaminated with Food and Drug Administration-controlled prescription drugs. The manufacturer is no longer in operation, and PC-SPES is no longer being made. There is evidence from both laboratory and animal studies to suggest that PC-SPES had some effect in inhibiting prostate cancer cell growth and prostate-specific antigen (PSA) expression, but it is not known whether these results were caused by adulterants such as diethylstilbestrol, which is an estrogenic compound, the herbs in PC-SPES, or their combination. In clinical trials, PC-SPES lowers PSA and testosterone levels in humans, but it is not known whether these results were caused by adulterants, the herbs in PC-SPES, or their combination. There is some evidence to suggest that PC-SPES has some anticancer effects that are not related to estrogen-like activity." There are products still on the market that claim to be substitutes for PC-SPES, but they are not the patented original formulation, and clinical trials on them have not been reported in peer-reviewed scientific journals. The information in the following illustrates the types of information that led to it being studied. More data are available at the National Cancer Institute website: http://www.cancer.gov/cancertopics/pdq/cam/pc-spes/HealthProfessional/

Supplementation with PC-SPES reduced ($\geq 50\%$) PSA levels in both hormone-responsive and HRPC patients [20]. The supplemental intake (2.88 g/day for 5 months) of PC-SPES was associated with a decline in PSA levels with no major side effects in men with advanced metastatic prostate cancer [21]. Similar inhibitory effects of PC-SPES on circulating PSA levels have been observed in HRPC patients [22], although in some subjects there were reports of estrogenic side effects [23]. Declines in PSA levels of $\geq 50\%$ were observed in 40% of androgen receptor (AR)-independent prostate cancer patients supplemented with PC-SPES (three capsules, three times per day). Conversely, discontinuation of PC-SPES led to a rapid rise of PSA in patients with advanced prostate carcinoma [24]. PC-SPES has been suspended from the market due to contaminations with other compounds including diethylstilbestrol (DES) and ethinyl estradiol [25]. Although PC-SPES is no longer available, in a small Phase I prospective study conducted in the United Kingdom with patients diagnosed with HRPC, the administration of PC-SPES-2, a quality-controlled PC-SPES formulation, induced in 7 out of 10 men a drop in PSA doubling time, which persisted after 3–6 months on trial [26].

These clinical studies suggest that characterization of the anticancer effects of each herbal component of PC-SPES might be useful to identify compounds for the prevention of prostate cancer. Several mechanisms contribute to the anti-prostate cancer activity of bioactive compounds found in PC-SPES herbs. In vitro studies with PC-3 cells found PC-SPES induced cell death accompanied by decreased expression of Bcl-2 and Bcl-xL, two anti-apoptotic proteins, and increased expression of Bax, a pro-apoptotic protein. Accordingly, the expression of the activated fragments of caspase-3 was increased by PC-SPES [27]. In LNCaP prostate cancer cells, PC-SPES reduced the expression of proteins necessary for microtubule polymerization, suggesting compounds in PC-SPES may interfere with cytoskeleton organization. Other anticancer mechanisms that may be activated by PC-SPES include inhibition of AR-activated binding to AR-response elements (ARE) harbored in the PSA gene, downregulation of expression of PSA, and activation of the JNK/c-Jun/AP-1 signal pathway leading to growth arrest and apoptosis [28]. For example, one of the eight herbal components of PC-SPES is *Rabdosia rubescens*. It contains oridonin which induced G0/G1 phase arrest, p53-dependent upregulation of p21, and apoptosis in LNCaP cells [29].

Saw palmetto (*Serenoa repens*), an herbal component of PC-SPES, was reported to induce growth arrest and apoptosis marked by increased expression of p53 and p21, while reducing nuclear levels of AR and phosphorylated STAT3. Similarly, Saw palmetto extracts were found to reduce growth of LNCaP tumor xenografts in Balb/c nude mice [30]. Another component of PC-SPES is *Scutellaria baicalensis*. It contains various flavone compounds (baicalein, wogonin, neobaicalein, and skullcapflavone) that inhibit the growth of prostate cancer cells, expression of AR and PSA [31], and production of prostaglandin E2 (PGE2) via suppression of cyclooxygenase-2 (COX-2) [32]. In vitro, extracts of *S. baicalensis* induced G1 phase arrest, and reduced cyclin D1 expression and COX-2 activity in LNCaP cells. In PC-3 cells, *S. baicalensis* preparations induced G2/M arrest accompanied by reduced cdk1 expression. Extracts of *S. baicalensis* were more effective than PC-SPES in reducing in vitro growth of PC-3 cells. In vivo, supplementation with extracts of *S. baicalensis* (200 mg/kg BW) or baicalein (20 mg/kg/day p.o.) to nude mice xenografted respectively with PC-3 or LNCaP cells reduced the tumor growth by ~50% [31,32].

Using combinations of herbal mixtures rather than individual herbs in prostate cancer therapies may help reducing doses of each individual herb due to additive or synergistic effects, but can also induce antagonistic effects. For example, combined extracts of *S. baicalensis* and *D. morifolium* or *D. morifolium* and *R. rubescens* inhibited synergistically or additively cell proliferation of prostate cancer cells [33]. In contrast, combinations of *S. baicalensis*, *G. uralensis*, and *P. notoginseng* exerted antagonistic effects in prostate cancer cells, suggesting that pharmacokinetics of various herbal components should be considered when designing strategies based on mixtures [33,34].

Some studies have reported adverse effects of herbal supplements in prostate cancer patients. For example, PC-SPES reduced the effectiveness of paclitaxel treatment in both androgen-sensitive and androgen-independent models of prostate cancer [35]. Dietary supplementation with a herbal preparation containing chrysin, a flavonoid found in *Pelargonium* sp., elk velvet antler, along with sex testosterone precursors induced manifestations of clinically aggressive prostate cancers, and in vitro growth stimulation of HRPC (DU-145, PC-3) and AR-responsive LNCaP cells [36]. Stimulation of urinary tract cancers was also reported for herbal products used in TCM and containing aristocholic acid, a carcinogen found in *Aristolochia fangchi* [37]. Clearly, more research is needed before herbal supplements can be recommended for prostate cancer therapy.

## LUNG CANCER

The prognosis for patients with lung cancer is generally poor with median survival less than 12 months and high death rate at 2 years [38]. Herbal supplements that have been used to prevent lung cancer include PC-SPES, which in non-small cell lung cancer (NSCLC) cells induced growth arrest and apoptosis, downregulated COX-2 and C/EBPβ expression, and inhibited NFkB activity [39]. These observations suggested compounds in PC-SPES may be useful for the prevention/treatment of inflammatory diseases of the lung. Pro-apoptotic effects in lung cancer (A549, GLC-82) cells were also reported for ponicidin, a diterpenoid derived from *R. rubescens* [40]. The latter is also a constituent of the herbal supplement PC-SPES. A rather remarkable example of effective herbal medicine was provided by a case report of regression of squamous cell carcinoma of the lung in a 51-year-old woman by a prescription of nine Chinese herbs (*Herba Hedyotis diffusae, Radix ophiopogonis, Herba taraxaci, Radix notoginseng, Pseudobulbus Cremastrae seu plaiones, Radix Panacis quinquefolii, Herba houttuyniae, Bulbus Fritillariae thunbergii, Rhizoma Pinelliae preparata*). Because spontaneous remission or regression is very rare in lung cancer, investigators concluded that compounds present in the herbal formulation were likely responsible for regression of the lung carcinoma [41]. Nevertheless, the generalizability of this report to prevention of squamous cell carcinoma of the lung remains to be demonstrated and adverse effects, if any, must also be documented.

*Viscum album* is known as a semi-parasite that grows on trees. It contains many compounds including lectins, viscotoxins, flavonoids, phytosterols, triterpines, and phenylpropanes. The anticarcinogenic effects of *V. album* extracts have been related to inhibition of inflammatory pathologies of the lung via selective reduction of COX-2 expression and PGE2 production without changes in COX-1 expression [42]. This selectivity toward COX-2 is of interest in cancer prevention since simultaneous inhibition of COX-1 and COX-2 by non-steroidal anti-inflammatory agents (NSAIDs) has been associated with unwanted side effects related to lower homeostatic levels of PGE2.

A review of 34 randomized studies representing 2815 patients revealed some tumor benefits associated with intake of *Astragalus*-based Chinese herbs in patients diagnosed with NSCLC and undergoing platinum-based chemotherapy [43]. Although investigators acknowledged the need for confirmation of results with controlled trials, purported anticancer benefits of *Astragalus* included reduced risk of death and improved tumor response. Wogonin, a naturally occurring plant flavonoid isolated from *S. baicalensis*, was reported to inhibit COX-2 expression in human lung cancer epithelial cells [44].

Herbs used in TCM vary depending on individual patient's syndrome [45]. A meta-analysis that evaluated 15 Chinese trials involving 862 subjects with NSCLC indicated studies are needed to confirm the effectiveness of Chinese herbal medicine. The same study highlighted that five herbs (*Astragali membranaceus, Angelica sinensis, Ophiopogon japonicas, Curcuma zedoaria,* and *Oldenlandia diffusa*) commonly used in TCM had anticancer properties [46]. These assertions also require documentation with more substantial evidence than that currently exists.

## ORAL AND GASTROINTESTINAL CANCERS

Reduced oral lesion size, vascular endothelial growth factor (VEGF), and cyclin D1 expression have been reported following intervention with tea preparations for patients at risk for oral cancer [47,48]. Colon cancer survival was improved by a combination of herbal medicine and vitamins compared to conventional therapy alone in a 10 year follow-up study with 193 colon cancer patients [49]. A case report of a 47-year-old man diagnosed with gastric B-cell lymphoma documented complete colon cancer regression possibly related to intake of large doses (60 capsules/day for 5 day) of *Ganodema lucidum* (Lingzhi), a TCM mushroom with anticancer properties [50]. Suggested mechanisms for the therapeutic effects of *G. lucidum* were stimulation of macrophage and T lymphocyte infiltration and production of various cytokines such as interleukin-1B (IL-1B), IL-6, tumor necrosis factor-α (TNF-α), and interferon-γ (IFN-γ).

In vitro investigations with colon cancer cell lines (SW480, SW620, DLD-1) documented PC-SPES (3 μL/mL) inhibited cell growth. Concentrations of 1.5 μL/mL induced ($\geq$60%) accumulation in G2-M phase of the cell cycle, which was accompanied by reduced expression of β-tubulin and stimulation of apoptosis. In vivo studies with the APC[Min] mouse model indicated supplementation with PC-SPES (250 mg/kg/day, 5 times/week for 10 weeks) via gavage reduced by 56% and 58% tumor load and number, respectively [51]. These data suggested bioactive compound in PC-SPES might have potent activity against colon cancer. But again more evidence is needed before its utility in cancer prevention can be determined.

*Melissa officinalis* is a traditional herb used in Mediterranean countries. Fifty percent ethanolic extracts of *M. officinalis* reduced proliferation (~60%) of colon cancer HCT-116 cells. Rosmarinic acid was identified as one of the compounds responsible for the antiproliferative effects of *M. officinalis* [52].

PHY906 is a TCM formulation of the four herbs *Glycyrrhiza uralensis* (Chinese licorice), *Paeonia lactiflora* (Chinese Peony), *S. baicalensis* (skullcaproot), and *Ziziphus jujube* (buckthorn tree). In female BDF-1 mice bearing subcutaneous colon tumors, supplementation with PHY906 enhanced the antitumor effects of the drug irinotecan [53], and decreased infiltration of neutrophils and macrophages, and TNF-α expression in the intestine [54]. Also, PHY906 induced expression of ASCL2, a component of the Wnt signaling pathway. Because the latter induces the expression of APC, a known tumor suppressor gene, compounds present in PHY906 may hold promise for the prevention of colon cancer. In a Phase I study, PHY906 did not alter the pharmacokinetics of irinotecan [55], suggesting combination therapies with PHY906 may not interfere with metabolism of cancer drugs. Conversely, evidence for potential herbal–drug or other interactions was documented for ginger-based preparations, which induced the expression of CYP1A2, CYP3A4, and MDR1, respectively, by 11.2-, 6.4-, and 5.4-fold in LS180 colon cancer cells [56].

Dietary supplementation with quercetin, curcumin, silymarin, and ginseng decreased the number of aberrant crypt foci (ACF) in an azoxymethane (AOM)-induced rat colon cancer model [57]. In colorectal cancer patients, intervention with tea extract tablets reduced the incidence of metachronous adenomas by 50% and the size of relapsed adenomas [58]. The hypothesized preventive effects of the tea extract were related to inhibition of angiogenesis and proliferation.

## BREAST CANCER

Although evidence on the effectiveness of CAM and herbal supplements for the treatment of early-stage breast cancer is inconclusive [59], a recent study with subjects 20–75 years of age enrolled in the Shanghai Breast Cancer Survival Study reported ~77% of patients used Chinese herbal medicine. Herbs most commonly used were *Ganoderma lucidum* (Lingzhi), sporophyte, and ginseng products [60]. A study that examined the use of specific herbs by patients receiving chemotherapy, of which 56% were women with breast cancer, reported participants were using herbs known to induce hormonal effects (black cohosh, ginseng, don quai), bleeding (e.g., garlic, gingko), or affecting the P450 metabolism of various drugs (e.g., cyclophosphamide, vincristine, and paclitaxel) [18]. The same study reported that ~28% of patients were at risk for detrimental herbal supplement–chemotherapy interactions. In a population of 763 disease-free breast cancer survivors in Los Angeles, herbs that were used frequently included garlic, gingko, and Echinacea [61].

Investigations of dietary supplement use by 435 women enrolled in the Women's Healthy Eating and Living (WHEL) study living in the western United States and who were at risk for breast cancer recurrence reported ~21% of subjects used herbal products [62] (Table 44.1).

A study with 998 breast cancer survivors enrolled in the Black Women's Health Study reported 68.2% had used either herbals or multivitamin supplements or both. The three most frequently used herbals were garlic (21.2%), gingko (12.0%), and Echinacea (9.4%) [63] (Table 44.2).

A blend of mushroom mycelia from the species *Agaricus blazei*, *Cordyceps sinensis*, *Coriolus versicolor*, *G. lucidum*, *Grifola frondosa*, and *Polyporus umbellatus* inhibited proliferation and induced cell cycle arrest at the G2/M phase of highly invasive human breast cancer MDA-MB-231 cells. Moreover, the mushroom preparation antagonized the metastatic behavior of MDA-MB-231 through inhibition of cell adhesion, cell migration, and cell invasion [64]. Extracts of soybean, *Gymnema sylvestre*, black cohosh, passion flower, and rutin strongly inhibited breast cancer resistance protein-mediated transport of methotrexate [65]. Conversely, a preparation (Essiac) containing four herbs, burdock, turkey rhubarb, sorrel, and slippery elm, was reported to stimulate growth of estrogen receptor (ER)-positive (T47-D) and ER-negative cancer cells as well as ER-dependent luciferase activity in ER-positive MCF-7 cells [66]. Clearly, caution should be exercised by breast cancer patients when using herbal supplements.

Although in vitro and animal studies suggested tea flavonoids may prevent breast cancer [67], a nested-control (144 cases and 288 controls) study in the Japan Public Health Center-based Prospective Study comprising 24,226 women aged 40–69 years found no significant associations between breast cancer risk and plasma levels of various tea catechins [68]. However, a study (353 cases, 701 controls) nested in the Shanghai Women's Health Study Cohort aged 40–70 years at baseline documented higher levels of urinary epicatechins may reduce the risk of breast cancer (OR = 0.59, 95%CI, 0.39–0.88) [69]. These observations support the notion herbal tea extracts may be a useful source of bioactive compounds that prevent breast cancer.

Ginseng is a perennial aromatic herb widely used in herbal remedies and dietary supplements. A recent 2 year study with male and female B6C3F1 rats conducted by the National Toxicology Program concluded that the administration of 5 g/kg of ginseng reduced the incidence of mammary gland fibroadenoma [70]. Similar evidence is lacking in humans, however.

## LEUKEMIA

Complete remission of chronic lymphocytic leukemia (CLL) was reported in a 57-year-old man after intake of a Chinese herbal extract, which also inhibited survival of primary CLL cells in vitro. However, the herbal composition of this mixture was not reported [71]. Subsequent studies by the same group revealed that the compound

## TABLE 44.2
## Use of Herbal Supplements in the Prevention and Treatment of Cancer in Human Studies

| Cancer | Reference | Herbal Supplement(s) | Outcome of Study |
|---|---|---|---|
| Multiple | Maggiore et al. [6] | Flaxseed, garlic, saw palmetto, aloe, cinnamon, Green tea extract, bilberry, curcumin, Echinacea | Consumption was more common in older adults with less advanced disease |
| | McCune et al. [18] | Ginkgo biloba, grapeseed oil, milk thistle, black cohosh, ginseng, dong quai, garlic, St. John's Wort | 78% patients used herbal supplements concurrently with chemotherapy, with 28% of patients at risk |
| | Walshe et al. [13] | Multiple | 8% used herbal supplements |
| | Ucan et al. [15] | Stinging nettle, pomegranate juice, raisins | 83% of cancer patients used herbals |
| | Molassiotis et al. [16] | Green tea, essiatic, Chinese herbs, sage, Echinacea, mistletoe, ginseng, gingko biloba, milk thistle | Use increased from 5 to ~14 after cancer diagnosis |
| | Shumay et al. [1] | Multiple | Use was associated with being female, Caucasian, education, and having breast cancer |
| | Ferrucci et al. [2] | Garlic, chamomille, Echinacea, ginseng, gingko biloba | ~70% of patients used supplements after cancer diagnosis |
| Stomach | Cheuk et al. [50] | *G. lucidum* (Lingzhi) | Regression of B-CLL |
| Blood | Battle et al. [71] | Herbal mixture | Associated with remission of CLL |
| | Shanafelt et al. [72] | Green tea extracts | EGCG-containing products were associated with tumor response in B-CLL patients |
| Skin | Kirsch [74] | *V. album* extract | Remission of liver metastasis |
| Breast | Newman et al. [62] | Alfalfa, barley sprouts, bee pollen, bilberry, don, Quai root, Echinacea, garlic, gingko biloba, ginseng, Gotu kola, red clover, silymarin, spirulina, blue green algae | ~21% of women diagnosed with breast cancer used herbal supplements |
| | Chen et al. [60] | *G. lucidum*, sporophyte, ginseng | CAM use among Chinese patients ~77% |
| Colorectal | Ohwada et al. [111] | *Corioulus versicolor* (mushroom) extract | Increased survival and reduced recurrence |
| | McCulloch et al. [49] | Pan-Asian Medicine and vitamins | Reduced risk of death by 95% in Stage I |
| Prostate | Small et al. [20] | PC-SPES[a] | Reduced PSA in hormone-responsive and HRPC subjects |
| | Oh et al. [24] | PC-SPES | Discontinuation of PC-SPES increased PSA |
| | Oh et al. [25] | PC-SPES | Reduced PSA levels by ≥50% in 40% patients |
| | Shabbir et al. [26] | PC-SPES2 | Reduced PSA doubling time in HRPC patients |
| | Pfeifer et al. [21] | PC-SPES | Declined PSA levels with no side effects |
| | de la Taille et al. [22] | PC-SPES | Decreased PSA levels |
| | Moyad et al. [23] | PC-SPES | Reduced PSA levels with estrogenic side effects |
| Lung | Liang et al. [41] | Mixture[b] | Associated with regression of SCC of the lung |
| | McCulloch et al. [43] | *Astragalus*-based meta-analysis | Improved NSCL cancer response |
| | Chen et al. [112] | *Astragalus*-based[c] meta-analysis | Inconclusive about cancer effects |
| | Guo et al. [45] | Mixture | Improved survival in Stage IV adenocarcinoma |

[a] PC-SPES, mixture of *Dendrantherma morifolium, Ganoderma lucidum, Glycyrrhiza glabra, Isatis indigotica, Panax pseudoginseng, Rabdopsia rubescens, S. baicalensis.*

[b] Mixture of *Herba Hedyotis diffusae, R. ophiopogonis, H. taraxaci, R. notoginseng, Radix Panacis quinquefolii, H. houttuyniae, Bulbus Fritillariae thunbergii, Rhizoma Pinelliae preparata.*

[c] Included *Radix Astragali membranaceus, Radix Angelica sinensis, Radix Ophiopogon japonicus, Radix Curcuma zedoaria, Herba Oldenlandia diffusa.*

honokiol, a major constituent of root and stem bark, induced caspase-3, -8, and -9 dependent apoptosis in B-CLL cells. This was accompanied by upregulation of Bax, and downregulation of the survival protein myeloid-cell leukemia sequence 1 (Mcl-1). A case report with four patients diagnosed with B-CLL who self-initiated intake of over-the-counter of epigallocatechin-gallate (EGCG)-containing products documented objective clinical responses [72]. However, no evidence from clinical trials supports the use of EGCG-based products for the prevention or treatment of leukemia.

## LIVER CANCER

Compounds in green tea may be effective in the prevention of liver cancer. For example, the administration of green tea polyphenols to high-risk individuals of liver cancer reduced urinary excretion of 8-hydroxydeoxyguanosine (8-OHdG), a biomarker of oxidative DNA damage, while inducing urinary levels of EGC and epicatechin (EC) [73]. These studies suggested urinary excretion of EGC/EC and 8-OHdG may serve as biomarkers of catechin intake and effect against liver cancer. However, a recent review by the European Food

Safety Agency (EFSA) did not support applications for health claims for green teas and cancer outcomes.

## SKIN CANCER

A case report of a man diagnosed with metastatic melanoma documented subcutaneous therapy with mistletoe extract (*V. album*) induced complete remission of liver metastasis [74]. Effectiveness of long-term treatment of primary intermediate-to-high risk malignant melanoma with fermented *V. album* preparations was reported in a cohort study with 686 cancer patients (329 receiving *V. album*, and 357 subjects as controls) in Germany and Switzerland. A significant longer survival related to tumor was observed in subjects assigned to treatment (two to three subcutaneous injections for 3 months) [75].

According to the National Cancer Institute (http://www.cancer.gov/cancertopics/pdq/cm/essiac/patient), Essiac "is an herbal tea mixture that contains burdock root, Indian rhubarb root, sheep sorrel, and slippery elm bark. It has been claimed to remove toxins from the body, make the immune system stronger, relieve pain, control diabetes, treat AIDS, reduce tumor size, increase cancer survival, and improve quality of life. No clinical trial using Essiac in humans has been reported in a peer-reviewed, scientific journal, and the FDA has not approved the use of Essiac for the treatment of any medical conditions." Essiac and Flor Essence are herbal tea mixtures that are sold worldwide as health tonics or herbal dietary supplements. Essiac was first promoted as a cancer treatment in the 1920s. Flor Essence was created a number of years later. "Supporters of Essiac and Flor Essence suggest that these products make the immune system stronger, have anti-inflammatory effects, and show anticancer activity." However, laboratory, animal, and clinical (human) studies with Essiac and Flor Essence have not reported clear evidence of an anticancer effect. The U.S. Food and Drug Administration has not approved Essiac or Flor Essence as a cancer treatment.

In summary, the evidence is mixed and inconclusive at present for these herbals and cancers. Objective, up to date sources of information include the websites of the National Cancer Institute, the National Center for Complementary and Alternative Medicine, the Office of Dietary Supplements at the National Institutes of Health, as well as the Food and Drug Administration and the European Food Safety Authority.

## FUTURE OF HERBAL RESEARCH AND NEEDS

Unequivocally, in many countries green and black tea are major dietary sources of herbal compounds of which flavan-3-ols catechins (green > black) are the most abundant [76]. Although a reduced risk or a trend for lower cancer risk have been documented for green tea against prostate [77,78], breast [79,80], lung [81], ovarian [82,83], liver [84], and gastric [85] cancer, no association have been found between tea consumption and risk of ovarian [86–88], gastric [89,90], and colon [91] cancer. Nor has EFSA found the data compelling for any of these teas and cancers. The anticancer

effects of herbal tea may be related to dose of intake. For example, some studies documented a protective effect for tea (~18%–25%) with 2 cups/day against lung [81] and endometrial [92] cancer, whereas protective effects against gastric cancer were observed only with consumption of ≥5 cups/day green tea [85]. Clearly much more research is needed.

A limited number of intervention trials have investigated the chemopreventive effects of tea compounds. Intervention trials with tea preparations suggested preventative effects against oral, lung, prostate, and colorectal cancer (reviewed in [93]). In preclinical models, the anticancer effects of EGCG have been related to activation of apoptosis, and inhibition of proliferation and angiogenesis [67]. Molecular targets of EGCG include epidermal growth factor (EGFR) and insulin-like growth factor-1 (IGF-1) receptor, MAPK signaling, and factors involved in apoptosis (p53, B-cell lymphoma 2 [Bcl-2]) and angiogenesis (VEGF). In combination with sulindac [94], EGCG protected against colon tumorigenesis. On the other hand, EGCG did not protect against mammary tumorigenesis [95] and even enhanced colonic inflammation [96]. Preclinical and clinical studies are needed to develop biomarkers of intake and efficacy for human cancer prevention by herbal tea.

Several factors have made estimation of herbal intake and efficacy difficult to make, including incorrect or underreporting; variations in formulations, chemical composition, and disposition; and differences in timing and dose of intake. Quality assurance is an important consideration when developing formulation for cancer applications. Cultivation of botanicals to be used for the preparation of herbal supplements should be standardized to reduce the effects of variations in cultivar and contamination, agricultural and processing practices on chemical composition and bioavailability. Studies of preclinical and clinical efficacy and toxicity are needed before herbal supplements can be recommended for cancer therapy [97].

## ACKNOWLEDGMENT

The authors are grateful to Dr. Johanna Dwyer for suggestions and critical review of the manuscript.

## REFERENCES

1. Shumay DM, Maskarinec G, Gotay CC, Heiby EM, Kakai H. Determinants of the degree of complementary and alternative medicine use among patients with cancer. *J Altern Complement Med* 2002;8(5):661–671.
2. Ferrucci LM, McCorkle R, Smith T, Stein KD, Cartmel B. Factors related to the use of dietary supplements by cancer survivors. *J Altern Complement Med* 2009;15(6):673–680.
3. Cassileth B, Yeung KS, Gubili J. Herbs and other botanicals in cancer patient care. *Curr Treat Options Oncol* 2008;9(2–3):109–116.
4. Naing A, Stephen SK, Frenkel M, Chandhasin C, Hong DS, Lei X, Falchook G, Wheler JJ, Fu S, Kurzrock R. Prevalence of complementary medicine use in a phase 1 clinical trials program: The MD Anderson Cancer Center Experience. *Cancer* 2011;117(22):5142–5150.

5. National Center for Complementary and Alternative Medicine. http://nccam.nih.gov. Accessed on June 01, 2012.

6. Maggiore RJ, Gross CP, Togawa K, Tew WP, Mohile SG, Owusu C, Klepin HD, Lichtman SM, Gajra A, Ramani R, Katheria V, Klapper SM, Hansen K, Hurria A; on behalf of the Cancer and Aging Research Group. Use of complementary medications among older adults with cancer. *Cancer* 2012;118(19):4815–4823. doi: 10.1002/cncr.27427.

7. Barnes PM, Bloom B, Nahin RL. Complementary and alternative medicine use among adults and children: United States, 2007. *Natl Health Stat Report* 2008;(12):1–23.

8. Anderson JG, Taylor AG. Use of complementary therapies for cancer symptom management: Results of the 2007 National Health Interview Survey. *J Altern Complement Med* 2012;18(3):235–241.

9. Smith ME, Bauer-Wu S. Traditional Chinese Medicine for cancer-related symptoms. *Semin Oncol Nurs* 2012;28(1):64–74.

10. Lam YC, Cheng CW, Peng H, Law CK, Huang X, Bian Z. Cancer patients' attitudes towards Chinese medicine: A Hong Kong survey. *Chin Med* 2009;4:25.

11. Baliga MS, Dsouza JJ. Amla (*Emblica officinalis* Gaertn), a wonder berry in the treatment and prevention of cancer. *Eur J Cancer Prev* 2011;20(3):225–239.

12. Baliga MS. Triphala, Ayurvedic formulation for treating and preventing cancer: A review. *J Altern Complement Med* 2010;16(12):1301–1308.

13. Walshe R, James EL, MacDonald-Wicks L, Boyes AW, Zucca A, Girgis A, Lecathelinais C. Socio-demographic and medical correlates of the use of biologically based complementary and alternative medicines amongst recent Australian cancer survivors. *Prev Med* 2012;54(1):23–26.

14. Adams J, Sibbritt D, Young AF. Naturopathy/herbalism consultations by mid-aged Australian women who have cancer. *Eur J Cancer Care (Engl)* 2005;14(5):443–447.

15. Ucan O, Pehlivan S, Ovayolu N, Sevinc A, Camci C. The use of complementary therapies in cancer patients: A questionnaire-based descriptive survey from southeastern Turkey. *Am J Clin Oncol* 2008;31(6):589–594.

16. Molassiotis A, Fernandez-Ortega P, Pud D, Ozden G, Scott JA, Panteli V, Margulies A et al. Use of complementary and alternative medicine in cancer patients: A European survey. *Ann Oncol* 2005;16(4):655–663.

17. European Medicines Agency. http://www.ema.europa.eu/ema. Accessed on June 18, 2012.

18. McCune JS, Hatfield AJ, Blackburn AA, Leith PO, Livingston RB, Ellis GK. Potential of chemotherapy-herb interactions in adult cancer patients. *Support Care Cancer* 2004;12(6):454–462.

19. Olaku O, White JD. Herbal therapy use by cancer patients: A literature review on case reports. *Eur J Cancer* 2011;47(4):508–514.

20. Small EJ, Frohlich MW, Bok R, Shinohara K, Grossfeld G, Rozenblat Z, Kelly WK, Corry M, Reese DM. Prospective trial of the herbal supplement PC-SPES in patients with progressive prostate cancer. *J Clin Oncol* 2000;18(21):3595–3603.

21. Pfeifer BL, Pirani JF, Hamann SR, Klippel KF. PC-SPES, a dietary supplement for the treatment of hormone-refractory prostate cancer. *BJU Int* 2000;85(4):481–485.

22. de la Taille A, Hayek OR, Burchardt M, Burchardt T, Katz AE. Role of herbal compounds (PC-SPES) in hormone-refractory prostate cancer: Two case reports. *J Altern Complement Med* 2000;6(5):449–451.

23. Moyad MA, Pienta KJ, Montie JE. Use of PC-SPES, a commercially available supplement for prostate cancer, in a patient with hormone-naive disease. *Urology* 1999;54(2):319–323.

24. Oh WK, George DJ, Kantoff PW. Rapid rise of serum prostate specific antigen levels after discontinuation of the herbal therapy PC-SPES in patients with advanced prostate carcinoma: Report of four cases. *Cancer* 2002;94(3):686–689.

25. Oh WK, Kantoff PW, Weinberg V, Jones G, Rini BI, Derynck MK, Bok R, Smith MR, Bubley GJ, Rosen RT, DiPaola RS, Small EJ. Prospective, multicenter, randomized phase II trial of the herbal supplement, PC-SPES, and diethylstilbestrol in patients with androgen-independent prostate cancer. *J Clin Oncol* 2004;22(18):3705–3712.

26. Shabbir M, Love J, Montgomery B. Phase I trial of PC-Spes2 in advanced hormone refractory prostate cancer. *Oncol Rep* 2008;19(3):831–835.

27. Du G, Zhang ZW, Zhang YK, Guo JM. Chinese herbal medicine PC-SPES II induces the apoptosis of androgen-independent prostate carcinoma cell line PC-3. *Zhonghua Nan Ke Xue* 2007;13(6):563–567.

28. Ikezoe T, Chen SS, Yang Y, Heber D, Taguchi H, Koeffler HP. PC-SPES: Molecular mechanism to induce apoptosis and down-regulate expression of PSA in LNCaP human prostate cancer cells. *Int J Oncol* 2003;23(5):1461–1470.

29. Ikezoe T, Chen SS, Tong XJ, Heber D, Taguchi H, Koeffler HP. Oridonin induces growth inhibition and apoptosis of a variety of human cancer cells. *Int J Oncol* 2003;23(4):1187–1193.

30. Yang Y, Ikezoe T, Zheng Z, Taguchi H, Koeffler HP, Zhu WG. Saw Palmetto induces growth arrest and apoptosis of androgen-dependent prostate cancer LNCaP cells via inactivation of STAT 3 and androgen receptor signaling. *Int J Oncol* 2007;31(3):593–600.

31. Bonham M, Posakony J, Coleman I, Montgomery B, Simon J, Nelson PS. Characterization of chemical constituents in *Scutellaria baicalensis* with antiandrogenic and growth-inhibitory activities toward prostate carcinoma. *Clin Cancer Res* 2005;11(10):3905–3914.

32. Ye F, Jiang S, Volshonok H, Wu J, Zhang DY. Molecular mechanism of anti-prostate cancer activity of *Scutellaria baicalensis* extract. *Nutr Cancer* 2007;57(1):100–110.

33. Adams LS, Seeram NP, Hardy ML, Carpenter C, Heber D. Analysis of the interactions of botanical extract combinations against the viability of prostate cancer cell lines. *Evid Based Complement Alternat Med* 2006;3(1):117–124.

34. Chung VQ, Tattersall M, Cheung HT. Interactions of a herbal combination that inhibits growth of prostate cancer cells. *Cancer Chemother Pharmacol* 2004;53(5):384–390.

35. Bonham MJ, Galkin A, Montgomery B, Stahl WL, Agus D, Nelson PS. Effects of the herbal extract PC-SPES on microtubule dynamics and paclitaxel-mediated prostate tumor growth inhibition. *J Natl Cancer Inst* 2002;94(21):1641–1647.

36. Shariat SF, Lamb DJ, Iyengar RG, Roehrborn CG, Slawin KM. Herbal/hormonal dietary supplement possibly associated with prostate cancer progression. *Clin Cancer Res* 2008;14(2):607–611.

37. Nortier JL, Martinez MC, Schmeiser HH, Arlt VM, Bieler CA, Petein M, Depierreux MF, De Pauw L, Abramowicz D, Vereerstraeten P, Vanherweghem JL. Urothelial carcinoma associated with the use of a Chinese herb (*Aristolochia fangchi*). *N Engl J Med* 2000;342(23):1686–1692.

38. Baak JP, Gyllenhaal C, Liu L, Guo H, Block KI. Prognostic proof and possible therapeutic mechanisms of herbal medicine in patients with metastatic lung and colon cancer. *Integr Cancer Ther* 2011;10(3):NP1–NP11.

39. Ikezoe T, Yang Y, Saitoh T, Heber D, McKenna R, Taguchi H, Koeffler HP. PC-SPES down-regulates COX-2 via inhibition of NF-kappaB and C/EBPbeta in non-small cell lung cancer cells. *Int J Oncol* 2006;29(2):453–461.

40. Liu JJ, Huang RW, Lin DJ, Peng J, Zhang M, Pan X, Hou M, Wu XY, Lin Q, Chen F. Ponicidin, an ent-kaurane diterpenoid derived from a constituent of the herbal supplement PC-SPES, *Rabdosia rubescens*, induces apoptosis by activation of caspase-3 and mitochondrial events in lung cancer cells in vitro. *Cancer Invest* 2006;24(2):136–148.

41. Liang HL, Xue CC, Li CG. Regression of squamous cell carcinoma of the lung by Chinese herbal medicine: A case with an 8-year follow-up. *Lung Cancer* 2004;43(3):355–360.

42. Hegde P, Maddur MS, Friboulet A, Bayry J, Kaveri SV. *Viscum album* exerts anti-inflammatory effect by selectively inhibiting cytokine-induced expression of cyclooxygenase-2. *PLoS ONE* 2011;6(10):e26312.

43. McCulloch M, See C, Shu XJ, Broffman M, Kramer A, Fan WY, Gao J, Lieb W, Shieh K, Colford JM Jr. *Astragalus*-based Chinese herbs and platinum-based chemotherapy for advanced non-small-cell lung cancer: Meta-analysis of randomized trials. *J Clin Oncol* 2006;24(3):419–430.

44. Chen LG, Hung LY, Tsai KW, Pan YS, Tsai YD, Li YZ, Liu YW. Wogonin, a bioactive flavonoid in herbal tea, inhibits inflammatory cyclooxygenase-2 gene expression in human lung epithelial cancer cells. *Mol Nutr Food Res* 2008;52(11):1349–1357.

45. Guo H, Liu JX, Xu L, Madebo T, Baak JP. Traditional Chinese medicine herbal treatment may have a relevant impact on the prognosis of patients with stage IV adenocarcinoma of the lung treated with platinum-based chemotherapy or combined targeted therapy and chemotherapy. *Integr Cancer Ther* 2011;10(2):127–137.

46. Hu YW, Liu CY, Du CM, Zhang J, Wu WQ, Gu ZL. Induction of apoptosis in human hepatocarcinoma SMMC-7721 cells in vitro by flavonoids from *Astragalus complanatus*. *J Ethnopharmacol* 2009;123(2):293–301.

47. Li N, Sun Z, Han C, Chen J. The chemopreventive effects of tea on human oral precancerous mucosa lesions. *Proc Soc Exp Biol Med* 1999;220(4):218–224.

48. Tsao AS, Liu D, Martin J, Tang XM, Lee JJ, El-Naggar AK et al. Phase II randomized, placebo-controlled trial of green tea extract in patients with high-risk oral premalignant lesions. *Cancer Prev Res* 2009;2(11):931–941.

49. McCulloch M, Broffman M, van der Laan M, Hubbard A, Kushi L, Abrams DI, Gao J, Colford JM Jr. Colon cancer survival with herbal medicine and vitamins combined with standard therapy in a whole-systems approach: Ten-year follow-up data analyzed with marginal structural models and propensity score methods. *Integr Cancer Ther* 2011;10(3):240–259.

50. Cheuk W, Chan JK, Nuovo G, Chan MK, Fok M. Regression of gastric large B-Cell lymphoma accompanied by a florid lymphoma-like T-cell reaction: Immunomodulatory effect of *Ganoderma lucidum* (Lingzhi)? *Int J Surg Pathol* 2007;15(2):180–186.

51. Huerta S, Arteaga JR, Irwin RW, Ikezoe T, Heber D, Koeffler HP. PC-SPES inhibits colon cancer growth in vitro and in vivo. *Cancer Res* 2002;62(18):5204–5209.

52. Encalada MA, Hoyos KM, Rehecho S, Berasategi I, de Ciriano MG, Ansorena D, Astiasarán I, Navarro-Blasco I, Cavero RY, Calvo MI. Anti-proliferative effect of *Melissa officinalis* on human colon cancer cell line. *Plant Foods Hum Nutr* 2011;66(4):328–334.

53. Wang E, Bussom S, Chen J, Quinn C, Bedognetti D, Lam W, Guan F, Jiang Z, Mark Y, Zhao Y, Stroncek DF, White J, Marincola FM, Cheng YC. Interaction of a traditional Chinese Medicine (PHY906) and CPT-11 on the inflammatory process in the tumor microenvironment. *BMC Med Genomics* 2011;4:38.

54. Lam W, Bussom S, Guan F, Jiang Z, Zhang W, Gullen EA, Liu SH, Cheng YC. The four-herb Chinese medicine PHY906 reduces chemotherapy-induced gastrointestinal toxicity. *Sci Transl Med* 2010;2(45):45ra59.

55. Kummar S, Copur MS, Rose M, Wadler S, Stephenson J, O'Rourke M, Brenckman W, Tilton R, Liu SH, Jiang Z, Su T, Cheng YC, Chu E. A phase I study of the Chinese herbal medicine PHY906 as a modulator of irinotecan-based chemotherapy in patients with advanced colorectal cancer. *Clin Colorectal Cancer* 2011;10(2):85–96.

56. Brandin H, Viitanen E, Myrberg O, Arvidsson AK. Effects of herbal medicinal products and food supplements on induction of CYP1A2, CYP3A4 and MDR1 in the human colon carcinoma cell line LS180. *Phytother Res* 2007;21(3):239–244.

57. Volate SR, Davenport DM, Muga SJ, Wargovich MJ. Modulation of aberrant crypt foci and apoptosis by dietary herbal supplements (quercetin, curcumin, silymarin, ginseng and rutin). *Carcinogenesis* 2005;26(8):1450–1456.

58. Shimizu M, Fukutomi Y, Ninomiya M, Nagura K, Kato T, Araki H et al. Green tea extracts for the prevention of metachronous colorectal adenomas: A pilot study. *Cancer Epidemiol Biomarkers Prev* 2008;17(11):3020–3025.

59. Gerber B, Scholz C, Reimer T, Briese V, Janni W. Complementary and alternative therapeutic approaches in patients with early breast cancer: A systematic review. *Breast Cancer Res Treat* 2006;95(3):199–209.

60. Chen Z, Gu K, Zheng Y, Zheng W, Lu W, Shu XO. The use of complementary and alternative medicine among Chinese women with breast cancer. *J Altern Complement Med* 2008;14(8):1049–1055.

61. Ganz PA, Desmond KA, Leedham B, Rowland JH, Meyerowitz BE, Belin TR. Quality of life in long-term, disease-free survivors of breast cancer: A follow-up study. *J Natl Cancer Inst* 2002;94(1):39–49. Erratum in: *J Natl Cancer Inst* 2002;94(6):463.

62. Newman V, Rock CL, Faerber S, Flatt SW, Wright FA, Pierce JP. Dietary supplement use by women at risk for breast cancer recurrence. The Women's Healthy Eating and Living Study Group. *J Am Diet Assoc* 1998;98(3):285–292.

63. Bright-Gbebry M, Makambi KH, Rohan JP, Llanos AA, Rosenberg L, Palmer JR, Adams-Campbell LL. Use of multivitamins, folic acid and herbal supplements among breast cancer survivors: The black women's health study. *BMC Complement Altern Med* 2011;11:30.

64. Jiang J, Sliva D. Novel medicinal mushroom blend suppresses growth and invasiveness of human breast cancer cells. *Int J Oncol.* 2010;37(6):1529–1536.

65. Tamaki H, Satoh H, Hori S, Ohtani H, Sawada Y. Inhibitory effects of herbal extracts on breast cancer resistance protein (BCRP) and structure-inhibitory potency relationship of isoflavonoids. *Drug Metab Pharmacokinet* 2010;25(2):170–179.

66. Kulp KS, Montgomery JL, Nelson DO, Cutter B, Latham ER, Shattuck DL, Klotz DM, Bennett LM. Essiac and Flor-Essence herbal tonics stimulate the in vitro growth of human breast cancer cells. *Breast Cancer Res Treat* 2006;98(3):249–259.

67. Yang CS, Wang H. Mechanistic issues concerning cancer prevention by tea catechins. *Mol Nutr Food Res.* 2011;55(6):819–831.

68. Iwasaki M, Inoue M, Sasazuki S, Miura T, Sawada N, Yamaji T et al. Plasma tea polyphenol levels and subsequent risk of breast cancer among Japanese women: A nested case-control study. *Breast Cancer Res Treat* 2010;124(3):827–834.

69. Luo J, Gao YT, Chow WH, Shu XO, Li H, Yang G et al. Urinary polyphenols and breast cancer risk: Results from the Shanghai Women's Health Study. *Breast Cancer Res Treat* 2010;120(3):693–702.

70. National Toxicology Program. Toxicology and carcinogenesis studies of ginseng (CAS No. 50647-08-0) in F344/N rats and B6C3F1 mice (gavage studies). *Natl Toxicol Program Tech Rep Ser* 2011;(567):1–149.

71. Battle TE, Castro-Malaspina H, Gribben JG, Frank DA. Sustained complete remission of CLL associated with the use of a Chinese herbal extract: Case report and mechanistic analysis. *Leuk Res* 2003;27(9):859–863.

72. Shanafelt TD, Lee YK, Call TG, Nowakowski GS, Dingli D, Zent CS, Kay NE. Clinical effects of oral green tea extracts in four patients with low grade B-cell malignancies. *Leuk Res* 2006;30(6):707–712.

73. Luo H, Tang L, Tang M, Billam M, Huang T, Yu J et al. Phase IIa chemoprevention trial of green tea polyphenols in high-risk individuals of liver cancer: Modulation of urinary excretion of green tea polyphenols and 8-hydroxydeoxyguanosine. *Carcinogenesis* 2006;27(2):262–268.

74. Kirsch A. Successful treatment of metastatic malignant melanoma with *Viscum album* extract (Iscador M). *J Altern Complement Med* 2007;13(4):443–445.

75. Augustin M, Bock PR, Hanisch J, Karasmann M, Schneider B. Safety and efficacy of the long-term adjuvant treatment of primary intermediate- to high-risk malignant melanoma (UICC/AJCC stage II and III) with a standardized fermented European mistletoe (*Viscum album* L.) extract. Results from a multi-center, comparative, epidemiological cohort study in Germany and Switzerland. *Arzneimittelforschung* 2005;55(1):38–49.

76. U.S. Department of Agriculture, Agricultural Research Service. 2007. USDA Database for the Flavonoid Content of Selected Foods, Release 2.1. Nutrient Data Laboratory Home Page: http://www.ars.usda.gov/nutrientdata. Accessed June 1, 2012.

77. Boehm K, Borrelli F, Ernst E, Habacher G, Hung SK, Milazzo S et al. Green tea (*Camellia sinensis*) for the prevention of cancer. *Cochrane Database Syst Rev* 2009;(3):CD005004.

78. Zheng J, Yang B, Huang T, Yu Y, Yang J, Li D. Green tea and black tea consumption and prostate cancer risk: An exploratory meta-analysis of observational studies. *Nutr Cancer* 2011;63(5):663–672.

79. Sun CL, Yuan JM, Koh WP, Yu MC. Green tea, black tea and breast cancer risk: A meta-analysis of epidemiological studies. *Carcinogenesis* 2006;27(7):1310–1315.

80. Seely D, Mills EJ, Wu P, Verma S, Guyatt GH. The effects of green tea consumption on incidence of breast cancer and recurrence of breast cancer: A systematic review and meta-analysis. *Integr Cancer Ther* 2005;4(2):144–155.

81. Tang N, Wu Y, Zhou B, Wang B, Yu R. Green tea, black tea consumption and risk of lung cancer: A meta-analysis. *Lung Cancer* 2009;65(3):274–283.

82. Nagle CM, Olsen CM, Bain CJ, Whiteman DC, Green AC, Webb PM. Tea consumption and risk of ovarian cancer. *Cancer Causes Control* 2010;21(9):1485–1491.

83. Butler LM, Wu AH. Green and black tea in relation to gynecologic cancers. *Mol Nutr Food Res* 2011;55(6):931–940.

84. Sing MF, Yang WS, Gao S, Gao J, Xiang YB. Epidemiological studies of the association between tea drinking and primary liver cancer: A meta-analysis. *Eur J Cancer Prev* 2011;20(3):157–165.

85. Kang H, Rha SY, Oh KW, Nam CM. Green tea consumption and stomach cancer risk: A meta-analysis. *Epidemiol Health* 2010;26;32:e2010001.

86. Braem MG, Onland-Moret NC, Schouten LJ, Tjonneland A, Hansen L, Dahm CC et al. Coffee and tea consumption and the risk of ovarian cancer: A prospective cohort study and updated meta-analysis. *Am J Clin Nutr* 2012;95(5):1172–1181.

87. Zhou B, Yang L, Wang L, Shi Y, Zhu H, Tang N, Wang B. The association of tea consumption with ovarian cancer risk: A metaanalysis. *Am J Obstet Gynecol* 2007;197(6):594.e1–e6.

88. Steevens J, Schouten LJ, Verhage BA, Goldbohm RA, van den Brandt PA. Tea and coffee drinking and ovarian cancer risk: Results from the Netherlands Cohort Study and a meta-analysis. *Br J Cancer* 2007;5;97(9):1291–1294.

89. Zhou Y, Li N, Zhuang W, Liu G, Wu T, Yao X et al. Green tea and gastric cancer risk: Meta-analysis of epidemiologic studies. *Asia Pac J Clin Nutr* 2008;17(1):159–165.

90. Myung SK, Bae WK, Oh SM, Kim Y, Ju W, Sung J et al. Green tea consumption and risk of stomach cancer: A meta-analysis of epidemiologic studies. *Int J Cancer* 2009;1;124(3):670–677. Erratum in: *Int J Cancer* 2009;15;124(6):1496.

91. Sun CL, Yuan JM, Koh WP, Yu MC. Green tea, black tea and colorectal cancer risk: A meta-analysis of epidemiologic studies. *Carcinogenesis* 2006;27(7):1301–1309.

92. Tang NP, Li H, Qiu YL, Zhou GM, Ma J. Tea consumption and risk of endometrial cancer: A metaanalysis. *Am J Obstet Gynecol* 2009;201(6):605.e1–e8.

93. Chow HH, Hakim IA. Pharmacokinetic and chemoprevention studies on tea in humans. *Pharmacol Res* 2011;64(2):105–112.

94. Orner GA, Dashwood WM, Blum CA, Diaz GD, Li Q, Dashwood RH. Suppression of tumorigenesis in the Apc(min) mouse: Down-regulation of beta-catenin signaling by a combination of tea plus sulindac. *Carcinogenesis* 2003;24(2):263–267.

95. Whitsett T, Carpenter M, Lamartiniere CA. Resveratrol, but not EGCG, in the diet suppresses DMBA-induced mammary cancer in rats. *J Carcinog* 2006;15:5–15.

96. Kim M, Murakami A, Miyamoto S, Tanaka T, Ohigashi H. The modifying effects of green tea polyphenols on acute colitis and inflammation-associated colon carcinogenesis in male ICR mice. *Biofactors* 2010;36(1):43–51.

97. Eng C. Are herbal medicines ripe for the cancer clinic? *Sci Transl Med* 2010;2(45):45ps41.

98. Ngamkitidechakul C, Jaijoy K, Hansakul P, Soonthornchareonnon N, Sireeratawong S. Antitumour effects of *Phyllanthus emblica* L.: Induction of cancer cell apoptosis and inhibition of in vivo tumour promotion and in vitro invasion of human cancer cells. *Phytother Res* 2010;24(9):1405–1413.

99. Yadav B, Bajaj A, Saxena M, Saxena AK. In vitro anticancer activity of the root, stem and leaves of *Withania somnifera* against various human cancer cell lines. *Indian J Pharm Sci* 2010;72(5):659–663.

100. Ryu B, Ro W, Park JW, Bu Y, Lee BJ, Lim S, Kim J, Yoon SW. Bojanggunbi-tang, a traditional Korean herbal prescription, ameliorates colonic inflammation induced by dextran sulfate sodium and 2,4,6-trinitrobenzene sulfonic acid in mice. *J Ethnopharmacol* 2011;135(2):582–585.

101. Yi W, Wetzstein HY. Anti-tumorigenic activity of five culinary and medicinal herbs grown under greenhouse conditions and their combination effects. *J Sci Food Agric* 2011;91(10):1849–1854.

102. Sze SC, Wong KL, Liu WK, Ng TB, Wong JH, Cheung HP, Yow CM, Chu ES, Qing Liu, Hu YM, Tsang KW, Lee WS, Yao Tong. Regulation of p21, MMP-1, and MDR-1 expression in human colon carcinoma HT29 cells by Tian Xian liquid, a Chinese medicinal formula, in vitro and in vivo. *Integr Cancer Ther* 2011;10(1):58–69.

103. Lee SJ, Park K, Ha SD, Kim WJ, Moon SK. *Gleditsia sinensis* thorn extract inhibits human colon cancer cells: The role of ERK1/2, G2/M-phase cell cycle arrest and p53 expression. *Phytother Res* 2010;24(12):1870–1876.

104. Yusup A, Upur H, Umar A, Berke B, Moore N. Ethanol extract of Abnormal Savda Munziq, a herbal preparation of traditional Uighur medicine, inhibits Caco-2 cells proliferation via cell cycle arrest and apoptosis. *Evid Based Complement Alternat Med* 2012;2012:926329.

105. Xu Y, Xu G, Liu L, Xu D, Liu J. Anti-invasion effect of rosmarinic acid via the extracellular signal-regulated kinase and oxidation-reduction pathway in Ls174-T cells. *J Cell Biochem* 2010;111(2):370–379.

106. Chia JS, Du JL, Hsu WB, Sun A, Chiang CP, Wang WB. Inhibition of metastasis, angiogenesis, and tumor growth by Chinese herbal cocktail Tien-Hsien Liquid. *BMC Cancer* 2010;10:175.

107. Tang YJ, Yang JS, Lin CF, Shyu WC, Tsuzuki M, Lu CC, Chen YF, Lai KC. *Houttuynia cordata* Thunb extract induces apoptosis through mitochondrial-dependent pathway in HT-29 human colon adenocarcinoma cells. *Oncol Rep* 2009;22(5):1051–1056.

108. Wang CZ, Li XL, Wang QF, Mehendale SR, Fishbein AB, Han AH, Sun S, Yuan CS. The mitochondrial pathway is involved in American ginseng-induced apoptosis of SW-480 colon cancer cells. *Oncol Rep* 2009;21(3):577–584.

109. Battle TE, Arbiser J, Frank DA. The natural product honokiol induces caspase-dependent apoptosis in B-cell chronic lymphocytic leukemia (B-CLL) cells. *Blood* 2005;106(2):690–697.

110. Jeong JC, Jang SW, Kim TH, Kwon CH, Kim YK. Mulberry fruit (*Moris fructus*) extracts induce human glioma cell death in vitro through ROS-dependent mitochondrial pathway and inhibits glioma tumor growth in vivo. *Nutr Cancer* 2010;62(3):402–412.

111. Ohwada S, Kawate S, Ikeya T, Yokomori T, Kusaba T, Roppongi T, Takahashi T, Nakamura S, Kawashima Y, Nakajima T, Morishita Y; Gunma Oncology Study Group (GOSG). Adjuvant therapy with protein-bound polysaccharide K and Tegafur uracil in patients with stage II or III colorectal cancer: Randomized, controlled trial. *Dis Colon Rectum* 2003;46(8):1060–1068.

112. Chen S, Flower A, Ritchie A, Liu J, Molassiotis A, Yu H, Lewith G. Oral Chinese herbal medicine (CHM) as an adjuvant treatment during chemotherapy for non-small cell lung cancer: A systematic review. *Lung Cancer* 2010;68(2):137–145.

# Part V

## Clinical Nutrition

# 45 Nutritional Assessment in the Clinical Setting

*Dong Wook Kim, Lalita Khaodhiar, and Caroline M. Apovian*

## CONTENTS

## INTRODUCTION

Nutrition assessment is the comprehensive approach used to identify patients' nutrition status and malnutrition and requires an integration of detailed medical and nutritional history, physical examination, anthropometric measurement, and laboratory tests (Table 45.1). In the clinical setting, many acute and chronic illnesses relate to the patients' nutritional status. Moreover, malnutrition is not uncommon and its prevalence in the hospital setting has been reported to be between 20% and 50%.[1] An appropriate nutrition assessment is necessary in identifying malnutrition, and it should be followed by intensive nutritional intervention in appropriate cases. Proper nutritional management will reduce complications associated with malnutrition and improve clinical outcomes in both the inpatient and the outpatient setting.

This chapter reviews the definition and classifications of malnutrition as well as nutritional assessment parameters, which include medical and nutritional history, physical examination, anthropometric measurement, and specific laboratory tests.

## DEFINITION AND CLASSIFICATIONS OF MALNUTRITION

Malnutrition is defined as an inadequate or imbalanced nutritional status, which includes both "undernutrition" and "overnutrition." Like undernutrition, overnutrition also increases morbidity and mortality, causes decreased function and quality of life, higher health care costs, and requires intensive nutritional intervention.[2] Undernutrition includes both micronutrient (vitamins, minerals, trace elements, essential fatty acids) deficiency and macronutrient deficiency, which is also called "protein energy malnutrition" (Figure 45.1).

Standardized definitions for the diagnosis and characterization of malnutrition did not exist until recently. The diagnostic approaches varied widely and had poor sensitivity and specificity, which caused confusion and misdiagnosis.[2]

In 2012, the Academy of Nutrition and Dietetics and the American Society for Parenteral and Enteral Nutrition (ASPEN) proposed etiologic-based definitions that take the degree of inflammatory response into consideration. These etiologic-based definitions were classified into three categories: starvation-related malnutrition, chronic disease–related malnutrition, and acute disease–related malnutrition.[2,3] As part of these three categories, six characteristics of malnutrition were further defined: insufficient energy intake, weight loss, loss of muscle mass, loss of subcutaneous fat, localized or generalized fluid accumulation, and diminished functional status as measured by hand grip strength. The identification of two or more of the six parameters is required for the malnutrition diagnosis (Table 45.2).

## MEDICAL AND NUTRITIONAL HISTORY

Obtaining a thorough medical history including hospitalizations, operations, major injuries, chronic illnesses, significant acute illnesses, alcohol intake, and clinical diagnoses is particularly useful in raising suspicion for the presence of malnutrition and the inflammatory response in any given patient. One of the strongest predictors of outcome is preadmission weight loss. Thus determining the patient's weight

**TABLE 45.1**

**Systematic Approach to Nutrition Assessment**

- History and clinical diagnosis can be a helpful guide to raise suspicion for the presence of inflammation and malnutrition
- Clinical signs and physical examination

   Clinical indicators of inflammation may include fever or hypothermia as well as other nonspecific signs of systemic inflammatory response such as tachycardia

   Physical examination can reveal signs of edema, weight gain/loss, and specific nutrient deficiencies
- Anthropometric data

   Weight loss and underweight status are well-validated indicators of malnutrition. Height, weight, skin-folds, circumferences, and other assessments of body composition are helpful
- Laboratory indicators of inflammatory response and possible protein malnutrition (serum albumin, prealbumin) should be interpreted with caution. Other useful laboratory indicators of inflammation can include elevated CRP, white blood cell count, and glucose. Negative nitrogen balance and elevated resting energy expenditure may also be used to support the presence of systemic inflammatory response
- Dietary data may be obtained in practical fashion using a modified diet history and/or 24 h recall
- Functional outcomes such as strength and physical performance may also be tested as additional supportive findings

*Source:*   Adapted from *A.S.P.E.N. Adult Nutrition Support Core Curriculum*, 3rd edn., A.S.P.E.N., Silver Spring, MD, 2012.

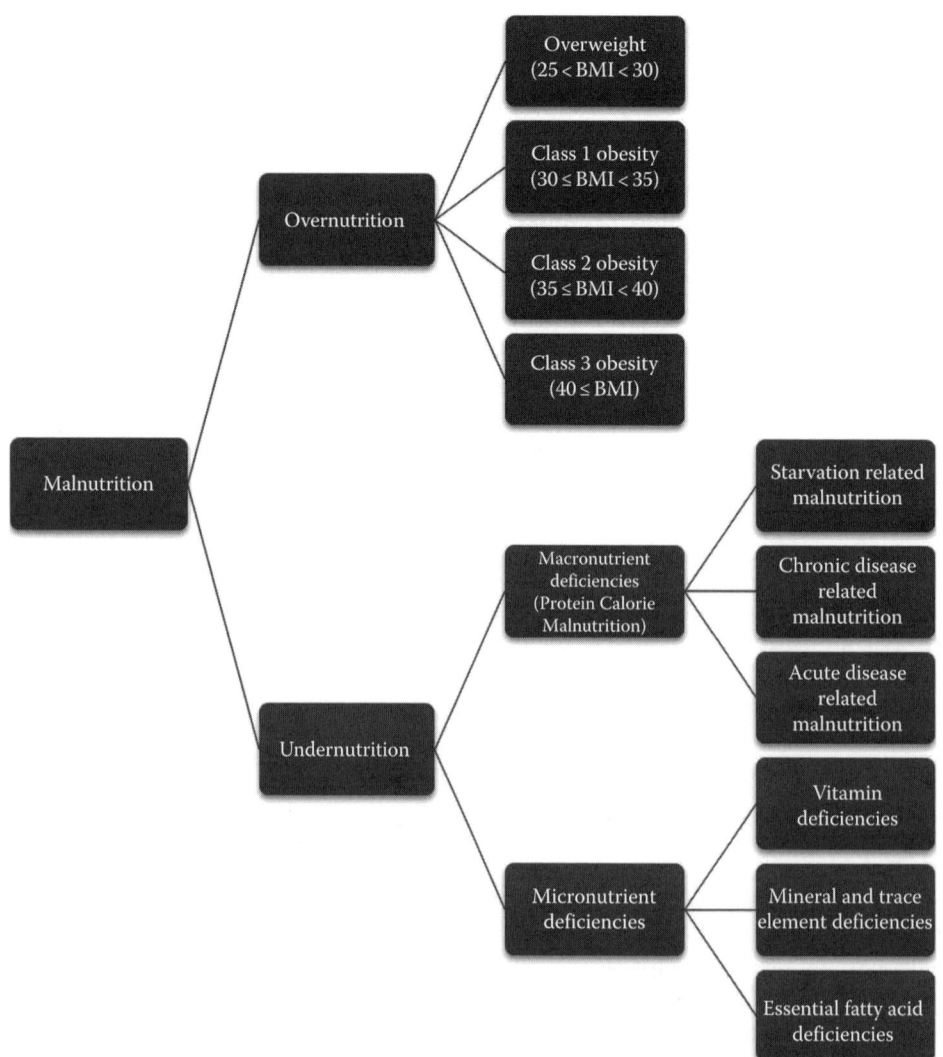

**FIGURE 45.1**   Classification of malnutrition.

**TABLE 45.2**

**Etiology-Based Malnutrition Definitions and Clinical Characteristics**

| Etiology-based malnutrition definitions | Starvation-related malnutrition | Chronic disease–related malnutrition | Acute disease–related malnutrition |
|---|---|---|---|
| Inflammation | None | Mild to moderate | Severe |
| Related disorders | Pure starvation, anorexia nervosa | Organ failure, cancer, rheumatoid disease, sarcopenic obesity | Sepsis, trauma, burns, closed head injury |
| Characteristics (identification of two or more) | Insufficient energy intake Weight loss Loss of muscle mass Loss of subcutaneous fat Localized or generalized fluid accumulation Diminished functional status as measured by hand grip strength | | |

*Source:* White, J.V. et al., *J. Parenter. Enteral. Nutr.*, 36, 275, 2012.

loss history is an essential nutrition assessment parameter.[4] It is also often a sign of an underlying occult disease or inflammatory condition. It is important to inquire about both the amount and the duration of weight loss. For example, a recent unintentional weight loss of 5% of body weight over the preceding 1 month or 10% over 6 months suggests severe malnutrition, whereas a loss of 30% of body weight over 6 months is usually life-threatening. Involuntary weight loss carries a greater nutritional risk than intentional weight loss, as long as the patient followed a weight loss plan based on sound nutritional practices. However, the current popularity of "fad diets" that provide inadequate nutrient content increases the likelihood that even intentional weight loss may be associated with nutritional deficiency and poor clinical outcome.

Several medical and surgical conditions and chronic diseases can place patients at increased risk for malnutrition.[4] Such conditions or diseases may contribute to malnutrition by increasing nutrition requirements or compromising nutrient intake and/or absorption. For example, conditions often characterized by severe acute inflammatory responses include critical illness, major infection/sepsis, adult respiratory distress syndrome, systemic inflammatory response syndrome, severe burns, major abdominal surgery, multiple traumas, and closed head injury. Many other conditions or diseases are more typically associated with a mild to moderate chronic inflammatory response (Table 45.3). Note that in hospitalized patients, acute inflammatory events are frequently superimposed on those with chronic conditions; for example, a patient with chronic obstructive pulmonary disease is admitted to the hospital with pneumonia and acute respiratory failure or a patient with diabetes mellitus develops a urinary tract infection and a hyperosmolar nonketotic state.

A thorough review of medications the patient is taking is an essential component of the nutrition assessment.

**TABLE 45.3**

**Association of Medical/Surgical Conditions and Chronic Diseases with Nutrition Risk and/or Inflammatory Response**

- Look for medical or surgical conditions or chronic disease that can place one at nutrition risk secondary to increased requirements, or compromised intake or assimilation such as critical illness, severe burns, major abdominal surgery, multitrauma, closed head injury, previous gastrointestinal surgery, severe gastrointestinal hemorrhage, enterocutaneous fistula, gastrointestinal obstruction, mesenteric ischemia, severe acute pancreatitis, chronic pancreatitis, inflammatory bowel disease, celiac disease, bacterial overgrowth, solid or hematologic malignancy, bone marrow transplant, acquired immune deficiency syndrome, and organ failure/transplant (kidney, liver, heart, lung, or gut).
- A number of conditions or diseases are often characterized by severe acute inflammatory response, including critical illness, major infection/sepsis, adult respiratory distress syndrome, systemic inflammatory response syndrome, severe burns, major abdominal surgery, multitrauma, and closed head injury.
- Many conditions or diseases are more typically associated with mild to moderate chronic inflammatory response. Examples include cardiovascular disease, congestive heart failure, cystic fibrosis, inflammatory bowel disease, celiac disease, chronic pancreatitis, sarcopenic obesity, diabetes mellitus, metabolic syndrome, cerebrovascular accident, rheumatoid arthritis, solid tumors, hematologic malignancies, neuromuscular disease, dementia, organ failure/transplant (kidney, liver, heart, lung, or gut), periodontal disease, pressure wounds, and chronic obstructive pulmonary disease. Note that acute exacerbations, infections, or other complications may superimpose acute inflammatory response on such conditions or diseases.
- Examples of starvation-associated conditions that generally have little or no inflammatory component include anorexia nervosa or compromised intake in the setting of major depression.

A detailed report of ingestion of multivitamins, minerals, laxatives, topical medications, over-the-counter medications and products such as nutrition supplements should be obtained. Clinicians should have knowledge of the potential drug–nutrient interactions of medications that they prescribe. Certain drugs may promote anorexia or interfere with the absorption, metabolism, and excretion of nutrients. Certain foods and alcoholic beverages may also modify drug absorption, metabolism, and excretion.

## DIETARY ASSESSMENT

The purpose of obtaining dietary information is to assess the patients' nutritional status, to identify patients with inadequate or imbalanced food or nutrient intakes and to help formulate a nutrition treatment plan. The most commonly used dietary assessment methods in clinical settings include the 24 h recall and diet history.[5] The diet history may be obtained from the patient, medical records, family, and caregivers. In hospitalized patients, calorie counts can be conducted by the nursing or dietary staff. The 24 h recall is an informal and qualitative method which elicits all the foods and beverages the patient has consumed in the preceding 24 h. Although diet information is easily obtained using this method, it may not be a true reflection of the patient's usual intake. A modified diet history is a retrospective measure of dietary information, and patients are asked to recall his or her typical daily intake including amounts of foods consumed and the frequency of consumption. This method provides more information about intake patterns than the others, and tends to reveal long-term dietary habits with greater accuracy. However, only limited information about actual quantities of foods and drinks consumed is obtained using this method. In addition, people who eat a wide variety of foods may find it difficult to describe their usual intake. It is important to specifically address dietary practices as well as the use of nutrition supplements. Since patients will often present with acute medical events superimposed on chronic health conditions, it is not unusual for them to have had compromised dietary intakes and malnutrition for prolonged periods prior to assessment. It is important not to overlook a prolonged period of inadequate intake so that appropriate intervention may be undertaken in a timely manner.

Dietary assessment must continue when enteral or parenteral feedings are initiated. It is important to monitor how much of the ordered formula is actually being administered to and received by the patient. It is not uncommon for enteral feedings to be interrupted or held for procedures, tolerance issues, feeding tube displacements, and other events.[6] Patients may be considerably underfed for protracted periods even in the hospital. Once a patient is being transitioned to oral feedings, amounts of food and/or supplements consumed as well as patient tolerance should continue to be closely monitored. Patients with an ongoing inflammatory response may suffer anorexia. Moreover, it is not unusual for patients to suffer multiple missed or delayed meals for tests or procedures.

## PHYSICAL EXAMINATION

The physical examination of a patient for nutritional assessment and diagnosis is helpful in terms of confirming the significance of findings that were ascertained by a medical and nutritional history. The systematic physical examination including general appearance, skin, hair, nail, mucous membranes, respiratory system, cardiovascular system, endocrine system, nervous system, and musculoskeletal system is required for the identification of nutritional deficiencies. Table 45.4 describes nutritional deficiencies and associated abnormal findings on the physical examination.

There are limitations to the ability of a physical examination to diagnose nutritional deficiencies. The physical findings and clinical symptoms of micronutrient deficiencies such as vitamins, essential fatty acids, and trace elements are relatively nonspecific. For example, the most representative physical finding of essential fatty acid deficiency is a generalized and scaly dermatitis, but this is also commonly seen in other micronutrient deficiencies such as vitamin C, pyridoxine, riboflavin, biotin, and zinc deficiencies.[7] Other systemic diseases such as fungal infection, HIV infection, heavy alcohol intake, and Parkinson's disease can have similar skin findings as well. Thus the physical signs need to be correlated with the medical and nutritional history and laboratory testing to confirm the nutritional diagnosis. In the clinical setting, it is uncommon to have an isolated micronutrient deficiency. Most cases of nutritional deficiencies are prone to be combined nutritional deficiencies, which make it more difficult to diagnose by physical examination and history alone. Even though a specific nutrient deficiency is suspected, a systematic physical examination is required to capture physical signs of other potential nutrient deficiencies.

## ANTHROPOMETRY

The word "anthropometry" originates from the Greek words "anthropos" and "metron" meaning "man" and "measure," respectively. Anthropometry is the measurement of the human individual in terms of the dimensions of bone, muscle, and adipose tissue, which provides information on body muscle mass and fat reserves. The commonly used measurements are body weight, height, triceps skin fold, and mid-arm muscle circumference.

The body weight measurement in pounds or kilograms is very simple, easily obtained, and provides one of the most useful nutritional parameters for assessing the patient's nutritional status. Comparison of a patient's current weight to their usual weight is generally used for the diagnosis of malnutrition, which correlates with the development of disease as well as prognosis. Intentional weight loss should be distinguished from unintentional weight loss and psychological disorders such as anorexia nervosa, compulsive overeating, or rumination syndrome. Fluid retention, which is caused by various medical and nutritional conditions such as cardiac failure, end-stage liver disease, kidney disease, and hypoalbuminemic malnutrition can confound weight assessment.

**TABLE 45.4**

## Physical Findings of Nutritional Disorders

| System | Findings | Nutritional Disorder |
|---|---|---|
| General | Wasting, loss of subcutaneous fat, generalized weakness | Macronutrient deficiency (chronic disease- and starvation-related malnutrition) |
| | Loss of appetite (anorexia) | Zinc deficiency |
| Skin | Petechiae, purpura | Vitamin C deficiency, vitamin K deficiency |
| | Poor wound healing, pressure ulcer | Zinc deficiency, vitamin C deficiency |
| | Pellagra type dermatitis (desquamation, erythema, scaling, and keratosis of sun-exposed areas | Niacin or tryptophan deficiency, leucine excess |
| | Eczematous scaling | Essential fatty acid, zinc, or biotin deficiency |
| Hair | Corkscrew hairs | Vitamin C deficiency |
| | Thin hair, hair loss | Zinc deficiency, essential fatty acid deficiency, macronutrient deficiency |
| Nail | Koilonychia (spoon nails) | Iron deficiency |
| Eyes | Night blindness, photophobia, blurring | Vitamin A deficiency, riboflavin deficiency |
| Oral | Angular stomatitis | Riboflavin, pyridoxine, niacin deficiency |
| | Cheilosis | Riboflavin, niacin deficiency |
| | Gingival enlargement, gum bleeding | Vitamin C deficiency |
| | Loss of lingual papillae | Riboflavin, niacin, folate deficiency |
| | Glossitis | Vitamin B12 deficiency, iron deficiency, riboflavin deficiency |
| Neck | Goiter | Iodine deficiency |
| Respiratory | Acute respiratory failure | Refeeding syndrome (most causes are non-nutritional) |
| Cardiovascular | Heart failure (cardiomyopathy) | Thiamine deficiency, refeeding syndrome, selenium deficiency, carnitine deficiency, pyridoxine deficiency |
| | Edema | Thiamine deficiency, macronutrient deficiency (acute illness–related malnutrition) |
| Gastrointestinal | Diarrhea | Niacin deficiency |
| | Hepatomegaly | Macronutrient deficiency (protein deficiency) |
| Musculoskeletal | Bone tenderness, joint pain | Vitamin D deficiency, vitamin C deficiency |
| | Muscle wasting | Macronutrient deficiency (chronic disease- or starvation-related malnutrition) |
| Neurologic | Confabulation, disorientation | Thiamine deficiency (Korsakoff syndrome) |
| | Dementia, degenerative neuropathy | Niacin deficiency, vitamin B12 deficiency, manganese excess |
| | Peripheral neuropathy | Thiamine deficiency, pyridoxine deficiency, vitamin B12 deficiency, copper deficiency, chromium deficiency |
| Hematologic | Signs of anemia (fatigue, pale skin, dizziness) | Iron deficiency, vitamin B12 deficiency, folate deficiency, copper deficiency |

Sudden weight changes caused by volume status change should not be used for nutritional assessment.

Height is another essential nutritional parameter, which is used for nutritional calculations such as ideal body weight and body mass index (BMI). Changes in height can also be an indicator of the presence of disease. For example, in the elderly height loss can be an indicator of a vertebral fracture and osteoporosis.[2] Direct measurement of height can be a challenge for patients who are wheel chair-bound or amputees. There are several indirect ways to measure height, such as arm span, summation of body parts, or knee height measurement, which can be used alternatively in situations where a direct measurement cannot be obtained.[8]

BMI, which is the weight in kilograms divided by the height in meters squared, is widely used in clinical practice to assess nutritional status. It is well known that elevated BMI is strongly correlated with cardiovascular disease, diabetes, obstructive sleep apnea, and hyperlipidemia, as well as an increase in mortality. Lower BMI (underweight) is also associated with increased risk of death, and the BMI/mortality association forms a j-shaped curve. However, the BMI measurement does not take into account ethnic variations. For example, among Indians and Bangladeshis, the risk of death is not increased with a higher BMI range between 25 and 32 kg/m$^2$, whereas East Asians and Caucasians do have increased mortality in that range of BMI.[9] Another limitation of the BMI is that it is not an accurate measure of body composition. For example, athletes with a disproportionate amount of muscle will have a high BMI, without the associated health risk.

Measurement of triceps skin fold is useful for estimating body fat stores and the mid-arm muscle circumference is used to estimate lean body mass. Because approximately 50% of body fat is subcutaneous, these measurements can be used as an indicator of fat stores and muscle mass. They are relatively simple and easy techniques to use. However, they are only standardized for the non-hospitalized population and not widely applicable to hospitalized patients. Depending on hydration status, they can be incorrectly measured.

There are more objective, accurate methods to measure the body composition such as underwater weighing, magnetic resonance imaging, and total body nitrogen and potassium analysis. Underwater weighing has been considered the gold standard for body composition studies. However, these techniques are currently used primarily for research only due to their high cost and complexity of testing. Bioelectrical impedance analysis (BIA) is a simple, noninvasive method to estimate lean body mass, but it is considered less accurate than the gold standard. BIA can analyze fluid volumes and fat-free body mass based on differences in resistance to an electrical current. However, it is not fully validated for use in disease states, and it is also affected by edema and fever. Dual-Energy X-ray Absorptiometry (DXA) is primarily used for measuring bone density. It can also be used to quantify the mineral, fat, and lean mass. It provides a higher degree of precision in only one measurement and has the ability to show exactly where fat is distributed throughout the body. DXA is relatively safe and presents little burden to the subject. Recently, DXA has become the new "reference standard" method to measure the body composition. However, clinical use DXA scanning in nutritional screening and assessment is still limited mainly by cost and availability.

## LABORATORY TESTING

Laboratory findings must be appropriately used in combination with other assessments to diagnose malnutrition. Additional evidence of malnutrition including insufficient energy intake, unintentional weight loss, loss of muscle mass and subcutaneous fat, fluid accumulation, or diminished functional status is warranted to make a well-informed diagnosis. In the outpatient setting, routine laboratory tests such as a complete blood count, blood glucose, and electrolyte levels and serum lipid profiles may provide valuable nutritional information. In hospitalized patients, the most widely used laboratory tests in the nutritional assessment are measurements of serum protein concentrations.

## SERUM PROTEINS

Despite the lack of specificity and sensitivity as indicators of nutrition status, measurement of serum proteins such as albumin and prealbumin levels remains the traditional standard method of nutritional assessment. Hypoalbuminemia is a strong predictor of risk of morbidity and mortality in both hospitalized and ambulatory patients. In most circumstances, hypoalbuminemia in hospitalized patients identifies those with recent or ongoing systemic inflammatory response. Low serum levels indicate that a patient is very ill and probably requires aggressive and closely monitored medical nutrition therapy.[10] Measurement of the acute-phase reactant, C-reactive protein (CRP) along with serum proteins may be helpful in confirming the presence of an elevated systemic inflammatory state. If the CRP is increased and serum albumin or prealbumin is decreased, then inflammation is likely to be a contributing factor.[11]

A serum albumin value of less than 3.5 g/dL is associated with a mild systemic inflammatory response. A value of less than 2.4 g/dL represents a severe systemic inflammatory response, reflecting systemic inflammation that produces

anorexia, increased protein catabolism, and acceleration of the development of protein energy malnutrition. Because the half-life for albumin is 18–20 days and the fractional replacement rate is about 10% per day, the return of serum albumin to normal levels takes about 2 weeks of feeding after the remission of the stress response. Adequate feeding will not increase the serum albumin concentration in the presence of ongoing systemic inflammation, although substantial nutritional benefit will occur in terms of immune function and wound healing.[12]

Other transport proteins such as transferrin, prealbumin, and retinol-binding protein have shorter half-lives of 7 days, 2 days, and half a day, respectively, and they also fall acutely with acute injury and systemic inflammation. Serum transferrin also depends on iron status, while serum prealbumin and retinol-binding protein vary with dietary carbohydrate and renal function. As a result, these proteins do not reliably identify the presence and severity of the systemic inflammatory response any better than does albumin, but they reflect the nutritional response more quickly when inflammation decreases.

## NITROGEN BALANCE

Nitrogen balance is used to evaluate the adequacy of protein intake by comparing nitrogen intake with nitrogen excretion. In patients with systemic inflammation, urea nitrogen urine concentration is significantly increased, reflecting catabolism of protein associated with this condition. Nutrition support and physical therapy, when feasible, may limit loss of muscle mass in acutely ill hospitalized patients.[13] Adjustments in protein intake can be made in an attempt to improve nitrogen economy and loss of lean tissue.

Nitrogen intake is determined by dividing protein intake (in grams) by 6.25. Most of the body's nitrogen is lost in the urine, and the analysis of a 24 h urine collection for urea nitrogen content (UUN) is required to calculate nitrogen balance. An additional 3–5 g of nitrogen is lost daily via feces, skin and sweat. The formula for calculating nitrogen balance is as follows:

$$\text{Nitrogen balance} = \text{Nitrogen intake} - \text{Nitrogen losses}$$

$$\text{Nitrogen intake} = \text{Protein intake in grams}/6.25$$

Nitrogen losses = Urinary urea nitrogen (UUN)
+ Non-urea urinary nitrogen (1–2 g)
+ Fecal nitrogen (1–2 g)
+ Miscellaneous losses from desquamation of skin, epithelial surfaces, sweat, etc. ($\sim$1 g or 0.1–0.5 g/m$^2$)

Nitrogen balance (in grams) = protein intake (in grams)/6.25 − (UUN excretion in grams + 3–5 g)

## NUTRIENT LEVELS

Although nutritional assessment does not routinely include measurement of micronutrient levels, clinical circumstances may warrant a more in-depth investigation of the status of specific nutrients. For example, iron studies should be performed in patients with a microcytic anemia. An evaluation of B12 and folate levels is warranted in the presence of peripheral neuropathy or macrocytic anemia. For patients with fat malabsorption, levels of the fat-soluble vitamins A, D, E, and K should be checked. In any case, information obtained from the patient's medical history and findings of the physical examination can guide the decision regarding the need for further laboratory testing (Table 45.3).

## MISCELLANEOUS SERUM ASSAYS

Levels of blood glucose, serum electrolyte concentrations, renal function, hepatic function, and blood gases are important parts of the nutrition support intervention. They will direct the fluid, energy, protein, and electrolyte prescription in patients requiring nutritional intervention. Hyperglycemia has been shown to increase mortality in critically ill patients. Severely hyperglycemic individuals should achieve reasonable glucose homeostasis before nutrition support is initiated.[14,15]

## CONCLUSION

Malnutrition is associated with increased morbidity and mortality rates in the hospital and other clinical settings. It also prolongs the length of hospital stay and increases treatment costs. The goal of malnutrition management is early detection based on an appropriate nutrition assessment followed by intensive nutritional intervention. Nutrition assessment is the first and essential step in malnutrition management. Therefore, it should be part of a comprehensive medical examination in order to detect malnutrition early and initiate proper treatment to avoid excess morbidity, mortality, and increased health care costs.

## REFERENCES

1. Norman, K, Pichard, C, Lochs, H, Pirlich, M. *Clin Nutr* 27:5;2008.
2. White, JV, Guenter, P, Jensen, G et al. *J Parenter Enteral Nutr* 36:275;2012.
3. Jensen, GL, Bistrian, B, Roubenoff, R, Heimburger, DC. *J Parenter Enteral Nutr* 33:710;2009.
4. Jensen, GL, Hsiao, PY, Wheeler, D. *J Parenter Enteral Nutr* 36:267;2012.
5. Hark, L, Bowman, M, Bellini, L. In: Morrison, G, Hark, L, eds. *Medical Nutrition and Disease*. Blackwell Science, Melden, MA, 1999, p. 3.
6. Kyle, UG, Genton, L, Heidegger, CP et al. *Clin Nutr* 25:727;2006.
7. Jeppesen, PB, Høy, CE, Mortensen, PB. *Am J Clin Nutr* 68:126;1998.
8. Russell, MK, Mueller, C. In: Gottschlich MM, ed. *The A.S.P.E.N. Nutrition Support Core Curriculum*. A.S.P.E.N., Silver Spring, MD, 2007, p. 163.
9. Zheng, W, McLerran, DF, Rolland, B et al. *N Engl J Med* 24:719;2011.
10. Fuhrman, MP, Charney, P, Mueller, CM. *J Am Diet Assoc* 104:1258;2004.
11. Robinson, MK, Trujillo, EB, Mogensen, KM et al. *J Parenter Enteral Nutr* 27:389;2003.
12. Bistrian, B. In: Goldman, L, Schafer, AI, eds. *Goldman's Cecil Medicine*. Saunders Elsevier, Philadelphia, PA, 2012, p. 1384.
13. Wray, CJ, Mammen, JM, Hasselgren, PO. *Nutrition* 18:971;2002.
14. Bagshaw, SM, Egi, M, George, C, Bellomo, R. *Crit Care Med* 37:463;2009.
15. Freire, AX, Bridges, L, Umpierrez, GE et al. *Chest* 128:3109;2005.

# 46 Metabolic Syndrome, Overweight, and Fatty Liver

*E.L. Thomas, J.A. Fitzpatrick, Gary Frost, and Jimmy D. Bell*

## CONTENTS

## INTRODUCTION

The advance of obesity across the Western population appears unabated, despite the increasing efforts by governments and international organizations. In the United Kingdom alone, it is estimated that by the year 2050, close to 80% of the population will be either overweight or obese.[1] Accompanying this increase in obesity are a plethora of comorbidities, including insulin resistance, diabetes, CVD, and some form of cancers, many of which are having catastrophic effects both on an individual's quality of life and on the country's economy.[2] This problem has now extended to the younger population in the United Kingdom, where ca. 23% and 33% of 4–5 and 10–11 year-old children, respectively, are overweight or obese.[3] Again, in many cases, childhood obesity is associated with insulin resistance and type II diabetes (T2D).[4] A similar trend is observed in women of childbearing age, the consequences of which are as yet unknown.

## METABOLIC SYNDROME

Modern humans have created for themselves the "perfect nutritional milieu" for the rampant development of obesity, T2D, and insulin resistance.[5] This is resulting in a reduction in life expectancy and a significant impact on the quality of life.

The "metabolic syndrome" is currently defined as central obesity plus two factors: raised triglycerides (TGs), reduced HDL, hypertension, and evidence of pathological insulin resistance, such as raised fasting plasma glucose (FPG, now defined as >5.6 mM) or previous diabetes.[6] Sources of oxidative stress appear to include cells overloaded with fat, both in adipose tissue and in the liver,[7–10] leading to "metabolically triggered inflammation,"[11] and is regarded as a metabolically inflexible phenotype, in which mitochondrial function and capacity may be critically compromised.[12,13]

The metabolic syndrome can be viewed as a continuum that sits at the opposite end of the oxidative stress spectrum to the calorie restriction phenotype.[14] A common feature of these two phenotypes is the involvement of the insulin/insulin-like growth factor axis.[15,16] In evolutionary terms, insulin resistance may be a positive process that ensures deposition of fat[17] and reduces oxidative redox signaling-induced stress.[18,19] Indeed, it has been proposed that different ethnic groups may show different level of predisposition to insulin resistance through epigenetic control.[20] Due to climate and geographical exposure, predisposition will vary across the globe, which in turn may be reflected by different fat distributions.[21–23]

## BMI DECONSTRUCTED

In recent years, we have seen a slow, but inexorable move toward the acquisition of more detailed phenotypic information from overweight/obese individuals, both for scientific purposes and to provide better advice to those trying to avoid or reverse the effects of increased body adiposity. For many decades, body mass index (BMI) has been the ubiquitous method to get a surrogate measure of body adiposity. Although at population level BMI has served extremely well as a tool to uncover the relationship between obesity and some life-threatening disorders, this has not been done without some reservations.[24] Since its introduction, BMI has been known to have considerable limitations, especially at the extremes of BMI, in children, athletes, and for different ethnic and age groups.[24,25] Based on the assumption that changes in body weight reflected changes in body fat, BMI was proposed as an estimate of obesity. But obesity is defined as excess body fat rather than body weight, and differences in body weight do not always go hand in hand with changes in body fat.[26] It is the very fact that BMI, waist-to-hip ratio (WHR), and waist

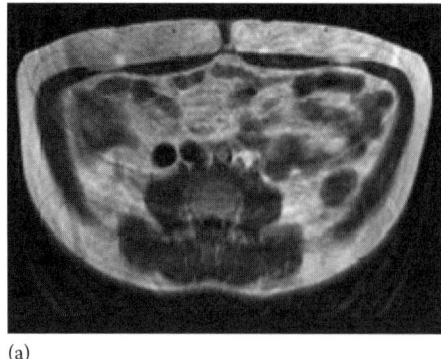
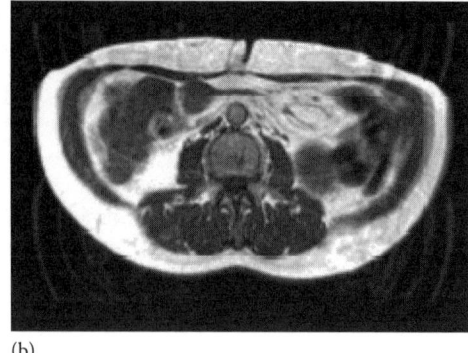

(a)                                                         (b)

**FIGURE 46.1** BMI is poorly predictive of adipose tissue content. Transverse MRI images taken at the level of the umbilicus from two male subjects ((a) and (b)) with a BMI of 26.2 kg/m². Total and regional adipose tissue content varies considerably between subjects despite the same BMI. (Total body fat content: Subject A 23.1 L, Subject B 21.8 L. Visceral fat content: Subject A 3.3 L, Subject B 2.7 L.)

circumference (WC) do not measure body fat directly, which led many to question the validity of these methods. After all, it is adipose tissue, a fully functional organ, which is the cause of the comorbid conditions. However, it was not until the advent of in vivo imaging techniques, including CT and magnetic resonance imaging (MRI) and spectroscopy (MRS), that the true extent of the limitations of BMI became clear, especially since the relationship between fat distribution (rather than fat content alone) became the center point of scientific interest.[27–30] Several alternative anthropometric (WHR and WC) and non-anthropometric methods (BodPod) have been developed (as adjunct to or to replace BMI altogether) in order to take into account fat distribution. But most of these do not

fare any better than BMI at an individual level (Figure 46.1).[31] Thus, direct measurement of individual fat depots, including ectopic fat (liver, pancreas, heart, and muscle), has become imperative for scientists trying to unravel the relationship between body fat and metabolic dysregulation. It is within this context that both CT and MRI have become the gold standard for the assessment of body fat content and distribution.

## LOOKING WITHIN

The two principal imaging techniques available for assessing body fat content and distribution are CT and MRI. The applicability of the former to the study of fat

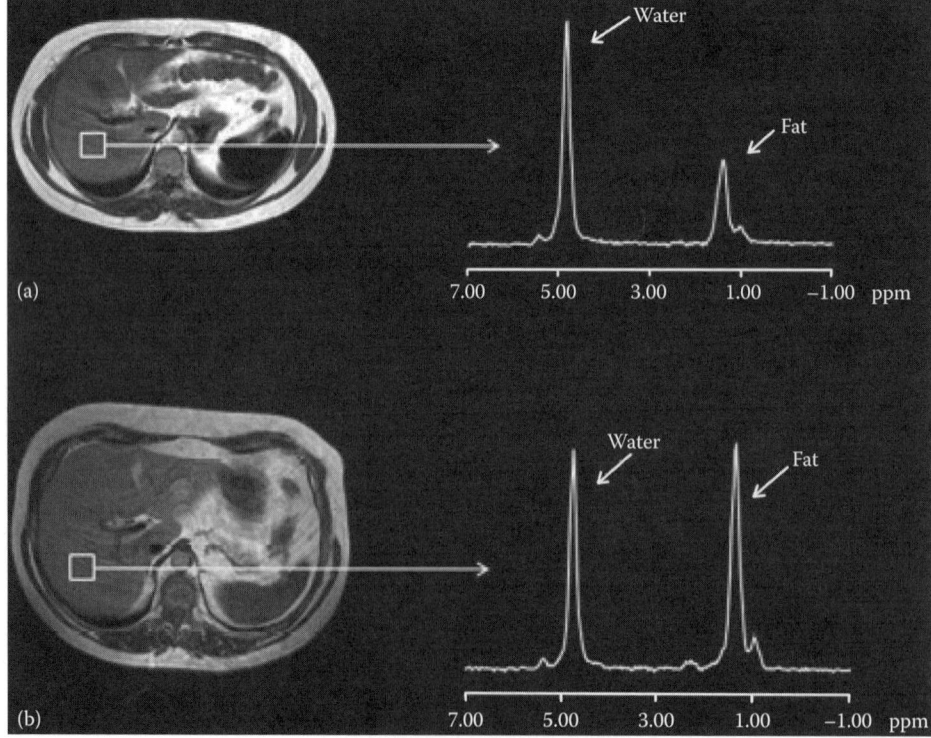

**FIGURE 46.2** Transverse MRI images taken at the level of the umbilicus from two male subjects ((a) and (b)) with different levels of visceral and liver fat. These differences in body adiposity are accompanied by the expected changes in insulin sensitivity and other risk factors associated with abdominal obesity.

in human volunteers has been hampered by the fact that ionizing radiation is required during the acquisition of the images, while the relative cost of an MRI examination has limited its applicability to large population studies. Despite this caveat, and given its accuracy and reproducibility, MRI/MRS has become the gold standard in the field of obesity.[32–34] This in turn has helped us to begin to understand the role of gene–environment interactions in the development of obesity, as well as giving new insight into the mode of action of emerging therapies. This has principally arisen from the fact that both visceral fat and liver fat have been recognized as being directly involved in the pathogenesis of comorbidities of obesity, including insulin resistance and T2D.[35] Examples of MR images and spectra from subjects with different levels of visceral and liver fat are shown in Figure 46.2. These differences in body adiposity are accompanied by the expected changes in insulin sensitivity and other risk factors associated with abdominal obesity.

## "FAT-FIT" AND MHOS

It has been reported, for well over two decades, that some obese subjects do not present the common cardiometabolic risk factors, including elevated blood pressure, elevated TGs, C-reactive protein, insulin resistance, elevated glucose levels/diabetes, or decreased HDL, despite their excess body fat.[36] Research groups in Europe and the United States have estimated that a significant number of overweight/obese subjects (20%–35%) are "metabolically healthy obese" (MHO) individuals.[37–40] In this subphenotype, there is a clear dissociation between the well-established relationship between body fat content and metabolic risk factors. A related subphenotype has also been reported, known as the "fat-fit" subjects, of which Sumo-wrestle are the best, but not the sole example, which again show a similar dissociation between body fat content and metabolic risk factors.[41–44] Figure 46.3 shows typical MR images from both "fat-fit" and "fat-unfit" subjects

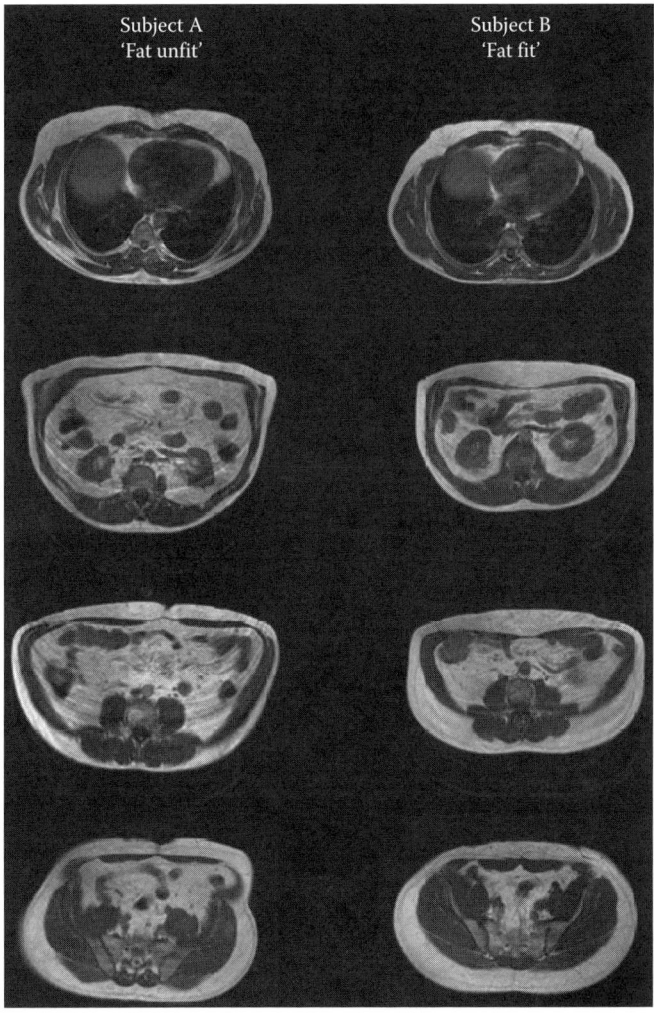

**FIGURE 46.3** MR images from two Caucasian male subjects. Subject A classified as "fat-unfit" with a $VO_{2max}$ of 31.5 mL/kg/min and Subject B "fat-fit" with a $VO_{2max}$ of 41.7 mL/kg/min. Despite a similar BMI (Subject A = 31.8 kg/m² and Subject B = 31.1 kg/m²), there are clear differences in fat distribution. Subject A has almost double the amount of visceral fat (8.84 L) compared with Subject B (4.29 L). A similar trend is seen in their liver fat content (Subjects A = 10.3% vs. Subject B 4.29).

with similar BMI. A clear difference in both visceral fat and liver fat can be observed between the two cohorts. Interestingly, subjects with Prader–Willi-syndrome also show a fascinating subphenotype, not dissimilar to the "fat-fit," where the levels of visceral fat depot and metabolic risk factors do not commensurate with their excessively large body fat content.[45]

The relationship between MHO and "fat-fit" subjects is unclear, but reduced levels of visceral and/or liver fat may be the common denominator.[43] Both of these fat depots have been not only shown to correlate with the development of obesity comorbidities, but more recently also implicated in the actual mechanism that leads to the development of insulin resistance and T2D. Indeed, liver fat, in combination with systemic inflammation, is rapidly being recognized as the main cause of insulin resistance in subjects with a variety of BMI and body fat content and distribution.[46] Recently, Stefan et al.[35] have proposed the existence of "metabolically benign and malignant fatty liver," emphasizing the importance of in-depth phenotyping in basic and clinical research. Moreover, the fact that exercise has been shown to have a significant impact on fat content, especially liver and visceral fat, reemphasizes the importance of these fat depots and begins to bring together different subphenotypes, which through different mechanisms or genetic propensities have arrived to highly favorable fat distribution, despite inhabiting an extremely obesogenic environment. Fatness and fitness may be able to coexist in specific environment, which may have given the bearer a definitive advantage during the process of evolution, where feast and famine were the norm for most organisms, including early humans.

## TOFI AND MONW

Given the earlier discussion, it is not surprising that an opposite phenotype to the "MHO/Fat-Fit" has been reported. Here, subjects with a BMI < 25 kg/m² were seen to have disproportionally high levels of many of the risk factors associated with the metabolic syndrome. These subjects have been defined as "metabolically-obese but normal-weight" (MONW) and further refined by the use of MRI as "thin-outside-fat-inside" (TOFI).[47–50] In general, these subjects have been described as being at higher risk of developing insulin resistance and T2D due to the fact that they have reduced physical activity/$VO_{2max}$, reduced insulin sensitivity and higher abdominal adiposity, and a more atherogenic lipid profile. Another important characteristic observed in this cohort of subjects is elevated levels of liver fat.[31] Once again, the combination of aberrant level of central obesity and liver fat appears to overwhelm whatever protective effect normal body weight/body fat may provide to most individuals. It is interesting to note that the TOFI subjects tend to lead a relatively sedentary life, with little physical activity, and appear to maintain their weight through control of their diet alone, rather than a more global approach to healthy living.

## EAT CLEVER, PLAY SMART

The identification of visceral fat and liver fat as fundamental contributors to the development of comorbidities of obesity has led to a frantic search for effective lifestyle and pharmacological/clinical intervention to contain/reduce their impact on a subject's health outcome. Thus, it is no longer acceptable to focus solely on body weight reduction as an outcome of interventional procedures; they have to lead to significant modulations of these key fat depots as well as markers of systemic inflammation. Caloric restriction, as well as gastric bypass, is known to reduce these body fat depots and improve insulin sensitivity.[50–52] However, and more importantly, changes in dietary composition appear to have similar effects. Increases in the consumption of resistant starches led to improvement in insulin sensitivity, while protein-rich diet reduces liver and visceral fat and improves insulin sensitivity.[53] Similarly, increase in physical activity, especially resistant exercise, alters fat volume in a depot-specific matter, leading to significant improvement in insulin sensitivity.[54–57]

In conclusion, there is increasing evidence of the existence of several subphenotypes of human subjects where there is a clear dissociation between body fat quantity and adverse metabolic risk factors. Much of this evidence points toward the importance of determining the level of individual fat depots, especially visceral and liver fat, and the value of targeted lifestyle interventions to modulate their effects on health.

## REFERENCES

1. Devaux, M, Sassi, F. *Eur J Pub Health* 23:1–5;2012.
2. Bray, GA. *Endocrinol Metab Clin North Am* 25:907;1996.
3. Statistics from Health Survey for England 2010, National Obesity Observatory, http://www.noo.org.uk/news.php, Accessed on July 05, 2012.
4. Chiarelli, F, Marcovecchio, ML. *Eur J Endocrinol* 159:S67;2008. Review.
5. Diet, nutrition and the prevention of chronic diseases. *World Health Organ Tech Rep Ser* 916:i-149;2003.
6. Zimmet, P, Magliano, D, Matsuzawa, Y et al. *J Atheroscler Thromb* 12:295;2005.
7. Fujita, K, Nishizawa, H, Funahashi, T et al. *Circ J* 70:1437;2006.
8. Furukawa, S, Fujita, T, Shimabukuro, M et al. *J Clin Invest* 114:1752;2004.
9. Jeong, SK, Kim, YK, Park, JW, *J Korean Med Sci* 23:789;2008.
10. van der Poorten, D, Milner, KL, Hui J et al. *Hepatology* 48:449;2008.
11. Hotamisligil, GS. *Nature* 444:860;2006.
12. Pasquali, R, Vicennati, V, Gambineri, A, Pagotto, U. *Int J Obes (Lond)* 32:1764;2008.
13. Storlien, L, Oakes, ND, Kelley, DE. *Proc Nutr Soc* 63:363;2004.
14. Guarente, L. *Nature* 444:868;2006.
15. Murphy, CT, McCarroll, SA, Bargmann, CI et al. *Nature* 424:277;2003.
16. Nakae, J, Biggs, WH III, Kitamura, T et al. *Nat Genet* 32:245;2002.
17. Dulloo, AG. *Horm Res* 65:90;2006.
18. Erol, A. *Bioessays* 29:811;2007.

19. Fridlyand, LE, Philipson, LH. *Diabetes Obes Metab* 8:136;2006.

20. Stoger, R. *Bioessays* 30:156;2008.

21. Sirikul, B, Gower, BA, Hunter, GR et al. *Am J Physiol Endocrinol Metab* 291:E724;2006.

22. Wu, CH, Heshka, S, Wang, J et al. *Int J Obes (Lond)* 31:1384;2007.

23. Fridlyand, LE, Philipson, LH. *Med Hypotheses* 67:1034;2006.

24. Prentice, AM, Jebb, SA. *Obes Rev* 2:141;2001.

25. Deurenberg, P, Deurenberg-Yap, M. *Forum Nutr* 56:299;2003.

26. Gallagher, D, Heymsfield, SB, Heo, M et al. *Am J Clin Nutr* 72:694;2000.

27. Kuk, JL, Katzmarzyk, PT, Nichaman, MZ et al. *Obesity (Silver Spring)* 14:336;2006.

28. Björntorp, P. *Diabetes Care* 14:1132;1991.

29. Matsuzawa, Y, Nakamura, T, Shimomura, I, Kotani, K. *Obes Res* 3:645S;1995.

30. Després, JP, Lemieux, I. *Nature* 14:881;2006.

31. Thomas, EL, Parkinson, JR, Frost, GS et al. *Obesity (Silver Spring)* 20:76;2012.

32. Tothill, P, Han, TS, Avenell, A et al. *Eur J Clin Nutr* 50:747;1996.

33. Thomas, EL, Saeed, N, Hajnal, JV et al. *J Appl Physiol* 85:1778;1998.

34. Sohlström, A, Wahlund, LO, Forsum, E. *Am J Clin Nutr* 58:830;1996.

35. Stefan, N, Häring, HU. *Diabetes* 60:2011;2011.

36. Karelis, AD, St-Pierre, DH, Conus, F, Rabasa-Lhoret, R, Poehlman, ET. *J Clin Endocrinol Metab* 89:2569;2004.

37. Stefan, N, Kantartzis, K, Machann, J et al. *Arch Intern Med* 168:1609;2008.

38. Wildman, RP, Muntner, P, Reynolds, K. *Arch Intern Med* 168:1617;2008.

39. McAuley, PA, Blair, SN. *J Sports Sci* 29:773;2011.

40. Pataky, Z, Makoundou, V, Nilsson, P et al. *Int J Obes (Lond)* 35:1208;2011.

41. Lee, CD, Blair, SN, Jackson, AS. *Am J Clin Nutr* 69:373;1999.

42. Wei, M, Kampert, JB, Barlow, CE et al. *JAMA* 27:1547;1999.

43. O'Donovan, G, Thomas, EL, McCarthy, JP et al. *Int J Obes (Lond)* 33:1356;2009.

44. Matsuzawa, Y. *Diabetes Metab Rev* 13:3;1997.

45. Goldstone, AP, Brynes, AE, Thomas, EL et al. *Am J Clin Nutr* 75:468;2002.

46. Fabbrini, E, Magkos, F, Mohammed, BS et al. *Proc Natl Acad Sci U S A* 106:15430;2009.

47. Ruderman, NB, Schneider, SH, Berchtold, P. *Am J Clin Nutr* 34:1617;1981.

48. Conus, F, Rabasa-Lhoret, R, Péronnet, F. *Appl Physiol Nutr Metab* 32:4;2007.

49. De Lorenzo A, Martinoli, R, Vaia, F, Di Renzo, L. *Nutr Metab Cardiovasc Dis* 16:513;2006.

50. Thomas, EL, Brynes, AE, Hamilton, G et al. *World J Gastroenterol* 12:5813;2008.

51. Gasteyger, C, Larsen, TM, Vercruysse, F et al. *Diabetes Obes Metab* 11:596;2009.

52. Janssen, I, Fortier, A, Hudson, R, Ross, R. *Diabetes Care* 25:431;2002.

53. So, PW, Yu, WS, Kuo, YT et al. *PLoS ONE* 2:e1309;2007.

54. Thomas, EL, Brynes, AE, McCarthy, J et al. *Lipids* 35:769;2000.

55. Ross, R, Janssen, I, Dawson, J et al. *Obes Res* 12:789;2001.

56. van der Heijden, GJ, Wang, ZJ, Chu, ZD et al. *Obesity (Silver Spring)* 18:384;2010.

57. Idoate, F, Ibañez, J, Gorostiaga, EM et al. *Int J Obes (Lond)* 35:700;2011.

# 47 The Malnourished Child

*Rikki S. Corniola, David L. Suskind, Leslie Lewinter-Suskind,
Krishna K. Murthy, and Robert M. Suskind*

## CONTENTS

In the last 20 years, there has been a tremendous effort worldwide to reduce the annual number of under-five deaths from nearly 12 million in 1990 to fewer than 7.6 million in 2010[1]. Despite this immense effort, that still equates to over 20,000 deaths per day of children under the age of five. These deaths represent, however, only a fraction of the children in developing countries who suffer from malnutrition, many of whom survive.[2–3] It is estimated that in 2011, 314 million children under the age of five were mildly, moderately, or severely stunted with another 258 million mildly, moderately, or severely underweight.[4] For these children who do survive, early malnutrition generates a long-term insult to their ultimate development and, consequently, to the community and world in which they must live.

The basis of childhood malnutrition, in much of the world, is socioeconomic,[5–10] often exacerbated by natural and political disasters.[8,11,12] In the United States, primary protein–energy malnutrition (PEM) is less commonly seen.[13] There is, however, an increasing awareness of the occurrence of malnutrition secondary to disease states[14] such as diarrhea,[15] chronic illnesses such as HIV and TB,[16] cancer,[17] intrauterine growth retardation,[18] and child abuse.[19] Although PEM is considered a direct cause of death, particular importance is given to the effects of nutritional status in the overall prognosis of a disease state.[20] This observation, together with the recognition of the long-term effects of malnutrition on growth and development, has highlighted the need for accurately determining deficiencies, for methods to discern their impact on disease states, and for effective programs for their prevention and treatment.[21–23]

## ANTHROPOMETRIC CLASSIFICATION OF PROTEIN–ENERGY MALNUTRITION

In 1956, Gomez et al.[24] used local standards to define malnutrition in terms of weight-for-age. Current classifications use internationally accepted standards derived from the weights and heights of healthy children from North America or Europe. Several studies support the use of such standards for all children. Habicht et al.[25] reviewed anthropometric data taken from several racial-ethnic groups and concluded that the differences among diverse well-nourished populations were small compared to the differences between socioeconomic classes of the same populations. They concluded that data drawn from studies of well-to-do populations could, therefore, be used as standards. Martorell[26] in Honduras showed a clear association between socioeconomic status and "stunting," that is, severe growth retardation, as well as correlations even within gradations of poverty to eventual height deficits.

Height-for-age and weight-for-height are basic indices for defining a child's nutritional status. A decreased weight-for-height indicates an acute state of malnutrition; a decreased height-for-age, on the other hand, indicates that the child has, at some period, been chronically malnourished.[27] Combined deficits of height-for-age and weight-for-height indicate long-term malnutrition as well as the existence of current nutritional deficits. The effect of malnutrition on linear growth may not in fact be apparent until approximately 4 months after its effect on changes in weight.[28]

Weight-for-height is classified as grades I, II, and III of 80%–90%, 70%–80%, and less than 70% of ideal weight-for-height, respectively.[29] Height-for-age classifications are grades I, II, and III of 90%–95%, 85%–90%, and less than 85% of height-for-age, respectively. Children in developing countries commonly become wasted between 1 and 2 years of age. By 3 and 4 years of age, when they are better able to procure their own food, wasting may be replaced by stunting.[29] The result is a short child with a normal weight-for-height.

Other anthropometric methods, such as arm circumference and triceps skin fold, are also used for determining the presence of malnutrition. Anderson et al.,[30] however, in a study of over 5000 Indian children, found arm circumference measurements unreliable for determining severe malnutrition. They concluded that, because of the possibility of misclassification of moderately to severely malnourished children, use of weight was preferable in determining nutritional status. Ross et al.[31] in Sudan found that weight-for-height measurements and mid-upper-arm circumference (MUAC) measurements did not always identify the same individual children as malnourished. Connor and Manary found that in children over 12 months old, changes in MUAC measurements significantly correlated with body mass measurements in the second month of home-based treatment for moderate malnutrition.[32] Keet et al.,[33] in an investigation of triceps skin-fold measurements, found that marasmic children had skin-fold values below the 3rd percentile for normal children of the same sex. Children with marasmus–kwashiorkor and kwashiorkor ranged from below the 3rd percentile to the 50th percentile. Ultrasonography has been used to assess muscle and fat in the arms and legs of malnourished children, and this, combined with anthropometric measurements, has been a useful tool in assessing children suspected of being malnourished.

## CLINICAL CLASSIFICATION OF PROTEIN–ENERGY MALNUTRITION

The three states of PEM are marasmus, marasmic-kwashiorkor, and kwashiorkor. They are compounded by a whole spectrum of nutritional disorders that include deficiencies

of one or more vitamins, minerals, and trace minerals. The three states of PEM can be differentiated most clearly on the basis of clinical findings.

Marasmus, which predominates in infancy, is characterized by severe weight reduction, gross wasting of muscle and subcutaneous tissue, no detectable edema and, if prolonged, marked stunting (Figure 47.1). Marasmus results from a severe deprivation, or impaired absorption, of protein, energy, vitamins, and minerals. The hair and skin changes and hepatomegaly resulting from fatty infiltration of the liver, which is seen in kwashiorkor, are not usually found in marasmus. The marasmic child, characteristically irritable and apathetic, is the skin-and-bones portrait of starvation. The term for this is *wasting*. When such malnutrition continues on a long-term basis in a young child, it results in stunting, a term introduced by Waterlow[27] to describe the profound effect of nutritional deprivation on linear growth.

Marasmic-kwashiorkor presents with clinical findings of both marasmus and kwashiorkor (Figure 47.2). The child with marasmus–kwashiorkor has edema, gross wasting, and is usually stunted. There may also be mild hair and skin changes and a palpable fatty-infiltrated liver. The child with marasmus–kwashiorkor is one who demonstrates the

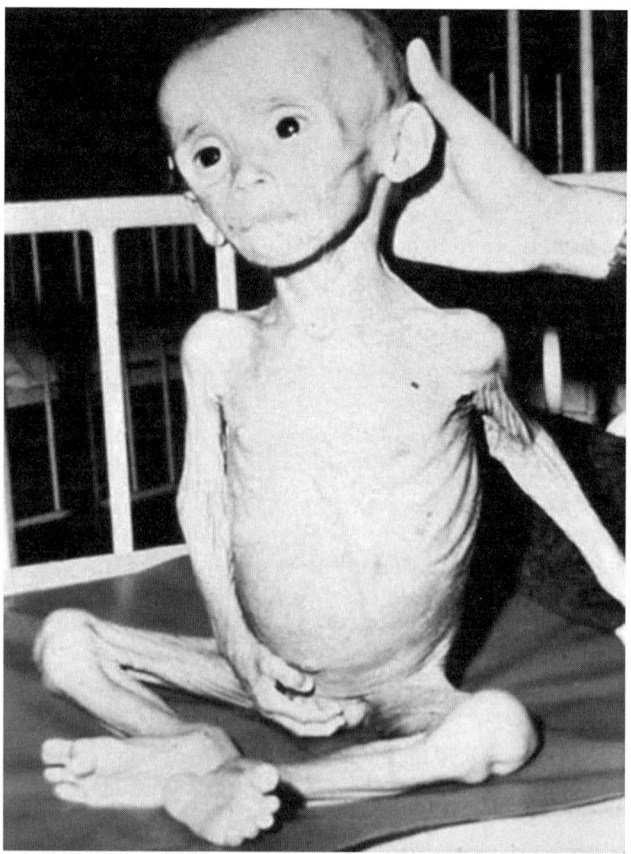

**FIGURE 47.1** Marasmic child (2 years old) with characteristic growth retardation, weight loss, muscular atrophy, and loss of subcutaneous tissue.

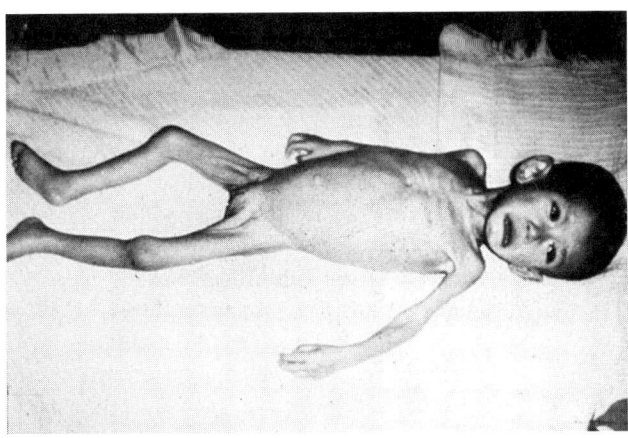

**FIGURE 47.2** Child (1.5 years old) with marasmic-kwashiorkor, with wasting, stunting, edema, and mild hepatomegaly.

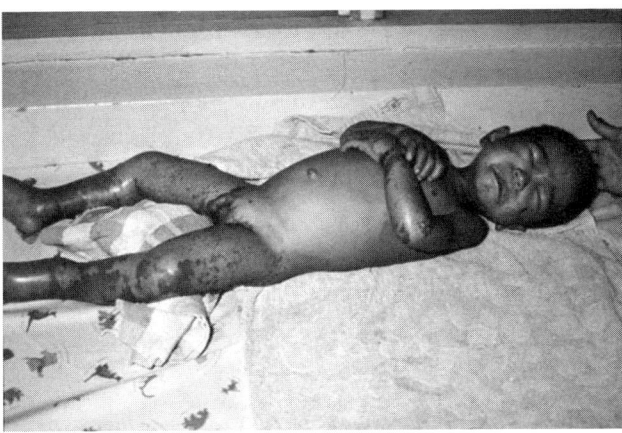

**FIGURE 47.3** Child (2.5 years old) with kwashiorkor, with evidence of edema, skin lesions, muscular atrophy, and enlarged liver.

combined effects of an inadequate intake of nutrients to meet requirements plus superimposed infection.

Kwashiorkor results from either inadequate protein intake or, more commonly, from an acute or chronic infection. It appears predominantly in older infants and young children. Clinically, it is characterized by edema, skin lesions, hair changes, apathy, anorexia, a large fatty liver, and decreased serum albumin (Figure 47.3). Weight loss is also usual, even without a decrease in energy intake. The edema of kwashiorkor can only partially be explained by the low serum albumin; other contributing factors include electrolyte abnormalities, increased capillary permeability, increased cortisol, antidiuretic hormone levels,[27] aldosterone levels,[34] and oxidative stress.[35]

## PROGNOSIS AND MORTALITY

Although mortality in the presence of severe PEM varies with the level of care, a study of over 2400 cases concluded that the worst prognostic factors were infection and water and electrolyte disturbances.[36] Garrow and

Pike[37] found that a decreased serum sodium and increased serum bilirubin were negative prognostic signs. Waterlow et al.[38] reported an increased mortality among children with gross hepatomegaly. Poor prognosis was also attributed to hypothermia, when the rectal temperature was less than 35°C, especially when accompanied by profound hypoglycemia.[39]

## PATHOGENESIS

Marasmus results from inadequate energy intake and kwashiorkor from the catabolic stress of infection and/or a deficiency of dietary protein. Gopalan,[40] in 1968, found that there was no essential difference between the protein/energy ratio in the diets of children with marasmus and those with kwashiorkor, and that each of the clinical syndromes appeared in different children for whom there was no demonstrable difference in diet. Instead Gopalan suggested that kwashiorkor was essentially a failure of adaptation occurring when sufficient food was consumed for energy maintenance but without sufficient dietary protein available for the synthesis of visceral proteins.[40] More recently, Keusch[20] described the mechanisms by which infection, as a result of the production of tumor necrosis factor (TNF) and interleukin-1 (IL-1) by macrophages, inhibited the production of visceral proteins and stimulated the release of acute phase reactants. Amino acids, for the most part, are diverted into the production of acute-phase reactants at the expense of visceral protein synthesis. As a result, the production of albumin and lipoproteins is decreased, leading to the development of hypoalbuminemia, edema, and fatty infiltration of the liver.

Marasmus, on the other hand, results from a lack of both energy and protein. The resulting "adaptation" produces increased cortisol levels and decreased insulin levels. Muscle provides the essential amino acids for the maintenance of visceral protein synthesis, which leads in turn to the production of adequate amounts of serum albumin and lipoproteins, avoiding edema and fatty infiltration of the liver.

When infection is superimposed on the marasmic state, essential amino acids are diverted to the production of acute-phase reactants, rather than to visceral proteins. Cortisol and growth hormone, rather than insulin, become the major contributors to the metabolic status of the patient. Growth hormone further contributes to the amino acid deficit by driving amino acids into the lean body mass so that they are no longer available for visceral protein synthesis.

Scrimshaw and Behar[41] developed a triangular model to describe the development of a spectrum of protein–energy-deficient states (Figure 47.4). Time is represented on the horizontal axis. The vertical axis demonstrates the rapid development of metabolic disorders leading to edema and fatty infiltration of the liver, seen in kwashiorkor; the hypotenuse reflects the overall slower process of wasting seen in marasmus. The typical patient falls somewhere in between.

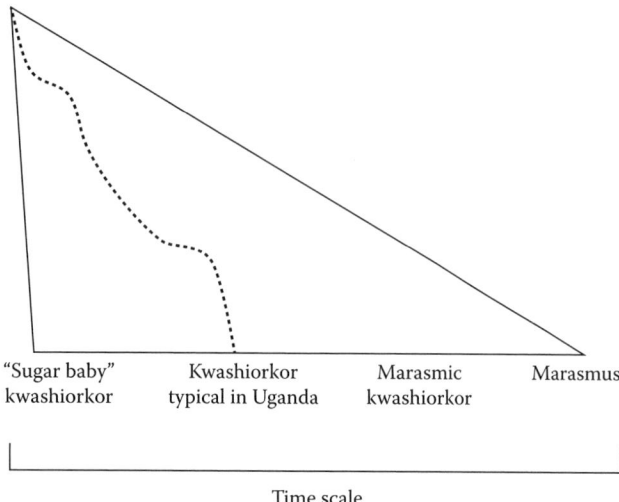

Time scale

**FIGURE 47.4** The development of PEM spectrum of diseases. (Adapted from Scrimshaw, N.S. and Behar, M., *Science*, 133, 2039, 1961.)

## INTERACTION OF INFECTION AND NUTRITION

Infections usually result in a predictable pattern of metabolic changes including dysregulation of hormones, cytokines, and pro-inflammatory mediators leading to hypermetabolism, a negative nitrogen balance, and increased gluconeogenesis and lipid oxidation.[42] These metabolic consequences of infectious disease states result in the development of marasmic-kwashiorkor or kwashiorkor.[43] The extrametabolic demands of the immune system are especially problematic for malnourished children, who not only are more susceptible to infection,[44] but also have limited capacity to mount the appropriate immune response.[45] The consequent interactions of infection with malnutrition are unquestionably some of the most important factors in the increased morbidity and mortality associated with PEM.

In 1973, Puffer and Serrano[46] demonstrated that nutritional deficiency was associated with 60.9% of the deaths from infectious diseases. Diarrhea and measles were the diseases with the greatest morbidity and mortality in which malnutrition was a factor.[47] Chronic illnesses such as HIV and TB exacerbate the malnourished state and further complicate treatment because of complex drug interactions and toxicities.[16]

The mechanisms by which infection leads to a malnourished state include (1) anorexia, (2) replacement of solid foods with a low-energy, low-protein diet; (3) decreased nutrient absorption resulting from diarrhea and intestinal parasites; and (4) increased urinary losses of nitrogen, potassium, magnesium, zinc, phosphate, sulfur, and vitamins A, C, and $B_2$.[44] Increased urinary nitrogen excretion, which exists in the mildest of infectious diseases, results from an increased mobilization of amino acids from skeletal muscle for gluconeogenesis in the liver with deamination and excretion of nitrogen in the form of urea.[48] Despite the mobilization of amino acids from peripheral muscle, there is also a decrease in whole-blood amino acids after exposure to an

infectious agent.[49] Without an increased dietary intake to compensate for losses, a kwashiorkor-like syndrome results, which presents with the decreased ability to mount a metabolic response to infection.[50] Furthermore, with infection, there is sequestration or diversion of the essential protein cofactors iron, copper, and zinc from normal metabolic pathways. Consequently, to balance the modest synthesis of acute-phase reactants, including haptoglobin, C-reactive protein, α1-antitrypsin, and α2-macrogolublin,[50,51] there is a concomitant decrease in visceral protein synthesis.[52] Each of these changes is felt to be mediated by TNF and IL-1.

Children with PEM may have either hypochromic microcytic or normochromic normocytic anemia.[53] In chronic infections, anemia may occur as a result of defective hemoglobin synthesis accompanied by inadequate bone marrow stores of iron[52] and vitamin A deficiency.[54] Infection also affects the endocrine system. Changes in hormone levels occur simultaneously with infection and precede the changes in amino acids and serum albumin levels.[27] With infection, there is a decrease in serum albumin and insulin levels as well as an increase in cortisol levels. In addition, decreased food intake results in negative nitrogen balance secondary to increased tissue catabolism.

Diarrhea and malnutrition are often seen simultaneously with one condition exacerbating the other. Diarrhea has been identified as a major indicator of death during severe acute malnutrition in young children.[55] There is a significant loss of potassium and magnesium in the stools, leading to a decrease in serum electrolytes.[56] There is also urinary loss of electrolytes as a result of increased muscle breakdown.[57] Iron absorption and metabolism are also affected by infection.[52,58] Infections such as malaria and typhoid may cause increased hemolysis and resultant acute hemolytic anemia.

## NUTRITION AND IMMUNITY

### CELLULAR IMMUNE RESPONSE

The cell-mediated response is compromised in malnourished children. This is illustrated by the fact that the mortality rate for measles among malnourished children is four times that of well-nourished children.[59] In addition, individuals given supplemental protein have a significantly lower incidence of tuberculosis than non-supplemented, poorly nourished individuals.[60]

Atrophy of the thymus was the first indication that malnutrition could affect cellular immunity in children who died from kwashiorkor.[61] In addition, the concentration of thymulin in the thymus of malnourished children has been found to be decreased.[62] Thymic atrophy, which occurs as a result of protein, energy, vitamin, and mineral deficiencies, especially zinc,[63] is associated with a decreased production of thymic hormone, an underlying T-cell deficiency,[64] and an increased susceptibility to disseminated infections.[65]

Lymph nodes, tonsils,[66] and spleen also appear to be smaller in malnourished children.[67] Children who are malnourished have a significantly higher percentage of false-negative skin teets than well-nourished children.[68] Further studies have confirmed this defective skin test responsiveness to antigens such as Monilia,[69] streptococcal antigen,[70] Trichophyton,[71] and mumps virus.[72] There is also a correlation between the degree of immune impairment and the degree of weight loss, with alterations in cellular immunity being normalized as nutritional status improves.[72,73]

Edelman et al.[74] performed a series of in vivo and in vitro experiments designed to evaluate the inflammatory, sensitizing, and recall limbs of the cell-mediated immune system, as well as the responsiveness of isolated lymphocytes. To evaluate T-lymphocyte function in vivo, there must be intact circulating thymus-derived T lymphocytes, which are capable of being sensitized to a foreign antigen. Sensitized lymphocytes must be able to identify the foreign antigen and release lymphokines, which, in turn, produce a local inflammatory response. In this study, dinitroflourobenzene, (DNFB) was applied to the forearms of 30 malnourished children. Only four (13%) had positive inflammatory responses, indicating that the inflammatory response is depressed in children with PEM.

Other investigators have found that isolated peripheral lymphocytes from malnourished children react poorly to stimulation with mitogens such as phytohemagglutinin (PHA)[66,71] and pokeweed.[72] The depression in lymphocyte transformation improved with nutritional recovery.[66,72] Sellmeyer et al.[75] also reported a profound depression of lymphocyte transformation in well-nourished children who had measles and gastroenteritis. Decreased T-cell response to mitogen or antigen stimulation has been attributed to an increase in cell cycle duration,[76] deficiency of a humoral factor required for optimum response of T-cells,[77] an inhibitory substance in the serum,[78] or increased levels of $\alpha$-fetoprotein.[79] In addition to the depressed in vitro responsiveness of isolated lymphocytes to antigenic and mitogenic stimulation,[80] circulating lymphocytes are numerically decreased in malnourished children,[80] particularly the helper phenotype,[81] which is replaced by a proportionate increase in "null" lymphoid cells.[81] Keusch et al.,[82] however, found that not all malnourished patients had decreased circulating T-cells, although all were clinically similar. This suggests that specific nutrient deficits associated with PEM may be important etiologic factors in the depressed cellular immune response.

## NATURAL KILLER CELLS

Natural killer (NK) cells are non-T, non-B large granular lymphoid cells that play a vital role in immune surveillance against virus-infected and cancer cells. Unlike cytotoxic T cells, which are antigen-specific and major histocompatibility complex (MHC)-restricted, NK cells act nonspecifically and in an unrestricted manner.[83] Depressed NK cell activity in children with PEM returned to normal levels with improved nutritional status.[84] Addition of exogenous interferon, a potent stimulator of NK cells in vitro, had variable effects on NK activity, depending on the degree of malnutrition. In well-nourished and nutritionally recovered children,

interferon-enhanced NK activity, although it had no effect on cells from marasmic children, had a suppressive effect on cells from kwashiorkor patients.

## INTERLEUKINS

ILs, a family of peptide/glycoprotein hormones or factors produced by activated leukocytes, act as autoparacrine signals for activation, differentiation, and proliferation of a variety of cell types participating in the immune response. A number of these factors have been studied extensively; genes for some have been cloned. Recombinant products are undergoing clinical trials.

The most extensively characterized ILs are IL-1 and IL-2, products primarily of macrophages and T cells, respectively. Macrophages also produce TNF or cachectin. IL-1 acts as an activation signal for T- and B-cell proliferation and participates in inflammatory responses as well. IL-2 is synthesized and secreted by activated helper T-cells with T4 or CD4 phenotype and acts as a potent stimulator of cytotoxic/suppressor T cells, NK cells, B cells, and lymphokine-activated killer cells. Helper T cells also produce interferon-$\alpha$, which has potent stimulatory effects on macrophages and NK cells.

The effect of malnutrition on synthesis and secretion of ILs is not well defined. A significant decrease in IL-1 activity was observed following in vitro stimulation of macrophages from children with severe malnutrition[85] as well as in a mouse model of protein malnutrition.[86] In addition, macrophages from children with kwashiorkor produced a suppressor factor(s) that inhibits the proliferation of murine thymocytes. The investigators suggest that a significant impairment of macrophage function may result in suppression of cell-mediated immunity in the malnourished child. Zinc has also been shown to enhance the activation and response of thymocytes to IL-1.[87] Addition of zinc to in vitro cultures of human peripheral blood T cells[88] or murine splenic T cells[89] resulted in the induction of interferon-$\alpha$ and IL-4 production, respectively. The other macrophage products, cachectin and TNF,[90,91] have been shown to be identical molecules based on bioactivity, on immunologic studies, and on amino acid sequence homology.[92–94] Increased serum cachectin levels have been reported in human patients with Gram-negative septic shock,[95] parasitism, and severe malnutrition.[96,97] Cachectin also appears to play an important role in the pathogenesis of the cerebral form of murine malaria[98,99] and in the early stages of graft-versus-host disease.[100]

Earlier studies suggested that severe malnutrition has a markedly suppressive and long-lasting effect on cell-mediated immunity, as reflected by defective T-cell function. Since T cells play a central role in the regulation of the duration and the magnitude of the immune response, one can expect a wide-ranging effect on different cell types participating in a protective immune response.[101] One study suggests that cell-mediated immunity may remain depressed for several years in small-for-gestation, low-birth-weight infants.[102] Paradoxically, overnutrition or obesity can also result in variable impairment of cell-mediated immune responses.[103,104]

Although there is little information available describing the relationship between IL-2 levels and human malnutrition, a single-nutrient deficiency, such as vitamin A or iron,[106,107] has been shown to result in decreased T-cell proliferation and IL-2 production in animals. Interestingly, even mild dietary zinc deficiency has been shown to reduce the function of Th1 cells due to decreased production of interferon-$\gamma$, IL-2, and TNF-$\alpha$.[108] Murthy[105] evaluated the effect of vitamin A deficiency in rats with regard to T-cell numbers and function. A decrease in the absolute number and percentage of T cells was observed, primarily reflecting the helper T-cell subset, which in turn resulted in altered helper/suppressor T-cell ratio. Furthermore, T cells from vitamin A-deficient rats had a significantly decreased proliferative response to PHA and produced significantly decreased levels of IL-2 when compared with pair-fed and normal control rats. Furthermore, Ahmed and others have recently suggested that levels of vitamin A sufficient to maintain normal vision are not adequate for maintaining measures of T-cell-mediated immunity, but supplementation can improve mitogen-stimulated IL-2, Il-4, and TNF-$\alpha$ measures compared to a non-supplemented group.[109] Severe iron deficiency in mice resulted in a decreased proliferative response of T cell to mitogens, such as concanavalin A, as well as suppressed levels of IL-2 production. Mild-to-moderate iron deficiency, on the other hand, does not appear to affect IL-2 production.[107]

These observations suggest that synthesis and secretion of various ILs produced by macrophages and T cells may be adversely affected by single-nutrient deficiencies. Severe PEM and/or deficiencies of essential vitamins and minerals are most likely to result in defective T-cell functions and, in turn, in a poor cell-mediated immune response to infections and vaccines.

One must also consider the possibility that certain factors such as $\alpha$1-globulin and C-reactive protein, which are elevated in response to infection,[66] may interfere with in vivo and in vitro cell-mediated immune response in malnourished children. All these influences may play roles of varying importance in the depressed cell-mediated immunity, which often improves long before the malnourished child has completely recovered nutritionally.[80]

## Humoral Immune Response

The B lymphocyte is responsible for immunoglobulin production. Determining if the humoral immune system has been altered is accomplished measuring various aspects of the humoral system, such as serum immunoglobulins, secretory immunoglobulins, the number of circulating B cells, and the antibody response to antigens.

In malnutrition, the number of B cells and the circulating immunoglobulin levels are normal or elevated.[110] These levels may be secondary to either a depressed suppressor T-cell population or an increased exposure to various antigens.[110] Although there are normal or increased levels of circulating immunoglobulins and B cells, one cannot assume competency of the humoral immune response to foreign antigens.

Antibody response to antigens appears to vary, depending on the specific antigen, in the malnourished children. Antibody response to antigens such as yellow fever[111] and typhoid vaccines,[112] for example, is markedly impaired, whereas the response to measles, poliovirus, tetanus, and diphtheria toxoid antigens is adequate.[113] There is also a decreased affinity of antibodies to tetanus toxoid and an increased incidence of circulating immune complexes.[114,115] The response to an antigenic stimulus constitutes a much more sensitive and reliable evaluation of the humoral immune system than does the level of circulating immunoglobulins. Although malnourished children have normal or elevated immunoglobulins, the fact that their antibody responses to several vaccines are depressed suggests that nutritional status does affect the humoral immune system. Recent evidence has also shown that vitamins A, $B_6$, $B_{12}$, D, E, and folic acid and the trace elements zinc, copper, and selenium work in synergy to support the protective activities of the immune cells and are essential in antibody production.[116]

The increased incidence of respiratory and gastrointestinal (GI) tract infections common to malnourished children may reflect a deficient secretory IgA system. A significant decrease in secretory IgA (sIgA) and secretory component levels associated with malnutrition has been reported.[117,118] Appropriate renutrition results in restoration of sIgA to normal levels. It is significant that, as the malnourished child's nutritional status improves, his antibody response to certain antigens improves.

## Polymorphonuclear Leukocyte Response

The polymorphonuclear (PMN) leukocyte, which is important in controlling bacterial infections, derives its energy for the phagocytosis and killing of bacteria from glycolysis. Malnourished and normally nourished children have the same total white cell count and the same proportion of PMNs. In malnourished children, however, there is impairment of leukocyte metabolism[119] that affects the activity of key enzymes needed to the completion of bactericidal action of the leukocyte.[120] There is, however, no defect in the phagocytizing ability of PMNs in the malnourished child, although the glycolytic phagocytizing ability of PMN as judged by lactate production is impaired.[121,122] There is also no apparent abnormality either in vacuole formation or in degranulation after phagocytosis by PMNs.[123] Studies of bactericidal activity of PMNs have produced conflicting results.[124,125] The PMNs in malnourished children respond appropriately to dermal injury, are able to phagocytize bacteria adequately, and are able to kill bacteria adequately in the majority of patients. The PMN appears to be the least affected component of the immune system in PEM.

## Complement System

Defects in the complement system have been associated with increased susceptibility to bacterial infection. Activation of the complement system leads to production of complement fragments that are involved in viral neutralization, chemotaxis of PMN leukocytes, monocytes, eosinophils, opsonization of fungi, endotoxin inactivation, lysis of virus-infected cells, and bacteriolysis.[126] Coovadia et al.[47] were the first to report reduced hemolytic activity in the serum of children with PEM. Many of the children they studied had C3 and C4 on the surface of the red blood cell as a result of activation of the complement system. Other investigators have found decreased complement values for malnourished children compared with those for well-nourished controls.[127,128] Suskind et al.[129] found that the hemolytic complement activity of children with malnutrition was significantly depressed, with a significant percentage of the children having anticomplementary activity in their serum. With recovery, the hemolytic activity of the patients' serum improved and the anticomplementary activity disappeared. In addition, about 40% of children had, at the time of admission, circulating endotoxin, which disappeared with treatment.[130]

The increased morbidity–mortality associated with infection and malnutrition is most likely a result of the effect of malnutrition on the immune response. Malnourished children also have an increased susceptibility to infectious agents. It is well established that this increased susceptibility to infection is secondary to the effect of severe PEM on the cell-mediated immune system, humoral immune system, and complement system, and is reversed with improvement in nutritional status. Studies also confirm that the PMN leukocyte system is relatively intact. In order to combat potentially lethal infection in undernourished children, both antibiotic and nutritional therapies are essential.

## TREATMENT OF THE MALNOURISHED CHILD

### DIAGNOSTIC STUDIES

It is important to document the deficiencies that are present in the newly admitted, severely malnourished child. These may include any one or a combination of deficits including protein, energy, vitamins, and minerals. Since nearly all seriously malnourished children are infected, it is essential to determine the site, etiologic agent, and antibiotic sensitivities to all identified pathogens. In addition to a thorough history and physical examination, each child requires a complete blood count and culture of nasopharynx, throat, ear exudate, blood, urine (by suprapubic aspiration), and stool. Cerebrospinal fluid is obtained when clinically indicated. An electrocardiogram and a chest film are routine. Serum electrolytes are measured on admission and throughout recovery. Plasma vitamin A and E levels and the plasma proteins, including serum albumin, should be measured on admission.

The prevalence of infection in malnourished children is significant.[131] Of greatest concern is the septic patient with a life-threatening infection. Signs that have been helpful in diagnosing the septic patient include hypothermia (rectal temperature, <36°C), hypotension (blood pressure, <60/40), leukocytosis with a marked shift to the left, petechiae, and a positive

blood culture. These clinical presentations are considered risk factors of mortality in severely malnourished children.[132]

### FLUID AND ELECTROLYTE THERAPY

Children with PEM have a significant increase in total body water. Active and passive transport of sodium and potassium is severely affected in malnourished children.[133] Normally, the patient presents with normal or low serum sodium, low potassium, low magnesium, and trace minerals.[134] The use of magnesium in the treatment of children with PEM is based on the work of Caddell et al. in Thailand[135] and in East and West Africa.[136]

Although these children have an increase in their total body water, they often show evidence of intravascular dehydration. This is especially true of children with a history of severe diarrhea. Once dehydration is assessed according to the WHO criteria, rehydration should be attempted orally. Some cases can be managed with rice-based solution (sodium 90 mmol/L, potassium 20, chloride 80, citrate 10; rice powder 50 g/L) 10 mL/kg/h for the first 2 h. Subsequently, children should be given 5 mL/kg/h for the next 10 h or until the deficit is corrected.[139] Additionally, children should be given 5–10 mL or oral rehydration solution after each watery stool. If a child is unable to drink due to weakness or vomiting, oral rehydration solution should be given via nasogastric tube.[139]

In cases of severe dehydration, intravenous rehydration is necessary. A severely dehydrated child may receive as much as 20 mL/kg of intravenous solution (2% of body weight) during the first hour of therapy to increase intravascular volume and therefore renal blood flow. Ahmed and others have proposed a standardized rehydration protocol including an initial rehydrating fluid (Na$^+$ 133 mmol/L, K$^+$ 20, Cl 98 acetate 48; plus 5% dextrose; solution A) 20 mL/kg for 1 h then 10 mL/kg for 1 h. After 1 h, oral rehydration solution 10 mL/kg/h is started and continued as with less-severe dehydration.[139] Patients showing evidence of severe potassium depletion may be given up to 6–7 mEq/kg of potassium through oral supplementation. The intravenous solution may contain up to 40 mEq/L of potassium. Infants younger than 2 months should receive a 50% diluted solution with potassium supplemented to 20 mmol/L and 5% added dextrose (solution B).[139] However, if vomiting persists after insertion of a nasogastric tube, solution B should be infused at 10 mL/kg/h for 2 h, and then at 5 mL/kg/h until either the child is able to drink or the deficit is corrected.[139]

B-complex vitamins are given parenterally for the several days of hospitalization (Table 47.1). Because of the marked decrease in total body potassium, the patient is given supplemental intravenous and oral potassium at a maintenance dose of 5 mEq/kg daily. Magnesium is given at a dose of 0.4 mEq/kg intramuscularly for 7 days followed by oral magnesium in a dosage of 1.4 mEq/kg/day. Once a patient has reached an oral intake of 175 kilocalories (kCal) and 4 g/kg/day of protein, their requirement for magnesium at oral dosages is met by the formula alone. No further oral supplementation is usually required.

**TABLE 47.1**

**Diet Composition**

**Macronutrient Composition of Formula (Per kg Body Weight)**

| Energy (Cal) | Protein (g) | Fat (g) | Carbohydrate (g) |
|---|---|---|---|
| 175 | 4 | 9.5 | 18.3 |

**Vitamin Supplementation**

| Vitamin | Unit | Daily Initial Therapy IM or IV for 3 Days Beginning on Day 2 | Daily Maintenance Therapy from the 5th Day Until the End of Week 10 |
|---|---|---|---|
| Thiamine | mg | 5.0 | Si 0.7 |
| Riboflavin | mg | 5.0 | 1.0 |
| Pyridoxine | mg | 2.5 | 1.0 |
| Nicotinamide | mg | 37.5 | 11.0 |
| Pantothenate | mg | 5.0 | 5.0 |
| Ascorbic acid | mg | 200 | 45.0 |
| Folic acid | mg | 1.5 | 0.1 |
| Vitamin B$_{12}$ | μg | 7.5 | 5.0 |
| Vitamin A | IU[a] | 5000 | 2500 |
| Vitamin D | IU[a] | 1000 | 400 |
| Vitamin E | IU | 50 | 10 |
| Vitamin K | μg[a] | 300 | 100 |

**Mineral Requirements/Day (Formula Plus Supplement)**

| Mineral | Unit | Dose |
|---|---|---|
| Sodium (Na) | mEq/kg | 2.0–3.0 |
| Potassium (K) | mEq/kg | 5.0 |
| Magnesium (Mg) | mEq/kg | 1.4 |
| Zinc (Zn) | mg/kg | 1.0–2.0 |
| Iron (Fe) | mg/kg | 6.0 |
| Calcium (Ca) | mg | 800.0 |
| Phosphorous (P) | mg | 800.0 |
| Fluorine (F) | mg | 0.5–1.5 |
| Manganese (Mn) | mg | 1.0–1.5 |
| Copper (Cu) | mg | 1.0–1.5 |
| Molybdenum (Mo) | mg | 0.05–0.1 |
| Chromium (Cr) | mg | 0.02–0.08 |
| Selenium (Se) | mg | 0.02–0.08 |
| Iodine (1) | mg | 0.07 |

[a] Therapeutic doses of the fat-soluble vitamins are given as indicated to combat overt deficiency disease.

## DIETARY THERAPY

During the famine in Ethiopia, Lindtjorn[137] found that although malnutrition did not increase the incidence of diarrheal disease, nutritional rehabilitation reduced the problem of diarrhea and led to a decreased mortality. Other research has shown that malnutrition is a significant factor in the duration, but not incidence, of diarrhea.[132] When diarrhea is severe, oral intake may be withheld for up to 24 h. The current standardized protocol for refeeding begins immediately on admission, when appropriate, with a liquid diet given every 2 h. Specifically, children with marasmus and marasmic-kwashiorkor are given 10 mL/kg/feed (80 kcal/kg/day) on day 1 and 12 mL/kg/feed (96 kcal/kg/day) on days 2 and 3.[139] If diarrhea is not present, a concentrated diet is given at 12 mL/kg (175 kcal/kg/day).[139] If the child is diagnosed with kwashiorkor, the treatment is started at 9 mL/kg/feed (72 kcal/kg/day) and continued through day 3. Then, if there is no diarrhea, the concentration is increased to 108 kcal/kg/day on day 4 onward.[109] Fjeld et al.[138] have suggested a method, using doubly labeled water, in which energy for maintenance activity, tissue synthesis, and storage are measured in patients to predict energy requirements necessary to achieve catch-up. Dietary intake is initiated at 50 Cal/kg and 1 g/kg of protein. Monitored care is essential until a patient has reached at least 90% of weight-for-height.

In early stages of PEM, feeding is more efficiently accomplished via a milk-based formula given by tube. Formulas

**TABLE 47.2**
**Antibiotics Used in Treating the Malnourished Child**

| Indications | Antibiotic | Dose (mg/kg day) |
|---|---|---|
| Pneumonia or otitis media | Ampicillin | 50–100 |
| | Penicillin | 50–100 |
| | Bactrim (TMP-SMZ) | 8–10 mg/k TMP |
| Staph pneumonia | Oxacillin | 100–200 |
| Genitourinary infection | Ampicillin | 100 |
| | Gantrisin | 150–200 |
| Sepsis | Systemic antibiotics | |
| | Ampicillin and | 200–300 |
| | Gentamycin, or | 3.0–7.5 |
| | Cefuroxime, or | 75–150 |
| | Ceftriaxone | 50–100 |
| GI antisepsis | Colistin (for aerobic organisms) | 5–10 |
| | Flagyl (for anaerobic organisms) | 35–50 |

supplemented with dextromaltose and corn oil do not seem to result in the prolonged diarrhea associated with lactose or monosaccharidic intolerance. Formulas should also contain appropriate supplementation of essential vitamins and minerals (Table 47.1). Children over the age of 1 year should be given 1 mL of a multivitamin supplement containing vitamin A (5000 IU), vitamin D (1000 IU), thiamine hydrochloride (1.6 mg), riboflavin (1 mg), pyridoxine hydrochloride (1 mg), nicotinamide (10 mg), calcium D-pantothenate (5 mg), ascorbic acid (50 mg), two times a day for at least 15 days. Infants less than 1 year of age should receive half of this dose.[139]

It is important to consider iron supplementation. Lynch et al.[140] have shown that iron absorption in PEM is decreased. Without supplementation, the decreased bone marrow iron stores seen in PEM patients on admission disappear completely within 4–6 weeks. Intramuscular iron produces an immediate increase in bone marrow stores. Because of the poor absorption of oral iron in PEM, parenteral iron or high doses of oral iron in the range of 6 mg/kg/day of elemental iron is recommended. Iron therapy should be initiated, however, only when the patient is on antibiotics and/or when the threat of infection has passed usually after about 1–2 weeks of hospitalization.

Zinc supplementation is also suggested. Investigators in Chile found that 2 mg/kg of elemental zinc as zinc acetate given to marasmic infants had significant positive effects on weight gain and host defense mechanisms.[141] Investigators in Bangladesh have also found zinc supplementation to be important in the recovery of malnourished children,[142,143] particularly in the treatment of those experiencing diarrhea.[144,145]

In addition to nutritional supplementation, several investigators have found that psycho-stimulation improves developmental catch-up in malnourished children.

**ANTIBIOTIC THERAPY**

Because several of the host defenses against infection are affected in PEM, survival is dependent on the immediate identification and treatment of infection. The use of antibiotics is associated with decreased morbidity and mortality in PEM, especially in the septic child (Table 47.2). For septic children, a regimen of ampicillin and gentamicin, or a cephalosporin, is standard. Gentamicin is often used because of the common occurrence of Pseudomonas sepsis.

Two drugs may be used for intestinal antisepsis against aerobic and anaerobic organisms (Table 47.2). They are considered because of the occurrence of small bowel overgrowth.[131] The GI tract is one of the major sources of endotoxin production, and an increased incidence of endotoxemia has been described in children with PEM.[146] If the GI tract is sterilized, a potential source of Gram-negative sepsis and endotoxic shock may be eliminated for the few days needed to regenerate an intact GI mucosa. GI antiseptics plus one broad-spectrum antibiotic is considerably less expensive than the traditional systemic antibiotics used for 7–10 days.

## LONG-TERM CONSEQUENCES OF PEM

### GROWTH

Children who survive malnutrition are generally stunted.[2,147] In one squatter colony in Cape Town, South Africa, 47.2% of preschool children were below the 3rd percentile for height-for-age—significant evidence of chronic malnutrition.[1] An estimated 32%–52% of preschool Ethiopian children in Sudanese refugee camps were less than 80% of reference standards for height and weight.[12] The mortality rate for these children was 22 per 10,000 per day.

The severity of the effects of malnutrition is correlated with the age of onset and duration; the most profound damage results when the period of deprivation occurs during the first 2 years of life.[148–151] Korean children who were adopted in the United States before 2 years of age had better catch-up than those adopted later.[152] Animal studies confirm the negative effects of early and prolonged nutritional deprivation.[153] In addition, there is some indication that this influence may begin as early as the first weeks after birth.[154]

As increasing numbers of children survive episodes of malnutrition, investigators have attempted to ascertain the potential for improving or reversing the deleterious effects.[153,155] Results of these studies generally indicate that, even under optimal circumstances, "catch-up," that is, attaining the growth and development of children who have not had early nutritional deprivation, is never complete. Malnourished rats demonstrated limited catch-up in height and weight when compared with controls.[156] Prolonged malnutrition in pigs during the suckling period produced long-term stunting even when rehabilitation included ad libitum food intake.[157] In Hyderabad, India, previously malnourished boys who were studied through adulthood demonstrated significant stunting of ultimate stature.[158] In addition, the severity of their stunting was proportional to the severity of the childhood malnutrition. The 240 malnourished Korean orphans adopted in the United States surpassed the standards of Korean children but were still significantly shorter and weighed less than well-nourished controls.[152] Bone age, an indicator of height potential, is also affected. Delayed bone maturation was seen in 17 of 20 kwashiorkor patients studied by Belli et al.[159] Alvear et al.[148] also correlated bone age to nutritional status. All studies on catch-up in humans do not reach the same conclusions, but these differences may well reflect differences in study design.[160,161]

Although ultimate catch-up is usually limited, recovering malnourished children often have accelerated growth compared to healthy controls.[162] In northern Thailand, infants between 6 and 18 months fed a high-protein diet grew at or above reference standards in height and weight, although they were not able to attain complete catch-up for age.[163]

The onset of puberty is also affected as a result of early malnutrition.[164] Cameron et al.[165] found that boys who had experienced kwashiorkor had significant delays to all pubertal stages. Galler et al.[162] reported that girls with histories of marasmus had significant delays in the onset of menarche compared to healthy controls.

Less easily measurable, but perhaps more important, is the effect of early malnutrition on psychological and behavioral development. Head circumference, because of its relationship to brain development, is an important growth parameter. Househam and de Villiers[166] performed computed tomography on the brains of eight kwashiorkor patients of 4 years of age and under and found severe cerebral atrophy in all children. Stoch and Smythe,[167] studying the effects of early malnutrition on intellectual development, reported that previously malnourished children were not able to catch up in head circumference. They concluded that since there was little growth in head circumference after 10 years of age, this effect was likely to be permanent. Chase and Martin[150] reported that a malnourished child who began renourishment at 5 months of age achieved the 50th percentile in height and weight after 3 years of age, but remained below the 3rd percentile in head circumference. A study of 150 preterm and full-term infants also found that catch-up growth of head circumference lagged behind that height.[168] Graham and Adrianzen,[169] on the other hand, found that head circumference paralleled the increase in stature in 13 malnourished Peruvian children.

Investigators have attempted to ascertain the extent of the effect of malnutrition on intellectual development.[167,170,171] Grantham-McGregor et al.[151] reported that the developmental delays found in severely malnourished children were associated with stunting, indicating a relationship with chronic deprivation rather than acute malnutrition. Agarwal et al.,[172] using the Wechsler Intelligence Scale for Indian Children and a series of Piagetian tasks, demonstrated a relationship between cognitive development and malnutrition in 1300 children between 6 and 8 years of age that was not influenced by other environmental factors. Galler et al.[170,171,173] found a significant impact of early malnutrition on later intellectual performance, fine motor skills, and classroom attention.

There is evidence, however, that by adding psycho-stimulation to a dietary rehabilitative program, the prognosis of these children greatly improves.[21,174,175] In addition, Carughi et al.[176] found, in studies on rats, that stimulation during nutritional rehabilitation enhanced dendritic branching and thickness of the occipital cortex.

## SUMMARY

Prognosis for the child with severe PEM is optimal with hospital treatment. Careful clinical and laboratory diagnosis must be complemented by an adequate hospital stay. Considerations include careful diagnosis of the type of deficiency disease, the extent of fluid and electrolyte imbalance, and the kind, site, and antibiotic sensitivity of existing infection(s). When the malnutrition is secondary to another disease state, consideration must be given to the impact of the disease state and its therapy on nutritional status as well as on nutritional interventions.

Immediate management of malnutrition includes fluid and electrolyte therapy, nutritional support, and antibiotic therapy. Ultimately, nutrition intake should provide at least 175 Cal/kg/day and 4 g protein/kg/day, plus appropriate vitamin and mineral supplementation. The problem of sepsis must be combated with vigorous antibiotic therapy.

Because of this relationship to eventual prognosis, it is important to recognize the prevalence of malnutrition secondary to disease states. For most of the world's children, however, the main cause of malnutrition is poverty and deprivation. Some of these children suffer severely enough to be hospitalized, but the majority survive with critical physical and developmental stunting. Improving the mortality from malnutrition is, of course, an important objective. It is, however, the long-term ramification of malnutrition, especially those that may prevent a child from developing intellectually and behaviorally, that accentuate the need for innovative and creative solutions to this critical problem.

## REFERENCES

1. You D, Rou New J, Wardlaw T. Levels and trends in child mortality: Report 2012. UNICEF, New York, 2012. Available online at: http://www.childmortality.org/files_v11/download/Levels%20and%20Trends%20in%20Child%20Mortality%20Report%202012.pdf
2. Bagenholm G, Nasher AA, Kristiansson B. *Eur J Clin Nutr* 44:425;1990.
3. Leichsenring M, Doehring-Schwerdtfeger E, Bremer HJ et al. *Eur J Pediatr* 148:155;1988.
4. Stevens GA, Finucane MM, Paciorek CJ et al. *Lancet* 380:824; 2012.
5. Coulter JB, Omer MI, Suliman GI et al. *Ann Trop Paediatr* 8:96;1988.
6. Victora CG, Barros FC, Vaughan JP et al. *Ann Hum Biol* 14:49;1987.
7. Brown KH, Solomons NW. *Infect Dis Clin North Am* 5:297;1991.
8. Lindtjorn B. *BMJ* 301:1123;1990.
9. Gillam SJ. *Trop Doct* 19:82;1989.
10. Lima M, Figueira F, Ebrahim GJ. *J Trop Pediatr* 36:14;1990.
11. Lindtjorn B. *Ann Trop Paediatr* 7:1;1987.
12. Shears P, Berry AM, Murphy R, Nabil MA. *Br Med J (Clin Res Ed)* 295:314;1987.
13. Avery ME, Rotch TM. *Acta Paediatr Hung* 31:149;1991.
14. Fuchs G. *Secondary Malnutrition in Children.* New York: Raven Press, 1990.
15. Sallon S, Deckelbaum RJ, Schmid, II et al. *Am J Dis Child* 142:312;1988.
16. Trehan I, O'Hare BA, Phiri A, Heikens GT. *AIDS Res Treat* 2012:790786;2012.
17. Smith DE, Stevens MC, Booth IW. *Eur J Pediatr* 150:318;1991.
18. Gayle HD, Dibley MJ, Marks JS, Trowbridge FL. *Am J Dis Child* 141:531;1987.
19. Karp RJ, Scholl TO, Decker E, Ebert E. *Clin Pediatr (Phila)* 28:317;1989.
20. Keusch GT. *Malnutrition, Infection and Immune Function.* New York: Raven; 1990.
21. Super CM, Herrera MG, Mora JO. *Child Dev* 61:29;1990.
22. Rivera JA, Habicht JP, Robson DS. *Am J Clin Nutr* 54:62;1991.
23. Latham MC. *J Environ Pathol Toxicol Oncol* 10:168;1990.
24. Gomez F, Ramos Galvan R, Frenk S et al. *Bull World Health Organ* 78:1275;2000.
25. Habicht JP, Martorell R, Yarbrough C et al. *Lancet* 1:611;1974.
26. Martorell R. *Poverty and Stature in Children.* New York: Raven Press; 1988.
27. Gardner LI. Endocrine aspects of malnutrition: Marasmus, kwashiorkor and psychosocial deprivation. In Amacher P. (Ed.), *Kroc Foundation Symposia, Number 1.* Santa Ynez: CA Kroc Foundation; 1973.
28. Bairagi R. *Am J Epidemiol* 126:258;1987.
29. Waterlow JC. *Lancet* 2:87;1973.
30. Anderson MA, Gopaldas T, Abbi R, Gujral S. *Indian Pediatr* 27:247;1990.
31. Ross DA, Taylor N, Hayes R, McLean M. *Int J Epidemiol* 19:636;1990.
32. Connor NE, Manary MJ. *Matern Child Health J* 15:980;2011.
33. Keet MP, Hansen JD, Truswell AS. *Pediatrics* 45:965;1970.
34. Ahmed T, Rahman S, Cravioto A. *Indian J Med Res* 130:651;2009.
35. Jahoor F, Badaloo A, Reid M, Forrester T. *Ann Trop Paediatr* 28:87;2008.
36. Calderon RR, Ga JM. *Am J Clin Nutr* 16:351;1965.
37. Garrow JS, Pike MC. *Br J Nutr* 21:155;1967.
38. Waterlow JC, Cravioto J, Stephen JM. *Adv Protein Chem* 15:131;1960.
39. Kahn E, Falcke HC. *J Pediatr* 49:37;1956.
40. Gopalan C. *Kwashiokor and Marasmus: Evolution and Distinguishing Features.* Boston, MA: Little Brown, 1968.
41. Scrimshaw NS, Behar M. *Science* 133:2039;1961.
42. Kurpad AV. *Indian J Med Res* 124:129;2006.
43. Morley DC. *Am J Dis Child* 103:230;1962.
44. Beisel WR. *Malnutrition as a Consequence of Stress.* New York: Raven Press, 1977.
45. Manary MJ, Broadhead RL, Yarasheski KE. *Am J Clin Nutr* 67:1205;1998.
46. Puffer RR, Serrano CV. *Bol Oficina Sanit Panam* 75:1;1973.
47. Coovadia HM, Parent MA, Loening WE et al. *Am J Clin Nutr* 27:665;1974.
48. Gamrin L, Essen P, Forsberg AM et al. *Crit Care Med* 24:575;1996.
49. Feigin RD, Klainer AS, Beisel WR, Hornick RB. *N Engl J Med* 278:293;1968.
50. Reid M, Badaloo A, Forrester T et al. *Am J Clin Nutr* 76:1409;2002.
51. Aslan Y, Erduran E, Gedik Y et al. *Cent Afr J Med* 42:179;1996.
52. Alleyne C. *Protein Energy Malnutrition.* London, U.K.: Edward Arnold, 1977.
53. Wickramasinghe SN, Akinyanju OO, Grange A. *Clin Lab Haematol* 10:135;1988.
54. George J, Yiannakis M, Main B et al. *J Nutr* 142:781;2012.
55. Irena AH, Mwambazi M, Mulenga V. *Nutr J* 10:110;2011.
56. Alleyne GA. *Br J Nutr* 24:205;1970.
57. Alleyne GA, Millward DJ, Scullard GH. *J Pediatr* 76:75;1970.
58. Beresford CH, Neale RJ, Brooks OG. *Lancet* 1:568;1971.
59. Gordon JE, Jansen AA, Ascoli W. *J Pediatr* 66:779;1965.
60. Leyton GB. *Lancet* 2:73;1946.
61. Vint FW. *East Afr Med J* 13:332;1937.
62. Jambon B, Ziegler O, Maire B et al. *Am J Clin Nutr* 48:335;1988.
63. Golden MH, Jackson AA, Golden BE. *Lancet* 2:1057;1977.
64. Chandra RK. *Clin Exp Immunol* 38:228;1979.
65. Purtilo DT, Connor DH. *Arch Dis Child* 50:149;1975.
66. Smythe PM, Brereton-Stiles GG, Grace HJ et al. *Lancet* 2:939;1971.
67. Mugerwa JW. *J Pathol* 105:105;1971.
68. Jayalakshmi VT, Gopalan C. *Indian J Med Res* 46:87;1958.
69. Feldman G, Gianantonio CA. *Medicina (B Aires)* 32:1;1972.
70. Work TH, Ifekwunigwe A, Jelliffe DB et al. *Ann Intern Med* 79:701;1973.
71. Chandra RK. *J Pediatr* 81:1194;1972.
72. Abbassy AS, el-Din MK, Hassan AI et al. *J Trop Med Hyg* 77:13;1974.
73. Law DK, Dudrick SJ, Abdou NI. *Ann Intern Med* 79:545;1973.
74. Edelman R, Suskind R, Olson RE, Sirisinha S. *Lancet* 1:506;1973.
75. Sellmeyer E, Bhettay E, Truswell AS et al. *Arch Dis Child* 47:429;1972.
76. Murthy PB, Rahiman MA, Tulpule PG. *Br J Nutr* 47:445;1982.
77. Beatty DW, Dowdle EB. *Clin Exp Immunol* 32:134;1978.
78. Salimonu LS, Johnson AO, Williams AI et al. *Clin Exp Immunol* 47:626;1982.
79. Chandra RK, Bhujwala RA. *Int Arch Allergy Appl Immunol* 1977;53:180;1977.
80. Kulapongs P. *In vitro Cell-Mediated Immune Response in Thai Children with PEM.* New York: Raven Press, 1977.
81. Chandra RK. *Acta Paediatr Scand* 68:841;1979.
82. Keusch GT, Cruz JR, Torun B et al. *J Pediatr Gastroenterol Nutr* 6:265;1987.

83. Ritz J, Schmidt RE, Michon J et al. *Adv Immunol* 42:181;1988.
84. Salimonu LS, Ojo-Amaize E, Johnson AO et al. *Cell Immunol* 82:210;1983.
85. Bhaskaram P, Sivakumar B. *Arch Dis Child* 61:182;1986.
86. Hassanein NM, Talaat RM, Bassiouny K, Hamed MR. *Egypt J Immunol* 13:49;2006.
87. Winchurch RA. *Clin Immunol Immunopathol* 47:174;1988.
88. Salas M, Kirchner H. *Clin Immunol Immunopathol* 45:139;1987.
89. Winchurch RA, Togo J, Adler WH. *Eur J Immunol* 17:127;1987.
90. Kawakami M, Cerami A. *J Exp Med* 154:631;1981.
91. Carswell EA, Old LJ, Kassel RL et al. *Proc Natl Acad Sci U S A* 72:3666;1975.
92. Beutler B, Mahoney J, Le Trang N et al. *J Exp Med* 161:984;1985.
93. Pennica D, Hayflick JS, Bringman TS et al. *Proc Natl Acad Sci U S A* 82:6060;1985.
94. Caput D, Beutler B, Hartog K et al. *Proc Natl Acad Sci U S A* 83:1670;1986.
95. Waage A, Halstensen A, Espevik T. *Lancet* 1:355;1987.
96. Scuderi P, Sterling KE, Lam KS et al. *Lancet* 2:1364;1986.
97. Cerami A, Ikeda Y, Le Trang N et al. *Immunol Lett* 11:173;1985.
98. Clark IA, Cowden WB, Butcher GA, Hunt NH. *Am J Pathol* 129:192;1987.
99. Grau GE, Fajardo LF, Piguet PF et al. *Science* 237:1210;1987.
100. Piguet PF, Grau GE, Allet B, Vassalli P. *J Exp Med* 166:1280;1987.
101. Chandra RK. *Acta Paediatr Scand* 68:137;1979.
102. Xanthou M. *Acta Paediatr Scand Suppl* 319:143;1985.
103. Chandra RK, Kutty KM. *Acta Paediatr Scand* 69:25;1980.
104. Chandra RK. *Cancer Res* 41:3795;1981.
105. Murthy KJ. *Vitamin A Deficiency and T Lymphocyte Function.* ASPEN: New Orleans, LA, 339, 1987.
106. Kuvibidila S, Nauss KM, Baliga BS, Suskind RM. *Am J Clin Nutr* 37:15;1983.
107. Kuvibidila SR, Baliga BS, Suskind RM. *Am J Clin Nutr* 34:2635;1981.
108. Beck FW, Prasad AS, Kaplan J et al. *Am J Physiol* 272:E1002;1997.
109. Ahmad SM, Haskell MJ, Raqib R, Stephenson CB. *Br J Nutr* 102:797;2009.
110. Suskind R. *Immunoglobulins and Antibody Response in Thai Children with PEM.* New York: Raven Press, 1977.
111. Brown RE, Katz M. *Trop Geogr Med* 18:125;1966.
112. Jose DG, Welch JS, Doherty PL. *Aust Paediatr J* 6:192;1970.
113. Brown RE, Katz M. *East Afr Med J* 42:221;1965.
114. Chandra RK, Chandra S, Gupta S. *Am J Clin Nutr* 40:131;1984.
115. Spurr GB, Barac-Nieto M, Reina JC, Ramirez R. *Am J Clin Nutr* 39:452;1984.
116. Maggini S, Wintergerst ES, Beveridge S, Hornig DH. *Br J Nutr* 98(Suppl 1):S29;2007.
117. Sirisinha S, Suskind R, Edelman R et al. *Pediatrics* 55:166;1975.
118. Watson RR, McMurray DN, Martin P, Reyes MA. *Am J Clin Nutr* 42:281;1985.
119. Selvaraj RJ, Bhat KS. *Am J Clin Nutr* 25:166;1972.
120. Selvaraj RJ, Bhat KS. *Biochem J* 127:255;1972.
121. Yoshida T, Metcoff J, Frenk S, De la Pena C. *Nature* 214:525;1967.
122. Seth V, Chandra RK. *Arch Dis Child* 47:282;1972.
123. Douglas SD SK. *The Phagocyte in Protein Energy Malnutrition.* New York: Raven Press, 1977.
124. Patrick J, Golden M. *Am J Clin Nutr* 30:1478;1977.
125. Tuck R, Burke V, Gracey M et al. *Arch Dis Child* 1979;54:445;1979.
126. Sirisinha S. *The Complement System in Protein-Calorie Malnutrition.* New York: Raven Press, 1977.
127. Neumann CG, Lawlor GJ, Jr., Stiehm ER et al. *Am J Clin Nutr* 28:89;1975.
128. Sirisinha S, Edelman R, Suskind R et al. *Lancet* 1:1016;1973.
129. Suskind R, Edelman R, Kulapongs P et al. *Am J Clin Nutr* 29:1089;1976.
130. Klein K. *Endotoxemia, a Possible Cause of Decreased Complement Activity in Malnourished Children.* New York: Raven Press, 1977.
131. Suskind R. *The Inpatient and Outpatient Treatment of the Child with Severe Protein-Calorie Malnutrition.* New York: Academic Press, 1975.
132. Roy SK, Buis M, Weersma R et al. *J Health Popul Nutr* 29:229;2011.
133. Willis JS, Golden MH. *Eur J Clin Nutr* 42:635;1988.
134. Garrow JS. *Electrolyte Metabolism in Severe Infantile Malnutrition.* Blackwell Publishing: Oxford, U.K., 1968.
135. Caddell JL, Suskind R, Sillup H, Olson RE. *J Pediatr* 83:129;1973.
136. Caddell JL, Goddard DR. *N Engl J Med* 276:533;1967.
137. Lindtjorn B. *Trop Geogr Med* 42:365;1990.
138. Fjeld CR, Schoeller DA, Brown KH. *Pediatr Res* 25:503;1989.
139. Ahmed T, Ali M, Ullah MM et al. *Lancet* 353:1919;1999.
140. Lynch SR, Becker D, Seftel H et al. *Am J Clin Nutr* 23:792;1970.
141. Castillo-Duran C, Heresi G, Fisberg M, Uauy R. *Am J Clin Nutr* 45:602;1987.
142. Khanum S, Alam AN, Anwar I et al. *Eur J Clin Nutr* 42:709;1988.
143. Simmer K, Khanum S, Carlsson L, Thompson RP. *Am J Clin Nutr* 47:1036;1988.
144. Roy SK, Tomkins AM, Akramuzzaman SM et al. *Arch Dis Child* 77:196;1997.
145. Roy SK, Tomkins AM, Haider R et al. *Eur J Clin Nutr* 53:529;1999.
146. Klein K, Fuchs GJ, Kulapongs P et al. *J Pediatr Gastroenterol Nutr* 7:225;1988.
147. Keller W, Fillmore CM. *World Health Stat Q* 36:129;1983.
148. Alvear J, Artaza C, Vial M et al. *Arch Dis Child* 61:257;1986.
149. Briers PJ, Hoorweg J, Stanfield JP. *Acta Paediatr Scand* 64:853;1975.
150. Chase HP, Martin HP. *N Engl J Med* 282:933;1970.
151. Grantham-McGregor S, Powell C, Fletcher P. *Eur J Clin Nutr* 43:403;1989.
152. Lien NM, Meyer KK, Winick M. *Am J Clin Nutr* 30:1734;1977.
153. Eberhardt MJ, Halas ES. *Physiol Behav* 41:309;1987.
154. Lucas A. *Acta Paediatr Scand Suppl* 365:58;1990.
155. Alleyne C. *The Effects of Protein Energy Malnutrition on Growth.* London, U.K.: Edward Arnold, 1977.
156. Smart JL, Massey RF, Nash SC, Tonkiss J. *Br J Nutr* 58:245;1987.
157. Widdowson M. *Changes in Pigs due to Undernutrition before Birth and for One, Two, and Three Years Afterwards, and the Effects of Rehabilitation.* New York: Plenum Press, 1974.
158. Satyanarayana K, Prasanna Krishna T, Narasinga Rao BS. *Hum Nutr Clin Nutr* 40:131;1986.
159. Belli L, Andreatta M, Reggiori A, Tragni C. *Radiol Med* 79:568;1990.
160. Waterlow JC, Buzina R, Keller W, Lane JM et al. *Bull World Health Organ* 55:489;1977.

161. Sutphen JL. *J Pediatr Gastroenterol Nutr* 4:169;1985.
162. Galler JR, Ramsey FC, Salt P, Archer E. *J Pediatr Gastroenterol Nutr* 6:841;1987.
163. Lewinter-Suskind L. Study on the effects of high protein supplement diets on children in northern Thailand. *Proceedings of the International Conference on Nutrition.* Chaingmai, Thailand, 1974.
164. Kulin HE, Bwibo N, Mutie D, Santner SJ. *Am J Clin Nutr* 36:527;1982.
165. Cameron N, Mitchell J, Meyer D et al. *Ann Hum Biol* 17:217;1990.
166. Househam KC, de Villiers JF. *Arch Dis Child* 62:589;1987.
167. Stoch MB, Smythe PM. *Arch Dis Child* 38:546;1963.
168. Brandt I. *Arztl Jugendkd* 81:321;1990.
169. Graham GG, Adrianzen, TB. *Pediat Res* 5:691;1971.
170. Galler JR, Ramsey FC, Forde V et al. *J Pediatr Gastroenterol Nutr* 6:847;1987.
171. Galler JR, Ramsey FC, Salt P, Archer E. *J Pediatr Gastroenterol Nutr* 6:855;1987.
172. Agarwal DK, Upadhyay SK, Agarwal KN. *Acta Paediatr Scand* 78:115;1989.
173. Galler JR, Ramsey FC, Morley DS et al. *Pediatr Res* 28:235;1990.
174. Grantham-McGregor S, Schofield W, Powell C. *Pediatrics* 79:247;1987.
175. Puentes-Rojas R, Winter-Elizalde A, Mateluna-Garate E et al. *Bol Med Hosp Infant Mex* 46:308;1989.
176. Carughi A, Carpenter KJ, Diamond MC. *J Nutr* 119:2005;1989.

# 48 Childhood Obesity

*David L. Suskind, Rikki S. Corniola, and Robert M. Suskind*

## CONTENTS

Obesity in childhood is the major health issue in pediatric health care today. The prevalence of obesity-related comorbidities has risen in parallel with that of obesity. Studies in the United States confirm the growing prevalence of obesity in children and adolescents.[1] Early detection and treatment of obesity are essential. The percentage of obese children who become obese adults is 14% at age 6 months,[2] 41% at age 7 years,[3] and about 70% at 10–13 years of age.[4] Conversely, if an obese child does not lose weight by the end of adolescence, the odds against his/her doing so as an adult are 28–1.[5]

The prevalence of childhood obesity in the United States is 17%,[6] which is more than three times higher than in the 1960s and 1970s. For boys and girls ages 2–20 years, a BMI $\geq$ 95th percentile defines obesity. Using that definition, the prevalence of obesity rose from about 5% before 1980 to 16.9% overall in 2007–2008.[6] Prevalence of overweight, defined as BMI 85th to 94.9th percentile, also increased, from about 10% to 14.8%. While obesity affects all pediatric populations, regardless of age, race, or gender, prevalence disparities are clear with Hispanic and African American youth having substantially higher rates of obesity (around 25%) than non-Hispanic white children. Age-related differences are also evident; the obesity prevalence in 2007–2008 among children 6–19 years of age was 18.7% in contrast to the prevalence of 10.4% in children 2–5 years of age.[6]

Exogenous obesity occurring during childhood is a result of a complex interaction between genetic and environmental factors. Studies implicating genetic influences include those showing differences in energy expenditure between offspring of obese and nonobese parents,[7-9] adoption studies demonstrating a significant relationship between adoptees and their biological parents,[10-12] overfeeding studies of identical twins,[13] and, at the cellular level, lipoprotein lipase activity studies in obese individuals.[14-16] In addition, mutations in genes associated with appetite regulation (leptin, pro-opiomelanocortin, brain-derived neurotrophic factor, FTO (fat-mass and obesity-associated gene), taste (TAS2R38-bitter taste sensitivity/preference for sweet), metabolism (PNPLA3), and adipocyte development are seen within populations with severe obesity.[17,18]

Environmental factors that have affected the prevalence of obesity include season, geographic region, population density,[19] socioeconomic factors[20-22] including education, income, family size,[23] and activity levels.[24] The environmental factors contribute to the development of obesity by affecting the opportunities for physical activity and access to healthy food options, as well as through cultural and social pressures. The environment characteristics that influence weight-related diet and physical activity behaviors particularly among the disadvantaged include supermarket access or food sources, places to exercise, and safety.[25,26] Culture influences perception of risk associated with obesity and behaviors associated with obesity development (i.e., feeding practices and engagement in physical activity).[27] There is also evidence to suggest that the development of obesity may extend and spread through social ties.[28] Incorporation of both genetic and environmental influences on obesity is required in efforts toward successful treatment of childhood obesity.

Although exogenous obesity accounts for the vast majority of cases of pediatric obesity, it is important to consider potential endogenous causes of obesity including endocrine disorders, hypothalamic defects, medication effects, and genetic disorders when evaluating an obese child. Obesity early in infancy raises concern for mutations of the leptin signaling pathway (extremely rare but potentially treatable by leptin replacement) or melanocortin-4-receptor abnormalities.[29,30] A short duration of obesity is suggestive of an endocrine, such as hypothyroidism, or a central cause of obesity. History of early hypotonia, feeding difficulties with hypogonadism during infancy followed by the onset of rapid weight gain in early childhood without acceleration in growth velocity raises clinical suspicion for the presence of Prader–Willi Syndrome. Other clinical features which should raise concerns for obesity-related genetic syndromes include developmental delays, short stature (due to endocrine abnormalities), digital abnormalities (polydactyly/syndactyly), visual impairment, deafness, and altered onset of pubertal development.[31]

Obesity is a medical condition that affects nearly every organ system, including the gastrointestinal, musculoskeletal, endocrine, reproductive, cardiovascular, and pulmonary systems. In particular, obese children and adolescents are at increased risk for a large number of medical disorders including tibia vara (Blount's disease), slipped capital femoral epiphysis, asthma, sleep-disordered breathing, pseudotumor cerebri, hypertension, type II diabetes mellitus, hyperlipidemia, hyperandrogenemia, and polycystic ovarian syndrome.[32–34] Obesity also predisposes to psychosocial dysfunction, reduced quality of life, and social isolation.[35,36] With regard to gastrointestinal disease, non-alcoholic fatty liver disease (NAFLD), non-alcoholic steatohepatitis (NASH), cirrhosis, and cholelithiasis[32] are related to obesity. These associated disease conditions result from both direct anthropometric changes as well as metabolic derangements related to increased fat mass and insulin resistance.[34]

Functional gastrointestinal complaints are common in the setting of childhood obesity, including constipation, gastroesophageal reflux disease (GERD), irritable bowel syndrome, encopresis, and functional abdominal pain.[37] Poor dietary habits in obese children and adolescents appear to be related to constipation and encopresis, while abnormal LES sphincter relaxation and elevated intra-abdominal pressure, a consequence of excess subcutaneous and visceral fat, contribute to increased GERD symptoms.

Psychosocial morbidity is also associated with childhood obesity. Negative, early stereotyping frequently sets up aberrant behavior and emotional responses in these children. Five- and six-year-old children characterize children with the endomorphic or obese body type as "lazy," "ugly," and "stupid."[38] Obese children have demonstrated significantly lower body self-esteem than normal-weight children.[39,40] Discrimination against overweight people is as common as discrimination based on sexual orientation, ethnicity, physical disability, and religion.[41] Despite the common prevalence of overweight and obesity, weight-based stigmatization remains a relatively acceptable societal norm. Evidence exists suggesting adult obese patients have an increased prevalence of psychiatric morbidity, most commonly depression, related to weight bias and particularly as a result of being bullied in school and the psychiatric morbidity carried over from childhood.[42]

Obesity is a risk factor for a number of nutritional and micronutrient deficiencies, including fat-soluble vitamins, minerals, and antioxidants.[37] Consumption of energy-dense, yet nutrient-poor foods likely contributes to the development of such nutritional deficiencies. In particular, increased consumption of sugar-sweetened beverages is linked with calcium and vitamin D deficiency (presumably via reduced milk intake).[43] In addition, multiple studies have shown an inverse relationship between BMI and serum vitamin D (25-OH) levels, possibly related to reduced activity level, decreased sun exposure, and increased storage in adipose tissue.[44] Serum levels of fat-soluble antioxidants, including beta-carotene (vitamin A) and alpha-tocopherol (vitamin E), are also significantly lower in obese children, potentially leading to increased LDL oxidation.[45] The relationship of dietary intake of fat to inadequate nutrient intake is less clear. Two pediatric studies have suggested that higher fat diets carry an increased risk of suboptimal intake of vitamins A, D, and folate.[46,47] Conversely, lower fat intake may also be associated with lower intake of calcium, magnesium, phosphorous, vitamin E, vitamin B12, thiamine, niacin, riboflavin, and zinc.[47]

The basis of successful obesity treatment is behavior change to improve energy balance. Successful treatment of obesity is predicated on a decreased caloric intake and increased energy expenditures. Success can be enhanced by nutrition education, behavior modification, physical activity, social support, and the patient's willingness to make changes. Weight loss in such programs is modest, especially in contrast to the dramatic change sought by patients, parents, and providers, but can be sustained.[48] The goals of a treatment program for childhood obesity should (1) be appropriate for the child's age and developmental status, (2) result in significant weight reduction to within 20% of the ideal weight-for-height, and (3) inculcate long-term appropriate eating and physical activity habits that result in weight maintenance but do not hinder growth and development. The treatment includes caloric intake reduced to below energy expenditure, increased physical activity, and modification of eating behavior. The type of diet depends on the age of the child and the severity of the obesity. Because growth is a factor in childhood obesity, diets must provide adequate protein, minerals, and vitamins to support lean body mass and linear growth.[49] Straightforward measures which the American Academy of pediatrics recommends for weight-reduction and maintenance behaviors for treatment of Child and Adolescent Overweight and Obesity include avoidance of sugar-sweetened beverages, reduced portion size, intake of five to nine fruit and vegetable servings per day, 1 h of moderate to vigorous physical activity daily, daily breakfast, maximum daily screen-time exposure of 2 h, and eating at home.[50]

## TREATMENT

### DIET

There are a number of dietary therapies which have been used for weight loss and weight management. A recent comparison trial of the various macronutrient weight-loss diets among adults concluded that reduced-calorie diets regardless of macronutrient composition result in clinically meaningful weight loss, although actual differences in macronutrient compositions between study diets were modest.[51] While data exist in general for adults in regards to the efficacy of varied nutritional regimens, data are often relatively sparse for children and adolescents. Available randomized controlled trial data examining diets exclusively among youth are few and have been limited by high attrition rates and relatively short-term follow-up periods. The pediatric section of the Diogenes (diet, obesity, and genes) study examined the effect of a 26-week dietary intervention on weight changes among families with at least one overweight parent/adult and one healthy child. Children were randomized (along with their overweight parent) to specific *ad libitum* diets (five low-fat [25%–30% fat by energy] diets were available: low protein [LP] and low glycemic index [LGI]; LP and high glycemic index [HGI]; high protein [HP] and LGI; HP and HGI; and control). Of the 800 children enrolled and randomized, 465 (58%) completed all assessments (baseline, 4 and 26 weeks). While neither glycemic index nor protein dietary content had an effect on body composition separately, the LP and HGI diet increased body fat (+1.5%), while the HP and LGI diet reduced the percentage of overweight or obese children (46.2% at baseline to 39.6% at 26 weeks) during the study period.[52] The high drop-out rate limits the validity of these findings.

Dietary therapy may also be considered for acute management of severe obesity, where the goal of therapy is to quickly reduce weight and associated morbidities. In particular, there are data to suggest that very low energy diets such as the protein-sparing modified fast are well tolerated with noteworthy metabolic, cardiovascular risk, and obstructive sleep apnea improvements.[53,54] However, such diets require close medical management and monitoring. Suskind et al. found that children who were enrolled in a comprehensive weight management program including a very low calorie/high protein diet, nutrition education, exercise, and behavior modification sustained weight loss over a 1-year period.[55]

## Protein-Sparing Modified Fast Diet

Very low calorie diets are effective in the medical management of childhood obesity. These diets are typically less than 800 kilocalories (kcal) per day, and contain high biological value protein, with added vitamins, minerals, and small amounts of carbohydrate.[56] One such diet developed by Blackburn and Bistrian for adults and modified by Merritt and Suskind for children[57] is the high-protein/low-calorie protein-sparing modified fast (PSMF) diet.[58–60]

Hospitalized adolescents have been studied metabolically while on the PSMF diet.[57,61–68] The diet was found to be safe and effective for children who lost weight while preserving lean body mass. In the weight reduction program at Children's Hospital of New Orleans, PSMF was compared with the traditional hypocaloric balanced diet.[69] The PSMF diet consists of 1.5–2.0 g of biologically high-quality protein per kilogram ideal body weight per day and provides

600–800 cal daily. Total dietary fat intake is low, ranging from 27 to 36 g per day. The protein sources of the PSMF diet include lean beef (fat-trimmed and unmarbled) such as round steak, chicken, and turkey (skin removed), fish (if canned, water-packed), and other food such as shrimp, crab, oysters, and clams. Four cups of raw or two cups of cooked nonstarchy vegetables are recommended daily. Free food (e.g., pickles, spices, lemon, lime, unsweetened gelatin, and artificial sweetener) are allowed *ad libitum*. Daily supplements include one multivitamin with minerals and iron, 25 mEq of potassium in the form of Morton Lite Salt (Morton Thiokol) or K-lyte (Mead Johnson Laboratories) and 800 mg elemental calcium as four tablets of Tums (Lewis-Howe). A 5 mg tablet of vitamin K, Mephyton (Merck, Sharp, and Dohme), is taken weekly. Additionally, children drink a minimum of 2 L/day of water or calorie-free fluids.

After 10 weeks of being on PSMF or after having reached 120% of ideal weight/height, the child is started on a balanced deficit diet of 1000–1200 cal. The child's intake is gradually increased during the next 2–3 months to provide for maintenance of weight loss and adequate growth.[55]

## Hypocaloric Liquid Diets and Meal Replacements

Liquid diets have become popular; many adults find it easier to drink a premade or easily mixed drink than to "count calories."[70–72] One study[62] with eight adolescents, however, revealed poor compliance and a high attrition rate. Further studies are needed to determine the role of hypocaloric liquid diets in the treatment of childhood obesity. Another study evaluated meal replacements (MR) as a method of weight loss. In a randomized control trial comparing three groups of obese adolescents: a 1300–1500 cal diets delivered via MR for 12 months versus MR for 4 months with conventional food diet (CFD) for 8 months versus CFD for 12 months. Among the 75 adolescents completing the trial, participants receiving MR had greater weight loss at month 4 (6.3% reduction in BMI versus 3.8% BMI reduction, MR versus CFD, $p = 0.01$) compared to CFD, but no differences in weight outcomes were seen between groups at 12 months. In fact, all groups increased their BMI in months 5–12 of the study. Thus, while MR improved short-term weight loss compared to CFD, continued use did not promote continued weight loss in the long-term.[73] In general, long-term diets must be palatable and adaptable to the typical lifestyle to maintain patient compliance with prescribed regimens.

## Safety Measures During Dietary Restriction

One advantage of the PSMF diet is that ketonuria, which occurs within 2 days, can be monitored daily to assess compliance. However, some subjects, under carefully controlled conditions, have had losses of nitrogen, lymphopenia, and decreases in transferrin and $C_3$.[57,63,66] Nitrogen losses are mitigated when carbohydrate is added to the diets.[63] These metabolic changes appear to have no clinical significance.

Hypocaloric diets may result in a temporary reduction in growth velocity.[74–76] Two studies using PSMF diet[61,62] have reported contradictory findings regarding its impact on linear growth. In one study, most of the children had growth velocities below the 50th percentile; the other reported that linear growth was maintained in all five children. Linear growth was not, however, compared to growth velocity standards for age and sex. No current data suggest that a temporary delay in linear growth velocity in obese children is associated with permanent stunting. Close monitoring of a child's growth during weight reduction is recommended.

## EXERCISE

Treatment programs are structured with either aerobic activities and/or a change in lifestyle activity. Aerobic activities are running, walking, cycling, or swimming, and they are done several times per week at a specific duration and intensity (Table 48.1). The goal is to increase caloric expenditure and improve fitness. Activity intensity is also important.

Lifestyle activity is less structured and does not require intensity. Although this program can be made isocaloric to an aerobic program, the intensity of the physical activity is likely to be lower and fitness effects may not be as pronounced. If the goal of the activity is to produce weight loss, then the energy expenditure, and not the physical activity intensity, is the important factor.

Many people do not sustain participation in physical activity programs.[77] The most important factor in predicting nonadherence is intensity; subjects adhere less to higher-intensity programs.[78] Thus, activity programs must be evaluated both in terms of weight change goals and potential adherence.

Fitness may be measured to assess comparative effects of programs, but fitness should not be considered an end point.[79] In addition, weight change itself has been shown to improve fitness when fitness is measured via treadmill or step tests.[79]

Physical activity programs[80] should incorporate (1) frequency—3–5 times per week; (2) intensity—50%–60% maximal ability (50%–60% maximal heart rate); (3) duration—15 min initially, building to 30–40 min; (4) mode—use of large muscles, such as walking, jogging, swimming, or cycling; (5) interest—patient-dependent, such as tennis, dancing, skating; (6) enjoyment—an important factor in adherence; (7) incorporation into functional activities, such as walking to school, taking stairs versus elevators, bicycles versus cars; and (8) reducing passive "activities" such as frequent TV watching, lying down after school or meals, spending time with friends who do not like active play.

## BEHAVIOR MODIFICATION

Obesity is a result of more than just the satisfaction of hunger. Habit and interpersonal relationships are important contributory factors. Understanding and treating childhood obesity must take these into consideration.[81–83] Decreasing caloric intake and increased physical activity through behavioral modification remains the cornerstone to treating obesity. As behavioral modification remains the key to success, healthcare providers must effectively counsel patients to adopt and maintain healthy weight-related behaviors.

Approaches that attempt to ameliorate obesity by modifying behavior must first analyze the discrete behaviors centered around eating, e.g., the type and frequency of food consumed as well as the behaviors antecedent and consequent to food consumption. When these behaviors are understood, programs to modify them can be designed.

Family-based approaches analyze the structure and function of impinging relationships, exploring behaviors that, explicitly or implicitly, influence fatness, activity, and food consumption. These two approaches, incorporated into a multidisciplinary childhood obesity program, increase long-term treatment effectiveness.

The two overall methods of behavior modification are the "gradual shift" (shaping) and "all or none" (replacement/omission) approaches. Techniques supporting these methods include diet and activity self-monitoring, goal setting, stimulus control, cue elimination, behavior substitution, exploration of alternatives to overeating, and parental support.

## TABLE 48.1
### Calories Expended in Various Physical Activities

| Exercises | Calories per Min | Time (min) |
|---|---|---|
| Archery | 3.5–5 | 45–60 |
| Backpacking | 6–13.5 | 30–45 |
| Badminton | 5–11 | 20–30 |
| Basketball (nongame) | 3.5–11 | 20–30 |
| Baseball | 4.7 | 45–60 |
| Bicycling | 3.5–10 | 20–30 |
| Bowling | 2.5–5 | 45–60 |
| Calisthenics (aerobic dancing) | 5 | 20–30 |
| Canoeing (2.5–4.0 mph) | 3.5–10 | 30.45 |
| Dancing (social, square) | 3.5–8 | 20–30 |
| Fencing | 7.5–12 | 30–40 |
| Fishing (stream, wading) | 6–8 | 30–45 |
| Football (touch) | 7–12 | 20–35 |
| Golf (walking) | 5–9 | 45–60 |
| Handball | 10–45 | 15–30 |
| Hiking | 3.5–8 | 30–45 |
| Horseback riding | 3.5–10 | 20–45 |
| Horseshoes | 2.5–3.5 | 60–90 |
| Judo and karate | 13 | 15–25 |
| Paddleball (racket) and squash | 10–15 | 30–60 |
| Rowing | 5–15 | 30–45 |
| Running | | |
| 12 min mile (5 mph) | 10 | 20–60 |
| 8 min mile (7.5 mph) | 15 | 15–30 |
| 6 min mile (10 mph) | 20 | 15–30 |
| 5 min mile (12 mph) | 25 | 15–30 |
| Sailing | 3–6 | 30–60 |
| Scuba diving | 6–10 | 30–60 |

1. *Diet and activity self-monitoring* requires the child to keep a daily diary of all foods eaten and activities undertaken. The goal is to help children and parents become aware of energy requirements and expenditures.
2. Children are also encouraged to *set weekly goals* for weight loss. Appropriate praise and material rewards are given for goal attainment.
3. *Stimulus control*, or the avoidance of situations that encourage overeating, is taught. An example is understanding the ways in which to cope with parties and ordering in restaurants.
4. *Cue elimination*, i.e., elimination of those foods that both tempt and induce obesity, is encouraged. An example is banning purchase of high-fat and high-calorie foods.
5. *Behavior substitution* is the technique of initiating a non-eating activity at a time when food would normally be consumed, e.g., going for a walk after school rather than heading for the kitchen to "snack." It also means becoming aware when overeating occurs as a result of boredom and learning to substitute other activities.
6. *Parental support*: Parents become part of the "team." They are instructed in weight-losing techniques, on setting up consistent enforceable limits, on how to provide positive reinforcement for weight-losing behaviors and how to ignore behaviors incompatible with weight loss.

Current guidelines advocate the use of patient-centered communication as a means to motivate families to change behaviors.[50] Motivational Interviewing (MI) is a client-centered approach used to enhance an individual's intrinsic motivation for behavior change by exploring ambivalence and taking steps to resolve it.[84] Suskind et al. found that a comprehensive program of MI, diet, education, exercise, and behavior modification provided to groups of 12–15 obese children was most effective in promoting significant weight loss among the children.[55]

An important element of MI is a sympathetic non-judgemental healthcare provider who understands that patient ambivalence is normal. Healthcare providers can use MI to guide patients toward health-related goals by allowing them to express their own motivations for change.[84] Reflective listening techniques and open-ended questions are important tools used during MI, which focuses communication toward change rather than maintenance of current behaviors.

Schwartz et al.[85] examined the practicability of implementation of MI by physicians and dietitians in the primary care setting. In general, results suggested promise for MI with parents reporting positive perceptions of the MI counseling approach with some indications of improvement in behavioral and weight parameters; however, the study was non-randomized and had a high drop-out rate which limits the interpretation of the results of the study.[85] Another study examined an MI-based intervention delivered in person and

via telephone to families seen at 10 pediatric practices via a cluster, randomized controlled trial.[86] While intervention participants did demonstrate greater decreases in television viewing, fast food and sugar-sweetened intake, and BMI as compared to control counterparts, only television viewing reductions achieved statistical significance. Further studies are required to determine the true efficacy of MI in behavioral change for the obese child and adolescent.

## DRUG THERAPY

Historically, major issues about safety and efficacy of drugs used for weight reduction have led to significant concerns about the role of pharmacological therapy in weight management. In order to meet criteria for labeling as a "weight loss" drug, an agent must induce ≥5% weight loss in clinical trials. This criterion is based upon medical reports demonstrating that weight reduction of 5% or more decreases the risk for diabetes and cardiovascular disease.[87] The only FDA-approved weight loss drug for long-term use in children is Orlistat (Xenical).[82] Orlistat causes fat malabsorption by inhibiting pancreatic lipase. Orlistat's efficacy in reducing weight has been meek; among adolescents taking Orlistat in conjunction with a lifestyle modification intervention, only 26% achieved more than 5% weight loss.[88] It has been linked to reduction in fat-soluble vitamins and beta-carotene as well as gastrointestinal side effects. A few noradrenergic drugs, such as phentermine, have been FDA-approved for adults for short-term use. These medications carry with them the potential for abuse, cardiovascular side effects, as well as questions regarding their long-term efficacy and safety. Metformin, used for obese children with type 2 diabetes mellitus, is not a weight loss treatment since the decrease in weight in clinical trials has been relatively small (BMI Z-score difference between metformin versus placebo = −0.07 among obese insulin-resistant children).[89]

## BARIATRIC SURGERY

Over the past decade, bariatric surgery has increased substantially in the adolescent populations, with the rate of weight loss surgery (WLS) among adolescents tripling between 2000 and 2003.[90] This reflects an increased awareness of severe morbid pediatric obesity and its associated health risks, as well as the difficulty in finding effective lifestyle and medication interventions for severe obesity. Adolescent WLS represented approximately 1% of overall bariatric surgery procedures in the United States, with roux-en-y gastric bypass (RYGB) comprising the majority of cases.[90] The adjustable gastric band (AGB), approved for use in patients years 18 years and older, has been studied in industry-sponsored studies in adolescents as young as 14 years. Although attractive due to its reduced short-term operative complication risk, AGB has a higher rate of re-operation compared to RYGB in both adults and adolescents.[91] Vertical sleeve gastrectomy (VSG) has gained increased interest as a stand-alone WLS, as it shows similar weight loss and comorbidity resolution when compared to RYGB, but long-term data (>5 years) are lacking. More aggressive malabsorptive weight loss procedures, such as biliopancreatic diversion with duodenal switch and jejunoileal bypass, are not recommended for adolescents.

All three surgical options (AGB, RYGB, VSG) result in clinically significant weight loss, with patients undergoing RYGB and VSG losing on average 50%–60% of excess weight, which appears to be sustainable in a majority of patients.[92,93] AGB results in comparable or slightly lower excess weight loss at a slower, more gradual rate.[94] A large prospective controlled study following long-term outcomes among adults who had undergone WLS (AGB, vertical banded gastroplasty, or RYGB)[95] demonstrated a range of 15%–25% mean weight loss at 15 years post-operative follow-up, although mean weight loss regressed from the maximal nadir at 1 year. However, of the 265 RYGB patients enrolled in this study, less than 25% ($n = 58$) were included in the 10-year follow-up measurement and only 4% ($n = 10$) in the 15-year follow-up.

Along with weight loss, significant post-surgical improvements in key comorbidities, such as diabetes, obstructive sleep apnea, depression, cardiovascular function, dyslipidemia, and quality of life, have been demonstrated.[96] Although progressive NASH has been proposed as a major indication for WLS in adolescents, there is a lack of controlled prospective data supporting the efficacy of WLS for the treatment of NASH, although a meta-analysis of retrospective data in adults suggests a 70% resolution of NASH with WLS.[97]

Short-term complications after RYGB and VSG may include leakage at anastomotic sites, wound infections and gastrojejunal strictures requiring endoscopic dilatation, small bowel obstruction, and development of cholelithiasis. Band slippage, gastric obstruction, and esophageal or gastric pouch dilation have been reported after AGB placement; and up to 30% of adult patients with AGB may require major re-operation.[98] The incidence of short-term operative complications for adolescents undergoing WLS in academic centers appears to be lower than that seen in adults, and no perioperative mortality has been reported.[90,99] Long-term complications appear to be primarily nutritional, due to deficient intake or absorption of iron, vitamin B12, vitamin D, and other key nutrients; and lifelong vitamin and mineral supplementation is recommended after all types of bariatric surgery. Adherence to supplementation may be particularly poor among adolescents, necessitating close follow-up to monitor serum levels and for symptoms of deficiencies.

## CLINIC- AND SCHOOL-BASED PROGRAMS

Multidisciplinary interventions have replaced one-on-one dietary instruction by a physician. These medically supervised programs usually use groups to teach dietary restriction, nutrition, exercise, behavior modification, and family lifestyle change. Such programs have demonstrated short-term success,[100] although some long-term studies indicate recidivism rates similar to those reported in adults. In two studies, 80%–100% of children returned to pre-clinic levels of obesity 7–9 years after treatment.[101,102] Other studies, however, reported more favorable results 5[103] and 10[104] years after treatment.

Intervention is usually clinic/hospital- or school-based. In either setting, the treatment team usually consists of a physician, dietitian, psychologist, and exercise physiologist. Therapy may be group or individual. Group intervention has the decided advantage of providing a support system beyond that of the therapeutic team. A school-based program provides an additional support group, i.e., peers who may provide moral support to a child who needs to lose weight. In addition, school resources and the environment are conducive to successful management of childhood obesity[3,105]; schools allow easy access to children providing continuity, concentrated contact, and cost-effectiveness. Intervention also takes place within the context of the child's natural environment, removing the stigma of hospital-based programs. In addition, schools provide the possibility of intervention before the obesity becomes severe; they are a unique place for the dissemination of information to children and their families.

The presence of both peer groups and significant adults in schools offers backup support for the obesity team. The physical layout of the school, including classrooms, gymnasium, and outdoor fields are excellent for the educational as well for as the physical activity components of the obesity programs.[105] Finally, because maintenance of weight loss requires long-term, sustained effort, the continuum of time provided through schools is invaluable, especially when weight control programs are started early and incorporated into the total school system.[106]

The four elements that are common among several school-based obesity programs[80] include (1) integration of behavior modification, nutrition education, physical activity, and familial support; (2) structured physical activities, four or five times per week, with encouragement and incentives to participate during nonschool hours; (3) team approach, including teachers, physical education instructors, school nurses, counselors, and/or lunchroom supervisors; (4) parent involvement for ensuring home support for the development of new behaviors.

## NUTRITION AND PHYSICAL EDUCATION PROGRAMS

Obese individuals generally know little about nutrition and are particularly vulnerable to popular food myths.[107] The most important factor the obese child must learn is that any diet that reduces caloric intake below caloric expenditure can produce weight loss. The most important thing the professional must learn is the patient's eating preferences. In that way, dietary design can incorporate foods that the patient can eat indefinitely.

In addition, when educating a family or patient, a nutrition program should include[80]: (1) teaching the critical aspects of quality nutrition, i.e., food groups, serving requirements, and variety; (2) developing an understanding of intake–expenditure balance; (3) teaching the impact of high-calorie, low-nutrition snacks on weight; (4) teaching selectivity in fast-food intake; (5) alerting children to the myths incorporated into media advertising; (6) teaching the way to read food labels.

Acquisitions of the skills as well as the positive attitude necessary for lifetime participation in physical activities are important components of weight maintenance. Although physical education programs may foster this, obese children often lack the motivation, self-confidence, stamina, and motor skills necessary to successfully join with their peers. Their frustration often leads to complete withdrawal from participation. This may be obviated by providing a separate physical education class designed exclusively for overweight children.

Optimally, schools could be used to support an integrated environment designed to promote a healthier lifestyle. Health education could teach students how to monitor diet and exercise behavior, how to recognize when changes are needed, how to initiate those changes, and how to monitor and maintain their successes. Nutrition courses could emphasize the long-term problems resulting from high-fat, high-calorie "snacking." School cafeterias could serve low-calorie, low-fat meals; and vending machines could offer snacks that have reduced fat, sugar, and sodium. Further research is needed to determine the most effective way schools could be used to have a significant impact on children's eating and physical activity behavior.

## Social Support

Success in treating childhood obesity is dependent on a complex support network that includes the family, the peer group, and health professionals. Parents exert a powerful influence on the eating, activity, and attitude patterns of their children. They determine what food enters the house, and they establish the emotional environment that may impinge on eating behavior. It is generally felt that the parental role in the treatment of a child's obesity needs to be most structured for younger children; adolescents may require more independence.

Family-based behavioral treatment for obese 6–12-year-old children was examined for its effect on weight and growth over 10 years.[104] Obese children and their parents were randomized to three groups, each of which was provided similar diet, exercise, and behavior modification training, but differed in reinforcement for weight loss and behavioral change. In one group, parents and children were reinforced for behavioral change and weight loss; in the second group, only children were reinforced for behavioral change and weight loss; in the control group, families were reinforced only for attendance. Children in the group in which both parent and child were reinforced showed significantly greater decreases in percent overweight after 5 and 10 years (−11.2% and −7.5%, respectively) than children in the control group (+7.9% and +14.3%, respectively). Children in the group that only reinforced children showed an increase in percent overweight after 5 and 10 years (+2.7% and +4.5%, respectively). Height, on the other hand, showed no difference among the three

groups. At 10 years, a child's height was correlated with the height of the parents of the same sex ($r = 0.78$); children were 1.8 cm taller than their parents.[104] This study provides evidence of the importance of family reinforcement in the long-term treatment of childhood obesity. It also satisfies concerns regarding the effect of weight regulation on linear growth.

Involvement of peers appears to be helpful in successful treatment of obese children. It is especially helpful when nonobese children learn not to tease a child for being overweight and to be openly supportive of changes in weight and eating patterns. Support of health professionals including the pediatrician, nutritionist, and psychologist is also an important factor in a child's success in losing weight.

## SUMMARY

The multidisciplinary approach to weight loss in children combines nutrition education, behavioral modification, psychosocial support, dietary restriction, and increased physical activity designed to gradually mobilize fat stores while preserving lean body mass. Hypocaloric diets promote rapid weight loss and a reduction in risk factors. They are not appropriate for weight maintenance programs. A more long-term approach stresses maintenance of weight loss, and includes exercise, behavior modification, and family and social involvement. Success is enhanced by family, peer group, and health professional support. Although schools have the potential of contributing to both treatment and prevention of childhood obesity, more research is needed to define and clarify their potential role.

The results of a 10-year follow-up of behavioral, family-based treatment program for obese children provide evidence that treatment of obesity in childhood can produce effects that persist into young adulthood. Although still overweight, the children in the treatment group showed significantly greater decreases in percent overweight than control children. Treatment, which was relatively conservative, involved a nutritious, low-fat diet with regular exercise.

Childhood obesity is an intellectual challenge, but it is not an intractable problem. Successful management of obesity can improve the quality of life and reduce the morbidity and mortality associated with childhood obesity. Obesity-prone people who wish to control their weight must learn to eat defensively and to maintain a relatively high level of physical activity.

## REFERENCES

1. Gortmaker SL, Dietz WH, Jr., Sobol AM, Wehler CA. *Am J Dis Child* 141: 535; 1987.
2. Charney E, Goodman HC, McBride M, Lyon B, Pratt R. *N Engl J Med* 295: 6; 1976.
3. Stark O, Atkins E, Wolff OH, Douglas JW. *Br Med J (Clin Res Ed)* 283: 13; 1981.
4. Abraham S, Collins G, Nordsieck M. *HSMHA Health Rep* 86: 273; 1971.
5. Stunkard A, Burt V. *Am J Psychiatry* 123: 1443; 1967.
6. Ogden CL, Carroll MD, Curtin LR, Lamb MM, Flegal KM. *JAMA* 303: 242; 2010.

7. Bogardus C, Lillioja S, Ravussin E et al. *N Engl J Med* 315: 96; 1986.
8. Ravussin E, Lillioja S, Knowler WC et al. *N Engl J Med* 318: 467; 1988.
9. Roberts SB, Savage J, Coward WA, Chew B, Lucas A. *N Engl J Med* 318: 461; 1988.
10. MacDonald A, Stunkard A. *N Engl J Med* 322: 1530; 1990.
11. Stunkard AJ, Harris JR, Pedersen NL, McClearn GE. *N Engl J Med* 322: 1483; 1990.
12. Stunkard AJ, Sorensen TI, Hanis C et al. *N Engl J Med* 314: 193; 1986.
13. Bouchard C, Tremblay A, Despres JP et al. *N Engl J Med* 322: 1477; 1990.
14. Maes HH, Neale MC, Eaves LJ. *Behav Genet* 27: 325; 1997.
15. Kern PA, Ong JM, Saffari B, Carty J. *N Engl J Med* 322: 1053; 1990.
16. Reitman JS, Kosmakos FC, Howard BV, Taskinen MR et al. *J Clin Invest* 70: 791; 1982.
17. Grimm ER, Steinle NI. *Nutr Rev* 69: 52; 2011.
18. Han JC, Lawlor DA, Kimm SY. *Lancet* 375: 1737; 2010.
19. Dietz WH, Jr., Gortmaker SL. *Am J Clin Nutr* 39: 619; 1984.
20. Garn SM, Bailey SM, Cole PE, Higgins IT. *Am J Clin Nutr* 30: 721; 1977.
21. Garn SM, Clark DC. *Pediatrics* 57: 443; 1976.
22. Goldblatt PB, Moore ME, Stunkard AJ. *JAMA* 192: 1039; 1965.
23. Ravelli GP, Belmont L. *Am J Epidemiol* 109: 66; 1979.
24. Dietz WH, Jr., Gortmaker SL. *Pediatrics* 75: 807; 1985.
25. Lovasi GS, Hutson MA, Guerra M, Neckerman KM. *Epidemiol Rev* 31: 7; 2009.
26. Jennings A, Welch A, Jones AP et al. *Am J Prev Med* 40: 405; 2011.
27. Caprio S, Daniels SR, Drewnowski A et al. *Obesity (Silver Spring)* 16: 2566; 2008.
28. Christakis NA, Fowler JH. *N Engl J Med* 357: 370; 2007.
29. Farooqi IS, Yeo GS, Keogh JM et al. *J Clin Invest* 106: 271; 2000.
30. Farooqi IS, Wangensteen T, Collins S et al. *N Engl J Med* 356: 237; 2007.
31. Farooqi IS, O'Rahilly S. *Int J Obes (Lond)* 29: 1149; 2005.
32. Fisberg M, Baur L, Chen W et al. *J Pediatr Gastroenterol Nutr* 39(Suppl 2): S678; 2004.
33. Sin DD, Sutherland ER. *Thorax* 63: 1018; 2008.
34. Abrams P, Levitt Katz LE. *Curr Opin Endocrinol Diabetes Obes* 18: 23; 2011.
35. Schwimmer JB, Burwinkle TM, Varni JW. *JAMA* 289: 1813; 2003.
36. Braet C, Mervielde I, Vandereycken W. *J Pediatr Psychol* 22: 59; 1997.
37. Teitelbaum JE, Sinha P, Micale M, Yeung S, Jaeger J. *J Pediatr* 154: 444; 2009.
38. Staffieri JR. *J Pers Soc Psychol* 7: 101; 1967.
39. Mendelson BK, Mendelson MJ, White DR. *J Pers Assess* 76: 90; 2001.
40. Mendelson BK, White DR. *Percept Mot Skills* 54: 899; 1982.
41. Puhl RM, Andreyeva T, Brownell KD. *Int J Obes (Lond)* 32: 992; 2008.
42. Vaidya V. *Adv Psychosom Med* 27: 73; 2006.
43. Xanthakos SA. *Pediatr Clin North Am* 56: 1105; 2009.
44. Jorde R, Sneve M, Emaus N et al. *Eur J Nutr* 49: 401; 2010.
45. Strauss RS. *J Pediatr* 134: 160; 1999.
46. Ballew C, Kuester S, Serdula M et al. *J Pediatr* 136: 181; 2000.
47. Obarzanek E, Hunsberger SA, Van Horn L et al. *Pediatrics* 100: 51; 1997.
48. Barton M. *Pediatrics* 125: 361; 2010.
49. American Academy of Pediatrics. Committee on Nutrition. *Pediatrics* 68: 880; 1981.
50. Barlow SE. *Pediatrics* 120(Suppl 4): S164; 2007.
51. Sacks FM, Bray GA, Carey VJ et al. *N Engl J Med* 360: 859; 2009.
52. Papadaki A, Linardakis M, Larsen TM et al. *Pediatrics* 126: e1143; 2010.
53. Johansson K, Hemmingsson E, Harlid R et al. *BMJ* 342: d3017; 2011.
54. Pekkarinen T, Takala I, Mustajoki P. *Int J Obes Relat Metab Disord* 22: 661; 1998.
55. Suskind RM, Blecker U, Udall JN, Jr. et al. *Pediatr Diabetes* 1: 23; 2000.
56. Wadden TA, Stunkard AJ, Brownell KD. *Ann Intern Med* 99: 675; 1983.
57. Merritt RJ, Bistrian BR, Blackburn GL, Suskind RM. *J Pediatr* 96: 13; 1980.
58. Bistrian BR, Blackburn GL, Flatt JP et al. *Diabetes* 25: 494; 1976.
59. Bistrian BR, Blackburn GL, Stanbury JB. *N Engl J Med* 296: 774; 1977.
60. Bistrian DR, Winterer J, Blackburn GL et al. *J Lab Clin Med* 89: 1030; 1977.
61. Archibald EH, Harrison JE, Pencharz PB. *Am J Dis Child* 137: 658; 1983.
62. Brown MR, Klish WJ, Hollander J et al. *Am J Clin Nutr* 38: 20; 1983.
63. Dietz WH, Jr., Schoeller DA. *J Pediatr* 100: 638; 1982.
64. Merritt RJ. *Int J Obes* 2: 207; 1978.
65. Pencharz PB, Clarke R, Archibald EH, Vaisman N. *Can J Physiol Pharmacol* 66: 1469; 1988.
66. Pencharz PB, Motil KJ, Parsons HG, Duffy BJ. *Clin Sci (Lond)* 59: 13; 1980.
67. Stallings VA, Archibald EH, Pencharz PB. *Am J Clin Nutr* 47: 220; 1988.
68. Stallings VA, Archibald EH, Pencharz PB et al. *Am J Clin Nutr* 48: 91; 1988.
69. Figueroa-Colon R, von Almen TK, Franklin FA et al. *Am J Dis Child* 147: 160; 1993.
70. Vertes V, Genuth SM, Hazelton IM. *JAMA* 238: 2151; 1977.
71. Genuth SM, Castro JH, Vertes V. *JAMA* 230: 987; 1974.
72. Vertes V, Genuth SM, Hazelton IM. *JAMA* 238: 2142; 1977.
73. Berkowitz RI, Wadden TA, Gehrman CA et al. *Obesity (Silver Spring)* 19: 1193; 2011.
74. Brook CG, Lloyd JK, Wolff OH. *Br Med J* 3: 44; 1974.
75. Dietz WH, Jr., Hartung R. *Am J Dis Child* 139: 705; 1985.
76. Wolff OH. *Q J Med* 24: 109; 1955.
77. Oldridge NB. *Prev Med* 11: 56; 1982.
78. Epstein LH, Wing RR, Thompson JK. *Addict Behav* 3: 185; 1978.
79. Epstein LH, Koeske R, Zidansek J, Wing RR. *Am J Dis Child* 137: 654; 1983.
80. Ward DS, Bar-Or O. *Pediatrician* 13: 44; 1986.
81. Dietz WH, Jr., *Ann NY Acad Sci* 499: 47; 1987.
82. Epstein LH, Valoski A, Koeske R, Wing RR. *J Am Diet Assoc* 86: 481; 1986.
83. Ganley RM. *Fam Process* 25: 437; 1986.
84. Miller WR, Rollnick S. *Motivational Interviewing: Preparing People for Change*, 2nd edn., New York: Guilford Press; 2002.
85. Schwartz RP, Hamre R, Dietz WH et al. *Arch Pediatr Adolesc Med* 161: 495; 2007.
86. Taveras EM, Gortmaker SL, Hohman KH et al. *Arch Pediatr Adolesc Med* 165: 714; 2011.

87. Douketis JD, Macie C, Thabane L, Williamson DF. *Int J Obes (Lond)* 29: 1153; 2005.
88. Chanoine JP, Hampl S, Jensen C et al. *JAMA* 293: 2873; 2005.
89. Yanovski JA, Krakoff J, Salaita CG et al. *Diabetes* 60: 477; 2011.
90. Tsai WS, Inge TH, Burd RS. *Arch Pediatr Adolesc Med* 161: 217; 2007.
91. Treadwell JR, Sun F, Schoelles K. *Ann Surg* 248: 763; 2008.
92. Inabnet WB 3rd, Belle SH, Bessler M et al. *Surg Obes Relat Dis* 6: 1; 2010.
93. Inge TH, Jenkins TM, Zeller M et al. *J Pediatr* 156: 103; 2010.
94. Nadler EP, Youn HA, Ren CJ, Fielding GA. *J Pediatr Surg* 43: 141; 2008.
95. Sjostrom L, Narbro K, Sjostrom CD et al. *N Engl J Med* 357: 741; 2007.
96. Holterman AX, Browne A, Tussing L et al. *J Pediatr Surg* 45: 74; 2010.
97. Mummadi RR, Kasturi KS, Chennareddygari S, Sood GK. *Clin Gastroenterol Hepatol* 6: 1396; 2008.
98. Balsiger BM, Ernst D, Giachino D et al. *J Gastrointest Surg* 11: 1470; 2007.
99. Varela JE, Hinojosa MW, Nguyen NT. *Surg Obes Relat Dis* 3: 537; 2007.
100. Epstein LH, Wing RR, Koeske R et al. *J Consult Clin Psychol* 49: 674; 1981.
101. Lloyd JK, Wolff OH. *Br Med J* 2: 145; 1961.
102. Ginsberg-Fellner F, Knittle JL. *Pediatr Res* 15: 1381; 1981.
103. Epstein LH, Wing RR, Koeske R, Valoski A. *J Consult Clin Psychol* 55: 91; 1987.
104. Epstein LH, Valoski A, Wing RR, McCurley J. *JAMA* 264: 2519; 1990.
105. Brownell KD, Kaye FS. *Am J Clin Nutr* 35: 277; 1982.
106. Collipp PJ. *J NY State Sch Nurse Teach Assoc* 5: 19; 1974.
107. Stunkard AJ. *Am J Clin Nutr* 45: 1142; 1987.

# 49 Eating Disorders

*Craig A. Johnston and John P. Foreyt*

## CONTENTS

The incidence of eating disorders is increasing, and health care professionals are faced with the difficult task of treating these refractory conditions.[1,2] Cases of weight loss and self-inflicted starvation have been dated back to at least the fourth century A.D.[3] For example, in literature from the Middle Ages, several cases were cited of religious women who reportedly existed on very little food over extended time periods only by virtue of spiritual power.[3–6] The first clinical description of anorexia nervosa (AN) was reported in 1694 and included symptoms such as decreased appetite, amenorrhea, food aversion, emaciation, and hyperactivity.[7] The actual term "anorexia nervosa" was used in 1874 to describe a condition beginning in adolescence, predominantly among females, with metabolic sequence associated with prolonged starvation and calorie depletion. The cognitive/perceptual body image distortions associated with the disorder was described during this time as well.[8] The initial treatments for this disorder included family participation; however, some argued that successful intervention required the patients to be separated from the family environment.[9]

The overall view of this disorder changed in the early 1900s when an autopsy performed on a malnourished patient revealed pituitary lesions on the patient's brain. Because of this finding, AN tended to be seen as a medical disorder caused by pituitary abnormalities. As psychoanalytic theory spread in the 1940s and 1950s, AN became increasingly differentiated from the medically based "Simmonds disease," and was reconceptualized as a psychiatric disorder characterized by an excessive drive for thinness, including purgative behaviors, body image disturbance, and denial of illness rooted in unconscious conflicts around oral-sadistic impulses, oral impregnation, and regressive fantasies.[10,11] Ultimately, the psychoanalytic viewpoint was challenged by the clinical studies of Hilde Bruch,[12] whose work stimulated a major reconceptualization of AN and its treatment. The emphasis for eating disorders became faulty developmental learning experiences, particularly discrimination of internal states and body boundaries, perceptions of ineffectiveness, and lack of autonomy. Thus, treatment was focused on promoting patient's self-efficacy and autonomy.

Whereas a fairly straightforward history is found for AN, the historical accounts of bulimic behavior are somewhat more difficult to trace. In early Roman accounts, "vomitoria" (public places where people went to vomit) were described.[13] The public nature of the vomiting, however, is not consistent with the secretiveness of the purging (and bingeing) included in current conceptualizations of bulimia nervosa (BN). The Babylonian Talmud written in about 400 A.D. describes bulimia as a symptom of various illnesses.[14] Patients with AN were also reported to have an occasional "voracious" appetite,[15] or a cluster of symptoms including vomiting, bulimia, and mood lability.[11,13,14,16] A clear case conceptualization of this disorder was first given in 1958 and included a description of extreme binge-purge cycles, laxative abuse, and dramatic vomiting in a woman who was not, but wished to be, underweight.[17]

## CLASSIFICATION

Although nosological or syndromal classification is the standard in mental health in general, some have suggested that eating disorders may not be distinct disorders. For example, patients with eating disorders experience a high frequency of comorbid psychological conditions, including mood, anxiety, and substance use disorders.[18–21] Possible reasons for these comorbidities include a large overlap of symptoms, poor inter-rater reliability, and a common biological pathway that has been implicated in these disorders.[22–25] Specifically, the neurotransmitter serotonin is thought to play a role in the etiology or maintenance of eating disorders, substance use disorders, depression, and obsessive-compulsive disorder.[22] Also, none of these disorders has a distinct and reliable biological marker that is not shared by one of the mentioned comorbid conditions.[23,26] Finally, many of the cognitive and behavioral features of each of these disorders are observationally and phenomenologically similar. Based on this evidence, some have concluded that eating disorders may be addictions or may exist on a continuum with obsessive-compulsive disorder.[23,27,28]

Although similarities exist, discontinuities between eating disorders and other disorders also have been highlighted. For instance, the frequency with which co-occurring medical and mood symptoms resolve with increased and/or better regulated food intake runs counter to the assumption that eating disorders simply represent atypical forms of other conditions.[29] AN and BN may share specific familial liability which is distinct from that involved in other comorbid problems, such as major depressive disorder and substance dependence.[30–33] Further, arguments that eating disorders are addictions are confounded by the fact that the central features of addiction (e.g., tolerance and withdrawal) do not apply to food.[21,34–38] Finally, eating disorders do not evolve into other conditions, providing robust support that these disorders are distinct.[39]

## DEFINITIONS

AN and BN are currently recognized by specific sets of symptoms, according to the *Diagnostic and Statistical Manual of Mental Disorders*, fourth edition, text revision DSM-IV-TR.[40] The central characteristic of AN is a "drive for thinness." This involves weight loss beyond the point of social desirability, attractiveness, and good health. Despite very low weights, individuals with AN deny that they are too thin and instead perceive themselves as having too much fat. Secondary characteristics include a preoccupation with food, amenorrhea, and a variety of psychological and physiological disturbances. In addition to curtailing food intake, high levels of exercise and purging may be used as weight control strategies.[40] AN is divided into either the restricting or the binge/purge types.

The salient characteristic of BN is an excessive intake of food (usually high in calories) over a relatively short period of time, accompanied by compensatory behaviors to prevent weight gain.[40] These compensatory behaviors take various forms including, but not limited to, self-induced vomiting, misuse of laxatives, severe caloric restriction, diuretics, and enemas. Because those with BN usually regard their binge eating as shameful and view their behavior as a loss of control, this behavior typically occurs in secret. AN and BN are sometimes considered to occur on a continuum of severity[29,33,41] because a substantial proportion of individuals with BN and AN either present with a history of the other disorder or develop time-limited symptoms of the other disorders.[29,39,42]

Given that binge eating also may occur in the absence of purging or other inappropriate compensatory behaviors, the DSM-IV-TR[40] has proposed binge eating disorder (BED) as a tentative diagnostic category worthy of further study and is currently included in its appendix. The salient characteristic of BED is an excessive intake of food (usually high in calories) over a relatively short period of time. Whereas compensatory behaviors are present with BN, these behaviors are not found in BED. This is the key distinction between these syndromes. BED has been heavily studied in eating behaviors of individuals who are obese.[43–45]

Under the DSM-IV[40] AN and BN are the two named eating disorders. However, the most common eating diagnosis given is Eating Disorder Not Otherwise Specified (EDNOS).[46] The EDNOS category becomes a "catchall" for situations in which severe eating disorder symptomotology is present, but full criteria for AN or BN are not met. Additionally, individuals with BED are given the diagnosis of EDNOS due to the lack of a specific BED diagnosis.[47] The fifth edition of the DSM is projected to be released in 2013. The eating disorder section will be significantly revised in order to reduce the over reliance on the EDNOS category. In order to achieve this, the diagnostic criteria of AN and BN will be broadened, and BED will be added as a specific eating disorder.[48]

Although not "officially" a disorder, night eating syndrome (NES) is characterized by morning anorexia, evening hyperphagia, and insomnia[49] and is often associated with obesity, though some studies have not supported this link.[50] NES was first described in 1955 and studied in a group of obese patients who were refractory to usual weight loss treatments.[51] NES is gaining greater recognition for its role in the growing numbers of obese adults.[50] In 2008, an expert committee developed the first set of diagnostic criteria. The proposed criteria include (1) at least 25% of food is consumed following the evening meal at least two times per week, (2) awareness and recall of night eating episodes, (3) one of the following: lack of desire to eat in the morning, insomnia in the form of sleep onset or sleep maintenance are present four or more nights per week, belief that one must eat in order to go to sleep or fall back asleep, or worsening mood in the evening, (4) significant impairment in functioning, (5) symptoms present for at least 3 months, (6) not resulting from substance abuse or dependence, medical disorder, medication, or another psychiatric disorder. NES is not to be confused with sleep-related eating disorder (SRED). In SRED, the nocturnal eating episodes occur during the main sleep phase, and individuals with SRED are unaware that the eating is taking place and the behavior is seen as involuntary.[49] See Table 49.1 for the diagnostic criteria for the disorders mentioned earlier.

## PREVALENCE

Peak age at onset may be somewhat earlier in AN than in BN. AN tends to begin in adolescence between the ages of 14 and 18.[40,52,53] The mean age of onset for BN is 17–19.[40,52,54–57] Both disorders occur predominantly in females with approximately 90% of the cases being found in this gender.[5,39,40,52,58–60] Although there have been indications of a somewhat less unequal socioeconomic distribution, AN has been most frequently noted in upper socioeconomic groups.[61–63]

The lifetime prevalence of AN for women is estimated at roughly 0.5%.[40,64] Epidemiological studies have reported ranges between 0.2% and 1.3% in female samples.[65–68] BN is somewhat more prevalent than AN, with estimates varying between 1% and 3%.[40,65,66,69] Some discrepancies occur in the prevalence rates of these disorders based on the restrictiveness of the diagnostic criteria utilized.[69,70] For example, between 4% and 19% of all young women may engage in clinically significant levels of bulimic behavior.[71–74]

Rates of AN and BN have increased in the recent past, particularly in younger age groups.[29,56,70,75–77] It is possible these increases reflect better screening and earlier detection efforts instead of an actual upsurge in rates.[2,39,70–78]

Although typically thought of as disorders affecting adolescents and adults, there is increasing evidence of early/childhood-onset AN. Overall, childhood-onset AN may not differ significantly from those with adolescent-onset AN in terms of psychopathology and key diagnostic features;[80,81] however, children may present symptoms somewhat differently from their adolescent counterparts.[82–84] Although differences are seen, they appear to be small.[84,85] Young participants in certain professional or recreational subcultures emphasizing conformance to rigid weight standards, such as dancers and some athletes, may be a particularly high risk for disordered eating.[60,83,85–88] All of this evidence suggests that the current nosology may underestimate eating disorders in prepubescent youths.[84]

A paucity of research exists on the natural history of AN and BN,[89,90] although there is some indication that symptoms of disordered eating occur early in life. Further, these symptoms may heighten risk at later developmental levels.[91] There is a clear need for additional prospective research in young populations to clarify the natural course of eating problems, as well as age-related changes in their manifestations.[89,90,92]

Lifetime prevalence of EDNOS is 4.78% in adolescents and 4.64% in adults. However, this diagnosis is not well defined and encompasses a wide range of symptomatology including BED.[46] Research on BED is still in its infancy and the development and maintenance of this disorder are still in large part unknown. Preliminary estimates indicate that the prevalence of

**TABLE 49.1**

**Diagnostic Criteria of Eating Disorders**

| Symptoms | Anorexia Nervosa[a] | Bulimia Nervosa[a] | Binge-Eating Disorder[a] | Night Eating Syndrome[b] |
|---|:---:|:---:|:---:|:---:|
| Refusal to maintain body weight at least at a minimally normal weight for age and height | × | | | |
| Intense fear of gaining weight or becoming fat, even though underweight | × | | | |
| Primary or secondary amenorrhea | × | | | |
| Body image disturbances | × | × | | |
| Occurs at least two times a week for 3 months | | × | | |
| Does not occur exclusively as a manifestation of AN | | × | | |
| During an episode, eating, within a certain time period, an amount of food that is larger than one that most people would eat | | × | × | |
| During an episode, there is a sense of lack of control over eating | | | | |
| Recurrent inappropriate compensatory behavior in order to prevent gaining weight | | × | × | |
| Occurs at least 2 days a week for 6 months | | | × | |
| Eating much more rapidly than usual | | | × | |
| Eating until uncomfortably full | | | × | |
| Eating large amounts of food even though not feeling hungry | | | × | |
| Eating alone because of embarrassment over food quantity | | | × | |
| During an episode, feeling disgusted, depressed, guilty, or ashamed after the binge | | | × | × |
| Marked distress | | | × | × |
| Eating excessive amounts of food in the late evening or night (a minimum of ¼ of daily caloric intake) | | | | × |
| Eating primarily carbohydrates at night | | | | × |
| Suffer from insomnia | | | | × |
| Not eating in the morning for several hours; first daily meal is often not until after noon | | | | × |
| Waking up with indigestion or heartburn | | | | × |

[a] All symptoms for these disorders have been adapted from the *Diagnostic and Statistical Manual of Mental Disorders*, 4th edn., text revision (DSM-IV-TR).

[b] Currently, this syndrome is not included in the DSM-IV-TR.

BED may range from less than 1% to approximately 4% in community samples and perhaps as much as 50% among patients at obesity clinics.[40,42,66,93] By comparison to both AN and BN, BED seems to emerge a bit later, typically in late adolescence or early adulthood, and to be somewhat more equally represented across genders and among ethnically diverse groups.[39,40,42,93–95] BED is not punctuated by compensatory behaviors associated with AN and BN, and as a result, obesity is a common comorbidity.[39,42,45,94,96,97] Some evidence suggests that binge eating problems may be more common than anticipated among children and adolescents in obesity treatment programs.[98]

The typical onset of NES is early adulthood and ranges from early teens to late twenties and appears to persist through adulthood.[50] There is evidence for the existence of a familial link with family members of individuals with NES being almost five times more likely to also have NES.[99] Others have hypothesized that NES may be associated with variations in the circadian rhythm gene; however, currently there is no empirical evidence to support this link.[100] NES is highly comorbid with other eating disorders, particularly BED.[49] Objective binge eating episodes are common to both BED and NES, though NES is proposed as a distinct diagnostic category from BED. While individuals with NES

experience anxiety which leads to night time eating episodes, the anxiety is in regards to being able to fall asleep, whereas, in patients with BED, there is little association between night time eating and anxiety over sleep onset or maintenance.[101]

Although much is known about the occurrence of eating disorders, research is still lacking with culturally diverse populations and in different countries.[26,63,102,103] Many of the conclusions drawn about the etiology and treatment outcome of eating disorders have been based on work with potentially biased samples (e.g., clinic-based inpatients, and ethnically homogenous groups), and little systematic epidemiological research has focused on cross-cultural groups and children, although research in this area is increasing.[2,103,104] For example, treatments are being developed for Asian American women that take cultural differences into account.[105]

### ASSOCIATED CONDITIONS

#### Psychological

A relationship between eating disorders and other psychological conditions has frequently been noted. Mood, anxiety, substance use, and personality disorders are among the most commonly reported comorbidities.[29,96,97,106] For example,

34% of women who meet criteria for borderline personality disorder also met criteria for an eating disorder.[107] Because many of these findings are based on cross-sectional studies with correlational data, the nature of these relationships is difficult to determine. For instance, it has been suggested that some of these associated disorders (e.g., mood problems) may be the result of severe calorie restriction and/or compensatory behaviors[29,108] or artifacts of self-report methodologies that tend to overestimate certain types of psychopathology.[108] In a therapeutic context, these commonly reoccurring conditions make the assessment and management of eating disorders much more complex.[2,96,107–111]

## Medical

Eating disorders are also associated with numerous medical complications in multiple body systems. For example, metabolic and structural brain abnormalities are common and include reversible brain atrophy and gray matter volume deficits, altered serotonin activity, and changes in cerebral blood flow.[112–118] Both structural and functional cardiac irregularities have been observed.[119–123] Dental issues including gingival changes and dermatological abnormalities on the hands of the patients who purge are also of concern.[124–128] Endocrinological manifestations may consist of osteopenia and osteoporosis, as well as a variety of metabolic irregularities.[129–135] Although amenorrhea is among the diagnostic criteria for AN, a wide variety of other gynecological complications may occur.[118,132,136] Gastrointestinal problems, such as gastric capacity, gastric emptying, gastrointestinal peptide releases, and occult gastrointestinal bleeding are often associated with eating disorders.[137–140] Many of these medical comorbidities are directly associated with poor nutrition,[29,112,120,141,142] and may subside when nutrition is improved. However, some (e.g., growth stunting,[143,144] long-term fracture risk)[135] may present continuing challenges even after average weight is attained.[145] Finally, the aggregate mortality rate for AN is approximately 5.6% per decade, including both suicide and death secondary to medical complications.[146] This is higher than the mortality rates associated for any other psychiatric condition. Taken together, these comorbidities highlight the importance of a biopsychosocial approach in the assessment and management of patients with eating disorders.[147,148]

## DIFFERENTIAL DIAGNOSIS

A variety of psychiatric disorders may be associated with changes in weight and/or eating behavior, but not all should be considered eating disorders. For example, changes in appetite and attitudes toward food are sometimes evident in conversion disorders, schizophrenia, and mood disorders. The distinguishing factors in these cases are the absence of an intense drive for thinness, a disturbed body image, and an increased activity level, which are specific indicators for AN.[68] Although individuals with AN and schizophrenia both may avoid specific foods, this avoidance generally occurs in very different contexts. Those with AN may refuse foods due to concerns about caloric content, whereas those with schizophrenia may avoid foods for reasons that are unrelated to fear of weight gain per se but consistent with broader disturbances in reality testing that characterize psychotic disorders, such as a belief that the food is "poisoned."[40,149] Similarly, even though body dysmorphic disorder (BDD) centers on an appearance preoccupation and desire for weight loss, these disorders usually are not characterized by a fear of becoming "fat" despite being underweight.[40,149] Likewise, overeating in depressive disorders occurs in the broader context of other mood symptoms and typically does not include the compensatory behaviors characteristic of BN.[40,149] As discussed, the diagnostic process is complicated by the fact that eating disorders are often comorbid with several other disorders (e.g., mood, anxiety, substance use, and personality disorders).[29,40]

An additional problem inherent in the study of the eating disorders is the continuing evolution of the diagnostic categories. The significant overlap of symptoms (i.e., 16%–47%) between AN and BN,[150,151] as assessed via the diagnostic criteria contained in the DSM-III-R,[152] resulted in the creation of two "types" of AN in the DSM-IV and DSM-IV-TR. Specifically, those individuals who previously would have been concurrently diagnosed with AN and BN would most likely qualify for the diagnosis of AN, binge eating/purging type.

Historically, average-weight and underweight persons with binge eating tend to be similar on a number of demographic, clinical, and psychometric variables and to differ from those with AN who do not binge.[153] Moreover, compared to their counterparts who do not engage in binge eating, individuals with AN who binge have long been described as more likely to have problems with mood, impulsive behavior, and self-control (e.g., affective lability, shoplifting, alcohol and other substance misuse, self-mutilation, sexual activity),[154] may be more extroverted,[155] have histories of obesity both personally and in their families, show greater childhood maladjustment, have higher rates of familial alcoholism and affective illness, and experience greater conflict and negativity in family relationships.[8] Because of these factors, the binge eating/purging subtype of AN has often been viewed as more difficult to treat and is associated with poorer outcomes.[154]

More recent evidence on the differences between the restricting and the binge eating/purging subtypes has been mixed, with some studies lending support to the distinction[156,157] and others casting doubt on it.[158,159] For instance, the frequently reported "crossover rate" between restricting AN and binge eating/purging AN,[158] as well as between AN and BN,[160,161] is often cited as evidence for a single shared eating disorder psychopathology in which restricting AN is only one "phase."[158,161] Clearly, additional work is warranted in this area.

## ETIOLOGY

Given that eating disorders generally begin during the adolescent years, most etiological theories are set against the backdrop of adolescence and its concomitants. In addition, culturally defined norms and influences, personality factors, and affective difficulties are often considered important causal factors.[162–165] The transition between childhood and adolescence involves numerous biopsychosocial changes requiring adaptation. These include shifts in body appearance and functioning, identity development, and the reorganization of social roles, supports, and family relationships. All of these occur within the escalating responsibility for independent functioning. These demands for readjustment and increasing maturity may interact with emerging competencies and predispositions in such a way as to lower the threshold for emotional distress and dysfunction.[166–168] Further, hormones (e.g., estrogen) and neurotransmitters (e.g., dopamine, serotonin) appear to play a significant role in the pathophysiology of eating disorders.[169,170] Other factors such as culture, family, negative life events, and personality traits have the potential to exacerbate or ameliorate the difficulties inherent in negotiating this developmental transition.[52,168,171]

## CULTURAL INFLUENCES

It is theorized that the traditional definition of femininity has much to do with the development of eating disorders.[162,172,173] Specifically, social norms shape women's motivational priorities by defining femininity and self-worth at least partially in terms of body size.[52,165,174] Because a woman's interpersonal relationships may be disproportionately influenced by the approximation of her physical appearance to that of the feminine cultural ideal (which currently is extremely thin), women may be more vulnerable than their male counterparts to develop a preoccupation with weight and fear of becoming "fat."[162,175,176] From a feminist perspective, women experiencing eating disorders may be especially sensitive to coercive pressure to conform to socially derived notions of beauty and femininity, which currently are skewed toward unrealistic thinness.[177] The persistence and pervasiveness of these messages (e.g., across different mass media categories) can have a corrosive impact on a young woman's emerging sense of competence. These social influences also reinforce and maintain the equation of thinness with self-worth and success.[172,174,178] Based on this, it has been theorized that eating disorders may evolve in some women under the interactive influence of additional developmental stressors at the societal, familial, and individual levels. To further complicate this, women may be under increased pressure to achieve in multiple domains of accomplishment, while the cultural messages regarding women's proper roles in Western culture and body image are often contradictory.[39,52,165,166,172,179,180]

The concept of a cultural desire for thinness does not appear to completely explain the development of eating disorders.[172] For example, in non-Western cultures, AN often occurs in individuals who do not manifest the "fat phobia" that is characteristic of AN in Western samples.[175,181,182] These cross-cultural findings raise the possibility that the application of culturally flexible diagnostic criteria may enhance both the validity and the utility of eating disorder categories[175] by focusing more attention on the factors of etiological significance in each culture.[182]

## PSYCHOSOCIAL INFLUENCES

Similar to etiological perspectives on AN, conceptualizations of BN and BED have emphasized both immediate and extended family relationships and transitions that include broad societal and cultural factors.[63,102,162,163,173,183–185] There is some evidence that the incidence of eating disorders appears to be on the rise,[76,77,162,173] and this increase corresponds to heightened social pressures, particularly for women, toward increasing thinness.[102,166,173,184,185]

Overall, concern about body weight and fairly reasonable weight control efforts and dieting tend to precede the development of eating disorders.[42,68,186] However, the precise etiological role of dieting in the development of eating disorders remains controversial.[187–190] Clearly, the etiology of eating disorders is complicated and an exclusive focus on one factor such as dieting may be misleading.[166] Although dieting figures prominently in many etiological models as one of many important facts,[39,191] it is generally conceptualized as insufficient as a complete explanation for these complex disorders.[41,187]

Similarly, the role of personality in the development of eating disorders also emphasizes their multifaceted nature.[192–194] Individuals with AN have been described as exhibiting constrictive, conforming, obsessive characteristics,[195,196] perfectionistic standards,[197,198] social inhibition, compliance, emotional constraint,[199] and "self-hate guilt."[200] Although personality traits associated with BN follow less consistent patterns, patients with BN have been characterized as manifesting poor impulse control, chronic depression, acting-out behaviors, low frustration tolerance, affective lability, difficult temperament, and inhibition.[196,199] Perfectionistic standards predict bulimic behavior in women who consider themselves overweight, but only in the context of low-self-esteem.[201] Finally, populations with eating disorders have been described as experiencing greater than typical rates of personality disorders, personality-disorder-related symptoms,[196,199] chronic low self-esteem,[202] and poor introspective awareness.[192]

Some differences in information-processing patterns have been observed in patients with AN and BN. Both deficiencies in emotional processing and attention biases have been associated with AN;[203,204] however, these differences may not be readily apparent.[205] BN may also be associated with attentional biases,[203] and bulimic behavior may serve as a cognitive avoidance strategy against unpleasant self-awareness in terms of emotion and threat processing.[206] Additional research in this area is warranted.

There are also reports suggesting that eating disorders may be triggered by traumatic separations, losses, and other adversities.[104,207–211] Examples of traumatic events include family discord and divorce, parental death, dysfunctional parental behavior, separations from the family of origin (e.g., for college or summer vacation), parental illness, sibling or parental pregnancy, and numerous other types of family difficulties.[104,151,209,210,212] Imagined or actual instances of personal failure have also been noted to precede AN.[58,213,214]

Specific traumas, such as childhood sexual abuse, have been suggested as potential etiological factors in the development of eating disorders,[104,215-217] although this literature has produced mixed results. For example, higher reported rates of childhood sexual abuse have been found in those with BN than in populations without eating disorders.[218] A meta-analytic review on the relationship between child sexual abuse and eating disorders concluded that although there was a small positive relationship overall, results varied according to the specific methodology.[219] Sexual abuse is clearly not an eating-disorder-specific risk factor, but is more often associated with increased risk for general psychiatric disturbance.[39,104,220,221] Because of this, it is possible that sexual abuse may indirectly influence the development of eating disorders by virtue of its relationship with other risk factors. Overall, if abuse is a factor of etiological significance in eating disorders, it is probably part of a complex interaction with other risk factors that are still not well understood.[104,220]

Although the majority of women do not develop eating disorders,[1,52] any etiological theory must account for the fact that AN and BN occur predominantly in women. Adolescence is a time of transition for males as well as females, but fewer males develop eating disorders. As discussed earlier, the converging social influences reinforcing the equation of thinness with feminine self-worth and success may constitute gender-linked risk factors for AN and BN. However, the assumption of gender-specific risk does not seem as compelling in the case of BED, where gender disparity is much less marked.[85] Ultimately, it is unlikely that gender differences in the internalization of cultural values completely account for the risk of eating disorders.[1,30]

## NEUROBIOLOGICAL/GENETIC INFLUENCES

Biological theories have focused on the hormonal changes accompanying puberty[8,222] and on differences in the central nervous system (CNS) and neurotransmitter functioning.[18,22,223-228] Relationships between eating and mood disorders in first-degree relatives suggest a possible genetic component to both types of disorders.[229,230] Twin studies estimated that genetic factors account for 50%–83% of the variance in eating disorders.[231-233] Although additional preliminary support for the potential role of genetic etiological factors has been reported for both AN and BN,[104,234-237] complex genetic environment interactions and genetically based vulnerabilities to psychopathology seem more in line with evidence compared to simple gene-behavior models.[104,193,194,235,238-240] Genetic data for eating disorders tend to be overinterpreted, as is the case in much of the behavioral genetics literature on psychological disorders.[238,241,242]

The relative efficacy of antidepressants in the treatment of BN has led to the development of a serotonin hypothesis.[22,226,243,244] Serotonin is linked to carbohydrate consumption and binge eating in both animals and humans,

and BN may be associated with lower endogenous levels of CNS serotonin.[274,745] In an effort to compensate for this deficiency, individuals with BN may consume foods high in tryptophan and relatively low in protein (typical of a high-carbohydrate meal). In this way, binge eating may serve as a form of mood regulation and self-medication, which can be ameliorated by the higher levels of serotonin brought about by the use of antidepressant medications.[227,246,247] Based in part on the relative ineffectiveness of medication interventions designed to raise the levels of serotonin available to the CNS in the treatment of AN,[246] the serotonergic hypothesis also suggests that AN may be associated with overactivity in CNS serotonergic activity.[22] This overactivity subsequently leads to decreased food intake and weight loss. In sum, serotonin dysregulation may play an important role in the etiology or maintenance of eating disorders.[22,30,104]

Disruptions in other neurotransmitter systems have also been implicated in the etiology of eating disorders.[248] Some studies have found alterations in noradrenergic and peptide neuromodulator activity in patients with BN as well as reduced levels of norepinephrine and serotonin metabolites in cerebrospinal fluid.[224,249]

Finally, eating disorders are also viewed as neuropsychological in origin. Differences have been noted between patients with eating disorders and controls in brain metabolic functions and hemispheric activity.[18,225,250] Although neurotransmitter dysregulation and neuropsychological dysfunctions may play a role in the etiology or maintenance of eating disorders, they do not point to the definitive causal role. It is possible that these neurochemical changes occur as a result of eating-disordered behavior and are not actually causal.[223,226] Specifically, these neurotransmitter derangements may be the consequence of extremes in dietary intake and purging or other compensatory behaviors. As such, they may be more important in the maintenance of eating-disordered behaviors and hindrance of recovery.[223,226]

Neurotransmitter and neuropeptide modulator alterations are also not specific to BN or to eating disorders in general. For example, similar alterations in serotonin regulation have been found in depression, impulsivity, substance use disorders, and obsessive-compulsive disorder.[22,244] Furthermore, decreased levels of cholecystokinin have been found in both patients with BN and patients with panic disorder.[251,252] Due to this lack of disorder-related specificity, it has been suggested that dysregulation in serotonin and other neurotransmitter systems may be a common pathway for many disorders, rather than a specific mechanism in eating disorders.[243]

Several prenatal, perinatal, and early childhood complications have been investigated as possible risk factors for eating disorders. For instance, early-onset AN may be associated with spring and early summer births.[253] Perinatal difficulties, such as very preterm birth among girls with low birth weight for gestational age, birth trauma, pediatric infectious disease, and postinfectious process have also been linked with AN.[254-257] Various other etiological influences have been investigated, including genetic risk factors. Specifically, these influences may be epigenetic due to damage to the brain caused by hypoxia.[258] Despite the general consensus that eating disorders have some familial component[241,259,260] and account for as much as 50% or more of the variance,[104,261] no specific genetic loci have yet been identified with certainty.[104,259,262] Unraveling genetic and environmental influences is complicated for a variety of reasons, ranging from the relatively low prevalence of AN and BN to difficulties inherent in genetic analyses and their interpretation.[104,238,241,259–261,263] The specific contributions of genetic versus environmental influences to eating disorders are unclear at present.[104,238,241]

One of the problems in determining the etiology of eating disorders is the lack of prospective and replication studies, adequate sampling and sample sizes, and appropriate analyses in determinant studies.[243] Some studies of biological determinants suffer from small sample sizes and uncorrected statistical analyses, which lead to illusory biological differences. Replications of results are surprisingly lacking. Some of the lack of reproducibility or reliability of findings may lie in the narrow nosological classification system currently in favor. A system of functional classification may help to alleviate this problem by making the psychological dysfunction the elementary unit of analysis, rather than a broader and potentially less reliable syndrome.[25] In fact, many biological variables that have low diagnostic specificity when syndromes are considered can be related very strongly to specific psychopathological dimensions. Future research should focus on these issues in order to adequately address the problem of eating disorders.

In sum, efforts to explain the etiology of eating disorders have focused on a wide variety of possible influences and mechanisms, with a particular emphasis on biological and genetic factors. An overemphasis on physiological mechanisms creates a false and outdated dichotomy between mind and body, which is inconsistent with more contemporary biopsychosocial approaches. It is doubtful that the occurrence of these complex disorders will be explained without an understanding of the many relevant interacting dimensions, including physiological, societal, familial, psychiatric, and psychological influences.[39,42,243] Furthermore, it is highly probable that no narrow definition of the psychological dimension will suffice. A behavioral-systems view should include a recognition and assessment of cognitive factors, emotional regulation, coping skills, and behavioral–environmental contingencies. Consideration of these multiple interacting factors holds promise for advancing our understanding of the etiological mechanisms involved in these disorders.

## ASSESSMENT

A detailed review of assessment instruments is beyond the scope of the present chapter; however, several general points are worth noting as a prelude to our focal discussion on intervention.

Given the complex nature of eating disorders, comprehensive, multimodal assessment is required.[29,264–268] There is a wide range of factors that currently seem relevant to these disorders. Accordingly, assessment should extend beyond eating behavior per se to include (1) self-regulation, particularly mood/affective regulation (including the identification and expression of feelings); (2) social competence and interpersonal relationships; (3) personal identity, self-esteem; (4) distorted beliefs and cognitions; (5) psychological comorbidities such as mood, anxiety, personality, and substance use disorders, as well as the history of other psychological problems and treatment; and (6) family functioning, especially when the patient is a child or adolescent.[29,161,266,269–271]

### ASSESSMENT OF THE FAMILY ENVIRONMENT

The family is perhaps the most critical context for the development of interpersonal roles and skills. Typically, as children grow, mature, and seek increasing independence, family roles shift accordingly resulting in exposure to expanded spheres of social influence, as well as opportunities to experiment with new roles and activities. Although the family continues to provide a secure base, its influence is increasingly replaced with other sources of stress and support as a youth makes the transition from middle adolescence to young adulthood.[167,168] Eating disorders may interfere with this developmental process by increasing parental concern and involvement in children's lives to levels consistent with those more appropriate at younger ages.[272]

The issue remains that some youths seem to have exceptional difficulty negotiating this developmental transition while others do not.[52,171] To address this, considerable attention has focused on the families of girls with eating disorders. Family characteristics and interaction patterns, such as parental overprotectiveness, indirect communication styles (especially around emotional-laden material), and certain conflict resolution strategies may differentiate families whose adolescents develop eating disorders from those who do not.[208,270,273–276] Early attachment and parent–child bonding difficulties,[277,278] parental eating/dieting, family history of dysfunctional eating, and family disparagement and/or teasing about a child's appearance[39] are also possible factors of significance.

Based on these findings, family characteristics should be included in the routine evaluation of young patients with eating disorders,[208,274] especially when the patient is younger than 18 and is still residing in the family home.[29,68,270,272] Additional aspects of family functioning commonly assessed include parental perceptions of the onset and details of the child's disordered eating, factors associated with problem onset, associated changes in the child's behavior, biopsychosocial developmental history, broader family difficulties, familial impact of the child's eating disorder, and parental expectations.[68,269,270,272,279] Of course, this information should be assessed with great sensitivity and with a clear recognition that family members often feel responsible for their child's disorder.[272] Because it will be important for the clinician to establish a working alliance with the family that enhances their participation,[2,68,269,272,279] it is widely recommended that the clinician take a solution-focused approach that avoids searching for a cause of the illness.[272]

## ASSESSMENT OF RELATIONSHIPS AND ENVIRONMENT OUTSIDE THE FAMILY

As discussed previously, during adolescence the family's influence gradually becomes eclipsed by that of other external sources of support (e.g., teachers, peers, colleagues), which gain importance as youths become increasingly mobile, independent, and involved in the world around them. These extrafamilial experiences provide critical opportunities for acquiring the key skills and competencies (e.g., social competence, identity formation) that support healthy adult functioning.[167,168] To the extent that eating disorders are marked by difficulties in negotiating this normative developmental process, these disorders may hinder timely psychosocial development as demonstrated by some individuals with AN and BN having serious interpersonal difficulties. These difficulties may persist even after eating disorder symptoms improve. One review found that only 47% of those with AN had married or were maintaining active partnerships.[280] Patients with BN reported that their problems with eating and weight significantly interfere with their social relationships (94%) and school or job performance (84%).[281] Bulimic behavior also may be associated with decreased social contact.[282] These findings demonstrate the importance of assessing the level and extent of patients' social functioning.

## MEDICAL ASSESSMENT

All patients with eating disorders should undergo medical assessment.[57,147,148,283–288] A standard medical assessment typically includes physical examination, laboratory tests, multiple-channel chemistry analysis, complete blood count, and urinalysis. In addition, endocrinological/metabolic, cardiovascular, renal, gastrointestinal, musculoskeletal, dermatological, hematological, and pulmonary systems usually are reviewed.[29,68,283,284] The clinician should be alert to complaints of weakness, tiredness, constipation, and depression as these can be produced by electrolyte abnormalities,[283,84,289] which are complications of vomiting and purgative abuse. The medical assessment is used, along with other measures, to determine whether hospitalization is necessary. Hospitalization is useful for nutritional rehabilitation and general medical care.[29,137,271,272,290,291]

## TREATMENT

The treatment of eating disorders is an active area of research with the scientific merit of many approaches needing to be further explored and established. Treatments include individual approaches (various forms of individual psychotherapy, as well as psychopharmacology), family therapy, group psychotherapy, and intensive programs involving all the preceding plus training in coping skills, assertiveness, women's issues, and nutritional education. Treatment can take place in inpatient settings, outpatient settings, or both. The primary

elements in each of these modalities, along with adjunctive techniques, are reviewed.

Although the following approaches and techniques are designed specifically for the treatment of AN, BN, and BED, some have been used with other target problems as well. As a rule, additional and better studies of the comparative efficacy of these techniques, either combined or used separately, continue to be warranted. The use of multicomponent, multidisciplinary approaches to the treatment of eating disorders is strongly advocated. Future research will be needed to refine the use of these techniques. Moreover, the numerous ethical issues surrounding assessment and treatment of patients with eating disorders have yet to be resolved.[292–297] Clinicians should not attempt to treat patients with eating disorders without specific training in these disorders.

## PSYCHOSOCIAL THERAPIES: GENERAL ISSUES

In individual psychotherapy, the cornerstones of the treatment, both philosophically and pragmatically, are flexibility and sensitivity. Tailoring the therapeutic program to the patient's specific timing, pacing, and stylistic needs is imperative. Specifically, treatments for eating disorders must be designed to integrate psychosocial interventions, medical management, and the appropriate dietary and rehabilitative services, as well as psychiatric medications when warranted.[269,270,298] In addition, the therapist should have the sensitivity and skill necessary to forge a positive therapeutic alliance that will provide a secure base from which the patient can actively engage and persist in treatment.[2,41,269,270,272,299] In this regard, building trust is key, particularly when the patient is ambivalent about treatment or perceives family pressure to participate.[2,41,300,301] Because treatment is often long term and may involve periodic relapses, the therapist must respond flexibly to changes in each patient's level of functioning and maturity.[302] Although developmentally appropriate levels of autonomy should be encouraged, the therapist should not overestimate the patients' abilities for self-sufficiency, which may be discordant with their chronological age in some cases.[272]

Other important aspects of therapy include (1) conducting a thorough initial assessment and continuing to gather information throughout the treatment, ranging from data on weight and amounts of food consumed to broader information about social and family functioning;[41,272,299] (2) providing the patient with an understanding of the treatment approach and realistic expectations about treatment outcome;[41,270,299] and (3) educating the patient regarding the physiology and psychology of disordered eating.[41,272,299]

## INPATIENT APPROACHES

Hospitalization is not so much an approach as it is a setting in which many therapeutic techniques and procedures can be conducted under close supervision. Indications for hospitalization may include a variety of factors,[29,137,270–272,290,299,303,304] such as weight 15%–25% below average or more (particularly if accompanied by evidence of dehydration or malnutrition), serious medical instabilities and metabolic abnormalities (e.g., hypokalemic alkalosis from bulimic complications), psychiatric emergencies (e.g., clinical depression and/or suicidal thoughts, intents, or gestures), and nonresponsiveness to outpatient treatment.

Most hospital programs are multidisciplinary and have many therapeutic components, including outpatient therapy and follow-up services. Psychiatry, psychology, nursing, dietetics, occupational therapy, physical therapy, social and general medicine services may be involved in an integrated team approach to treatment.[305–307] Although each member of the interdisciplinary team contributes to the patient's care within his or her scope of practice, professional roles are not neatly dictated by discipline. That is, programs take different approaches to the question of which professions or disciplines are represented on the team and what roles various professionals play.

For patients with AN, refeeding tends to begin with a diet of 1000–1600 cal/day, which is gradually increased to 3000–3600 cal/day.[29,270,308] It is important to develop a consensus at the outset of treatment among the patient, family, and treatment team about the timing and pace of refeeding. Patient involvement in meal planning is also encouraged.[305,306] It is common to set limits on the duration of meals, after which time patients may be given a supplement or liquid meal.[304,305,308,309] There is general agreement that nasogastric tube feedings are rarely required with most patients,[29,137,296,304] consistent with the general philosophy of care emphasizing patient-team collaboration.[305,306,310] Multiple publications have provided a more thorough review of inpatient care.[311,312]

## Goal Weights

During inpatient weight stabilization of patients with AN, it is important to establish reasonable weight goals and predictable weight gain milestones, broken down into achievable weekly targets—usually between 1 and 3 lb/week.[29,269] However, decisions about specific goal weights are complex and must be tailored to the unique needs of each patient considering such factors as medical necessity, body mass index, weight history, anticipated length of stay, fear of weight gain, and tolerance of increases in food consumption.[270] Given the matrix of biopsychosocial dynamics involved, these kinds of decisions are best formulated from a multidisciplinary perspective.[29,270,310]

## Special Problems

Special problems that may complicate inpatient treatment include the following: (1) Patients may not be completely convinced that their weight and eating behaviors are sufficiently serious to require treatment and hospitalization; (2) Inherent in any hospitalization is some loss of autonomous functioning and control; (3) Serious comorbid conditions, such as severe depression and medical problems, may hinder treatment; (4) Some patients may be especially responsive to the inadvertent reinforcement contingencies in some

units, whereby the most seriously ill patients receive the most staff attention; (5) Interactions among patients with different eating disorders may not always be harmonious, particularly when some patients with medical emergencies (such as those with AN) may require more staff time and attention.[2,68,269,270,303,313]

Despite considerable variability, typical durations of hospitalization range from fewer than 7–26 days.[308,314–316] In the context of shorter hospital stays, inpatient treatment increasingly emphasizes stabilization of the patient's immediate medical condition.[29,269,270,272,316–318]

In an effort to address patient needs more efficiently in the context of diminishing inpatient resources, an increasing number of programs have developed continuum models providing a broader spectrum of services emphasizing continuity across levels of care.[306,308,317,319] In these comprehensive treatment programs, patients typically are evaluated and then assigned to one of several levels of care on the basis of specified criteria. Results of the initial assessment guide patients to the least restrictive alternative that is appropriate in each case. In cases where inpatient treatment is initially indicated, patients can make the transition to less intensive care as soon as it is warranted.[270,306] The transition between inpatient and outpatient treatment modalities is supported by communication between these providers and may be important with respect to retention.[312]

## MULTICOMPONENT OUTPATIENT TREATMENT PROGRAMS

Intensive, multicomponent outpatient treatment programs are frequently used for the treatment of AN, BN, and BED.[57,269,320–322] These programs typically combine educational seminars with group, individual, family, and body image therapy, incorporating many of the themes discussed earlier and utilizing many of the techniques outlined later. These approaches may also be utilized in conjunction with pharmacological interventions.[323] Nevertheless, the bulk of the treatment outcome research tends to center on specific strategies.

## PSYCHOTHERAPY TECHNIQUES AND THERAPY COMPONENTS

Comparisons of therapeutic processes and techniques have failed to identify a clear choice among approaches that works best *for all eating disorders*. Specifically, reviews of the literature tend to find that behavioral, cognitive, cognitive-behavioral, and interpersonal therapeutic approaches perform significantly better than either no treatment or pharmacological interventions alone.[324,325] Yet there is no consistent, clear-cut pattern of differential performance among the above-mentioned theoretical approaches in the scientific literature *for all eating disorders*. In fact, reviews of the literature indicate that numerous types of therapeutic technique have been attempted with eating disorders, and that virtually all have shown some efficacy.[29,324,326,327]

One major exception is in the treatment of BN, where cognitive-behavior therapy (CBT) is currently recommended

## Behavioral Therapies and Techniques

### Exposure Plus Response Prevention

There has been some controversy about the role of exposure plus response prevention (ERP) procedures in the treatment of bulimic behaviors. The basic process of ERP is as follows. Vomiting can be viewed as a response to overeating that decreases anxiety related to fear of gaining weight.[331] As a result, individuals learn that vomiting after eating leads to anxiety reduction. Therefore, binge eating might not occur if an individual with BN was prevented from vomiting afterwards.[331] Although some research has supported the use of ERP procedures,[332–336] several of these studies lacked adequate controls and had small samples. Controlled studies have found that ERP procedures added no benefit to, and potentially detracted from, the efficacy of CBT.[337] In a study comparing ERP alone to CBT alone, 1-year follow-up data indicated that patients assigned to the ERP-alone condition experienced significantly greater relapse, whereas patients in the CBT-alone group maintained or slightly improved their scores on measures of bulimia-specific psychopathology and more general measures of psychological functioning.[19]

### Operant Conditioning Techniques

Operant conditioning techniques have been used to facilitate weight gain in hospital settings. These techniques use positive and negative contingencies (e.g., social praise, recreational activities, visiting privileges, hospital rewards, bed rest, and/or earlier or later discharge) in association with a performance criterion such as eating or weight gain.[270,338–342] In the case of AN, this criterion is generally a predetermined weight or weight increase. Given that the use of operant techniques presupposes the ability to control the environmental contingencies, this approach has been used primarily in inpatient settings. Although this type of contingency management can produce initial and rapid weight gains, these procedures have not been shown to be more effective than other treatments in terms of extended weight maintenance, including simpler hospital programs with discharge contingent on weight gains.[343] Research utilizing operant approaches suggests that in terms of treatment efficacy, they are not superior to CBT techniques.[325] These findings are consistent with the more traditional assertion that operant conditioning techniques are helpful when part of a comprehensive treatment program, but inadequate when used alone.[344,345] Additionally, patients with eating disorders, especially AN, may be more likely to discontinue treatment when behavior therapy alone is used.[346]

### Response Delay

Response delay procedures are based on the theory that impulses are more easily delayed than resisted. It is hypothesized that during the delay period, the event sequence will be altered causing the urge to subside and become more manageable. Ultimately, the impulses will yield to resistance efforts. The delay tactic can involve allowing some predetermined length of time to pass or engaging in some alternative activity.[347] For instance, a client with BN may choose to wait 20 min before bingeing or, alternatively, call a friend, walk the dog, or take a leisurely bath. It is important that the activity be selected ahead of time and involves something of the client's choice that is experienced as pleasurable, esteem-building, and/or self-nurturing. Garner and Bemis[348] recommended that some clients (particularly those who have not yet made a commitment to stop vomiting) prepare a "mnemonic card" listing prebinge delay tactics for consultation on those occasions when urges to binge seem irresistible. Response delay strategies are commonly included in multicomponent behavioral programs. As such, they are presently considered one well-accepted strategy routinely incorporated into broader treatment packages, which may explain the dearth of current research specifically focused on response delay per se.

### Self-Monitoring Techniques

Self-monitoring techniques are generally recognized as helpful, particularly when patients binge. Although formats differ, patients are typically encouraged to record the context and parameters of their binge eating, associated and preceding thoughts, feelings, events, and the presence or absence of others.[41,299] Self-monitoring can be used as a vehicle for the clients and therapist to explore options to increase self-control over eating and decreasing food avoidance.[349] Although self-monitoring alone has been shown to be effective, outcomes are significantly improved when used in conjunction with a CBT package.[337] Overall, self-monitoring should be viewed as one meaningful component of CBT and not as a "treatment" in and of itself.

### Social Skills Training

Social skills training has been used to help correct the deficits in social competencies, assertiveness, interpersonal communication, and basic problem-solving capabilities frequently observed in those with eating disorders. Social skills training has also been used to modify the social isolation and interpersonal anxiety associated with AN.[350] Although social skills training has shown no better outcomes in terms of weight at 1 year compared to a placebo condition, it did result in greater treatment retention and a more rapid decrease in their levels of anxiety, depression, and fear of negative evaluation.[350] Incorporating the typical targets of social skills training interventions into inpatient interventions for AN appears to enhance overall effectiveness and generalization of treatment.[303] It is common for social skills to be addressed within the broader context of comprehensive treatment packages.[270] As such, little current research has focused specifically on the value added by social skills training.

### Stimulus Control Strategies

Stimulus control strategies are used routinely in the multicomponent treatment of eating disorders to minimize or neutralize environmental cues that lead to inappropriate eating.[44,299] These strategies include reducing household binge triggers (e.g., favorite binge foods), structuring the environment to promote healthful eating practices (e.g., by replacing countertop candy with fresh fruit), and avoiding high-risk eating situations (e.g., buffets). Stimulus control procedures emphasizing minimal therapist contact, in the absence of cognitive therapy, have been shown to successfully reduce vomiting frequency of BN.[351] However, no strong conclusions can be drawn about the efficacy or generalizability of these procedures as these results were based on a case study. Given that stimulus control procedures are ubiquitous in CBT programs, these strategies should be further evaluated in larger, controlled investigations to assess their specific contribution to the overall efficacy of comprehensive treatment programs.

### Systematic Desensitization

Systematic desensitization has been used to decrease anxiety related to fears of gaining weight and/or being criticized,[340,352,353] self-deprecating thoughts,[354] and changes in physical appearance concomitant with weight gain.[355] Unfortunately, in recent years, little attention has focused on systematic desensitization in the treatment of eating disorders.

## Cognitive/Cognitive-Behavioral Techniques

Cognitive retraining or restructuring techniques combat distorted body image, erroneous beliefs and assumptions, and misinterpretations of environmental messages.[356] Individuals with AN or BN may be especially prone to evaluate their self-worth in terms of shape and weight. Based on an overgeneralization and incorporation of very real social pressures, such individuals may hold a variety of dysfunctional beliefs, such as equating overweight with unworthiness, weakness, and a dismal future, as well as the corollary that being thin is associated with improved self-worth and success.[178,299,357,358] Therapy consequently involves questioning these social values, identifying the ways patients may apply them in their lives, and learning to challenge them on their own.[359]

CBT has been well established as an empirically supported treatment for BN.[39,41,329,330,360–362] Research utilizing approaches that combine cognitive and behavioral interventions (i.e., CBT) has demonstrated meaningful levels of clinical improvement.[359,363] CBT has been found to be mildly superior to supportive-expressive treatment on measures of vomiting frequency in patients with BN, but the results were much stronger when other symptoms were examined (e.g., concern about eating and weight, depression, and self-esteem).[364] CBT techniques alone and used in combination with pharmacological interventions tend to be superior to pharmacological interventions alone in reducing the primary symptoms of BN.[365–370]

Although CBT also seems promising in the treatment of AN[325,371,372] and BED,[373–375] one of the most significant issues in the treatment of eating disorders is the growing recognition that a narrow behavioral focus on disordered eating may not address important core issues that play a role in etiology and maintenance. Primary in this area is a recognition that dysfunctional interpersonal relationships and sociocultural pressure may be at the heart of eating disorders. Thus, there is a need to determine whether focusing on interpersonal relationships might be more effective than a sole focus on disordered eating per se. Although IPT did not lead to further improvements in patients who did not respond to CBT,[376] IPT has been found to be as effective as CBT for nonpurging BN.[377] Some attempts have been made to broaden the focus of CBT to include interpersonal difficulties as one of several additional treatment modules.[161] Specifically, in the case of treatment for BED in adolescents, CBT is the treatment of choice.[362]

## Interpersonal Psychotherapy

IPT is focused on helping the client understand and change maladaptive interpersonal interactions.[378] For the treatment of BN, IPT has been found to be as effective as CBT, but IPT appears to work somewhat more slowly.[160,161,364,375,379] It is possible that IPT may address secondary mechanisms (e.g., dissatisfaction with social relationships, difficulties with social functioning, negative affect, and low self-esteem) implicated in the development and maintenance of BN.[41,380] Research on the efficacy of IPT for patients with BED who have not responded to CBT has not found it effective,[376] suggesting that patients benefiting from CBT may not be significantly different from those who benefit from IPT.[376] Clearly, this issue deserves further investigation.

## Dialectical and Behavior Therapy

Although eating disorders are relatively rare, about 34% of people with an eating disorder also meet criteria for borderline personality disorder.[107] Eating disorders are challenging to treat when they occur on their own. Treatment is further compounded when there is a comorbid personality disorder.[107] Dialectical Behavior Therapy (DBT) is an empirically supported cognitive-behavioral based therapy developed for the treatment of borderline personality disorder and recurrent self-harm or parasuicidal behaviors.[381] Borderline personality disorder is characterized by emotional dysregulation and associated problem behaviors (e.g., self-harm, impulsive behaviors, unstable self-image, and mood lability).[382] Likewise, eating disordered behaviors such as binging, purging, restriction, and excessive exercise are also thought to be associated with emotional dysregulation.[383] Due to the common need to address problem behaviors associated with emotional dysregulation and high prevalence of comorbid eating disorders and borderline personality disorder, DBT has been adapted for the treatment of AN, BN, and BED.[383] DBT appears to be effective in reducing eating disorder behaviors when compared to a wait-list control condition.[384–386] When compared to an active treatment control group, DBT showed significant decreases in binge eating post treatment, though these differences were no longer present at 12-month follow-up.[385] Further randomized controlled trials comparing DBT to other empirically supported treatments for eating disorders, such as CBT and IPT, are needed.

## Supportive-Expressive Therapy

Supportive-expressive therapy, originally developed as a brief psychoanalytic approach,[387] has also been applied in the treatment of eating disorders. Supportive-expressive therapy posits that eating disorder symptoms disguise underlying interpersonal problems. Therapy is nondirective and interpretive, with a focus on listening to the patient, promoting expression of feelings, and identifying problems and solutions. A primary task during therapy is to explore the past in order to illuminate interpersonal difficulties and establish core conflictual relationship themes that underlie eating disorder symptoms. Supportive-expressive therapy has been found to be slightly less effective than CBT in reducing the frequency of self-induced vomiting, but CBT was significantly more effective in ameliorating dysfunctional attitudes about eating and weight, depression, poor self-esteem, and general psychological distress.[364]

## Body Image Work

Body image work helps patients become more aware and accepting of their bodies. Photographs, videotapes, various types of role playing, cognitive restructuring, movement, expressive art, and guided imagery therapies are often employed.[322] A body-image-oriented form of CBT with patients diagnosed with BED produced significant decreases in body image disturbance compared to no-treatment controls.[388] In addition, remission was achieved in 82% of treated patients at termination and 77% of cases at follow-up.[388] Although these cognitive-behavioral methods are integrated routinely into current treatment programs for eating disorders,[70,269,299] few empirical investigations have focused specifically on body image work. More research on the additive value of body image work would be helpful in guiding decisions about incorporating these approaches into broader multicomponent treatment packages.

## Family Therapy

Family therapy ranges from supportive, informational counseling to more intensive work focused on changing a family's structural and/or functional patterns. Family therapy has been used as a treatment by itself[389] and as an element of multicomponent treatment packages.[279,390] As a primary treatment, family therapy generally encourages a patient with AN to disengage gradually from the family, progress toward adolescence and adulthood, and realign family roles and boundaries along more developmentally appropriate and adaptive lines.[272] The agenda of family therapy as an element of a treatment package[322] includes helping the patient find a way to achieve age-appropriate separation from the family without the feared loss of all family connectedness, express personal needs and feelings clearly, and enhance communication between the parents, so that the patient is not needed as a facilitator.[322]

Adolescents receiving family intervention for AN were shown to outperform those receiving individual treatment on measures of maintained body weight at a 5-year follow-up.[391] Family therapy has also been shown to be superior to individual supportive therapy in patients whose eating disorders started before age 19 and whose eating disorders were not chronic.[392] Family therapy has also been demonstrated to be an important component of combined therapy in patients with AN.[393] Treatment protocols that include family therapy have been found to be superior to no-treatment conditions on measures of weight gain, return of menstruation, and aspects of social and sexual adjustment.[393–395] By contrast, an evaluation of behavioral-family systems therapy (BFST; see later) for AN with adolescent females found that family therapy and ego-oriented individual therapy, which focuses on improving a patient's ego strength, coping skills, and individuation from the family, were equivalent in producing improvements in eating attitudes, body dissatisfaction, interoceptive awareness, depression, and family conflict.[396,397] In addition, many of these improvements are maintained 1 year after treatment termination. In fact, the only difference in outcome between the two therapy approaches was that BFST produced greater changes in body mass index. Similarly, few differences were found in a study that compared a family therapy to separate counseling for the patient and parent.[398]

Although there is a paucity of controlled evaluations, family involvement is considered a key component of comprehensive treatment for an eating disorder, especially when the patient is a legal minor or still resides with the family of origin.[269,270,272,399,400] A manualized, family-based intervention for AN[272] has shown preliminary promise in the treatment of adolescents[401] and has been adapted for BN.[402] Both adolescents and their families perceived this treatment to be effective and acceptable.[403]

Another family approach to treating AN, BFST combines components of behavior modification, cognitive therapy, and family systems therapy.[404] As discussed earlier, comparisons of BFST with ego-oriented individual therapy[396] have found generally equivalent efficacy in adolescent females, with a majority of patients in the BFST group attaining their target weights by a 1-year follow-up.[405] These preliminary data suggest that BFST may be a potentially efficacious treatment for adolescents and their families.

## Feminist Approaches to Treatment

Although the definition of a "feminist approach" with respect to psychological interventions is continually evolving and somewhat difficult to articulate, a brief description of the ideas that fall under the umbrella of the term is warranted. Primarily, it is important to consider the social and cultural context of patients with eating disorders.[406] Feminist therapists attempt to broaden the focus from blaming the individual with an eating disorder to examining the pathological social factors beyond the patient. In contrast to traditional techniques (which may be rooted in many of the same cultural biases and pressures that contribute to women's eating problems), feminist approaches are designed to empower patients, in order to minimize the risk of revictimization in the course of treatment.[165] They also consider the potential impact of sexual abuse on the development of eating disorders in children[407] and adults.[215] Unfortunately, these approaches have rarely been subjected to empirical testing.

## Group Therapy

### Group Approaches for AN

Compared to group approaches for patients with BN or BED, group therapy has traditionally been much less common in the treatment of AN.[408] However, group work may be beneficial for those patients whose medical conditions have been stabilized. For instance, several group therapy protocols have been developed for young patients with AN, including a body image group, a meal-planning/nutritional education group, a family group, and an adolescent group.[270] Several group treatments for AN have shown potential promise, such as a group CBT program with four phases (motivation, day patient, outpatient, and separation),[409] as well as an 8-week nutrition and behavior change group conducted by a multidisciplinary team.[410] Specific factors that are relevant to the group treatment of eating disorders include group size, composition, climate,[411,412] structure through various treatment stages,[408,409] and members' readiness to change.[413]

### Group Approaches for BN

Experiential group therapy has been advocated for the treatment of average-weight women with BN. This type of therapy may incorporate a feminist perspective, taking the position that eating disorders are caused in part by the conflicting role demands placed on women. From this perspective, BN is considered to be related to the pressure to achieve a stereotypically perfect female image.[414] Treatment consequently questions these standards.[415] Some evidence supports the efficacy of this treatment.[414,415] Unfortunately, as a group, studies examining this approach suffer from being statistically underpowered, which is a problem plaguing research on many of the treatment approaches to eating disorders. Both CBT and IPT (discussed earlier as empirically supported treatments) have been delivered in group formats. Both approaches have shown efficacy in group settings for patients with BN and BED.[375,416] Differences in outcomes between individual and group CBT appear to be minor with significant cost effectiveness benefits associated with a group approach.[417]

## Lifestyle Activity

Moderate exercise (walking, stretching) is thought to promote a healthy distribution of weight gain and a balanced view of physical activity as part of a healthy lifestyle.[291,418,419] As such, lifestyle activity is often included as one facet of multicomponent treatment packages. For instance, adjunctive exercise has been shown to enhance extended CBT for BED.[420] There is also some preliminary evidence that adapted physical activity/graded exercise may be a valuable component in comprehensive interventions for AN.[291,418,419] However, the exact role of graded exercise in the treatment of AN remains unclear. For instance, the inclusion of a graded exercise program beneficially impacted compliance, but it did not affect body composition in the short term.[421]

## Psychoeducational Approaches

Based on the idea that maladaptive beliefs and behaviors develop as the result of erroneous or insufficient information, psychoeducational approaches have been viewed as an important part of treatment for eating disorders.[422] Psychoeducation typically consists of providing information to patients about the nature of their disorders and methods for overcoming them with the intention of promoting attitudinal and behavior change. In addition, psychoeducational programs tend to focus on a coaching model of treatment. Because the patient is empowered with information and methods, the locus of change is within the patient.[422,423] Psychoeducational programs cover a wide range of topics, depending on the treatment population and professionals involved. For eating disorders, topics may include the multidimensional etiology of AN, BN, and BED, the negative consequences of dieting, nutritional information, set-point theory, the effects of starvation on behavior, the cultural context of eating disorders, body image and self-esteem issues, cognitive and behavior change strategies, medical complications, and relapse prevention.[422,423] Finally, psychoeducational programs most often are provided to patients (and in some cases family members) in group formats that facilitate interaction and support.

Olmsted and colleagues[424] utilized a sequential cohort design to compare the relative effectiveness of an 18-week CBT intervention for BN with that of a 4-week (five-session) group psychoeducational protocol. CBT was found to be significantly more effective for the most seriously ill patients (32% of the sample who reported bingeing more than 42 times in the month prior to treatment) on measures of vomiting frequency. For less severely ill patients, no significant difference on measures of vomiting frequency between CBT and the psychoeducational intervention was detected. A similar but less robust finding was reported for scores on the Drive for Thinness and Maturity Fears scales included in this study. A self-help book has also been shown to reduce binging and purging symptoms.[425] Additionally, family therapy and family group psychoeducation have both been associated with weight restoration in adolescents with AN.[426] Taken together, this pattern of results highlights the relative effectiveness of psychoeducational interventions for the delivery of efficient and cost-effective treatment of eating disorders for some patients.[427,428]

## Innovative Methods of Treatment Delivery

Increasingly, new technologies are being used in the management of eating disorders, including computer-based methods of learning to eat and recognize satiety,[429] adjunctive e-mail in the outpatient treatment of AN,[430,431] and the delivery of family therapy for AN via telehealth.[432] CBT delivered via telehealth has shown significant promise for individuals with limited access to specialized centers.[433] Although many of the issues surrounding the use of these approaches have yet to be fully explored and resolved,[430,431] these innovative methods deserve more systematic investigation.

## Psychosocial Treatments: Conclusions

Despite the vast array of psychosocial treatments potentially available for the treatment of eating disorders, none address all symptoms of all eating disorders in all patients. For example, although CBT substantially improves symptoms of BN and BED, not all patients benefit.[161,361,376] In fact, as noted earlier, the evidence for many psychosocial therapies is weak or equivocal at this time, especially in the case of interventions with children and adolescents. Across developmental levels, patients with eating disorders appear to have high rates of relapse, regardless of the treatment modality.[345,434-436] This suggests that current psychosocial treatments are not adequate, and that future efforts should focus on optimizing empirically supported treatments, evaluating other existing therapies, and developing new approaches.[1,2] In addition, existing therapies that have shown promise in the treatment of other disorders (e.g., motivation enhancement and dialectical behavioral therapies) have been applied to eating disorders with some success.[110,383,437] A CBT approach that focuses on the psychopathology of the eating disorders rather than the diagnosis is also under investigation.[438] Efforts such as these, as well as up-and-coming theories and strategies, are essential to advancing the state of the science.

## PHARMACOLOGICAL TREATMENT

### Anorexia Nervosa

Pharmacological treatment has typically been explored as one component of multicomponent programs for AN. The medications used have included neuroleptic antidepressants[439] and anti-anxiety medications. Small amounts of benzodiazepine (e.g., Iorezapam) before meals may be helpful for some highly anxious patients with AN,[440] although others have argued that the use of medications to stimulate appetite is misguided.[137] They argue that antidepressant medications should not be used until patients have attained average weight, and then used only if a patient meets the criteria for major depressive disorder.

Other drugs such as olanzapine (an atypical neuroleptic) were first explored in preliminary case, retrospective, and open-label studies with very small numbers of participants as possibly promoting weight gain among patients with AN.[255,441-443] A 10-week randomized controlled trial using olanzapine resulted in decreased obsessional symptoms and increased rate of weight gain.[444] Fluoxetine has also demonstrated long-term results in symptom improvement.[445] Reports on the use of citalopram[446] and tramadol,[447] zinc and cyproheptadine[448] have also been published. Although these results seemed promising, interpretation of these findings is difficult until more controlled studies with larger numbers of participants have been reported.

The current consensus based on the accumulation of empirical results to date seems to have coalesced around the view that pharmacological treatments are not generally effective in the acute treatment of patients with AN, although they may be helpful in mitigating relapse after healthy weight has been achieved in some patients within the broader context of a comprehensive treatment program.[366,370,449-452]

### Bulimia Nervosa

Pharmacological treatments for BN have been associated with more positive outcomes than those for AN. Antidepressants have been associated most consistently with the short-term amelioration of binge-eating and purging behaviors.[366,370] However, pharmacotherapy has generally not been linked with durable long-term improvements without psychotherapy, and it has not been shown to be more effective than CBT alone.[39,366,370,452]

Various types of antidepressants, as well as anticonvulsant medication (phenytoin sodium), have been explored in the treatment of binge eating. In a review of the efficacy of antidepressants, tricyclic antidepressants significantly reduced binge eating and/or vomiting compared to placebo.[453] The reduction in binge eating ranged from 47% to 91%. Overall, antidepressant medications typically used included releasing agents and reuptake inhibitors, such as imipramine, amitriptyline, and desipramine.

In conjunction with the serotonin etiological theory discussed earlier in this chapter, the selective serotonin reuptake inhibitor (SSRI), fluoxetine, has also shown efficacy in the treatment of BN[454]. Two studies utilizing fluoxetine with small samples reported significant short-term improvement in bingeing and vomiting, along with long-term maintenance of gains.[246] Patients treated with fluoxetine for 16 weeks demonstrated significant reduction in binge-eating and vomiting episodes, compared to patients treated with placebo.[455] Fluoxetine treatment alone has produced results similar to the combination of psychodynamically oriented supportive psychotherapy and fluoxetine.[456] When compared to CBT, however, fluoxetine alone produced poorer outcomes and the combination of both was only marginally better than CBT alone.[369,456]

Monoamine oxidase (MAOI) antidepressants have been used because of data suggesting a link between BN and mood disorders.[453,457,458] Results have been mixed. Some evidence has shown that these antidepressants have no effect on eating behavior,[459] whereas other evidence demonstrated dramatic improvement in both mood and eating behavior in women meeting the DSM-II-R criteria for BN.[458] Unfortunately in these studies there was no control group, the sample size was small, the method for measuring improvement was not specified, and follow-up data were not presented. Overall, MAOIs should not be considered as the first line of treatment for BN.

Desipramine, a tricyclic, has fewer side effects than the MAOIs. An advantage of desipramine is that it does not require that patients be placed on diets with rigid restrictions. Furthermore, desipramine hydrochloride was shown to reduce binge frequency by 91% whereas the placebo group showed a 19% increase in binge frequency.[460] Of the 22 patients on the drug, 15 attained complete abstinence from bingeing and purging after 6 weeks of treatment. However, questions about the endurance of these improvements remain to be fully explored.[2,370] Moreover, because tricyclic antidepressants may have potentially adverse side effects, individuals (especially youths) who are prescribed these drugs should be carefully monitored, and medication should be discontinued when problems arise.[461–464]

Anticonvulsant medications, such as phenytoin sodium, have been used in the treatment of eating disorders, based on the hypothesis that binge eating may be a symptom of epileptic convulsions. Abnormal electroencephalograms have been found in some individuals with compulsive eating disorders.[465,466] Treatment successes as high as 90% have been reported with phenytoin.[465] However, the criteria for improvement were unclear, and there were no controls for placebo effects. Other studies on the effects of anticonvulsant medication on compulsive eating indicated a lack of response to medication.[68,468] Preliminary evidence is also available for the use of topirimate, desipramine, fluvoxamine, trazodone, ondasetron, and brofamine.[442,454]

In sum, reviews of the literature have concluded that antidepressants generally have been shown useful in the short-term treatment of BN, with various types of antidepressants appearing roughly comparable.[469] No drugs, other than antidepressants, are recommended for BN.[470] However, pharmacotherapy alone has been associated with substantial relapse and less overall effectiveness than CBT.[39,366,370,452,464]

## Binge Eating Disorder

The success with antidepressants in the treatment of BN has led to the use of this class of drugs in the treatment of BED. SSRIs are the most commonly studied. Randomized controlled trials have been conducted with fluoxetine, fluvoxamine, sertraline, citalopram, and escitalopram.[471–477] Although there are some inconsistencies in the findings from these studies, the majority of them resulted in significant improvements compared to a placebo. Other drugs that were being used to treat obesity such as sibutramine, topiramate, and zonisamide have also been found to reduce binge eating symptoms.[478–480] Although all of these medications have outperformed placebo control groups, there is little to no evidence that medication is superior to the use of CBT strategies.[472,481]

## Night Eating Syndrome

SSRIs have been shown to be helpful in the treatment of NES, and bright light therapy has shown some success in case studies.[50] Allison et al.[49] have developed a cognitive behavioral self-help book based on clinical experience in treating NES. The treatment involves psychoeducation, eating modification, self-monitoring of food intake, eating schedule, stimulus control, exposure and response prevention for craved foods, relaxation, sleep hygiene, cognitive restructuring, physical activity, social support, and medication referral. While this is thought to be a promising treatment for NES, a randomized controlled trial is needed to evaluate its efficacy. Research concerning the diagnostic criteria of NES and potential treatments of NES is still in its infancy, though NES may play an important role in the increasing prevalence of obesity in adults.[50]

## Limitations to Pharmacotherapy

Medications are frequently promoted as a primary treatment modality, due to the tendency to view eating disorders as caused by biological deficiencies. This occurs despite the weak evidence for a biological etiology, and the fact that eating disorders occur disproportionately in women and in cultures emphasizing thinness as a value. Although the rewarding effects of eating can be inhibited by opiate antagonists[482] and binge eating and vomiting can be reduced through the administration of SSRIs,[455] medications do not address many patients' problems of social isolation and perceived lack of nurturance from interpersonal relationships. Use of prescription medications for the treatment of eating disorders may inappropriately replace needed therapy. Further research is crucial to evaluate whether and to what extent medications add to the effectiveness of empirically supported psychological approaches, as well as to determine how such medication regimens can be administered in controlled, ethical ways.

## INTEGRATION OF PSYCHOLOGY AND PHARMACOLOGY

The efficacy of combining pharmacological and psychological interventions remains an area of focus for eating disorder research.[367,368,370,483] However, the cumulative results to date raise questions about whether medications (e.g., antidepressants) enhance treatment effects over and above those associated with CBT alone, especially over the long term when medication is withdrawn.[2,370] For instance, the combination of CBT and the antidepressant desipramine has been compared to CBT alone and antidepressant medication alone in the treatment of BN.[484] In this study, participants were randomly assigned to one of the following groups: desipramine withdrawn at 16 weeks; desipramine withdrawn at 24 weeks; combined treatment (medication withdrawn at either 16 or 24 weeks); and 15 sessions of CBT. In general, CBT and the antidepressant–CBT combination both outperformed medication alone on measures of binge eating and purging. Most interestingly, the results of this study suggested that continued use of CBT prevented relapse in subjects withdrawn from medication at 16 weeks.

In a study combining group-administered CBT with tricyclic antidepressant medication, subjects in the combined condition showed a 51% abstinence rate in bulimic behaviors, compared to a 16% abstinence rate in the medication-only condition.[485] By contrast, in a study of the treatment of binge eating as a method of facilitating weight loss in obese patients, the use of desipramine did not lead to greater improvements in binge-eating symptoms than CBT alone did. Neither CBT nor the combination of CBT with desipramine improved overall weight loss at the end of treatment or follow-up.[320] These contradictory findings suggest that the value of augmenting CBT with drug treatment for patients with BN or BED is still unclear and should be further studied.[39,365,370,486] Given the paucity of research focused on young samples, empirically supported conclusions about adjunctive pharmacotherapy with children and adolescents are premature at present.[2]

## PREDICTION OF OUTCOME

With the notable exception of the empirical support for CBT and IPT, there are very few data suggesting that different treatments have better or worse outcomes, and few differential outcome data based on treatment and symptom characteristics. Overall, BN is associated with improved remission rates 10 or more years following intake and lower mortality rates compared to AN.[487] For the most part, treatment effectiveness has been explored in relationship to *patient,* not *treatment,* characteristics.

Favorable long-term prognosis has been related to early age at onset of illness.[15,58,488–492] Poor outcomes have been associated with longer duration of illness and previous hospitalizations[343,489–491,493–496]; very low weight during illness[213,489,490,496]; and the presence of bulimic symptoms, such as vomiting and laxative abuse.[436,488,489,496–498] Less commonly mentioned negative prognosticators include overestimation of body size[343,499]; premorbid personality and family relationship difficulties[213,436,489,490]; depressive and obsessive-compulsive symptoms[436,500–504]; high rates of physical complaints[500]; and neuroticism.[213,436,491] Although some research has suggested that lower socioeconomic status may be associated with a less favorable outcome,[343,489,494,500] others raise questions about the predictive value of socioeconomic factors.[436]

The most common difficulty at follow-up is subsyndromal bulimia, followed by full BN. In general, after CBT, approximately 50% of patients with BN were asymptomatic at 2–10 years follow-up.[505] Average-weight patients with BN did not tend to develop AN, and their rate of obesity was found to be lower than that of the general population. Percentage of body weight increase and type of eating disorder appear to be important variables associated with outcome during a 1-year follow-up.[506] Specifically, patients diagnosed with BN tended to fare better than those diagnosed with either AN or both BN and AN (by DSM-III-R criteria). With respect to body weight, each 10% increase in percentage of body weight was associated with an 18% increase in hazard. Finally, symptom duration at baseline and substance use history appear to be unfavorable prognostic indicators.[507]

Rorty, Yager, and Rossotto[508] examined the factors that former patients with BN felt were especially instrumental in their recovery. Responses from 40 female participants suggested several such factors, including a sense of being "fed up" with the disorder, the desire to have a better life, the importance/difficulty of cognitive change, and the development of empathic and caring relationships with others. Factors perceived by the former patients as making recovery more difficult included lack of understanding by important others, insufficient acknowledgement or activity by therapists, and the sabotage of the healing process by family members or others.

Although not focused specifically on treatment outcome, a study on the natural course of BN and BED in community women[509] highlighted the differential outcome of these two disorders. Over a 5-year period, the majority of those with BED were considered to have recovered, but the course of those with BN was more variable, punctuated by higher relapse rates and marked by less positive overall outcome.

## TREATMENT DIFFICULTIES

The treatment of eating disorders is known to be difficult and, in many cases, resistant to treatment.[487] The problem can be further compounded by physician attitudes toward patient groups with particular diagnoses, as negative attitudes can interfere with the development of rapport and may also affect treatment outcomes.[510] A study investigating clinicians' reactions to eating disordered patients found that these reactions could be classified into four categories: frustrated, helpless, incompetent, and worried.[510] In general, physicians reported feeling a lack of competence in treating eating disordered patients. A lack of observed improvement in patients, a belief that eating disordered behavior was a personal choice, and patients' comorbid personality disorders accentuated physicians' feelings of incompetence. Inexperienced clinicians were more likely to report feelings of incompetence while more experienced specialists did not report these same reactions. Further research is needed to address this concern in the training of medical students, professionals, and early career clinicians.

## PREVENTION

Public health measures are vital to help prevent the development of eating disorders. Unfortunately, there is a serious dearth of information about effective prevention programming. This is in part due to the complex nature of eating disorders.[166,511–513] Additional research on cultural factors that may predispose some women to develop eating disorders, as well as on strategies for helping women resist unhealthy social pressures, is imperative.[166,513–515] Moreover, there is a clear need for targeted prevention efforts for high-risk populations, such as athletes and women with a family history of eating disorders. For example, an extended prevention program in a residential ballet school focused on changing the sociocultural climate including peer relations, faculty–student interactions, the inculcation of health habits and system-wide norms has shown preliminary promise.[513] Other innovative efforts to target high-risk women have included Internet-based psychoeducation self-help programs[516] and multistage models for reaching high-risk women within college campus communities.[517]

Although limited, there is a growing body of research on efficacious prevention strategies and models.[518] Interventions that address attitudinal risk factors, promote healthy weight control behaviors, and body acceptance have encouraging support.[518] Characteristics that are associated with successful programs include interactive multisession designs that are delivered by professionals.[518] Outcomes associated with programs of this type include a reduction of eating disorder risk factors (elevated perceived pressure to be thin, internalization of the thin ideal standard of beauty, body mass, body dissatisfaction, and negative affect) and current or future eating pathology.[518]

The optimal combination sequencing and targeting of preventive efforts have yet to be identified.[519] There are indications that some preventive interventions may be associated with unintended negative consequences. For instance, Mann et al.[520] found that combining primary and secondary prevention efforts not only was ineffective in ameliorating dysfunctional eating but also resulted in a small increase in symptoms. Reflecting on these results, the authors reasoned that reducing the stigma of eating disorders during intervention may have normalized disordered eating behaviors.[520] Similarly, given that obesity poses serious health risks to an increasing proportion of the population,[521] it will be challenging to titrate a broad public health message to motivate the initiation and maintenance of healthful weight control practices without promoting the maladaptive excesses associated with cultural pressures toward thinness.

By comparison to the emphasis on risk factors, the relative neglect of health-related competencies continues to represent a strategic oversight, considering that certain healthful practices (e.g., regular appropriate exercise) may attenuate some of the factors associated with disordered eating, including stress and other negative mood states.[92] Overall, there is an important need for a more balanced focus in both research and preventive intervention efforts.[92,166] Although there will always be a role for treatment of the tertiary level, primary prevention efforts hold considerable promise for truly addressing and reducing the tremendous social impact of eating disorders.

Considering the cost of eating disorders makes the need for prevention even more salient. In addition to the health and personal toll, eating disorders are significant economic concerns. For example, based on a comparison of treatment costs for eating disorders to those for other psychiatric conditions, the therapy expenditures for AN exceed those for schizophrenia, and the costs of treating BN and BED are at least comparable to and perhaps in excess of those attributable to obsessive-compulsive disorder.[146] BED's link with overweight and obesity further heightens the risk for additional medical complications (e.g., hypertension, type 2 diabetes, dyslipidemia), thereby adding to its social and economic impact.[521] In addition, the discrimination and stigmatization attendant to overweight and obesity are well known.[521]

## CONCLUSIONS

In spite of a large literature on the etiology of eating disorders, with a particular focus on physiological and personality factors, the results of treatment outcome studies for eating disorders are less than satisfying. Patients with eating disorders appear to have high relapse rates, experience their disorders for long periods of time, and often suffer from several other comorbid psychiatric conditions.[1,39,436,522] The continued emphasis on internal-deficits models, rather than a focus on social and cultural risk factors, is puzzling.[103,165,241] Research has consistently reaffirmed the role of individual-specific

environmental factors[104,241] and the importance of complicated gene-environment transactions, in which polygenic diatheses may be protean in their manifestation across different environmental contexts.[104,238,241] If we are to generate the new perspectives necessary to effectively prevent and treat eating disorders, there is a clear need for truly integrated biopsychosocial perspectives highlighting which aspects of the environment may be particularly hazardous[523] for which individuals.[104,238,241]

In summary, this chapter has reviewed the considerable controversy and complexity surrounding the treatment of the eating disorders (i.e., AN, BN, and BED). The field is one of intense activity and interest. Yet few questions about these disorders have been answered definitively. The importance of cultural factors (such as changing nature of women's roles) is increasing at the same time that biological factors (such as neurological functioning) are being explored.

## ACKNOWLEDGMENTS

The authors would like to thank Lisa Terre, Walker S. Carols Poston II, Jill K. McGavin, and Allen A. Winebarger for their contributions to earlier editions of this chapter. Preparation of this manuscript was supported, in part, by a grant form the United States Department of Agriculture (USDA ARS 2533759358).

## REFERENCES

1. Ben-Tovim, D. *Curr Opin Psychiatr* 16:65; 2003.
2. Gowers, S, Bryant-Waugh, R. *J Child Psychol Psych* 45:63; 2004.
3. Lacey, JH. *Brit Med J* 285:1816 1982.
4. Bell, RM. *Holy Anorexia*. University of Chicago Press, Chicago, IL, 1985.
5. Halmi, KA. *Psychiatr Clin North Am* 5:371; 1982.
6. Hammond, WA. *Fasting Girls: Their Physiology and Pathology*. Putnam, New York, 1879.
7. Powers, PS, Fernandez, RC. In: Powers, PS, Fernandez, RC eds. *Current Treatment of Anorexia Nervosa and Bulimia*. Karger, Basel, Switzerland, 1984.
8. Strober, M. In: Browell, KD, Foreyt, JP eds. *Handbook of Eating Disorders: Physiology, Psychology, and Treatment of Obesity, Anorexia, and Bulimia*. Guilford Press, New York, 1986.
9. Playfair, WS. *Lancet* 1: 817; 1888.
10. Sheehan, HL, Summers, VK. *Q J Med* 18:319; 1949.
11. Stunkard, A. In: Fairburn, CG, Wilson, GT eds. *Binge Eating: Nature, Assessment and Treatment*. Guilford Press, New York, 1993.
12. Bruch, H. *Obesity, Anorexia Nervosa and the Person within*. Basic Books, New York, 1973.
13. Lowenberg, M, Todhunter, E, Wilson, E et al. *Food and Man*. Wiley, New York, 1974.
14. Kaplan, AS, Garfinkel, AH. *Am J Psychiatry* 141:721; 1984.
15. Gull, WW. *Trans Clin Soc Lond* 7:22; 1874.
16. Janet, P. *Les obsessions et la psychasthenie*. Alcan, Paris, 1919.
17. Binswanger, L. In: May, R, Angel, E, Ellenberger, HF eds. *Existence: A New Dimension in Psychiatry and Psychology*. Basic Books, New York, 1958.

18. Braun, CMJ, Chouinard, MJ. *Neuropsychol Rev* 3:171; 1992.
19. Cooper, PJ, Steere, J. *Behav Res Ther* 33.875, 1995.
20. Holderness, CC, Brooks-Gunn, J, Warren, MP. *Int J Eat Disord* 16:1; 1994.
21. Wilson, GT In: Brownell, KD, Fairburn, CG eds. *Eating Disorders and Obesity: A Comprehensive Handbook*. Guilford Press, New York, 1995.
22. Brewerton, TD. *Psychoneuroendocrino* 20:561; 1995.
23. Jarry, JL, Vaccarino, FJ. *J Psychiatry Neurosci* 21:36; 1996.
24. Kaye, WH, Weltzin, TE, Hsu, LKG, Bulik, CM. *Clin Psychiat* 52:464; 1991.
25. Van Praag, HM. *Make-Believes in Psychiatry or the Perils of Progress*. Brunner/Mazel, New York, 1993.
26. Gillberg, C. *Brit J Hosp Med* 51:209; 1994.
27. Gold, MS. In: Ferrari, E, Brambilla, D, Solerte, SB eds. *Primary and Secondary Eating Disorders: A Psychoneuroendocrine and Metabolic Approach*. Pergamon Press, New York, 1993.
28. Parham, ES. In: VanItallie, TB, Simonpoulos, AP, Gullo, SP, Futterweit, W eds. *Obesity: New Directions in Assessment and Management*. Charles Press, Philadelphia, PA, 1995.
29. American Psychiatric Association (APA). *Practice Guidelines*. American Psychiatric Association, Washington, DC, 1996.
30. Kaye, W, Strober, M, Stein, D, Gendall, K. *Biol Psychiat* 45:1285; 1999.
31. Lilenfeld, L, Kaye, W, Greeno, C et al. *Arch Gen Psychiatry* 55:603; 1998.
32. Strober, M, Lampert, C, Morrell, W et al. *Int J Eat Disord* 9:239; 1990.
33. Strober, M, Freeman, R, Lampert, C et al. *Am J Psychiatry* 157:393; 2000.
34. Goodrick, GK. In: Poston, WSC, Haddock, C eds. *Food as a Drug*. Haworth Press, New York, 2000.
35. Haddock, C, Dill, P. In: Poston, WSC, Haddock, C eds. *Food as a Drug*. Haworth Press, New York, 2000.
36. Wilson, GT. *Adv Behav Res Ther* 13:27; 1991.
37. Wilson, GT. In: Poston, WSC, Haddock, C eds. *Food as a Drug*. Haworth Press, New York, 2000.
38. Poston, WSC, Haddock, C. *Food as a Drug*. Haworth Press, New York, 2000.
39. Fairburn, CG, Harrison, PJ. *Lancet* 361:407; 2003.
40. American Psychiatric Association (APA). *Diagnostic and Statistical Manual of Mental Disorders Text Revision*. American Psychiatric Association, Washington, DC, 2000.
41. Wilson, GT, Pike, K. In: Barlow, DH ed. *Clinical Handbook of Psychological Disorders*. Guilford Press, New York, 2001.
42. Walsh, B, Devlin, M. *Science* 280:1387; 1998.
43. Brody, ML, Walsh, BT, Devlin, M. *J Consult Clin Psych* 62:381; 1994.
44. Cooper, Z, Fairburn, CG, Hawker, DM. *Cognitiv-Behavioral Treatment of Obesity: A Clinician's Guide*. Guilford Press, New York, 2003.
45. Stunkard, A, Allison, K. *Int J Obes Relat Metab Disord* 27:1; 2003.
46. Le Grange, D, Swanson, SA, Crow, SJ. www.onlinelibrary.wiley.com.ezproxyhost.library.tmc.edu/doi/10.1002/eat.22006/pdf. Accessed June 6, 2012.
47. Grave, RO. *Eur J Intern Med* 22:153; 2011.
48. Smink, FRE, van Hoeken, D, Hock, HW. www.springerlink.com.ezproxyhost.library.tmc.edu/content/g8514k1766j6r4n4/fulltext.pdf. Accessed June 6, 2012.
49. Allison, KC, Lundgren, JD, O'Reardon, JP et al. *Int J Eat Disord* 43:241; 2010.
50. Vander Wal, JS. *Clin Psychol Rev* 32:49; 2012.
51. Stunkard, AJ, Grace, WJ, Wolf, HG. *Am J Med* 19:78; 1955.
52. Bulik, C. *Child Adolesc Psychiatr Clin* 11:201; 2002.
53. Halmi, KA, Casper, RC, Eckert, EC et al. *Psychiatr Res* 1:290; 1979.
54. Agras, WS, Kirkley, BG. In: Brownell, KD, Foreyt, JP eds. *Handbook of Eating Disorders: Physiology, Psychology, and Treatment of Obesity, Anorexia, and Bulimia*. Basic Books, New York, 1986.
55. Fairburn, CG, Cooper, PJ. *Brit Med J* 284:1153; 1982.
56. Mehler, PS. *N Engl J Med* 349:875; 2003.
57. Mitchell, JE, Hatsukami, D, Eckert, ED, Pyle, RL. *Am J Psychiatry* 142:482; 1985.
58. Halmi, KA. *Psychosom Med* 36:18; 1974.
59. Hay, GG, Leonard, JC. *Lancet* ii:574; 1979.
60. Ricciardelli, LA, McCabe, MP. *Psychol Bull* 130:179; 2004.
61. Eckert, ED. In: Mitchell, JE ed. *Anorexia Nervosa and Bulimia: Diagnosis and Treatment*. University of Minnesota Press, Minneapolis, MN, 1985.
62. McClelland, L, Crisp, A. *Int J Eat Disord* 29:150; 2001.
63. Wildes, J, Emery, R, Simons, A. *Clin Psychol Rev* 21:521; 2001.
64. Hudson, JI, Hiripi, E, Pope, HG, Jr., Kessler, RC. *Biol Psychiatry* 61:348; 2007.
65. Hoek, HW. In: Brownell, KD, Fairburn, CG eds. *Eating Disorders and Obesity: A Comprehensive Handbook*. Guilford Press, New York, 1995.
66. Hoek, HW, van Hoeken, D. *Int J Eat Disord* 34:383; 2003.
67. Wakeling, A. *Psychiatry Res* 63:202; 1996.
68. Woodside, DB. *Curr Probl Pediatr* 25:67; 1995.
69. Hsu, LK. *Psychiatr Clin North Am* 19:6814; 1996.
70. Edwards, MD, Kerry, I. *Clin Nutr* 77:899; 1993.
71. Halmi, KA, Falk, JR, Schwartz, E. *Psychol Med* 11:697; 1981.
72. Kaltiala-Heino, R, Rissanen, A, Rimpela, M, Rantanen, P. *Acta Psychiatr Scand* 100:33; 1999.
73. Pyle, RL, Mitchell, JE, Eckert, EE et al. *Int J Eat Disord* 2:75; 1983.
74. Strangler, RS, Printz, AM. *Am J Psychiatry* 137:937; 1980.
75. Ash, JB, Piazza, E. *Int J Eat Disord* 18:27; 1995.
76. Jones, DJ, Fox, MM, Babigian, HM, Hutton, HE. *Psychosom Med* 42:551; 1980.
77. Willi, J, Grossman, S. *Am J Psychiatry* 140:564; 1983.
78. Fombonne, E. *Br J Psychiatry* 166:462; 1995.
79. Pawluck, D, Gorey, K. *Int J Eat Disord* 23:347; 1998.
80. Cooper, PJ, Watkins, B, Bryant-Waugh, R, Lask, B. *Psychol Med* 32:873; 2002.
81. Watkins, B, Lask, B. *Child Adolesc Psychiatr Clin N Am* 11:185; 2002.
82. Rosen, DS. *Adolesc Med* 14:49; 2003.
83. Powers, PS, Santana, CA. *Child Adolesc Psychiatr Clin N Am* 11:219; 2002.
84. Robin, AL, Gilroy, M, Dennis, A. *Clin Psychol Rev* 18:421; 1998.
85. Robb, A, Dadson, M. *Child Adolesc Psychiatr Clin N Am* 11:399; 2002.
86. Bettle, N, Bettle, O, Neumarker, U, Neumarker, K. *Psychopathology* 31:153; 1998.
87. Byrne, S, McLean, N. *J Sci Med Sport* 4:145; 2001.
88. Hulley, A, Hill, A. *Int J Eat Disord* 30:312; 2001.
89. Brewerton, TD. *Child Adolesc Psychiatr Clin* 11:237; 2002.
90. Steiner, H, Lock, J. *J Am Acad Child Adolesc Psychiatry* 37:352; 1998.
91. Kotler, L, Cohen, P, Davies M et al. *J Am Acad Child Adolesc Psychiatry* 40:1434; 2001.
92. Terre, L. *Adv Med Psychother* 6:151; 1993.

93. Striegel-Moore, R, Franko, D. *Int J Eat Disord* 34:S19; 2003.
94. Pike, K, Dohm, F, Striegel-Moore, R et al. *Am J Psychiatry* 158:1455; 2001.
95. Striegel-Moore, R, Dohm, F, Kraemer, H et al. *Am J Psychiatry* 160:1326; 2003.
96. deZwaan, M. *Int J Obes Relat Metab Disord* 25:S51;2001.
97. Dingemans, AE, Bruna, MJ, van Furth, EF. *Int J Obes Relat Metab Disord* 26:299; 2002.
98. Decaluwe, V, Braet, C, Fairburn, C. *Int J Eat Disord* 33:78; 2003.
99. Lundgren, JD, Allison, KC, Stunkard, AJ. *Int J Eat Disord* 39:516; 2006.
100. Gallant, AR, Lundgren, J, Drapeau, V. *Obes Rev* 13:528; 2012.
101. Sassaroli, S, Ruggiero, GM, Vinai, P et al. *Eat Disord* 17:140; 2009.
102. Keel, PK, Klump, KL. *Psychol Bull* 129:747; 2003.
103. Pate, JE, Pumariega, AJ, Hester, C, Garner, DM. *J Am Acad Child Adolesc Psychiatry* 31:802; 1992.
104. Jacobi, C, Hayward, C, deZwaan, M et al. *Psychol Bull* 130:19; 2004.
105. Smart, R. *Eat Disord* 18:58; 2010.
106. Calero-Elvira, A, Krug, I, Davis, K et al. *Eur Eat Disord* 17:243; 2009.
107. Zanarini, MC, Frankenburg, FR, Hennen, J et al. *Am J Psychiatry* 161:2108; 2004.
108. O'Brien, K, Vincent, *N Clin Psychol Rev* 23:57; 2003.
109. Haas, H, Clopton, J. *Int J Eat Disord* 33:412; 2003.
110. Kotler, L, Boudreau, G, Delvin, M. *J Pediatr Prat* 9:431; 2003.
111. Rosenvinge, J, Martinussen, M, Ostensen, E. *Eat Weight Disord* 5:52; 2000.
112. Drevelengas, A, Chourmouzi, D, Pitsavas, G et al. *Neuroradiology* 43:838; 2001.
113. Frank, G, Kaye, W, Weltzin, T et al. *Int J Eat Disord* 30:57; 2001.
114. Hirano, H, Tomura, N, Okane, K et al. *J Comput Assist Tomo* 23:280; 1999.
115. Lambe, E, Katzman D, Mikulis, D et al. *Arch Gen Psychiatry* 54:537; 1997.
116. Rastam, M, Bjure, J, Vestergren, E et al. *Dev Med Child Neurol* 43:239; 2001.
117. Roser, W, Bubl, R, Buergin, D et al. *Int J Eat Disord* 26:119; 1999.
118. Rome, ES. *Curr Probl Pediatr Adolesc Health Care* 42:28; 2012.
119. Eidem, B, Cetta, F, Webb, J et al. *J Adolescent Health* 29:267; 2001.
120. Mont, L, Castro, J, Herreros, B et al. *J Am Acad Child Adolesc Psychiatry* 42:808; 2003.
121. Panagiotopoulos, C, McCrindle, B, Hick, K, Katzman, D. *Pediatrics* 105:1100; 2000.
122. Swenne, I. *Acta Paediatr* 89:447; 2000.
123. Swenne, L, Larsson, P. *Acta Paediatr* 88:304; 1999.
124. Daluiski, A, Rahbar, B, Meals, R. *Clin Orthop Relat R* 343:107; 1997.
125. Hediger, C, Rost, B, Itin, P. *J Suisse Med* 130:565; 2000.
126. Schulze, U, Pettke-Rank, C, Kreienkamp, M et al. *Pediatr Dermatol* 16:90; 1999.
127. Strumia, R, Varotti, E, Manzato, E, Gualandi, M. *Dermatology* 203:314;2001.
128. Studen-Pavlovich, D, Elliott, M. *Dent Clin North Am* 45:491; 2001.
129. Golden, N. *Adolesc Med State Art Rev* 14:97; 2003.

130. Levine, R. *Adolesc Med State Art Rev* 13:129; 2002.
131. Mehler, PS. *Int J Eat Disord* 33:113; 2003.
132. Seidenfeld, M, Rickert, V. *Am Fam Physician* 64:445; 2001.
133. Slupik, R. *Int J Fertil Womens Med* 44:125; 1999.
134. Stoving, R, Hangaard, J, Hansen-Nord, M, Hagen, C. *J Psychiatr Res* 33:139; 1999.
135. Mehler, PS, Cleary, BS, Gaudiani, JL. *Curr Probl Pediatr Adolesc Health Care* 19:194; 2011.
136. Key, A, Mason, H, Allan, R, Lask, B. *Int J Eat Disord* 32:319; 2002.
137. Andersen, AE, Bowers, W, Evans, K. In: Garner, DM, Garfinkel, PE eds. *Handbook of Treatment for Eating Disorders.* Guilford Press, New York, 1997.
138. Baranowska, B, Radzikowska, M, Wasilewsk-Dziubinska, E et al. *Diabetes Obes Metab* 2:99; 2000.
139. Ferron, S. *Am J Psychiat* 156:801; 1999.
140. Jeejeebhoy, K. *Semin Gastrointest Dis* 9:183; 1998.
141. Abella, E, Feliu, E, Granada, I et al. *Am J Clin Pathol* 118:582; 2002.
142. McLoughlin, D, Wassif, W, Morton, J et al. *Nutrition* 16:192; 2000.
143. Lantzouni, E, Frank, G, Golden, N, Shenker, R. *J Adol Health* 31:162; 2002.
144. Modan-Moses, D, Yarloslavsky, A, Novikov, I et al. *Int J Eat Disord* 111:270; 2003.
145. Lucas, A, Melton, L, Crowson, C, O'Fallon, W. *Mayo Clin Proc* 74:972; 1999.
146. Agras, WS. *Pschiatr Clin North Am* 24:371; 2001.
147. Caruso, D, Klein, H. *Semin Gastrointest Dis* 9:176; 1998.
148. Kreipe, R, Birndorf, S. *Med Clin N Am* 84:1027; 2000.
149. First, M, Frances, A, Pincus, H. *DSM-IV-TR Handbook of Differential Diagnosis.* American Psychiatric Publishing, Washington, DC, 2002.
150. Casper, RC, Eckert, ED, Halmi, KA et al. *Arch Gen Psychiatry* 37:1030; 1980.
151. Theander, S. *Acta Psychiatr Scand* 65:1; 1970.
152. American Psychiatric Association (APA). *Diagnostic and Statistical Manual of Mental Disorders.* American Psychiatric Association, Washington, DC, 1987.
153. Garner, DM, Garfinkel, PE, O'Shaughnessy, M. Understanding anorexia nervosa and bulimia. Report of Fourth Ross Conference on Medical Research. Ross Laboratories, Columbus, OH, 1983.
154. Garfinkel, PE, Moldofsky, H, Garner, DM. *Arch Gen Psychiatry* 37:1036; 1980.
155. Beumont, PJV. *Aust N Z J Psychiatry* 11:223; 1977.
156. Fassino, S, Amianto, F, Gramaglia, C et al. *Eat Weight Disord* 9:81; 2004.
157. Vervaet, M, van Heeringen, C, Audenaert, K. *Compr Psychiatry* 45:37; 2004.
158. Eddy, K, Keel, P, Doer, D et al. *Int J Eat Disord* 31:191; 2002.
159. Pryor, T, Wiederman, M, McGilley, B. *Int J Eat Disord* 19:371; 1996.
160. Agras, WS, Walsh, BT, Fairburn, CG et al. *Arch Gen Psychiatry* 57:459; 2000.
161. Fairburn, CG, Cooper, Z, Shafran, R *Behav Res Ther* 41:509; 2003.
162. Iancu, I, Spivak, B, Ratzoni, G et al. *Psychopathology* 27:29; 1994.
163. Markey, CN. *J Treat Prevent* 12:139; 2004.
164. Polivy, J, Herman, CP. *J Soc Clin Psychol* 23:1; 2004.
165. Striegel-Moore, RH. In: Brownell, KD, Fairburn, CG eds. *Eating Disorders and Obesity: A Comprehensive Handbook.* Guilford Press, New York, 1995.

166. Steiner, H, Kwan, W, Shaffer, T et al. *Eur Child Adolesc Psychiatry* 12:138; 2003.

167. Terre, L, Burkhart, B. In: Blau, G, Gullotta, T eds. *Adolescent Dysfunctional Behavior*. Sage, Thousand Oaks, CA, 1996.

168. Terre, L, Ghiselli, W. *J Psychosom Res* 42:197; 1997.

169. Kaye, WH, Fudge, JL, Paulus, M. *Nat Rev Neurosci* 10:573; 2009.

170. Neufang, S, Specht, K, Hausmann, M et al. *Cereb Cortex* 19:464; 2009.

171. Fornari, V, Dancyger, I. *Adolesc Med State Art Rev* 14:61; 2003.

172. Gilbert, S, Thompson, JK. *Clin Psyhol* (New York) 3:183; 1996.

173. Wilfley, DE, Rodin, J. In: Brownell, KD, Fairburn, CG eds. *Eating Disorders and Obesity: A Comprehensive Handbook*. Guilford Press, New York, 1995.

174. Williamson, L. *Soc Work Health Care* 28:61; 1998.

175. Lee, S. *Soc Sci Med* 41:25; 1995.

176. Wiederman, M, Pryor, T. *Int J Eat Disord* 27:90; 2000.

177. Schwartz, MB, Chambliss H, Brownell, K et al. *Obes Res* 11:1033; 2003.

178. Fairburn, CG, Shafran, R, Cooper, Z. *Behav Res Ther* 37:1; 1999.

179. Heinberg, LJ. In: Thompson, JK ed. *Body Image, Eating Disorders, and Obesity: An Integrative Guide for Assessment and Treatment*. American Psychological Association, Washington, DC, 1996.

180. Striegel-Moore, RH. In: Fairburn, CG, Wilson, GT eds. *Binge Eating: Nature, Assessment, and Treatment*. Guilford Press, New York, 1993.

181. Ngai, E, Lee, S, Lee, A. *Acta Psychiatr Scand* 102:314; 2000.

182. Simpson, K. *J Psychiatr Ment Health Nurs* 9:65; 2002.

183. Crisp, AH, Palmer, RL, Kalucy, RS. *Br J Psychiatry* 218:549; 1976.

184. Malson, H, Swann, C. *J Community Appl Soc Psychol* 9:397; 1999.

185. Schwartz, DM, Thompson, MG, Johnson, CL. *Int J Eat Disord* 1:20; 1982.

186. Beumont, PJV, Booth, AL, Abraham, SF et al. In: Darby, PL, Garfinkle, PE, Garner, DM, Coscina, DV eds. *Anorexia Nervosa: Recent Developments in Research*. Liss, New York, 1983.

187. Fairburn, CG, Cooper, Z, Doll, H, Welch, S. *Arch Gen Psychiatry* 56:468; 1999.

188. Fairburn, CG, Welch, S, Doll, H et al. *Arch Gen Psychiatry* 54:509; 1997.

189. Halmi, KA. *Arch Gen Psychiatry* 54:507; 1997.

190. Howard, C, Porzelius, L. *Clin Psychol Rev* 19:25; 1999.

191. Halmi, KA. *J Pediatr Endocr Met* 15:1379; 2002.

192. Leon, GR, Fulkerson, JA, Perry, CL, Early-Zald, MB. *J Abnorm Psychol* 104:140; 1995.

193. Strober, M. *J Clin Psychiatry* 52:9; 1991.

194. Strober, M. In: Brownell, KD, Fairburn, CG eds. *Eating Disorders and Obesity: A Comprehensive Handbook*. Guilford Press, New York, 1995.

195. Sohlberg, S, Strober, M. *Acta Psychiatr Scand* 89:1; 1994.

196. Vitousek, K, Manke, F. *J Abnorm Psychol* 103:137; 1994.

197. Halmi, KA, Sunday, S, Strober, M et al. *Am J Psychiat* 157:1799; 2000.

198. Tyrka, A, Waldron, I, Graber, J, Brook-Gunnn, J. *Int J Eat Disord* 32:282; 2002.

199. Wonderliche, SA, Fullerton, D, Swift, W, Klein, MH. *Int J Eat Disord* 15:233; 1994.

200. Berghold, K, Lock, J. *Am J Psychother* 56:378; 2002.

201. Vohs, K, Bardone, A, Joiner, T et al. *J Abnorm Psychol* 108:695; 1999.

202. Silverstone, PH. *Med Hypotheses* 39:311; 1992.

203. Dobson, K, Dozols, D. *Clin Psychol Rev* 23:1001; 2001.

204. Zonnnevijlle-Bender, M, van Goozen, S, Cohen-Kettenis, P et al. *Eur Child Adolesc Psychiatry* 11:38; 2002.

205. Mendlewicz, L, Nef, F, Simon, Y. *Neuropsychobiology* 44:59; 2001.

206. Ainsworth, C, Waller, G, Kennedy, F. *Clin Psychol Rev* 22:1155; 2002.

207. Garner, DM, Garfinkel, PE, Schwartz, D, Thompson, M. *Psychol Rep* 47:483; 1980.

208. Hodes, M, Le Grange, D. *Int J Eat Disord* 34:383; 2003.

209. Johnson, J, Cohen, P, Kasen, S, Brook, J. *Am J Psychiatr* 159:394; 2002.

210. Kalucy, RS, Crisp, AH, Harding, B. *Br J Med Psychol* 50:381; 1977.

211. Strober, M. *Int J Eat Disord* 1:28; 1981.

212. Beumont, PJV, Abraham, SF, Argall, WJ et al. *Aust N Z J Psychiatry* 12:145; 1978.

213. Dally, PD. *Anorexia Nervosa*. Grune & Stratton, New York, 1969.

214. Rowland, CV, Jr. *Int Psychiatr Clin* 7:37; 1970.

215. Everill, JT, Waller, G. *Int J Eat Disord* 18:1:1995.

216. Waller, G. *Int J Eat Disord* 23:213; 1998.

217. Wonderliche, SA, Brewerton, TD, Jocic, Z et al. *J Am Acad Child Adolesc Psychiatry* 36:1107;1997.

218. Rorty, M, Yager, J, Rossotto, E. *Am J Psychiatry* 151:1122; 1994.

219. Smolak, L, Murnen, S. *Int J Eat Disord* 31:136; 2002.

220. Vize, CM, Cooper, PJ. *Br J Psychiatry* 167:80; 1995.

221. Welch, SL, Fairburn, CG. *Am J Psychiatry* 151:402; 1994.

222. Garfinkel, PE, Garner, DM. Anorexia Nervosa: A Multidimensional Perspective. Brunner/Mazel, New York, 1982.

223. Bailer, U, Kaye, W. *Curr Drug Targets CNS Neurol Disord* 2:53; 2003.

224. Brambilla, F. *CNS Drug* 15:119; 2001.

225. Chowdhury, U, Gordon, I, Lask, B et al. *Int J Eat Disord* 33:388; 2003.

226. Kaye, WH, Weltzin, TE. *J Clin Psychiat* 52:21; 1991.

227. Wolfe, B, Metzger, E, Jimerson, D. *Psychopharmacol Bull* 33:345; 1997.

228. Wurtman, RJ, Wirtman, JJ. In: Stunkard, AJ, Stellar, E eds. *Eating and its Disorders*. Guilford Press, New York, 1984.

229. Hudson, JI, Pope, HG, Jonas, JM, Yurgelun-Todd, D. *Br J Psychiatry* 142:133; 1983.

230. Steiger, H, Stotland, S, Ghadirian, AM, Whitehead, V. *Int J Eat Disord* 18:107; 1995.

231. Javaras, KN, Laird, NM, Reichborn-Kjennerud, T et al. *Int J Eat Disord* 41:174; 2008.

232. Bulik, CM, Slof-Op't Landt, MC, van Furth, ED, Sullivan, PF. *Annu Rev Nutr* 27:263; 2007.

233. Bulik, CM, Tozzi, F. *Drugs Today* (Barc) 40:741; 2004.

234. Fichter, MM, Noegel, R. *Int J Eat Disord* 9:255; 1990.

235. Holland, AJ, Sicotte, N, Treasure, J. *J Psychosom Res* 32:561; 1988.

236. Hsu, LK, Chesler, BE, Santhouse, R. *Int J Eat Disord* 9:275; 1990.

237. Treasure, J, Holland, A. In: Szmukler, GI, Dare, C, Treasure, J eds. *Handbook of Eating Disorders: Theory, Treatment and Research*. Wiley, Chichester, U.K., 1995.

238. Kendler, KS. *Arch Gen Psychiatry* 58:1005; 2001.

239. Kendler, KS, MacLean, C, Neale, M et al. *Am J Psychiatry* 148:1627; 1991.

240. Clark, TK, Weiss, AR, Berrettini, WH. *Clin Pharmacol Ther* 91:181; 2012.

241. Bulik, C, Sullivan, P, Wade, T, Kendler, K. *Int J Eat Disord* 27:1; 2000.
242. Poston, WSC, Winebarger, AA. *J Prim Prev* 17:133; 1996.
243. Ericsson, M, Poston, WS, Foreyt, JP. *Addict Behav* 21:733; 1996.
244. Weltzin,TE, Feernstrom, MH, Kaye, WH. *Nutr Rev* 52:399; 1994.
245. Jimerson, DC, Wolfe, BE, Metzger, E et al. *Arch Gen Psychiatry* 54:529; 1997.
246. Advokat, C, Kutlesic, V. *Neurosci Biobehav R* 19:59; 1995.
247. Craighead, LW, Agras, WS. *J Consult Clin Psych* 59:115; 1991.
248. Mauri, MC, Rudelli, R, Somaschinin, E et al. *Prog Neuropsychopharmacol Biol Psychiatry* 20:207; 1996.
249. Kaye, WH, Ballenger, JC, Lydiard, B et al. *Am J Psychiat* 147:225; 1990.
250. Maggia, G, Bianchi, B. *Eat Weight Disord* 3:100; 1998.
251. Brambilla, F, Bellodi, L, Perna, G et al. *Am J Psychiatry* 150:1111; 1993.
252. Lydiard, RB, Brewerton, TD, Fossey, MD et al. *Am J Psychiatry* 150:1099; 1993.
253. Watkins, B, Willoughby, K, Waller, G et al. *Int J Eat Disord* 32:11; 2002.
254. Cnnattingius, S, Hultman, C, Dahl, M, Sparen, P. *Arch Gen Psychiatry* 56:634; 1999.
255. Powers, PS, Santana, CA, Bannon, YS. *Int J Eat Disord* 32:146; 2002.
256. Sokol, M. *J Child Adolesc Psychopharmacol* 10:133; 2000.
257. Sokol, M, Ward, P, Tamiya, H et al. *Am J Psychiatry* 159:1430; 2002.
258. Campbell, IC, Mill, J, Uher, R, Schmidt, U. *Neurosci Biobehav Rev* 35:784; 2011.
259. Costa, J, Brennen, M, Hochgeschwender, U. *Child Adolesc Psychiatr Clin* 11:387; 2002.
260. Waters, E, Kendler, K. *Am J Psychiatry* 152:64; 1995.
261. Klump, K, Miller, K, Keel, P et al. *Psychol Med* 31:737; 2001.
262. The Price Foundation Collaborative Group. *Psychol Med* 31:635; 2001.
263. Karwautz, A, Rabe-Hesketh, S, Hu, X et al. *Psychol Med* 31:317:2001.
264. Devlin, MJ. *Psychiatr Clin North Am* 19:761; 1996.
265. Foreyt, JP, McGavin, JK. In: Mash, EJ, Terdal, LG eds. *Behavioral Assessment of Childhood Disorders*. Guilford Press, New York, 1988.
266. Foreyt, JP, Mikhail, C. In: Mash, EJ, Terdal, LG eds. *Assessment of Childhood Disorders*. Guilford Press, New Yqrk, 1997.
267. Lee, MI, Miltenberger, RG. *Behav Modif* 21:159; 1997.
268. Tobin, DL, Johnson, C, Steinnberg, S et al. *J Abnorm Psychol* 100:14; 1991.
269. Weltzin, TE, Bolton, BG. In: VanHasselt, V, Hersen, M eds. Handbook of psychological treatment protocols for children and adolescents Erlbaum, Mahwah, NJ; 1998.
270. Williamson, DA, Duchmann, E, Barker, S, Bruno, R. In: VanHasselt, V, Hersen, M eds. *Handbook of Psychological Treatment Protocols for Children and Adolescents*. Erlbaum, Mahwah, NJ, 1998.
271. Williamson, SA, Zucker, N, Martin, C, Smeets, M. In: Adams, H, Sutker, P eds. *Comprehensive Handbook of Psychopathology*. Kluwer, New York, 2001.
272. Lock, J, Le Grange, D, Agras, W, Dare, C. *Treatment Manual for Anorexia Nervosa: A Family-Based Approach*. Guilford Press, New York, 2001.
273. Casper, RC, Troiani, M. *Int J Eat Disord* 30:338; 2001.
274. Johnson, J, Pure, DL In: Brownell, KD, Foreyt, JP eds. *Handbook of Eating Disorders: Physiology, Psychology, and Treatment of Obesity, Anorexia, and Bulimia*. Basic Books, New York, 1986.
275. Laliberte, M, Boland, F, Leichner, P. *J Clin Psychol* 55:1021; 1999.
276. Shoebridge, P, Gowers, S. *Br J Psychiatry* 176:132; 2000.
277. Leung, N, Thomas, G, Waller, G. *Br J Clin Psychol* 39:205; 2000.
278. Ward, A, Ramsay, R, Turnbull, S et al. *Br J Med Psychol* 74:497; 2001.
279. Strober, M, Yager, J. In: Garner, DM, Garfinkel, PE eds. *Handbook of Psychotherapy For Anorexia Nervosa and Bulimia*. Guilford Press, New York, 1985.
280. Schwartz, DM, Thompson, MG. *Am J Psychiatry* 138:319; 1981.
281. Leon, GE, Carroll, KK, Chernyk, B, Finn, S. *Int J Eat Disord* 4:43; 1985.
282. Johnson, C, Larson, R. *Psychosom Med* 44:341; 1982.
283. McGilley, B, Pryor, T. *Am Fam Physician* 57:2743; 1998.
284. Mehler, PS. *Ann Intern Med* 134:1048; 2001.
285. Mitchell, JE. In: Brownell, KD, Foreyt, JP eds. *Handbook of Eating Disorders: Physiology, Psychology, and Treatment of Obesity, Anorexia, and Bulimia*. Basic Books, New York, 1986.
286. Kaplan, AS, Garfinkel, PE. *Medical Issues and the Eating Disorders: The Interface*. Brunner/Mazel, New York, 1993.
287. Powers, PS, Santana, CA. *Prim Care* 29:81; 2002.
288. Walsh, JM, Wheat, ME, Freund, K. *J Gen Intern Med* 15:577; 2000.
289. Webb, WL, Gehi, M. *Psychosomatics* 22:199; 1981.
290. Andersen, AE. In: Brownell, KD, Foreyt, JP eds. *Handbook of Eating Disorders: Physiology, Psychology, and Treatment of Obesity, Anorexia, And Bulimia*. Basic Books, New York, 1986.
291. Powers, PS. In: Powers, PS, Fernandez, RC eds. *Current Treatment of Anorexia Nerovos and Bulimia*. Karger, Basel, Switzerland, 1984.
292. Bartholomew, T, Paxton, S. *J Law Med* 10:308; 2003.
293. Draper, H. *Bioethics* 14:120; 2000.
294. English, A. *Curr Womens Health Rep* 2:442; 2002.
295. MacDonald, C. *Can J Psychiatry* 47:267; 2002.
296. Robb, A, Silber, T, Orrell-Valente, J et al. *Am J Psychiatry* 159:1347; 2002.
297. Watson, T, Bowers, W, Andersen, A. *Am J Psychiatry* 157:1806; 2000.
298. Yager, J. In: Brownell, KD, Fairburn, CG eds. *Eating Disorders and Obesity: A Comprehensive Handbook*. Guilford Press, New York, 1995.
299. Fairburn, CG, Marcus, MD, Wilson, GT. In: Fairburn, CG, Wilson, GT eds. *Binge Eating: Nature, Assessment, and Treatment*. Guilford Press, New York, 1993.
300. Bruch, H. *Handbook of Psychotherapy for Anorexia Nervosa and Bulimia*. Guilford Press, New York, 1985.
301. Levenkron, S. *Treating and Overcoming Anorexia Nervosa*. Warner Books, New York, 1983.
302. Goodsitt, A. In: Garner, DM, Garfinke, PE eds. *Handbook of Treatment for Eating Disorders*. Guilford Press, New York, 1997.
303. Fichter, MM. In: Brownell, KD, Fairburn, CG eds. *Eating Disorders and Obesity: A Comprehensive Handbook*. Guilford Press, New York, 1995.
304. Powers, PS, Powers, HP. *Psychosomatics* 25:512; 1984.
305. Breiner, S. *J Pediatr Nurs* 18:75; 2003.

306. Cummings, M, Waller, D, Johnson, C et al. *J Child Adolesc Psychiatr Nurs* 14:167; 2001.
307. Kohn, M, Golden, N. *Paediatr Drugs* 3:91; 2001.
308. Anzai, N, Lindsey-Dudley, K, Bidwell, R. *Child Adol Psych Clin* 11:279; 2002.
309. Imbierowicz, K, Braks, K, Jacoby, G et al. *Int J Eat Disord* 32:135; 2002.
310. Matusevich, D, Garcia, A, Gutt, S et al. *Eat Weight Disord* 7:196; 2002.
311. Sylvester, CJ, Forman, SF. *Curr Opin Pediatr* 20:390; 2008.
312. Weaver, L, Sit, L, Liebman, R. *Psychiatry Rep* 14:96; 2012.
313. Garfinkel, PE, Garner, DM, Kennedy, S. In: Garner, DM, Garfinkel, PE eds. *Handbook of Psychotherapy for Anorexia Nervosa and Bulimia*. Guilford Press, New York, 1985.
314. Kaczynski, J, Denison, H, Wiknertz, A et al. *Lakartidningen* 97:2734; 2000.
315. Striegel-Moore, R, Leslie, D, Petrill, S et al. *Int J Eat Disord* 27:381; 2000.
316. Wiseman, C, Sunday, S, Klapper, F et al. *Int J Eat Disord* 30:69; 2001.
317. Fennig, S, Fennig, S, Roe, D. *Gen Hosp Psychiatry* 24:87; 2002.
318. Patel, D, Pratt, H, Greydanus, D. *J Adolesc Res* 18:244; 2003.
319. Grigoriadis, S, Kaplan, A, Carter, J, Woodside, B. *Eat Weight Disord* 6:115; 2001.
320. Agras, WS, Telch, CF, Arnow, B et al. *Behav Ther* 25:225; 1994.
321. Lacey, JH. In: Garner, DM, Garfinkel, PE eds. *Handbook of Psychotherapy for Anorexia Nervosa and Bulimia*. Guilford Press, New York, 1985.
322. Wooley, SC, Kearney-Cooke, A. In: Brownell, KD, Foreyt, JP eds. *Handbook of Eating Disorders: Physiology, Psychology, and Treatment of Obesity, Anorexia, and Bulimia*. Basic Books, New York, 1986.
323. Yager, J. *Psychiatry* 57:153; 1994.
324. Richards, P, Baldwin, B, Frost, H et al. *Eat Disord* 8:189; 2000.
325. Wilson, GT, Fairburn, CG. *J Consult Clin Psychol* 61:261; 1993.
326. Garner, DM, Garfinkel, PE. *Handbook of Psychotherapy and Anorexia Nervosa and Bulimia*. Guilford Press, New York, 1985.
327. Garner, DM, Garfinkel, PE. *Handbook of Treatment for Eating Disorders*. Guilford Press, New York, 1997.
328. Chambless, D, Baker, M, Baucom, D et al. *Clin Psychol* 51:3; 1998.
329. Dalle-Grave, R, Ricca, V, Todesco, T. *Eat Weight Disord* 6:81; 2001.
330. Wilson, GT. *Behav Res Ther* 37:S79; 1999.
331. Rosen, JC, Leitenberg, H. *Behav Ther* 13:117; 1982.
332. Gray, JJ, Hoage, CM. *Psychol Rep* 66:667; 1990.
333. Kennedy, SH, Katz, R, Neitzert, CS et al. *Behav Res Ther* 33:685; 1995.
334. Leitenberg, H, Rosen, J, Gross, J et al. *J Consult Clin Psych* 56:535; 1988.
335. Williamson, DA, Prather, RC, Bennett, SM et al. *Behav Modif* 13:340; 1989.
336. Wilson, GT, Rossiter, E, Kleinfield, EI, Lindholm, L. *Behav Res Ther* 24:277; 1986.
337. Agras, WS, Schneider, JA, Arnow, B et al. *J Consult Clin Psychol* 57:215; 1989.
338. Bachrach, AJ, Erwin, WJ, Mohr, PJ In: Ullmann, L, Krasner, L eds. *Case Studies in Behavior Modification*. Holt, Rinehart & Winston, New York, 1965.
339. Griffiths, R, Gross, G, Russell, J et al. *Int J Eat Disord* 23:443; 1998.
340. Lang, PJ In: Ullmann, LP, Krasner, L eds. *Case Studies in Behavior Modification*. Holt, Rinehart & Winston, New York, 1965.
341. Leitenberg, H, Agras, WS, Thompson, LE. *Behav Res Ther* 6:211; 1968.
342. Steinhausen, HC. In: Brownell, KD, Fairburn, CG eds. *Eating Disorders and Obesity: A Comprehensive Handbook*. Guilford Press, New York, 1995.
343. Garfinkel, PE, Moldofsky, H, Garner, DM In: Vigersky, RA ed. *Anorexia Nervosa*. Raven Press, New York, 1977.
344. Bemis, KM. *Psychol Bull* 85:593; 1978.
345. Steinhausen, HC. *Horm Res* 43:168; 1995.
346. Fairburn, CG, Jones, R, Peveler, RC et al. *Arch Gen Psychiatry* 50:419; 1993.
347. Garner, DM, Vitousek, KM, Pike, KM. In: Garner, DM, Garfinkel, PE eds. *Handbook of Treatment for Eating Disorders*. Guilford Press, New York, 1997.
348. Garner, DM, Bemis, KM. In: Garner, DM, Garfinkel, PE eds. *Handbook of Psychotherapy for Anorexia Nervosa and Bulimia*. Guilford Press, New York, 1985.
349. Fairburn, CG. *J Psychsom Res* 24:193; 1980.
350. Pillay, M, Crisp, AH. *J Psychiatry* 139:533; 1981.
351. Viens, MJ, Hrannchuk, K. *J Behav Ther Exp Psychiatry* 23:313; 1993.
352. Hallsten, EA. *Behav Res Ther* 3:87; 1965.
353. Ollendick, TH. *Behav Modif* 3:124; 1979.
354. Monti, PM, McCrady, BS, Barlow, DH. *Behav Ther* 8:258; 1977.
355. Schnurer, AT, Rubin, RR, Roy, A. *J Behav Ther Exp Psychiatry* 4:149; 1973.
356. Beck, A. *Cognitive Therapy and the Emotional Disorders*. International Universities Press, New York, 1976.
357. Fairburn, CG, Cooper, Z, Cooper, PJ. In: Brownell, KD, Foreyt, JP eds. *Handbook of Eating Disorders: Physiology, Psychology, and Treatment of Obesity, Anorexia, and Bulimia*. Basic Books, New York, 1986.
358. Tuschen, B, Bents, H. In: Brownell, KD, Fairburn, CG eds. *Eating Disorders and Obesity: A Comprehensive Handbook*. Guilford Press, New York, 1995.
359. Pike, KM, Loeb, K, Vitousek, K. In: Thompson, JK ed. *Body Image, Eating Disorders, and Obesity: An Integrative Guide for Assessment and Treatment*. American Psychological Association, Washington, DC, 1996.
360. Anderson, D, Maloney, K. *Clin Psychol Rev* 21:971; 2001.
361. Thompson-Brenner, H, Glass, S, Westen, D. *Clin Psychol (New York)* 10:269; 2003.
362. Wilfley, DE, Kolko, RP, Kass, AE. *Child Adolesc Psychiatr Clin N Am* 20:271; 2011.
363. Mitchell, JE, Hoberman, HN, Petersonn, CB et al. *Int J Eat Disord* 20:219; 1996.
364. Garner, DM, Rockert, W, Davis, R et al. *Am J Psychiatry* 150:37; 1993.
365. Agras, WS. *Drugs Today* 33:405; 1997.
366. Casper, RC. *Psychopharmacol Bull* 36:88; 2002.
367. Crow, SJ, Mitchell, JE. In: Thompson, JK ed. *Body Image, Eating Disorders, and Obesity: An Integrative Guide for Assessment and Treatment*. American Psychological Association, Washington, DC, 1996.
368. Crow, SJ, Mitchell, JE. *Psychiatr Clin North Am* 19:755; 1966.
369. Goldbloom, DS, Olmsted, M, Davis, R et al. *Behav Res Ther* 35:803; 1997.

370. Mitchell, JE, deZwaan, M, Roerig, J. *Curr Drug Targets CNS Neurol Disord* 2:17; 2003.

371. Bowers, W. *Pschiatr Clin North Am* 24:293; 2001.

372. Serfaty, M, Turkington, D, Heap, M et al. *Eur Eat Disord Rev* 7:334; 1999.

373. Ricca, V, Mannucci, E, Zucchi, T et al. *Psychother Psychosom* 69:287; 2000.

374. Wilfley, DE, Cohen, LR. *Psychopharmacol Bull* 33:437; 1997.

375. Wilfley, DE, Welch, R, Stein, R et al. *Arch Gen Psychiatry* 59:713; 2002.

376. Agras, WS, Telch, CF, Arnow, B et al. *J Consult Clin Psych* 63:356; 1995.

377. Wilfley, DE, Agras, WS, Telch, CF et al. *J Consult Clin Psychol* 61:296; 1993.

378. Gillies, L. In: Barlow, D ed. *Clinical Handbook of Psychological Disorders: A Step-by-Step Manual.* Guilford Press, New York, 2001.

379. Fairburn, CG, Norman, PA, Welch, SL et al. *Arch Gen Psychiatry* 52:304; 1995.

380. Agras, WS. *J Clin Psychiat* 52:29; 1991.

381. Linehan, MM. *Cognitive-Behavioral Treatment of Borderline Personality Disorder.* Guilford Press, New York, 1993.

382. Chen, EY, Safer, DL. In: Grilo, CM, Mitchell, JE eds. *The Treatment of Eating Disorders: A Clinical Handbook.* Guilford Press, New York, 2012.

383. Bankoff, SM, Karpel, MG, Forbes, HE, Pantalone, DW. *Eat Disord* 20:196; 2012.

384. Hill, DM, Craighead, LM, Safer, DL. *Int J Eat Disord* 44:249; 2011.

385. Safer, DL, Telch, CF, Agras, WS. *Am J Psychiatry* 158:632; 2001.

386. Telch, CF, Agras, WS, Linehan, MM. *J Consult Clin Psychol* 69:1061; 2001.

387. Luborksy, I. *Principles of Psychoanalytic Psychotherapy: A Manual for Supportive-Expressive Treatment.* Basic Books, New York, 1984.

388. Rosen, JC, Reiter, J, Orosan, P. *J Consult Clin Psychol* 63:263; 1995.

389. Minuchin, S, Rosman, BL, Baker, L. *Psychosomatic Families: Anorexia Nervosa in Context.* Harvard University Press, Cambridge, MA, 1978.

390. Dare, C, Eisler, I. In: Garner, DM, Garfinkel, PE eds. *Handbook of Treatment for Eating Disorders.* Guilford Press, New York, 1997.

391. Dare, C, Eisler, I. In: Brownell, KD, Fairburn, CG eds. *Eating Disorders and Obesity: A Comprehensive Handbook.* Guilford Press, New York, 1995.

392. Russell, GFM, Szmukler, GI, Dare, C, Eisler, I. *Arch Gen Psychiatry* 44:1047; 1987.

393. Crisp, AH, Norton, K, Gowers, S et al. *Br J Psychiatry* 159:325; 1991.

394. Lock, H, Le Grange, D. *Child Adolesc Psychiatr Clin N Am* 11:331; 2002.

395. Lock, H, Le Grange, D. *Int J Eat Disord* 37:S64; 2005.

396. Robin, AL, Siegel, PT, Koepke, T et al. *J Dev Behav Pediatr* 15:111; 1994.

397. Robin, AL, Siegel, PT, Moye, A. *Int J Eat Disord* 17:313; 1995.

398. Le Grange, D, Eisler, I, Dare, C, Russell, GFM. *Int J Eat Disord* 12:347; 1992.

399. Lemmon, C, Josephson, A. *Child Adolesc Psychol Clin* 10:519; 2001.

400. Loeb, KL, Le Grange, D. *Int J Child Adolesc Health* 2:243; 2009.

401. Lock, H, Le Grange, D. *J Psychother Pract Res* 10:253; 2001.

402. Le Grange, D, Lock, J. *Treating Bulimia in Adolescents: A Family-Based Approach.* Guilford Press, New York, 2007.

403. Krautter, T, Lock, J. *J Fam Ther* 26:66; 2004.

404. Robin, AL, Bedway, M, Siegel, P, Gilroy, M. In: Hibbs, ED, Jensen, PS eds. *Psychosocial Treatments for Child and Adolescent Disorders: Empirically Based Strategies for Clinical Practice.* American Psychological Association. Washington, DC, 1996.

405. Robin, AL, Siegel, P, Moye, A et al. *J Am Acad Child Adolesc Psychiatry* 38:1482; 1999.

406. Wooley, SC In: Brownell, KD, Fairburn, CG eds. *Eating Disorders and Obesity: A Comprehensive Handbook.* Guilford Press, New York, 1995.

407. Kearney-Cooke, A, Striegel-Moore, R. *Int J Eat Disord* 15:305; 1994.

408. Hall, A. In: Garner, DM, Garfinkel, PE eds. *Handbook of Psychotherapy for Anorexia Nervosa and Bulimia,* Guilford Press, New York, 1985.

409. Gerlinghoff, M, Gross, G, Backmund, H. *Eur Child Adolsc Psychiatry* 12:72; 2003.

410. Waisberg, J, Woods, M. *Can J Diet Pract Res* 63:202; 2002.

411. Polivy, J, Gederoff, I. In: Garner, DM, Garfinkel, PE eds. *Handbook of Treatment for Eating Disorder.* Guilford Press, New York, 1997.

412. Tasca, G, Flynn, C, Bissada, H. *Int J Group Psychother* 52:409; 2002.

413. Gusella, J, Butler, G, Nichols, L, Bird, D. *Eur Eat Disord Rev* 11:58; 2003.

414. White, WC, Boskind-White, M. *Psychotherapy (Chic)* 18:501; 1981.

415. Boskind-Lodahl, M, White, WC. *J Am Coll Health* 27:84; 1978.

416. Leung, N, Waller, G, Glyn, T. *Behav Res Ther* 38:145; 2000.

417. Katzman, MA, Bara-Carril, N, Rabe-Hesketh, S et al. *Psychosom Med* 72:656; 2010.

418. Carraro, A, Cognolato, S, Bernardis, A. *Eat Weight Disord* 3:110:1998.

419. Duesund, L, Skarderud, F. *Clin Child Psychol Psychiatry* 8:53; 2003.

420. Pendleton, VR, Goodrick, GK, Poston, WS et al. *Int J Eat Disord* 31:172; 2002.

421. Thien, V, Thomas, A, Markin, D, Birmingham, C. *Int J Eat Disord* 28:101; 2000.

422. Olmsted, MP, Kaplan, AS. In: Brownell, KD, Fairburn, CG eds. *Eating Disorders and Obesity: A Comprehensive Handbook.* Guilford Press, New York, 1995.

423. Garner, DM. In: Garner, DM, Garfinkel, PE eds. *Handbook of Treatment for Eating Disorders.* Guilford Press, NewYork, 1997.

424. Olmstead, MP, Davis, R, Rockert, W et al. *Behav Res Ther* 29:71; 1991.

425. Allen, S, Dalton, WT, III. *J Health Psychol* 16:1165; 2011.

426. Geist, R. *Can J Psychiatr* 45:173; 2000.

427. Stice, E, Ragan, J. *Int J Eat Disord* 31:159; 2002.

428. Wiseman, C, Sunday, S, Klapper, F et al. *Eat Disord J Treat Prev* 10:313; 2002.

429. Bergh, C, Brodin, U, Lindberg, G, Sodersten, P. *P Natl Acad Sci U S A* 99:9486; 2002.

430. Bailey, R, Yager, J, Jenson, J. *Am J Psychiat* 159:1298; 2002.

431. Yager, J. *Int J Eat Disord* 29:125; 2001.

432. Goldfield, G, Boachie, A. *Telemed J E Health* 9:111; 2003.

433. Crow, SJ, Mitchell, JE, Crosby, RD et al. *Behav Res Ther* 47:451; 2009.

434. Fisher, M. *Adolesc Med State Art Rev* 14:149; 2003.
435. Keller, MB, Herzog, DB, Lavori, PW et al. *Int J Eat Disord* 12:1; 1992.
436. Steinhausen, HC. *Am J Psychiatry* 159:1284; 2002.
437. Wanden-Berghe, RG, Sanz-Valero, J, Wanden-Berghe, C. *Eat Disord* 19:34; 2011.
438. Murphy, R, Straebler, S, Cooper, Z, Fairburn, CG. *Psychiatr Clin North Am* 33:611; 2010.
439. Hoffman, L, Halmi, K. *Psychiatr Clin North Am* 16:767; 1993.
440. Garfinkel, PE, Walsh, BT. In: Garner, DM, Garfinkel, PE eds. *Handbook of Treatment for Eating Disorders*. Guilford Press, New York, 1997.
441. Malina, A, Gaskill, J, McConaha, C et al. *Int J Eat Disord* 33:234; 2003.
442. Golden, NH, Attia, E. *Pediatr Clin North Am* 58:121; 2011.
443. Mehler, C, Wewetzerk, C, Schulze, U et al. *Eur Child Adolesc Psychiatry* 10:151; 2001.
444. Bissada, H, Tasca, GA, Barber, AM et al. *Am J Psychol* 165:1281; 2008.
445. Walsh, BT, Kaplan, AS, Attia, E et al. *JAMA* 295:2605; 2006.
446. Fassino, S, Leombruni, P, Daga, G et al. *Eur Neuropsychopharm* 12:453; 2002.
447. Mendelson, S. *Am J Psychiatry* 158:963; 2001.
448. Bulik, CM, Berkman, ND, Brownley, KA, et al. *Int J Eat Disord* 40:310; 2007.
449. Attia, E, Mayer, L, Killory, E. *J Psychiatr Pract* 7:157; 2001.
450. Kotler, L, Walsh, B. *Eur Child Adolesc Psychiatry* 9:I108; 2000.
451. Krueger, S, Kennedy, S. *J Psychiatr Neurosci* 25:497; 2000.
452. Zhu, A, Walsh, B. *Can J Psychiatry* 47:227; 2002.
453. Mitchell, JE, Raymond, N, Specker, S. *Int J Eat Disord* 14:229; 1993.
454. Shapiro, JR, Berkman, NK, Brownley, KA et al. *Int J Eat Disord* 40:321; 2007.
455. Goldstein, DJ, Wilson, MG, Thompson, VL et al. *Br J Psychiatry* 166:660; 1995.
456. Walsh, BT, Wilsonn, GT, Loeb, KL et al. *Am J Psychiatry* 154:523; 1997.
457. Hudson, JI, Laffer, PS, Pope, HG. *Am J Psychiatry* 139:685; 1982.
458. Walsh BT, Stewart, JW, Wright, L et al. *Am J Psychiatry* 139:1629; 1982.
459. Russell, GFM. *Psychol Med* 9:429; 1979.
460. Hughes, PL, Wells, LA, Cunningham, CJ, Ilstrup, DM. *Treating Bulimia with Despramine: A Double-Blind Placebo-Controlled Study*. American Psychiatric Association, Los Angeles, CA, 1984.
461. Diler, R, Avci, A. *Swiss Med Wkly* 132:470; 2002.
462. Gorman, J, Kent, J. *J Clin Psychiatry* 60:33; 1999.
463. Srinivasan, K, Ashok, M, Vaz, M, Yeragani, V. *Pediatr Cardiol* 25:20; 2004.
464. Tingelstad, J. *J Am Acad Child Adolesc Psychiatry* 30:845; 1991.
465. Green, RS, Rau, JH. *Am J Psychiatry* 131:428; 1974.
466. Rau, JH, Green, RS. *Compr Psychiatry* 16:223; 1975.
467. Weiss, T, Levitz, L. *Am J Psychiatry* 133:1093; 1976.
468. Greenway, FL, Dahms, WT, Bray, GA. *Curr Ther Res* 21:338; 1977.
469. Balcaltchuk, J, Hay, P, Mari, H. *Aust N Z J Psychiatry* 34:310; 2000.
470. Wilson, GT, Shafran, R. *Lancet* 365:79; 2005.
471. Arnold, LM, McElroy, SL, Hudson, JI et al. *J Clin Psychiatry* 63:1028; 2002.
472. Grilo, CM, Masheb, RM, Wilson, GT. *Biol Psychiatry* 57:301; 2005.
473. Hudson, JI, McElroy, SL, Raymond, NC et al. *Am J Psychiatry* 155:1756; 1998.
474. Pearlstein, T, Spurell, E, Hohlstein, LA et al. *Arch Womens Ment Health* 6:147; 2003.
475. McElroy, SL, Casuto, LS, Nelson, EB et al. *Am J Psychiatry* 157:104; 2000.
476. McElroy, SL, Hudson, JI, Malhotra, S et al. *J Clin Psychiatry* 64:807; 2003.
477. Guerdjikova, AL, McElroy, SL, Kotwal, R et al. *Hum Psychopharmacol* 23:1; 2008.
478. Appolinario, JC, Bacaltchuk, J, Sichieri, R et al. *Arch Gen Psychiatry* 60:1109; 2003.
479. Milano, W, Petrella, C, Casella, A et al. *Adv Ther* 22:25; 2005.
480. Wilfley, DE, Crow, SJ, Hudson, JI et al. *Am J Psychiatry* 165; 51; 2008.
481. Ricca, V, Mannucci, E, Mezzaini, B et al. *Psychother Psychosom* 70:298; 2001.
482. Marrazzi, MA, Markham, KM, Kinzie, J, Luby, ED. *Int J Obesity* 19:143; 1995.
483. Mitchell, JE, Peterson, CB, Myers, T, Wonderlich, S. *Psychiatr Clin North Am* 24:315; 2001.
484. Agras, WS, Rossiter, EM, Arnow, B et al. *Am J Psychiatry* 149:82; 1992.
485. Mitchell, JE, Pyler, RL, Eckert, ED et al. *Arch Gen Psychiatry* 47:149; 1990.
486. Crow, SJ, Mitchell, JE. *Drugs* 48:372; 1994.
487. Keel, PK, Brown, TA. *Int J Eat Disord* 43:195; 2010.
488. Halmi, KA, Brodland, G, Rigas, C. *Life Hist Res Psychopathology* 4:290; 1975.
489. Hsu, LK, Crisp, AH, Harding, B. *Lancet* 1:61; 1979.
490. Morgan, HG, Russell, GFM. *Psychol Med* 5:355; 1975.
491. Pierloot, R, Wellens, W, Houben, M. *Psychother Psychosom* 36:101; 1975.
492. Sturzenberger, S, Cantwell, PD, Burroughs, J et al. *J Am Acad Child Psychiatry* 16:703; 1977.
493. Howard, W, Evans, K, Quintero-Howard, C et al. *Am J Psychiatry* 156:1697; 1999.
494. Seidensticher, JF, Tzagournis, M. *J Chronic Dis* 21:361; 1968.
495. Steinhausen, H, Boyadjieva, S, Grigoroiu-Serbanescu, M et al. *Acta Psychiatr Scand* 101:60;2000.
496. Zipfel, S, Lowe, B, Reas, D et al. *Lancet* 355:721; 2000.
497. Fichter, MM, Quadflieg, N. *Int J Eat Disord* 26:359; 1999.
498. Ostuzzi, R, Didonna, F, Micciolo, R. *Eat Weight Disord* 4:194; 1999.
499. Kalucy, RS, Crisp, AH, Lacey, JH, Harding, B. *Aust N Z J Psychiatry* 11:251; 1977.
500. Halmi, KA, Brodland, G, Loney, J. *Ann Intern Med* 78:907; 1973.
501. Nilsson, E, Gillberg, C, Gillberg, I, Rastam, M. *J Am Acad Child Adolesc Psychiatry* 38:1389; 1999.
502. Rastam, M, Gillberg, C, Wentz, E. *Eur Child Adolesc Psychiatry* 12:I78; 2003.
503. Signorini, A, Bellini, O, Pasanisi, F et al. *Eat Weight Disord* 8:168; 2003.
504. Wentz, E, Gillberg, C, Gillberg, I, Rastam, M. *J Child Psychol Psychiatry* 42:613; 2001.
505. Hsu, LK. In: Brownell, KD, Fairburn, CG eds. *Eating Disorders and Obesity: A Comprehensive Handbook*. Guilford Press, New York, 1995.
506. Herzog, DB, Sacks, NR, Keller, MB et al. *J Am Acad Child Adolesc Psychiatry* 32:835; 1993.

507. Keel, PK, Mitchell, JE, Miller, KB et al. *Arch Gen Psychiatry* 56:63; 1999.

508. Rorty, M, Yager, J, Rossotto, E. *Int J Eat Disord* 14:249; 1993.

509. Fairburn, CG, Cooper, Z, Doll, H et al. *Arch Gen Psychiatry* 57:659; 2000.

510. Thompson-Brenner, H, Satir, DA, Franko, DL, Herzog, DB. *Psychiatr Serv* 63:73; 2012.

511. Fairburn, CG. In: Brownell, KD, Fairburn, CG eds. *Eating Disorders and Obesity: A Comprehensive Handbook.* Guilford Press, New York, 1995.

512. Huon, G, Braganza, C, Brown, L et al. *Int J Eat Disord* 23:455; 1998.

513. Piran, N. *J Prim Prev* 20:75; 1999.

514. Battle, EK, Brownell, KD. *Addict Behav* 21:755; 1996.

515. Foreyt, JP, Poston, WS, Goodrick, GK. *Addict Behav* 21:767; 1996.

516. Zabinski, M, Pung, M, Wilfley, D et al. *Int J Eat Disord* 29:401; 2001.

517. Schwitzer, A, Bergholz, K, Dore, T, Salimi, L. *J Am Coll Health* 46:199; 1998.

518. Shaw, H, Stice, E, Becker, CB. *Child Adolesc Psychiatr Clin N Am* 18:199; 2009.

519. Stice, E, Shaw, H. *Psychol Bull* 130:206; 2004.

520. Mann, T, Nolen-Hoeksema, S, Huang, K et al. *Health Psychol* 16:215; 1997.

521. Terre, L, Poston, WS, Foreyt, J. In: Goldstein, J ed. *The Management of Eating Disorders and Obesity,* Humana Press, Totowa, NJ; 2005.

522. Kirschenbaum, DS, Fitzgibbon, ML. *Behav Ther* 26:43; 1995.

523. Horgen, K, Brownell, K. In: Wadden, TA, Stunkard, AJ eds. *Handbook of Obesity and Treatment.* Guilford Press, New York, 2002.

# 50 Food Addiction and Obesity

*Catherine L. Carpenter*

## CONTENTS

## INTRODUCTION

Studies about determinants of obesity have primarily focused on poor nutrition and lack of exercise. Addictive behaviors, in relationship to overeating and food craving, may however represent an important pathway to obesity that has received little study until recently. The lack of research can partially be explained by conflicting acceptance about the role of addiction in development of obesity.[1–4] The following chapter will provide an overview about addictive behavior, what parts of the brain promote addiction, the potential interrelationships between brain regions that influence eating and addiction, and segments of the population that may be predisposed to food addiction and overeating. Differing views and evidence about whether food addiction can be considered a determinant of obesity or a consequence of obesity will be presented throughout this chapter.

## WHAT IS ADDICTION?

There is some controversy about when substance use becomes an addiction. Addiction starts with the taking of substances such as heroin or behaviors such as gambling that activate brain reward circuits.[5] Activation of these circuits motivates behavior. Most individuals enjoy the experience without feeling compelled to repeat it. For some (usually a small percentage), the experience produces strong conditioned associations to environmental cues that signal availability of the drug or the behavior.[5] Activation of reward circuits becomes involuntary, with a very rapid onset, and the addict is compelled to repeat administration of the substance or repeat the behavior. Food addiction has behavioral and neurological characteristics in common with substance abuse and dependence, most notably increased craving for food or food-related substances leading to a state of heightened pleasure, energy, or excitement.[6]

Obese individuals behave differently than normal-weighted individuals in relationship to food stimuli and reward.[7–10] In brain scanning studies, elicitation of activation localizes the brain area involved in response to stimuli. The gustatory cortex (anterior and mid-insula, frontal operculum) and the location of subjective emotional feeling and task control[11,12] were activated to a greater degree in obese compared to normal-weighted subjects. The activation occurred as a result of anticipation of a food reward and in actual consumption of the food.[9] In the same study, it was further determined that emotional eaters, during a negative mood state, experienced an even greater anticipation and feeling of reward from consumption of food.[9]

The reward pathway, most often associated with dopamine, is modulated by the strength of dopamine binding to the dopamine receptor, which can be influenced by changes in dopamine level, receptor density, or receptor affinity.[13] Dopamine release may be initiated by food stimuli. Food pictures elicited an increase of extracellular dopamine in the dorsal striatum that was significantly correlated with increases in self-reports of hunger and desire for food,[7] demonstrating a link between dopamine and motivation to eat.

The expectation of reward may cause overcompensation in terms of eating beyond satiation. Obese individuals appear to be especially sensitive to the palatability of food and, once food is consumed, will experience reduced reward that could drive overeating as a compensatory reaction.[8,9] Leptin replacement decreases brain activation in response to food cues in genetically leptin-deficient adults,[10] further suggesting that once food is consumed and leptin levels rise in healthy individuals, interest in food cues is diminished. These mechanisms may not operate, however, in obese individuals who lack sensitivity to leptin. Among leptin-insensitive individuals, brain activation to food cues may remain during eating such that satiety signals may be overcome or even ignored.

There are multiple etiologic pathways to obesity. Many investigators concur that food addiction is associated with development of obesity in certain individuals.[14] However, not all obese individuals gain weight because they are addicted to food. Other individuals that are not predisposed to food addiction can, for instance, develop obesity through modest energy imbalances over a sustained period of time.[15] The numerous factors that can cause weight gain pose complex challenges to the investigation of obesity determinants. The study of food addiction in a population-based sample will undoubtedly include individuals that are not addicted to food, and therefore, a mixture of studies with positive and negative associations between food addiction and obesity are to be expected.

Obesity may promote food addiction among individuals who were not addicted to food prior to weight gain. That is, the obese state can alter neurologic functioning and endocrine secretion, such that food addictions could be acquired during weight gain.[2] Neuroimaging studies using PET and MRI have shown that aberrant eating behaviors and obesity have altered the brain function as well as neuroanatomy.[6] Inflammation, resulting from excess adipose tissue and unhealthy dietary patterns, may enhance addictive patterns in general and addiction to food in particular.[16]

Weight-loss studies are especially important in terms of providing insight about whether obesity-related characteristics such as food craving change as a function of weight loss or whether these characteristics remain constant in spite of weight loss, suggesting an existence, prior to becoming obese.[2] In a family-based study of weight loss in relationship to eating and exercise perception, obese children lost weight, reduced their liking of foods high in fat and/or sugar, and increased their preference for foods lower in fat and sugar, compared to lean children who had no change in weight or food preference. These results provide evidence of high-fat and sugar preferences diminishing because of weight loss.[17] In a small clinical study of bariatric surgery patients, dopamine type 2 receptor–binding potentials decreased after surgery, with a suggested concomitant increase in extracellular dopamine levels competing with the radioligand,[18] providing further evidence for dopamine functioning changing as a result of weight loss. Some risk factors and behaviors can occur prior to obesity and nonetheless change as a function of weight loss, suggesting that determining when food addiction occurs in relationship to obesity is a complex question that has not yet been fully addressed.

## WHAT PARTS OF THE BRAIN ARE AFFECTED BY FOOD CRAVING AND ADDICTION?

Feeding behaviors have evolved over millions of years, and their neurological components are some of most powerful stimuli–reward mechanisms found in living multicellular organisms.[19] Drug abuse and addiction as well as certain types of obesity can be understood as resulting from repetitive habits that become increasingly more difficult to control despite the knowledge that the behavior has harmful consequences.[20] Feeding and drug use involve learned habits and preferences that are ingrained by the reinforcing properties of powerful and repetitive rewards.[21]

## DOPAMINE REWARD SYSTEM

The reward center of the brain, located in the primitive brainstem area, is called the ventral tegmental area (VTA). The VTA has a high density of dopamine neurons that are activated by rewards that are unanticipated. When the reward becomes learned and attached to other stimuli, the dopamine neurons increase their firing rate in the presence of the conditioned stimuli. If a reward is predicted but not awarded, the dopamine neurons are inhibited and become silent.[22] Addictive drugs that directly increase dopamine levels produce strong reinforcement signals that can thwart the normal stimulus–reward system.

The dopamine reward system is most characteristically linked to "wanting" rather than "liking" of food.[23,24] "Wanting" of food and food-related reward is modulated by dopamine release in the mesolimbic region of the brain,[25] and fluctuation of dopamine dramatically changes "wanting" or craving for food, while "liking" of food remains relatively constant.[26]

Dopamine also plays an inhibitory role in relationship to food intake. Disruption of the capacity to inhibit one's urges can promote overeating as well as increase the frequency of eating. In a small study of morbidly obese subjects compared to controls, PET scanning was used to assess regional brain glucose metabolism. Results showed lower dopamine receptor availability among obese subjects compared to controls, with patterns of activity occurring in multiple regions (dorsolateral prefrontal, medial orbitofrontal, anterior cingulate gyrus, and somatosensory cortices) among the obese subjects.[27] The multiregional brain activity suggests a relationship between striatal dopamine D2 receptors and metabolism in the somatosensory cortex region that processes palatability of food, providing a possible mechanism for dopamine regulation of the reinforcing properties of food. In addition, the hyporesponsiveness of the dopamine reward circuitry may promote overeating to compensate.[27]

## TASTE AND SOMATOSENSORY SYSTEM

The somatosensory cortex, a region associated with sensation in the mouth, lips, and tongue, is related to pleasure derived from the taste of food and may lead to overeating as a result. The sensation of taste serves as primary reinforcement and provides immediate reward or punishment for food consumption.[28] Obese relative to lean individuals showed greater resting metabolic activity in the oral somatosensory cortex, suggesting that obese subjects could be more sensitive to the rewarding properties of food related to palatability.[8] Anticipation of food has also been linked to the somatosensory region. Obese relative to lean adolescent girls showed greater activation bilaterally in the gustatory cortex and in the somatosensory regions in response to both an anticipated intake of a chocolate milk shake compared to a tasteless solution and in response to the actual consumption of the milk shake.[9] In a later study by the same authors, normal-weighted adolescents at high risk for obesity (both parents were obese) showed an elevated somatosensory response to consumption of food (chocolate milk shake) compared to normal-weighted adolescents at low risk (two lean parents), although there were no significant differences for anticipation of food.[29] Not all studies are consistent in relationship to somatosensory activation for anticipation and actual intake of food. In a functional MRI (fMRI) study of obese and lean women, obese relative to lean women showed greater activation in the somatosensory cortex in response to intake and anticipated intake of a milk shake.[30]

Intake of particular foods may influence somatosensory cortical activity. fMRI was used to assess brain response among 18 healthy normal-weighted subjects to isoviscous, isosweet fat emulsions of increasing fat concentration. Significant responses that positively correlated with increasing fat concentration were found in the anterior insula, frontal operculum, and secondary somatosensory cortex, anterior cingulate cortex, and amygdala. The study further evaluated brain response according to identified "taster" status using a continuous scale based on ranking of the fat concentration tastes. Taster status was significantly correlated with self-reported preference of the samples and with cortical response in somatosensory area and secondarily in the anterior insula, amygdala, and orbitofrontal cortex.[31] Targeted perception of fat taste was localized to the somatosensory cortex, the same region whose response was shown to vary according to obesity and high risk for obesity.

## FOOD CRAVING

Food craving is an intense desire to eat a particular food that exceeds the normal feelings of hunger.[32,33] There are several aspects of food craving that distinguish it from ordinary food choices. The desire for the food is intense, and only the specific food that is craved will satisfy the urge.[32] Foods that elicit craving have distinct tastes and generate sensations that most humans and other warm-blooded animals find rewarding.[24]

Much of the preclinical work on "food addiction" has focused on animal models of sugar craving and dependence.[34] In one model of sweet craving, rats binged on sweet solutions after food restriction that gradually increased in total daily intake to eventually drinking as much sweet solution in a 12 h access period as ad libitum–fed rats do in 24 h.[35] Other animal models of craving have shown that, in some instances, the craving for intense sweetness exceeds the craving for cocaine among rats given the choice of cocaine or water sweetened with saccharin.[36] Similar connections between sweet craving and drug abuse have been observed in humans.[32] In a study of opiate addicts who were currently abstinent compared to randomly sampled controls, the addicts showed a heightened and significant preference for and/or intake of sweets, compared to controls.[37] Likewise there is evidence linking the consumption of sweets to alcohol intake in both animals and humans.[38] In a study of healthy subjects with no history of alcoholism or drug dependence, sweet taste preference was associated with having alcohol-related problems.[39]

Carbohydrate craving has also been linked to depression and depressed mood. Carbohydrate cravers are thought to learn that negative mood can be alleviated by self-administering snacks that are high in carbohydrate and low in protein, resulting in obesity.[40] In a double-blinded placebo-controlled trial, overweight women who craved carbohydrates were given a carbohydrate beverage or a taste and calorie-matched protein-rich balanced nutrient beverage. When rendered mildly dysphoric (unhappy), carbohydrate cravers chose the carbohydrate beverage significantly more often than the protein-rich beverage.[41] With the strong evidence linking increased consumption of sugar-sweetened beverages and weight gain,[42] carbohydrate craving could represent an important underlying determinant of obesity in some individuals.

## MU-OPIOID RECEPTORS AND HEDONIC EATING

The biological purpose of hunger is to signal the need for nutritional intake. However, humans tend to eat until their "plate is empty" and often eat beyond feeling satiated. The phenomenon of eating beyond one's nutritional needs has multiple determinants including pursuit of reward and feelings of pleasure.[43] The striatal opioid network evolved a specialized capacity to promote overeating of energy-dense foods beyond acute homeostatic needs, to ensure an energy reserve for potential future famine and the likelihood of starvation.[44]

There are two concepts that classify the different types of motivating behaviors with regard to addiction. "Liking," in contrast to wanting, refers to the pleasurable feeling associated with the receipt and consumption of a reward.[4] The neural substrate of "liking" has been localized to the nucleus accumbens, the ventral palladium, and the orbitofrontal cortex, involving GABAergic, opioid, and endocannabinoid neurotransmissions.[26] In the early stages of addiction, motivation to consume the substance is often driven by the pursuit of pleasure. Certain addicts no longer "like" but "need" drugs of abuse, although reduction in the pleasure or hedonic properties of the drug varies depending on the drug.[45] The chronic overuse of drugs alters neural pathways underlying reward and motivation so that exposure to drug-related stimuli leads to habitual patterns and behaviors of drug seeking that are no longer voluntary or goal directed.[43] Overconsumption could be likened to addiction if the food consumption patterns become habitual and the ability to control overeating becomes lost.

The opioid receptor system regulates intake of palatable food. Drugs such as heroin, morphine, alcohol, and cannabinoids interact with the opioid system, providing evidence for common neural substrates between food and drug reward with regard to the brain's opioid system.[46] In a study of the effects of intra-accumbens opioids on macronutrient selection among rats, administration of mu-receptor agonists markedly enhanced the intake of fat or carbohydrate when diets were presented individually, with the intake of fat much greater in magnitude than carbohydrates.[47] Additional evidence for the localization of mu-receptor activity and food consumption is provided by a study of rats that were overfed with a high-fat diet compared to rats fed with a control diet. The rats on high-fat diets had a greater mu-receptor density in the hypothalamus, compared to control rats.[48] Human studies show a connection between opioid receptor activity and obesity. In a randomized placebo- and monotherapy-controlled double blind study of 419 patients, percent weight change from baseline was greater for a combined opioid receptor antagonist (naltrexone plus bupropion) compared to placebo and monotherapy.[49] If the opioid receptor system, designed to promote overeating as a protective mechanism against future starvation, becomes dysregulated, then there may be great potential for weight gain and obesity.

## SUSCEPTIBILITY TO FOOD ADDICTION AND OBESITY

Environmental change, in combination with genetic susceptibility, is most likely responsible for the obesity prevalence increases observed over the past three decades.[50] Since consuming food is critical to survival, it is perfectly reasonable that this activity would be highly valued within our inherited biological control mechanisms that evolved over the centuries of food scarcity and insecurity.[16] Only in recent times has there been a surplus of calories available to all Americans including those in the lower socioeconomic strata. Internalized motivation to consume sugar and fat supported by societal pressures activate reward and pleasure circuits in the brain that, if repeated over time, can lead to food addiction and obesity in susceptible individuals.

## DOPAMINE RECEPTOR D2 GENE (DRD2)

Dysregulation of binding of dopamine to the dopamine receptor could result in the malfunctioning of human stimulus–reward system. While many studies have linked the DRD2 to classical addictions such as cocaine,[51] alcohol,[52,53] nicotine,[54,55] and opioids,[56] fewer studies have shown associations between DRD2 and obesity.[57–59] The Taq1A polymorphism, the most frequently studied polymorphism, is located more than 10 kbp downstream from the coding region of the DRD2 at chromosome 11q23. Recent studies have further localized the coding region of Taq1A within the coding region of a neighboring gene, ANKK1.[60] Evidence indicates that individuals carrying this allele have reduced brain DRD2 density compared with other individuals.[61–64] It has been suggested

that persistent substance abuse in individuals with the A1 allele may be a form of self-stimulatory behavior that compensates for insufficient dopamine activity.[65] The availability of DRD2 is decreased in obese individuals in proportion to their BMI,[66] and the reduced density of the DRD2 is suspected to underlie the effect of having the A1 allele of TaqI polymorphism.[61]

## MU-OPIOID RECEPTOR GENE (OPRM1)

The mu-opioid receptor gene (OPRM1, located on chromosome 6q24) is one of four genes whose protein products bind to endogenous opioids. OPRM1 is a member of the large family of transmembrane G-protein-coupled receptors. It is widely expressed in both brain and periphery.[67] The mu-opioid receptor is the primary site of action for the most commonly used opioids, including morphine, heroin, fentanyl, and methadone.[22] Five different single-nucleotide polymorphisms (SNPs) in the coding region of the OPRM1 were identified from 113 former heroin addicts in methadone maintenance and 39 controls with no history of drug abuse. The most prevalent SNP was a nucleotide substitution at position 118 (A118G), predicting an amino acid change at a putative N-glycosylation site. This SNP displayed an allelic frequency of approximately 10% in the study population. Significant differences in allele distribution were observed among ethnic groups studied.[68] In a targeted study of food addiction among obese subjects, the functional A118G polymorphism of the OPRM1 was found to be associated with binge-eating disorders, and individuals with the combination of DRD2 Taq 1 allele and A118G polymorphism were much more likely to engage in binge eating. Overeating characterized by binge eating may be influenced by both dopamine and opioid receptor pathways.[58] Receptor dysfunction in both the dopamine and the opioid pathways may render individuals especially susceptible to food addiction and obesity.

## SUMMARY

There are multiple etiologic pathways to obesity. Many investigators concur that food addiction is associated with development of obesity in certain individuals. However, not all obese individuals gain weight because they are addicted to food. Determining when food addiction occurs in relationship to obesity is a complex question that has not yet been fully addressed.

Drug abuse and addiction as well as certain types of obesity can be understood as resulting from repetitive habits that become increasingly more difficult to control despite the knowledge that the behavior has harmful consequences. Dopamine plays both stimulatory and inhibitory roles in relationship to food intake with dopamine linked to "wanting" and craving for food as well as inhibiting the capacity to control overeating.

The somatosensory cortex, a region associated with sensation in the mouth, lips, and tongue, is related to pleasure derived from the taste of food and may lead to overeating as a result. The sensation of taste serves as primary reinforcement and provides immediate reward or punishment for food consumption.

Food craving is an intense desire to eat a particular food that exceeds the normal feelings of hunger. Foods such as sugar and fat have distinct tastes and generate sensations that most humans and other warm-blooded animals find rewarding. Individuals who crave foods, however, have intense desire for particular foods, and only the specific food that is craved will satisfy their urges. With the strong evidence linking increased consumption of sugar-sweetened beverages and weight gain, carbohydrate craving, in particular, could represent an important underlying determinant of obesity in some individuals.

The phenomenon of eating beyond one's nutritional needs has multiple determinants including pursuit of reward and feelings of pleasure. The opioid receptor system regulates intake of palatable food. If the opioid receptor system, designed to promote overeating as a protective mechanism against future starvation, becomes dysregulated, then there may be great potential for weight gain and obesity.

Since consuming food is critical to survival, we have inherited strong control mechanisms that evolved over the centuries of food scarcity and insecurity that include dopamine reward, somatosensory taste mechanisms, and overeating to ensure survival. Polymorphic variants in the dopamine and mu-opioid receptor pathways appear to render individuals especially susceptible to food addiction and obesity.

## REFERENCES

1. Ziauddeen, HJ, Farooqi, S, Fletcher, PC. *Nat Rev Neurosci* 13: 279; 2012.
2. Berthoud, H-R, Zheng H. *Physiol Behav* 107: 527; 2012.
3. Allen, P, Batra, P, Geiger, BM et al. *Physiol Behav* 107: 126; 2012.
4. Corsica, JA, Pelchat, ML. *Curr Opin Gastroenterol* 26: 165; 2010.
5. Kalivas, PW, O'Brien, C. *Neuropsychophamacology Rev* 33: 166; 2008.
6. Zhang, Y, van Deneen, KM, Tian J et al. *Pharm Des* 17: 1149; 2011.
7. Volkow, ND, Wang, G-J, Fowler, JS et al. *Synapse* 44: 175; 2002.
8. Wang, G-J, Volkow, ND, Felder, C et al. *Neuroreport* 13: 1151; 2002.
9. Stice, E, Spoor, S, Bohon, C et al. *J Abnorm Psychol* 117: 924; 2008.
10. Baicy, K, London, ED, Monterosso, J et al. *Proc Natl Acad Sci USA* 104: 18276; 2007.
11. Craig, AD. *Ann NY Acad Sci* 1225: 72; 2011.
12. Higo, T, Mars, RB, Boorman, ED et al. *Proc Natl Acad Sci USA* 108: 4230; 2011.
13. Jackson, DM, Westlind-Danielsson, A. *Pharmacol Ther* 64: 291; 1994.
14. Davis, C, Curtis, C, Levitan, RD et al. *Appetite* 57: 711; 2011.
15. Hall, KD, Sack, SG, Chandramohan D et al. *Lancet* 378: 826; 2011.
16. Heber, D, Carpenter, CL. *Mol Neurobiol* 44: 160; 2011.
17. Epstein, LH, Valoski, A, Wing, RR et al. *Appetite* 12: 105; 1989
18. Dunn, JP, Cowan, RL, Volkow, ND et al. *Brain Res* 1350: 123; 2010.
19. Kelley, AE, Berridge, KC. *J Neurosci* 22: 3306; 2002.
20. Volkow, ND, Wang, G-J, Fowler, JS et al. *Phil Trans R Soc* 363: 3191; 2008.
21. Volkow, ND, Wise, RA. *Nat Neurosci* 8: 555; 2005.
22. Luscher, C. In: Katzung BG, Masters SB, and Trevor AJ (eds.), *Basic and Clinical Pharmacology*, 12th edn., McGraw-Hill, New York. http://www.accessmedicine.com/content.aspx?aID=55826407. Accessed June 12, 2012.
23. Nasser, J. *Obes Rev* 2: 213; 2001.
24. Berridge, KC. *Neurosci Biobehav Rev* 20: 1; 1995.
25. Martel, P, Fantino, M. *Pharmacol Biochem Behav* 55: 297; 1996.
26. Berridge, KC, Ho, CY, Richard, JM et al. *Brain Res* 1350: 43; 2010.
27. Volkow, ND, Wang, GJ, Telang, F et al. *Neuroimage* 42: 1537; 2008.
28. Rolls, ET. *Int J Obes* 35: 550; 2011.
29. Stice, E, Yokum, S, Burger, KS et al. *J Neurosci* 31: 4360; 2011.
30. Ng, J, Stice, E, Yokum, S et al. *Appetite* 57: 65–72; 2011.
31. Eldeghaidy, S, Marcian, IL. McGlone, F et al. *J Neurophysiol* 105: 2573; 2011.
32. Pelchat, ML. *Physiol Behav* 76: 347; 2002.
33. White, MA, Whisenhunt, BL, Williamson, DA et al. *Obes Res* 10: 107; 2002.
34. Avena, NM, Novstdly, MR, Hoebel, BG. In, Kobeissy FH (ed.), *Psychiatric Disorders: Methods and Protocols*. Human Press, New York, p. 829; 2012.
35. Avena, NM, Hoebel, RP, Hoebel, BG. *Neurosci Biobehav Rev* 32: 20; 2008.
36. Lenoir, M, Serre, F, Cantin, L et al. *PLoS One* 2: e698; 2007.
37. Morabia, A, Fabre, J, Chee, E et al. *Br J Nutr* 84: 173; 1989.
38. Leggio, L, Addolorato, G, Cippitelli, A et al. *Alcohol Clin Exp Res* 35: 194; 2011.
39. Lange, LA, Kampov-Polevoy, AB, Garbutt, JC. *Alcohol* 45: 431; 2010.
40. Spring, B, Schneider, K, Smith, M et al. *Psychopharmacology* 197: 637; 2008.
41. Corsica, JA, Spring, BJ. *Eating Behav* 9: 447; 2008.
42. Malik, VS, Popkin, BM, Bray, GA et al. *Circulation* 121: 1356; 2010.
43. Pandit, R, deJong, JW, Vanderschuren, LJMJ et al. *Eur J Phamacol* 660: 28; 2011.
44. Kelley, AE, Baldo, BA, Pratt, WE et al. *Physio Behav* 86: 773; 2005.
45. Lambert, NM, McLeod, M, Schenk, S. *Addiction* 101: 713; 2006.
46. Kelley, AE, Bakshi, VP, Haber, SN et al. *Physio Behav* 76: 365; 2002.
47. Zhang, M, Gosnell, BA, Kelley, AE. *J Pharm Exp Ther* 285: 908; 1998.
48. Barnes, MJ, Lapanowski, K, Conley, A et al. *Brain Res Bull* 61: 511; 2003.
49. Greenway, FL, Dunayevich, E, Tollefson, G et al. *J Clin Endocrinol Metab* 94: 4898; 2009.
50. Speakman, JR, Levitsky, DA, Allison, DB et al. *Dis Model Mech* 4: 733; 2011.
51. Noble, EP, Blum, K, Khalsa, ME et al. *Drug Alcohol Depend* 33: 271; 1993.

52. Blum, K, Noble, EP, Sheridan, PJ et al. *JAMA* 263: 2055; 1990.

53. Munafò, MR, Matheson, IJ, Flint, *J Mol Psychiatry* 12: 454; 2007.

54. Munafò, M, Clark, T, Johnstone, E et al. *Nicotine Tob Res* 6: 583; 2004.

55. Gelernter, J, Yu, Y, Weiss, R et al. *Hum Mol Genet* 15: 3498; 2006.

56. Lawford, BR, Young, RM, Noble, EP et al. *Am J Med Genet* 96: 592; 2000.

57. Blum, K, Braverman, ER, Wood, RC et al. *Pharmacogenetics* 6: 297; 1996.

58. Davis, CA, Levitan, RD, Reid, C et al. *Obesity* 17: 1220; 2009.

59. Epstein, LH, Temple, JL, Neaderhiser, BJ et al. *Behav Neurosci* 121: 877; 2007.

60. Neville, MJ. Johnstone, EC, Walton, RT. *Hum Mutat* 23: 540; 2004.

61. Jönsson, EG, Nöthen, MM, Gründhage, F et al. *Mol Psychiatry* 4: 290; 1999.

62. Noble, EP, Blum, K, Ritchie, T et al. *Arch Gen Psychiatry* 48: 648; 1991.

63. Pohjalainen, T, Rinne, JO, Nagren, K et al. *Mol Psychiatry* 3: 256; 1998.

64. Thompson, J, Thomas, N, Singleton, A et al. *Pharmacogenetics* 7: 479; 1997.

65. Comings, DE, Blum, K. *Prog Brain Res* 126: 325; 2000.

66. Wang, GJ, Volkow, ND, Logan, J et al. *Lancet* 357: 354; 2001.

67. Berettini, W. *Clin Neurosci Res* 5: 69; 2005.

68. Bond, C, LaForge, KS, Tian, M et al. *Proc Natl Acad Sci U S A* 95: 9608; 1998.

# 51 Nutrition and Liver Disease

*Sammy Saab and David Heber*

## CONTENTS

## INTRODUCTION AND BRIEF OVERVIEW OF LIVER DISEASES

The liver supports almost every organ in the body and is vital for survival. Because of its strategic location and multidimensional functions, the liver is also prone to injuries, affected directly or indirectly by nutrition. The most common causes of liver injury include acute and chronic viral infections (hepatitis A, B, C), alcohol damage, fatty liver, cirrhosis, and cancer. Much less common are drug-induced liver injuries due to direct toxicity or less well-defined immunoallergic reactions. What is remarkable is the emerging commonality of nutritional factors in liver disease. For example, fatty liver interacts with both alcohol and hepatitis C in increasing the risk of cirrhosis. For this reason, nonalcoholic fatty liver disease (NAFLD) is the first topic covered, and then nutritional factors are mentioned throughout the discussion of the other etiological factors in liver disease.

Many liver diseases are accompanied by jaundice secondary to increased levels of bilirubin in blood and in tissues. The increased bilirubin results from the breakup of the hemoglobin of dead red blood cells. Normally, the liver removes bilirubin from the blood and excretes it through the bile. Diseases that interfere with liver function will lead to derangement of these processes. However, the liver has a great capacity to regenerate and has a large reserve capacity. In most cases, the liver only produces symptoms after extensive damage.

The classic symptoms of liver damage include the following: (1) Pale stools occur when stercobilin, a brown pigment, is absent from the stool. Stercobilin is derived from bilirubin metabolites produced in the liver; (2) dark urine occurs when bilirubin mixes with urine; (3) jaundice is the yellowing of the skin and whites of the eyes due to bilirubin deposits. Pruritus is a common presenting complaint with liver failure even in patients without jaundice. Often this pruritus cannot be relieved by drugs; (4) swelling of the abdomen, ankles, and feet occurs because the liver fails to make albumin, leading to osmotic flow of fluids into extracellular space

and peritoneal fluid; (5) fatigue occurs as the result of malnutrition associated with nausea and anorexia; (6) bruising and easy bleeding result from reduced liver synthesis of clotting proteins. Liver diseases can be diagnosed by physical examination, imaging, and liver-associated laboratory tests. The liver function tests, which are commonly used for AST, ALT, bilirubin, and alkaline phosphatase and LDH measurements, are not measures of liver function, but rather reflect biochemical functions of the liver or the release of liver enzymes into the bloodstream due to damage to liver cells. These liver-associated tests can be used in the overall evaluation of liver function but sometimes can be normal even in the face of liver cirrhosis or liver failure. When infections are suspected, serologic studies can be informative, and when trace minerals are suspected, chemical testing can be performed.

## NONALCOHOLIC FATTY LIVER DISEASES

NAFLD is a common but broad category of often silent disease due to the accumulation of triglycerides in the liver and by definition occurs in individuals who do not have excess alcohol consumption.[1–3] The histological lesions found in the liver can range from simple fat deposits in the liver called steatosis to nonalcoholic steatohepatitis (NASH) characterized by liver inflammation to fibrosis, cirrhosis, and hepatocellular carcinoma.[4,5] While only a small percentage of those individuals with fatty liver progress to cirrhosis, there are so many individuals with obesity and fatty liver that this etiology is now the third most common cause for liver transplantation behind hepatitis and alcoholism.

NAFLD is currently considered the hepatic manifestation of metabolic syndrome that affects about half of all Americans between 45 and 65.[6–8] Growing evidence suggests that the fast-growing and alarming epidemic of NAFLD is closely intertwined with the Westernization of dietary patterns with an increasing intake of simple sugars, especially fructose. In addition, insulin resistance is related to fat deposition in the liver and so contributes to the worldwide epidemic of type 2 diabetes.[9–14]

Fructose is an isomer of glucose[15] but is metabolized very differently from glucose. Recent decades have witnessed an enormous rise in fructose consumption. Studies on ancient diets have shown that at the dawn of agriculture 8500 years ago, the intake of fructose per capita was around 2 kg/year from fruits and vegetables. The industrialization of sugar production from plantations in the seventeenth century converted a rare spice from the orient into an expensive staple item used in baked goods and candies. Significant increases in consumption occurred following the abolition of sugar taxes in the 1870s. By 1950, annual consumption had increased to 45 kg/person/year, and by 1997, nearly 20 years after the introduction of high-fructose corn syrup into the food supply, consumption had risen to 69 kg/year.[13,16] Fructose is used in a wide variety of food products due to its sweeter taste and its lack of inhibition of satiety compared with other sugars.[16] From a metabolic standpoint, fructose is absorbed by the small intestine and is transported across the epithelial barrier into cells and the bloodstream by the fructose-specific GLUT5 transporter.[17] Entry of fructose into cells is not insulin dependent and does not promote insulin secretion unlike glucose. Absorbed fructose is transported in plasma via the hepatic portal vein to the liver where fructose is predominantly metabolized via its phosphorylation; only a small amount of fructose is metabolized by hexokinase in muscle and adipose tissue.[13,16]

Starting in the 1960s, a number of animal and human studies have reported associations with excessive fructose consumption and adverse metabolic effects, which may have important hepatic consequences (including the development of NAFLD). The potential role of fructose in the pathogenesis of NAFLD has recently gained increased attention.[9–17] Fructose can lead to NAFLD by promoting an increase in fasting and postprandial triglycerides, which can in turn result in liver fat deposition.[18–29] In addition, hypertriglyceridemia secondary to excess fructose consumption under conditions of positive calorie balance has been shown to promote insulin resistance.[21,22] Chronic fructose consumption causes hyperinsulinemia due to insulin resistance.[21]

Continuous fructose ingestion may impose a metabolic burden on the liver through the induction of fructokinase and fatty acid synthase. In the liver, fructose is metabolized to fructose-1-phosphate by fructokinase, which consumes ATP.[13,16] As a consequence, a massive incorporation of fructose into liver metabolism can lead to high levels of metabolic stress via ATP depletion. In an experimental study in the rat, Vilà et al.[23] have shown that fructose-induced fructokinase hyperexpression in the liver can be reduced (by 0.6-fold) by the hydroxymethyl-glutaryl-CoA reductase inhibitor atorvastatin (Lipitor®). Of note, clinical studies have shown that atorvastatin can improve liver injury in NAFLD patients with hyperlipidemia.[24,25] Fatty acid synthase catalyzes the last step in the fatty acid biosynthetic pathway and is a key determinant of the maximal capacity of the liver to synthesize fatty acids by de novo lipogenesis.[26] In a clinical study, increased fructose consumption in patients with NAFLD was associated with hyperexpression of hepatic mRNA for

fatty acid synthase, suggesting that this molecular derangement could play a crucial role in fructose-induced fatty liver infiltration.[27]

In fatty liver disease, some evidence exists supporting the use of vitamin E. Vitamin E was studied in 167 adult patients with NASH and without diabetes who received either vitamin E at a dose of 800 IU daily (84 subjects) or placebo (83 subjects) for 96 weeks.[38] The primary outcome was an improvement in histological features of NASH, as assessed with the use of a composite of standardized scores for steatosis, lobular inflammation, hepatocellular ballooning, and fibrosis. There was an improvement in histological features in 43% of those who received vitamin E compared to 19% of those receiving placebo. Additional studies are necessary to confirm these findings.

Omega-3 fatty acids are approved in the United States to treat hypertriglyceridemia. They are also available over the counter as dietary supplements. There has been a significant interest in exploring the effects of omega-3 fatty acids in animal models of fatty liver as well as in humans with NAFLD. Many of the human trials have been in small numbers of individuals treated for varying times. In one study of 144 NAFLD patients with dyslipidemia given either 2 g of omega-3 fatty acids from seal oils or placebo for 24 weeks, omega-3 fatty acid supplementation was associated with significant improvement in serum aminotransferases, serum triglycerides, and hepatic steatosis at 24 weeks.[39] There is an ongoing phase 3, multicenter, randomized, controlled trial of eicosapentaenoic acid (EPA) in patients with biopsy-proven NASH in the United States, and its results are expected to shed further light on the role of omega-3 fatty acids in the management of NAFLD (ClinicalTrials.gov Identifier: NCT01154985).

Coffee consumption has been associated with benefits in liver disease for unclear reasons, with some proposing that aromatic extracts isolated from coffee beans may be beneficial.[30] Coffee oils, called diterpenes, have been evaluated. The diterpenes, kahweol and cafestol, have been shown to have beneficial effects on glutathione metabolism.[31] However, the idea of diterprene effects on liver health may be mitigated by the fact that most of these fats are trapped by the filter paper used to make traditional American coffee by the drip method. They survive in coffee made by the French press method. Nonetheless, it is also possible that caffeine itself may have antioxidant activity providing a beneficial effect. [42]

The majority of patients with NAFLD are overweight and obese, lead relatively sedentary lifestyles, and have underlying insulin resistance. Treatment aimed at improving body weight and activity should be the basis of approaches to combating this disease. Evidence suggests that diets low in processed carbohydrates and saturated fats with a goal to achieve a 500–1000 cal/day deficit improve insulin sensitivity, reduce serum aminotransferases, and decrease hepatic steatosis. Improvements are seen with as little as a 5% reduction in body weight. Weight loss through total caloric restriction results in improved parameters of insulin sensitivity and regression of hepatic steatosis.[33] Data regarding the utility of specific dietary regimens may be debated, but it appears that diets consisting of a reduction in processed carbohydrates and saturated fats to effect a caloric deficit of 500–1000 cal/day may be beneficial and can be recommended in overweight or obese patients with NAFLD4.[34] Histopathologic parameters of steatohepatitis also appear to improve with weight loss. Antioxidant supplementation, specifically with vitamin E, may be considered as adjunctive therapy. Larger confirmatory studies are needed to ensure they are safe and beneficial in patients with NASH. For patients failing to achieve weight-loss goals, future approaches are likely to consist of combination therapy targeting insulin resistance, oxidative stress, and fibrogenesis.

## ALCOHOL AND LIVER DISEASE

Alcohol remains one of the most common causes of both acute and chronic liver diseases in the United States.[35] In Western countries, up to 50% of cases of end-stage liver disease are related primarily to alcohol.[36] Excessive alcohol consumption is the third leading preventable cause of death in the United States. Alcohol-related deaths, excluding accidents/homicides, accounted for 24,518 deaths in the United States in 2009 with 15,183 of those specifically attributed to ALD.[37]

Prevalence ratios were measured for the co-occurrence of obesity (i.e., body mass index ≥ 30.0 kg/m² or waist circumference ≥ 102 cm in men and ≥88 cm in women) and specific patterns of alcohol use (i.e., nondrinkers, non-excessive drinkers, and excessive drinkers) as a predictor of elevations in serum ALT and AST in 8373 adults aged ≥20 years who participated in the 2005–2008 National Health and Nutrition Examination Survey.[38] Approximately 34.7% of adult men and 38.6% of adult women in the United States had co-occurrence of obesity and any alcohol use, including 16.4% of men and 9.8% of women who had co-occurrence of obesity and excessive drinking during 2005–2008. When compared to male nondrinkers without obesity after multivariate adjustment, male excessive drinkers with obesity were 3 times more likely to have elevated ALT and 2.4 times more likely to have elevated AST. Similarly, when compared to female nondrinkers without obesity, female excessive drinkers with obesity were 2.4 times more likely to have elevated serum ALT and 3.4 times more likely to have elevated serum AST. The co-occurrence of obesity and excessive drinking may place adults at an increased risk for potential liver injury.[38]

The mortality from alcoholic cirrhosis is higher than that of nonalcoholic cirrhosis with a survival rate at 5 and 10 years of only 23% and 7%, respectively.[39] Therefore, the mortality of ALD is more than that of many major forms of cancer, such as breast, colon, and prostate.[40] Alcohol represents a major financial burden on the overall economy as well, with an estimated cost of 185 billion dollars annually including estimated lost productivity and motor vehicle accidents.[51]

There are several factors involved in the development of ALD. Daily intake of alcohol for 10–12 years with doses in excess of 40–80 g/day for males and of 20–40 g/day for females is generally needed to cause ALD.[42–45] Because different types of alcoholic beverages have varying alcohol content, the threshold is different for each type of beverage. As a reference, the amount of alcohol in 8 ounces of wine, 1 ounce of hard liquor, and 12 ounces of beer is approximately the same. It has been estimated from survey data that daily drinking of 3–6 cans (12 oz each) of beer/day for males or 1.5–3 cans of beer/day for females for 10 years or longer can cause ALD.[46]

Despite reaching the required amounts of alcohol intake listed earlier, only 10%–35% of heavy alcohol drinkers will develop alcoholic hepatitis, and only 8%–20% will develop cirrhosis.[47] Therefore, host factors including gender and polymorphism(s) of alcohol-metabolizing enzymes may play a role. Furthermore, coexisting external factors including obesity and hepatitis C infection can increase the likelihood of developing ALD. There are several studies demonstrating that women develop liver disease after exposure to lower quantities of alcohol and over shorter time periods.[43,44]

Alcohol-induced liver injury represents a wide spectrum of pathologic abnormalities: from mild steatosis to hepatocellular carcinoma in the setting of cirrhosis.[48] Macrovesicular steatosis represents the first and the most common pathologic change seen with chronic alcohol ingestion (in up to 90% of heavy alcohol users).[49] Macrovesicular change also represents an easily reversible finding when abstinence from alcohol is achieved. Hepatocyte death by apoptosis as well as areas of microvesicular steatosis can also be seen, although more commonly in steatohepatitis. Ballooning degeneration of hepatocytes, infiltrating neutrophils, Mallory bodies, and fibrosis represent a more concerning collection of pathologic findings indicative of steatohepatitis (alcoholic hepatitis).[48]

The clinical relevance of alcoholic hepatitis is twofold: Severe alcoholic hepatitis is associated with a 40% 6-month mortality, and progression to cirrhosis is nine times greater than in those with steatosis alone.[50] Hepatocellular cancer develops in 5%–15% of those with alcoholic cirrhosis, most commonly in individuals with macronodular cirrhosis.[48] It has been recognized that the most important clinical risk factor for the development of hepatocellular carcinoma is cirrhosis. In Western countries, about 70%–90% of hepatocellular carcinomas develop in patients with macronodular cirrhosis that is characterized by large nodules varying in size surrounded by fibrosis. Alcohol and hepatitis C interact to increase the risk of hepatocellular carcinoma such that when both are present, relative risk is increased 100-fold. However, to put alcoholism itself into perspective as a potential causative factor for hepatocellular carcinoma, it must be realized that among the main risk factors for hepatocellular carcinoma, chronic infections of hepatitis B virus (HBV) and hepatitis C virus (HCV) are the most important in humans, accounting for more than 70% of HCC cases worldwide.[51] Obesity with NASH is increasing in incidence, and as these lead to more cases of cirrhosis, it is anticipated that NASH will contribute to cirrhosis and then to hepatocellular carcinoma as well in larger numbers of individuals.

Addressing the underlying addiction to alcohol is the paramount step in managing ALD. Abstinence from alcohol leads to resolution of alcoholic fatty liver disease (benign steatosis), and abstinence improves survival in alcoholic cirrhotic patients, even those with decompensated liver function. Furthermore, reducing alcohol consumption, but not completely stopping, has been shown to improve survival in patients with ALD.[35–37] While there is no question regarding the benefit of abstinence, motivating patients to follow this treatment regimen, monitoring their compliance, and preventing relapse remain major obstacles to the treatment of ALD. Certainly, inpatient and outpatient rehabilitation programs have demonstrated effectiveness in assisting patients to achieve and maintain sobriety.[51] Referral to and communication with an addiction specialist and encouraging active participation in Alcoholics Anonymous represent the best method of assisting patients with alcoholism and concomitant ALD. While this may not be available to all patients, studies indicate that heavy drinkers who receive brief interventions (less than 1 h in length and incorporating motivational counseling techniques) are twice as likely as control patients to have modified their drinking habits 6–12 months after the intervention.[52] Recognition and treatment of comorbid psychiatric conditions is also a useful step in assisting patients with alcohol dependence.[53]

Pharmacotherapy in combination with psychosocial interventions can aid patients in maintaining abstinence from alcohol. Naltrexone and acamprosate have been shown to assist in reducing or eliminating alcohol intake in chronic heavy drinkers.[54] Disulfiram, which has long been approved by the Food and Drug Administration (FDA) for the treatment of alcoholism, is still widely used but less clearly supported by clinical trial evidence.[55] Disulfiram is still believed to have a role in alcoholism treatment, and it is hypothesized that under supervised administration, disulfiram can have favorable outcomes for patients.[56] Topiramate has demonstrated safety and efficacy in multiple clinical trials in decreasing both craving and withdrawal symptoms and increasing quality of life measures among alcohol-dependent individuals.[57] Finally, baclofen has proven effective in promoting alcohol abstinence in alcohol-dependent patients with liver cirrhosis.[58] Given the high likelihood of chronic, heavy alcohol use, the consequent difficulty in achieving/maintaining sobriety, and the low margin for error in patients with ALD, the coordination of both pharmacotherapy and psychosocial intervention is best handled by an addiction specialist.

Other lifestyle modifications, such as smoking cessation and weight loss, if applicable, are also crucial to improving the outcome of those suffering from ALD. Smoking is an independent risk factor for advancement of hepatic fibrosis that can lead to more severe ALD and may be linked to the development of HCC.[59,60] Obesity, which can also cause fatty liver, NASH, and cirrhosis, may be an independent risk factor for the progression of ALD.[72]

It has long been established that patients with ALD are nearly all malnourished, and the degree of malnutrition correlates with disease severity.[62,63] In addition, complications of ALD (e.g., infections, encephalopathy, ascites, and variceal bleeding) have been shown to be strongly associated with protein–calorie malnutrition (PCM).[63,64] Micronutrient deficiencies of folate, vitamin B6, vitamin A, and thiamin are among the most commonly encountered. Mineral/element (e.g., selenium, zinc, copper, and magnesium) levels are often altered in ALD and, in some instances, are thought to be involved in its pathogenesis.[62] In particular, zinc is decreased in patients with ALD. In animal models, zinc supplementation has been shown to improve, attenuate, and/or prevent ALD through a variety of mechanisms.[65]

Patients with ALD can have varying nutritional status, from morbid obesity to profound underweight and malnutrition. Given the high caloric content of alcohol (7.1 kcal/g), patients with ALD and concomitant high-calorie diets can expect to develop truncal obesity and resultant progression of ALD.[64,66] Given similar mechanisms of pathogenesis (e.g., oxidative stress, cytokines, cytochrome P450), patients with the metabolic syndrome/insulin resistance and concomitant ALD would be expected to have more severe disease with a quicker progression to fibrosis.[67] The possibility of concomitant ALD and obesity-related liver disease (including their combined effect on the rising incidence of HCC) is an active area of hepatology research. This interaction of obesity-associated fatty liver and alcohol may account for a significant pathophysiological pathway in ALD.

At the other end of the nutritional spectrum, several mechanisms are hypothesized to contribute to ALD-associated malnutrition in ALD. Decreased caloric intake (secondary to anorexia and reduced intake of nonalcohol calories); decreased intestinal absorption/digestion of nutrients (secondary to altered gut integrity, pancreatic insufficiency, decreased bile excretion, and a decrease in intestinal enzymes); and decreased processing and storage of nutrients (secondary to decreased functional liver mass, abnormal oxidation of fat, and preferential metabolism of alcohol) are all thought to be involved in the malnutrition associated with ALD.[68] Increased catabolism of skeletal muscle and visceral proteins leading to a hypermetabolic state in alcoholic hepatitis is also a key component in the development of PCM in ALD.[69]

With so many mechanisms at play, the diagnosis and treatment of malnutrition in patients with ALD is sometimes difficult. The laboratory tests most commonly used to assess nutritional status (e.g., anthropometry and serum albumin concentration) are often affected by concomitant liver disease. In order to obtain valid data on the prevalence and degree of malnutrition among alcoholics with alcoholic liver disease, reliable and sensitive methods to assess nutritional status are required. Easily applicable techniques include anthropometric measurements such as body mass index, triceps skinfold thickness, and mid-arm muscle area. Other approaches include the bioelectric impedance analysis for assessing body composition and the determination of resting energy expenditure by indirect calorimetry. Each technique has limitations and may give erroneous results in alcoholic cirrhotics. For metabolic studies, direct measurements are needed.

In a recent study, different methods for the assessment of body composition in patients with liver cirrhosis were compared.[63] All applied techniques, including bioelectric impedance analysis, total body nitrogen content, dual x-ray absorptiometry, and four-site skinfold measurements, could detect advanced protein malnutrition but differed significantly in patients with high volumes of extracellular fluid such as ascites and peripheral edema. Although these mistakes may be avoided with more precise approaches, such as in vivo neutron activation analysis and isotope dilution techniques,[64] application of these methods is time consuming and restricted to the research setting. Based on the available data demonstrating the prevalence of malnutrition in ALD and the difficulty in diagnosis, patients with severe forms of ALD should be considered malnourished and treated as such.

Nutritional support for patients with ALD depends on the severity of liver disease, the concomitant factors leading to malnutrition (e.g., anorexia and pancreatic insufficiency), and the presence of obesity. Obese patients with less severe liver injury should be referred to a dietician and advised concerning dietary restriction and regular exercise. In outpatient therapy for patients with ALD, nutritional support in alcoholic cirrhotic patients improves nutritional status and cell-mediated immunity, as well as decreases infectious complications and consequent hospitalizations.[70,71] Another study of cirrhotics (not exclusively ALD) demonstrated that a late-evening nutritional supplement over a 12-month period improved body protein stores in patients with cirrhosis.[72] Without question, there are limited data regarding outpatient nutritional therapy in patients with ALD. While more study is warranted, our general practice is to encourage bedtime nutritional supplements in outpatients with severe ALD (e.g., ASH and cirrhosis).

Veterans Administration Cooperative Studies Program[73–77] included over 600 patients hospitalized with ALD. PCM was present in nearly all patients with severe ALD. The degree of malnutrition correlated with the development of serious complications such as encephalopathy, ascites, and hepatorenal syndrome. Moreover, nutritional support improved nutritional and metabolic parameters, severity of liver injury, and, most importantly, mortality in patients with moderate malnutrition and ALD. A major multicenter study demonstrated that enteral nutrition, when compared to corticosteroids, has similar short-term mortality rates, improved 1-year mortality rates, and reduced infectious complications.[78] An additional study demonstrated the benefit of tube-fed nutrition (improved PSE scores, bilirubin, and antipyrine clearance) compared with a regular diet in ALD.[91] Parenteral nutrition for patients with ALD is rarely indicated but appears to improve liver function and nitrogen balance. However, it fails to convey a survival benefit over standard therapy.[79,80]

The American College of Gastroenterology (ACG) and the American Association for the Study of Liver Diseases (AASLD) guidelines recommend 1.2–1.5 g/kg of protein and 35–40 kcal/kg of body weight per day in patients with ALD.[81] The available clinical trials vary considerably regarding the composition of the nutritional support utilized.[68] One randomized trial comparing long-term nutritional supplementation with oral BCAA improved surrogate markers and perceived health status and decreased hospitalizations in patients with advanced cirrhosis by comparison to lact-albumin or maltodextrins.[82] Another study demonstrated that long-term BCAA supplementation is associated with decreased frequency of hepatic failure and overall complication frequency.[83] Other studies have not been as clear in establishing a benefit.[84]

While some studies have failed to demonstrate a clear survival benefit for all patients with severe ALD receiving enteral nutrition,[68,78,85] the implementation of aggressive nutritional support in these patients is generally performed since at a minimum nutritional support will improve metabolic status.

Oxidative stress is thought to play a key role in the pathogenesis of ALD. Alcohol mediates oxidative stress in a number of ways including lipid peroxidation, production of reactive oxygen species, and depletion of endogenous antioxidant capabilities.[86,87] Vitamin E deficiency has been well documented in ALD.[46] Vitamin E has experimentally proven hepatoprotective capabilities including membrane stabilization, reduced NFκB activation and TNF production, and inhibition of hepatic stellate cell activation.[88–90] The first study examining vitamin E supplementation (500 mg) in decompensated ambulatory alcoholic cirrhotics failed to show benefit at 1-year follow-up.[91] In a study of patients with mild to moderate alcoholic hepatitis, 1000 IU of vitamin E per day improved serum hyaluronic acid but had no beneficial effects on tests of liver function or mortality when compared with placebo.[92] Clinical trials examining antioxidant therapy in ALD have not yet been definitive in establishing a benefit.

Lecithin, a mixture of phospholipids from plant sources, may have a role to play in ALD, but to date, the human studies have not demonstrated clear benefits. Lecithin has been demonstrated to prevent alcoholic liver cirrhosis in baboons[93] and appears to have anti-inflammatory, anti-apoptotic, and antifibrotic effects.[94,95] However, a VA Cooperative Study evaluating lecithin in humans with early ALD[96] failed to show definitive benefit. It has been proposed that the results were compromised by patients decreasing their alcohol use markedly during the trial.

*Silybum Marianum* (milk thistle) is a popular dietary supplement for patients wishing to maintain liver health. In animal models, hepatoprotective effects of milk thistle in several forms of liver injury (toxic hepatitis, fatty liver, cirrhosis, ischemic injury, radiation toxicity, and viral hepatitis) have been shown. Mechanisms including anti-inflammatory, anti-oxidative, antifibrotic, and immunomodulating effects are thought to explain the benefit of silymarin in liver disease.[97] A randomized double-blind control evaluating placebo versus silymarin in alcohol- and nonalcohol-induced cirrhosis showed a 39% versus 58% 4-year survival, respectively.[98] However, similar trials have failed to show outcome benefit in ALD.[99,100] Meta-analyses have failed to demonstrate a benefit for silymarin in ALD, but trials analyzed had numerous flaws making any interpretation difficult.[101]

In alcoholic hepatitis and cirrhosis, abnormal hepatic gene expression of methyl donor metabolism specifically in methionine and glutathione metabolism occurs and often contributes to decreased hepatic *S*-adenosylmethionine (SAM), cysteine, and glutathione levels.[102] Rodent and primate studies demonstrate that SAM depletion occurs in early stages of fatty liver infiltration in ALD and decreased SAM concentration, liver injury, and mitochondrial damage can be reversed with SAM supplementation.[103] SAM appears to attenuate oxidative stress and hepatic stellate cell activation in an ethanol-LPS-induced fibrotic rat model.[104] Clinical trial evidence is lacking. Betaine (trimethylglycine) is a key nutrient for humans similar in function to choline and can be obtained from a variety of foods and nutritional supplements.[105] In the liver, betaine can transfer one methyl group to homocysteine to form methionine. This process removes toxic metabolites (homocysteine and *S*-adenosylhomocysteine), restores SAM levels, reverses steatosis, prevents apoptosis, and reduces both damaged protein accumulation and oxidative stress.[106,107] Betaine also appears to attenuate alcoholic steatosis by restoring phosphatidylcholine generation via the phosphatidylethanolamine methyltransferase pathway.[107] Studies suggest that betaine offers hepatic protection against ethanol-induced oxidative stress by decreasing sulfur-containing amino acid breakdown as well.[108] Betaine supplementation is promising, but there are further clinical studies needed.

## NUTRITION IN VIRAL HEPATITIS

Viral hepatitis comprises five different diseases caused by five different viral agents: hepatitis A, B, C, D, and E viruses. Hepatitis E is rarely found in the United States. All five forms can cause acute hepatitis; only hepatitis B, C, and D can lead to chronic hepatitis.[109,110]

In acute viral hepatitis, jaundice is a common presentation that follows a pre-icteric period of 5–10 days, deepens for 1–2 weeks, and then levels off and decreases. Convalescence requires 3 weeks to 3 months, and optimal care during this time is essential.[111] The mainstay of treatment for AVH is supportive care, as most cases are self-limited. General measures in all types of viral hepatitis include bed rest if the patient is very symptomatic, high-calorie diet, avoidance of hepatotoxic medications, and abstinence from alcohol.[112] Optimal nutrition provides the foundation for recovery of injured liver cells and overall regain of strength, which is a major aspect of basic care.[113]

There are no specific diet recommendations that have been shown to be helpful in AVH. Fever and infection increase the nutrient requirements, and a well-balanced diet is recommended during the illness. While it is known that low-fat diets high in refined carbohydrates are associated with extended and complicated illness,[114] such diets are still widely used that could lengthen patient hospitalization and contribute to additional costs.

Viral hepatitis classically presents in the form of loss of appetite, nausea, vomiting, fatigue, and jaundice and usually recovers spontaneously with hepatocellular regeneration. Treatment of acute hepatitis is largely supportive. However, hospitalization is needed for patients whose nausea, vomiting, malaise, and fever place them at risk for dehydration.[110,115]

The dietary treatment of viral hepatitis has passed through various phases of evolution with conclusions drawn from small, observational studies to extensive studies among army personnel that have shown that patients on a diet supplying high calories and proteins, supplemented with vitamins, improved more rapidly than those who ate only what they chose.[113,114] It is likely that nausea, vomiting, and loss of appetite contribute to poor nutrition during acute viral hepatitis. In acute hepatitis, it is clear that adequate nutrition is important and a well-balanced normal diet with increased calories and proteins needs to be taken to meet the energy demands of the tissue regeneration process.[116,117]

Chronic viral hepatitis is a progressive liver disease leading to the development of cirrhosis in about 20%–30% of patients.[118–122] Several host or viral factors, such as age, gender, consumption of alcohol, duration of infection, and viral coinfections,[118,120,122] have been associated with histological severity and rate of fibrosis progression. Recently, there is increasing interest for hepatic steatosis, which has been found to be related to the extent of fibrosis in patients with chronic hepatitis C.[123,124]

Diabetes mellitus is a common disorder in the general population, but its prevalence is particularly high among cirrhotic patients.[125–127] Data from several studies have suggested that the prevalence of diabetes mellitus is also high among patients with chronic hepatitis C with or without coexisting cirrhosis.[128–130] Moreover, diabetes has been reported to be present more frequently in patients with HCV- than HBV-related chronic liver disease in most but not all studies.[128,130–132]

The possible effect of diabetes mellitus on the histological progression of chronic viral hepatitis has been infrequently studied to date. Diabetes is a comorbid condition of chronic liver disease, mostly NAFLD,[133–135] and biochemical evidence of ongoing liver damage, as expressed by increased aminotransferases activity, may be detected in a large proportion of diabetic patients.[136,137] Moreover, progression to cirrhosis has been documented in several patients with diabetes mellitus and NASH.[138,139] In addition, recent studies have suggested that the presence of diabetes mellitus or even of insulin resistance may be associated with increased fibrosis progression in patients with chronic hepatitis C.[140–143]

## DRUG-INDUCED LIVER INJURY AND NUTRITION

Nutrition is clearly involved in NAFLD and ALD and plays an important role in the support of the patient with viral hepatitis. Given the commonality of nutrition-related liver disorders, the identification of a drug-induced liver injury (DILI) can be difficult and requires a prior understanding of the very common nutrition-related liver disorders that may accompany DILI and complicate its diagnosis. Hepatocellular injury may be associated with hepatic fatty infiltration (steatosis). Histological features of drug-induced steatohepatitis can be similar to alcoholic liver disease or nonalcoholic fatty liver. Drugs associated with this type of injury include amiodarone, methotrexate, valproic acid, tamoxifen, total parenteral nutrition, and nifedipine.

All drugs have the potential to cause injury, but there is an individualistic predisposition to this relatively rare complication of drug administration that remains poorly understood. The liver is particularly susceptible to drug-induced injury because of its inherent role in the clearance, the biotransformation, and the excretion of medications. DILI is now the most common cause of acute liver failure (ALF); it has in fact surpassed acute viral hepatitis in this regard. It is the cause of 25% of hospitalizations for jaundice and accounts for 10% of cases of acute hepatitis. One hepatotoxic drug, acetaminophen, is responsible for over 40% of all incidents of ALF in the United States today.

Despite the strong association of drugs and ALF, the majority of patients with symptomatic acute DILI are expected to completely recover with supportive care after discontinuation of the suspect drug or medicinal herb. In addition, patients with milder episodes of DILI that may be unrecognized are also expected to recover without residual clinical, laboratory, radiological, or histological evidence of liver disease.

Accurate data on the frequency of DILI are not readily available as most cases are asymptomatic with only mild elevations of liver enzymes. For instance, commonly used medications such as nonsteroidal anti-inflammatory drugs (NSAIDs), statins, antidepressants, several antibiotics, and quinidine often cause asymptomatic elevations of transaminase levels. With continued use, adaptation and normalization of the elevated liver enzymes may occur. Fortunately, clinically significant DILI is uncommon—it happens in less than 1 per 1000 patients taking meds at therapeutic doses. Because of this rarity, it is uncommon for a hepatotoxic drug to be identified during clinical trials, which may involve only a few thousand people. Quite often, the potential for liver injury is only recognized after many thousands of patients have been exposed to a medication.

Hepatotoxicity may be intrinsic (predictable) or idiosyncratic (unpredictable) in nature. Intrinsically hepatotoxic agents have dose-related effects. Typically, toxicity becomes evident shortly after exposure. Toxic effects are similar in animals, and the incidence is relatively high. As a result, these drugs may be identified as hepatotoxic long before they are introduced to the market. Idiosyncratic hepatotoxins, however, have an unpredictable effect that is not reproducible in animals and is not dose dependent. With this kind of drug, liver injury may not be evident for many weeks after exposure. Although less common, idiosyncratic reactions are more likely to progress to ALF. Acetaminophen is an example of an intrinsically hepatotoxic agent, while isoniazid and halothane exhibit idiosyncratic hepatotoxicity.

An observation, called "Hy's rule," an observation by the late Dr. Hyman Zimmerman, is frequently used by regulatory agencies in assessing the hepatotoxic potential of drugs being tested in clinical trials. Idiosyncratic hepatocellular injury leading to ALF is a rare form of DILI with a characteristic clinical presentation that includes an acute onset after uneventful treatment with drug for weeks to months. Serum alanine aminotransferase (ALT) rises to very high levels, and the appearance of jaundice indicates a high mortality even if the therapy is discontinued. Drugs that can cause this type of injury almost always are associated with frequent (2%–15% of all treated patients) and minor serum aminotransferase elevations. These elevations are believed to reflect true liver injury but often reverse even if drug therapy is continued. The basis for this "adaptation" is not known, as is why some patients do not adapt and develop progressive liver injury. Understanding how drugs cause severe idiosyncratic hepatocellular toxicity has been frustrated by the lack of good preclinical models. Indeed, because these events occur so rarely, the vast majority of humans are not good models. Registry studies from Sweden, Spain, and the United States have confirmed the validity of Hy's rule by demonstrating a 9%–12% mortality rate in consecutive DILI patients. In patients with suspected DILI, the causative agent should be immediately discontinued, and hospitalized patients with severe coagulopathy or encephalopathy should be referred for potential liver transplantation. Recent studies have shown that DILI can infrequently evolve into chronic liver injury including cirrhosis and even liver-related morbidity and mortality in a minority of patients.[144–146] Conversely, the majority of patients even with serious DILI will recover completely once drug administration is discontinued. For example, 712 of 784 (90.8%) DILI patients with jaundice recovered, and only 72 (9.2%) died or underwent liver transplant surgery.[145] In contrast, the prognosis of patients with severe DILI who progress to ALF with concomitant coagulopathy (i.e., international normalized ratio [INR] > 1.5) and encephalopathy is usually poor.[146,147]

In most Western countries, acetaminophen overdose is the most frequently identified etiology of ALF.[146–149] Fortunately, prognosis is generally better in acetaminophen-induced liver failure patients treated with N-acetylcysteine than in ALF patients with idiosyncratic DILI (i.e., 60%–80% versus 20%–40%, respectively, transplant-free survival).[146,147,149] In the largest prospective series of U.S. ALF patients with idiosyncratic DILI, only 25% recovered once encephalopathy developed.[146] Independent predictors of outcome in ALF due to DILI have not been reported.[146,147]

Recently, the U.S. Acute Liver Failure Study Group demonstrated that the antioxidant N-acetylcysteine may benefit patients with ALF due to DILI, hepatitis B, and other etiologies, particularly in those with early-stage encephalopathy when given intravenously.[150] However, use of corticosteroids in ALF due to DILI is not recommended due to the lack of benefit in previously reported studies.[151,152] Overall, it is recommended to refer all hospitalized patients with severe

DILI to a transplant center in light of their potential for poor outcomes.[153]

DILI is a relatively uncommon adverse drug reaction; it is often not possible to confidently identify the specific culprit when DILI is suspected in a patient who is being treated with multiple medications.[154] Drugs cause liver injuries by many different mechanisms. These injuries resemble almost all-known liver diseases, and there are no pathognomonic findings, even upon liver biopsy, which make diagnosis of DILI certain. Therefore, when possible DILI is suspected, it is essential to gather additional clinical and laboratory information necessary for differential diagnosis of the cause. It is important to observe the time course of the injury and to seek alternative causes of the liver injury, such as acute viral hepatitis A, B, or C; concomitant use of a hepatotoxic drug or exposure to hepatotoxins, autoimmune or alcoholic hepatitis, biliary tract disorders, and circulatory problems of hypotension or right heart congestive failure may cause ischemic or hypoxic hepatopathy. It is also prudent to assess the subject for previously existing liver disease, such as chronic hepatitis C or NASH, which may or may not have been recognized before exposure to the experimental drug.

It should be recognized that DILI may occur also in persons with preexisting liver disease as a superimposed problem. Because available clinical laboratory tests are not ideal biomarkers, the diagnosis of DILI remains generally one of exclusion and thus is typically time and resource intensive. In the context of medical treatment, a biomarker has been defined as "a characteristic that is objectively measured and evaluated as an indicator of … responses to a therapeutic intervention."[145] DILI will often resolve despite continuing treatment with the offending drug(s) due to a process termed adaptation.[146] No current biomarkers can distinguish between patients who are capable of adaptation with continued treatment and patients who will experience progressive liver injury unless treatment is discontinued. Biomarkers that could predict adaptation would be very useful in the treatment of conditions such as tuberculosis, in which DILI is a relatively common occurrence but for which there are limited treatment options.

Drug-induced hepatic injury is the most common reason cited for withdrawal of an approved drug. Early detection can decrease the severity of hepatotoxicity if the drug is discontinued. The manifestations of drug-induced hepatotoxicity are highly variable, ranging from asymptomatic elevation of liver enzymes to fulminant hepatic failure. Knowledge of the commonly implicated agents and high index of suspicion are essential in diagnosis.

In the last few years, the U.S. FDA has withdrawn two drugs from the market for causing severe liver injury: bromfenac and troglitazone. Bromfenac (Duract), an NSAID, was introduced in 1997 as a short-term analgesic for orthopedic patients. Although approved for a dosing period of less than 10 days, patients used it for longer periods. This resulted in more than 50 cases of severe hepatic injury, and the drug had to be withdrawn in 1998. Troglitazone (Rezulin) is a thiazolidinedione and was approved in 1997 as an antidiabetic agent. Over 3 years, more than 90 cases of hepatotoxicity were reported, which resulted in withdrawal of this drug. Pemoline (Cylert), used for attention-deficit disorder and narcolepsy, is no longer available in the United States. The FDA concluded that the overall risk of liver toxicity from pemoline outweighs the benefits. In May 2005, Abbott chose to stop sales and marketing of their brand of pemoline (Cylert) in the United States. In October 2005, all companies that produced generic versions of pemoline also agreed to stop sales and marketing of pemoline. Other drugs that have significant limitations of use because of their hepatotoxic effects are felbamate (Felbatol), an antiepileptic used for complex partial seizures; zileuton (Zyflo), indicated for asthma; tolcapone (Tasmar), used for Parkinson disease; trovafloxacin (Trovan), an antibiotic; benoxaprofen, an NSAID; and tienilic acid, a diuretic.

In April 2010, the U.S. FDA had added a boxed warning, the strongest warning issued by the FDA, to the prescribing information for propylthiouracil (PTU). The boxed warning emphasizes the risk for severe liver injury and ALF, some of which have been fatal. The boxed warning also states that PTU should be reserved for use in those who cannot tolerate other treatments such as methimazole, radioactive iodine, or surgery. The decision to include a boxed warning was based on the FDA's review of post-marketing safety reports and meetings held with the American Thyroid Association, the National Institute of Child Health and Human Development, and the pediatric endocrine clinical community. In June 2009, the FDA issued a report that identified 32 cases (22 adult and 10 pediatric) of serious liver injury associated with PTU. Of the adults, 12 deaths and 5 liver transplants occurred, and among the pediatric patients, 1 death and 6 liver transplants occurred. PTU is indicated for hyperthyroidism due to Graves disease. These reports suggest an increased risk for liver toxicity with PTU compared with methimazole. Serious liver injury has been identified with methimazole in five cases (three resulting in death). PTU is considered as a second-line drug therapy, except in patients who are allergic or intolerant to methimazole or for women who are in the first trimester of pregnancy. Rare cases of embryopathy, including aplasia cutis, have been reported with methimazole during pregnancy. DILI mechanism is classified into two general categories: (1) intrinsic or predictable drug reactions. Drugs that fall into this category cause reproducible injuries in animals, and the injury is dose related. The injury can be due to the drug itself or to a metabolite.

Acetaminophen is a classic example of a known intrinsic or predictable hepatotoxin at super-therapeutic doses. Another classic example is carbon tetrachloride. (2) Idiosyncratic drug reactions can be subdivided into those that are classified as hypersensitivity or immunoallergic and those that are metabolic–idiosyncratic. For hypersensitivity, phenytoin is a classic, if not common, cause of hypersensitivity reactions. The response is characterized by fever, rash, and eosinophilia and is an immune-related response with a typical short latency period of 1–4 weeks. Acetaminophen is the most common drug ingredient in America. It is found in more than 600 different over-the-counter and prescription medicines, including generic and store brand pain relievers, fever reducers, and sleep aids as well as cough, cold, and allergy medicines. Many over-the-counter and prescription medicines may have store brand or generic versions. For example, there are many store brand products that are similar to brands like Tylenol®, NyQuil®, and Robitussin®. Prescription medicines that come in generic form may list the ingredients in place of a drug name. (For example, "hydrocodone and acetaminophen" appear on the generic version of "Vicodin.") A prescription label may list the ingredients, the brand name, or both.

Metabolic–idiosyncratic or immunoallergic reactions may occur through an indirect metabolite of the offending drug. Unlike intrinsic hepatotoxins, the response rate is variable and can occur within a week or up to 1 year later. It occurs in a minority of patients taking the drug, and no clinical manifestations of hypersensitivity are noted. INH toxicity is considered to fall into this class. Not all drugs fall neatly into one of these categories, and overlapping mechanisms may occur with some drugs (e.g., halothane). A large number of these cases remain idiosyncratic and idiopathic in that no offending agent is ever identified.

Reliably establishing whether liver disease has been caused by a drug or a dietary supplement requires the exclusion of other plausible causes and the search for a clinical drug signature. The drug signature consists of the pattern of liver test abnormality, the duration of latency to symptomatic presentation, the presence or absence of immune-mediated hypersensitivity, and the response to drug withdrawal. Assigning causality in DILI due to a particular medication or herbal and dietary supplement relies on clinical history, exclusion of competing causes, prior reports of DILI, and judgment—no objective laboratory or histological tests exist to confirm a diagnosis of suspected DILI. Current causality assessment instruments are based on algorithmic scoring systems but are not widely used. Expert opinion remains the gold standard, but is cumbersome and has limited reproducibility. The lack of a valid and widely available causality assessment method hinders the identification of genetic and biochemical markers that may help better define DILI. Emerging technologies in pharmacogenomics and toxicogenomics may identify such markers if well-defined DILI cases and controls can provide tissue samples for analysis.[155]

Determination of causality also includes an evaluation of individual susceptibility to DILI. This susceptibility is governed by both genetic and environmental factors. Components of the drug signature in conjunction with certain risk factors have been incorporated into formal scoring systems that are predictive of the likelihood of DILI. The most validated scoring system is the Roussel Uclaf causality assessment method, which nonetheless retains certain imperfections.

Mitigating the potential for DILI is achieved by the identification of toxicity signals during clinical trials and the monitoring of liver tests in clinical practice. There are three signals of liver toxicity in clinical trials: (1) a statistically significant doubling (or more) in the incidence of serum ALT elevation >3 × the upper limit of normal (ULN), (2) any incidence of serum ALT elevation >8 to 10 × ULN, and (3) any incidence of serum ALT elevation >3 × ULN accompanied

by a serum bilirubin elevation >2 × ULN. Monitoring of liver tests in clinical practice has shown unconvincing efficacy, but where a benefit–risk analysis would favor continued therapy, monthly monitoring may have some benefit compared with no monitoring at all.[156]

With rare exception, treatment of DILI is principally supportive. Drug toxicity is the most common cause of ALF, defined as a prolonged prothrombin time (INR ≥ 1.5) and any degree of mental alteration occurring <26 weeks after the onset of illness in a patient without preexisting cirrhosis. A patient who meets these criteria must be evaluated for liver transplantation. The pathogenesis of DILI can be examined on the basis of the two principal patterns of injury. The hepatocellular pattern is characterized by a predominant rise in the level of transaminases and results from the demise of hepatocytes by means of either apoptosis or necrosis. The cholestatic pattern is characterized by a predominant rise of the serum alkaline phosphatase level and usually results from injury to the bile ductular cells either directly by the drug or its metabolite or indirectly by an adaptive immune response.

Although uncommon, DILI can be a severe and sometimes life-threatening complication of drug therapy. Physicians need to know which medications have the highest risk of causing liver toxicity and which patients are most susceptible. Whenever possible, choose the drug with the superior safety profile, particularly for people at high risk for DILI. In patients with evidence of unexplained liver injury, seek a history of prescriptions, illicit drugs, over-the-counter medications, and specific herbal medications. Finally, health-care professionals need to be aware of the large number of combination medications that contain acetaminophen, raising the possibility that individuals receiving multiple agents may inadvertently overdose.

## MALNUTRITION IN CIRRHOSIS

The opposite situation to obesity and associated fatty liver is the malnutrition encountered in liver cirrhosis or end-stage liver disease. Liver failure results in over 26,000 deaths per year, making it the twelfth leading cause of death in the United States. Patients with compensated chronic liver failure (without ascites, variceal bleeding, encephalopathy, or jaundice) have a median survival of 12 years. After decompensation, median survival drops to ~2 years. A validated index called the CPT (Child–Turcotte–Pugh) predicts prognosis for patients without liver transplantation (see Table 51.1).

Patients are grouped into three classes based on the total CTP score, which is simply the sum of the scores for each of the 5 variables. Patients scoring 5–6 points are considered to have "class A" failure; their 1- and 2-year median survivals are 95% and 90%, respectively. A score of 7–9 is considered class B with median survivals of 80% at 1 year and 70% at 2 years. Class C patients (10–15) have far greater mortality: 1-year median survival is 45%, and 2 year is 38%. Variations in the timing and subjectivity inherent in the scoring of the CTP (e.g., in grading ascites or encephalopathy) are its major limitations. In addition,

**TABLE 51.1**

**CTP Score Includes Five Variables, Each Scored 1–3**

| | Numerical Value | | |
|---|---|---|---|
| Ascites | None | Slight | Moderate/severe |
| Encephalopathy | None | Grade 1–2 | Grade 3–4 |
| Bilirubin (mg/dL) | < 2.0 | 2.0–3.0 | >3.0 |
| Albumin (mg/L) | > 3.5 | 2.8–3.5 | <2.8 |
| Increase in seconds from normal prothrombin time | 1–3 | 4–6 | >6.0 |

the scale does not include renal function, an important prognostic factor in liver failure. The model for end-stage liver disease (MELD) score was developed in 2000 to overcome the previously mentioned limitations and determine survival benefit from transjugular intrahepatic portosystemic shunting. It is currently used to help determine organ allocation for liver transplantation, and there is increasing evidence that it can also be used generally to predict survival in patients with chronic liver failure.[157,158] The MELD score relies on laboratory values alone (serum creatinine, total bilirubin, and INR). An additional benefit over CTP is that it can predict prognosis on the order of months with more precision—making it helpful for determining hospice eligibility in the United States. The formula to calculate MELD score is complex, and a calculator can be found at http://www.unos.org/resources/meldPeldCalculator.asp.

Malnutrition in patients with cirrhosis is prevalent and is found in 25% of patients with CTP class A up to 80% in patients with CTP class C. Most cirrhotic patients have inadequate caloric intake due to multiple factors[159–161] including early satiety related to impaired gastric relaxation and ascites in addition to poor appetite thought related to the high level of cytokines such as TNF-alpha. Furthermore, many of them have nutrient malabsorption due to portal hypertension.[162] Moreover, due to the poor capacity of the liver to store glucose in the form of glycogen, the cirrhotic patient switches to gluconeogenesis from amino acids after an overnight fast. This is observed in noncirrhotic patients only after 3 days of fasting. This in addition leads to poor utilization of proteins after a meal and predisposes the cirrhotic patient to being in negative nitrogen balance and PCM.[163] PCM is also a very strong predictor of morbidity and mortality[164,165] even after controlling for other factors.[166] In one report with 50 patients with cirrhosis, it was found that uncontrolled ascites, hepatic encephalopathy, spontaneous bacterial peritonitis, and hepatorenal syndrome developed in 65.5% of malnourished patients versus 11.8% of well-nourished ones and among the PCM patients, 20% were dead at 1 year versus none in the non-PCM group.[164] In another report that looked at 212 patients, nutrition was an important predictor of survival, and after controlling for other factors, survival at 1 year was less than 65% in severely malnourished cirrhotic patients compared to over 85% in patients with better nutrition.[166]

## REFERENCES

1. Clark JM, Diehl AM. *JAMA* 289:3000;2003.
2. Law K, Brunt EM. *Clin Liver Dis* 14:591;2010.
3. Vernon G, Baranova A, Younossi ZM. *Aliment Pharmacol Ther* 34:274;2011.
4. Dowman JK, Tomlinson JW, Newsome PN. *Aliment Pharmacol Ther* 33:525;2011.
5. Smith BW, Adams LA. *Crit Rev Clin Lab Sci* 48:97;2011.
6. Vanni E, Bugianesi E, Kotronen A et al. *Dig Liver Dis* 42:320;2010.
7. Bugianesi E, Moscatiello S, Ciaravella MF, Marchesini G. *Curr Pharm Des* 16:1941;2010.
8. McCullough AJ. *J Clin Gastroenterol* 40:S17;2006.
9. Nomura K, Yamanouchi T. *J Nutr Biochem* 23:203;2012.
10. Castro GS, Cardoso JF, Vannucchi H et al. *Acta Cir Bras* 26:45;2011.
11. Anania FA. *J Hepatol* 55:218;2011.
12. Alisi A, Manco M, Pezzullo M, Nobili V. *Hepatology* 53:372;2011.
13. Lim JS, Mietus-Snyder M, Valente A et al. *Nat Rev Gastroenterol Hepatol* 7:251;2010.
14. Nseir W, Nassar F, Assy N. *World J Gastroenterol* 16:2579;2010.
15. Stanhope KL, Havel PJ. *Ann N Y Acad Sci* 1190:15;2010.
16. Lustig RH. *J Am Diet Assoc* 110:1307;2010.
17. Tappy L, Lê KA, Tran C, Paquot N. *Nutrition* 26:1044;2010.
18. Gallagher EJ, Leroith D, Karnieli E. *Med Clin North Am* 95:855;2011.
19. McCullough AJ. *J Dig Dis* 12:333;2011.
20. Moore JB. *Proc Nutr Soc* 69:211;2010.
21. Gallagher EJ, Leroith D, Karnieli E. *Mt Sinai J Med* 77:511;2010.
22. Huang D, Dhawan T, Young S et al. *Lipids Health Dis* 10:20;2011.
23. Vilà L, Rebollo A, Adalsteisson GS et al. *Toxicol Appl Pharmacol* 251:32;2011.
24. Teff KL, Elliott SS, Tschöp M et al. *J Clin Endocrinol Metab* 89:2963;2004.
25. Lê KA, Tappy L. *Curr Opin Clin Nutr Metab Care* 9:469;2006.
26. D'Angelo G, Elmarakby AA, Pollock DM, Stepp DW. *Hypertension* 46:806;2005.
27. Ackerman Z, Oron-Herman M, Grozovski M et al. *Hypertension* 45:1012;2005.
28. Sanyal A, Chalasani N, Kowdley K et al. *NEJM* 362:1675;2010.
29. Zhu FS, Liu S, Chen XM et al. *World J Gastroenterol* 14:6395;2008.
30. Huber W, Scharf G, Rossmanith W et al. *Arch Toxicol* 75:685;2002.
31. Scharf G, Prustomersky S, Huber W. *Adv Exp Med Biol* 500:535;2001.
32. Lee C. *Clinica Chimica Acta* 295:141;2000.
33. Petersen KF, Dufour S, Befroy D et al. *Diabetes* 54:603;2005.
34. Paredes AH, Torres DM, Harrison SA. *Clin Liver Dis* 16:397;2012.
35. Sofair AN, Barry V, Manos MM et al. *J Clin Gastroenterol* 44:301;2010.
36. Orholm M, Sorensen TI, Bentsen, K et al. *Liver* 5:253;1985.
37. DiMartini A, Crone C, Dew MA. *Clin Liver Dis* 15:727;2011.
38. Kochanek KD, Xu J, Murphy SL et al. National Vital Statistics Reports. Centers for Disease Control and Prevention, Vol. 60, p. 38, 2011.

39. Propst A, Propst T, Zangerl G et al. *Dig Dis Sci* 40:1805;1995.
40. Chedid A, Mendenhall CL, Gartside P et al. *Am J Gastroenterol* 86:210;1991.
41. Kim, WR, Brown Jr., RS, Terrault NA, El-Serag H. *Hepatology* 36:227;2002.
42. Thun MJ, Peto R, Lopez AD et al. *N Engl J Med* 337:1705;1997.
43. Becker U, Deis A, Sorensen TI et al. *Hepatology* 23:1025;1996.
44. Fuchs CS, Stampfer MJ, Colditz GA et al. *N Engl J Med* 332:1245;1995.
45. Grant BF, Dufour MC, Harford TC. *Semin Liver Dis* 8:12;1988.
46. Arteel G, Marsano L, Mendez C et al. *Best Pract Res Clin Gastroenterol* 17:625;2003.
47. Espinoza P, Ducot B, Pelletier G et al. *Dig Dis Sci* 32:244;1987.
48. Lefkowitch JH. *Clin Liver Dis* 9:37;2005.
49. Mathurin P, Beuzin F, Louvet A et al. *Aliment Pharmacol Ther* 25:1047;2007.
50. Lucey MR, Mathurin P, Morgan TR. *N Engl J Med* 360:2758;2009.
51. Miller WR, Walters ST, Bennett ME. *J Stud Alcohol* 62:211;2001.
52. Kaner EF, Dickinson HO, Beyer F et al. *Drug Alcohol Rev* 28:301;2009.
53. Moos RH, King MJ, Patterson MA. *Psychiatr Serv* 47:68;1996.
54. Bouza C, Angeles M, Munoz A, Amate JM. *Addiction* 99:811;2004.
55. Williams SH. *Am Fam Physician* 72:1775;2005.
56. Garbutt JC, West SL, Carey TS et al. *JAMA* 281:1318;1999.
57. Kenna GA, Lomastro TL, Schiesl A et al. *Curr Drug Abuse Rev* 2:135;2009.
58. Addolorato G, Leggio L, Ferrulli A et al. *Lancet* 370:1915;2007.
59. Corrao G, Lepore AR, Torchio P et al. *Eur J Epidemiol* 10:657;1994.
60. Klatsky AL, Armstrong MA. *Am J Epidemiol* 136:1248;1992.
61. Naveau S, Giraud V, Borotto E et al. *Hepatology* 25:108;1997.
62. Halsted, CH. *Semin Liver Dis* 24:289;2004.
63. Prijatmoko D, Strauss BJG, Lambert JR et al. *Gastroenterology* 103:1839;1993.
64. Nielsen K, Kondrup J, Martinsen L et al. *Br J Nutr* 69:665;1993.
65. Kang YJ, Zhou Z. *Mol Aspects Med* 26:391;2005.
66. Raynard B, Balian A, Fallik D et al. *Hepatology* 35:635;2002.
67. Lieber CS. *Hepatol Res* 28:1;2004.
68. Griffith CM, Schenker S. *Alcohol Res Health* 29:296;2006.
69. John WJ, Phillips R, Ott L et al. *J Parenter Enteral Nutr* 13:124;1989.
70. Hirsch S, Bunout D, de la Maza P et al. *J Parenter Enteral Nutr* 17:119;1993.
71. Hirsch S, de la Maza MP, Gattas V et al. *J Am Coll Nutr* 18:434;1999.
72. Plank LD, Gane EJ, Peng S et al. *Hepatology* 48:557;2008.
73. Mendenhall CL, Moritz TE, Roselle GA et al. *J Parenter Enteral Nutr* 19:258;1995.
74. Mendenhall CL, Moritz TE, Roselle GA et al. *Hepatology* 17:564;1993.
75. Mendenhall CL, Anderson S, Weesner RE et al. *Am J Med* 76:211;1984.
76. Mendenhall C, Bongiovanni G, Goldberg S et al. *J Parenter Enteral Nutr* 9:590;1985.
77. Mendenhall CL, Tosch T, Weesner RE et al. *Am J Clin Nutr* 43:213;1986.
78. Cabre E, Rodriguez-Iglesias P, Caballeria J et al. *Hepatology* 32:36;2000.
79. Kearns PJ, Young H, Garcia G et al. *Gastroenterology* 102:200;1992.
80. Simon D, Galambos JT. *J Hepatol* 7:200;1988.
81. McCullough AJ, O'Connor JF. *Am J Gastroenterol* 93:2022;1998.
82. Marchesini G, Bianchi G, Merli M et al. *Gastroenterology* 124:1792;2003.
83. Charlton, M. *J Nutr* 136:295S;2006.
84. Calvey H, Davis M, Williams R. *J Hepatol* 1:141;1985.
85. Tan HH, Virmani S, Martin P. *Mt Sinai J Med* 76:484;2009.
86. Dey A, Cederbaum AI. *Hepatology* 43:S63;2006.
87. Szuster-Ciesielska A, Daniluk J, Kandefer-Szerszen M. *Med Sci Monit* 8:CR419;2002.
88. Hill DB, Devalaraja R, Joshi-Barve S et al. *Clin Biochem* 32:563;1999.
89. Evstigneeva RP, Volkov IM, Chudinova VV. *Membr Cell Biol* 12:151;1998.
90. Lee KS, Buck M, Houglum K, Chojkier, M. *J Clin Invest* 96:2461;1995.
91. de la Maza MP, Petermann M, Bunout D, Hirsch. *S J Am Coll Nutr* 14:192;1995.
92. Mezey E, Potter JJ, Rennie-Tankersley L et al. *J Hepatol* 40:40;2004.
93. Lieber CS, Robins SJ, Li J et al. *Gastroenterology* 106:152;1994.
94. Okiyama W, Tanaka N, Nakajima T et al. *J Hepatol* 50:1236;2009.
95. Cao Q, Mak KM, Lieber CS. *J Lab Clin Med* 139:202;2002.
96. Lieber CS, Weiss DG, Groszmann R et al. *Alcohol Clin Exp Res* 27:1765;2003.
97. Lieber CS, Leo MA, Cao Q et al. *J Clin Gastroenterol* 37:336;2003.
98. Ferenci P, Dragosics B, Dittrich H et al. *J Hepatol* 9:105;1989.
99. Lucena MI, Andrade RJ, de la Cruz JP et al. *Int J Clin Pharmacol Ther* 40:2;2002.
100. Pares A, Planas R, Torres M et al. *J Hepatol* 28:615;1998.
101. Rambaldi A, Gluud C. *Cochrane Database Syst Rev* 2:CD002235;2006.
102. Lee TD, Sadda MR, Mendler MH et al. *Alcohol Clin Exp Res* 28:173;2004.
103. Lieber CS. *Alcohol* 27:173;2002.
104. Karaa A, Thompson KJ, McKillop IH et al. *Shock* 30:197;2008.
105. Purohit V, Abdelmalek MF, Barve S et al. *Am J Clin Nutr* 86:14;2007.
106. Kharbanda KK. *Semin Liver Dis* 29:155;2009.
107. Kharbanda KK, Mailliard ME, Baldwin CR et al. *J Hepatol* 46:314;2007.
108. Kim SJ, Jung YS, Kwon do Y, Kim YC. *Biochem Biophys Res Commun* 368:893;2008.
109. Aggarwal R, Indian J. *Gastroenterol* 26(Editorial):3;2007.
110. Aggarwal R, Shahi H, Naik S et al. *J Hepatol* 26:1425;1997.
111. Williams SR. Diseases of the liver, gall bladder and pancreas. In: Smith JM, ed. *Diet Therapy*, 2nd edn. Mosby Publications, London, U.K., p. 119, 1995.
112. Han S-HB, Saab S, Martin P. *Curr Treat Options Gastroenterol* 3:481;2000.
113. Antia EP, Abraham P. In: Galanter M, ed. *Clinical Dietetics and Nutrition*, 4th edn. Oxford University Press, New York, p. 298, 2005.

114. Leone NC, Ratner F, Diefnbach WCL. *Ann N Y Acad Sci* 57:948;1954.
115. Koff RS. Acute viral hepatitis. In: Lawrence SF, Emmet BK, eds. *Handbook of Liver Disease*, 2nd edn. Elsevier Publications, New Delhi, India, p. 35, 2005.
116. Schaffner F. *Can Med Accos J* 106:505;1972.
117. Iber FL, Mendeloff AL. *Arch Intern Med* 109:110;1962.
118. Fattovich G, Brollo L, Giustina G et al. *Gut* 32:294;1991.
119. Tong MJ, EI-Farra NS, Reikes AR, Co RL. *N Engl J Med* 332:1463;1995.
120. Poynard T, Bedossa P, Opolon P. *Lancet* 349:825;1997.
121. Niederau C, Lange S, Heintges T et al. *Hepatology* 28:1687;1998.
122. Papatheodoridis GV, Manesis E, Hadziyannis SJ. *J Hepatol* 34:306;2001.
123. Hourigan LF, Macdonald GA, Purdie D et al. *Hepatology* 29:1215;1999.
124. Clouston A, Jonsson JR, Purdie DM et al. *J Hepatol* 34:314;2001.
125. Megeysi C, Samols E, Marks V. *Lancet* 2:1051;1967.
126. Petrides AS, Vogt C, Schulze-Berge D et al. *Hepatology* 19:616;1994.
127. Han SH, Martin P. *J Clin Gastroenterol* 30:227;2000.
128. Mason AL, Lau JY, Hoang N et al. *Hepatology* 29:328;1999.
129. Knobler H, Schihmanter R, Zifroni A et al. *Mayo Clin Proc* 75:355;2000.
130. Mehta SH, Brancati FL, Sulkowski MS et al. *Ann Intern Med* 133:592;2000.
131. Caronia S, Taylor K, Pagliaro L et al. *Hepatology* 30:1059;1999.
132. Mangia A, Schiavone G, Lezzi G et al. *Am J Gastroenterol* 93:2363;1998.
133. Clark JM, Brancati FL, Diehl AM. *Gastroenterology* 122:1649;2002.
134. James OF, Day CP. *J Hepatol* 29:495;1998.
135. El-Serag HB, Tran T, Everhart JE. *Gastroenterology* 126:460;2004.
136. Marchesini G, Brizi M, Morselli-Labate AM et al. *Am J Med* 107:450;1999.
137. Falck-Ytter Y, Younossi ZM, Marchesini G, McCullough AJ. *Semin Liver Dis* 21:17;2001.
138. Falchuk K, Fiske SC, Haggitt RC et al. *Gastroenterology* 78:535;1980.
139. Katbamna BH, Petrelli M, McCullough AJ. The liver in diabetes mellitus and hyperlipidemia. In: Gitlin N, ed. *The Liver and Systemic Disease*. Churchill Livingstone, New York, p. 73, 1997.
140. Ong JP, Younossi ZM, Speer C et al. *Liver* 21:266;2001.
141. Monto A, Alonzo J, Watson JJ et al. *Hepatology* 36:729;2002.
142. Ortiz V, Berenguer M, Rayon JM et al. *Am J Gastroenterol* 97:2408;2002.
143. Hui JM, Sud A, Farrell GC et al. *Gastroenterology* 125:1695;2003.
144. Zimmerman H. Hepatotoxicity: The Adverse Effects of Drugs and Other Chemicals on the Liver. 2nd edn. Lippincott Williams & Wilkins, Philadelphia, PA, 1999.
145. Björnsson E, Olsson R. *Hepatology* 42:481;2005.
146. Ostapowicz G, Fontana RJ, Schiødt FV et al. *Ann Intern Med* 137:947;2002.
147. Wei G, Bergquist A, Broomé U et al. *J Intern Med* 262:393;2007.
148. Larson AM, Polson J, Fontana RJ et al. *Hepatology* 42:1364;2005.
149. Chun LJ, Tong MJ, Busuttil RW, Hiatt JR. *J Clin Gastroenterol* 43:342;2009.
150. Lee WM, Hynan LS, Rossaro L et al. *Gastroenterology* 137:856;2009.
151. Bacardi R. *Gut* 20:620;1979.
152. Dechene A, Treichel U, Gerken G et al. *Hepatology* 42:358A;2005.
153. Fontana RJ. *Semin Liver Dis* 28:175;2008.
154. Hayashi PH. *Semin Liver Dis* 29:348;2009.
155. Biomarkers Definitions Working Group. *Clin Pharmacol Ther* 69:89;2001.
156. Watkins PB, Seeff LB. *Hepatology* 43:618;2006.
157. Cholongitas E, Papatheodoridis GV, Vangeli M et al. *Aliment Pharmacol Ther* 22:1079;2005.
158. Said A, Williams J, Holden J et al. *J Hepatology* 40:897;2004.
159. Minino AM, Heron MP, Smith BL et al. National Vital Statistics Reports, Vol. 54, p. 1, 2006.
160. D'Amico G, Garcia-Tsao G, Pagliaro L. *J Hepatology* 44:217;2006.
161. Diehl A. Alcoholic and nonalcoholic steatohepatitis. In: Goldman L, Ausiello D, eds. *Cecil Textbook of Medicine*. 22nd edn., Saunders, Philadelphia, PA, p. 935, 2004.
162. Tsiaousi ET, Hatzitolios AI, Trygonis SK et al. *J Gastroenterol Hepatol* 23:527;2008.
163. Kondrup J. *Best Pract Res Clin Gastroenterol* 20:547;2006.
164. Alvares-da-Silva MR, Reverbel da Silveira T. *Nutrition* 21:113;2005.
165. Gunsar F, Raimondo ML, Jones S et al. *Aliment Pharmacol Ther* 24:563;2006.
166. Alberino F, Gatta A, Amodio P et al. *Nutrition* 17:445;2001.

# 52 Food Allergy and Food Intolerance

*David Heber*

## CONTENTS

## INTRODUCTION

During the last 20 years, the reported prevalence of food allergies has significantly increased. However, it is not clear whether the prevalence of allergy has actually increased over the years or whether the increased reporting of this entity is merely a reflection of an increased public awareness or even based on false perceptions.[1,2] There are striking differences between the reported prevalence of allergy based on self-reporting and based on objective criteria. Among well-designed studies that were population based and utilized an oral food challenge for diagnosis, a wide range of prevalence was noted for cow's milk[3,4] and peanut allergy[4,5] (0.5% vs. 5.6% and 0.15% vs. 3.0%, respectively). While genetic differences fail to explain the disparities, the timing of exposure, the confounding environmental factors, and the interpretation of oral food challenge results may each account in part for the large variations in reported incidences.

Food intolerances are instances where symptoms such as fatigue, irritable bowel syndrome, weight gain, and migraine headache are ascribed to food allergies. These disorders are far more common than food allergies. A recent phenomenon has been the issue of gluten intolerance rather than confirmed gluten enteropathy or celiac disease. Such individuals ascribe symptoms and weight gain to their ingestion of gluten-containing grains. They may lose weight on a gluten-free diet because they eliminate refined carbohydrate calories without replacing them.

The correct diagnosis of food allergy is crucial not only to avoid inadvertent exposure and subsequent risk of anaphylaxis in a truly food allergic patient but also, at the other end of the spectrum, to prevent misdiagnosis in nonallergic individuals. The latter may lead to unnecessary dietary restrictions leading to malnutrition.[6] The gold standard for the diagnosis of a food allergy is the oral food challenge. However, this procedure is expensive, time and labor consuming, and not readily available for all patients.

Individuals may attribute a variety of illnesses or symptoms to a "food allergy." Surveys of adults have shown that 18%–22% believe that they have a food allergy and 28% of parents suspect a food allergy in their infants and young children.[7–9] However, true food allergy affects 6%–8% of children and approximately 3.5% of adults.[9–12] The way in which food allergy is defined may, in part, explain the discrepancy between suspected and true food allergy. A food allergy is an adverse *immune response* directed toward protein in food. This is in contrast to a larger number of nonimmune-mediated adverse reactions to food.[13] The nonimmune-mediated reactions include those caused by toxins in foods, such as spoiled foods, which would affect anyone ingesting the tainted food, pharmacological responses, and adverse reactions caused by a particular condition of the affected individual, such as a digestive problem (*food intolerance*).

Examples of food intolerance and non-immunological toxic or adverse reactions to foods include (1) lactose intolerance manifested as bloating and diarrhea from an inability to digest lactose. This may be dose related. There is a loss of lactase in aging, while others have loss of lactase due to intestinal injury or genetic absence or reduction in intestinal lactase; (2) tyramine sensitivity due to the presence of tyramine in hard cheeses can trigger a migraine headache; (3) histamine released from spoiled dark meat fish such as tuna can result in oral pruritus, flushing, vomiting, and hives; and (4) caffeine can cause heart palpitations and rapid pulse at high doses or in individuals not accustomed to caffeine consumption.

## PHYSIOLOGY OF FOOD ALLERGIES

A large number of potentially immunoreactive food proteins pass through the gut, but the normal response to these foreign proteins is to recognize but ignore them, a process termed "oral tolerance."[14] The gastrointestinal component of immune reactivity has a daunting task of identifying gut pathogens and eliminating them while allowing certain bacteria, gut flora, to remain while simultaneously avoiding adverse immune responses to dietary nutrients. Approximately 2% of ingested food enters the bloodstream in an immunologically intact form but causes no symptoms in the normal individual. It remains unclear why some individuals develop food allergies, but a genetic predisposition toward allergic responses plays a role.[15] For those individuals predisposed to food allergies, food allergens can elicit specific responses in several ways.

Allergic reactions that occur promptly following ingestion of a causal food protein typically are the result of the generation of IgE antibodies, an immune protein that recognizes and binds the triggering food protein.[11,16]

Despite the low pH in the stomach and the presence of proteolytic enzymes that can degrade nutrients in the upper gastrointestinal tract, some food components are resistant to degradation, and immunogenic material enters the intestinal lumen. Orally administered antigen (Ag) has been detected in the gut epithelium and the lamina propria within minutes after feeding[17] and Ag-loaded CD11c + cells in the lamina propria 30–60 min after feeding mice labeled as dextran or ovalbumin.[18] How luminal Ag gains access to dendritic cells to activate immune responses through the supposedly impermeable epithelial (Ep) barrier remains something of a mystery. Material of low molecular weight, such as haptens and polypeptides, may pass directly across the epithelium by paracellular diffusion through pores in the tight junctions connecting Ep cells. Conversely, larger molecular complexes can be taken across enterocytes by transcytosis after fluid phase uptake at the apical membrane.

When a protein enters the intestine, immune cells, termed dendritic cells, act to present the Ag by processing the protein (usually a glycoprotein) and presenting a small portion of the protein to T cells, a type of lymphocyte that specifically recognizes the protein fragment. In the normal setting, lower Ag exposure results from an intact Ep barrier, IgA production, and other innate immune defense

mechanisms, and a Th3 predominates with secretion of IL-10 and TGF-β. No specific IgE is produced, and eosinophils and mast cells (MCs) remain in a resting state. This results in a state of controlled inflammation that characterizes the normal gut mucosa. In contrast, altered Ep permeability leads to an increased Ag load and certain forms of Ag-presenting cells (APCs), including Ep CD86⁺ cells and dendritic cell type 2 (DC2), result in activation of B lymphocytes producing IgE (B ∈ cell) and a bias toward a Th2 form of immune response with IL-4, IL-5, and IL-13 production. MC activation leads to the release of various factors, including TNF-α, and secondary recruitment and activation of eosinophils and neutrophils. Together, these events lead to altered gut function, inflammation, and clinical manifestations of GI food allergy (see Figure 52.1).

Chronic disease attributed to food allergy, for example, rashes (atopic dermatitis [AD]) or gastrointestinal disorders, involves an immune response to food protein but may not involve the generation of IgE antibody (non-IgE mediated).[11,16,20] In this case, the T cell may, through direct interaction with specific receptors on the cells, elaborate mediators (cytokines) with direct effects. An example is the release of tumor necrosis factor alpha that causes gut edema in certain forms of cow's milk allergy (CMA).[21] Further research is under way to better delineate the mechanisms of non-IgE-mediated food allergy.

## FOOD ALLERGENS

A rather short list of foods/food groups accounts for the majority (85%–90%) of food allergic reactions: chicken egg, cow's milk, wheat, soybean, peanut, tree nuts (e.g., walnut, cashew), fish (e.g., tuna, salmon, cod), and shellfish (e.g., shrimp, crab).[9,10,22] However, virtually any food protein could elicit an allergic response.[23] Many of the allergenic food proteins have been characterized and are generally heat-stable, water-soluble glycoproteins from 10 to 70 kD in size. For many of these proteins, the particular allergenic epitopes that bind IgE or T cell receptors have been mapped.[24,25]

## FOOD ALLERGY VERSUS FOOD INTOLERANCE

The target organs of food allergy include the skin and the gastrointestinal and respiratory tracts. The pathophysiological basis of the disorders may be IgE mediated, non-IgE mediated, or both.[16] Disorders with an acute onset occurring within minutes to an hour after food ingestion are typically mediated by IgE antibody, while those that are more chronic and occur hours after ingestion are usually not IgE mediated.

A variety of symptoms and medical problems have been attributed to food allergy, for example, headaches, seizures, behavioral disorders, fatigue, and arthritis, but many of these are either false associations or adverse reactions that are not immunological in nature.[26] Food allergy may play a role in a minority of patients with migraine

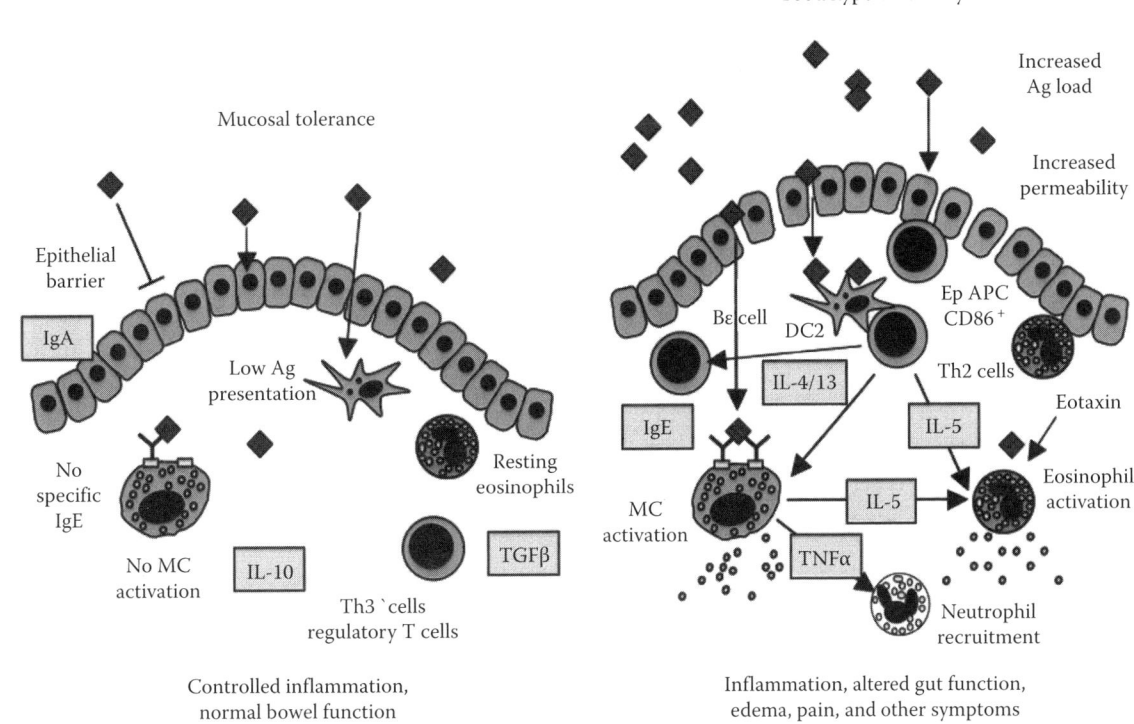

**FIGURE 52.1** Mechanisms leading to mucosal tolerance or hypersensitivity to food Ags in the GI tract. (From Bischoff, S. and Crowe, S.E., *Gastroenterology*, 128, 1089, 2005. With permission.)

headaches,[27] although the pharmacological activity of certain chemicals that are found in some foods (i.e., tyramine in cheeses) is more often responsible.

The role of food allergy in childhood behavioral disorders is also controversial. Although a subset of patients with behavioral disorders may be affected by food dyes,[28] there is no convincing evidence that food allergy per se plays a direct role in these disorders and children are not allergic to "sugar."[29] On the other hand, for individuals with these ailments who also have bona fide allergies, treatment to relieve symptoms of asthma, AD, and hay fever should be pursued in parallel to treatment directed at the unrelated disorder.

## SKIN REACTIONS

Urticaria or "hives" are characterized by transient pruritic and erythematous raised lesions with central clearing and a surrounding area of erythema, similar in appearance to a mosquito bite. The rash should leave no residual lesions after resolution. Hives may sometimes be accompanied by localized swelling (angioedema). Although there are many causes of acute urticaria, food allergy accounts for up to 20% of episodes.[30] The immediate onset of hives is mediated by specific IgE to food protein. Lesions usually occur within an hour of ingestion or skin contact with the causal food. Chronic urticaria resulting from food allergies is characterized by periods of hives that continue to occur over 6 weeks. Only 1.4% of chronic/persistent urticaria is associated with food allergy,[31] so a search for a causative food in the initial

evaluation of this illness is often negative. In some cases, topical exposure to a food (e.g., on the skin of the face) can cause a local reaction either through irritation or through specific immune mechanisms.[32] This may be observed when young children are eating a food they tolerate but develop hives around the lips.

AD is a chronic and relapsing rash characterized by a typical distribution on the extensor surfaces and face of infants or creases in older children and adults and extreme pruritus.[33] It is often associated with allergic disorders (asthma and allergic rhinitis) and with a family history of allergy. Both IgE-antibody-mediated and non-IgE-mediated (cellular) food allergic mechanisms have been identified in disorder.[34–36] Clinical studies utilizing double-blind, placebo-controlled food challenges (DBPCFC) have shown that one-third of children with moderate to severe AD have food allergy.[33,37] The more severe the rash, the more likely that food allergy is associated.[38] However, AD is rarely associated with food allergy in adults.[39]

Dermatitis herpetiformis (DH) is a chronic papulovesicular skin disorder with lesions distributed over the extensor surfaces of the elbows, knees, and buttocks.[40] Immunohistological examination of the lesions reveals the deposition of granular IgA antibody at the dermoepidermal junction. The disorder is associated with a specific non-IgE-mediated immune response to gluten (a protein found in grains such as wheat, barley, and rye). Although related to celiac disease, there may be no associated gastrointestinal complaints. The rash abates with the elimination of gluten from the diet.

## GASTROINTESTINAL REACTIONS

Immediate gastrointestinal hypersensitivity involves an immediate onset of gastrointestinal symptoms following the ingestion of a triggering food protein varying from minutes up to 2 h. Symptoms may include nausea, vomiting, abdominal pain, and diarrhea. This reaction is more commonly associated with reactions in other organ systems, such as during systemic anaphylaxis in patients with other atopic diseases.[26] For example, children with AD undergoing oral food challenges with foods to which they have specific IgE antibody will sometimes manifest only gastrointestinal symptoms.[41]

A pollen-like food allergy reaction to ingestion includes pruritus and angioedema of the lips, tongue, and palate. These symptoms occur while eating certain fresh fruits and vegetables.[42,43] The reaction occurs primarily in adults with pollen allergy (hay fever) sensitized to cross-reacting proteins in particular fruits and vegetables.[44,45] For example, (1) ragweed pollen cross-reacts with proteins found in melons; (2) grass pollen cross-reacts with proteins found in peaches, potato, tomato, and cherries; and (3) birch pollen cross-reacts with apple, carrot, cherry, apricot, plum, and celery. The proteins are labile, and cooked forms of the fruits and vegetables generally do not usually induce symptoms.

Food allergy is a possible cause of rectal bleeding due to colitis in infants. Infants with this disorder are typically healthy but have streaks of blood mixed with mucus in their stool. The most common causal food is cow's milk or soy, and breast-fed infants can develop this reaction from small amounts of protein passed through breast milk in mothers ingesting the causal protein. Tests for food allergy are usually negative. Maternal avoidance of the causal protein will usually resolve symptoms for the breast-fed infant. In infants fed with cow's milk or soy formula, substitution with a protein hydrolysate formula generally leads to cessation of obvious bleeding within 72 h. The majority of infants who develop this condition while ingesting protein hydrolysate formulas will experience resolution of bleeding with the substitution of an amino-acid-based formula.

Infants or young children with food-induced protein enteropathy may experience failure to thrive, diarrhea, emesis, and hypoproteinemia usually related to an immunological reaction to cow's milk protein.[46,47] The syndrome may also occur following infectious gastroenteritis in infants. Patchy villous atrophy with cellular infiltrate on biopsy is a characteristic. Diagnosis is based upon the combined findings from endoscopy/biopsy, allergen elimination, and challenge. While this syndrome resembles celiac disease, resolution generally occurs in 1–2 years, and there is no association with neoplasia.

Initially described and defined by Powell,[48,49] a protein-induced enterocolitis syndrome is characterized by a symptom complex of profuse vomiting and diarrhea diagnosed in infancy during chronic ingestion of the causal food protein, usually cow's milk or soy. Since both small and large bowels are involved, the term "enterocolitis" is used. When the causal protein is reintroduced after a period of avoidance, symptoms characteristically develop after a delay of 2 h, with profuse vomiting and later diarrhea. There is also an accompanying increase in the peripheral polymorphonuclear leukocyte count, and in about 20% of episodes, severe acidosis and dehydration may occur. Confirmation of the allergy includes a negative search for other causes, an improvement when not ingesting the causal protein, and a positive oral challenge resulting in the characteristic symptoms/signs. Approximately half of the infants react to both cow's milk and soy. Sensitivity to milk is lost in 60% and to soy in 25% of the patients after 2 years from the time of presentation.[50] Treatment with a hydrolyzed cow's milk formula is advised, although some patients may react to the residual peptides in these formulas, requiring an amino-acid-based formula.[51] Solid foods, particularly oat and rice, may also induce food-protein-induced enterocolitis syndrome (FPIES).[52]

An infiltration of esophagus, gastric or intestinal walls with eosinophils, peripheral eosinophilia (in 50%–75%), and absence of vasculitis[53–58] occurs with allergic eosinophilic gastroenteritis (AEG). Patients with AEG present with postprandial nausea, abdominal pain, vomiting, diarrhea, protein-losing enteropathy, and weight loss, and depending on the depth of infiltration, abdominal bloating, obstruction, and ascites can also develop. Those with allergic eosinophilic esophagitis may present with symptoms of severe reflux disease and typically with pain while food is being swallowed. The diagnosis requires a biopsy showing eosinophilic infiltration, although there may be patchy disease and infiltration may be missed. In children with allergic eosinophilic esophagitis, significant success from dietary elimination has been achieved.[59,60] The disorder has been associated with positive tests for food-specific IgE antibody in some of the children, but most with this disorder do not have IgE-mediated food allergy.

Celiac disease is a dietary protein enteropathy characterized by an extensive loss of absorptive villi and hyperplasia of the crypts leading to malabsorption, chronic diarrhea, steatorrhea, abdominal distention, flatulence, and weight loss or failure to thrive.[61,62] As the disease represents an immune response to a food protein, it may be considered a food allergic disorder. It is associated with human leukocyte Ag (HLA)-DQ2, which is present in over 90% of patients.[62] Patients with celiac disease are sensitive to gliadin, the alcohol-soluble portion of gluten found in wheat, oat, rye, and barley. Endoscopy typically reveals total villous atrophy and extensive cellular infiltrate. Chronic ingestion of gluten-containing grains in celiac patients is associated with increased risk of malignancy, especially T cell lymphoma.

Ingestion of whole cow's milk by infants less than 6 months of age may lead to occult blood loss from the gastrointestinal tract and iron-deficiency anemia.[63] The use of infant formulas generally results in resolution of symptoms. There is limited evidence that *infantile colic* is associated with food (cow's milk) allergy in a subset of patients.[64]

## RESPIRATORY TRACT REACTIONS

Hay fever is characterized by symptoms of congestion, rhinorrhea, and nasal pruritus. These symptoms are usually associated with hypersensitivity to airborne allergens, not foods. Rarely, isolated nasal symptoms may occur as a result of IgE-mediated allergy to ingested food proteins.[65] The prevalence of this illness, even among patients referred to allergy clinics, appears to be under 1%. On the other hand, 25%–80% of patients with documented IgE-mediated food allergy experience nasal symptoms during oral food challenges that result in systemic symptoms. In contrast to immune-mediated rhinitis, *gustatory rhinitis* refers to rhinorrhea caused by spicy foods. This reaction is mediated by neurological mechanisms.[66]

Isolated wheezing, cough, and dyspnea induced by lower airway inflammation and bronchoconstriction can be related to food allergy but more commonly is related to airborne allergens and viral infections. Asthma reactions may occur based on IgE-mediated reactions from ingestion of the causative food or from inhalation of vapors released during cooking or in occupational settings.[67,68] The prevalence of food-related asthma in the general population is unknown, but studies report a prevalence of 5.7% among children with asthma,[69] 11% among children with AD,[67] and 24% among children with a history of food-induced wheezing.[70] The prevalence of food-induced wheezing among adults with asthma is under 2%.[71]

## ANAPHYLAXIS

Allergic reactions that affect more than one organ system, or are severe in nature, are termed anaphylactic reactions.[72] Food is the most common cause of out of hospital anaphylaxis. Symptoms may affect the skin, respiratory tract, and gastrointestinal tract. Symptoms can be severe, progressive, and potentially fatal. When blood circulation is impaired, the term *anaphylactic shock* is used. Fatal food-induced anaphylaxis appears to be more common among teenaged patients with underlying asthma.[73,74] In addition, patients who experienced fatal or near-fatal anaphylaxis were unaware that they had ingested the incriminated food, had almost immediate symptoms, and had a delay in receiving emergency treatment with epinephrine, a medication that reverses many of the severe symptoms of anaphylaxis, and in about half of the cases, there was a period of quiescence prior to a respiratory decompensation. The foods most often responsible for food-induced anaphylaxis are peanut, tree nuts, and shellfish.

## FOOD-ASSOCIATED, EXERCISE-INDUCED ANAPHYLAXIS

This uncommon disorder refers to patients who are able to ingest a particular food or exercise without a reaction.[75,76] However, when exercise follows the ingestion of a particular food, anaphylaxis results. Wheat is a common trigger.

In some cases, exercise after any meal results in a reaction. Treatment depends on elimination of the causal food for 12 h prior to exercise.

## DIAGNOSTIC METHODS IN FOOD ALLERGY

Arguably, the medical history is the most important diagnostic test for food allergy. For example, a diagnosis is apparent when there is an acute onset of typical symptoms, such as hives and wheezing, following the isolated ingestion of a suspected food with confirmatory laboratory studies indicating the presence of specific IgE antibody to the suspected food.[26,77] However, the diagnosis is more complicated when multiple foods are implicated or when chronic diseases, such as asthma or AD, are evaluated. The diagnosis of food allergy and identification of the particular foods responsible is also problematic when reactions are not mediated by IgE antibody, as is the case with a number of gastrointestinal food allergies. In these latter circumstances, well-devised elimination diets followed by physician-supervised oral food challenges are critical in the identification and proper treatment of these disorders.

A history and physical examination should review general medical concerns to exclude non-immunological adverse reactions to foods or to consider other allergic causes for symptoms, for example, another type of allergy such as a cat allergy causing asthma. In relation to foods, a careful history should focus on the symptoms attributed to food ingestion (type, acute vs. chronic), the foods involved, the consistency of reactions, the quantity of food required to elicit symptoms, the timing between ingestion and onset of symptoms, the most recent reaction/patterns of reactivity, and any ancillary associated activity that may play a role (i.e., exercise, alcohol ingestion). The information gathered is used to determine the best mode of diagnosis or may lead to dismissal of the problem based upon the history alone.

If the symptoms being evaluated are typical of IgE-mediated reaction, for example, urticaria and wheezing, and if the symptoms follow soon after a food ingestion, that history may clearly implicate a particular food. In this circumstance, a positive test for specific IgE antibody to the suspected food would be confirmatory. If the ingestion was of mixed foods and the causal food was uncertain, for example, fruit salad, the history may help to eliminate some of the foods—those frequently ingested without symptoms—and specific tests for IgE may help to further narrow the possibilities. In chronic disorders such as AD or asthma, it is more difficult to pinpoint causal foods. The approach to diagnosis in these chronic disorders usually requires elimination diets and oral food challenges to confirm suspected associations. This is particularly the case for the non-IgE-mediated reactions or those attributed to food dyes/preservatives in which ancillary laboratory testing is not helpful.

For IgE-mediated food allergy, specific tests can help to identify, or exclude, responsible foods. One method to determine the presence of specific IgE antibody is prick–puncture skin testing. While the patient is not taking antihistamines, a device, such as a bifurcated needle, plastic probe, or lancet, is used to puncture the skin through a glycerinated extract of a food and the appropriate positive (histamine) and negative (saline–glycerin) controls. A local wheal and flare response indicates the presence of food-specific IgE antibody (a wheal >3 mm is considered positive). Prick skin tests are most valuable when they are negative since the negative predictive value of the tests is very high (over 95%).[78,79] Unfortunately, the positive predictive value is on the order of only 50%. Thus, a positive skin test in isolation cannot be considered proof of clinically relevant hypersensitivity. These test limitations indicate that screening for food allergy with large batteries of tests is not a useful approach. Rather, directed testing for foods suspected to be a problem, identified by a careful medical history and knowledge of the epidemiology of the disorder, is a more efficient approach. The protein in commercial extracts of some fruits and vegetables is prone to degradation, so fresh extracts of these foods may be more reliable, and the "prick–prick" manner of testing may be indicated where the probe is used to first pierce the food being tested (to obtain liquid) and then the skin of the patient.[80]

Blood tests are often employed to detect food-specific IgE antibodies. These tests are often called radioallergosorbent test (RAST) though the modern tests do not use radioactivity. Unlike skin tests, serum tests for IgE antibodies can be used, while the patient is taking antihistamines and does not depend on having an area of rash-free skin for testing. Like skin tests, a negative result is very reliable in ruling out an IgE-mediated reaction to a particular food, but a positive result has low specificity. For many allergens, the blood test is considered slightly less sensitive than allergy skin tests.

The stronger an individual's food-specific IgE antibody response, the more likely it is that the person would have an allergic reaction to the tested food. The degree of response may be determined by the size of a skin test response or concentration of food-specific IgE antibody.[81–83] Although it is counterintuitive, the degree of IgE response does not generally correlate with severity of an allergic reaction. Tests must be interpreted according to age, clinical history, and the food being tested. Test results are also influenced by the presence of less clinically relevant cross-reactive proteins. For example, most peanut-allergic patients will have positive skin tests to at least a few of the other members of the legume family, but only 5% will have clinical reactions to more than one legume.[84,85] Tests for IgE antibodies do not help in diagnosing food allergies that are not associated with IgE. Studies are under way for improved tests for these disorders, including the use of a skin patch test where an area of skin is exposed to food protein for 24–48 h and the area is examined for the development of a rash in the ensuing days.[35,36] Pending improved tests for non-IgE-antibody-mediated food allergies, further testing with oral challenges, if the history does not resolve the issue, would be required. Lastly, one should be wary of tests such as measurement of IgG₄ antibody, provocation–neutralization, cytotoxicity, and applied kinesiology, among other unproved methods that are not useful.[86,87]

As an adjunct to testing, the first step to prove a cause and effect relationship with a particular illness and food allergy (whether IgE mediated or not) is to show resolution of symptoms with elimination of the suspected foods. In many cases, one or several foods are eliminated, which may be the obvious course of action when an isolated food ingestion (i.e., peanut) causes a sudden acute reaction and there is a positive test for IgE to the food. This would also represent a therapeutic intervention. However, eliminating one or a few suspected foods from the diet when the diagnosis is not so clear (asthma, AD, and chronic urticaria) can be a crucial step in determining if food is causal in the disease process. If symptoms persist, the eliminated food(s) is (are) excluded as a cause of symptoms. Alternatively, and as is more likely the case for evaluating chronic disorders without acute reactions, eliminating a large number of foods suspected to cause a chronic problem (usually including those that are common causes of food allergic reactions as described earlier) and giving a list of "allowed foods" may be the preferred approach. The primary disadvantage of this approach is that if symptoms persist, the cause could still be attributed to foods left in the diet. Thus, a third type of elimination diet is an elemental diet in which calories are obtained from a hydrolyzed formula or, preferably, from an amino-acid-based formula. A variation is to include a few foods likely to be tolerated (but, again, this adds the possibility that persistent symptoms are caused by these foods). This diet is extremely difficult to maintain in patients beyond infancy. In extreme cases, nasogastric feeding of the amino-acid-based formula can be achieved, although some patients can tolerate the taste of these formulas with the use of flavoring agents provided by the manufacturers. This diet may be required when the diets mentioned earlier fail to resolve symptoms, but suspicion for food-related illness remains high. It is also required in disorders associated with multiple food allergies such as AEG. With AEG, prolonged dietary elimination for 3–6 weeks is sometimes needed to determine if resolution of symptoms will occur.[59]

## ORAL FOOD CHALLENGE TESTS: THE GOLD STANDARD

Oral food challenges are performed by feeding the patient the suspected food under physician observation. There are several settings in which physician-supervised oral food challenges are required for diagnosis of food allergic disease. Because food challenges may elicit severe reactions, they are usually conducted under physician supervision with emergency medications to treat anaphylaxis immediately available. Challenges can be performed "openly" with the patient ingesting the food in its native form, "single blind" with the food masked and the patient unaware if they are receiving the test food, or as DBPCFC, where neither patient nor physician knows which challenges contain the food being tested. While open and single-blind challenges are open to patient or observer bias, the DBPCFC is considered the "gold standard" for diagnosis since bias is removed.[26]

To reduce the risk of a severe allergic reaction, the food is given in gradually increasing amounts that may be individualized in both dose and timing depending on the patient's history. For most IgE-mediated reactions, experts suggest giving 8–10 g of the dry food or 100 mL of wet food (double amount for meat/fish) at 10–15 min intervals over about 90 min followed by a larger, meal size portion of food a few hours later.[88] Starting doses may be a minute amount applied to the inner lip followed by 1% of the total challenge followed by gradually increasing amounts (4%, 10%, 20%, etc.). However, challenges may be individualized to parallel the clinical history (i.e., feeding over consecutive days for chronic disorders with delayed symptoms). Similarly, higher-risk challenges may start at extremely low doses with very gradual increases over longer time intervals. The person undergoing an oral food challenge is monitored for symptoms. Challenges are terminated when a reaction becomes apparent and emergency medications are given, as needed. Generally, antihistamines are given at the earliest sign of a reaction with epinephrine and other treatments given if there is progression of symptoms or any potentially life-threatening symptoms.

The practical issues in preparing food challenges include palatability and masking foods in appropriate vehicles, with placebos for DBPCFCs. In many cases, dry forms of the food (flour, powdered egg whites, etc.) can be hidden in puddings or liquids. Bulkier foods may be hidden in pancakes or ground beef. Flavoring agents such as mint can be added for further masking.[89] Hiding the food in opaque capsules is a convenient method to administer blinded challenges for patients who are able to ingest these capsules.

Non-IgE-mediated reactions (e.g., AEG, enterocolitis) are more difficult to diagnose since there are no specific laboratory tests to identify particular foods that may be responsible for these illnesses. In many cases, a biopsy may be needed (e.g., AEG) to establish an initial diagnosis. Elimination diets with gradual reintroduction of foods and supervised oral food challenges are often needed to identify whether diet plays a role in the disorder and to identify the causal foods. Specific challenge protocols have been advised for food-induced enterocolitis syndrome.[90] Oral challenges can be used to evaluate reactions to food additives (coloring and flavoring agents and preservatives) or virtually any complaint associated with foods. When used to evaluate behavioral disorders or other complaints not convincingly associated with food allergy, DBPCFCs are advised to avoid bias.

## CURRENT TREATMENT METHODS FOR FOOD ALLERGY

Treatment for food allergy requires dietary elimination of the offending food. The elimination of particular dietary food proteins is not a simple task. A primary pitfall in avoidance has been the ambiguity of food labeling practices. For example, terms such as natural flavors could be on a label without indicating the flavor is an allergen, such as milk, or

the term casein or whey, which are milk proteins, could be used, but these scientific terms may not be familiar to lay persons. Many of these problems have been addressed by the Food Allergen Labeling and Consumer Protection Act (FALCPA) of 2004 that came into effect January 2006. The law requires that the eight major allergens or allergenic food groups—milk, egg, fish, shellfish, tree nuts, wheat, peanut, and soy—be declared on ingredient labels using plain English words. The law applies to all types of packaged foods except for meat, egg, and poultry products and raw agricultural foods such as fruits and vegetables in their natural state. The plain English words used to identify the foods may be placed within the ingredient list or as a separate statement "contains." The law does not exclude using more scientific terms for food allergens as long as the label indicates, in some location, the plain English term for the food. In addition, the law requires that the specific type of allergen, in regard to grouped allergens such as fish or shellfish, be named. For example, walnut, salmon, or lobster would be named specifically.

There are a number of limitations to the legislation. First, only the eight major allergenic groups are considered. This means if an individual is allergic to mustard, the label may not indicate that the ingredient should, terms such as natural flavor or spice, be used. The manufacturer would have to be called to learn more about the actual ingredients. Second, the FALCPA legislation has also not considered how much of a food protein in a given product may make it unsafe. This "threshold" ambiguity is problematic because a trace amount may not pose an allergenic risk, but may be labeled as containing an allergen. However, purified oils, such as soy oil that does not contain appreciable soy protein, may not need to be labeled as containing soy. Prior to the law, processing aids such as soy lecithin were not declared on foods. Soy lecithin is a fatty derivative of soy, which contains a very small amount of soy protein. The amount of soy protein in soy lecithin that most experts would agree is unlikely to cause an allergic reaction. Soy lecithin is used as an antistick agent in many baked products. For example, soy lecithin may keep cookies from sticking to a pan. In other cases, soy lecithin is added directly to the food. The legislation does not differentiate this, and a food product may be listed as "contains soy" even though most experts would believe that this would be a safe product.

The legislation does not add regulations about possible inclusion of an allergen. Therefore, companies may voluntarily use terms such as "may contain" an allergen at their discretion. The specific requirements of the law may change, and updates are available at the website of the Center for Food Safety and Applied Nutrition (www.cfsan.fda.gov).

In regard to avoidance, patients and parents must also be made aware that the food protein, as opposed to sugar or fat, is the ingredient being eliminated. For example, lactose-free cow's milk contains cow's milk protein, and many egg substitutes contain chicken egg proteins. Conversely, peanut oil and soy oil do not generally contain the food protein, unless the processing method is one in which the protein is not completely eliminated (as with cold-pressed or "extruded" oil). Patients and families undertaking an avoidance diet must also be taught about avoidance in a variety of settings, such as in obtaining restaurant meals where issues of cross contact during food preparation may pose dangers.[91] There are easily missed pitfalls in attempts to avoid food allergens including the following: (1) Natural flavors or spices listed on a label may contain allergens; (2) cross contamination can occur in food processing leading to allergens being present in adequate amounts to trigger an allergic reaction; and (3) hidden ingredients not declared on a food label may be allergenic (e.g., peanut butter in sauces or egg whites applied to baked goods).

Lay organizations such as The Food Allergy & Anaphylaxis Network (800–929–4040; www.foodallergy.org) assist families and physicians in the difficult task of eliminating the allergenic foods. When multiple foods are eliminated from the diet, it is prudent to enlist the aid of a dietitian in formulating a nutritionally balanced diet.

For life-threatening food allergies, an emergency plan must be in place to treat reactions caused by accidental ingestions. Injectable epinephrine and oral antihistamine should be readily available and administered without delay to treat patients at risk for severe reactions. Caregivers must be familiarized with indications for the use and method of administration of these medications.[92]

Most children outgrow their allergies to milk, egg, wheat, and soy by age 3–5 years.[93] However, patients allergic to peanuts, tree nuts, fish, and shellfish are much less likely to lose their clinical reactivity, and these sensitivities may persist into adulthood. Nonetheless, about 20% of very young children outgrow a peanut allergy by school age, and 8% outgrow a tree-nut allergy.[94] Elevated concentrations of food-specific IgE may indicate a lower likelihood of developing tolerance in the subsequent few years.[95] However, tests for food-specific IgE antibody (prick skin tests and serum-food-specific IgE) remain positive for years after the food allergy has resolved and cannot be followed as the sole indicator of tolerance. Thus, it is recommended that patients with chronic disease such as AD be rechallenged intermittently (e.g., egg [every 2–3 years]; milk, soy, and wheat [every 1–2 years]; peanut, nuts, fish, and shellfish [if tolerance is suspected]; and other foods [every 1–2 years]) to determine whether their food allergy persists if their test results are favorable so that restriction diets may be discontinued as soon as possible.

## PREVENTION OF FOOD ALLERGY

Approaches to delay or prevent allergy through dietary manipulation have been the subject of reviews and consensus statements.[96,97] Studies suggest a beneficial role for exclusive breast-feeding infants at "high risk" for atopic disease for the first 3–6 months of life and avoiding supplementation with cow's milk or soy formulas in favor of hypoallergenic formulas, if breast feeding is not possible. There are currently no conclusive studies indicating that the manipulation

of the mother's diet during pregnancy or breast feeding or the restriction of allergenic foods from the infants diet will prevent the development of food allergy.[96,98] Currently, the American Academy of Pediatrics recommends a conservative approach, including that mothers of "high-risk" infants avoid allergens such as peanuts and nuts during lactation and that major allergens such as peanuts, nuts, and seafood be introduced after 3 years of age.[97]

## ORAL TOLERANCE TO FOOD ANTIGENS

The intestine is exposed continuously to vast amounts of foreign antigenic material. As well as ingesting >100 g of foreign protein per day in our diet, the intestine is colonized by a dense community of commensal microbes, referred to as the microbiome. The density of these microbes increases along the gastrointestinal tract, reaching up to 10–12 bacteria per gram of gut content in the colon. At the same time, the mucosal barriers are thin and very vulnerable to pathogenic infection, meaning that the intestinal immune system has to discriminate between generating protective immunity against harmful Ags and tolerance against harmless materials. Active immune responses directed against the colonic bacteria can result in inflammatory bowel diseases such as Crohn's disease and ulcerative colitis. The incidence of Crohn's disease and ulcerative colitis is increasing throughout the world and in some countries can affect up to 0.6% of the population.[99]

Failure to induce tolerance to food protein is thought to result in food allergy and celiac disease, which is the most prevalent food-induced pathology.[100] As with other food allergies, there is a more widespread impression of gluten sensitivity leading to celiac disease than it actually exists in the general population.

The ability of orally administered Ag to suppress subsequent immune responses, both in the gut and in the systemic immune system, was first described 100 years ago and has been studied widely since.[101,102] This phenomenon is referred to as "oral tolerance," and its effects on systemic immunity have led to attempts to exploit it therapeutically to prevent or treat autoimmune diseases. However, there is an important difference between tolerance to gut bacteria and tolerance to food proteins. Tolerance to food protein induced via the small intestine affects local and systemic immune responses; tolerance to gut bacteria in the colon does not attenuate systemic responses.

Oral tolerance has been demonstrated extensively in rodents using many different model Ags including purified proteins, cellular Ags, and small haptens, and it has also been shown in humans.[103–105] The effects of oral tolerance are measured typically as reductions in systemic delayed-type hypersensitivity, T cell proliferation, and cytokine production. Serum antibody responses can also be suppressed, particularly IgE and T helper type 1–dependent IgG2a production, as can mucosal T cell and immunoglobulin A responses. Moreover, oral tolerance has been shown to suppress immunopathology in experimental models of autoimmune encephalitis,[106] collagen-induced arthritis,[107] type 1 diabetes,[108] and others (see Ref. [109] for review). Thus, oral tolerance attenuates a broad range of immune responses and appears to play a central role in immune homeostasis.

## FUTURE FOOD ALLERGY PREVENTION STRATEGIES

Food allergies are common. Currently, strict avoidance of causal foods and treatment of accidental ingestions are the only available therapy for food allergy.[110] Immunotherapy ("allergy shots") has not proven practical for treatment except in the case of the oral allergy syndrome in which immunotherapy with the pollens responsible for the cross-reactivity may provide relief. Unfortunately, many patients accidentally ingest allergenic foods, which can result in severe anaphylactic reactions. Several immunotherapies are being developed for food allergies; these involve oral, sublingual, epicutaneous, or subcutaneous administration of small amounts of native or modified allergens to induce immune tolerance. Oral immunotherapy seems to be the most promising approach based on results from small uncontrolled and controlled studies. However, it is a challenge to compare results among immunotherapy trials because of differences in protocols. Studies conducted thus far have tested the most prevalent food allergens: it is not clear whether their results can be extended to other allergens. Sublingual administration of immunotherapy has shown some efficacy and fewer side effects than oral administration in some trials, yet neither approach can be recommended for routine practice. Controlled studies with larger numbers of subjects are needed to determine short- and long-term efficacy and side effects. Until that time, standard avoidance of causal foods and provision of emergency measures remain the established modes of treatment outside of research settings.

## REFERENCES

1. Fleischer, DM, Bock, SA, Spears, GC et al. *J Pediatr* 158:578;2011.
2. Rona, RJ, Keil, T, Summers, C et al. *J Allergy Clin Immunol* 120:638;2007.
3. Katz, Y, Rajuan, N, Goldberg, MR et al. *J Allergy Clin Immunol* 126:77;2010.
4. Osborne, NJ, Koplin, JJ, Martin, PE et al. *J Allergy Clin Immunol* 127:668;2011.
5. Du Toit, G, Katz, Y, Sasieni, P et al. *J Allergy Clin Immunol* 122:978;2008.
6. Vieira, MC, Morais, MB, Spolidoro, JV et al. *BMC Pediatr* 23:25;2010.
7. Altman, DR, Chiaramonte, L. *J Allergy Clin Immunol* 97:1247;1996.
8. Sloan, AE, Powers, ME. *J Allergy Clin Immunol* 78:127;1986.
9. Bock, SA. *Pediatrics* 79:683;1987.
10. Sicherer, SH, Munoz-Furlong, A, Sampson, HA. *J Allergy Clin Immunol* 114:159;2004.
11. Sampson, HA. *J Allergy Clin Immunol* 113: 805;2004.
12. Young, E, Stoneham, MD, Petruckevitch, A et al. *Lancet* 343:1127;1994.
13. Johansson, SG, Bieber, T, Dahl, R et al. *J Allergy Clin Immunol* 113.832,2004.
14. Chehade, M, Mayer, L. *J Allergy Clin Immunol* 115:3;2005.
15. Sicherer, SH, Furlong, TJ, Maes, HH et al. *J Allergy Clin Immunol* 106:53;2000.
16. Sicherer, SH. *Lancet* 360:701;2002.
17. Goubier, A et al. *Immunity* 29:464;2008.
18. Chirdo, FG, Millington, OR, Beacock-Sharp, H, Mowat, AM. *Eur J Immunol* 35:1831;2005.
19. Bischoff, S, Crowe, SE. *Gastroenterology* 128:1089;2005.
20. Sampson, HA, Anderson, JA. *J Pediatr Gastroenterol Nutr* 94:S87;2000.
21. Chung, HL, Hwang, JB, Park, JJ, Kim, SG. *J Allergy Clin Immunol* 109:150; 2002.
22. Sicherer, SH, Munoz-Furlong, A, Sampson, HA. *J Allergy Clin Immunol* 112:1203;2003.
23. Hefle, SL, Nordlee, JA, Taylor, SL. *Crit Rev Food Sci Nutr* 36:S69;1996.
24. Shek, LP, Soderstrom, L, Ahlstedt, S et al. *J Allergy Clin Immunol* 114:387;2004.
25. Shreffler, WG, Beyer, K, Chu, TH et al. *J Allergy Clin Immunol* 113:776;2004.
26. Sicherer, SH, Teuber, S. *J Allergy Clin Immunol* 114: 1146;2004.
27. Weber, RW, Vaughan, TR. *Immunol Allergy Clin North Am* 11:831;1991.
28. Bateman, B, Warner, JO, Hutchinson, E et al. *Arch Dis Child* 89:506; 2004.
29. Wolraich, ML, Lindgren, SD, Stumbo, PJ et al. *N Engl J Med* 330:301;1994.
30. Sehgal, VN, Rege, VL. *Ann Allergy* 31:279;1973.
31. Champion, RH. *Br J Dermatol* 119:427;1988.
32. Hanifin, JM. *J Dermatol* 24:495;1997.
33. Leung, DY, Nicklas, RA, Li, JT et al. *Ann Allergy Asthma Immunol* 93:S1;2004.
34. Eigenmann, PA, Sicherer, SH, Borkowski, TA et al. *Pediatrics* 101:E8;1998.
35. Niggemann, B, Reibel, S, Wahn, U. *Allergy* 55:281;2000.
36. Isolauri, E, Turjanmaa, K. *J Allergy Clin Immunol* 97:9;1996.
37. Sicherer, SH, Sampson, HA. *J Allergy Clin Immunol* 104:S114;1999.
38. Guillet, G, Guillet, MH. *Arch Dermatol* 128:187;1992.
39. de-Maat, BF, Bruijnzeel, KC. *Monogr Allergy* 32:157;996.
40. Nicolas, ME, Krause, PK, Gibson, LE. *Int J Dermatol* 42:588;2003.
41. Sampson, HA, Scanlon, SM. *J Pediatr* 115:23;1989.
42. Ma, S, Sicherer, SH, Nowak-Wegrzyn, A. *J Allergy Clin Immunol* 112:784;2003.
43. Sicherer, SH. *Pediatrics* 111:1609;2003.
44. Rodriguez, J, Crespo, JF, Lopez-Rubio, A et al. *J Allergy Clin Immunol* 106:183;2000.
45. Ortolani, C, Ispano, M, Pastorello, E et al. *Ann Allergy* 61:47;1988.
46. Iyngkaran, N, Yadav, M, Boey, C et al. *J Pediatr Gastroenterol Nutr* 8:667;1988.
47. Walker-Smith, JA. *Clin Gastroenterol* 15:55;1986.
48. Powell, GK. *J Pediatr* 93:553;1978.
49. Powell, G. *Comprehen Ther* 12:28;1986.
50. Sicherer, SH, Eigenmann, PA, Sampson, HA. *J Pediatr* 133:214;1998.
51. de Boijjieu, D, Matarazzo, P, Dupont, C. *J Pediatr* 131:744;1997.
52. Nowak-Wegrzyn, A, Sampson, HA, Wood, RA et al. *Pediatrics* 111:829;2003.

53. Talley, NJ, Shorter, RG, Phillips, SF et al. *Gut* 31:54;1990.
54. Justinich, C, Katz, A, Gurbindo, C et al. *J Pediatr Gastroenterol Nutr* 23:81;1996.
55. Liacouras, CA, Wenner, WJ, Brown, K et al. *J Pediatr Gastroenterol Nutr* 26:380;1998.
56. Rothenberg, ME. *J Allergy Clin Immunol* 113:11;2004.
57. Straumann, A, Simon, HU. *J Allergy Clin Immunol* 115:418;2005.
58. Teitelbaum, JE. *J Pediatr Gastroenterol Nutr* 38:358;2004.
59. Kelly, KJ, Lazenby, AJ, Rowe, PC et al. *Gastroenterol* 109:1503;1995.
60. Spergel, JM, Beausoleil, JL, Mascarenhas, M et al. *J Allergy Clin Immunol* 109:363;2002.
61. Ciclitira, PJ, King, AL, Fraser, JS. *Gastroenterol* 120:1526;2001.
62. Farrell, RJ, Kelly, CP. *N Engl J Med* 346:180;2002.
63. Zeigler, RE, Fomon, SJ, Nelson, SE et al. *J Pediatr* 116:11;1990.
64. Hill, DJ, Hosking, CS. *J Pediatr Gastroenterol Nutr* 30:S67;2000.
65. Sampson, H, Eigenmann, PA. *Rhinitis: Mechanisms and Management*, Marcel Dekker, Inc.: New York, Chapter 6, p. 95, 1999.
66. Raphael, G, Raphael, M, Kaliner, M. *J Allergy Clin Immunol* 83:110;1989.
67. James, JM, Bernhisel-Broadbent, J, Sampson, HA. *Am J Respir Crit Care Med* 149:59;1994.
68. Roberts, G, Golder, N, Lack, G. *Allergy* 57:713;2002.
69. Novembre, E, de Martino, M, Vierucci, A. *J Allergy Clin Immunol* 81:1059;1988.
70. Bock, SA. *Pediatr Allergy Immunol* 3:188;1992.
71. Onorato, J, Merland, N, Terral, C et al. *J Allergy Clin Immunol* 78:1139;1986.
72. Joint Task Force on Practice Parameters. *J Allergy Clin Immunol* 115:S483;2005.
73. Bock, SA, Munoz-Furlong, A, Sampson, HA. *J Allergy Clin Immunol* 107:191;2001.
74. Sampson, HA, Mendelson, LM, Rosen, JP. *N Engl J Med* 327:380;1992.
75. Palosuo, K, Alenius, H, Varjonen, E et al. *J Allergy Clin Immunol* 103:912;1999.
76. Romano, A, Di Fonso, M, Giuffreda, F et al. *Int Arch Allergy Immunol* 125:264;2001.
77. Sicherer, SH. *Pediatr Allergy Immunol* 10:226;1999.
78. Sampson, HA, Albergo, R. *J Allergy Clin Immunol* 74:26;1984.
79. Bock, S, Buckley, J, Holst, A et al. *Clin Allergy* 8:559;1978.
80. Ortolani, C, Ispano, M, Pastorello, EA et al. *J Allergy Clin Immunol* 83:683;1989.
81. Sampson, HA. *J Allergy Clin Immunol* 107:891;2001.
82. Sporik, R, Hill, DJ, Hosking, CS. *Clin Exp Allergy* 30:1541;2000.
83. Crespo, JF, Pascual, C, Ferrer, A et al. *Allergy Proc* 15:73;1994.
84. Bernhisel-Broadbent, J, Sampson, HA. *J Allergy Clin Immunol* 83:435;1989.
85. Sicherer, SH. *J Allergy Clin Immunol* 108:881;2001.
86. Bernstein, IL, Storms, WW. *Ann Allergy Asthma Immunol* 75:543;1995.
87. Beyer, K, Teuber, SS. *Curr Opin Allergy Clin Immunol* 5:261;2005.
88. Bock, SA, Sampson, HA, Atkins, FM et al. *J Allergy Clin Immunol* 82:986;1988.
89. Vlieg-Boerstra, BJ, Bijleveld, CM, Van Der, HS et al. *J Allergy Clin Immunol* 113:341;2004.
90. Sicherer, SH. *J Allergy Clin Immunol* 115:149;2005.
91. Furlong, TJ, DeSimone, J, Sicherer, SH. *J Allergy Clin Immunol* 108:867;2001.
92. Sicherer, SH, Simons, FE. *J Allergy Clin Immunol* 115:575;2005.
93. Wood, RA. *Pediatrics* 111:1631;2003.
94. Skolnick, HS, Conover-Walker, MK, Koerner, CB et al. *J Allergy Clin Immunol* 107:367;2001.
95. Perry, TT, Matsui, EC, Kay Conover-Walker, M et al. *J Allergy Clin Immunol* 114:44;2004.
96. Muraro, A, Dreborg, S, Halken, S et al. *Pediatr Allergy Immunol* 15:291;2004.
97. Committee on Nutrition, American Academy of Pediatrics. *Pediatrics* 106:346;2000.
98. Lack, G, Fox, D, Northstone, K et al. *N Engl J Med* 348:977;2003.
99. Molodecky, NA et al. *Gastroenterology* 142:46;2011.
100. Meresse, B, Ripoche, J, Heyman, M, Cerf-Bensussan, N. *Mucosal Immunol* 2:8;2009.
101. Wells, HG, Osborne, TB. *J Infect Dis* 8:66;1911.
102. Weiner, HL, da Cunha, AP, Quintana, F, Wu, H. *Immunol Rev* 241:241;2011.
103. Kapp, K et al. *Eur J Immunol* 40:3128;2010.
104. Kraus, TA, Toy, L, Chan, L et al. *Gastroenterology* 126:1771;2004.
105. Husby, S, Mestecky, J, Moldoveanu, Z et al. *J Immunol* 152:4663;1994.
106. Higgins, PJ, Weiner, HL. *J Immunol* 140:440;1988.
107. Nagler-Anderson, C, Bober, LA, Robinson, ME et al. *Proc Natl Acad Sci USA* 83:7443;1986.
108. Zhang, ZJ, Davidson, L, Eisenbarth, G, Weiner, HL. *Proc Natl Acad Sci U S A* 88:10252;1991.
109. Faria, AM, Weiner, HL. *Clin Dev Immunol* 13:143;2006.
110. Nowak-Wegrzyn, A, Sampson, HA. *Immunol Allergy Clin North Am* 24:705;2004.

# 53 Nutrition and Immune Function

*David Heber*

## CONTENTS

## INTRODUCTION

Over the last century, the intricate interaction between immunity and metabolism has been recognized and investigated extensively.[1] Indeed, it has been demonstrated that adipose tissue is not merely the site of energy storage, but can be considered as an "immune-related" organ producing a series of molecules named "adipocytokines." Nutritional depletion, specific deficiencies, and kwashiorkor-like malnutrition suppress immune function.

The cloning of the obese gene (ob) and identification of its protein product, leptin, has provided fundamental insight into the hypothalamic regulation of body weight. Circulating levels of this adipocyte-derived hormone are proportional to fat mass but may be lowered rapidly by fasting or increased by inflammatory mediators. The impaired T-cell immunity of mice, now known to be defective in leptin (ob/ob) or its receptor (db/db), is related to absence of functional leptin signaling due to the absence of a functional leptin protein (ob/ob) or the leptin receptor protein (db/db).[2] Impaired cell-mediated immunity and reduced levels of leptin are both features of low body weight in humans. Indeed, malnutrition predisposes to death from infectious diseases and the impaired immune function resulting from protein–energy malnutrition (PEM) and HIV infection is well documented.[3] On an evolutionary basis, the ability to fight off infection and the ability to store fat in cells were both critical to survival. While the adaptation to starvation and associated gradual weight loss does not impair immune function, rapid weight loss does.[4] Moreover, the close interrelationship of immune function and nutrition has been confirmed with modern molecular nutrition tools.

The immune system during adapted starvation is a fail-safe system until it decompensates. On the other hand, staying with the theme that humans are well adapted to starvation but poorly adapted to overnutrition, there is chronic low-grade inflammation associated with overweight and obesity, mediated by intra-abdominal fat-resident immune cells that cause a systemic inflammation. In order to understand these two poles of the interaction of nutrition and immune function, it is necessary to understand the difference between innate and adaptive immune mechanisms.

## INNATE IMMUNE SYSTEM

The innate immune system consists of the cells and mechanisms that defend the host from infection by other organisms, in a nonspecific manner. This means that the cells of the innate system recognize and respond to pathogens in a generic way, but unlike the adaptive immune system, it does not confer long-lasting or protective immunity to the host. Innate immune systems provide immediate defense against infection and are the dominant immune system found in plants, fungi, insects, and in primitive multicellular organisms. It is thought to be an older evolutionary development than the adaptive immune system. The innate immune system is activated by "danger signals" and can be likened to firemen playing cards in the fire station until the alarm goes off and they all jump down the pole and onto fire trucks to put out the fire. A fresh perspective in approaching the immune system is offered by the premises laid down by Polly Matzinger in her "danger model."[5,6] Even today, more than a decade after its emergence, this model offers a fundamentally different interpretation of classic and newly emerging concepts in immunology.

The innate immune system in humans carries out the following functions: (1) recruitment of immune cells to sites of infection, through the production of chemical factors, including specialized chemical mediators, called cytokines and chemokines; (2) activation of the complement cascade to identify bacteria, activate cells and promote clearance of dead cells or antibody complexes; (3) identification and removal of foreign substances present in organs, tissues, the blood and lymph, by specialized white blood cells (WBCs);

and (4) activation of the adaptive immune system through a process known as antigen presentation.

The activation of the innate immune system is accompanied by inflammation (Latin, *inflammatio*, "setting on fire"), a complex biological response of vascular tissues to harmful stimuli, such as pathogens, damaged cells, or irritants. The inflammatory response is characterized by the following symptoms: redness (rubor), heat (calor), swelling (tumor), and pain (dolor). Inflammation is a protective attempt by the organism to remove the injuring stimulus as well as initiate the healing process for the tissue.

Inflammation can be classified as either acute or chronic. Acute inflammation is the initial response of the body to harmful stimuli and is achieved by the increased movement of plasma and leukocytes from the blood into the injured tissues. A cascade of biochemical events propagates and matures the inflammatory response, involving the local vascular system, the immune system, and various cells within the injured tissue.[7] Prolonged inflammation, known as chronic inflammation, leads to a progressive shift in the type of cells that are present at the site of inflammation and is characterized by simultaneous destruction and healing of the tissue from the inflammatory process. Chronic inflammation is associated with many diseases including heart disease, diabetes, and common forms of cancer. So while acute inflammation and healing is a lifesaving adaptation analogous to the ability to store energy as fat, prolonged inflammation damages critical tissues and organs in the body. Obesity is associated with increased chronic inflammation while starvation is associated with impaired immune function.

In the absence of inflammation, wounds and infections would never heal and progressive destruction of the tissue would compromise the survival of the organism.[8] However, chronic inflammation can also lead to a host of diseases, such as hay fever, atherosclerosis, and rheumatoid arthritis. It is for that reason that inflammation is normally closely regulated by the body.

WBCs are called leukocytes and are able to move freely through the circulation, lymphatics, and tissues in order to capture cellular breakdown products, foreign materials, or invading pathogens. Most leukocytes cannot divide or reproduce on their own, but are the products of stem cells found in the bone marrow that develop into one or another type of white cell. Leukemia is the unregulated overproduction of cells from one step of the process, such as promyelocytic leukemia where the promyelocyte crowds out the development of other white cells leading to infection, other red cells leading to anemia, or platelets leading to bleeding. The different leukocytes of the innate immune system include natural killer cells (NK cells), mast cells, eosinophils, basophils, and the phagocytic cells including macrophages, neutrophils, and dendritic cells (DCs), and function within the immune system by identifying and eliminating pathogens that might cause infection.

When activated, mast cells rapidly release characteristic granules, rich in histamine and heparin, along with various hormonal mediators, and chemokines, or chemotactic cytokines, into the environment. Histamine dilates blood vessels, causing the characteristic signs of inflammation, and recruits neutrophils and macrophages. Macrophages, neutrophils, and DCs are called phagocytic cells because they engulf and internalize foreign matter, cell debris, or pathogens.

Macrophages, from the Greek, meaning "large eating cells," are large phagocytic WBCs that move outside of the vascular system across the cell membranes of capillary vessels and enter the areas between cells in response to "danger signals" from invading pathogens, foreign materials, or dying cells. In tissues, organ-specific macrophages are differentiated from phagocytic cells present in the blood called monocytes. Macrophages are the most efficient phagocytes and can engulf and digest substantial numbers of bacteria, cellular material, or microbes. The binding of molecules to receptors on the surface of a macrophage triggers it to engulf and destroy its "meal" through the generation of a "respiratory burst," causing the release of reactive oxygen species. The stimulated macrophage also produces chemokines, proteins that summon other cells to the site of infection or injury.

Neutrophils, along with eosinophils and basophils, are known as granulocytes due to the presence of granules in their cytoplasm. Polymorphonuclear cells (PMNs) are white cells with distinctive lobed nuclei. Neutrophil granules contain a variety of toxic substances that kill or inhibit growth of bacteria and fungi. Similar to macrophages, neutrophils attack pathogens by activating a respiratory burst. The main products of the neutrophil respiratory burst are strong oxidizing agents including hydrogen peroxide, free oxygen radicals, and hypochlorite. Neutrophils are the most abundant type of phagocytes, normally representing 50%–60% of the total circulating leukocytes, and are usually the first cells to arrive at the site of an infection. The bone marrow of a normal healthy adult produces more than 100 billion neutrophils per day and more than 10 times that many per day during acute inflammation.

Basophils and eosinophils are similar to the neutrophils in containing granules. When activated by a pathogen encounter, basophils release histamine, which is important in defending against parasites and plays a role in allergic reactions (such as asthma). Upon activation, eosinophils secrete a range of highly toxic proteins and free radicals that are highly effective in killing bacteria and parasites, but are also responsible for tissue damage occurring during allergic reactions. Activation and toxin release by eosinophils is therefore tightly regulated to prevent any inappropriate tissue destruction.

NK cells are a component of the innate immune system that does not directly attack invading microbes. Rather, NK cells destroy compromised host cells, such as tumor cells or virus-infected cells, recognizing such cells by a condition known as "missing self." This term describes cells with low levels of a cell-surface marker called MHC I (major histocompatibility complex)—a situation that can arise in viral infections of host cells. They were named "natural killer" because of the initial notion that they do not require activation in order to kill cells that are "missing self."

DCs are phagocytic cells present in tissues that are in contact with the external environment, mainly the skin (where they are often called Langerhans cells) and the inner mucosal lining of the nose, lungs, stomach, and intestines. They are named for their resemblance to neuronal dendrites, but DCs are not connected to the nervous system. DCs are very important in the process of antigen presentation and serve as a link between the innate and adaptive immune systems.

DCs are present in all tissues, where they gather antigens from the local environment but are not in an immunostimulatory state. In Janeway's "stranger" model, antigen-presenting cells (APCs) (later appreciated to be DCs) were endowed with pattern-recognition receptors (PRRs) that recognize the unique features of microbial molecules (pathogen-associated molecular patterns, PAMPs). When PAMPs were present—for example, from an infection or adjuvant—then DCs were stimulated to migrate to lymphoid tissues and present both antigen and co-stimulatory molecules (CD80 and/or CD86) to T cells. In Matzinger's "danger" model,[5,6] the crucial event controlling the initiation of an immune response was not infection, but the production of danger signals known as damage-associated molecular patterns (DAMPs) from cells stressed, damaged, and/or dying in the local tissue. These were postulated to act on DCs in a manner that also caused them to migrate to lymphoid tissue and present antigens to T cells in an immunostimulatory manner. It has been speculated that DAMPs might be produced in response to PAMPs and therefore that DAMPs might be the final mediator promoting immune responses in all situations, including infection. This might occur; however, it is also possible, and in our view probable, that DAMPs and PAMPs can alert the immune system to a problem independently and possibly even in a synergistic manner.

## ADAPTIVE IMMUNE SYSTEM

The adaptive immune response provides the immune system with the ability to recognize and remember specific pathogens (to generate immunity) and to mount stronger attacks each time the pathogen is encountered.[9] It is adaptive immunity because the body's immune system prepares itself for future challenges. It is believed to have evolved at the time of the first vertebrates with jaws including various types of fish, reptiles, and amphibians. One can speculate that eating led to potential repeat exposure to toxic substances requiring a specific memory for antigens and the ability to mount a more robust response to eliminate threatening substances.

This immune response system is highly adaptable because of a process of accelerated somatic mutations, and irreversible genetic recombinations of antigen receptor gene segments. This mechanism allows a small number of genes to generate a vast number of different antigen receptors, which are then uniquely expressed on each individual lymphocyte. Because the gene rearrangement leads to an irreversible change in the DNA of each cell, all of the offspring of that cell will then

inherit genes encoding the same receptor specificity, including the memory B cells and memory T cells that are the keys to long-lived specific immunity.

The host's cells express "self" antigens. These antigens are different from those on the surface of bacteria ("nonself" antigens) or on the surface of virally infected host cells ("missing self"). The adaptive response is triggered by recognizing nonself and missing-self antigens.

With the exception of nonnucleated cells (including red blood cells), all cells are capable of presenting antigen and of activating the adaptive response. Some cells are specially equipped to present antigen and to prime naive T cells. DCs and B cells (and to a lesser extent macrophages) are equipped with special immunostimulatory receptors that allow for enhanced activation of T cells and are termed professional APCs. Several T-cell subgroups can be activated by professional APCs, and each type of T cell is specially equipped to deal with each unique toxin or bacterial and viral pathogen. The type of T cell activated, and the type of response generated, depends, in part, on the context in which the APC first encountered the antigen.

## MALNUTRITION AND IMMUNE FUNCTION

Nutrient deficiencies can impair immune function, and nutrient supplementation can restore normal immune capacity.[10] The association of malnutrition and infection has been recorded in ancient historical accounts. For example, an examination of church records in England in the twelfth century shows an interesting association between consecutive years of famine and epidemics of pestilence or communicable diseases. Recent epidemiologic studies in the Americas and Asia have confirmed that infection, often added on malnutrition, is a major cause of morbidity and is responsible for about two-thirds of all deaths among children under 5 years of age. In 1968, Scrimshaw summarized the human and animal data on interactions, often synergistic but occasionally antagonistic, between nutritional deficiencies and infectious illness.[1]

Careful observations showed a correlation between nutritional status and morbidity and mortality largely due to infections.[11] It was shown that the risk of death increased from ~0.1% in the well nourished to as much as 18% in severely malnourished infants. The number of episodes of diarrhea increased by 40%, and the duration of each episode increased by more than twofold. The effect of malnutrition on different infections is variable. For some organisms, for example, measles, tuberculosis, and Pneumocystis carinii, there is little doubt that nutritional deficiencies enhance susceptibility and worsen prognosis. For others, such as yellow fever and poliomyelitis, nutrition does not appear to have a major influence on natural history and outcome.

PEM causes widespread atrophy of lymphoid tissues, especially in children. The thymus, spleen, tonsils, and lymph nodes are all affected, with histological evidence of atrophy being greatest in the T lymphocyte areas of these tissues. Lymphocytes and eosinophils show lowered blood counts,

NK cells show reduced activity,[12] and cultured blood lymphocytes react poorly to mitogens. Production of thymic hormones is reduced, as is a patient's ability to fend off and recover from infectious illnesses. These closely linked events can initiate a "downhill spiral" or a "vicious cycle" that leads inexorably to death. PEM causes a marked repression of cell-mediated immunity and the function of T lymphocytes. Malnourished children show dermal anergy, with loss of delayed dermal hypersensitivity (DDH) reactions, decrease or reversal of the T helper/suppressor cell ratio, and loss of the ability of killer lymphocytes to recognize and destroy foreign tissues. In contrast, B lymphocyte numbers and functions generally appear to be maintained. While existing antibody production is conserved or even increased during generalized malnutrition, new primary antibody responses to T-cell-dependent antigens and antibody affinity are impaired.

Research conducted in military personnel has shown immune dysregulation caused by stress that is similar to the immune dysregulation noted in the elderly (e.g., anergy and decreased proliferative response).[13]

## IMMUNE FUNCTION IN OBESITY

As abdominal fat expands in response to positive energy balance, there is a need for new blood vessel formation. However, these new vessels can often not keep up with the metabolic needs of expanding abdominal fat, leading to the death of adipocytes. As these adipocytes die, they release cellular debris that results in the activation of macrophages that release cytokines resulting in insulin resistance in fat cells as well as a systemic inflammation. The macrophages collect in circular collections and engulf the fat released from dead adipose cells in both abdominal fat and subcutaneous fat tissue.[14]

This systemic inflammation leads to an increase in innate immune function and defects in adaptive immunity. These defects have been identified in mice fed with high-fat diets to induce obesity. Mice fed a 70% fat diet develop obesity and specific defects in the ability of DCs to present antigens to the immune system leading to defects in adaptive immunity.[15]

There are a number of chronic diseases that are impacted by the enhanced innate immune function and inflammation. Since inflammation is a common mechanism across many different chronic diseases of aging, obesity-associated changes in immune function are critical in mediating the obesity-associated increased risks of heart disease, diabetes, common forms of cancer, asthma, and connective tissue diseases.

## MACROPHAGE RECEPTORS FOR OMEGA-3 FATTY ACIDS

As noted previously, chronic activation of inflammatory pathways plays an important role in the pathogenesis of insulin resistance, and the macrophage/adipocyte nexus provides a key mechanism underlying many common chronic diseases associated with excess body fat.[16] Migration of macrophages

to adipose tissue (including intramuscular fat depots) and liver with subsequent activation of macrophage pro-inflammatory pathways and cytokine secretion is the critical link between overnutrition and inflammation.

Omega-3 fatty acids (ω-3 FAs), DHA and EPA, exert anti-inflammatory effects, but the mechanisms are poorly understood. Recently it was discovered that the G protein–coupled receptor 120 (GPR120) functions as an ω-3 FA receptor/sensor.[17] Stimulation of GPR120 with ω-3 FAs or a chemical agonist caused broad anti-inflammatory effects in monocytes (RAW 264.7 cells) and in macrophages obtained from the intraperitoneal fluid. All of these effects were abrogated by GPR120 knockdown, demonstrating that the GPR120 membrane protein functions as an ω-3 FA receptor/sensor in pro-inflammatory macrophages and mature adipocytes. Moreover, GPR120 is highly expressed in pro-inflammatory macrophages and functions as an ω-3 FA receptor, mediating the anti-inflammatory effects of this class of FAs to inhibit both the TLR2/3/4 and the TNF-α response pathways and cause systemic insulin sensitization. Therefore, the in vivo anti-inflammatory and insulin-sensitizing effects of ω-3 FAs are dependent on expression of GPR120, as demonstrated in studies of obese GPR120 KO animals and WT littermates.

The worldwide diversity of dietary intakes of n-6 and n-3 FAs influences tissue compositions of ω-3 long-chain fatty acids (LCFAs: EPA, DHA, and docosapentaenoic acid) and risks of cardiovascular and mental illnesses[18] via inflammatory mechanisms mediated by eicosanoids synthesized from arachidonic acid and other long-chain ω-6 FAs. By increasing ω-3 FA intake from fish and fish oil or algae oil supplements and decreasing ω-6 FA consumption from vegetable oils and processed foods, it is possible to change tissue and plasma FA balance. More research is needed to connect these changes to changes in immune function, but there is evidence from epidemiological studies[19] that increases in the ratio of ω-6:ω-3. PUFA are associated with increases in chronic inflammatory diseases such as nonalcoholic fatty liver disease (NAFLD), cardiovascular disease, obesity, inflammatory bowel disease (IBD), rheumatoid arthritis, and Alzheimer's disease (AD). By increasing the ratio of ω-6:ω-3 PUFA in the Western diet, reductions may be achieved in the incidence of these chronic inflammatory diseases.

## IMMUNE FUNCTION AND VITAMIN AND MINERAL BALANCE

Vitamin A deficiency has long been known to be associated with increased susceptibility to viral infections such as mumps. While it has long been recognized that vitamin A and its metabolites have immune-regulatory roles, the mechanisms of action have not been known. Recently, there has been a significant progress in elucidating the functions of retinoic acid in regulation of immune cell development.[20] Retinoic acid (all-*trans* and 9-*cis* retinoic acid) is produced from the cells of the intestine such as DCs and provides an intestine-specific environmental cue to differentiating immune cells. When T cells and B cells are activated in the intestine and associated lymphoid tissues, gut-homing receptors are induced on the cells in a retinoic acid and antigen-dependent manner. Retinoic acid, produced by gut DCs, is also an important signal that induces IgA-producing B cells. The gut-homing T cells and B cells play essential roles in protecting the digestive tract from pathogens. Retinoic acid is required also for production of mature phagocytes in bone marrow. On the other hand, retinoic acid induces a subset of FoxP3+ regulatory T cells that is important for maintaining immune tolerance in the gut. Therefore, retinoids provide both positive and negative regulatory signals to fine control the mucosal immune system.

Although the best-known actions of vitamin D involve its regulation of bone mineral homeostasis, vitamin D exerts its influence on many physiologic processes. One of these processes is the immune system. Both the adaptive and innate immune systems are impacted by the active metabolite of vitamin D, 1,25(OH)(2)D. These observations have been proposed as potential mechanisms mediating the predisposition of individuals with vitamin D deficiency to infectious diseases such as tuberculosis as well as to autoimmune diseases such as type 1 diabetes mellitus and multiple sclerosis.[21]

Selenium (Se) is an essential trace element needed for the biosynthesis of a small number of mammalian selenoproteins. Selenium intake and personal selenium status are implicated in widespread human pathologies including cancer, cardiovascular disease, and neurodegeneration.[22] Positive effects of selenium supplementation have been observed in a number of clinical trials with patients suffering from sepsis, HIV infection, or autoimmune thyroid disease.[23] Most importantly, the lower the selenium status during critical illness, the more likely that the patients will not survive.[24] Supplementation with trace elements in some individuals with nutritional deficiency to correct a selenium deficiency has been shown to enhance antibody titers to influenza vaccination and shows a trend toward fewer subjects with respiratory tract infections. Another study reported better immune responsiveness and "fewer infection-related illnesses" with a multivitamin supplement than with a placebo in apparently healthy, independent-living elderly.[25] Other researchers have supplemented the diets of seniors with poor eating habits and found no immunological benefit or reduction in acute respiratory tract infections. The reason for the variability of results is likely related to the adaptation to starvation that can maintain immune function until late in the process as long as multivitamin and mineral intake is normal. Some, but not all, clinical trials have proven effective in improving the outcome of critically ill patients by selenium supplementation, but the best application regimen, most suitable selenium compound, and the mechanisms of action are not yet established.

A randomized, double-blind, placebo-controlled trial was carried out to investigate the effects of micronutrients supplementation on immunity and the incidence of common infections in type 2 diabetic outpatients.[26] A total of 196 type 2 diabetic outpatients were randomized to receive tablets of micronutrients (n = 97) or placebo (n = 99) for 6 months.

Individualized dietary energy intake and daily physical activity were recommended. Anthropometric measurements, blood biochemical variables, and the incidence of common infections were measured at baseline and at 6 months. Data on diet, exercise, and infection (upper respiratory tract infection, skin infection, urinary and genital tract infections, other infections) were recorded 1 month before the study and every month during the study. Blood concentrations of total protein, iron (Fe), folic acid, and hemoglobin increased, and unsaturated iron-binding capacity (UIBC) levels were decreased in the micronutrients supplementation group compared to the placebo group at 6 months. Moreover, at 6 months, compared to the placebo group, the blood concentrations of IgE, CD4+, CD4+/CD8+, WBC, lymphocyte counts, and basophilic leukocyte increased and CD8+ count decreased in the supplementation group, and the levels of IgA, IgM, and IgG and complements C3 and C4 did not differ. The incidence of upper respiratory infection, vaginitis, urinary tract infection, gingivitis, and dental ulcer were lower, and body temperature and duration of fever greatly improved in the supplementation than the placebo group. These data suggest that supplementation of micronutrients might increase immune function and reduce the incidence of common infections in type 2 diabetic outpatients.

In addition, deficiencies of vitamins B6 and folate are associated with reduced immunocompetence.[25] Trace elements modulate immune responses through their critical role in enzyme activity. Although dietary requirements of most of these elements are met by a balanced diet, there are certain population groups and specific disease states that are likely to be associated with deficiency of one or more of these essential elements. The role of trace elements in maintenance of immune function and their causal role in secondary immunodeficiency are increasingly being recognized. There is growing research concerning the role of zinc, copper, selenium, and other elements in immunity and the mechanisms that underlie such roles. The problem of interaction of trace elements and immunity is a complex one because of the frequently associated other nutritional deficiencies, the presence of clinical or subclinical infections that in themselves have a significant effect on immunity, and finally the altered metabolism due to the underlying disease.[25]

## PRACTICAL CONSIDERATIONS FOR MODULATING IMMUNE FUNCTION

The practical applications of the interaction of immune function and nutrition are fourfold. First, it is important to achieve and maintain optimal intra-abdominal fat depots that do not trigger chronic inflammation. The growing global epidemic of obesity and type 2 diabetes associated with the adoption of Western diets and lifestyles has significant implications for immune function but in an opposite direction to that associated with malnutrition. Chronic inflammation is associated with numerous age-related chronic diseases. Improved immune function in these individuals is achieved through a balanced diet and a healthy active lifestyle.

It is clear that malnutrition, especially PEM associated with kwashiorkor-like findings in children in the developed world or in hospitalized patients, can impair immune function. Therefore, recognizing and treating malnutrition is a critical component of maintaining normal immune function in hospitalized patients, the elderly, and in military personnel working under stressed conditions.

Finally, in addition to calorie and protein balance, micronutrients and lipid balance of ω-3 and ω-6 are critical. These needs can be met through a balanced diet, but in at-risk groups including the elderly, individuals consuming unbalanced diets, and in military personnel under stress, it may be advisable to include a multivitamin/multimineral dietary supplement to support healthy immune function. For balancing ω-3 and ω-6 FAs in cells, it is important to both increase the intake of DHA and EPA from fish or supplements while also reducing the intake of ω-6 FAs from foods containing vegetable oils.

## REFERENCES

1. Scrimshaw, NS, Taylor, CE, Gordon, JE. *Monogr Ser World Health Organ* 57:3;1968.
2. Faggioni, R, Feingold, KR, Grunfeld, C. *FASEB J* 15:2565;2001.
3. Thea, DM, Porat R, Khondi, N. et al. *Ann Int Med* 124:757;1996.
4. Scrimshaw, NS, Taylor, CE, Gordon, JE. *Am J Med Sci* 237:367;1959.
5. Matzinger P. *Ann N Y Acad Sci* 961:341;2002.
6. Matzinger P. *Science* 296:301; 2002.
7. Ingersoll, MA, Platt, AM, Potteaux, S, Randolph, GJ. *Trends Immunol* 32:470;2011.
8. Serhan, CN. *Ann Rev Immunol* 25:101;2007.
9. Medzhitov, R, Janeway CA Jr. *Cold Spring Harb Symp Quant Biol* 64:429;1999.
10. Bhaskaram, P. *Nutr Rev* 60:S40;2002.
11. O'Neill, SM, Fitzgerald, A, Briend, A, Van den Broeck, J. *J Nutr* 142:520;2012.
12. Salimonu, LS. *Afr J Med Sci* 21:55;1992.
13. Castell, LM, Thake, CD, Ensign W. *Mil Med* 175:158;2010.
14. Lê, KA, Mahurkar, S, Alderete, TL et al. *Diabetes* 60:2802;2011.
15. Smith, AG, Sheridan, PA, Harp, JB, Beck, MA. *J Nutr* 137:1236;2007.
16. Schenk, S, Saberi, M, Olefsky, JM. *J Clin Invest* 118:2992;2008.
17. Oh, DY, Talukdar, S, Bae, EJ et al. *Cell* 142:687;2010.
18. Hibbeln, JR, Nieminen, LR, Blasbalg, TL et al. *Am J Clin Nutr* 83:1483S;2006.
19. Patterson, E, Wall, R, Fitzgerald, GF et al. *J Nutr Metab* 2012:539426;2012 (Epub April 5, 2012).
20. Kim, CH. *Endocr Metab Immune Disord Drug Targets* 8:289;2008.
21. Bikle, DD. *Vitam Horm* 86:1;2011.
22. Papp, LV, Lu, J, Holmgren, A, Khanna, KK. *Antioxid Redox Signal* 9:775;2007.
23. Broome, CS, McArdle, F, Kyle, JA et al. *Am J Clin Nutr* 80:154;2004.
24. Manzanares, W, Biestro, A, Galusso, F et al. *Intensive Care Med* 35:882;2009.
25. Chandra, S, Chandra RK. *Prog Food Nutr Sci* 10:1;1986.
26. Liu. Y, Jing. H, Wang. J et al. *Asia Pac J Clin Nutr* 20:375;2011.

# 54 Nutrition and Dental Health

*Wenyuan Shi and David Heber*

## CONTENTS

## INTRODUCTION AND PUBLIC HEALTH IMPLICATIONS

Dental care is estimated to cost approximately 60 billion dollars per year, making it the third largest expenditure of health-care dollars in the United States.[1] Nutrition is intimately involved in the prevention and etiology of both dental caries or tooth decay and periodontal disease, which are the major dental disorders. Furthermore, gingivitis and periodontal disease can be risk factors for cardiovascular (CV) disease as well as being closely associated with type 2 diabetes mellitus (DM). Recent research has demonstrated that certain polyphenols from fruits and vegetables as well as botanicals can inhibit biofilm formation and may have a role to play in the prevention of dental diseases beyond current proven practices of fluoridation and regular dental hygiene. In many populations, dental caries has been identified as one of the most prevalent chronic conditions affecting from 60% to 90% of children. In children in industrialized countries, dental caries are up to five times more prevalent than the second most prevalent chronic condition in children, asthma.[2] Dental caries are a major cause of pain and infection that can have severe consequences for the quality of life of the affected children and their families.[3] The second important characteristic is that dental caries in children are mostly preventable.[4–6]

A significant decrease of the onset of tooth decay has been observed, especially in the western part of the world[7] in nations like Germany,[8] England, United States, Scandinavia, Scotland,[9] Norway,[10] and Australia.[11] This diminution of dental caries levels could be due to the use of different fluoride-releasing vehicles and other preventive systems.[9,10,12] However, recent research demonstrated that dental caries distribution was nonhomogeneous through different geographical areas and there were many variations within nations. In fact, several population groups still have a high caries incidence and a need for reducing dental caries and prevention of tooth decay.[13–15]

Periodontal diseases are inflammatory diseases affecting the supporting tissues of the tooth. The American Academy of Periodontology (AAP) has classified periodontitis into aggressive periodontitis (AgP), chronic periodontitis (CP), and periodontitis as a manifestation of systemic diseases.[16] Both AgP and CP have a multifactorial etiology with dental plaque as the initiating factor.[17] However, the initiation and progression of periodontitis are influenced by other factors including microbiologic, social and behavioral, systemic, and genetic factors.[18] The prevalence of periodontal diseases varies in different regions of the world according to the definition of periodontitis and study population, and there are indications that they may be more prevalent in developing than in developed countries.[19,20] The National Health and Nutrition Examination Survey III (NHANES III) conducted in the United States between 1988 and 1994[21] has demonstrated that 50% of the adult population has gingival inflammation. The prevalence of AgP in the United States ranges between 0.6% in Whites and 2.6% in African-Americans.[22]

Diabetes mellitus (DM) is closely associated with obesity and many chronic diseases, including liver disease and kidney disease, but diabetes is also a risk factor for periodontal disease, especially when it is not well controlled.[23] Conversely, the presence of CP in diabetic patients is associated with worse glycemic control,[24] and the induction of periodontitis in rodents leads to glucose intolerance and diabetes.[25] Therefore, diabetes and periodontal disease may interact in a vicious cycle, promoting each other. These close associations with diabetes make the prevention of diabetes and obesity highly relevant to the prevention of periodontal disease.

Gingivitis and CP are inflammatory diseases of the periodontium. They are associated with local inflammation, which manifests itself as pain and bleeding and slowly leads to the weakening and loosening of periodontal structures and subsequent loss of teeth. Recent data suggest that bacteria and bacterial products present in dental plaque and crevicular fluid can stimulate immune cells to produce and release a number of inflammatory mediators.[26] They play a role in the local destruction of gingiva and bone, but are also released to the bloodstream, and their serum concentration is regarded as a marker of periodontal disease. This is true in particular for serum C-reactive protein (CRP) concentration, in the general as well as in some specific populations,[27–29] but also for other cytokines.[30] According to current knowledge, inflammation is responsible for the development of atherosclerosis. It has been found that markers of inflammation are predictors of CV mortality and morbidity in the general population.[31,32] Therefore, CP-induced, low-grade systemic inflammation may play a specific role in the pathogenesis of atherosclerosis. Bacteria causing periodontal diseases, such as *Porphyromonas gingivalis* and *Treponema denticola*, have also been found in atherosclerotic plaques,[33] provoking speculation regarding their direct role in the pathogenesis of atherosclerosis. CP (as well as diabetes itself) is associated with an increased risk of CV complications.[23] It seems possible that atherosclerotic processes may be initiated or accelerated by periodontal disease-associated inflammation and/or bacteria.[33]

## DENTAL CARIES AND NUTRITION

Dental caries is a dynamic process that involves a susceptible tooth, cariogenic bacteria in dental plaque such as *Streptococcus mutans*, and a fermentable carbohydrate. Other contributing factors also include absence of fluoride, salivary gland hypofunction, and poor oral hygiene. Fermentable carbohydrates are commonly considered to be primarily sucrose (table sugar). However, all simple sugars are potentially cariogenic. The universal sweetener in use today, high-fructose corn syrup, is made from the simple sugars, glucose and fructose. The frequency of sugar eaten is the primary factor involved in the caries process. Sugary foods or liquids consumed 20 min apart allow for separate opportunities for bacteria to feed and produce acid. When the pH of the dental plaque falls below 5.5, the caries process begins. Form and composition of a fermentable carbohydrate plays a secondary role depending on how long it takes for a food or drink to clear the oral cavity. Liquids clear faster than soft, sticky foods.

Sugar alcohols such as xylitol and sorbitol are not fermentable in the mouth and so are used in gums and other products intended to reduce the tendency of foods to cause dental caries.

Dentists and other oral health professionals are concerned about the record numbers of sugar-sweetened beverages such as soft drinks being consumed by America's youth.[34,35] Preliminary data suggest that frequent consumption of these beverages can lead to enamel erosion and tooth decay. The data are limited, however, and the gaps leave many questions about the extent to which these beverages singularly cause or contribute to tooth decay. One 12 oz soda contains 10 teaspoons of sugar as well as acid. Diet soda includes both citric and phosphoric acid, which may cause direct demineralization of the tooth enamel. While clinical study data are lacking, common recommendations to reduce the impact of soft drinks include rinsing the mouth with water, bypassing the teeth by using a straw, or drinking soft drinks together with a meal to help reduce the negative effects of the liquid fermentable carbohydrates. Protective factors from specific foods and diet sequencing may also be utilized in order to reduce the destructive influence of fermentable carbohydrates. Fats and proteins consumed in a meal help coat the tooth surface to protect it from sugars. Fluoride in both food and water can also help remineralize the enamel. Diet and periodontal disease are not as clearly connected as diet and dental caries. Overall nutritional status can affect host susceptibility and influence disease progression especially in type 2 diabetes. Good nutrition can be protective by helping increase resistance to periodontal infection and help minimize its severity, while malnutrition can reduce resistance to periodontal infection through effects of malnutrition on immune function. The physical consistency of food has a direct effect on periodontal health. Crunchy, fibrous foods increase salivary flow, and saliva has antibacterial properties.

## ORAL MICROBIAL ENVIRONMENT AND BACTERIAL INTERACTIONS

Several hundred different taxa of bacteria contribute to the complex ecosystem in the oral cavity[36–39] and form highly structured, multispecies communities that are responsible for two major human oral diseases: caries (tooth decay) and gingivitis/periodontitis (gum diseases).[40–42]

The resident bacteria of the oral microbial community carry out a plethora of interactions at various levels to form sophisticated, multispecies biofilm structures, perform physiological functions, and induce microbial pathogenesis.[43–55] The development of these oral microbial communities, especially the sequence of adherence to host tissue by the early bacterial colonizers, as well as the subsequent recruitment of intermediate and late colonizers to the already attached microbes through coadhesion, has been investigated.[43,45] These studies have developed information from in vivo observations of biofilm formation and its architecture as well as in vitro investigation of single bacterial adherence events between single bacterial species.[43,45,47,48]

Importantly, during the development of highly structured microbial communities, the incoming bacteria must be able to attach to resident members of the extracellular matrix and, more importantly, overcome the invasion resistance in order to integrate into the community.[49] It has been shown, for example, that the predominantly gram-positive oral microbiota of mice develops invasion resistance and responds to the presence of *Escherichia coli* isolated from gut bacteria by producing hydrogen peroxide ($H_2O_2$). *E. coli* cells are more sensitive to this bactericidal agent than the oral isolates comprising the gram positives, leading to selective killing of the gram-negative foreign intruder.[50] Further analysis revealed that the lipopolysaccharides (LPS) of *E. coli* were the main determinant responsible for triggering the $H_2O_2$ production by oral communities.[50]

## CRANBERRIES AND ORAL HEALTH

In recent years, several researchers have tried to identify edible, nontoxic compounds that could interfere with formation of the cariogenic biofilm. In this regard, it has been demonstrated that certain constituents of cranberries may limit dental caries by inhibiting the production of organic acids by cariogenic bacteria, the formation of biofilms by S. mutans and Streptococcus sobrinus, and the adhesion and coaggregation of a considerable number of other oral species of Streptococcus.

The cranberry is a native North American fruit for which a number of studies have reported beneficial properties for human health. Cranberries are particularly rich in various polyphenolic compounds, including flavonoids, phenolic acids, and complex phenolic polymers. It has been reported that high-molecular-mass proanthocyanidins (condensed tannins) from cranberry juice inhibit the adherence of uropathogenic fimbriated E. coli and thus protect against urinary tract infections. Furthermore, a high-molecular-weight cranberry fraction was also reported to inhibit the sialic acid–specific adhesion of Helicobacter pylori to human gastric mucosa, a critical step for gastric ulcer development. In the area of dental research, it has been reported that a nondialyzable material (NDM) prepared from cranberry juice concentrate inhibits the coaggregation of many oral bacteria and prevents mutans streptococci (MS) (S. mutans and S. sobrinus) biofilm formation.

Yamanaka and colleagues[51] assessed the effect of cranberry juice on the ability of several oral species of Streptococcus to adhere to hydroxyapatite pellets that had been pretreated with saliva. When the bacteria were exposed to cranberry juice, their adhesion to the pellets decreased significantly. Furthermore, the hydrophobicity of the cells declined with increasing concentration of cranberry juice. In the same study, the authors found that the NDM fraction of cranberry juice inhibited 80%–95% of biofilm formation among the streptococci studied (S. sobrinus, S. mutans, Streptococcus criceti, Streptococcus sanguinis, Streptococcus oralis, and Streptococcus mitis). Other groups[52,53] subsequently confirmed the ability of cranberry extracts to prevent the formation of biofilms by cariogenic streptococci. It has also been reported that the polyphenols in cranberries led to the desorption of S. sobrinus from an artificial dental biofilm.[54] These observations suggest that cranberry polyphenols can inhibit the colonization of dental surfaces by oral streptococci and thereby slow the development of cariogenic dental plaque.

In a clinical study, Weiss and colleagues[55] investigated the effect on oral health of a mouthwash supplemented with the NDM fraction of cranberries. After 6 weeks of daily use of the mouthwash, total microflora, notably S. mutans, was significantly reduced. In support of these in vivo results, in vitro studies showed that the NDM fraction inhibited the adhesion of S. sobrinus to a hydroxyapatite surface pretreated with saliva.[55]

The polysaccharides glucan and fructan play a primary role in the adhesion of bacteria to dental surfaces and in the maturation of the biofilm. Various groups have demonstrated that the ability of cranberry to inhibit the adhesion of S. mutans to the dental biofilm depends on inactivation of glucosyltransferase and fructosyltransferase, two extracellular enzymes produced by S. mutans that catalyze the formation of glucan and fructan, respectively.[52,56] The proteins binding the glucans on the surface of S. mutans also contribute to the formation of the biofilm. Koo and colleagues,[57] using hydroxyapatite surfaces pretreated with glucans, found that cranberry juice significantly blocked the adhesion of S. mutans to glucan-binding sites.[58] Therefore, the polyphenols in cranberries may influence the formation of dental caries by affecting the colonization of dental surfaces and the production of acids by cariogenic bacteria.

The colonization of subgingival sites by periodontopathogenic bacteria is an essential stage in the initiation of periodontal disease. The capacity of these bacteria to form a biofilm and adhere to host tissues therefore plays a major role in periodontitis. The NDM fraction of cranberries inhibits the formation of biofilm by P. gingivalis[59] and Fusobacterium nucleatum,[60] two species of bacteria associated with CP. The NDM fraction may also inhibit the adhesion of P. gingivalis to various proteins, including type I collagen,[59] and may reduce bacterial coaggregation involving periodontopathogenic bacteria.[55]

The strong proteolytic activities of the red complex bacteria described by Socransky and colleagues[17] (i.e., P. gingivalis, T. denticola, and Tannerella forsythia) are important in the destruction of periodontal tissue. Bodet and colleagues[61] reported that the NDM fraction in cranberries inhibited the proteolytic activities of all three species. More specifically, the polyphenols acted on the gingipain activity of P. gingivalis, the trypsin-like activity of T. forsythia and the chymotrypsin-like activity of T. denticola. These observations suggest that the NDM fraction has the potential to limit the multiplication of these bacterial species in periodontal pockets by limiting the availability of the amino acids and peptides on which their growth depends; it may also reduce the destruction of tissues mediated by the action of bacterial proteinases. Host cell production of cytokines such as TNF-alpha and interleukin-1-beta causes progression of periodontitis, and it has been shown that the NDM fraction of cranberry juice can inhibit subcellular signaling molecules such as AP-1 essential to the secretion of cytokines.[62]

Several studies have supported the premise that matrix metalloproteinases (MMPs) secreted by the host's cells play a key role in periodontitis. In fact, periodontal disease is characterized by a high concentration of MMPs in the gingival crevicular fluid, which leads to loss of gingival collagen, degradation of the periodontal ligament, and resorption of alveolar bone.[63] The NDM fraction of cranberries inhibits the secretion of MMP-3 and MMP-9 by the gingival fibroblasts and macrophages following stimulation by the LPS of Aggregatibacter actinomycetemcomitans.[64]

The polyphenols of cranberries, specifically the proanthocyanidins in the NDM fraction isolated from cranberry juice, appear to have potential for preventing and/or treating dental caries and periodontal disease. However, results obtained in vitro are difficult to transpose to the in vivo situation, since the oral environment could interfere with the biological properties of these molecules. Aside from the study by Weiss and colleagues,[55] which demonstrated that a polyphenolic fraction integrated into a mouthwash led to a significant reduction in *S. mutans*, no clinical studies involving substantial numbers of participants have been conducted. Clinical studies in this area are therefore warranted.

It is unlikely that the consumption of cranberry juice on its own can benefit oral health, given the insufficient contact time between the oral tissues (the teeth and gingiva) and the cranberry polyphenols. In addition, the sugar that is added to cranberry drinks, as well as the acidity of these beverages, may have the counterproductive effect of contributing to the demineralization of tooth enamel. Studies to isolate and characterize the bioactive molecules in cranberry extracts are therefore necessary. These molecules could then be integrated into oral hygiene products, which could be tested for their potential benefits in preventing oral diseases. In addition, localized application of these bioactive substances to diseased periodontal sites, through irrigation or insertion of a resorbable fiber, could allow for modulation of the host response through inhibition of the enzymes that destroy the extracellular matrix and attenuation of the virulence of the periodontopathogens. In such situations, cranberry polyphenols could allow reductions in the use of antibiotics, thereby preventing the development of bacterial resistance.

## GREEN TEA AND ORAL HEALTH

Tea is the most popular beverage in the world after water, and green tea is made from the leaves of *Camellia sinensis*. Once picked, the leaves are steamed or heated to inactivate endogenous oxidative enzymes. If left to ferment without enzyme inactivation, the oxidative enzymes cause polymerization of catechins and either oolong or black tea is formed, depending on the degree of fermentation that is allowed to proceed. Drinking green tea as a health beverage was recommended in China 5000 years ago. Eighty percent of global tea consumption today is black tea, and it is the most popular beverage in Europe and North America. However, there is a growing interest in green tea in the Western world due to scientific findings that demonstrate the health potential of the beverage. Many studies have tested the qualities of green tea as an antioxidant, antimutagenic, and anticarcinogenic and its role in hypertension prevention, CV risk modification, ultraviolet radiation protection, weight management, and oral health improvement.

Green tea has a unique composition, which includes proteins (15%–20% of dry weight), with enzymes making up a considerable portion; carbohydrates (5%–7% of dry weight) such as cellulose, pectin, glucose, fructose, and sucrose; and lipid components including linoleic and linolenic acids and sterols such as stigmasterol. Besides macronutrients, green tea also includes vitamins (B, C, E), xanthic bases such as caffeine (27 mg/240 mL tea infusion) and theophylline; pigments such as chlorophyll and carotenoids; volatile components such as aldehydes and alcohols; and minerals and trace elements such as Ca, Mg, Cr, Mn, Fe, Cu, Zn, Mo, Se, Na,

P, Co, Sr, Ni, K, F, and Al. Polyphenols constitute the most interesting group of green tea components. The main polyphenols in green tea are catechins (flavan-3-ols). The four main catechins are epigallocatechin 3 gallate (EGCG) that constitutes about 59% of total catechins, epigallocatechin (EGC) about 19%, epicatechin 3 gallate (ECG) about 13.6%, and epicatechin (EC) about 6.4%.

Oral pathologies such as dental caries, periodontal diseases, and tooth loss can greatly influence human health. Among those, dental caries is caused as a result of infectious diseases caused by numerous factors related to nutrition and bacterial infections. There are reports that tea consumption may decrease dental caries in humans and laboratory animals.[65] Magalhaes et al.[66] found that rinsing the mouth with green tea extract (0.61%) protected from erosion and abrasion of the tooth dentine similarly to rinsing with fluoride extract (250 ppm) or chlorhexidine extract (0.06% as found in oral hygiene products). In addition, 1 week of mouthwash with green tea (1.6 g of pulverized green tea in 40 mL DDW, three times a day) was able to significantly reduce the salivary levels of the virulent cariogenic pathogens *Streptococcus mutans* and lactobacilli. Such reduction of those pathogen levels will very likely decrease the susceptibility to dental caries.[67] Another study failed to demonstrate the antibacterial effect of green tea catechins on *S. mutans*.[68] The reason for the conflicting evidence might be that green tea has indirect antibacterial activity through mediation of protective saliva components such as secretory immunoglobulins, lysozyme, lactoferrin, oral peroxidases, histatins, and mucins.

Zhang and Kashket[69] showed that tea extract reduced α-amylase activity in human saliva. Therefore, tea consumption is likely to be an anticariogenic agent that lessens the cariogenic potential of starch-containing foods like crackers and cakes. It might lead to less maltose release that causes mineral depletion from tooth enamel. Dental enamel contains mainly hydroxyapatite $Ca_{10}(PO_4)_6(OH)_2$. With every pH unit decrease, the solubility of hydroxyapatite raises by tenfold; therefore, pH decrease in the vicinity of tooth enamel is harmful.[70] In a study that checked acid production from bacterial plaque in humans, it was found that EGCG extract given before sucrose administration caused reduction in acid production and impaired the pH decrease by a mechanism inhibiting the enzyme lactate dehydrogenase that leads to the formation of lactic acid from pyruvate.[71] In addition, tea polyphenols significantly blocked the adhesion of oral bacteria in the glycoprotein layer in a model that stimulated defensive saliva.[72] Prevention of pH decrease in the vicinity of teeth enamel and blocking bacterial adhesion are additional mechanisms explaining the anticariogenic properties of tea.

## CHINESE HERBS FOR PREVENTION OF CARIES: A GLIMPSE INTO THE FUTURE

Research on botanical dietary supplements is still immature with mechanistic research being highly prominent and clinical trial evidence relatively scant. Nonetheless, in many areas of medicine including dental health, there is active clinical research including some funded by the National Institutes of Health through the National Center for Complementary and Alternative Medicine. In many instances, the original ideas come from traditional medical practices leading to the identification of single ingredients and ultimately phytochemicals that can be studied using advanced scientific methods. This is also true for dental research.

In traditional Chinese medicine (TCM) practice, a group of herbs has been widely used for a specific therapeutic application defined as Qing Re Jie Du or "alleviating heat and relieving the symptoms caused by toxins."[73,74] Many herbs in this category have been found to have antimicrobial activities. One of the authors (W-Y S) and coworkers screened over 1000 Chinese medicinal herbal extracts for inhibitory activities against *S. mutans* and other pathogens.[75] This process led to the identification of an extract made from *Sophora flavescens* with potent antimicrobial activity against *S. mutans*.[76]

*S. flavescens* is a perennial shrub found in Northeast Asia. It grows in sandy soils on mountain slopes or river valleys. In spring or autumn, the roots are collected, cleaned, sliced, and air-dried. The processed root of *S. flavescens* is also known as "ku shen," which means "a precious medicinal root with bitter taste." In more than 1000 years of TCM practice, it has been used to treat pyretic and analgesic symptoms. Although a variety of bioactive compounds have been recently isolated from *S. flavescens* for the treatment of inflammation, cancer, and CV disorders,[77] and antibacterial activity,[78] biologically directed fractionation led to identification of kurarinone, a known compound isolated from *S. flavescens* as a major bioactive substance.[77–80] Several bioactivities of kurarinone have been previously reported, including antifungal activities against *Candida albicans* and *Cladosporium cucumerinum*,[81] antimalarial activity,[82] cytotoxic activity against human tumor cells (myeloid leukemia HL-60 cells),[77] and COX-1 inhibitory activity. At the current stage, the molecular mechanisms of its actions in bacteria and in mammalian cells remain to be established. Kurarinone was effective against both *S. mutans* and multidrug-resistant strains (MRSA and VRE) at the same minimum inhibitory concentration of 2 µg/mL. While these data suggest a potential application of kurarinone for the prevention and treatment of dental caries, further work in animals and ultimately in humans with a clinical end point must be carried out.

Using the same systematic screen of herbs with Qing Re Jie Du function for the inhibitory activities against *S. mutans,* antimicrobial activity was also found for extracts of *Glycyrrhiza uralensis* Fisch. ex DC (Chinese name "Gancao" or Chinese licorice).[83] This is one of the most frequently used traditional medicines in China.

Moreover, a novel compound, glycyrrhizol A, was found to be responsible for this bioactivity using biodirected fractionation of the herbal extract. After producing the effective herbal extract in large quantity, it was used to develop a sugar-free lollipop to effectively kill cavity-causing bacteria like *S. mutans* in vitro. Safety, toxicity, stability, and in vivo efficacy studies were conducted to test the usefulness of this lollipop in killing cavity-causing bacteria in humans. Safety and

toxicity studies enabled the conduct of two pilot human studies, indicating that a brief application of these lollipops (twice a day for 10 days) led to marked reduction of cavity-causing bacteria in oral cavity among most of the human subjects tested. A lollipop was used rather than a mouthwash to prolong the time of contact of the active antimicrobials with the oral microflora. If successful in clinical trials, a lollipop could be used to control or prevent tooth decay, making it a novel tool to promote oral health as a functional food for special dietary use. However, the anticavity effect must be demonstrated clinically beyond the microbiology end point used in this pilot study.

The effect of magnolia bark extract (MBE)[84] on different variables related to caries and gingivitis was tested following daily administration through a sugar-free chewing gum. The study was performed with healthy adult volunteers at high risk for caries as a randomized double-blind interventional study.[85] A total of 120 subjects with a salivary MS concentration $\geq 10^5$ CFU/mL and presence of bleeding on probing classified as >25% were enrolled and divided into three groups to receive magnolia, xylitol, or control gums. The study design included examinations at baseline, after 7 days, after 30 days of gum use, and 7 days after the end of gum use. Plaque pH was assessed using the strip method following a sucrose challenge. Area under the curve (AUC 5.7 and AUC 6.2) was recorded. Whole saliva was collected and the number of salivary MS (CFU/mL) was counted. Bleeding on probing was recorded as a proxy of dental plaque. Data were analyzed using ANOVA repeated measures. Magnolia gum significantly reduced plaque acidogenicity, MS salivary concentration, and gingival bleeding.

These interesting studies give a glimpse into the future of preventive dentistry. While the application of an herbal lollipop or sugarless chewing gum may help to promote oral health, it is not likely that either of these methods could currently replace dental preventive strategies including tooth brushing and fluoride application.

## GENERAL NUTRITION AND DENTAL HEALTH

The oral cavity is the site of a complex microbiome maintained by host tissues including the gums. The blood supply of oxygen and nutrition to the gums is critical in maintaining dental health. Smoking cigarettes or other forms of tobacco impairs blood flow to the gums and has been associated with periodontal disease.[86] Cigarette smokers without prediabetes exhibit significantly severe periodontal disease compared to nonsmokers. In smokers with prediabetes, the severity of periodontal disease due to tobacco seems to be overshadowed by the hyperglycemic state, obscuring the effect of habitual smoking.

Both the foods eaten and timing of eating can affect dental health. Vitamin deficiencies can express themselves in oral disease as with scurvy and B vitamin deficiencies discussed elsewhere in this text. For this reason, it is advisable to eat a balanced diet providing necessary macronutrients and micronutrients and to take dietary supplements. It is also important to limit between-meal snacking on high-sugar/high-fat foods not only for dental health but also to avoid overweight and obesity.

The American Dental Association advises when choosing meals and snacks to (1) drink plenty of water and (2) eat a variety of foods from each of the five major food groups, including whole grains; fruits; vegetables; lean sources of protein such as lean beef, skinless poultry, and fish; dry beans, peas, and other legumes; and low-fat and fat-free dairy foods. Foods that are eaten as part of a meal cause less harm to teeth than when they are eaten as small snacks throughout the day, because more saliva is released during a meal. Saliva helps wash foods from the mouth and lessens the effects of acids, which can harm teeth and cause cavities. Finally, brushing twice a day with fluoride toothpaste that has the American Dental Association Seal of Acceptance, flossing daily, and visiting a dentist regularly are integral parts of any dental health program. With regular dental care, dentists can prevent oral problems from occurring in the first place and catch those that do occur in the early stages, while they are easy to treat.

The future of dental health research includes a new focus on the oral microbiome, the factors governing the interaction of the bacteria in biofilms, and the formation of plaque. Natural products from foods such as berries and from botanicals including many used in TCM hold the potential of natural modulation of the oral microbiome. As with the gastrointestinal microbiome, the effects of prebiotics and probiotics on the dental microflora may also provide additional approaches to dental health through nutrition.

## REFERENCES

1. Cohen JW, Machlin SR, Zuvekas SH et al. *Health Care Expenses in the United States, 1996. Rockville, MD: Agency for Healthcare Research and Quality*, 2000; MEPS Research Findings 12. AHRQ Pub. No. 01-0009.
2. USDHHS (2000). *Oral Health in America: A Report of the Surgeon General. Rockville, MD, USA: Department of Health and Human Services.* National Institute of Dental and Craniofacial Research, National Institutes of Health.
3. Casamassimo PS, Thikkurissy S, Edelstein BL, Maiorini E. *J Am Dent Assoc* 140:650;2009.
4. Fejerskov O. *Caries Res* 38:182;2004.
5. Fisher-Owens SA, Gansky SA, Platt LJ et al. *Pediatrics* 120:e510;2007.
6. Selwitz RH, Ismail AI, Pitts NB. Dental caries. *Lancet* 369:51;2007.
7. Petersen PE. *Community Dent Oral Epidemiol* 31(Suppl 1):3;2003.
8. Schulte AG, Momeni A, Pieper K. *Community Dent Health* 23:197;2006.
9. Petersson HG, Bratthall D. *Eur J Oral Sci* 104:436;1996.
10. Birkeland JM, Haugejorden O, Fehr FR. *Acta Odontol Scand* 60:281;2002.
11. Davies MJ, Spencer AJ, Slade GD. *Aust Dent J* 42:389;1997.
12. Birkeland JM, Haugejorden O, Fehr FR. *Caries Res* 34:109;2000.
13. Pitts NB, Evans DJ, Nugent ZJ, Pine CM. *Community Dent Health* 19:46;2002.
14. Traebert J, Suárez CS, Onofri DA, Marcenes W. *Cad Saude Publica* 18:817;2002.
15. Traebert JL, Peres MA, Galesso ER et al. *Rev Saude Publica* 35(3):283;2001.
16. Armitage GC. *Ann Periodontol* 4:1;1999.
17. Offenbacher S, Schroeder HE, Seymour GJ, Kornman KS. *Periodontol* 14:216;1997.
18. Brown LF, Beck JD, Rozier RG. *J Periodontol* 65:316;1994.
19. Baelum V, Fejerskov O, Karring T. *J Periodontal Res* 21:221;1986.
20. Stoltenberg JL, Osborn JB, Pihlström BL et al. *J Periodontol* 64:853;1993.
21. Albandar JM, Kingman A. *J Periodontol* 70:30;1999.
22. Albandar JM, Brown LJ, Brunelle JA, Löe H. *J Periodontol* 67:953;1996.
23. Ryan ME, Carnu O, Kamer A. *J Am Dent Assoc* 134:34S;2003.
24. Taylor GW, Borgnakke WS. *Oral Diseases* 14:191;2008.
25. Watanabe K, Petro BJ, Shlimon AE, Untermann TG. *J Periodontol* 79:1208;2008.
26. Bodet C, Chandad F, Grenier D. *Clin Exp Immunol* 143:50;2006.
27. Ebersole JL, Machen RL, Steffen MJ, Willmann DE. *Clin Exp Immunol* 107:347;1997.
28. Franek E, Blaschyk R, Kolonko A et al. *J Nephrol* 19:346;2006.
29. Czerniuk MR, Gorska R, Filipiak J, Opolski G. *J Periodontol* 33:415;2006.
30. Offenbacher S, Barros SP, Beck JD. *J Periodontol* 79:1577;2008.
31. Bassuk SS, Rifai N, Ridker PM. *Curr Probl Cardiol* 29:439;2004.
32. Rattazzi M, Puato M, Faggin E et al. *J Hypertens* 21:1787;2003.
33. Zaremba M, Gorska R, Suwalski P, Kowalski J. *J Periodontol* 78:322;2007.
34. Enns CW, Mickel SJ, Goldman JD. *Fam Econ Nutr Rev* 15:15;2003.
35. Nielsen SJ, Popkin BM. *Am J Prev Med* 27:205;2004.
36. Aas JA, Paster BJ, Stokes LN et al. *J Clin Microbiol* 43:5721;2005.
37. Paster BJ, Boches SK, Galvin JL et al. *J Bacteriol* 183:3770;2001.
38. Paster BJ, Olsen I, Aas JA, Dewhirst FE. *Periodontol* 2000(42):80;2006.
39. Dewhirst FE, Chen T, Izard J et al. *J Bacteriol* 192:5002;2010.
40. Dahlén G. *Adv Dent Res* 7:163;1993.
41. Marsh PD *Adv Dent Res* 8:263;1994.
42. Nishihara T, Koseki T. *Periodontol* 2000(36):14;2004.
43. Kolenbrander PE. *Annu Rev Microbiol* 54:413;2000.
44. Kolenbrander PE, Andersen RN, Blehert DS et al. *Microbiol Mol Biol Rev* 66:486;2002.
45. Kolenbrander PE, Palmer RJ, Periasamy S, Jakubovics NS. *Nat Rev Micro* 8:471;2010.
46. Kuramitsu HK, He X, Lux R et al. *Microbiol Mol Biol Rev* 71:653;2007.
47. Kolenbrander PE, Egland PG, Diaz PI, Palmer RJ Jr. *Trends Microbiol* 13:11;2005.
48. Zijnge V, van Leeuwen MBM, Degener JE et al. *PLoS One* 5:e9321;2010.
49. Vollaard E, Clasener H. *Antimicrob Agents Chemother* 38:409;1994.
50. He X, Tian Y, Guo L et al. *Microb Ecol* 60:655;2010.
51. Yamanaka A, Kimizuka R, Kato T, Okuda K. *Oral Microbiol Immunol* 19:150;2004.

52. Duarte S, Gregoire S, Singh AP et al. *FEMS Microbiol Lett.* 257:50;2006.

53. Yamanaka-Okada A, Sato E, Kouchi T et al. *Bull Tokyo Dent Coll* 49(3):107;2008.

54. Steinberg D, Feldman M, Ofek I, Weiss EI. *Int J Antimicrob Agents* 25:247;2005.

55. Weiss EI, Kozlovsky A, Steinberg D et al. *FEMS Microbiol Lett* 232:89;2004.

56. Steinberg D, Feldman M, Ofek I, Weiss EI. *J Antimicrob Chemother* 54:86;2004.

57. Banas JA, Vickerman MM. *Crit Rev Oral Biol Med* 14:89;2003.

58. Koo H, Nino de Guzman P, Schobel BD et al. *Caries Res* 40:20;2006.

59. Labrecque J, Bodet C, Chandad F, Grenier D. *J Antimicrob Chemother* 58:439;2006.

60. Yamanaka A, Kouchi T, Kasai K et al. *J Periodontal Res* 42:589;2007.

61. Bodet C, Piché M, Chandad F, Grenier D. *J Antimicrob Chemother* 57:685;2006.

62. Bodet C, Chandad F, Grenier D. *Eur J Oral Sci* 115:64;2007.

63. Sorsa T, Tjäderhane L, Konttinen YT et al. *Ann Med* 38:306;2006.

64. Bodet C, Chandad F, Grenier D. *J Periodontal Res* 42:159;2007.

65. Wu CD, Wei GX. *Nutrition* 18:443;2002.

66. Magalhaes AC, Wiegand A, Rios D et al. *J Dent* 37:994;2009.

67. Ferrazzano GF, Roberto L, Amato I et al. *J Med Food* 14:907;2011.

68. Hirao K, Yumoto H, Nakanishi T et al. *Life Sci* 86:654;2010.

69. Zhang J, Kashket S. *Caries Res* 32:233;1998.

70. Dawes C. *J Can Dent Assoc* 69:722;2003.

71. Hirasawa M, Takada K, Otake S. *Caries Res* 40:265;2006.

72. Xiao Y, Liu T, Zhan L, Zhou X. *Hua Xi Kou Qiang Yi Xue Za Zhi* 18:340;2000.

73. Chen Q. *Pharmacology and Clinical Applications of Classical TCM Formulas.* People's Publisher, Beijing, People's Republic of China; 1998.

74. Huang TK. *A Handbook of the Composition and Pharmacology of Common Chinese Drugs.* China Medical Science and Technology, Beijing, People's Republic of China;1994.

75. Chen L, Ma L, Park NH, Shi WJ. *Microbiol* 39:3009;2001.

76. Chen L, Cheng X, Shi W et al. *J Clin Microbiol* 43:3574;2005.

77. Kang TH, Jeong SJ, Ko WG et al. *J Nat Prod* 63:680;2000.

78. Kuroyanagi M, Arakawa T, Hirayama Y, Hayashi T. *J Nat Prod* 62:1595;1999.

79. Lee HO, Park NK, Jeong SI et al. *Yakhak Hoe Chi* 45:588;2001.

80. Zheng Y, Yao J, Shao X, Muralee N. *Nongyaoxue Xuebao* 1:91;1999.

81. Tan RX, Wolfender JL, Zhang LX et al. *Phytochemistry* 42:1305;1996.

82. Kim YC, Kim HS, Wataya Y et al. *Biol Pharm Bull* 27:748;2004.

83. He J, Chen L, Heber D et al. *J Nat Prod* 69:121;2006.

84. Greenberg M, Urnezis P, Tian M. *J Agric Food Chem* 55:9465;2007.

85. Campus G, Cagetti MG, Cocco F et al. *Caries Res* 45:393;2011.

86. Javed F, Al-Askar M, Samaranayake LP, AL-Hezaimi K. *Am J Med Sci* 345(2):94;2013.

# 55 Protein Nutrition, Meal Timing, and Muscle Health

*Donald K. Layman*

## CONTENTS

## INTRODUCTION

The past decade witnessed an emergence of dietary protein in the popular press and nutrition research. Rediscovery of protein as a critical dietary component has been fueled by three distinct areas of research. One area driving intense interest is use of higher-protein diets for weight loss; a second area evolved from concern about sarcopenia—age-related loss of muscle; and the third area emerged from characterizing the unique role of the branched-chain amino acid (BCAA) leucine as a translation initiation signal for muscle protein synthesis (mPS). These three areas of research are beginning to converge as a unified concept for adult protein needs that emphasizes the quantity and quality of protein necessary at individual meals instead of conventional dietary guidelines focused on minimum protein requirements defined as net daily intake in proportion to body weight or as a percentage of energy intake.[1,2]

Historically, protein requirements have been based on the minimum amount of dietary protein necessary to prevent deficiencies or to achieve efficient growth.[3] For adults, growth has ended and acute deficiencies are rare. Instead, adult requirements are defined as the minimum amount of protein necessary for nitrogen balance. Nitrogen balance studies are performed mostly in young healthy adults with controlled feeding conditions for 7–14 days. The new areas of protein research shift the emphasis from whole body nitrogen balance to functional outcomes related to body composition and specifically muscle mass and function.[4] These outcomes are changing the philosophy about protein needs from minimum daily requirements to specific meal thresholds for essential amino acids (EAA). This review will summarize these areas of research and develop the perspective that optimum protein intake for adults should be built around individual meals providing at least 30 g of high-quality protein and the unique role of the amino acid leucine in defining the meal threshold.[1,2]

## ROLE OF PROTEIN DURING WEIGHT LOSS

The initial evidence that higher-protein intakes could spare lean tissue during weight loss was demonstrated in the 1970s.[5,6] During food restriction, the body is forced to modify the balance of metabolic fuels. There is a shift away from use of carbohydrate to use of stored fatty acids. Likewise, lean tissues are degraded to maintain a constant supply of amino acids for hepatic gluconeogenesis and for synthesis of essential proteins in plasma and organs. These researchers demonstrated that providing a diet enriched in high-quality proteins would minimize degradation of lean tissues and reduce nitrogen loss. They found that protein intakes up to 1.5 g/kg/day could achieve net protein anabolism even during dietary energy restriction.[6]

Since the late 1990s, there have been numerous weight loss studies using higher-protein diets.[7–9] Diets with protein >1.4 g/kg/day produce greater weight loss,[7–9] increased loss of body fat with sparing of lean tissue,[8,10–12] and improved glycemic regulations including reduced postprandial hyperinsulinemia[10,13] and reductions in blood triglycerides.[14] Multiple mechanisms have been proposed to explain the apparent metabolic advantages of higher-protein diets. Some of the mechanisms relate to direct effects of protein to enhance satiety, increase thermogenesis, and reduce loss of metabolically active skeletal muscle, while other potential mechanisms focus on parallel reductions in carbohydrates that improve glycemic regulations resulting in lower postmeal insulin levels and reduced potential for fat storage.[15,16] However, the most consistent benefit of higher-protein diets during weight loss is improved body composition with protection of lean body mass and partitioning energy loss to use of stored fat.[17,18]

While the majority of weight loss studies support use of higher-protein diets, other randomized controlled trials (RCTs) reported no differences in weight loss or body composition among diets with different macronutrient compositions.[19–21] These studies concluded that the critical factor in weight loss was calorie intake and specifically the energy deficit created by the diet. However, on further inspection of these large clinical trials, a confounding factor was diet compliance. In most large RCTs, subjects tend to relapse toward preexisting diet behaviors. Hence, the conclusion that all diets are equal is essentially a discovery that most subjects fail to follow the new diets. This behavior pattern begs the fundamental question of the efficacy of individual diets and highlights the importance of nutrition education for long-term dietary compliance. Appropriate nutrition education is particularly important for incorporating protein into the diet. Major factors determining efficacy of higher-protein diets are the goals for the quantity and distribution of protein at individual meals.

## PROTEIN THRESHOLD FOR MEALS: THE SARCOPENIA STORY

The importance of the meal dose of protein for adults has been demonstrated in research focused on aging and sarcopenia.[1,4,22] Aging reflects development of anabolic resistance to hormones and amino acid substrates, progressive decline in mPS, and loss of strength. The decline in muscle mass and function leads to increased likelihood of falls and injury, loss of bone density, reduced glucose tolerance, and increased risk for obesity.

Muscle protein turnover, the balance between synthesis and breakdown, is not a static process but a pulsatory pattern with anabolic periods occurring after meals and catabolic periods during postabsorptive times.[23] The anabolic periods after meals are driven by a rapid stimulation of protein synthesis with small changes in protein breakdown. The catabolic period between meals occurs with a decline in protein synthesis, while protein breakdown is maintained at higher rates. The net balance between the anabolic versus catabolic periods determines changes in muscle mass. During periods of immobility such as bed rest, during acute energy restriction, or during chronic undernutrition, protein turnover is negative, resulting in loss of muscle mass and function. There is general consensus that protein synthesis and the post-meal anabolic periods determine changes in muscle mass.[23]

Mechanisms to explain anabolic resistance and net loss of muscle mass during aging remain unclear. Research from Volpi et al.[24–26] demonstrates that age-related changes that originate from translation regulations versus defects in DNA or transcription. In a series of studies, these researchers found that mPS responds similarly in elderly subjects (>68-year old) and young adults (<30-year old) given a large bolus of amino acids demonstrating that older adults maintain mPS capacity if adequate EAA are available. For aging adults, amino acid availability can be limited by dietary supply, modified by visceral metabolism, or limited by blood flow to tissues. However, studies have shown that providing additional amino acids eliminates the anabolic resistance. Elderly subjects provided a drink containing 40 g mixture of amino acids (18 g EAA + 22 g non-EAA) stimulate mPS similar to young adults.[24] Further, the anabolic response could be duplicated with a drink containing solely the EAA. These investigators also discovered that supplementing the amino acid mixture with 40 g of glucose increased plasma insulin and mPS in young adults, while the glucose supplement inhibited mPS in the elderly.[25] This negative effect of glucose (or insulin) was confirmed in a subsequent study.[27] Insulin is now thought to function in a permissive but not regulatory role in adults.[28] These findings demonstrate that high-carbohydrate diets contribute to the anabolic resistance seen in elderly but the age-related decline in mPS can be overcome with higher amounts of EAA.

Cuthbertson et al.[28] proposed that the age-related decline in mPS is due to a deficit in anabolic signaling that increases the threshold for EAA required to trigger translation initiation. They provided drinks containing 5, 10, 20, or 40 g of EAA to young (~28-year old) and older (~70-year old) adults. With 10 g of EAA, mPS was more than 50% greater in the young subjects compared with elderly, and the increase was associated with greater activation of translation factors (i.e., mTORC1, p70S6K, and eIF4F). The young subjects exhibited a dose-dependent increase in mPS from 5 to 10 g of EAA with no additional increase from 10 to 20 g. At 20 g of EAA, the older subjects exhibited increased mPS and activation of translation factors equivalent to the young subjects consuming 10 g of EAA. The older subjects had no additional stimulation with increasing intake from 20 to 40 g of EAA. These findings demonstrate that the anabolic resistance of aging is associated with defects in translation signaling that can be overcome with additional EAA. Further, once the translation signal is fully activated to trigger mPS, further doubling of EAA intake had no additional effects on mPS.

These studies using whole proteins are consistent with a meal-based threshold for EAA to stimulate mPS.[29,30] EAA make up approximately 40%–50% of the weight of plant and animal proteins. Multiple studies have shown that single meals require about 30–35 g of high-quality protein to achieve maximum mPS in older adults. Protein intakes at individual meals less than 20 g (<9 g EAA) produce little or no stimulation of mPS[1] or impact on nitrogen balance.[31] Likewise, meals containing more than 40 g of protein (>18 g EAA) exceed the necessary threshold and produce no additional stimulation of mPS. Collectively, these studies demonstrate that adults have a minimum threshold for protein or specifically EAA required to generate a post-meal anabolic response in skeletal muscle.

## PROTEIN THRESHOLD FOR MEALS: THE LEUCINE STORY

While complete diets with complete mixtures of EAA are necessary to achieve positive long-term effects on body composition and muscle mass, a single amino acid—leucine—appears to be the essential factor accounting for the meal threshold for protein. Dietary protein provides nine essential (indispensable) and 11 nonessential (dispensable) amino acids that serve as the building blocks for body structures, enzymes, hormones, and nitrogen-based compounds required for every function of the body. Among the nine EAA, the three BCAA, leucine, valine, and isoleucine, are a unique family of amino acids because of their chemistry, basic biology, and roles in metabolism. The BCAA are relatively small amino acids with aliphatic side chains that are hydrophobic and allow them to exist in tightly coiled positions within proteins. These characteristics allowed the BCAA to evolve as predominant amino acids in structural proteins such as myosin, fibrinogen, and keratin; in transcription factors known as leucine zipper proteins; and in globular proteins that require both water-soluble and hydrophobic characteristics such as hemoglobin and myoglobin. In total, the BCAA account for over 20% of the amino acids in all proteins, and leucine alone accounts for over 8% of all amino acids.[32]

Beyond the chemical and structural characteristics, leucine has evolved to have unique roles in metabolism including a specific role in initiating the anabolic response after a meal. All amino acids are required as substrates for assembly of new peptides, but leucine serves a second role, particularly in skeletal muscle, as a nutrient signal to initiate mPS. Leucine functions in tandem with hormones including insulin to activate key elements of translation initiation, the first step in synthesis of a new protein. With increasing age, the contribution of anabolic hormones to initiate translation declines,[28,33] increasing the importance of leucine as a post-meal anabolic signal.[34,35] Only leucine has the capacity to initiate the post-meal anabolic response.[36]

The unique metabolic attributes of leucine are, at least in part, associated with the absence of the branched-chain aminotransferase (BCAT) in the liver.[15] BCAT is the first step in degradation of the three BCAA. The liver has the capacity to produce urea and is the principal location for degradation of all amino acids except for the BCAA. Absence of BCAT in the liver results in an enriched supply of the BCAA appearing in the blood after a protein-containing meal. The three BCAA account for >50% of total splanchnic output of amino acids after a meal. Leucine in the plasma reaches peripheral tissues in direct proportion to dietary intakes. This pattern of interorgan movement of amino acids allows leucine to serve as a nutrient signal of diet quality to skeletal muscle.

The principal regulatory site for leucine action in skeletal muscle is a kinase in the insulin-signaling cascade identified as mTORC1 (*m*ammalian *t*arget *o*f *r*apamycin *c*omplex 1).[37,38] The mTORC1 signal coordinates initiating the translation phase of protein synthesis (Figure 55.1). Translation requires assembly and organization of the ribosome, mRNA, tRNAs, and more than a dozen protein factors necessary to link together amino acids into a peptide. Increases in leucine stimulate the mTORC1 kinase to activate two of the key protein factors—the S6 ribosomal protein (rpS6) and eIF4F initiation complex (composed of eIF4E, eIF4G, and eIF4A). The active form of the rpS6 protein binds to the ribosome and directs the ribosome to selectively locate mRNA that code for proteins to increase the capacity for protein synthesis, while the eIF4F complex binds to an mRNA, allowing it to unfold and prepare for initiating protein synthesis. Specifically,

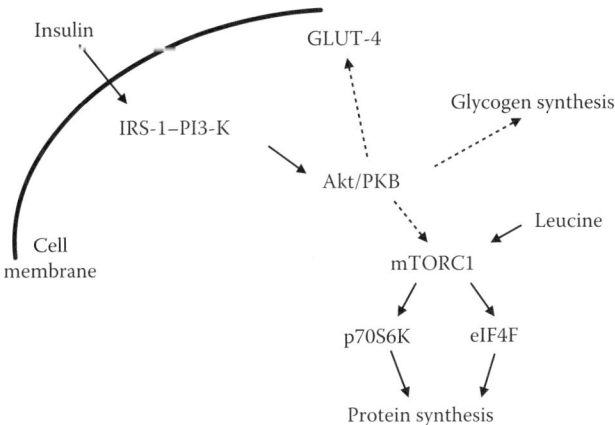

**FIGURE 55.1**   Insulin and leucine signaling in muscle.

leucine acting through mTORC1 stimulates phosphorylation of the inhibitory binding protein 4E-BP1, causing the binding protein to dissociate from eIF4E. Leucine also stimulates activation of the initiation factor eIF4G through an mTORC1-independent kinase. Phosphorylated eIF4G binds with free eIF4E and eIF4A to form the active eIF4F initiation complex. Further, leucine via mTORC1 activates p70S6 kinase, leading to phosphorylation of the rpS6. Together the active eIF4F and rpS6 factors serve to trigger mPS. Mechanisms for translational regulations by leucine have been previously reviewed.[37,38]

The role of leucine to facilitate assembly of the initiation complex and trigger mPS has been studied with free leucine and leucine present in EAA mixtures[39,40] and observed with both animal[35,41] and human[30,42] studies. These studies establish the potential for leucine to generate a postprandial initiation signal and stimulate a post-meal anabolic response. Likewise, leucine supplementation stimulates recovery of mPS after exercise.[42,43]

Anthony et al.[44,45] examined the time course of the anabolic response to an oral bolus of free leucine. They found that translation factors and mPS increased and peaked ~60 min after the oral dose. They also reported that insulin had an additive effect on mPS but insulin was not required for leucine stimulation of either initiation factors or mPS.[45] Crozier et al.[39] extended these findings by examining meal responses to different leucine doses ranging from zero up to 100% of the normal daily leucine intake. They found that the maximum response of mPS required sufficient dietary leucine to approximately double the plasma leucine concentration above the fasting baseline. This leucine dose appears to fully trigger the initiation process. They also found that additional dietary leucine increasing plasma leucine up to 10-fold higher than the fasting baseline had no additional effects on activation of translation initiation factors or mPS.

Similar results have been reported for leucine contained within proteins and consumed as part of a complete meal.[35,41] For leucine derived from proteins, digestion and absorption slows the rate of appearance of leucine into the blood; however, activation of translation factors and stimulation of mPS still require doubling of plasma leucine concentration.

Because of the importance of increasing plasma leucine to trigger the anabolic response, proteins such as whey protein that have higher leucine content and rapid digestion rates appear to be most effective in stimulation of mPS.[41,46] This finding suggests that protein quality defined by leucine content is an important consideration in designing small meals when the total amount of protein is limited.

To test the physiological significance of a leucine threshold, we designed a meal-feeding protocol with adult rats.[46] Meals were patterned after American eating habits with a small breakfast meal providing 20% of daily energy and a diet containing 16% of energy as protein. Based on previous research,[41] we estimated the precise amount of leucine required to achieve the initiation signal threshold at a meal for adult rats and then selected four proteins that provided a range of leucine contents to bracket the proposed leucine threshold (wheat gluten 6.8% leucine w/w, soy protein isolate 8.0%, egg white protein 8.8%, whey protein isolate 10.9%). As predicted, the whey and egg proteins provided sufficient leucine to increase plasma leucine concentrations, activate translation factors rpS6 and eIF4F, and stimulate mPS. To further test the hypothesis, we used the same protocol and supplemented the wheat gluten group with additional leucine to be equivalent to the whey group. The initiation response and mPS in the wheat plus leucine group was equivalent to the whey group. This finding provides additional proof that leucine is a limiting factor in initiating mPS and is consistent with other reports demonstrating that leucine supplements can enhance meals with low protein content or poor protein quality.[47,48]

The importance of leucine for stimulation of mPS has also been established with human studies.[30,34,49–51] These studies demonstrate that after a protein meal, there is a strong correlation of plasma leucine concentration with mPS requiring approximately doubling of plasma leucine to stimulate an anabolic response. Similar to the animal studies, supplemental leucine can also be used to achieve the amino acid threshold and enhance the response to a low-protein diet.[34,50] The range of leucine to initiate mPS at a meal is ~2.5 to 3.5 g. Normal food choices generally contain a mixture of high- and low-quality proteins, with animal and plant proteins providing approximately 70% and 30% of total protein, respectively, in American diet. This mixture of proteins has an average leucine content of ~8%, suggesting that the meal threshold for protein should be 30–40 g, consistent with findings from aging studies.[1,2]

While evidence is accumulating in support of a leucine threshold for stimulation of mPS, other studies found no response of mPS to supplemental leucine.[52–54] While these findings appear contradictory, the studies added leucine to preexisting meal patterns of free-living subjects. These studies appear to have used baseline diets that already exceeded the leucine threshold, and the leucine supplement had no additional effect. This is consistent with animal studies that show once the leucine threshold is achieved and the active translation complex assembled, additional leucine supplements have minimal effects.[39,41] For further support of this interpretation, amino acid supplements without adequate leucine have no potential to stimulate mPS.[36]

## APPLYING THE MEAL THRESHOLD TO WEIGHT MANAGEMENT

A new paradigm for dietary protein is evolving from the role of leucine in muscle health with a shift of the diet focus to meal composition.[1,2] Current nutrition guidelines define the protein requirement as the daily need for grams of protein per kilogram of body weight (g/kg/day). This expression implies that protein needs are a net daily sum that can be met at any time similar to vitamins or minerals. Further, protein needs are often characterized as a percentage of energy intake relegating protein to a role as a minor component of daily energy needs.[55] These guidelines for dietary protein imply that protein is relatively unimportant in adult meal planning. The body of evidence is growing that these definitions are inadequate to characterize protein needs for adults.[1,2,4] The new paradigm makes protein the centerpiece of meal planning defined by the specific amount of protein required to activate mPS.

While the meal-based protein threshold is backed by numerous short-term well-controlled studies, the long-term physiological impact of redefining the dose and distribution of dietary protein remains to be established. Initial studies applying the new paradigm to weight management support the hypothesis that the meal content of protein is a key factor for outcomes related to body composition, energy expenditure via thermogenesis, and satiety.[10,12,56–58]

*Body Composition.* Using the protein threshold, we conducted three clinical weight loss trials with diets designed to provide 10 g/day of leucine (~125 g/day of dietary protein) and a minimum of 2.5 g of leucine (i.e., 30 g of protein) at each of three meals.[10,12,56,57] To maintain equal energy intakes and minimize postprandial insulin response, protein was increased at meals at the expense of dietary carbohydrates. The control diet was a high-carbohydrate, low-protein diet following the guidelines of the USDA Food Guide Pyramid and meeting the minimum protein requirement of the RDA (0.8 g/kg/day). Subjects consuming the protein-rich diets lost more weight and were more effective in correcting body composition during weight loss. Consumption of the protein-rich diet resulted in greater loss of body fat and attenuated loss of lean tissue consistent with a protein-sparing mechanism derived from leucine. Similar findings have been reported by other research groups.[58,59]

Our first study was a 10-week highly controlled feeding study designed to minimize behavioral aspects of diet compliance. Participants were assigned diets with defined meal composition with a required 14-day menu rotation; all of the breakfast and lunch meals were prepared at our food research center to ensure compliance with the protein threshold at the first two meals each day. The higher-protein diet resulted in increased fat loss, attenuated loss of lean mass, reduced triacylglycerides (TAG), and increased HDL cholesterol (HDL-C).[10,56]

The second study was a 16-week evaluation of the same diets with or without exercise.[12] The primary diet outcomes of increased fat loss, attenuated loss of lean mass, reduced

TAG, and increased HDL-C were consistent with study 1. Addition of exercise further increased fat loss and attenuated loss of lean mass, and the body composition effects of exercise were significantly greater with the higher-protein diet. Exercise alone is well established to protect lean tissue during weight loss,[60] and higher-protein diets combined with resistance exercise appear to produce synergistic effects for correction of body composition.[59,61] The interactive effects of protein and exercise have also been observed in studies of aging and sarcopenia.[1]

Our third study was a multicenter 12-month weight loss program with free-living subjects.[57] That study highlights the difference between dietary compliance and diet efficacy. After 4 months, all subjects lost weight and the higher-protein groups lost 17% more body weight and 22% more body fat. After 12 months, mean weight loss in the protein group was 23% higher than the high-carbohydrate diet group, but the means were not significantly different due to a wide range of compliance. Individual weight losses ranged from 0.6 to 30.8 kg within the higher-protein group and 1.7–23.2 kg for the higher-carbohydrate group. These findings support the view that the most critical factor for weight loss is energy intake.[19–21] However, a secondary analysis selecting subjects who maintained compliance with energy restriction goals revealed that the higher-protein group had significantly greater weight loss and fat loss while protecting lean tissues. These findings illustrate that both energy restriction and the protein dose and distribution are important to optimize weight loss and body composition.

*Thermogenesis.* An added mechanism by which protein may confer its beneficial body composition effects involves increased diet-induced thermogenesis.[62] Thermic values for carbohydrates and fats contribute <10% to energy expenditure, while estimates for protein are 20%–30% and may account for 5%–10% of total daily energy expenditure.[63] The conventional view held that protein induced a systemic thermogenic effect owing to the large energy cost of protein digestion, amino acid absorption/transport, and nitrogen metabolism;[64] however, an alternate theory suggests the thermic effect of protein may be associated with the high energy costs of postprandial protein synthesis.[65–67] Leucine-induced stimulation of mPS represents a high energy demand on muscle metabolism with elevated ATP consumption and increased mitochondrial biogenesis.[67–69] Maintaining the metabolic role of skeletal muscle for energy expenditure is considered a major factor contributing to long-term weight management.[70]

*Satiety.* Protein has greater satiety value than either carbohydrates or fats and has the potential to reduce food intake at subsequent meals.[62,71] Short-term studies repeatedly reveal that subjects consuming higher-protein meals consistently feel fuller longer and with less quantity of food than individuals eating lower-protein, higher-carbohydrate meals.[72] Although these data are derived from acute treatments (i.e., a single higher-protein meal), a higher-protein breakfast meal (>30 g protein) consistently has the greatest effect on satiety and daily energy intake.[72,73] The common American meal pattern of limiting protein intake to a single large meal late in the day reduces satiety benefits of dietary protein.[73]

Two studies to date have shown satiety effects in the long term resulting in reduced body weight and improved body composition.[58,74] Controversy arises with attempts to explain mechanisms of protein's effect on satiety. Many have investigated the effect of protein on gut hormones including as ghrelin, GLP-1, and PYY as potential mechanisms, yet results are inconclusive.[58,62,75]

Evidence is emerging to suggest a role for the leucine component of higher-protein diets in triggering satiety. In one recent finding, leucine stimulation of mTORC1 was found in the hypothalamus and resulted in decreased food intake.[76] This may implicate a direct effect of leucine on the brain rather than an indirect effect on gut hormones as has been previously studied. Interestingly, leucine may also confer its effect by stimulating mTORC1 in adipose tissue. This effect has been shown to stimulate leptin secretion—an effect attenuated by rapamycin treatment, an inhibitor of mTORC1.[77]

## SUMMARY

Maintenance of body composition and particularly skeletal muscle is essential for adult health. But acute weight loss, immobility, undernutrition, and aging result in loss of muscle mass and function. These changes contribute to the age-related loss of muscle termed sarcopenia. Muscle mass is determined by the net balance between the anabolic periods occurring after a meal and the catabolic periods during the postabsorptive times between meals. For children and young adults, the anabolic period is enhanced by hormones (i.e., insulin, IGF-1, and growth hormone) that assure efficient use of dietary amino acids and energy. However, older adults develop anabolic resistance associated with loss of sensitivity to growth hormones. New research demonstrates that the anabolic resistance of aging can be overcome by enriching meals with EAA.

Anabolic resistance appears to be associated with a change in regulation of the initiation phase of mPS. A key enzyme in regulation of translation is mTORC1 that is sensitive to plasma insulin and the EAA leucine. In older adults, the anabolic influence of the insulin signal declines, and the mTORC1 signal pathway becomes largely directed by leucine. Increasing the post-meal plasma and tissue concentrations of leucine appears to represent an essential dietary signal to initiate the translation process to build new proteins. In the absence of adequate leucine at a meal, skeletal muscle remains in a catabolic period.

Discovery of the leucine signal for mPS has led to a new understanding about the amount of dietary protein necessary to produce an anabolic response for adults. Current dietary guidelines define protein needs for adults as g/kg/day or as percentage of dietary energy. These guidelines make no mention of the amount or timing of protein at individual meals. The new protein perspective recognizes that adults have a meal threshold for optimum intake to maintain skeletal muscle. The protein threshold requires at least 30 g of high-quality protein at each meal to provide adequate leucine to trigger mPS. The concept of a protein threshold emphasizes that the meal distribution of protein should be an essential component of understanding adult protein needs.

## REFERENCES

1. Paddon-Jones D, Rasmussen BB, *Curr Opin Clin Nutr Metab Care* 12:86;2009.
2. Layman DK, *Nutr Metab* 6:12;2009.
3. Institute of Medicine, *Food and Nutrition Board: Dietary Reference Intakes*. Washington, DC: National Academy Press, 2002.
4. Wolfe RR, *Am J Clin Nutr* 84:475;2006.
5. Flatt J-P, Blackburn GL, *Am J Clin Nutr* 27:175;1974.
6. Bistrian BR, Winterer, J, Blackburn, GL et al., *J Lab Clin Med* 89:1030;1977.
7. Skov AR, Toubro S, Ronn B et al., *Int J Obes Relat Metab Disord* 23:528;1999.
8. Parker B, Noakes M, Luscombe N et al., *Diabetes Care* 25:425;2002.
9. Foster GD, Wyatt HR, Hill JO et al., *N Engl J Med* 348:2082;2003.
133:411;2003.
11. Farnsworth E, Luscombe ND, Noakes M et al., *Am J Clin Nutr* 78:31;2003.
12. Layman DK, Evans E, Baum JI et al., *J Nutr* 135:1903;2005.
13. Piatti PM, Monti F, Fermo I et al., *Metabolism* 43:1481;1994.
14. Volek JS, Sharman MJ, *Obes Res* 12:115S;2004.
15. Layman DK, *J Nutr* 133:261S;2003.
16. Layman DK, Baum JI, *J Nutr* 134:968S;2004.
17. Krieger JW, Sitren HS, Daniels MJ, Langkamp-Henken B, *Am J Clin Nutr* 83:260;2006.
18. Devkota S, Layman DK, *Curr Opin Clin Nutr Metab Care* 13:403;2010.
19. Stern L, Iqbal N, Seshadri P et al., *Ann Intern Med* 140:778;2004.
20. Gardner CD, Kiazand A, Alhassan S et al., *JAMA* 297:969;2007.
21. Sacks FM, Bray GA, Carey VJ et al., *N Engl J Med* 360:859;2009.
22. Bopp MJ, Houston DK, Lenchik L et al., *J Am Diet Assoc* 108:1216;2008.
23. Phillips SM, Glover EI, Rennie MJ, *J Appl Physiol* 107:645;2009.
24. Volpi E, Mittendorfer B, Wolf SE, Wolfe RR, *Am J Physiol* 277:E513;1999.
25. Volpi E, Mittendorfer B, Rasmussen BB, Wolfe RR, *J Clin Endocrinol Metab* 85:4481:2000.
26. Volpi E, Kobayashi H, Sheffield-Moore M et al., *Am J Clin Nutr* 78:250;2003.
27. Guillet C, Prod'homme M, Balage M et al., *FASEB J* 18:1586;2004.
28. Cuthbertson D, Smith K, Babraj J et al., *FASEB J* 19:422;2005.
29. Symons TB, Schutzler SE, Cocke TL, et al., *Am J Clin Nutr* 86:451;2007.
30. Pennings B, Groen B, Lange A et al., *Am J Physiol* 302:E992;2012.
31. Arnal MA, Mosoni L, Boirie Y et al., *Am J Clin Nutr* 69:1202;1999.
32. Brosnan JT, Brosnan ME, *J Nutr* 136:207S;2006.
33. Rasmussen BB, Fujita S, Wolfe RR et al., *FASEB J* 20:768;2006.
34. Katsanos CS, Kobayashi H, Sheffield-Moore M et al., *Am J Physiol* 291:E381;2006.
35. Rieu I, Balage M, Sornet C et al., *Nutrition* 23:323;2007.
36. Garlick PJ, *J Nutr* 135:1553S;2005.
37. Kimball SR, Jefferson LS, *Curr Opin Clin Nutr Metab Care* 7:39;2004.
38. Vary TC, Lynch CJ, *Am J Physiol* 290:631;2006.
39. Crozier SJ, Kimball SR, Emmert SW et al., *J Nutr* 135:376;2005.
40. Escobar J, Frank JW, Suryawan A et al., *Am J Physiol* 293:E1615;2007.
41. Norton LE, Layman DK, Bunpo P et al., *J Nutr* 139:1103;2009.
42. Tang JE, Moore DR, Kujbida GW et al., *J Appl Physiol* 107:987;2009.
43. Norton LE, Layman DK, *J Nutr* 136:533S;2006.
44. Anthony JC, Anthony TG, Kimball SR et al., *J Nutr* 130:139;2000.
45. Anthony JC, Lang CH, Crozier SJ et al., *Am J Physiol* 282:E1092;2002.
46. Norton LE, Wilson GJ, Layman DK et al., *Nutr Metab* 9:67;2012.
47. Torrazza RM, Suryawan A, Gazzaneo MC et al., *J Nutr* 140:2145;2010.
48. Rieu I, Sornet C, Bayle G et al., *J Nutr* 133:1198;2003.
49. Koopman R, Wagenmakers AJM, Manders RJF et al., *Am J Physiol* 288:E653;2005.
50. Rieu I, Balage M, Sornet C et al., *J Physiol* 575:305;2006.
51. West DWD, Burd NA, Coffey VG et al., *Am J Clin Nutr* 94:795;2011.
52. Debras E, Prod'homme M, Rieu I et al., *Nutrition* 23:267;2007.
53. Koopman R, Verdijk LB, Beelen M et al., *Brit J Nutr* 99:571;2008.
54. Tipton KD, Elliott TA, Ferrando AA et al., *Appl Physiol Nutr Metab* 34:151;2009.
55. Millward DJ, *J Nutr* 134:1588S;2004.
56. Layman DK, Shiue H, Sather C et al., *J Nutr* 133:403;2003.
57. Layman DK, Evans EM, Erickson D et al., *J Nutr* 139:514;2009.
58. Leidy HJ, Carnell NS, Mattes, RD, Campbell WW, *Obesity* 15:421;2007.
59. Josse AR, Atkinson SA, Tarnopolsky MA, Phillips SM, *J Nutr* 141:1626;2011.
60. Jakicic JM, Clark, Coleman K, Donnelly E et al., *Med Sci Sports Exerc* 33:2145;2001.
61. Atherton PJ, Babraj JA, Smith K et al., *FASEB J* 19:786;2005.
62. Westerterp-Plantenga MS, Luscombe-March N, Lejeune MPGM et al., *Int J Obes* 30:S16;2006.
63. Tappy L, *Reprod Nutr Dev* 36:391;1996.
64. Buchholz AC, Schoeller DA, *Am J Clin Nutr* 79:S899;2004.
65. Tessari P, Kiwanuka E, Zanetti M et al., *Am J Physiol* 284:E1037;2003.
66. van Milgen J, *J Nutr* 132:3195;2002.
67. Wilson GJ, Layman DK, Moulton CJ et al., *Am J Physiol* 301:E1236;2011.
68. She P, Reid TM, Bronson SK et al., *Cell Metab* 6:181;2007.
69. Sun X, Zemel MB, *Nutr Metab* 6:26;2009.

70. Wing RR, Hill JO, *Annu Rev Nutr* 21:323;2001.
71. Rolls BJ, Hetherington M, Burley VJ, *Physiol Behav* 43:145;1988.
72. Veldhorst M, Smeets A, Soenen S et al., *Physiol Behav* 94:300;2008.
73. de Castro JM, *J Nutr* 134:104;2004.
74. Weigle DS, Breen PA, Matthys CC et al., *Am J Clin Nutr* 82:41;2005.
75. Smeets AJ, Soenen S, Luscombe-Marsh ND et al., *J Nutr* 138:698;2008.
76. Cota D, Proulx K, Smith KA et al., *Science* 312:927;2006.
77. Lynch CJ, Gern B, Lloyd C et al., *Am J Physiol* 291:E621;2006.

# 56 Micronutrient and Macronutrient Supplementation

*David Heber and Jeffrey Blumberg*

## CONTENTS

## INTRODUCTION

While it is generally taught that nutrients should first be obtained from whole foods, nutritional surveys demonstrate that in the modern diets of industrialized nations, which consist primarily of processed foods with limited amounts of fruits, vegetables, and whole grains, macronutrients and micronutrients are being consumed in amounts that fall short of meeting recommended intakes.

Blood and urine levels of biochemical indicators can help in assessing the adequacy of intake of many micronutrients over a limited period of time. These measurements reflect the sum of intakes from foods (some fortified with micronutrients) and from dietary supplements. However, biochemical indicators of nutritional status can also be influenced by factors other than diet, such as disease states and drug use. Dietary deficiencies have characteristic signs and symptoms, which have been well documented in the last century. However, more recent studies have determined that less than optimal biochemical levels can also be associated with risks of adverse health outcomes, including cardiovascular disease, stroke, impaired cognitive function, cancer, eye diseases, and poor bone health. Conversely, the consumption of excess amounts of certain nutrients can also be toxic.

The U.S. Centers for Disease Control and Prevention issued its Second Nutrition Report in 2012,[1] which summarized findings of blood and urine analyses on samples obtained in the National Health and Nutrition Examination Surveys (NHANES) conducted by the U.S. Centers for Disease Control and Prevention. In NHANES 2003–2006, 10% or less of the general U.S. population had nutrition deficiencies for selected indicators. However, for most nutrition indicators, the prevalence varied by age, gender, or ethnicity. For example, children and adolescents were rarely deficient in vitamin $B_{12}$ (<1%), while older adults were more likely to be deficient (4%). Men were more likely to be vitamin C deficient (7%) compared to women (5%). Non-Hispanic black (31%) and Mexican-Americans (12%) were more likely to be vitamin D deficient compared to non-Hispanic whites (3%). Vitamin $B_6$ (serum pyridoxal-5′-phosphate < 20 nmol/L), iron (serum body iron < 0 mg/kg), and vitamin D (serum 25-hydroxyvitamin D < 30 nmol/L) are the three nutrients assessed in this latest report with the highest prevalence of deficiency at 10.1%, 9.5%, and 8.1%, respectively.

After 1998, blood folate levels increased by about 50% across race/ethnic groups with the fortification of processed flour with folic acid. From 1999–2002 to 2003–2006, blood folate levels decreased slightly (<10%) in each race/ethnic group, likely as a result of the intentional small reduction in the amount of fortification of foods during this time period.

Healthy people can certainly meet most of their basic needs for almost all vitamins and minerals by eating a balanced diet rich in fruit and vegetables and whole grains and sources of good protein and fat. But most people do not come even close to meeting this goal, well described by the 2010 Dietary Guidelines for Americans, so that over 75% of adults in the United States fail to meet the recommended dietary allowance (RDA) for vitamins A, D, and E.[2] Similarly, between 50% and 75% of this population are not consuming the 90 and 75 mg of vitamin C daily recommended for men and women, respectively, by the U.S. Institute of Medicine (IOM). A lower but still concerning 25%–50% of women are falling short of their required intake for riboflavin and folic acid. And these overall figures do not address the gaps between actual and recommended nutrient intakes in vulnerable groups like pregnant women (and women likely to become pregnant), the elderly, and those with diseases associated with increased nutrient requirements or taking medications that interfere with nutrient absorption and metabolism.[3] Dietary supplements present one approach to dealing with these problems.

Dietary supplements have been popular, over-the-counter products for the past 60 years, first as multivitamins and later as an array of formulations containing multiple combinations of macronutrients and micronutrients, sometimes including botanical ingredients and phytochemicals. As defined by Congress in the Dietary Supplement and Health Education Act of 1994,[4] a dietary supplement is any product (other than tobacco) that (1) is intended to supplement the diet; (2) contains one or more dietary ingredients (including vitamins, minerals, herbs, or other botanicals; amino acids; and other substances) or their constituents; (3) is intended to be taken by mouth as a pill, capsule, tablet, or liquid; and (4) is labeled on the front panel as being a dietary supplement. This chapter focuses on both micronutrient (vitamins and minerals) and selected macronutrient (protein and fish oil) supplementation, while bioactive substances and botanical dietary supplements will be discussed in the following chapter.

The RDA was developed during World War II by a committee of the U.S. National Academy of Sciences in order to investigate issues of nutrition that might "affect national defense."[5] The committee was renamed the Food and Nutrition Board (FNB) in 1941, after which it began to deliberate on a set of recommendations of a standard daily allowance for each essential nutrient. The standards would be used for nutrition recommendations for the armed forces, for civilians, and for overseas population who might need food relief. The RDAs were meant to provide superior nutrition for civilians and military personnel, so they included a "margin of safety." Because of food rationing during the war, the food guides created by government agencies to direct citizens' nutritional intake also took food availability into account. The FNB subsequently revised the RDAs every 5–10 years. In the early 1950s, the U.S. Department of Agriculture nutritionists made a new set of guidelines that also included the number of servings of each food group in order to make it easier for people to obtain the RDA of each nutrient.

The current Dietary Reference Intake (DRI) recommendation for selected micronutrients[6–8] is composed of the following: (1) Estimated Average Requirements (EAR), expected to satisfy the needs of 50% of the people in that age group based on a review of the scientific literature; (2) RDA, the daily dietary intake level of a nutrient considered sufficient by the FNB to meet the requirements of nearly all (97%–98%) healthy individuals in each age/life stage and gender group (the RDA is calculated based on the EAR and is usually approximately 20% higher than the EAR); (3) an Adequate Intake (AI) is determined when an RDA has not been established due to insufficient data and represents an amount estimated to be adequate for everyone in the demographic group, and (4) tolerable upper intake level (UL) to caution against an excessive intake of each nutrient that can be harmful in large amounts. This is the highest level of daily consumption that current data have shown to cause no adverse effects in humans when used indefinitely without medical supervision. The Daily Value (DV) is a term used on food and supplement labels and based on the RDAs published in 1968; as the RDAs are periodically updated, there are some discrepancies between the current RDAs and the DVs.

## COMMON COMBINATION SUPPLEMENTS

### MULTIVITAMINS

Multivitamin supplements are commonly provided in combination with dietary minerals and are the most popular form of dietary supplement. While no regulatory or legal definition has been promulgated for multivitamin/mineral (MVM) supplements, they have been described by the National Institutes of Health (NIH) as a supplement containing three or more vitamins and minerals, and that does not include herbs, hormones, or drugs, where each vitamin and mineral is included at a dose below the UL.[5] However, generally speaking, an MVM supplement is a dietary supplement that is formulated at about 100% of the DV of most vitamins and essential minerals. No single MVM dosage form contains the DV for calcium, magnesium, potassium, and phosphorus since the resulting product would be too large to swallow. Many MVMs are formulated or labeled to differentiate consumer sectors, such as prenatal, children, mature or 50+, men, women, diabetic, or stress. Consumer MVM formulas are available as tablets, capsules, bulk powder, or liquid. Most MVMs are intended to be taken once or twice daily, although some formulations are designed for a greater frequency of consumption. MVMs generally contain the lipid-soluble vitamins, A, D, E, and K; the water-soluble vitamins, thiamin (vitamin $B_1$), riboflavin (vitamin $B_2$), vitamin $B_6$, vitamin $B_{12}$, vitamin C, folic acid, niacin, pantothenic acid, and biotin; and essential minerals, including calcium, phosphorus, iron, iodine, magnesium, manganese, copper, and zinc. Folic acid is usually provided at 400 µg, which is the legal limit for inclusion in an MVM, where it is always accompanied by vitamin $B_{12}$. In prenatal multivitamins, 800 µg folic acid is typically provided. However, folic acid should not be taken in large quantities in the absence of vitamin $B_{12}$ as this can lead to subacute combined degeneration of the spinal cord and irreversible paralysis. Zinc is always included in combination with copper as consumption of large amounts of zinc (above 50 mg) without copper can lead to a copper-deficiency anemia, since these two minerals share a common transporter.

While there is some controversy about the impact of MVM on the risk for chronic disease, there is general agreement that specific groups of people benefit from MVM, including women of childbearing age and pregnant women to assure AI of folic acid and reduce the risk of neural tube defects in newborns.[9] Dietary imbalances result from restrictive diets and those who cannot or will not eat a nutritious diet including many elderly. Some medications also affect micronutrient bioavailability and/or metabolism, so MVMs are indicated where there is a significant risk of drug-induced nutrient deficiencies. MVM intake is generally considered beneficial and safe in these vulnerable groups when taken as indicated.

While the evidence is mixed, data, which suggest a health benefit from the regular use of MVM, come largely from prospective cohort studies, which evaluate differences in health outcomes between cohorts that take MVM versus cohorts that do not.[10] Associations derived from such studies may not result from MVM themselves but may reflect underlying characteristics of MVM users. For example, it has been suggested that MVM users may, overall, have more underlying diseases, thus making MVM appear as less beneficial.[8] On the other hand, it has also been suggested that MVM users may, overall, be more health conscious, thus making MVM appear as more beneficial.[11,12] For example, subjects who enroll in prospective studies such as the Harvard Physician Health Study have markedly better (48% reduction in overall mortality) health statistics than the general population.

### CALCIUM AND VITAMIN D SUPPLEMENTS

Calcium supplements are recommended for individuals who do not obtain their need for this mineral from foods. With the reduced consumption of dairy products in the last few decades, more Americans, particularly postmenopausal women, are supplementing their diet with calcium in addition to consuming an MVM.

Most calcium supplements are best taken with food since stomach acid enhances dissolution of the tablets. As the fractional absorption of calcium decreases with increasing amounts, doses should be spread across the day and limited to not more than 600 mg at a time. Recommended daily calcium intake for adults is 1200 mg from supplements and foods but is increased to 1500 mg in women over 50 years due to decreased absorption of calcium. Vitamin D is formulated into most calcium supplements. Proper vitamin D status is critical to calcium status because it induces the synthesis of intestinal proteins responsible for calcium absorption.[13]

In contrast to claims by the dairy industry in the 1980s, the absorption of calcium from most food and commonly used dietary supplements is similar.[14] Soy and other vegetable milks are often sold with calcium added so that their calcium concentration is comparable to milk. A number of fruit juices are now fortified with calcium. Calcium carbonate is the most common and least expensive calcium supplement. It should be taken with food as its absorption is dependent on low pH in the intestine.[15] The absorption of calcium from calcium carbonate is similar to the absorption of calcium from milk.[16] While most people digest calcium carbonate well, some complain of gastrointestinal discomfort or gas. Taking magnesium concurrently can help to avoid constipation. Calcium carbonate is 40% elemental calcium, so 1000 mg provides 400 mg of calcium. However, supplement labels typically indicate how much calcium is present in each serving, not how much calcium carbonate is present.

Antacids frequently contain calcium carbonate and are a commonly used, inexpensive calcium supplement. Calcium citrate can be taken without food and is the supplement of choice for individuals with achlorhydria or who are taking histamine-2 blockers or proton-pump inhibitors.[17]

Calcium citrate is about 21% elemental calcium, so 1000 mg will provide 210 mg of calcium. It is more expensive than calcium carbonate and more of it must be taken to get the same amount of calcium.

## B-COMPLEX SUPPLEMENTS

B vitamins are a group of water-soluble vitamins that play important roles in cell metabolism. The B vitamins were once thought to be a single vitamin, referred to as vitamin B, but later research showed that B vitamins are chemically distinct vitamins that often coexist in the same foods. In general, supplements containing all or most all eight B vitamins are referred to as a vitamin B complex. Individual B vitamin supplements are referred to by the specific name of each vitamin as follows: vitamin $B_1$ (thiamin), vitamin $B_2$ (riboflavin), vitamin $B_3$ (niacin or niacinamide), vitamin $B_5$ (pantothenic acid), vitamin $B_6$ (pyridoxine, pyridoxal, pyridoxamine, or pyridoxinehydrochloride), vitamin $B_7$ (biotin), vitamin $B_9$ (folic acid), and vitamin $B_{12}$ (including various cobalamins, most commonly cyanocobalamin).

A commonly used combination of B vitamins has been formulated to reduce homocysteine levels and consists of vitamins $B_6$, $B_{12}$, and folic acid ($B_9$). While this combination of B vitamins does lower total plasma homocysteine, its impact on cardiovascular events is equivocal,[18] though meta-analyses suggest that only long-term supplementation with these B vitamins at doses sufficient to achieve at least a 20% reduction in homocysteine may be effective in reducing the risk of stroke.[19]

## INDIVIDUAL VITAMINS

### VITAMIN A

Dietary vitamin A refers to vitamin A in all its forms. Preformed vitamin A can be consumed from animal foods or metabolically converted from carotenoid precursors found in plant foods. Preformed vitamin A in dietary supplements is commercially produced in the form of esters such as retinyl acetate or palmitate. In foods of animal origin, the major form of vitamin A is an ester, primarily retinyl palmitate, which is converted to the retinol, an alcohol, in the small intestine. Retinol functions as a storage form of the vitamin and can be converted to and from its visually active aldehyde form, retinal. The associated acid (retinoic acid), a metabolite that can be irreversibly synthesized from vitamin A, has only partial vitamin A activity and does not function in the retina for the visual cycle.

Four carotenoids found in plant foods, including alpha-carotene, beta-carotene, gamma-carotene, and beta-cryptoxanthin, can be converted to retinal via the activity of beta-carotene 15,15′-monooxygenase.

In 2001, the IOM recommended a new unit for assessing the contribution of carotenoids to vitamin A activity, the retinol activity equivalent (RAE). Each μg RAE corresponds to 1 μg retinol, 2 μg of β-carotene in oil, 12 μg of "dietary" β-carotene, or 24 μg of the three other dietary provitamin A carotenoids.[20]

Because the conversion of retinol from provitamin carotenoids is actively regulated by the amount of retinol available to the body, there is no risk of vitamin A toxicity from carotenoid consumption (although carotenoderma can be an untoward side effect). The calculated rates of conversion apply strictly only for vitamin A-deficient humans. The absorption of carotenoids depends greatly on the amount of lipids ingested with them as lipids increase the uptake of carotenoids. A sample vegan diet for 1 day that provides sufficient vitamin A has been published by the FNB.[20] On the other hand, reference values for retinol or its equivalents, provided by the IOM, have decreased. The RDA (for men) of 1968 was 5000 IU (1500 μg retinol). In 1974, the RDA was set to 1000 RE (1000 μg retinol), whereas the 2000 RDA is 900 RAE (900 μg or 3000 IU retinol). This is equivalent to 1,800 μg of β-carotene supplement (3,000 IU) or 10,800 μg of β-carotene in food (18,000 IU).

Night blindness is still prevalent in countries where little meat or vitamin A-fortified foods are available. The role of vitamin A in the visual cycle is specifically related to the retinal form. Within the eye, 11-*cis*-retinal is bound to rhodopsin (rods) and iodopsin (cones) at conserved lysine residues. As light enters the eye, the 11-*cis*-retinal is isomerized to the all-*trans* form. The all-*trans* retinal dissociates from the opsin in a series of steps called photobleaching. This isomerization induces a nervous signal along the optic nerve to the visual center of the brain. After separating from opsin, the all-*trans*-retinal is recycled and converted back to the 11-*cis*-retinal form by a series of enzymatic reactions. In addition, some of the all-*trans* retinal may be converted to all-*trans* retinol form and then transported with an interphotoreceptor retinol-binding protein (IRBP) to the pigment epithelial cells. Further esterification into all-*trans* retinyl esters allows for storage of all-*trans*-retinol within the pigment epithelial cells to be reused when needed.[13] The final stage is conversion of 11-*cis*-retinal to form rhodopsin in the retina. Rhodopsin is needed to see in low light as well as for night vision. It is for this reason that a deficiency in vitamin A will inhibit the reformation of rhodopsin and lead to one of the first symptoms, night blindness.

Vitamin A deficiency is estimated to affect approximately one-third of children under the age of 5 around the world. It is estimated to claim the lives of 670,000 children under 5 annually.[21] Approximately 250,000–500,000 children in developing countries become blind each year owing to vitamin A deficiency, with the highest prevalence in Southeast Asia and Africa. Vitamin A deficiency can be considered a nutritionally acquired immunodeficiency disease. Even children who are only mildly deficient in vitamin A have a higher incidence of respiratory disease and diarrhea as well as a higher rate of mortality from infectious disease compared to children who consume sufficient vitamin A.[22] Vitamin A supplementation has been found to decrease both the severity and incidence of deaths related to diarrhea and measles in developing countries, where vitamin A deficiency is common.[23] The onset of infection reduces blood retinol levels very rapidly. This phenomenon is generally believed to be related to decreased synthesis of retinol-binding protein (RBP) by the liver. In this manner, infection stimulates a vicious cycle, because inadequate vitamin A nutritional status is related to increased severity and likelihood of death from infectious disease. Therapeutic doses for severe disease include 60,000 µg (200,000 IU), which has been shown to reduce child mortality rates by 35%–70%. Some countries where vitamin A deficiency is a public health problem address its elimination with national programs of vitamin A supplementation. However, as the benefit of this regimen of high-dose vitamin A supplementation lasts only 4–6 months, repeated treatments are required.

Vitamin A deficiency can occur as either a primary or a secondary deficiency. A primary vitamin A deficiency occurs among children and adults who do not consume an AI of provitamin A carotenoids from fruits and vegetables or preformed vitamin A from animal and dairy products. Early weaning from breast milk can also increase the risk of vitamin A deficiency.

Secondary vitamin A deficiency is associated with chronic malabsorption of lipids, impaired bile production and release, and chronic exposure to oxidants, such as cigarette smoke and chronic alcoholism.

Results of some prospective studies suggest that long-term intakes of preformed vitamin A in excess of 1500 µg/day (5000 IU/day) are associated with increased risk of osteoporotic fracture and decreased bone mineral density (BMD) in older men and women. Although this level of intake is greater than the RDA of 700–900 µg (2,300–3,000 IU), it is substantially lower than the UL of 3,000 µg (10,000 IU). Only excess intakes of preformed vitamin A (retinol), not β-carotene, have been associated with adverse effects on bone health. Although these observational studies cannot provide the underlying mechanism(s) of action for the association between excess retinol intake and osteoporosis, limited experimental data suggest that excess retinol may stimulate bone resorption or interfere with the ability of vitamin D to maintain calcium balance.[24] In a prospective, population-based cohort study, the overall risk of fracture was substantially increased among men with high levels of serum retinol. Retinol is released in target cells and converted to retinoic acid, which exerts its effects by binding to specific nuclear receptors. Retinoid receptors have been identified in both osteoblasts and osteoclasts. Retinoic acid suppresses osteoblast activity and stimulates osteoclast formation in vitro. This study suggests that serum levels higher than 86 µg/dL (3 µmol/L) may increase the risk of fracture. The normal level of serum retinol appears to be highly regulated within a range of 20.1–80.2 µg/dL (0.7–2.8 µmol/L).

In the United States, retinol intakes in excess of 5000 IU/day can be easily attained by those who regularly consume MVM and fortified foods, including some breakfast cereals. In contrast, a significant number of elderly have insufficient vitamin A intakes, which have also been associated with decreased bone density. Until supplements and fortified foods are reformulated to reflect the current RDA for vitamin A, it is prudent to use MVMs that contain 2500 IU of vitamin A as retinyl palmitate or 5000 IU of vitamin A, of which at least 50% comes from β-carotene.

## VITAMIN B₁ (THIAMIN)

Thiamin occurs in the human body as free thiamin and as a monophosphate, thiamin triphosphate, and thiamin pyrophosphate (also known as thiamin diphosphate). The RDA for adults is 1.1 mg for women and 1.2 mg for men.[25] A deficiency of thiamin can result from one or more of the following factors: (1) inadequate thiamin intake, (2) an increased requirement for thiamin, (3) excessive loss of thiamin from the body, (4) consumption of antithiamin factors found in foods, or (5) a combination of these four different factors. Antithiamin factors are found in tea leaves and betel nuts, and thiamin depletion in humans has been associated with the consumption of large amounts of tea and coffee (including decaffeinated), as well as chewing tea leaves and betel nuts. Thiaminase enzymes can be found in certain raw freshwater fish, raw shellfish, and ferns and can break down thiamin found in food. Individuals who habitually eat these foods are at increased risk of thiamin deficiency. However, if the foods are eaten after cooking, the thiaminase enzymes will be heat inactivated and deficiency will not occur.

Beriberi is the deficiency disease resulting from thiamin deficiency as described in Asia due to consumption of polished white rice as a primary food source. Beriberi occurs in two forms called the wet and the dry form. Wet beriberi is a form of heart failure in which edema and swelling are common. On the other hand, dry beriberi is characterized by burning sensations and muscle weakness due to nerve damage. In the brain and central nervous system, thiamin deficiency is called Wernicke's syndrome. Wernicke–Korsakoff syndrome occurs most commonly in alcoholics and is accompanied by amnesia, fabrication, as well as eye movement and gait disorders. This disorder is sometimes also seen with severe malnutrition secondary to cancer and AIDS. Intravenous vitamin B complex is administered routinely to alcoholics in the hospital or emergency room since some of the oxidative damage to the brain is irreversible, making it critical to provide adequate thiamin as a preventive measure if there is any suspicion of malnutrition in an alcoholic or evidence of advanced malnutrition in a cancer or AIDS patient.[26]

## VITAMIN B₂ (RIBOFLAVIN)

Riboflavin is involved in energy metabolism in the mitochondria and is a critical part of the coenzymes flavin adenine dinucleotide (FAD) and flavin mononucleotide (FMN). The FAD molecule consists of riboflavin bound to the phosphate group of an adenine diphosphate (ADP) molecule. A carbon-nitrogen bond binds the flavin group to ribitol, a sugar alcohol. Due to this type of chemical bond, riboflavin is not a nucleotide despite being named FAD. The transfer of electrons within the mitochondria depends critically on flavocoenzymes, which participate in these reactions in numerous metabolic pathways and are critical for the metabolism of carbohydrates, fats, and proteins. FAD is part of the mitochondrial electron transport chain, which carries out oxidative phosphorylation resulting in the formation of ATP. Flavocoenzymes also participate in the metabolism of drugs and toxins in conjunction with cytochrome oxidases.[27]

Glutathione is a key antioxidant in the cell and FAD is required to generate reduced glutathione from its oxidized form. The oxidized form links two glutathiones so the reduction results in the formation of two glutathione molecules. Glutathione deficiency may explain why riboflavin deficiency has been associated with evidence of increased oxidative damage.[28] Riboflavin status is commonly assessed by measuring glutathione reductase activity in red blood cells.[29] Uric acid is formed by the action of xanthine oxidase, another FAD-dependent enzyme, which enables the oxidation of hypoxanthine and xanthine to uric acid. Due to its high concentration in the blood, uric acid is an important antioxidant in the circulation. With riboflavin deficiency, there could be reduced blood uric acid levels promoting oxidant stress as well.[30]

FMN is required for pyridoxine 5′-phosphate oxidase, which converts vitamin $B_6$ found in foods to its coenzyme form, pyridoxal 5′-phosphate (PLP).

Interactions of vitamin $B_6$ and riboflavin nutritional adequacy have been found in elderly individuals.[31] With severe riboflavin deficiency, the conversion of tryptophan to nicotinamide adenine dinucleotide (NAD) and nicotinamide adenine dinucleotide phosphate (NADP) can be impaired, increasing the risk of niacin deficiency. An FAD-dependent enzyme, methylenetetrahydrofolate reductase (MTHFR), is required in the complex metabolic pathways resulting in the formation of methionine from homocysteine. The niacin-containing coenzymes, NAD and NADP, from the amino acid tryptophan, depend on the FAD-dependent enzyme, kynurenine monooxygenase for synthesis. Riboflavin and other B vitamins have been associated with decreased plasma homocysteine levels.[32] In individuals, homozygous for the C677T polymorphism of the MTHFR gene and in individuals with low folate intake, this has been clearly demonstrated.[33]

Since riboflavin is found together with other B vitamins, it is rare to find isolated riboflavin deficiency. Riboflavin deficiency is characterized by glossitis, an inflammation and redness of the tongue; redness and swelling of the mouth and throat; and dry cracked lips or cheilosis including sores at the corners of the mouth called angular stomatitis. Other symptoms may include vascularization of the cornea and seborrheic dermatitis. Anemia occurs with riboflavin deficiency and is characterized by decreased red blood cell counts, although the cells are of normal size and hemoglobin concentration is also normal.

Riboflavin and riboflavin 5′-monophosphate are available as supplements, but riboflavin is most often found in MVM and vitamin B-complex preparations. There are no known toxic or adverse effects of high riboflavin intake. A varied diet will supply adequate riboflavin amounting to between 1.5 and 2 mg/day. MVMs containing 100% of the DV provide 1.7 mg of riboflavin or sometimes more. The RDA for riboflavin is 1.3 mg for men and 1.1 mg for women, which should prevent deficiency in most individuals and is easily obtained in a varied diet.

## VITAMIN $B_3$ (NIACIN)

It is estimated that one-sixth to one-quarter of all elderly individuals do not consume the recommended 16 mg in men and 14 mg in women needed to meet the RDA. Niacin is found both as nicotinic acid and nicotinamide so niacin equivalents, or NE, are used in the RDA. Since niacin intake goes down between the ages of 60 and 90, the elderly should consume 20 mg of supplemental niacin in addition to consuming niacin from foods.[34,35] Adverse events include flushing of the skin primarily on the face, arms, and chest, which is a common side effect of nicotinic acid consumption of 30 mg/day or more. Flushing from nicotinamide is rare. However, the FNB does not distinguish between nicotinamide and nicotinic acid, setting the UL for both at 35 mg/day based on the adverse event of flushing, which only occurs with nicotinic acid.[36] The flushing associated with nicotinic acid is a common accompaniment of treatment of hyperlipidemias characterized by high triglycerides under the supervision of a physician.

## VITAMIN $B_5$ (PANTOTHENIC ACID)

Pantothenic acid is naturally found in a wide variety of foods and deficiency is rare outside the setting of severe malnutrition. Pantothenic acid given to prisoners of war in the Second World War relieved symptoms of numbness, burning, and tingling of the feet ascribed to pantothenic acid deficiency.[37] The FNB has set an AI of 5 mg of pantothenic acid for adults in the absence of adequate evidence to establish an RDA. Coenzyme A (CoA), which is critical to cellular energy production from dietary fat, carbohydrates, and proteins, requires pantothenic acid as an integral component. CoA is involved in the synthesis of cholesterol, steroid hormones, acetylcholine, melatonin, and the oxygen-binding heme in the hemoglobin protein. The liver requires CoA to metabolize a number of drugs and toxins.[38] In animal models, it is possible to demonstrate effects of pantothenic acid supplementation, but human intervention studies have not demonstrated benefits of supplementation with vitamin $B_5$. Dietary supplements are available over the counter with as much as 1000 mg of pantothenic acid. There is no evidence of toxicity in humans and no UL has been set.

## VITAMIN $B_6$

Vitamin $B_6$ occurs in three different forms: pyridoxal, pyridoxine, and pyridoxamine. PLP is the major form utilized as a coenzyme and is the most significant in human physiology. PLP is involved in the function of 100 essential enzymes in the body.

Epidemiological studies have established an association between low vitamin $B_6$ intake, increased homocysteine levels, and increased risk of cardiovascular disease. The relative risk of heart disease in women who consumed an average of 4.6 mg of vitamin $B_6$ per day was about two-thirds of the risk of women who consumed 1.1 mg/day.[39] Higher plasma PLP levels have been associated with a decreased risk of cardiovascular disease independent of homocysteine concentrations,[40] while other studies have suggested that low plasma PLP levels are associated with increased risks for heart disease.[41–43] While vitamin $B_6$ supplementation alone does not lower homocysteine levels, plasma homocysteine is reduced by vitamin $B_6$ supplementation during an oral methionine load test.[44] Based on these results, vitamin $B_6$ most likely plays a role in homocysteine metabolism.

The RDA for vitamin $B_6$ in adults is between 1.3 and 1.7 mg and the UL is 100 mg. Elderly individuals may require greater amounts of vitamin $B_6$. The elderly may benefit from the B6 in an MVM.

## VITAMIN $B_7$ (BIOTIN)

Biotin can be found in many foods in small amounts. Therefore, biotin deficiency is only seen in patients who receive parenteral nutrition without biotin supplementation or who consume raw egg whites. Egg whites contain a protein called avidin, which binds biotin and prevents intestinal absorption. Cooking the eggs inactivates avidin so only raw egg whites can contribute to biotin deficiency. Vitamin $B_6$ is synthesized by bacteria, yeasts, molds, algae, and some plant species, but not humans.[45] The FNB established an AI of 30 μg as there is not enough information to establish an RDA. There is no UL since there is no evidence of toxicity.

## VITAMIN $B_9$ (FOLIC ACID)

The root of the word folic acid comes from the Latin for leaf, and folate is indeed found in green leafy vegetables. As a vitamin, folic acid functions within the pathways denoted as methyl donor reactions. Together with coenzymes, folic acid acts as a methyl group or "one carbon" acceptor and donor in amino acid and nucleic acid metabolism. In DNA metabolism, folate coenzymes are critical for the synthesis of DNA from thymidine and purine precursors of methionine.

The amino acid methionine is utilized in the synthesis of S-adenosylmethionine (SAM). SAM is used in many biological methylation reactions, including the methylation of a number of DNA sites regulating gene transcription. In promoter regions like CpG islands or other functional regions, methylation of DNA modulates gene expression. Epigenetic control of gene expression is mediated by methylation as well as histone protein acetylation and deacetylation. Both folate- and vitamin $B_{12}$-dependent enzymes are involved in the synthesis of methionine from homocysteine. With folate deficiency, plasma homocysteine levels increase, possibly increasing the risk of cardiovascular diseases.

Reduced intake of dark green leafy vegetables is the most common cause of relative folate deficiency, which prompted public health actions such as the fortification of flour with folic acid. Chronic alcoholism is associated with both low dietary intake and diminished absorption of folate. The natural forms of folate in foods include tetrahydrofolate, 5-methyl tetrahydrofolate, and 10-methyl tetrahydrofolate. Folic acid is the form used in dietary supplements and fortified foods and has a higher bioavailability than naturally occurring folates. In order to account for the differences in bioavailability between synthetic folic acid and the multiple folates found in foods, the FNB established the dietary folate equivalent (DFE).[46] In this unit expression, 1 μg of food folate equals 1 μg of DFE, 1 μg of folic acid taken with meals or as fortified food equals 1.7 μg of DFE, and 1 μg of folic acid taken as a supplement on an empty stomach is counted as 2 μg of DFE. The RDA for adult males and females is 400 μg using the DFE criteria earlier. The RDA for pregnant women is 600 μg.

In a widely quoted example of genetic heterogeneity, the C677T polymorphism of MTHFR affects the interaction of folic acid and homocysteine. When folate intake is low, individuals who are T/T homozygotes for this gene have lower levels of the MTHFR enzyme and, thus, higher concentrations of circulating homocysteine. When folate intake is high, the polymorphism is masked as high folate concentrations stabilize the MTHFR enzyme and homocysteine levels are reduced. This common polymorphism is inherited in the heterozygous (C/T) form in up to 50% of a given population, while between 5% and 25% can have the homozygous T/T polymorphism.[47]

Folic acid is available as a dietary supplement by itself and in combination with other B vitamins as B-complex supplements and MVM. Many MVMs contain 400 μg of folic acid. Doses greater than 1 mg of folic acid require a prescription.

## VITAMIN $B_{12}$ (CYANOCOBALAMIN)

Only small amounts of vitamin $B_{12}$ are required in the diet, so the most common causes of deficiency of this vitamin are the result of autoimmune destruction of gastric mucosa, surgical removal of the stomach, or severe malabsorption of nutrients in the small intestine. Most likely as the result of decreased stomach acid production, Vitamin $B_{12}$ deficiency can be found in 10%–15% of individuals over 60 years of age.[48] Digestion of food in the stomach frees vitamin $B_{12}$ from food, allowing it to bind to R proteins.[49] In the small intestine, R proteins are degraded by pancreatic enzymes, freeing vitamin $B_{12}$ to bind to intrinsic factor (IF), a protein secreted by specialized cells in the stomach. Receptors on the surface of the distal small intestine take up the IF-$B_{12}$ complex.[50] While vitamin $B_{12}$ is inefficiently absorbed by passive diffusion through mucosal membranes, so little is needed that the 1% efficiency of this diffusion process still yields a practical method of supplementation that is more convenient than intramuscular injection.[51]

Methylmalonic acid (MMA) is a biomarker that can be used to detect subclinical vitamin $B_{12}$ deficiency as the result of impairment of the activities of $B_{12}$-requiring enzymes, including L-methylmalonyl-CoA mutase, resulting in increased levels of this metabolite typically detected in urine samples. Elevated homocysteine levels may also be observed.[52]

The major form of vitamin $B_{12}$ in supplements is cyanocobalamin, but methylcobalamin is also used in some formulations. This supplement is available by prescription in an injectable form and as a nasal gel for the treatment of pernicious anemia. These supplements are required for those patients who have undergone a Roux-en-Y gastric bypass operation for obesity since the gastric mucosa no longer is available to produce IF. Cyanocobalamin is also found in small amounts in vitamin B complexes, MVM, and as a vitamin $B_{12}$ supplement in various doses.[53]

## VITAMIN C

It is believed that humans lost the ability to synthesize vitamin C as the result of its plentiful presence in the plant-based diets of ancient mankind. In common with other water-soluble vitamins, vitamin C must be taken relatively frequently to avoid deficiency with about 3% of stored vitamin C lost daily in the urine. British sailors in the eighteenth century would spend long periods of time at sea and suffered from scurvy characterized by bleeding and easy bruising, hair and tooth loss, and joint pain and swelling. By conducting clinical experiments in the 1700s, Dr. James Lind developed the theory that citrus fruits cured scurvy. He argued for the health benefits of better ventilation aboard naval ships, the improved cleanliness of sailors' bodies, clothing and bedding, and below-deck fumigation with sulfur and arsenic. He also proposed that fresh water could be obtained by distilling sea water. His work did much to advance the practice of preventive medicine and improved nutrition in the Royal Navy. The term "limeys" was used to describe British sailors as a result of this dietary habit. Vitamin C was not identified as a vitamin until the early 1930s and then its function in the synthesis of collagen was discovered, which explained that the bleeding and bruising were secondary to weakening of connective tissues and blood vessels. The RDA for vitamin C was increased in 2000 from the previous recommendation of 60 mg daily for men and women to 90 mg for men and 75 mg for women. The recommended intake for smokers is 35 mg/day higher than for nonsmokers, since smokers are under increased oxidative stress from the toxins in cigarette smoke and have reduced blood levels of vitamin C.[7] Nutrition experts have suggested that the RDA for vitamin C be increased to 200 mg to encourage greater intake of fruits and vegetables containing this popular vitamin.[54] Vitamin C is one of the most widely consumed vitamins and is available at doses up to 1000 mg. Individuals with a predisposition to oxalate kidney stones may wish to monitor their intake of vitamin C as it is metabolized to oxalate in the urine.

## VITAMIN D

While listed as a vitamin, vitamin D is more appropriately considered a steroid hormone in the same family as testosterone, estrogen, thyroid hormone, and cortisol. Prior to World War II, rickets or bowing of the bones of the lower extremity was the most common presentation of vitamin D deficiency. Since the advent of vitamin D fortification of foods, rickets is rare, but the role of vitamin D in numerous chronic diseases including common forms of cancer has developed a large field of research outside the scope of this chapter. However, Michael Holick and his coworkers have pioneered research into the benefits of vitamin D supplements beyond bone health and at levels about the current RDA.[55] The current RDA for vitamin D is 400 IU for children younger than 1 year, 600 IU for children at least 1 year of age and adults up to 70 years, and 800 IU/day for older adults. The IOM concluded that serum 25-hydroxyvitamin D [25(OH)D] of 20 ng/mL or more covers the requirements of 97.5% of the population. This form of vitamin D is present in the blood as the result of hepatic hydroxylation of vitamin D at the 1-position. However, the active form of vitamin D is 1,25 dihydroxyvitamin D and this second hydroxylation step takes place in the kidney under the control of calcium, phosphorus, and parathyroid hormone. An inactive 24,25 dihydroxyvitamin D can also be formed in the kidney to dispose of excess vitamin D. The 1-hydroxylase enzyme has been identified in breast and prostate tissues where it may have a role in maintaining normal cellular function. Vitamin D is also formed in the skin from 7-dehydrocholesterol, but less sun exposure due to sedentary occupations has led to increased awareness that subclinical vitamin D deficiency may be more common especially in northern latitudes.

In contrast to the RDA, the Clinical Practice Guidelines of the U.S. Endocrine Society recommend 400–1000 IU for children younger than 1 year, 600–1000 IU for children over 1 year, and 1500–2000 IU for adults aged 19 years or more to maintain 25(OH)D above 30 ng/mL. Since the average daily intake of vitamin D in the United States ranges from 145 to 275 IU for women and 200 to 300 IU for men, supplementation of vitamin D is needed to reach the RDA. Moreover, higher amounts may be required in patients with inflammatory bowel disease or a history of gastric bypass surgery due to malabsorption of vitamin D. Differences in the recommendations from the IOM and the Endocrine Society reflect different goals and views on current evidence, and future research may further alter these recommendations. Vitamin D is contained in the flesh of fatty fish and fish liver oils such as cod liver oil, which was a common supplement in the early twentieth century until the fortification of dairy foods after World War II. Today the primary food source of vitamin D in the American diet is fortified milk, which contains 100 IU/cup.

## VITAMIN E

Dietary vitamin E comprises eight fat-soluble antioxidants found in foods. There are four tocopherols and four tocotrienols, each denoted as alpha, beta, gamma, and delta.

Both tocopherols and tocotrienols are essential to maintain membrane integrity of plant cells, but the tocotrienols are found in the seeds of plants. Palm oil-derived tocotrienols from the seeds of the palm tree have been processed into tocotrienol supplements. The scavenging of singlet oxygen by α-tocopherol provides protection for chloroplasts exposed to ultraviolet light and oxidant stress.[56]

Tocotrienols and tocopherols prevent the propagation of lipid peroxidation in membranes. Through what is known as the Antioxidant Network popularized by Dr. Lester Packer, the oxidation products of vitamin E are reduced back to their antioxidant forms through the actions of vitamin C, thioredoxins, and other antioxidants. Tocopherols and tocotrienols protect cellular lipids in numerous organelles by directly quenching singlet oxygen.

Alpha-tocopherol transfer protein is synthesized in the liver and protein preferentially incorporates alpha-tocopherol into lipoproteins, delivering them via the circulation to tissues. Therefore, alpha-tocopherol is the form of vitamin E found in the highest concentrations in the circulation and in tissues. The RDA for vitamin E is based on alpha-tocopherol.

Synthetic alpha-tocopherol, which is labeled all-racemic (*all-rac*)- or *dl*-alpha-tocopherol, has about one-half the biological activity of naturally occurring *RRR*-alpha-tocopherol. Vitamin E in fortified foods is typically the synthetic *all-rac*-alpha-tocopherol, while the form of alpha-tocopherol naturally found in foods is *RRR*-alpha-tocopherol also referred to as "natural" or *d*-alpha-tocopherol. The most plentiful form of vitamin E in the American diet is gamma-tocopherol, found in vegetable oils. In the blood, the levels of gamma-tocopherol are about one-tenth that of alpha-tocopherol due to the actions of the alpha-tocopherol transfer protein. Moreover, metabolites of gamma tocopherols are detected in urine in greater amounts than those of alpha-tocopherol and not retained by the body.[57] Some test-tube research suggests that gamma-tocopherol or its metabolites may have functions within the cell as antioxidants or through cell signaling pathways.[58]

Tocotrienols are less well studied and are not as popular as dietary supplements as tocopherols. However, studies demonstrate that tocotrienols decrease hepatic cholesterol production and reduce plasma cholesterol levels in animals. Delta- and gamma-tocotrienols inhibit the mevalonate pathway in mammalian cells by posttranscriptional suppression of HMG-CoA reductase and appear to specifically modulate the intracellular mechanism for controlled degradation of the HMG-CoA reductase protein, an activity similar to isoprenoids derived from mevalonate.[59,60] Tocotrienols provide an exciting area for future nutritional research.

The UL has been established by the FNB at 1000 mg of alpha-tocopherol in any form (equivalent to 1500 IU *RRR*-alpha-tocopherol or 1100 IU *all-rac*-alpha-tocopherol). The rationale that any form of alpha-tocopherol can be absorbed and thus could be potentially harmful is the basis for a UL that refers to all forms of alpha-tocopherol.

A meta-analysis reported that adults who took supplements of 400 IU/day or more were 6% more likely to die from any cause than those who did not take vitamin E supplements.[59] This study combined the results of 19 clinical trials of vitamin E supplementation for various diseases, including heart disease, end-stage renal failure, and Alzheimer's disease, but further breakdown of the risk by vitamin E dose and adjustment for other vitamin and mineral supplements revealed that the increased risk of death was statistically significant only at a dose of 2000 IU/day, which is higher than the UL for adults. On the other hand, a different meta-analysis of 68 randomized trials found that supplemental vitamin E, singly or in combination with other antioxidant supplements, did not significantly alter risk of all-cause mortality.[61,62] At present, there is no convincing evidence that vitamin E supplementation up to 800 IU/day increases the risk of death from any cause including cardiovascular disease.

The RDA for vitamin E is 15 mg for adults. In the United States, over 90% of individuals over 2 years of age do not meet the daily requirement for vitamin E from food sources alone. Most daily MVMs contain 30 IU of *all-rac*-alpha-tocopherol, or 90% of the RDA, and higher doses are commonly consumed as single supplements at a dose of 400 IU/day. While there is no conclusive evidence that vitamin E supplementation at higher doses than found in most foods lowers chronic disease risk, improved methods of testing the effects of vitamin E and other antioxidant supplements have been suggested.[63] Tocotrienols derived from palm oil and rice bran oil are sold as supplements and are being actively studied for their effects on chronic disease risk including heart disease and common forms of cancer.

## MINERALS AND TRACE MINERALS

### MAGNESIUM

Magnesium is abundant in the cells of both plants and animals. Furthermore, the kidneys are able to limit urinary excretion of magnesium when intake is low. Therefore, magnesium deficiency is rare in healthy individuals eating a varied diet.[64] Chronic alcoholics with poor diets, gastrointestinal disorders, and urinary loss of magnesium frequently have evidence of magnesium deficiency. Magnesium deficiency can also occur in those with prolonged diarrhea or malabsorption of magnesium due to celiac disease, loss of a portion of the intestine due to surgery or trauma, or intestinal inflammation secondary to radiation. Urinary loss of magnesium secondary to diabetes mellitus and long-term use of certain diuretics can result in magnesium deficiency as can medications that cause renal magnesium wasting.[65] Poor dietary intake of magnesium in the elderly, increased urinary excretion of magnesium with age, and malabsorption may increase the risk of magnesium deficiency.[66]

Magnesium has a reputation as a dietary supplement useful in the control of blood pressure. However, many foods high in magnesium (fruits, vegetables, whole grains) are also frequently high in potassium and dietary fiber. Therefore, it is difficult to evaluate independent effects of magnesium on blood pressure in studies, which have examined the effects of fruits and vegetables on blood pressure. Epidemiological studies have found an inverse association of dietary fiber, potassium, and magnesium with the incidence of hypertension prospectively over a 4-year period.[67] Dietary fiber and dietary magnesium were each inversely associated with systolic and diastolic blood pressures in 40,000 nurses who did not develop hypertension over the 4-year study period. However, neither dietary fiber nor magnesium reduced the risk of developing hypertension.[68] Dietary magnesium intake was examined in the Atherosclerosis Risk in Communities (ARIC) study along with magnesium blood levels and the risk of developing hypertension in 7731 men and women over a 6-year period.[69] Although the investigators found no association between dietary magnesium and the incidence of hypertension, they suggested that low serum magnesium levels may play a modest role in the development of hypertension.

Magnesium dietary supplements are sold as magnesium oxide, gluconate, chloride, and citrate as well as in the form of amino acid chelates. Magnesium hydroxide is used in antacid formulas.[53] The RDA for adult males over 30 years of age is 420 mg, and for females over 30 years of age, it is 320 mg. MVMs typically provide about 100 mg of magnesium. Because magnesium is plentiful in foods, eating a varied diet that includes fruits, vegetables, and whole grains should provide the balance of the magnesium requirement for most individuals.

## POTASSIUM

Potassium is plentiful in many foods, including fruits and vegetables, where the ratio to sodium is favorable and may oppose some of the negative effects of excess sodium. Increased potassium can be fatal by causing cardiac arrest, and so potassium supplements are only available by prescription and require monitoring of blood potassium levels to be sure that they are in the range of 3.5–5.0 milliequivalents per liter. Some potassium-sparing diuretics or inadequate kidney function can lead to elevated levels of potassium in the circulation. During very-low-calorie diets (<1000 cal/day), potassium is supplemented to avoid low potassium levels due to urinary losses. A diet supplying at least 4.7 g of potassium daily has been associated with decreased risk of stroke, hypertension, osteoporosis, and kidney stones. However, fruits and vegetables are among the richest sources of dietary potassium, and a great deal of evidence supports an association between the increased consumption of fruits and vegetables with a reduced risk of cardiovascular disease.[70,71] Therefore, it is difficult to assign the observed health benefits to potassium alone.

## PHOSPHORUS

Phosphorus is essential for many intracellular processes, notably glycolysis, membrane maintenance, oxygen transport, muscle contraction, and protection from oxidative damage. Next to calcium, phosphorus is the most abundant mineral in the body. About 85% of phosphorus in the body can be found in bones and teeth, but it is also present in cells and tissues throughout the body. A varied diet provides adequate phosphorus for most people to meet the RDA for phosphorus, which is 700 mg for adults. Acute phosphorus deficiency is a clinical problem in children with gastrointestinal diseases and malnutrition who are fed too rapidly. This was also seen in prisoners of war who overate on being liberated. The rapid entry of glucose into cells reduces extracellular potassium, leading to life-threatening hemolytic anemia as red cells are incapacitated. A high-fructose diet can also increase urinary loss of phosphorus and is more marked when the diet is low in magnesium.[72] Fructose consumption in the United States has been increasing rapidly since the introduction of high-fructose corn syrup in 1970, while magnesium intake has decreased over the past century. As fructose enters liver cells, it is phosphorylated in the 1-position. The subsequent phosphorylation in the 6-position is regulated by the energy of the hepatocyte and the ADP/ATP ratio, while 1-phosphorylation is not. As phosphorus depletion continues, there is an accumulation of IMP and uric acid. Hyperuricemia has been related to fructose intake and this phosphorylation trapping phenomenon has been implicated.

## TRACE MINERALS

### Iodine

Iodine is needed to synthesize thyroid hormone and deficiency is uncommon in the United States due to the iodine fortification of salt and the use of periodate in bleaching white flour. Individuals moving from low-iodine areas, such as mountainous areas of Peru, Mexico, and Southeast Asia, frequently suffer from thyroid disease when immigrating to the United States due to the increase in dietary iodide. Potassium iodide is available as a nutritional supplement, typically in combination products, such as MVM, which typically contain 100% of the DV or 150 µg.[73] People living in northern coastal areas of Japan eat large amounts of seaweed and as a result ingest between 50,000 and 80,000 µg of iodine/day.[73] Therefore, the body can adapt to very different dietary intakes of iodine from very low to very high. However, with migration, many of these metabolic adaptations cannot be rapidly reversed leading to thyroid diseases. While most individuals get all the iodine they need from the diet, it is unlikely that an additional 150 µg/day will cause any adverse effects.

### Iron

Iron deficiency is common among premenopausal and pregnant women in the United States.

Average dietary iron intakes vary from 16 to 18 mg/day in men to 12 mg in pre- and postmenopausal women and 15 mg in pregnant women.[6] Thus, the majority of premenopausal and pregnant women in the United States consume less than the RDA for iron and may need supplementation. On the other hand, many men consume more than the RDA. Fortunately, iron absorption is regulated by the body so that when stores are high, oral absorption is reduced. With the exception of one of 250 men with hemochromatosis, most men will not develop iron deposits despite exceeding the RDA. The amount of iron from dietary supplements that is absorbed is also influenced by the body stores of iron. In particular, individuals with anemia have been shown to absorb more iron than individuals with normal blood counts.[74] Vitamin C is known to enhance the bioavailability of iron by reducing dietary iron from the ferric ($Fe^{3+}$) form to the ferrous ($Fe^{2+}$) form of iron. MVMs typically provide 18 mg iron for the general population and have reduced amounts in their mature or 50-plus formulations ranging from no iron to 10 mg per dose.

## Selenium

Selenium is incorporated into over 100 selenoproteins including numerous enzymes, which are selenium dependent.[75] Selenium is incorporated into the amino acid cysteine in place of sulfur, forming selenocysteine. Selenocysteine is then incorporated into an enzyme at a specific location in the amino acid sequence. Selenium from the soil is incorporated into organic selenium by plants and selenium-enriched forms of some foods such as garlic are available. Inorganic selenium supplements are available as sodium selenite and sodium selenate. Selenite is better absorbed than selenate but is only about 50% bioavailable. Organic selenium, in the form of selenomethionine in foods, is 90% absorbed.[6] Selenomethionine and selenium-enriched yeast are available as dietary supplements. Both inorganic and organic forms of selenium are incorporated into selenocysteine by the body and utilized to synthesize selenoproteins.

## Chromium

Chromium has a historic reputation as a trace mineral that helps in controlling blood glucose. Chromium supplementation improved some measures of glucose metabolism and blood lipid profiles in studies of individuals with impaired glucose tolerance and hyperlipidemia.[76] MVMs containing 100% of the DV generally contain 60–120 μg chromium. This is greater, the AI of 20–25 μg for adult women and 30–35 μg for adult men established by the FNB in the absence of adequate data to establish an RDA.

## Zinc

Zinc participates in key aspects of cell function important for normal growth and development, immune function, and reproduction. Zinc deficiency in humans was first described in 1961 in Egypt, when the consumption of diets high in phytic acid from cereals reduced zinc absorption leading to "adolescent nutritional dwarfism."[6] Zinc deficiency is an important public health issue in many developing countries. Clinically, zinc deficiency occurs in patients with prolonged or repeated bouts of diarrhea due to gastrointestinal diseases. The RDA for zinc is 8 mg for adult women and 11 mg for adult men. MVM containing 100% of the DV of most nutrients will generally provide 15–20 mg of zinc together with copper. High doses of zinc in the absence of

copper will lead to copper-deficiency anemia since copper and zinc share a common transport mechanism in the intestine.

## Manganese

Manganese deficiency has not occurred in humans eating typical diets. In the absence of adequate data to establish an RDA, an AI for manganese is based on average dietary intakes of manganese determined from the Total Diet Study, documenting the content of representative American diets.[6] Supplements of manganese are available as manganese gluconate, sulfate, or ascorbate, as well as amino acid chelates. Manganese is available in combination products or as a single supplement.[53]

## Molybdenum

Molybdenum deficiency is rare. Acquired molybdenum deficiency was demonstrated in a patient with Crohn's disease receiving long-term total parenteral nutrition (TPN) without molybdenum added to the TPN solution.[77] He demonstrated biochemical signs of molybdenum deficiency, including low plasma uric acid levels, decreased urinary excretion of uric acid and sulfate, and increased urinary excretion of sulfite. The patient also developed rapid heart and respiratory rates, headache, and night blindness and ultimately became comatose. These symptoms and signs disappeared following molybdenum administration. The RDA for molybdenum is 45 μg for adults. MVMs formulated at about 100% of the DV for most nutrients typically provide 75 μg molybdenum. Although the amount of molybdenum presently found in most MVM is higher than the RDA, it is well below the UL of 2000 μg.

## MACRONUTRIENT SUPPLEMENTS

### PROTEIN

#### Protein Requirements

The RDA for protein of high biological value for adults is based on body weight at 0.8 g/kg.[5] In a recent report concerning DRIs, the acceptable macronutrient distribution range (AMDR) was set at 10%–35% of total calories from protein. The AMDR is defined as the acceptable range of intakes for protein associated with reduced risk of chronic disease while providing intakes of essential nutrients.[78] This range was largely set so that the intake of other macronutrients in the diet would be in an acceptable range.

Daily protein consumption ranges from 88 to 92 g for men and from 63 to 66 g for women.[79] Animal products provide 75% of the essential amino acids in the food supply, followed by dairy products, cereal products, eggs, legumes, fruits, and vegetables.[79]

There are many conditions in which extra protein is needed, including periods of growth, pregnancy, lactation, intense strength and endurance training and other forms of physical activity, and possibly in the elderly.[80] Additionally, protein appears to play an important role in the regulation of long-term energy balance, maintenance of body weight, and satiety.

Given the variation in the needs for protein throughout the life cycle, there is an individual optimum intake that exists based on lean body mass and activity levels. However, optimal intakes are difficult to determine based on the existing science base in nutrition. In 1977, Garza et al.[81] studied a small number of healthy volunteers and found that 0.8 g/kg/day resulted in positive nitrogen balance. Subsequent studies in endurance athletes found that more than 1 g/kg/day was required for positive nitrogen balance,[82] and studies in weight lifters indicated that more than 2 g/kg/day were needed to achieve positive nitrogen balance.[83] Therefore, while the RDA is set at 56 g/day for men consistent with the 1977 study, the allowable range of macronutrient intake is broad (10%–35% of total calories), enabling some individual adjustment for optimal intakes both to control hunger and to provide support to lean tissues.

### Protein and Satiety

Researchers in the Netherlands[84] have investigated the effects of protein on hunger perceptions by studying two groups of subjects in a whole-body energy chamber under controlled conditions for over 24 h. Subjects were fed isocaloric diets, which were either high protein/high carbohydrate (protein/carbohydrate/fat, percentage of calories 30/60/10) or high fat (protein/carbohydrate/fat, percentage of calories 10/30/60). Significantly more satiety was reported by subjects on the high-protein/high-carbohydrate diet. At the same time, hunger, appetite, desire to eat, and estimated quantity of food eaten were significantly lower in this group, with less hunger both during and after the high-protein meals. The level of protein in the diet may also impact maintenance of body weight after weight loss. After following a very-low-energy diet for 4 weeks, subjects who consumed a 20% higher intake of protein than controls (15% vs. 18% of energy) showed a 50% lower body weight regain, only consisting of fat-free mass, with increased satiety and decreased energy efficiency during a 3-month maintenance period.[85]

Similar studies have reported improved weight loss and fat loss in subjects consuming a high-protein diet versus a control diet (25% vs. 12% energy from protein) *ad libitum*, due to a reduction in daily calorie intake of approximately 16%,[86] and improved utilization of body fat with maintenance of lean body mass in subjects consuming 32% of energy from protein compared with controls who consumed 15% of calories as protein.[87] A similar study comparing diets with 15% versus 30% of calories from protein found that while weight loss in the two groups was similar over the 6-week trial, diet satisfaction was significantly greater in those consuming the higher-protein diet.[88]

A meta-analysis of such studies[89] concluded that, on average, high-protein diets were associated with a 9% decrease in total calorie intake. While the role of protein in affecting overall calorie intake and in body weight regulation in comparison to fat and carbohydrate requires further investigation, there is compelling evidence that protein affects hunger signaling mechanisms in the brain, induces thermogenesis, and contributes to the building and maintenance of lean body mass.

Protein supplements are provided as pure protein powder or as meal replacements. The meal replacements typically contain a percentage of the RDA of most common vitamins and minerals (20%–35%) as well as some carbohydrate and flavoring. Many are used together with milk or soy milk, which adds additional protein, but they are also available in liquid or water mixable forms.

Protein-enriched meal replacements incorporated in a diet providing 30% of energy from protein compared to 15% of energy from protein have demonstrated greater retention of lean mass. Flechtner-Mors et al.[90] demonstrated greater weight loss, lean body mass retention, and greater fat loss in 34 subjects with metabolic syndrome consuming a protein-rich diet compared to 43 subjects consuming a conventional protein for 1 year. In this study, increased protein intake from meal replacements and food was also associated with greater reduction in waist circumference, sagittal diameter, hemoglobin A1c, and triglycerides.

These studies demonstrate that the metabolic and satiety factors demonstrated in controlled feeding studies can also be detected in studies of free-living subjects.

## FISH OIL SUPPLEMENTS

The n-3 (also called omega-3) fatty acids in fish oil are long-chain fatty acids, which compete with n-6 fatty acids found in many foods and vegetable oils for common sites on enzymes and receptors in the body. The diversity of dietary intakes of n-6 and n-3 fatty acids in diets internationally leads to a wide difference in the fatty acid compositions of n-3 long-chain fatty acids, specifically eicosapentaenoic, docosapentaenoic, and docosahexaenoic acids. Observational studies indicate an inverse association between the intake of n-3 fatty acids and the risk of cardiovascular disease and some forms of mental illnesses.[91] Potential mechanisms underlying this benefit appear to be through anti-inflammatory pathways involving the modulation of eicosanoids synthesized from arachidonic acid and other long-chain n-6 fatty acids. By increasing n-3 fatty acid intake from fish and fish oil or algae oil supplements and decreasing n-6 fatty acid consumption from vegetable oils and processed foods, it is possible to change tissue and plasma fatty acid balance. While more research is needed to connect these changes to alterations in immune function, there is evidence from observational studies[92] that increases in the ratio of (n-6):(n-3) polyunsaturated fatty acids are associated with increases in chronic inflammatory diseases such as nonalcoholic fatty liver disease, cardiovascular disease, obesity, inflammatory bowel disease, rheumatoid arthritis, and Alzheimer's disease. By increasing the ratio of (n-3):(n-6) polyunsaturated fatty acids in the Western diet, reductions might be achieved in the incidence of these chronic inflammatory diseases. Fish oil supplements have been studied in a wide variety of other conditions, including clinical depression,[93,94] anxiety,[95–97] cancer, and age-related macular degeneration, although a clear benefit of n-3 fatty acid supplementation in these conditions remains to be proven.

## CONCLUSION

A recent national survey found that one-third of Americans ages 1 year and older take an MVM.[98] Dietary supplement use was found to be generally more prevalent among females, non-Hispanic whites, older adults, and individuals with greater than a high school education and less common among obese individuals.[98] Other studies have reported similar trends in use.[99–104] Additionally, a few studies have found that individuals taking a daily MVM are more likely to have healthier diets[105,106] or rate their health as excellent or very good,[101,104] suggesting that those who are not taking these supplements may be the ones who would benefit the most from supplementation as they are likely to have poorer diets.

Although there is no consensus that MVM use by the general population reduces the risk of major chronic diseases, they do contribute to the intake of essential micronutrients and help fill the gap between actual intakes and those recommended by the RDA. While some concern exists about the potential for excessive intake of single micronutrients from high doses of single supplements, MVMs formulated at about 100% of the DVs are generally considered as safe in healthy individuals. In 2007, the U.S. Food and Drug Administration established standards of current good manufacturing practices (CGMPs) to ensure dietary supplements meet quality standards with respect to identity, purity, strength, and composition.[107] All U.S. and foreign companies were required to comply with the CGMPs by 2010. In addition to these government regulations, at least three independent organizations evaluate the quality of dietary supplements on a fee basis: NSF International, U.S. Pharmacopeia, and ConsumerLab.com. Supplement labels of approved products can bear the certification mark of these organizations. However, many products that are in full compliance do not carry such seals of approval on their labels, and absence of such verification does not indicate lack of adherence to CGMPs or other regulations.

National surveys indicate that many Americans are not getting enough micronutrients from the diet, possibly increasing their risk for several common chronic diseases that have been significantly associated with dietary patterns and nutritional status. Further, marginal or subclinical micronutrient deficiencies have been linked to general fatigue,[108] impaired immunity,[109,110] and adverse effects on cognition.[111] Nutrition education campaigns such as the Dietary Guidelines for Americans have yet to have an impact on consumer behaviors with regard to selecting and/or preparing more nutrient dense foods, including fruits, vegetables, whole grains, and healthful sources of protein. Instead, there is a prevalent pattern for consumption of energy-rich, nutrient-poor diets of processed foods with hidden fats and sugars.[112] Consequently, micronutrient inadequacies are widespread in the United States and around the world. Together with some evidence that intakes of micronutrients at and, in some cases, above the RDA or AI are associated with the promotion of health and reduction in the risk of chronic disease, it has been proposed that taking a daily MVM can be a prudent and cost-effective recommendation for public health.[34,35]

In 2006, an NIH State-of-the-Science Conference on MVM and chronic disease prevention concluded that there was insufficient evidence to recommend in favor or against taking an MVM.[113] This conclusion was drawn exclusively from evidence derived from the conduct of randomized clinical trials (RCTs) because they have traditionally been accepted as the "gold standard" for establishing cause-and-effect relationships. However, the foundation of RCTs for drugs in evidence-based medicine has distinct differences with that needed for the development of nutrient requirements and dietary guidance.[114,115] There is a need to better define the types of evidence necessary for developing dietary guidelines and recommending nutrient interventions than that used for drug efficacy and safety. For example, unlike drugs, nutrients and other bioactive dietary components work in complex networks, are homeostatically controlled, and cannot be contrasted to a true placebo group. Although RCTs present one approach toward understanding the efficacy of nutrient interventions, the innate complexities of nutrient actions and interactions cannot always be adequately addressed through a single research design. There are several other concerns with RCTs, such as selection of subjects, compliance during a long-term study, the need to recruit a large number of subjects, trial cost, and confounding with dietary intake of nutrients.[116] Thus, it is not realistic to expect that many long-term RCTs will be undertaken or would even provide definitive results on whether MVM and other dietary supplements are effective in chronic disease prevention. Thus, new approaches to evidence-based nutrition that examine the totality of basic and human studies, including observational data and short-term RCTs that assess relevant intermediary biomarkers of chronic disease, present a practical methods to help inform decisions about the use of dietary supplements from personal, medical, and public health perspectives.[116]

## REFERENCES

1. Centers for Disease Control and Prevention Second Nutrition Report, 2012 http://www.cdc.gov/nutritionreport/pdf/ExeSummary_Web_032612.pdf#zoom = 100 (accessed July 5, 2012).
2. Troesch, B, Hoeft, B, McBurney, M et al. *Brit J Nutr* 1–7, 2012; doi:10.1017/S0007114512001808 (epub ahead of print).
3. Troesch, B, Eggersdorfer, M, Weber, P. *J Nutr* 142:979;2012.
4. Dietary Supplement Health and Education Act of 1994. Public Law 103–417, *103rd Congress*. http://www.fda.gov/opacom/laws/dshea.html (accessed July 5, 2012).
5. National Research Council. *Food and Nutrition Board Recommended Dietary Allowances*. 10th edn. National Academy Press, Washington, DC, 1989.
6. Institute of Medicine. *Dietary Reference Intakes: The Essential Guide to Nutrient Requirements*. National Academies Press, Washington, DC, 2006.

7. Food and Nutrition Board, Institute of Medicine. *Dietary Reference Intakes for Vitamin A, Vitamin K, Boron, Chromium, Copper, Iodine, Iron, Manganese, Molybdenum, Nickel, Silicon, Vanadium and Zinc.* National Academies Press, Washington, DC, 2001.

8. Food and Nutrition Board, Institute of Medicine. *Dietary Reference Intakes for Vitamin C, Vitamin E, Selenium, and Carotenoids.* National Academies Press, Washington, DC, 2000.

9. Kennedy, D, Koren, G. *Can Fam Physician* 58:394;2012.

10. Li, K, Kaaks, R, Linseisen, J, Rohrmann, S. *Eur J Nutrition* 51:407;2012.

11. Seddon, JM, Christen, WG, Manson, JE et al. *Am J Pub Health* 84:788;1994.

12. Neuhouser, ML, Wassertheil-Smoller, S, Thomson, C et al. *Arch Intern Med* 169:294;2009.

13. Combs, G. *The Vitamins.* Academic Press, New York 2008.

14. Weaver, CM. *Calcium.* In Barbara AB and Robert MR (eds). *Present Knowledge in Nutrition,* 9th edn. ILSI Press, Washington, DC, p. 377, 2006.

15. Remington, JR. *The Science and Practice of Pharmacy.* Lippincott Williams & Wilkins, Baltimore, MD, 1338, 2005.

16. Zhao, Y, Martin, BR, Weaver, CM. *J Nutr* 135:2379;2005.

17. Straub, DA. *Nutrition Clin Pract* 22:286;2007.

18. Lonn, E, Yusuf, S, Arnold, MJ et al. *N Engl J Med* 354:1567;2006.

19. Lee, M, Hong, K-S, Chang, S-C, Saver, JL. *Stroke* 41:1205;2010.

20. National Academy of Sciences, Institute of Medicine, Food and Nutrition Board. *Dietary Reference Intakes for Vitamin A, Vitamin K, Arsenic, Boron, Chromium, Copper, Iodine, Iron, Manganese, Molybdenum, Nickel, Silicon, Vanadium, and Zinc.* National Academy Press, Washington, DC 2001.

21. Black, RE, Allen, LH, Bhutta, ZA et al. *Lancet* 371:243;2008.

22. Field, CJ, Johnson, IR, Schley, PD. *J Leukoc Biol* 71:16;2002.

23. West, CE. *Nutr Rev* 58:46;2000.

24. Binkley, N, Krueger, BS. *Nutr Rev* 58:138;2000.

25. Tanphaichitr, V.Thiamin. In Shils M, Olson JA, Shike M, Ross AC, eds. *Modern Nutrition in Health and Disease,* 9th edn. Lippincott Williams & Wilkins, Baltimore, MD, p. 381, 1999.

26. Todd, K, Butterworth, RF. *Ann NY Acad Sci* 893:404;1999.

27. Metzler, DE. *Biochemistry. The Chemical Reactions of Living Cells,* 2nd edn. Harcourt, San Diego, CA, 2001.

28. Powers, HJ. *Proc Nutr Soc* 58:435;1999.

29. Rivlin, RS. Riboflavin. In Ziegler EE, Filer LJ, eds. *Present Knowledge in Nutrition,* 7th edn. ILSI Press, Washington, DC, p. 167, 1996.

30. Bohles, H. *Int J Vitamin Nutr Res* 67:321;1997.

31. Russell, RM. *Am J Clin Nutr* 71:878;2000.

32. Christian, P, West, KP Jr. *Am J Clin Nutr* 68:435S;1998.

33. Suharno, D, West, CE, Karyadi D et al. *Lancet* 342:1325;1993.

34. Fairfield, KM, Fletcher, RH. *JAMA* 287:3116;2002.

35. Fletcher, RH, Fairfield, KM. *JAMA* 287:3127;2002.

36. Food and Nutrition Board, Institute of Medicine. *Niacin. Dietary Reference Intakes: Thiamin, Riboflavin, Niacin, Vitamin $B_6$,* Vitamin $B_{12}$, Pantothenic Acid, Biotin, and Choline. National Academy Press, Washington, DC, p. 123, 1998.

37. Plesofsky-Vig, N. Pantothenic acid. In Shils ME, Olson JA, Shike M, Ross AC, eds. *Modern Nutrition in Health and Disease,* 9th edn. Lippincott Williams & Wilkins, Philadelphia, PA, p. 423, 1999.

38. Brody, T. *Nutritional Biochemistry,* 2nd edn. Academic Press, San Diego 1999.

39. Rimm, EB, Willett, WC, Hu, FB et al. *JAMA* 279:359;1998.

40. Folsom, AR, Nieto, FJ, McGovern, PG et al. *Circulation* 98:204;1998.

41. Robinson, K, Arheart, K, Refsum, H et al. *Circulation* 97:437;1998.

42. Robinson, K, Mayer, EL, Miller, DP et al. *Circulation* 92:2825;1995.

43. Lin, PT, Cheng, CH, Liaw, YP et al. *Nutrition* 22:1146;2006.

44. Ubbink, JB, Vermaak, WJ, van der Merwe, A et al. *J Nutr* 124:1927;1994.

45. Mock, DM. Biotin. In Shils ME, Olson JA, Shike M, Ross AC, eds. *Modern Nutrition in Health and Disease,* 9th edn. Lippincott Williams & Wilkins, Baltimore, MD, p. 459, 1999.

46. Bailey, LB. *Nutr Rev* 56:294;1998.

47. Kauwell, GP, Wilsky, CE, Cerda, JJ et al. *Metabolism* 49:1440;2000.

48. Baik, HW, Russell, RM. *Ann Rev Nutr* 19:357;1999.

49. Shane, B. Folic acid, vitamin B-12, and vitamin B-6. In Stipanuk M, ed. *Biochemical and Physiological Aspects of Human Nutrition.* W.B. Saunders Co., Philadelphia, PA, p. 483, 2000.

50. Herbert, V. Vitamin B-12. In Ziegler EE, Filer LJ, eds. *Present Knowledge in Nutrition,* 7th edn. ILSI Press, Washington, DC, p. 191, 1996.

51. Carmel, R. Cobalamin (Vitamin B-12). In Shils ME, Shike M, Ross AC, Caballero B, Cousins RJ, eds. *Modern Nutrition in Health and Disease.* Lippincott Williams & Wilkins. Philadelphia, PA, p. 482, 2006.

52. Weir, DG, Scott, JM. Vitamin $B_{12}$ Cobalamin. In Shils M, ed. *Nutrition in Health and Disease,* 9th edn. Williams & Wilkins, Baltimore, MD, p. 447, 1999.

53. Hendler, SS, Rorvik, DR, eds. *PDR for Nutritional Supplements.* Medical Economics Company, Inc., Montvale, NJ, 2001.

54. Frei, B, Birlouez-Aragon, I, Lykkesfeldt, J. *Crit Rev Food Sci Nutr* 52:815;2012.

55. Pramyothin, P, Holick, MF. *Curr Opin Gastroenterol* 28:139;2012.

56. Munné-Bosch, S, Alegre, L. *Critical Rev Plant Sci* 21:31;2002.

57. Traber, MG, Elsner, A, Brigelius-Flohe, R. *FEBS Lett* 437:145;1998.

58. Li, D, Saldeen, T, Mehta, JL. *Biochem Biophys Res Commun* 259:157;1999.

59. Miller, ER, Pastor-Barriuso, R, Dalal D et al. *Ann Intern Med* 142:37;2005.

60. Song, BL, DeBose-Boyd, RA. *J Biol Chem* 281:25054;2006.

61. Bjelakovic, G, Nikolova, D, Gluud, LL et al. *JAMA* 297:842;2007.

62. Biesalski, HK, Grune, T, Tinz, J et al. *Nutrients* 2:929;2010.

63. Blumberg, JB, Frei, B. *Free Radic Biol Med* 43:1374;2007.

64. Shils, ME. Magnesium. In: O'Dell BL, Sunde RA, eds. *Handbook of Nutritionally Essential Minerals.* Marcel Dekker, Inc., New York, p. 117, 1997.

65. Rude, RK, Shils, ME. Magnesium. In: Shils ME, Shike M, Ross AC, Caballero B, Cousins RJ, eds. *Modern Nutrition in Health and Disease.* 10th edn. Lippincott Williams & Wilkins, Baltimore, MD p. 223;2006.

66. Rosanoff, A, Weaver, CM, Rude, RK. *Nutr Rev* 70:153;2012.

67. Ascherio, A, Rimm, EB, Giovannucci, EL et al. *Circulation* 86:1475;1992.

68. Ascherio, A, Hennekens, C, Willett, WC et al. *Hypertension* 27:1065;1996.

69. Peacock, JM, Folsom, AR, Arnett, DK et al. *Ann Epidemiol* 9:159;1999.

70. Liu, S, Manson, JE, Lee, IM et al. *Am J Clin Nutr* 72:922;2000.

71. Joshipura, KJ, Ascherio, A, Manson, JE et al. *JAMA* 282:1233;1999.
72. Milne, DB, Nielsen, FH. *J Am Coll Nutr* 19:31;2000.
73. Hetzel, BS, Clugston, GA. Iodine. In Shils M, Olson JA, Shike M, Ross AC, eds. *Modern Nutrition in Health and Disease*, 9th edn. Williams & Wilkins, Baltimore, MD, p. 253, 1999.
74. Lynch, SR. *Nutr Rev* 55:102;1997.
75. Rayman, MP. *Lancet* 356:233;2000.
76. Mertz, W. *J Nutr* 123:626;1993.
77. Abumrad, NN, Schneider, AJ, Steel, D, Rogers, LS. *Am J Clin Nutr* 34:2551;1981.
78. Barr, SI, Murphy, SP, Agurs-Collins, TD, Poos, MI. *Nutr Rev* 61:352;2003.
79. McDowell, M, Briefel, R, Alaimo, K et al. Energy and macronutrient intakes of persons ages 2 months and over in the United States: Third National Health and Nutrition Examination Survey, Phase 1, 1988–1991. U.S. Government Printing Office, Vital and Health Statistics, Washington, DC, 1994.
80. Campbell, WW, Crim, MC, Dallal, GE et al. *Am J Clin Nutr* 60:501;1994.
81. Garza, C, Scrimshaw, NS, Young, VR. *J Nutr* 107:335;1977.
82. Tarnopolsky, M. *Nutrition* 20:662;2004.
83. Tarnopolsky, MA, Atkinson, SA, MacDougall, JD et al. *J Appl Physiol* 73:1986;1992.
84. Westerterp-Plantenga, MS, Rolland, V, Wilson, SAJ, Westerterp, KR. *Eur J Clin Nutr* 53:495;1999.
85. Westerterp-Plantenga, MS, Lejeune, MP, Nihs, I et al. *Int J Obes Relat Metab Disord* 28:57;2004.
86. Skov, AR, Toubros, S, Ronn, B et al. *Int J Obes Relat Metab Disord* 23:528;1999.
87. Layman, DK, Boileau, RA, Erickson, DJ et al. *J Nutr* 133:411;2003.
88. Johnston, CS, Tjonn, SL, Swan, PD. *J Nutr* 134:586;2004.
89. Eisenstein, J, Roberts, SB, Dallal, G, Saltzman, E. *Nutr Rev* 60:189;2002.
90. Flechtner-Mors, M, Ditschuneit, H, Johnson, TD et al. *Obes Res* 8:399;2000.
91. Hibbeln, JR, Nieminen, LR, Blasbalg, TL et al. *Am J Clin Nutr* 83:1483S;2006.
92. Patterson, E, Wall, R, Fitzgerald, GF et al. *J Nutr Metab* 2012:539426. Epub 2012 April 5.
93. Su, KP, Huang, S-Yi, Chiu, C-C et al. *Eur Neuropsychopharm* 13:267;2003.
94. Naliwaiko, K, Araújo, RLF, Da Fonseca, RV et al. *Nutr Neuroscience* 7:91;2004.
95. Green, P, Hermesh, H, Monselise, A et al. *Eur Neuropsychopharmacol* 16:107;2006.
96. Yehuda, S, Rabinovitz, S, Mostofsky, DI. *Nutr Neuroscience* 8:265;2005.
97. Nemets, B, Stahl, Z, Belmaker, RH. *Am J Psychiatry* 159:477;2002.
98. Bailey, RL, Gahche, JJ, Lentino, CV et al. *J Nutr* 141:261;2011.
99. Satia-Abouta J, Kristal, AR, Patterson, RE et al. *Am J Prev Med* 24:43;2003.
100. Archer, SL, Stamler, J, Moag-Stahlberg, A et al. *J Am Diet Assoc* 105:1106;2005.
101. Sullivan, KM, Ford, ES, Azrak, MF, Mokdad, AH. *Public Health Rep* 124:384;2009.
102. Park, SY, Murphy, SP, Martin, CL, Kolonel, LN. *J Am Diet Assoc* 108:529;2008.
103. Shelton, RC, Puleo, E, Syngal, S, Emmons, KM. *Cancer Causes Control* 20:1271;2009.
104. Radimer, K, Bindewald, B, Hughes, J et al. *Am J Epidemiol* 160:339;2004.
105. Rock, CL. *Am J Clin Nutr* 85:277S;2007.
106. Foote, JA, Murphy, SP, Wilkens, LR et al. *Am J Epidemiol* 157:888;2003.
107. U.S. Food and Drug Administration Dietary supplement current good manufacturing practices (CGMPs) and interim final rule (IFR) facts. http://www.fda.gov/Food/DietarySupplements/GuidanceComplianceRegulatoryInformation/RegulationsLaws/ucm110858.htm (accessed July 5, 2012).
108. Huskisson, E, Maggini, S, Ruf, M. *J Int Med Res* 35:277;2007.
109. Ibs, K-H, Rink, L. Zinc. In: Hughes DA, Darlington LG, Bendich A, eds. *Diet and Human Immune Function*. Human Press Inc., Towata, p. 241, 2004.
110. Bhaskaram, P. *Br J Nutr* 85:S75;2001.
111. Eussen, SJ, de Groot, LC, Joosten, LW et al. *Am J Clin Nutr* 84:361;2006.
112. Centers for Disease Control and Prevention. State indicator report on fruits and vegetables, 2009. http://www.fruitsandveggiesmatter.gov/indicatorreport (accessed July 5, 2012).
113. National Institutes of Health State-of-the-Science Panel. *Am J Clin Nutr* 85:257S;2007.
114. Heaney, RP. *J Nutr* 138:1591;2008.
115. Blumberg, J, Heaney, RP, Huncharek, M et al. *Nutr Rev* 68:478;2010.
116. Ames, BN, McCann, JC, Stampfer, MJ, Willett, WC. *Am J Clin Nutr* 86:522;2007.

# 57 Bioactive Substances and Botanical Dietary Supplements

*David Heber*

## CONTENTS

## INTRODUCTION

The recommended dietary allowances, dietary guidelines, and many government licensing and regulatory policies are based on the early twentieth century science that identified classical nutritional deficiency diseases for vitamins and minerals. In the 1990s, nutrient recommendations for foods were broadened as dietary reference intakes (DRIs) and population reference intakes (PRIs) that now incorporate a tolerable upper intake level (UL) below which no adverse effects are noted.[1–3] As discussed in the last chapter, these guidelines are not designed to deal with any substances beyond those recognized to be essential to human health based on some demonstration of function or an instance of deficiency. Attempting to move beyond a deficiency model, this effort extended to establishing macronutrient ranges for protein, carbohydrate, and fat and provided information for a very limited number of trace minerals where the evidence of essentiality was weak.

Over several decades of the late twentieth century, nutritional science has uncovered new groups of substances that we will classify as bioactive substances and botanical dietary supplements. Many plant-based foods with a wide range of traditional intakes, such as green tea, have functions in population studies, in animal and cell culture models, and in limited clinical intervention studies suggesting major health benefits for the public. Many bioactive substances are found within dietary supplements in the nutritional range where they have immunomodulatory activity and little risk of toxicity. When taken in pharmacological doses, these supplements can have potential drug–nutrient interactions and other toxicities.

At the present time, there are general opinions and some strong biases among nutritional scientists about the benefits and the potential hazards of botanical dietary supplements and even traditional multivitamin/multimineral supplements. There is clearly a need to develop a scientific framework to communicate the potential benefits of bioactive substances to the public that establishes reasonable certainty of benefits while also providing assurance of safety.

This chapter will review the definitions and present knowledge on bioactive substances and botanical dietary supplements. It is not possible to discuss all bioactive substances or even to scratch the surface on the large number of botanical dietary supplements. Therefore, a selected number of substances in each category will be reviewed.

## BIOACTIVE SUBSTANCES

Bioactive substances have been defined as "extranutritional constituents that typically occur in small quantities in foods."[4] Many bioactive compounds have been discovered but represent a much smaller universe than the botanical dietary supplements to be discussed later in this chapter. Bioactive substances vary widely in chemical structure and function and are grouped by structure or by their occurrence in commonly eaten foods.

In the chemical classification, one of the largest categories is that of phenolic compounds, which includes the subcategory of over 5000 flavonoids. These are present in all plants and have been studied extensively in cereals, legumes, nuts, olive oil, vegetables, fruits, tea, and red wine. Many phenolic compounds have antioxidant properties, and some studies have demonstrated favorable effects on thrombosis and tumor growth in animal models. The epidemiologic literature is limited and inconsistent in its ability to uncover associations of specific bioactive substances and health, but many studies have reported protective associations between overall fruit and vegetable intakes with regard to heart disease and common forms of cancer.

Numerous bioactive compounds appear to have beneficial health effects. Hydroxytyrosol, one of many phenolics in olives and olive oil, is a potent antioxidant. Resveratrol, found in nuts and red wine, has antioxidant, antithrombotic, and anti-inflammatory properties and inhibits carcinogenesis. Lycopene, a potent antioxidant carotenoid in tomatoes and other fruits, is thought to protect against prostate and other cancers and inhibits tumor cell growth in animals. Organosulfur compounds in garlic and onions, isothiocyanates in cruciferous vegetables, and monoterpenes in citrus fruits, cherries, and herbs have anticarcinogenic actions in experimental models, as well as cardioprotective effects.

However, the vast amount of scientific information has not been accepted by the government bodies or the Institute of Medicine as adequate for science-based dietary recommendations beyond the very few health claims approved by the U.S. Food and Drug Administration (FDA) for foods. Despite this, there is sufficient evidence to recommend consuming food sources rich in bioactive compounds. From a practical perspective, this translates to recommending a diet rich in a variety of fruits, vegetables, whole grains, legumes, oils, and nuts.

## POLYPHENOLS

Polyphenols are present in all plants and, thus, are in the diet.[5,6] There are over 8000 phenolic structures that have been identified that vary structurally from being simple molecules to large polymers (e.g., hydrolysable tannins). There are more than 10 classes of polyphenols that have been defined on the basis of their chemistry.[6] The flavonoids are the most common polyphenols present in plant food. Based on an analysis of specific flavonoids in fruits and vegetables grown in the United States and the Netherlands,[7] flavonoids can be categorized into 13 classes including over 5000 different compounds. The most common flavonoids are flavones, flavonols, and their glycosides.[6]

The primary phenols in cereals and legumes are flavonoids, phenolic acids, and tannins. The major polyphenols in wine include phenolic acids, anthocyanins, tannins, and other flavonoids. The most abundant phenolic compound in fruits is flavonol. Nuts are rich in tannins. Olive oil contains both phenolic acids and hydrolysable tannins as does pomegranate juice. The predominant flavonoid in onions is quercetin glycoside, whereas in tea and apples, it is quercetin-3-rutinoside.[6]

Although polyphenols are present in virtually all plant foods, their levels vary enormously among diets depending on the type and quantity of plant foods in the diet. For example, some plant foods and beverages that are particularly rich in polyphenols are pomegranate juice, red wine, grape juice, and legumes. Commonly used spices are also rich in polyphenols, and their antioxidant activity is directly related to their content of phenolic groups.[8] There also can be marked variability in the polyphenol content within the same food or food category due to genetic factors and environmental conditions. For example, market basket studies of broccoli have found several fold differences in glucosinolate content.

The consumption data for dietary polyphenols, although limited, indicate that the intake reported is highly variable among the population groups studied.[9] Moreover, these surveys may underestimate intake due to the omission of many polyphenols from nutrient databases. Nonetheless, although we presently have a poor understanding of the intake of total polyphenols as well as the specific classes and individual polyphenols, it is clear that a diet rich in plant foods and polyphenol-rich beverages combine to provide a high level of dietary polyphenols compared to populations not eating these foods. Several population studies have reported an inverse association between flavonoid intake and risk of coronary disease and cancer.[10–13] In the Zutphen Elderly Study,[10] a high intake of flavonoids (approximately 30 mg/day) was associated with approximately a 50% reduction in cardiovascular diseases.

## FRUITS AND VEGETABLES

Numerous epidemiologic studies indicate that an increase in the consumption of fruits and vegetables is associated with a decrease in the incidence of cardiovascular disease.[14–21] Results from the Nurses' Health Study and the Health Professionals' Follow-up Study indicate that persons in the highest quintile of fruit and vegetable intake (8.0 servings/day) had a relative risk (RR) for coronary heart disease of 0.80 (95% confidence interval (CI), 0.69–0.93) compared with those in the lowest quintile of intake (3.0 servings/day), after adjustment for standard cardiovascular risk factors. These results were also equivalent to a 4% reduction in heart disease for every 1-serving/day increase in the intake of fruits and vegetables.[16] Green leafy vegetables and vitamin C–rich fruits and vegetables contributed the most to the apparent protective effect of total fruit and vegetable intake, with RR of 0.77 (95% CI, 0.64–0.93) and 0.94 (95% CI, 0.88–0.99), respectively, for every 1-serving/day increase. Similar results have been reported from the Women's Health Study[20] and the Physicians' Health Study.[17] In addition, comparable data have been reported from studies conducted in Japan[19] and China.[20] Bazzano et al.[14] reported that frequency of fruit and vegetable intake was inversely associated with stroke incidence, stroke mortality, ischemic heart disease mortality, and cardiovascular disease mortality. The incidence of stroke was greatly reduced (RR 0.73; 95% CI, 0.57–0.95) for individuals consuming ≥3 servings/day of fruits and vegetables, compared with the reference group of ≥1 serving/day. In addition, stroke mortality was also greatly reduced (RR 0.58; 95% CI, 0.33–1.02), from the highest quintile to the lowest.[22]

More than 200 studies have examined the relation between the consumption of fruits and vegetables and the risk of various cancers. A meta-analysis of 26 studies by Gandini et al.[23] found an association between risk of breast cancer and intake of fruits and vegetables. When high consumption versus low consumption was compared in these studies, an RR of 0.75 (95% CI, 0.66–0.85; P ≤ 0.001) was observed from 17 studies on consumption of vegetables, whereas 12 studies involving fruit consumption resulted in an RR of 0.94 (95% CI, 0.79–1.11; P ≤ 0.001). A multiethnic case-control study involving 1619 African American, white, Japanese, and Chinese men with confirmed prostate cancer and 1618 control subjects examined the protective effects of fruit and vegetable intake on prostate cancer.[24] Whereas risk of prostate cancer was not related to fruit consumption, both cruciferous and yellow-orange vegetable intakes were inversely related to prostate cancer. This association was strongest for advanced cases of prostate cancer with an odds ratio (OR) of 0.67 (P for trend ≤ 0.01) for the highest quintile of yellow-orange vegetable intake and an OR of 0.61 (P for trend ≤ 0.006) for the highest quintile of cruciferous vegetable intake.

Overall, the population studies reviewed evaluating associations between intakes of a variety of plant-based foods indicate a protective effect, both on cardiovascular disease and on common forms of cancers. While not the totality of studies in the literature, there are enough studies to support recommending an increase in the intake of fruits and vegetables. Our group has utilized color linked to phytochemical families as a way to accomplish the translation of complex chemistry to the public and to the patients counseled to enhance their intake of bioactive substances from fruits and vegetables.[25]

Most Americans eat only two to three servings of fruits and vegetables per day without regard to the phytochemical contents of the foods being eaten. Certain phytochemicals give fruits and vegetables their colors and also indicate their unique physiological roles. All of the colored phytochemicals that absorb light in the visible spectrum have antioxidant properties. In artificial membrane systems, it is possible to show synergistic interactions of lutein and lycopene in antioxidant capacity, and there are well-known antioxidant interactions of vitamin C and vitamin E based on their solubilities in hydrophilic and hydrophobic compartments of cells.

However, many phytochemicals have other functions beyond acting as antioxidants. For example, lycopene stabilizes the connexin 43 gene product that is essential for gap junction communication[26] while also interacting with vitamin D in the differentiation of HL-60 leukemia cells.[27] In breast cancer cells, lycopene can interfere with insulin-like growth factor 1–stimulated tumor cell proliferation.[28] Lycopene levels in the blood are associated with a reduced risk of prostate cancer,[29] and lycopene administration may reduce proliferation and increase apoptosis in human prostate tissue where lycopene is the predominant carotenoid.[30] Lutein is concentrated in the retina, where it may help prevent macular degeneration, the most common preventable form of age-related blindness.[31] Other studies have found that lycopene, α-carotene, and β-carotene are associated with a reduced risk of lung cancer.[32]

On the basis of a recent review of functional properties of foods[33] and a research from our laboratories demonstrating that it is relatively simple to influence circulating levels of lycopene with administration of only 177 mL (6 fluid ounces) of mixed vegetable juice daily,[34] we developed a color code for a book aimed at helping consumers to change dietary patterns to include more fruits and vegetables by including one serving from each of the seven color groups each day: (1) red (lycopene family) including tomatoes and tomato products such as juice, soups, and pasta sauces; (2) red purple (anthocyanins, hydrolysable tannins, and polyphenols) including grapes, blackberries, pomegranates, red wine, raspberries, and blueberries; (3) orange (alpha- and beta-carotene) including carrots, mangos, and pumpkin; (4) orange yellow (beta-cryptoxanthin and flavonoids) including cantaloupe, peaches, tangerines, papaya, and oranges; (5) yellow green (lutein and zeaxanthin) including spinach, avocado, and honeydew melon; (6) green (glucosinolates and indoles) including broccoli, bok choi, kale, and cabbages; and (7) white green (allyl sulfides) including leeks, garlic, onion, and chives.

The color concept was incorporated into a number of public health messages including those from the National Cancer Institute.[35] While the color method may be superior to the current system of simply encouraging increased fruit and vegetable intakes by increasing variety, it does not account for actual phytochemical delivery to the consumer. Today, there is no labeling law that enables fruit and vegetable manufacturers to list the phytochemicals in their products. Fruits and vegetables are developed and grown less for their flavor and nutritional content and more to accommodate the need to transport these products over long distances and extend their shelf life once they get to market. Finally, research in this area needs to continue on the phytochemicals provided by fruits and vegetables including those that do not have color, such as isoprenoids.[36] These important phytochemicals are widely distributed among different plant species, but the delivery of phytochemicals and their effects on biomarkers relevant to cancer prevention need to be documented.

## ISOFLAVONES FROM SOY FOODS

Because soy foods are the most significant dietary source of isoflavones, many studies with humans and nonhuman primates have been conducted evaluating the effects of soy foods and the constituents of soy foods on numerous heart disease risk factors. Soy foods have been shown to have favorable effects on plasma lipids and lipoproteins. A meta-analysis of 38 clinical studies reported that total cholesterol was decreased by 9%, low-density lipoprotein (LDL) cholesterol by 13%, and triglycerides by 11% when an average of 47 g of soybean protein was consumed[37] with a greater response observed in subjects having a higher baseline cholesterol level. High-density lipoprotein (HDL) cholesterol was increased modestly (i.e., 2.4%; not significant). The active components of soy protein that are thought to account for these effects are the isoflavones genistein and daidzein. Crouse et al.[38] found that soy protein containing isoflavones significantly reduced total and LDL cholesterol levels by 4% and 6%, respectively, in hypercholesterolemic subjects (LDL cholesterol, 140–200 mg/dL). Moreover, when the soy protein was stripped of isoflavones by ethanol extraction, the cholesterol-lowering effect was lost. It is important to note that isoflavone bioavailability is dependent on gut microflora activity. Thus, isoflavone absorption and its beneficial effects may be highly variable and could explain discrepant study results.[39]

Research to date shows multiple beneficial effects of soy that appear to be the result of isoflavones, and there is an approved U.S. heart health claim for foods containing more than 6.25 g of soy protein per serving. Soy isoflavones possess antioxidant properties and have been shown to suppress tumor promoter–induced hydrogen peroxide and superoxide anion formation.[40–42] In addition to its own antioxidant actions, genistein also enhances the activity of a number of antioxidant enzymes, including catalase, glutathione peroxidase, glutathione reductase, and superoxide dismutase.[40] The current evidence suggests that isoflavones may play a role in the prevention and treatment of several types of cancer. Many of these effects are considered to be protective in nature, although a few potentially adverse effects have been reported. Of note is that many of the effects, positive and negative, have been shown with very high concentrations and not at levels likely to be achieved by eating foods containing phytoestrogens.[40,42] Additionally, the role of such factors as bioavailability, absorption, duration of exposure, and potential influence of other dietary components remains to be established.

## GREEN TEA AND BLACK TEA

Tea is a rich source of antioxidant polyphenols (i.e., catechins, flavonols, theaflavins, and thearubigins). The primary sources of polyphenols in green tea (35%–52%) are catechins and flavonols, which include epicatechin, epicatechin-3-gallate, epigallocatechin, and epigallocatechin-3-gallate.[43,44] In addition, tea contains smaller concentrations of quercetin and theaflavins (black tea).[45] Thearubigens are the major fraction of black tea polyphenols and account for >20% of the solids in brewed tea.[46] Human studies have established that these antioxidant polyphenols, in particular epigallocatechin-3-gallate, protect against carcinogenesis.[44] In animals, green tea significantly increased activity of antioxidants and detoxifying enzymes, such as glutathione S-transferase, catalase, and quinone reductase, in lungs, liver, and small intestine.[44] Topical administration of epigallocatechin-3-gallate, subsequent to ultraviolet radiation, significantly reduced tumor induction in mice.

Whether tea has preventive effects for common forms of cancer remains to be established. In a Japanese prospective cohort study of 8552 individuals, consumption of >10 cups of green tea a day was associated with delayed onset of cancer by 8.7 years in women and 3.0 years in men compared with those who consumed <3 cups/day.[43] In addition, a lower RR was observed for lung, colon, and liver cancers. Likewise, a prospective study in postmenopausal women found that those who consumed ≥2 cups of tea (primarily black tea) had a slightly lower risk for all cancers compared with women who never or only occasionally consumed tea.[47] On the other hand, Nagano et al.[48] found no protective relationship between tea consumption and cancer (all sites) in 38,540 Japanese men and women.

## PHYTOSTEROLS

Plants do not synthesize cholesterol but do produce phytosterols that are chemically similar to cholesterol with the exception of some sterol side chain substitutions at the C24 position. Phytosterols are not synthesized by humans and are poorly absorbed. However, they interfere with intestinal absorption of cholesterol both from the diet and from the recirculating bile in the enterohepatic circulation. The primary plant sterols in the diet are sitosterol, stigmasterol, and campesterol. Typical consumption of plant sterols is approximately 200–400 mg/day. The most abundant plant sterol in Western diets is β-sitosterol.[49]

Studies with sitosterol or mixtures of plant sterols (approximately 1 g/day) have shown that they reduce serum cholesterol levels in humans by approximately 10%.[50] There is some emerging evidence that the sterols present in the unsaponifiable fraction of rice bran oil, oryzanols (a group of ferulate esters of triterpene alcohols and phytosterols), decrease plasma cholesterol levels.[51]

## CINNAMON

Spices are not only active as antioxidants, but some have specifically physiological effects. Among the best studied of the spices is cinnamon. Cinnamon polyphenols are bioactive, appearing to mimic the effect of insulin through increased glucose uptake in adipocytes and skeletal muscles.[51–53] There are numerous human clinical trials demonstrating these effects with cinnamon spice as well as water extracts of cinnamon.[54–59] As such, cinnamon polyphenols are exemplary bioactive substances.

## ISOTHIOCYANATES

Isothiocyanates are toxic substances found as glucosinolates in over 450 species of plants including a number of commonly eaten cruciferous vegetables, including broccoli, Brussels sprouts, cabbage, and cauliflower. The isothiocyanate is released with chewing or crushing of the cells, which activates myrosinase enzymes that act upon the glucosinolates to liberate isothiocyanates.[60] It has been shown that uptake of isothiocyanates is markedly reduced when the vegetables are cooked because of inactivation of myrosinase.[61] The anticarcinogenic potential of cruciferous vegetables requires further study because most are consumed in the cooked form. Some naturally occurring forms of this phytochemical include

2-phenethyl isothiocyanate, benzyl isothiocyanate, and sulforaphanes.[62] These compounds have marked chemopreventive potency in animals and human cell cultures. α-Naphthyl, β-naphthyl, 2-phenethyl isothiocyanate, benzyl isothiocyanate, and other arylalkyl isothiocyanates have been reported to protect against tumorigenesis in the lung, breast, liver, stomach, and esophagus.[63]

## BOTANICAL DIETARY SUPPLEMENTS

A botanical is a plant or plant part valued for its medicinal or therapeutic properties, flavor, and/or scent. Herbs are a subset of botanicals. Products made from botanicals that are used to maintain or improve health may be called herbal products, botanical products, or phytomedicines. To be classified as a dietary supplement, a botanical must meet the definition defined by Congress in the Dietary Supplement Health and Education Act, which became law in 1994. A dietary supplement is a product (other than tobacco) that (1) is intended to supplement the diet; (2) contains one or more dietary ingredients (including vitamins, minerals, herbs or other botanicals, amino acids, and other substances) or their constituents; (3) is intended to be taken by mouth as a pill, capsule, tablet, or liquid; and (4) is labeled on the front panel as being a dietary supplement.

Based on this official legal definition, it is evident that there is a significant overlap of dietary supplements, in general, with the vitamin and mineral supplements discussed in the prior chapter. There is also an overlap with the bioactive substances discussed in this chapter depending on whether the substance occurs in a food or is provided as a separate capsule, pill, or tablet. This section will be concerned with products that are both botanicals and dietary supplements.

Botanical dietary supplements can be prepared as teas, decoctions, tinctures, and extracts. A tea, also known as an infusion, is made by adding boiling water to fresh or dried botanicals and steeping them. The tea may be drunk either hot or cold. Some roots, bark, and berries require more forceful treatment to extract their desired ingredients. They are simmered in boiling water for longer periods than teas, making a decoction, which also may be drunk hot or cold. A tincture is made by soaking a botanical in a solution of alcohol and water. Tinctures are sold as liquids and are used for concentrating and preserving a botanical. They are made in different strengths that are expressed as botanical-to-extract ratios (i.e., ratios of the weight of the dried botanical to the volume or weight of the finished product). An extract is made by soaking the botanical in a liquid that removes specific types of chemicals. The liquid can be used as is or evaporated to make a dry extract for use in capsules or tablets.

Dietary supplements are not required to be standardized in the United States. In fact, no legal or regulatory definition exists for standardization in the United States as it applies to botanical dietary supplements. Because of this, the term "standardization" may mean many different things. Some manufacturers use the term standardization incorrectly to refer to uniform manufacturing practices. Ideally, the chemical markers chosen for standardization would also be the constituents that are responsible for a botanical's effect in the body. In this way, each lot of the product would have a consistent health effect. However, the components responsible for the effects of most botanicals have not been identified or clearly defined. For example, the sennosides in the botanical senna are known to be responsible for the laxative effect of the plant, but the active compounds in saw palmetto are poorly defined so that fatty acid profiles are used for standardization.

The use of herbal and alternative medicines has increased in the last two decades in the United States and is now the subject of clinical and basic science investigations supported by the NIH Office of Dietary Supplements Research and the National Center for Complementary and Alternative Medicine. The Dietary Supplement Health Education Act (DSHEA) of 1994 enables manufacturers to market these approaches without proving efficacy or safety prior to marketing. It is difficult to determine the quality of a botanical dietary supplement product from its label. The degree of quality control depends on the manufacturer, the supplier, and others in the production process. In 2007, the FDA issued good manufacturing practices (GMPs) for dietary supplements, a set of requirements and expectations by which dietary supplements must be manufactured, prepared, and stored to ensure quality. Manufacturers are now expected to guarantee the identity, purity, strength, and composition of their dietary supplements. For example, the GMPs aim to prevent the inclusion of the wrong ingredients, the addition of too much or too little of a dietary ingredient, the possibility of contamination (by pesticides, heavy metals such as lead, bacteria), and the improper packaging and labeling of a product.

While the agency has recently increased its vigilance over claims, it has limited resources for policing advertising claims. These practices engender significant challenges to scientists attempting to examine the benefits of a particular herbal or alternative approach or to evaluate any relationship of reported adverse events to consumption of an herbal product.

## CHINESE RED YEAST RICE: A CASE STUDY

The example of Chinese red yeast rice (RYR) is a case study illustrating the fine points of defining a product as a drug or a botanical dietary supplement. RYR is used to color a wide variety of food products, including pickled tofu, red rice vinegar, char siu, Peking duck, and Chinese pastries that require red food coloring. It is also traditionally used in the production of several types of Chinese wine, Japanese sake (akaisake), and Korean rice wine (hongju), imparting a reddish color to these wines. Although used mainly for its color in cuisine, RYR imparts a subtle but pleasant taste to food and is commonly used in the cuisine of Fujian regions of China. In addition to its culinary use, RYR is also used in traditional Chinese medicine. Its use has been documented as far back as the Tang dynasty in China in 800 AD where it was taken internally to invigorate the body, aid in digestion, and revitalize the blood. A more complete description is in the traditional Chinese pharmacopoeia, *Ben Cao Gang Mu-Dan Shi Bu Yi*, from the Ming dynasty (1378–1644).

In the late 1970s, researchers in the United States and Japan were isolating lovastatin from Aspergillus and monacolins from Monascus, respectively, the latter being the same fungus used to make RYR but cultured under carefully controlled conditions. Chemical analysis soon showed that lovastatin and monacolin K, one of the several different monacolins in Chinese RYR, were chemically identical. The article "The origin of statins" summarizes how the two isolations, documentations, and patent applications were just months apart.[64] Lovastatin became the patented, prescription drug Mevacor for Merck & Co. RYR went on to become a contentious nonprescription dietary supplement in the United States and other countries.

Lovastatin and other prescription "statin" drugs inhibit cholesterol synthesis by blocking action of the enzyme HMG-CoA reductase. As a consequence, circulating total cholesterol and LDL cholesterol are lowered. In a meta-analysis of 91 randomized clinical trials of ≥12 weeks duration, totaling 68,485 participants, LDL cholesterol was lowered by 24%–49% depending on the statin.[65] Different strains of Monascus fungus will produce different amounts of monacolins. The "Went" strain of Monascus purpureus (purpureus = purple in Latin), when properly fermented and processed, will yield a dried RYR powder that is approximately 0.4% monacolins, of which roughly half will be monacolin K (identical to lovastatin). Monacolin content of an RYR product is described in a 2008 clinical trial report.[66]

The position of the U.S. FDA is that RYR products that contain monacolin K, that is, lovastatin, are identical to a drug and, thus, subject to regulation as a drug. In 1998, the FDA initiated action to ban a product (Cholestin) containing RYR extract. The U.S. District Court in Utah allowed the product to be sold without restriction. This decision was reversed on appeal to the U.S. District Court.

Two reviews confirm that the monacolin content of RYR dietary supplements can vary over a wide range, with some containing negligible monacolins.[67,68] In 2007, the FDA sent warning letters to two dietary supplement companies. One was making a monacolin content claim about its RYR product, and the other was not, but the FDA noted that both products contained monacolins. Both products were withdrawn. The FDA also issued a warning press release. The key message in the release was that consumers should "… not buy or eat red yeast rice products … may contain an unauthorized drug that could be harmful to health." The rationale for "… harmful to health …" was that consumers might not understand that the dangers of monacolin-containing RYR might be the same as those of prescription statin drugs.

The amount typically used in clinical trials was 1200–2400 mg/day of RYR containing approximately 10 mg total monacolins with the balance being the rice on which the yeast strain was fermented. About a half to three quarters of the monacolins are monacolin K. This finding suggests that other monacolins and non-monacolin compounds (e.g., phytosterols, fatty acids) in the products may contribute to the cholesterol-lowering activity of Chinese RYR, as the monacolin K content is lower than what is usually considered effective for lovastatin (20–80 mg/day). In 2006, Liu et al. published a meta-analysis of clinical trials. The article cited 93 published, controlled clinical trials (91 published in Chinese). Total cholesterol decreased by 35 mg/dL, LDL cholesterol by 28 mg/dL, and triglycerides by 35 mg/dL, and HDL cholesterol increased by 6 mg/dL. The incidence of reported adverse effects ranged from 1.3% to 36%.[69] Of the clinical trials reviewed in the meta-analysis, the only study conducted in the United States was that conducted by our group at UCLA, which reported a 22% reduction of LDL cholesterol after 12 weeks.[70]

Subsequent to the 2006 meta-analysis, there developed a number of articles reporting on a massive trial conducted in China: the China Coronary Secondary Prevention Study (CCSPS). Close to 5000 post-heart-attack patients were enrolled for an average of 4.5 years to receive either a placebo or an RYR product named Xuezhikang. This is a patented process (the U.S. patent #6,046,022), ethanol extract of RYR, with a total monacolins content of approximately 0.8%. It is also sold as Lipascor. In the treated group, risk of subsequent heart attacks was reduced by 45%, cardio deaths by 31%, and all-cause deaths by 33%.[71]

A recent study reported on its use in clinical practice in statin-intolerant patients. Muscle pain is a common complaint among patients taking statins. Investigators reviewed 1400 clinical charts and identified 25 patients treated with RYR for at least 4 weeks who had experienced myalgias (68%), gastrointestinal intolerance (16%), and/or elevated alanine aminotransferase levels (8%) with previous use of other lipid-lowering drugs. The total cholesterol decreased 15% (−37 ± 26 mg/dL, P < 0.001), and the LDL cholesterol decreased 21% (−35 ± 25 mg/dL, P < 0.001) during 74 ± 39 days of treatment. Most (92%) patients tolerated the treatment, and many (56%) achieved their LDL cholesterol goal. In patients unable to tolerate daily statin use, the total cholesterol level decreased 13% (−33 ± 10 mg/dL, P < 0.001), and the LDL cholesterol decreased 19% (−31 ± 4 mg/dL, P < 0.001). Therefore, Chinese RYR modestly decreased total and LDL cholesterol, was well tolerated, and was an acceptable alternative in patients intolerant of other lipid-lowering medications.[72]

Beginning in 2003, RYR products began to reappear in the U.S. market. As of 2012, there are at least 30 brands available. Many of these avoid the FDA restriction by not having any appreciable monacolin content. Their labels and websites say no more than "fermented according to traditional Asian methods" or "similar to that used in culinary applications." The labeling on these products often says nothing about cholesterol. If they do not contain lovastatin, do not claim to contain lovastatin, and do not make a claim to lower cholesterol, they are not subject to FDA action.

The European Food Safety Authority (EFSA) based it on positive opinion about Chinese RYR on two clinical trials, including our own[70] concluding that "Monacolin K from red yeast rice contributes to the maintenance of normal blood cholesterol concentrations."[73]

The story of Chinese RYR indicates how the provision in the DSHEA prohibiting substances previously approved as drugs from appearing in botanical dietary supplements affects what is available to the public. The patents for statins were issued to Merck in 1987, and the DSHEA law was passed in 1994. It is interesting to speculate as to what would be available to consumers today if these two dates were reversed. The challenges for manufacturers of botanical dietary supplements are to provide supplements that have scientifically sound results but do not make a claim that could be construed as preventing, treating, or mitigating a disease condition that would make the supplement a drug as in the case of Chinese RYR. There is another pathway in which a substance can be defined as botanical drug for an indicated medical condition. To date, only one such application for genital warts has been approved as the process is nearly as difficult as obtaining a drug approval and does not provide the same degree of patent protection as FDA grants to prescription drugs.

## CONCLUSIONS

This review by its nature must be incomplete, as a complete review would require an entire textbook devoted to these two large categories. Bioactive substances and botanical dietary supplements remain of great interest to the public and to scientists but are a perplexing topic for government regulators. The old adage of Hippocrates "Let food be your medicine, and medicine be your food" has inspired a great wave of interest in natural remedies and healthy foods by the public. This interest resulted in the funding of the DSHEA legislation and the Office of Dietary Supplement Research at the NIH. Much of the research that has emerged has been inconclusive (interpreted as negative) and has been used to attempt to diminish hope for these categories ever obtaining scientific credibility. There is a great need for research on both bioactive substances and botanical dietary supplements, but the long-term commitment of government agencies to this task is hampered by a lack of research funding and an industry that is not prepared to spend the research dollars needed to unravel the scientific challenges facing these two large categories of nutritional substances that hold the promise of better health through nutrition.

## REFERENCES

1. Institute of Medicine. *Dietary Reference Intakes: The Essential Guide to Nutrient Requirements*. Washington, DC: National Academies Press, 2006.
2. Food and Nutrition Board, Institute of Medicine. *Dietary Reference Intakes for Vitamin A, Vitamin K, Boron, Chromium, Copper, Iodine, Iron, Manganese, Molybdenum, Nickel, Silicon, Vanadium and Zinc*. Washington, DC: National Academies Press, 2001.
3. Food and Nutrition Board, Institute of Medicine. *Dietary Reference Intakes for Vitamin C, Vitamin E, Selenium, and Carotenoids*. Washington, DC: National Academies Press, 2000.
4. Kitts, DD. *Can J Physiol Pharmacol* 72:423;1994.
5. Kris-Etherton, PM, Hecker, KD, Bonanome, A et al. *Am J Med* 30:71S;2002.
6. Bravo, L. *Nutr Rev* 56:317;1998.
7. Sampson, L, Rimm, E, Hollman, PCH et al. *J Am Diet Assoc* 102:1414;2002.
8. Kim, IS, Yang, MR, Lee, OH, Kang, SN. *Int J Mol Sci* 12:4120;2011.
9. Peterson, J, Dwyer, J. *Nutr Res* 18:1995;1998.
10. Hertog, MGL, Feskens, EJM, Hollman, PCH et al. *Lancet* 342:1007;1993.
11. Hertog, MGL, Kromhout D, Aravanis, C et al. *Arch Intern Med* 155:381;1995.
12. Knekt, P, Jarvinen, R, Reunanen, A, Maatela, J. *BMJ* 312:478;1996.
13. Yochum, L, Kushi, LH, Meyer, K, Folsom, AR. *Am J Epidemiol*. 149:943;1999.
14. Bazzano, LA, He, J, Ogden, LG et al. *Am J Clin Nutr* 76:93;2002.
15. Gillman, MW, Cupples, LA, Gagnon, D et al. *JAMA* 273:1113;1995.
16. Joshipura, KJ, Hu, FB, Manson, JE et al. *Ann Intern Med* 134:1106;2001.
17. Liu, S, Lee, I-M, Ajani, U. *Int J Epidemiol* 30:130;2001.
18. Liu, S, Manson, JE, Lee, I-M et al. *Am J Clin Nutr* 72:922;2000.
19. Sasazuki, S. *Jpn Circ J* 65:200;2001.
20. Zhao, W, Chen, J. *Asia Pacific J Clin Nutr* 10:146;2001.
21. Menotti, A, Kromhout, D, Blackburn, H et al. *Eur J Epidemiol* 15:507;1999.
22. Rosengren, A, Stegmayr, B, Johansson, I et al. *J Intern Med* 246:577;1999.
23. Gandini, S, Merzenich, H, Robertson, C, Boyle, P. *Eur J Cancer* 36:636;2000.
24. Kolonel, LN, Hankin, JH, Whittemore, AS et al. *Cancer Epidemiol Biomark Prev* 9:795;2000.
25. Heber, D, Bowerman S. *J Nutr* 131(11 Suppl):3078S;2001.
26. Stahl, W, von Laar, J, Martin, HD et al. *Arch Biochem Biophys* 373:271;2000.
27. Amir, H, Karas, M, Giat, J et al. *Nutr Cancer* 33:105;1999.
28. Karas, M, Amir, H, Fishman, D et al. *Nutr Cancer* 36:101;2000.
29. Gann, PH, Ma, J, Giovannucci, E et al. *Cancer Res* 59:1225;1999.
30. Kucuk, O, Sarkar, FH, Sakr, W et al. *Cancer Epidemiol Biomarkers Prev* 10:861;2001.
31. Mares-Perlman, JA, Fisher, AI, Klein, R et al. *Am J Epidemiol* 153:424;2001.
32. Heber, D. *Am J Clin Nutr* 72:901;2000.
33. Milner, J. *Am J Clin Nutr* 71(suppl):1654S;2000.
34. Heber, D, Yip, I, Go, VLW et al. *FASEB J* 14:A719;2000.
35. Sample the Spectrum. National Cancer Institute. Available at http://www.5aday.gov (Accessed August 8, 2001).
36. Elson, C. *Adv Exp Med Biol* 399:71;1996.
37. Anderson, JW, Johnstone, BM, Cook-Newell, ME. *N Engl J Med* 333:276;1995.
38. Crouse, JR III, Morgan, T, Terry, JG et al. *Arch Intern Med* 159:2070;1999.
39. Xu, X, Harris, KS, Wang, HJ et al. *J Nutr* 125:2307;1995.
40. Kurzer, MS, Xu, X. *Annu Rev Nutr* 17:353;1997.
41. Setchell, KDR, Cassidy A. *J Nutr* 129:758S;1999.
42. Bingham, SA, Atkinson, C, Liggins, J et al. *Br J Nutr* 79:393;1998.

43. Fujiki, H, Suganuma, M, Okabe S et al. *Mutat Res* 402:307;1998.
44. Bushman, JL. *Nutr Cancer* 31:151;1998.
45. Yang, CS, Chung, JY, Yang, G et al. *J Nutr* 130:472S;2000.
46. Yang, CS, Landau, JM. *J Nutr* 130:2409;2000.
47. Zheng, W, Doyle, TJ, Kushi LH et al. *Am J Epidemiol* 144:175;1996.
48. Nagano, J, Kono, S, Preston, DL et al. *Cancer Causes Control* 112:501;2001.
49. Ling, WH, Jones, PJ. *Life Sci* 57:195;1995.
50. Vahouny, GV, Kritchevsky D. Plant and marine sterols and cholesterol metabolism. In: Spiller GA, ed. *Nutritional Pharmacology* Alan R. Liss, New York, p. 31 1981.
51. Anderson RA. *Proc Nutr Soc* 67:48;2008.
52. Broadhurst, CL, Polansky MM, Anderson RA. *J Agric Food Chem* 48:849;2000.
53. Cao, H, Polansky, MM, Anderson, RA. *Arch Biochem Biophys* 459:214;2007.
54. Baker, WL, Gutierrez-Williams, G, White, CM et al. *Diabetes Care* 31:41;2008.
55. Kirkham, S, Akilen, R, Sharma, S, Tsiami A. *Diabetes Obes Metab* 11:1100;2009.
56. Pham, AQ, Kourlas, H, Pham, DQ. *Pharmacotherapy* 27:595;2007.
57. Hlebowicz, J, Hlebowicz, A, Lindstedt, S et al. *Am J Clin Nutr* 89:815;2009.
58. Hlebowicz, J, Darwiche, G, Bjorgell, O, Almer LO. *Am J Clin Nutr* 85:1552;2007.
59. Solomon, TP, Blannin, AK. *Eur J Appl Physiol* 105:969;2009.
60. Hecht, SS. *J Nutr* 129:768S;1999.
61. Getahun, SM, Chung, FL. *Cancer Epidemiol Biomarkers Prev* 8:447;1999.
62. Zhang, Y, Talalay, P. *Cancer Res* 54:1976S;1994.
63. Hecht, SS. *Drug Metab Rev* 32:395;2000.
64. Endo, A. *Atheroscler Suppl* 5:125;2004.
65. Edwards, JE, Moore, RA. *BMC Fam Pract* 4:18;2006.
66. Becker, DJ, Gordon, RY, Morris, PB et al. *Mayo Clin Proc* 83:758;2008.
67. Li, YG, Zhang, F, Wang, ZT, Hu, ZB. *J Pharm Biomed Anal* 35:1101;2004.
68. Heber, D, Lembertas, A, Lu, QY et al. *J Altern Complement Med* 7:133;2001.
69. Liu, J, Zhang, J, Shi, Y et al. *Chin Med* 1:4;2006.
70. Heber, D, Yip, I, Ashley, JM et al. *Am J Clin Nutr* 69:231;1999.
71. Lu, ZL. *Zhonghua Xin Xue Guan Bing Za Zhi* 33:109;2005.
72. Venero, CV, Venero, JV, Wortham, DC et al. *Am J Cardiol* 105:664;2010.
73. EFSA Panel on Dietetic Products, Nutrition and Alergies (NDA). Scientific Opinion on the substantiation of health claims related to monacolin K from red yeast rice and maintenance of normal blood LDL-cholesterol concentrations (ID 1648, 1700) pursuant to Article 13(1) of Regulation (EC) No 1924/2006 *EFSA Journal* 2011:9(7);2304.

# 58 Nutrition and Diabetes

*Zhaoping Li and David Heber*

## CONTENTS

## INTRODUCTION

Nutrition is central to the prevention and treatment of diabetes mellitus (DM), but the approaches to type 1 DM (T1DM) and type 2 DM (T2DM) are different. T1DM results from an autoimmune destruction of insulin-secreting cells in the pancreas and requires insulin replacement and matching of the diet to the insulin provided.[1] On the other hand, T2DM is closely associated with excess adiposity and requires primary attention to weight management in prevention and treatment until the late stages of T2DM when insulin stores are depleted.[2] This chapter will begin by outlining the history and evolution of diabetes as a public health problem. Given the prevalence of T2DM, weight reduction and weight management in T2DM will be discussed first followed by sections on the various foods that can have a role in controlling blood sugar in patients with either T1DM or T2DM. Controlling blood sugar is an important component of treatment, but not the sole aspect of improving the quality of life of diabetes patients. Overall lifestyle change can help control risk factors for cardiovascular disease that is heightened by inflammation, oxidative stress, and lipid abnormalities that frequently accompany poor control of blood glucose.

## HISTORY AND PUBLIC HEALTH IMPACT

DM literally means sweet urine as doctors actually tasted urine to make the diagnosis prior to the availability of chemical testing.[3] Diabetes was well known in ancient times, and in Hindu literature, the word diabetes literally meant "one whose urine attracts ants." With the discovery that insulin could restore life to a dog whose pancreas was removed surgically, Banting and Best in the early twentieth century focused on the treatment of T1DM with insulin.[4] This disease that usually occurred in children and adolescents results from the autoimmune destruction of pancreatic beta-cells that normally secrete insulin. In these individuals, replacing insulin is critical to survival, and the clinical challenge is to match their food intake to the insulin administered to eliminate both hyperglycemia and hypoglycemia. In the absence of any insulin, these individuals suffer from acute ketoacidosis, a condition that is life threatening and requires immediate treatment. In this condition, the absence of insulin permits runaway production of fat-derived ketone bodies leading to a loss of fluid and electrolytes. Replacement of fluid and electrolytes and small amounts of insulin predictably corrects this condition that is often the result of children and adolescents acting out in response to stress. Into the 1970s, the primary focus of diabetologists was the treatment of T1DM in adults and children.

Adult-onset diabetes was less well understood and was thought to be due to senescence of the beta-cell, but the central concept of treating this disease was to control blood sugar as with T1DM. The close connection of obesity and T2DM via increased abdominal fat was discovered and investigated thoroughly over the last 30 years. It is now clear that the inflammation associated with T2DM and obesity plays an important role in the development of cardiovascular disease and renal failure in these patients. The observation that hyperlipidemia and hypertension as well as hyperglycemia are characteristic of T2DM has led to a new understanding of the prevention and treatment of T2DM.

Diabetes affects an estimated 25.8 million people in the United States (90%–95% have T2DM); 18.8 million have been diagnosed, but 7 million are unaware they have the disease. According to the American Diabetes Association and the CDC, those affected include 12.6 million U.S. women (10.8% of all women age 20 or older), 13 million U.S. men (11.8% of all men age 20 or older), 215,000 people younger than age 20, 10.9 million adults older than age 65, 4.9 million non-Hispanic African Americans (18.7% of all African Americans age 20 or older), and 15.7 million Caucasian Americans (10.2% of all Caucasian Americans age 20 or older). According to the most recent statistics, diabetes was the sixth leading cause of death and the fifth leading cause of death from disease. Diabetes costs $116 billion annually in direct medical costs. Diabetes costs $58 billion annually in indirect costs (loss of work, disability, loss of life).[5] Increasingly, this is becoming a worldwide problem as the result of the global spread of Western diets called the global nutrition transition.[6]

Controlling blood sugar still remains an important component of the treatment of T2DM, but it is possible that control blood glucose may not deal with the underlying factors promoting progression of T2DM. While the difference between T1DM and T2DM was typically said to be that there was lack of insulin in type 1 and excess insulin with insulin resistance in T2DM. Studies have clearly shown an evolution of insulin secretion from excess to deficient over a period of 10 years.[7] There are several theories to explain this phenomenon including the idea that a protein called insulin-associated polypeptide (IAPP) is secreted in excess amounts with insulin and taken up into the endoplasmic reticulum where it results in amyloid accumulation in the endoplasmic reticulum leading to protein overload and cell death.[8] At autopsy, patients with T2DM have burned out beta-cells and are deficient in pancreatic insulin.[9]

## WEIGHT MANAGEMENT AND WEIGHT REDUCTION IN TYPE 2 DIABETES

The vast majority of patients with T2DM have excess body fat, and about 36% are medically obese.[10] Since obesity is more common in underserved minority populations, so is T2DM.[10] T2DM results primarily from insulin resistance and increased body fat both of which result from a gene–environment interaction.[11,12] While hyperglycemia is the hallmark of T2DM, the increased risk of cardiovascular mortality is associated with hyperlipidemia and hypertension that occur more commonly in patients with T2DM than in the general population.[13]

Because weight reduction can decrease insulin resistance and demands on the pancreatic beta-cell to secrete insulin, weight loss is an integral and necessary component of treatment for obese individuals with T2DM. Weight loss in patients with T2DM is associated with decreased insulin

resistance, improved measures of glycemia, reduced serum lipids, and reduced blood pressure.[14–16]

However, long-term data assessing to which extent weight loss is maintained in patients with diabetes are not available. In studies of weight loss in type 2 diabetic subjects,[17–19] the most successful long-term weight loss from diet was reported in the Diabetes Treatment Study[19] with weight loss of 9 kg maintained over 6 years. To accomplish this required long-term access to therapeutic contact.

The Diabetes Prevention Program (DPP) demonstrated long-term benefit in people with glucose intolerance from structured, intensive lifestyle programs.[20,21] In the DPP, participants randomly assigned to an intensive lifestyle intervention that included low-fat diet, increased physical activity, educational sessions, and frequent follow-up were able to lose 7% of body weight in the first year and sustain a 5% weight loss over an average follow-up period of 3 years. DPP program participants received training in diet, exercise, and behavior modification from case managers who met with them for at least 16 sessions in the first 24 weeks and monthly thereafter. With intensive lifestyle intervention, the risk of developing diabetes was reduced by 58% relative to standard care. Wing et al.[20] demonstrated a 2.5 kg weight loss, and Tuomilehto et al.[22] documented a 3.5 kg weight loss at 2 years with such programs and also demonstrated that lifestyle changes reduce the risk of developing diabetes.

Meal replacements are a viable strategy for weight reduction in patients with T2DM, resulting in beneficial changes in measures of glycemic control and reduction of medications.[23] Structured meal replacements provide a defined amount of energy (usually 200–300 cal), often as prepackaged meal, snack bar, or formula product. Most of the energy is derived from protein and carbohydrate. Vitamins, minerals, and fiber may also be included. Use of meal replacements once or twice daily to replace a usual meal can result in significant weight loss.[24–28] Presumably the meal replacement causes a reduction in energy intake by eliminating the choice of type and amount of food. Weight loss can be as much as 11% of starting weight at 2 years, but meal replacement therapy must be continued if weight loss is to be maintained; attrition may occur in about 33% of patients.[26]

Very-low-calorie diets (VLCDs) provide 800 or fewer calories daily, primarily from protein and carbohydrate, with mineral and vitamin supplementation. These diets can produce substantial weight loss and rapid improvements in glycemia and lipemia in patients with T2DM.[15,29] Of note, reductions in glycemia occur before significant weight loss, suggesting that caloric restriction plays an important role in correcting hyperglycemia. Unfortunately, when VLCDs are stopped and self-selected meals are reintroduced, weight gain is common.[30,31] Most people treated with VLCDs are not able to maintain long-term weight loss. Thus, VLCDs appear to have limited utility in the treatment of T2DM and should be considered only in conjunction with a structured weight-maintenance program.

Dietary fat is often hidden, and reducing dietary fat restricts calorie intake especially from processed foods.

Spontaneous food consumption and total energy intake are increased when the diet is high in fat and decreases when the diet is low in fat.[32,33]

Exercise improves insulin sensitivity, can acutely lower blood glucose in patients with diabetes, and may also improve cardiovascular status. Exercise by itself has only a modest effect on weight.[34] Exercise is to be encouraged but like behavioral therapies, may be most useful as an adjunct to other weight-loss strategies, such as dietary fat reduction. Exercise is, however, important in long-term maintenance of weight loss.[35,36]

Behavioral approaches to weight loss include strategies such as self-monitoring of food intake and exercise, nutrition education, stimulus control, preplanning of food intake, and self-reinforcement. Weight loss with behavioral therapy alone has been modest.[37,38] It is clear that behavioral approaches are most useful as an adjunct to other weight-loss strategies.[39]

## PREVENTION OF TYPE 2 DIABETES THROUGH DIET AND LIFESTYLE

Excess body fat is perhaps the most notable modifiable risk factor for the development of T2DM.[40] It is estimated that the risk of T2DM attributable to obesity is as much as 75%.[41] A striking increase in the prevalence of obesity, as well as diabetes, was reported between NHANES II and NHANES III. As the prevalence of obesity continues to increase globally, it is expected that the prevalence of diabetes in the world's population will also increase.

Numerous interventions focusing on weight loss through hypocaloric, low-fat diets; increased physical activity; and a variety of behavior change strategies have emerged.[20,21] Several studies have demonstrated the potential for moderate, sustained weight loss to substantially reduce risk for T2DM.[42–44] The risk for T2DM has been observed to be increased in men who gained weight over a 12-year period of follow-up,[45] while overweight men who lost weight had a reduced risk of diabetes. In the Framingham Study cohort, sustained weight loss over two consecutive 8-year periods led to a 37% lower risk of diabetes; however, those who regained the lost weight failed to experience any reduction in diabetes.

The Finnish Diabetes Prevention Study[22] included 522 overweight individuals with impaired glucose tolerance randomized to control or intensive lifestyle intervention, which included weight reduction (5% or more), reduction of total and saturated fat (to less than 30% and 10% of calories, respectively), increased fiber (>15 g/1000 kcal), and increased physical activity (>4 h/week). The risk of diabetes was reduced by 58% in the intervention group, an outcome directly associated with changes in lifestyle.

In the United States, the DPP study tested the safety and efficacy of pharmacological therapy and lifestyle modification of weight management and physical activity.[21] However, in this trial for the first time, a lifestyle intervention was more effective than pharmacological intervention with metformin alone. The relatively small weight loss induced

with an intensive intervention of 5%–7% was achieved with 30 min/day of exercise and dietitian instruction on a whole food diet. Participants randomly assigned to intensive lifestyle reduced their risk of developing T2DM by 58% over nearly 3 years of follow-up. Significant risk reduction was observed across subgroups of ethnicity, age, gender, body mass index (BMI), and fasting glucose. Among individuals over age 60 years, the risk reduction was 71%. Moreover, metformin was relatively ineffective in the older volunteers and in those who were less overweight.

Recently, the DPP Outcomes Study[46] examined participants who returned to normal glucose regulation at least once during the DPP compared with those who consistently met criteria for prediabetes. The study demonstrated that prediabetes is a high-risk state for diabetes, especially in patients who remain with prediabetes despite intensive lifestyle intervention. Reversion to normal glucose regulation, even if transient, is associated with a significantly reduced risk of future diabetes independent of previous treatment group.

A healthy active lifestyle through biological effects of physical activity independent of its effects in promoting weight loss may prevent or delay the development of T2DM. This has been demonstrated in a number of prospective studies.[47–50] Physical activity may provide some protection against mortality at all levels of glucose tolerance, as has been demonstrated in middle-aged men.[51,52] Of interest in this regard is a large prospective observational study demonstrating that cardiorespiratory fitness levels in men influence the effects of obesity on health.[53] No elevated mortality risk in obese men was observed if they were physically fit, and lean men had increased longevity only if they were physically fit. In middle age, physical activity provides important protection against the onset of T2DM; a recent meta-analysis reported that even moderate-intensity leisure-time activity or brisk walking reduced diabetes incidence by 30%.[54] Moderate-to-high cardiorespiratory fitness may reduce mortality risk across all categories of body composition.

Thus, there is clearly strong evidence that comprehensive lifestyle interventions reduce the incidence of T2DM. Additional work in the area of increasing adherence and long-term success of intervention strategies for sustained lifestyle change is needed.

## FOOD EFFECTS ON DIABETES

### GLYCEMIC INDEX

The usefulness of low-glycemic-index (GI) diets in individuals with diabetes is controversial.[55] Thomas and Elliott[56] assessed randomized controlled trials (RCT) with interventions >4 weeks that compared a low-GI diet with a higher-GI diet for T1DM or T2DM. Twelve RCT (n 612) were identified. There was a significant decrease in glycated Hb (HbA1c) with low-GI diet than with the control diet, indicating improved glycemic control (seven trials, n 457, weighted mean difference (WMD): 0.4% HbA1c; 95% confidence interval (CI) (0.7, 0.20; P = 0.001). In four studies reporting the results for glycemic control as fructosamine, three of which were 6 weeks or less in duration, pooled data showed a decrease in fructosamine (WMD: 0.23 mmol/L, 95% CI 0.47, 0.00; P = 0.05), n 141, with low-GI diet than with high-GI diet. Glycosylated albumin levels decreased significantly with low-GI diet, but not with high-GI diet, in one study that reported this outcome. Lowering the GI of the diet may contribute to improved glycemic control in diabetes.

After the meta-analysis, in a cross-sectional study of 2810 people with T1DM from the EURODIAB IDDM Complications Study,[57] the GI calculated from 3 day food records was examined for its relation to HbA$_{1c}$ and serum lipid concentrations. HbA$_{1c}$ levels were lower in the lowest GI quartile compared with the highest quartile. Of the serum lipids, only high-density lipoprotein (HDL) cholesterol was independently related to the GI. Interestingly, the consumption of bread and pasta had the biggest effect on the overall GI. The effects on lipids after low-GI diets—compared to high-GI diets—appear to be minimal. In a recent study of 146 pediatric patients with T1DM,[58] patients that had good glycemic control consumed diets with significantly (Tukey test, P = 0.000) lower GI/GL (54.8 ± 2.7/118.3 ± 29.8) than the ones with intermediate (60.1 ± 3.8/142.5 ± 27.3) and poor (60.3 ± 4.1/153.7 ± 40.7) glycemic control. The diet consumed by 75.5% of diabetics with good glycemic control was classified as medium GL, suggesting that the consumption of medium GL diet may favor an adequate glycemic control. The low-GI diet consumed by these participants also presented higher protein content, which might have contributed to the attenuation of the postprandial glycemic response and better glycemic control of these patients. In this study, the intake of a reduced GI/GL diet favored the glycemic control of the studied population.

In the Canadian Trial of Carbohydrates in Diabetes (CCD), a 1 year controlled trial of low-GI dietary carbohydrate in subjects with T2DM managed by diet alone with optimal glycemic control, long-term HbA1c was not affected by altering the GI or the amount of dietary carbohydrate. Differences in total cholesterol to HDL cholesterol among diets had disappeared by 6 month. However, because of sustained reductions in postprandial glucose and CRP, a low-GI diet may be preferred for the dietary management of T2DM.

Epidemiologic studies have provided suggestive evidence that a diet in which carbohydrate-rich foods with high fiber and low GI are predominant may contribute to diabetes prevention. In the Nurses' Health Study, which includes 65,173 women followed for 6 years,[59] the dietary GI was positively associated with risk of diabetes after adjustment for age, BMI, smoking, physical activity, family history of diabetes, alcohol and cereal fiber intake, and total energy intake. Comparing the highest with the lowest quintile, the relative risk (RR) of diabetes was 1.37 (95% CI 1.09–1.71; P trend = 0.005). The glycemic load (GL) was also positively associated with diabetes (RR = 1.47; 95% CI 1.16–1.86; P trend = 0.003). These results were confirmed in the Health Professionals' Follow-Up Study.[60] However, no intervention studies have so far evaluated the potential of low-GI, high-fiber diets to

reduce the risk of diabetes or to prevent cardiovascular disease in diabetic patients; moreover, the results of the few available intervention studies evaluating the effects of GI on the cardiovascular disease risk factor profile are not always concordant.

## Fiber

With large amounts of fiber (>30 g/day) in suboptimal controlled type 1 subjects,[61–63] there is a positive effect of fiber on glycemia. In subjects being treated with two or more injections of insulin per day and HbA$_{1c}$ levels of 7%–10% consuming either a high-fiber (50 g/day), low-GI diet or a low-fiber (15 g/day), high-GI diet for 24 weeks, the high-fiber diet significantly reduced the mean daily blood glucose concentration (P < 0.05), the number of hypoglycemic events (P < 0.01), and, in the subgroup of patients compliant to diet, the HbA$_{1c}$ (P < 0.05), but had no beneficial effect on cholesterol, HDL cholesterol, or triglyceride concentrations.[64]

On the other hand, a cross-sectional analysis of dietary fiber in T1DM patients enrolled in the EURODIAB IDDM Complications Study revealed that a higher intake of total fiber (grams per day) was independently associated with higher levels of HDL cholesterol in both men and women and lower LDL cholesterol levels in men but not women.[65] No substantial differences were observed between soluble fiber and insoluble fiber intakes. Mean total fiber intake was 18.5 g/day in men and 16.2 g/day in women.

In a randomized, crossover study, 13 patients with T2DM were assigned to follow a diet containing moderate amounts of fiber (total, 24 g; 8 g of soluble fiber and 16 g of insoluble fiber) and a high-fiber diet (total, 50 g; 25 g of soluble fiber and 25 g of insoluble fiber), containing foods not fortified with fiber (unfortified foods) each for 6 weeks. A high intake of dietary fiber, particularly of the soluble type, above the level recommended by the ADA, improves glycemic control, decreases hyperinsulinemia, and lowers plasma lipid concentrations.[66]

A recent meta-analysis of 45 prospective cohort studies and 21 RCT between 1966 and February 2012 using random effects models found that compared with never/rare consumers of whole grains, those consuming 48–80 g whole grain/day (3–5 serving/day) had a ~26% lower risk of T2D (RR = 0.74) (95% CI 0.69, 0.80).[67]

## Resistant Starch

Resistant starch (nondigestible oligosaccharides and the starch amylose) is not digested and therefore not absorbed as glucose in the small intestine. It is, however, almost completely fermented in the colon and produces about 2 kcal/g of energy.[68] It is estimated that resistant starch and unabsorbed starch represent <10 g/day of the total starch ingested in the average Western diet.[69] Legumes are the major food source of resistant starch in the diet, containing 2–3 g resistant starch per 100 g cooked legumes. Uncooked cornstarch contains about 6 g resistant starch per 100 g dry weight.[70] It has been suggested that ingestion of resistant starch produces a lesser increase in postprandial glucose than digestible starch and correspondingly lower insulin levels. As a result, it has been proposed that food containing naturally occurring resistant starch (cornstarch) or food modified to contain more resistant starch (high-amylose cornstarch) may modify postprandial glycemic response, prevent hypoglycemia, and reduce hyperglycemia; these effects may explain differences in the GIs of some food.[71]

There have been several one-meal[72–74] and second-meal studies[75–77] in nondiabetic subjects, comparing subjects' physical response to food high in resistant starch and their response to food with an equivalent amount of digestible starch. All studies found some reduction in postprandial glucose and insulin responses to the first meal but observed mixed results after the second meal. Long-term studies have not consistently confirmed these results.[78–82] Published studies involving people with diabetes have focused on uncooked cornstarch and its potential to prevent nighttime hypoglycemia.[78,83,84,85] In uncontrolled studies, evening cornstarch in specific dosages or dosages based on g/kg body weight resulted in less hypoglycemia around 2:00 a.m. in all groups.[92,93] It has not been established that bedtime cornstarch snacks are more effective in preventing nocturnal hypoglycemia than other types of carbohydrate.

## Sucrose

Historically, the most widely held belief about nutrition and diabetes was that added sugars caused the disease. It was called "sugar diabetes," and patients were advised to avoid added sugars and that naturally occurring sugars be restricted. This belief was based on the assumption that sucrose and other sugars were more rapidly digested and absorbed then starch-containing food and thereby aggravated hyperglycemia. However, scientific evidence does not support this assumption. The available evidence from clinical studies demonstrates that dietary sucrose does not increase glycemia more than isocaloric amounts of starch.[85–88] Thus, the intake of sucrose and sucrose-containing food in diabetic individuals need not be restricted because of a concern about aggravating hyperglycemia. If sucrose is part of the food/meal plan, it should be substituted for other carbohydrate sources or, if added, should be adequately covered with insulin or other glucose-lowering medication. In addition, the intake of other nutrients (such as fat) often ingested with sucrose-containing foods must be taken into account. In one study, when individuals with T2DM were taught how to incorporate sucrose in their daily meal plan, no negative impact on dietary habits or metabolic control was observed.[89]

Since sucrose is composed of glucose and fructose as a disaccharide, the association of fructose with an increased incidence of obesity-associated diseases has implications for the intake of sucrose in both T1DM and T2DM. The majority of dietary fructose comes from two sweeteners, sucrose and high-fructose corn syrup (HFCS), which are commonly used in manufactured foods and beverages. Specifically, the increase in fructose consumption is primarily due to the increased use of HFCS in the Western diet. Based upon disappearance data, the annual per capita intake of HFCS from 1967 to 2006 increased from 0.03 to 58.2 lb, whereas sucrose decreased from 98.5 to 62.3 lb.[90]

In a recent study,[91] 40 men and women consumed 24 oz of HFCS or sucrose-sweetened beverages in a randomized crossover design study. Blood and urine samples were collected over 6 h. Blood pressure, heart rate, fructose, and a variety of other metabolic biomarkers were measured. Fructose area under the curve and maximum concentration, dose-normalized glucose area under the curve and maximum concentration, relative bioavailability of glucose, changes in postprandial concentrations of serum uric acid, and systolic blood pressure maximum levels were higher when HFCS-sweetened beverages were consumed as compared with sucrose-sweetened beverages. Compared with sucrose, HFCS led to greater fructose systemic exposure and significantly different acute metabolic effects compared to sucrose.

## Fructose

Fructose is naturally occurring as a monosaccharide in fruits and vegetables and accounts for about 9% of average energy intake in the United States.[92] Fructose is somewhat sweeter than sucrose. It has been estimated that one-third of dietary fructose comes from fruits, vegetables, and other natural sources in the diet and two-thirds comes from food and beverages to which fructose has been added as fructose or HFCS.[93] However, with the increased intake of HFCS, these estimates may have to be revised.

In several studies in diabetic subjects, fructose produced a reduction in postprandial glycemia when it replaced sucrose or starch as a carbohydrate source.[94–97] Thus, fructose might be a good sweetening agent in the diabetic diet. However, this potential benefit is tempered by the concern that fructose may have adverse effects on plasma lipids. Consumption of large amounts of fructose (15%–20% of daily energy intake [90th percentile of usual intake]) has been shown to increase fasting total and LDL cholesterol in subjects with diabetes[94] and fasting total and LDL cholesterol and triglycerides in nondiabetic subjects.[98–100]

## MONOUNSATURATED FATS

Diets high in monounsaturated fat[101–104] result in improvements in glucose tolerance and lipids compared with diets high in saturated fat. A meta-analysis has found that high-MUFA diets reduce fasting glucose in patients with T2DM.[105] Diets enriched with monounsaturated fat may also reduce insulin resistance.[104] There is, however, a concern that when high monounsaturated fat diets are eaten ad libitum outside of a controlled setting, they may result in increased energy intake and weight gain.[106] A recent meta-analysis of nine randomized controlled intervention trials with a total of 1547 participants and a running time of at least 6 months compared high diet versus low diet in MUFA among adults with abnormal glucose metabolism (T2D, impaired glucose tolerance, and insulin resistant), being overweight or obese. It was found that high-MUFA diets appear to be effective in reducing HbA1c and therefore should be recommended in the dietary regimes of T2D.[107] More studies comparing diets high in monounsaturated fat with diets high in carbohydrate with ad libitum energy intake are needed to evaluate the efficacy of these diets and determine effects of MUFA in reducing cardiovascular risk in diabetes.

## OMEGA-3 FATTY ACIDS

The relationship between omega-3 polyunsaturated fatty acids (n-3 PUFA) from seafood sources (eicosapentaenoic acid, EPA; docosahexaenoic acid, DHA) or plant sources (alpha-linolenic acid, ALA) and risk of T2DM remains unclear. A meta-analysis searched multiple literature databases through June 2011, did not support either major harms or benefits of fish/seafood or EPA+DHA on development of DM, and suggests that ALA may be associated with modestly lower risk.[108]

A multicenter, randomized, double-blind, placebo-controlled study evaluated the possible worsening of glycemic control after a moderate daily intake of n-3 fatty acid ethyl esters in patients with hypertriglyceridemia with and without glucose intolerance or diabetes.[109] Plasma triacylglycerol concentrations decreased significantly, up to 21.53% at 6 month compared with baseline (decreased 15% compared with placebo), with a tendency toward a progressive reduction with time. There was no evidence for a different response in patients with either NIDDM or impaired glucose tolerance. Among NIDDM patients, the triacylglycerol reduction was greater in those with HDL cholesterol ≤0.91 mmol/L. There was no alteration in the major GIs: fasting glucose, HbA1c, insulinemia, and oral glucose tolerance in patients with impaired glucose tolerance or NIDDM after treatment with n-3 ethyl esters.

In a pooled analysis with 23 RCT and 1075 participants, omega-3 PUFA supplementation in T2DM lowers triglycerides and VLDL cholesterol but may raise LDL cholesterol (although results were nonsignificant in subgroups) and has no statistically significant effect on glycemic control or fasting insulin.[110]

## PROTEIN

Abnormalities of protein metabolism are assumed to be less affected by insulin deficiency and insulin resistance than abnormalities of glucose metabolism.[111] However, moderate hyperglycemia may contribute to increased turnover of protein in type 2 diabetic subjects. During moderate hyperglycemia, obese subjects with T2DM, compared to nondiabetic obese subjects, demonstrate an increase in whole-body nitrogen flux and a higher rate of protein synthesis and breakdown.[112,113] A high-quality protein (95 g protein/day), very-low-energy diet capable of maintaining nitrogen balance in obese subjects without diabetes did not prevent negative nitrogen balance in diabetic subjects, despite weight loss and improved glycemic control.[113] This increased protein turnover was restored to normal only with oral glucose-lowering agents or exogenous insulin sufficient to achieve euglycemia and with increased protein intake.[113,114] These study results suggest that people

with T2DM have an increased need for protein during moderate hyperglycemia and an altered adaptive mechanism for protein sparing during weight loss. Thus, with energy restriction, the protein requirements of people with diabetes may be greater than the recommended dietary allowance (RDA) of 0.8 g protein/kg body wt, and increased amounts of protein may aid in weight management efforts through effects on satiety and maintenance of lean body mass.[115]

## MICRONUTRIENTS

Selected micronutrients may affect glucose and insulin metabolism, but the data are scarce or inconsistent. Vitamin D deficiency has been associated with impaired human insulin action, suggesting a role in the pathogenesis of T2DM. In a prospective interventional study, vitamin D3 (2000 IU) supplementation affected the metabolic profiles of Saudi T2DM. Over an 18-month period, circulating 25-hydroxyvitamin D levels remained below normal 18 months after the onset of treatment. Yet, this "suboptimal" supplementation significantly improved lipid profile with a favorable change in HDL/LDL ratio and HOMA-beta function, which were more pronounced in T2DM females.[116]

Vitamin E has also been studied with regard to T2DM. Within the range that can be obtained from food intake, men with higher plasma concentrations of alpha-tocopherol experienced reduced risk for diabetes compared to men with lower concentrations of alpha-tocopherol.[117] Results of studies that evaluated effects of vitamin E on insulin sensitivity have been equivocal.[118–120] Insufficient intake of magnesium, zinc, and chromium has been implicated as possible risk factors for the development of diabetes.[59,121–125] However, the efficacy of supplemented intake has not been established.

The positive effects of chromium on glucose metabolism have been recognized since the observation that brewer's yeast improved glycemic control in the 1920s. In 1957, chromium was identified to be the active component of glucose tolerance factor from brewer's yeast.[126,127] Two recent studies did not show an improvement in either glycemia or lipid parameters.[128,129] Western populations, which showed a negative result with chromium supplementation, were chromium sufficient, in contrast to Asian populations such as Chinese and Asian Indians who tend to be chromium deficient. These differences as well as ethnic variations may account for the disparate results in different studies from various geographical and ethnic regions. Cefalu et al.[130] conducted a comprehensive evaluation of chromium supplementation on metabolic parameters in a cohort of T2DM subjects representing a wide phenotype range and to evaluate changes in "responders" and "nonresponders." After preintervention testing to assess glycemia, insulin sensitivity (assessed by euglycemic clamps), chromium status, and body composition, subjects were randomized in a double-blind fashion to placebo or 1000 μg chromium. There was not a consistent effect of chromium supplementation to improve insulin action across all phenotypes, but "response" to chromium was more likely in insulin-resistant individuals who had more elevated fasting glucose and $A_{1c}$ levels.

## CONCLUSION

Patients with T2DM are part of a global epidemic requiring a combined diet and lifestyle approach. The evidence for the effects of nutrition including specific macronutrient and micronutrients is emerging, but the clarion call to action against obesity and T2DM cannot await further investigation. It is clear from the studies presented that weight management is critical to the prevention and treatment of T2DM. At the last stages of T2DM when the beta-cell mass in the pancreas is exhausted or in T1DM, there is evidence that some macronutrients, fiber, and micronutrients may help in achieving optimal glucose control.

## REFERENCES

1. Hahr, AJ, Molitch, ME. *Am J Ther* 15:543;2008.
2. Wycherley, TP, Noakes, M, Clifton, PM et al. *Diabetes Care* 33:969;2010.
3. Eknoyan, G, Nagy, J. *Adv Chronic Kidney Dis* 12:223;2005.
4. Bliss, M. *Horm Res* 64(Suppl 2):98–102;2005.
5. Roberts, H, Jiles, R, Mokdad, A et al. *Ethn Dis* 19:276;2009.
6. Danaei, G, Finucane, MM, Lu, Y et al. *Lancet* 378:31;2011.
7. Prentki, M, Nolan, CJ. *J Clin Invest* 116:1802;2006.
8. Daval, M, Bedrood, S, Gurlo, T et al. *Amyloid* 17:118;2010.
9. Butler, AE, Janson, J, Bonner-Weir, S et al. *Diabetes* 52:102;2003.
10. Cowie, CC, Harris, MI, Eberhardt, MS. *Diabetes Care* 17:1158;1994.
11. Olefsky, JM, Kolterman, OG, Scarlett JA. *Am J Physiol* 243:E15;1982.
12. Campbell, PJ, Gerich, JE. *J Clin Endocrinol Metab* 70:1114;1990.
13. Albu, J, Konnaaarides, C, Pi-Sunyer, FX. *Diabetes Rev* 3:335;1995.
14. Amatruda, JM, Richeson, JF, Welle, SL et al. *Arch Intern Med* 148:873;1988.
15. Henry, RR, Wiest-Kent, TA, Scheaffer, L et al. *Diabetes* 35:155;1986.
16. Hughes, TA, Gwynne, JT, Switzer, BR. *Am J Med* 77:7–17;1984.
17. Laitinen, JH, Ahola, IE, Sarkkinen, ES et al. *J Am Diet Assoc* 93:276;1993.
18. Hanefeld, M, Fischer, S, Schmechel, H et al. *Diabetes Care* 14:308;1991.
19. Hadden, DR, Blair, AL, Wilson, EA et al. *Q J Med* 59:579;1986.
20. Wing, RR, Venditti, E, Jakicic, JM et al. *Diabetes Care* 21:350;1998.
21. The Diabetes Prevention Program. *Diabetes Care* 22:623;1999.
22. Tuomilehto, J, Lindstrom, J, Eriksson, JG et al. *N Engl J Med* 344:1343;2001.
23. Li, Z, Hong, K, Saltsman, P et al. *Eur J Clin Nutr* 59:411;2005.
24. Rothacker, DQ, Staniszewski, BA, Ellis, PK. *J Am Diet Assoc* 101:345;2001.
25. Metz, JA, Stern, JS, Kris-Etherton, P et al. *Arch Intern Med* 160:2150;2000.
26. Ditschuneit, HH, Flechtner-Mors, M, Johnson, TD, Adler, G. *Am J Clin Nutr* 69:198;1999.
27. Ashley, JM, St. Jeor, ST, Schrage, JP et al. *Arch Intern Med* 161:1599;2001.
28. Quinn, RD. *Nutrition* 16:344;2000.
29. Wing, RR, Marcus, MD, Salata, R et al. *Arch Intern Med* 151:1334;1991.
30. Henry, RR, Gumbiner B. *Diabetes Care* 14:802;1991.
31. Wing RR. *J Am Diet Assoc* 95:569;1995.
32. Kendall, A, Levitsky, DA, Strupp, BJ, Lissner L. *Am J Clin Nutr* 53:1124;1991.
33. Lissner, L, Levitsky, DA, Strupp, BJ et al. *Am J Clin Nutr* 46:886;1987.
34. Bouchard, C, Depres, JP, Tremblay, A. *Obes Res* 1:133;1993.
35. Maggio, CA, Pi-Sunyer, FX. *Diabetes Care* 20:1744;1997.
36. Pavlou, KN, Krey, S, Steffee, WP. *Am J Clin Nutr* 49:1115;1989.
37. Brown, SA, Upchurch, S, Anding, R et al. *Diabetes Care* 19:613;1996.
38. Foreyt, JP, Goodrick, GK. *Ann Intern Med* 119:698;1993.
39. Butryn, ML, Webb, V, Wadden, TA. *Psychiatr Clin North Am* 34:841;2011.
40. Edelstein, SL, Knowler, WC, Bain, RP et al. *Diabetes* 46:701;1997.
41. Manson, JE, Spelsberg, A. *Am J Prev Med* 10:172;1994.
42. Viswanathan, M, Snehalatha, C, Viswanathan, V et al. *Diabetes Res Clin Pract* 35:107;1997.
43. Pan, XR, Li, GW, Hu, YH et al. *Diabetes Care* 20:537;1997.
44. Eriksson, KF, Lindgarde, F. *Diabetologia* 34:891;1991.
45. Wannamethee, SG, Shaper, AG. *Diabetes Care* 22:1266;1999.
46. Perreault, L, Pan, Q, Mather, KJ et al. *Lancet* 379:2243;2012.
47. Manson, JE, Rimm, EB, Stampfer, MJ et al. *Lancet* 338:774;1991.
48. Helmrich, SP, Ragland, DR, Leung, RW, Paffenbarger, RS, Jr. *N Engl J Med* 325:147;1991.
49. Frisch, RE, Wyshak, G, Albright, TE et al. *Diabetes* 35:1101;1986.
50. Perry, IJ, Wannamethee, SG, Walker, MK, T et al. *BMJ* 310:560;1995.
51. Wei, M, Gibbons, LW, Mitchell, TL et al. *Ann Intern Med* 130:89;1999.
52. Kohl, HW, Gordon, NF, Villegas, JA, Blair SN. *Diabetes Care* 15:184;1992.
53. Lee, CD, Blair, SN, Jackson, AS. *Am J Clin Nutr* 69:373;1999.
54. Jeon, CY, Lokken, RP, Hu, FB, van Dam, RM. *Diabetes Care* 30:744;2007.
55. Pi-Sunyer, FX. *Am J Clin Nutr* 76:290S;2002.
56. Thomas, DE, Elliott, EJ. *Br J Nutr* 104:797;2010.
57. Buyken, AE, Toeller, M, Heitkamp, G et al. *Am J Clin Nutr* 73:574;2001.
58. Queiroz, KC, Novato, SI, de Cassia Goncalves, AR. *Nutr Hosp* 27:510;2012.
59. Salmeron, J, Manson, JE, Stampfer, MJ et al. *JAMA* 277:472;1997.
60. Salmeron, J, Ascherio, A, Rimm, EB et al. *Diabetes Care* 20:545;1997.
61. Chenon, D, Phaka, M, Monnier, LH et al. *Am J Clin Nutr* 40:58;1984.
62. Riccardi, G, Rivellese, A, Pacioni, D et al. *Diabetologia* 26:116;1984.
63. Vaaler, S, Hanssen, KF, Aagenaes, O. *Acta Med Scand* 208:389;1980.
64. Giacco, R, Parillo, M, Rivellese, AA et al. *Diabetes Care* 23:1461;2000.
65. Toeller, M, Buyken, AE, Heitkamp, G et al. *Diabetes Care* 22(Suppl 2):B21;1999.
66. Chandalia, M, Garg, A, Lutjohann, D et al. *N Engl J Med* 342:1392;2000.

67. Yen, EQ, Chackon, SA, Choun, EL et al. *J Nutr* 142:1304;2012.
68. Joint FAO/WHO Expert Consultation. *FAO Food Nutr Pap* 66:1;1998.
69. Wursch, P. *World Rev Nutr Diet* 60:199;1989.
70. Englyst, HN, Veenstra, J, Hudson, GJ. *Br J Nutr* 75:327;1996.
71. Brennan, CS. *Mol Nutr Food Res* 49:560;2005.
72. Hoebler, C, Karinthi, A, Chiron, HC et al. *Eur J Clin Nutr* 53:360;1999.
73. Granfeldt, Y, Drews, A, Bjorck, I. *J Nutr* 125:459;1995.
74. Raben, A, Tagliabue, A, Christensen, NJ et al. *Am J Clin Nutr* 60:544;1994.
75. Achour, L, Flourie, B, Briet, F et al. *Am J Clin Nutr* 66:1151;1997.
76. Heijnen, ML, Deurenberg, P, van Amelsvoort, JM, Beynen, AC. *Br J Nutr* 73:423;1995.
77. Liljeberg, HG, Akerberg, AK, Bjorck, IM. *Am J Clin Nutr* 69:647;1999.
78. Axelsen, M, Wesslau, C, Lonnroth, P et al. *J Intern Med* 245:229;1999.
79. Jenkins, DJ, Vuksan, V, Kendall, CW et al. *J Am Coll Nutr* 17:609;1998.
80. Noakes, M, Clifton, PM, Nestel, PJ et al. *Am J Clin Nutr* 64:944;1996.
81. Luo, J, Rizkalla, SW, Alamowitch, C et al. *Am J Clin Nutr* 63:939;1996.
82. Behall, KM, Howe, JC. *Am J Clin Nutr* 61:334;1995.
83. Axelsen, M, Lonnroth, P, Lenner, RA et al. *Am J Clin Nutr* 71:1108;2000.
84. Axelsen, M, Lonnroth, P, Arvidsson, LR, Smith, U. *Eur J Clin Invest* 27:157;1997.
85. Kaufman, FR, Halvorson, M, Kaufman, ND. *Diabetes Res Clin Pract* 30:205;1995.
86. Bantle, JP, Swanson, JE, Thomas, W, Laine, DC. *Diabetes Care* 16:1301;1993.
87. Abraira, C, Derler, J. *Am J Med* 84:193;1988.
88. Jellish, WS, Emanuele, MA, Abraira, C. *Am J Med* 77:1015;1984.
89. Nadeau, J, Koski, KG, Strychar, I, Yale, JF. *Diabetes Care* 24:222;2001.
90. Bray, GA, Nielsen, SJ, Popkin, BM. *Am J Clin Nutr* 79:537;2004.
91. Le, MT, Frye, RF, Rivard, CJ et al. *Metabolism* 61:641;2012.
92. Gibney, M, Sigman-Grant, M, Stanton, JL, Jr., Keast, DR. *Am J Clin Nutr* 62:178S;1995.
93. Park, YK, Yetley, EA. *Am J Clin Nutr* 58:737S;1993.
94. Bantle, JP, Swanson, JE, Thomas, W, Laine, DC. *Diabetes Care* 15:1468;1992.
95. Bantle, JP, Laine, DC, Thomas, JW. *JAMA* 256:3241;1986.
96. Crapo, PA, Kolterman, OG, Henry, RR. *Diabetes Care* 9:111;1986.
97. Malerbi, DA, Paiva, ES, Duarte, AL, Wajchenberg, BL. *Diabetes Care* 19:1249;1996.
98. Bantle, JP, Raatz, SK, Thomas, W, Georgopoulos, A. *Am J Clin Nutr* 72:1128;2000.
99. Swanson, JE, Laine, DC, Thomas, W, Bantle, JP. *Am J Clin Nutr* 55:851;1992.
100. Reiser, S, Powell, AS, Scholfield, DJ et al. *Am J Clin Nutr* 49:832;1989.
101. Walker, KZ, O'Dea, K, Johnson, L et al. *Am J Clin Nutr* 63:254;1996.
102. Campbell, LV, Marmot, PE, Dyer, JA et al. *Diabetes Care* 17:177;1994.
103. Rasmussen, OW, Thomsen, C, Hansen, KW et al. *Diabetes Care* 16:1565;1993.
104. Parillo, M, Rivellese, AA, Ciardullo, AV et al. *Metabolism* 41:1373;1992.
105. Schwingshackl, L, Strasser, B. *Ann Nutr Metab* 60:33;2012.
106. Yu-Poth, S, Zhao, G, Etherton, T et al. *Am J Clin Nutr* 69:632;1999.
107. Schwingshackl, L, Strasser, B, Hoffmann, G. *Ann Nutr Metab* 58:290;2011.
108. Wu, JH, Micha, R, Imamura, F et al. *Br J Nutr* 107(Suppl 2):S214;2012.
109. Sirtori, CR, Paoletti, R, Mancini, M et al. *Am J Clin Nutr* 65:1874;1997.
110. Hartweg, J, Perera, R, Montori, V et al. *Cochrane Database Syst Rev* CD003205;2008.
111. Henry, RR. *Diabetes Care* 17:1502;1994.
112. Gougeon, R, Marliss, EB, Jones, PJ et al. *Int J Obes Relat Metab Disord* 22:250;1998.
113. Gougeon, R, Pencharz, PB, Sigal, RJ. *Am J Clin Nutr* 65:861;1997.
114. Gougeon, R, Styhler, K, Morais, JA et al. *Diabetes Care* 23:1;2000.
115. Flechtner-Mors, M, Boehm, BO, Wittmann, R et al. *Diabetes Metab Res Rev* 26:393;2010.
116. Al-Daghri, NM, Alkharfy, KM, Al-Othman, A et al. *Cardiovasc Diabetol* 11:85;2012.
117. Salonen, JT, Nyyssonen, K, Tuomainen,TP et al. *BMJ* 311:1124;1995.
118. Sanchez-Lugo, L, Mayer-Davis, EJ, Howard, G et al. *Am J Clin Nutr* 66:1224;1997.
119. Paolisso, G, D'Amore, A, Giugliano, D et al. *Am J Clin Nutr* 57:650;1993.
120. Reunanen, A, Knekt, P, Aaran, R-K, Aromaa, A. *Eur J Clin Nutr* 52:89–93;1998.
121. Meyer, KA, Kushi, LH, Jacobs, DR Jr. et al. *Am J Clin Nutr* 71:921;2000.
122. Lukaksi, HC. *Am J Clin Nutr* 72(Suppl):585S;2000.
123. Singh, RB, Niaz, MA, Rastogi, SS et al. *J Am Coll Nutr* 17:564;1998.
124. Anderson, RA. *Nutr Rev* 56:266;1998.
125. Anderson, RA. *Diabetes Metab* 26:22;2000.
126. Chowdhury, S, Pandit, K, Roychowdury, P, Bhattacharya, B. *J Assoc Physicians India* 51:701;2003.
127. Mertz, W. *J Am Coll Nutr* 17:544;1998.
128. Ali, A, Ma, Y, Reynolds, J et al. *Endocr Pract* 17:16;2011.
129. Kleefstra, N, Houweling, ST, Jansman, FG et al. *Diabetes Care* 29:521;2006.
130. Cefalu, WT, Rood, J, Pinsonat, P et al. *Metabolism* 59:755;2010.

# 59 Nutrition in Renal Disease and Hypertension

*David Martins, Keith Norris, and David Heber*

## CONTENTS

## INTRODUCTION

Chronic renal insufficiency is the ninth leading cause of death in the United States, according to the Centers for Disease Control.[1] In this disease, the kidneys are damaged and cannot filter blood effectively. This damage can cause wastes to build up in the body and lead to other health problems, including cardiovascular disease (CVD), anemia, and bone disease. People with early chronic kidney disease (CKD) tend not to feel any symptoms. The only ways to detect CKD are through a blood test to estimate kidney function and a urine test to assess kidney damage. If left untreated, chronic renal insufficiency leads to renal failure.

The most common cause of chronic renal insufficiency is diabetes.[2] After 10–20 years of diabetes mellitus, approximately 20% of patients with either type 1 diabetes mellitus (T1DM) or type 2 diabetes mellitus (T2DM) develop diabetic nephropathy, making diabetes mellitus the leading cause of end-stage renal disease (ESRD). Both genetic and environmental factors determine which patients eventually develop diabetic nephropathy, and there remains a need for research to better understand the pathophysiology and molecular pathways that lead from the onset of hyperglycemia to renal failure. Changes in the vasculature and the glomerulus, including those to mesangial cells, the filtration barrier, and podocytes, play important roles in the pathophysiology of the diabetic kidney. High blood pressure (BP) is the second most common cause of chronic renal insufficiency and is often associated with metabolic syndrome and obesity. However, the exact mechanism of the development of hypertension in obesity remains to be established.[3]

Polycystic kidney disease is the most common inherited kidney disease.[4] It causes cyst formation in the kidneys. If the cysts are numerous and large enough, they may prevent the kidneys from carrying out their normal functions. Kidney stones can also lead to chronic renal insufficiency. When kidney stones[4] become too numerous and too big, they can interfere with normal kidney functions, causing chronic renal insufficiency. Having one kidney stone puts a patient at a 50% increased risk of having another within 5–7 years. Treatment of kidney stones is essential in preventing chronic renal insufficiency. Urinary infections, if long lasting, can lead to chronic renal insufficiency.[5] Urinary infections mostly affect the bladder but can also spread to the kidneys. If the glomeruli in the kidneys become infected, they can no longer eliminate excess fluid and waste at the rate that is necessary to keep the body healthy. Urinary infections, if treated successfully, can prevent chronic renal insufficiency. Once renal function declines so that metabolic derangements including electrolyte balance and uremia become prominent, then protein restriction is used to increase interdialysis intervals.[6]

Restriction of dietary protein intake has been a relevant part of the management of CKD for more than 100 years, but even today, the principal goal of protein-restricted regimens is to decrease the accumulation of nitrogen waste products, hydrogen ions, phosphates, and inorganic ions while maintaining an adequate nutritional status to avoid secondary problems such as metabolic acidosis, bone disease, and insulin resistance, as well as proteinuria and deterioration of renal function. A large multicenter study proved that providing essential amino acids rather than a mixture of essential and nonessential amino acids does not affect the progression of renal disease.[7]

## OVERVIEW AND PUBLIC HEALTH IMPLICATIONS

Nutrition plays a most prominent role in the prevention of renal disease through the treatment of hypertension and diabetes. CKD has become more common over the last 20 years in association with increases in the prevalence of metabolic syndrome, hypertension, diabetes, and obesity. It was reported to affect over 13% of the U.S. population in 2004.[8] In 2010, it was reported by the Centers for Disease Control that more than 35% of people aged 20 years or older with diabetes have CKD and more than 20% of people aged 20 years or older with hypertension have CKD.[9] The rise in incidence of CKD has been attributed to an aging populace and increases in hypertension (HTN), diabetes, and obesity within the U.S. population, conditions affected by diet. CKD is associated with electrolyte imbalances, mineral and bone disorders, anemia, dyslipidemia, and HTN. Furthermore, reduced glomerular filtration rate (GFR) and albuminuria are independently associated with an increase in cardiovascular and all-cause mortality.[10,11]

From another viewpoint, HTN has been reported to occur in 85%–95% of patients with CKD (stages 3–5).[12] The relationship between HTN and CKD is cyclic in nature. Uncontrolled HTN is a risk factor for developing CKD, and HTN is associated with a more rapid progression of CKD and is the second leading cause of ESRD in the United States.[13,14] Meanwhile, progressive renal disease can exacerbate uncontrolled HTN due to volume expansion and increased systemic vascular resistance. Multiple guidelines discuss the importance of lowering BP to slow the progression of renal disease and reduce cardiovascular morbidity and mortality.[15–17] However, in order to achieve and maintain adequate BP control, most patients with CKD require combinations of antihypertensive agents; often up to three or four medication classes may need to be employed.[18]

## HYPERTENSION AND CHRONIC KIDNEY DISEASE

HTN is one of the leading causes of CKD due to the deleterious effects that increased BP has on kidney vasculature. Long-term, uncontrolled, high BP leads to high intraglomerular pressure, impairing glomerular filtration.[19,20] Damage to the glomeruli leads to an increase in protein filtration, resulting in abnormally increased amounts of protein in the urine (microalbuminuria or proteinuria).[19,20] Microalbuminuria is the presence of small amounts of albumin in the urine and is often the first sign of CKD. Proteinuria (protein-to-creatinine ratio ≥ 200 mg/g) develops as CKD progresses and is associated with a poor prognosis for both kidney disease and CVD.[10,11,21]

The estimated GFR, which helps clinicians determine how well the kidneys are filtering waste, is used in the staging of CKD. The National Kidney Foundation defines CKD

### TABLE 59.1
### Staging of CKD

| Stage | Description | GFR (mL/min/1.73 m²) |
|-------|-------------|----------------------|
| 1 | Kidney damage with normal or increased GFR | ≥90 |
| 2 | Kidney damage with mildly decreased GFR | 60–90 |
| 3 | Moderately decreased GFR | 30–59 |
| 4 | Severely decreased GFR | 15–29 |
| 5 | Kidney failure | <15 or on dialysis |

*Source:* Collins, A.J. et al., *Am. J. Kidney Dis.,* 59, evii, 2012.
*Note:* GFR, glomerular filtration rate.

as either kidney damage, identified by markers in the urine or blood or by imaging, with or without changes in the GFR, or GFR <60 mL/min/1.73 m² for a minimum of 3 months.[16] Table 59.1 depicts the staging criteria as determined by the Kidney Disease Outcomes Quality Initiative (KDOQI) guidelines.[16]

Patients with nondiabetic and diabetic CKD should have a target BP goal of <130/80 mmHg.[15–17] Ultimately, the rationale for lowering BP in all patients with CKD is to reduce both renal and cardiovascular morbidity and mortality. Maintaining BP control and minimizing proteinuria in patients with CKD and HTN is essential for the prevention of the progression of kidney disease and the development or worsening of CVD.[15,16]

Recent literature suggests that BP targets in diabetic and nondiabetic CKD may need to be individualized based on the presence of proteinuria. Some trials have failed to show a reduction in cardiovascular or renal outcomes in diabetic and nondiabetic patients with CKD when a BP target of <130/80 mmHg is achieved compared to lowering BP to <140/90 mmHg.[22,23] However, patients who have proteinuria are less likely to experience a decline in renal function, kidney failure, or death when the lower BP target is achieved.[22,24] It is likely that future guidelines may include a lower BP goal, <130/80 mmHg, for patients with proteinuria, but maintain a goal of <140/90 mmHg for patients without proteinuria.

## NUTRITIONAL APPROACHES TO KIDNEY DISEASE PREVENTION

Increased physical activity, weight loss, and dietary modifications are recommended for all patients with HTN. Lifestyle modification remains a critical component of therapy for HTN, regardless of whether patients require medications to achieve their BP goal. The dietary approaches to stop HTN (DASH) diet emphasizes an increased consumption of fruits and vegetables, an inclusion of low-fat dairy and lean protein, and a restriction of saturated fats; this meal plan has been shown to significantly lower systolic BP nearly equivalent to the reduction achieved by antihypertensive monotherapy.

In addition, decreasing sodium and alcohol intake has been established as an effective intervention toward decreasing BP. Initiating these healthy dietary practices while increasing daily activity augments the benefit received from antihypertensive therapy and can play an essential role in achieving BP goals.

The interrelationship of CKD and HTN leads to further emphasis on the importance of achieving BP control and decreasing proteinuria, if present. Agents that reduce proteinuria in addition to BP are generally first line, but patients may often require three to four antihypertensive agents in order to achieve their goals and minimize their risk for CVD and ESRD. A discussion of the pharmacotherapy for HTN is outside the scope of this chapter.

## HYPERTENSION CONTROL AND PREVENTION OF RENAL DISEASE

HTN affects one in three adult Americans and contributes to nearly half of all cardiovascular deaths in the United States.[25] Although the diagnosis of HTN is made at a sustained BP level of 140/90 mmHg, the risk of cardiovascular death with elevated BP is actually a continuum of risk that doubles for every 20/10 mmHg rise in BP above 115/75 mmHg.[26] Hence, the creation of the new category of "pre-HTN" in the HTN classification scheme for BP (levels 120–139/80–89 mmHg) promotes the adoption of lifestyle changes that have been shown to lower BP prior to the onset of HTN (Table 59.2).

## CARDIOVASCULAR DISEASE BURDEN AND RISK ASSESSMENT

The morbidity and mortality of HTN stem in part from the tendency of elevated BP to occur together with other CVD risk factors and a cluster of metabolic disorders known as metabolic syndrome (see Chapter 20 for the discussion of metabolic syndrome).

Since the risk of cardiovascular death at any given level of BP depends on the number of concurrent CVD risk factors, a comprehensive clinical and laboratory cardiovascular risk assessment is needed to establish the CVD burden

### TABLE 59.2
### BP Classification and Staging of HTN (Adults 18 Years and Older)

| BP Category | Systolic BP, mmHg | Diastolic BP, mmHg |
|---|---|---|
| Normal | <120 | <80 |
| Prehypertension | 120–139 | 80–89 |
| Stage 1 hypertension | 140–159 | 90–99 |
| Stage 2 hypertension | ≥160 | ≥100 |

*Source:* The Seventh Report of the Joint National Committee on Prevention, Detection, Evaluation, and Treatment of High Blood Pressure (JNC 7), *Hypertension*, 42, 1206, 2003.

and determine the scope of lifestyle changes and/or need for pharmaceutical intervention in patients with HTN.

## LIFESTYLE CHANGES

Many of the CVD risk factors are behavioral and modifiable by lifestyle changes. Although the potential therapeutic impact of established lifestyle changes on BP varies across the spectrum, they have all been shown to lower BP and/or mitigate the risk of cardiovascular death in a dose- and time-dependent fashion.

## DIETARY PATTERNS AND POPULATION BLOOD PRESSURE

BP varies from population to population and from person to person in the same population for wide variety of reasons.[27] Vegetarian populations exhibit lower BPs than nonvegetarians, and dietary patterns plentiful in whole grains, fruits, and vegetables have been associated with lower BPs.[28] There is a natural tendency for BP to increase with age that is attenuated by a high intake of fruits and vegetables in both men and women.[29,30] The intake of as little as three or more servings of fruits and vegetables a day was associated with a 42% lower stroke mortality and a 27% lower CVD mortality over 19 years follow-up, after adjustment for established CVD risk factors.[31] The choices of food and number of daily servings utilized in the DASH study shown in Table 59.3 were associated with about 11.4 mmHg decrease in systolic BP and about 5.5 mmHg decrease in diastolic BP after 8 weeks.[32]

## DASH DIETARY PATTERN

The DASH diet plan promotes the liberal intake of whole grains, fruits, and vegetables and the limitation of sweets and saturated fats. Fruits and vegetables are high in dietary fibers and minerals, including potassium. High potassium intake has long been associated with low BP and was actually once advocated for the treatment and prevention of HTN.[33] The intake of 60 mmol (2340 mg) or more of potassium a day was associated with a decrease of about 4.4 mmHg in systolic BP and 2.5 mmHg in diastolic BP.[34] The potassium content of selected potassium-rich fruits and vegetables are shown in Table 59.4.

Although the DASH diet is not designed to promote weight loss, the calorie limit of the diet can be manipulated in overweight and obese adults to achieve weight loss. A 2000 cal a day diet in an inactive adult male that measures 74 in. and weighs 250 lb will lead to an estimated daily deficit of about 1000 cal that will translate to a 2 lb weight loss/week on the DASH diet. The high prevalence of overweight and obesity in the United States has been attributed in part to excessive intake of sweets and saturated fats.[35] The limitation of sweets and saturated fats in persons with a strong appetite for these calorie-dense foods will create an additional calorie deficit that will facilitate weight loss. A daily deficit of 500 cal

**TABLE 59.3**
**DASH Diet**

| Food Group | Daily Servings | Serving Sizes | Examples for a Typical American Diet | Significance of Each Food Group to the DASH Diet[a] |
|---|---|---|---|---|
| Grains and grain products | 7–8 | 1 slice bread<br>1 c (0.24 L) ready- to-eat cereal[b]<br>½ c (12 L) cooked rice, pasta, or cereal | Bread, biscuit, corn bread, cereals, oatmeal, grits, rice, pasta, crackers, unsalted pretzels | Major sources of energy and fiber |
| Vegetables | 4–5 | 1 c raw leafy vegetable<br>½ c cooked vegetable<br>6 oz (180 mL) vegetable juice | Fresh, canned, or frozen vegetables: tomatoes, corn, potatoes, greens (e.g., collards, kale, turnip greens, spinach), yams, squash, carrots, okra | Rich sources of potassium, magnesium, and fiber |
| Fruits | 4–5 | 1 medium-size fruit, 1/2 c dried fruit, ½ c fresh, frozen, or canned fruit, 6 oz fruit juice | Bananas, grapes, apples, oranges, unsweetened fruit juices, grapefruit, mangoes, melons, peaches, dried fruit | Important source of potassium, magnesium, and fiber |
| Low-fat or fat-free dairy foods | 2–3 | 6 oz fruit juice, 8 oz (240 mL) milk, 1 c yogurt, 11/2 oz (42 g) cheese | Fat-free (skim) or low-fat (1%) milk, fat-free cheeses, low-fat yogurt, low-fat ice cream, or frozen yogurt | Major sources of calcium and protein |
| Lean meats, poultry, and fish | ≤ 2 | 3 oz (84 g) cooked lean meats, poultry (remove skin), or fish Broil or roast, rather than fry | Chicken, turkey, ground turkey or chicken, chicken sausage, lean pork, or beef, fish and seafood: haddock, halibut, flounder, catfish, salmon, shrimp, crab, oyster, calms | Rich sources of protein and magnesium |
| Nuts, seeds, and beans | 4–5/week | 1/3 c (0.08 L) or 1 ½ oz (42 g) nuts, 1 tbsp (15 mL) or ½ oz (14 g) seeds, ½ c cooked dry beans | Black beans, kidney beans, navy beans, pigeon peas, pinto beans, split peas, peanuts (roasted or boiled), almonds, pecans, walnuts, hazelnuts | Rich sources of energy, magnesium, potassium, protein, and fiber |
| Fats and oils[c] | 2–3 | 1 tbsp low-fat mayonnaise, 2 tbsp (30) light salad dressing, 1 tsp vegetable oil | Margarine, low-fat mayonnaise, light salad dressing, vegetable oil (olive, corn, canola, or safflower) | Reduced fat from typical diet (>30% of total calories) to 27% of total calories |
| Sweets | 5/week | 1 tsp vegetable oil, 1 tbsp sugar, 1 tbsp jelly or jam, ½ oz jelly beans, 8 oz lemonade | Sugar, jelly, jam, honey, molasses, hard candy, fruit juices | Sweets should be those that are low in fat |

[a]  The DASH dietary plan shown here is based on 2000 cal a day. The number of daily servings may vary according to the individual's daily caloric requirements.
[b]  Serving size should be based on the product's nutrition label.
[c]  Fat content may change serving counts for fats and oils: For example, 1 tbsp of regular salad dressing equals 1 serving; 1 tbsp of a low-fat dressing equals one-half serving; 1 tbsp of fat-free dressing equals 0 serving.

**TABLE 59.4**
**Potassium Content of Selected Fruits and Vegetables**

| Fruits | | | Vegetables | | |
|---|---|---|---|---|---|
| Fruit | Serving Size | Potassium Content, mg | Vegetable | Serving Size | Potassium Content, mg |
| Orange | One small or 1/2 a cup of orange juice | 236 mg (6 mmol) | Carrots | 1/2 cup fresh | 177 mg (4.5 mmol) |
| Mango | One medium | 323 mg (8 mmol) | Green beans | 1/2 cup Fresh | 187 mg (4.8 mmol) |
| Raisins | 1/3 of a cup | 363 mg (9 mmol) | Mushroom | 1/2 cup cooked | 277 mg (7 mmol) |
| Banana | One small | 467 mg (12 mmol) | Tomato | One cup | 400 mg (10.2 mmol) |
| Prune | One cup of prune juice | 707 mg (18 mmol) | Potato | 1/2 medium with skin | 422 mg (10.8 mmol) |
| Papaya | One medium | 781 mg (20 mmol) | Avocado | 1/2 of a medium | 450 mg (11.5 mmol) |

*Source:*  U.S. Department of Agriculture, Agricultural Research Service, *USDA National Nutrient Database for Standard Reference*, Release 25. Nutrient Data Laboratory, Beltsville, MD, 2012, http://www.ars.usda.gov/ba/bhnrc/ndl

## TABLE 59.5
### Calorie Content of a Select List of Sweet Drinks and Snacks

| | Drinks | | | Snacks | |
|---|---|---|---|---|---|
| Drink | Serving Size | Calorie Content | Snack | Calorie Content/100 g | |
| Apple juice | 1 cup | 117 | Apple pie | 411 | |
| Soft drink | 12 fl oz can | 140–150 | Cookies | 458 | |
| Orange juice | 1 cup | 112 | Cupcakes | 369 | |
| Grape juice | 1 cup | 154 | Brownie | 379 | |

*Source:* U.S. Department of Agriculture, Agricultural Research Service, *USDA National Nutrient Database for Standard Reference*, Release 25. Nutrient Data Laboratory, Beltsville, MD, 2012, http://www.ars.usda.gov/ba/bhnrc/ndl

## TABLE 59.6
### Sodium Content of Common Food Items

| Sodium Content/100 g (3.2 oz) Portion (mg) | | Sodium Content/100 g (3.2 oz) Portion (mg) | |
|---|---|---|---|
| Doughnuts | 500 | Lasagna | 490 |
| Canned soups | 350–450 | Tuna in oil | 800 |
| Biscuits | 630 | Pork sausage | 958 |
| Potato chips | 1000 | Canned crabmeat | 1000 |
| Saltine crackers | 1100 | Cooked bacon | 1021 |
| Commercial cereals | 700–1100 | Pork canned ham | 1100 |
| Salted popcorn | 1940 | Corned beef | 1740 |

*Note:* These estimates vary with portion sizes and brands. More accurate values are given in the nutritional information on the package of most products, in the form of mg of sodium per serving.

resulting from the limitation of sweets and saturated fats will lead to an additional weight loss of about 1 lb/week on the DASH diet. The potential calorie deficit from the limitation of a select list of sweet drinks and snacks is shown in Table 59.5.

## DIETARY SODIUM AND BLOOD PRESSURE

The prevalence of HTN and its associated cardiovascular mortality across populations is strongly influenced by the amount of sodium in the diet. High levels of dietary sodium predispose to the higher levels of BPs at any given age and to a steeper rise in the BP with age.[36] The high prevalence of HTN in Western and industrialized populations has been attributed in part to the high levels of sodium in the diet. The amount of sodium in the standard American diet is currently estimated to be about 10 g (435 mmol) a day. Most of the excess sodium is consumed in precooked and prepackaged food items with added sodium chloride as a preservative during processing and preparation to prolong shelf life. Net dietary sodium reductions of 44 mmol/24 h and 33 mmol/24 h over 10–15 years were associated with a 25% reduction in the risk of cardiovascular events in two randomized controlled clinical trials with more than 3000 prehypertensive adults aged 30–54 years.[37] The sodium content of some of the common prepackaged food items is shown in Table 59.6.

Small reductions in sodium intake could have significant impact on the levels of BP and the prevalence of HTN. About 50% of the BP lowering effect of the DASH diet has been attributed directly to the 2300 mg dietary sodium limit in the high-sodium DASH diet. Dietary sodium reduction lowers BP among adults with normal as well as elevated BPs.[38] The lower the dietary sodium intake, the lower the BP, regardless of the baseline BP level. The 77 mmol (1.8 g) difference between high- and low-sodium DASH diet was associated with a respective additional reduction of 6.7 and 3.5 mmHg in the systolic and diastolic BPs.[39] In addition, the limitation of the average dietary sodium intake in the United States to no more than 2300 mg, or 100 mmol, a day has been projected to reduce the number of cases of HTN by about 11 million.[40]

## DIETARY BARRIERS TO BLOOD PRESSURE CONTROL

In addition to the determination of the BP level, dietary sodium intake modulates BP response to antihypertensive medications. The use of non-diuretic antihypertensive medications is usually associated with the activation of physiological mechanisms that engender sodium and water retention to compensate for the reduction in BP. Diuretics or "water pills" are usually prescribed to patients on more than one antihypertensive medication to disrupt this compensatory mechanism and maintain BP control. The efficacy of diuretics, however, is contingent upon the ability of the patient to reduce dietary sodium intake and maintain a net sodium loss in the urine on the treatment, and this can be assessed by the measurement of urinary sodium excretion. High dietary sodium intake impairs sodium loss on diuretic therapy and may account, in part, for the poor BP control in almost half of the people on BP medications.[41] Although the high intake of potassium associated with the adequate consumption of fruits and vegetables has been shown to mitigate some of the effects of high sodium intake on BP, two-thirds of adult Americans still consume less than two to three servings of fruits and vegetables a day. This suboptimal intake of fruits and vegetables is also apt to predispose patients on diuretic treatment to low serum potassium and precipitate numbness and muscle cramps that could interfere with medication adherence and BP control. High-sodium, low-potassium dietary patterns also tend to be plentiful in sweets and saturated fats. This Standard American Dietary (SAD) pattern constitutes a major dietary barrier to BP control. The complementary role of nutrition to BP control cannot be overemphasized. The comparative effectiveness of nutrition and medications for BP control needs to be given more emphasis in the health profession educational curriculum. The ability of patients to increase the intake of potassium needs to be enhanced by ensuring that fresh fruits and vegetables are readily accessible and affordable to the patients. Policies and procedures that limit and monitor the amount of sodium allowed in precooked and prepackaged food items will protect the consumers and afford the food industry an opportunity to revise their strategies and align making profit with protecting the health of the nation at the same time.

## NUTRITION IN CHRONIC KIDNEY DISEASE AND END-STAGE RENAL DISEASE

Patients with CKD, and particularly those with stage 5 CKD, have protein wasting with sarcopenia resulting in fatigue and weakness. Moreover, due to aggravation of metabolic and hormonal parameters, protein wasting in these individuals is associated with increased morbidity and mortality.[42–45] It has not been established whether protein depletion itself or secondary comorbidities including cardiovascular risk factors such as elevated triglycerides and inflammatory cytokines that often accompany renal failure may be the cause of protein depletion.[46–48] Protein restriction is established as a standard component of the nutritional management of patients with advanced renal disease, since high-protein diets lead to the accumulation of potentially toxic metabolites of protein metabolism as well as potassium, fat, and pro-inflammatory fatty acids. Thus, the balancing of protein intake is a complex undertaking, particularly as anorexia and other comorbid conditions often influence what patients can or will eat.

Numerous clinical studies of the effects of low protein intake on progression of the CKD were carried out in the 1970s and 1980s. Subsequently, the National Institutes of Health supported the largest and the most comprehensive multicenter trial of protein in renal disease ever conducted—the modification of diet in renal disease (MDRD) study. This randomized prospective controlled trial was undertaken to test the effects of low-protein diet (LPD) and low-phosphorus diet and strict BP control on the progression of renal disease.[49] The MDRD study investigated the effects of three levels of dietary protein and phosphorus intakes and two BP goals on the progression of CKD. Eight hundred forty (840) adults with various renal diseases except for insulin-dependent diabetes mellitus were studied. Study A included 585 patients who had a GFR, measured by 125 I-iothalamate clearances, of 25–55 mL/min/1.73 m². These persons were randomly assigned to 1.3 g protein/kg standard body weight (BW)/day and 16–20 mg phosphorus/kg/day or to 0.58 g protein/kg/day and 5–10 mg phosphorus/kg/day. They were also assigned to a mean arterial BP goal of either 107 mmHg (113 mmHg for those with 61 years of age or older) or 92 mmHg (98 mmHg for those with 61 years of age or older).

In MDRD study B, 255 patients with a baseline GFR of 13–24 mL/min/1.73 m² were randomly assigned to a 0.28 g protein/kg/day and 4–9 mg phosphorus/kg/day diet supplemented with 0.28 g/kg/day of ketoacids and amino acids or to 0.58 g protein/kg/day with 5–10 mg phosphorus/kg/day. They were also randomly assigned to either the above modest or the strict BP control groups. Progression of renal failure was measured periodically for an average of 2.2 years. There were no differences between the groups in the decline in GFR

in study A. In study B, there was a borderline significantly greater rate of decline in GFR with the 0.58 gm protein/kg/day diet than with the very-low-protein ketoacid/amino acid diet (p = 0.07). In the 12-year follow-up analysis of study A, during the first 6 years after the initiation of dietary protein prescription, there was a significantly lower adjusted hazard ratio of reaching ESRD or combination of either ESRD or mortality in those assigned to the 0.58 g protein/kg/day diet compared with those assigned to the 1.3 g protein/kg/day diet.[50]

During the second 6-year period of follow-up, this difference tended to reverse itself. In the study B patients, there was a significantly greater adjusted hazard ratio for death after they developed ESRD in those given the ketoacid-supplemented diet. This increase in hazard ratio was seen during the 12 years after initiation of ketoacid-supplemented diet prescription. It is important to appreciate that after an average of 2.2 years of follow-up, the patients were discharged to be followed up with their various primary care physicians and therefore probably had little or no aggressive dietary therapy; ketoacids were almost certainly unavailable to them, and essentially no clinical follow-up data were available to accept for the times of onset of their dialysis therapy and mortality.

The following characteristics of the MDRD study may limit interpretation of the findings. (1) The follow-up period was only 2.2 years, and the p-value with ketoacid diet was <0.07 that is not statistically significant. (2) Benefits from the intervention may have been delayed and missed in the MDRD, since in the Diabetes Complications and Control Trial (DCCT), which evaluated the results of tight vs. conventional glucose control in patients with insulin-dependent diabetes mellitus,[51] a reduced occurrence of microalbuminuria, albuminuria, and diabetic retinopathy and neuropathy benefits generally only became apparent 2.5–3.0 years after the onset of the clinical trial. (3) Twenty-five percentage of enrolled patients had polycystic kidney disease, which is a disease known to have a slow progression and may be particularly refractory to LPD therapy. (4) There was no comparison between the ketoacid-supplemented diet and a more normal protein intake. (5) The tryptophan content of the VLPD was augmented in the MDRD study to reduce the possibility of deficiency.[49] Recent evidence indicates that some metabolites of tryptophan may be nephrotoxic.[52]

A secondary analysis by Levey et al.[53,54] indicated that the patients with baseline GFRs between 13 and 24 mL/min/1.73 m² responded to a 0.2 g/kg/day protein intake with a 1.15 mL/min/year slower mean decline in GFR, which was equivalent to 29% of the mean GFR decline. The GFR tended to decrease more slowly as the actual (not prescribed) protein intake fell progressively to about 0.75 g/kg/day.[53,54] In long-term follow-up of the MDRD study, assignment to a very LPD did not delay progression to kidney failure, but appeared to increase the risk of death.[7]

Probably the major safety issue concerning LPD is the risk of protein-energy wasting. This concern is especially important when individuals are prescribed as little as 0.6 g protein/kg/day. This concern is based on two related issues. The fact that the LPD of 0.6 g/kg/day is close to the dietary requirement for clinically stable individuals who are normal or have CKD indicates that some people may be at increased risk for protein malnutrition. In contrast, rather extensive research indicates that such diets provide adequate daily protein for almost all clinically stable CKD patients.[55]

The other issue is that with such restriction in protein intake, it often becomes more difficult to meet the average daily energy needs of the patient. This is particularly true because in order to provide adequate quantities of essential amino acids with these protein-restricted diets, a large proportion of the protein must be of high biological value, that is animal protein. In contrast, it is often the foods higher in lower-quality protein that provide the most calories (e.g., bread, rolls, pasta, biscuits, cakes). This is the case because high-calorie butter, jam, cream cheese, sauces, etc., can be readily added to these latter foods. A solution to this dilemma is to frequently monitor the protein-energy status of the patient. If evidence for protein malnutrition emerges, the protein intake may be increased up to 0.80 g protein/kg/day. Evidence for energy malnutrition may be treated with dietary counseling, by increasing the protein intake, as this will increase the availability of low-quality proteins that can be ingested with a consequent increase in energy intake or with the oral or parenteral high-energy supplements.

In a recent review of literature, Eyre and Attman analyzed 14 studies with a total of 666 subjects with CKD (GFR ≤ 20 mL/min) who were prescribed a dietary protein intake from 0.3 g/kg/day (supplemented with ketoacids/amino acids) to 0.5 g/kg/day for more than 12 months.[56] All but two studies concluded that the LPD were not associated with deterioration in body composition. Other recent studies have reported similar findings.[57]

There is no clear evidence base on which to recommend a dietary protein intake for patients with stage 1 or 2 CKD. Published trials to a large extent have examined the effect of protein intake on the progression of renal failure in individuals with stages 3–5 CKD. Since the published data so far have not been definitive, consent should be obtained from the patient after a discussion of the evidence and the side effects of LPD. This can then be followed with a diet providing 0.60–0.75 g protein/kg/day can be prescribed. To ensure an adequate intake of essential amino acids, this diet should provide at least 50% of the protein as high biological value. This amount of protein intake normally will maintain neutral or positive nitrogen balance.[58]

For stages 4 and 5 CKD, the potential advantages of LPD and low-phosphorus diet at this degree of renal insufficiency are more compelling. The rationale for an LPD at this stage is that toxic products of nitrogen metabolism begin to accumulate in significant amounts at these levels of renal insufficiency. LPD generate less nitrogenous compounds (e.g., guanidines, acids, minerals), which have potentially toxic effects on the patient. Hence, LPD will reduce the risk of uremic symptoms.

Patients can suffer from anorexia and nausea which leads to very little protein intake. These patients are at increased risk of malnutrition. Encouragement and specific training to follow the prescribed diet may increase the likelihood that they do not ingest less than the recommended intake of proteins or other nutrients. To maintain neutral or positive nitrogen balance, patients should be prescribed 0.60 g protein/kg/day. For individuals who are unable to maintain adequate dietary energy intake with such a diet or who will not accept this diet, an intake of up to 0.75 or 0.80 g protein/kg/day may be recommended. This latter protein intake is easier for most people to adhere to and, as indicated earlier, frequently enables people to more readily ingest a higher dietary energy intake. The MDRD study describes a more rapid loss of GFR in people ingesting dietary protein intakes >0.75 g/kg/day.[50] As stated before, at least 50% of the protein should be of high biological value.

Nephrotic syndrome is a nonspecific disorder in which the kidneys are damaged, causing them to leak large amounts of protein. The prescribed protein intake in nephrotic patients is not increased unless their proteinuria exceeds 5.0 g/day. Above 5.0 g proteinuria/day, the prescribed diet, is increased by 1 g/day of high biological value protein for each additional g/day of proteinuria. Proteinuria is monitored periodically; if urinary protein excretion changes, the dietary protein intake can be modified accordingly. This approach is based upon the adverse consequences observed in CKD patients who are protein wasted.[59]

Clinical practice guidelines for nutrition in CKD from the National Kidney Foundation recommend a protein intake of 1.2–1.3 g protein/kg/day for clinically stable chronic peritoneal dialysis (CPD) patients.[60] Dietary protein requirements in patients undergoing automated peritoneal dialysis appear to be similar.[61] Patients undergoing hemodialysis lose protein in the dialysate. Nitrogen balance studies suggest that to maintain normal total body protein and protein balance, some maintenance hemodialysis patients require more than 1.0 g of protein/kg/day.

Clinical practice guidelines[60] on nutrition in CKD patients recommend 1.2 g of protein/kg BW/day for clinically stable patients; half of the dietary protein should be of high biological value.

During maintenance hemodialysis, monitoring nitrogen balance requires a consideration of total nitrogen appearance (TNA), which is defined as the sum of dialysate, urine, fecal nitrogen losses, and (in dialysis patients) post-dialysis increment in body urea-nitrogen content.[61] As nitrogen is rather expensive to measure, and there are few commercial laboratories that measure nitrogen, urea is usually measured instead. Urea is the major nitrogenous product of protein and amino acid degradation, and, unlike nitrogen, it can be both precisely and inexpensively measured. TNA usually can be estimated accurately by measuring urea-nitrogen appearance (UNA). UNA is the amount of urea nitrogen that appears or accumulates in body fluids and all outputs (most commonly, urine and dialysate).

Clinically stable people who are at zero nitrogen balance should theoretically have a total nitrogen output that is equal to nitrogen intake minus about 0.5 g nitrogen/day from such unmeasured losses as sweat, blood drawing, growth of nails, and replacement of exfoliated skin. Nitrogen output therefore should closely correlate with nitrogen intake in these individuals and can be used to estimate dietary nitrogen output, and therefore, dietary protein needs to maintain balance. In stable CKD patients, both TNA and UNA are in balance with dietary nitrogen and protein intake.[36]

For the purpose of estimation, dietary proteins are assumed to have 6.25 g of N per gram of protein. UNA is calculated as follows:

UNA (g/day) = UUN + DUN + change in body UN all in units of g/day, where body UN is the body urea nitrogen and DUN is the dialysate urea nitrogen. The change in body urea nitrogen (g/day) is different than blood urea nitrogen (BUN) and is calculated by subtracting the final BUN after dialysis from the initial BUN. Since BUN goes down during dialysis, this is expressed as BUN (final) minus BUN (initial) as a positive number. This difference is then multiplied by the body water volume estimated as 0.6 times BW. You have now accounted for the change in BUN during dialysis from the point of view of BUN, but you also must correct for the change in body water that occurs as the result of dialysis. This is calculated by multiplying 0.6 times the difference between the final BW and the initial BW and then multiplying this result by the final BUN in g/L. The final BW will be greater than the initial BW or body water, and by multiplying by the final BUN, you have accounted for this change during dialysis.

Mathematically, the formulas can be summarized as follows:

$$UNA = UUN + DUN + \Delta \text{ body UN}$$

$$\Delta \text{ body UN} = ([BUN(final) - BUN(initial)] \times 0.6 \text{ BW})$$
$$+ ([BW(final) - BW(initial)] \times BUN(final)])$$

The calculation is made to reflect the time between dialysis intervals and then normalized to 24 h. The estimate that BW times 0.6 estimates body water is valid for average body composition. In edematous or lean patients, the estimated proportion of BW that is water is increased, and in the obese or the very young, it is decreased.

Although there are not yet any systematically collected data on which to recommend protein requirements in maintenance hemodialysis patients receiving more frequent dialysis treatments, this dietary intake is estimated to provide adequate protein nutrition.

Alterations in dietary protein intake have an important role in prevention and management of CKD. Using soy protein instead of animal protein reduces development of kidney disease in animals.[62] Reducing protein intake preserves kidney function in persons with early diabetic kidney disease. These observations lead to the potential for substitution of soy protein for animal protein to result in less hyperfiltration and glomerular HTN with resulting protection from diabetic nephropathy. Specific components of soy protein may lead to the benefits including specific peptides, amino acids, and isoflavones. Substituting soy protein for animal protein usually

decreases hyperfiltration in diabetic subjects and may reduce urine albumin excretion. Limited data are available on effects of soy peptides, isoflavones, and other soy components on renal function in diabetes. Further studies are required to discern the specific benefits of soy protein and its components on renal function in diabetic subjects.[62]

Studies clearly indicate that people prescribed with special diets are much more likely to adhere if they are periodically monitored, educated, and encouraged to follow their dietary prescription.[63] In order to maximize compliance, physicians and dietitians should schedule frequent, often monthly, visits with patients who have CKD stage 5 and often stage 4. Less-frequent visits may be convened with patients who have stable and less-severe renal insufficiency, as long as evidence indicates that they are adequately compliant.

## REFERENCES

1. Centers for Disease Control Summary Health Statistics for U.S. Adults: National Health Interview Survey, 2010. Series 10, Number 252, January 2012.
2. Vallon, V, Thomson, SC *Annu Rev Physiol* 74:351;2012.
3. Hall, JE, Brands, MW, Hildebrandt, DA, Mizelle, HL. *Hypertension* 19:I45;1992.
4. Nishiura, JL, Neves, RF, Eloi, SR et al. *Clin J Am Soc Nephrol* 4:838;2009.
5. Heikkilä, J, Holmberg, C, Kyllönen, L et al. *J Urol* 186:2392;2011.
6. Aparicio, M, Bellizzi, V, Chauveau, P et al. *J Ren Nutr* 22:S1;2012.
7. Menon, V, Kopple, JD, Wang, X et al. *Am J Kidney Dis* 53:208;2009.
8. Coresh, J, Selvin, E, Stevens, LA et al. *JAMA* 298:2038;2007.
9. Collins, AJ, Foley, RN, Chavers, B et al. *Am J Kidney Dis* 59(Suppl 1):evii;2012.
10. Matsushita, K, van der Velde, M, Astor, BC et al. *Lancet* 375:2073;2010.
11. Rashidi, A, Sehgal, AR, Rahman, M. *Am J Cardiol* 102:1668;2008.
12. Rao, MV, Qiu, Y, Wang, C et al. *Am J Kidney Dis* 51(Suppl 2):S30;2008.
13. Botdorf, J, Chaudhary, K, Whaley-Connell, A. *Cardiorenal Med* 1:183;2011.
14. Segura, J, Ruilope, L. *Adv Chronic Kidney Dis* 18:23;2011.
15. Chobanian, AV, Bakris, GL, Black, HR et al. *JAMA* 289:2560;2003.
16. National Kidney Foundation. *Am J Kidney Dis* 39(Suppl 1):S1;2002.
17. American Diabetes Association. *Diabetes Care* 35(Suppl 1):S1;2012.
18. Bakris, GL, Williams, M, Dworkin, L. et al *Am J Kidney Dis* 36:646;2000.
19. Keane, WF, Eknoyan, G. *Am J Kidney Dis* 33:1004;1999.
20. Yoshioka, T, Rennke, HG, Salant, DJ et al. *Circ Res* 61:531;1987.
21. Sarnak, M, Levey, A, Schoolwerth, A et al. *Circulation* 108:2154;2003.
22. Upadhyay, A, Earley, A, Haynes, SM, Uhlig, K. *Ann Intern Med* 154:541;2011.
23. Cushman, C, Evan, GW, Byington, RP et al. *N Engl J Med* 363:1575;2010.

24. Brenner, BM, Cooper, ME, De Zeeuw, D et al. *N Engl J Med* 345:861–869.
25. Egan, BM, Zhao, Y, Axon, RN. *JAMA* 303:2043;2010.
26. Chobanian, AV, Bakris, GL, Black, HR et al. *The Seventh Report of the Joint National Committee on Prevention, Detection, Evaluation, and Treatment of High Blood Pressure (JNC 7). Hypertension* 42:1206;2003.
27. Blackburn, H, Prineas, R. *Prog Biochem Pharmacol* 19:31;1983.
28. Ascherio, A, Hennekens, C, Willett, WC et al. *Hypertension* 27:1065;1996.
29. Ascherio, A, Rimm, EB, Giovannucci, EL et al. *Circulation* 86:1475;1992.
30. Bazzano, LA, He, J, Ogden, LG et al. *Am J Clin Nutr* 76:93;2002.
31. Appel, LJ, Moore, TJ, Obarzanek, E et al. *New Engl J Med* 336:1117;1997.
32. National High Blood Pressure Education Program Working Group. *Arch Intern Med* 153:186;1993.
33. Whelton, PK, He, J, Cutler, JA et al. *JAMA* 277:1624;1997.
34. Swinburn, B. *European Congress on Obesity*, May 6–9, 2009, Amsterdam, the Netherlands. Abstract T1:RS3.3.
35. INTERSALT Cooperative Group. *BMJ* 297:319;1988.
36. Cook, NR, Cutler, JA, Obarzanek, E et al. *BMJ* 334:885;2007.
37. Chobanian, AV, Hill, M. *Hypertension* 35:858;2000.
38. Sacks, FM, Svetkey, LP, Vollmer, WM et al. *N Engl J Med* 344:3;2001.
39. Palar, K, Sturm, R. *Am J Health Promot* 24:49;2009.
40. Centers for Disease Control and Prevention (CDC). *MMWR Morb Mortal Wkly Rep* 60:103;2011.
41. Centers for Disease Control and Prevention (CDC). *MMWR Morb Mortal Wkly Rep* 56:213;2007.
42. Weiner, DE, Tighiouart, H, Elsayed, EF et al. *Am J Kidney Dis* 51:212;2008.
43. Muntner, P, He, J, Astor, BC et al. *J Am Soc Nephrol* 16:529;2005.
44. Menon, V, Greene, T, Wang, X et al. *Kidney Int* 68:766;2005.
45. Kalantar-Zadeh, K, Kilpatrick, RD, Kuwae, N et al. *Nephrol Dial Transplant* 20:1880;2005.
46. Kopple, JD, Zhu, X, Lew, NL et al. *Kidney Int* 56:1136;1999.
47. Kopple, JD. *Am J Clin Nutr* 65:1544;1997.
48. Kalantar-Zadeh, K, Kopple, JD. *Am J Kidney Dis* 38:1343;2001.
49. Klahr, S, Levey, AS, Beck, GJ et al. *N Engl J Med* 330:877;1994.
50. Levey, AS, Greene, T, Sarnak, MJ et al. *Am J Kidney Dis* 48:879;2006.
51. The Diabetes Control and Complications Trial Research Group. *N Engl J Med* 329:977;1993.
52. Enomoto, A, Takeda, M, Tojo, A et al. *J Am Soc Nephrol* 13:1711;2002.
53. Levey, AS, Adler, S, Caggiula, AW et al. *Am J Kidney Dis* 27:652;1996.
54. Levey, AS, Greene, T, Beck, GJ et al. *J Am Soc Nephrol* 10:2426;1999.
55. Eyre, S, Attman, PO. *J Ren Nutr* 18:167;2008.
56. Fouque, D, Wang, P, Laville, M et al. *Cochrane Database Syst Rev* CD001892;2000.
57. Chauveau, P, Vendrely, B, El Haggan, W et al. *J Ren Nutr* 13:282;2003.
58. Kopple, JD. *J Nutr* 129:247S;1999.
59. Rambod, M, Bross, R, Zitterkoph, J et al. *Am J Kidney Dis* 53:298;2009.
60. NKFK/DOQI. *Am J Kidney Dis* 35(Suppl. 2):S1;2000.
61. Westra, WM, Kopple, JD, Krediet, RT. *Perit Dial Int* 27:192;2007.
62. Anderson, JW. *Asia Pac J Clin Nutr* 17(Suppl 1):324;2008.
63. Appel, LJ, Champagne, CM, Harsha, DW et al. *JAMA* 289:2083;2003.
64. U.S. Department of Agriculture, Agricultural Research Service, *USDA National Nutrient Database for Standard Reference*, Release 25. Nutrient Data Laboratory, Beltsville, MD, 2013. http://www.ars.usda.gov/ba/bhnrc/ndl

# 60 Diet–Gene Interactions

*Carolyn D. Berdanier*

## CONTENTS

It has long been understood that humans as well as other creatures can vary in their health status. In part, this variation is attributable to variation in the environment and in part is due to variation in the genetic heritage of the individual. A well-nourished individual is far more likely to be healthy than is a poorly nourished individual, yet people do develop unhealthy conditions due in part to their genetic heritage. There is a large list of disorders that are attributable to mutations in specific genes in the metabolic pathways.[1–4] For the most part, these disorders are infrequent. Some of them are manageable with appropriate dietary maneuvers. Table 60.1 lists a number of these disorders and associated mutation(s). This is a partial list, and not all of the genetic diseases are listed. For some of the disorders, there is more than one mutation associated with the disease. For example, there are a number of genetic mutations in the code for red cell glucose-6-phosphate dehydrogenase. The code is carried as a recessive trait on the X chromosome, and thus only males are affected. These mutations are usually silent. That is, the male, having a defective red cell glucose-6-phosphate dehydrogenase, does not know he has the problem unless his cells are tested or unless he is given a drug such as quinine or one of the sulfur antibiotics that increases the oxidation of NADPH+H+. When this happens, NADPH+H+ is depleted and is not available to reduce oxidized glutathione. In turn, the red cell ruptures (hemolytic anemia). In almost all cases, the affected male has sufficient enzyme activity to meet the normal demands for NADPH+H+. It is only when stressed by these drugs that a problem develops.

There are other genomic defects that are silent as well. For example, people unable to metabolize the pentoses found in plums and cherries are unaware of their condition. It may come to light if a non-glucose-specific screening test is used just after the individual has consumed these fruits. There may appear to be an elevated level of sugar in the blood and urine. If a specific assay for glucose (glucokinase) is used rather than a nonspecific test, the mistake in diabetes diagnosis will not be made. The pentose is not metabolized and is excreted in the urine. This defect is thus innocuous and poses no harm to the affected individual.

Some individuals may be intolerant of exercise, because they are unable to use the glycogen in their muscles for fuel. Unless forced to exercise, these people might not be aware of their metabolic defect. They may have adopted a very sedentary lifestyle by unconscious realization of their intolerance. Again, the defect although potentially harmful is avoided because of an unconscious selection of lifestyle by the affected individual.

Unconscious food selection has been observed in children with some of the macronutrient intolerances. Children who are lactose intolerant may refuse to consume milk; those who are gluten intolerant may avoid wheat-containing products and so forth. There may be an instinctive avoidance that helps the individual enjoy their food without serious consequences.

Many of the disorders listed in Table 60.1 have no cure, and many are characterized by a shortened life span. However, for some as indicated earlier, there are nutrition and lifestyle strategies that may be helpful. Diseases associated with the malabsorption of carbohydrate that is lactose intolerance, galactose intolerance, etc., can be managed by the omission of these carbohydrates from the diet. Some of the amino acid disorders can be managed by the reduction of the dietary intakes of the particular amino acid in question. For example, phenylketonuria can be managed by a reduction in the phenylalanine content of the diet. This is rather tricky, since enough of this essential amino acid must be provided but not too much, so that there is a surplus that cannot be appropriately metabolized. In addition, since phenylalanine is used to make tyrosine, this amino acid must then be provided in the diet in sufficient amounts to meet the need. Considerable skill is needed to design a diet that will meet the amino acid needs of the individual but not exceed that need.

**TABLE 60.1**

**Genetic Disorders in Nutrient Metabolism[1,4]**

| Disease | Mutated Gene | Characteristics |
|---|---|---|
| *Amino Acid Diseases* | | |
| Maple syrup urine disease | Branched-chain keto acid dehydrogenase | Elevated levels of a-keto acids and their metabolites in blood and urine, mental retardation, keto acidosis, and early death |
| Homocysteinemia | Cystathionine synthase | Absence of cross-linked collagen, eye malformations, osteoporosis, mental retardation, thromboembolism, and vascular occlusions |
| Phenylketonuria | Phenylalanine hydroxylase | Mental retardation, decreased neurotransmitter production, shortened life span, and six mutations in this gene have been reported |
| Tyrosinemia | Tyrosine transaminase | Eye and skin lesions, mental retardation |
| | Fumarylacetoacetate | Normocytic anemia, leukocytosis, and increased serum bilirubin |
| | Hydroxylase | Increased hepatic enzymes and prolonged prothrombin time |
| Albinism | Tyrosinase | Lack of melanin production and sensitivity to sunlight |
| Alcaptonuria | Homogentisate oxidase | Elevated homogentisate levels in blood, bones, and internal organs; increased susceptibility to viruses and arthritis |
| Histidinemia | Histidase | Elevated blood and urine levels of histidine and decreased histamine |
| Hyperprolinemia | Proline oxidase 2 mutations | Mental retardation and seizures |
| Hyperornithinemia | Ornithine-δ-aminotransferase | Increased levels of ornithine in blood, progression vision loss, and increased urine loss of ornithine |
| Urea cycle defects | Arginase | Progressive lethargy, mental retardation, and urea cycle failure |
| | Carbamoyl phosphate synthase | Symptoms of ammonia toxicity and early death |
| | Ornithine transcarbamylase | |
| | Argininosuccinate synthase | |
| | Argininosuccinase | |
| Hyperlysinemia | α-Aminoadipic semialdehyde synthase | Elevated levels of lysine in blood and urine; condition is generally benign. |
| Hypermethioninemia | Methionine adenyltransferase | Benign |
| Nonketotic hyperglycemia | Glycine cleavage system (3 mutations) | Early death, hypoglycemia, mental retardation, and seizures |
| Gout | ? | Excess uric acid production, renal uric acid stones; uric acid crystals accumulate in joints. |
| Lesch–Nyhan | Hypoxanthine phosphoribosyltransferase | Hyperuricemia, choreoathetosis, spasticity, mental retardation, self-mutilation, and gouty arthritis |
| *Lipid Diseases Other than Those Relating to Lipemia* | | |
| Tay–Sachs | Hexosaminidase A | Early death, CNS degeneration, and ganglioside GM2 accumulation |
| Gaucher's | Glucocerebrosidase | Hepatomegaly, splenomegaly, erosion of long bones and pelvis, mental retardation, and glucocerebroside accumulation |
| Fabry's | α-Galactosidase A | Skin rash, renal failure, pain in legs, and ceramide trihexoside accumulation |
| Niemann–Pick | Sphingomyelinase | Enlarged liver and spleen, mental retardation, and sphingomyelin accumulation |
| Krabbe's | Galactocerebroside | Mental retardation, and absence of myelin |
| Gangliosidosis | Ganglioside: β galactosidase | Enlarged liver, mental retardation |
| Sandhoff–Jatzkewitz | Hexosaminidase A and B | Same as Tay-Sachs but develops quicker |
| Fucosidosis | aL-Fucosidase | Cerebral degeneration, spastic muscles, and thick skin |
| Refsum's | α-Hydroxylating enzyme | Neurological problems: deafness, blindness, and cerebellar ataxia |
| *Carbohydrate-Related Disorders* | | |
| Lactose intolerance | Lactase | Chronic or intermittent diarrhea, flatulence, nausea, vomiting, and growth failure in young children |
| Sucrose intolerance | Sucrase | Diarrhea, flatulence, nausea, and poor growth in infants |
| Galactose intolerance | Galactose carrier | Diarrhea, growth failure in infants, stools contain large amounts of glucose, galactose, and lactic acid |
| Galactosemia | Three genes: galactose-1-P-uridyl transferase | Increased cellular content of galactose-1-phosphate, eye cataracts, mental retardation, and cell galactitol; 3 mutations in this gene |
| | Galactokinase | Cataracts, cellular accumulation of galactose, and galactitol |
| | Galactoepimerase | No severe symptoms; 2 mutations in this gene |

TABLE 60.1 (continued)

## Genetic Disorders in Nutrient Metabolism[1,4]

| Disease | Mutated Gene | Characteristics |
|---|---|---|
| *Carbohydrate-Related Disorders* | | |
| Fructosemia | Fructokinase | Fructosuria, fructosemia |
| | Fructose-1-P-aldolase | Hypoglycemia, vomiting after a fructose load, fructosemia, and fructosuria |
| | | In children: poor growth, jaundice, hyperbilirubinemia, albuminuria, and amino aciduria |
| | Fructose 1,6-diphosphatase | Hypoglycemia, hepatomegaly, poor muscle tone, and increased blood lactate |
| Pentosuria | NADP-linked xylitol dehydrogenase | Elevated levels of pentose in urine |
| Hemolytic anemia | Red cell glucose-6-phosphate dehydrogenase | Low red cell NADPH and hemolysis of red cell especially with quinine treatment |
| | Pyruvate kinase | Nonspherocytic anemia and accumulation of glucose metabolites in red cells |
| | | Jaundice in the newborn |
| Type VII glycogen storage disease | Phosphofructokinase | Intolerance to exercise, elevated muscle glycogen levels, and accumulation of hexose monophosphates in muscle |
| Von Gierke's (type I glycogen storage) | Glucose-6-phosphatase | Hypoglycemia, hyperlipemia, brain damage in some pts, excess liver glycogen, shortened life span, and increased glycerol utilization |
| Amylopectinosis (type IV glycogenosis) | Branching enzyme, hepatic amylo-(1,4 → 1,6)transglucosidase | Tissue accumulation of long-chain glycogen that is poorly branched and intolerance to exercise |
| Pompe's (type II glycogenosis) | Lysosomal a-1,4-glucosidase (acid maltase) | Generalized glycogen excess in viscera and muscles, nervous system muscle weakness, hepatomegaly, and enlarged heart |
| | Amylo-1,6-glucosidase (debranching enzyme) | Generalized glycogen excess in viscera, nervous system, and muscles; hepatomegaly; and enlarged heart |
| Forbes (type III glycogenosis) | Muscle phosphorylase | Tissue accumulation of highly branched glycogen, hypoglycemia, acidosis muscle weakness, and enlarged heart |
| McArdle's (type V glycogenosis) | Liver phosphorylase | Intolerance to exercise |
| Hers (type VI glycogenosis) | Phosphorylase kinase | Hepatomegaly, increased liver glycogen content, elevated serum lipids, growth retardation |
| *Micronutrient-Related Disorders* | | |
| Porphyria | Uroporphyrinogen III cosynthase | Increased red cell porphyrin, excess excretion of δ-aminolevulinic acid (urine), and porphobilinogen (stool); photosensitivity |
| | Ferrochelatase | Excess protoporphyrin in stool; photosensitivity |
| | ALA dehydratase | Neurovisceral symptoms; excess δ-aminolevulinic acid in urine |
| | Porphobilinogen deaminase | Neurovisceral symptoms; excess δ-aminolevulinic acid and porphobilinogen in urine |
| | Coproporphyrinogen oxidase | Photosensitivity, neurovisceral symptoms, excess δ-aminolevulinic acid, porphobilinogen, and coproporphyrin in urine |
| | Protoporphyrinogen oxidase | Photosensitivity, neurovisceral symptoms, excess δ-aminolevulinic acid, porphobilinogen and coproporphyrin in urine, and coproporphyrin and protophyrin in feces |
| | Uroporphyrinogen decarboxylate (2 mutations) | Photosensitivity, uroporphyrin and 7-carboxylate porphyrin in urine, and isocoproporphyrin in feces |
| Wilson's | ? | Reduction in the rate of incorporation of copper into ceruloplasmin |
| | | Reduction in the biliary excretion of copper, increased urinary copper, excess hepatic copper, and liver disease |
| Menkes | Intestinal copper carrier | Symptoms of copper deficiency and deficient copper-dependent enzymes |
| Hemochromatosis | ? | Excess serum iron, excess liver iron, and excess serum ferritin |
| Molybdenum | ? | Mental retardation, deficient sulfite oxidase, and xanthine dehydrogenase activity |
| Cofactor deficiency | Neuronal loss and demyelination; early death | |
| Rickets | 25(OH)$_2$ D hydroxylase | Vitamin D–deficient rickets |
| | D receptor resistance (5 mutations) | Vitamin D–deficient rickets |

*Note:* The question mark in the table indicates that the frequency of the problems not fully known.

## MUTATIONS IN GENES THAT ARE IMPORTANT TO MICRONUTRIENT METABOLISM

Just as there are important interactions between genetic signatures and diet with respect to the macronutrients, there are also instances of interactions between the micronutrients and genes. Both vitamins and minerals have been identified that interact with specific genes, and when mutated, these genes affect metabolic function.

There are two genetic disorders that have assisted scientists in understanding the function and metabolism of copper. In one, Menkes syndrome, copper absorption is faulty. Intestinal cells absorb the copper but cannot release it into the circulation. Parenteral copper corrects most of the condition, which resembles copper deficiency, but care must be exercised in its administration. Too much can be toxic. In addition, parenterally administered copper does not reach the brain and cannot prevent the cerebral degeneration and premature death characteristic of patients with Menkes disease. Another genetic disorder in copper status is Wilson's disease. This condition is also associated with premature death and is due to an impaired incorporation of copper into ceruloplasmin and decreased biliary excretion of copper. This results in an accumulation of copper in the liver and brain. Early signs of Wilson's disease include liver dysfunction, neurological disease, and deposits of copper in the cornea manifested as a ring that looks like a halo around the pupil. This lesion is called the Kayser–Fleischer ring. Renal stones, renal aciduria, neurological deficits, and osteoporosis also characterize Wilson's disease. Periodic bleeding, which removes some of the excess copper, can be helpful in managing Wilson's disease, as can treatment with copper-chelating agents such as D-penicillamine and by increasing the intake of zinc, which interferes with copper absorption.

Iron is an essential mineral for hemoglobin formation. However, there are a number of genetic reasons why excess iron and subsequent problems are encountered. These are the porphyrias and hemochromatosis. In the latter, excess iron accumulates, and in the former, there are abnormalities in porphyrin metabolism. Some of these disorders are devastating, while others are less so. Vitamin D and the uptake of calcium and phosphate are linked. In the absence of active vitamin D, rickets develops. Some individuals are unable to activate the vitamin. That is, they do not have a normal activity of the renal enzyme, $25(OH)_2D$ hydroxylase. As a result, these individuals develop vitamin D rickets. The bones are not appropriately mineralized, because there is a deficiency of the active vitamin. This can be managed by providing the active form of the vitamin. In addition, there is also a resistance to the activity of active vitamin D. The genetic problem here is a deficiency in the receptor for the vitamin. Five different mutations have been reported that accounts for this problem. Patients with these genetic problems also develop rickets and are collectively referred to as having vitamin D–resistant rickets. Lastly, there are a couple of complex disorders that affect more pathways in addition to those of vitamin D. These include the Fanconi syndrome, X-linked

hypophosphatemia, and pseudohypoparathyroidism. In each of these, there is a disturbed mineralization of the skeletal system as well as disturbed regulation of calcium status, phosphorus status, and soft tissue mineralization.

Although many of these disorders are uncommon (and some are very rare), most of these are disorders that appear early in life. An individual with galactose intolerance, for example, shows that intolerance as soon as he/she is exposed to galactose. Phenotypic expression of a genotype where the mutation is a key component of a metabolic pathway is early and consistent with the importance of the gene.

In contrast, there is a large list of phenotypic disorders that are chronic in nature and for whom the genetic signature is being slowly elucidated. Many of these disorders have both a diet and a genetic component. They include all those diseases or genetic disorders referred to as lipemia, diabetes, heart disease, and others.

## GENETIC BASIS FOR LIPOPROTEINEMIA

Hyperlipemia is fairly common in western nations. However, there is no single cause. As with some of the less well-known genetic disorders, more than one mutation has been found that is associated with this characteristic.[5–7] Table 60.2 lists the proteins involved in lipid transport as well as mutations (and their estimated frequencies) that result in lipid transport abnormalities. Not all of the genetic diseases of lipid transport are associated with atherosclerosis nor are all associated with elevated serum lipid levels. The genes for the transport proteins, apo A-I, apo A-II, apo A-IV, apo (a), apo B, apo D, apo C-I, apo C-II, apo C-III, apo D, and apo E, have been identified. In addition to these transport proteins, we have: (1) proteins that are the important rate-limiting enzymes, (2) receptors that are involved in lipoprotein processing, (3) the peripheral lipoprotein lipase (LPL) and the hepatic LPL, (4) the lipoprotein receptors on the plasma membrane of the cells that receive and oxidize or store the transported lipids, and (5) the rate-limiting enzymes of lipid synthesis and use. Included in this last category are the fatty acid enzymes of lipid synthesis and use: the fatty acid synthase complex, acetyl CoA carboxylase, HMG CoA reductase, HMG CoA synthase, cholesterol ester transfer protein (CETP), fatty-acid-binding protein (FABP), lecithin–cholesterol acyltransferase (LCAT), cholesterol 7-hydroxylase, and the high-density-lipoprotein-binding protein (HDLBP). Many of these proteins have been isolated and studied in detail. Several of their cognate genes have been identified and mapped.

LPL is synthesized by these target cells but is anchored on the outside of the cells by a polysaccharide chain on the endothelial wall of the surrounding capillaries. Should this LPL be missing or genetically aberrant (type I lipemia or chylomicronemia), so that the chylomicrons cannot be hydrolyzed, these chylomicrons accumulate, and the individual would have a lipemia characterized by elevated levels of triacylglyceride and cholesterol-containing chylomicrons.

## TABLE 60.2
## Mutations of Genes Involved in Lipoprotein Metabolism[1,5–7]

| Gene | Chromosome Location | Characteristics of Mutation | Frequency of Mutation |
|---|---|---|---|
| Apo A-II | 1 | Transport protein in HDL | ? |
| Apo B 48 | 2 p 23–24 | Hypobetalipoproteinemia | 1:1,000,000 |
| HDLBP | 2 q 37 | | ? |
| Apo D | 3 | Transport protein similar to retinol-binding protein | ? |
| Apo (a) | 6 | Abnormal transport protein for LDL | ? |
| LPL | 8 p 22 | Defective chylomicron clearance | 1:1,000,000 |
| Apo A-I | 11 | Defective HDL production (Tangier disease) | 1:1,000,000 |
| Apo C-III | 11 | | ? |
| Apo A-IV | 11 | | ? |
| Hepatic LPL (HTGL) | 15 q 21 | Defective IDL clearance | ? |
| CETP | 16 q 22.1 | | ? |
| LCAT | 16 q 22.1 | Familial lecithin: cholesterol transferase deficiency: 2 types | Rare |
| LDL receptor | 19 | Familial hypercholesterolemia | 1:500 |
| Apo B 100 | 2 | Familial defective apo B 100 | 1:500–501:1000 |
| Apo E | 19 | Type III hyperlipoproteinemia | 1:5000 |
| Apo C-I | 19 | Transport protein for VLDL | ? |
| Apo C-II | 19 | Defective chylomicron clearance | 1:1,000,000 |

*Note:* The question mark in the table indicates that the frequency of the problems not fully known.

Also, characteristic of this condition is the presence of an enlarged liver and spleen, considerable abdominal discomfort, and the presence of subcutaneous xanthomas (clusters of hard saturated fatty acid and cholesterol-rich nodules). Like familial hypolipoproteinemia, this condition is rare. Of interest is the observation that, despite the very high blood lipid levels of these people, few die of coronary vessel disease. Their shortened life span is due to an inappropriate lipid deposition in all of the vital organs that, in turn, has a negative effect on organ function and life span.

Failure to appropriately edit the apo B gene in the intestinal cell will result in a disorder called *familial hypobetalipoproteinemia*. In this disorder, there will be a total or partial (depending on the genetic mutation) absence of lipoproteins in the blood. Hypobetalipoproteinemia can also develop, should there be base substitutions in the gene for the apo B protein. In addition to very low blood lipids, patients with this disorder also have fat malabsorption (steatorrhea). The feces contain an abnormally large amount of fat and have a characteristic peculiar odor. In this disorder, not only is the triacylglyceride absorption affected but also are the fat-soluble vitamins. Without the ability to absorb these energy-rich food components and the vital fat-soluble vitamins, the patient does not thrive and survive. Fortunately, this genetic mutation is not very common. It is inherited as an autosomal recessive trait.

Defects in exogenous fat transport are manifested in several ways. As described earlier, defective chylomicron formation due to mutations in either the apo B gene or its editing leads to and is characterized by fat malabsorption. This includes the malabsorption of fat-soluble vitamins as well. Twenty different mutations have been identified in the gene for the apo B protein. These mutations are inherited via an autosomal recessive mode and are characterized not only by fat malabsorption but also by acanthocytes, retinitis pigmentosa, and muscular neuropathies. To a large extent, these symptoms can be attributed to a relative deficiency of the fat-soluble vitamins due to malabsorption. While a defect in the apo B gene can account for defective fat absorption, there may be another mutation (in the microsomal triglyceride transfer protein) that also might result in fat malabsorption. This transfer protein is essential for apo B translocation and subsequent synthesis of chylomicrons. Defects in this transfer protein would impair apo B availability and chylomicron formation. In these defects, very low levels of chylomicrons are found in the blood. Persons with this disorder are rare (one in a million). In this circumstance, the severity of the disease is related to the size of the mutated gene product and whether it can associate with the lipids it must carry. The size of the truncated apo B can vary from apo B-9 (41 residues) to apo B-89 (4487 residues). Except in the case of the apo B-25, the result of a deletion of the entire exon 21, all the truncated forms reported to date are C–T transitions or base deletions. These deletions can involve misaligned pairing-deletion mechanisms. Frameshift mutation can be compensated by a reading frame restoration of the apo B gene.

Familial hyperchylomicronemia is characterized by elevations in chylomicrons having both triglycerides and cholesterol. Hyperchylomicronemia was found to be due to mutations in the genes that encode the enzyme LPL needed for the hydrolysis of chylomicrons. This enzyme is a glycoprotein having an apparent monomeric molecular weight of about 60,000 Da on SDS gel electrophoresis and 48,300 Da by sedimentation–equilibrium ultracentrifugation. The enzyme is linked to the endothelial cells of the capillary system. LPL is quite similar to hepatic triglyceride lipase, an enzyme found in the hepatic sinusoids. The main difference between the two lipases is that the interstitial lipase has a requirement for the lipid-carrying protein, apo C-II, for full activity, whereas hepatic LPL does not. Mutations in the gene for apo C-II can result in aberrant lipase activity because apo C-II serves as a cofactor in the LPL-catalyzed reaction. Hepatic triglyceride lipase has no such requirement. Aberrations in the hepatic triglyceride lipase result in an accumulation of very-low-density lipoproteins (VLDL), rather than accumulations of chylomicrons. Mutations in the genes for LPL and apo C-II are very rare, occurring at a frequency of one in a million. The gene for LPL has been mapped to chromosome 8, while that for apo C-II has been mapped to chromosome 19 and the hepatic LPL to chromosome 15. Other features of these disorders include an inflammation of the exocrine pancreas and eruptive xanthomas. Chylomicronemia does not appear to be atherogenic. The mutations in the LPL gene appear to be insertions or deletions or due to aberrant splicing, while those in the apo C-II gene seem to be due to splice site mutations or small deletions. Twenty-two mutations in the apo C-II gene have been reported. With respect to the aberrant splicing of the LPL gene in three unrelated humans, Holzl et al. reported a C → A mutation in position −3 of the acceptor splice site of intron 6, which caused aberrant splicing. The major transcript showed a deletion of exons 6 through 9 and amounted to about 3% of normal. Trace amounts of both a normally spliced LPL mRNA and a second aberrant transcript devoid of exon 7 were found. In one of these patients, Holzl et al. found a three-splice mutation on one allele, while on the other allele they found a missense mutation resulting in Gly 188 → Glu substitution. All three subjects were classed as hyperchylomicronemic due to LPL deficiency.

The absence of LPL activity in certain tissues or in certain individuals can be attributed to mutations in LPL promoter region. Studies of tissue-specific expression of LPL showed that cis-acting elements located within −1824 bp of the five flanking regions were required for the expression of LPL. These include nuclear factors recognizing both the CCAAT box and the octamer sequence immediately flanking the transcriptional start site. Those tissues that have no LPL activity lack this promoter region. Since humans and mice have identical CCAAT and octamer sequences, one could suppose that humans having an intact LPL gene of normal sequence but lacking LPL activity might have a deficient or mutated promoter region; proof that this might occur is presently lacking.

Mutations in the gene for hepatic LPL result in elevated blood levels of triglycerides and cholesterol, and these elevations are related to an increased risk for atherosclerosis. Hepatic LPL must be secreted by the hepatocyte into the sinusoids to function as a catalyst for the hydrolysis of core triglycerides (TG) and surface phospholipids of chylomicron remnants, high density lipoprotein (HDL), and intermediate density lipoprotein (IDL). Through its activity, it augments the uptake of HDL cholesterol by the liver (reverse cholesterol transport) and is involved in the reduction of HDL size from $HDL_2$ to $HDL_3$. Hepatic LPL aids in the clearance of chylomicron remnants by exposing the apo E epitopes for enzymatic action. Missense mutations in the hepatic LPL gene include substitutions of serine for phenylalanine at amino acid position 267, threonine for methionine at position 383, and asparagine for serine at position 291. These mutations result in poorly secreted enzyme, and thus the phenotypic expression of the mutation is low hepatic lipase activity. The frequency of the Asn 291 Ser mutation in a population having premature CVD has been reported as 5.2%.

Defects in chylomicron remnant clearance are much more common than any of the previously mentioned mutations. Defective clearance due to mutations in the apo E gene results in a lipemia known as type III hyperlipoproteinemia. It is associated with premature atherosclerosis, and patients with these defects have high serum triglyceride as well as high serum cholesterol levels. Xanthomas are found in nearly three-quarters of the population with these defects. The lipemia is responsive to energy restriction using diets that have 40% of energy from carbohydrate, 40% from fat, and 20% from protein. Weight loss is efficacious for most people with this defect. The apo E gene codes for the protein on the surface of the chylomicron remnant that is the ligand for receptor-mediated clearance of this particle. A number of mutations in the apo E gene have been reported, and the phenotypes of these mutations are grouped into three general groups labeled $E_2$, $E_3$, and $E_4$. Those of the $E_2$ groups fail to bind the particles to the cell surface receptor for the chylomicron remnant. Those of the $E_3$ and $E_4$ groups have generally low remnant clearance rates. The apo E allele and phenotype frequency vary. The $E_2$ frequency is about 8%, the $E_3$ about 77%, and the $E_4$ about 15% of the total population with an apo E mutation. The incidence of apo E gene mutations is about 1% of the population. Since apo E is involved in both endogenous and exogenous lipid transport and clearance, a faulty apo E gene is devastating. Mature human apo E is a 299 amino acid polypeptide. Apo E genes as well as other apolipoproteins contain 11 or 22 amino acid repeated sequences as one of their key features. These appear to encode largely amphipathic helices, which are needed for lipid binding. There is a high degree of conservation among species of nucleotide sequences in the gene fragment that encodes the amino acid repeats. The gene for apo E has been mapped to chromosome 19, as have the genes for apo C-I, apo C-II, and LDLR. There appears to be a tight linkage among these genes, which coordinates their expression. Among the common mutations are amino acid substitutions at positions 112 and 158, while less-frequent substitutions occur at other positions in the polypeptide chain. Several of these involve the exchange of neutral amino acids for acidic amino acids with the net result of alterations in polypeptide charge and subsequent inadequate binding to the appropriate cell surface receptors. In a rare form of the disorder, the mutation is such that no useful apo E is formed. Transgenic mice have been constructed with an apo E mutation that mimics apo E deficiency. These mice, like humans, develop hypercholesterolemia and increased susceptibility to atherosclerosis. When these mice were fed diets low (5%) or high (16%) in fat, a differential serum cholesterol pattern was observed: those fed the high-fat diet had significantly higher levels of cholesterol and VLDL and LDL than those fed a low-fat or stock diet. The transgenic mice even when fed the stock diet had significantly higher levels of cholesterol and VLDL and LDL than the normal control mice. There was a gender difference as well. Male transgenic mice were less diet responsive in terms of their cholesterol levels than female transgenic mice. As mentioned, there is some sequence homology between humans and mice in the apo E DNA, and one could infer that these responses to dietary fat intake in mice could be observed in humans as well. While the earlier transgenic approach used the gene knockout paradigm (an extreme in the variants of apo E mutants), it nonetheless suggests that variation in the apo E genes could determine the responsiveness of humans with apo E defects to dietary manipulation. Indeed, such nutrient–gene interactions have been reported. The dietary fat clearance in normal subjects appears to be regulated by the genetic variance in apo E sequence, and this, in turn, is related to fat intake. Not only is triacylglycerol clearance affected but also is cholesterol clearance. One study reported that the apo E genotype declares the response to cholesterol intake with respect to blood cholesterol levels and that this genotype influences cholesterol synthesis. Those subjects who respond poorly to an oral cholesterol challenge vis-à-vis blood cholesterol clearance had higher rates of cholesterol synthesis than those who could rapidly clear their blood of cholesterol after an oral challenge. One of the more interesting variants of the apo E is called the *Milano variant*. In this variant, blood lipid levels are elevated, but these elevations are not associated with an increased risk of atherosclerosis.

Cholesterol traffic is also controlled by the LDL receptor and the transport protein, apo B-100. Mutations in the gene for the LDL receptor or in the gene for apo B-100, the ligand for the LDL receptor, result in high serum levels of cholesterol. The former results in the disorder called familial hypercholesterolemia and occurs with a frequency of about 1 in 500. Familial hypercholesterolemia is associated with early death from atherosclerosis in man and related primates. Dietary fat saturation affects transcription of LDL receptor mRNA in that feeding a diet containing saturated fat results in decreased LDL receptor mRNA compared to feeding an unsaturated-fat diet. These results suggest that unsaturated

fatty acids may interact with proteins that in turn serve as either *cis*- or *trans*-acting elements for this gene in much the same way as polyunsaturated fatty acids affect fatty acid synthetase gene expression.

Familial defective apo B-100 hypercholesterolemia is due to a mutation in the coding sequence of the apo B gene at bp 3500 that changes the base sequence such that glutamine is substituted for arginine. This is in the LDL receptor-binding region of the apo B protein and results in a binding affinity of less than 4% of normal. Polymorphic variation in the genes for both the LDL receptor and the apo B-100 has been reported for mice, and this variation has provided the opportunity to identify the genetic and molecular constraints of lipoprotein gene expression. Both apo B and apo E serve as ligands for the LDL receptor. In contrast to apo E, apo B has little homology with the other apolipoproteins. Apo B in mice is quite variable, and this variation imparts or confers a diet-responsive characteristic in inbred mouse strains vis-a-vis polypeptide sequence and activity. That is, some mouse strains have reduced levels of plasma apo B when fed a high-fat diet compared to controls fed a stock diet, while other mouse strains are unresponsive to diet vis-à-vis their plasma apo B-100 levels. Such polymorphism also exists in humans. Apo B has been mapped to chromosome 2 and produces two gene products, apo B-100 and B-48. In the intestine, the apo B primary transcript is co- or post-transcriptionally modified. This modification converts codon 2153 from a glutamine (CAA) to an in-frame, premature termination codon (UAA), thereby causing translation to terminate after amino acid 2152. This mRNA editing thus explains the difference in size of these two proteins. If more of the apo B gene is deleted, hypocholesterolemia is observed. This is because apo B-48 is required for the transport of chylomicrons from the intestine. If lacking, chylomicron formation is impaired, and low serum cholesterol levels are observed. Both familial defective apo B-100 and familial hypercholesterolemia are characterized by high levels of LDL. Both are associated with CVD, but only the familial hypercholesterolemia is characterized by tendon xanthomas. Both are inherited as autosomal dominant disorders. Collectively, these mutations have a cumulative frequency of 1 in 250. However, because polymorphism in the apo B gene can and does occur, there is the possibility that the frequency is collectively much greater, perhaps as high as 1 in 5. If this is the case, then the population variation in plasma cholesterol levels could be explained based on these genetic differences alone, apart from those mutations that are associated with the rest of the genes that encode components of the lipid transport system.

Genetically determined abnormalities in LDL metabolism may also be due to mutation in the large glycoprotein, apo (a). Apo (a) is a highly variable, disulfide protein bonded to the apo B-100. It is thought to resemble plasminogen. In fact, the genes that encode Lp (a) and plasminogen are very close to each other on the long arm of chromosome 6. In general, LDLs containing apo (a) do not bind well to the LPL receptor, and people having significant amounts of apo

(a) have a two- to threefold increase in CVD risk. Many individuals have little or no apo (a), and it has been suggested that those who have it are abnormal with respect to LPL activity.

Several mutations in the genes that encode the endogenous lipid transport have been reported. The reverse cholesterol transport pathway is part of this endogenous lipid transport system. It involves the movement of cholesterol from peripheral tissues to the liver. The peripheral tissues cannot oxidize cholesterol and so must send it to the liver, whereupon it is prepared for excretion, via cholesterol 7 α hydroxylase, as bile acids. This pathway uses the HDL to shuttle the cholesterol in this direction. HDL consists primarily of apo A-1 and cholesterol, which is esterified by the enzyme lecithin: cholesterol acyl transferase (LCAT). Mutations in the LCAT gene have been reported and result in one of two diseases: familial LCAT deficiency and fisheye disease. Thirteen different mutations have been identified, and in one, a single T → A transversion in codon 252 in exon 6, converting met (ATG) to Lys (AAG), was observed. Three unrelated families were found to have this mutation; however, the severity of their disease varied. In these families, no other mutation in LCAT was observed. Of the remaining 12 LCAT mutations, 10 were point mutations, three were frameshifts, and one consisted of a three-base insertion, which maintained its reading frame. For fish-eye disease, three mutations have been reported. This disorder is less serious than familial LCAT deficiency and is characterized by dyslipoproteinemia and corneal opacity. LCAT activity is 15% of normal, and there is a reduced level of HDL in the plasma. In contrast, familial LCAT deficiency is characterized by a variety of symptoms including lipoprotein abnormalities, renal failure, premature atherosclerosis, reduced levels of plasma cholesterol esters, and high plasma levels of cholesterol and lecithin.

The LCAT enzyme requires apo A-I as a cofactor. If there is a mutation in the gene for apo A-I, defective HDL production results. This is a rare mutation, and its frequency is estimated as one in a million. Individuals with this defect have premature CVD, corneal clouding, and very low HDL levels. Plasma apo A-I has a variety of charge isoforms with similar antigenicity and amino acid composition. Humans, baboons, African green monkeys, and cynomolgus monkeys have been studied, and there are species differences in hepatic and intestinal apo A-I production. In all instances, the differences in apo A-I were reported between intestine and liver. In the liver, there was a twofold higher level of apo A-I mRNA than in the intestine, and the abundance of this mRNA was species-specific. The apo A-I gene is regulated at the level of transcription, and a portion of the species-specific difference-in apo A-I gene expression is due to a sequence divergence in the 5′ regulatory region including the exon/intron 1 of the apo A-I gene. The capacity to produce HDLs is both genetically controlled and tissue-specific and probably explains why some genotypes respond

normally to a high-fat diet by producing more HDL, while other genotypes become hypercholesterolemic under these same conditions. Attempts to create a transgenic mouse expressing a human apo A-I gene have not been fully successful but have provided additional information about the relationship of apo A-I to HDL size. The human apo A-I gene was inserted into the mouse and in these mice; both the mouse and the human genes were expressed. This dual expression suggests a species difference in the control of this expression. In other words, the control points differed, and this resulted in a broader spectrum of HDL particles.

Defective HDL metabolism due to a mutation in the apo A-I gene results in a rare autosomal dominant disorder described in a small group of villagers in Italy. Affected individuals have reduced levels of HDL cholesterol and apo A-I levels but have no increased risk of CVD. The disorder, named Apo A-I Milano, is due to a point mutation in the apo A-I gene changing codon 173, so that cysteine is used instead of arginine. Normal apo A-I has no cysteine so this change has effects (because of the sulfide group in the cysteine) on the apo A-I structure.

Defective lipoprotein processing has already been discussed with respect to LDP, LCAP, and apo C-II deficiencies. A deficient cholesterol ester transport protein (CETP) has been reported due to a mutation of the gene for this protein located on chromosome 16. A mutation in this gene has been used to explain the atherogenicity of high-fat diets in primates, but to date no evidence of such a mutation in humans has been put forward.

## NUTRIENT–GENE INTERACTIONS IN LIPID TRANSPORT

Nutrients can sometimes affect the expression of the previously described genetic factors.[5–21] This suggests that CVD could develop as a result of a nutrient–gene interaction. The diet influence involves not only the amount of fat consumed but also the type of fat and the amount and type of carbohydrate. For example, the editing of the apo B gene is enhanced by dietary carbohydrate. A number of genes have carbohydrate response elements, and it is possible that this gene has this element in its promoter region. A carbohydrate response element has also been identified in the apo E gene. Carbohydrate influences mRNA stability and RNA processing of this gene. Similarly, the gene that encodes the seven-enzyme complex of mammalian fatty acid synthetase has a fatty acid response unit in its promoter. The expression of this gene is downregulated by dietary polyunsaturated fatty acids. The lipid transport genes might also have a lipid response element.

Dietary lipids, even in the absence of direct effects on transcription and translation, do influence the phenotypic expression of specific genotypes either because of overconsumption or because they have effects on certain of the hormones, that is, insulin or the steroid hormones, or the catabolic hormones that regulate or influence lipid synthesis, oxidation, and storage.

The level of cholesterol in the blood depends on the diet consumed and how much cholesterol is being synthesized. The cholesterol content of the gut LDL of a person on a low-cholesterol diet might run as low as 7%–10% of the total lipid in the lipoprotein, while the hepatic LPL of this same individual might be as high as 58% of total lipid. People consuming a low-cholesterol-low-saturated-fat diet may reduce the contribution of the diet to the blood cholesterol while increasing the hepatic de novo cholesterol synthesis. Persons having an LPL receptor deficiency are characterized by high serum cholesterol levels and, in some cases, by high serum triacylglycerides. The reason these blood lipids are elevated is that the individuals cannot utilize the lipids carried by the LPL due to the error(s) in the receptor molecule. Further, because these circulating lipids do not enter into the adipose and hepatic cell in normal amounts, the synthesis of triacylglycerides and cholesterol is not appropriately downregulated. Hence, this individual has elevated serum lipids not only because the LPL lipid is not appropriately cleared from the blood but also because of high rates of endogenous lipid synthesis. Individuals with this disorder have lipid deposits in unusual places such as immediately under the skin, around the eyes, on the tendons, and in the vascular tree. It is this last feature that probably accounts for the shortened life span of these people with the cause of death being cardiovascular disease. As can be seen from the metabolic characteristics of this disorder, low-cholesterol diets are probably useless in reducing serum cholesterol levels since de novo synthesis of cholesterol from nonlipid precursors can and does occur. Treatment with lipid adsorbents (high-fiber diets and the drug cholestyramine) will help reduce the cholesterol (but not triacylglycerides) coming from the intestine, and there are drugs (statins and fibrates) that can safely lower de novo cholesterol synthesis as well as increase intracellular lipid oxidation. All of these therapies may help reduce the serum lipid levels, but even doing this only treats the symptoms, not the genetic disorder. For that, gene therapy is needed to correct the genetic disorder that is the basic underlying cause of the symptoms.

Heart disease in its various forms is associated with elevated levels of the VLDL. In addition to the earlier descriptions of lipemias, some of which are associated with heart disease, there are other genetically determined forms of heart disease (Table 60.3). Chapter 61 discusses cardiovascular disease in depth. The lipemia-associated disorders have been subdivided into three general categories. In one, patients are characterized by elevated serum cholesterol, phospholipid, and triacylglyceride levels; elevated VLDL levels (and sometimes LDL levels); fatty deposits on the tendons and in areas on the arms just under the skin; vascular atheromas; and ischemic heart disease. This type of lipemia is inherited as an autosomal dominant trait in one person in 5000. Another lipemia occurs in patients having a normal cholesterol level but an elevated triacylglyceride level and elevated VLDL levels. These characteristics are associated with ischemic heart disease and premature atherosclerosis. It is frequently seen in obese patients with type 2 diabetes. People with diabetes mellitus have five times the risk of

## TABLE 60.3
## Mutations That Phenotype as Heart Disease[5–21]

| Mutation | Characteristics |
|---|---|
| LPL 3 mutations | High plasma TG—heart disease |
| MTHR gene 26 different mutations | Elevated homocysteine levels in blood and urine |
| 4p16.1 (between D4S2957 and D4S827) | Cardiac malformations |
| 9q31 (Tangier disease) 5 mutations | Premature CAD |
| LDL receptor 36 different mutations | Hypercholesterolemia, premature CAD or CVD |
| Elastin synthesis 7q11.23 4 mutations | Supravalvular aortic stenosis and congenital heart and vascular disease |
| Leu 54 to Met in paraoxonase | CVD |
| Troponin T 6 mutations | Hypertrophic cardiomyopathy |
| α-Tropomyosin | Hypertrophic cardiomyopathy |
| Myosin | Hypertrophic cardiomyopathy |
| ApoB gene 4 mutations | Hypercholesterolemia, peripheral vascular disease, CAD |
| 11 BHSD 6 mutations | Hypertension |
| hBENaC | Hypertension |
| Bradykinin receptor (14q32) 8 mutations | Cardiovascular disease |
| Transcription factor NKX2–5 3 mutations | Congenital heart disease |

people without diabetes of developing premature atherosclerosis and its associated coronary events. Cardiovascular disease, followed by renal disease, is the leading causes of death for people with diabetes mellitus. Diabetes mellitus is also a group of disorders with both genetic and nutritional components (Table 60.4).[22–46] Diabetes mellitus is roughly divided into two types: type 1 patients are those who develop the disease due to pancreatic deficiency. They need insulin replacement therapy to manage their blood glucose levels. Type 1 patients comprise about 10% of all the people with diabetes. Type 2 patients are those whose disease can be managed through diet, exercise, and oral medication (see Chapter 58 for more information on nutrition and diabetes mellitus). Many of these people progress to hormone replacement therapy, but they start out not needing it. In both obesity and diabetes, metabolic problems associated with aberrant glucose transporters have been reported. Table 60.5 gives a list of these transporters and their function. Should there be a problem in these transporters, glucose entry into the cell is reduced, and this of course means that there is a decrease in glucose uptake, a typical sign of diabetes.

There is a third group of people with diabetes who develop their disease as a result of a mutation in the mitochondrial genome. We do not know how many people have this form of the disease. The estimates vary from 0.1% to 9% of the population with diabetes. These people have other metabolic problems that are also related to their mitochondrial dysfunction.

Both heart disease risk and diabetes risk increase with an increase in body fat. Obesity per se is a health risk for

**TABLE 60.4**

**Mutations That Associate with Type 1 and Type 2 Diabetes Mellitus[22–46]**

| Gene | Comments |
|---|---|
| *Nuclear DNA* | |
| Hepatic nuclear transcription factor 4α (MODY 1) | Impaired insulin secretion |
| Glucokinase (MODY 2) | Impaired insulin secretion; 44 different mutations in this gene have been reported. |
| Hepatic transcription factor 1α (MODY 3) | Subjects are generally nonobese. |
| Glycogen synthase | Hypertension and type 2 are found in this genotype, which is polymorphic. Activation of the enzyme is impaired. |
| Glucagon receptor | Susceptibility to type 2 is variable among different population groups. |
| Insulin receptor | Associated with peripheral insulin resistance in some type 2 subjects |
| Insulin receptor substrate (IRS-1) | Results in a signal transmission defect associated with insulin resistance |
| Mitochondrial α glycerol 3 phosphate dehydrogenase | Associated with type 2 and with impaired mitochondrial function |
| Mobile glucose transporters (GLUT 1-5) | Associated with both obesity and type 2 |
| *Mitochondrial DNA (heteroplasmic[a])* | |
| tRNA[leu] | 7 mutations have been found that associate with diabetes. |
| ND 1 | 11 mutations have been reported. |
| ND 2, ND 3, ND 4 | 1 mutation in each of these genes has been reported. |
| tRNA[Cys,Ser,Lys] | 1 mutation in each of these genes has been reported. |
| tRNA[thr] | 4 mutations have been found. |
| D-Loop[b] | 3 mutations have been reported. |
| COX II | 2 mutations have been reported. |
| ATPase 6,8 | 4 mutations have been reported. |

[a] Mutations in the mitochondrial genome that associate with diabetes are heteroplasmic, that is, there is mixture of normal and abnormal DNA in each cell. The percentage of the abnormal determines the degree to which the function of that cell is impaired.

[b] Promoter regions for the 13 structural genes found in the mitochondrial genome are found here.

**TABLE 60.5**

**Aberrant Mobile Glucose Transports and Their Consequences[1]**

| Protein | Consequences of an Error |
|---|---|
| GLUT 1 | Minimal changes in glucose uptake by all tissues that use glucose |
| GLUT 2 | Liver—glucose metabolic pathways suppressed; increased gluconeogenic activity |
| | β cell—pancreas unresponsive to glucose stimulation |
| | Kidney—increased gluconeogenic activity |
| GLUT 3 | Minimal changes in glucose uptake and metabolism |
| GLUT 4 | Adipose tissue—decrease glucose use by fat cell; compensatory increase in hepatic glucose use; increase hepatic lipogenesis and lipid output; increase hepatic glycogen store |
| | Heart, muscle—decrease glucose use by muscle could be lethal if compensatory use of fatty acids and ketones is insufficient. |

a number of other conditions as well. Chapters 46, 48, and 63 address some of the issues with obesity. Table 60.6 provides a list of mutations that associate with obesity.[22–24,47–55] Most of these associate with extreme obesity or obesity that develops in early childhood. Whether mild obesity or somewhat overweight is a genetic trait is questionable.

For some people who habitually overeat and underexercise, this excess food is converted to body fat stores. It has been postulated that loss of food intake control could be a genetic trait as well. See Chapters 8, 49, and 50 for more information on food intake control. Certainly, mutations in the leptin gene, the leptin receptor gene, and the genes for several other neuronal signals that are involved in food intake regulation suggest that genetics plays a role in excess food consumption. Should this behavior be suppressed, excess body fat is reduced.

**GENETIC SCREENING**

In addition to the problems associated with obesity, diabetes, heart disease, and the lipemias, there is a vast array of other diseases that have a genetic link as well. Reports on the many diseases called cancer have indicated that there can be a genetic susceptibility to one of the many forms of cancer as well. The whole concept of an interaction between genetic susceptibility and environmental influences has suggested that it should be possible to screen people for their genotype so as to then develop strategies to prevent or delay the phenotypic expression of a particular genotype.

While scientists have sequenced the human genome and have steadily been able to map it and identify genes of importance to tissue function, mapping is not complete. That is, although we know the sequence of the bases in the human

**TABLE 60.6**

**Mutations That Phenotype as Obesity**[22–24,47–55]

| Mutation | Characteristics |
|---|---|
| Estrogen receptor B 4 mutations | Obesity |
| Proopiomelanocortin 6 mutations | Extreme childhood and adolescent obesity |
| Leptin 3 mutations | Hyperphasia, obesity |
| Leptin receptor | Hyperphasia, obesity |
| Uncoupling protein 1 5 mutations | Obesity |
| Uncoupling protein 2 | Obesity |
| Uncoupling protein 3 | Obesity |
| MC3 receptor | Obesity |
| Neuropeptide Y receptor | Obesity |
| MSTN | Obesity |
| CCKAR | Obesity |
| Chromosome 2p12–13 (Alstrom syndrome) | Retinal pigment degeneration, neurogenic deafness, infantile obesity, hyperlipidemia, type 2 diabetes, hyperglycemia, and hyperlipidemia |
| Gs α 2 mutations | Albright hereditary osteodystrophy: skeletal abnormalities and obesity |
| Peroxisome proliferator α 2 | Obesity |
| Insulin receptor substrate | Type 2 diabetes, obesity |
| β3-adrenergic receptor | Type 2 diabetes, obesity |
| OB D75514—D7S530 insulin receptor gene | Type 2 diabetes, obesity, hypertension, and insulin resistance |
| Tumor necrosis factor | Obesity |
| 4p16.3 (Achondroplasia) | Obesity |
| 20q11 (posterior polymorphous) | Obesity, corneal dystrophy |
| 15q11.2–q12 (Prader–Willi syndrome) | Hyperphasia, early onset obesity |
| 12q23–q24.1 (Schinzel syndrome) | Obesity |
| 11q13 (Bardet–Biedl syndrome) | Obesity |
| 16q21 | Obesity |
| 3p13–p12 | Obesity |
| 15q22.3–q23 | Obesity |
| 8q22–q23 (Cohen syndrome) | Obesity |
| Xq26–q27 (X-linked) (Borjeson–Forssman–Lehmann syndrome) | Obesity |
| Xq21.1–q22 (X-linked) (Wilson–Turner syndrome) | Obesity |
| Xq26 (X-linked) (Simpson–Golabi–Behmel syndrome) | Obesity |
| HSD3B1 (1p13.1) | Obesity |
| ATP1A2 (1q21–q23) | Obesity |
| ACP1 (2p25) | Obesity |
| APOB (2p24–p23) | Obesity |
| APOD (3q27–qter) | Obesity |
| TNFir24 (6p21.3) | Obesity |
| LPL (8p22) | Obesity |
| ADRB3 (8p12–p11.1) | Obesity |
| SUR (11p15.1) | Obesity |
| DRD2 (11q22.2–q22.3) | Obesity |
| APOA4 (11q23–qter) | Obesity |
| LDLR (19p13.2) | Obesity |

genome, we do not know where all the codes are that dictate the synthesis and function of all the resultant proteins. Further, we do not know all the variations that can associate with a given metabolic or pathologic characteristic. Lifestyle choices, environmental conditions, economic well-being, social systems, food choices, and food availability all influence whether and how the phenotype of a genotype is expressed. For example, a normally black-haired child who is protein malnourished might have a reddish hair color instead of his/her genetically determined and expected black hair color. This child has not been given an adequate diet, and this inadequacy has influenced the phenotypic expression of his/her genotype. When adequately nourished, the hair color changes and becomes black. Another example, a person with a genotype for obesity might not become obese if the food supply is inadequate, and/or the person must be very physically active in order to survive. In the instance of diabetes, this is particularly apparent. A person with one of the more than 100 genetic messages associated with type 2 diabetes might not develop the disease if that person is physically active and controls his/her food intake so as to remain slim. The American Diabetes Association has noted that likely twice as many people have a diabetes genotype than actually develop the disease.[56] Again, this speaks to the importance of environmental factors in the phenotypic expression of one's genotype. Many of the chronic diseases that afflict mankind develop as a result of an interaction between an individual's genotype and his environment. The question that now arises is can one be screened for genotypes that are associated with specific diseases? The answer to this question is both a yes and a no. A number of single gene mutations affecting single reaction sequences have been identified. Many of these are listed in Table 60.1. Screening tests are available to detect the presence of mutations that result in metabolic malfunction. The success of such screening depends largely on the identification and careful description of the phenotype. It is not possible to simultaneously screen for all known mutations or polymorphisms in the human genome. The development of screening tests for the polygenic chronic diseases has been fraught with difficulty. Probably the most difficult task is the identification of those base sequences that associate with a very carefully described clinical disorder. The second problem is identifying the base sequence before the disorder is developed. Third, there is the problem of knowing with certainty that the genotype will positively lead to a specific phenotype. As mentioned, there can be polymorphisms (specific base sequences) that have no clinical significance, others that relate to specific clinical characteristics and still others whose clinical importance has yet to be discovered. The challenge for scientists seeking to understand the genetics of specific phenotypes is to develop discrete screening tools that will predict with certainty, specific disorders. For some of the rare single gene disorders in Table 60.1, excellent screening tests are available. However, for those diseases that are chronic in nature and (perhaps) slow in developing, screening is not as simple. This is because we do not know with certainty that a suspect base sequence is the root cause of the phenotype. For some diseases, a generic phenotype, that is, diabetes, can have many genotypes as shown in Table 60.4. There are many more mutations in addition to those in Table 60.4, and an updated list of these can be found in the Online Mendelian Inheritance in Man (OMIM) website maintained by NIH. Similarly, the collection of diseases called cancer has a long list of mutations associated with it. Even if one were to subdivide the list according to where the cancer began (and one was sure of this origin), one would discover that there are many mutations associated with each of these different cancers. Cancer is characterized by abnormal cell growth in a specific location. There is lung cancer, pancreatic cancer, breast cancer, and so forth. Each of these is associated with one or more mutations/polymorphisms in specific areas of the DNA.

Reports of associations between specific diseases and gene mutations have been accumulated and listed on a website maintained by NIH. One can consult this website, OMIM, (http://www.ncbi.nlm.nih.gov/omim) to learn of these associations. Table 60.7 provides a partial list of common disorders

**TABLE 60.7**
**Genetic Linkages in Human Disease**

| Disease | Number of Entries in OMIM[a] |
|---|---|
| Cancer | 2366 |
| Diabetes mellitus | 394 |
| Cardiovascular disease | 614 |
| Osteoporosis | 229 |
| Measles | 19 |
| Mumps | 7 |
| Polio | 8 |
| Bipolar disease | 75 |
| Manic depression | 6 |
| Schizophrenia | 189 |
| Alzheimer's disease | 298 |
| Parkinson's disease | 82 |
| Muscular dystrophy | 332 |
| Arthritis | 340 |
| Renal disease | 835 |
| Obesity | 443 |
| Hypertension | 548 |

[a] OMIM: Online Mendelian Inheritance in Man. A website maintained by NIH.

and the number of entries into the OMIM data bank.[57–59] Some areas have far more entries than other areas. In part, this is due to the broad spectrum of disorders that phenotype as the listed disorder and in part because some areas have received more research attention than have other areas.

As mentioned earlier, cancer is not a single disease but a collection of diseases that the OMIM groups all together. There has been tremendous interest both in finding a cure for cancer and in developing ways of determining who is at risk for which one of these diseases and how genetics can influence the efficacy of the treatments used. The number of entries into the OMIM for cancer reflects this interest. Some of the entries are duplicates. For example, entry # 604370 to the OMIM for cancer reports familial susceptibility to breast cancer at gene locus 17q21, 14q32.3, 6q25.2q27, and 3q26.3. Entry #114480 reports these same loci and 15 other loci. The numbers and letter refer to the location of the mutation at a specific site on the DNA. The first number in the loci identification indicates chromosome number. This number is followed by a letter that indicates the region in the chromosome. The chromosome is divided into regions and given an alphabetical designation. This is then followed by a number that indicates a more specific region of the chromosomal DNA. For some of these mutations, there are screening tests to determine whether the individual carries these mutations. For other mutations, there is no screening test. The OMIM website gives this information as well as where such testing can be done. As noted earlier, it is very important to have a complete description of the phenotype before genotyping is done to assure that the screening is reliable and useful. It is also important to have a knowledgeable individual interpret the results of such screening.

On the Internet, one can find advertisements for home genetic testing kits. The advertisements suggest that one can test oneself for the presence of gene mutations that in turn can predict the risk for developing a number of diseases. These tests can screen for the presence of specific genotypes but cannot be all inclusive of all the genotypes that associate with all of the human disorders.[57–59] Herein lies the problem for these tests. It can give the user a false sense of security thinking that specific genetic signature of one form of a disease is not present. The user might not know that this disease has many genetic signatures. With this false sense of security, the user then might indulge in lifestyle choices that could in turn potentiate the phenotypic expression of another genotype for that same disease, a genotype that was not included in the home test. As mentioned previously, it is not possible to develop a test that will screen for all possible genetic aberrations that are disease related! The Food and Drug Administration (FDA), the Federal Trade Commission (FTC), and the Centers for Disease Control (CDC) all caution the consumer to have a healthy dose of skepticism when using these tests for many of the same reasons: lack of knowledge of the phenotype, lack of knowledge in the interpretation of the results, lack of completeness of the test, and lack of clearly defined results that are of use to the consumer.[59]

Of concern to nutritionists are the tests that are advertised in association with advertisements for specific foods, food products, or supplements that the consumer is urged to buy based on the results of these screening tests. Again, the FTC, the FDA, and the CDC are concerned that unscrupulous advertisers might take advantage of the unsophisticated consumer who is convinced by these advertisements to buy items that would not be useful in terms of the phenotypic expression of his/her unknown or only partially known genotype. Our present knowledge in nutrition has not progressed to the point where we can make these recommendations, so it is highly unlikely that a company can promise such in its advertisements.

## SUMMARY

A number of the chronic diseases that affect humans have both genetic and nutritional linkages. In some, the genetic linkage is very strong, and, likely, in people with these mutations, the disease will develop regardless of dietary influence. In other disorders, a combination of genetic and dietary factors is needed before the disease manifests itself. Paramount to successful delay or avoidance of some of these disorders is an early identification of mutations and their associated phenotypes. Genetic screening may be valuable in developing successful strategies that can forestall disease development.

## REFERENCES

1. Berdanier, CD. *Advanced Nutrition: Macronutrients*, 2nd edn. CRC Press, Boca Raton, FL, 327p., 2000.
2. Berdanier, CD. *Advanced Nutrition: Micronutrients*. CRC Press, Boca Raton, FL, 236p., 1998.
3. Murray, RK, Granner, DK, Mayes, PA, Rodwell, VW. *Harpers Biochemistry*. Appleton & Lange, Stamford, CT, 359p., 2004.
4. Scriver, CR, Beaudet, AL, Sly, WS, Valle, D. *The Metabolic Basis of Inherited Disease*. McGraw Hill, New York, 3006.p, 1989.
5. Julieen, P, Vohl, MC, Gaudet, D et al. *Diabetes* 46, 2063, 1997.
6. Eckstrom, U, Abrahamson, M, Wallmark, A et al. *Eur J Clin Invest* 28, 740, 1998.
7. Sun, XM, Patel, DD, Knight, BL, Soutar, AK. *Atherosclerosis* 136, 175, 1998.
8. Kluijtmans, LA, van den Heuvel, LP, Boers, GH et al. *Am J Hum Genet* 58, 35, 1996.
9. Goyette, P, Christensen, AE, Rosenblatt, DS, Rozen, R. *Am J Hum Genet* 59, 1268, 1996.
10. Howard, TD, Guttmacher, AE, McKinnon, W et al. *Am J Hum Genet* 61, 1405, 1997.
11. Soutar, AK. *J Intern Med* 231, 633, 1992.
12. Folsom, AR, Nieto, FL, McGovern, PG et al. *J Clin Invest* 98, 204, 1998.
13. Keating, MT. *Circulation* 92, 142, 1995.
14. Garin, MC, James RW, Dussoix, P et al. *J Clin Invest* 99, 62, 1997.
15. Watkins, H, McKenna, WI, Thierfelder, HJ et al. *N Eng J Med* 332, 1058, 1995.
16. Pullinger, CR, Hennessy, LK, Chatterton, JE et al. *J Clin Invest* 95, 1225, 1995.
17. Genest, JJ, Ordovas, JM, McNamara, JR et al. *Atherosclerosis* 82, 7, 1990.
18. Mune, T, Roggerson, RM, Nikkila, H et al. *Nat Genet* 10, 394, 1995.
19. Shimkets, RA, Warnock, DG, Bositis, CM. *Cell* 79, 407, 1994.
20. Erdmann, J, Hegemann, N, Weidemann, A et al. *Am J Med Genet* 80, 521, 1998.
21. Schott, JJ, Benson, DW, Basson, CT et al. *Science* 281, 108, 1998.
22. Utsunomiya, N, Ohagi, S, Sanke, T et al. *Diabetologia* 41, 701, 1996.
23. Hani, EH, Boutin, P, Durand, E et al. *Diabetologia* 41, 1511, 1998.
24. Cama, A, Sierra, ML, Ottini, L. *J Clin Endocrinol Metab* 73, 894, 1991.
25. Jackson, RS, Creemers, JW, Ohagi, S et al. *Nat Genet* 16, 303, 1997.
26. Froguel, P, Vaxillaire, M, Velho, G. *Diabetes Rev* 5, 123, 1997.
27. Velho, G, Blanche, H, Vaxillaire, M et al. *Diabetologia* 40, 217, 1997.
28. Vionnet, N, Stoffel, M, Takeda, J et al. *Nature* 356, 721, 1992.
29. Shimada, F, Makino, H, Hashimoto, H. *Diabetologia* 36, 433, 1993.
30. Hattersley, AT, Turner, RC, Permutt, MA. *Lancet* 339, 1307, 1993.
31. Shitani, M, Ikegami, H, Yamato, E et al. *Diabetologia* 39, 1398, 1996.
32. Taylor, SI, Kadowaki, H, Accili, D et al. *Diabetes Care* 13, 257, 1990.
33. Kadowaki, T, Kadowaki, H, Rechler, MM. *J Clin Invest* 86, 254, 1990.
34. Odawara, M, Kadowaki, T, Yaamamotto, R. *Science* 245, 66, 1989.
35. Taylor, ST, Cama, A, Accili, D et al. *Endocr Rev* 13, 566, 1992.
36. Chevre, JC, Hani, EH, Boutin, P et al. *Diabetologia* 41, 1017, 1998.
37. Velho, G, Froguel, P. *Endocrinology* 138, 233, 1998.

38. Vaxillaire, M, Rouard, M, Yamagata, K et al. *Hum Mol Genet* 6, 583, 1997.
39. Frayling, TMTM, Bulamn, MP, Ellard, S et al. *Diabetes* 46, 720, 1997.
40. Hansen, T, Eiberg, H, Rouard, M et al. *Diabetes* 46, 726, 1997.
41. Yagui, K, Shimada, F, Mimura, M et al. *Diabetologia* 41, 1024, 1998.
42. Steiner, DF, Tager, HS, Chan, SJ et al. *Diabetes Care* 13, 600, 1990.
43. DeFronzo, RA. *Diabetes Rev* 5, 177, 1997.
44. Strom, TM, Hortnagel, K, Hofmann, S et al. *Hum Mol Genet* 7, 2021, 1998.
45. van den Ouweland, JMW, Lempkes, HHPJ, Ruitenbeck, W et al. *Nat Genet* 1, 368, 1992.
46. Mathews, CE, Berdanier, CD. *Proc Soc Exp Biol Med* 219, 97, 1998.
47. Rosenkranz, K, Hinney, A, Zeigler, A et al. *J Clin Endocrinol Metab* 83, 4524, 1998.
48. Hinney, A, Becker, I, Heibut, O et al. *J Endocrinol Metab* 83, 3737, 1998.
49. Karvonen, MK, Pesonen, U, Heinonen, P et al. *J Endocrinol Metab* 83, 3239, 1998.
50. Comuzzie, AG, Allison, DB. *Science* 280, 1374, 1998.
51. Urhammer, SA, Fridberg, M, Sorenson, TI et al. *J Clin Endocrinol Metab* 82, 4069, 1997.
52. Macari, F, Lautier, C, Girardet, A. *Hum Genet* 103, 658, 1998.
53. Warner, DR, Weng, G, Yu, S et al. *J Biol Chem* 273, 23976, 1998.
54. Ristow, M, Muller-Wieland, D, Pfeiffer, A et al. *N Eng J Med* 339, 953, 1998.
55. Perusse, L, Chagnon, YC, Dionne, FT, Bouchard, C. *Obesity Res* 5, 1225, 1996.
56. Diagnosis and Classification of Diabetes Mellitus. *Diabetes Care* 34S, S62, 2011
57. NCIB. http://www.ncbi.nih.gov/omim, accessed May 29, 2012.
58. NLM. http://www.nlm.nih.gov/medlineplus/genetictesting.html, accessed May 31, 2012.
59. FTC. http://www.ftc.gov/bcp/edu/pubs/consumer/health/hea0.2.shtm, accessed May 31, 2012.

# 61 Diet, Nutrition, and the Prevention of Cardiovascular Disease

*Annie Ferland and Robert H. Eckel*

## CONTENTS

## INTRODUCTION

The increasing prevalence of obesity and cardiovascular disease (CVD) worldwide is a cause of great concern both for the health of individuals and for the associated medical and economic costs to societies. The recent Heart Disease and Stroke Statistics published in 2011[1] identified that coronary heart disease (CHD) caused ≈1 of every 6 deaths in the United States in 2007. Figure 61.1 portrays the prevalence of CVD, including CHD, heart failure, stroke, and hypertension, in the U.S. adult population over 20 years, by age and sex.[1]

As a causal effect, sedentary lifestyle, poor food choices, and increased energy intake are incriminated. This is leading to weight gain, positive energy balance, obesity, and health-related comorbidities. Thus, this increases the public interest in dietary strategies to reduce body weight and thereby reduce CVD risk.

The relationship between diet and CVD has been studied intensively for over a 100 years. For a long time, the consensus was to reduce serum total cholesterol levels to prevent heart disease.[2] The origin of this premise was that diet, serum cholesterol, and CVD were closely linked. Evidence appeared as early as 1908, when Ignatowski produced an animal model of atherosclerosis, by feeding rabbits with animal protein from meat, milk, and eggs.[3] Twenty-five years later, Anitschkow concluded that cholesterol in the food we eat is transported into the bloodstream. When cholesterol is deposed in the arteries supplying the heart, the ultimate consequence of its accumulation is a heart attack.[3] However, it was the rapid increase in the incidence and prevalence of CVD and of other clinical manifestations of atherosclerosis

in the 1940s and 1950s in the United States that led to a more intensive investigation of its etiology. Meanwhile, discoveries from epidemiological studies as well as from cohorts from low- to high-risk countries suggested a main role of dietary cholesterol and saturated fat in the cause of atherosclerosis and CVD in humans.[4] This assumption was part of what was commonly referred as the diet–heart hypothesis. Over time, this was found to be simplistic because diet may mediate CVD through multiple biological mechanisms other than only serum total cholesterol or what we now know as low-density lipoprotein cholesterol (LDL-C).[4] Indeed, various dietary factors, such as the type of fat, dietary cholesterol, omega-3 fatty acids, *trans*-fatty acids, carbohydrates, glycemic index (GI), fiber, folate, and dietary patterns, can all potentially influence CVD risk (Figure 61.2). Thus, identification of the dietary changes that most effectively prevent CVD is critical.

## ASSESSMENT OF THE PATIENT'S RISK STATUS

The assessment of the patient's risk is primordial to determine the intensity of a clinical intervention. Some obesity-associated diseases and CVD risk factors classified patients in a very high-risk category for subsequent mortality. Consequently, patients classified in the high-risk category require aggressive modifications of their risk factors, in addition to the clinical management of the disease.

The measurement of body weight alone is helpful but at times inconclusive for the clinical assessment of body fatness.[5] Thus, the Center for Disease Control and Prevention has adopted the Quetelet-Kaup index, or

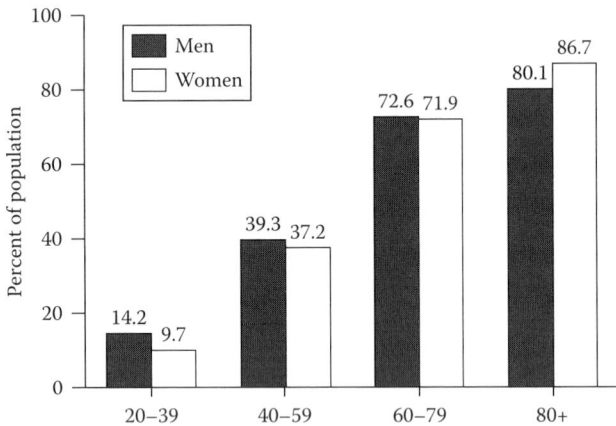

**FIGURE 61.1** Prevalence of cardiovascular disease in adults ≥20 years of age by age and sex (National Health and Nutrition Examination Survey: 2005–2008). (From National Center for Health Statistics and National Heart, Lung, and Blood Institute.) These data include CHD, heart failure, stroke, and Hypertension. (Adapted from Roger, V.L. et al., *Circulation*, 123(4), e18, 2011.)

body mass index (BMI), as an indicator to assess excess adiposity and classify people as normal, overweight, or obese, as summarized in Table 61.1.[6]

BMI is calculated as weight in kilograms divided by height in meters squared and is expressed in $kg/m^2$. Obesity is defined by a BMI >30.0 $kg/m^2$ and overweight by a BMI between 25.0 and 29.9 $kg/m^2$, with a separate classification for the degree of obesity. A BMI from 30.0 to 34.9 $kg/m^2$ is class 1 or mild obesity, 35.0–39.9 $kg/m^2$ is class 2 or moderate obesity, and 40.0 $kg/m^2$ is class 3 or severe obesity. BMI should also be assessed in association with waist circumference, which rather evaluates the distribution of body fat.[5] Although BMI and waist circumference are interrelated,

increased waist circumference can be a better predictor of CVD risk and mortality in adults who are categorized as normal or overweight in terms of BMI.[7,8] In accordance to the BMI and waist circumference definition from the Practical Guide for Identification, Evaluation, and Treatment of Overweight and Obesity, adults aged 18 years or more with a BMI between 25.0 and 34.9 $kg/m^2$ and a waist circumference of ≥102 cm for men and ≥88 cm for women have an increased risk for cardiovascular comorbidity.[9] Moreover, considering that waist circumference is closely correlated to visceral adipose tissue and metabolic complications, simultaneous measurement of simple variables such as waist circumference and fasting plasma triglycerides levels has also been suggested to be used as an inexpensive screening tool to identify men and women with high CAD risk.[10,11]

## NATIONAL DIETARY GUIDELINES IN THE PRESENCE OF CVD

Changes in deleterious lifestyle habits are considered the most efficient and the least expensive way to reduce CVD risk. The INTERHEART study identified nine modifiable risk factors, which predicts 90% of myocardial infarction worldwide in both sexes: lipoprotein profile, smoking, hypertension, diabetes, abdominal obesity, psychosocial factors, consumption of fruits and vegetables, alcohol intake, and regular physical activity.[12] Since numerous patients with CVD are overweight or obese, and present high-risk waist circumference,[13] weight loss should be one of the first-line therapy prescribed by health professionals.[14,15] This approach can also improve insulin sensitivity and influence positively most of the metabolic abnormality (i.e., hypertension, diabetes, lipid disorder, or preexisting CVD). Several methods and strategies are available, and it is

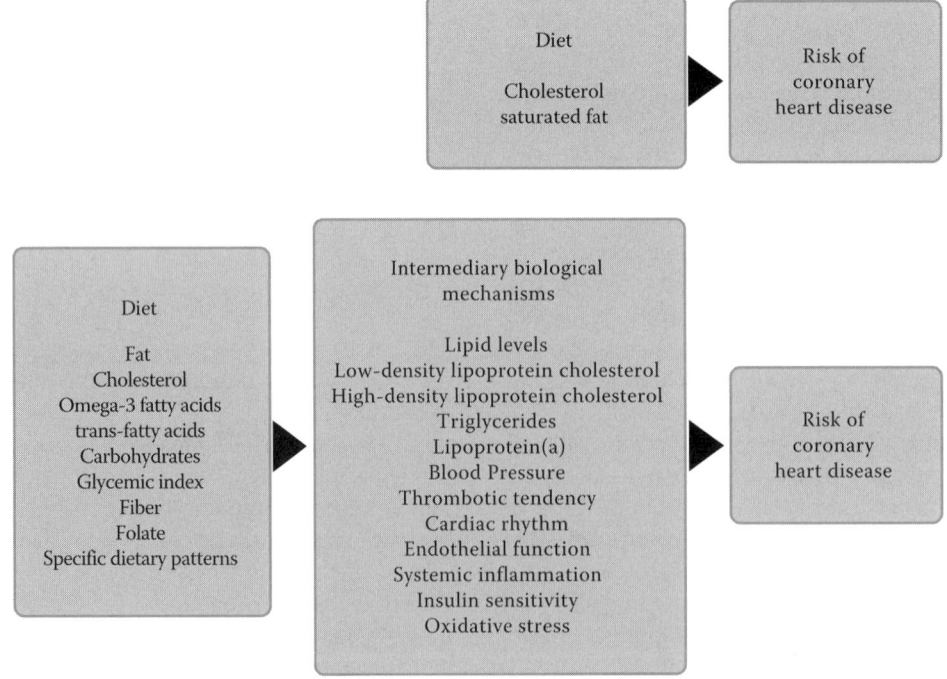

**FIGURE 61.2** Dietary factors that can potentially influence CVD risk.

**TABLE 61.1**

**Classification of Overweight and Obesity by BMI, Waist Circumference, Percent Body Fat, and Associated Disease Risk**

| | BMI (kg/m²) | Obesity Class | Disease Risk[a] (Relative to Normal Weight and Weight Circumference) | |
|---|---|---|---|---|
| | | | Men ≤ 40 in (≤102 cm) Women ≤ 35 in (≤88 cm) | Men > 40 in (>102 cm) Women > 35 in (>102 cm) |
| Underweight | <18.5 | | | |
| Normal | 18.5–24.9 | | | |
| Overweight | 25.0–29.9 | | Increased | High |
| Mild obesity | 30.0–34.9 | I | High | Very high |
| Moderate obesity | 35.0–39.9 | II | Very high | Very high |
| Severe obesity | ≥40.0 | III | Extremely high | Extremely high |

*Source:* National Institutes of Health, *The Practical Guide to the Identification, Evaluation, and Treatment of Overweight and Obesity in Adults*, U.S. Department of Health and Human Services, Public Health Services, National Heart, Lung, and Blood Institute, Bethesda, MD, 2000, NIH publication No. 00-4084.

[a] Disease risk for CVD, hypertension, and type 2 diabetes.

**TABLE 61.2**

**Major Risk Factors for CHD**

| | | |
|---|---|---|
| **Non-modifiable Risk Factors** | Age | Men > 45 Years; Women > 55 Years |
| | Male gender | |
| | Family history of premature CHD | CHD in male first-degree relative <55 years; CHD in female first-degree relative <65 years |
| **Modifiable Risk Factors** | High levels of LDL-C | |
| **(With a Relationship with Diet)** | Low high-density lipoprotein cholesterol | <40 mg/dL |
| | High blood pressure (hypertension) | >140/90 mm Hg |
| | Diabetes | |
| | Obesity (especially abdominal obesity) | BMI >30 kg/m²; Waist circumference >102 cm in men and >88 cm in women |
| | An "atherogenic" diet | High in saturated fats and cholesterol, low in vegetables, fruits, and whole grains |
| **Modifiable Risk Factors** | Physical inactivity | |
| | Cigarette smoking | Or any smoking in past year |

*Source:* Adapted from Third Report of the National Cholesterol Education Program (NCEP) Expert Panel on Detection, Evaluation, and Treatment of High Blood Cholesterol in Adults (Adult Treatment Panel III) Final Report, *Circulation*, 106(25), 3143, 2002.

important to target the right approach in order to achieve and maintain optimal body weight. The awareness of foods and overall eating patterns must be emphasized. Table 61.2 presents the major modifiable and non-modifiable risk factors for CVD.

Elevated LDL-C is one of the primary risk factors implicated in the development of atherosclerotic CVD. Both the American Heart Association (AHA) and the National Cholesterol Education Program (NCEP-ATP III) emphasize dietary measures to achieve LDL-C goals, since reduction in LDL-C levels is associated with reduced CAD risk.[15,16] The NCEP-ATP III report has updated the recommendations for clinical management of high blood cholesterol, considering LDL-C as the primary target of cholesterol-lowering intervention.[16,17] Therapeutic modalities for LDL-C lowering include both therapeutic lifestyle changes (TLCs) and drug therapies. TLC includes (1) reduced intakes of saturated fat and cholesterol, (2) therapeutic options for enhancing LDL lowering such as plant stanols/sterols (2 g/day) and increased soluble fiber (10–25 g), (3) increased physical activity, and (4) weight control, to lower population cholesterol levels and reduce CVD risk. It is recommended to reduce intakes of saturated fat to <7% of total calories and dietary cholesterol to <200 mg/day, respectively (Table 61.3).

**TABLE 61.3**

**Macronutrient Composition Suggested by the AHA Diet and Lifestyle Recommendations, the Therapeutic Lifestyle Changes by the NCEP-ATP III, the DASH Study, and the Lyon Heart Study**

| | AHA Diet and Lifestyle Recommendations | TLC Diet (NCEP-ATP III) | DASH | Mediterranean Style (Lyon Heart Study) |
|---|---|---|---|---|
| Total fat (% kcal) | 25–35 | 25–35 | 27 | 31 |
| Saturated fat | <7 | <7 | 6 | 8 |
| *Trans*-fatty acid | <1 | As low as possible | — | 4 |
| Polyunsaturated | >10 | >10 | 8 | 5 |
| ω-6 Linoleic acid | — | — | — | 4 |
| ω-9 Oleic acid | — | — | — | 1 |
| Monounsaturated | >15 | >20 | 13 | 13 |
| Cholesterol (mg) | <200 | <200 | 150 | 200 |
| Carbohydrate (% kcal) | ≥55 | 50–60 | 55 | 53 |
| Protein (% kcal) | 15 | 15 | 18 | 16 |
| Fiber (g) | 20–30 | 20–30 | >30 | 19 |
| Sodium (mmol) | 100 | 100 | <100 | <100 |
| Alcohol | Women: ≤1 drink/day Men: ≤2 drink/day | — | — | 6% kcal |
| Total calories | Maintain energy balance Achieve a healthy body weight | Prevent weight gain Maintain ideal body weight | Maintain ideal body weight | |

*Sources:* Adapted from Lichtenstein, A.L. et al., *Circulation*, 114(1), 86, 2006; Third Report of the National Cholesterol Education Program (NCEP) Expert Panel on Detection, Evaluation, and Treatment of High Blood Cholesterol in Adults (Adult Treatment Panel III) Final Report, *Circulation*, 106(25), 3143, 2002; Appel, L.J. et al. *Hypertension*, 47(2), 296, 2006; de Lorgeril, M. et al., *Circulation*, 99(6), 779, 1999.

Dietary recommendations also emphasize the consumption of monounsaturated (MUFAs) and polyunsaturated fatty acids (PUFAs), and to consume more fruits, vegetables, and whole grain products.[15] These recommendations apply particularly to patients who are overweight or obese, but the clinical approach is more intensive for higher-risk persons. Accordingly, the LDL-C goals in primary prevention are also lower in individuals with a higher level of risk.

Six weeks after the initiation of the TLC diet, the LDL-C response must be reassessed. Other therapeutic options to lower LDL-C can be added, such as plant stanols/sterols and soluble fiber. The NCEP-ATP III recommendations about the optimal cholesterol target are to maintain total cholesterol below 5.2 mmol/L (203 mg/dL) and raise HDL-cholesterol to the highest extent possible.[16] It is generally advised to modify LDL-C target in accordance with the presence of one or more risk factors such as cigarette smoking, high blood pressure (≥140/90 mm Hg), low HDL-C (<1.03 mmol/L | <40 mg/dL), and family history of early CAD (aged ≤45 years for men and ≤55 years for women). In the absence of risk factors or the presence of only one risk factor, one is permitted to target an LDL-C below 4.14 mmol/L (<160 mg/dL). The presence of two or more risk factors suggests targeting an LDL-C level below 3.36 mmol/L (<130 mg/dL). The ultimate category considered at very high risk is the one associated with the presence of CVD or diabetes. These patients should attain the lowest range of LDL-C (<2.59 mmol/L | <100 mg/dL). Of note, sustained weight loss is an important issue regarding LDL-C management in overweight and obese individuals, as well as in persons with the metabolic

syndrome. If the LDL-C goal is not achieved 6 weeks after the intensification of the LDL lowering therapy, a statin should be added. Other drugs include cholesterol absorption inhibitors, bile acid sequestrants, nicotinic acid, and fibrates but in general, all of these classes are less efficacious than statins and less well proven or not proven to reduce CVD events.

The AHA Diet and Lifestyle Recommendations have established guidelines for reducing the risk of CVD by dietary and other lifestyle practices.[15,17] The energy balance should be maintained by matching the intake of energy to overall energy expenditure to achieve a healthy body weight. Patients must include a variety of fruits, vegetables, whole grains and cereal products, low-fat dairy products, low saturated fat, fish, and lean meats while eating adequate amounts of essential nutrients. Table 61.3 presents the macronutrient composition suggested by the AHA diet. Portion number and size should be monitored, and consumption of foods and beverages with low nutritional quality, high caloric density, and added sugars should be limited.

Multiple evidence indicates that lowering dietary sodium intake helps lower blood pressure.[18–20] In fact, reducing sodium intake by 1800 mg/day or achieving an average daily consumption of 2400 mg is associated with systolic and diastolic blood pressure reductions.[18] Of note, the average intake of sodium in the United States is approximately 3400 mg/day.[21] Reducing sodium intake by choosing foods low in sodium and limiting the amount of sodium added to food are also an important target. Moreover, alcohol consumption should not exceed more than two drinks per day for men and one drink per day for women.

The practical guideline for identification, evaluation, and treatment of overweight and obesity in adults recommends low-calorie diet to induce weight loss in overweight and obese patients.[9] Weight loss from 5% to 10% through 6 months may reduce several risk factors for heart disease and stroke in people who are overweight or obese with comorbidities, even if optimal weight is not attained. A reduction around 500–1000 kcal/day is recommended to achieve weight reduction and to produce a recommended weight loss of 1–2 lb/week. In general, diets containing 1000–1200 kcal/day should be recommended to most women. Diets between 1200 and 1600 kcal/day should be selected for men and for women who weigh 75 kg or more. Of importance, the optimal weight loss diet must have adequate nutritional composition to reduce risk factors.

## RECOMMENDED DIETARY PATTERNS IN PRESENCE OF CVD

Current dietary guidelines advocate food-based diets for optimal health and prevention of chronic disease. Such dietary approaches showed to effectively benefit hypercholesterolemia and hypertension and significantly reduce CVD risk. However, dietary recommendations often focus on particular nutrients in a way that is sometimes difficult to translate into clinical practice. Changing the diet is about changing the pattern, not simply an avoidance of a particular nutrient. Thus, pattern analysis provides information about the relationship between the whole diet and disease risk. This is a more comprehensive approach because it focuses on the entire diet rather than on just one food or nutrient.[22] Considerable research showed that people following the Dietary Approaches to Stop Hypertension (DASH) or the Mediterranean style eating patterns have a lower risk of CVD and lower likelihood of developing hypertension. Other studies have evaluated the relation of overall dietary pattern to the CVD risk.

*The DASH dietary pattern*: Major goals of the dietary recommendations in the presence of CVD are to lower blood pressure in addition to improve serum lipids. The DASH eating pattern is a carbohydrate-rich diet, currently advocated in several scientific dietary reports and guidelines for the prevention and treatment of blood pressure.[15,18,20,21] The DASH diet emphasized vegetables, fruits and low-fat dairy products, whole grains, poultry, fish and nuts, and a limited amount of red meat, sweets, and sugar-containing beverages, and limits the amounts of total fat, saturated fat, and cholesterol. This dietary pattern can substantially lower mean systolic blood pressure from 7.1 mm Hg in people without hypertension to 11.5 mm Hg in people with hypertension.[19,20] The Seventh Report of the Joint National Committee on Prevention, Detection, Evaluation, and Treatment of High Blood Pressure (JNC7) also recommends several lifestyle modifications and the adoption of the DASH eating pattern in order to manage hypertension. The major lifestyle modifications that have shown to lower BP include weight reduction, which may reduce systolic BP by 5–20 mm Hg/10 kg weight loss, and reducing the daily dietary sodium intake to no more than 2400 mg of dietary sodium.[23] More so, the alcohol

consumption should be limited to no more than two drinks in most men and no more than one drink per day in women and lighter-weight individuals. It is well known that high sodium intake, obesity, and alcohol consumption can influence arterial blood pressure. Of interest, an increase of 1 mm Hg of systolic BP is associated with an increase risk of 1%–2% of cardiovascular complications after myocardial infarction.[24]

*The Mediterranean food pattern*: There are several definitions of the Mediterranean-style eating pattern. Each region from Spain to the Middle East, which includes at least 16 countries that border the Mediterranean Sea, customizes the basic Mediterranean-style dietary pattern. These diets take advantage of the regional food availability and cultural preferences. Similarities include daily consumption of unrefined cereals and cereal products, vegetables, fruits, dairy products, and red or white wine, and olive oil is the most important fat source. A weekly consumption of potatoes, fish, olives, nuts, eggs, and sweets is also suggested. Fish and poultry are consumed in low to moderate amounts, eggs are consumed up to four times weekly, and red meat and meat products are limited to a monthly consumption. Most of the foods consumed are fresh, seasonal whole foods, and the preparation methods are simple. Convincing evidence for the protective role of the Mediterranean diet in reducing traditional risk factors and the rate of cardiovascular complications after myocardial infarction comes from the Lyon Diet Heart Study.[25] A Mediterranean diet + a supplement of α-linolenic margarine was compared with standard advice after a first myocardial infarction. At 27 months, a reduction in the rate of coronary events of 76% was seen in the Mediterranean diet group, and the decision was made to stop the trial. Even 4 years after the myocardial infarction, the final follow-up still showed the protective effect of the diet.[24] Other randomized controlled trials such as the Heart Institute of Spokane Diet Intervention and Evaluation Trial (THIS-DIET) and the *Prevencion con Dieta Mediterranea* Study also support the role of the Mediterranean diet in the prevention of CVD.[26,27]

Short-term studies (12 weeks) found that promoting the Mediterranean-style food pattern with a more specific increase in the consumption of legumes, nuts, and seeds and a decrease in the consumption of sweets was associated with a reduction in body weight (–10.5 kg), waist circumference (–1.2 cm), and a decrease in circulating oxidized LDL (–11.3%).[28,29] The adoption of a Mediterranean diet can also lower LDL-C by 5%–10% even in the absence of weight loss.[30] Moreover, further improvements in systolic and diastolic blood pressure, triglycerides, and glucose control can be achieved with a clinically meaningful reduction in body weight (10%). Shai et al. have shown in a 2-year trial of a calorie-restricted Mediterranean-style dietary pattern that despite maximal weight loss at 6 months and partial weight rebound, there were significant improvements in the levels of HDL-C and LDL-C during a 7–24-month weight maintenance period.[31] More so, a recent meta-analysis showed that a Mediterranean diet is more effective compared to a low-fat diet in improving their body weight, BMI, systolic and diastolic blood pressure, fasting plasma glucose, total cholesterol, and C-reactive protein after 2 years of follow-up.[32] Thus, the adoption of a Mediterranean style dietary pattern appears to be effective in inducing clinically relevant short- and long-term changes in CVD risk factors.

*Other dietary patterns*: Dietary patterns can be defined using a score-based approach (or diet indexes) or can be empirically derived using principal component analysis or cluster analysis. For example, the Healthy Eating Index (HEI) was developed to measure how well American diets conform to the major recommendations of the Food Guide Pyramid or the Dietary Guidelines for Americans. Accordingly, a higher HEI to the Dietary Guidelines for Americans was associated with a 28% lower risk of CVD (RR = 0.72; 95% CI: 0.60–0.88; p < 0.001).[33] Another method used is the diet quality score, which is based on the sum of the number of foods recommended by current dietary guidelines. This Recommended Food Score was associated with a lower risk of CVD mortality (RR = 0.67; 95% CI: 0.47–0.95; p < 0.001).[34] In addition to diet scores based on diet quality, scores were also developed to measure the adherence to specific recommendations. The "low-carbohydrate-diet score" was created to classify women according to the relative intakes for fat, protein, and carbohydrate. During the 20 years of follow-up, the RR of CVD comparing the highest to the lowest group of the "low-carbohydrate-diet score" was 0.70 (95% CI: 0.56–0.88; p = 0.002) when adjusted for vegetable sources of protein and fat.[35] Meanwhile, a diet score reflecting a diet low in *trans*-fatty acids and glycemic load, high in cereal, fiber, omega-3 fatty acids, and folate, with a high ratio of PUFA:SFA, strongly predicted a reduced risk of CVD (RR = 0.43; 95% CI: 0.33–0.55; p < 0.001).[36]

Observational studies have also examined the associations between empiric dietary patterns and CVD. The Seven Countries study found that participants in a dietary cluster characterized by high alcohol intake had the highest mortality from CVD or stroke (14.4 deaths per 100 in 15 years) in contrast with those in a cluster with high intake of PUFA with the lowest mortality (5.4 deaths per 100 in 15 years).[37] However, one of the main limitations is that these results were adjusted only for age and geographical area. In the Whitehall II study, four clusters were identified: (1) unhealthy, characterized by white bread, processed meat, French fries, and full-cream milk; (2) sweets, characterized

by white bread, biscuits, cakes, processed meat, and high-fat dairy products; (3) Mediterranean-like, defined by fruits, vegetables, rice, pasta, and wine; and (4) healthy, with high intake of fruits, vegetables, whole-meal bread, and low-fat dairy, and low intake of alcohol. Compared to the unhealthy cluster, the healthy cluster was associated with a 29% reduction in the risk of fatal CVD and nonfatal myocardial infarction after adjustment for confounding factors.[38] Five different clusters were also identified in the Framingham Nutrition studies: (1) heart healthy, (2) light eating, (3) wine and moderate eating, (4) high fat, and (5) empty calorie clusters. Women who consumed a heart-healthy diet and who had never smoked had more than 80% lower odds for subclinical heart disease compared with those with the less-heart healthy cluster (OR = 0.17; 95% CI: 0.07–0.36; P = 0.0001).[39]

Most studies that used factor analysis have focused on two major patterns: (1) "healthy or prudent," which is characterized by vegetables, fruits, legumes, fish, poultry, and whole grains, and (2) "Western" characterized by red meat, processed meat, refined grains, French fries, and sweets/dessert. In most studies, the prudent pattern was associated with reduced risk for CVD, while the Western pattern was associated with a significantly increased risk.[22,36] In the Nurses' cohort, the prudent diet was also associated with a 28% lower CVD mortality.[40] In general, patterns identified by cluster of factor analysis showed numerous associations with CVD risk factors, including a better lipid profile, in contrast with the Westernized patterns.

## IMPACT OF DIETARY MACRONUTRIENT COMPOSITION FOR THE PREVENTION OF CVD

The optimal diets for prevention of CVD are sill subject of debate. Early reports showed that saturated fatty acids increase and PUFAs decrease total and LDL-C, respectively. Several meta-analyses have also developed predictive equations to summarize the effects of different dietary fatty acids on serum cholesterol levels. In general, the regression equation shows that when saturated and monounsaturated fat are substituted for carbohydrate under isocaloric conditions increases in HDL-C are seen, whereas PUFAs have a neutral effect.[41] Figure 61.3 shows the predicted changes in serum lipids and lipoproteins when 5%

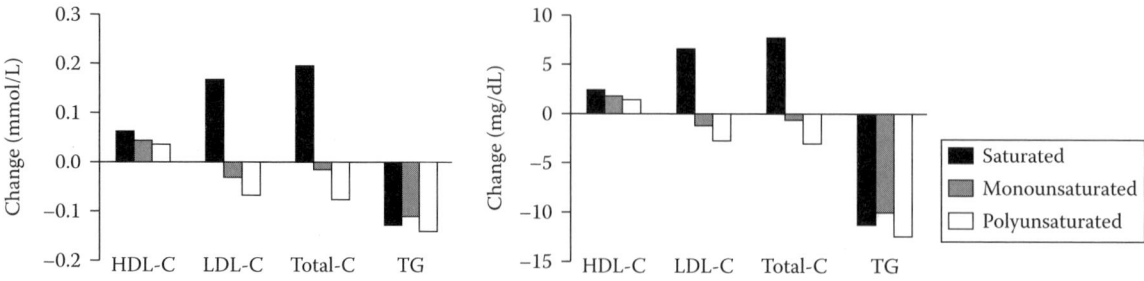

**FIGURE 61.3**  Predicted changes in serum lipids and lipoproteins when 5% of energy as carbohydrate is replaced by fatty acids of a particular class under isocaloric conditions. (Adapted from Mensink, R.P. et al., *Arterio Thrombol*, 12(8), 911, 1992.)

of energy as carbohydrate is replaced by fatty acids of a particular class under isocaloric conditions. Moreover, the replacement of carbohydrate by fat lowered serum triglycerides, independent of the nature of the fat. Replacement of saturated fatty acids by unsaturated fat raised the HDL-C to LDL-C cholesterol ratio, whereas replacement by carbohydrates had no effect.[41]

The reduction of saturated fat is widely recommended to reduce CVD risk, but the type of macronutrients that should replace it is still subject of debate. The 11-year report of the Oslo Diet–Heart Study showed a decrease in myocardial infarction mortality when following a diet reduced in saturated fat and increased in PUFA.[42] When MUFAs or PUFAs replace saturated fat, LDL-C decreases and HDL-C changes only slightly. On the other hand, substituting polyunsaturated for saturated fat may have beneficial effects on insulin sensitivity[43] and type 2 diabetes.[44] The randomized, crossover Omni Heart Trial has addressed this issue in evaluating the optimal macronutrient substitutions for saturated fat (carbohydrate, protein, or unsaturated fat).[45] Three different diet interventions were evaluated, such as a high-carbohydrate diet (similar to the DASH diet), a high-protein diet (10% higher in protein than the two other diets), and a diet high in unsaturated fat (10% higher in unsaturated fat sources such as olive oil, canola, and safflower oil). Interestingly, partial substitution of carbohydrate with either protein or monounsaturated fat can further help lower blood pressure, improve lipid levels, and reduce the 10-year risk of CVD. A recent expert panel reviewed the evidence in the reduction of saturated fat to prevent CVD.[46] It was found that replacing only 1% of energy from saturated fat with PUFA in those people consuming a Westernized diet can lower LDL-C and produce only a modest reduction in CVD of 2%–3%. Also considered was that insufficient evidence exists to judge the effect of replacing saturated fat with MUFA on CVD risk.

Trans-fatty acids are found in stick margarine, vegetable shortenings, and commercial bakery and deep-fried foods. Numerous controlled metabolic studies showed that trans-fatty acids raise LDL-C and maintain or lower HDL-C relative to unsaturated fatty acids and may promote insulin resistance and increase the risk of type 2 diabetes.[47–50] In the Nurses' Health Study cohort, it was found that a higher intake of trans-fat and, to a smaller extend, saturated fat was associated with increased risk of CVD.[51] Within the same study, the opposite effect was found with higher intakes of PUFA and MUFA.

*Omega-3 fatty acids and CVD*: An increase in dietary intake of n-3 PUFAs seems to be a preventive approach to reduce the risk of both sudden death and death from CVD, either in animal models or in patients with and without CAD.[52] It is estimated that the requirement for n-6 and n-3 fatty acids in adults is 1.0% and 0.2% of daily energy intake, respectively.[53] Ideally, this should be associated with an acceptable macronutrient distribution range for eicosapentaenoic acid (EPA) and docosahexaenoic acid (DHA) of 0.25–2.0 g/day. The potential mechanisms by which higher

quantities of ingested n-3 fatty acids may reduce the risk of CVD are not well defined but may include (1) reduced susceptibility to ventricular arrhythmia, (2) antithrombogenic effects, (3) increased nitric oxide and endothelial relaxation, (4) slow atherosclerotic plaque growth, (5) lower triglycerides, and (6) lower blood pressure.[54] Many of these effects, however, are seen only at higher levels of intake.

In the early 1990s, the DART trial reported a 29% reduction in all-cause mortality over a 2-year period following the increased intake of fatty fish to 200–400 g/week in individuals with previous myocardial infarction.[55] Subsequently, the Gruppo Italiano per lo Studio della Sopravvivenza nell'Infarto Miocardico (GISSI)-Prevenzione trial reported a 15% reduction in the composite primary end point of death, nonfatal myocardial infarction, or nonfatal stroke, with a 20% reduction in overall mortality and a 45% reduction in sudden death after 3.5 years using a 850 mg dose of EPA and DHA n-3 fatty acid supplementation (either with and without vitamin E) in subjects with preexisting CVD.[56,57] The GISSI Heart Failure trial also confirmed the reduction in mortality in a population of patients with symptomatic chronic heart failure, as seen in the GISSI-Prevenzione trial, although the extent of the reduction was smaller.[58] The long-term use of EPA was also tested in the open-label Japan EPA Acid Lipid Intervention Study.[59] At mean follow-up of 4.6 years, a major coronary event occurred in 2.8% of hypercholesterolemic patients treated with 1800 mg of EPA daily with statins compared to 3.5% in the statins group. This study also showed a 19% relative reduction in major coronary events and a significant reduction in stroke. Interestingly, the level of LDL-C after treatment decreased similarly in both groups.

In contrast to the growing body of evidence supporting a protective effect of omega-3 fatty acids in secondary prevention, the recent Alpha Omega trial showed major cardiovascular event in 13.9% of patient during the median follow-up of 3.7 year.[60] Neither the EPA-DHA nor the ALA supplemented margarines reduced the rate of major fatal or nonfatal cardiovascular events and cardiac interventions in a cohort of patients with previous myocardial infarction. Another study reported no effect of 3.5 g/day of DHA+EPA versus corn oil on cardiac events in post-MI patients after 1.5 years of intervention.[61] The Dart 2 trial also reported no benefit of oily fish and an apparent adverse effect of fish oil supplements on CVD mortality.[62] Risk for death from CVD and for sudden cardiac death was actually higher among subjects advised to consume oily fish (HR = 1.26; 95% CI: 1.00–1.58; P = 0.047) compared with the control group (HR = 1.54; 95% CI: 1.06–2.23; P = 0.025). The adverse effect of the advice to eat oily fish was observed primarily in those assigned to fish oil supplements (n = 462). Thus, further research is needed to confirm the role of omega-3 fatty acid supplements for secondary prevention of coronary disease.

In general, major clinical trials in secondary prevention of CVD showed an inverse association with n-3 fatty acids and morbidity or mortality from CVD. However, conflicting results have been reported in patients with an implantable cardioverter defibrillator assigned to receive n-3 supplement, showing either protective or no effect on arrhythmic and cardiac death.[63–65] More so, a study has also shown that fish oil supplementation does not reduce the risk of ventricular tachycardia or ventricular fibrillation in this population and may be pro-arrhythmic in some patients.[63]

In general, LDL-C and HDL-C are not changes. However, Harris et al. reported that high doses of omega-3 fatty acids can decrease triglycerides levels by 25%–30% with an associated increase of 1%–3% in HDL-cholesterol and a 5%–10% increase in LDL-cholesterol.[66] Current guidelines recommend at least two servings of fatty fish per week (such as mackerel, lake trout, herring, sardines, albacore tuna, and salmon) in conjunction with the inclusion of vegetable oils and food sources high in α-linolenic acids (canola, soybean oils, flaxseed, walnuts) for most individuals.[15,52] In patients with documented CVD, EPA and DHA supplements could be considered in addition to the consumption of 1 g daily of EPA + DHA from varied fatty fish. In patients with high levels of TG, 2–4 g of EPA + DHA daily are sometimes recommended, ideally from supplements under medical supervision. Thus, diets using PUFA as the predominant form of dietary fat, whole grains as the main form of carbohydrate, an abundance of fruits and vegetables, and adequate intake of omega-3 fatty acids can offer significant protection against CVD.

## CARBOHYDRATE INTAKE AND GLYCEMIC INDEX

The replacement of saturated fat with carbohydrates reduces both LDL-C and HDL-C and, thus, has little effect on the LDL:HDL ratio.[41] Also, triglyceride levels increase when carbohydrates replace fats. These changes in diet would be expected to have minimal benefit on CVD risk. However, there might be a benefit if the carbohydrate is unrefined and has a low GI.[46]

Although controversial, the GI of foods is still a popular approach. David J. A. Jenkins has proposed the first table of GI of foods in 1981.[67] He has suggested that the proposed GI list may reflect the physiological effect of foods, since different carbohydrate foods with the same macronutrient composition can induce a different glycemic response. Per gram of carbohydrate, foods with a high GI produce a higher peak in postprandial blood glucose and a greater overall blood glucose response during the first 2 h following the consumption of the carbohydrate-rich food than do foods with a low GI. According to Jenkins, the GI of food is calculated using the area under the positive blood glucose response curve in response to the consumption of 50 g of carbohydrate provided by the proposed food divided by the area under the blood glucose response curve following the consumption of 50 g of carbohydrate provided by the control foods, generally white bread or sucrose.[67] Many food factors can influence the measure and the reproducibility of GI: (1) the type and the amount of protein and fat (decreases the blood glucose response), (2) the type and the amount

of carbohydrate (ratio of amylose and amylopectin in the selected food) and fiber (fiber reduces the rate of absorption of glucose from the gut), (3) food processing and cooking (rise in blood glucose and insulin following the consumption of cooked as opposed to raw foods, and increased time of cooking is associated with an increase in glycemic response), (4) the ripeness of the food (changes in composition of the fruits as they ripen can increase the glycemic response), and (5) food processing (grinding, extruding, and flaking can increase glycemic response).[68,69] And perhaps most important foods are typically eaten together, and the GI is variably affected by overall content of the consumption. It is reported that consuming low-GI index meals can increase HDL-cholesterol concentrations, decrease LDL-cholesterol and triglycerides concentrations, and increase satiety.[70,71] Moreover, an observational study showed that the chronic consumption of a diet with a high glycemic load (GI × dietary carbohydrate content) is independently associated with an increase risk of CVD.[72] Accordingly, the EPIC-MORGEN study showed that a high GI and glycemic load, and high carbohydrate and starch intake were associated with increased risk of CVD in men.[73] Moreover, consumption of sugar-sweetened beverages was associated with increased risk of CVD and some adverse changes in lipids, inflammatory factors, and leptin in men.[74]

The low-GI foods include the majority of fruits and vegetables, legumes, and whole wheat bread, whereas high-GI foods include refined cereal products such as white bread, potatoes, and rice. In general, when glucose is used as the standard for the GI measure, it is recommended to consume most often foods having a low-GI, equal or lower than 55, to consume periodically foods having a GI between 56 and 69 and avoid those that are higher than 70.[75] However, it is generally agreed that there is a need for long-term clinical trials to establish the clinical relevance and the use of GI in relation to weight regulation, obesity, type 2 diabetes, and CVD.

## CARDIOVASCULAR EFFECT OF NONCONVENTIONAL (POPULAR) DIETS

Considering the alarming increase in the incidence and the prevalence of obesity and diabetes, it has been noted that a large proportion of people experiment popular diets that promote spectacular weight loss without efforts advocating important changes in carbohydrate and lipid consumption. Many of these diets restrain consumption of carbohydrate and increase lipid consumption in order to restrict daily caloric consumption and increase satiety. Only a few important studies, mostly randomized controlled trials, have compared such diets and evaluated their impact on CVD risk factors. The adherence rate and the effectiveness of four popular diets (Atkins, Zone, Weight Watcher, and Ornish) were compared in the study of Dansinger et al.[76] They observed only a modest reduction in body weight at 1 year, without any differences between diets. All diets decrease LDL-C except for the Atkins diet (very low-carbohydrate diet) and all diets increased HDL-C except for the Ornish diet (very low-fat diet). None had an impact on triglycerides, blood pressure, or fasting glucose over 1 year. Changes in body weight, in lipid profile, in fasting glucose and in blood pressure were compared between four popular weight-loss diets (Atkins, Zone, Ornish, and LEARN) in a cohort of overweight/obese premenopausal women. Weight loss in the Atkins group was significantly greater compared to the other diets. More so, these diets induce the greater decrease in HDL-C, in triglycerides, and in systolic blood pressure. In general, evidence indicates that very low-carbohydrate diets (<20–30 g CHO per day) can be better in terms of short-term weight loss and improvement of some CVD risk factors (within 6 months) relative to traditional low-fat diets. However, these differences dissipated after 12 months, and important dropouts were observed (20%–40% of the study population). Overall, these popular diets induce only modest changes in body weight and CVD risk factors, and adherence to the dietary changes difficult to follow in the long run.[77]

## PHYSICAL ACTIVITY

Increasing levels of physical activity is also essential to achieve cardiovascular fitness and to induce weight loss. Moreover, physical activity helps reduce the risk for all-cause mortality, CVD, stroke, hypertension, and type 2 diabetes in adults and older adults.[78] Both the American College of Sports Medicine and the U.S. Physical Activity Guidelines Advisory Committee generally support 30–60 min/day of moderate to vigorous intensity physical activity in sedentary individuals on most if not all days of the week.[78,79] The amount of moderate to vigorous intensity activity most consistently associated with the prevention of unhealthy weight gain or significant weight loss by physical activity alone is in the range of 3–5 h/week.

## DIETARY PLANT STEROLS AND THEIR IMPACT ON LIPID PROFILE

Dietary phytosterols or plant sterols collectively imply plant-derived sterols and stanols. They have been documented to be effective in reducing total and LDL-C in normocholesterolemic and hypercholesterolemic subjects and thereby reduce cardiovascular risk.[80] However, dietary plant sterols do not generally affect HDL-C or triglycerides. Recent observations from animal and human studies have demonstrated reductions in the levels of pro-inflammatory cytokines, including c-reactive protein, after consumption of plant sterols.[81–83] The mechanism explaining cholesterol-lowering effects of plant sterols is by interference with the intestinal tract uptake of both dietary and biliary cholesterol in humans.[82] The NCEP-ATPIII recommends the addition of 2 g/day of plant sterols to the diet in patients at risk of CVD.[84] Plant sterols can be provided in small quantities in many fruits, vegetables, nuts, seeds, cereals, legumes, and other plant sources or incorporated into food products.

Moreover, the effectiveness of plant sterol added to foods such as margarine has reported up to a 15% reduction in total and LDL-C (181–184). The intake of 2–3 g of plant sterols per day was shown to decrease total and LDL-C by 9%–20% respectively, without altering HDL-C.[85–88]

Considering the potential of functional ingredients recognized by the AHA and the NCEP-ATPIII, which now advocate the use of viscous fibers and plant sterols, soy protein, and nuts, Jenkins et al. have compared the effectiveness of these functional ingredients to the traditional first-generation statin treatment (lovastatin) on lipid profile.[15,16,89] The "portfolio" diet reduced LDL-C (30%) and induced clinically significant reductions in the CVD risk. Interestingly, the dietary combinations of these functional ingredients may not differ from the effect of first-generation statin regarding the achieved lipid targets.[89]

## SOY PROTEIN, ISOFLAVONES, AND CHOLESTEROL LEVELS

Soy protein has been associated with a lowering effect of 5%–6% in LDL-C levels in response to protein substitution (animal for soy protein).[90] A meta-analysis showed that consuming a high-vegetable-protein diet in replacement of animal protein products can lower total cholesterol, LDL-C, and triglycerides by 4%–7% without affecting HDL-C.[91] However, these effects were more important when baseline total cholesterol levels were ≥230 mg/dL. Studies have examined dietary soy protein in the form of whole foods such as tofu, "soymilk," or as soy protein added to foods. Hence, others have focused on the specific components of soy, such as the soy phytoestrogen isoflavones. Somehow, the effects on HDL-C levels were inconsistent.[92,93] In moderately hypercholesterolemic men, the consumption of 20–50 g of soy protein per day induced a 3.0%–4.5% decrease in non-HDL-C concentration.[94] Moreover, phytoestrogen isoflavones have been largely associated with cholesterol reduction.[93] In this study, Crouse et al. demonstrated that 62 mg of isoflavones (which corresponded to approximately 30 g of whole soy) can decrease total cholesterol (9%) and LDL-C (10%) in hypercholesterolemic individuals compared to a casein diet. The related effects in reducing total and LDL-C may be explained by the substitution of soy products, which are naturally low in saturated fat and cholesterol, for animal protein, which are high in these constituents.

## CONCLUSION

Lifestyle and dietary modifications are important strategies in the management of CVD. Achieving a normal lipoprotein profile, body weight, and blood pressure is primordial in the prevention and treatment of CVD. Conventional dietary guidelines provide nutritional recommendations together with other healthy practices to reduce health complications. In conjunction with a suitable energy intake for maintaining a normal body weight, a dietary pattern that contains an optimal carbohydrate, protein, and fat dietary ratio should be consumed to improve lipid profiles and blood pressure. Evidence from metabolic studies, prospective cohort studies, and clinical trials indicates that diets using nonhydrogenated unsaturated fats as the predominant form of dietary fat, whole grains as the main form of carbohydrate (with a low-GI), an abundance of fruits and vegetables, and adequate ometa-3 fatty acids can offer significant protection against CVD. The ideal treatment for long-term abdominal obesity, hypertension, and CVD should be individualized, intensive, and under the supervision of qualified health-care professionals. Moreover, people should emphasize an intervention that aims to modify the whole dietary pattern, such as the Mediterranean style or the DASH eating pattern. Thus, the adoption of an optimal dietary pattern together with regular physical activity, maintenance of a healthy body weight, and avoidance of smoking may prevent the majority of CVD in Western populations.

## ACKNOWLEDGMENT

Annie Ferland is a recipient of a postdoctoral scholar from the Fond de la recherché en Santé du Québec (FRSQ).

## REFERENCES

1. Roger, VL, Go, AS, Lloyd-Jones, DM et al. *Circulation* 123:e18;2011.
2. Consensus conference. *JAMA* 253:2080;1985.
3. Gordon, T. *Am J Epidemiol* 127:220;1988.
4. Hu, FB, Willett, WC. *JAMA* 288:2569;2002.
5. Cornier, MA, Desprès, JP, Davis, N, et al. *Circulation* 124:1996;2011.
6. Center for Diseases Control and Prevention. Body mass index. http://www.cdc.gov/healthyweight/assessing/bmi/index.html. Accessed October 26, 2011.
7. Dagenais, GR, Yi, Q, Mann, JF et al. *Am Heart J* 149:54;2005.
8. de Koning, L, Merchant, AT, Pogue, J et al. *Eur Heart J* 28:850;2007.
9. National Institutes of Health. *The Practical Guide to the Identification, Evaluation, and Treatment of Overweight and Obesity in Adults*. NIH, Rockville, MD, 2002.
10. Pouliot, MC, Desprès, JP, Nadeau, A et al. *Diabetes* 41:826;1992.
11. Lemieux, I, Pascot, A, Couillard, C et al. *Circulation* 102:179;2000.
12. Yusuf, S, Hawken, S, Ounpuu, S et al. *Lancet* 364:937;2004.
13. Desprès, JP. *A Can J Cardiol* 8:561;1992.
14. Eckel, RH, Krauss, RM. *Circulation* 97:2099;1998.
15. Lichtenstein, AH, Appel, LJ, Brands, M et al. *Circulation* 114:82;2006.
16. Third Report of the National Cholesterol Education Program (NCEP) Expert Panel on Detection, Evaluation, and Treatment of High Blood Cholesterol in Adults (Adult Treatment Panel III) final report. *Circulation* 106:3143;2002.
17. Klein, S, Burke, LE, Bray, GA et al. *Circulation* 110:2952;2004.
18. Appel, LJ, Moore, TJ, Obarzanek, E et al. *New Engl J Med* 336:1117;1997.
19. Vollmer, WM, Sacks, FM, Ard, J et al. *Ann Intern Med* 135:1019;2001.
20. Sacks, FM, Svetkey, LP, Vollmer, WM et al. *New Engl J Med* 344:3;2001.
21. U.S. Department of Health and Human Services. *Dietary Guidelines for Americans*, Washington, DC, 2010.
22. Fung, TT, Willett, WC, Stampfer, MJ et al. *Arch Intern Med* 161:1857;2001.
23. Chobanian, AV, Bakris, GL, Black, HR et al. *JAMA* 289:2560;2003.
24. de Lorgeril, M, Salen, P, Martin, JL et al. *Circulation* 99:779;1999.
25. De Lorgeril, M, Salen, P, Martin, JL et al. *J Am Coll Cardiol* 28:1103;1996.
26. Tuttle, KR, Shuler, LA, Packard, DP et al. *Am J Cardiol* 101:1523;2008.
27. Estruch, R, Martinez-Gonzalez, MA, Corella, D et al. *Ann Intern Med* 145:1;2006.
28. Goulet, J, Lapointe, A, Lamarche, B et al. *Eur J Clin Nutr* 61:1293;2007.
29. Lapointe, A, Goulet, J, Couillard, C et al. *J Nutr* 135:410;2005.
30. Richard, C, Couture, P, Desroches, S et al. *Nutr Metab Cardiovasc Dis* 21:628;2011.
31. Shai, I, Schwarzfuchs, D, Henkin, Y et al. *New Engl J Med* 359:229;2008.
32. Nordmann, AJ, Suter-Zimmermann, K, Bucher, HC et al. *Am J Med* 124:841;2011.
33. McCullough, ML, Feskanich, D, Rimm, EB et al. *Am J Clin Nutr* 72:1223;2000.
34. Kant, AK, Schatzkin, A, Graubard, BI et al. *JAMA* 283:2109;2000.
35. Halton, TL, Willett, WC, Liu, S et al. *New Engl J Med* 355:1991;2006.
36. Stampfer, MJ, Hu, FB, Manson, JE et al. *New Engl J Med* 343:16;2000.
37. Farchi, G, Mariotti, S, Menotti, A et al. *Am J Clin Nutr* 50:1095;1989.
38. Brunner, EJ, Mosdol, A, Witte, DR et al. *Am J Clin Nutr* 87:1414;2008.
39. Millen, BE, Quatromoni, PA, Nam, BH et al. *J Am Diet Ass* 104:208;2004.
40. Heidemann, C, Schulze, MB, Franco, OH et al. *Circulation* 118:230;2008.
41. Mensink, RP, Katan, MB. *Arterio Thrombol* 12:911;1992.
42. Leren, P. *Circulation* 42:935;1970.
43. Hu, FB, van Dam, RM, Liu, S. *Diabetologia* 44:805;2001.
44. Salmeron, J, Hu, FB, Manson, JE et al. *Am J Clin Nutr* 73:1019;2001.
45. Appel, LJ, Sacks, FM, Carey, VJ et al. *JAMA* 294:2455;2005.
46. Astrup, A, Dyerberg, J, Elwood, P et al. *Am J Clin Nutr* 93:684;2011.
47. Mensink, RP, Katan, MB. *N Engl J Med* 323:439;1990.
48. Judd, JT, Baer, DJ, Clevidence, BA et al. *Lipids* 37:123;2002.
49. Judd, JT, Clevidence, BA, Muesing, RA et al. *Am J Clin Nutr* 59:861;1994.
50. Lichtenstein, AH, Ausman, LM, Jalbert, SM et al. *N Engl J Med* 340:1933;1999.
51. Hu, FB, Stampfer, MJ, Manson, JE et al. *N Engl J Med* 337:1491;1997.
52. Kris-Etherton, PM, Harris, WS, Appel, LJ. *Circulation* 106:2747;2002.
53. De Caterina, R. n-3 Fatty acids in cardiovascular disease. *N Engl J Med* 364:2439;2011.
54. Connor, WE. *Am J Clin Nutr* 71:171S;2000.
55. Burr, ML, Fehily, AM, Gilbert, JF et al. *Lancet* 2:757;1989.

56. Gruppo Italiano per lo Studio della Sopravvivenza nell'Infarto miocardico. *Lancet* 354:447;1999.
57. Marchioli, R, Barzi, F, Bomba, E et al. *Circulation* 105:1897;2002.
58. Tavazzi, L, Maggioni, AP, Marchioli, R et al. *Lancet* 372:1223;2008.
59. Yokoyama, M, Origasa, H, Matsuzaki, M et al. *Lancet* 369:1090;2007.
60. Kromhout, D, Giltay, EJ, Geleijnse, JM. *N Engl J Med* 3(63):2015;2010.
61. Nilsen, DW, Albrektsen, G, Landmark, K et al. *Am J Clin Nutr* 74:50;2001.
62. Burr, ML, Ashfield-Watt, PA, Dunstan, FD et al. *Eur J Clin Nutr* 57:193;2003.
63. Raitt, MH, Connor, WE, Morris, C et al. *JAMA* 293:2884;2005.
64. Brouwer, IA, Zock, PL, Wever, EF et al. *Eur J Clin Nutr* 57:1323;2003.
65. Christensen, JH, Riahi, S, Schmidt, EB et al. *Cardiology* 7:338;2005.
66. Harris, WS. *Lipids* 31:243;1996.
67. Jenkins, DJ, Wolever, TM, Taylor, RH et al. *Am J Clin Nutr* 34:362;1981.
68. Pi-Sunyer, FX. *Am J Clin Nutr* 76:290S;2002.
69. Brand, JC, Nicholson, PL, Thorburn, AW et al. *Am J Clin Nutr* 42:1192;1985.
70. Ford, ES, Liu, S. *Arch Intern Med* 161:572;2001.
71. Jenkins, DJ, Wolever, TM, Kalmusky, J et al. *Am J Clin Nutr* 42:604;1985.
72. Liu, S, Willett, WC, Stampfer, MJ et al. *Am J Clin Nutr* 71:1455;2000.
73. Burger, KN, Beulens, JW, Boer, JM et al. *PloS one* 6:e25955;2011.
74. de Koning, L, Malik, VS, Kellogg, MD et al. *Circulation* 12:2012.
75. Foster-Powell, K, Holt, SH, Brand-Miller, JC. *Am J Clin Nutr* 76:5;2002.
76. Dansinger, ML, Gleason, JA, Griffith, JL et al. *JAMA* 293.43,2005.
77. Gardner, CD, Kiazand, A, Alhassan, S, et al. *JAMA* 297:969;2007.
78. Haskell, WL, Lee, IM, Pate, RR et al. *PMed Sci Sports Exerc* 39:1423;2007.
79. U.S. Department of Health and Human Services. Physical activity guidelines advisory committee report, Washington, DC, 2008.
80. Abumweis, SS, Barake, R, Jones, PJ. *Food Nutr Res* 52:2008.
81. Devaraj, S, Autret, BC, Jialal, I. *Am J Clin Nutr* 84:756;2006.
82. Jones, PJ, Demonty, I, Chan, YM et al. *Lipids* 6:28;2007.
83. Nashed, B, Yeganeh, B, HayGlass, KT et al. *J Nutr* 135:2438;2005.
84. Grundy, SM. *Am J Cardiol* 96:47D;2005.
85. Miettinen, TA, Puska, P, Gylling, H et al. *N Engl J Med* 333:1308;1995.
86. Gylling, H, Miettinen, TA. *Diabetologia* 37:773;1994.
87. Patch, CS, Tapsell, LC, Williams, PG. *J Am Coll Nutr* 105:46;2005.
88. Cater, NB, Garcia-Garcia, AB, Vega, GL et al. *Am J Cardiol* 96:23D;2005.
89. Jenkins, DJ, Kendall, CW, Marchie, A et al. *Eur J Clin Nutr* 59:851;2005.
90. Sacks, FM, Lichtenstein, A, Van Horn, L et al. *Circulation* 113:1034;2006.
91. Anderson, JW, Johnstone, BM, Cook-Newell, ME. *N Engl J Med* 333:276;1995.
92. Wong, WW, Smith, EO, Stuff, JE et al. *Am J Clin Nutr* 68:1385S;1998.
93. Crouse, JR, 3rd, Morgan, T, Terry, JG et al. *Arch Intern Med* 159:2070;1999.
94. Teixeira, SR, Potter, SM, Weigel, R et al. *Am J Clin Nutr* 71:1077;2000.
95. Appel, LJ et al. *Hypertension* 47(2):296;2006.

# 62 Nutrition and the Gastrointestinal Tract

*Harry L. Greene*

## CONTENTS

## INTRODUCTION

No organ is more essential to the maintenance of adequate nutrition than the gastrointestinal (GI) tract. The lining of the GI tract consists of a single layer of highly specialized columnar epithelial cells that interface between the external and internal environments. Its primary function is the transfer of dietary constituents from the bowel lumen into the circulation. Consequently, the GI tract must convert the varied physical and chemical forms of food into simple molecules that can be easily transferred across cell membranes. This process requires coordinated motor activity and secretion of digestive enzymes that alter chemical properties of food. Subsequently, intact transport mechanisms across cell membranes are necessary to accomplish the final transfer of vital nutrients into the blood or lymphatics. Finally, assimilation of essential nutrients must be done from food sources alien, and often hostile, to the body. Failure of any of these processes can result in malabsorption, immune dysfunction, or bacterial invasion.

Advances in our understanding of basic anatomy, physiology, and biochemistry, as well as clinical nutrition, have fostered the development of "ideally" digestible and utilizable foods. The purpose of these foods is to provide a diet in a form that will provide optimal nutritional support during periods of illness when there is damage to one or more of the GI functions. A review of the basic mechanisms involved in digestion and absorption of nutrients and how these mechanisms are affected by various diseases is the topic of this chapter.

## ANATOMY AND PHYSIOLOGY

### Esophagus

The esophagus is a hollow tube of striated and smooth muscle with a length of 25–35 cm in the adult. A specialized arrangement of semicircular muscle fibers at the lower end of the esophagus termed the *gastroesophageal ring* represents the lower esophageal sphincter (LES). The function of the LES is to allow the passage of material coming from the mouth and the prevention of regurgitation of gastric contents back into the low-pressure area of the esophagus. The LES relaxation in response to swallowing is mediated primarily by the vagus nerve; however, a number of humoral agents can alter the LES pressure. Among the agents that raise LES pressure are gastrin, histamine, metoclopramide, cholinergic drugs (such as bethanecol), diazepam, and a protein meal.[1] Examples of agents that lower LES pressure are glucagon, estrogens and progesterone, isoproterenol, atropine, alcohol, and fats; smoking is also known to lower LES pressure. Increasing numbers of infants, children, adults, and the aging population have abnormalities in the LES and suffer from acid erosions in the lower esophagus.

### Stomach

The two main functions of the stomach relate to its secretory function that aids digestion and its motor activity.

### Secretory Function

The stomach secretes sodium, potassium, hydrochloric acid, pepsinogen, intrinsic factor, and mucus into the gastric lumen and gastrin into the blood. These highly acidic secretions participate in the breakdown of proteins (pepsinogen is activated to the proteolytic enzyme pepsin), but most importantly they dissolve soluble foods and bring the ingested material close to the osmolality of plasma. Bactericidal action is prominent, as gastric juice has a pH of about 1.0. Intrinsic factor, which is essential for absorption of vitamin $B_{12}$ in the ileum, is secreted in relatively large amounts by the gastric mucosa.

#### Acid Secretion

The major physiological stimulant to acid secretion by the oxyntic, or parietal, cells is the ingestion of meals. Two factors are known to be operative when food is present in the stomach: gastric distention and chemical stimulation of gastrin release. Distention of the stomach results in a small but significant stimulation of acid secretion. When various food components were studied for acid-stimulating activity, amino acids and partially digested protein were found to be effective, while glucose and fat caused no stimulation.[2] The increase in gastrin accounted for most of the observed acid secretory response. Phenylalanine and tryptophan were the most potent of amino acids in release of gastrin and stimulants of acid secretion in humans. Chemical stimulation, however, is not entirely mediated by gastrin; caffeine and alcohol stimulate acid secretion without an increase in gastrin.

Histamine is another of the best-defined chemical messengers that regulate acid secretion. It appears to act at a separate receptor on the *oxyntic* cells, and potentiating interactions have been reported to occur with the other secretagogues. All the factors regulating histamine release have not been defined, but the reduction in acid secretion following $H_2$-receptor antagonists leaves little doubt that histamine has an important role in acid secretion.

#### Pepsin

Pepsinogen is secreted by gastric peptic (or chief) cells as a precursor to pepsin. The inactive pepsinogen released is activated by gastric acid and the optimal pH is 2. In addition, pepsin itself activates pepsinogen. Pepsin digestion of protein is incomplete, cleaving at aromatic amino acid residues to yield various peptides. As stomach contents pass into the duodenum, pepsin is inactivated by the more alkaline pH present there.

### Motor Functions

The stomach is required to adapt to an ingested meal in two ways: It must relax to receive a volume sometimes exceeding a liter in a matter of minutes, and it must initiate and maintain coordinated peristaltic activity to mix and slowly empty its contents into the small intestine.

Proximal gastric relaxation occurs with each swallow as well as in response to distention during filling. This response leads to an increase in volume with little rise in intragastric pressure. Gastrin can increase motility; however, activity is decreased by vagotomy, catecholamines, and secretin. The midpoint of the greater curvature is considered to behave like the pacemaker of the stomach. The coordination of phase lag assures that the peristaltic waves will proceed smoothly from greater curvature to the pylorus.

After ingestion of a liquid meal, the normal stomach empties in an exponential pattern, as regulated by the proximal stomach. When emptying of discrete solid particles is examined, emptying patterns are approximately linear with time and are regulated by the antrum. Thus, with a mixed meal containing both solid and liquid components, there are two patterns of emptying, with the liquid emptying more rapidly than the solid. The following are other factors that may also influence gastric emptying.

### Osmolality

Osmoreceptors that appear to be situated in the jejunum rather than in the duodenum affect gastric emptying rate. Solutions that are either hyperosmolar or hypo-osmolar to extracellular physiological tonicity cause slower gastric emptying than the corresponding isotonic solution.

### Acid

Intraduodenal acid retards gastric emptying, the magnitude of the effect being proportional to the concentration of the acid.

### Fats

Fatty acids with chain lengths of 12 and 14 carbon atoms are potent inhibitors of gastric emptying. Less slowing is brought about by fatty acids with a chain length of 16–18 carbon atoms. Unsaturated fats retard emptying more than do saturated fats.[3]

### Amino Acids

Although recent work has suggested that tryptophan is a potent inhibitor of gastric emptying, the effect of other amino acids appears to be related more to osmotic changes than to a specific action of the amino acid.

### Energy Density

Higher energy density promotes slower gastric emptying. Whether or not this is controlled by a sensory system is unclear.

### Temperature

The rate of emptying of solutions that are colder or warmer than body temperature reduces gastric emptying.

### Posture

Posture influences gastric emptying to some extent. Liquids are emptied more rapidly when a subject is in a sitting position or is lying on the right side. With a solid meal, emptying in normal subjects is much the same as in the erect or recumbent position.

## SMALL INTESTINE

### Histology

The length of the small intestine in the newborn infant is about 200 cm. It elongates with age, so that by adulthood the length ranges from 700 to 800 cm. While the intestine grows in length, it also grows in diameter. Therefore, at birth, the calculated surface area of the intestine is about 950 cm$^2$ and increases to about 7600 cm$^2$ by adulthood. A normal 4 kg infant ingests about 500 cal/day. If the average adult requires 2200 cal of intake, simple mathematics shows that an infant has only 2 cm$^2$ of small intestine to absorb 1 cal, whereas the adult has about 3.5 cm$^2$. This difference accounts for what can be called the *intestinal reserve capacity* of an adult. Almost half of an adult's intestine can be removed before the efficiency of absorption approximates that of the infant's intestine. For this reason, infants do not tolerate intestinal surgery as well as adults. On the other hand, the infant, by virtue of his growth potential, has the ability to greatly increase the length and diameter of the intestine, whereas the adult has a greatly limited capacity for this adaptation. The adult who has 90% of his gut removed surgically may not survive, whereas the infant will increase the length of the remaining segment as he grows in height, and eventually, a relatively efficient intestinal tract can develop.[4]

The luminal surface of the small intestine is so organized that the surface area available for contact with intestinal contents is greatly amplified by readily visible spiral or circular concentric folds called *plicae circulares*, most prominent in the distal duodenum and proximal jejunum. The plicae are covered by another series of infoldings called *villi* that in turn are covered by a single layer of epithelial cells. At low magnifications in the scanning electron microscope, the overall villous pattern can be seen (Figure 62.1). While finger villi are regarded as the norm, leaf-shaped and tongue-shaped villi are not unusual. Epithelial cells migrate from the crypts to the tip of the villi, and as migration progresses, maturation and differentiation of cell functions occur. The principal cells of the villi, generally termed *enterocytes*, have as their most distinctive feature the apical striated border composed of microvilli. This striated border provides the vast digestive–absorptive surface area essential for nutrition. Of particular note is the fact that only one layer of cells separates the external environment from the blood, yet bacteria are effectively excluded.

### Digestive–Absorptive Sequence

Digestion is the process by which the large molecules in the diet are broken down into smaller ones acceptable to the enterocytes. In the case of fat, it also includes converting water-insoluble substances into water-miscible ones. Absorption is the process by which the contents of the small bowel enter the mucosal epithelial cells and eventually the portal vein or the lymphatics.

Substances that cross the membrane of the enterocyte may do so by one of three mechanisms: simple diffusion,

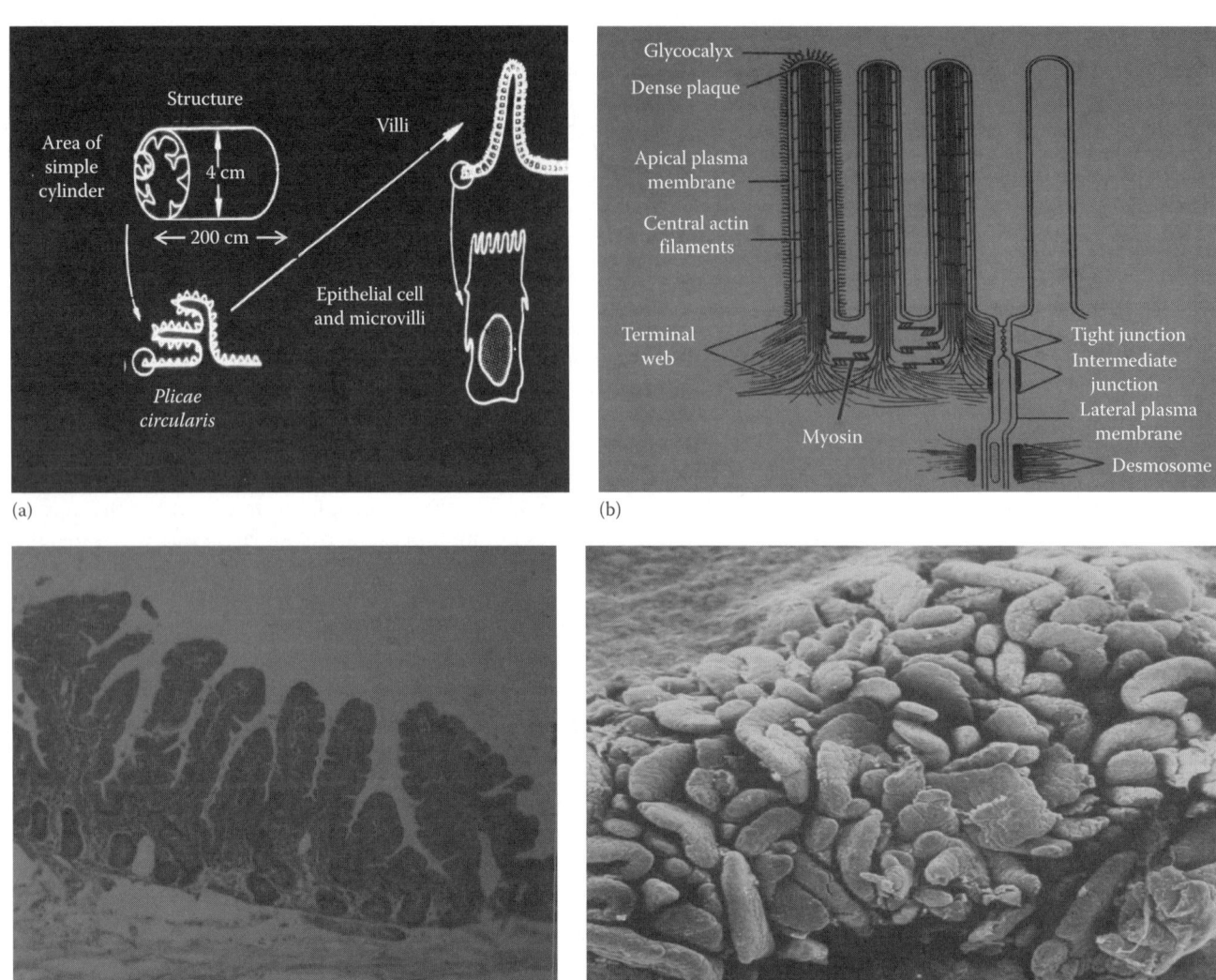

**FIGURE 62.1** (a) Diagram depicting the folds of the intestine as well as the microvilli of individual cells. (b) Diagram of the structure of microvilli and tight junction between cells. (c) Normal light microscopy of a normal jejuna biopsy (hematoxylin and eosin, ×100). (d) Scanning electron micrograph (about 100×) of normal jejunal biopsy specimen showing a normal villus pattern with both fingerlike projections as well as broader villus projections.

facilitated diffusion, or active transport. The importance of these mechanisms is related to the transport kinetics—that is, an active transport mechanism is capable of saturation and sensitive to competition. Thus, if an actively absorbed substance is present in excess, the mechanism becomes overloaded and the actual absorption site then moves distally. Also, if two substances that are actively absorbed by the same mechanism are present simultaneously, competition will cause each to be absorbed less efficiently and, again, the absorption site moves distally.

Some of the other factors that determine where and how much is absorbed are its physicochemical state, molecular weight, osmolality, and blood flow to the bowel. Exceptions are vitamin $B_{12}$ and bile acids, which are absorbed in the distal ileum. In addition, it has been found that adjacent to all biologic membranes, there is a layer of relatively unstirred water, through which movement of solute molecules is

determined only by diffusional forces. Such a layer exerts a major portion of the total resistance encountered by molecules during its passage from the intestinal lumen into the cell interior and constitutes the rate-limiting step to uptake of long-chain fatty acids and cholesterol by the enterocyte.[5]

**Intestinal Immune System**

As only a lining of single cells must assimilate essential nutrients from food, it must also prevent invasion by bacteria and other potentially noxious agents. It is not surprising that the immune system is so evident in the GI tract. Elements of the intestinal immune system include (1) lymphocytes scattered between the cells of the GI epithelium, (2) lymphocytes and macrophages scattered diffusely in the lamina propria of the stomach and intestine, and (3) differentiated lymphoid structures located along the course of the GI tract. The latter, which include the tonsils, the Peyer's patches, and the lymphoid structures of the appendix, are the initial site of interaction between many antigens and the immune system. The overlying epithelial surface contains T-lymphocytes, which appear to facilitate the binding and entry of antigens. Memory cells produced in response to antigens migrate to other parts of the body and the intestine via the general circulation. Reexposure to antigens leads to differentiation of these memory cells into plasma cells that produce type-specific IgA or IgE.[6]

Plasma cells in the lamina propria of the gut synthesize and secrete immunoglobulins including antibodies directed against antigens present in the gut lumen. Plasma cells produce IgA in contrast to other lymphoid tissues where IgG is the predominants immunoglobulin produced. IgA enters the intestinal lumen with two additional peptide chains: one of these, the secretory component, protects the IgA from luminal digestion: the second facilitates polymerization. Secretory IgA may prevent bacterial adherence to the mucosal surfaces, but it does not appear to fix complement.[7]

**Factors Affecting Gastrointestinal Function**

*Maturation*

The newborn GI tract undergoes many maturational changes during the first months of life. During the first 3–4 months, sucking reflexes are present, while extrusion reflexes protect against introduction of potentially indigestible solids. Esophageal motility is present at birth, but coordination of propulsive waves does not develop until after 4 months of postnatal life. LES pressure remains low, and the intragastric pressure often exceeds the esophageal and LES pressure. This results in a high incidence of "spitting" of gastric contents for the first 3–6 months of life. Gastric motility is poorly coordinated for 3–4 months, which leads to poor antral mixing and therefore less digestion of solid foods than after 4 months of age. Usually at 12 weeks, intestinal peristalsis of a type seen in older children and adults develops, but it is approximately one-third slower. The slower transit may serve to increase exposure time to the intestinal mucosa and thereby improve nutrient digestions and absorption. The motor function in the large intestine appears to be fully mature at birth.

Intestinal mucosal permeability is greatest during the neonatal period, and many large molecules, including proteins such as immunoglobulins, tend to be absorbed intact. This process provides a mechanism for passive transfer of antibodies from mother's milk but also permits the passage of whole proteins with a potential to provoke allergic responses. The relationship between ingestion of whole cow's milk and anemia from chronic intestinal blood loss during the first few months of life appears to result from this mechanism. Other nonhuman protein foods may also cause changes in the first 6 months of life.

*Secretory and Absorptive Functions*

These functions of the intestine mature during the first 2 years of life. In general, animal fat is less well digested and absorbed than vegetable oils by infants. The intestinal mucosal alpha-glucosidases (sucrose, maltase, isomaltase)

are well developed by 32 weeks of gestation and are present at near-adult levels at the time of the term delivery. By contract, the beta-galactosidase, lactase, develops late in fetal life and does not reach maximal activity until feeding begins. In spite of the relatively low lactase activity, formulas containing lactose are well tolerated by term infants and many infants over 34 weeks' gestation. For extremely premature infants (27–32 weeks' gestation), formulas with less than 60% of total carbohydrate calories as lactose are generally best tolerated.

*Senescence*

Age-related changes in intestinal function occur simultaneously with loss of lean body mass. Impaired glucose homeostasis, decreased clearance of drugs, variability in temperature control, and deterioration in immunologic function also occur with the alteration in GI function. Other changes include loss of dentition, reduced taste and smell acuity, esophageal dysmotility and delayed gastric emptying, hypochlorhydria, a tendency to ischemia, and intestinal amyloidosis. These factors and the frequent use of medication in the elderly may all contribute to impaired GI tract function and an increased tendency toward malnutrition. Many of the physiological changes observed with aging (immune senescence, reduction in visceral protein levels, decreased lean body mass) are similar to those observed in malnutrition in younger subjects,[8] although normal aging alone does not appear to impair protein-energy absorption substantially. Gastric emptying and intestinal transit are slowed, and the efficiency of absorption, particularly of vitamin A, may be improved as a result. On the other hand, absorption of vitamin $B_{12}$, calcium, and zinc seems to be impaired in the elderly.

*Adaptation*

The GI tract is capable of extensive adaptation, particularly in children. Where intestinal function is marginal (as may occur after extensive resection), the residual intestine is capable of considerable dilation, increase in rugosity, and hypertrophy of villi and microvilli. Increased surface area and absorptive capacity result. Cell turnover and enzyme activities increase. These adaptive changes can be maximized by mucosal exposure to nutrients, pancreatic and biliary secretions, and by certain hormonal factors that remain unidentified. The search for trophic hormones has important therapeutic implication, but no candidates have shown conclusive growth-stimulating activity in the small intestine. Gastrin's trophic action affects primarily the esophagus, stomach, colon, and pancreas and may play some role in adaptation of the small intestine. Cholecystokinin and secretion are mildly trophic to the small intestine, but this reaction may be due to their stimulation of bile and pancreatic secretions. Factors that limit intestinal adaptation include inadequate blood supply, poor nutritional status, and the presence of residual disease. The ileum is better able to adapt than the jejunum, which cannot assume certain specialized functions of the ileum such as active absorption of vitamin $B_{12}$ and bile salts. Slower transit in the ileum may improve absorptive capacity but conversely provides a better milieu for bacterial overgrowth.

## DISEASE AND IATROGENIC FACTORS

### DISEASE FACTORS

Abnormalities of GI function may produce manifestations that vary in nutritional importance from the mild discomfort of colonic spasm or heartburn to the debilitating or fatal consequences of regional enteritis or cancer. Many disorders affect more than one facet of gut activity, but in assessing the nutritional significance of any disorder, it is beneficial to consider its impact on each stage of assimilation (ingestion, luminal digestion, motility, brush border activity, transport, and intestinal vascular supply).

Congenital anomalies are usually manifested during infancy or early childhood and are composed primarily of atresias, abnormalities of rotation, duplications, and ano-rectal anomalies. Congenital enzyme deficiencies (disaccharidase, enterokinase, or lipase deficiencies and transport disorders) may also cause malabsorption. Reduction in biliary and pancreatic secretions produces severe fat malabsorption and less severe malabsorption of other nutrients. Immune deficiency syndromes frequently are associated with malabsorption, pernicious anemia, and increased GI infections. Enteropathy caused by sensitivity to cow's milk protein or soy protein and eosinophilic gastroenteritis (EGE) are examples of abnormal responses of the intestinal epithelium to whole-food proteins.[9] Abnormalities of motility that prevent appropriate delivery of food (achalasia, pyloric stenosis) or affect intestinal transit, producing bacterial overgrowth (pseudo-obstruction, diabetic neuropathy), may result in bacterial deconjugation of bile salts and associated steatorrhea with severe nutrient deficiencies. Peptide-secreting endocrine tumors may result in watery diarrhea and malabsorption. Diseases involving the bowel wall (Whipple's disease, inflammatory bowel disease [IBD], scleroderma) may cause abnormalities of motility, secretion, digestion, and absorption with attendant malabsorption and diarrhea. In addition, vascular insufficiency, endocrine disorders (hypopituitarism, thyrotoxicosis), malignant tumors, and other remote conditions frequently compromise gut function.

### SURGERY

The surgical procedures that most commonly have impact on nutritional status are those performed for peptic ulcer disease and those involving small bowel resection. Approximately 10%–25% of postgastrectomy patients have disabling symptoms of nausea, vomiting, or diarrhea. Weight loss of 10–15 lb and mild steatorrhea are almost universal after partial gastrectomy, as is lactose intolerance. Malabsorption of vitamin B$_{12}$, iron, and calcium may produce symptoms but usually responds to supplementation. The bacterial overgrowth that is common to some degree often responds to broad-spectrum antibiotics. Symptoms due to dumping can usually be handled with dietary restriction of foods with high osmolarity (i.e., reduction of simple carbohydrate load, juices, and certain soups). Although resection of up to 50% of the small bowel is well tolerated, adverse prognostic factors include loss of ileum, rather than jejunum; loss of the ileocecal valve; residual disease of the intestine, liver, or pancreas; advanced age; and massive resection.

### RADIATION

The severity of radiotherapy-induced damage to the GI tract depends upon the total dose given and the time elapsed between exposures. Intestinal fibrosis due to small vessel ischemia results in mucosal dysfunction, disordered motility with bacterial overgrowth, and, at times, severe malabsorption.

### MEDICATIONS

Many medications interact luminally with specific nutrients to alter availability for absorption or to affect their actions or metabolism. Some directly affect gut function and impair nutrient absorption. Examples of commonly used drugs that affect nutrition are neomycin, colchicines, sulfasalazine, diphenylhydantoin, alcohol, and cytotoxic agents.

With dietary guidance, nutrient supplementation, and adequate treatment of the primary disease, the GI tract can withstand considerable insult and yet maintain acceptable nutritional status and activity. In cases of failure of the GI tract, a temporary period of total parenteral nutrition (TPN) can enable some patients to recover GI function. If no functional return is possible, permanent home parenteral nutrition may be provided.

## MOTOR DISORDERS THAT IMPAIR NUTRIENT DIGESTION/ABSORPTION

### DISORDERS OF SMOOTH MUSCLE

#### Primary Visceral Myopathy

A heterogeneous group of disorders (many described only recently) remains so poorly understood that it is best referred by the generic term primary visceral myopathy.[10] Smooth muscle, in these syndromes, shows various degrees of damage ranging from vacuolization to replacement with collagen. Some cases are familial: families with both dominant and recessive transmission have been reported. Most cases, however, are sporadic: the patients give no history of affected relatives. Various parts of the gut may be selectively affected in patterns that are unpredictable, even in the familial syndromes. When the muscularis propria of the small intestine and stomach are diseased, nutrient delivery is severely impaired. Treatment in these extensive cases is limited to parenteral alimentation, which, though expensive, can be effective in prolonging life.

#### Scleroderma

The term scleroderma is used in a general sense to name a heterogeneous group of disorders characterized by occlusion of small vessels in the extremities and by changes that are probably secondary to occlusion, including cutaneous fibrosis, resorption of bone in the digits, pulmonary fibrosis, renal insufficiency, and fibrosis of visceral muscle. The classic form is the CREST syndrome, characterized by subcutaneous calcinosis, Reynaud's phenomenon, esophageal motor dysfunction, sclerodactyly, and cutaneous telangiectasia. In one rare form of the disease, localized scleroderma or morphea, visceral myopathy does not occur. Although the visceral myopathy can be the first evidence of the disease, it usually is not manifested clinically until other systems are involved. The muscular fibrosis is variable in extent but most commonly involved the esophagus. The muscle of the stomach, small intestine, and colon is less commonly affected. Malnutrition may be severe, and it can be treated only by parenteral alimentation.

## DISORDERS OF STRIATED MUSCLE

### Myotonic Dystrophy

Myotonic dystrophy is a dominant hereditary disorder characterized by dysfunction of the somatic musculature, premature balding, cataracts, and a variety of other disorders. The striated muscle of the pharynx and esophagus may be involved, giving rise to minor degrees of dysphagia, which, however, does not usually compromise nutrition. In some cases, there is also dysfunction of smooth muscle of the esophagus, stomach, and small intestine, but this is rarely severe and has received little study.

### Myasthenic Syndromes

In myasthenia, whether primary or secondary, the weakness of the striated musculature is often most severe in muscle innervated by the cranial nerves, including that of the pharynx and esophagus. The threat of aspiration pneumonia and the oropharyngeal dysphagia makes eating both difficult and dangerous, and nutritional impairment is common.

## DISORDERS OF NERVES

### Achalasia

The commonest and best studied visceral neuropathy is that in achalasia, a disorder confined to the nerves that supply the smooth muscle of the esophagus. The LES fails to relax and the smooth muscle of the distal esophagus fails to contract after a swallow. Food is retained in the flaccid esophagus, which may become enormously distended, and escapes into the stomach by hydrostatic force when that force is sufficient to breach the constantly contracted sphincter. Because this slow rate of flow into the stomach limits the rate at which nutrients are delivered to the intestine, impaired nutrition is a constant feature of the disease. The myenteric plexus of the esophagus in achalasia is depleted of ganglion cells. The pathogenesis of this selective neuropathy is unknown.

### Visceral Neuropathy of Diabetes

Severe motor dysfunction is found in some cases of diabetes mellitus, especially in diabetics who have developed vascular and peripheral neural complications. The motor functions of smooth muscle in the esophagus, stomach, and intestine are affected, but the problem of greatest clinical importance is delay in gastric emptying. This delay impairs nutrition

because of slow delivery of food to the intestine and because the gastric retention often leads to vomiting. "Tight" control of the diabetes is difficult because of the abnormal rate at which nutrients are delivered to the intestine. Although the problem is usually regarded as a visceral neuropathy, it has not been characterized anatomically. The seat of the lesion may be in the myenteric plexus itself, but some evidence suggests that the major defect is demyelination of the preganglionic nerves in the extrinsic nerve supply to the gut.

## DISORDERS OF UNKNOWN CAUSE

### Reflux Esophagitis and Its Consequences

Reflux of gastric contents into the esophagus is a common problem. Depending on its severity and duration, the reflux may lead to diffuse esophagitis, esophageal ulceration, and esophageal carcinoma. The physiological abnormalities that contribute to a pathological degree of reflux include defective contraction of the LES, defective peristalsis in the distal esophagus, and defective gastric emptying. Whether these disorders arise from dysfunction of muscle, nerves, or both is unclear.

### Anorexia Nervosa

Anorexia nervosa is usually considered to be a psychogenic derangement of unknown mechanisms of appetite and satiety. Recently, however, a physiological disturbance was detected in the form of delayed gastric emptying and depressed gastric secretion in anorexia nervosa. Whether these abnormalities of gastric function contribute to the cause of the anorexia or reflect a consequence of severe malnutrition is unclear.

## SPECIFIC DISORDERS THAT MAY AFFECT NUTRITION

### MALABSORPTION AND MALDIGESTION OF CARBOHYDRATES

In essence, the assimilation of carbohydrate depends on a series of sequential processes beginning with luminal hydrolysis (in the case of starch), followed by intestinal surface membrane digestion of all oligosaccharides, and terminating in the final transport of the released monosaccharides into and across the intestinal cell.[11] A defect in any stage of overall hydrolysis or transport may result in malassimilation of carbohydrate. Patients with severe pancreatic insufficiency may have mild maldigestion of starch because of greatly reduced amounts of pancreatic amylase. However, even 10% of the normal quantity of amylase appears to be sufficient to catalyze the digestion of starch to its final products because of the tremendous overabundance of pancreatic α-amylase present in the intestine under normal circumstances.

### Lactase Deficiency

Deficiencies of intestinal disaccharidases are relatively common. Indeed, more than half the world's population has lactase deficiency in adulthood resulting in a distinct symptom complex of abdominal fullness, bloating, mild nausea, and distention that occurs 15–30 min after ingestion of milk products containing lactose. Thirty minutes to 3 h later, individuals with lactase deficiency typically complain of cramping abdominal pain and passage of watery bowel movements. Notably, the absence of lactase in the intestinal surface membrane allows the lactose to remain in the intestinal lumen, where it is eventually metabolized by bacteria in the lower ileum and the colon to two- and three-carbon acids, hydrogen gas, and $CO_2$. These products produce both a marked osmotic effect and increased volumes of intraintestinal gasses. Increased fluid retained by osmotic forces produces distention of intestinal walls that in turn may stimulate motor activity and further augment the watery diarrhea. At times, secondary malabsorption of other nutrients and drugs also may occur.

Newborns of all racial groups have an abundance of intestinal lactase, and the acquired type of deficiency that has a genetic basis develops between the ages of 4 and 18 in population groups that are particularly susceptible. Whereas either an abundance of lactase or the absence of the enzyme may have provided a selective advantage in past generations, there is little evidence that large sections of the world's population were ever dependent on the intake of large amounts of milk to maintain adequate nutrition.

It has been well established that lactase is a relatively fragile digestive enzyme, which is depressed more readily by intestinal diseases than is the case with its companion oligosaccharidases. For example, studies of in vivo rates of hydrolysis in patients with generalized intestinal dysfunction caused by tropical sprue revealed that hydrolysis of sucrose and maltose is lowered by 40%–50%, whereas hydrolysis of lactose is depressed by 75%. This is particularly important because lactose hydrolysis is rate limiting for overall assimilation of this disaccharide in normal individuals. In addition to its relative sensitivity to intestinal injury, lactase often remains depressed longer after an intestinal insult than does either sucrose or maltase.[12]

In patients with untreated sprue, both lactase and sucrose typically are depressed; however, lactase is more severely affected, and consequently the sucrose:lactose (S:L) ratio is elevated. When the patient is treated, the generalized intestinal symptoms and biochemical tests of malabsorption respond dramatically within 1–2 months. Yet, paradoxically, the S:L ratio in such patients becomes even more elevated during the early treatment period because a rapid increase in sucrose activity to normal levels is not matched by a parallel improvement in lactase. Many months later, lactase activity does respond in most patients, and the S:L ratios approach those in normal individuals. In some patients who probably had acquired lactase deficiency before contracting tropical sprue, S:L ratios are extremely high at the outset because of an almost complete absence of lactase, and successful treatment of the sprue does not ameliorate the lactase deficiency. This longitudinal clinical study illustrates both the sensitivity and prolonged depression of lactase in intestinal disease.

## Sucrase–Isomaltase Deficiency

Intolerance to dietary sucrose has been observed in many areas of the world, and although originally thought to be rare, sucrose–dextrinase deficiency has been found in 10% of Greenland Eskimos and may be present in as many as 0.2% of North Americans. The defect appears to be inherited as an autosomal recessive gene, and as yet, no means of identifying heterozygotes has been developed. Symptoms occur in early childhood when sucrose is ingested and are indistinguishable from those of lactase deficiency, expect that sucrose is the offending sugar. Starch is usually well tolerated, probably because only amylopectin has the α1,6 branching links that require dextrinase activity. Amylose, having only α1,4 linkages, can be readily hydrolyzed by glucoamylase.[13]

## Glucose–Galactose Malabsorption

Because all dietary carbohydrate has either glucose or galactose as a monosaccharide component, intolerance to all ingested carbohydrates may occur when the glucose–galactose transporter is defective. This rare, recessively inherited malady has been identified, particularly in children from Scandinavia. It is usually associated with a benign glycosuria caused by the same defect in renal tubular brush borders. Furthermore, because no significant rise in blood sugar concentration occurs after ingestion of a glucose–galactose mixture, the malady can be distinguished from the more common oligosaccharidase deficiencies. Although elimination of all dietary carbohydrates may be required, sucrose may be tolerated better than other carbohydrates because one of its monosaccharide products, fructose, can be absorbed normally.

## PROTRACTED DIARRHEA OF INFANCY

During the early and mid-twentieth century, it was not uncommon to see specialized hospital wards crowded with malnourished infants secondary to chronic diarrhea. During the 1950s, the first major advance in technology was to provide intravenous fluids and electrolytes. Most infants were able to recover. However, those who had developed marasmus were never able to absorb sufficient nutrients to recover. These unfortunate infants were given the diagnosis of "intractable diarrhea and malnutrition of infancy."

During the late 1960s, a second major advance in technology was the advent of TPN, which provided not only fluid and electrolytes but also sufficient calories, protein, vitamins, and minerals sufficient for growth.[14] In the majority of instances, the infants with "intractable diarrhea" were able to recover and with time resume a normal diet.

During the 1970s, a third technology is small bowel biopsy, for histology and enzyme measurement and pancreatic secretions for measurement of enzyme activities and bacterial colony count. This technology provided the basis for understanding the pathophysiology of how the small bowel responds to malnutrition as well as how it can recover following the injury from malnutrition and bacterial invasion associated with the condition.

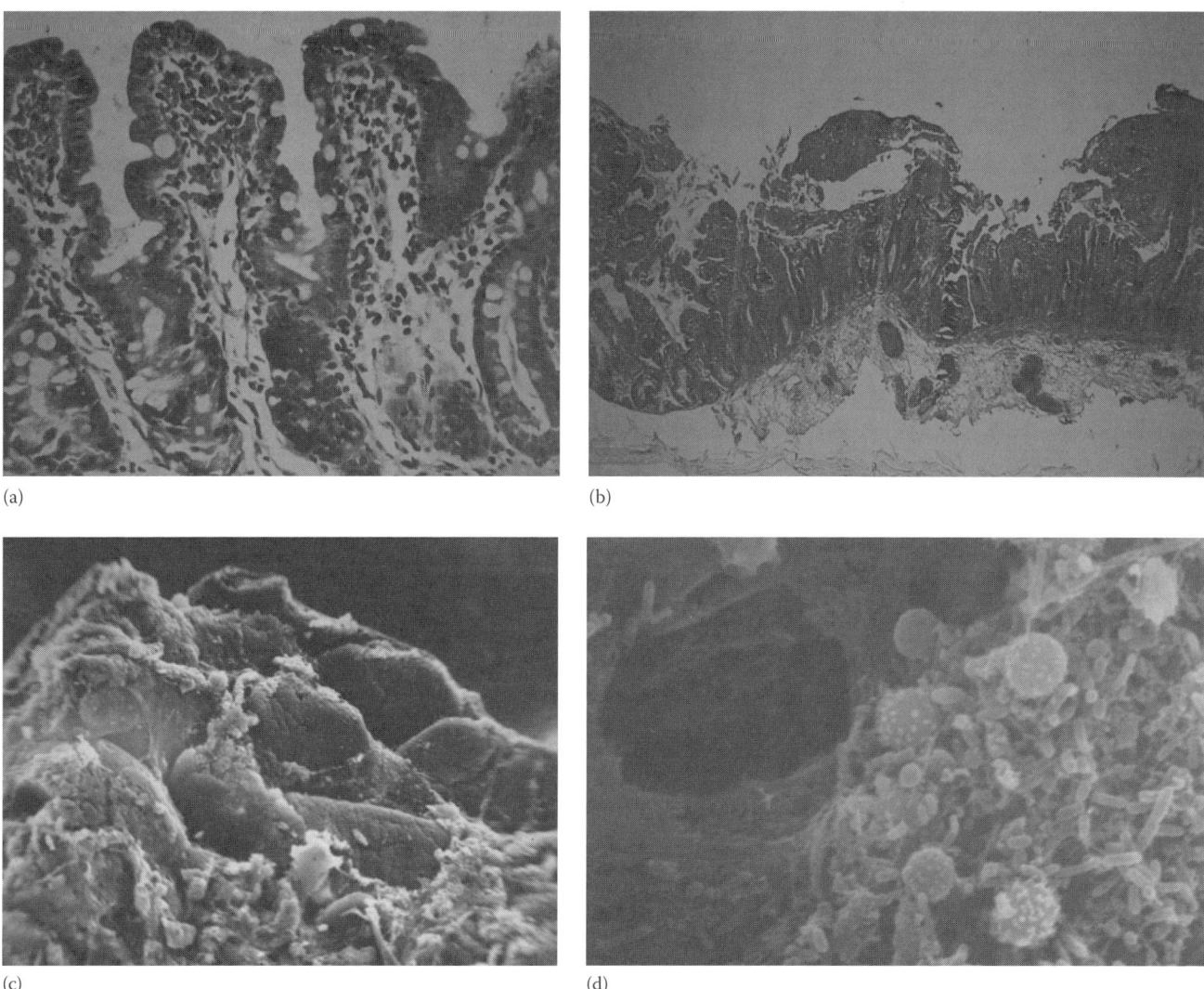

(a)

(b)

(c)

(d)

**FIGURE 62.2** (a) Demonstrates the following points: (1) the ratio of villus height to crypt depth (normally 4:1) is about to 1:1 (hematoxylin and eosin, ×100). (2) The number of mitotic figures in the crypts is substantially reduced and the crypt cells show a reduction in cytoplasm. (3) The villus epithelium is more cuboidal rather than the typical columnar appearance. (4) The epithelium and lamina propria has a larger number of inflammatory cells than normal. (b) This section was taken at the same time as A and shows that adjacent to intact mucosa are focal areas of ulceration (hematoxylin and eosin, ×200). (c) (about 100×) and (d) (about 1000×) depict scanning electron micrograph (SEM) sections from those shown in the H and E sections in A and B earlier. Of note is the number of bacteria adjacent to the crypt opening.

Understanding the pathophysiology then provided the framework for developing new nutritional formulations, which have been useful in the treatment and prevention of malabsorptive diarrhea and malnutrition.[15]

Anatomical changes in the jejunum of patients with intractable diarrhea and malnutrition are depicted in Figure 62.2. The figure shows that the ratio of villus height is markedly shortened, which significantly reduces the surface area for nutrient assimilation and absorption. The villus epithelial cells are cuboidal rather than columnar and the number of mitotic figures in the crypts is substantially reduced with a reduction in cytoplasm. These changes in morphology suggest that cell turnover and migration from crypt to villus is severely depressed, a suggestion later confirmed by radiolabeled cellular turnover studies.

In addition to the morphologic abnormalities, the brush border digestive enzymes are severely depressed. Lactase activity is barely detectable in some instances. Pancreatic enzyme amylase, lipase, and trypsin activities from intestinal aspirates are substantially depressed. Aerobic bacterial cultures of jejunal aspirates show a 10-fold increase, although none of the bacteria are considered "pathologic." Despite the lack of "pathologic" bacteria, many infants show a patchy breakdown of the intestinal barrier with ulcerations and bacterial infiltrates seen by scanning electron microscopy (see Figure 62.2d). Also gastric emptying is increased, whereas intestinal motility is depressed.[16]

Treatment of these infants with TPN, oral, and systemic antibiotics resulted in an apparent complete healing of the mucosa as well as improvement in brush border and pancreatic enzyme activities. However, maximal enzymatic activities were achieved only after resumption of formula feedings. Subsequent to the treatment with TPN, the histological, enzymatic, and bacterial cultures suggested that some infants could be successfully managed with simple fluid and electrolyte replacement coupled with formula modifications to circumvent the morphologic and enzymatic abnormalities. First, to address the issue of gastric emptying and abnormal motility, continuous feeding via nasogastric tube is initiated. Second, lactose was removed from the formula and replaced with dextrin and sucrose (since pancreatic amylase and brush border glucoamylase and sucrose were present. The protein was hydrolyzed to 30%–40% amino acids and the remainder as peptides. The amount of osmotically active ingredients was adjusted to provide an osmolality of 200–300 osmoles. Vitamin and mineral content was included to meet 100% daily values. The tube feedings were gradually increased as tolerated (first in volume to meet fluid/electrolyte requirements and then in concentration to meet calorie/protein requirements).

The infant formula industry has utilized the data from the earlier findings to develop specialized infant formulas, which when used early in the course of diarrhea have virtually eliminated the problem of chronic diarrhea, malabsorption, and malnutrition in developed countries.

## ALTERED IMMUNE FUNCTION IN INTESTINAL DISEASE

### Celiac Disease

Celiac disease—also known as gluten-sensitive enteropathy, celiac sprue, or nontropical sprue—is characterized by damage to the small intestinal mucosa and by malabsorption of most nutrients. The disease is activated by the dietary ingestion of wheat, rye, barley, and possibly oats. The onset of symptoms often occurs in the first 3 years of life after weaning and the introduction of cereals in the diet. A second peak incidence occurs in the third decade.

Clinical manifestations of celiac disease reflect the consequences of malabsorption. The small intestinal lesion is most marked in the proximal intestine and reveals profound infiltration of the lamina propria with lymphocytes and plasma cells and a marked increase of intraepithelial lymphocytes (Figure 62.3). The disease has a striking genetic component, and humoral-antibody and cell-mediated immune mechanisms appear to play a major role in the pathogenesis of tissue damage. Treatment consists of withdrawal of wheat gluten and similar proteins in rye, barley, and oats from the diet.

A 33 amino acid peptide fraction was identified from the 266 amino acid, gliadin that triggers the destructive inflammatory response in celiac disease. The disease is more common than generally thought and treatment has focused on dietary restriction of gluten-containing foods. However patient compliance may be problematic. Thus, several investigations show promise as possible alternative therapies[17]: (1) engineering gluten-free grains; (2) decreasing intestinal permeability by blocking the epithelial zonulin receptor; (3) inducing oral tolerance to gluten with a therapeutic vaccine; (4) degrading immunodominant gliadin peptides using probiotics with endopeptidases or transglutaminase inhibitors. These treatment options have shown encouraging preliminary results in clinical trials and may offer an improved therapy. However in the meantime dietary restriction of gluten-containing foods is the mainstay of therapy.

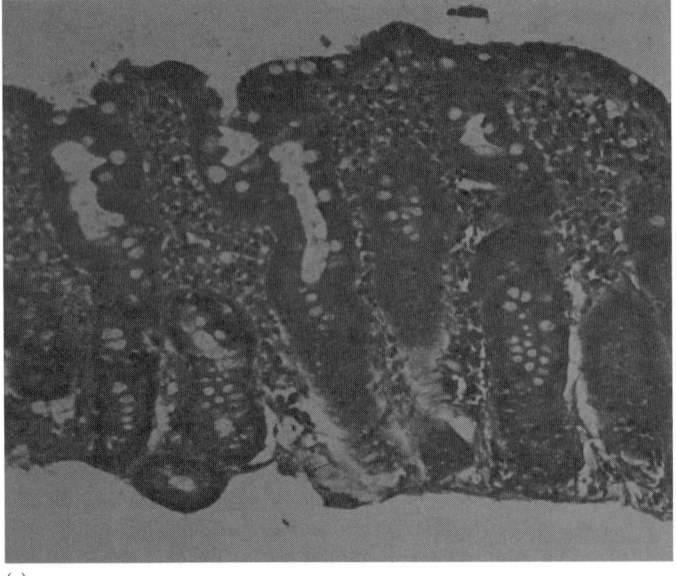

(a)

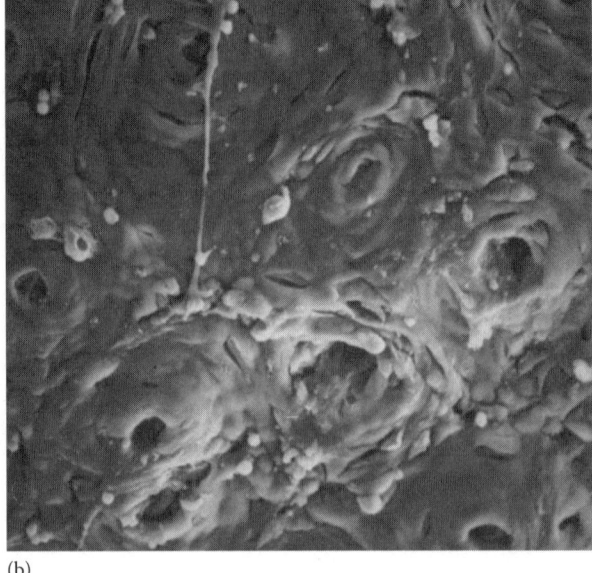

(b)

**FIGURE 62.3** (a) Jejunal histology of a patient with untreated celiac disease showing marked infiltration of plasma cells and other inflammatory cells in the lamina propria. The villi are shortened and the crypts are elongated with extensive mitoses in the crypt cells; (b) shows a scanning electron micrograph from the same patient demonstrating the complete lack of villi and only crypt areas remaining. A gluten-free diet for 6 months resulted in almost complete recovery of the intestinal mucosa.

## Eosinophilic Esophagitis

Esophageal eosinophils were once considered to be a hallmark of gastroesophageal reflux disease. However, it has become apparent that the esophagus, which is normally devoid of eosinophils, is an immunologically active organ that is capable of recruiting eosinophils in response to a variety of stimuli. Eosinophilic esophagitis (EoE) has been described in association with eosinophilic gastroenteritis (EGE), an uncommon condition that can cause a range of symptoms, including malabsorption, dysmotility, and ascites, depending upon the layer of the intestinal tract that is involved. EoE predominantly affects men between the ages of 20 and 40, but cases in women and in younger and older patients have also been reported. Recent systematic reviews found a male-to-female ratio of approximately 3:1. More than 90% of adults with EoE present with intermittent difficulty swallowing solids, while food impaction occurs in more than 60%. Heartburn is the only manifestation in 24% of patients. Noncardiac chest pain, vomiting, and abdominal pain have also been seen but less frequently.

Up to 80% of patients with EoE have a history of atopic disease such as asthma, allergic rhinitis, or allergies to food or medicine. One-third to one-half of patients have peripheral eosinophilia, and up to 55% have increased serum levels of immunoglobulin E (IgE). In children, presenting symptoms vary with age and include feeding disorders, vomiting, abdominal pain, and dysphagia. Moreover, children with EoE have a higher frequency of atopic symptoms and peripheral eosinophilia than do adults.

Although no single endoscopic feature of EoE is pathognomonic, the esophagus shows mucosal fragility in 59% of cases, a corrugated or ringed appearance in 49%, strictures in 40%, whitish papules in 16%, and a narrow caliber in 5%. Many of these features, including longitudinal furrows, are subtle and can be missed. Between 9% and 32% of patients with symptoms suggesting EoE have normal endoscopic findings. Motor abnormalities are common in patients with EoE (up to 40% of patients have esophageal manometric abnormalities, including uncoordinated contractions and ineffective peristalsis), and esophageal manometry is of limited diagnostic value and so is not recommended as a routine test.

A panel of experts defined EoE as "a chronic, immune/antigen-mediated, esophageal disease characterized clinically by symptoms related to esophageal dysfunction and histologically by eosinophil-predominant inflammation." It is important to differentiate between EoE, which is a clinicopathologic diagnosis, and esophageal eosinophilia in the absence of characteristic symptoms, which can be seen in association with multiple conditions. Acid reflux does not appear to be a causative factor in most patients. However, reflux may play a secondary role, as some patients have experienced symptomatic, endoscopic, and histological resolution of EoE after treatment with a proton pump inhibitor.

Studies in children suggest that food allergies are a major contributor to EoE. In children, a strict amino acid elemental diet has led to complete resolution of symptoms and a marked decrease in esophageal eosinophils. However, symptoms tend to recur once patients resume a regular diet.

The current consensus definition for EoE is

- Clinical symptoms of esophageal dysfunction (e.g., dysphagia, food impaction)
- At least 15 eosinophils per high-power field
- Either no response to a high-dose proton pump inhibitor or normal results on pH monitoring of the distal esophagus

Other features such as basal zone hyperplasia, edema, and papillary elongation are seen to a greater extent in patients with EoE than in patients with GERD (see Figure 62.4).[17]

Studies in children suggest that food allergies are a major contributor to EoE. In children, a strict amino acid elemental diet has led to complete resolution of symptoms and a marked decrease in esophageal eosinophils. However, symptoms tend to recur once patients resume a regular diet.[18] It is unclear if dietary modification is effective in adults. In six adults with EoE and a history of wheat and rye allergies, symptoms did not improve when these foods were eliminated and did not worsen when they were reintroduced. EoE has also been responsive to budesonide.[19]

## Eosinophilic Gastroenteritis

EGE is an uncommon GI disease affecting both children and adults. EGE is characterized by the following:

- The presence of abnormal GI symptoms, most often abdominal pain.
- Eosinophilic infiltration in one or more areas of the GI tract, defined as 20 or more eosinophils per high-power field.
- The absence of an identified cause of eosinophilia.
- The exclusion of eosinophilic involvement in organs other than the GI tract.
- A history of atopy or food allergies is often present.

Clinical symptoms are determined by the anatomical locations of eosinophilic infiltrates and the depth of GI involvement. Kaijser was probably the first to report a patient with EGE in 1937; since then, the number of case reports has increased. Treatments are often unsatisfactory, although some benefits have been reported with elemental diets as well as elimination diets. Recently, reports suggest that budesonide may be of some benefit; however, long-term outcomes are uncertain.[19]

Although the disease is idiopathic, recent investigations support the role of eosinophils, T helper 2 (Th2) cytokines (interleukin [IL]-3, IL-4, IL-5, and IL-13), and eotaxin as the critical factors in the pathogenesis of EGE. Atopy is present in a subset of patients, as these patients demonstrate increased total IgE on food-specific IgE radioallergosorbent assay test (RAST) or skin tests. Furthermore, lamina propria T cells from the duodenum of these patients proliferated in response to milk proteins and secreted Th2 cytokines (IL-13). However, other studies suggest a non–IgE-mediated mechanism. Death from EGE has been

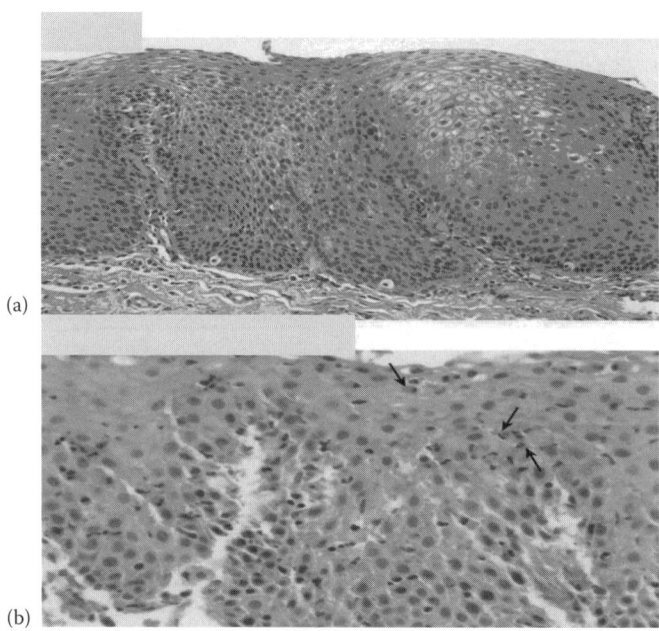

**FIGURE 62.4** (a) Esophageal biopsy with changes of gastroesophageal reflux disease (GERD). Characteristic findings include squamous hyperplasia wherein the basal cell layer accounts for greater than 15% of the mucosal thickness; the subepithelial papillae reach greater than two-thirds of the mucosal thickness; and a variety of inflammatory cells may be present including eosinophils, lymphocytes, and neutrophils (hematoxylin and eosin, ×100). (b) Esophageal biopsy from a patient with Eosinophilic esophagitis (EoE) showing numerous intraepithelial eosinophils (>15 per high-power field) and superficial eosinophilic microabscesses (arrows). Squamous hyperplasia is seen as well, with elongation of the subepithelial papillae and an expanded basal cell layer (hematoxylin and eosin, ×400).

reported only rarely. Morbidity includes malnutrition and intestinal obstruction and perforation.

## Inflammatory Bowel Disease

Two major forms of IBD are Crohn's disease and ulcerative colitis (UC). Usual onset is between ages 15–30, but there are many younger patients as well as older. The cause of IBD is unknown but appears to involve the interaction of host microflora, genetic predisposition, and abnormal immune responses in the intestinal wall.

### Crohn's Disease

*Crohn's disease* is a chronic, relapsing inflammatory disease of the GI tract. It may involve any part of the GI tract although distal ileum and colon are most frequently involved. In addition, normal epithelium may be located between two areas of involvement or an affected area between two normal areas. The inflammation affects all layers of the GI tract, and ulcerations, abscesses, and fistulas may develop. Submucosal thickening and scarring may lead to narrowing with localized strictures and subsequent partial or complete bowel obstruction.[20]

Treatment consists of medical management with occasional surgery to repair fistulas, obstructions, or other complications. Complete removal of diseased bowel will usually provide clinical recovery within 1–4 years, but recurrence is the rule. Medical management of the more complex cases is generally best left to gastroenterologists, since the newer drugs require clinical experience. The two primary agents

are aminosalicylate anti-inflammatory agents (sulfasalazine and mesalazine) and corticosteroids (most often prednisone), which could be considered a second-tier treatment because of its long-term complications. Other second-tier treatment is mercaptopurine immunosuppressing drugs (most commonly azathioprine and 6-mercaptopurine). They are prescribed for four categories: (1) maintenance of remission for people who are steroid dependent, (2) fistulizing disease, (3) induction of remission in steroid refractory cases, and (4) maintenance of remission after surgical resection.

A relatively new class of drugs are the tumor necrosis factor (TNF) inhibitors. Infliximab and adalimumab are antibodies that target TNF to reduce inflammatory symptoms. Both drugs have black box warnings and require care in prescribing. Natalizumab is an anti-integrin monoclonal antibody. It was approved by the FDA in 2008 and appears to have some utility in increasing the rate of remission.[21]

Diet and lifestyle have been effective in reducing symptoms in some patients, although certain foods have been found to aggravate symptoms. A low residue, low lactose is usually recommended and patients are encouraged to keep a diary in an effort to identify offending foods. In extreme cases, TPN may be useful to relieve symptoms. Because fat and vitamin malabsorption is often an issue, supplements of vitamin $B_{12}$, A, D, E, and K as well as folate are recommended. Hookworm therapy has been linked to diseases of an overactive immune system and there is at least one randomized trial ongoing, which is to evaluate the therapy in Crohn's disease.

**TABLE 62.1**

**Findings in Diagnostic Workup of Crohn's Disease versus UC**

| Sign | Crohn's Disease | UC |
|---|---|---|
| Color involvement | Usually | Always |
| Terminal ileum | Commonly | Seldom |
| Rectum involvement | Seldom | Usually |
| Anal involvement | Common | Seldom |
| Bile duct involvement | No increase in rate of primary sclerosing cholangitis | Higher rate |
| Distribution of disease inflammation | Patchy area of inflammation with skip lesions | Continuous areas of inflammation |
| Endoscopy | Deep geographic and snakelike inflammation/ulcerations | Continuous |
| Depth of inflammation | Transmural, deep penetration | Shallow mucosal |
| Stenosis | Common | Seldom |
| Granulomas | May have nonnecrotizing peri-intestinal crypt granulomas | Not seen |

*Ulcerative Colitis*

*UC* is similar in many respects to Crohn's disease in that it is a chronic, relapsing, and inflammatory disease of unknown cause. By contrast, it only involves the colon, mucosa, and submucosa, and between periods of relapse, the patient may be completely symptom-free with little if any morphologic changes in the colon. Table 62.1 lists major differences between Crohn's disease and UC. In unusual cases, it is difficult to distinguish between Crohn's disease and UC on clinical and radiological grounds. Treatment is similar to Crohn's disease with anti-inflammatory drugs, immunosuppression, and biologic therapy targeting specific components of the immune response. Colectomy (partial or total removal of the large bowel through surgery) is occasionally necessary and is considered to be a cure for the disease.

## Common Variable Immunodeficiency Syndromes

The common variable immunodeficiency syndromes are a collection of immune disorders rather than a single disease. Patients with these disorders have a variable reduction of serum immunoglobulins and impaired antibody responses. Onset is after infancy, most commonly in the second and third decade. Plasma cells are usually absent or markedly reduced in lymphoid sites, including the intestinal lamina propria. Chronic GI disorders, especially diarrhea, occur in as many as 60% of patients. Twenty percent to thirty percent of patients have mild to moderate malabsorption, frequently associated with infestation by the protozoan parasite *Giardia lamblia*[22].

## REFERENCES

1. Pope, CE II. The esophagus. In: Gitnick, GL ed., *Current Gastroenterology*, Vol. I. Boston, MA: Houghton Mifflin Medical Division, p. 1; 1980.
2. Richardson, CT, Walsh, JH, Hicks, MI et al. *J Clin Invest* 58:623;1976.
3. Hunt, JN, Know, MT. *J Physiol (Lond)* 914:327;1968.
4. Klish, WJ, Putnam, TC. *Am J Dis Child* 135:1056;1981.
5. Dietschy, JM In: *Disturbances in Lipid and Lipoprotein Metabolism*, Dietschy, JM, Gotto, AM, Ontko, JA. Bethesda, MD: American Physiological Society, p. 1, 1977.
6. Doe, WF, Hapel, AJ. *Clin Gastroenterol* 12:415;1983.
7. Kagnoff, MF. In: Green, M, Greene, HL eds. *The Role of the Gastrointestinal Tract in Nutrient Delivery*, New York: Academic Press, p. 239, 1984.
8. Costa, M, Patel, Y, Furness, JB et al. *Neurosci Lett* 6:215;1977.
9. Walker, A In: Johnson, LR ed. *Physiology of the Gastrointestinal Tract*, New York: Raven Press, p. 128, 1981.
10. Christensen, J In: Green, M, Greene, HL eds. *The Role of the Gastrointestinal Tract in Nutrient Delivery*, New York: Academic Press, p. 84, 1984.
11. Gray, GM In: Green, M, Greene, HL eds. *The Role of the Gastrointestinal Track in Nutrient Delivery*, New York: Academic Press, p. 133, 1984.
12. Shaukat, A *Ann Intern Med* 152:797;2010.
13. Gray, GM, Townley, RRW, Conklin, KA. *N Engl J Med* 296:750;1976.
14. Schwachman, H, Lloyd-Still, JD, Khaw, KT et al. *Am J Dis Child* 125:365;1973.
15. Greene, HL, McCabe, DR, Merenstein, GB *J Pediatr* 87:695;1975.
16. Greene, HL. In: Winters, RW, Greene, HL eds. *Nutritional Support of the Seriously Ill Patient*, New York: Academic Press, p. 181, 1983.
17. Bakshi, A, Stephen, S, Borum, ML, et al. Gastroenterology & Hepatology 8:582;2012.
18. Spergel, JM, Shuker, M. *Gastrointest Endosc Clin N Am* 18(1):179;2008.
19. Aceves, SS, Bastian, JF, Newbury, RO et al. *Am J Gastroenterol* 102(10):2271;2007.
20. Podolsky, DK. *N Eng J Med* 347:417;2002.
21. Rutgeets, P. *Gastroenterology* 136:1182;2009.
22. Katz, AJ, Rosen, FS. *Ciba Found Symp* 1977(46):243; 1977.

# 63 Nutritional Management of the Bariatric Surgery Patient

*Thai Pham, Hsiao C. Li, Edward H. Livingston, and Sergio Huerta*

## CONTENTS

## INTRODUCTION

The nutritional imbalance of patients submitting to weight reduction surgery begins prior to the operation and continues throughout life. Understanding where the patient starts, the sequelae and magnitude of the deficiency depending on the procedure performed as well as follow-up and compliance issues are paramount in counseling patients regarding their nutritional requirements following bariatric surgery. In addition to these challenges, the health-care provider needs to consider the lack of sufficient level I evidence and the unavailability of long-term data as well as the need to individualize patient care based on the specific patient population.

The following discussion will address the nutritional deficiencies and their management following the three most common bariatric operations performed in the United States: the laparoscopic adjustable band (LAB), the Roux-en-Y gastric bypass (RYGB), and the sleeve gastrectomy (SG). Other bypass operations performed in Europe such as the biliopancreatic diversion (BPD) are not common in the United States.[1]

## NUTRITIONAL ASSESSMENT

Adequate care of the bariatric patient begins in the preoperative consultation. Bariatric surgery should not be performed in the absence of a strongly structured multidisciplinary bariatric program, which includes dietitians, psychologists, and exercise specialists. Data on this aspect of bariatric surgery does not require type I evidence as it is common sense.

Original guidelines for nutritional assessment of the bariatric patient were published by the National Institute of Health in 1991 in the consensus report on Gastrointestinal Surgery for Severe Obesity.[2] Substantial data have accumulated since then and the SG seems to be gaining popularity in the United States as a single stage operation for the management of morbid obesity. Since then, guidelines for the management of the bariatric patient have been published by the American Society of Metabolic and Bariatric Surgery (ASMBS) in 2008[3] and the American Association of Clinical Endocrinologists, the Obesity Society, and American Society for Metabolic and Bariatric Surgery, AACE/TOS/ASMBS, also in 2008.[4] In general, recommendations from the AACE/TOS/ASMBS are more stringent and are similar for both the RYGB and the LAB patient. It is reasonable to assume that they could apply similarly to the SG.

The ASMBS has included suggestions from history taking to postoperative follow-up to biochemical monitoring of nutritional status culminating in suggested postoperative vitamin supplementation. The AACE/TOS/ASMBS provides a comprehensive review of all aspects of bariatric surgery with specific recommendations and level of evidence for each.[4]

## PREOPERATIVE PATIENT

The ASMBS guidelines suggest a thorough history and physical exam during the preoperative evaluation of the bariatric patient that includes (1) anthropometrics, (2) weight history, (3) past medical history, social history and a review of available laboratory values, (4) dietary history, (5) a history of physical activity, and (6) a psychosocial history. Preoperative nutrition education is also suggested by the ASMBS.[3] Similar recommendations are provided by the AACE/TOS/ASMBS guidelines and include a list of potential members of a bariatric surgery team with the specific recommendation of a registered dietitian.[4]

The goals of dietary treatment are to understand, educate, and provide tools to effect lifelong changes in the nutritional behavior of the obese patient. Dietary assessment using 24 h recall, food frequency questionnaires, or a food diary begins in the preoperative period. This will provide information on eating patterns, type and amounts of food eaten, food intolerances, and estimation of macro- and micronutrients. A thorough clinical history is important as symptoms of persistent nausea, vomiting, diarrhea, or abdominal pain should be evaluated by a physician. This detailed investigation into the patient's dietary patterns will provide necessary data to help the dietitian modify and promote good eating behavior in order to maximize weight loss, maintain a healthy weight, and treat nutritional deficiencies following bariatric surgery.

Ironically, studies indicate that a majority of obese patients have nutritional deficiencies prior to undergoing bariatric surgery despite their high caloric diets.[5] Obese patients often present with deficiencies of vitamins A, E, and D as well as carotenoids, zinc, selenium, and thiamin.[6] The incidence of iron[7] and vitamin D[8] deficiencies in morbidly obese patients is more of a rule rather than an exception, occurring in up to 80% and 50% of the of preoperative subjects, respectively.[3] The higher the BMI, the more profound the deficiency.[9] $B_{12}$ deficiency occurred with an incidence of 13% in a small cohort of patient prior to bariatric surgery.[10] Folic acid deficiency is observed in more than half of preoperative bariatric surgery patients.[11] In a small cohort of patients considering RYGB, 23% were deficient in vitamin E.[11] A similar study reported zinc deficiency in 28% of preoperative patients.[10] These studies further suggest that these deficiencies are exacerbated following bariatric surgery. Thus, careful preoperative evaluation and dietary education and supplementation to correct the deficiencies are necessary prior to and following bariatric surgery. Table 63.1 depicts typical baseline guidelines.

Because of the metabolic mechanisms of the body to adapt to starvation, protein deficiency in the preoperative patients is rare. However, routine laboratory assessment should be undertaken including albumin, transferrin, and lymphocyte count. If protein malnutrition is present, it should prompt investigation of multiple vitamin and mineral deficiencies. Bypass operations should not be undertaken in these cases.

In order to understand how bariatric surgery causes weight loss and leads to vitamin and mineral deficiency, the surgical anatomy of the three most common bariatric procedures is depicted in Figure 63.1. In RYGB, the stomach size is restricted with the creation of a small 30–60 mL gastric pouch, and intestinal absorption is reduced by bypassing the proximal segment

**TABLE 63.1**
**Screening of Various Deficiencies**

|  | **ASMBS** | **AACE/TOS/ASMBS for RYGB** |
|---|---|---|
|  | Screening Levels | Screening Levels |
| $B_1$ (thiamin) | Serum thiamin | First year and thereafter |
| $B_6$ (pyridoxine) | PLP | laboratory tests |
| $B_{12}$ (cobalamin) | [a]Serum $B_{12}$ | Every 3–6 months annually |
| Folic acid | RBC folate | CBC, platelets |
| Iron | Ferritin | Electrolytes |
| Vitamin A | Plasma retinol | Glucose |
| Vitamin D | 25(OH) vitamin D | Iron studies, ferritin |
| Vitamin E | Plasma α-tocopherol | Vitamin $B_{12}$ ([a]MMA) |
| Vitamin K | Prothrombin time | Liver function, lipid profile |
| Zinc | Plasma zinc | 25 (OH) vitamin D |
| Protein | Serum albumin/total protein | Optional: PTH, thiamin, RBC folate |

[a] The MMA assay is a better marker than $B_{12}$ serum levels. Up to one-third of patients with $B_{12}$ deficiency may be missed with serum levels alone.

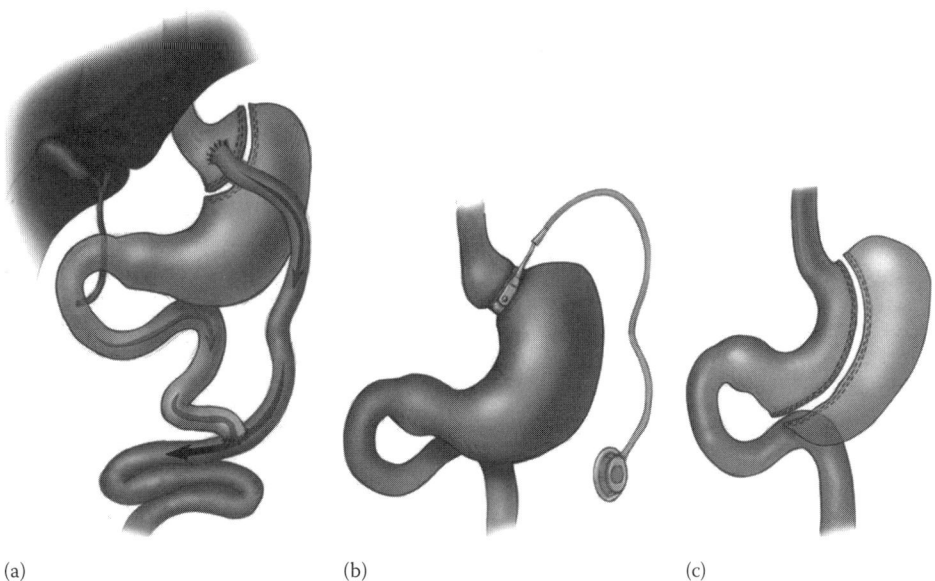

(a)                                    (b)                                    (c)

**FIGURE 63.1**  Common operations performed in the United States. (a) The RYGB involves a restrictive and a bypass component. (b) The LAB and (c) the SG are purely restrictive operations.

of the small intestine (Figure 63.1a). The LAB attempts to create stomach restriction by placement of an inflatable band around the proximal stomach just below the junction of the esophagus and stomach (Figure 63.1b). SG reduces the stomach size by removing the greater curvature of the stomach, thus creating a thin tubular stomach (Figure 63.1c).

Figure 63.2 depicts the typical sites for absorption for vitamins and minerals for an RYGB with a line also drawn to illustrate the typical anatomy following an SG.[12] As depicted in Figure 63.2, the surgical anatomy of the bariatric procedure has significant effect on the absorption of nutrients, with RYGB having the most significant effect on nutrient absorption as a result of the bypassed duodenum and a significant portion of the jejunum.

Most of the data available to assess the effects of weight reduction surgery emanates from our experience with the RYGB. Extrapolation of this data has been extended to the LAB with some exceptions and almost entirely with regard to the SG. While deficiencies might be specific to the type of operation performed, some occur in all forms of weight reduction surgery. For instance, fat-soluble vitamin deficiencies might occur following a BPD or a duodenal switch, but are uncommon with the RYGB or LAB. Iron, vitamin D, and vitamin $B_{12}$ deficiencies are common following RYGB. Folic acid deficiency is well documented in LAB.[13] Thiamin deficiency is common in all weight reduction operations emanating primarily from postoperative vomiting that might occur after any form of surgery as a result of the restrictive component of the procedure. The discussion as follows emphasizes nutritional deficiencies on the type of operation performed. These data is primarily derived from type II evidence.

### Roux-en-Y Gastric Bypass

In contrast to the LAB and the SG, the RYGB leads to weight reduction via two mechanisms: reduction of stomach size by creation of a small gastric pouch and limitation of intestinal absorption by the bypass of the proximal small intestine (see Figure 63.1a). RYGB has the longest follow-up data on weight loss and nutritional deficiencies. Level II evidence indicates that RYGB patients most commonly develop deficiencies of iron, calcium, $B_{12}$, folic acid, and vitamin D.[14,15] However, nutritional deficiencies of thiamin, $B_6$, magnesium, copper, selenium, vitamin A, and zinc might also occur. More than half of patients subjected to an RYGB demonstrate iron deficiency anemia.[14] Vitamin D deficiency might occur in up to 80% of patients following an RYGB, and this, compounded with a decrease in calcium absorption, leads to secondary hyperparathyroidism and a high rate of bone fractures.[16] Folic acid deficiency has been reported with a wide range of incidence, but is thought to occur in up to 40% of patients following RYGB. $B_{12}$ levels might drop by 70% in patients after an RYGB.[6] Thiamin deficiency leading to Wernicke's encephalopathy has been commonly reported following RYGB.[17]

RYGB impairs production of intrinsic factor (IF), a protein made in the distal stomach that is required for $B_{12}$ absorption in the terminal ileum. Thus, $B_{12}$ deficiency is not uncommon following RYGB, occurring at a rate of 35%, typically within 1 year following surgical intervention[18] and with an increasing frequency every year thereafter.[19] Both homocysteine levels and methylmalonic acid (MMA) are good surrogates to assess $B_{12}$ levels.[20,21]

A wide range of deficiency in folic acid has been cited in the literature following RYGB (6%–65%).[22] The most recent data suggest it occurs in only 10%–35% of patients following RYGB.[23] Because deficiency of folic acid might occur even when supplementation is provided, it is important to monitor levels. Folic acid found in multivitamins typically corrects the deficit in patient with RYGB if compliance is adequate.

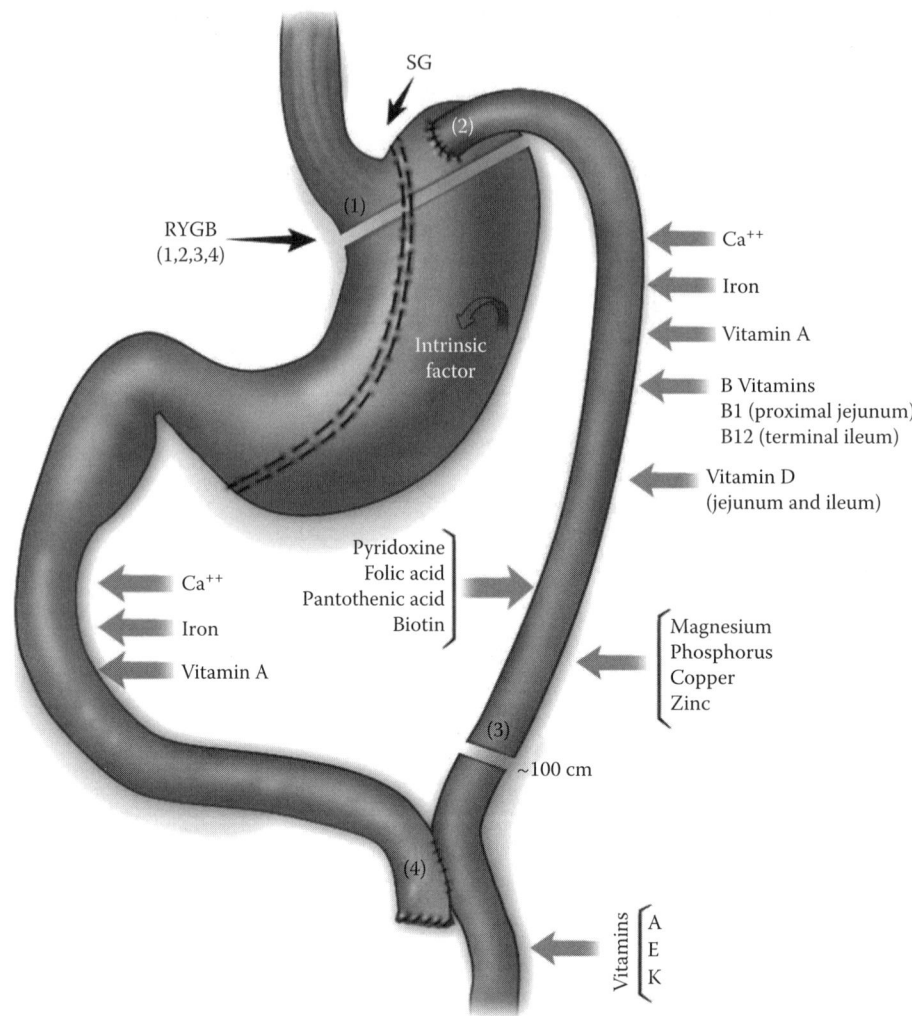

**FIGURE 63.2**  Depicts the typical sites for absorption for vitamins and minerals for an RYGB with a line also drawn to illustrate the typical anatomy following an SG. Sleeve gastrectomy is depicted by the stapled line indicated by the arrow SG (1) Gastric pouch for RYGB and segment of SG. (2) Alimentary limb of RYGB. (3) Bypassed segment of RYGB. (4) Anastomosis to of the biliopancreatic limb of the RYGB. (Adapted from Rhode, B.M. and MacLean, L.D., in: Deitel, M. and Cowan, J.R., eds., *UPDATE: Surgery for the Morbidly Obese Patient*, FD-Communications Inc., Toronto, Canada, p. 161, 2000, Figure 1.)

Because the proximal intestinal segment most responsible for iron absorption is bypassed with an RYGB, iron deficiency anemia is likely to occur. This is compounded by the decreased consumption of iron-rich foods, including red meat, which decrease substantially following weight reduction surgery. There are a large number of studies investigating iron deficiency in multiple cohorts subjected to RYGB. A higher rate of iron deficiency was reported in women and super obese patients (BMI > 50 kg/m[2]) with an incidence of over 50% in both groups.[18,24]

Although more common in patients with long-alimentary-limb bypass operations, vitamin A, E, and K deficiencies might occur after RYGB (52.5% for vitamin A[25] and 36% for zinc 1 year post-RYGB[10]).

RYGB restricts food intake and induces malabsorption of nutrients, therefore micronutrient deficiencies are to be expected and must be closely monitored both in the preoperative and the postoperative patient. Close monitoring is required for folic acid, iron, vitamin B$_{12}$, and calcium

deficiencies. Typical supplementation guidelines are outlined in Table 63.2. Management of known deficiencies in vitamins and minerals is depicted on Table 63.3.

## LAB

In the LAB, because there is no intestinal diversion, the observed nutritional deficiencies are the result of the change in eating habits following surgical intervention or from pre-existing deficiencies prior to surgery. Iron deficiency anemia has been attributed to the change in dietary habits of patient following LAB as the amount of red meat consumption decreases substantially.[6] Using homocysteine levels as a surrogate for folic acid and B$_{12}$, the levels of homocystine were found to be altered in patients following LAB in a 2-year follow-up study inclusive of 293 subjects.[26] Folic acid deficiency might decrease up to 44% in 2 years following LAB.[13] A few studies have failed to demonstrate alterations in calcium and vitamin D following LAB.[27,28] However, these studies have shown a high rate of bone remodeling in these patients,

## TABLE 63.2
## Recommended Vitamin and Mineral Supplementation

| | RYGB | | LAB | |
|---|---|---|---|---|
| | **ASMBS** | **AACE/TOS/ASMBS** | **ASMBS** | **AACE/TOS/ASMBS** |
| Protein (g/day) | None | 60–120 | None | 60–120 |
| Iron[a] (mg/day) | 18–27 | 40–65 | None | 40–65 |
| Calcium (mg/day) | 1500–2000 | 1200–2000 | 1500 | 1200–2000 |
| $B_{12}$ | | | | |
| Oral (μg/day) | 350–500 | 350 | None | 350 |
| IM (μg/month—3 months/ 6 months) | 1000 | 1000–3000 | None | 1000–3000 |
| Intranasal (μg/week) | None | 500 | None | 500 |
| Vitamin D (IUD) | None | 400–800 | None | 400–800 |
| MVA (2 X day) | 200% DV | MVA with folic acid | 100% DV | MVA with minerals |

*Note:* MVA, multivitamin; DV, daily value.

[a] Menstruating women and adolescents submitting to weight reduction surgery might need further supplementation.

## TABLE 63.3
## Treatment of Vitamin and Mineral Deficiencies

$B_1$ (thiamin)
- Early symptoms — 20–30 mg/day PO
- Advanced symptoms — 20–30 mg/day IV or IM
- With hyperemesis — 100 mg/day parenteral followed by 50 mg/day until recovery
- WKS[a] — 100 mg/day IV

$B_6$ (pyridoxine)
- Treatment — 50 mg/day or 100–200 mg when deficiency is related to medications

$B_{12}$ (cobalamin)
- Known deficiency — 1000 mg/week IM × 8 weeks, followed by 1000 mg/month for life or 350–500 mg/day PO

Folic acid
- Treatment — >1000 mg/day

Iron[b]
- Treatment — 300 mg/day PO with severe symptoms use IV

Vitamin D
- Treatment — 50,000 IU ergocalciferol/week PO X 8 weeks

Vitamin A
- No corneal changes — 10,000–25,000 IU/day PO for 1–2 weeks until symptoms improve
- Corneal changes — 50,000–100,000 IU/day IM for 2 weeks

Vitamin K
- 10 mg parenteral
- Chronic deficiency — 1–2 mg PO a day or weekly parenterally

Vitamin E
- Supplemental vitamin E 100–100 IU/day

Zinc
- 60 mg elemental zinc PO X 2/day

[a] Women and adolescents submitting to weight reduction surgery might need further supplementation.
[b] WKS Wenicke's encephalopathy.

indicating calcium and vitamin D alterations that are unde- tected and could be attributed to PTH changes stimulated by estradiol and cortisol, which occurs after this operation.[29,30]

Although more common in patients with long-alimentary- limb bypass operations (i.e., BPD or duodenal switch), defi- ciencies of vitamins A, E, and K might occur after LAB. For instance, vitamin A deficiency has been documented to occur a rate of 25.5% after a LAB.[25] Thus, close monitor- ing of these nutrients is necessary following LAB. Unlike RYGB, the lack of intestinal diversion of LAB means that most of these nutrient deficiencies can be readily treated with oral supplementation with daily multivitamins (Table 63.2). Compliance is, therefore, paramount. Management of known deficiencies is outlined in Table 63.3.

## SG

The goal of the SG procedure is to reduce gastric size by removing the greater curvature of the stomach (Figure 63.1c). Similar to what is seen in LAB, nutritional deficiencies seen in this patient population stem from preexisting deficien- cies or from substantial dietary changes following surgery. Over the past 5 years, SG has gained popularity as a primary weight reduction procedure due to its low procedural morbid- ity profile.[5,31] Thus, it has the least long-term data published in terms of durability of weight loss and nutritional follow- up. However, the few studies that have assessed nutritional deficiencies in this population show that SG can exacerbate preexisting micronutrient deficiencies. A small observational study showed that 51% of patients undergoing SG had at least one or more deficiencies of micronutrients such as vitamins A, E, D, $B_6$, $B_{12}$, folate, iron, calcium, and/or potassium.[5] The same study showed that following SG, these deficiencies were modestly worse at 1-year of follow-up. A second study found that while deficiencies occurred in the preoperative set- ting, nutrient levels normalized in patients submitting to SG at a 5-year follow-up.[31]

Other reports have documented iron deficiency anemia in up to 14% of patients at 1 year of follow-up after SG.[6] While folic acid and $B_{12}$ have been found to be normal in patients 2 years following SG, a quarter of these patients had elevated levels of homocysteine,[31] which makes it likely that there is a mild defi- ciency which might become evident with much longer follow-up though data are lacking at this time. In a prospective compari- son of SG versus RYGB patients, RYGB patients experienced greater deficiencies of vitamins $B_{12}$ and D compared to SG.[32]

A case of acute post-gastric reduction surgery syndrome (see description later) was reported in a patient 5 months fol- lowing SG. However, in this case, it is likely that the patient had substantial preoperative deficiencies prior to surgery that precipitated the syndrome following inability to eat and poor follow-up. This patient's BMI was 70 kg/m². He developed intractable vomiting following the operation and presented with a 49 kg weight loss accompanied by weakness and par- esthesias of the lower extremities leading to an inability to walk.[33] This case illustrates the fact that preoperative defi- ciencies might be profound and that follow-up is essential in these patients.

In general, micronutrient deficiencies are not common fol- lowing SG, but lifelong oral supplementation with daily mul- tivitamins can minimize risk. While specific guidelines for vitamin and mineral supplementation are currently lacking for patients with SG, it is reasonable to apply the recommen- dations for the LAB (Table 63.2). Similarly, known deficien- cies can be treated according to the same management as for LAB and RYGB (Table 63.3).

### Post-Bariatric Surgery Diet Progression

Table 63.4 outlines the typical dietary progression following bariatric surgery. Early in the dietary progression, particu- lar emphasis is placed on small meals, consuming enough liquids to avoid dehydration, and consuming enough protein to allow for adequate wound healing. Typically patients are kept without any form of oral intake overnight after the sur- gery, except for LAB. On postoperative days one and/or two, a clear liquid diet is initiated with progress to a full liquid diet by postoperative day two. Because a clear liquid diet is devoid of nutrients, this should not be continued beyond 48 h and some form of supplementation must be instituted (i.e., low-residue diet or a clear liquid diet with nutritional supplements).

For patients undergoing weight reduction surgery, they should be discharged on a full liquid diet (i.e., milk or milk products) with high-protein supplementation, for 2 weeks. Diets that have been blended or liquefied with adequate fluid (pureed diets) can be implemented if full liquid diets are well tolerated. At week three, following bariatric sur- gery, patients should be advanced to a diet that is likely to be adopted for the rest of life. It is important to emphasize that bariatric surgery should serve as a staging platform for a lifestyle change that includes healthy eating habits.

## TABLE 63.4
### Diet Progression Following Bariatric Surgery

| Duration of Diet After Surgery | Diet Type | Important Nutrients |
|---|---|---|
| 1–2 Days post-surgery | Clear liquids | |
| 1–2 Weeks post-surgery | Full liquids | Protein and fluids |
| 3–4 Weeks post-surgery | Pureed diet | Protein and fluids; multivitamins; supplementation of micronutrients such as B vitamins, iron, calcium |
| >4 Weeks post-surgery | Regular diet | Continue micronutrient supplementation |

A diet history diary is important to achieve a good goal for dietary changes following bariatric surgery. It is best for bariatric patients to follow a well-established weight reduction surgery pathway.[34]

## VITAMIN AND MINERALS KNOWN TO BE DEFICIENT FOLLOWING WEIGHT REDUCTION SURGERY

### B Vitamins

### B₁ (Thiamin)

Thiamin is absorbed in the *proximal jejunum*, has a half-life of 9–18 days, and can be rapidly depleted if a patient has inadequate intake and is profoundly exacerbated by vomiting. Preoperative deficiency of $B_1$ occurs in 15%–29% of patients, and it is more commonly seen in African Americans and Hispanics compared to Caucasians.[7,35]

Thiamin deficiency and its complications have been documented for RYGB and LAB, and it is more likely to occur in the early postoperative period as a result of surgically induced–intractable vomiting[7,35] While routine screening for thiamin deficiency is not required, patients presenting with intractable vomiting should be assessed for possible $B_1$ deficit.

Symptoms of thiamin deficiency can occur with mild deficiency (early) and severe deficiency. Early symptoms are related to mild central nervous system manifestations including anorexia, gait ataxia, and irritability. Muscle cramps and paresthesias may also occur. Severe thiamin deficiency leads to beriberi and in severe cases to Wernicke's encephalopathy and Korsakoff's psychoses.[36]

Thiamin supplementation should be required of all patients submitting to weight reduction surgery and can be accomplished by adequate intake of multivitamins. Patients with persistent vomiting or with symptoms of thiamin deficiency should be immediately treated with intramuscular or intravenous thiamin. Hospitalized patients receiving intravenous fluids should include thiamin to prevent depletion (Table 63.3).

### B₆ (Pyridoxal Phosphate)

There is a wide range of findings in the levels of $B_6$ in patients submitting to weight reduction surgery. Some studies have documented a deficiency in 64% of patients prior to surgical intervention.[11] Serum levels of $B_6$ do not correlate with deficiency of this vitamin,[37] which indicates that supplementation has to be higher than the recommended amounts to prevent deficiency in bariatric patients. Signs and symptoms of this deficiency include changes in the epithelial layers, central nervous system dysfunction including confusion and depression, and blood and platelet abnormalities such as microcytic anemia and platelet dysfunction. Severe deficiency might lead to neuropathy. Deficiency can be corrected with vitamin $B_6$ 50 mg/day, or 100–200 mg/day if deficiency is related to medications (Table 63.2).

### B₁₂ (Cobalamin)

Protein-bound cobalamin requires pepsin for its release. Patients with achlorhydria have decreased levels of active pepsin leading to poor $B_{12}$ absorption.[38] Because $B_{12}$ requires IF to be absorbed in the *terminal ileum* and both IF and acid production are reduced in the RYGB, the 3–5-year body stores are likely, be depleted if no supplementation is provided. Cobalamin deficiency is less common in LAB or SG patients.

Factors other than surgery are known to affect $B_{12}$ absorption and include metformin[39] and proton pump inhibitors, owing to the decrease in acid production.

$B_{12}$ deficiency typically causes megaloblastic anemia, but neurological symptoms can occur including polyneuropathy, paresthesia, and permanent neural impairment as well as psychosis.[20,40] Supplementation is required in patients submitting to weight reduction surgery to prevent deficiency (Table 63.2). Known deficiencies should be aggressively treated (Table 63.3).

### Folic Acid

Most folic acid absorption takes place in the *proximal jejunum*. But following adaptation after surgery, absorption can occur throughout the small bowel. Anticonvulsants, oral contraceptives, and chemotherapeutic agents might lead to folic acid deficiency.[3]

Patients with folic acid deficiency might present with neurological symptoms including forgetfulness, irritability, and paranoia.[41] Appropriate supplementation with MVA (200% DV, Table 63.2) prevents depletion, and deficiency can be treated with more than 1000 µg/day (Table 63.3).

### Iron

Iron absorption occurs in the *duodenum and proximal jejunum*. Symptoms of iron deficiency include anemia-related symptoms (i.e., fatigue, tachycardia, and impaired learning ability), dysphagia, koilonychia, and enteropathy. Five stages of deficiency are described: Stages I and II are related to low levels of ferritin. In stages III and IV, anemia occurs without and with microcytosis, respectively. Symptoms occur in stage V. Duration for the development of iron deficiency and anemia vary widely in the literature, but seems to occur within 2 years after weight reduction surgery, even in patients receiving supplementation.[42] Iron supplementation should be provided after bariatric surgery (Table 63.2), and patients should be treated with intravenous iron if severe symptoms develop (Table 63.3).

### Calcium and Vitamin D

Calcium absorption occurs in the *duodenum* and *proximal jejunum*. Signs and symptoms of deficiency are leg cramping and tetany as well as neuromuscular hyperexcitability. Secondary hyperparathyroidism might develop and if untreated, might lead to osteoporosis. Available evidence suggests that the preferred form of supplementation is calcium citrate over calcium carbonate owing to better absorption of the former.[43] Supplementation is recommended for patients following surgery (Table 63.2), and deficiency in vitamin D should be treated with 50,000 IU ergocalciferol by mouth weekly for 8 weeks (Table 63.3).[7]

## Fat-Soluble Vitamins (A, E, K) and Zinc

Deficiency in vitamins A, E, and K are more commonly reported following an operation not typically performed in the United States such as the BPD or its analog, the duodenal switch. These deficiencies occur in more than half of patients 1 year after the operation[44] and develop because most of the absorption takes place in the distal small intestine after mixture of these vitamins with bile.[45] While passive absorption of A, E, and K vitamins also occurs in the proximal intestine, deficiencies after long-limb bypass operations suggest that fat-absorptive mechanisms are impaired more distally in the intestine. This is also supported by the fact that RYGB with longer Roux-Y limbs are more likely to lead to deficiencies of these vitamins.[24]

A myriad of case reports populate the literature that describe vitamin A deficiency leading to ophthalmologic disorders in patients following weight reduction surgery and even in their progeny many years after the operation.[46] Severe deficiency can cause blindness and loss of taste. Skin abnormalities and poor wound healing have also been noted. Multivitamins provide adequate supplementation if compliance is adequate, and treatment should be aggressively addressed with high oral or intramuscular formulations (Table 63.3). Routine vitamin A supplementation is not recommended after RYGB or restrictive procedures.[4] Iron and copper deficiencies should be evaluated as vitamin A is being corrected.

Vitamin K deficiency was suggested in RYGB patients compared to LAB where the prothrombin time served as a surrogate.[25] Vitamin K deficiency manifests as problems with coagulation, easy bruising, and osteoporosis. Multivitamins prevent deficiency following bariatric surgery, and deficiency should be corrected with parenteral administration (10 mg). Chronic deficiency should be treated with 1–2 mg/day orally or the same dose parenterally once a week (Table 63.3).

While vitamin E deficiency has been noted to occur preoperatively in patients considering weight reduction surgery, appropriate vitamin supplementation corrects this deficiency postoperatively.[11] Neurological manifestations of vitamin E deficiency include altered proprioception, hyporeflexia, and gait disturbances. Ophthalmoplegia, nyctalopia, erythrocyte hemolysis, and nystagmus might also occur. Supplemental vitamin E prevents and corrects deficiency (Table 63.2).

Zinc's absorption is dependent on fats. While plasma levels of zinc might be normal in patients following RYGB, erythrocyte and urinary levels have been found to be decreased in these patients.[47] Plasma zinc levels are particularly unreliable in the presence of systemic inflammation. Alterations of taste and smell occur; poor appetite, irritability, alopecia,

dermatitis, loss of muscle mass, diarrhea, impaired wound healing, and dermatitis might also occur with zinc deficiency. Supplementation is not recommended for RYGB or restrictive operations. Deficiency can be treated with elemental zinc orally (Table 63.3). Red meat intolerance in these patients might account for the observed deficiency in patients following an RYGB.

Suggested recommendation for vitamins A, E, K, as well as zinc can be appropriately provided in multivitamins Table 63.2. Compliance remains the issue of major concern in patients submitting to weight reduction surgery.

## Copper

Copper deficiency has rarely been reported in the literature. Symptoms of copper deficiency following RYGB might mimic $B_{12}$ abnormalities such ataxia and paresthesia.[48,49] While copper is absorbed by the bypassed stomach and the proximal intestine, it is surprising that deficiency of this mineral only occurs rarely in patients following an RYGB. Copper deficiency also causes anemia and neutropenia. Copper deficiency can be exacerbated by abnormal high levels of zinc supplementation.[50]

## Selenium, Magnesium, and Potassium

These minerals have also been found to be altered in patients following RYGB.[10,51,52] Selenium is an antioxidant and deficiency is rare in RYGB. In other bariatric procedures, selenium deficiency did not result in clinical manifestations.[53] Magnesium is absorbed throughout the small bowel. Hypomagnesemia might cause neuromuscular, intestinal, and cardiovascular abnormalities. Hypomagnesemia is uncommon following RYGB with long-limb bypasses and is associated with severe diarrhea.[53] Multivitamin supplementation has been found to correct these deficiencies.

## Protein

All weight reduction procedures have the theoretical risk of leading to protein malnutrition. However, as a result of the powerful adaptation of the body to starvation, protein deficiency is not common. If present, this is a marker for multivitamin and mineral deficiencies. Iron, folic acid, as well as copper deficiency anemia is commonly found in patients with protein alterations. Vitamin $B_6$, thiamin, and zinc deficits might also be found in these patients. While no strict guidelines exist for protein supplementation, 60–120 g/day of total protein that includes estimated average requirements of essential and nonessential amino acids is recommended for patients following weight reduction surgery.

As with protein deficiency *hypophosphatemia* is a marker of severe malnutrition. Rapid nutrition administration in a severely malnourished patient might lead to depletion of phosphorus from the serum leading to the "refeeding syndrome."[54] Careful nutritional support is therefore required in the severely malnourished bariatric patient. Hypophosphatemia can lead to rhabdomyolysis, respiratory abnormalities, and central nervous system dysfunction.

*Acute post-gastric reduction syndrome* is a complication of weight reduction surgery involving systemic and central nervous system symptoms that are characterized by intractable vomiting, weakness, and hyporeflexia.[55] Other symptoms include pain, incontinence, visual impairment associated with diplopia and numbness. While less common, dysphonia and delirium as well as memory, attention, and hearing loss might occur. Physical exam typically demonstrates gaze-evoked nystagmus and severe proximal extremity weakness. Diagnostic studies are characterized by axonal sensory motor polyneuropathy of the lower extremities involving the quadriceps. Nerve biopsies have demonstrated multifocal myelinated fiber loss and lack of inflammatory cells. Treatment requires aggressive multivitamin administration and nutritional support. Intravenous administration of gamma globulin has also been provided to these patients.[56] This syndrome should be considered a marker of multiple vitamin and mineral deficiencies.

## KEY ISSUES

1. Lifelong surveillance is required for all patients submitting to weight reduction surgery—guidelines are provided by the ASMBS and the AACE/TOS/ASMBS.[3,4]

2. Nutritional deficiencies are best documented for the RYGB, and some small studies have shown evidence for the LAB. There is minimal data today with regard to the SG. However, the available evidence suggests that nutritional deficiencies occur in the following order: RYGB > LAB > SG.

3. Compliance with vitamin and mineral supplementation remains a major issue of concern in patients submitting to weight reduction surgery.

4. There are some common deficiencies noted in all types of weight reduction operations such as thiamin, folic acid, iron, and vitamin D. Vitamin $B_6$, copper, selenium, magnesium, and potassium have only been documented in case reports following RYGB.

5. Fat-soluble vitamins (A, E, K) and zinc are more commonly observed following long-limb bypass surgery such as the BPD and duodenal switch but might occur occasionally with the RYGB and rarely with LAB and SG.

6. The SG requires much more long-term data, but currently supplementation should be provided as with the LAB.

7. The cornerstone of a successful bariatric surgery program is a multidisciplinary approach with preoperative, intraoperative, and postoperative care.

## REFERENCES

1. Livingston, EH. *Ann Intern Med* 155:329;2011.
2. National Institutes of Health Consensus Development Conference Statement. *Am J Clin Nutr* 55:615S;1992.
3. Aills, L, Blankenship, J, Buffington, C et al. *Surg Obes Relat Dis* 4:S73;2008.
4. Mechanick, JI, Kushner, RF, Sugerman, HJ et al. *Surg Obes Relat Dis* 4:S109;2008
5. Damms-Machado, A, Friedrich, A, Kramer, KM et al. *Obes Surg* 22:881;2012.
6. Jacques, J, Dixon, J. In: Deitel M, Gagner M, Dixon J, Himpens J, Madan A, eds *Handbook of Obesity Surgery: Current Concepts and Therapy of Morbid Obesity and Related Disease FD-Communications Inc*. Toronto, Canada, p. 326;2010.
7. Flancbaum, L, Belsley S, Drake V et al. *J Gastrointest Surg* 10:1033;2006.
8. Carlin, AM, Rao, DS, Meslemani, AM et al. *Surg Obes Relat Dis* 2:98;2006.
9. Buffington, C, Walker, B, Cowan, GS, Jr., Scruggs D. *Obes Surg* 3:421;1993.
10. Madan, AK, Orth, WS, Tichansky, DS, Ternovits CA. *Obes Surg* 16:603;2006.
11. Boylan, LM, Sugerman, HJ, Driskell, JA. *J Am Diet Assoc* 88:579;1988.
12. Rhode, BM, MacLean, LD. In: Deitel M, Cowan JR, eds. *UPDATE: Surgery for the Morbidly Obese Patient*. FD-Communications Inc, Toronto, Canada, p. 161, 2000.
13. Gasteyger, C, Suter, M, Calmes, JM et al. *Obes Surg* 16:243;2006.
14. Shikora, SA, Kim, JJ, Tarnoff ME. *Nutr Clin Pract* 22:29;2007.
15. Malinowski, SS. *Am J Med Sci* 331:219;2006.
16. Newbury, L, Dolan, K, Hatzifotis, M et al *Obes Surg* 13:893;2003.
17. Loh, Y, Watson, WD, Verma, A et al. *Obes Surg* 14:129;2004.
18. Brolin, RE, Gorman, JH, Gorman, RC et al. *J Gastrointest Surg* 2:436;1998.
19. Fujioka, K. *Diabetes Care* 28:481;2005.
20. Crowley, LV, Olson RW. *Am J Gastroenterol* 78:406;1983.
21. Sumner, AE, Chin, MM, Abrahm, JL et al. *Ann Intern Med* 124:469;1996.
22. MacLean, LD, Rhode, BM, Shizgal, HM. *Ann Surg* 198:347;1983.
23. Faintuch, J, Matsuda, M, Cruz, ME et al. *Obes Surg* 14:175;2004.
24. Brolin, RE, LaMarca, LB, Kenler, HA, Cody RP. *J Gastrointest Surg* 6:195;2002.
25. Ledoux, S, Msika, S, Moussa, F et al. *Obes Surg* 16:1041;2006.
26. Dixon, JB, Dixon, ME, O'Brien et al. *Int J Obes Relat Metab Disord* 25:219;2001.
27. Giusti, V, Gasteyger, C, Suter, M et al. *Int J Obes (Lond)* 29:1429;2005.
28. Pugnale, N, Giusti, V, Suter, M et al. *Int J Obes Relat Metab Disord* 27:110;2003.
29. Guney, E, Kisakol, G, Ozgen, G et al. *Obes Surg* 13:383;2003.
30. Riedt, CS, Cifuentes, M, Stahl, TC et al. *J Bone Miner Res* 20:455;2005.
31. Saif, T, Strain, GW, Dakin, G et al. *Surg Obes Relat Dis Feb*, 8:542;2012.
32. Gehrer, S, Kern B, Peters T et al. *Obes Surg* 20:447;2010.
33. Ramos-De la Medina, A, Noguera-Rojas, W, Anitua-Valdovinos, MM et al. *Surg Obes Relat Dis* 7:119;2011.
34. Huerta, S, Heber, D, Sawicki MP et al. *Am Surg* 67:1128;2001.
35. Carrodeguas, L, Kaidar-Person, O, Szomstein, S et al. *Surg Obes Relat Dis* 1:517;2005.
36. Nautiyal, A, Singh, S, Alaimo, DJ. *Am J Med* 117:804;2004.
37. Turkki, PR, Ingerman, L, Schroeder, LA et al. *J Am Coll Nutr* 11:272;1992.
38. Ponsky, TA, Brody, F, Pucci, E. *J Am Coll Surg* 201:125;2005.

39. Bauman, WA, Shaw, S, Jayatilleke, E et al. *Diabetes Care* 23:1227;2000.
40. Smith, CD, Herkes, SB, Behrns, KE et al. *Ann Surg* 218:91;1993.
41. Alvarez-Leite, JI. *Curr Opin Clin Nutr Metab Care* 7:569;2004.
42. Brolin, RE, Gorman, RC, Milgrim, LM, Kenler, HA. *Int J Obes* 15:661;1991.
43. Sakhaee, K, Bhuket, T, Adams-Huet, B, Rao, DS. *Am J Ther* 6:313;1999.
44. Dolan, K, Hatzifotis, M, Newbury, L et al. *Ann Surg* 240:51;2004.
45. Slater, GH, Ren, CJ, Siegel, N et al. *J Gastrointest Surg* 8:48;2004.
46. Huerta, S, Rogers, LM, Li, Z et al. *Am J Clin Nutr* 76:426;2002.
47. Cominetti, C, Garrido, AB, Jr., Cozzolino, SM. *Obes Surg* 16:448;2006.
48. Kumar, N, McEvoy, KM, Ahlskog, JE. *Arch Neurol* 60:1782;2003.
49. Kumar, N, Ahlskog, JE, Gross, JB, Jr. *Clin Gastroenterol Hepatol* 2:1074;2004.
50. Willis, MS, Monaghan, SA, Miller, ML et al. *Am J Clin Pathol* 123:125;2005.
51. Crowley, LV, Seay, J, Mullin, G. *Am J Gastroenterol* 79:850;1984.
52. Schauer, PR, Ikramuddin, S, Gourash, W et al. *Ann Surg* 232:515;2000.
53. Dolan, K, Hatzifotis, M, Newbury, L, Fielding, G. *Obes Surg* 14:165;2004.
54. Apovian, CM, McMahon, MM, Bistrian, BR. *Crit Care Med* 18:1030;1990.
55. Akhtar, M, Collins, MP, Kissel, JT. *Neurology* 58:2002.
56. Chang, CG, Adams-Huet, B, Provost DA. *Obes Surg* 14:182;2004.

# 64 Dietary Factors Related to Frailty and Reduced Functional Capacity

*William J. Evans*

## CONTENTS

Aging is associated with an astonishing number of changes and adaptive responses. The challenge of scientists and clinicians has been to separate true biological aging from genetic and environmental adaptations. For example, a reduction in lean body mass and an increase in fat mass is one of the most striking and consistent changes associated with advancing age. Skeletal muscle[1] and bone mass are the principal (if not exclusive) components of lean body mass to decline with age. These changes in body composition appear to occur throughout life and have important functional and metabolic consequences.

The loss of skeletal muscle mass occurs under a wide variety of conditions. Sarcopenia is the age-associated loss of skeletal muscle mass and function and is a universal phenomenon. Myopenia refers to the general loss of skeletal muscle mass that may result from a number of conditions including disuse (atrophy), malnutrition, or cachexia. There is a remarkable overlap among each of these conditions that result in loss of muscle. Sarcopenia is associated with a number of factors including, reduced level of physical activity, loss of motor units, decreased androgen production, insulin resistance, inadequate dietary protein, and inflammation. However, loss of skeletal muscle as the principal feature of sarcopenia has evolved. While the loss of muscle amount appears to be a universal phenomenon of aging and is associated with risk of disability, it is the age-associated loss of strength that is more strongly associated with risk of mobility disability.[2,3] Longitudinal trials also reveal that rate of age-associated loss of muscle strength is greater than that of loss of muscle mass. In a longitudinal aging study, Goodpaster et al.[4] demonstrated that although the loss of muscle mass was associated with the decline in strength in older adults, the strength decline was much more rapid than the concomitant loss of muscle mass, suggesting a decline in muscle quality. They also reported that maintaining or gaining muscle mass does not prevent aging-associated declines in muscle strength.

Changes in muscle force production may be independent of skeletal muscle mass. Fiatarone et al.[5] examined the relationship between amount of muscle and muscle strength in a group of 89 extremely old and frail nursing home residents. They showed a significant correlation, however, after controlling for gender, r = 0.25, demonstrating that muscle mass explained only a very small amount (only 6%) of the variability in muscle strength. This lack of a strong relationship between muscle mass and force production in very old people may result from a number of factors. Muscle strength is a function of muscle mass, muscle quality, and neurological recruitment of motor units. Motor unit recruitment patterns are unlikely to be responsive to nutritional interventions; however, low skeletal muscle amount and poor quality may be a result of changing diet and nutritional needs with advancing age.

The term "frailty" has been used for decades to describe elderly patients who have multiple chronic diseases, limited activities of daily living, and increased risk of disability and loss of independence. The concept of frailty was much used but poorly understood. But it was not until Fried et al.[6] provided an operational definition of frailty that factors which may contribute to this syndrome could be described and understood. Frailty is increasingly recognized as a geriatric syndrome that compromises the ability to maintain a stable homeostasis and is associated with an increased risk for multiple adverse health-related outcomes, including falls, fractures, disability, institutionalization, and death.[6,7] Frailty is considered a continuum rather than a discrete process, where several stages or degrees of severity can be reversed with appropriate interventions.[8] The components of frailty described by Fried et al.[6] consist of weight loss, fatigue, slow gait speed, weakness, and low activity levels. According to this model, those individuals with one or two of these conditions would be considered "pre-frail," and those with three or more are considered to be frail.

Low muscle mass or function may be an important contributor to each of the frailty categories. Changes in skeletal muscle loss include three categories: cachexia, sarcopenia, and inactivity (atrophy).[9] While there is overlap with each of these potential causes of loss of muscle, it is important to understand the etiology of this loss to determine the appropriate treatment. Each of these conditions results in a metabolic adaptation of increased protein degradation (cachexia), decreased rate of muscle protein synthesis (inactivity), or an alteration in both (sarcopenia). Cachexia is characterized by loss of skeletal muscle and body weight and is considered a metabolic condition associated with an underlying illness and inflammation.[10] Sarcopenia is the age-associated loss of skeletal muscle and function.[11] Sarcopenia is a complex syndrome that may also be associated with muscle mass loss alone or in combination with increased fat mass. The causes of sarcopenia are multifactorial and can include disuse, changing endocrine function, chronic diseases, inflammation, insulin resistance, and nutritional deficiencies. Sarcopenia is considered a major component in the pathway leading to frailty.[6,12,13] Unlike that seen in any other group of people, in older people, functional capacity is a powerful predictor of morbidity and mortality. Habitual gait speed, measured over a 3 or 4 m course, is an easy to assess index of functional status,[14,15] and slow habitual gait speed is associated with mortality, risk of hospitalization and institutionalization. Indeed, Studenski et al.[16] accumulated data from a number of studies that measured habitual gait speed and reported a striking relationship between walking speed and mortality. They concluded that "gait speed may be a simple and accessible indicator of the health of an older person." Sarcopenia will be diagnosed not only based on low muscle mass, but based on those with a slow habitual gait speed.[11]

## DIETARY FACTORS

Basal metabolic rate (BMR) declines with advancing age, and the cause of this changing BMR is saropenia.[1] Declining BMR and reduced levels of overall activity contribute to decreased energy requirements in older people. Increased fatness in older individuals results from a continuing reduction in energy needs and a lack of matched decrease in energy intake. Increasing body fatness is strongly associated with risk of mobility disability in older people. Goodpaster et al.[17] examined thigh CT scans from 2627 men and women between 70 and 79 years. By examination of the CT attenuation score, they determined the amount of intramyocellular fat and demonstrated that lipid accumulation increased with increasing BMI and with advancing age. Higher muscle attenuation values (indicating greater amount of muscle lipid) were also associated with greater specific force production (r = 0.26, P < 0.01). Multivariate regression analysis revealed that the attenuation coefficient of muscle was independently associated with muscle strength after adjustment for muscle cross-sectional area and mid-thigh adipose tissue in men and women. Increased body fatness in older people is also associated with increased markers of inflammation which may have a direct effect on skeletal muscle protein metabolism and result in decreased muscle mass and/or quality.[18]

## WEIGHT LOSS

Body fatness contributes to risk of chronic diseases such as type 2 diabetes, hypertension and stroke, and chronic kidney disease. The accumulation of fat in skeletal muscle also results in insulin resistance and reduced muscle quality (decreased force produced/cross-sectional area). In addition, older people with insulin resistance or type 2 diabetes experience an accelerated rate of sarcopenia and experience reduced muscle quality compared with age-match individuals with normal glucose tolerance.[19] However, weight loss to decrease body fatness in elderly people may be problematic. Newman et al.[20] reported that the composition of weight gain in elderly people is almost entirely fat and during weight loss older people experience an exaggerated loss of skeletal muscle mass. They concluded that "these findings suggest that weight loss, even with regain, could accelerate sarcopenia in older adults." Ensrud et al.[21] examined the effects of weight gain, weight stability, or weight loss on changes in bone density and fracture risk in 6785 older women over an average of 5.7 years. They reported that women who lost weight had 1.8 times the risk of a subsequent hip fracture than those women who were weight stable or had gained weight irrespective of current weight or intention to lose weight. They concluded that even voluntary weight loss in overweight women increases the risk of hip fracture. Villareal et al.[22] examined the effects of caloric restriction with and without a regular exercise program in postmenopausal women. They showed that the women who lost weight and did not exercise decreased bone mineral density over a 1 year time, and those who exercised showed no change in bone density.

Weight loss in elderly people is difficult to achieve. As described previously, declining BMR and physical activity levels result in a low energy requirement. In very older nursing home residents, average kcal intake to achieve energy balance was 1675 ± 297 for men and 1358 ± 236 for women.[23] These estimates were determined from weighing meals before and after serving an individual. With energy intake this low, a 200–300 energy deficit would be very difficult to achieve and would compromise nutrition status.

One potential dietary intervention that has been demonstrated to result in significant weight loss in older people is a shift in dietary macronutrient intake away from fat and increased carbohydrate (CHO) and protein intake. Hays et al. examined the response of overweight elderly men and women with impaired glucose tolerance to a diet that consisted of 20% of energy from fat, 60% of energy from CHO, and 20% from protein. They provided the diet ad libitum with each subject provided 150% of estimated energy requirement and measured food intake by weighing the food provided and uneaten food returned. The subjects were randomly assigned to the low-fat diet, the low-fat diet + aerobic exercise (3 days/week), or a control group that provided 40% of energy from fat, 45% CHO, and 15% from protein. Subjects in both dietary groups did not change their total dietary energy intake;

however, those consuming the lower-fat diet lost a significant amount of weight, while those consuming the higher fat intake showed no change in weight (low fat + exercise, −4.8 ± 0.9 kg [P = 0.003], and low fat no exercise, −3.2 ± 1.2 kg [P = 0.02]) and a higher percentage of body fat (−3.5% ± 0.7% [P = 0.01] and −2.2% +/−1.2% [P = 0.049]) than controls (−0.1 ± 0.6 kg and 0.2% ± 0.6%). None of the groups demonstrated a decrease in BMR, which is a common adaptation to a hypocaloric diet. Using a hyper-insulinemic, euglcycemic glucose clamp, these investigators[24] also demonstrated that the subjects on the low-fat diet increased their rate of glucose disposal. In one of the largest dietary intervention studies,[25] the Women's Health Initiative Dietary Modification trial randomly assigned >48,000 postmenopausal women to an intervention or control group. The intervention included group and individual sessions to promote a decrease in fat intake and increases in vegetable, fruit, and grain consumption and did not include weight loss or caloric restriction goals. The control group received diet-related education materials. The women in the intervention group lost weight (those in the control group did not), and those who maintained a fat intake that was >10% below baseline intake retained their significant weight loss for up to 7 years. This study also demonstrated that the greater the decrease in dietary fat intake, the greater the amount of weight loss and maintenance of that loss in weight. In commenting on this study, Bray[26] wrote that "those who adhered to a low-fat diet maintaining their initial reduction in body fat much more effectively than those who did not … long-term success in reducing intake of dietary fat may be an important strategy for weight maintenance."

## DIETARY PROTEIN

Taken together, these studies indicate that a shift in macronutrient intake away from fat may be an important, safe, and effective strategy for elderly people to lose body fat and maintain a low BMI. Both CHO and protein increase thermogenesis (increased metabolic rate), while dietary fat has almost no thermic effect.[27] Dietary protein is more thermogenic than is CHO such that a diet that is rich in protein may result in a prolonged increase in metabolic rate and have a significant effect on energy balance. Acheson et al.[28] examined the postprandial increase in metabolic rate following protein and CHO intake. They reported a 14% increase in metabolic rate following ingestion of whey protein that was significantly greater than that seen following an equivalent casein or soy protein intake. The rise in thermogenesis was greater for any protein source than that following ingestion of glucose.

Increased dietary protein coupled with a decrease in fat intake may have a number of important benefits. A growing body of literature demonstrates that aging is associated with an increased need for dietary protein and an increase in dietary protein intake in older people has been associated with improved functional capacity and bone health.[29]

Campbell et al.[30] reported that when healthy older (n = 12, 56–80 years) people were provided the U.S. recommended dietary allowance (USRDA) for protein of 0.8 g × kg⁻¹ × day⁻¹, they remained in negative nitrogen balance for almost 10 days. They argued that these data and a reexamination of previous studies examining protein requirements in older people was a strong indication that the current USRDA for protein was inadequate to meet the needs for most older people. A subsequent longitudinal study[31] examined the adaptations that older men and women made to 3 months of consuming 0.8 g protein × kg⁻¹ × day⁻¹. The subjects in this study were initially in negative nitrogen balance and accommodated to the protein intake by a gradual improvement in N balance. The accommodation occurred at the expense of muscle mass as there was a significant reduction of thigh muscle cross-sectional area. These data provide strong evidence that the current USRDA for protein is inadequate for older people and long-term consumption of a diet providing this amount of protein will result in accelerated sarcopenia, even if an individual consumes high-quality protein and maintains his/her body weight. Any weight loss would further increase the need for dietary protein. In support of these clinical trials,[32] a longitudinal, observational study of 2066 men and women between 70 and 79 examined dietary protein intake, and changes in FFM over 3 years were measured by using dual-energy x-ray absorptiometry. After adjustment for potential confounders and using an energy-adjusted protein intake, the investigators reported that participants in the highest quintile of protein intake lost approximately 40% less lean mass (LM) and aLM (appendicular LM) than did those in the lowest quintile of protein intake. Beasley et al.[33] prospectively examined a cohort of 24,417 women aged 65–79 years who were free of frailty at baseline. After 3 years of follow-up, the investigators measured those exhibiting symptoms of frailty using the Fried criteria[6] and reported that a 20% increase in protein intake was associated with a 32% (95% CI = 23%–50%) lower risk of frailty. They concluded that "Incorporating more protein into the diet may be an intervention target for frailty prevention."

The age-associated increase in the need for dietary protein is very likely a result of a number metabolic, hormonal, and lifestyle changes that occur with advancing age. Hormonal changes include decreases in testosterone, estrogen, growth hormone and IGF1, and insulin resistance. Each of these changes has been demonstrated to reduce the rate of muscle protein synthesis. Decreased levels of physical activity result in decreased muscle protein synthetic rate and loss of muscle mass.[34] A greatly reduced level of physical activity is common among elderly people. For older people, hospitalization can result in reduced bone density, orthostatic intolerance, increased thrombotic effects, reduced cognitive function, and reduced functional capacity.[35] Length of stay in a hospital is longer for older people compared with young patients and is increased more if an elderly individual enters the hospital with type 2 diabetes.

In addition to the detrimental effects of reduced physical activity in older patients, reduced food intake during hospitalization increases morbidity and mortality. Sullivan et al.[36] examined 497 patients 65 years and older admitted to a VA hospital. They reported that 21% of these patients had an average daily in-hospital nutrient intake of less than 50% of their calculated maintenance energy requirements. These patients had a significantly higher in-hospital mortality rate as well as 90 day post-discharge mortality compared with those patients with adequate intake. These investigators showed that the principal reason for reduced food intake is that many of these patients were provided substantially lower amounts of food because these patients were frequently ordered to have nothing by mouth and were not fed by another route. The data demonstrated that nutrition status among elderly hospitalized patients has a powerful effect on outcomes that is independent of diagnosis. Kortebein et al.[37] examined the responses of healthy older men and women to 10 days of complete bed rest. Subjects consumed a eucaloric diet (no change in body weight) that provided the USRDA for protein before and during the bed rest period. Interestingly, these subjects were in negative N balance prior to bed rest providing more evidence for inadequacy of the protein RDA for elderly people. During the bed rest period, all subjects experienced a substantial decrease in N balance accompanied by an average 1.5 kg decrease in whole-body LM and a 0.95 kg decrease in aLM. The loss of muscle mass was due to a striking decrease in the fractional rate of muscle protein synthesis (FSR). The subjects experienced a 15.1% reduction in $VO_{2peak}$ and a similar reduction in strength. Despite the fact that these subjects were healthy with no functional deficits when they started the bed rest period, there average level of physical activity was reduced (almost 8% reduction in PA) when they returned home. Ferrando et al.[38] tested the effects of providing a mixture of essential amino acids (EAA) in older people during 10 days of bed rest in older subjects. Subjects were given a placebo (n = 12, 68 ± 5 (SD) years, 83 ± 19 kg) or 15 g of EAA (n = 10, 71 ± 6, 72 ± 8 kg) three times per day throughout 10 days of bed rest and showed that the supplemented group preserved pre–bed rest protein FSR and LM. This study strongly suggests that increasing dietary protein intake during bed rest, hospitalization, or substantial reductions in physical activity may help to preserve muscle mass and functional status.

## CONCLUSIONS

Loss of skeletal muscle mass is central to the development of frailty in older people. Sarcopenia is common with advancing age and the rate of sarcopenia is responsive to nutritional status, particularly dietary protein. Healthy older people consuming the current USRDA for protein are at risk of losing skeletal muscle at an accelerated rate

and developing frailty. Increased dietary protein intake will preserve or increase muscle mass and function, particularly during periods of extreme inactivity such as prolonged bed rest during hospitalization. Another common feature of aging is an increase in body fatness. Body fat is an independent predictor of disability and poor functional status; however, caloric restriction to lose body weight results in substantial loss of muscle mass and bone density. Strategies for weight loss for older people should include exercise to help preserve LM and a shift in macronutrient intake toward a lower-fat and higher protein and carbohydrate intake to maintain nutritional status.

## REFERENCES

1. Tzankoff SP, Norris AH. *J Appl Physiol* 33:536;1978.
2. Newman AB, Kupelian V, Visser M et al. *J Am Geriatr Soc* 51:1602;2003.
3. Newman AB, Kupelian V, Visser M et al. *J Gerontol A Biol Sci Med Sci* 61:72;2006.
4. Goodpaster BH, Park SW, Harris TB et al. *J Gerontol A Biol Sci Med Sci* 61:1059;2006.
5. Fiatarone MA, O'Neill EF, Ryan ND et al. *N Engl J Med* 330:1769;1994.
6. Fried LP, Tangen CM, Walston J et al. *J Gerontol A Biol Sci Med Sci* 56:M146;2001.
7. Bandeen-Roche K, Xue QL, Ferrucci L et al. *J Gerontol A Biol Sci Med Sci* 61:262;2006.
8. Walston J, Hadley EC, Ferrucci L et al. *J Am Geriatr Soc* 54:991;2006.
9. Evans WJ. *Am J Clin Nutr* 91:1123S;2010.
10. Evans WJ, Morley JE, Argiles J et al. *Clin Nutr* 27:793;2008.
11. Fielding RA, Vellas B, Evans WJ et al. *J Am Med Dir Assoc* 12:249;2011.
12. Evans WJ. *J Gerontol A Biol Sci Med Sci* 50:5;1995.
13. Evans WJ, Campbell WW. *J Nutr* 123:465;1993.
14. Guralnik JM, Ferrucci L, Pieper CF et al. *J Gerontol A Biol Sci Med Sci* 55:M221;2000.
15. Guralnik JM, Ferrucci L, Simonsick EM et al. *N Engl J Med* 332:556;1995.
16. Studenski S, Perera S, Patel K et al. *JAMA* 305:50;2011.
17. Goodpaster BH, Carlson CL, Visser M et al. *J Appl Physiol* 90:2157;2001.
18. Schrager MA, Metter EJ, Simonsick E et al. *J Appl Physiol* 102:919;2007.
19. Park SW, Goodpaster BH, Strotmeyer ES et al. *Diabetes* 55:1813;2006.
20. Newman AB, Lee JS, Visser M et al. *Am J Clin Nutr* 82:872;2005.
21. Ensrud KE, Ewing SK, Stone KL et al. *J Am Geriatr Soc* 51:1740;2003.
22. Villareal DT, Fontana L, Weiss EP et al. *Arch Intern Med* 166:2502;2006.
23. Bernstein M, Tucker KL, Ryan ND et al. *J Am Diet Assoc* 102:1096;2002.
24. Hays NP, Starling RD, Sullivan DH et al. *J Gerontol A Biol Sci Med Sci* 61:299;2006.
25. Howard BV, Manson JE, Stefanick ML et al. *JAMA* 295:9;2006.
26. Bray GA. *Am J Clin Nutr* 93:481;2011.

27. Jequier E, Tappy L. *Physiol Rev* 79:451;1999.
28. Acheson KJ, Blondel-Lubrano A, Oguey Araymon S et al. *Am J Clin Nutr* 93:525;2011.
29. Wolfe RR, Miller SL, Miller KB. *Clin Nutr* 27:675;2008.
30. Campbell WW, Crim MC, Dallal GE et al. *Am J Clin Nutr* 60:167;1994.
31. Campbell WW, Trappe TA, Wolfe RR et al. *J Gerontol A Biol Sci Med Sci* 56:M373;2001.
32. Houston DK, Nicklas BJ, Ding J et al. *Am J Clin Nutr* 87:150;2008.
33. Beasley JM, LaCroix AZ, Neuhouser ML et al. *J Am Geriatr Soc* 58:1063;2010.
34. Ferrando AA, Lane HW, Stuart CA et al. *Am J Physiol* 270:E627;1996.
35. Creditor MC. *Ann Intern Med* 118:219;1993.
36. Sullivan DH, Sun S, Walls RC. *JAMA* 281:2013;1999.
37. Kortebein P, Ferrando A, Lombeida J et al. *JAMA* 297:1772;2007.
38. Ferrando AA, Paddon-Jones D, Hays NP et al. *Clin Nutr* 29:18;2010.

# 65 Enteral and Parenteral Nutrition

*Zhaoping Li and David Heber*

## CONTENTS

## INTRODUCTION

While humans are well adapted to uncomplicated starvation with the ability to survive for up to 6 months with adequate fluid and electrolytes, acute or chronic critical illness can activate the immune system and impair the adaptation to starvation leading to various nutritional deficits, including sarcopenia and weakness, impaired immune function, and premature death.[1–5] In fact, the loss of greater than 50% of pre-illness lean body mass is incompatible with life due to the immune impairment that accompanies this protein loss, leading to complicating infections and sepsis often from bacteria or viruses that could be removed if immune function were intact. A prominent cause of death in severely malnourished patients and one of the most common causes of death in adults and especially in children under the age of 5 years in developing countries is infection secondary to malnutrition. Up to 50% of patients hospitalized in general medical and surgical wards are also malnourished, but often do not display the outward signs of reduced body weight so typical of malnutrition in free-living adults. As discussed elsewhere in this text, evidence of protein–calorie malnutrition such as hypoalbuminemia is a harbinger of poor survival from a wide range of medical conditions in hospitalized patients and increasingly in community or home settings as patients are provided nutritional support outside the hospital. The early assessment of nutritional status leading to the early provision of nutrients is key in the multidisciplinary management of malnutrition in illness.

A survey of over 500 international health professionals found that early specialized nutrition support is an accepted practice. More than 90% of physicians and dietitians around the world strongly recommended the initiation of either enteral (EN) or parenteral nutrition (PN) within 24–48 h after a patient is admitted to an intensive care unit (ICU). However, there is a significant gap between this perception and the actual practice of initiating nutritional support.[6] There are still unsettled issues about the timing of initiating PN when EN either is impossible or does not meet the nutritional goals of the patient. The recommendations contained in current guidelines from different medical specialty societies are not universally accepted as yet and are largely based on expert opinions and data from limited clinical investigations.[2,4] This chapter will review the appropriate use of EN and PN in detail with some discussion of the transition or choice between the two methods of providing nutrition support to patients unable to obtain adequate nutrition from food alone.

### ENTERAL VERSUS PARENTERAL NUTRITION

Over the past two decades, EN has generally been preferred over total PN (TPN) for several reasons, including lower morbidity, lower costs, a shorter length of hospital stay, and the preservation of both the mucosal barrier and maintenance of immune function.[7,8] The dictum "If the gut works, use it" has become a standard part of medical and surgical training mantra. There was great enthusiasm for the wide application of TPN in the 1970s and early 1980s due to a general belief that aggressive nutritional support could reverse or delay the progression of such serious disorders as cancer cachexia and AIDS. The enthusiasm for TPN waned with the discovery of the predominant role of tumor or viral proliferation and systemic inflammation in the progression of these diseases. Concomitant with the disappointment over the failure of TPN to reverse the progression of underlying disease conditions, evidence of significant adverse metabolic conditions associated with TPN became apparent. In fact, most of these reported complications were due to the administration of hypercaloric PN with hyperglycemia and hypercapnia leading to detrimental clinical outcomes.[9] Therefore, the prescription of less-caloric PN, which includes parenteral lipid emulsions as well as amino acids and glucose, has been adopted by various critical care facilities to avoid the risks of overloading syndrome. Some recent randomized trials[10] and meta-analyses[11] have shown that PN adjusted to lower calories and proper macronutrient composition is as reliable as EN for critically ill patients. Significant differences remain with EN being less costly than PN and utilizing the systems related to the gastrointestinal (GI) tract more effectively including the immune system. Therefore, the use of EN will be discussed first followed by PN including TPN.

## EARLY INITIATION OF ENTERAL NUTRITION

Clinical guidelines recommend the initiation of EN as soon as possible in critically ill patients[1–3,5] based on substantial evidence and expert opinion.[11–13] In the past, EN has been withheld after surgeries such as gastric resection until bowel movements appeared, and then EN would be initiated. However, the initiation of EN is now recommended regardless of the presence of traditional clinical milestones of improved GI function such as the presence of bowel sounds and flatus.[12] In the critically ill patient, early EN at or near 100% of the calories prescribed via the gut can reduce mortality, particularly in malnourished patients who have undergone medical or surgical procedures.[14] Underfeeding is common in critically ill patients, mainly because of GI dysmotility resulting in diarrhea or comorbid complications including hemodynamic conditions.[15] EN increases hemodynamic demands on the splanchnic circulation, and if it is compromised due to vascular disease or trauma, then EN can lead to lethal complications such as non-occlusive bowel necrosis. Fortunately, this complication is infrequent with an estimated incidence of 0.3%–8.5% in the ICU. However, non-occlusive bowel necrosis may occur even in young patients who previously tolerated EN.[16,17]

On the positive side, there is substantial and consistent evidence that early EN postoperatively is both safe and is associated with enhanced recovery and fewer complications.[18–20] A meta-analysis of 15 randomized trials and 1240 patients undergoing GI tract resection found that on balance early postoperative EN is associated with a significant reduction in total complications compared with traditional postoperative feeding practices.[19] A significant reduction of 45% in all postoperative complications was seen when early postoperative feeding was administered. One potential explanation is that the provision of EN may protect the gut's barrier function and maintain gut-associated lymphoid tissue (GALT) mass and function. The GALT is the largest component of the immune system, and maintaining its function through EN may be important in maintaining immune function. Another new area that will receive attention in the future is the effect of EN on the microbial flora or microbiome of the gut. The early use of EN was also supported by another meta-analysis of results from three randomized trials that included 126 trauma patients admitted to a critical care setting. Early provision of EN was associated with reduced mortality in this meta-analysis as well.[21]

EN formulations have changed over the years. An elemental diet was used in the beginning era of early postoperative feeding during the early 1980s.[22] A progressive advance toward either a polymeric or a partially hydrolyzed diet occurred during the next decade.[23,24] Two meta-analyses showed that the perioperative prescription of immune-enhancing nutrients, especially arginine, is advantageous compared with a standard diet when attempting to reduce the risk of infectious complications and anastomotic dehiscence.[25,26] Arginine-supplemented diets can overcome arginine deficiency, which can occur after surgical trauma. The perioperative administration of enteral arginine supplementation together with omega-3 ($\omega$-3) fats may restore T-lymphocyte function, including CD4 count, and may thus beneficially affect the surgical patient. Furthermore, arginine metabolism via arginase-1 may improve healing by increasing the production of polyamines.[27] One of the aims of nutritional support in critical illness is to minimize the loss of lean body mass that occurs rapidly after trauma or sepsis. Most authorities advocate the avoidance of either prolonged hypocaloric or hypercaloric feeding.[28–32]

## ENTERAL FORMULAS

Enteral formulas in general can be divided into two basic categories: (1) polymeric formulas or (2) elemental formulas and semi-elemental formulas. These categories can be further divided into standard, disease-specific, and immune-enhancing formulas. Numerous enteral formulas exist in each category, with each company making different beneficial claims for its products. These products do not currently require Food and Drug Administration (FDA) approval for their proposed clinical implications and are regulated as food supplements. Polymeric standard formulas contain nutrient profiles that approach a typical diet that meets general dietary recommendations. Most nutritionally complete commercial formulas contain adequate vitamins and minerals when a sufficient volume of formula to meet energy and macronutrient needs is provided. Some disease-specific formulas are nutritionally incomplete in relation to vitamin and mineral content (e.g., hepatic formulas).

Liquid vitamin and mineral supplements may be indicated for patients receiving nutritionally incomplete or diluted formulas for prolonged periods of time. Fat-soluble vitamin supplementation such as vitamin K may be indicated for patients with fat malabsorption or for patients with vitamin K deficiency; most commercial formulas include vitamin K. The quantity of water in enteral formulas is often described as water content or moisture content. The quantity of water is usually reported in milliliters of water either per 1000 mL of formula or per liter of formula. Most enteral formulas contain water in the general range of 690–860 mL/1000 mL of enteral formula. This must be considered when making fluid recommendations.

Standard polymeric enteral formulas are the most widely used in patients requiring EN, ranging from hospitalized patients and nursing home residents to home-care patients. Some popular formulas are also available over the counter without a prescription. In order to manage patients who may require more concentrated nutrition or who have specific fluid restrictions, polymeric formulas are available in concentrations varying from 1 to 2 kcal/mL. Formulas concentrated to deliver 2 kcal/mL are used in patients requiring fluid restriction such as those with congestive heart failure, renal failure, ascites or edema, hyponatremia due to fluid overload, or retention of water due to the endocrine abnormality of inappropriate secretion of antidiuretic hormone. Another use for these formulas is the delivery of smaller volumes to meet calorie requirements of the patients who have high caloric requirements or who require cyclic feeding, nocturnal feeding, or bolus feeding because only smaller volumes are tolerated. The use of concentrated formulas must be accompanied by additional water flushes of nasogastric or intragastric tubes, intravenous fluids, or some oral water intake in order to avoid hypernatremia due to dehydration. Major contributors to the renal solute load that must be excreted are the protein, sodium, potassium, and chloride in enteral formulas. Adequate hydration is necessary for glomerular filtration in the kidney and normal clearance of these solutes.

GI tolerance (e.g., gastric retention, abdominal distention, diarrhea, nausea, and vomiting) is influenced by the osmolality of enteral formulas that is obviously increased in the more hypercaloric versions. This problem is especially relevant in critically ill patients. Administering hypertonic formulas at a slow, continuous rate initially (10–20 cc/h) with a gradual titration to the final volume while monitoring for GI complications can reduce the incidence of GI intolerance and allow these formulas to be administered at full strength without problems. What may be more important than the osmolality of the enteral formula is the osmotic contribution from liquid medications either infused with the enteral formula or infused through the feeding tube. The average osmolality range of commercially prepared liquid medications is reported to be 450–10,950 mOsm/kg.[67] The osmolality of enteral formulas ranges from 270 to 700 mOsm/kg.

The method for enteral tube feeding is limited to the type and site of enteral feeding access. The formula delivery method selected for the patient also depends on the patient's hemodynamic stability, gastric emptying rate, GI tolerance to tube feeding, type of formula selected, nutrient needs, patient mobility, and ease of administration. The main methods of tube feeding are by continuous, intermittent, or bolus delivery.

Each institution should have an established protocol for the initiation and advancement of enteral feedings. Bolus feedings involve the delivery of larger amounts of formula over short periods of time, usually 5 min or less. The bolus method should only be used with gastric delivery. The stomach can act as a reservoir to handle relatively large volumes of formula (e.g., 400 mL) over a short time as opposed to the small intestine. The feedings are usually administered via a gastrostomy tube, owing to the large lumen, but they can also be given through a small-bore nasogastric tube. Usually a syringe or bulb is used to push 200–500 mL of formula into the feeding tube several times a day. A patient should demonstrate adequate gastric emptying and the ability to protect his/her airway (i.e., an intact gag reflex) prior to initiating bolus feedings, especially in the critical care setting, to decrease the risk of aspiration. The ability to absorb nutrients using this type of feeding depends on the access site and the functional capability of the gut.

Bolus feedings are considered the most physiologic method of administration as the gut can rest between feedings and allow for normal hormonal fluctuations. They are the easiest to administer as a pump is not required. Bolus feedings also allow for increased patient mobility as they are delivered intermittently and do not require a pump. For these reasons, this method of feeding is most desirable for stable patients who are going home or to an extended care facility with tube feedings.

Intermittent feeding requires the formula to be infused over a 20–30 min period. A feeding container and gravity drip are usually used for this method. Intermittent feedings are less likely to cause GI side effects than bolus feeding, as the formula is administered over a longer interval. Depending on the volume delivered, this method may be used for gastric, as well as small bowel, formula delivery.

Continuous formula delivery is usually the enteral delivery method best tolerated. Continuous feedings are delivered slowly over 12–24 h, typically with an infusion pump. In order to avoid accidental bolus delivery, continuous infusion is preferred over gravity, as a constant infusion rate can be sustained. Postpyloric feedings require continuous infusion. The small bowel does not act as a reservoir for large volumes of fluid within a short time, and GI complications usually arise if feedings are delivered in this manner. Initiation and progression of continuous feedings should be individualized and based on the patient's clinical condition and feeding tolerance. Typically, feedings may be initiated at 10–50 mL/h, with lower range for the critically ill. Progression of tube feedings may range from 10 to 25 mL/h every 4–24 h, depending on the patient's tolerance, until the desired goal rate is achieved. As a patient begins to transition to oral intake, the tube feedings may be cycled to allow for appetite stimulation or to allow for bowel rest and time away from the pump. The feedings may be administered at night and held back during the day to allow for patient mobility and an opportunity to eat.

Enteral formulas meet the RDA but lack important phytochemicals found in a healthy diet. While an emerging area of research, these phytochemicals have potential benefits in several organ systems. Therefore, patients requiring long-term EN and their caregivers may at some point wish to use the so-called natural EN where foods are blended. As an example, a commercial formula called Compleat Pediatric (Nestle, Inc.) contains blended chicken, peas, carrots, tomatoes, and cranberry juice. For patients and health-care workers who want to prepare natural EN, recipes have been developed and published that can be used for guidance.[33] Potential issues in using homemade EN include risk of foodborne infections, proper blenderizing to avoid clogging feeding tubes, and the inclusion of adequate macronutrients and micronutrients to meet dietary needs.

Meeting protein goals for nutritional support includes a consideration of nonprotein calories that must be administered together with protein to provide adequate energy for incorporation into the body of the administered protein. In general, the average healthy adult requires a nonprotein calorie to gram of nitrogen (npc:g N) ratio of 150–250:1. In a catabolic state, the body catabolizes lean body mass as a nitrogen and energy source. To minimize this process, it is recommended to provide an npc:g N of 100–150:1. This protein content of enteral formulas becomes extremely important in patients who require healing of wounds due to trauma, burns, metabolic stress, and infection and increased wound-healing requirements.

Standard polymeric formulas with added fiber are used to help decrease diarrhea and prevent constipation especially in patients requiring long-term EN. However, the effects of fiber-containing formulas on diarrhea remain to be established. The Adequate Intake of the Dietary Reference Intake recommendation for fiber is between 25 and 38 g/d based on total caloric requirement. Currently, the enteral formula with the greatest amount of fiber has only 18 g/L at a calorie concentration of 1.2 kcal/mL. It would require 1800 calories of this formula to provide 27 g of fiber. From a practical standpoint, it is difficult to meet the recommended amount of fiber from fiber-containing enteral formulas, especially in the acute care setting where most patients do not receive 100% of prescribed EN.[34–37]

Fiber-enriched shakes using both soluble and insoluble fibers have been offered to promote digestive health through the prebiotic effects of fiber on colonic microflora. Undigestible fibers such as fructo-oligosaccharides are delivered to the large bowel where they are metabolized by the colonic microflora. There are limited data on this potential benefit and its significance, but one clinical trial in patients requiring long-term EN in which such fibers were used[38] demonstrated a significant increase in short-chain fatty acids and a change in the microflora. In the hospitalized, critically ill patient population, there are no such data available. Fiber also may enhance glycemic control in patients with impaired glucose tolerance by slowing transit time, but this has not been adequately tested. The data from studies on fiber-containing formulas do not yet demonstrate significant effects on digestive health or glycemic control in the ICU or in patients receiving long-term EN. It is not generally harmful to provide fiber-containing formulas to long-term home EN patients as long as there is adequate attention to fluid intake and the prevention of constipation. Fiber-containing formulas may need to be avoided in hypotensive patients at high risk for developing ischemic bowel,[39] and there have been case reports of bowel obstruction associated with the use of fiber-containing formula in the burn and trauma patients.[40]

Elemental and semi-elemental enteral formulas are designed to deliver protein as free amino acids or dipeptides and tripeptides and fat as medium-chain triglycerides (TGs) with the concept that providing more easily absorbed forms of protein and fat will require minimal digestive efforts for absorption in patients who have either malabsorption or pancreatic insufficiency. Limited trials have been conducted comparing free amino acid and peptide-based formulas to a standard formula. When compared to standard enteral formulas, semi-elemental and elemental formulas demonstrate no advantage for patients with Crohn's disease or in critically ill patients in terms of mortality, infectious complications, or diarrhea. There is very little clinical evidence to support the use of elemental or semi-elemental formulas, even in patients with pancreatic insufficiency and maldigestion. In summary, for most patients with malabsorption and/or maldigestion unable to be managed with a standard formula and exogenous pancreatic enzymes, an elemental or semi-elemental formula may be an alternative option. In cases of maldigestion with intestinal villous atrophy, a progressive program of advancing from elemental to semi-elemental to standard formulas is a common practice, but there are no clinical trial data to support this logical approach.

## DISEASE–SPECIFIC FORMULATIONS

### DIABETES FORMULAS

Enteral formulas for diabetes have been developed as medical foods with the potential benefit of improved glycemic control. Enteral formulas designed for glycemic control typically include a mixture of soluble and insoluble fibers, as well as 42%–49% fat with a reduction in carbohydrates from typical polymeric formulas to the range of 31%–40% of total calories. Formulas have been further modified to include increased amounts of monounsaturated fatty acids (MUFA) and less polyunsaturated and saturated fatty acids based on the research from the nutritional literature on MUFA and type 2 diabetes mellitus. The use of these formulas in hospitalized patients has not been beneficial. A study of 50 ICU patients with glucose intolerance receiving continuous insulin infusions was randomized to receive either a standard enteral formula or an isocaloric diabetes formula. Although the patients who received the diabetes formula had improved glycemic control and decreased insulin requirements, no significant differences were found between groups in infectious complications, ICU length of stay, ventilator duration, or mortality.[41] When glycemic control in hospitalized patients with type 2 diabetes was studied using a diabetes formula higher in fat content (50% fat with 33.3% MUFA) versus another diabetes formula higher in carbohydrate content (starch and fructose based), blood glucose was significantly higher at day 8 in the group that received the high-carbohydrate diabetes formula when compared with baseline ($P = 0.006$) but not in the group that received the high-fat formula. By days 8 and 15, mean blood glucose was equally high (>200 mg/dL) in both groups indicating that neither formula was helpful in controlling blood glucose.[42] While glycemic control and decreased insulin requirements were demonstrated in one other study of diabetes formulas,[43] the clinical significance of the results was not evident.

The clinical benefits of using a diabetes formula remain unclear based on current evidence. Diabetes enteral formulas now include higher amounts of MUFA, which is consistent with the American Diabetes Association recommendations.[44] The evidence that these formulas are clinically important has not been gathered. One potential caution in using these formulas relates to the delayed gastric emptying known to occur in diabetes. Symptoms of nausea and vomiting related to poor gastric motility might be exacerbated with a high-fat, fiber-containing diabetes enteral formula.

## RENAL FORMULAS

Renal disease–specific enteral formulas have lower protein and electrolyte concentrations than standard formulas. Potassium, phosphorus, and magnesium concentrations are also reduced in renal formulas. These two changes have been incorporated to decrease the buildup of toxins as well as electrolytes in patients with chronic kidney disease. No comparative clinical trials to date have been conducted to assess the efficacy and clinical outcomes of renal formulas when compared with standard formulas.

Commercially available renal disease–specific enteral formulas contain between 7% and 18% protein. In end-stage renal disease, low-protein formulas are used to attempt to avoid dialysis, and thus the intake of protein and electrolytes should be limited. On the other hand, the increased protein needs in patients undergoing dialysis are often unrecognized by clinicians. Chronic kidney disease is associated with hypermetabolism and catabolism of lean body mass.[45] Dialysis is associated with heat loss, increasing energy expenditure via shivering thermogenesis to compensate for the heat loss. Moreover, a stress response occurs during dialysis that further increases catabolism.[46] While dialysis is beneficial in clearing the blood of accumulated electrolytes and toxins, nutrients are lost during dialysis, including the loss of approximately 0.2 g of protein per liter of filtrate.[47,48] Protein breakdown has been measured in patients with chronic kidney

disease, and it is elevated amounting to 1.4–1.8 of protein per kg of body weight per day.[49] Specific formulas for calculating protein needs have been developed, and the Kidney Disease Outcomes Quality Initiative (KDOQI) guidelines suggest that patients on maintenance dialysis receive 1.2–1.3 g of protein per kg of body weight. It is difficult to meet this guideline with low-protein enteral formulas.[50] As discussed elsewhere in this text in detail, protein should be provided in amounts as high as 2.5 g/kg of body weight to maintain nitrogen balance in patients on maintenance dialysis.[51] Either a standard or high-protein formula should be used to limit the loss of lean body mass in patients receiving chronic dialysis and in cases of acute renal failure. It remains a clinical art to use protein restriction in the management of renal failure patients at early stages when it can delay dialysis while using protein to replace losses as best as possible during dialysis. Renal enteral formulas are more useful for the former and less useful in the latter scenarios.

## LIVER DISEASE–SPECIFIC FORMULAS

Enteral formulas designed for patients with liver disease have increased amounts of branched-chain amino acids (BCAAs) and decreased amounts of aromatic amino acids (AAAs) to offset an imbalanced ratio of BCAA:AAA that has been implicated in hepatic encephalopathy. It has been suggested but not proven that plasma amino acids cross the blood–brain barrier where they act as neurotransmitters resulting in hepatic encephalopathy.[52] Unfortunately, carefully controlled clinical studies show no benefit of these special BCAA-enriched formulas in preventing hepatic encephalopathy.[53] In a multicenter, randomized study that compared long-term BCAA supplementation with either an isocaloric or an isocaloric–isonitrogenous enteral supplement for a year in 174 cirrhotic patients, BCAA supplementation was shown to significantly reduce progression of liver failure and deaths when compared with the isocaloric–isonitrogenous formula but not when compared with isocaloric supplement. Although mortality was improved, the finding of encephalopathy did not differ between the BCAA group and other supplementation groups. Therefore, the evidence justifying the use of BCAA-enriched formulas in this population is not yet available. Since patients with end-stage liver disease also typically suffer from protein–calorie malnutrition, it is difficult to justify the use of these formulas that have less protein and cost 10-fold more than standard formulas.

## PULMONARY DISEASE–SPECIFIC FORMULAS

Enteral formulas for patients with pulmonary disease have increased ratios of fat to carbohydrates, with the goal of minimizing total carbon dioxide production since respiratory clearance of carbon dioxide is limited in certain types of chronic lung disease. The protein provided by these formulas is comparable or higher than standard formulas with the concept of maintaining lean body mass in the face of increased energy expenditure from respirations dependent on the diaphragmatic muscle. Originally, these formulas were designed to enable earlier weaning of patients with chronic pulmonary disease from respirators. Unfortunately, while the respiratory quotient changes slightly with the use of these formulas, in one study there was no difference in carbon dioxide production evident with the use of these formulas.[54] Other studies demonstrate expected differences in pulmonary parameters, such as RQ, $VCO_2$, minute ventilation, and end-tidal $CO_2$, when using a high-fat, low-carbohydrate formula, but find no difference in days on mechanical ventilation comparing the special formulas to the standard formulas.[55–58] In one carefully conducted study of a high-fat, low-carbohydrate enteral formula and an isocaloric, isonitrogenous standard formula, the group that received the high-fat, low-carbohydrate formula experienced a decrease in arterial $pCO_2$ and duration of mechanical ventilation.[59] In a critical study, it was shown that hypercaloric feeding in pulmonary disease patients was a more potent factor in correlating with carbon dioxide production than the ratio of carbohydrate and fat.[60]

Specialized enteral formulas for these patients with similar macronutrient ratio as the traditional pulmonary formula and a higher ω-3:ω-6 (omgega-6) fatty acid ratio and antioxidants have been developed for patients with acute lung injury and acute respiratory distress syndrome (ARDS). These formulas are based on the notion that inflammation secondary to arachidonic acid metabolites promotes damage to lung epithelium.[61] An enteral formula enriched with eicosapentaenoic acid (EPA), gamma-linolenic acid (GLA), and antioxidants developed for patients with acute lung injury or ARDS has been studied in comparison with a standard pulmonary formula with similar macronutrients. Compared with the control group, decreases in pulmonary inflammation, improved oxygenation from baseline to day 4 and 7, decreased days of ventilatory support, decreased ICU length of stay, and decreased incidence of new organ failure were observed.[62] These findings have been confirmed in two other studies.[63,64] Based on these studies, a pulmonary enteral formula enriched with a high ω-3:ω-6 fatty acid ratio with additional antioxidants may be useful in the treatment of patients with acute lung injury and ARDS.

## IMMUNONUTRITION AND IMMUNE-ENHANCING FORMULAS

Since immune function is impaired with malnutrition and increased inflammation is a hallmark of many chronic diseases in hospitalized and ICU patients, immune-enhancing enteral formulas have been developed to support immune function by reducing inflammatory processes and enhancing the preservation of GI cells. These goals are accomplished by adding the following four ingredients. First, ω-3 fatty acids have been shown to balance the inflammatory cascade by competing with arachidonic acid for the conversion to eicosanoids. Second, glutamine is supplemented as it is often depleted in ill patients.[65,66] Glutamine is the most abundant amino acid in the body and in normal situations is considered

a nonessential amino acid (NEAA). It can be synthesized in many tissues of the body, predominantly skeletal muscle, and is the primary fuel for rapidly dividing tissues such as the small bowel. It is also a precursor to the antioxidant glutathione. Glutamine has beneficial effects on the GALT, since it is a fuel for intestinal enterocytes and protects the integrity of the gut mucosal barrier.[67] At a cellular level, glutamine has been found to attenuate cytokine release.[66] Third, arginine is a precursor to nitric oxide as well as important in cell growth and wound healing via effects on collagen synthesis. Various aspects of immune function are enhanced through nitric oxide formation.[46] Fourth, nucleotides consumed as RNA are essential in DNA and RNA production, making them important during the high turnover of DNA and RNA observed in ill patients.[67] Finally, antioxidants are often added given the general concept that oxidant stress and inflammation are closely linked, with oxidant stress inducing inflammation and inflammation being amplified through further oxidant stress.

A meta-analysis of studies utilizing a formula supplemented with arginine, ω-3 fatty acids, and nucleotides in elective surgical patients found reduced hospital length of stay; a decrease in infectious complications such as abdominal abscess, wound infection, and pneumonia; and a decrease in complications associated with anastomotic leak by comparison to patients receiving standard formulas.[48] In studies of different immune-enhancing enteral formulas compared to standard formulas in patients undergoing surgery for either head and neck or upper GI cancer, outcomes such as ICU and hospital length of stay, infectious complications, mechanical ventilation, and noninfectious complications were not uniformly improved.[25,68–77] This group of studies may be difficult to interpret due to the heterogeneity of the patients and the formulas studied, and they do not establish the efficacy of these formulas.

Clinical trials of arginine-containing formulas have resulted in inconsistent findings, with some suggestive of increased mortality associated with the use of arginine supplementation in septic patients.[78,79] In extensive meta-analyses and in clinical guideline committee deliberations, the use of arginine in ICU patients was found to have no benefits for mortality, length of stay, or infectious complications. Nitric oxide has beneficial effects on vascular function but is also produced by macrophages with immune activation. Nitric oxide has a short half-life and at higher doses may act as a prooxidant.

Glutamine supplementation has been found to reduce infectious complications in burn and trauma patients and to reduce mortality in burn patients.[3,80] In a meta-analysis that combined assessments of parenteral and enteral glutamine, benefits were shown. However, the preponderance of studies using parenteral glutamine resulted in no further support for the use of glutamine in enteral formulas.[81]

In nonsurgical patients requiring long-term EN, a formula supplemented with arginine, ω-3 fatty acids, and nucleotides had no significant effects after 12 weeks on leukocyte or lymphocyte count or immune function as assessed by levels of interleukin-6, prealbumin, transferrin, and retinol-binding protein by comparison to a standard enteral formula.[82]

In summary, the evidence in favor of immune-enhancing formulas is mixed with many studies in small numbers of subjects and with different formulas being combined to attempt to draw conclusions. At the present time, more research is needed to establish the benefits of these specialized enteral formulas.

## SUMMARY OF ENTERAL FEEDING SECTION

Although EN is the preferred route of nutrient provision in those individuals unable to consume adequate nutrients orally, it is not without complications. Compared with PN, EN complications are less serious. Most of the complications with EN are minor; however, occasionally serious complications can develop. Most complications can be prevented or at least be made less severe. Appropriate patient assessment for needs and risks, proper feeding route, and formula selection, in addition to appropriate monitoring of the EN feeding regimen, can increase the success of enteral feeding. The most common complications can be categorized as mechanical, metabolic, and GI.

It is very important to continuously monitor patients for signs of formula intolerance, hydration and electrolyte status, and nutritional status. Physical indicators that should be monitored include incidence of vomiting, stool frequency, diarrhea, abdominal cramps, bloating, signs of edema or dehydration, and weight changes. In addition, several laboratory parameters should be monitored daily with the initiation of enteral feeding and tapered as the patient stabilizes and demonstrates tolerance.

Enteral feeding is the preferred method of providing nutrition in those who cannot consume adequate nutrients orally. Enteral feeding has many advantages over PN, including preservation of the structure and function of the GI tract, more efficient nutrient utilization, fewer infections and metabolic complications, greater ease of administration, and lower cost. In order for EN to be successful, patient assessment for the optimal access site, appropriate formula selection, nutrient requirements, monitoring, and troubleshooting complications are required.

## PARENTERAL NUTRITION

PN was developed to provide nutrition to those unable to take complete nutrition via the GI tract due to an inability to digest or absorb nutrients. A nonfunctioning GI tract and failure to tolerate EN still remain the primary reasons for PN. Certain accompanying conditions also need consideration, such as a patient being nutritionally at risk, and projected inability to consume anything by mouth for at least 7–14 days. Situations that indicate the need for PN include short bowel syndrome and malabsorption, bowel obstruction, intractable diarrhea or vomiting, prolonged ileus, and high-output GI fistulas.[83]

Multidisciplinary nutrition support teams (NSTs) have reduced the inappropriate overuse of total PN based on

early enthusiasm for this aggressive method of nutrition to reverse cancer cachexia or to place the bowel at rest in cases of regional enteritis. The effectiveness of adult NSTs was studied from February 1999 through June 2002, at a university hospital.[84] The NST was given authority to discontinue inappropriate TPN orders evaluating the indications for TPN based on the American Society for Parenteral and Enteral Nutrition (ASPEN) standards. These standards included short gut, severe pancreatitis, severe malnutrition/catabolism with inability to enterally feed for more than 5 days and inability to enterally feed greater than 50% of nutritional needs for more than 9 days, enterocutaneous fistula, intra-abdominal leak, bowel obstruction, chylothorax, ischemic bowel, hemodynamic instability, massive GI bleed, and lack of abdominal wall integrity. The number of inappropriate TPN orders declined from 62/194 (32.0%) in the first 11 months of the study to 22/168 (13.1%) in the second 11 months ($P < 0.0001$). This number further declined to 17/215 (7.9%) in the final 12 months of data collection. The involvement of a multidisciplinary NST was associated with a marked reduction in inappropriate TPN orders, and these are now standard in most large medical centers where TPN is performed.

Another important specialized application of PN is in bone marrow transplant patients who suffer from graft versus host disease. This disease commonly affects the skin, liver, and digestive tract. Clinical symptoms of the digestive tract include diarrhea, abdominal pain and cramps, nausea and vomiting, GI bleeding, dysphagia, and weight loss. Studies show that graft versus host disease is often associated with malnutrition; protein losing enteropathy; magnesium derangements; and deficiencies of zinc, vitamin $B_{12}$, and vitamin D. While there is evidence of beneficial effects of ω-3 polyunsaturated fatty acids and pancreatic enzyme replacement therapy, most experts recommend providing at least 1.5 g protein/kg body weight, supplied by TPN in cases with severe diarrhea. When diarrhea is <500 mL a day, a stepwise enteral diet can be followed. No studies exist on dietary fiber and immunonutrition in these patients. Future research is needed on absorption capacity, vitamin and mineral status, and nutritional support strategies including prebiotics and probiotics.[85]

Prior to initiating PN, vascular access is obtained. Determination of venous access is based upon the duration of therapy, patient limitations, and availability of equipment and facilities. Central or peripheral veins may be used for the provision of PN. Peripheral access with conventional needles that use the small veins of the extremities, typically the hands and forearms, is called peripheral PN (PPN). Since small veins are easily sclerosed by hypertonic parenteral solutions, it is recommended that peripheral PPN solutions have osmolalities ≤ 900 mOsm/1.5 L. Even with appropriate PPN, intravenous sites may need frequent changing to maintain venous patency. The increased volume requirement necessary to minimize the PPN solution's osmolality limits nutrient provision as well as the clinical utility of PPN.[86] PPN solutions vary considerably delivering only dextrose with electrolytes, vitamins, and minerals or also including some lipids and amino acids to increase the provision of calories and protein. PPN formulations composed of carbohydrate, amino acids, and lipid generally provide 1000–1200 kcal/day. However, PPN may be useful when the long-term plan for nutrition is uncertain and the patient requires interim nutrition intervention in which the GI tract is temporarily nonfunctional, such as with prolonged ileus or hyperemesis gravidarum. The combined use of EN and PPN is sometimes called transitional feeding.

TPN must be provided via large central veins that can accommodate the pH and increased osmolality of the parenteral feeding solutions. The initial site most commonly used is the subclavian vein, but there are eight sites of large veins in the trunk that can be potential venous sites. The most common venipuncture sites include the subclavian, internal jugular, femoral, cephalic, and basilic veins. The primary indications for central venous access include chemotherapy, antibiotic administration, and risk of tissue necrosis with vesicant medications. Access is obtained with specialized catheters, with the distal tip placed into the vena cava or right atrial area. Several varieties of central venous catheters are available, the most common being polyurethane and silicone. Most catheters are available in a variety of external diameters, lengths, and number of portals or lumens. Multilumen versions provide for simultaneous infusion of TPN with multiple or incompatible drugs.

Physiologic, functional, psychological, and social factors all need consideration prior to determining the type and location of catheter placement. If the patient is in the acute care setting and unlikely to be discharged with TPN, the physiologic factors are of primary concern. However, if a patient is to receive PN in an alternate care setting such as the home, several other factors must be taken into account for optimal patient adherence to the difficult regimen required with home PN (HPN) including impaired vision, developmental disability, frailty, and the availability of adequate support systems for catheter care. HPN is a safe treatment with a high probability of survival. The risk of death during HPN is increased by the absence of a specialist team and appears greater during the early period of treatment. Survival probability is decreased in patients with age >40 or <2 years, very short bowel remnant, presence of a stoma, chronic intestinal pseudo-obstruction of myopathic origin, systemic sclerosis, radiation enteritis, intra-abdominal desmoids, necrotizing enterocolitis, and congenital mucosal diseases. Liver failure is the HPN-related complication with the greatest risk of death.[87] Its cause remains unclear, although recent studies suggest that the omega-6 polyunsaturated fatty acids in plant oil–based lipid emulsions and the associated phytosterols contribute to the development of hepatotoxicity. In contrast, fish oil–based lipid emulsions are composed mainly of ω-3 polyunsaturated fatty acids and are hypothesized to be hepatoprotective.[88] In several animal models of parenteral nutrition–associated liver disease (PNALD), the use of an intravenous fish oil–based lipid emulsion improved PN-associated cholestasis without resultant essential fatty

acid (EFA) deficiency or growth impairment. Following these results and preliminary human data, an open trial for compassionate use was initiated, followed by a randomized controlled trial to evaluate the current management of pediatric PNALD. To date, more than 130 children with PNALD have been treated with Omegaven, a fish oil–based emulsion, with improved liver function among most patients.[89] While the evidence is still early in its development, it appears that the use of a fish oil–based emulsion is efficacious and hepatoprotective.

Carbohydrate serves as the primary energy source in parenteral solutions. The amount of carbohydrate provided is based upon the patient's individual nutrient requirements and glucose oxidation rate. Although the exact requirement is individualized, guidelines are available. A minimum of 100 g/day is often used as the obligate need for the central nervous system, white blood cells, red blood cells, and renal medulla. The maximum rate of glucose oxidation in adults is 4–6 mg/kg/min, or 300–500 g for a 70 kg person, with the lower range suggested for critically ill patients secondary to endogenous glucose production. Excessive carbohydrate provision is associated with hyperglycemia, excessive carbon dioxide production, and hepatic steatosis.

Carbohydrate is provided almost exclusively as dextrose monohydrate in parenteral solutions. Each gram of hydrated dextrose provides 3.4 kcal/g. Commercial dextrose preparations are available in concentrations from 5% to 70%. Dextrose solutions have an acidic pH (3.5–5.5) and are stable after autoclave sterilization. Sterilization also increases the shelf life of dextrose solutions so that they can be stored for extended periods at room temperature.

Glycerol is a naturally occurring 3-carbon glycolytic intermediate. Glycerol yields 4.3 kcal/g when oxidized to carbon dioxide and water and does not require insulin for cellular uptake. When provided in low concentrations (3%) with amino acids, it has been found to be protein sparing. Because of these advantages, glycerol is used as an alternative source of calories in some parenteral formulations, primarily in PPN.

Since the introduction of intravenous lipids in Europe in the mid-1960s, lipid emulsions have been extensively used as a nutrient source in PN. The aqueous lipid emulsions available in the United States as of 2006 consist of long-chain triacylglycerols (TAG) manufactured from soybean and safflower oil. Therefore, the lipid emulsions not only provide a source of kilocalories but also EFA. These products contain egg yolk phospholipid as an emulsifying agent and glycerin, which make the products nearly isotonic. The glycerol raises the caloric concentration of the 10% emulsion to 1.1 kcal/mL and the 20% emulsion to 2.0 kcal/mL. The phospholipid may contribute to the phosphorus intake of patients who receive large amounts of lipids (>500 mL/day). Combinations of long- and medium-chain TAG emulsions have been available in Europe for several years. In most of the non-U.S. markets, lipids of various origin and mixtures are available including fish oil, olive oil, and medium-chain TGs.

Most patients tolerate daily infusion of lipids provided as an intermittent or continuous infusion, often as part of a TNA.

Continuous delivery with a moderate dose is favored over intermittent infusion due to decreased fluctuations in serum TAG levels and improved fat oxidation.[29] The requirement of a test dose is usually eliminated with continuous delivery, as the administration rate tends to be less than that with the test dose. Patients should still be monitored for fever, chills, headache, and back pain during the first dose of intravenous lipid. Absolute contraindications to intravenous fat emulsions include pathologic hyperlipidemia, lipoid nephrosis, severe egg allergy, and acute pancreatitis when associated with severe hypertriglyceridemia. Caution should be taken in delivery to patients with severe liver disease, adult respiratory distress syndrome, or severe metabolic or catabolic stress. If serum TAG levels are greater than 500 mg/dL, lipids should be held with only the minimal requirements for EFA provided to avoid further metabolic complications.

Lipid requirements are met by providing at least 4% of energy as EFA or approximately 10% of energy as a commercial lipid emulsion from safflower oil to prevent EFA deficiency. Since lipid emulsions vary in their composition of EFA depending on the oil source, the minimum amount provided is based upon the EFA content rather than a percentage of total energy. Recommendations for optimal lipid delivery have evolved over the years. Historically, it once was common practice to provide 40%–60% of energy as lipid due to its concentrated energy source when allowed for decreased volume delivery. However, over the years, concerns that soy-based lipid emulsions currently available in the United States are proinflammatory and impair neutrophil function, endotoxin clearance, and complement synthesis have resulted in the recommendation to limit lipid administration to 1 g/kg/day or 25%–30% of total energy.[90]

Protein is a critical nutrient needed to maintain nitrogen balance to help minimize loss of lean body mass and protein degradation for gluconeogenesis. The nitrogen source utilized for PN is in the form of crystalline amino acids. Parenteral amino acid products can be divided into standard and modified (disease-specific). Standard amino acid products are suitable for the majority of patients. They contain a balanced mixture of essential and NEAAs in which the ratios are based on FAO/WHO recommendations for optimal proportions of essential amino acids. Standard formulations are available in a range of concentrations from 3% to 15%. Most institutions stock 10% and 15% concentrations, since more dilute solutions can be made readily by adding sterile water with an automated compounder.

Modified amino acid solutions are designed for patients with disease- or age-specific amino acid requirements. Formulations are marketed for adults with hepatic failure, renal dysfunction, metabolic stress, and for neonates with special requirements for growth and development. These modified formulations are significantly more costly than the standard formulations and may not always prove as cost-effective; therefore, strict criteria should be established for their use.

Patients with hepatic failure develop multiple metabolic abnormalities including electrolyte disturbances and alterations in amino acid metabolism. In severe liver disease, hepatic encephalopathy can occur, which is associated with decreased BCAA serum levels and elevated AAA and methionine serum levels. Patients with hepatic disease without encephalopathy may be provided with moderate levels of standard amino acids with close monitoring of their mental status. When hepatic encephalopathy is severe (≥grade II), a modified hepatic protein formulation may be beneficial in decreasing the clinical course of encephalopathy. These formulations have high concentrations of BCAA (~45% of protein) and low concentrations of AAA and methionine. Improvement in hepatic encephalopathy and variable influence in lower mortality have been found in some patients who received this formulation.[91]

Modified formulations are marketed for patients with renal failure. These formulas contain mainly essential amino acids and were designed on the premise that endogenous urea could be used as a nitrogen source to synthesize NEAAs via transamination reactions. The clinical benefit of these solutions has been challenged. Prospective, randomized, and controlled studies have demonstrated that standard amino acids are as effective as modified amino acids in patients who have renal failure and who require PN.[92,93] Intravenous renal failure formulations have limited usefulness currently secondary to the relative ease at which patients now undergo beside dialysis or hemofiltration. Thus, patients with severe renal failure may be given standard amino acids as part of PN in most clinical situations.

A parenteral formulation with an enhanced BCAA formulation is marketed for patients with metabolic stress such as that caused by trauma, burns, and sepsis. Metabolic stress causes an efflux of amino acids from skeletal muscle and the gut to the liver for gluconeogenesis and support of acute phase protein synthesis. Metabolically stressed patients have also been shown to have increased serum levels of AAA and decreased BCAA levels. Therefore, the rationale of using a high BCAA formula in these patients is to provide the preferential fuel to the body and normalize the patient's amino acid patterns. Multiple studies have evaluated the benefits of high BCAA formulations in metabolic stress. Some studies have shown positive benefits when using these formulations, such as nitrogen retention, improved visceral protein levels, and reversal of skin test anergy, but there were no differences in morbidity or mortality.[94] Other studies have failed to exhibit significant outcome advantages of BCAAs over standard amino acid formulas in metabolic stress.[95] Therefore, since the cost-effectiveness of high BCAA solutions has not been clearly demonstrated, initiation of nutrition support with a standard amino acid solution is recommended in patients with metabolic stress.

Parenteral protein requirements are based upon the patient's clinical condition. In the critically ill population, a range of 1.5–2.0 g/kg/day is appropriate. For patients with renal or hepatic disease, protein recommendations vary according to the disease stage and its intervention. For those with renal disease on peritoneal dialysis, 1.2–1.5 g/kg/day of ideal body weight is recommended for maintenance or repletion.

For hemodialysis, 1.1–1.4 g/kg of ideal body weight per day is recommended for maintenance or repletion. For patients with uncomplicated hepatic dysfunction, 0.8–1.5 g/kg dry weight is suggested, for end-stage liver disease with encephalopathy, 0.5–0.7 g/kg; if a high BCAA formula is used, then 0.8–1.2 g/kg/day is suggested.

Electrolytes are added to parenteral solutions based upon individual need. The amount added daily varies based upon the patient's weight, disease state, renal and hepatic function, nutrition status, pharmacotherapy, acid–base status, and overall electrolyte balance. Extrarenal electrolyte losses may be a result of diarrhea, ostomy output, vomiting, fistulas, or nasogastric suctioning. As patients become anabolic during parenteral nutrient delivery, they may experience increased requirements for the major intracellular electrolytes (potassium, phosphorus, and magnesium). During refeeding of undernourished patients, these electrolytes should be monitored frequently and replenished accordingly.

For calcium provision, calcium gluconate is the preferred form for parenteral formulations due to its stability in solution and decreased chance of dissociating and forming a precipitate with phosphorus. Whether to provide an electrolyte as a chloride or an acetate salt depends on the patient's acid–base status. Generally, acid–base balance is maintained with providing chloride and acetate in a 1:1 ratio. If a patient has altered acid–base status with skewed electrolyte levels, then the chloride to acetate ratio can be adjusted to facilitate correction. Acetate and chloride are also present in the base amino acid solutions in various amounts, and should be considered when attempting electrolyte homeostasis.

Electrolytes increase the osmolarity of the parenteral solution; however, large amounts can be added to solutions with amino acids and dextrose without affecting the stability. The solubility of calcium and phosphorus varies with the volume of the solution, its pH, the type of calcium preparation, the temperature at which the solutions are stored, and the order of admixture.[1] Solutions can be prepared with a range of calcium and phosphorus contents as long as the product of calcium (in mEq) and phosphorus (in mmol) is less than 200. When lipids are added to the parenteral solutions, caution is needed when adding electrolytes, as there are limitations and hazards. An insoluble precipitate can form when there are excess cations in the parenteral solutions, as with calcium and phosphate, which may not be visualized in TNAs. Crystal formation in the lungs with subsequent death was reported in patients as a result of precipitate formation in TPN solutions.[96]

Vitamins are typically added to every parenteral formulation in doses consistent with the American Medical Association Nutrition Advisory Group's recommendations.[97] Guidelines are established for the 12 essential vitamins. Most institutions use a commercially available multiple-entity product, which contains 12 essential vitamins for adults (MVI-12). Most multivitamin preparations for adults do not contain vitamin K because it antagonizes the effects of coumadin in patients receiving this medication. In adults, vitamin K may be administered by adding 1–2 mg/day to the parenteral solution or by giving 5–10 mg/week intramuscularly or subcutaneously. Individual vitamin preparations are also available and are used to supplement the multivitamin doses when a deficiency state exists or with increased needs due to disease or medical condition.

Trace minerals are essential to normal metabolism and growth, and serve as metabolic cofactors essential for the proper functioning of several enzyme systems. Although the requirements are minute, deficiency states can develop fairly rapidly secondary to increased metabolic demands or excessive losses. Most clinicians add these micronutrients daily; however, there are clinical conditions necessitating trace mineral restriction and therefore adjustments in the daily intakes. The Nutrition Advisory Group of the American Medical Association (AMA) has also published guidelines for four trace elements known to be important in human nutrition.[98]

Since the original recommendations, it has become more evident that selenium also is essential, and many clinicians add this element to the parenteral solution daily along with the other four. Most institutions use a commercially available multiple-entity product, but there are also single-entity mineral solutions available for use during times of increased requirements or when certain minerals are contraindicated. Zinc requirements are increased during metabolic stress due to increased urinary losses and with excessive GI losses as with diarrhea, external biliary or fistula drainage, and increased ostomy output. Manganese and copper are excreted through the biliary tract, whereas zinc, chromium, and selenium are excreted via the kidney. Therefore, copper and manganese should be restricted or withheld from PN in patients with cholestatic liver disease. Selenium depletion has been found in patients receiving long-term TPN, as well as with thermal injury, acquired immunodeficiency syndrome, liver failure, and critical illness.

## USE OF INSULIN IN TPN

Even with care to avoid excess carbohydrate delivery, patients receiving TPN often become hyperglycemic. One method of achieving desired blood glucose control with continuous TPN infusions is by adding regular insulin to the TPN solution. For patients with diabetes mellitus, stress hyperglycemia, steroids, or risk for refeeding syndrome, dextrose should be restricted initially to approximately 100–150 g/day. For other patients with normal glucose tolerance, dextrose may be initiated at 200–250 g/day. If after 24 h serum glucose levels are acceptable, then the dextrose may be advanced to goal over the next 24–48 h as indicated. Capillary glucose measurements should be obtained three to four times daily until the values are normal for two consecutive days. Regular insulin may be administered according to a sliding scale. A continuous intravenous insulin infusion or drip may be substituted for sliding scale if serum glucose levels are consistently elevated beyond suggested levels. The importance of glucose control cannot be overemphasized. Recent work by Van den Berghe has reported a major decrease in numerous ICU-related complications including mortality when tight glycemic control is maintained.[59] Insulin may also be added to the TPN solution; however, one needs to remember that providing insulin in this manner confines the delivery over the time period of the TPN mixture, and if the hyperglycemia resolves, then the TPN bag must be discontinued to avoid inadvertent hypoglycemia. For patients requiring insulin prior to TPN institution, approximately half of the established insulin requirement may be included as regular insulin in the initial bag of TPN formula.[1] If blood glucose levels are less than 200 mg/dL, approximately two-thirds of the previous day's subcutaneous insulin dose may be added to the TPN as regular insulin.[99]

The proof-of-concept Leuven studies assessed causality and revealed that targeting strict normoglycemia (80–110 mg/dL) with insulin improved outcome compared with tolerating hyperglycemia to the renal threshold (215 mg/dL). A large multicenter trial (NICE-SUGAR [Normoglycaemia in Intensive Care Evaluation and Survival Using Glucose Algorithm Regulation]) found an intermediate blood glucose target (140–180 mg/dL) safer than targeting normoglycemia. Differences in design and in execution of glycemic control at the bedside may have contributed to these results. In NICE-SUGAR, the blood glucose target range in the control group was lower, there were problems to reach and maintain normoglycemia in the intervention group, and inaccurate handheld blood glucose meters and variable blood sampling sites were allowed. Inaccurate tools led to insulin-dosing errors with consequently (undetected) hypoglycemia and unacceptable blood glucose variability. Also, the studies were done superimposed upon different nutritional strategies. Thus, such differences do not allow simple, evidence-based recommendations for daily practice, but an intermediate blood glucose target may be preferable while awaiting better tools to facilitate safely reaching normoglycemia.[100]

A few studies have suggested that absorbance of insulin to glass bottles, polyvinyl chloride bags, and tubing occurs, with the greatest loss occurring during the first hour of infusion. So, when adding insulin to TPN solutions to optimize blood glucose control, it is important to remember that the patient may have an increased insulin requirement due to absorbance.

### PROVIDING OTHER MEDICATIONS IN TPN

Many patients receiving TPN are also receiving multiple medications, leading to the desire to add the medications to the TPN solutions. Using TPN as a drug delivery vehicle is very tempting, as it may allow for continuous medication infusion in addition to minimizing fluid volume delivery by eliminating the need for a separate diluent for each medication administered. However, scrutiny is needed prior to adding medications to the TPN solution, as there is potential for drug–drug and drug–nutrient interactions. Issues needing consideration include medication compatibility with TPN constituents, the effect of pH changes on TPN compatibility, and drug effectiveness, whether the infusion schedule of the TPN is appropriate to achieve therapeutic levels of the drug or the potential for interactions among the drugs if more than one is added. The complexity of these issues usually leads to consultation with a pharmacist experienced in TPN compounding and compatibility, reference to the institution's policy and procedure manual, or contact with the drug manufacturers. Medications most frequently added to TPN include albumin, aminophylline, cimetidine, famotidine, ranitidine, heparin, hydrochloric acid, and regular insulin.

Stress ulcer prophylaxis with the addition of H2-receptor blockers is common practice with patients on TPN who are not receiving any gastric luminal nutrients. This may be achieved by adding the H2-receptor blockers to the TPN solution. Famotidine (20 and 40 mg/L) and ranitidine hydrochloride have been shown to be stable in PN solutions and three-in-one admixtures.

In order to reduce the complications of catheter occlusion related to fibrin formation around the catheter tip, heparin may be added to the TPN solution. Adding up to 1000 units of heparin per liter reduces the incidence of catheter occlusion without exhibiting anticoagulant effects on serum.[1] Larger amounts of heparin may be used for peripheral PN.

## MONITORING OF TPN

Serious complications with TPN may develop if careful initiation and monitoring are not followed. TPN solutions may be infused continuously over a 24 h period or cycled over shorter time intervals. If a patient is critically ill or just beginning to receive TPN, it is suggested to infuse it over a 24 h period until patient tolerance is demonstrated. TPN should not be initiated at goal levels of nutrients, as many patients may not tolerate this prescription. Proportional increases in carbohydrate-dependent electrolytes such as magnesium and phosphorus, in protein-dependent electrolytes such as potassium, and in volume-dependent electrolytes such as sodium should be made as the macronutrients are increased.

Lipids may be infused for up to 24 h, and may reduce the adverse effect of lipids on the reticuloendothelial system. Lipids can be given with the first TPN infusion unless serum TG levels are elevated. It is suggested to maintain TG levels at ≤400 mg/dL, while lipids are being infused. If TG levels exceed the recommended level, lipids should be held until levels normalize. As this occurs, patients may be provided with lipids in amounts to prevent EFA deficiency. For persistent or severe hypertriglyceridemia or for patients with egg allergy, small amounts of enterally delivered EFA can usually be administered to alleviate the symptoms of EFA deficiency. Critically ill patients may also be receiving significant amounts of lipid from lipid-based medications, which may predispose them to hypertriglyceridemia prior to TPN infusion. The amount of lipid from medications should be considered in the final TPN formulation to avoid providing excess long-chain TG.

In most acute care settings, PN is usually provided over a 24 h continuous rate. In patients who require TPN for an extended period, it may also be delivered in a cyclic pattern.

During TPN, circulating insulin levels remain elevated, reducing the amount of carbohydrate that enters the cell, thus favoring hepatic lipogenesis. Cyclic TPN with periods free from intravenous nutrient delivery allows for patient mobility, and therefore, it is usually utilized with ambulatory patients. For individuals with limited vascular access, cyclic infusion may be required in order to administer necessary medications or blood products. Conversion from 24 h continuous infusion to cyclic infusion can be accomplished in 2–3 days. The largest concern is with the initiation and discontinuation of the carbohydrate infusion and potential for hyperglycemia and rebound hypoglycemia. Another concern is with the increased volume delivery over a shorter time frame. Most stable patients with adequate renal function and cardiac reserves can tolerate cyclic TPN over 8–14 h.

## TRANSITION FROM TPN TO ENTERAL FEEDING

In a transition from TPN to enteral feeding, GI function should be evaluated and TPN should be decreased as the enteral intake and tolerance improves to avoid overfeeding. TPN may be discontinued once the patient is tolerating approximately 65%–75% of goal nutrients. For patients who are eating, TPN may be reduced and stopped over a 24–48 h period. If TPN is inadvertently but abruptly discontinued in patients who are not eating, all insulin should be stopped and blood glucose levels should be monitored for 60 min after discontinuation of TPN. Based upon the blood glucose levels, appropriate therapy should be implemented. Lastly, if the TPN was used as a vehicle for medication or electrolyte administration, an alternate plan should be made once it is discontinued. Attempting to switch medications to the enteral route is usually employed. Consultation with a pharmacist can help facilitate this transition.

## COMPLICATIONS OF PARENTERAL NUTRITION

Complications of PN have been widely reported. However, TPN can be safe with minimal complications when it is managed and monitored by a multidisciplinary team of trained professionals. The type of complications that may arise are diverse but for simplicity be divided into mechanical, infectious, and metabolic categories.

Mechanical complications of catheter insertion include pneumothorax, hydrothorax, and great vessel injury. The catheter malposition may result in venous thrombosis, causing head, neck, or arm swelling, or possibly a pulmonary embolus. To minimize morbidity, placing lines with portable ultrasound and obtaining a chest radiograph before using a new central line for TPN is important to ensure correct line placement and absence of internal injuries that may have occurred during insertion.

Catheter-related infections can carry a high risk for increasing the morbidity and potential mortality rate as well as significantly increasing the medical costs. A catheter infection rate of less than 3% is desirable.[5] Appropriate use of aseptic technique by trained personnel is essential to maintain an acceptable catheter infection rate. Nursing protocols should be established for dressing changes and line manipulation. Dressings should be changed every 48 h and should include local sterilizing ointment and an occlusive dressing. Since gram-positive catheter-related sepsis may be treated with antibiotics, removal of the catheter is not always necessary. Catheter removal is usually necessary with gram-negative organisms.

With close monitoring of TPN, avoidance of metabolic complications is possible. Refeeding syndrome may be defined as a constellation of fluid, micronutrient, electrolyte, and vitamin imbalances that occur within the first few days after refeeding a starved patient. Refeeding syndrome may involve hemolytic anemia, respiratory distress, paresthesias, tetany, and cardiac arrhythmias. Typical biochemical findings include hypokalemia, hypophosphatemia, and hypomagnesemia. Proposed risk factors for refeeding include alcoholism, anorexia nervosa, marasmus, rapid refeeding, and excessive dextrose infusion. In order to prevent the syndrome from occurring, it is suggested to replete serum potassium, phosphorus, and magnesium concentrations prior to beginning TPN; limit initial carbohydrate to 150 g/day, fluid to 800 mL, and sodium intake to no more than 20 mEq/day in at-risk patients; include adequate amounts of potassium, magnesium, phosphorus, and vitamins in the TPN solution; and increase carbohydrate-dependent minerals in proportion to increases in carbohydrate when TPN is advanced.

Hyperglycemia (nonfasting blood glucose >220 mg/dL) is a common metabolic complication of TPN. Risk factors include metabolic stress, medications, obesity, diabetes, and excess dextrose administration. Careful glucose monitoring, especially in the first few days of TPN administration, can help guide advancement of dextrose to goal. Administration of dextrose in amounts less than the maximum glucose oxidation rate (4–7 mg/kg/min) and initiating dextrose in reduced amounts (100–150 g/day) in at-risk patients may help minimize the occurrence of hyperglycemia.

Patients receiving TPN may also experience fluid and electrolyte abnormalities. The etiology of the abnormalities may be related to several factors, including the patient's medical condition and treatment, medications, or excessive or inadequate free water provision. Fluid balance and electrolyte status should be monitored closely, with corrections in abnormalities made accordingly.

## SUMMARY

PN has been one of the major advancements in clinical nutrition over the past several decades. Its institution has saved countless lives of people who would have otherwise died of malnutrition and its complications due to loss of GI function. The early enthusiasm for TPN as aggressive nutrition to reverse cancer cachexia, regional enteritis, and other chronic diseases has given way to the careful selection, implementation, and monitoring of PN for nutritional supplementation in numerous diseases.

## REFERENCES

1. Weimann A, Braga M, Harsanyi L et al. *Clin Nutr* 25:224;2006.
2. American Society for Parenteral and Enteral Nutrition (ASPEN) Board of Directors. *J Parenter Enteral Nutr* 33:255;2009.
3. Heyland DK, Dhaliwal R, Drover JW et al. *J Parenter Enteral Nutr* 27:355;2003.
4. Singer P, Berger MM, Van den Berghe G et al. *Clin Nutr* 28:387;2009.
5. Kreymann KG, Berger MM, Deutz NE et al. *Clin Nutr* 25:210;2006.
6. Cahill NE, Narasimhan S, Dhaliwal R, Heyland DK. *J Parenter Enteral Nutr* 34:685;2010.
7. Moore FA, Moore EE, Jones TN et al. *J Trauma* 29:916;1989.
8. Kudsk KA, Croce MA, Fabian TC et al. *Ann Surg* 215:503;1992.
9. Van den Berghe G, Wouters P, Weekers F et al. *N Engl J Med* 345:1359;2001.
10. Seike J, Tangoku A, Yuasa Y et al. *J Med Invest* 58:75;2011.
11. Simpson F, Doig GS. *Intensive Care Med* 31:12;2005.
12. Martindale RG, McClave SA, Vanek VW et al. *Crit Care Med* 37:1757;2009.
13. Gramlich L, Kichian K, Pinilla J et al. *Nutrition* 20:843;2004.
14. Alberda C, Gramlich L, Jones N et al. *Intensive Care Med* 35:1728;2009.
15. Ridley EJ, Davies AR. *Nutrition* 27:509;2011.
16. Spalding DR, Behranwala KA, Straker P et al. *Ann R Coll Surg Engl* 91:477;2009.
17. de Aguilar-Nascimento JE, Dock-Nascimento DB, Bragagnolo R. *Nutrition* 26:354;2010.
18. Lewis SJ, Andersen HK, Thomas S. *J Gastrointest Surg* 13:569;2009.
19. Andersen HK, Lewis SJ, Thomas S. *Cochrane Database Syst Rev* October 18:CD004080;2006.
20. Osland E, Yunus RM, Khan S, Memon MA. *J Parenter Enteral Nutr* 35:473;2011.
21. Doig GS, Heighes PT, Simpson F, Sweetman EA. *Injury* 42:50;2011.
22. Ryan JA Jr., Page CP, Babcock L. *Am Surg* 47:393;1981.
23. Han-Geurts IJ, Hop WC, Kok NF et al. *Br J Surg* 94:555;2007.
24. Delaney CP, Zutshi M, Senagore AJ et al. *Dis Colon Rectum* 46:851;2003.
25. Waitzberg DL, Saito H, Plank LD et al. *World J Surg* 30:1592;2006.
26. Drover JW, Dhaliwal R, Weitzel L et al. *J Am Coll Surg* 212:385;2011.
27. Debats IB, Wolfs TG, Gotoh T et al. *Nitric Oxide* 21:175;2009.
28. Stapleton RD, Jones N, Heyland DK. *Crit Care Med* 35:S535;2007.
29. Dickerson RN. *Nutr Clin Pract* 26:48;2011.
30. Zaloga GP, Roberts P. *New Horiz* 2:257;1994.
31. McCowen KC, Friel C, Sternberg J et al. *Crit Care Med* 28:3606;2000.
32. Arabi YM, Tamim HM, Dhar GS et al. *Am J Clin Nutr* 93:569;2011.
33. Malone A. *Pract Gastroenterol* 29:44;2005.
34. Alpern EH, Stutz L, Peterson S et al. *Am J Crit Care* 13:221;2004.
35. O'Leary-Kelley CM, Puntillo KA, Barr J et al. *Am J Crit Care* 14:222;2005.
36. Rice TW, Swope T, Bozeman S, Wheeler AP. *Nutrition* 21:786;2005.
37. O'Meara D, Mireles-Cabodevila E, Frame F et al. *Am J Crit Care* 17:53;2008.
38. Schneider SM, Girard-Pipau F, Anty R et al. *Clin Nutr* 25:82;2006.
39. McClave SA, Chang WK. *Nutr Clin Pract* 18:279;2003.
40. Scaife CL, Saffle JR, Morris SE. *J Trauma* 47:859;1999.
41. Mesejo A, Acosta JA, Ortega C et al. *Clin Nutr* 22:295;2003.
42. León-Sanz M, García-Luna PP, Planas M et al. *J Parenter Enteral Nutr* 29:21;2005.
43. Pohl M, Mayr P, Mertl-Roetzer M et al. *Eur J Clin Nutr* 59:1121;2005.
44. American Diabetes Association. *Diabetes Care* 30(suppl 1):S48;2007.
45. Druml W, Mitch WE. *Sem Dial* 9:484;1996.
46. Druml W. *Int J Artif Organs* 19:118;1996.
47. Frankenfield DC, Badellino MM, Reynolds HN et al. *J Parenter Enteral Nutr* 17:551;1993.
48. Bergström J. *Miner Electrolyte Metab* 18:280;1992.
49. Macias WL, Alaka KJ, Murphy MH et al. *J Parenter Enteral Nutr* 50:56;1996.
50. Kopple JD. *Am J Kidney Dis* 37(1 suppl 12):S66;2001.
51. Btaiche IF, Mohammad RA, Alaniz C, Mueller BA. *Pharmacotherapy* 28:600;2008.
52. Als-Nielsen B, Koretz RL, Kjaergard LL, Gluud C. *Cochrane Database Syst Rev* 2:CD001939;2003.
53. Marchesini G, Bianchi G, Merli M et al. *Gastroenterology* 124:1792;2003.
54. Vermeeren MA, Wouters EF, Nelissen LH et al. *Am J Clin Nutr* 73:295;2001.
55. van den Berg B, Bogaard JM, Hop WC. *Intensive Care Med* 20:470;1994.
56. Angelillo VA, Bedi S, Durfee D et al. *Ann Intern Med* 103:883;1985.
57. Kuo CD, Shiao GM, Lee JD. *Chest* 104:189;1993.
58. Cai B, Zhu Y, Ma Y et al. *Nutrition* 15:290;1989.
59. al-Saady NM, Blackmore CM, Bennett ED. *Intensive Care Med* 15:290;1989.
60. Talpers SS, Romberger DJ, Bunce SB, Pingleton SK. *Chest* 102:551;1992.
61. Parsons PE, Eisner MD, Thompson BT et al. *Crit Care Med* 33:1;2005.
62. Gadek JE, DeMichele SJ, Karlstad MD et al. *Crit Care Med* 27:1409;1999.
63. Singer P, Theilla M, Fisher H et al. *Crit Care Med* 34:1033;2006.
64. Pontes-Arruda A, Aragão AM, Albuquerque JD. *Crit Care Med* 34:2325;2006.
65. Mayer K, Seeger W. *Curr Opin Clin Nutr Metab Care* 11:121;2008.
66. Wischmeyer PE. *Crit Care Med* 35(9 Suppl):S541;2007.
67. Vermeulen MA, van de Poll MC, Ligthart-Melis GC et al. *Crit Care Med* 35(9 Suppl):S568;2007.
68. Kieft H, Roos AN, van Drunen JDE et al. *Intensive Care Med* 31:524;2005.
69. Casas-Rodera P, Gómez-Candela C, Benítez S et al. *Nutr Hosp* 23:105;2008.
70. Aiko S, Yoshizumi Y, Ishizuka T et al. *Dis Esophagus* 21:619;2000.
71. Chen DW, Fei ZW, Zhang YC et al. *Asian J Surg* 28:121;2005.
72. de Luis D, Izaola O, Cuellar L et al. *Eur J Clin Nutr* 57:96;2003.

73. de Luis D, Izaola O, Cuellar L et al. *Eur J Clin Nutr* 58:1505;2004.
74. de Luis D, Izaola O, Cuellar L et al. *Eur J Clin Nutr* 61:200;2007.
75. Farreras N, Artigas V, Cardona D et al. *Clin Nutr* 24:55;2005.
76. Sakurai Y, Masui T, Yoshida I et al. *World J Surg* 31:2150;2007.
77. Takeuchi H, Shunji I, Kawaguchi Y et al. *World J Surg* 31:2160;2007.
78. Bower RH, Cerra FB, Bershadsky B et al. *Crit Care Med* 23:436;1995.
79. Dent D, Heyland D, Levy H. *Crit Care Med* 30:A17;2003.
80. Marik PE, Zaloga GP. *Intensive Care Med* 34:1980;2008.
81. Wischmeyer PE. *Curr Opin Gastroenterol* 24:190;2008.
82. Sakurai Y, Oh-oka Y, Kato S et al. *Nutrition* 22:713;2006.
83. Dickerson R, Brown R, Whithe, K. In: *Clinical Nutrition: Parenteral Nutrition*. WB Saunders, Philadelphia, PA, 1993.
84. Saalwachter AR, Evans HL, Willcutts KF et al. *Am Surg* 70:1107;2004.
85. van der Meij BS, de Graaf P, Wierdsma NJ et al. *Bone Marrow Transplant* 2012. Doi: 10.1038/bmt.2012.124 [epub ahead of print].
86. Brogden BJ. *Br J Nurs* 13:1068;2004.
87. Pironi L, Goulet O, Buchman A et al. *Clin Nutr* 31:831;2012.
88. Fallon EM, Le HD, Puder M. *Curr Opin Organ Transplant* 15:334;2010.
89. Le HD, de Meijer VE, Robinson EM et al. *Am J Clin Nutr* 94:749;2011.
90. Vanek VW, Seidner DL, Allen P et al. *Nutr Clin Pract* 27:150;2012.
91. Cerra FB, Cheung NK, Fischer JE et al. *J Parenter Enteral Nutr* 9:288;1985.
92. Lau MT. *J Infus Nurs* 34:315;2011.
93. Feinstein EI, Blumenkrantz MJ, Healy M et al. *Medicine* (Baltimore) 60:124;1981.
94. Cerra FB, Mazuski J, Teasley K et al. *Crit Care Med* 11:775;1983.
95. Bower RH, Muggia-Sullam M, Vallgren S et al. *Ann Surg* 203:13;1986.
96. Lumpkin MM, Burlington DB. *FDA Safety Alert: Hazards of Precipitation Associated with Parenteral Nutrition*. U.S. Food and Drug Administration, Rockville, MD, 1994.
97. American Medical Association Department of Foods and Nutrition. *J Parent Enteral Nutr* 3:258;1979.
98. Guidelines for essential trace element preparations for parenteral use: A statement by the Nutrition Advisory Group. *J Parent Enteral Nutr* 3:263;1979.
99. Egi M, Bellomo R, Stachowski E et al. *Crit Care Med* 36:2249;2008.
100. Mesotten D, Van den Berghe G. *Curr Diab Rep* 12:101;2012.

# 66 Mechanisms Accounting for the Cancer Protective Effects of Bioactive Dietary Components in Fruits and Vegetables

*Cindy D. Davis and John A. Milner*

## CONTENTS

Dietary behavior is one of the most important and modifiable determinants for the risk of developing cancer. Recommendations to consume larger quantities of fruits and vegetables for protection from chronic diseases, including cancer, come principally from epidemiologic investigations and from a variety of animal and cell culture studies. Collectively, epidemiologic studies suggest that increased consumption of fruits, vegetables, and whole grains may reduce cancer risk, yet it is evident that considerable inconsistencies exist in the literature.[1-3] This discrepancy is illustrated in Table 66.1, which highlights some of the epidemiologic studies investigating the relationship between vegetable intake and colon cancer. Recent meta-analysis of prospective studies and colorectal cancer risk suggest a small protective effect (RR = 0.91, 95% CI = 0.86–0.96) of the highest versus lowest intake of vegetables and a linear dose–response (RR = 0.98, 95% CI = 0.97–0.99) per 100 g/day.[24]

In 2007, the American Institute for Cancer Research and the World Cancer Research Fund evaluated over 7000 studies which investigated the relationship between diet, physical activity, and cancer.[25] They concluded that nonstarchy vegetables probably protect against cancers of the mouth, pharynx, and larynx, and those of the esophagus and stomach.[25] Limited evidence also suggests that they may protect against cancers of the nasopharynx, lung, colorectum, ovary, and endometrium.[25] Fruits probably protect against cancers of the mouth, pharynx, and larynx, and those of the esophagus, lung, and stomach.[25] The possibility that fruits may also protect against cancers of the nasopharynx, pancreas, liver, and colorectum has also surfaced.[25] Based on these conclusions, they recommended that individuals eat at least five portions/servings (at least 400 g or 14 oz) of a variety of vegetables and fruits every day. Moreover, these recommendations for consumption tend to exclude starchy vegetables such as potato, yam, sweet potato, and cassava. While these relationships are based upon the epidemiologic literature, it must be pointed out that there are a number of limitations/considerations that are specific to the analysis of dietary intake of fruits and vegetables. These include: most studies of consumption of dietary fruits and vegetables have been conducted in populations with relatively homogeneous diets, smokers consume fewer fruits and vegetables than nonsmokers, fat intake inversely correlates with fruit and vegetable intake in the United States, and studies using self-reporting tend to over-report vegetable and fruit consumption. Thus, it is not surprising that uncertainty exists about the relationship between plant-based diets and cancer prevention.

Fruits and vegetables contain as many as 25,000 different bioactive food components, many of which may influence cancer under specific circumstances, including several nonessential components (Table 66.2) such as isothiocyanates, allyl sulfides, flavonoids/isoflavones, and monoterpenes, various essential minerals (e.g., selenium, zinc, iodine, calcium), and several vitamins (e.g., C, D, E, and folic acid).[26,28] The phytochemical composition of fruits and vegetables depends both on the species and subtype, as well as the environmental, cultivation, growing, harvesting, and storage conditions.

**TABLE 66.1**
**Vegetable Intake and Colon Cancer Risk**

| Type of Study | Population | Intake | Risk Modification (Highest vs. Lowest Intake) | Reference |
|---|---|---|---|---|
| Prospective | 47,605 subjects, Japan | ≤245 vs. ≥313 g/day; total vegetables | RR = 1.24, NS[a] | [4] |
| | 45,181 men, 62,643 women, Japan | 0–2 serving/week vs. every day, green leafy vegetables | HR = 1.19, NS | [5] |
| | 62,509 men, 70,554 women, the United States | 0.9 vs. 4.1 serving/day men; 1.0 vs. 4.1 serving/day women total vegetables | RR = .63, $p < 0.02$ for trend men, RR =.74, NS women | [6] |
| | 58,279 men, 62,573 women, the Netherlands | 165 vs. 210 g/day men; 166 vs. 209 g/day women total vegetables | RR =.89, NS men; RR = .80, NS women | [7] |
| | 519,978 subjects, Europe | <1.4 vs. >5.2 g/day fiber from vegetables | HR = .94, NS | [8] |
| | 120,852 subjects, the Netherlands | <150.6 vs. ≥225.6 g/day total vegetables | OR = 0.86 for hHMLH1- tumors, NS; OR = 0.04 for hMLH1 + tumors, NS | [9] |
| | 291,094 men, 196,949 women, the United States | 1.4 vs. 5.2 servings/1000 kcal men; 1.8 vs. 6.5 servings/1000 kcal women | RR = 0.82 men, NS RR = 1.12 women, NS | [10] |
| | 85,903 men, 105,108 women, the United States | 71.9 vs. 236.2 g/1000 kcal men; 85.5 vs. 286.5 g/1000 kcal women | RR = 0.85 men, NS RR = 0.94 women, NS | [11] |
| | 288,109 men, 195,229 women, the United States | <0.56 vs. >1.43 cup equivalents/1000 kcal | RR = 0.87, NS | [12] |
| | 131,985 men, 320,770 women, Europe | <95.1 vs. >284.4 g/day | HR = 0.92, NS | [13] |
| Case-control | 59 cases, 291 controls, India | ≤21 vs. ≥21 serving/week nonfried vegetables | OR = 0.40, $p < 0.05$ | [14] |
| | 613 cases, 996 controls, the United States | Mean intake 17.7 serving/week Caucasians, 13.9 serving/week African–Americans, total vegetables | OR = 0.50, $p < 0.006$ for trend both Caucasian and African–Americans | [15] |
| | 352 cases, 736 controls, Taiwan | ≤2 vs. ≥4 serving/day total vegetables | OR = 0.36 | [16] |
| | 184 cases, 259 controls, the Netherlands | ≤166 vs. >223 g/day | OR = 0.4, $p < 0.01$ for trend | [17] |
| | 931 cases (462 male and 469 female), 1552 controls (851 male and 701 female), China | ≤68 vs. ≥122 serving/week men; ≤67 vs. ≥119 serving/week women total vegetables | OR = 0.8, $p < 0.04$ for trend, men; OR = 1.0, NS women | [18] |
| | 484 cases, 1452 controls, Uruguay | | OR = 0.7, $p < 0.04$ trend all vegetables, OR = 1.2, NS cruciferous vegetables | [19] |
| | 223 cases, 491 controls, Switzerland | ≤5.5 vs. >9 serving/week raw vegetables; ≤5.25 vs. >8.75 serving/week cooked vegetables | OR = 0.55, $p < 0.05$ for trend raw vegetables; OR = 0.43, $p < 0.01$ for trend cooked vegetables | [20] |
| | 488 cases, 488 controls, the United States | Median of 9 vs. 45.5 serving/week total vegetables | OR = 0.47, $p < 0.001$ for trend | [21] |
| | 232 cases, 259 controls, the Netherlands | <142 vs. >247 g/day | OR = 0.4, $p < 0.0004$ for trend | [22] |
| | 834 cases, 939 controls, Australia | <4.13 vs. >7.36 servings/day | OR = 0.88, NS | [23] |

[a] NS, not significant.

Microbial and cellular metabolism of several bioactive food compounds can generate a multitude of metabolites with varying degrees of effects on the overall cancer process.

It is logical to believe that all fruits and vegetables are not equivalent in their ability to influence health. Thus, it is not that surprising that some types of vegetables surface more frequently as protective against cancer, including carrots and green, cruciferous, and allium vegetables.[26,27] For example, allium vegetables, which include onions and garlic, are a rich source of organosulfur compounds, and appear to have protective effects against stomach and colorectal cancer.[25]

Folate-rich foods may protect against pancreatic cancer, and at least some evidence suggests that these foods also protect against esophageal and colorectal cancers.[25] Foods with higher amounts of carotenoids may reduce the risk of the mouth, pharynx, and larynx and lung cancer.[25] Foods containing β-carotene or vitamin C seem to protect against esophageal cancer; and foods containing lycopene possibly protect against prostate cancer.[25] There is limited evidence to suggest that foods containing quercetin protect against lung cancer.[25] Similarly, foods containing selenium are linked to reduced prostate cancer, and there is some evidence suggesting that

**TABLE 66.2**

**Phytochemicals Present in Vegetables and Fruits That May Be Protective against Cancer**

| Groups | Phytochemicals | Food Sources |
|---|---|---|
| Carotenoids | Carotene, lutein, lycopene | Citrus fruit, carrots, squash, tomato |
| Flavonoids | Quercetin, kaempferol, tangerin, rutin | Citrus fruit |
| Glucosinolates | Glucobrassinin, indole-3-carbinol, sinigrin | Cruciferous vegetables |
| Isothiocyanates | Sulforaphane, phenylethylisothiocyanate | Cruciferous vegetables |
| Phenols | Resveratrol, coumarin, ellagic acid, catechins | Grape, citrus fruit, berries, green tea |
| Sulfides | Allyl sulfur, dithiolethiones | Garlic, broccoli |

they also protect against stomach and colorectal cancers.[25] Food sources of pyridoxine and/or vitamin E may also protect against esophageal and prostate cancers.[25] Overall, these findings suggest multiple foods can be involved with protection, but the response appears to be tissue-specific rather than a general metabolic response.

Finally, not all individuals should be expected to respond identically to dietary components since their attributions likely reflect their ability to influence specific molecular targets that can be influenced by a host of environmental and genetic factors.[29] Collectively, the magnitude of the response to fruits and vegetables is probably influenced by many factors, including the type, quantity, and duration of consumption of these foods, the consumer's genetic background, and a host of environmental factors.[30,31]

## VEGETABLE INTAKE, GENETIC POLYMORPHISMS, AND CANCER RISK

Human genetic variation is one of the factors modifying the response to constituents of plant foods in population-based studies. Some common single nucleotide polymorphisms (SNPs) in genes involved in nutrient metabolism, metabolic activation, and/or detoxification could establish the magnitude or whether there is a positive or negative response to vegetables for cancer risk. For example, the glutathione S-transferase (GST) family of enzymes, which includes four major classes (alpha, mu, theta, and pi), are involved in the metabolism of environmental carcinogens and reactive oxygen species (ROS). Polymorphisms in the *GSTM1* and *GSTT1* genes result in the absence of the corresponding GST protein and enzyme activity.[32,33] Depending on the population, 27%–53% of people are homozygous for deletion of the *GSTM1* gene and 20%–47% are homozygous for deletion of the *GSTT1* gene.[34] It has been hypothesized that individuals with the GST-null genotypes are at higher risk for cancer because of reduced capacity to dispose of activated carcinogens.[35] Epidemiological evidence supports that individuals possessing these genotypes are predisposed to a number of cancers including breast, prostate, liver, and colon (Table 66.3).[36] However, isothiocyanates are metabolized by GST, thus polymorphisms associated with reduced GST activity may result in longer circulating half-lives of isothiocyanates and potentially greater chemoprotective effects of cruciferous vegetables.

A pharmacokinetic study of sulforaphane disposition showed that *GSTM1*-null individuals compared to GSTM1 positive individuals had greater areas under the curve for plasma sulforaphane metabolite concentrations, faster rates of urinary sulforaphane metabolite excretion in the first 6 h after consumption, and higher total excretion over 24 h.[37] Several epidemiologic studies provide evidence that GST polymorphisms in conjunction with cruciferous vegetable intake are critical risk factors for cancer or precancerous lesions (Table 66.3).[38–51] For example, those with the highest quartile of broccoli intake had the lowest risk for colorectal adenomas compared with individuals who reportedly never ate broccoli; this inverse association was observed only in those individuals with the *GSTM1*-null genotype.[52,53] Similarly, colon cancer risk was altered by cruciferous vegetable intake in individuals with the *GSTM1*-null genotype.[41] Associations have also been investigated in relation to lung cancer risk, for which carcinogen exposure is a known risk factor, and found that the detoxifying effects of the GSTs may play a more decisive role. Isothiocyanate intake in combination with the *GSTM1*-null genotype was protective against lung cancer in current, but not former, smokers. However, among never-smokers, higher isothiocyanate intake was also associated with reduced risk of lung cancer in *GSTM1*- and/or *GSTT1*-null individuals, suggesting that the protective effects of isothioycanates are not limited to their capacity to alter the metabolism of tobacco-related carcinogens.[39] In contrast, Wang et al.[38] observed that among individuals with the *GSTM1*-present genotype, higher dietary intake of cruciferous vegetables was associated with a 40% reduction in lung cancer risk, whereas among individuals with the *GSTM1*-null genotype higher cruciferous intake was associated with a slight increase or no change in risk. Combination effects between dietary isothiocyantes and *GSTP1* genotype can modulate the age of disease onset; in men, there was a clinically significant difference of 17 years in the age of onset of oral cancer between *GSTP1* present and low isothiocyanate intake and *GSTP1* null and high isothiocyante intake ($P = 0.001$).[54] Possible explanations for the discrepancies in the literature about whether or not cruciferous vegetables are more beneficial for individuals with the GST-null or present genotypes may reflect differences in exposure to natural or synthetic cancer-promoting agents, differences in the amounts of cruciferous vegetables or isothiocyantes consumed, and/or variation caused by other gene polymorphisms.

**TABLE 66.3**

**Genetic Polymorphisms and Vegetable Intake: Representative Epidemiologic Studies with Significant Interactions for Cancer Risk Modification**

| Gene | Genotype | Cancer Site | Risk Modification | Reference |
|------|----------|-------------|-------------------|-----------|
| Glutathione S-transferase | GSTM1 null or present | Lung | High cruciferous vegetable intake (>3.01 servings/week) reduced cancer risk (OR = 0.61) only among individuals with GSTM1 present | [38] |
| | GSTM1 null or present | Lung | High isothiocyanate intake (>53 μmol/week) reduced cancer risk (OR = 0.55) only among individuals with GSTM1 absent | [39] |
| | GSTM1 null or present | Prostate | High broccoli intake (>339 g/month) reduced cancer risk (OR = 0.49) only among individuals with GSTM1 present | [40] |
| | GSTM1 or GSTT1 null or present | Colon | High isothiocyanate intake (>5.16 μmol/1000 kcal) decreased cancer risk (OR = 0.31) only among individuals with both GSTM1 and GSTT1 absent | [41] |
| | GSTT1 null or present | Colorectal | High fruit and vegetable consumption reduced cancer risk more when GSTT1 is present (OR = 0.32 men, .53 women) | [42] |
| | GSTM1, GSTT1 or GSTM1/T1 null or present | Lung | Intake of carotenoid-rich red and yellow vegetables was inversely associated with cancer risk in carriers of the GSTM1 ($p = 0.04$), GSTT1 ($p = 0.03$), or GSTM1/T1 ($p = 0.04$) positive genotypes | [43] |
| | GSTM1, GSTT1 or GSTM1/T1 null or present | Gastric | High isothiocyanate excretion (>3.32 μmol/g creatinine) reduced cancer risk more when GSTM1 (OR = 0.50), GSTT1 (OR = 0.47), or GSTM1/T1 (OR = 0.44) was absent | [44] |
| | GSTM1, GSTT1 or GSTM1/T1 null or present | Colorectal | Isothiocyanate excretion was inversely associated with cancer risk (OR = 0.51) in individuals that were both GSTM1 and GSTT1 null | [45] |
| | GSTM1 null or present | Lung | High isothiocyante intake (>80 μmol/week) reduced cancer risk more when GSTM1 null (OR = 0.52) | [46] |
| | A to G at base 1578 | Colorectal | High fruit and vegetable consumption reduced risk (OR = 0.40) only among men with A/A genotype | [42] |
| Methylenetetrahydrofolate reductase | C to T at base 677 | Breast | Low green vegetable intake (<1/week) increased risk (OR = 5.6) in women with TT genotype | [47] |
| | C to T at base 677 | Colorectal | High vegetable intake (>21 servings/week) decreased risk (OR = 0.49) only in individuals with CC genotype | [48] |
| | C to T at base 677 | Colorectal | High fruit and vegetable consumption (>2 servings/day) increased risk (OR = 2.18) in individuals with the TT genotype | [50] |
| X-ray repair cross-complementing group 1 | Arg to Trp at codon 194 | Breast | High fruit and vegetable consumption (>35 servings/week) reduced risk (OR = 0.58) only among women with Arg/Trp or Trp/Trp genotypes | [48] |
| O6-Methylguanine DNA methyl-transferase | A to G at codon 143 | Breast | High fruit and vegetable consumption (>35 servings/week) reduced risk (OR = 0.6) among women with AG or GG genotypes | [49] |
| Myeloperoxidase | G to A at base −463 | Breast | High fruit and vegetable consumption (>29 servings/week) reduced risk (OR = 0.75) among women with GA or AA genotypes | [51] |

Folate from vegetables, particularly green, leafy vegetables, has also been implicated as cancer protective. Polymorphisms in folate-metabolizing enzymes may also affect the relationship between folate/vegetable intake and cancer risk (Table 66.3). A polymorphism in the methylenetetrahydrofolate reductase (MTHFR) gene, which causes the substitution of C to T at nucleotide 677, is the most important common variant known in folate metabolic pathways. This polymorphism, which occurs in 5%–20% of the population worldwide,[55] results in reduced conversion of 5,10-methylenetetrahydrofolate to

5-methylenetetrahydrofolate, the form of folate that circulates in plasma. Individuals with this polymorphism appear to have increased dietary folate and riboflavin requirements.[56–58] Although there have been only a few studies analyzing this polymorphism, vegetable intake, and cancer risk, it appears to alter the relationship between folate status and colorectal cancer susceptibility.[59–61] As compared with subjects with the CC or CT genotype having low folate levels, those with the TT genotype showed a decreased risk of colorectal adenomas when they had high levels of plasma folate (adjusted

OR = 0.58), and an increased risk when they had low folate levels (adjusted OR = 2.13).[59] Thus, since there was no clear relationship between plasma folate and colorectal adenomas among those with the CC or CT genotype, only a subset of the population may benefit from exaggerated folate intakes. Furthermore, it remains unclear if this nutrigenetic response is constant across tissues. For example, the TT polymorphism of MTHFR has been linked to enhanced endometrial, ovarian, and breast cancers.[62–65] Moreover, compared to CC individuals with high folate intake, elevation of breast cancer risk was most pronounced among women with the TT genotype who consumed the lowest levels of dietary folate (OR = 1.83) or total folate intake (OR = 1.71).[65] Thus, in order to provide the best dietary recommendations for everyone for cancer prevention, it may be necessary to include the impact of genetic variation and to consider requirements for supplements that reflect a specific genomic profile and tissue of interest. Undeniably, a better understanding of the mechanisms whereby folate and other dietary bioactive components inhibit the cancer process will help clarify which gene polymorphisms are important in determining the magnitude of the response.

## MECHANISMS OF DIETARY CANCER PREVENTION

Carcinogenesis is generally recognized as a multistep process in which distinct molecular and cellular alterations occur. A multitude of sites within the cancer process may be influenced by bioactive food components. Figure 66.1 illustrates different steps where information exists that specific bioactive food components present in fruits and vegetables can interact with cellular processes involved with carcinogenesis. These include carcinogen metabolism, DNA repair, cell proliferation/apoptosis, inflammation, differentiation, oxidant/antioxidant balance, and angiogenesis. These various processes will be briefly described later and the effect of specific dietary bioactive components on these processes will be addressed later in the chapter. The response is complicated since multiple steps in the cancer process can be modified simultaneously. Thus, a better understanding of how the response relates to exposures and which process is

most involved in bringing about a change in tumor incidence and/or tumor behavior is essential. Furthermore, since many of these processes are likely influenced by several food components, it is necessary to obtain a better understanding about nutrient–nutrient interactions.

Virtually, all dietary or environmental pollutants/carcinogens to which humans are exposed require enzymatic biotransformation (metabolic activation) to become carcinogenic. Biotransformation enzymes, also referred to as xenobiotic- or drug-metabolizing enzymes, have a major role in regulating the mutagenic and neoplastic effects of chemical carcinogens, as well as metabolizing other drugs and endogenous compounds such as steroid hormones. The drug-metabolizing enzyme system comprises Phase I (oxidation, reduction, and hydrolysis) usually catalyzed by cytochrome P-450 enzymes and Phase II (glucuronidation, sulfation, acetylation, methylation, and conjugation with glutathione) enzymes. The induction of Phase II enzymes is largely mediated by the antioxidant response element (ARE), which is located in the promoter region of specific genes.[66] Generally, the transcription factor, nuclear factor E2-related factor 2 (Nrf2), binds to the ARE sequence to initiate gene expression. Many enzyme inducers, including dietary components, also lead to the activation of several signal transduction pathways, such as the mitogen-activated protein kinases (MAPK), protein kinase C (PKC), and phosphatidylinositol 3-kinase (PI3K) pathways. The consequences of the activation of these signaling cascades are dissociation of Nrf2 from another cytosolic protein, Keap1, nuclear translocation, and accumulation of Nrf2 protein, which leads to increased expression of detoxifying enzymes through activation of ARE. Bioactive components present in fruits and vegetables can prevent carcinogenesis by blocking metabolic activation, increasing detoxification, or by providing alternative targets for electrophilic metabolites.

Activated carcinogens exert their biological effects by forming covalent adducts with the individual nucleic acids of DNA or RNA. First, they distort the shape of the DNA molecule, potentially causing mistranslation of the DNA sequence. Second, when the DNA replicates, an adducted base that persists unrepaired can be misread, producing mutations in critical genes such as oncogenes and tumor suppressor genes.

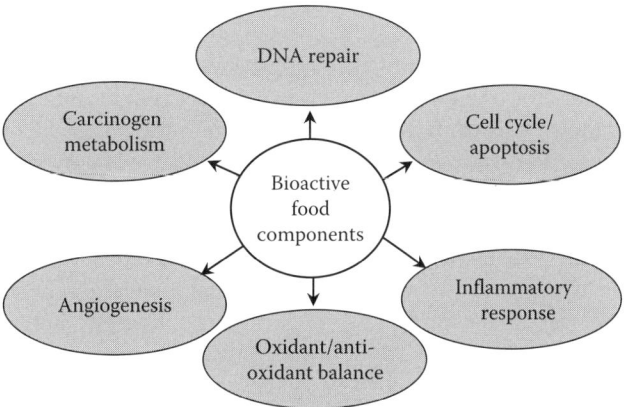

**FIGURE 66.1**  Bioactive food components influence multiple biological processes that are important for carcinogenesis.

Third, repair of bulky adducts can result in breakages of the DNA strand which can, in turn, result in mutations or deletions of genetic material.[25] Numerous DNA repair pathways exist to prevent the persistence of damage, and are integral to the maintenance of genome stability, and prevention of cancer.[67] DNA repair mechanisms include direct repair, base excision repair, nucleotide excision repair, double-strand break repair, and repair of interstrand cross-links.[68] DNA damage can also arrest cell cycle progression to allow for repair and prevention of the alteration to become permanent or activate apoptosis to eliminate cells with potentially catastrophic mutations.[68] Alterations in DNA repair, cell cycle progression, and apoptosis are all important molecular targets for dietary components in cancer prevention.

One of the hallmarks of cancer is aggressive proliferation of cells. In normal cells, proliferation is a finely controlled balance between growth-promoting and growth-inhibiting signals. However, cancer cells often acquire the capability of not only generating their own growth signals but also becoming insensitive to growth-suppressing signals.[69] Several proteins are recognized to be critical for cell cycle regulation including the cyclins, cyclin-dependent kinases (CDKs), CDK inhibitors (CDKIs), regulatory proteins (retinoblastoma [Rb] and p53), and the E2F transcription factor. The progression of the cell cycle from one phase to the next is regulated by sequential activation and inactivation of "check points" that monitor the cell's status.[70] These "check points" are mechanisms whereby the cell actively halts progression through the cell cycle until it can ensure that an earlier process, such as DNA replication or mitosis, is complete. In response to DNA damage, check points can also trigger the induction of necessary repair genes or cause the cells to undergo programmed cell death or apoptosis. The DNA damage check point arrests cells in the G1, S, or G2 phase depending upon the cell cycle status of the cell at the time damage was incurred.[71]

Apoptosis, interchangeably referred to as programmed cell death, is a key pathway for regulating homeostasis, that in Greek literally means "falling away." It is a natural, organized process that accounts for approximately three billion cell deaths in the human body every minute. It helps maintain a natural balance between cell death and cell renewal by destroying excess, damaged, or abnormal cells. Apoptosis is one of the most potent defenses against cancer since this process eliminates potentially deleterious, mutated cells. Triggers for apoptosis induction include DNA damage, disruption of the cell cycle, hypoxia, detachment of cells from their surrounding tissue, and loss of trophic signaling.[72] It is characterized by cell shrinkage, chromatin condensation, and fragmentation of the cell into compact membrane-enclosed structures, called "apoptotic-bodies" that are engulfed by macrophages and removed from the tissue in a controlled manner.[73] These morphological changes are a result of characteristic molecular and biochemical events occurring in the cell, most notably the activation of proteolytic enzymes. Proteolytic cleavage of procaspases is an important step leading to caspase activation, which in turn is amplified by the cleavage and activation of other downstream caspases in the apoptosis

cascade. Caspases are a family of cysteinyl aspartate-specific proteases involved in apoptosis and subdivided into initiation (8, 9, and 10) and executioner (3, 6, and 7) caspases. There are two main pathways of apoptosis: the extrinsic pathway (death receptor pathway) and the intrinsic pathway (mitochondrial pathway), which are activated by caspase-8 and caspase-9, respectively. A critical common element to both pathways is the involvement of caspase-3, which results in cleavage and inactivation of key cellular proteins including the DNA repair enzyme poly(-ADP-ribose) polymerase (PARP). In addition, mitogenic and stress-responsive pathways are involved in the regulation of apoptotic signaling.

Compelling evidence exists that bioactive dietary components can trigger apoptosis through numerous intracellular molecular targets in both apoptotic pathways in vitro. Distinct from the apoptotic events in the normal physiological process, which are mediated mainly by the interaction between death receptors and their relevant ligands,[74] many bioactive dietary components appear to induce apoptosis through the mitochondria-mediated pathway by activating p53 and its target genes. Dietary compounds generally induce oxidative stress, which downregulates anti-apoptotic molecules such as Bcl-2 or Bcl-x and upregulates pro-apoptotic molecules such as Bax or Bak.[65] The imbalance between anti-apoptotic and pro-apoptotic proteins elicits the release of cytochrome c from the mitochondrial membrane, which forms a complex with caspase-9 with the subsequent activation of caspases-3, -6, and -7.[76] The activated caspases degrade important intracellular proteins, leading to the morphological changes and the phenotype of apoptotic cells.[77] To enhance this mitochondria-mediated apoptosis, dietary components also activate pro-apoptotic c-Jun N-terminal kinase (JNK) and inhibit anti-apoptotic NF-κB signaling pathways.[75] Thus, the cytotoxic effects of dietary components on cells can be monitored by measuring their effects on mitochondria, caspases, and other apoptosis-related proteins.

Inflammation represents a physiological response to invading microorganisms, trauma, chemical irritation, or foreign tissues. Although acute inflammation is usually beneficial, chronic inflammation is often detrimental to the host. Epidemiologic data show an association between chronic inflammatory conditions and subsequent malignant transformation in the inflamed tissue.[78] Evidence indicates that there are multiple mechanisms linking inflammation to cancer, and that there are multiple targets for cancer prevention by bioactive dietary components. At the molecular level, free radicals and aldehydes produced during chronic inflammation can induce gene mutations and post-translational modifications of key cancer-related proteins.[79] Other products of inflammation, including cytokines (peptide hormones that mediate the inflammatory response such as interleukins or IL-1, IL-4, IL-6, IL-10, interferon (and tumor necrosis factor α), growth factors, and transcription factors such as NF-κB, control the expression of oncogenes and tumor suppressor genes and key inflammatory enzymes such as inducible nitric oxide synthase (iNOS) and cyclooxygenase-2 (COX-2). These enzymes, in turn, directly influence ROS and eicosanoid levels.

Chronic inflammation results in increased DNA damage, cellular proliferation, disruption of DNA repair pathways, inhibition of apoptosis, and the promotion of angiogenesis and invasion[78]; all of which are important during the cancer process. Several of these mechanisms are amenable to influence by dietary constituents.

The generation of ROS is a result of normal cellular metabolism. ROS profoundly affects numerous critical cellular functions, and the absence of efficient cellular detoxification mechanisms which remove these radicals can increase cancer risk.[80] All ROS have the potential to interact with cellular components including DNA bases or the deoxyribosyl backbone of DNA to produce damaged bases or strand breaks.[81] Thus, ROS can act as DNA-damaging agents, effectively increasing the mutation rate within cells and thus promoting oncogenic transformation.[82] ROS can also specifically activate certain intracellular signaling cascades and thus contribute to tumor development and metastasis through the regulation of cellular phenotypes such as proliferation, death, and motility.[81] The effect of ROS is balanced by antioxidant enzymes and the antioxidant action of dietary bioactive components present in fruits and vegetables.[83] The so-called nutritional antioxidants act at least partially through multiple mechanisms and in different cellular compartments, but possibly as free radical scavengers that neutralize free radicals, reduce peroxide concentrations, promote the repair of oxidized membranes, and/or quench iron to decrease ROS production.[84]

Angiogenesis is a normal physiological process where new blood vessels grow from preexisting ones. While angiogenesis occurs during growth and wound healing, it can also indicate that a tumor has possibly changed from a benign to a malignant state. While enhanced angiogenesis promotes tumor growth by increasing oxygen and nutrient delivery, increasing evidence suggest that this process occurs early in cancer development and thus occurs as a result of signals arising from transformed cells. Angiogenesis in malignant tumors is a complex process that involves the tight interplay of cancerous cells and their microenvironment including surrounding endothelial cells, phagocytes, and their pro- and inhibitory secreted factors. Premalignant and malignant cells both exhibit increasing levels of cellular and molecular angiogenic dysregulation, advancing their malignant phenotypes. This contributes to their ability to produce pro-angiogenic molecules, as well as the surrounding stroma that initiates pathologic-angiogenesis through paracrine microenvironmental on endothelial cells. Endothelial cells are stimulated and are attracted to the site where the new blood supply is needed by various chemoattractants including growth factors such as vascular endothelial growth factor (VEGF), fibroblast growth factor (FGF), and insulin-like growth factor-1 (IGF-1), and inflammatory molecules including IL-8, COX-2, and iNOS.[85,86] Chemotactic migration is potentiated by the degradation of extracellular matrix components.[87] This is accomplished via matrix-metalloproteinases (MMPs).[88,89] MMPs include collagenases (MMP-1, MMP-8, and MMP-13), gelatinases (MMP-2 and MMP-9), stromelysins (MMP-3, MMP-10, and MMP-7), and elastase (MMP-12).[90]

The expression of matrix metalloproteinases is predominately regulated by the AP-1 transcription complex, which can be activated by several mechanisms involving growth factors, cell–cell interactions, and interactions among cells and matrix.[91] In addition, there are natural MMP inhibitors (tissue inhibitors of metalloproteinases, TIMPs), which are also involved in regulating the activation and activity of these enzymes. MMPs are involved in many physiological processes involving matrix remodeling, and appear to be critical in angiogenesis, tumor cell invasion, and metastasis. In addition to removing physical barriers to migration through degradation of the extracellular matrix, MMPs can modulate cell adhesion, and generate extracellular matrix degradation products that are chemotactic for endothelial cells.

An inhibition of angiogenesis serves two primary functions: (1) it limits tumor size by restricting oxygen and nutrients, and (2) it decreases the opportunities for metastatic cells to enter the circulatory system. Several dietary components have surfaced as inhibitors of angiogenesis in various animal and cell culture models.[92–94] Specifically, they appear to possess a wide range of angiopreventive properties by modifying pro-angiogenic stimuli including inflammation, cytokine and growth factor production, endothelial cell function, and/or intracellular and extracellular communications.

## VITAMIN A AND CAROTENOIDS

Vitamin A or retinol is a fat-soluble vitamin with an unsaturated aliphatic chain. It has a role in cell differentiation, in the protein metabolism of cells originating from the ectoderm, and in the formation of the chromosphere component of visual cycle chromoproteins. Experimentally, there is evidence that retinoids (vitamin A and its derivatives) can influence cancer biology, especially because they influence growth and differentiation.[95] Because lack of proper differentiation is a feature of cancer cells, adequate vitamin A may allow normal cell differentiation and thus avoid the development of cancer.[96] Experimental and clinical studies with retinoids reveal that they can inhibit or reverse the carcinogenic process in some organs, including hematological malignancy, as well as premalignant and malignant lesions in the oral cavity, head and neck, breast, skin, liver, and cerivix,[95–98] but may increase prostate cancer risk.[99] Supplemental vitamin A can also decrease the number of hepatic metastasis resulting from colon cancer.[100] Except for the occurrence in milk fat, egg yolk, and liver of mammals, most vitamin A is usually obtained from carotenoids. Carotenoids constitute a class of over 600 natural compounds occurring predominantly in fruits and vegetables. These precursors to vitamin A occur in common green, yellow/red, and yellow/orange vegetables and fruits.[101] They include lutein, cryptoxanthin, lycopene, β-carotene, α-carotene, and zeaxanthin (Figure 66.2).

Numerous epidemiologic studies indicate that individuals who consume diets with a relatively large amount of fruits and vegetables rich in carotenoids and/or high levels of serum β-carotene are at a lower risk for cancer at several tumor sites, including lung, colon, and breast.[101–110] Further evidence

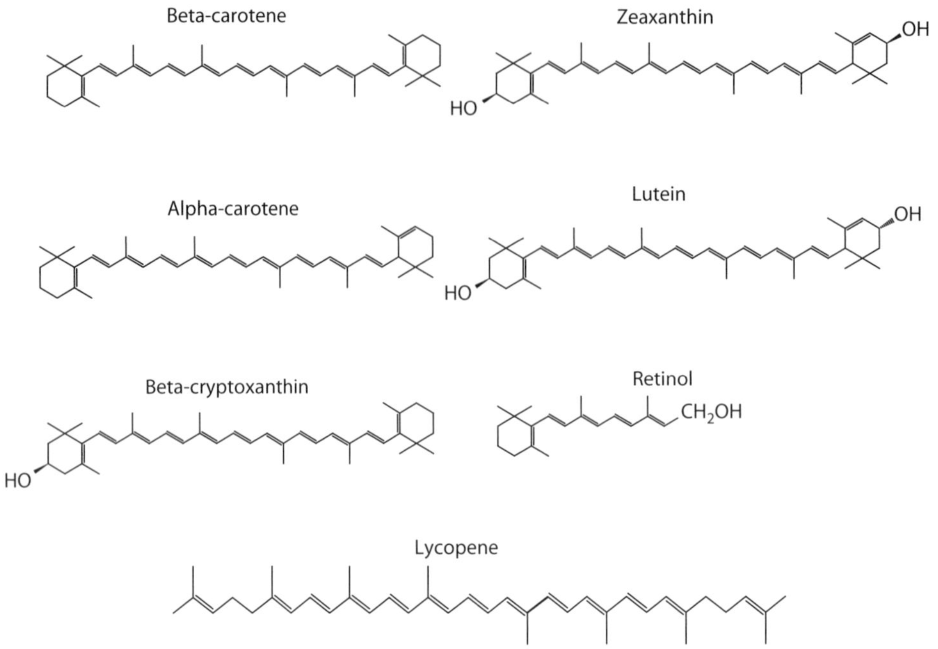

**FIGURE 66.2** Structures of carotenoids.

from cell culture and animal experiments suggested that β-carotene, the carotenoid with the greatest pro-vitamin A activity, could be the compound responsible for this association.[111] On the basis of this evidence, four randomized intervention trials were conducted to test the effect of β-carotene supplements on cancer—the α-Tocopherol β-Carotene Study (ATBC Study),[112] the Physician's Health Study (PHS),[113] the β-Carotene and Retinol Efficacy Trial (CARET),[114] and the Women's Health Study[115] (Table 66.4). Unexpectedly, results from the ATBC and CARET studies showed adverse treatment effects in terms of increased lung cancer incidence in high-risk subjects.[116] These studies suggest that in high-risk individuals β-carotene may have an adverse effect on cancer risk. This is supported by a recent French study that found high β-carotene intake was inversely associated with risk of tobacco-related cancers among nonsmokers whereas high β-carotene intake was directly associated with risk among

smokers.[117] Molecular analysis of the normal lung epithelium from subjects in the ATBC trial demonstrated that β-carotene supplementation increased cyclin D1 expression, suggesting aberrant cell proliferation.[118]

The different results obtained in supplementation trials compared to cohort studies may reflect that, in addition to β-carotene, fruits and vegetables contain numerous other compounds that may be protective against cancer such as folic acid, other carotenoids, and polyphenols. In fact, β-carotene may simply be a marker for the actual protective substances in fruits and vegetables. Alternately, β-carotene may have different effects when consumed as a supplement rather than in the food supply. The ATBC, CARET, and PHS studies illustrate that definitive evidence of both safety and efficacy is required for individual fruit and vegetable constituents before dietary guidelines, beyond simply greater consumption, can be proposed. Because β-carotene is the major source of vitamin A

**TABLE 66.4**

**Human Supplementation Trials with β-Carotene**

| Study | Population | Intervention | Duration | Cancer Outcome |
|---|---|---|---|---|
| ATBC[112] | 29,133 Finnish male smokers (50–69 years of age) | β-Carotene, 20 mg/day Vitamin E, 50 mg/day | 5–8 years | 18% increase in lung cancer 8% increase in mortality |
| CARET[114] | 18,314 men and women and asbestos workers (25–74 years of age) | β-Carotene, 30 mg/day Vitamin A, 25,000 IU | <4 years | 28% increase in lung cancer 17% increase in deaths |
| PHS[113] | 22,071 U.S. male physicians (40–84 years of age) | β-Carotene, 50 mg on alternate days | 12 years | No effect of supplement on cancer incidence |
| Women's Health[115] | 39,876 female health professionals (>45 years of age) | β-Carotene, 50 mg on alternate days | 4.1 years | No effect of supplement on cancer incidence |

*Abbreviations:* ATBC, α-Tocopherol β-Carotene Study; CARET, β-Carotene and Retinol Efficacy Trial; PHS, the Physician's Health Study.

for much of the world's population, it is critical to define its safe intake from foods and supplements.[119] The CARET study also demonstrates the importance of large-scale primary prevention trials because the differences observed (lung cancer incidence of 4.6 and 5.9 per 1000 in the placebo and treatment groups, respectively) would not be detected in smaller studies.[114] These studies also may suggest that the effect of β-carotene may depend on the dose consumed. In a recent study in Finland, men in the highest tertile of serum concentrations of β-carotene had a 2.3-fold higher risk of prostate cancer compared to those in the lowest tertile (RR = 2.29, 95% CI = 1.12–4.66).[120] In animals models, low doses of β-carotene inhibit carcinogen-induced aberrant crypt formation; however, very high doses augment aberrant crypt incidence.[121]

β-Carotene mediates its cancer protective and cancer-promoting effects through modulation of intracellular redox status. Through this mechanism, it affects redox-sensitive molecular pathways involved in the regulation of cell cycle progression and apoptosis.[122] At low concentrations, the carotenoid may serve as an antioxidant inhibiting free radical production,[123,124] while at relatively high concentrations and/or in the presence of a chronic oxidative stress (i.e., smoke) it may behave as a pro-oxidant, propagating free radical–induced reactions, consuming endogenous antioxidants and inducing DNA oxidative damage.[125–127] These effects may be mediated by carotenoid breakdown products.[125] In this context, β-carotene may regulate cell growth and death by the modulation of redox-sensitive genes and transcription factors.[122,128] Wang et al.[129] have used the ferret to model β-carotene/tobacco interactions in lung and noted a relative lack of both retinoic acid and retinoic acid receptor β expression in the lungs of smoke-exposed ferrets given high-dose β-carotene. The authors suggested that oxidative metabolites of β-carotene might cause diminished retinoid signaling and thus increase tumorigenesis. In contrast with a pharmacologic dose of β-carotene, a physiological dose in smoke-exposed ferrets had no detrimental effects and afforded weak protection against lung damage induced by cigarette smoke.[130]

Although lycopene is not a vitamin A precursor, it is another carotenoid that has been proposed to have anticancer properties.[131–135] Lycopene is present in tomatoes, watermelon, pink grapefruit, and guava. Like other carotenoids, lycopene can serve as a potent antioxidant, and thereby influence exposure to ROS.[136] Interestingly, at physiological concentrations it can also retard the growth of human cancer cells, possibly by influencing growth factor receptor signals and altering cell cycle progression.[137–139] Lycopene can sometimes upregulate the gene connexin 43, which may account for changes in intercellular gap junctional communications.[140] Evidence also exists that lycopene may upregulate the expression of the urokinase plasminogen activator receptor and facilitate invasion.[141] Recent evidence also suggests that lycopene can increase the expression of Phase II enzymes with an ARE via Nrf2 translocation from the cytosol to the nucleus.[142] Lycopene shows potent redox properties by which it decreases

the ROS generated by smoke and modulates redox-sensitive cell targets, including protein tyrosine phosphatases, protein kinases, MAPKs, and transcription factors.[143] Moreover, it counteracts the effects of smoke on carcinogen-bioactivating enzymes and on molecular pathways involved in cell proliferation, apoptosis, and inflammation.[143] In mice, high-dose (14 mg/kg) lycopene, can significantly decrease vascular endothelial growth factor levels in plasma.[144] As with many bioactive food components, a better understanding of molecular targets will assist in identification of those individuals who might benefit and those who might be placed at risk as a result of dietary intervention.[145]

## VITAMIN C

Vitamin C is the most abundant water-soluble antioxidant in the body. There are two chemical forms of vitamin C: the reduced form (ascorbic acid) and the oxidized form (dehydro-ascorbic acid). Vitamin C is unique in that it can be regenerated after it becomes oxidized. The reduced form is the more predominant chemical structure in the body and is involved in many biochemical and biological functions. Specific food sources include citrus fruits, mangoes, papaya, banana, strawberries, melon, broccoli, cabbage and other green leafy vegetables, peppers, tomatoes, pumpkin, and yams. Epidemiologic evidence indicates that high intakes of vitamin C-rich fruits and vegetables and high vitamin C concentrations in serum are inversely associated with the risk of some cancers.[146] Hensen et al.[147] analyzed 46 epidemiologic studies on the protective effects of vitamin C against various types of cancers; 33 of these studies found a significant link between vitamin C intake and a reduced incidence of cancer. Of the 44 published in vivo studies examining oxidative damage after supplementation with vitamin C, 38 found a decrease in the number of markers of oxidative damage to DNA, lipid, or protein; 14 showed no changes; and only 6 reported an increase.[148] Case-control data indicate a risk reduction of 40%–60% for gastric cancer[149] and 66% for oral/pharyngeal cancer,[150] and cohort data indicate a risk reduction of 23% for lung cancer in men for the highest versus lowest intake of vitamin C.[151] The World Cancer Research Fund report concluded that there is a substantial amount of consistent evidence, from both cohort and case-control studies, that foods containing vitamin C probably protect against esophageal cancer.[25] Vitamin C concentration in plasma has also been shown to have an inverse association with cancer-related mortality.[152]

In animal studies, high exposures vitamin C has been reported to be protective against skin, mammary, liver, and kidney cancer.[153–155] Vitamin C inhibits primary tumor growth and exhibits the ability to inhibit metastases through attenuated tumor invasion and proliferation.[156] A murine model has been generated that lacks the enzyme required for ascorbic acid synthesis (l-gulono-δ-lactone oxidase). In these mice, ascorbate supplementation inhibited melanoma cell growth and decreased serum inflammatory cytokines (IL-6 by 90% and IL-1β by 62%) compared to the levels in knockout mice deprived of ascorbate.[157] Ascorbate supplementation in these mice also improved survival after injection with ovarian cancer cells via modulation of natural killer cell cytotoxicity.[158] Proteomic analysis of tumor tissue in CT-26 colon cancer cells implanted into mice after treatment with ascorbic acid suggested a previously undefined role of ascorbic acid in the regulation of cytoskeleton remodeling in tumor tissues.[159] However, other studies have suggested that high doses of vitamin C can have adverse effects on skin and lung cancers,[160,161] thus suggesting that the response may be dose dependent. Pharmacologic doses of ascorbic acid can repress specificity protein transcription factors and specificity protein-regulated genes in colon cancer cells.[162] Nevertheless, vitamin C's ability to scavenge of free radicals to prevent oxidative-induced DNA damage and its ability to be a competitive inhibitor of nitrosamine formation from nitrate and amines in vivo may account for some of its reported anticancer properties.[163–165] Studies with cultured cells have shown that vitamin C can affect apoptosis and gene expression and this appears to be mediated by its redox effects.[166–170]

## FOLATE

Folate (folic acid) is so-called because it is abundant in foliage (green leafy vegetables). Epidemiologic and clinical studies indicate that dietary folate intake and blood folate concentrations are inversely associated with the risk of colon, lung, head and neck, breast, and cervical cancers.[171–177] Collectively, studies suggest an ~40% reduction in the risk of colorectal cancer in individuals with the highest dietary folate intake compared with those with the lowest intake.[178] Rates of childhood cancer including Wilms tumor, primitive neuroectodermal tumors, and ependymomas have decreased significantly following mandatory folic acid supplementation.[179] As mentioned previously, studies of folate and cancer are of particular interest as they not only demonstrate that this vitamin may exert a cancer-protective effect but also demonstrate the importance of nutrigenetic studies since functional polymorphisms in folate-metabolizing genes, especially MTHFR, are capable of modifying the relationship between it and colorectal cancer risk. Observational studies show that individuals with the homozygous genotype for the MTHFR 677C to T polymorphism are at increased risk for colon,[176] ovarian,[180] and esophageal[181] cancer when folate intake or status is low. Again, since there was no clear relationship between plasma folate and colorectal adenomas among those with the CC or CT genotype, only a subset of the population may benefit from supplemental folate for colon cancer prevention.

Animal studies using chemical and genetically predisposed models have provided considerable support for a causal relationship between folate depletion and increased cancer incidence, as well as a dose-dependent protective effect of folate supplementation.[178,182–187] However, animal studies have also shown that the dose and timing of folate intervention are critical in providing safe and effective cancer prevention.[178] In the APC[Min/+] mouse, a genetic model of colon cancer, a review of the published literature indicated that nutritional modulation of folate was shown to have different effects on

intestinal cancer depending on the dosage, duration and timing of intervention, and interaction of the APC[Min/+] genotype with other genetic factors affecting folate metabolism.[188] Although some studies demonstrated that folate deficiency before tumorigenesis increases the risk of tumor development, there are studies which demonstrate excess folate postweaning or after tumor initiation also increases intestinal tumor burden.[188] Exceptionally high supplemental folate levels and folate intervention after microscopic neoplastic foci established in the colorectal mucosa have been reported to promote rather than suppress colorectal carcinogenesis.[178] These results suggest that the optimal dose of folate for cancer prevention may vary among individuals and may depend on whether or not microscopic lesions are present. The results of a recent randomized trial of folic acid in the prevention of colorectal adenomas in humans are consistent with such an effect.[189] This study, which enrolled subjects with a history of prior adenomas, did not observe a modulation of recurrence rates after the first follow-up colonoscopy at 3 years. However, at that time of second follow-up, 6–8 years after initial randomization, a significant 2.3-fold increase in the multiplicity of recurrent adenomas occurred among those receiving folic acid supplements.[189]

The possibility of paradoxical effect of excessive quantities of folate promoting cancer may also apply to other human cancers. In a recent prospective cohort study among approximately 25,000 postmenopausal women, the risk of developing breast cancer was significantly increased among those taking folic acid supplements (a group whose consumption was > 853 μg of folate per day).[190] Like colorectal cancer, the promoting effect of folic acid has also been observed to occur in an animal model of breast carcinogenesis.[191] A meta-analysis of six randomized controlled trials of folic acid supplementation and prostate cancer incidence showed an RR = 1.24 (95%CI = 1.03–1.49) for men receiving folic acid compared to controls.[192]

The mechanisms by which dietary folate can modulate carcinogenesis are related to the sole biochemical function of folate mediating the transfer of one-carbon moieties (Figure 66.3). Folate is an essential cofactor for the de novo biosynthesis of purines and thymidylate. 5,10-Methylenetetrahydrofolate, an intracellular co-enzymatic form of folate, is required for conversion of deoxyuridylate to thymidylate and can be oxidized to 10-formyltetrahydrofolate for de novo purine synthesis. In this role, folate is an important factor in DNA synthesis, stability, integrity, and repair. A growing body of evidence from cell culture, animal and human studies indicates that folate deficiency is associated with DNA strand breaks, impaired DNA repair, and increased mutations, and that folate supplementation can correct some of these deficiency defects.[178,193–196] The central role of folate as a cofactor in nucleotide synthesis also means that abundant availability of the vitamin can facilitate the proliferation of rapidly dividing cells.[197]

Folate also has an essential role in one-carbon transfer involving remethylation of homocysteine to methionine, thereby ensuring the provision of S-adenosylmethionine, the primary methyl group donor for most biological methylation

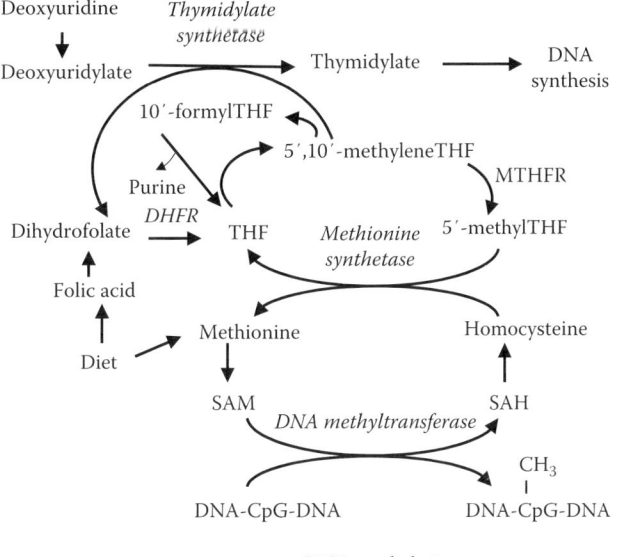

**FIGURE 66.3** Simplified version of methyl metabolism. Folate, in the form of 5-methyltetrahydrofolate, is involved in remethylation of homocysteine to methionine, which is a precursor of SAM, the primary methyl group donor for most biological methylation reactions including that of DNA. 5,10 Methylenetetrafhydrofolate is required for conversion of deoxyrudiylate to thymidylate for DNA synthesis. Abbreviations used: CH₃, methyl group; CpG, cytosine-guanine dinucleotide sequence; DHFR, dihydrofolate reductase; MTHFR, methylenetetrahydrofolate reductase; SAH, S-adenosylhomocysteine; SAM, S-adenosylmethionine; THF, tetrahydrofolate.

reactions including DNA methylation (Figure 66.3).[178] DNA methylation is an important epigenetic determinant of gene expression, maintenance of DNA integrity and stability, chromosomal modifications, and development of mutations. Aberrant patterns and dysregulation of DNA methylation are mechanistically related to carcinogenesis. Evidence from cell culture, animal and human studies suggest that folate deficiency and supplementation can influence DNA methylation.[198–201] DNA methylation at promoter CpG islands silences transcription, and hence inactivates the function of a wide array of tumor suppressor and cancer-related genes.[202] Folic acid supplementation is able to reverse preexisting global DNA hypomethylation and increase the extent of global DNA methylation above the preexisting level, thereby reducing the risk of neoplastic transformation.[202] In contrast, folic acid supplementation may cause de novo methylation of CpG islands of tumor suppressor genes, with consequent gene inactivation leading to tumor development and progression.[203]

## VITAMIN E

Vitamin E comes primarily from dietary vegetables oils (including safflower, corn, cottonseed, and soy bean oils), nuts, and green vegetables. Vitamin E is a collective term used to refer to a number of structurally and functionally different compounds that function, at least in part, as lipid-soluble antioxidants which can protect against the adverse effects of free radicals.[204] There are eight different isoforms that belong to two categories: four saturated analogs (α, β, γ, and δ) called tocopherols and four unsaturated analogs (α, β, γ, and δ) referred to as tocotrienols (Figure 66.4).

Few epidemiologic studies have investigated the association of cancer risk with diets providing large amounts of vitamin E. The World Cancer Research Fund concluded that there is limited evidence that foods containing vitamin E protect against esophageal and prostate cancer.[25] Other reviews have found no relationship between vitamin E and cancer risk.[205–207] However, one recent review of the epidemiological data suggests that vitamin E from food offers some protection against breast cancer, while vitamin E supplements do not.[204] This again raises the issue that other food components in the food matrix may be important in determining the response.

Owing to its high bioavailability, α-tocopherol is the best characterized vitamin E isomer and has been examined in a number of randomized clinical trials. For example, in the Women's Health Study with 39,876 healthy U.S. women, the administration of 600 IU of α-tocopherol on alternate days did not significantly affect the incidence of colon, lung, or total cancer.[115] In the Physician's Health Study II Randomized Control Trial, supplementation with vitamin E (400 IU of α-tocopherol every other day) for 8 years did not reduce the risk of prostate cancer or all other cancers.[208] Similarly, in the Cancer Prevention Study II Nutrition Cohort, the intake of vitamin E supplements was not associated with overall risk of prostate cancer or with risk of advanced prostate cancer.[209] However, in the α-Tocopherol and β-Carotene Prevention Study (ATBC), 34% fewer cases of prostate cancer and 16% fewer of colorectal cancer were diagnosed among male cigarette smokers who received daily vitamin E supplements compared to those given a placebo.[112] Further analysis indicated an association of high serum tocopherol with low prostate cancer risk.[210] These results encouraged the launching of the Selenium and Vitamin E Cancer Prevention Trial (SELECT),

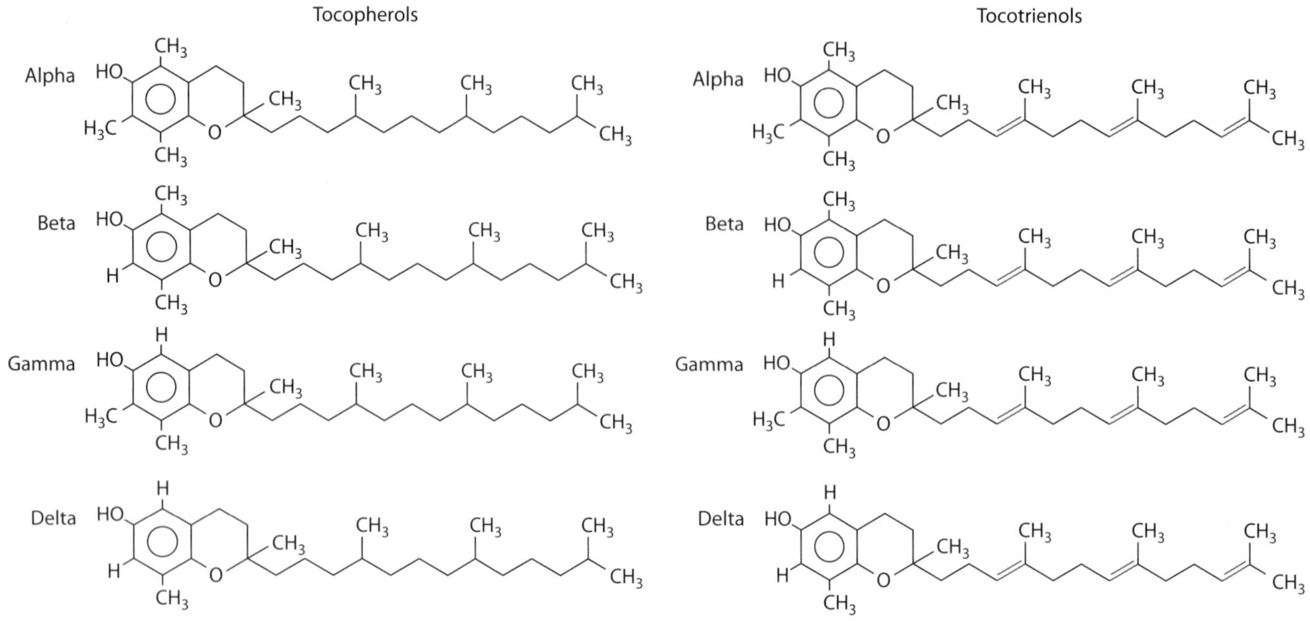

**FIGURE 66.4**  Structures of tocopherols and tocotrienols.

in which 35,533 men were randomized into four groups and took 400 IU α-tocopherol acetate or 200 μg selenium from selenomethionine daily, in a two-by-two design for an average of 5.5 years.[211] However, based on the recommendations of the Data Safety and Monitoring Committee, SELECT was terminated early due to lack of efficacy. Of concern, and described in a more recent report from SELECT, is the statistically significant increased risk of prostate cancer in the vitamin E alone arm (HR = 1.17, 95% CI = 1.004–1.36).[212]

In preclinical models, α-tocopherol is protective against colon, liver, lung, skin, and pancreatic cancer,[213–218] but the data are not consistent.[219] Cell culture studies suggest that vitamin E functions by scavenging oxygen radicals and terminating free radical chain reactions.[220,221] Vitamin E is able to inhibit cell proliferation and induce apoptosis in a variety of human malignant cell lines.[222–232] Vitamin E may also prevent cancer progression by increasing production of humoral antibodies and enhancing cell-mediated immunity.[233] Studies have also suggested that vitamin E may alter the cellular response to estrogen.[234] A number of explanations have been suggested for the increased prostate cancer risk observed with α-tocopherol in the SELECT study. First, supplementation of a nutrient to individuals who already have adequate intake may not produce any beneficial effect. Another explanation is that other tocopherols in our diet, such as γ or δ, are exerting cancer protective effects. Many studies have shown that γ-tocopherol is more effective than α-tocopherol in trapping reactive nitrogen species, in generating an inflammatory response, and in inhibiting cancer cell growth and apoptosis.[230,235–244] Recent studies also suggest that γ- and δ- tocopherol are more efficacious in inhibiting lung[243] and colon[244] carcinogenesis than α-tocopherol in animal models. In addition, high doses of α-tocopherol have been shown to decrease the blood and tissue levels of γ-tocopherol.[245,246] It should be noted that γ-tocopherol is more prominent than α-tocopherol

in the American diet.[247] Thus, speciation of the vitamin E molecule and likely other bioactive food components must be considered when evaluating diet and cancer interrelationships.

While the tocopherols have been investigated extensively, little is known about the tocotrienols. Recent studies suggest that the molecular targets of tocotrienols are distinct from those of tocopherols and may make them particularly effective for cancer prevention.[248] These include the inhibition of epithelial-to-mesenchymal transitions, the suppression of vascular endothelial growth factor and tumor angiogenesis, unique apoptotic targets, and the induction of antitumor immunity.[249–261] In addition, tocotrienol, but not tocopherol, has been shown to selectively target cancer stem cells by likely blocking their self-renewal properties.[249]

## SELENIUM

Selenium enters the food chain through plants and its concentration in foods is subject to several factors that are directly related to the amount and bioavailability of selenium in the soil.[262] Evidence for the cancer protective effects of selenium in humans was initially obtained by means of ecological and correlational studies which found an inverse relationship between selenium status and mortality from cancer of the colon, rectum, prostate, breast, ovary, lung and leukemia.[263] Data from most case-control and cohort studies indicate selenium's possible protective relationship with lung and prostate cancer, but data are not overly convincing for other cancer sites, including breast and colon/rectum.[25,264] A recent meta-analysis suggests that selenium supplementation may afford some protection against lung cancer in populations where average selenium levels are traditionally low.[265] Evidence suggests that toenail Se may be a useful predictor of status.[265] Cohort studies also have identified low baseline serum or toenail selenium concentrations as a risk factor for prostate cancer.[266,267] The World

Cancer Research Fund Continuous Update Project conducted a meta-analysis of toenail selenium and cancer risk, which indicated a reduction in prostate cancer risk (RR = 0.29, 95% CI = 0.14–0.61) with a toenail selenium concentration between 0.85 and 0.94 µg/g.[268]

Because epidemiologic studies have failed to consistently link low Se status with increased risk of cancer, meta-analyses and systematic reviews have been done to quantitatively summarize the existing epidemiologic literature. Forty-nine prospective observational studies with over one million participants were included in a Cochrane review.[269] They found that the epidemiologic data supported a reduced cancer incidence (OR = 0.69, 95% CI = 0.53–0.91) and mortality (OR = 0.55, 95% CI = 0.36–0.83) with higher Se exposure. This effect was more pronounced in men (OR = 0.66, 95% CI = 0.42–1.05) than in women (OR = 0.90, 95% CI = 0.45–1.77). However, it was not possible from these studies to determine that Se levels or Se intake was a surrogate for some other factor which lowered cancer risk.

The Nutritional Prevention of Cancer (NPC) Study provides the strongest evidence for the protective effects of selenium against cancer. This randomized controlled trial was designed to test selenium as a deterrent to the development of basal or squamous skin carcinomas. Secondary end-point analyses showed that the mineral resulted in a significant reduction in total cancer mortality (RR = 0.5), total cancer incidence (RR = 0.63), and incidence of lung (RR = 0.54), colorectal (RR = 0.42), and prostate (RR = 0.37) cancer.[270] Participants with baseline plasma selenium concentrations in the lowest two tertiles (<121.6 ng/mL) experienced reductions in total cancer incidence, whereas those in the highest tertile showed an elevated incidence (HR = 1.20, 95% CI = 0.77–1.86).[271] Re-analysis of incidence data through the end of the blinded clinical trial indicated that supplementation significantly reduced lung[272] and prostate[273] cancer only in individuals with the lowest baseline selenium concentrations. These results suggest that there may be a narrow window for the most beneficial dose of selenium. In contrast, the SELECT trial which was discussed in the section on vitamin E found no benefit of selenium supplementation on prostate cancer. Similarly, a recent trial in Canada of 303 men with high-grade prostatic intraepithelial neoplasia randomized to Se (200 µg/day, form not specified), vitamin E (800 IU/day), and soy (40 g/day) also found no effect of supplementation on prostate cancer development (HR = 1.03, 95% CI = 0.67–1.60) versus placebo.[274] On the basis of these outcomes, many scientists believe that selenium supplementation may not be efficacious for prostate cancer prevention in those consuming a Western-style diet with adequate selenium exposures.

Rather than considering this trial a failure, scientists should consider why the SELECT trial gave different results from the NPC study and use this information to better understand who might benefit from selenium supplementation and who might be placed at risk. Differences in baseline selenium status or formulation of the selenium supplement may have contributed to the differences observed between the two studies. In fact, in the SELECT trial, median baseline serum levels were 135 ng/mL compared to 114 ng/mL observed in the NPC trial, and 78% of subjects in the SELECT trial would have been classified as being in the upper tertile of baseline selenium in the NPC trial (the group that had a nonsignficant increased cancer risk with selenium supplementation). Another important difference between the two studies is the form of selenium provided. The NPC trial utilized selenium-enriched yeast whereas the SELECT trial used selenomethionine. Although Se-enriched yeast is predominantly selenomethionine, minor Se compounds in the yeast, such as Se-methyl-selenocysteine, but not selenomethionine, can be metabolized to alpha-keto acids which function as histone deacetylase inhibitors and lead to de-repression of silenced tumor-suppressor proteins.[275] These data suggest that different metabolites may have different biological effects. Moreover, a later analytical study reported that the selenomethionine distribution in the selenium-enriched yeast utilized in the NPC trial only accounted for 27% of the total selenium.[276] Thus, it is possible that the effect of selenium in the NPC trial was not caused by selenomethionine, but rather by other selenium compounds or the combination of selenium-containing compounds in the yeast. A better understanding of who might benefit from selenium supplementation and who might be placed at risk based on baseline selenium status, genetic polymorphisms in selenoproteins or in cancer-related processes, cancer site, dose and form of selenium is needed. Finally, it must be noted that because the number of cancer cases in the NPC was low, the statistical relationship may have been chance.

Extensive experimental evidence indicates that selenium supplementation reduces the incidence of cancer in animals.[277] Selenium supplementation in the diet or drinking water inhibits initiation and/or post-initiation stages of liver, esophageal, pancreatic, colon and mammary carcinogenesis,[278–290] and spontaneous liver and mammary tumorigenesis.[291,292] Studies have also suggested that selenium has beneficial effects against tumor promotion/progression. High-dose selenium supplementation (3 ppm in the drinking water) inhibits the progression of hormone refractory prostate cancer and the development of retroperitoneal lymph node metastases through an inhibition of angiogenesis.[293] Similarly, high-selenium soy protein had a greater inhibitory effect than low-selenium soy protein on pulmonary metastasis of melanoma cells in mice.[294] Nevertheless, it is difficult to extrapolate data in experimental animals to humans, as animal studies have generally used doses at least 10 times greater than those required to prevent clinical signs of deficiency, which, on a per unit body weight basis, are considerably higher exposures than those which occur in most humans.

Male beagle dogs, a species that spontaneously develops prostate cancer, more closely reflects the human situation. Studies in these dogs revealed that supplementation with selenium as selenomethionine or high-selenium yeast for 7 months significantly reduced DNA damage and unregulated epithelial-cell apoptosis in the prostate compared to dogs with unsupplemented diets.[295] However, a "u-shaped" dose response was evident and those dogs with high selenium status to beginning of treatment had an adverse response to increased selenomethionine exposure.[296] Further study of the process of carcinogenesis within the prostate of animal species vulnerable to spontaneous cancer development may provide important insights into the putative anticancer mechanisms of selenium and identify biomarkers that predict the prostate's response to selenium.

The cellular responses induced by selenium compounds are very diverse and are influenced by both the chemical form and the dose of selenium. Selenium appears to exert its cancer protective effects via changes in carcinogen metabolism and DNA adduct formation, regulation of apoptosis and cell cycle arrest, and/or inhibition of angiogenesis (Table 66.5).[281,290,293,297–333] However, these effects are often dependent on the concentration and chemical form of selenium. Different chemical forms of selenium are metabolized differently and exert different biochemical effects. Selenium-enriched foods often contain mixtures of different selenium compounds, and thus can affect multiple pathways to inhibit carcinogenesis.

## ISOTHIOCYANATES

The cancer protective properties of cruciferous vegetables, such as broccoli, watercress, Brussels sprouts, cabbage, and cauliflower, might be attributed to their high content of glucosinolates ($\beta$-thioglucoside $N$-hydroxysulfates), which are also responsible for their pungent odor and taste. The composition of glucosinolates among cruciferous vegetables varies, depending on the species, climate, and other agricultural conditions.[334] At least 120 different glucosinolates have been identified.[335] Physical stress such as chewing or chopping ruptures the plant cell wall and releases the plant-specific enzyme myrosinase, which cleaves the glucose moiety from the glucosinolates producing isothiocyanates. However, glucosinolates that escape the plant myrosinase may also be hydrolyzed in the intestinal tract, as the microflora are known to possess myrosinase activity.[36] Isothiocyanates are then metabolized in vivo through conjugation with glutathione, which is promoted by glutathione transferases (GST).[336,337] As discussed previously, polymorphisms associated with reduced GST activity may result in longer circulating half-lives of isothiocyanates and potentially greater cancer protective effects of cruciferous vegetables.[36]

Numerous studies in preclinical models have documented the cancer-preventive activity of a significant number of isothiocyanates; this protection is not organ-specific and has been seen in lung, esophagus, stomach, colon, mammary gland, bladder, pancreas, and skin.[338–344] Most notable is the inhibition of lung and esophagus cancers induced by tobacco products.[345–348] In addition, the isothiocyanates inhibit growth of human tumor cells in xenograft models of PC-3 prostate,[349] colorectal,[350] Barrett esophageal,[351] and breast[352] cancer. Several epidemiological studies have also shown that dietary consumption of isothiocyanates inversely correlates with the risk of developing lung, breast, and colon cancers.[353–355] This effect can be modified by genetic polymorphisms.

There are multiple mechanisms for the cancer protective effects of isothiocyanates. These include alterations in carcinogen metabolism due to changes in the activities of drug-metabolizing enzymes, induction of cell cycle arrest and apoptosis; inhibition of angiogenesis and metastasis, changes in histone acetylation status, and antioxidant and anti-inflammatory activities (Table 66.6).[356–399] Isothiocyanates are able to induce Phase II enzymes and inhibit Phase I enzymes. Induction of Phase II cellular enzymes is largely mediated by the ARE, which is regulated by the transcription factor Nrf2.

The term epigenetics refers to heritable changes in gene function that occur without a change in DNA sequence. Epigenetic changes have been implicated in the deregulation of gene expression during cancer development. Epigenetic changes can affect both the DNA methylation status and the pattern of histone post-translational modification in cancer cells. Histone acetylation typically results in an open chromatin configuration that facilitates transcription factor access to DNA and gene transcription, but the reverse scenario can silence tumor suppressor genes in cancer cells. The deacetylation of histones is catalyzed by the enzymes histone deacetylases (HDAC). Sulforaphane has been shown to inhibit HDAC activity and concomitant increases in acetylated histones in human embryonic kidney 293 cells, HCT116 human colorectal cancer cells, and various prostate epithelial cells lines (BPH-1, LnCaP, and PC-3).[400] The increased histone acetylation induced by sulforaphane caused the cells to undergo $G_2/M$ cell cycle arrest and increased apoptosis.[400] These effects were associated with increased acetylated histone H4 in the *p21* promoter and increased p21 protein expression.[401] Sulforaphane (443 mg/kg diet) was also found to suppress tumor development in *Apc*[min] mice. This was accompanied by an increase in acetylated histones in the polyps, including acetylated histones specifically associated with the promoter region of the *p21* and *bax* genes.[402] Phenethyl isothiocyanate can inhibit the level and activity of HDACs in prostate cancer cells, induce selective histone acetylation and methylation for chromatin unfolding.[403] Inhibition of HDAC activity following intake of broccoli sprouts was also reported in white blood cells of healthy human subjects.[349] These studies demonstrate that isothiocyanates can inhibit HDAC activity in vivo and suggest that this inhibition might contribute to the cancer protective effects of cruciferous vegetables.

## FLAVONOIDS

Flavonoids are a large group of plant products that have a common structure consisting of two phenolic benzene rings linked to a heterocyclic pyran or pyrone. Over 5000 flavonoids exist and can generally be grouped into one of the following subclasses: flavonols, flavonones, isoflavones, flavins, and anthocyanidins (Figure 66.5), which are present in many different fruits and vegetables (Table 66.7). This section will focus on flavonoids present in fruits and vegetables and will not discuss isoflavones or catechins, such as those in soy and green tea, respectively.

**TABLE 66.5**

**Examples of the Effects of Selenium on Cellular Processes Associated with Carcinogenesis**

| Cellular Process | Compound | Model System(s) | Effect |
|---|---|---|---|
| Carcinogen metabolism | Selenite | HepG2 cells[294] | Decreased CYP1A1 |
| | Selenocysteine Se-conjugates | Purified human enzymes[297] | Inhibited CYP1A1, 2C9, 2C19, and 2D6 activities |
| | Selenocysteine | Primary rat hepatocytes and H35 cells[298] | Increased GST α and B mRNA expression |
| | Selenite | TGF-α /c-Myc transgenic mice[299] | Increased GST α and J, increased CYP2D13, 7B1, and 8B1 expression |
| | Selenite | Rat liver[300] | Decreased GST and UDPGT activities and decreased glutathione-metabolizing enzyme activities |
| | Selenium-enriched garlic | Rat liver and mammary gland[301] | Inhibited GST and UDPGT activities and decreased carcinogen–DNA adducts |
| | Selenite, selenate, and selenomethionine | Rat colon[302] | Inhibited carcinogen–DNA adduct formation |
| DNA repair | Selenite | U2OS cells[303] | Decreased transcription coupled repair after exposure to irradiation |
| | Selenomethionine | Normal human fibroblasts[305] | Induced DNA repair |
| | Selenomethionine | LNCaP cells[306] | Increased oxidative DNA repair after exposure to irradiation or hydrogen peroxide |
| Cell proliferation | Selenomethionine | SNU-1 cells[307] | Low concentrations increased cell proliferation via MAPK phosphorylation and activation, but higher concentrations inhibited cell proliferation |
| | Methylseleninic acid | PC-3 cells[314] | Inhibited cell proliferation, decreased cyclin D1, cyclin D2, c-Myc, and PCNA expression |
| | Methylseleninic acid | PC-3 cells[307] | Inhibited cell proliferation via p53 activation of p21, and downregulated CDK 1 and 2 |
| | Methylselenol | HCT116 cells[308] | Increased G1 and G2 cell cycle arrest via inhibition of ERK1/2 phosphorylation and p38MAPK |
| | Selenite | Muc2/p21 knockout mice[309] | Inhibition of beta-catenin signaling |
| | Methylselenol | HT1080 cells[310] | Inhibition of ERK1/2 activation and c-Myc expression |
| | Methylseleninic acid | DU145 cells[311] | G1 arrest from p21Cip1 induction |
| | Selenite | Melanoma cells[312] | G0/G1 arrest; suppression of CDK2.CDK4 |
| | Methylseleninic acid | EC9706 and KYSE150 esophageal cells[313] | Inhibition of beta-catenin/TCF pathway |
| Apoptosis | Selenite | Murine lymphoma cells[315] | Increased apoptosis via inhibition of cytosol to membrane translocation of PKC and activity |
| | Methylseleninic acid | DU145 and LNCaP cells[316] | Increased apoptosis via ERK1/2 activation of caspases |
| | Selenite | NB4 cells[317] | Increased apoptosis via caspase-3 activation and Bcl-2 cleavage |
| | Methylseleninic acid | LNCaP cells[318] | Increased apoptosis via blocking TRAIL-mediated Bad phosphorylation and increasing cytochrome c release |
| | Selenite | HSC-3 cells[323] | Increased apoptosis via modulation of mitochondrial redox equilibrium and increased caspase-3 and -9 activities |
| | Selenite | HeLa cells[319] | Activation of ROS-mediated mitochondrial pathway |
| | Selenite | SW480 cells[320] | Increased apoptosis via decreased Bcl-xL, increased Bax, Bad, and Bim |
| | Selenium-enriched broccoli sprouts | LNCaP cells[321] | Increased apoptosis via downregulation of the survival Akt/mTOR pathway |
| | Selenite | HCT116 and SW480 cells[322] | Increased apoptosis via activation of AKT |

(continued)

**TABLE 66.5 (continued)**
**Examples of the Effects of Selenium on Cellular Processes Associated with Carcinogenesis**

| Cellular Process | Compound | Model System(s) | Effect |
|---|---|---|---|
| Oxidant/antioxidant balance | Selenium | Human peripheral blood mononuclear cells[324] | Increased superoxide dismutase, glutathione peroxidase, and catalase activities |
| | Selenium-enriched yeast | Human leukocytes[325] | Decreased DNA damage |
| | Diphenylmethyl-selenocyanate | Mouse skin[281] | Inhibited lipid peroxidation and nitric oxide production |
| | Selenite | Rat liver[326] | Increased oxidative DNA damage |
| | Selenite | J774A.1cells[328] | Decreased LPS-induced ROS and NO production |
| | Selenite | Rat liver[327] | Increased antioxidant activity, decreased conjugated dienes and malondialdehyde |
| Inflammation | Selenium | Human serum concentrations[329] | High concentrations decreased 8-iso-prostaglandin F2$\alpha$ and PGFF2$\alpha$ |
| | Selenium | Mice[330] | Deficiency abrogates inflammation-dependent plasma cell tumors |
| Angiogenesis | Selenate | Nude mice[293] | Inhibited angiogenesis of PC-3 tumors |
| | Methylseleninic acid and methylselenocyanate | HUVEC cells[331] | Inhibited MMP-2 and VEGF |
| | Selenium-enriched garlic, selenite and selenium- methylselenocysteine | Rat mammary tumors[331] | Inhibited intratumoral microvessel density |
| | Methylseleninic acid | MDA-MB-231 cells[332] | Inhibited angiopoietin and VEGF protein; decreased microvascular density |
| | Methylselninic acid | Large B-cell lymphoma cell lines[333] | Inhibited HIF-1$\alpha$ expression, VEGF secretion, inhibition of HDAC activity |

It is extremely difficult to estimate the daily human intake of flavonoids, especially because of the lack of standardized methods.[404] It is also quite complex to assess and quantify the bioavailability of flavonoids.[405] In 2004, Neuhouser[406] reviewed the epidemiologic literature from four cohort studies and six case-control studies which had examined associations between flavonoid intake and cancer risk. The data suggest that there is consistent evidence from these studies that flavonoids, especially quercetin, may reduce the risk of lung cancer.[406] A study in Italy compared intake of the six principal classes of flavonoids (i.e., flavones, flavan-3-ols, flavonols, flavones, anthocyanidins, and isoflavones) in breast cancer patients versus controls. After allowance for major confounding factors and energy intake, a reduced risk of breast cancer was found for increasing intake of flavones (OR = 0.81 for the highest versus the lowest quintile, $p < 0.02$ for trend) and flavonols (OR = 0.80, $p < 0.05$ for trend), but not for the other flavonoids.[407] More recent epidemiologic studies confirmed the protective role of a high flavonoids intake against colorectal[408–410] and lung[411] cancers. In fact, a meta-analysis indicated a significant association between the highest flavonoids intake and the reduced risk of developing lung cancer (RR = 0.76, 95% CI = 0.63–0.02).[412] Furthermore, an increase in flavonoids intake of 20 mg/day was associated with a 10% decreased risk of developing lung cancer (RR = 0.90, 95% CI = 0.83–0.97).[412] These observations suggest that various flavonoids are protective against cancer in epidemiological studies.

Studies with animal models of carcinogenesis have suggested that flavonoids have cancer-preventing activity, but results have been mixed. For example, it was reported that 2% dietary quercetin inhibited azoxymethane-induced hyperproliferation, focal dysplasia, and aberrant crypt foci formation in mice.[413,414] Quercetin also reduced tumor incidence by 76% and tumor multiplicity by 48%; however, no inhibitory effects were observed in APC[min] mice treated with quercetin.[415] Although quercetin inhibited local, UVB light-induced immunosuppression in SKH-1 hairless mice, it had no effect on skin tumorigenesis.[416] Quercetin did inhibit N-nitrosodiethylamine-induced lung tumorigenesis in mice when administered during the initiation phase.[417] Moreover, in utero quercetin exposure resulted in significantly enhanced gene expression of cytochrome P4501A1 and 1B1, NADPH quinine oxidoreductase, and UDP-glucuronyltransferase 1A6 in the liver of the fetuses and in their livers and lungs when they were adults, suggesting that in utero exposure to quercetin could affect adult cancer susceptibility.[418] Other dietary flavonoids have also been shown to inhibit tumor growth in experimental animals. For example, naringenin inhibited sarcoma S-180 cells implanted mice.[419] Additionally, cyanidine-3-glycoside suppressed the incidence and multiplicity of colorectal adenomas and carcinomas,[420] as well as small intestinal adenoma number in APC[Min] mice.[421] Both apigenin and naringenin can suppress carcinogen-induced aberrant crypt formation.[422] Apigenin can also inhibit oral cancer in hamsters[423] and prostate cancer in mice.[424] Nobiletin inhibited colon cancer[425] and anthocyanins have been shown to prevent skin cancer in rodents.[426]

**TABLE 66.6**

**Examples of Effects of Isothiocyanates on Cellular Processes Associated with Carcinogenesis**

| Cellular Process | Compound | Model System(s) | Effect |
|---|---|---|---|
| Carcinogen metabolism | PEITC | Rat liver[356] | Inhibited CYP2E1, but increased CYP2B1 activity |
| | SF | Rat lung[357] | Increased CYP1A1, 1A2, 2B1/2, 2C11, and 3A1/2 activities |
| | PEITC | Rat liver, colon, prostate, and blood[358] | Induced glutathione transferase, UDP-glucuronosyltransferase, sulfotransferase, and quinine reductase activities and carcinogen–DNA adduct formation |
| | AITC, iberverin, erucin, iberin, and SF | Rat duodenum, forestomach, and bladder[359] | Induced glutathione transferase and quinine reductase activities |
| | SF | Human jejunum and Caco-2 cells[360] | Induced glutathione transferase A1 and UDP glucuronosyltransferase |
| | SF | LNCaP, MDA PCa, PC-3, and TSU-Pr1 cells[361] | Induced quinone reductase activity |
| | SF | Human hepatocytes and HepG2 cells[362] | Induced glutathione transferase A1 and UDP-glucuronosyltransferase mRNA expression and inhibited PhIP–DNA adduct formation |
| | Japanese Daikon | Rat liver and lung[363] | Induced glutathione transferase activity, increased protein expression of GSTα, GSTμ, and GSTπ |
| Cell proliferation | AITC, BITC, PEITC, PPITC, PBITC, PHITC, SF, TMITC, TBITC | UM-UC3 and T24 cells[364] | Blocked cell-cycle progression at the G2-M or S phases |
| | SF | MCF-7 cells[365] | Blocked cell-cycle progression at G2-M phase via increased cyclin B1, histone H1 phosphorylation, and disrupted polymerization of mitotic microtubules |
| | SF | DU145 cells[366] | Blocked cell-cycle progression at G2-M phase via JNK-mediated signaling |
| | AITC | UM-UC-3 and AY-27 cells[367] | Inhibited cell proliferation, decreased α- and β-tubulin |
| | SF | SCC-13 and US-OS cells[368,371] | Blocked cell-cycle progression at G2-M phase via decreased cyclin B1, cyclin A, CDK1, and CDK2 |
| | PEITC | DU 145 cells[369] | Blocked cell-cycle progression at G2-M phase via increased p53 and WEE, and reduced CDC25C |
| | BEITC | BxPC-3 and PanC-1 cells[370] | Inhibited cell proliferation via decreased phosphorylation of P13K, AKT, PDK1, mTOR, FOXO1, and FOXO3a |
| | BITC | L9881 cells[372] | Blocked cell cycle at G2-M phase via MAPK/AP-1 pathway |
| Apoptosis | AITC, BITC, PEITC, PPITC, PBITC, PHITC, SF, TMITC, TBITC | UM-UC3 and T24 cells[364] | Increased apoptosis via induction of caspases -3, -8, and -9 and poly(ADP-ribose) polymerase |
| | SF | SV-40 transformed mouse embryonic fibroblasts[373,374] | Increased apoptosis via increased Bax and Bak |
| | SF | DAOY cells[375] | Increased apoptosis via induction of caspases -3, -8, and -9 and poly(ADP-ribose) polymerase |
| | PEITC | HepG2 cells[376] | Increased apoptosis via increased Bax translocation |
| | PEITC | T24 and Jurkat T cells[377] | Increased apoptosis via modification of intracellular thiol proteins |
| | BITC | A375.S2 cells[378] | Increased apoptosis through ER stress- and mitochondrial-dependent death receptor-mediated signaling |
| | PEITC | BRI-JMO4 cells[380] | Increased apoptosis through upregulation of Bas, PUMA, and BIM, downregulation of Bcl-xL and Bcl-2 |
| | PEITC | HEp-2 and KB cells[381] | Increased apoptosis through induction of death receptors DR4 and DR5 |
| | SF and PEITC | Human myeloma cells[382] | Induced apoptosis via depletion of mitochondrial membrane potential; cleavage of PARP and caspases-3 and -9. |

*(continued)*

**TABLE 66.6 (continued)**

**Examples of Effects of Isothiocyanates on Cellular Processes Associated with Carcinogenesis**

| Cellular Process | Compound | Model System(s) | Effect |
|---|---|---|---|
| Oxidant/ antioxidant balance | SF | PC-3 and DU145 cells[378] | Increased apoptosis is initiated by generation of ROS |
| | BITC and PEITC | HL-60 cells[384,385] | Inhibits superoxide generation |
| | SF | ARPE-19, HaCaT, and L1210 cells[386] | Decreased cytotoxicity of menadione, *tert*-butyl hydroperoxide, 4-hydroxynonenal, and peroxynitrite |
| | BITC and SF | Hepa 1c1c7 cells[387] | Glutathione depletion |
| | BITC | RL34 cells[388] | Increased ROS |
| Inflammation | SF and PEITC | Raw 264.7 cells[389] | Inhibited LPS-induced secretion of nitric oxide, prostaglandin $E_2$, and TNF-$\alpha$ |
| | AITC and BITC | J744A.1 cells[390] | Inhibited LPS-induced nitric oxide production and TNF-$\alpha$ |
| Differentiation | AITC and BITC | HL-60 cells[391] | Increased differentiation |
| | AITC | DS19 cells[392] | Stimulated histone acetylation which increases differentiation |
| DNA damage | SF and RPS | Mesenchymal stem cells[393] | Low concentrations protected, but high concentrations increased DNA damage induced by peroxides |
| | Mustard | Human WBC[394] | Decreased DNA damage and micronucleus formation induced by hydrogen peroxide or benzo(a)pyrene |
| Angiogenesis | BITC | Panc-1 cells[395] | Reduced phosphorylation of VEGFR2 and expression of HIF-$\alpha$ |
| Metastasis | PEITC | LNCaP, PC-3, DU-45, and PrEC cells[396] | Cleavage and increased transcriptional activity of Notch1 and Notch2, induction of Jagged1 and Jagged2 |
| | BITC | MDA-MB-231 cells[397] | Reduced urokinase-type plasminogen activator activity |
| | SF | Oral carcinoma cells[398] | Decreased MMP-1 and MMP-2 expression |
| Autophagy | PEITC | TRAMP mice[399] | Induction of autophagy via increased p62 and LC3 protein expression |

*Abbreviations:* AITC, allyl isothiocyanate; BITC, benzyl isothiocyanate; PBITC, phenylbutyl isothiocyanate; PEITC, phenylethylisothiocyanate; PHITC, phenylhexylisothiocyanate; PPITC, phenylpropyl isothiocyanate; RPS, raphasatin; SF, sulforaphane; TBITC, thienylbutyl isothiocyanate; TMITC, thienylmethyl isothiocyanate.

**TABLE 66.7**

**Some Common Sources of Flavonoids**

| Flavonoid | Major Food Sources |
|---|---|
| Apigenin (flavone) | Celery, parsley, thyme, sweet red pepper |
| Cyanidin (anthocyanidin) | Cherries, black grapes |
| EGCG (flavonol or catechin) | Apples, plums, cocoa, green tea, black tea |
| Genistein, daidzein (isoflavone) | Soybeans, chickpeas, legumes |
| Hesperetin, narigenin (flavanone) | Oranges, lemons, prunes |
| Quercetin, kaempferol, myricetin (flavonol) | Onions, broccoli, kale, apples, plums, cherries, strawberries, grapes, tea |

Flavonoids have a wide variety of biological effects, many of which are important in cancer prevention. Representative studies demonstrating some of the biological effects of isolated flavonoids on cellular processes associated with carcinogenesis are shown in Table 66.8.[360,427–480] Their cancer prevention activity in animal and cell culture experiments may result from their inhibition of Phase I and induce Phase II carcinogen-metabolizing enzymes, inhibition of cell proliferation, stimulation of apoptosis, inhibition of inflammation, and suppression of angiogenesis. The free radical scavenging ability of flavonoids has been fairly well characterized in experimental systems. Furthermore, some studies have reported the impairment of in vivo angiogenesis by dietary flavonoids.[481]

Epithelial–mesenchymal transition (EMT) is a process that converts an epithelial cell to a mesenchymal cell by promoting the loss of cell–cell adhesion, leading to the cells' release from the surrounding tissues; as a result, these cells acquire the migratory capability to invade. Therefore, EMT can be regarded as in the initiation of metastasis. Recent studies have suggested that flavonoids can inhibit EMT. Quercetin decreased the invasive ability of A431 epidermal cells by increasing EGF-depressed E-cadherin, down-regualting EMT markers and MMP-9, and reversing the EMT transition.[482] Luteolin has similar biological effects in A431 cells.[483]

## ALLIUM COMPOUNDS

The allium genus includes approximately 500 species.[485] Some commonly used allium vegetables include garlic, onion, leeks, chives, and scallions. These are used throughout the

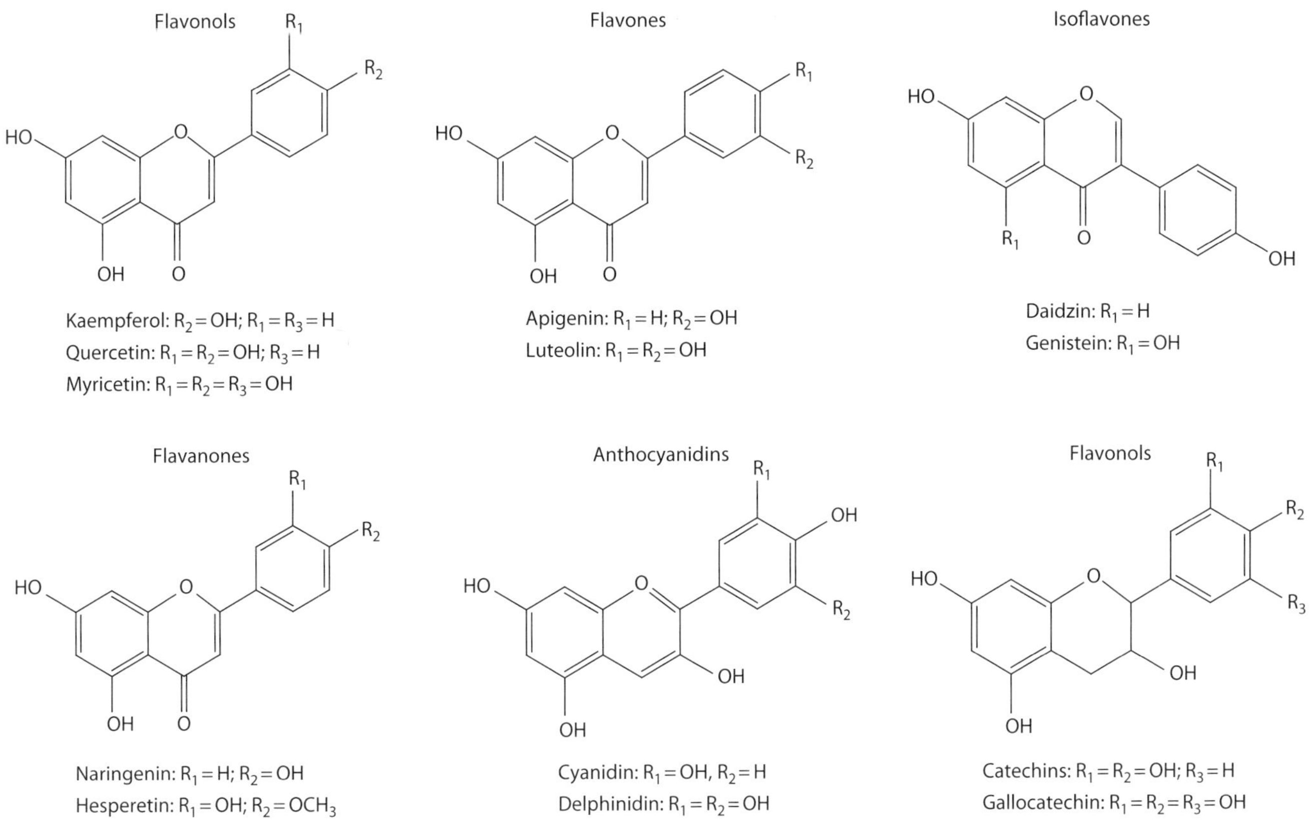

Flavonols

Kaempferol: R₂=OH; R₁=R₃=H
Quercetin: R₁=R₂=OH; R₃=H
Myricetin: R₁=R₂=R₃=OH

Flavones

Apigenin: R₁=H; R₂=OH
Luteolin: R₁=R₂=OH

Isoflavones

Daidzin: R₁=H
Genistein: R₁=OH

Flavanones

Naringenin: R₁=H; R₂=OH
Hesperetin: R₁=OH; R₂=OCH₃

Anthocyanidins

Cyanidin: R₁=OH, R₂=H
Delphinidin: R₁=R₂=OH

Flavonols

Catechins: R₁=R₂=OH; R₃=H
Gallocatechin: R₁=R₂=R₃=OH

**FIGURE 66.5** Structures of flavonoids.

world for their sensory characteristics, as well as their apparent health benefits. Health benefits of allium vegetables are attributed to sulfur-containing compounds, which are generated upon processing (cutting or chewing) (Figure 66.6). Garlic, in particular, has been shown to be protective against cancer.[485] The primary sulfur-containing constituents in garlic are the (γ-glutamyl-S-alk(en)yl-L-cysteines and S-alk(en)yl-L cysteine sulfoxides, including alliin.[293] The characteristic odor of garlic arises from allicin and other oil-soluble sulfur components. Typical volatiles in crushed garlic and garlic oil include diallyl sulfide (DAS), diallyl disulfide (DADS), diallyl trisulfide (DATS), methyl allyl disulfide (MADS), methyl allyl trisulfide (MATS), 2-vinyl-1-dithiin, and 3-vinyl-1,2-dithiin (Figure 66.6).

Epidemiologic findings and preclinical studies with cancer models appear to provide evidence that garlic and related sulfur constituents can suppress cancer risk and alter the biological behavior of tumors. Results from the Iowa Women's Health Study, a prospective cohort study, found that the strongest association among fruits and vegetables for colon cancer risk reduction was for garlic consumption, with an approximate 50% lesser risk of distal colon cancer associated with high consumption.[486] Fleisschauer and Arab summarized the epidemiologic literature related to garlic and cancer risk.[487] Nineteen studies reported relative risk estimates for garlic consumption and cancer incidence. Site-specific case-control studies of stomach and colorectal cancer suggested the protective effect of high intake of raw and/or cooked material. Cohort

studies confirmed this inverse association with colorectal cancer. However, the reliability of epidemiologic results may be limited since total vegetable consumption or other known risk factors were generally not considered.[485] In a double-blind, randomized study of Japanese patients with colorectal adenomas, a higher dose of aged garlic extract was shown to reduce the risk of new colorectal adenomas compared to a lower dose garlic extract.[488] Meta-analysis of case-control data in the World Cancer Research Fund report revealed a 20% decreased risk of cancer per 50 g allium vegetables/day and a 59% decreased risk per serving of garlic/day.[25]

Preclinical studies provide some of the strongest evidence that garlic and/or its related organosulfur compounds suppress cancer risk and alter the behavior of tumors. Garlic and its associated sulfur compounds have been found to inhibit mammary, colon, skin, uterine, esophagus, lung, renal, forestomach, and liver cancer incidence in animal models.[489–506] The protection of tumor incidence by garlic may arise from several mechanisms including altered formation and bioactivation of carcinogens, enhanced DNA repair, reduced cell proliferation, induction of apoptosis, inhibition of inflammation, and suppression of angiogenesis (Table 66.9).[507–559] It is likely that many of these processes are modified simultaneously. Furthermore, cancer progression is probably also highly dependent on epigenetic changes. There is evidence that some garlic constituents can influence histone homeostasis.[388] For example, Duesne et al. reported that DADS

**TABLE 66.8**

**Examples of Effects of Flavonoids on Cellular Processes Associated with Carcinogenesis**

| Cellular Process | Compound | Model System(s) | Effect |
|---|---|---|---|
| Carcinogen metabolism | Quercetin | Rat liver[427] | Induces CYP2B |
| | Quercetin | Purified enzyme[428] | Inhibits CYP1A1 and 1A2 activities |
| | Quercetin | Human liver,[429,430] human duodenum,[429,431] rat liver[432] | Inhibits sulfotransferase activity |
| | Quercetin | Rat liver,[433] rat intestine,[433] human jejunum,[360] Caco-2 cells[434] | Inhibits glucuronosyltransferase activity |
| | Quercetin | HL-60 cells[435] | Inhibits N-acetyltransferase activity |
| | Quercetin | HepG2 cells,[366] human lymphocytes[436] | Inhibits carcinogen–DNA adduct formation |
| | Kaempferol | MCF-7 cells[437] | Inhibit CYP1A1 transcription |
| | Kaempferol | Human liver and duodenum[438] | Inhibits sulfotransferase activity |
| | Naringenin, naringin, rutin | *Salmonella typhimurium* TA98[439] | Inhibits mutagenicity |
| Cell proliferation | Quercetin | PC-3 cells[440] | Cell-cycle arrest via block at G2/M phase, increased p21 expression |
| | Quercetin | HK1 and CNE2 nasopharyngeal cells[441] | Increased Rb gene expression resulting in block at G2/M or G0/G1 phases |
| | Quercetin | PC-3 and LnCap cells[442] | Inhibited cell proliferation and DNA synthesis via decreased cyclin D1, ErbB-2, and ErbB-3 expression |
| | Quercetin | T98G and U87 cells[443] | Inhibited Rb phosphorylation and increased cyclin D1 |
| | Quercetin | 253J cells[444] | Increased in calcium-activated potassium channels |
| | Quercetin and kaempferol | HuTu-80, Caco-2, and PMC42 cells[445] | Inhibited cell proliferation, decreased PCNA and Ki67 expression |
| | Apigenin | SW480 cells[446] | Cell-cycle arrest via block at G2/M phase |
| | Apigenin | Human multiple myeloma cells[447] | Inhibited CK2 kinase activity, decreased phosphorylation of Cdc37 |
| Apoptosis | Quercetin | PC-3,[448] HT-29,[449] BGC-823,[450] A-549,[457] and DLD-1[453] cells | Increased apoptosis via decreased Bcl-2 and Bcl-x and increased Bax and caspase-3 |
| | Quercetin | A549 cells[454] | Increased apoptosis via inactivation of Akt-1 and activation of MEK-ERK pathway |
| | Quercetin | HCT-116 cells[455] | Increased apoptosis via Inhibition of AMPK activity |
| | Quercetin and kaempferol | Prostate and breast cancer cells[456] | Increased apoptosis associated with ability to inhibit fatty acid synthase |
| | Kaempferol | U-2 OS cells[457] | Increased apoptosis via ER stress, decreased mitochondrial membrane potential |
| | Kaempferol | A2780 and OVCAR cells[458] | Increased apoptosis via increased p53, Bad, and Bax |
| | Naringenin | THP-1,[459] C6,[460] and DR-5[461] cells | Increased apoptosis via decreased Bcl-2 and Bcl-x and increased Bax and caspase-3 |
| | Apigenin | H460 cells[462] | Increased apoptosis via decreased Bid, Bcl-2, caspase-8; increased Bax, caspase-3, AIF, cytochrome c, and GADD 153 |
| | Apigenin | PC-3 and 22Rv1 cells[463] | Decreased HADC activity, increased histone acetylation, increased p21 and Bax |
| Inflammation | Quercetin and kaempferol | Human umbilical cord blood-derived cultured mast cells[465] | Inhibited release of IL-6, IL-8, and TNF-α |
| | Quercetin | Bone marrow-derived macrophages[465] | Inhibited cytokines and iNOS through inhibition of NF-κ B |
| | Naringenin, fisetin | RAW264.7 macrophages, human peripheral blood mononuclear cells[466] | Inhibited nitric oxide, TNF-α, and IL-2 production |
| | Apigenin, kaempferol | J744A.2 macrophages[467] | Inhibited TNF-α and IL-1β gene expression |
| | Quercetin, myricetin, apigenin | Peritoneal ecudate murine macrophages[468] | Reduced lipopolysaccharide-induced TNF-α production |

## TABLE 66.8 (continued)
## Examples of Effects of Flavonoids on Cellular Processes Associated with Carcinogenesis

| Cellular Process | Compound | Model System(s) | Effect |
|---|---|---|---|
| Oxidant/ antioxidant balance | Quercetin | Human lymphocytes,[437] Caco-2,[469] and V79 cells[470] | Protected against hydrogen peroxide-induced DNA damage |
| | Quercetin and kaempferol | Sperm and human lymphocytes[471] | Reduced DNA damage produced by estrogenic compounds |
| | Quercetin, naringin, and rutin | C3H10T1/2 cells[472] | Inhibited UVA-induced DNA strand breaks |
| | Quercetin | Human neutrophils[473] | Inhibited superoxide generation induced by arachidonic acid |
| | Naringin | HepG2 cells[474] | Inhibited iron-induced DNA oxidation, increased antioxidant enzymes |
| Angiogenesis | Quercetin | Human blood[475] | Inhibited TIMP-1 gene transcription and plasma protein concentrations |
| | Quercetin | Severe combined immune deficient mice inoculated with CWR22 prostate cells[476] | Reduced VEGF121 and VEGF165 mRNA and microvessel density |
| | Tangeretin, rutin | B16F10 cells[477] | Decreased number of metastatic nodules |
| | Kaempferol | OVCAR-3 and A270 cells[478,479] | Inhibited VEGF and HIF-1α expression |
| | Apigenin | CD-18 and S2 cells[480] | Inhibited VEGF and HIF-1α expression |

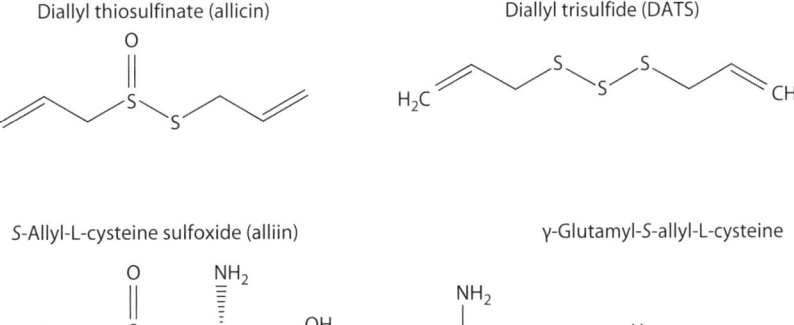

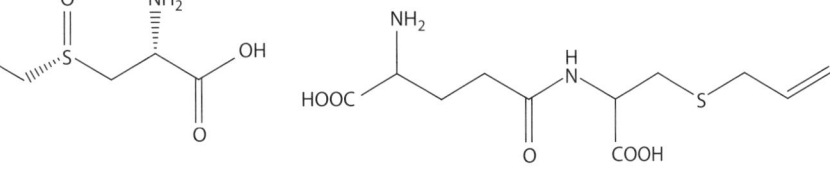

**FIGURE 66.6** Structures of allium compounds.

**TABLE 66.9**

**Examples of Effects of Allium Compounds on Cellular Processes Associated with Carcinogenesis**

| Cellular Process | Compound | Model Systems(s) | Effect |
|---|---|---|---|
| Carcinogen metabolism | Garlic | Human[507] | Blocked the enhanced urinary excretion of nitrosoproline |
| | DADS and DAS | Rat esophageal microsomes, purified rat, and human enzymes[508] | Inhibited rat and human CYP2E1 and rat CYP2A3 activity |
| | Garlic powder | Rat liver[509] | Inhibited CYP2E1 activity |
| | Garlic oil, DADS, DAS, and DATS | Rat liver[510] | Inhibited CYP2E1 activity, but increased CYP1A1, CYP2B1, and CYP3A1 activities |
| | Garlic powder | Rat liver[511,512] | Increased ethoxyresorufin deethylase, GST, and UDP-glucuronosyltransferase activities |
| | DADS, DAS, and DATS | Rat tissues[513] | Increased quinine reductase and glutathione transferase activities |
| | DADS | CE81T/VGH cells[514] | Inhibited N-acetyltransferase activity |
| | DADS, DAS, and DATS | HepG2 cells[515] | Induced Phase II gene expression through activation of ARE and Nrf2 protein accumulation |
| | SAC and DADS | Rat mammary gland[507] | Inhibited carcinogen–DNA adduct formation |
| | Crushed garlic | Rat liver[516] | Inhibited carcinogen–DNA adduct formation |
| | DAS | Rat liver[517] | Inhibited carcinogen–DNA adduct formation |
| DNA repair | DADS and SAC | Salmonella TA100[518] | Decreased mutagenicity of N-nitromorpholine |
| | Garlic extract | Human fibroblasts[519] | Stimulated DNA repair |
| Cell proliferation | DADS | Human A549 lung cells[520] and PC-3 cells[521] | Induced cell-cycle arrest at G2/M phase |
| | DATS | PC-3 and DU145 cells[522,523] | Induced cell-cycle arrest at G2/M phase by inhibition of CDK1 and hyperphosphorylation of Cdc25C |
| | DADS, DAS, and DATS | J5 cells[524] | Induced cell-cycle arrest at G2/M phase by inhibiting CDK7 and increasing cyclin B1 |
| | DADS | HCT-15 cells[525] | Induced cell-cycle arrest at G2/M phase by inhibiting cdc2 kinase activation and increased cyclin B1 |
| Apoptosis | DADS | T24[526] and B16F-10[527] cells | Apoptosis induced via caspase-3 activity |
| | Allicin | SiHA, L929 and SW480 cells[528] SGC-7901[529] | Apoptosis induced via caspases-3, -8, and -9 activation and cleavage of poly(ADP-ribose) polymerase |
| | SAMC and DADS | SW480 cells[530] | Apoptosis induced via caspase-3 activation and cleavage of poly (ADP-ribose) polymerase |
| | SAMC | SW480 and NIH3T3 cells[531] | Apoptosis induced via caspase-3 activation and JNK1 signaling pathway |
| | Water-soluble extract | MDA-MB-435 cells[532] | Apoptosis induced via increased translocation of BimEL to mitochondria |
| | Garlic | Hamster buccal pouch[533] | Apoptosis induced by downregulation of Bcl-2 and upregulation of Bax, Bim, p53, and caspases-3 and -8 |
| | DATS | PC-3 and DU145 cells[534,535] | Apoptosis induced via inactivation of Akt signaling |
| | Allicin | Human gastric epithelial cells[536] | Apoptosis induced via mitochondrial release of AIF and PKA |
| | DATS | DU145 and LNCaP cells[537] | Apoptosis induced by suppression of STAT3 phosphorylation |
| | DAS | HeLa cells[538] | Apoptosis induced through induction of p53, caspases, and mitochondria-dependent pathways |
| | Allicin | El-4 T-lymphocytes[539] | Apoptosis induced by activation of caspase-3, -12, and cytochrome c; increased ration of Bax/Bcl-2 |
| | SAC | PC-3 cells[540] | Apoptosis induced by increased caspase-8 and Bax, decreased Bcl-2 |
| | DADS | AGS cells[541] | Apoptosis induced by increased caspase-3, Fas, Bax, and decreased Bcl-2 |
| | Allicin | U87MG cells[542] | Apoptosis induced by activation of MAPK/ERK signaling |
| | DATS | A549 cells[543] | Apoptosis induced by activation of caspase-3, -8, and -9. |

**TABLE 66.9 (continued)**

**Examples of Effects of Allium Compounds on Cellular Processes Associated with Carcinogenesis**

| Cellular Process | Compound | Model Systems(s) | Effect |
|---|---|---|---|
| Inflammation | Allicin | HT-29 and Caco-2 cells[544] | Inhibited spontaneous and TNF-α-induced secretion of IL-1, IL-8, IP-10, and MIG |
| | Aqueous garlic extract | Rat thymocytes and splenocytes[545] | Decreased IL-2 production |
| | Aged garlic extract | Human peripheral blood lymphocytes[546] | Increased cytotoxicity against both NK-sensitive and resistant M14 cell lines |
| | Garlic extract | Balb/c mice[547] | Increased NK activity |
| | Fresh garlic and tablet | Balb/c mice[548] | Augmented delayed-type hypersensitivity |
| | AMS, DADS, and DAS | RAW 264.7 cells[549,550] | DADS inhibited iNOS, decreased TNF-α, IL-10, and increased IL-1 and IL-6. AMS increased IL-10. DAS inhibited COX-2 |
| | Allicin and ajoene | Raw 264.7 cells[551] | Decreased iNOS |
| | DAS | HEK 293T cells[552] | Inhibited COX-2 |
| | Aqueous garlic suspension | Sprague–Dawley rat colon[553] | Inhibited COX-2 expression |
| Oxidant/antioxidant balance | Aqueous garlic extract | Balb/c mouse liver, kidney, lung, and brain[554] | Ameliorated oxidative organ injury due to naphthalene toxicity |
| | SAMC | Rat kidney[555] | Scavenged hydroxyl radicals and singlet oxygen, ameliorated oxidative and nitrosative stress |
| | Aqueous garlic extract | Wistar rats liver and blood[556] | Decreased lipid peroxidation |
| Angiogenesis | DAS | Swiss albino mice injected with ehrlich ascites cells[557] | Decreased angiogenesis |
| Metastasis | DADS | AGS cells[558] | Decreased metastasis through inhibition of MMP-2 and -9; increased TIM-1 and -2. |
| | DAS, DADS, and DATS | Colo 205 cells[559] | Inhibition of metastasis through inhibition of MMP-2, -7, and -9, decreased expression of P13K, Ras, MEKK3, ERK1/2, and JNK1/2 |

*Abbreviations:* AMS, allyl methyl sulfide; DADS, diallyl disulfide; DAS, diallyl sulfide; DATS, diallyl trisulfide; SAC, *S*-allyl cysteine; SAMC, *S*-allylmercaptocysteine.

effectively increased histone H3 acetylation in cultured Caco-2 and HT-29 cells by reducing histone deacetylase activity.[560] This change in hyperacetylation was accompanied by an increase in p21(waf1/cip1) expression, demonstrating that epigenetic events can influence subsequent gene expression patterns and lead to the accumulation of cells in the G2 phase of the cell cycle.[560]

## MONOTERPENES

Monoterpenes are natural plant products found in the essential oils of many commonly consumed fruits and vegetables and are largely responsible for the pleasant fragrances of the fruits and plants. Limonene, the simplest monocyclic monoterpene, is the major constituent of several citrus oils (orange, lemon, lime, and grapefruit). Limonene and perillyl alcohol, a hydroxylated limonene analog, have demonstrated cancer protective and chemotherapeutic activity against mammary, skin, lung, pancreas, kidney, esophagus, liver, and colon tumors in rodent models,[561–571] but did not protect against carcinogen and testosterone-induced prostate

tumors.[573] They are capable of increasing tumor latency, decreasing tumor multiplicity, and causing regression of mammary carcinomas.[573,574] Limonene also increased the survival of lymphoma-bearing mice.[575]

One epidemiolical study reported that people without epithelial cell carcinomas consumed significantly more citrus peel, rich in limonene, than those having epithelial cell carcinomas.[576] Moreover, a dose–response relationship was observed between higher citrus peel in the diet and reduced risk of skin cancer.[576] Preliminary results of Phase I and Phase II clinical trials of limonene and perillyl alcohol demonstrate that these agents are well tolerated in cancer patients and may be useful as potential chemotherapeutic agents.[577–581] Results of larger human clinical trials are necessary to clarify whether or not monoterpenes are effective against cancer in humans.

Several mechanisms appear to account for the cancer protective effects of monoterpenes in preclinical models (Table 66.10).[575,581–591] These include modulation of carcinogen metabolism, inhibition of tumor cell proliferation, increased apoptosis, and induction of tumor cell differentiation.

**TABLE 66.10**

**Examples of Effects of Monoterpenes on Cellular Processes Associated with Carcinogenesis**

| Cellular Process | Compound | Model System(s) | Effect |
|---|---|---|---|
| Carcinogen metabolism | Limonene | Liver, spleen, kidney, and lung of rats[581] | Increased CYP2B and 2C and epoxide hydrolase activities, decreased carcinogen–DNA adduct formation |
| | Limonene | Liver and intestine of rats[582] | Increased UDP-glucuronosyltransferase activity |
| Cell proliferation | Perillyl alcohol | KPL-1, MCF-7, MKL-F, and MDA-MB-231 cells[583] | Induced growth arrest at G1 phase via decreased cyclin D1 and E and increased p21 |
| | Perillyl alcohol | HTB-43, SCC-25, and BroTo cells[584] | Induced cell-cycle arrest |
| Apoptosis | Perillyl alcohol | Diethylnitrosamine-induced rat liver tumors[585] | Increased apoptosis |
| | Citral | HL-60, BS24-1, RL-12, U937, 293, and MCF-7 cells[586] | Increased apoptosis via increased caspase-3 activity |
| | Perillyl alcohol | U87 and A172 cells and primary culture derived from human gliobastoma[587] | Increased apoptosis |
| | Perillyl alcohol | H322 and H838 cells[588] | Increased apoptosis via increased caspase-3 activity and PARP cleavage |
| | Limonene | K562 and HL60 cells[575] | Increased apoptosis via increased caspase-9, cleaved caspase-3, Bax, and cytochrome c release |
| | Limonene | Lymphoma cells[589] | Increased apoptosis by production of $H_2O_2$ and ERK pathway activation |
| Inflammation | Limonene | Balb/c mice with lymphoma[590] | Delayed hypersensitivity reaction to dinitroflourobenzene, phagocytosis, and microbicidal activity. Increased nitric oxide production by macrophages |
| Angiogenesis | Perillyl alcohol | Endothelial cells[591] | Inhibited angiogenesis by decreased VEGF and increased angiopoietin 2 expression |
| | Limonene | Gastric cancer cells in nude mice[566] | Inhibited angiogenesis and metastasis by decreased VEGF expression |

## SUMMARY

The research highlighted here is only a small part of the large body of striking evidence linking fruit and vegetable intake with cancer risk and tumor behavior. Variation in response among individuals likely depends on individual genetic polymorphisms and/or interactions among dietary components that influence absorption, metabolism, or site of action. Evidence suggests that the cancer protective effects of fruits and vegetables may result from additive or synergistic effects of various vitamins, minerals, phenolic phytochemicals, isothiocyanates, and allium compounds rather than from the effect of a single ingredient. Thus, the diet as a whole may play a more important role than individual components. A better understanding of physiologically important interactions is needed. Furthermore, the response is complicated since multiple steps in the cancer process can be modified simultaneously, including sites such as drug metabolism, DNA repair, cell proliferation, apoptosis, inflammation, differentiation, and angiogenesis. Since current evidence suggests that bioactive food components can typically influence more than one process, a better understanding of how the response relates to exposures and which process is most involved in bringing about a change in tumor incidence and/or tumor behavior is essential. Additional research is needed to determine the critical intake, duration, and when it should be provided to optimize the desired physiological response. Further research is also needed on the molecular targets for bioactive components and whether genetic and epigenetic events dictate the direction and magnitude of the response.

## REFERENCES

1. Kris-Etherton, P.M. et al. *Am. J. Med.*, 113, 71s, 2002.
2. Keck, A.S. and Finley, J.W. *Integr. Cancer Ther.*, 3, 5, 2004.
3. Demark-Wahnefried, W. and Rock, C.L. *Semin. Oncol.*, 30, 789, 2003.
4. Sato, Y. et al. *Public Health Nutr.*, 8, 309, 2004.
5. Kojima, M. et al. *Nutr. Cancer*, 50, 23, 2004.
6. McCullough, M.L. et al. *Cancer Causes Control*, 14, 959, 2003.
7. Voorrips, L.E. et al. *Am. J. Epidemiol.*, 152, 1081, 2000.
8. Bingham, S.A. et al. *Cancer Epidemiol. Biomark. Prev.*, 14, 1552, 2005.
9. Wark, P.A. et al. *Cancer Epidemiol. Biomark. Prev.*, 14, 1619, 2005.
10. Park, Y. et al. *Am. J. Epidemiol*, 166, 170, 2007.
11. Nomura, A.M.Y. et al. *Am. J. Clin. Nutr.*, 88, 730, 2008.
12. George, S.M. et al. *Am. J. Clin. Nutr.*, 89, 347, 2009.
13. van Duijnhoven, F.J.B. *Am. J. Clin. Nutr.*, 89, 1441, 2009.
14. Wang, J. et al. *Int. J. Cancer*, 118, 991, 2006.
15. Satia-Abouta, J. et al. *Int. J. Cancer*, 109, 728, 2004.
16. Yeh, C.C. et al. *J. Formos. Med. Assoc.*, 102, 305, 2003.

17. Diergaarde, B. et al. *Carcinogenesis*, 24, 283, 2003.
18. Chiu, B.C.-H. et al. *Cancer Epidemiol. Biomark. Prev.*, 12, 210, 2003.
19. Deneo-Pellegrini, H. et al. *Eur. J. Cancer Prev.*, 11, 369, 2002.
20. Levi, F. et al. *Br. J. Cancer*, 79, 1283, 1999.
21. Witte, J.S. et al. *Am. J. Epidemiol.*, 144, 1015, 1996.
22. Kampman, E. et al. *Cancer Causes Control*, 6, 225, 1995.
23. Annema, N. et al. *J. Am. Diet. Assoc.*, 111, 1479, 2011.
24. Aune, D. et al. *Gastroenterology*, 141, 106, 2011.
25. World Cancer Research Fund/American Institute for Cancer Research. *Food, Nutrition, Physical Activity and the Prevention of Cancer: A Global Perspective*. Washington, DC, 2007.
26. Michaud, D.S. et al. *Br. J. Cancer*, 87, 960, 2002.
27. Steinmetz, K.A. and Potter, J.D. *J. Am. Diet. Assoc.*, 96, 1027, 1996.
28. Milner, J.A. *J. Nutr.*, 133, 3820s, 2003.
29. Davis, C.D. and Milner, J.A. *Mutat. Res.*, 551, 51, 2004.
30. Mathew, A. et al. *Int. J. Cancer*, 108, 287, 2004.
31. Davis, C.D. and Milner, J.A. *Nutritional Health: Strategies for Disease Prevention*, 2nd edn., Humana Press Inc., Totowa, NJ, 2005, p. 151.
32. Zhong, S. et al. *Carcinogenesis*, 12, 1533, 1991.
33. Pemble, S.E. et al. *Biochem. J.*, 300, 271, 1994.
34. Seow, A. et al. *Mutat. Res.*, 592, 58, 2005.
35. Hayes, J.D., Flanagan, J.U., and Jowsey, I.R. *Ann. Res. Pharmacol. Toxicol.*, 45, 51, 2005.
36. Lampe, J.W. and Peterson, S. *J. Nutr.*, 132, 2991, 2002.
37. Gasper, A.V. et al. *Am. J. Clin. Nutr.*, 82, 1283, 2005.
38. Wang, L.I. et al. *Cancer Causes Control*, 15, 977, 2004.
39. Zhao, B. et al. *Cancer Epidemiol. Biomark. Prev.*, 10, 1063, 2001.
40. Joseph, M.A. et al. *Nutr. Cancer*, 50, 206, 2004.
41. Seow, A. et al. *Carcinogenesis*, 23, 2055, 2002.
42. Yeh, C.-C. et al. *World J. Gastronenterol.*, 11, 1473, 2005.
43. Gervasini, G. et al. *Nutr. Cancer*, 62, 750, 2010.
44. Moy, K.A. et al. *Int. J. Cancer*, 125, 2652, 2009.
45. Yang, G. et al. *Am. J. Clin. Nutr.*, 91, 704, 2010.
46. Carpenter, C.L., Yu, M.C., and London, S.J. *Nutr. Cancer*, 61, 492, 2009.
47. Lee, S.-A. et al. *Exp. Molec. Med.*, 36, 116, 2004.
48. Shen, J. et al. *Cancer Epidemiol. Biomark. Prev.*, 14, 336, 2005.
49. Shen, J. et al. *Carcinogenesis*, 26, 2131, 2005.
50. Boccia, S. et al. *Biomarkers*, 12, 635, 2007.
51. Ahn, J. et al. *Cancer Res.*, 64, 7634, 2004.
52. Lin, H.J. et al. *Cancer Epidemiol. Biomark. Prev.*, 7, 647, 1998.
53. Slattery, M.L. et al. *Cancer Causes Control*, 11, 1, 2000.
54. Karen-Ng, L.P. *Asian Pac. J. Cancer Prev.*, 12, 1161, 2011.
55. Molloy, A.M. *World Rev. Nutr. Diet*, 93, 153, 2004.
56. Bailey, L.B. and Gregory, J.F. *J. Nutr.*, 129, 919, 1999.
57. Chen, J., Giovannucci, E.L., and Hunter, D.J. *J. Nutr.*, 129, 560s, 1999.
58. Frost, P. et al. *Nat. Genet.*, 10, 111, 1995.
59. Margate, T. et al. *Int. J. Epidemiol.*, 32, 64, 2003.
60. Le Marchand, L. et al. *Cancer Epidemiol. Biomarkers Prev.*, 14, 1198, 2005.
61. Jiang, Q. et al. *Cancer Detect. Prev.*, 29, 146, 2005.
62. Esteller, M. et al. *Carcinogenesis*, 12, 2307, 1997.
63. Gershoni-Baruch, R. et al. *Eur. J. Cancer*, 18, 2313, 2000.
64. Campbell, I.G. et al. *Breast Cancer Res.*, R14, 1, 2002.
65. Chen, J. et al. *Cancer Res.*, 65, 1606, 2005.
66. Lee, J.S. and Surh, Y.J. *Cancer Lett.*, 224, 171, 2005.
67. Cooke, M.S. et al. *Mutat. Res.*, 574, 58, 2005.
68. Sancar, A. et al. *Ann. Rev. Biochem.*, 73, 39, 2004.
69. Hanahan, D. and Weinburg, R.A. *Cell*, 100, 57, 2000.
70. Meeran, S.M. and Katiyar, S.K. *Frontiers Biosci.*, 13, 2191, 2008.
71. Mailand, N. et al. *Science*, 288, 1425, 2000.
72. Sun, S.Y., Hail, N., and Lotan, R. *J. Natl. Cancer Inst.*, 96, 662, 2004.
73. Rodriguez, M. and Schaper, J. *J. Mol. Cell Cardiol.*, 38, 15, 2005.
74. Krammer, P.H. *Nature*, 407, 789, 2000.
75. Chen, C. and Kong, A.-N.T. *TRENDS Pharmacol. Sci.*, 26, 318, 2005.
76. Li, P. et al. *Cell*, 91, 479, 1997.
77. Thornberry, N.A. and Lazebnki, Y. *Science*, 281, 1312, 1998.
78. Hofseth, L.J. and Ying, L. *Biochim. Biophys. Acta*, 1765, 74, 2006.
79. Hussain, S.P., Hofseth, L.J., and Harris, C.C. *Nat. Rev. Cancer*, 3, 276, 2003.
80. Storz, P. *Front. Biosci.*, 10, 1881, 2005.
81. Bartsch, H. *Mut. Res. Rev. Genet. Toxicol.*, 340, 67, 1996.
82. Jackson, A.L. and Loeb, L.A. *Mutat. Res.*, 477, 7, 2001.
83. Valko, M. et al. *Molec. Cell. Biochem.*, 266, 37, 2004.
84. Berger, M.M. *Clin. Nutr.*, 24, 172, 2005.
85. Presta, M. et al. *Cytokine Growth Factor Rev.*, 16, 159, 2005.
86. Albini, A., Tosetti, F., Benelli, R., Noonan, D.M. *Cancer Res.*, 65, 10637, 2005.
87. Pfeffer, U. et al. *Int. J. Biol. Markers*, 18, 70, 2003.
88. Cockett, M.I. et al. *Biochem. Soc. Symp.*, 63, 295, 1998.
89. Ii, M. et al. *Exp. Biol. Med.*, 31, 20, 2006.
90. Bisacchi, D. et al. *Cancer Detect. Prev.*, 27, 229, 2008.
91. Westermarck, J. and Kahari, V.M. *FASEB J.*, 13, 781, 1999.
92. Singh, R.P. and Agarwal, R. *Curr. Cancer Drug Targets*, 7, 475, 2007.
93. Bhat, T.A. and Singh, R.P. *Food Chem. Toxicol.*, 46, 1334, 2008.
94. Dulak, J. *J. Physiol. Pharmacol.*, 56, 51, 2005.
95. Okuno, M. et al. *Curr. Cancer Drug Targets*, 4, 285, 2004.
96. Khera, P. and Koo, J.Y. *J. Drugs Dermatol.*, 4, 432, 2005.
97. Zhang, X., Dai, B., Zhang, B., and Wang, Z. *Gynecol. Oncol.*, 124, 366, 2012.
98. Fulan, H. et al. *Cancer Causes Control*, 22, 1383, 2011.
99. Mondul, A.M. et al. *Am. J. Epidemiol.*, 173, 813, 2011.
100. Park, E.Y., Pinali, D., Lindley, K., and Lane, M.A. *Nutr. Cancer*, 64, 372, 2012.
101. Yang, Y. et al. *Biomed. Environ. Sci.*, 9, 386, 1996.
102. Ziegler, R.G., Mayne, S.T., and Swanson, C.A. *Cancer Causes Control*, 7, 157, 1996.
103. Tapiero, H., Townsend, D.M., and Tew, K.D. *Biomed. Pharmacother.*, 58, 100, 2004.
104. Cooper, D.A., Eldridge, A.L., and Peters, I.C. *Nutr. Rev.*, 57, 133, 1999.
105. Rock, C.L. et al. *J. Clin. Oncol.*, 23, 6631, 2005.
106. Tamimi, R.M. et al. *Am. J. Epidemiol.*, 161, 153, 2005.
107. Steck-Scott, S. et al. *Int. J. Cancer*, 112, 295, 2004.
108. Zhang, X., et al. *Am. J. Clin. Nutr.*, 95, 713, 2012.
109. Kabat, G.C. et al., *Eur. J. Clin. Nutr.*, 66, 549, 2012.
110. Hu, F. et al. *Breast Cancer Res. Treat.*, 131, 239, 2012.
111. Krinsky, N.I. *Ann. Rev. Nutr.*, 13, 561, 1993.
112. Heinonen, O.P. et al. *N. Engl. J. Med.*, 330, 1029, 1994.
113. Hennekens, C.H. et al. *N. Engl. J. Med.*, 334, 1145, 1996.
114. Omenn, O.S. et al. *N. Engl. J. Med.*, 334, 1150, 1996.
115. Lee, I.M. et al. *J. Natl. Cancer Inst.*, 91, 2102, 1999.

116. Mannisto, S. et al. *Canc. Epidemiol. Biomarkers Prev.*, 13, 40, 2004.
117. Touvier, M. et al. *J. Natl. Cancer Inst.*, 97, 1338, 2005.
118. Wright, M.E. et al. *Cancer Prev. Res.*, 3, 745, 2010.
119. Bendich, A. *J. Nutr.*, 134, 225s, 2004.
120. Karppi, J., Kurl, S., Laukkanen, J.A., and Kauhanen, J. *Nutr. Cancer*, 64, 367, 2012.
121. Raju, J. et al. *Int. J. Cancer*, 113, 798, 2005.
122. Palozza, P. *Biochim. Biophys. Acta*, 1740, 215, 2005.
123. Hosotani, K. et al. *Biofactors*, 21, 241, 2004.
124. Palozza, P. et al. *J. Nutr.*, 135, 129, 2005.
125. Siems, W. et al. *J. Nutr. Biochem.*, 16, 385, 2005.
126. Palozza, P. et al. *Carcinogenesis*, 25, 1315, 2004.
127. Palozza, P. et al. *Arch. Biochem. Biophys.*, 430, 104, 2004.
128. Dulinska, J. et al. *Biochem. Biophys. Acta*, 1740, 189, 2005.
129. Wang, X.D. et al. *J. Natl. Cancer Inst.*, 91, 60, 1999.
130. Liu, C. et al. *Carcinogenesis*, 21, 2245, 2000.
131. Nkondjock, A. et al. *J. Nutr.*, 135, 592, 2005.
132. Davis, C.D. et al. *J. Nutr.*, 135, 2014s, 2005.
133. Giovannucci, E. *J. Nutr.*, 135, 2030s, 2005.
134. Almushatat, A.S. et al. *Int. J. Cancer*, 118, 1051, 2006.
135. Ito, Y. et al. *Asian Pac. J. Cancer Prev.*, 6, 10, 2005.
136. Heber, D. and Lu, Q.Y. *Exp. Biol. Med.*, 227, 920, 2002.
137. Hwang, E.S. and Bowen, P.E. *Biofactors*, 23, 75, 2005.
138. Hwang, E.S. and Bowen, P.E. *Biofactors*, 23, 97, 2005.
139. Palozza, P. et al. *Apoptosis*, 10, 1445, 2005.
140. Livny, O. et al. *J. Nutr.*, 132, 3754, 2002.
141. Forbes, K., Gillette, K., and Sehgal, I. *Exp. Biol. Med.*, 228, 967, 2003.
142. Ben-Dor, A. et al. *Mol. Cancer Ther.*, 4, 177, 2005.
143. Palozza, P. et al. *Curr. Cancer Drug Targets*, 12, 640, 2012.
144. Yang, C.M., Yen, Y.T., Huang, C.S., and Hu, M.L. *Mol. Nutr. Food Res.*, 55, 606, 2011.
145. Davis, C.D. *J. Nutr.*, 135, 2074s, 2005.
146. Li, K.W. et al. *Am. J. Clin. Nutr.*, 78, 1074, 2003.
147. Henssen, D.E., Block, G., and Levine, M. *J. Natl. Cancer Inst.*, 83, 547, 1991.
148. Carr, A. and Frei, B. *FASEB J.*, 13, 1007, 1999.
149. Estrom, A.M. et al. *Int. J. Cancer*, 87, 133, 2000.
150. Negri, E. et al. *Int. J. Cancer*, 86, 122, 2000.
151. Vorrips, L.E., Goldbohm, R.A., and Brants, H.A. *Cancer Epidemiol. Biomark. Prev.*, 9, 357, 2000.
152. Khaw, K.T., Bingham, S., and Welch, A. *Lancet*, 357, 657, 2001.
153. Lin, J.Y. et al. *J. Am. Acad. Dermatol.*, 48, 866, 2003.
154. Tsao, C.S. *Am. J. Clin. Nutr.*, 54, 1274s, 1991.
155. Surjyo, B. and Anisuir, K.B. *Indian J. Cancer*, 41, 72, 2004.
156. Chen, M.F. et al. *Nutr. Cancer*, 63, 1063, 2011.
157. Cha, J. et al. *Exp. Oncol.*, 33, 226, 2011.
158. Kim, J.E. et al. *Immunobiology*, 217, 873, 2012.
159. Lee, J. et al. *Cell. Mol. Biol. Lett.*, 17, 62, 2012.
160. D'Agostini, F. et al. *Carcinogenesis*, 26, 657, 2005.
161. Fiala, E.S. et al. *Carcinogenesis*, 26, 605, 2005.
162. Pathi, S.S. et al. *Nutr. Cancer*, 63, 1133, 2011.
163. Golde, D.W. *Integr. Cancer Ther.*, 2, 158, 2003.
164. Oliveira, C.P. *World J. Gastronenterol.*, 9, 446, 2003.
165. Zhang, Z.W. and Farthing, M.J.G. *Chinese J. Dig. Diseases*, 6, 53, 2005.
166. Kang, J.S. et al. *J. Cell. Physiol.*, 204, 192, 2005.
167. Han, S.S. *J. Cell. Biochem.*, 93, 257, 2004.
168. Cho, D. et al. *Melanoma Res.*, 13, 549, 2003.
169. Sagun, K.C., Carcamo, J.M., and Golde, D.W. *FASEB J.*, 19, 1657, 2005.
170. Duarte, T.L. and Lunec, J. *Free Radic. Res.*, 39, 671, 2005.
171. Kane, M.A. *Cancer Detect. Prev.*, 29, 46, 2005.
172. Piyanthilake, G.C. et al. *Cancer Res.*, 64, 8788, 2004.
173. Baglietto, L. et al. *BMJ.*, 331, 807, 2005.
174. Martinex, M.E., Henning, S.M., and Alberts, D.S. *Am. J. Clin. Nutr.*, 79, 691, 2004.
175. Shen, H. et al. *Cancer Epidemiol. Biomarkers Prev.*, 12, 980, 2003.
176. Strohle, A., Wolters, M., and Hahn, A. *Int. J. Oncol.*, 26, 1449, 2005.
177. Wei, E.K. et al. *J. Natl. Cancer Inst.*, 97, 684, 2005.
178. Kim, Y.I. *Environ. Mol. Mutagen*, 44, 10, 2004.
179. Linabery, A.M., Johnson, K.J., and Ross, J.A. *Pediatrics*, 129, 1125, 2012.
180. Zhang, L. et al. *Int. J. Mol. Sci.*, 13, 4009, 2012.
181. Zhao, P. *Asian Pac. J. Cancer Prev.*, 12, 2019, 2011.
182. Porigbny, J.P. et al. *Mutat. Res.*, 548, 53, 2004.
183. Carrier, J. et al. *Cancer Epidemiol. Biomarkers Prev.*, 12, 1262, 2003.
184. James, S.J. et al. *J. Nutr.*, 133, 3740s, 2003.
185. Davis, C.D. and Uthus, E.O. *J. Nutr.*, 133, 2907, 2003.
186. Kotsopoulos, J. et al. *Carcinogenesis*, 24, 937, 2003.
187. Trasler, J. et al. *Carcinogenesis*, 24, 39, 2003.
188. Teh, A.H. *Mutat. Rev.*, 751, 64, 2012.
189. Cole, B.F. et al. *JAMA*, 297, 2351, 2007.
190. Stolzenberg-Solomon, R.Z. et al. *Am. J. Clin. Nutr.*, 83, 895, 2006.
191. Kotsopoulos, J. et al. *Carcinogenesis*, 26, 1603, 2005.
192. Wien, T.N. et al. *BMJ Open*, 12, e000653, 2012.
193. Ames, B.N. *Mutat. Res.*, 475, 7, 2001.
194. Choi, S.W. and Mason, J.B. *J. Nutr.*, 132, 2413, 2002.
195. Fennech, M. *Mutat. Res.*, 475, 57, 2001.
196. Lamprecht, S.A. and Lipking, M. *Nat. Rev. Cancer*, 3, 601, 2003.
197. Mason, J.B. *Biofactors*, 37, 253, 2011.
198. Pufulete, M. et al. *Gut*, 54, 579, 2005.
199. Pufulete, M. et al. *Br. J. Cancer*, 92, 838, 2005.
200. Choi, S.W. et al. *Br. J. Cancer*, 93, 31, 2005.
201. Stempak, J.M. et al. *Carcinogenesis*, 26, 981, 2005.
202. Ly, A., Hoyt, L., Crowell, J., and Kim, Y.I., *Antioxid. Redox Signal.*, 17, 302, 2012.
203. Kim, Y.I. *Mol. Nutr. Food Res.*, 51, 267, 2007.
204. Kline, K. et al. *J. Marrary Gland Biol. Neoplasia*, 8, 91, 2003.
205. Pham, D.Q. and Plakogiannis, R. *Ann. Pharmacother.*, 39, 1870, 2005.
206. Lonn, E. et al. *J. Urol.*, 174, 1823, 2005.
207. Cho, E. et al. *Int. J. Cancer*, 118, 970, 2005.
208. Gaziano, J.M. *JAMA*, 301, 52, 2009.
209. Rodriguez, C. et al. *Cancer Epidemiol. Biomarkers Prev.*, 13, 378, 2004.
210. Weinstein, S.J. et al. *J. Natl. Cancer Inst.*, 97, 396, 2005.
211. Lippman, S.M. et al. *JAMA*, 301, 39, 2009.
212. Klein, E.A. et al. *JAMA*, 306, 1549, 2011.
213. Exon, J.H. et al. *Nutr. Cancer*, 49, 72, 2004.
214. Calvisi, D.F. et al. *J. Hepatol.*, 41, 815, 2004.
215. Quin, J. et al. *J. Surg. Res.*, 127, 139, 2005.
216. Uddin, A.N., Burns, F.J., and Rossman, T.G. *Carcinogenesis*, 26, 2179, 2005.
217. Heukamp, I. et al. *Pancreatology*, 5, 403, 2005.
218. Bansal, A.K. et al. *Chem. Biol. Interact.*, 156, 101, 2005.
219. Ju, J. *Carcinogenesis*, 31, 533, 2010.
220. Fantappie, O. et al. *Free Radic. Res.*, 38, 751, 2004.
221. Stapelberg, M. et al. *J. Biol. Chem.*, 280, 25369, 2005.
222. Shah, S.J. and Sylvester, P.W. *Biochem. Cell Biol.*, 83, 86, 2005.

223. Wang, X.F. et al. *Biochem. Biophys. Res. Commun.*, 326, 282, 2005.
224. Zu, K., Hawthorn, L., and Ip, C. *Mol. Cancer Ther.*, 4, 43, 2005.
225. Kang, Y.H. *Int. J. Cancer*, 112, 385, 2004.
226. Shah, S. and Sylvester, P.W. *Exp. Biol. Med.*, 229, 745, 2004.
227. Sakai, M. et al. *Anticancer Res.*, 24, 1683, 2004.
228. Jiang, Q. et al. *Proc. Natl. Acad. Sci. USA*, 101, 17825, 2004.
229. Shah, S.J. and Sylvester, P.W. *Exp. Boil. Med.*, 230, 235, 2005.
230. Jiang, Q., Wong, J., and Ames, B.N. *Ann. N.Y. Acad. Sci.*, 1031, 399, 2004.
231. Sylvester, P.W., Shah, S.J., and Samant, G.V. *J. Plant Physiol.*, 162, 803, 2005.
232. Alleva, R. et al. *Biochem. Biophys. Res. Commun.*, 331, 1515, 2005.
233. Meydani, S.N. et al. *J. Am. Med. Assoc.*, 277, 1380, 1997.
234. Chamras, H. et al. *Nutr. Cancer*, 52, 43, 2005.
235. Cooney, R.V. et al. *Proc. Natl. Acad. Sci. USA*, 90, 1771, 1993.
236. Cooney, R.V. et al. *Free Radic. Biol. Med.*, 19, 259, 1995.
237. Gysin, R., Azzi, A., and Visarius, T. *FASEB J.*, 16, 1952, 2002.
238. Jiang, Q. et al. *Am. J. Clin. Nutr.*, 74, 714, 2001.
239. Campbell, S., Stone, W., Whaley, S., and Krishnan, K. *Crit. Rev. Oncol. Hematol.*, 47, 249, 2003.
240. Hensley, K. et al. *Free Radic. Biol. Med.*, 36, 1, 2004.
241. Devaraj, S. et al. *Free Radic. Biol. Med.*, 44, 1203, 2008.
242. Ju, J. et al. *Cancer Prev. Res.*, 2, 143, 2009.
243. Li, G.X. et al. *Cancer Prev. Res.*, 4, 404, 2011.
244. Guan, F. et al. *Cancer Prev. Res.*, 5, 644, 2012.
245. Handelman, G.C. et al. *J. Nutr.*, 115, 807, 1985.
246. Huang, H.Y. and Appel, L.J. *J. Nutr.*, 133, 3137, 2003.
247. Traber, M.G. *Annu. Rev. Nutr.*, 27, 347, 2007.
248. Aggarwal, B.B., Sundaram, C., Prasad, S., and Kannappan, R. *Biochem. Pharmacol.*, 80, 1613, 2010.
249. Ling, M.T., Luk, S.U., Al-Ejeh, F., and Khanna, K.K. *Carcinogenesis*, 33, 233, 2012.
250. Wong, R.S., Radhakrishnan, A.K., Ibrahim, T.A., and Cheong, S.K. *Microsc. Microanal.*, 18, 462, 2012.
251. Kannappan, R., Gupta, S.C., Kim, J.H., and Aggarwal, B.H. *Genes Nutr.*, 7, 43, 2012.
252. Ayoub, N.M., Bachawal, S.V., and Sylvester, P.W. *Cell Prolif.*, 44, 516, 2011.
253. Shin-Kang, S. et al. *Free. Radic. Biol. Med.*, 51, 1164, 2011.
254. Inoue, A. et al. *Nutr. Cancer*, 63, 763, 2011.
255. Nesaretnam, K., Meganathan, P., Veerasenan, S.D., and Selvaduray, K.R. *Genes Nutr.*, 7, 3, 2012.
256. Jiang, Q. et al. *Int. J. Cancer*, 130, 685, 2012.
257. Campbell, S.E. et al. *Free Radic. Biol. Med.*, 50, 1344, 2011.
258. Rajendran, P. et al. *Br. J. Pharmacol*, 163, 283, 2011.
259. Fernandes, N.V., Guntipalli, P.K., and Mo, H. *Anticancer Res.*, 30, 4937, 2010.
260. Hsieh, T.C., Elangovan, S., and Wu, J.M. *Anticancer Res.*, 30, 2869, 2010.
261. Kannappan, R. et al. *Mol. Cancer Ther.*, 9, 2196, 2010.
262. Rayman, M.P. *Br. J. Nutr.*, 92, 557, 2004.
263. Schrauzer, G.N., White, D.A., and Schneider, C.I. *Bioinorg. Chem.*, 7, 23, 1997.
264. Etminan, M. et al. *Cancer Causes Control*, 16, 1125, 2005.
265. Zhuo, H., Smith, A.H., and Steinmaus, C. *Cancer Epidemiol. Biomarkers Prev.*, 13, 771, 2004.
266. Klein, E.A. *J. Urol.*, 171, S50, 2004.
267. Li, H. et al. *J. Natl. Cancer Inst.*, 96, 696, 2004.
268. Hurst, R. et al. *Am. J. Clin. Nutr.*, 96, 111, 2012.
269. Dennett, G. et al. *Cochrane Database Syst. Rev.*, 8, CD005195, 2011.
270. Clark, L.C. et al. *JAMA*, 276, 1957, 1996.
271. Duffield-Lillico, A.J. et al. *Cancer Epidemiol. Biomarkers Prev.*, 11, 630, 2002.
272. Reid, M.J. et al. *Cancer Epidemiol. Biomarkers Prev.*, 11, 1285, 2002.
273. Duffield-Lillico, A.J. et al. *BJU Int.*, 91, 608, 2003.
274. Fleschner, N.E. et al. *J. Clin. Oncol.*, 29, 2386, 2011.
275. Lee, J.I. et al. *Cancer Prev. Res.*, 2, 683, 2009.
276. Larsen, E.H. et al. *J. AOAC Int.*, 87, 225, 2004.
277. Davis, C.D. and Irons, R. *Current Nutr. Food Sci.*, 1, 201, 2005.
278. Baines, A.T. et al. *Cancer Lett.*, 160, 193, 2000.
279. Birt, D.F. et al. *J. Natl. Cancer Inst.*, 77, 1281, 1986.
280. Bjorkhem-Bergman, L. et al. *Carcinogenesis*, 26, 125, 2005.
281. Das, R.K. and Bhattacharya, S. *Asian Pac. J. Cancer Prev.*, 5, 151, 2004.
282. El-Bayoumy, K. and Sinha, R. *Mutat. Res.*, 551, 181, 2004.
283. Chen, X. et al. *Carcinogenesis*, 21, 1531, 2000.
284. Finley, J.W. et al. *J. Agric. Food Chem.*, 49, 2679, 2001.
285. Dias, D.F. et al. *Breast J.*, 6, 14, 2000.
286. Griffin, A.C. and Jacobs, M.M. *Cancer Lett.*, 3, 177, 1977.
287. Ip, C., Lisk, D.J., and Ganther, H.E. *Anticancer Res.*, 20, 4179, 2000.
288. Ip, C. et al. *J. Agric. Food Chem.*, 48, 2062, 2000.
289. McIntosh, G.H., Scherer, B., and Royle, P.J. *Asian P. J. Clin. Nutr.*, 13, s93, 2004.
290. Thirunavukkarasu, C. et al. *Cell Biochem. Funct.*, 20, 347, 2002.
291. Popova, N.V. *Cancer Lett.*, 179, 39, 2002.
292. Schrauzer, G.N., White, D.A., and Schneider, C.J. *Bioinorg. Chem.*, 8, 387, 1978.
293. Corcoran, N.M., Najdovska, M., and Costello, A.J. *J. Urol.*, 171, 907, 2004.
294. Li, D. et al. *J. Nutr.*, 134, 1536, 2004.
295. Waters, D.J. et al. *J. Natl. Cancer Inst.*, 95, 237, 2003.
296. Chinag, E.C. et al. *Dose Response*, 8, 285, 2009.
297. Morgan, K.T. et al. *Toxicol. Pathol.*, 30, 435, 2002.
298. Venhorst, J. *Xenobiotica*, 33, 57, 2003.
299. Hoen, P.A. et al. *Biochem. Pharmacol.*, 63, 1843, 2002.
300. Novoselov, S.V. et al. *Oncogene*, 24, 803, 2005.
301. Ip, C. and Lisk, D.J. *Nutr. Cancer*, 28, 184, 1997.
302. Davis, C.D. et al. *J. Nutr.*, 129, 63, 1999.
303. Abul-Hassan, K.S. et al. *Mutat. Res.*, 565, 45, 2004.
304. de Rosa, V. et al. *Free Radic. Res.*, 46, 105, 2012.
305. Seo, Y.R., Sweeney, C., and Smith, M.L. *Oncogene*, 21, 3663, 2002.
306. Verma, A. et al. *Nutr. Cancer*, 49, 184, 2004.
307. Dong, Y. et al. *Cancer Res.*, 63, 52, 2003.
308. Zeng, H., Briske-Anderson, M., Wu, M., and Moyer, M.P. *Nutr. Cancer*, 64, 128, 2012.
309. Fang, W. et al. *Int. J. Cancer*, 127, 32, 2010.
310. Zeng, H., Wu, M., and Botnen, J.H. *J. Nutr.*, 139, 1613, 2009.
311. Wang, Z. et al. *Curr. Cancer Drug Targets*, 10, 307, 2010.
312. Song, H. et al. *Immune Netw.* 9, 236, 2009.
313. Zhang, W. et al. *Cancer Lett.*, 296, 113, 2010.
314. Zu, K. et al. *Oncogene*, 25, 546, 2006.
315. Gopee, N.V., Johnson, V.J., and Sharma, R.P. *Toxicol. Sci.*, 78, 204, 2004.
316. Hu, H. et al. *Carcinogenesis*, 26, 1374, 2005.
317. Zuo, L. et al. *Ann. Hematol.*, 83, 751, 2004.

318. Yamaguchi, K. et al. *Oncogene*, 24, 5868, 2005.
319. Fu, L., Liu, Q., Shen, L., and Wang, Y. *J. Trace Elem. Med. Biol.*, 25, 130, 2011.
320. Yang, Y. et al. *Oncol. Res.*, 18, 1, 2009.
321. Abdulah, R. et al. *BMC Cancer*, 9, 414, 2009.
322. Luo, H. et al. *Cancer Lett.*, 315, 78, 2012.
323. Takahashi, M. et al. *Int. J. Oncol.*, 27, 489, 2005.
324. Kuppusamy, U.R. et al. *Biol. Trace Elem. Res.*, 106, 29, 2005.
325. Karunasinghe, N. et al. *Cancer Epidemiol. Biomarkers Prev.*, 13, 391, 2004.
326. Wycherly, B.J., Moak, M.A., and Christensen, M.J. *Nutr. Cancer*, 48, 78, 2004.
327. Mohamed, J. et al. *Pak. J. Biol. Sci.*, 14, 1055, 2011.
328. Kim, S.H. et al. *Exp. Biol. Med.*, 229, 203, 2004.
329. Helmersson, J. et al. *Free Radic Res.*, 39, 763, 2005.
330. Felix, K. et al. *Cancer Res.*, 64, 2910, 2004.
331. Jiang, C., Ganther, H., and Lu, J. *Mol. Carcinog.*, 29, 236, 2000.
332. Wu, X. et al. *BMC Cancer*, 12, 192, 2012.
333. Kassam, S. et al. *Cancer Chemother. Pharmacol.*, 68, 815, 2011.
334. Keum, Y.K., Jeong, W.S., and Kong, A.N.T. *Mutat. Res.*, 555, 191, 2004.
335. Fahey, J.W., Zalcmann, A.T., and Talalay, P. *Phytochemistry*, 56, 5, 2001.
336. Zhange, Y. et al. *Biochem. Biophys. Res. Commun.*, 206, 748, 1995.
337. Kolm, R.H. et al. *Biochem. J.*, 311, 450, 1995.
338. Sugie, S. et al. *Int. J. Cancer*, 115, 346, 2005.
339. Manesh, C. and Kuttan, G. *Fitoterapia*, 74, 355, 2003.
340. Smith, T.K., Mithen, R., and Johnson, I.T. *Carcinogenesis*, 24, 491, 2003.
341. Singh, A.V. et al. *Carcinogenesis*, 25, 83, 2004.
342. Pham, N.A. et al. *Mol. Cancer Ther.*, 3, 1239, 2004.
343. Nishikawa, A. et al. *Curr. Cancer Drug Targets*, 4, 373, 2004.
344. Nishikawa, A., Morse, M.A., and Chung, F.L. *Cancer Lett.*, 193, 11, 2003.
345. Hecht, S.S. et al. *Carcinogenesis*, 23, 1455, 2002.
346. Solt, D.B. et al. *Cancer Lett.*, 202, 147, 2003.
347. Hecht, S.S. et al. *Cancer Lett.*, 187, 87, 2002.
348. Witschi, H. et al. *Carcinogenesis*, 23, 289, 2002.
349. Myzak, M.C. et al. *Exp. Biol. Med.*, 232, 227, 2011.
350. Chen, M.J. et al. *Evid. Based Complement. Alternat. Med.*, 415, 231, 2012.
351. Qazi, A. et al. *Transl. Oncol.*, 3, 389, 2010.
352. Kanematsu, S. et al. *Oncol. Rep.*, 26, 603, 2011.
353. Fowke, J.H. et al. *Cancer Res.*, 63, 3980, 2003.
354. London, S.J. et al. *Lancet*, 356, 724, 2000.
355. Spitz, M.R. et al. *Cancer Epidemiol. Biomark. Prev.*, 9, 1017, 2001.
356. Guo, Z. et al. *Carcinogenesis*, 13, 2205, 1992.
357. Paolini, M. et al., *Carcinogenesis*, 25, 61, 2004.
358. Dingley, K.H. et al. *Nutr. Cancer*, 46, 212, 2003.
359. Munday, R. and Munday, C.M. *J. Agric. Food Chem.*, 52, 1867, 2004.
360. Petri, N. et al. *Drug Metab. Dispo.*, 31, 805, 2003.
361. Brooks, J.D., Paton, V.G., and Vidanes, G. *Cancer Epidemiol. Biomarkers Prev.*, 10, 949, 2001.
362. Bacon, J.R. et al. *Carcinogenesis*, 24, 1903, 2003.
363. Abdull Razis, A.F. et al. *Eur. J. Nutr.*, Epub, 2012.
364. Tang, L. and Zhang, Y. *J. Nutr.*, 134, 2004, 2004.
365. Jackson, S.J. and Singletary, K.W. *J. Nutr.*, 134, 2229, 2004.
366. Cho, S.D. et al. *Nutr. Cancer*, 52, 213, 2005.
367. Bhattacharya, A. et al. *Carcinogenesis*, 33, 394, 2012.
368. Balasubramanian, S., Chew, Y.C., and Eckert, R.L., *Mol. Pharmacol.*, 80, 870, 2011.
369. Tang, N.Y. et al. *Anticancer Res.*, 31, 1691, 2011.
370. Boreddy, S.R., Pramanik, K.C., and Srivastava, S.K. *Clin. Cancer Res.*, 17, 1784, 2011.
371. Kim, M.R., Zhou, L., Park, B.H., and Kim, J.R. *Mol. Med. Rep.*, 4, 929, 2011.
372. Yan, H. et al. *Br. J. Nutr.*, 106, 1779, 2011.
373. Choi, S. and Singh, S.V. *Cancer Res.*, 65, 2035, 2005.
374. Xiao, D. et al. *Clin. Cancer Res.*, 11, 2670, 2005.
375. Gingras, D. et al. *Cancer Lett.*, 203, 35, 2004.
376. Rose, P. et al. *Int. J. Biochem. Cell Biol.*, 37, 100, 2005.
377. Pullar, J.M. et al. *Carcinogenesis*, 25, 765, 2004.
378. Singh, S.V. et al. *J. Biol. Chem.*, 280, 19911, 2005.
379. Huang, S.H. et al. *J. Agric. Food Chem.*, 60, 665, 2012.
380. Xiao, Z., Mi, L., Chung, F.L., and Veenstra, T.D. *J. Nutr.*, 142, 1337S, 2012.
381. Hahm, E.R. and Sign, S.V. *Mol. Carcinog.*, 51, 465, 2012.
382. Huong, D. et al. *J. Agric. Food Chem.*, 59, 8124, 2011.
383. Jakubikova, J. et al. *Haematologica*, 96, 1170, 2011.
384. Miyoshi, N. et al. *Carcinogenesis*, 25, 567, 2004.
385. Gerhauser, C. et al. *Mutat. Res.*, 523/524, 163, 2003.
386. Gao, X. et al. *Proc. Natl. Acad. Sci. USA*, 98, 15221, 2001.
387. Zhang, Y. *Carcinogenesis*, 21, 1175, 2000.
388. Zhang, Y. et al. *Biochem. Biophys. Res. Commun.*, 206, 748, 1995.
389. Heiss, E. et al. *J. Biol. Chem.*, 276, 32008, 2001.
390. Ippoushi, K. et al. *Life Sci.*, 71, 411, 2002.
391. Zhang, Y. et al. *Mol. Cancer Ther.*, 2, 1045, 2003.
392. Lea, M.A. et al. *Int. J. Cancer*, 92, 784, 2001.
393. Zanichelli, F. et al. *Apoptosis*, 17, 964, 2012.
394. Lamy, E. et al. *Eur. J. Cancer Prev.*, 21, 400, 2012.
395. Boreddy, S.R., Sahu, R.P., and Srivastava, S.K. *PLoS One*, 6, e25799, 2011.
396. Kim, S.H. et al. *PLoS One*, 6, e26615, 2011.
397. Kim, E.J. et al. *Mol. Cell. Biochem.*, 359, 431, 2012.
398. Jee, H.G. et al. *Phytother. Res.*, 25, 1623, 2011.
399. Powolny, A.A. et al. *J. Natl. Cancer Inst.*, 6, 571, 2011.
400. Myzak, M.C. and Dashwood, R.H. *Curr. Drug Targets*, 7, 443, 2006.
401. Myzak, M.C., Karplus, A., Chung, F.-L., and Dashwood, R.H. *Cancer Res.*, 64, 5767, 2004.
402. Myzak, M.C. et al. *FASEB J.*, 20, 506, 2006.
403. Wang, L.G. et al., *Mol. Carcinog.*, 2006.
404. Scalbert, A. and Williamson, G. *J. Nutr.*, 130, 2073s, 2000.
405. Russo, G.L. *Pharm. Rep.*, 61, 67, 2009.
406. Neuhouser, M.L. *Nutr. Cancer*, 50, 1, 2004.
407. Bosetti, C. et al. *Cancer Epidemiol. Biomarkers Prev.*, 14, 805, 2005.
408. Djuric, Z., Severson, R.K., and Kato, I. *Nutr. Cancer*, 64, 351, 2012.
409. Lin, J. et al. *Am. J. Epidemiol.*, 164, 644, 2006.
410. Theodoratou, E. et al. *Cancer Epidemiol. Biomarkers Prev.*, 16, 684, 2007.
411. Cui, Y. et al. *Cancer*, 112, 2241, 2008.
412. Tang, N.P. et al. *Jpn. J. Clin. Oncol.*, 39, 352, 2009.
413. Deschner, E.E. et al. *Carcinogenesis*, 12, 1193, 1991.
414. Volate, S.R. et al. *Carcinogenesis*, 26, 1450, 2005.
415. Mahmoud, N.N. et al. *Carcinogenesis*, 21, 921, 2000.
416. Steerenberg, P.A. et al. *Cancer Lett.*, 114, 187, 1997.
417. Khanduja, K.L. et al. *Food Chem. Toxicol.*, 37, 313, 1999.
418. Vanhees, K. et al. *Mutagenesis*, 27, 445, 2012.
419. Kanno, S. et al. *Biol. Pharm. Bull.*, 28, 527, 2005.
420. Miyata, M. et al. *Cancer Lett.*, 183, 17, 2000.

421. Cooke, D. et al. *Eur. J. Cancer*, 41, 1931, 2005.
422. Leonardi, T. et al. *Exp. Biol. Med.*, 235, 717, 2010.
423. Silvan, S. et al. *Eur. J. Pharmacol.*, 670, 571, 2011.
424. Shukla, S., Maclennan, G.T., Fu, P., and Gupta, S. *Pharm. Res.*, 29, 1506, 2012.
425. Suzuki, R. et al. *Biofactors*, 22, 111, 2004.
426. Afaq, F. et al. *Int. J. Cancer*, 113, 423, 2005.
427. Rahden-Staron, I., Czeczot, H., and Szumilo, M. *Mutat. Res.*, 498, 57, 2001.
428. Schwarz, D., Kisselev, P., and Roots, I. *Eur. J. Cancer*, 41, 151, 2005.
429. Rossi, A.M. et al. *Int. J. Clin. Pharmacol. Ther.*, 42, 561, 2004.
430. De Santi, C. et al. *Xenobiotica*, 32, 363, 2002.
431. Marchetti, F. et al. *Xenobiotica*, 31, 841, 2001.
432. Mesia-Vela, S. and Kauffman, F.C. *Xenobiotica*, 33, 1211, 2003.
433. van der Logt, E.M. et al. *Carcinogenesis*, 24, 1651, 2003.
434. Galijatovic, A., Walle, U.K., and Walle, T. *Pharm. Res.*, 17, 21, 2000.
435. Kuo, H.M. et al. *Phytomedicine*, 9, 625, 2002.
436. Wilms, L.C. et al. *Mutat. Res.*, 582, 155, 2005.
437. Ciolino, H.P., Daschner, P.J., and Yeh, G.C. *Biochem. J.*, 340, 715, 1999.
438. De Santi, C. et al. *Xenobiotica*, 30, 857, 2000.
439. Bear, W.L. and Tell, R.W. *Anticancer Res.*, 20, 3609, 2000.
440. Vijayababu, M.R. et al. *J. Cancer Res. Clin. Oncol.*, 131, 765, 2005
441. Ong, C.S. et al. *Oncol. Rep.*, 11, 727, 2004.
442. Huynh, H. et al. *Int. J. Oncol.*, 23, 821, 2003.
443. Michaud-Levesque, J., Bousquet-Gagnon, N., and Beliveau, R. *Exp. Cell Res.*, 318, 925, 2012.
444. Kim, Y., Kim, W.J., and Chae, E.J. *Koerean J. Physiol. Pharmacol.*, 15, 279, 2011.
445. Ackland, M.L., van de Waarsenburg, S., and Jones, R. *In Vivo*, 19, 69, 2005.
446. Wang, W. et al. *Nutr. Cancer*, 48, 106, 2004.
447. Zhao, M. et al. *Mol. Cancer*, 29, 104, 2011.
448. Liu, K.C. et al. *Environ. Toxicol.*, Epub, 2012.
449. Kim, W.K. et al. *J. Nutr. Biochem.*, 16, 155, 2005.
450. Wang, P. et al. *Toxicol. In Vitro*, 26, 221, 2012.
451. Zheng, S.Y. et al. *Mol. Med. Rep.*, 5, 822, 2012.
452. Nguyen, T.T. et al. *Carcinogenesis*, 25, 647, 2004.
453. Bulzomi, P. et al. *J. Cell Physiol.*, 227, 1891, 2012.
454. Brusselmans, K. et al. *J. Biol. Chem.*, 280, 5636, 2005.
455. Kim, H.S. et al. *Apoptosis*, Epub, 2012.
456. Kempuraj, D. et al. *Br. J. Pharmacol.*, 145, 934, 2005.
457. Huang, W.W. et al. *Mol. Nutr. Food Res.*, 54, 1585, 2010.
458. Luo, H. et al. *Food Chem.*, 128, 513, 2011.
459. Park, J.H. et al. *Food Chem. Toxicol.*, 46, 3684, 2008.
460. Sabarinathan, D., Mahalakshmi, P., Vanisree, A.J. *Mol. Cell. Biochem.*, 345, 215, 2010.
461. Jin, C.Y. et al. *Mol. Nutr. Food Res.*, 55, 300, 2011.
462. Lu, H.F. et al. *Hum. Exp. Toxicol.*, 30, 1053, 2011.
463. Pandey, M. et al. *Mol. Carcinogen.*, Epub, 2011.
464. Kandare-Grzybowska, K. et al. *Br. J. Pharmacol.*, 148, 208, 2006.
465. Comalada, M. et al., *Eur. J. Immunol.*, 35, 584, 2005.
466. Lyu, S.Y. and Park, W.B. *Arch. Pharm. Res.*, 28, 573, 2005.
467. Kowalski, J. et al. *Pharmacol. Rep.*, 57, 390, 2005.
468. Ueda, H., Yamazaki, C., and Yamazaki, M. *Biosci. Biotechnol. Biochem.*, 68, 119, 2004.
469. Duthie, S.J. and Dobson, V.L. *Eur. J. Nutr.*, 38, 28, 1999.
470. Aherne, S.A. and O'Brien, N.M. *Nutr. Cancer*, 38, 106, 2000.
471. Cemeli, E., Schmid, T.E., and Anderson, D. *Environ. Mol. Mutag.*, 44, 420, 2004.
472. Yeh, S.L. et al. *J. Nutr. Biochem.*, 16, 729, 2005.
473. Lu, H.W. et al. *Arch. Biochem. Biophys.*, 393, 73, 2001.
474. Jagetia, G.C. et al. *Clin. Chim. Acta*, 347, 189, 2004.
475. Morrow, D.M. et al. *Mutat. Res.*, 480–481, 269, 2001.
476. Ma, Z.S. et al. *Int. J. Oncol.*, 24, 1297, 2004.
477. Martinez, C.C. et al. *J. Agric. Food Chem.*, 53, 6791, 2005.
478. Luo, H. et al. *Food Chem.*, 130, 321, 2012.
479. Lui, H. et al. *Nutr. Cancer*, 61, 554, 2009.
480. Melstron, L.G. et al. *J. Surg. Res.*, 167, 173, 2011.
481. Kanadaswami, E. et al. *In Vivo*, 19, 895, 2005.
482. Lin, Y.S. et al. *Cancer Sci.*, 102, 1829, 2011.
483. Lin, C.W. et al. *J. Cell. Physiol.*, 225, 472, 2010.
484. Sengupta, A., Ghosh, S., and Bhattacharjee, S. *Asian Pac. J. Cancer Prev.*, 5, 229, 2004.
485. Park, E.J. and Pezzuto, J.M. *Cancer Metastasis Rev.*, 21, 231, 2002.
486. Steinmetz, K.A. et al. *Am. J. Epidemiol.*, 139, 1, 1994.
487. Fleischauer, A.T. and Arab, L. *J. Nutr.*, 131, 1032S, 2001.
488. Tanaka, S. et al. *Hiroshima J. Med. Sci.*, 53, 39, 2004.
489. Singh, A. and Shukla, Y. *Cancer Lett.*, 131, 209, 1998.
490. Ip, C., Lisk, D.J., and Stoewsand, G.S. *Nutr. Cancer*, 17, 279, 1992.
491. Wargovich, M.J. *Carcinogenesis*, 8, 487, 1987.
492. Hussain, S.P., Jannu, L.N., and Rao, A.R. *Cancer Lett.*, 49, 175, 1990.
493. Wargovich, M.J. et al. *Cancer Res.*, 48, 6872, 1988.
494. Hong, J.Y. et al. *Carcinogenesis*, 13, 901, 1992.
495. Takahashi, S. et al. *Carcinogenesis*, 13, 1513, 1992.
496. Nagabhushan, M. et al. *Cancer Lett.*, 66, 207, 1992.
497. Park, K.A., Kweon, S., and Choi, H. *J. Biochem. Mol. Biol.*, 35, 615, 2002.
498. Wargovich, M.J. et al. *Cancer Epidemiol. Biomarkers Prev.*, 5, 355, 1996.
499. Wargovich, M.J. et al. *Carcinogenesis*, 21, 1149, 2000.
500. Milner, J.A. *J. Nutr.*, 131, 1027s, 2001.
501. Ross, S.A., Finley, J.W., and Milner, J.A. *J. Nutr.*, 136, 852s, 2006.
502. Wang, X. et al. *Mol. Med. Report*, 5, 66, 2012.
503. Lee, Y., Kim, H., Lee, J., and Kim, K. *Biol. Pharm. Bull.*, 34, 677, 2011.
504. Wu, P.P. et al. *Phytomedicine*, 18, 672, 2011.
505. Chihara, T. et al. *Asian Pac. J. Cancer Prev.*, 11, 1301, 2010.
506. Pai, M.H., Kuo, Y.H., Chiang, E.P., Tang, F.Y. *Br. J. Nutr.*, 20, 1, 2011.
507. Schaffer, E.M. et al. *Cancer Lett.*, 102, 199, 1996.
508. Mei, X. et al. *Acta Nutrim. Sin.*, 11, 141, 1989.
509. Morris, C.R. et al. *Nutr. Cancer*, 48, 54, 2004.
510. Wu, C.C. et al. *J. Agric. Food Chem.*, 50, 378, 2002.
511. Berges, R. et al. *Carcinogenesis*, 25, 1953, 2004.
512. Le Bon, A.M. et al. *J. Agric. Food Chem.*, 51, 7617, 2003.
513. Munday, R. and Munday, C.M. *Nutr. Cancer*, 40, 205, 2001.
514. Yu, F.S. et al. *Food Chem. Toxicol.*, 43, 1029, 2005.
515. Chen, C. et al. *Free Radic. Biol. Med.*, 37, 1578, 2004.
516. Zhou, L. and Mirvish, S.S. *Nutr. Cancer*, 51, 68, 2005.
517. Green, M. et al. *Oncol. Rep.*, 10, 767, 2003.
518. Dion, M.E., Agler, M., and Milner, J.A. *Nutr. Cancer*, 28, 1, 1997.
519. L'vova, G.N. and Zasukhina, G.D. *Genetika*, 38, 306, 2002.
520. Xu, X.J., Kassie, F., and Mersch-Sundermann, V. *Mutat. Res.*, Epub, 2005.
521. Arunkumar, A. et al. *Biol. Pharm. Bull.*, 28, 740, 2005.

522. Herman-Antosiewicz, A. and Singh, S.V. *J. Biol. Chem.*, 280, 28519, 2005.
523. Herman-Antosiewicz, A. et al. *Pharm. Res.*, 27, 1072, 2010.
524. Wu, C.C. et al. *Food Chem. Toxicol.*, 42, 1937, 2004.
525. Knowles, L.M. and Milner, J.A. *Carcinogenesis*, 21, 1129, 2000.
526. Lu, H.F. et al. *Food Chem. Toxicol.*, 42, 1543, 2004.
527. Bratheeshkumar, P., Thejass, P., and Kutan, G. *J. Environ. Pathol. Toxicol. Oncol.*, 29, 113, 2010.
528. Oommen, S. et al. *Eur. J. Pharmacol.*, 485, 97, 2004.
529. Zhang, W. et al. *Oncol. Rep.*, 24, 1585, 2010.
530. Xiao, D. et al. *Mol. Cancer Ther.*, 4, 1388, 2005.
531. Xiao, D. et al. *Cancer Res.*, 63, 6825, 2003.
532. Lund, T. et al. *Br. J. Cancer*, 92, 1773, 2005.
533. Bhuvaneswari, V., Rao, K.S., and Nagini, S. *Clin. Chim. Acta*, 350, 65, 2004.
534. Xiao, D. et al. *Oncogene*, 23, 5594, 2004.
535. Xiao, D. and Singh, S.V. *Carcinogenesis*, 27, 533, 2006.
536. Park, S.Y. et al. *Cancer Lett.*, 224, 123, 2005.
537. Chandra-Kuntal, K. and Singh, S.V. *Cancer Prev. Res.*, 3, 1473, 2010.
538. Wu, P.P. et al. *Int. J. Oncol.*, 38, 1605, 2011.
539. Wang, Z., Liu, Z., Cao, Z., and Li, L. *Nat. Prod. Res.*, 26, 1033, 2012.
540. Liu, Z. et al. *Nol. Med. Report*, 5, 439, 2012.
541. Lee, J.E., Lee, R.A., Kim, K.H., and Lee, J.H. *K. Korean Surg. Soc.*, 81, 85, 2011.
542. Cha, J.H. et al. *Oncol. Rep.*, 28, 41, 2012.
543. Li, W. et al. *Acta Biochim. Biophys. Sin*, 44, 577, 2012.
544. Lang, A. et al. *Clin. Nutr.*, 23, 1199, 2004.
545. Colic, M. et al. *Phytomedicine*, 9, 117, 2002.
546. Morioka, N. et al. *Cancer Immunol. Immunother.*, 37, 316, 1993.
547. Hassan, Z.M. et al. *Int. Immunopharmacol.*, 3, 1483, 2003.
548. Ghazanfari, T., Hassan, Z.M., and Ebrahimi, M. *Int. Immunopharmacol.*, 2, 1541, 2002.
549. Chang, H.P., Huang, S.Y., and Chen, Y.H. *J. Agric. Food Chem.*, 53, 2530, 2005.
550. Chang, H.P. and Chen, Y.H. *Nutrition*, 21, 530, 2005.
551. Dirsch, V.M. et al. *Atherosclerosis*, 139, 333, 1998.
552. Elango, E.M. et al. *J. Appl. Genet.*, 45, 469, 2004.
553. Sengupta, A., Ghosh, S., and Das, S. *Cancer Lett.*, 208, 127, 2004.
554. Omurtag, G.Z. et al. *J. Pharm. Pharmacol.*, 57, 623, 2005.
555. Pedraza-Chaverri, J. et al. *BMC Clin. Pharmacol.*, 4, 5, 2004.
556. Arivazhagan, S. et al. *J. Med. Food*, 7, 2334, 2004.
557. Shukla, Y., Arora, A., and Singh, A. *Biomed. Environ. Sci.*, 15, 41, 2002.
558. Park, H.S. et al. *J. Food Sci.*, 76, T105, 2011.
559. Lai, K.C. et al, *Environ. Toxicol.*, Epub, 2011.
560. Druesne, N. et al. *Carcinogenesis*, 25: 1227, 2004.
561. Crowell, P.L. and Gould, M.N. *Crit. Rev. Oncog.*, 5, 1, 1994.
562. Wattenberg, L.W. and Coccia, J.B. *Carcinogenesis*, 12, 115, 1991.
563. Stark, M.J. et al. *Cancer Lett.*, 96, 15, 1995.
564. Reddy, B.S. et al. *Cancer Res.*, 57, 420, 1997.
565. Liston, B.W. et al. *Cancer Res.*, 63, 2399, 2003.
566. Lu, X.G. et al. *World J. Gastroenterol.*, 10, 2140, 2004.
567. Raphael, T.J. and Kuttan, G. *J. Exp. Clin. Cancer Res.*, 22, 419, 2003.
568. Asamato, M. et al. *Jpn. J. Cancer Res.*, 93, 32, 2002.
569. Kaji, I. et al. *Int. J. Cancer*, 93, 441, 2001.
570. Chaudhary, S.C., Alam, M.S., Siddiqui, M.S., and Athar, M. *Chem. Biol. Interact.*, 179, 145, 2009.
571. Chaudhary, S.C., Siddiqui, M.S., Athar, M., and Alam, M.S. *Hum. Exp. Toxicol.*, 31, 798, 2012.
572. Wilson, M.J., Lidgren, B.R., and Sinha, A.A. *Exp. Mol. Pathol.*, 85, 83, 2008.
573. Haag, J.D., Lindstrom, M.J., and Gould, M.N. *Cancer Res.*, 52, 4021, 1992.
574. Haag, J.D. and Gould, M.N. *Cancer Chemother. Pharmacol.*, 34, 477, 1994.
575. Del Toro-Arreola, S. et al. *Int. Immunopharmacol*, 5, 829, 2005.
576. Haskim, I.A., Harris, R.B., and Ritenbaugh, C. *Nutr. Cancer*, 37, 161, 2000.
577. Sterarns, V. et al. *Clin. Cancer Res.*, 10, 7583, 2004.
578. Bailey, H.H. et al. *Gynecol. Oncol.*, 85, 464, 2002.
579. Hudes, G.R. et al. *Clin. Cancer Res.*, 6, 3071, 2000.
580. Matos, J.M. et al. *J. Surg. Res.*, 147, 194, 2008.
581. Maltzman, T.H. et al. *Carcinogenesis*, 12, 2081, 1991.
582. Van der Logt, E.M. et al. *Anticancer Res.*, 24, 843, 2004.
583. Yuri, T. et al. *Breast Cancer Res. Treat.*, 84, 251, 2004.
584. Samaila, D. et al. *Anticancer Res.*, 24, 3089, 2004.
585. Mills, J.J. et al. *Cancer Res.*, 55, 979, 1995.
586. Dudai, N. et al. *Planta Med.*, 71, 484, 2005.
587. Fernandes, J. et al. *Oncol. Rep.*, 13, 943, 2005.
588. Xu, M. et al. *Toxicol. Appl. Pharmacol.*, 195, 232, 2004.
589. Manuela, M.G. et al. *Cancer Invest.*, 28, 135, 2010.
590. Ji, J. et al. *Leuk. Lymphoma*, 47, 2617, 2006.
591. Loutrari, H. et al. *J. Pharmacol. Exp. Ther.*, 11, 568, 2004.

# 67 Nutrition and Cancer Treatment

*David Heber and Susan Bowerman*

## CONTENTS

## INTRODUCTION

Malnutrition is a frequent and serious problem in patients with cancer. Patients with lung, prostate, head and neck, and gastric cancers are more frequently affected, but the overall incidence of malnutrition ranges between 30% and 85% of different populations studied.[1,2] The advanced starvation state resulting from decreased food intake and hormonal/metabolic abnormalities characteristic of the interaction between tumor and host has been called cancer cachexia,[3] characterized by progressive, involuntary weight loss with depletion of lean body mass, muscle wasting and weakness, edema, impaired immune response, and declines in motor and mental function. Weight loss of greater than 10% of prediagnosis weight is seen in approximately 45% of patients.[2,4] Cancer-associated malnutrition and cachexia are related to considerable morbidity and mortality, including decreased quality of life,[5] impaired response to chemotherapy,[5] impaired muscle function,[6] and higher incidence of postoperative complications.[7–9] The goals of nutritional support are to provide the patient with energy and nutrients to maintain or improve their nutritional status and immune function, minimize gastrointestinal (GI) symptoms, and improve quality of life. Early intervention in adequately nourished patients or those with early signs of nutritional decline can delay the progression of malnutrition,[10] but a vicious cycle of cachexia can develop in which the effects of the disease lead to nutritional decline, predisposing the patient to increased complications and more severe disease, which promotes further decline.

While nutritional rehabilitation can be demonstrated in selected patients who respond to antineoplastic therapy, the application of parenteral and enteral nutrition as an adjunct to chemotherapy in cancer patients has not resulted in increased survival or predictable weight gain.[11,12] The pathophysiology of cancer-associated malnutrition is complex and cannot be explained on the basis of poor nutrient intake alone, suggesting that simply increasing nutrient intake is not sufficient to prevent or reverse malnutrition. Both tumor-derived and systemic factors, such as hormones and inflammatory cytokines produced by the host in response to the tumor, have been implicated in the pathophysiology of cancer cachexia, and there is increasing evidence that these factors are associated with malnutrition.[13–15]

## METABOLIC ABNORMALITIES IN THE CANCER PATIENT

Since predictable renutrition of the cancer patient has not been possible, a great deal of research has been conducted concerning specific hormonal and metabolic abnormalities that could interfere with renutrition. Research on the basic pathophysiology of cancer cachexia has resulted in the definition of several metabolic and hormonal abnormalities in malnourished cancer patients. These abnormalities are listed in Table 67.1.

### ENERGY BALANCE IN THE CANCER PATIENT

Based on autopsy studies performed in the 1920s[25,26] and animal studies done in the 1950s,[27] it was postulated that tumors acted to siphon off needed energy and protein from the host. In the 1970s and 1980s, specific abnormalities of intermediary metabolism were identified in cancer patients that could account for the common observation that such patients lost weight even in the face of apparently adequate nutrition. Studies conducted in a number of laboratories, including our own, have demonstrated that maladaptive metabolic abnormalities occur frequently in patients with cancer. In 1983,

## TABLE 67.1
### Metabolic Abnormalities in Cancer Patients

1. Hypogonadism in male cancer patients[16]
2. Increased glucose production[17,18]
3. Increased protein catabolism[19,20]
4. Increased lipolysis and fatty acid oxidation[21,22]
5. Insulin resistance[23,24]

we demonstrated that adequate calories and protein administered to six patients with active localized head and neck cancer via forced continuous enteral alimentation under metabolic ward conditions for 29 days failed to lead to significant weight gain.[28] The observed failure of these patients to gain weight despite adequate caloric intake under metabolic ward conditions supports the concept that malnourished cancer patients are hypermetabolic.

If metabolic abnormalities promote the development of malnutrition or interfere with renutrition, then there should be some evidence of abnormally increased energy expenditure. A number of investigators have used indirect calorimetry and the abbreviated Weir formula to calculate energy expenditure at rest and then compared this to the basal energy expenditure (BEE) determined using the Harris–Benedict formulas. Long et al.[29] demonstrated a mean difference of 2% when this comparison was performed in 20 normal controls. In 1980, Bozetti[30] found that 60% of a group of patients with advanced cancer had basal metabolic rates (BMRs) increased 20% above predicted. In 1983, Dempsey et al.[31] studied energy expenditure in a group of 173 malnourished GI cancer patients. Of these, 58% had abnormal resting energy expenditure (REE) by indirect calorimetry compared to BEE, but a greater percentage was hypometabolic rather than hypermetabolic (36% vs. 22%). Knox et al.[32] studied 200 patients with a variety of cancers and found abnormal energy metabolism in 59% but found more hypometabolic than hypermetabolic individuals (33% vs. 26%). While standard formulae accurately predict metabolic rate in normal individuals, the measured metabolic rates in patients with cancer have a much wider distribution. Controversy remains concerning the importance of REE in cancer-associated malnutrition; however, tumor resection has been shown to normalize REE in hypermetabolic patients.[33] Elevated REE and its role in the pathogenesis of cancer-associated malnutrition may depend upon the individual patient and disease characteristics.[4]

Lean body mass rather than fat mass correlates with the individual variations observed in measured REE. The hypothesis that the malnourished cancer patient may be hypermetabolic relative to the amount of lean body mass remaining has been examined. Peacock et al.[34] studied REE in noncachectic patients with sarcomas. These patients had no prior treatment, had large localized sarcomas, and had no weight loss or history of decreased food intake. REE corrected for body cell mass (BCM) determined by total body potassium counting or body surface area was significantly

greater in male sarcoma patients compared to controls. This difference was due to both a decrease in BCM and an increase in REE in these patients before the onset of weight loss.

## GLUCOSE AND PROTEIN METABOLISM

Changes in carbohydrate metabolism, similar to those seen in type 2 diabetes, are common in patients with cancer-associated malnutrition. Although glucose turnover is increased, glucose is poorly utilized by peripheral tissues due to insulin resistance and glucose insensitivity.[35,36] Tumors have been demonstrated to increase the rate of glucose utilization in a number of tissues, acting as metabolic traps.[37,38] Since there are only 1200 kcal stored in the body as liver and muscle glycogen, blood glucose levels would be expected to fall. This does not occur since there is also an increase in hepatic glucose production in cachectic and anorectic tumor-bearing animals and humans. The regulation of protein metabolism is tightly linked to carbohydrate metabolism, since these processes are critical to the normal adaptation to starvation or underfeeding. During starvation, there is a decrease in glucose production, protein synthesis, and protein catabolism. The decrease in glucose production occurs as fat-derived fuels, primarily ketone bodies, are used for energy production. While there are 54,000 kcal of protein stored in the BCM, only about half of these are available for energy production. In fact, depletion below 50% of body protein stores is incompatible with life.

Increased turnover of liver and muscle proteins and gluconeogenesis from amino acids of muscle origin are thought to contribute to rapid muscle wasting seen in cancer-associated malnutrition.[36,39] Whole-body protein breakdown is increased in lung cancer patients and has been shown to correlate with the degree of malnutrition such that more malnourished patients have greater elevations of their whole-body protein breakdown rates expressed per kg of body weight.[20] The results of metabolic studies in lung cancer patients compared to healthy controls are shown in Table 67.2. Muscle catabolism, measured by 3-methylhistidine excretion, was increased in lung cancer patients compared to that of healthy controls. Methylhistidine excretion rates did not correlate with weight loss, percentage of ideal body weight, or age in the lung cancer patients studied. Glucose production rates were markedly increased in lung cancer patients compared with healthy controls, and changes in glucose production rates in the cancer patients studied did not correlate with weight loss, percent of ideal body weight, or age.

Hydrazine sulfate is a noncompetitive inhibitor of gluconeogenesis. When this drug is administered to lung cancer patients, not only does whole-body glucose production decrease as expected, but there is also a decrease in whole-body protein breakdown rates.[40] Increases in glucose production are directly and quantitatively linked to increased protein breakdown and changes in the circulating levels of individual glucogenic amino acids. Table 67.3 shows the influence of hydrazine sulfate on lysine flux. At 1 month, there was a significant reduction in the hydrazine group and a nonsignificant increase in the placebo group.

## TABLE 67.2

## Total Body Protein Turnover, Glucose Production, and 3-Methylhistidine Excretion in the Fasting State on Day 5 of Constant Nitrogen and Calorie Intake in Lung Cancer Patients Compared to Healthy Controls

| Group | Protein Turnover (g/kg Day) | Glucose Production (mg/kg min) | 3-Methylhistidine Excretion (μmol/g Creatinine Day) |
|---|---|---|---|
| Control | 2.12 ± 0.38 | 2.18 ± 0.06 | 71 ± 8 |
| Lung cancer | 3.15 ± 0.51[a,b] | 2.84 ± 0.16[a] | 106 ± 11[a] |

[a] $p < 0.05$ versus control subjects.
[b] Mean ± SD.

## TABLE 67.3

## Whole-Body Lysine Flux in Lung Cancer Patients

| Placebo Group | Lysine Flux (μmol/h) | |
|---|---|---|
| | Baseline | 1 Month |
| 1 | 2172 | 2812 |
| 2 | 1869 | 2959 |
| 3 | 2373 | 2674 |
| 4 | 2772 | 2269 |
| 5 | 2758 | 3195 |
| 6 | 3542 | 3585 |
| Mean (SD) | 2580 (580) | 2920 (450)[a,b] |
| Hydrazine treated | | |
| 7 | 2675 | 1146 |
| 8 | 2522 | 2119 |
| 9 | 2666 | 3129 |
| 10 | 1808 | 1217 |
| 11 | 2264 | 1438 |
| 12 | 3114 | 2006 |
| Mean (SD) | 2510 (440) | 1840 (750)[b,c] |

[a] $p = 0.08$.
[b] $p < 0.05$, paired $t$-tests with baseline.
[c] $p < 0.01$ by combined paired $t$-test both groups.

## TUMOR AND HOST FACTORS

Inflammation is seen in many forms of cancer in various tissues, and both tumor and host factors are released locally and into the circulation during this process. These factors can promote profound metabolic abnormalities that lead to anorexia, malnutrition, and cachexia. These factors are cytokines and include tumor necrosis factor-alpha (TNFα), interleukins (IL-1, IL-6), and interferon-gamma (IFN-γ), which are produced by tumor, immune, and stromal cells and can promote angiogenesis and tumor growth and survival[41] and in many cases provide one means of intercellular communication between tumor cells and the cells of the microenvironment in which they grow. There is also increasing evidence supporting the role for chronic production of these factors

in the pathogenesis of cancer-associated malnutrition.[42,43] While an exclusive role for any single cytokine in cancer-associated malnutrition has not been defined, there is growing evidence that the host inflammatory response to a tumor supports the progression to cachexia.

Weight loss in cancer patients is due to depletion of both adipose tissue and skeletal muscle mass, while the nonmuscle protein compartment is relatively preserved, thus distinguishing cachexia from simple starvation.[44] The loss of both adipose tissue and skeletal muscle mass can be extensive. Studies of the body composition of lung cancer patients who had lost 32% of their preillness stable weight, compared with a group of controls, matched for age, sex, height, and preillness stable weight of the cancer patients. Although the overall weight loss was 32%, the cachectic patients had lost 85% of their total body fat and 75% of their skeletal muscle, and there was also a significant decrease in mineral content, suggesting erosion of bone. This marked loss of skeletal muscle explains why patients with cachexia have a reduced mobility and thus quality of life, together with a shorter life span, since loss of respiratory muscle function will lead to death from hypostatic pneumonia (Winsdor and Hill). Death of patients occurs with 25%–30% total body weight loss.[45] A similar situation is found in patients with acquired immunodeficiency syndrome (AIDS), where death is imminent when they have lost 34% of their ideal body weight.[46] Respiratory failure has been found to be responsible for the death of 48% of cancer patients[47].

One group of investigators has been studying short-term fasting as a means of enhancing sensitivity of tumors to chemotherapy so as to sensitize target tumor cells while having relatively low toxicity directed at normal cells and tissues.[48] This approach is still experimental and should only be considered within the context of a controlled clinical trial. However, the concept is novel and worthy of consideration. Longo et al. have proposed that changes in the levels of glucose, IGF-I, IGFBP-1, and in other proteins caused by fasting have the potential to improve the efficacy of chemotherapy against tumors by protecting normal cells and tissues and possibly by diminishing multidrug resistance in malignant cells.[49] Starvation sensitized yeast cells (*Saccharomyces cerevisiae*) expressing the oncogene-like RAS2(val19) to oxidative stress, and 15 of 17 mammalian cancer cell lines were sensitized to chemotherapeutic agents. Short-term starvation (or fasting) protects normal cells and tumor-bearing mice from the harmful side effects of a variety of chemotherapy drugs. Cycles of starvation were as effective as chemotherapeutic agents in delaying progression of different tumors and increased the effectiveness of chemotherapy drugs against melanoma, glioma, and breast cancer cells. In mouse models of neuroblastoma, fasting cycles plus chemotherapy drugs—but not either treatment alone—resulted in long-term cancer-free survival. In 4T1 breast cancer cells, short-term starvation resulted in increased phosphorylation of the stress-sensitizing Akt and S6 kinases, increased oxidative stress, caspase-3 cleavage, DNA damage, and apoptosis. These studies suggest that multiple cycles of fasting promote differential stress sensitization in a wide range of tumors and could potentially replace or augment the efficacy of certain chemotherapy drugs in the treatment of various cancers while reducing side effects of therapy in cancer patients. This counterintuitive idea of using short-term fasting prior to chemotherapy has yet to be tested and proven in humans.[50]

## MOLECULAR UNDERSTANDING OF METABOLIC ABNORMALITIES IN CANCER CELLS

Cancer cells simultaneously exhibit glycolysis with lactate secretion and mitochondrial respiration even in the presence of oxygen, a phenomenon known as the Warburg effect. The maintenance of this mixed metabolic phenotype is seemingly counterintuitive given that glycolysis produces only 2 mol of ATP per mole of glucose, far less than the 36 generated by mitochondrial respiration. A metabolic shift from oxidative phosphorylation in the mitochondria to glycolysis in the cytosol in cancer was first described over 80 years ago by Otto Warburg, who later considered such metabolic changes as "the origin of cancer" resulting from mitochondrial respiration injury.[51] It is now recognized that elevated glycolysis is a characteristic metabolism in many cancer cells. In fact, active glucose uptake by cancer cells constitutes the basis for fluorodeoxyglucose-positron emission tomography (FDG-PET), an imaging technology commonly used in cancer diagnosis.[52] In addition, cancer cells exhibit elevated generation of reactive oxygen species (ROS), which disturb redox balance leading to oxidative stress.[53] However, despite these long-standing observations and clinical relevance, the biochemical/molecular mechanisms responsible for such metabolic alterations and their relationship with mitochondrial respiratory dysfunction remain elusive.

Several hypotheses have been proposed for the Warburg effect in cancer cells. At the cellular level, mitochondrial respiration malfunction and enhancement of glycolysis are thought to be a metabolic advantage under the intermittent hypoxia conditions experienced by premalignant and malignant tumor cells.[54,55] However, aerobic glycolysis is not found exclusively in cancer cells but is also observed in rapidly dividing normal cells even under conditions of normoxia.[56] It is also widely believed that the glycolysis rate increases in order to match the increased anabolic needs of the rapidly proliferating cells for precursor metabolites.[57]

The actual molecular mechanisms that lead to the enhanced aerobic glycolysis are increasingly well understood. Under physiological condition, for example, PI3K/Akt signaling pathways play a critical role in promoting aerobic glycolysis in activated T cells in response to growth factors or cytokine stimulation.[58] In the pathophysiological condition of tumorigenesis, malfunction of mitochondrial respiration due to mitochondrial DNA mutations/deletions is an important contributing factor.[59–62] Also, p53, one of the most frequently mutated genes in cancers, is both a positive regulator of mitochondrial respiration[63] and a negative regulator of glycolysis.[64] These, together with the activation of hypoxia-inducible factor (HIF), a transcription factor that is activated by hypoxic stress but also by oncogenic, metabolic, and oxidative stress, often lead to the overexpression of the glucose transporters and various glycolysis pathway enzymes or isozyme subtypes explaining the increased glucose uptake and altered utilization.[65,66] The evidence accumulated so far thus indicates that the presence of aerobic glycolysis is a common characteristic of rapidly proliferating cells and that it may offer a growth advantage to rapidly proliferating normal cells, for example, during development and tissue regeneration, and to cancer cells in tumor formation.

## ASSESSMENT OF THE CANCER PATIENT'S NUTRITIONAL STATUS

The risk of malnutrition and its severity are affected by the tumor type, the stage of the disease, and the therapy being applied.[67] Cancer-associated malnutrition can affect the patient's response to therapy[68] and is also associated with reduced wound healing, reduced muscle function, and poor skin turgor that can lead to skin breakdown.[69] Early assessment and intervention are critical in order for nutritional support to improve outcome,[10] with nutritional screening as the first step. For hospitalized patients, initial screening should be performed as soon as possible following admission, or during hospital visits for outpatients, and at regular visits thereafter to identify nutritional decline as early as possible.[70] There are several nutritional assessment factors specific to the cancer patient, and these are listed in Table 67.4. Involuntary weight loss is a key indicator of undernutrition, and it is often a sign associated with a poorer prognosis and survival. The rate of weight loss is also important. Patients should be asked their usual weight, if they have had unintentional weight loss or if

**TABLE 67.4**
**Nutritional Assessment Factors in the Cancer Patient**

Involuntary weight loss

Comparison to usual, pre-illness, or ideal body weight

Anorexia and food intake

Anthropometric measures

Biochemical and cellular biomarkers

they have been eating less than usual. It is accepted that an involuntary weight loss of 10% of the patient's usual body weight over a period of 6 months or less indicates undernutrition in patients with cancer.[71] The body mass index (BMI) is an expression of weight relative to height (weight [in kg]/height$^2$ [in m]), and this value can be compared with established cutoff points that classify individuals as severely underweight, underweight, normal, overweight, obese, and morbidly obese (Table 67.5). However, these cutoff points are based on healthy adults and may not be appropriate in cancer patients. One complicating factor in cancer patients is the development of edema or ascites; these should be kept in mind when interpreting weight data. Tumor mass could also mask loss of weight and lean body mass. Assessment of weight changes over time may be a more appropriate indicator of nutritional decline, with rapid weight loss indicative of more severe malnutrition.[39]

Ideal body weight is the weight associated with optimal survivorship in populations studied by life insurance companies. A commonly used reference is the 1983 Metropolitan Life Insurance Tables. With these tables, ideal weight range is calculated based on height, body frame size, and sex, but no adjustments are made for age. Studies undertaken at the Gerontology Research Center (GRC), however, indicate that age significantly affects ideal body weight, while sex differences are not significant.[72] For a given height, older subjects have a higher ideal body weight range than younger individuals. Importantly, both tables are based on the same database, except that age is introduced as a variable only by the more recent GRC tables. Since cancer affects both the young and the aged, with the majority of patients being in the older age groups,[73] it is more appropriate to utilize the age-adjusted tables to calculate ideal body weight range. Serious shortcomings still exist since there is no correction for disease-related changes in height, and no guidelines are provided in these tables for patients 70 years or older.

Current weight compared to the expected or ideal body weight range can help to determine the patient's nutritional status. An additional variable for consideration is usual or preillness weight. Therefore, both information on percent ideal weight and percent usual or preillness weight should be collected on all patients. There are healthy individuals who are below their projected weight for many years. From a clinical standpoint, stable weight and an adequate diet often

equate with good nutrition even if the individual is below the ideal body weight range.

Anorexia and decreased food intake have long been recognized as key causes of undernutrition in patients with malignancies.[74,75] Anorexia is a treatable symptom of cancer, which, if left untreated, leads to significant patient discomfort in addition to malnutrition.[76]

A thorough dietary assessment should include current food and fluid intake, previous intake, and any recent changes. This information can be obtained initially by questioning the patient about a subjective loss of appetite and decrease in food intake. In order to further quantify these changes, the patient can be asked to rate his or her appetite level from 0 to 7 (0 = no appetite, 1 = very poor, 2 = poor, 3 = fair, 4 = good, 5 = very good, 6 = excellent, 7 = always hungry). From a report of usual intake, an indication of the patient's macro- and micronutrient intakes can be gained. The assessment should also aim to detect food aversions, intolerances, and any problems with feeding, such as taste changes.[77] Several screening tools have been developed specifically for cancer patients, including the oncology screening tool,[78] which screens patients for weight loss and includes a 2-week history of decreased food intake, nausea/vomiting, diarrhea, mouth sores, or difficulty with chewing and swallowing.

Detailed anthropometric measurements (such as mid-arm circumference and triceps skin fold) have long been utilized to determine skeletal muscle mass and nutritional status.[79] Although the value of these measurements can be limited if done in the hospital setting, serial measurements by the same professional in the outpatient clinic can help assess the patient's ongoing nutritional state. Problems with these measurements include interobserver variability and interference by edema or patient positioning. The decision to do these measurements should often be individualized according to the acuteness of the underlying process, the availability of trained personnel, and the goals of interventions. It should be noted that muscle wasting and loss of adipose tissue reserves seen on physical examination are important but late signs of undernutrition. Ideally, early diagnosis and intervention should be directed at avoiding this advanced stage of undernutrition or cachexia.

The most common biochemical measurements used to assess nutritional status are blood parameters such as serum albumin, prealbumin, and iron levels. However, these parameters are subject to homeostatic mechanisms and may be altered by underlying disease and treatment. These and other tests can be useful to assess protein depletion but are difficult to interpret in patients with advanced cancer who often have metastases to visceral sites with organ dysfunction as well as metabolic and immunologic derangements due to cancer therapy.

Routine chemistry panels include albumin levels, which can be a useful indication of nutritional state. Albumin has a half-life in the circulation of about 3 weeks. Hypoalbuminemia can result from malnutrition but is also associated with liver disease, disseminated malignancies,

**TABLE 67.5**
**BMI Cutoff Points**

| BMI (kg/m$^2$) | Interpretation |
| --- | --- |
| <16 | Severely underweight |
| 16–19 | Underweight |
| 20–25 | Normal |
| 26–30 | Overweight |
| 31–41 | Obese |
| >40 | Morbidly obese |

protein-losing enteropathy, nephrotic syndrome, and conditions leading to expanded plasma volume such as congestive heart failure.

Prealbumin has a half-life of just under 2 days and its level may increase with the use of steroid hormones and can be decreased by liver disease, disseminated malignancies, nephrotic syndrome, inflammatory bowel disease, the use of salicylates, or malnutrition.[80,81]

Transferrin can be measured by the transferrin antigen assay; the iron-binding capacity provides roughly equivalent results. Transferrin has a half-life of about 1 week and it may increase with storage iron depletion or the use of hormonal agents, while it may decrease with infection, malignancy, inflammation, liver disease, nephrotic syndrome, or malnutrition.[82]

Absolute lymphocyte counts can be reduced by malnutrition as well as a variety of other factors. More sophisticated tests (bioimpedance, total body K, BMR, and others) are clinical research procedures.[83]

In many instances, a brief clinical nutritional assessment based on the degree of weight loss from usual or preillness weight, current weight as a percentage of usual and ideal body weight, and dietary history is sufficient to determine the clinical situation and consider potential interventions. We therefore reserve the use of anthropometric and laboratory evaluations to specific individual situations. Interpretations of these evaluations should be based on an assessment of the clinical context.

A number of associated conditions are prevalent in older patients and can affect their food intake and nutrition. Mucositis, as a side effect of chemotherapy or radiation therapy, is common. Oral pain and dryness, poor dentition, periodontal disease, and ill-fitting dentures are also common. Other problems requiring consideration are dysphagia, alteration in taste, fatigue, nausea, vomiting, and diarrhea or constipation. Pain and other symptoms such as dyspnea can also interfere with nutrition. Depression is a well-known cause of weight loss, and depression can worsen due to the stress of coping with cancer. Feelings of isolation and actual social isolation are not uncommon, especially in those patients who do not have strong family support. Socioeconomic and living conditions must be taken into account because they may affect food availability and preparation. These can all be very serious problems for patients with cancer and require a multidisciplinary effort for proper management. Quality of life assessment provides valuable information regarding the patient's perception of his or her health. The European Organisation for Research and Treatment of Cancer Core Quality of Life Questionnaire (EORTC QLQ-30) is a validated measure of quality of life in cancer patients with five functional scales, three symptoms scales, and one global scale.[84] Other questionnaires have been developed for specific cancers.[85,86]

An understanding of the frequency and severity of malnutrition among cancer patients is necessary to better plan preventive, diagnostic, and therapeutic approaches including the allocation of a variety of resources. To this end and as part of a more comprehensive effort, we studied nutrition-related clinical variables in 644 consecutive oncology patients, regardless of type, status, or stage of cancer. The characteristics of these patients are shown in Table 67.6.

The majority was seen as outpatients. We divided patients by age (<65 vs. ≥65), and we analyzed the entire group as well as the subset of patients who had metastatic disease. Ideal body weight range was calculated using the GRC tables. The vast majority of the patients sustained the weight loss shown within a period of 6 months from cancer diagnosis.

As can be seen in Table 67.7, the incidence of weight loss is very high in all patients but particularly in those over the age of 65. Thus, 72% of all patients 65 years or older with metastatic cancer had some degree of weight loss, 56% were underweight, 54% had decreased appetite, and 61% reported a decrease in food intake. Also, 38% of patients 65 years or older with metastatic disease had weight loss of 10% or more of their usual body weight. These data suggest that undernutrition at various stages is highly prevalent among oncology patients, particularly in the older population. Attention to the nutritional status of patients may afford the clinician opportunities for early diagnosis and intervention.

**TABLE 67.6**
**Patient Characteristics in 644 Consecutive Cancer Patients[a]**

| Characteristic | Percent of Patients |
|---|---|
| Age: median (range) in years: 66 (22–91) | |
| <65 | 45 |
| ≥65 | 55 |
| Sex | |
| Women | 53 |
| Men | 47 |
| Type of cancer | |
| Breast | 16 |
| Colon/rectum | 14 |
| Leukemia/lymphoma | 13 |
| Lung/nonsmall cell | 14 |
| Prostate | 5 |
| Stomach | 4 |
| Head/neck squamous | 4 |
| Ovary | 3 |
| Kidney/urinary bladder | 3 |
| Lung/small cell | 2 |
| All others | 22 |
| Stage of cancer | |
| Metastatic | 52 |
| Nonmetastatic | 48 |

[a] Seen at Pacific Shores Medical Group and St. Mary Medical Center, Long Beach, California.

## TABLE 67.7
### Nutritional Variables in 644 Consecutive Cancer Patients[a]

| Variable | All Patients (n = 644) (%) | Patients with Metastases (n = 377) (%) |
|---|---|---|
| Decreased appetite | 54 | 59 |
| Decreased food intake | 61 | 67 |
| Underweight | 49 | 54 |
| Normal weight | 37 | 33 |
| Overweight | 14 | 13 |
| Weight loss | | |
| Any | 74 | 76 |
| Up to 5% | 15 | 15 |
| >5% to <10% | 22 | 20 |
| 10%–20% | 26 | 27 |
| None | 26 | 24 |

[a] Seen at Pacific Shores Medical Group and St. Mary Medical Center, Long Beach, California.

## NUTRITIONAL THERAPY OF ANOREXIA AND CACHEXIA

### COUNSELING

In patients with cancer, there is an association between poor nutritional parameters and worse overall morbidity and quality of life.[87] The benefits of initial and follow-up evaluations and counseling by a registered dietitian, preferably in the context of a team approach, can be enormous, although difficult to quantify.[88] However, recent studies indicate improved nutritional intake and quality of life after individualized dietary counseling.[89,90] The main benefits relate to patient satisfaction, nutrition improvement or maintenance, compliance with team or institutional management protocols and guidelines, and a judicious use of risky and expensive treatments. The costs of nutritional counseling are modest when compared to other interventions. Table 67.8 shows the benefits, methodology, and risks of common nutrition interventions. Nutritional evaluation and counseling, usually undertaken by a registered dietitian, is a first and important step. Ideally, a dietitian should be an integral part of the cancer care team. Compliance with dietary advice can be promoted by regular

## TABLE 67.8
### Benefits, Methodology, and Risks of Nutrition Interventions

| | Benefits | Methodology | Risks |
|---|---|---|---|
| 1. Counseling | Patient satisfaction, nutrition maintenance, and adherence to protocols | One initial and two follow-up visits by dietitian | None |
| 2. Food supplements | Nutrition maintenance | | Limited risks: diarrhea, nausea |
| a. Homemade | Avoid or delay need for more expensive therapy | a. Three 8 oz servings = 750 kcal/day | a. Diarrhea with lactose intolerance |
| b. Commercial | | b. Three 8 oz servings = 750–1080 kcal/day | b. Patients may not like taste. |
| 3. Appetite stimulants | | | |
| a. Megestrol acetate oral suspension | a. Improved appetite, weight, well-being, and quality of life | a. 200 mg/day, 1-month supply; 400 mg/day, 1-month supply; 800 mg/day, 1-month supply | a. Impotence, vaginal bleeding, and deep vein thrombosis |
| b. Dronabinol | b. Improved appetite and no significant weight change | b. 2.5 mg/day, 1-month supply; 5 mg/day, 1-month supply | b. Euphoria, somnolence, dizziness, and confusion |
| c. Prednisone | c. Short-term (4 weeks) appetite stimulation (see text) | c. 40 mg/day, 1-month supply | c. Hypokalemia, muscle weakness, cushingoid features, hyperglycemia, and immune suppression |
| 4. Enteral nutrition | Maintenance of nutrition via enteral route when oral route is not possible | Requires nasogastric, gastrostomy, or jejunostomy tube placement | Aspiration, diarrhea, nausea, bloating, infection, and bleeding |
| 5. Home parenteral nutrition | Maintenance of nutrition when no other alternative is appropriate. No evidence of improved survival in end-stage cancer | Central catheter surgically placed. Parenteral infusion equipment and parenteral formulas: dextrose (20%–25% w/w), crystalline amino acids (2%–4% w/w), and lipid emulsions (500 cc/day → 500 cc/week) | Catheter-related pneumothorax, sepsis, thrombosis, and bleeding. Hepatic dysfunction, fluid and electrolyte imbalance |

contact between the health-care provider and the patient, including regular nutritional assessments and advice.[91]

In addition to assessing the clinical nutritional parameters previously outlined, it is our practice to first determine, through the dietary history, whether the patient is consuming a "balanced diet." Nutritional assessment serves to confirm the presence, extent, degree, or severity and type of malnutrition and to determine the nutritional needs of the patient and nutritional support required. The dietitian obtains a 24–72 h recall diet history either verbally or, preferably, recorded at home. The diet record is then examined to assess the adequacy of calories and protein utilizing food analysis tables as compared to estimated energy and protein needs. In addition to assessing current food and fluid intake, any recent changes should be noted, along with food aversions, intolerances, or problems with feeding, such as taste changes.[77]

Energy requirements should be based on individual needs. Usually a weight maintenance diet depends on the BEE and is calculated based on the Harris–Benedict formula[24] that, on an average, results in a daily requirement of 20–25 kcal/kg of body weight. However, the addition of a stress factor may be necessary depending on weight change or the disease process. For example, a stress factor of between 0% and 20% has been suggested for patients with solid tumors.[92–94] Alterations in protein metabolism are common in the course of cancer, including whole-body protein turnover, increased protein synthesis and catabolism, as well as an increase in skeletal muscle breakdown. To account for the stress induced by the disease and treatment, protein requirements of cancer patients can be determined by adjusting the estimated requirement for healthy individuals to account for the stress induced by the disease and treatment.[95] Estimated protein requirements range from 1.2 to 2.0 g/kg body weight/day depending on the state of malnutrition and metabolic stress.[36,39]

One goal of nutrition education and counseling is to have the patient increase consumption of nutrient-dense foods to correct nutritional imbalances and deficiencies in order to achieve and maintain a desirable weight. Nutrient-dense foods are those with a high content in calories, protein, fat, and vitamins relative to their volume. Liquid supplements are the most common types of nutritional supplements and are readily available for patient consumption and are effective when patients are unable to meet requirements with normal foods alone, despite dietary counseling.[89] Patients may be anorectic due to illness or be affected by disabling factors such as difficulty in chewing, inability to prepare foods for themselves, visual difficulties, decreased energy level, or poor access to foods. Nutritional supplements may be homemade and are usually milk based, or they are commercially prepared and packaged. Although somewhat expensive, commercial supplements provide balanced and fortified (vitamin and mineral enriched) nutrition that require little or no preparation.

Not all cancer patients have the same requirements for nutrition. One major difference is whether patients are losing weight or have been treated successfully and are trying to prevent a recurrence through healthful nutrition. In the former case, calorically dense foods including those with low nutrient density can be used to increase the efficiency of calorie conversion to body fat stores. One limitation of this approach is that malnourished patients often are limited in their ability to absorb and digest fat due to the effects of malnutrition or enteritis due to radiation or chemotherapy. Therefore, over-prescription of high-fat foods can in some cases lead to GI distress. Foods containing refined sugar can also be used in these patients, as long as the patient has normal glucose tolerance. Since diabetes is not an uncommon comorbid condition in cancer patients, this is a practical consideration. Listed in Table 67.9 are calorically dense foods and strategies for these types of patients.

## TABLE 67.9
### Foods Recommended to Increase Calorie and Protein Intake of the Patient with Cancer

| Food Group | Recommendations |
| --- | --- |
| Fruits and vegetables | Fruit juice added to canned fruit; pureed fruit added to milk, cereals, pudding, ice cream, and gelatin; gelatin made with fruit juice to replace water; tender, cooked vegetables (mashed white or sweet potatoes, squash, spinach, and carrots); vegetables added to soups and sauces; vegetables in cream or cheese sauces |
| Grains | Hot cereals prepared with milk instead of water; high-protein noodles; noodles or rice in casseroles and soups; breaded and floured meats; bread or rice pudding; dense breads (i.e., bagels) and dense cereals (granolas, mueslis) |
| Beverages | Milk beverages; shakes made with fruit juices and sherbet when milk is not tolerated |
| Milk and calcium equivalents | Custards; milkshakes; ice cream; yogurt; cheeses; cheesecake; double strength milk (1 quart fluid milk mixed with 1 cup nonfat dry milk powder); cottage cheese; flavored milk; pudding; commercial eggnog; cream soups; nonfat dry milk powder added to puddings, soups, sauces and gravies, casseroles, and mixed dishes |
| Meat and protein equivalents | Diced or ground meat; casseroles; smooth peanut butter; cheese; egg and egg dishes; chopped, diced, or pureed meats mixed with soups, sauces, and gravies; fish, poultry, and vegetable protein meat substitutes; tuna, meat, or cheese in cream sauces |
| Fats | Margarine or oil added to vegetables, hot cereals, and casseroles; cream used in place of milk or added to fruits and desserts; sour cream; salad dressings; mayonnaise mixed with tuna, egg, and chicken salad |
| Sweets | Desserts made with dry milk powder, peanut butter, or eggs |

## FOOD SUPPLEMENTS

Liquid concentrated food supplements providing high calorie and protein, low-volume nutrients, and oral supplementation are the simplest, most natural, and least invasive method of increasing nutrient intake. The benefits of oral supplementation include increased appetite and weight gain, decreased GI toxicity, and improved performance status.[96–98] These products are particularly helpful when patients cannot maintain an adequate intake through a regular diet but are able to swallow and have a relatively intact GI tract.

Dietitians can help patients select products based on tolerance and palatability. Commercially prepared supplements are available in a variety of flavors (including unflavored) and in a variety of nutrient compositions. Most commercially prepared supplements are available in ready-to-drink cans or boxes and are usually lactose free, which for the patient is often more acceptable due to the increased incidence of perceived milk intolerance in this population. Vitamin and mineral fortified protein meal replacements designed to be mixed with milk provide an inexpensive and generally well-tolerated alternative for those who are not lactose intolerant. These supplements have vitamin, mineral, calorie, fat, carbohydrate, and protein content similar to most commercially prepared supplements.

Most 8 oz commercial supplements supply 1.0–1.5 kcal/mL, 8–15 g of protein, and 5–12 g of fat and are fortified with vitamins and minerals. When patients have difficulty in consuming adequate volumes of enteral supplement, then a high-caloric supplement containing 2 kcal/mL, for example, Novasource 2.0 (Novartis Pharmaceuticals) or TwoCal HN (Abbott Laboratories), can be used. The success of supplementation depends on sufficient quantities being consumed over an extended period of time. Acceptability and palatability of the supplement are key, and flavor, texture, and volume are all important.[99]

The volume and choice of supplement are based on patient's individual nutrient needs and preferences and GI tolerance. Supplements with fiber, generally soy or oat fiber, are available and may be beneficial to the patient who has diarrhea or constipation. Nutritional supplements are generally well accepted and may offer relief to a patient who has difficulty eating solid food. Tolerability can be enhanced by starting with small quantities and by diluting the supplement with water or ice to decrease osmolality. A patient will usually accept one to three 8 oz supplements per day, but there is great individual variability. Variety in supplements will help patients avoid taste fatigue, which is one main drawback to oral supplementation.[100] Patients who have alterations in taste or nausea may better tolerate an unflavored supplement.

A common concern of patients and families is whether adding vitamins and other micronutrients to the patient's diet is beneficial. An analysis of the dietary record for the recommended number of servings from the basic four food groups (milk, meat and meat substitutes, vegetable and fruit, and grain) helps establish whether the minimum vitamin and mineral requirements are met. A computerized diet analysis program can help to quickly and accurately assess the nutrient content including vitamins and minerals. When intake is inadequate, we prescribe a daily multivitamin.

Patients should be provided with practical dietary advice about how to improve daily caloric intake, and the following are some simple tips to increase food intake:

- Avoid favorite foods after highly emetogenic chemotherapy to prevent the development of food aversions.
- Emphasize consumption of higher-calorie foods that are still "nutrient-dense" foods as part of main meals or snacks, that is, fruit juices, cheeses, whole milk, and yogurt.
- Avoid the "Why don't you eat?" complaint. The patient should not be psychologically punished by the cancer care team or the family for not eating but rather should be supported to overcome anorexia and other problems that lead to decreased food intake.
- Emphasize the pleasurable as well as social aspects of meals. Encourage patients to have their meals in a relaxed, friendly, and familiar atmosphere.
- Moderate alcohol intake is usually compatible with treatments and should be allowed before meals unless contraindicated.
- Avoid odors that can cause nausea. A short walk outside while meals are being prepared is advisable.
- Encourage food supplements and snacks between meals without being concerned that they may affect intake at mealtime.

Patients are often deeply interested in the topic of nutrition as an unproven treatment. However, many will not bring up this topic unless encouraged and listened to in a nonjudgmental fashion. Open discussion and patient education may help prevent untoward effects of unbalanced diets and introduce nutrition-related issues into the mainstream of oncology care.

## OTHER THERAPIES

A number of alternative therapies are being used by cancer patients in addition to standard medical oncology therapy,[101] and these are listed in Table 67.10. For this chapter, the nutrition alternatives will be outlined without reference to acupuncture or other nonnutritional therapies. Often patients fail to indicate that they are using these nutritional therapies. A number of potential side effects and concerns, listed in Table 67.11, may arise and need to be addressed.

Until recently, most vitamin and herb preparations were thought to be nontoxic. Recent animal studies suggest that antioxidants may affect tumor biology. The α-Tocopherol β-Carotene Cancer Prevention Study (ATBC) and β-Carotene and Retinol Efficacy Trial (CARET) trials[99] in smokers demonstrated an increased incidence of lung cancer following the

**TABLE 67.10**

**Alternative Nutritional Therapies Being Used by Cancer Patients**

Multivitamins and single-vitamin supplements

Low-fat-, high-fiber-, and soy-protein-supplemented diets

Specific macrobiotic diets

Vegetable and grass juicing

Herbal supplements (green tea extract, antioxidants)

Chinese herbal medicine (mushrooms, teas, roots)

**TABLE 67.11**

**Potential Side Effects and Concerns**

Vitamin toxicities (e.g., vitamin A > 5000 IU/day)

Possible vitamin effects on tumor biology (apoptosis, proliferation)

Vitamin imbalances and conditioned deficiencies

Drug–nutrient interactions

administration of β-carotene at a dose of 30 mg/day. There were no cancer-stimulatory effects noted with these doses of β-carotene in nonsmokers in a large heart disease prevention trial. However, there remains real uncertainty as to the safety of vitamins and mineral supplementation during chemotherapy or radiation therapy. For the large numbers of patients being diagnosed today with early cancers of the breast and prostate, vitamin supplementation is as safe as in the general population once the treatment has been completed, and nutritional intervention may prevent or delay cancer recurrence. However, the possibility of antioxidant effects on tumor biology or the effectiveness of antitumor drugs on radiation therapy requires much more research before general recommendations can be made. Administration of cytotoxic drugs results in oxidative stress, which may interfere with cytotoxic effects or contribute to side effects. Antioxidants may enhance the anticancer effects of chemotherapy by detoxifying ROS.[102–105]

Accumulating evidence supporting a role for inflammatory mediators in the pathogenesis of cancer-associated malnutrition has led to the suggestion that dietary supplement with anti-inflammatory properties may be beneficial.[106] Eicosapentaenoic acid (EPA) is an essential long-chain n-3 polyunsaturated fatty acid. Individual studies have indicated that EPA can attenuate cancer-related wasting, improve immune function, halt or reverse weight loss, modulate the acute-phase response, or prolong survival in some patients.[107–109] However, results are not consistent for all cancer populations, and further studies would serve to confirm these studies in different cancer groups. At this time, each patient and each oncologist must decide on the advisability of a given regimen for a given cancer patient based on clinical criteria without the benefit of a large scientific basis of controlled trials.

## REFERENCES

1. Laviano, A. and Meguid, M.M. *Nutrition* 12: 358; 1996.
2. Bozzetti, F. In: Grimble. G. and Silk, D. eds. *Artificial Nutrition Support in Clinical Practice*, 2nd edn., Payne-James J. (ed.), GMM, London, U.K., p. 639, 2001.
3. Brennan, M.F. *Cancer Res* 58: 1867; 1977.
4. Bosaeus, I. et al. *Intl J Cancer* 93: 380; 2001.
5. Andreyev, H.J. et al. *Eur J Cancer* 34: 503; 1998.
6. Zeiderman, M.R. and McMahon, M.J. *Clin Nutr* 8: 161; 1989.
7. Meguid, M.M. et al. *Surg Clin North Am* 66: 1167; 1986.
8. van Bokhorst-de van der Schueren, M.A. et al. *Clin Nutr* 19: 437; 1997.
9. Jagoe, R.T., Goodship, T.H. and Gibson, G.J. *Ann Thoracic Surg* 71: 936; 2001.
10. MacDonald, N. *J Supportive Oncol* 1: 279; 2003.
11. Brennan, M.F. *New Engl J Med* 305: 375; 1981.
12. Shike, M. et al. *Ann Int Med* 101: 303; 1984.
13. Argiles, J.M. et al. *Drug Discov Today* 8: 838; 2003.
14. Argiles, J.M. et al. *Curr Opin Clin Nutr Metab Care* 6: 401; 2003.
15. Argiles, J.M. et al. *Int J Biochem Cell Biol* 35: 405; 2003.
16. Chlebowski, R.T. and Heber, D. *Cancer Res* 42: 2495; 1982.
17. Holroyde, C.P. et al. *Cancer Res* 35: 3710; 1975.
18. Chlebowski, R.T. and Heber, D. *Surg Clin North Am* 66: 957; 1986.
19. Burt, M.E. et al. *Cancer* 53: 1246; 1984.
20. Heber, D. et al. *Cancer Res* 42: 4815; 1982.
21. Jeevanandam, M. et al. *Metabolism* 35: 304; 1986.
22. Shaw, J.H.F. and Wolfe, R.R. *Ann Surg* 205: 368; 1987.
23. Bennegard, K., Lundgren, F. and Lundholm, K. *Clin Physiol* 6: 539; 1986.
24. Byerley, L.O. et al. *Cancer* 67: 2900; 1991.
25. Warren, S. *Am J Med Sci* 184: 610;1932.
26. Terepka, A.R. and Waterhouse, C. *Am J Med* 20: 225; 1956.
27. Fenninger, L.D. and Mider, G.B. *Adv Cancer Res* 2: 229; 1954.
28. Heber, D. et al. *Cancer* 58: 1867; 1986.
29. Long, C.L. et al. *J Parent Ent Nutr* 5: 366; 1981.
30. Bozzetti, F., Pagnoni, A.M. and Del Vecchio, M. *Surg Gynecol Obst* 150: 229; 1980.
31. Dempsey, D.T. et al. *Cancer* 53: 1265; 1984.
32. Knox, L.S., Crosby, L.O., Feurer, I.D. et al. *Ann Surg* 197: 152; 1983.
33. Fredrix, E.W., Staal-van den Brekel, A.J. and Wouters, E.F. *Cancer* 79: 717; 1997.
34. Peacock, J.L. et al. *Surgery* 102: 465; 1987.
35. Rofe, A.M. et al. *Anticancer Res* 14: 647; 1994.
36. Mutlu, E.A. and Mobarhan, S. *Nutr Clin Care* 3: 3; 2000.
37. Argiles, J.M. and Azcon-Bieto, J. *J Mol Cell Biochem* 81: 3; 1988.
38. Heber, D. *Nutrition* 5: 135; 1989.
39. Nitenberg, G. and Raynard, B. *Crit Rev Oncol Hematol* 34: 137; 2000.
40. Tayek, J., Heber, D. and Chlebowski, R.T. *Lancet* 2: 241; 1987.
41. Robinson, S.C. and Coussens, L.M. *Adv Cancer Res* 93: 159; 2005.
42. Strassmann, G. and Kambayashi, T. *Cytok Mol Ther* 1: 107; 1995.
43. Plata-Salaman, C.R. *Nutrition* 16: 1009;2000.
44. Fearon, K.C.H. *Proc Nutr Soc* 51: 251;1992.
45. Wigmore, S.J., Plester, C.E., Richardson, R.A. and Fearon, K.C.H. *Br J Cancer* 75: 106; 1997.

46. Kotler, D.P., Tierney, A.R., Culpepper-Morgan, J.A. et al. *J Parent Enteral Nutr* 14. 454, 1990.
47. Houten, L., Reilly, A.A., *J Surg Oncol* 13: 111; 1980.
48. Safdie, F.M., Dorff, T., Quinn, D. et al. *Aging* (Albany, NY) 1: 988; 2009.
49. Lee, C., Raffaghello, L., Longo, V.D. *Drug Resist Updat* 15: 114; 2012.
50. Lee, C., Raffaghello, L., Brandhorst, S. et al. *Sci Transl Med* 4: 124; 2012.
51. Warburg, O. *Science* 123: 309; 1956.
52. Herrmann, K., Benz, M.R., Czernin, J. et al. *Clin Cancer Res* 18: 2024; 2012.
53. Trachootham, D., Alexandre, J. and Huang, P. *Nat Rev Drug Discov* 8: 579; 2009.
54. Brahimi-Horn, M.C., Chiche, J. and Poyssegur, J. *Curr Opin Cell Biol* 19: 223; 2007.
55. Gatenby, R.A. and Gillies, R.J. *Nat Rev Cancer* 4: 891; 2004.
56. Zu, X.L. and Guppy, M. *Biochem Biophys Res Commun* 313: 459; 2004.
57. Heiden, M.G., Cantley, L.C. and Thompson, C.B. *Science* 324: 1029; 2009.
58. Wieman, H.L., Wofford, J.A. and Rathmell, J.C. *Mol Biol Cell* 18: 1437; 2007.
59. Copeland, W.C., Wachsman, J.T., Johnson, F.M. and Penta, J.S. *Cancer Invest* 20: 557; 2002.
60. Nomoto, S., Sanchez-Cespedes, M. and Sidransky, D. *Methods Mol Biol* 197: 107; 2002.
61. Carew, JS, Zhou, Y., Albitar, M. et al. *Leukemia* 17: 1427; 2003.
62. Pelicano, H, Xu, R.H., Du, M. et al. *J Cell Biol* 175: 913; 2006.
63. Matoba, S., Kang, J.G., Patino, W.D. et al. *Science* 312: 1650; 2006.
64. Bensaad, K., Tsuruta, A., Selak, M.A. et al. *Cell* 126: 117; 2006.
65. Kroemer, G., Pouyssegur, J. *Cancer Cell* 13: 472; 2008.
66. Christofk, H.R., Heiden, M.G., Harris, M.H. et al. *Nature* 452: 230; 2008.
67. Shike, M. and Brenna, M.F. In: DeVita, V.T.R., Hellman, S. and Rosenberg, S.A., eds. *Cancer: Principles and Practice of Oncology*, JB Lippincott, Philadelphia, PA, p. 2029, 1989.
68. DeWys, W.D. et al. *Am J Med* 69: 491; 1980.
68. Langer, C.J., Hoffman, J.P. and Ottery, F.D. *Nutrition* 17: 1S; 2001.
69. Holder, H. *Br J Nursing* 12: 667; 2003.
70. Blackburn, G. et al. *JPEN* 1: 11; 1977.
71. Andres, R. et al. *Ann Intern Med* 103: 1030; 1985.
72. Boring, C., Squires, T. and Tong, T. *CA: A Cancer J Clin* 41: 19; 1991.
73. DeWys, W. *Semin Oncol* 12: 452; 1985.
74. Theologides, A. *Cancer* 43: 2013; 1979.
75. Tchekmedyian, N.S. et al. *Oncology* 4: 185; 1990.
76. Baker, F. et al. *Psycho-oncology* 11: 273; 2002.
77. MSKCC Adult Oncology Screening Tool, Clinical Dietitian Staff 1994–1995, Food Service Department, Memorial Sloan-Kettering Cancer Center.
78. Chumlea, W.C. and Baumgartner, R.N. *Am J Clin Nutr* 50: 1158; 1989.
79. Henry, J.B. Clinical chemistry. In: *Clinical Diagnosis and Management by Laboratory Methods*, 18th edn., WD Saunders Co., Philadelphia, PA, 316, 1991.
80. Sacherk, R.A., McPhersonk, R.A. and Campos, J.M. Serum proteins of diagnostic significance. In: *Widmann's Clinical Interpreter of Laboratory Tests*, 10th edn., Table 9–11, FA Davis Company, Philadelphia, PA, 352, 1991.
81. Brittenham, G.M. Disorders of iron metabolism: Iron deficiency and overload. In: *Hematology: Basic Principles and Practice*, Hoffman R. (ed.), Churchill Livingstone Inc., New York, 334, 1991.
82. Harrisk, J.A. and Benedict, F.G. *Biometric Studies of Basal Metabolism in Man*. Publication No. 279. Carnegie Institute of Washington, Washington, DC, 1919.
83. Aaronsonk, N.K. et al. *J Natl Cancer Inst* 85: 365–376; 1993.
84. Kaptein, A.A., Morita, S. and Sakamoto, J. *World J Gastroenterol* 11: 3189; 2005.
85. Avis, N.E., Crawford, S. and Manuel, J. *J Clin Oncology* 23: 3322; 2005.
86. Ravasco, P.M. et al. *Support Care Cancer* 12: 246; 2004.
87. Chlebowski, R.T. et al. *Cancer* 58: 183; 1986.
88. Ravasco, P.M., Monteiro-Grillo, I. and Camilo, M.E. *Radiother Oncol* 67: 213; 2003.
89. Ravasco, P.M. et al. *J Clin Oncol* 23: 1341; 2005.
90. Wickham, R.S. et al. *Oncol Nurs Forum* 26: 697; 1999.
91. Parenteral and Enteral Nutrition Group of the British Dietetic Association (PEN group). *A Pocket Guide to Clinical Nutrition*, 3rd edn., The British Dietetic Association, Birmingham, U.K., 2004.
92. Hyltander, A. et al. *Eur J Cancer* 27: 9; 1991.
93. Barak, N., Wall-Alonso, E. and Sitrin, M.D. *J Parenteral Ent Nutr* 26: 231; 2002.
94. McAtear, C.A., Arrowsmith, H. and McWhirter, J. Current perspectives on enteral nutrition in adults. A report by the Working Party of the British Association for Parenteral and Enteral Nutrition (BAPEN), Maidenhead, U.K., 1999.
95. Bounous, G., Gentile, J.M. and Hugon, J. *Can J Surg* 14: 312; 1971.
96. Nayel, H., el-Ghoneimy, E. and el-Haddad, S. *Nutrition* 8: 13; 1992.
97. Ovesen, L. and Allingstrup, L. *J Parenteral Enteral Nutr* 16: 275; 1992.
98. Bell, E.A., Roe, L.W. and Rolls, B.J. *Physiol Behav* 78: 593; 2003.
99. Rivadeneiera, D.E. et al. *CA: A Cancer J Clin* 48: 69; 1998.
100. Wargovich, M.J. *Curr Opin Gastroenterol* 15: 177; 1999.
101. Prasad, K.N. et al. *J Am Coll Nutr* 18: 13; 1999.
102. Conklin, K.A. *Nutr Cancer* 37: 1; 2000.
103. Lamson, D.W. and Brignall, M.S. *Altern Med Rev* 5: 152; 2000.
104. Lamson, D.W. and Brignall, M.S. *Altern Med Rev* 5: 196; 2000.
105. McCarthy, D.O. *Biol Res Nurs* 5: 3; 2003.
106. Tisdale, M.J. *Nutrition* 12: 31S; 1996.
107. Gogos, C.A. et al. *Cancer* 15: 395; 1998.
108. Barber, M.D. et al. *J Nutr* 129: 1120; 1999.
109. Fearon, K.C. et al. *Gut* 52: 1479; 2003.

# 68 Nutrition and Age Related Eye Diseases

*Rohini Vishwanathan and Elizabeth J. Johnson*

## CONTENTS

## INTRODUCTION

Vision loss among the elderly is an important health problem. Approximately one person in three has some form of vision-reducing eye disease by the age of 65.[1] Age-related cataract, age-related macular degeneration (AMD), diabetic retinopathy, and glaucoma are the major diseases resulting in visual impairment and blindness in the aging U.S. population.[1–7]

A healthy lifestyle is implicated in the decreased risk of all of these age-related eye diseases. Of particular interest is the possibility that nutritional counseling or intervention might reduce the incidence or retard the progression of these diseases. The aim of this chapter is to review the clinical and epidemiological evidence to support a role for nutrition in age-related eye diseases.

## CATARACTS

Age-related cataract is the major cause of visual impairment and blindness in the aging U.S. population. In the United States, age-related cataract affects about one in every six people over the age of 40 years or about 22 million people.[3] Cataract removal accompanied by intraocular lens implant is the most commonly performed surgeries, with more than a million surgeries performed every year.[3,8] Although cataract can be treated with lens implantation, the procedure is costly, accounting for approximately $6.8 billion in direct medical costs for outpatient, inpatient, and prescription drugs.[3,8,9]

Cataract type is defined by location in the lens. The most common form is nuclear cataracts, which is found in the center (nucleus) of the lens. Nuclear cataracts are usually associated with advancing age. Cortical cataract begins as whitish, wedge-shaped opacities at the edges of the lens (cortex) and progresses toward the center. Cortical cataract is often associated with farsightedness, diabetes, and natural aging. Subcapsular cataract is found in the back of the lens in the membrane that envelops the lens (capsule). Subcapsular cataract is usually seen in patients who use steroids or who suffer from diabetes or extreme nearsightedness.

## ANTIOXIDANT VITAMINS

The lens is particularly vulnerable to oxidative damage due to its exposure to light. Oxidative damage can lead to denaturation of the lens protein to result in loss of transparency and increased light scattering in the lens. The antioxidant vitamins C and E may reduce the risk of cataracts through their role as an antioxidant.

*Vitamin C.* Results from several epidemiological studies find an inverse association between vitamin C intake from both diet and supplement and at least one type of cataract.[10–20] For example, observations from the Nurses Health Study's Nutrition and Vision Project, a prospective, observational study, found that vitamin C intake ≥362 mg/day for 10 years or longer in women below the age of 60 was associated with a 57% lower incidence of nuclear cataracts.[20] However, such a relationship was not always found in those using vitamin C supplements for ≥10 years.[10,15,21–25] Others have reported that vitamin C intake had no effect on cortical cataract and cataract extraction in women aged ≥60 years.[26,27] Furthermore, observations from two studies suggest that intake of high doses of vitamin C may increase the risk of cataract. There was an increased risk of cortical cataract in older women (≥60 years) who consumed vitamin C supplements for 5–9 years compared to the those taking vitamin C for 1–4 years and ≥10 years and those who never used vitamin C supplements.[26] Similarly, in a population-based, prospective study involving 24,593 women (≥65 years), a significantly higher risk of cataract was observed in those consuming ~1000 mg vitamin C supplements but not among those consuming multivitamin, which contain much lower levels of vitamin C.[28]

Reports on a possible association between plasma vitamin C concentrations and cataract risk have also been somewhat inconsistent. There are many reports of an inverse relationship between plasma ascorbic acid concentrations and the prevalence of cataract.[11,29–33] For example, the National Health and Nutrition Examination Survey II (NHANES II) correlated a 1 mg/dL increase in plasma ascorbate with a 26% decreased risk of cataracts in older (62–70 years) Americans.[31] However, others have observed that plasma vitamin C concentrations were not associated with risk of nuclear or cortical cataract.[25,34] Furthermore, the India–United States case-control study of age-related cataracts found an increased prevalence of posterior subcapsular (PSC) and nuclear cataracts with increased plasma vitamin C concentrations.[35] In this study, however, when vitamin C status was combined with other indicators of

antioxidant status (glutathione peroxidase [GPx], vitamin E, and glucose-6-phosphate dehydrogenase), the relationship became protective.

*Vitamin E.* The role of vitamin E, from food and supplements, in the development and progression of cataracts has been evaluated in several epidemiological studies. Two studies have observed that those in the highest quintile for vitamin E intake had a 40%–50% less at risk for cataract compared to those in the lowest quintile.[14,24] Others have[15] observed a lower prevalence of nuclear cataract in the highest quintile category of total vitamin E intake relative to those in the lowest quintile, but this relationship was observed in men only. In 3271 subjects (≥40 years) in Australia, vitamin E intake was related to 47% increased risk for PSC cataract.[36] However, there are several reports of no differences between persons with high and low vitamin E intakes.[10,11,37]

In the Women's Health Study cohort, those in the highest quintile for vitamin E intake had a significantly reduced risk of cataract. In this study, 70% of the women consumed vitamin E supplements; the median intake was 262 mg/day.[38] In a longitudinal study, it was found that regular vitamin E supplement users and persons with high plasma vitamin E had approximately 50% lower risk of nuclear cataract.[27] The use of vitamin E supplements for ≥10 years was found to slow the nuclear opacification during a 5-year follow-up in the Nurses' Health Study cohort.[39] However, in another study involving participants from this same study, vitamin E intake from the diet and supplements was not associated with cortical and PSC cataract.[20] In participants of the Vitamin E and Cataract Prevention Study (VECAT),[40] use of vitamin E supplementation was significantly associated with absence of cortical cataract, but not with nuclear cataract. Others[17] reported that the prevalence of cataract was 56% lower in persons who were using vitamin E supplement compared to persons not using supplements.

There has been only one randomized, double-masked, placebo-controlled trial evaluating a vitamin E intervention and cataract prevention. Pharmacological doses of vitamin E (500 IU) for 4 years was reported to reduce the incidence of or progression of nuclear, cortical, or PSC cataracts in subjects aged 55–80 years.[41] This may provide the best evidence for a role for vitamin E in cataract prevention.

The majority of studies that examined the relationship between plasma vitamin E and cataract report that an increased plasma vitamin E was protective against the risk of cataract.[25,27,34,42–44] One of these studies observed that cataract risk was not related to plasma vitamin E concentrations.[45] In contrast, studies have found increased levels of plasma α-tocopherol to be a risk factor for nuclear,[46] cortical,[23,33] and PSC cataracts.[23]

## CAROTENOIDS

The majority of the epidemiological data suggest that dietary carotenoids function in cataract prevention. This may be due to their role as antioxidants. Taylor et al.[20]

reported an 81% reduced rate of PSC cataract in female nonsmokers in the highest versus lowest quintile for total carotenoid intake and a 59% reduced rate in those with the highest plasma total carotenoids concentration. The Melbourne Visual Impairment Study, an observational study of >3000 over the age of 40 years, reported an inverse correlation between high lutein and zeaxanthin intake and the risk of nuclear cataracts.[47] Delcourt et al.[48] observed a 75% lower risk of nuclear cataracts among individuals with high plasma zeaxanthin, but not lutein, in a prospective study of 899 aged ≥60 years.

Among the carotenoids, lutein and zeaxanthin are the only ones to be found in the lens.[49] Lower intake of lutein-rich foods, for example, green leafy vegetables, was reported to be related to an increased rate of cataract extraction.[10] Similarly, it was observed that women in the highest quintile of lutein intake had a 27% lower prevalence of nuclear cataract than those in the lowest quintile of lutein intake.[50] In this study, this was not observed in men. In the Nurses' Health Study, those with the highest quintile of intake of lutein and zeaxanthin had a 22% decreased risk of cataract surgery and nuclear cataract compared with those in the lowest quintile after adjusting for other risk factors.[13,51] The intake of other dietary carotenoids were not associated with nuclear cataract.[13] Similar findings were observed in the U.S. male health professional's prospective study, in which men in the highest fifth of lutein and zeaxanthin intake had a 19% lower risk of cataract surgery relative to men in the lowest fifth. There was no relationship observed with the other carotenoids.[52] The Beaver Dam Eye Study found that the incidence of nuclear cataract in subjects in the highest quintile of lutein intake was half of that found in those in the lowest quintile.[37] Data from an observational study of 372 volunteers found that the risk of PSC cataract was lowest in those with highest plasma concentrations of lutein, whereas the risk of nuclear cataract and cortical cataract was lowest in subjects with the highest plasma concentration of α-carotene or β-carotene and lycopene, respectively.[45] In this study, there was no relationship between plasma lutein and zeaxanthin and cortical and PSC cataract. In a prospective observational study, higher intakes of lutein and zeaxanthin from both food and supplements were significantly related to a 20% decreased risk of cataract, but there was no association between dietary or plasma β-carotene.[38] Retrospective data from the Beaver Dam Eye Study cohort found a 71% reduced rate of nuclear cataract in men with the highest intake of β-carotene intake compared to those with the lowest intake but a 2.8-fold higher rate of nuclear cataract in women with the highest compared to the lowest serum β-carotene concentration.[15,37,53,54]

There has been only one randomized, double-masked, placebo-controlled trial involving a single carotenoid intervention and cataract. In this study, U.S. male physicians showed no overall effect of β-carotene supplementation (50 mg/day on alternate days for 12 years) on the incidence or cataract surgery.[55] However, β-carotene supplementation was related to reduce the risk of cataract by about 25% in smokers.

## B Vitamins

The B vitamins may have a protective role in cataract prevention through their involvement in homocysteine metabolism.[56–58] Hyperhomocysteinemia produces oxidative stress by generating reactive oxygen species spontaneously.[59] The B vitamins have been found to be folate, and vitamin $B_2$, $B_6$, or $B_{12}$ insufficiency was associated with hyperhomocysteinemia.[60] The Blue Mountains Eye Study reported that use of thiamin and folate supplements was associated with reduced prevalence of nuclear and cortical cataracts with a statistically significant trend for dose. This study also found that use of riboflavin, niacin, and vitamin $B_{12}$ supplements was related to a decreased risk of cortical cataract.[61] In the Linxian trials, supplementation with riboflavin (3 mg) and niacin (40 mg) for 5–6 years significantly lowered risk of nuclear cataract in a rural Chinese population.[62] However, a significant increased risk of PSC was also observed with riboflavin/niacin supplementation, although the numbers or cases were small. In the Nurses' Health Study cohort, higher intake of riboflavin and thiamin was associated with a lower prevalence and a slower progression of nuclear cataract over a 5-year period.[13,39] This study also reported that women with higher baseline cataract and higher niacin intake had a smaller increase in nuclear cataract. In the Blue Mountains Eye Study,[63] riboflavin and thiamin intakes were also observed to have a protective effect. Higher dietary intake of riboflavin and folate was related to reduced nuclear sclerosis in the Beaver Dam Eye Study.[15] Riboflavin and niacin intakes were also associated with reduced prevalence of cortical cataract in the Lens Opacities Case-Control Study.[14,15]

Not all studies have reported a protective effect of the B vitamins. A null effect of dietary or supplemental intake of riboflavin and niacin on cataract has also been reported.[10,61]

## Zinc

Zinc has a structural role in antioxidant enzymes and loss of zinc from biological membranes increases their susceptibility to oxidative damage and impairs their function.[64,65] Therefore, zinc has been evaluated for its possible role in cataract prevention. Epidemiological data from the Blue Mountains Eye Follow-up Study found that participants with zinc intakes above the median in combination with vitamins C and E and β-carotene were associated with reduced incidence of nuclear cataract, but not cortical and PSC cataract.[18]

## N3 Fatty Acids

High intakes of dietary n3 polyunsaturated fatty acids were shown to reduce the incidence of nuclear cataract in the Blue Mountains Eye Study cohort.[66] In a prospective study examining the relationship between dietary fat and cataract extraction in women (n = 71,083, 16-year follow-up), women in the highest quintile of long-chain n3 fatty acids (0.21% of energy) had a 12% lower risk of cataract extraction compared to those in the lowest quintile (0.03% of energy) (relative risk = 0.88;

95% confidence interval [CI], 0.79–0.98; P for trend = 0.02).[67] Both Arnarsson et al.[68] and Cumming et al.[63] report that there was no association between the intake of foods or oils containing n3 fatty acids and age-related cataract prevalence.

## INTERVENTION TRIALS EVALUATING MULTIVITAMIN/ MINERAL SUPPLEMENTATION

Several randomized placebo-controlled clinical trials have evaluated interventions with combinations of vitamins and minerals on cataract risk. The Linxian trial[62] used 14 vitamins and 12 minerals, which was reported to decrease the risk of nuclear cataract by 36%. However, the population examined had suboptimal nutrient intakes at the start of the study and the effect may have been due to an improved status of certain nutrients. The Age-Related Eye Disease Study (AREDS) reported that a combination of high-dose antioxidants (vitamins C, 500 mg; vitamin E, 400 IU; β-carotene, 15 mg; zinc, 80 mg; and copper, 2 mg) had no effect on the 7-year risk of development or progression of age-related cataract or visual acuity loss.[69] The Roche European-American Cataract Trial (REACT) examined the effect of daily supplementation with β-carotene (18 mg), vitamin C (750 mg), and vitamin E (600 mg) on the progression of age-related cataract.[70] This was carried out in the United States and the United Kingdom and was a double-masked randomized placebo-controlled 3-year trial in 445 patients. The study intervention was found to significantly decrease the progression of cataracts after 3 years for both U.S. and U.K. patients, but no effect for the U.K. patients alone. The Antioxidants in Prevention of Cataracts Study was a 5-year, randomized, triple-masked, placebo-controlled study that evaluated these same nutrients.[26] This study found no effect of a vitamin C (500 mg), β-carotene (15 mg), and vitamin E (400 IU) intervention on cataract progression. The Italian-American Clinical Trial of Nutrition Supplements and Age-Related Cataract (CTNS) was a 13 year study designed to evaluate the use of a vitamin–mineral supplement (Centrum®) in preventing age-related cataract or delaying its progression. This study found that a 9-year multivitamin/mineral intervention reduced the risk of age-related cataract, with a significant decrease in development or progression of nuclear cataract.[71] However, a significant increase in the development or progression of PSC opacities was also observed. In the Alpha-Tocopherol Beta-Carotene (ATBC) trial, alpha-tocopherol (50 mg/day) and β-carotene (20 mg/day) supplementation over 5–8 years had no effect on the rates of cataract extraction or prevalence of lens opacities, nuclear, cortical, or PSC cataract in male Finnish smokers.[72] In the Physician's Health Study, a prospective study examining the reported use of vitamin supplements and risk of cataract and cataract extraction, men who used multivitamin supplements had a marginally significant decreased in risk of incident cataract compared to nonsupplement users. Multivitamin users who also used supplements containing only vitamins C and/or E had a risk of incident cataract similar to users of multivitamin only. In this study, use of vitamin C and/ or E was not related to a reduced risk.[22] In summary, the majority of studies examining multivitamin and antioxidant supplement usage have found no benefit in reducing the risk of cataracts.

## AGE-RELATED MACULAR DEGENERATION

AMD is the leading cause of blindness among the elderly in industrialized countries. Unlike cataract, there is no cure for AMD with no treatment that can reverse the damage due to AMD. The greatest risk factor for AMD is aging with the prevalence increasing dramatically with increasing age. Nearly 24% of Americans over the age of 80 have intermediate signs of AMD and 12% have advanced disease, whereas the respective prevalence among people 40–49 years is 2% and 0.1%.[73]

AMD is an eye disease that affects the central area of the retina, known as the macula, resulting in loss of central vision. In the early stages of the disease, lipid material, known as drusen, accumulates in deposits underneath the retinal pigment epithelium (RPE). Drusen appears as pale yellow spots on the retina. This accumulation is thought to be due to a loss of RPE's ability to transport nutrients and metabolic products. The early stages of AMD are generally asymptomatic. In later states of AMD, the RPE may develop areas of hyperpigmentation and hypopigmentation. In the later stages, the RPE may become completely atrophied. In some cases, new blood vessels grow under the RPE and sometimes into the subretinal space (wet, exudative, or neovascular AMD). Hemorrhage can occur and result in scarring of the retina. In the later stages, there may be distortion of vision or complete loss of visual function, particularly central vision.[74] The pathogenesis of AMD is not completely understood. However, chemical- and light-induced oxidative damage to the photoreceptors is thought to be involved. The retina is susceptible to oxidative damage because of its high consumption of oxygen, its high concentrations of the polyunsaturated fatty acids (which are highly oxidizable), and its exposure to visible light.

Inflammation has also been implicated as a potential risk factor for AMD.[75–78] A major proportion of AMD cases have been identified in several cohorts to specific polymorphisms in the complement regulatory gene CFH[79,80] and implicate local inflammation and activation of the complement cascade, an event in the host immunologic defense in the development of drusen.[81] Additional evidence for the role of inflammation in AMD pathogenesis comes from reports of associations of AMD with other gene loci involved with the alternative complement pathway (factor B) or in regions of genes suspected to be involved in cellular immunity[80] and by enhanced AMD risk among persons with markers of chronic or acute inflammation.[82] Given that oxidative and light damage are implicated in the etiology of AMD, antioxidant and anti-inflammatory nutrients have been explored as providing benefit in decreasing the risk of AMD.

## Vitamin C

Vitamin C has been suggested to have a role in AMD prevention because of its role as antioxidant. However, there are several reports of no relationship between dietary or plasma concentrations of vitamin C and risk of AMD.[83–86]

## Vitamin E

Vitamin E is a major dietary antioxidant. In a study examining vitamin E supplement use,[85] the prevalence of AMD was also similar between those who took vitamin E supplement for >2 years and those who never took vitamin E supplements. Three double-blinded, placebo-controlled primary prevention trials have been published on AMD and high doses of vitamin E.[87–89] The results of these studies found that there was no association of treatment group with any sign of AMD. In studies involving measures of vitamin E in plasma, a protective effect of increased plasma vitamin E against AMD has been found in some studies,[84,86] but not in others.[46,90]

## Carotenoids

Carotenoids also function as antioxidants. Particular attention has been given to lutein and zeaxanthin because, compared to the other carotenoids, they selectively and exclusively accumulate in the macula[91] where they are referred to as macular pigment (MP). Findings from several case-control studies suggest that high intakes of carotenoid, particularly lutein and zeaxanthin, are related to lower risk of advanced neovascular AMD.[84,85,92] A relationship between carotenoids status and age-related eye disease risk was evaluated in the Carotenoids in Age-Related Eye Disease Study (CAREDS), a cross-sectional study of 1678 women (54–86 years).[93] In CAREDS, high dietary lutein and zeaxanthin were related to a decreased risk of intermediate AMD in women <75 years, but not in women ≥75 years.[94] Similarly, the Blue Mountain Eye Study found that high intake of lutein/zeaxanthin was related to a reduced risk of incident neovascular AMD and indistinct soft or reticular drusen over 5 and 10 years.[95] In AREDS, lutein/zeaxanthin intake was associated with a decreased risk of prevalent neovascular AMD and large or extensive intermediate drusen when comparing the highest and lowest quintiles of intakes.[83] However, a nested case-control study from the Beaver Dam Eye Study found no difference in serum levels of lutein/zeaxanthin between early AMD and age-, sex-, and smoking-matched controls.[46]

Evidence that high MP concentrations may lower the risk of AMD comes from analysis of retinas from donors with AMD and controls for lutein and zeaxanthin.[96] Concentrations of lutein and zeaxanthin in retinal tissue were less, on average, for the AMD donors than for the controls. MP can be measured noninvasively in vivo.[97] In the evaluation of MP density in subjects (21–81 years) with healthy eyes and in healthy eyes of subjects known to be at high risk

of AMD due to advanced disease in the fellow eye. Healthy eyes at risk for AMD had significantly less MP than eyes at no risk.[98] In another study, MP in the eyes of AMD patients was 32% lower than that in healthy eyes.[99] In a prospective study in patients with early and late AMD, their children, and normal controls, it was found that MP density was reduced in late AMD.[100] In contrast, in CAREDS, MP density was not related to AMD.[101] This may be due to the cross-sectional study design, suggesting that prospective studies are needed to determine if there is a relationship between AMD risk and MP density.

## B Vitamins

Vitamin $B_{12}$ and folate are essential coenzymes in homocysteine metabolism. Hyperhomocysteinemia has been associated with risk of AMD.[102–109] Treatment with folate, vitamin $B_6$, and vitamin $B_{12}$ has shown to reduce plasma homocysteine levels and has hence been explored as a treatment option for AMD. In a population-based cross-sectional analysis of data from the Blue Mountains Eye Study, participants with low serum vitamin $B_{12}$ had a twofold increased risk of AMD.[108] No association was observed with serum folate. Furthermore, in patients with serum homocysteine ≤15 μmol/L, low plasma $B_{12}$ was related to four times higher odds of AMD. However, others have reported that plasma vitamin $B_{12}$ and RBC and plasma folate were not different between patients with wet AMD and controls.[107] Blood concentrations of homocysteine were not related to RBC folate and serum vitamin $B_{12}$ in AMD patients aged ≥40 years in NHANES III.[104] The absence of any association was attributed to limited information on change in diet and lifestyle, exclusion of persons in older age group due to missing data and differences in fasting status at the time of blood draw. An inverse association was observed between RBC folate concentration and soft drusen in non-Hispanic Blacks in this population. A randomized, double-blinded, placebo-controlled study (Women's Antioxidant and Folic Acid Cardiovascular Study) showed that women at a high risk of cardiovascular disease, supplemented daily with folic acid (2.5 mg), vitamin $B_6$ (50 mg), and vitamin $B_{12}$ (1 mg) for an average of 7.3 years, had a statistically significant 35%–40% decreased risk of AMD.[110] In a subset of 300 participants analyzed for blood levels of homocysteine, the decreased risk was partially due to a significant reduction in plasma homocysteine concentrations. However, these results may not be applied to the general public given that in this study the AMD diagnosis was self-reported and the subjects were women with a high risk of cardiovascular disease.

Niacin has been evaluated in the treatment of AMD due to because of its actions as a vasodialator.[111–113] Several reports have suggested that choroidal blood flow is reduced in AMD.[114–119] In studies in AMD patients, niacin treatment was shown to produce vasodilatation of retinal arterioles and modified choroidal circulation.[120,121]

## ZINC

There are several reasons to support the role of zinc in the development of AMD. The zinc concentration in the retina is one of the highest levels in the body, suggesting a special role in the eye.[122] Zinc is a known cofactor for many antioxidant enzymes, including superoxide dismutase (SOD) and catalase, which is important for protection against oxidative damage.[123] Retinal dehydrogenase also requires zinc as a cofactor in the metabolism of vitamin A and in rhodopsin synthesis.[123] Elderly patients are at higher risk of zinc deficiency.[124–126] However, scientific evidence that zinc intake is associated with the development or progression of AMD is limited. A recent study found zinc levels in the RPE and choroid to be reduced significantly by 24% in AMD eyes compared to normal eyes, lending support to the possible importance of zinc in AMD.[127]

The Blue Mountain Eye Study was a population-based study, in which 2454 patients were evaluated for AMD at baseline, 5 and 10 years after initial enrollment and energy-adjusted nutrient intakes were assessed for relationships with AMD risk. For total zinc intake, the relative risk comparing the top decile intake (≥15.8 mg/day) with the remaining population was 0.56 (95% CI, 0.32–0.97) for all forms of AMD and 0.54 (95% CI, 0.30–0.97) for early AMD. However, in two large prospective studies (Nurses' Health Study and the Health Professionals Follow-up Study) involving men and women (n = 72,489) with no diagnosis of AMD at baseline, zinc intake, either in food or in supplements, was not associated with a reduced risk of AMD.[128] Furthermore, no association was observed between zinc intake and prevalence of AMD-related drusen in the cohort of the Nurses' Health Study who also participated in the Nutrition and Vision Project.[129]

Zinc supplementation (100 mg zinc sulfate for 12–24 months) given to elderly people with early stages of AMD resulted in better maintenance of visual acuity than in those receiving placebo.[130] A more recent randomized, placebo-controlled study showed supplementation with 50 mg/day for 6 months of zinc monocysteine significantly improved macular function in persons with dry AMD.[131] The beneficial effect of zinc supplementation may have been due to the presence of cysteine. Cysteine can be metabolized into other sulfur-containing compounds such as glutathione, which is an important antioxidant in the eye. However, patients with wet AMD in one eye had no positive effect on the other eye diagnosed with drusen after 200 mg/day zinc supplementation for 2 years.[132]

A protective effect of zinc is contrasted by the findings of high concentrations in sub-RPE deposits, with levels being particularly high in eyes with AMD.[133] Therefore, zinc supplementation may be beneficial in combination with other antioxidants but not in isolation.[134]

## N3 FATTY ACIDS

Due to their anti-inflammatory actions, n fatty acids[135] have been implicated in having a role in AMD prevention.[136] Rod outer segments of the retina have a high concentration of docosahexaenoic acid (DHA).[137] Epidemiological studies examining the relationship of n3 fatty acids or fish intake (a major source of n3 fatty acids) with AMD suggest a trend toward a protective relationship.

A meta-analysis, including nine prospective studies and three randomized clinical trials, reported that a high dietary intake of n3 fatty acids was associated with a 38% reduction in the risk of late AMD.[138] Fish intake at least twice a week was associated with a 24% reduced risk for early AMD and 33% reduced risk for late AMD (pooled odds ratio [OR], 0.67; 95% CI, 0.53–0.85). In a prospective follow-up study of the Nurses' Health Study and the Health Professionals Follow-up Study, odds of AMD decreased with increased DHA intake. Consumption of >4 servings of fish/week was associated with a 35% lower risk of AMD compared with ≤3 servings/month in pooled multivariate analysis.[139] Of the individual fish types examined, a significant inverse association was found only with tuna intake.

The Dietary Ancillary Study of the Eye Disease Case-Control Study[84] reported results for participants with neovascular AMD and control subjects without AMD.[140] In demographically adjusted analyses, increasing intake of linoleic acid (an unsaturated n6 fatty acid) was significantly associated with higher prevalence of AMD (P for trend = 0.004). This association remained in multivariate analyses (P for trend = 0.02). However, intake of n3 fatty acids was not associated with AMD after controlling for confounding variables. When the study population was stratified by linoleic acid intake (≤5.5 or ≥5.6 g/day), the risk for AMD significantly decreased with high intake of n3 fatty acids only among those with low linoleic acid intake (P for trend = 0.05; P for continuous variable = 0.03). A prospective cohort study reported similar findings. In this study, 261 persons aged 60 years or older at baseline with an average follow-up of 4.6 years were evaluated for progression to late AMD. Higher fish intake was associated with a 64% lower risk of progression to advanced AMD among subjects with lower linoleic acid intake.[141] Others have also observed a benefit of a high n3 fatty acid intake with low intake of linoleic acid.[142] These findings indicate an interaction or competition between n3 and n6 fatty acids such that both the levels of n3 fatty acids and its ratio to the n6 acids may be important when considering the risk/benefit to AMD.

The Blue Mountains Eye Study was a population-based survey of vision, common eye diseases, and diet in an urban population aged ≥49 years.[143] In the 2915 subjects, more frequent consumption of fish was related to a decreased risk of late ARM, after adjusting for age, sex, and smoking. The protective effect of fish intake was observed at a relatively low consumption (1–3 times/month compared with intake <1 time/month. The OR for intake >5 times/week compared with <1 time/month was 0.46 (95% CI, 0.12–1.68). There was little evidence of a decreased risk for early AMD with increased fish intake. A prospective cohort study from the AREDS trial found that increased intakes of n3 fatty acids reduced the risk by 30% of developing central geographic atrophy and neovascular AMD.[144]

In the Beaver Dam Eye Study, a retrospective population-based study, a relationship between fish intake neovascular AMD or geographic atrophy was not found. A null finding may be due to the observation that fish intakes were very low[145] and not varied enough to measure a difference in risk for AMD. NHANES III consuming fish more than once a week compared with once a month or less was not associated with either early or late AMD.[146]

The current AREDS 2 clinical trial is evaluating the benefit of 1 g eicosahexaenoic acid + DHA (2:1) on the progression to late AMD.

## Vitamin D

There is considerable scientific evidence that 1,25-dihydroxyvitamin D has a variety of effects on immune system function.[147] There are several reports of an inverse relationship between vitamin D plasma levels and several chronic conditions associated with inflammation.[148–151] The vitamin D receptor is expressed on cells of the human immune system and 1,25-dihydroxyvitamin D has been shown to suppress pro-inflammatory cytokines in vitro, perhaps in part by altering T-cell function toward a T-helper 2 (anti-inflammatory) rather than a T-helper 1 (pro-inflammatory) response.[152,153] A possible role of vitamin D in ocular functioning is supported by evidence that the vitamin D receptor is located in retinal tissue.[154,155] Given this and the role that inflammation may have in the development of AMD, vitamin D has been suggested to be related to a decrease risk of AMD.

Evidence for such a role comes from observations in human studies. The relationship between serum 25-hydroxyvitamin D (25[OH]D) concentrations and the prevalence of early AMD was recently investigated in participants of the CAREDS study. In this retrospective cohort study or 1313 women, there was no significant relationship observed between early AMD and 25(OH)D. A significant age interaction (P = 0.002) suggested selective mortality bias in women aged ≥75 years. Serum 25(OH)D was associated with decreased odds of early AMD in women <75 years (n = 968) and increased odds in women aged 75 years or older (n = 319) (OR for quintile 5 vs. 1, 0.52; 95% CI, 0.29–0.91; P for trend =.02 and OR, 1.76; 95% CI, 0.77–4.13; P for trend = 0.05, respectively). Further adjustment for body mass index and physical activity, predictors of 25(OH)D, attenuated the association in women <75 years. Among women <75 years, intake of vitamin D from both foods and supplements was related to decreased odds of early AMD in multivariate analysis.

In a cross-sectional study of 7752 subjects ≥60 years from NHANES III, levels of serum vitamin D were inversely associated with early AMD but not advanced AMD.[156] The OR and 95% CI for early AMD among participants in the highest versus lowest quintile of serum vitamin D was 0.64 (95% CI, 0.5–0.8; P trend < 0.001). Additional analyses of associations with food and supplemental sources of vitamin D found that milk intake was inversely associated with early AMD (OR, 0.75; 95% CI, 0.6–0.9). Fish intake was inversely associated with advanced AMD (OR, 0.41; 95% CI, 0.2–0.9).

Furthermore, it was observed that consistent use of vitamin D supplements was inversely associated with early AMD only in those who did not consume milk daily (early AMD: OR, 0.67; 95% CI, 0.5–0.9). Other studies evaluated the association of fish intake to AMD and found that higher fish intake was associated with a lower risk of AMD development and progression.[140,141,145,157]

However, in a cross-sectional study involving participants >60 years, there was no association between serum vitamin D levels and the presence of AMD.[158] Unlike the previous studies evaluating the relationship between vitamin D status and AMD risk, this study did not adjust for potential confounders, for example age, smoking, body mass index, in the statistical analysis.

### Intervention Trials

It is likely that a protective effect of an individual nutrient is through interactions with other protective nutrients, as suggested by the results of several intervention trials. The Rotterdam Study reported that high dietary intake of vitamins C and E, β-carotene, and zinc was associated with a 35% reduction in incident AMD risk in older adults.[159] AREDS was designed to evaluate the benefit of supplementation with these same nutrients in delaying the progression of advanced AMD. This double-blind, placebo-controlled clinical trial followed approximately 3600 participants with varying stages of AMD. The intervention consisted of daily supplementation of vitamin C (500 mg), vitamin E (400 IU), β-carotene (15 mg), zinc (as zinc oxide, 80 mg), and copper (as copper oxide, 2 mg) for approximately 5 years. It was found that people at high risk for developing advanced stages of AMD (intermediate or advanced AMD in one eye but not the other eye) lowered the risk of progression of the disease by about 25% when treated with these nutrients.[160] In the same high-risk group, the risk of vision loss caused by advance AMD was reduced by about 19%. For those subjects who had either no AMD or early AMD, the nutrients did not provide benefit. This is similar to two recent systematic reviews found that randomized clinical trials did not show that antioxidant supplements prevented early AMD.[161,162] These results showed that key nutrients may be of benefit in people at risk for developing advanced AMD but perhaps not early AMD.

AREDS 2 has begun and aims to refine the findings of AREDS by including lutein, zeaxanthin, and n3 fatty acids into the test formulation of the first AREDS trial.

## DIABETIC RETINOPATHY

Diabetic retinopathy is a leading cause of visual impairment in persons with diabetes. Diabetic retinopathy accounts for approximately 5% of the global prevalence of blindness and about 15%–17% in developed countries.[4] Long-term control of blood glucose concentrations[163,164] and optimal blood pressure levels[165] play key roles in the delay or prevention of retinopathy. Microvascular complications are involved in diabetic retinopathy. Micronutrients that have been studied for a role in vascularization are vitamin C, vitamin E, and magnesium.[166] Vitamins C and E have also been evaluated because of the increased levels of oxidative stress in the vascular endothelium of diabetic patients.[167,168]

## VITAMIN C

Five cross-sectional studies consistently reported that plasma/serum levels of vitamin C were lower in diabetic patients with retinopathy than those without retinopathy.[169–173] However, a cross-sectional analysis of NHANES III found no association between serum vitamin C level and the prevalence of diabetic retinopathy (OR, 1.3; 95% CI, 0.8–2.3), comparing the 1st and 4th quartiles of serum vitamin C.[174] Similarly, a prospective analysis of the Atherosclerosis Risk in Communities Study did not find an association between dietary vitamin C intake and risk of diabetic retinopathy (OR, 1.1; 95% CI, 0.7–1.9, 1st vs. 4th quartiles of intake).[175] In addition, the San Luis Valley Diabetes Study did not observe an inverse association between dietary vitamin C and the prevalence of diabetic retinopathy when comparing the 1st and 10th deciles of intake.[176] A recent systematic review concluded that the evidence suggests dietary intake or plasma levels of vitamin C do not seem to be associated with diabetic retinopathy.[177]

## VITAMIN E

Two population-based studies found vitamin E intake to be not related to a decreased risk of diabetic retinopathy. The Atherosclerosis Risk in Communities Study found no association when comparing the 1st and 4th quartiles of dietary vitamin E intake (OR, 1.3; 95% CI, 0.8–2.2).[175] NHANES reported an OR of 2.7; 95% CI, 1.6–4.6 when comparing extreme quartiles of serum vitamin E level (P for trend <0.14).[174–176] In the San Louis Valley Diabetes Study,[176] comparison of the 1st and 9th decile for intake found an increased risk for increased severity of diabetic retinopathy (OR = 2.21, P = 0.01). However, an increased risk was not observed for the 10th decile. One study observed significantly higher plasma vitamin E levels in patients with retinopathy than in those without retinopathy,[169] whereas two studies showed no difference in plasma/serum vitamin E levels between diabetic patients with or without retinopathy.[178,179]

There are several studies that have evaluated supplementation with vitamin E on measures of oxidative stress, plasma levels of glucose, lipids, HbALc, and insulin in patients with diabetes. The results have been inconsistent.[180–182] Ble-Castillo et al. found no effect on HbA1c, glucose, lipids, and lipoproteins in the serum, or Cu, Zn SOD in diabetic patients given 800 IU/day vitamin E for 6 weeks.[183] No effect on HbA1c, fasting blood glucose, or glycated plasma proteins was found with supplementation with α-tocopherol (1 g/day, 10 weeks), although a significant positive effect on oxidation of LDL-cholesterol was measured.[184] Gazis et al. reported that 1600 IU α-tocopherol given to diabetic patient for 8 weeks had no effect on endothelial function.[185] Supplementation with 200 IU/day of vitamin E for 27 weeks had no effect

on fasting blood glucose, serum insulin, or HbA1c levels.[186] However, one study reported that supplementation with 900 mg/day over 3 months had a positive effect on HbA1c.[187] A recent systematic review concluded that the evidence suggests that dietary intake or plasma levels of vitamin E do not seem to be associated with diabetic retinopathy.[177]

## MAGNESIUM

Studies on the association between serum/plasma levels of magnesium and diabetic retinopathy have been inconsistent. Compared to those without diabetic retinopathy, both lower and higher plasma/serum magnesium concentrations have been reported in those with diabetic retinopathy.[188–191] However, a single prospective cohort study demonstrated an inverse association of plasma magnesium with the progression of diabetic retinopathy.[192] The significant association remained after adjusting for potential confounders, including hemoglobin. A recent systematic review concluded that the evidence suggests dietary intake or plasma levels of magnesium do not seem to be associated with diabetic retinopathy.[177]

In summary, the evidence to date does not consistently support or refute a role for nutrients in the prevention or delay in progression of diabetic retinopathy. However, this may be due to the lack of randomized controlled trials designed to evaluate this.

## GLAUCOMA

Glaucoma is the deterioration of the optic nerve that may cause the loss of vision. It is the second leading cause of blindness worldwide, affecting more than 60 million people, and is increasing because of the aging population.[5] In 2002, more than 2.2 million in the United States aged 40 years and older had primary open-angle glaucoma (POAG).[193] POAG is the most common form of glaucoma. Pseudoexfoliation syndrome glaucoma (PEXG) is an age-related, generalize disorder of the extracellular matrix characterized by the multifocal production of progressive accumulation of a fibrillar extracellular material in intra- and extraocular tissue, which is the result of either an excessive production or insufficient breakdown of both.[194] The pathogenesis of glaucoma is still not well understood. It had been suggested that oxidative stress plays a role in glaucoma.[195] Elevated intraocular pressure (IOP) is considered a major risk factor for POAG.[196] However, glaucoma can develop without elevated IOP[197,198] suggesting that other factors play a role in the pathogenesis of glaucoma. Like AMD, the blindness resulting from glaucoma cannot be cured. IOP is a modifiable risk factor. Given the oxidative factor to glaucoma, antioxidant nutrients have been suggested to play a role in the prevention of glaucoma.

### FRUITS AND VEGETABLES

Fruits and vegetables are rich sources of dietary antioxidants. Coleman et al. investigated the association between glaucoma and the consumption of specific fruits and vegetables in a cohort of women aged 65 and older participating in the Study of Osteoporotic Fractures.[199] In this cross-sectional cohort study of 1155 women, the odds of glaucoma risk were decreased by 69% (OR, 0.31; 95% CI, 0.11–0.91) in those who consumed at least one serving per month of green collards and kale compared with those who consumed fewer than one serving per month, by 64% (OR, 0.36; 95% CI, 0.17–0.77) in women who consumed more than two servings per week of carrots compared with those who consumed fewer than one serving per week, and by 47% (OR, 0.53; 95% CI, 0.29–0.97) in women who consumed at least one serving per week of canned or dried peaches compared with those who consumed fewer than one serving per month.

In the prospective study by Kang et al.,[200] no relationship was found between the risk of POAG and six food groups (citrus foods, cruciferous vegetables, yellow vegetables, green leafy vegetables, all fruits combined, and all vegetables combined). The authors showed a 32% decreased risk of POAG after 4 years in subjects in the highest quintiles of lutein and vitamin E intake. In the pooled 4-year data, there was a 32% reduction in the risk of glaucoma in all subjects in the third quintile of vitamin C intake.

The exact mechanism in which fruits and vegetables and antioxidants may affect glaucoma presence is unknown. It may not be one factor alone having a beneficial effect. Food components contained in fruits and vegetables may be acting synergistically.

## DIETARY FAT

The essential fatty acids, linoleic acid (n6 fatty acid) and linolenic acid (n3 fatty acid), are competitive substrates for the endogenous ophthalmic enzymes that generate arachidonic acid, the precursor of prostaglandin F2-a. Analogs of prostaglandin F2-a are potent hypotensive agents.[201] Dietary fat intake might modulate the availability of intraocular prostaglandins, altering IOP to influence the risk of POAG. N3 fatty acids are important for systemic and are essential for the health of neurologic tissues including the retina.[202] Kang et al. evaluated the relation between dietary fat intake and POAG.[203] Total dietary intake of fats was not related to POAG risk. However, a diet with higher n6:n3 ratio was inversely associated with a risk of POAG, particularly among the high-tension subtype. Other studies suggest that high intake of n3 fatty acids may be beneficial for reducing the risk of glaucoma. Ren et al. found that patients with POAG have lower circulating n3 fatty acid concentrations than their unaffected siblings.[204]

## B VITAMINS

Homocysteine has toxic effects such as apoptosis of retinal ganglion cells,[205] extracellular matrix alterations,[206] oxidative stress,[207] and ischemic vascular dysregulation, all of which have been implicated in the pathology of glaucoma.[208] Although not entirely consistent,[209] many studies on PEXG have shown a relationship with homocysteine,[210–217]

while only a few studies have reported a relationship with POAG.[213,218,219] The metabolism of homocysteine is dependent on vitamins $B_{12}$ and $B_6$ and folate.[220] These vitamins are major determinants of homocysteine levels, and a deficiency of any one of these vitamins will elevate homocysteine levels. Therefore, it has been proposed that homocysteine may also be responsible for the induction of pathologic changes leading to glaucomatous optic nerve damage, and therefore, these vitamins may play a role in glaucoma prevention.

In a prospective controlled trial of 48 patients with normal tension glaucoma, 38 patients with PEXG, and 34 patients with POAG,[217] the mean homocysteine level of the PEXG group was significantly higher (P = 0.03) than that of the control group. There were no statistical differences in serum vitamin $B_{12}$ and folate levels among control subjects and glaucoma groups. It was found that the mean plasma vitamin $B_6$ level was significantly higher in subjects with normal tension glaucoma (P = 0.03) and POAG (0.025) versus controls. These results are somewhat differing to the work of Rossler et al.[221] In an investigation of a possible association between homocysteine and B vitamins and normal tension glaucoma, plasma levels of these components were determined in 42 patients with normal tension glaucoma and in 42 age-matched and sex-matched controls.[221] No significant difference was found between these groups for homocysteine, vitamin $B_6$, or folate. However, there was a trend toward a significant difference for plasma $B_{12}$ (P = 0.052). The authors concluded that a role of homocysteine as a modifiable risk factor in the pathogenesis of normal tension glaucoma is not likely.

In a similar study of 36 patients with PEXG, 40 with POAG, and 40 age-matched healthy subjects, plasma homocysteine was reported to be significantly higher in PEXG compared with POAG and controls (P = 0.03 and P = 0.0007, respectively).[222] However, there were no statistical differences in serum vitamin $B_{12}$ and folic acid levels among PEXG, POAG, and control subjects (P > 0.05). A moderate, although statistically significant, relationship between homocysteine and folic acid levels was found in the PEXG group (R2 = 0.23, P = 0.003). Furthermore, homocysteine levels were found not to be related with folic acid or vitamin $B_{12}$ in either POAG or control subjects. The authors concluded that elevated homocysteine might play a role in the pathogenesis of PEXG, being an independent factor stressing vasculopathy in addition to pseudoexfoliation, and therefore may be a modifiable risk factor for PEXG.

In conclusion, the studies to date suggest that homocysteine may be involved in the pathogenesis of glaucoma. However, this is based in large part on cross-sectional data. The effectiveness of a B vitamin intervention remains to be determined, requiring randomized clinical trials.

## VITAMIN C

Oxidative stress may contribute to glaucoma etiology and progress.[223–225] Therefore, vitamin C has been suggested to be protective against the risk of glaucoma. Two recent studies found that serum concentrations of vitamin C were significantly lower in glaucoma patients than in healthy controls.[226,227] This is contrast to an earlier report of no differences in the intake of plasma levels of vitamin C in glaucoma patients and controls.[228] Furthermore, in two prospective cohort studies data from two large prospective cohorts, there was little evidence that intake of vitamin C substantially reduced the risk of developing POAG.[200] Therefore, these inconsistent results make it difficult to draw conclusions on the role of vitamin C in the prevention or progression of glaucoma, and randomized clinical trials may be warranted.

## VITAMIN E

Similar to vitamin C, vitamin E may be protective against glaucoma because of its role as an antioxidant. In a multicenter case-control study of 31 healthy individuals and 160 glaucoma patients with no known additional abnormalities were analyzed for biochemical measures of antioxidants and serum oxidative stress markers as oxidation degradation products.[229] Measures included malonyldialdehyde (MDA), advanced oxidation protein products (AOPP), antioxidants, vitamins E and A, serine (Ser), SOD, GPx, transferrin (TF), and total antioxidant capacity (TADA). TADA, AOPP, SOD, and GPx were found to be decreased, and MDA, Ser, TF, vitamins A and E increased in the patient group. All data, excluding AOPP, varied significantly. Vitamin E was the most consistent parameter. The authors suggested that vitamin E is a significantly protective against glaucoma. In contrast, Kang et al. reported that in prospective cohort studies data from two large prospective cohorts, there was little evidence that intake of vitamin E substantially reduced the risk of developing POAG.[200]

## SELENIUM

Selenium is an essential trace element incorporated into selenoproteins, which are important antioxidant enzymes.[230] In a study evaluating participants undergoing either cataract or trabeculectomy surgery (n = 101), data were collected on the use of dietary supplements and the ingestion of high-selenium-containing foods. Cases were defined as subjects with POAG and controls were subjects without POAG. Aqueous humor and plasma samples were collected at the onset of surgery and analysis of total selenium. There was no significant difference between the glaucoma and control groups in the plasma selenium levels or the aqueous humor selenium levels. However, when the data were analyzed by the intertertile intervals of plasma and aqueous humor concentrations of selenium (based on the control group distribution of selenium) some differences between the glaucoma and control group were found. The OR for glaucoma was lowest with the middle third of aqueous selenium levels (OR = 0.06 and 0.41 for the middle and highest thirds, respectively), suggesting a protective effect with higher aqueous humor selenium

levels and a greater risk with higher plasma selenium levels (OR = 4.6 and 11.3 for the middle and highest thirds, respectively).The IOP in glaucoma subjects was independently significantly associated with plasma selenium level. In this study, the mean plasma selenium of glaucomatous subjects was 209 ng/mL, while those subjects without glaucoma average 194 ng/mL. Plasma selenium concentrations of approximately 100 ng/mL or more fully saturate the body's GPx pools.[231] These investigators suggested that the glutathione peroxide pools in the study participants were fully saturated, leaving excess selenium in the body system. It was suggested that excessive plasma selenium concentrations could have damage potential before being excreted. Bruhn et al.[232] also speculate that the observations regarding glaucoma development in relation to aqueous humor levels of selenium suggest a protective effect of aqueous humor selenium for glaucoma. From these observations, it is difficult to determine if selenium is involved in the prevention or development of glaucoma.

## SUMMARY

There is biological plausibility for a relationship between certain nutrients and certain age-related eye diseases. Supporting evidence comes from epidemiology of dietary intakes and serum/plasma concentrations and risk of disease. Intervention trials have been inconsistent in terms of benefit of supplementation with the exception of AREDS for AMD.

## FUTURE DIRECTIONS

Discussion on the need for future research needs to take into consideration that a nutrient benefit may be related to the stage at which damage occurs. Studies evaluating dietary patterns are few and more are needed given that it is likely that nutrients are acting synergistically to provide protection. The inconsistencies among studies in terms of the amount of nutrient required for protection against eye disease make it difficult to make specific recommendations for dietary intakes of some of these nutrients. Therefore, it may be more practical to recommend specific food choices rich in vitamins C and E, B vitamins, lutein and zeaxanthin, n3 fatty acids, zinc, and possibly selenium, thereby benefiting from possible effects of the components in food that may also be important. Further trials are warranted to address the usefulness of nutrient supplementation in eye disease prevention. It is likely that some eye diseases, particularly those that are age related, develop over many years, and the etiology is due to many factors. There are likely to be differences in the potential protective effect of nutrient depending on the stage of the disease.

## REFERENCES

1. Congdon N, O'Colmain B, Klaver CCW et al., *Arch Ophthalmol* 122:477;2004.
2. World Health Organization, *B World Health Organ* 69:657;1991.

3. Vision Problems in the U.S., Prevent Blindness in the U.S., National Eye Institute, National Institutes of Health. www.nei.hin.gov/eyedata/pdf/VPUS/pdf (accessed on July 12, 2012).
4. Resnikoff S, Pascolini D, Eyta'ale D et al., *B World Health Organ* 82:844;2004.
5. Quigley HA, Broman AT. *Brit J Ophthalmol* 9:262;2006.
6. Thylefors B, Negrel AD, Pararajasegaram R, Dadzie KY, *B World Health Organ* 69:115;1995.
7. Congdon N, Vingerling JR, Klein BEK et al., *Arch Ophthalmol* 122:487;2004.
8. Javitt JC. *Arch Ophthalmol* 111:1329;1993.
9. Steinberg EP, Javitt JC, Sharkey PK et al., *Arch Ophthalmol* 111:1041;1992.
10. Hankinson SE, Stampfer MJ, Seddon JM et al., *BMJ* 305:244;1992.
11. Jacques PF, Chylack PF Jr., *Am J Clin Nutr* 53:353S;1991.
12. Jacques PF, Taylor A, Hankinson SE et al., *Am J Clin Nutr* 66:911;1997.
13. Jacques PF, Taylor A, Moeller S et al., *Arch Ophthalmol* 119:1009;2001.
14. Leske MC, Chylack LT Jr., Wu SY, *Arch Ophthalmol* 109:244;1991.
15. Mares-Perlman JA, Brady WE, Klein BE et al., *Am J Epidemiol* 141:322;1995.
16. Mares-Perlman JA, Lyle BJ, Klein R et al., *Arch Ophthalmol* 118:556;2000.
17. Robertson JM, Donner AP, Trevithick, JR. *Ann NY Acad Sci* 570:372;1989.
18. Tan AG, Mitchell PL, Flood VM et al., *Am J Clin Nutr* 87:1899;2008.
19. Taylor A, Hobbs M., *Nutrition* 17:845;2001.
20. Taylor A, Jacques PF, Chalack LT Jr. et al., *Am J Clin Nutr* 75:540;2002.
21. Chasan-Taber L, Willett WC, Seddon JM et al., *Epidemiology* 10:679;1999.
22. Seddon, JM, Christen, WG, Manson, JE et al., *Amer J Public Health* 84:788;1992.
23. The Italian-American Cataract Study Group, *Am J Epidemiol* 133:541;1991.
24. Tavani A, Negri E, LaVeccia C, *Ann Physiol* 6:41;1996.
25. Vitale S, West S, Hallfrisch J et al., *Epidemiology* 4:195;1993.
26. Gritz DC, Srinivasan M., Smith ED et al., *Br J Ophthalmol* 90:847;2006.
27. Leske, M.C. et al., *Ophthalmology* 105:831;1998.
28. Rautiainen S, Lindblad, BE, Morgenstern R, Wolk, A, *Am J Clin Nutr* 91:487;2010.
29. Dherani, M, Murthy GVS, Gupta SK et al., *IOVS* 49:3328:2008.
30. Jalal D, Koorosh F, Fereidoun H. *Curr Eye Res* 34:118;2009.
31. Simon JA, Hudes ES, *J Clin Epidemiol* 52:1207;1999.
32. Valero MP, Fletcher, AE, DeStavola BL et al., *J Nutr* 132:1299;2002.
33. Ferrigno L, Aldigeri R., Rosmini F et al., *Ophthalmic Epidemiol* 12:71;2005.
34. Nourmohammadi I, Modarress M, Khanaki K, Shaabani M, *Ann Nutr Metab* 52:296;2008.
35. Moha, M, Sperduto RD, Angra SK et al., *Arch Ophthalmol* 107:670;1989.
36. McCarty CA, Mukesh BN, Fu CL, Taylor HR, *Am J Ophthalmol* 128:446;1999.
37. Lyle BJ, Mares-Perlman JA, Klein BE et al., *Am J Epidemiol* 149:801;1999.
38. Christen WG, Liu S, Glynn RJ et al., *D Arch Ophthalmol* 126:102;2008.
39. Jacques PF, Taylor A, Moeller S et al., *Arch Ophthalmol* 123:517;2005.
40. Nadalin G, Robman LD, McCarty CA et al., *Ophthal Epidemiol* 6:105;1999.
41. McNeil JJ, Robman L, Tikellis B. et al., *Ophthalmology* 111:75;2004.
42. Knekt P, Heliovarra M, Rissenen A et al., *BMJ* 304:1392;1992.
43. Leske MC, Wu SY, Hyman L et al., *Arch Ophthalmol* 113:1113;1995.
44. Rouhiainen P, Rouhiainen H, Saloneen JT, *Am J Epidemiol* 114:496;1996.
45. Gale CR, Hall NF, Phillips DIK, Martyn CN. *Ophthalmology* 108:1992;2001.
46. Mares-Perlman JA, Brady WE, Klein R et al. *Arch Ophthalmol* 113:518;1995.
47. Vu HTV, Robman L, Hodge A et al., *IOVS* 47:3783;2006.
48. Delcourt C, Carriere I, Delage M et al., *IOVS* 47:2329;2006.
49. Yeum KJ, Taylor A, Tang G, Russell RM, *IOVS* 36:2756;1995.
50. Mares-Perlman JA, Klein BEK, Klein R, Ritter LL, *Ophthalmology* 101:315;1994.
51. Chasan-Taber L, Willett WE, Seddon JM et al. *Am J Clin Nutr* 70:517;1999.
52. Brown L, Rimm EB, Seddon JM et al., *Am J Clin Nutr* 70:517;1999.
53. Lyle BJ, Mares-Perlman, JA, Klein BE et al., *Am J Clin Nutr* 69:272;1999.
54. Mares-Perlman, JA, Brady WE, Klein BE et al., *IOVS* 36:276;1995.
55. Christen WG, Manson JE, Glunn RJ et al., *Arch Ophthalmol* 121:372;2003.
56. Jacques PF, Bostom AG, Wilson PW et al., *Amer J Clin Nutr* 73:613;2001.
57. Jacques PF, Kalmbach R, Bagley PJ et al., *J Nutr*, 132:283;2002.
58. Kang SS, Wong PW, Norusis M, *Metab: Clin Exp* 36:458;1987.
59. Heinecke JW, Rosen J, Suzuki LA, Chait A, *J Biol Chem* 262:10098;1987.
60. Chen K.-J, Pam W-H, Yang F-L, et al. *Asia Pacific J Clin Nutr* 14:250;2005.
61. Kuzniarz M, Mitchel P, Cumming RG, Flood VM. *Am J Ophthalmol.* 132:19;2001.
62. Sperduto RD, Hu TS, Milton RC et al., *Arch Ophthalmol* 111:1246;1993.
63. Cumming RG, Mitchell P, Smith W. *Ophthalmol* 107:450;2000.
64. O'Dell BL. *J Nutr* 130:1432S;2000.
65. Food and Nutrition Board, *Dietary Reference Intakes for Vitamin A, Vitamin K, Arsenic, Boron, Chromium, Copper, Iodine, Iron, Manganese, Molybdenum, Nickel, Silicon, Vanadium, and Zinc. Institute of Medicine*, Washington, DC: National Academy Press; 2001.
66. Townend BS, Townend ME, Flood V et al., *Am J Ophthalmol* 143:932;2007.
67. Lu M, Cho E, Taylor A et al., *Am J Epidemiol* 6:948;2005.
68. Arnarsson A, Jonasson F, Sasaki H et al., *Dev Ophthalmol* 35:12;2002.
69. Age-Related Eye Disease Study Research Group, *Arch Ophthalmol* 119:1439;2001.

70. Chylack, LT Jr., Brown NB, Bron A et al., *Ophthal Epidemiol* 9:49;2002.
71. Clinical Trial of Nutritional Supplements and Age-Related Cataract Study Group, *Ophthalmology* 15:599;2008.
72. Teikari JM, Virtamo J, Rautalahti M et al., *Acta Ophthalmol Scand* 75:634;1997.
73. Prevalence of Blindness Data Tables (NEI Statistics and Data). National Eye Institute, National Institute of Health, 2004. www.nei.nih.gov/eyedata/pbd_tables.asp (accessed on June 4, 2012).
74. Snodderly DM. *Am J Clin Nutr* 62:1448S;1995.
75. Johnson LV, Ozaki S, Staples MK et al., *Exp Eye Res* 70:441;2000.
76. Johnson LV, Leitner WP, Staples MK, Anderson DH, *Exp Eye Res* 73:887;2001.
77. Wirostko E, Wirostko WJ, *Wirostko Acta Ophthalmol Scand* 82:243;2004.
78. Klein R, Klein BEK, Tomany SC, Crickshanks KJ, *Arch Ophthalmol* 2:674;2003.
79. Haddad S, Chen CA, Santangelo SL, Seddon JM, *Survey Ophthalmol* 1:316;2006.
80. Gorin MB, *Arch Ophthalmol* 125:21;2007.
81. Hageman GS, Anderson DH, Johnson LV et al., *Proc Nat Acad Sci U S A* 102:7227;2005.
82. Despriet DDG, Klaver CCW, Witteman JCM et al., *JAMA* 296:301;2006.
83. Age-Related Eye Disease Study Research Group, *Arch Ophthalmol* 125:1225;2007.
84. Eye Disease Case-Control Study Group and (EDCCSG), *Arch Ophthalmol* 111:104;1993.
85. Seddon JM, Ajani UA, Sperduto RD et al., *JAMA* 272:1413;1994.
86. West S, Vitale S, Hallifrisch J et al., *Arch Ophthalmol* 112:222;1994.
87. Christen WG, Glynn RJ, Chew EY, Buring JE, *Ophthalmology* 117:1163;2010.
88. Taylor HR, Tikellis G, Robman LD et al., *BMJ* 325:11;2002.
89. Teikari JM, Rautalahti M, Haukka J et al., *Acta Ophthalmol Scand* 76:224;1998.
90. Sanders TAB, Haines AP, Warmald R et al., *Am J Clin Nutr* 57:428;1993.
91. Bone RA, Landrum JT, Tarsis SL, *Vision Res* 25:1531;1985.
92. Snellen EL, Verbeek AL, Van Den Hoogen GW et al., *Acta Ophthalmol Scand* 0:368;2002.
93. Moeller SM, Voland R, Tinker L et al., *Arch Ophthalmol* 126:354;2008.
94. Moeller SM, Parekh N, Tinker L et al., *Arch Ophthalmol* 124:1151;2006.
95. Tan JSL, Wang JJ, Flood V et al., *Ophthalmol* 115:334;2008.
96. Bone RA, Landrum JT, Mayne ST, Gomez CM et al., *IOVS* 42:235;2001.
97. Wooten BR, Hammond BR, Land RI, Snodderly DM, *IOVS* 40:2481;1999.
98. Beatty S, Murray IJ, Henson DB, Carden D et al., *IOVS* 42:439;2001.
99. Bernstein PS, Shao D-Y, Wintch SW, *Ophthalmology* 109:1780;2002.
100. Schweitzer D, Lang GE, Remsch H et al., *Ophthalmology* 97:84–90;2000.
101. LaRowe TL, Mares JA, Snodderly DM et al., *Ophthalmology* 115:876;2008.
102. Axer-Siegel R, Bourla D, Ehrlich R et al., *Am J Ophthalmol* 137:84;2004.
103. Coral K, Raman R, Rathi S et al., *Eye* 20:203;2006.
104. Heuberger RA, Fisher AI, Jacques PF et al., *Am J Clin Nutr* 76:897;2002.
105. Kamburoglu G, Gumus K, Kadayifcilar S, Eldem B. *Graefes Arch Clin Exp Ophthalmol* 244:56;2006.
106. Krishnadev N, Meleth AAD, Chew EY. *Curr Opin Ophthalmol* 21:184;2010.
107. Nowak M, Swietochowska E, Wielkoszynski T et al., *Eur J Ophthalmol* 15:764–767;2005.
108. Rochtchina E, Wang JJ, Flood VM, Mitchell P, *Am J Ophthalmol* 143:344;2007.
109. Vine AK, Stader J, Branham K et al., *Ophthalmology* 112:2076;2005.
110. Christen WG, Glynn RJ, Chew EY et al., *Arch Int Med* 169:335;2009.
111. Benjo AM, Maranhao RC, Coimbra SR et al., *Atherosclerosis* 187:116;2006.
112. Hamilton SJ, Chew GT, Davis TME, Watts GF, *Diab Vasc Dis Res* 7:96;2010.
113. Warnholtz A, Wild P, Ostad MA et al., *Atherosclerosis* 204:216;2009.
114. Boker T, Fang T, Steinmetz, German R, *J Ophthalmol* 2:10;1993.
115. Friedman E, Krupsky S, Lane AM et al., *Ophthalmology* 102:640;1995.
116. Holz FG, Wolfensberger TJ, Piguet B et al., *Ophthalmology* 10:1522;1994.
117. Pauleikhoff D, Chen JC, Chisholm IH, Bird AC, *Am J Ophthalmol* 109:11;1990.
118. Sarks JP, Sarks SH, Killingsworth MC. *Eye* 2:552;1988.
119. Sark, SH. *Br J Ophthalmol* 60:324;1976.
120. Barakat MR, Metelitsina TI, DuPont JC, Grunwald JE, *Curr Eye Res* 31:629;2006.
121. Metelitsina TI, Grunwald JE, DuPont JC, Ying GS. *Br J Ophthalmol* 88:1568;2004.
122. Newsome DA, Oliver PD, Deupree DM et al., *Curr Eye Res* 11:213;1992.
123. Grahn BH, Paterson PG, Gottschall-Pass KT, Zhang Z, *J Am Coll Nutr* 20:106;2001.
124. Vasto S, Mocchegiani E, Candore G et al., *Biogerontology* 7:315;2006.
125. Marcellini F, Giuli C, Papa R et al., *Biogerontology* 7:339;2006.
126. Marian, E, Cornacchiola V, Polidori MC et al., *Biogerontology* 7:391;2006.
127. Erie JC, Good JA, Butz JA, Pulido JS, *Am J Ophthalmol* 147:276;2009.
128. Cho E, Seddon JM, Rosner B et al., *Ann Epidemiol* 11:328;2001.
129. Morris MS, Jacques PF, Chylack LT et al., *Ophthal Epidemiol* 14:288;2007.
130. Newsome DA, Swartz M, Leone NC et al., *Arch Ophthalmol* 106:192;1988.
131. Newsome DA. *Curr Eye Res* 33:598;2008.
132. Stur, M, Tittl M, Reitner A, Meisinger V, *IOVS* 37:225;1996.
133. Lengyel I, Flynn JM, Peto T et al., *Exp Eye Res* 84:772;2007.
134. Wood JPM, Osborne NN, *Neurochem Res* 28:1525;2003.
135. Adkins Y, Kelley DS, *J Nutr Biochem* 2:781;2010.
136. Bazan NG, Molina MF, Gordon WC, *Ann Rev Nutr* 31:321;2010.
137. Neuringer M, Anderson GJ, Connor WE, *Annu Rev Nutr* 8:517;1988.
138. Chong EWT, Kreis AJ, Wong TY et al., *Arch Ophthal* 126:826;2008.
139. Cho E, Hung S, Willett WE et al., *Am J Clin Nutr* 73:209;2001.

140. Seddon JM, Rosner B, Sperduto RD et al., *Arch Ophthalmol* 119:1191;2001.
141. Seddon JM, Cote J, Rosner B, *Arch Ophthalmol* 121:1728;2003.
142. Tan JSL, Wang JJ, Flood V, Mitchell P, *Arch Ophthalmol* 127:656;2009.
143. Smith W, Mitchell P, Leeder SR, *Arch Ophthalmol* 118:401;2000.
144. Sangiovanni JP, Agron E, Meleth AD et al., *Am J Clin Nutr* 90:1601;2009.
145. Mares-Perlman JA, Brady WE, Klein R et al., *Arch Ophthalmol* 113:743;1995.
146. Heuberger RA, Mares-Perlman JA, Klein R et al., *Arch Ophthalmol* 119:1833;2001.
147. Griffin MD, Xing N, Kumar R, *Ann Rev Nutr* 23:117;2003.
148. Holick MF, *Am J Clin Nutr* 79:62;2004.
149. Hayes CE, Nashold FE, Spach KM, Pedersen LB, *Cell Mol Biol* 49:277;2003.
150. Merlino LA, Curis J, Mikuls, TR et al., *Arthr Rheumat* 50:72;2004.
151. Timms PM, Mannan N, Hitman GA et al., *QJM* 95:787;2002.
152. Mora JR, Iwata M, von Andrian UH, *Nat Rev Immunol* 8:685;2008.
153. Mullin GE, Dobs A, *Nutr Clin Pract* 22:305;2007.
154. Craig TA, Sommer S, Sussman CR et al., *J Bone Min Res* 23:2008.
155. Bidmon HJ, Stumpf WE. *Histochemical* J 27:516;1995.
156. Parekh N, Chappell RJ, Millen AE et al., *Arch Ophthalmol* 125:661;2007.
157. Seddon JM, George S, Rosner B, *Arch Ophthalmol* 124:995;2006.
158. Golan S, Shalev V, Treister G et al., *Eye* 25:1122;2011.
159. van Leeuwen R, Boekhoorn S, Vingerling JR et al., *JAMA* 294:3101;2005.
160. Age-Related Eye Disease Study Research Group, *Arch Ophthalmol* 119:1417;2001.
161. Chong EWT, Wong TY, Kreis AJ et al., *BMJ* 335:755;2007.
162. Evans JR, Henshaw K, *Cochrane Database Syst Rev* (1): CD000253;2008.
163. Nathan DM, Cleary PA, Backlund JYC et al., *New Engl J Med* 353:2643;2005.
164. Holman RR, Paul SK, Bethel MA et al., *New Engl J Med* 359:1577;2008.
165. Klein R, Klein DE, Moss SE, Cruickshanks KJ, *Ophthalmology* 5:1801;1998.
166. Wirostko B, Wong TY, Simo R, *Prog Retinal Eye Res* 27:608;2008.
167. Baynes JW, Thorpe SR, *Diabetes* 48:1;1999.
168. Giugliano D, Ceriello A, Paolisso G, *Diabetes Care* 19:257;1996.
169. Rema M, Mohan V, Bhaskar A, Shanmugasundaram KR, *Indian J Ophthalmol* 43:17;1995.
170. Ali SM, Chakraborty SK, *Bangladesh Med Res Counc Bull* 15:7;1989.
171. Sinclair AJ, Girling AJ, Gray L et al., *Gerontology* 38:68;1992.
172. Gurler B, Vural J, Yilmaz N et al., *Eye* 14 Pt 5:730;2000.
173. Gupta MM, Char S, *Indian J Physiol Pharmacol* 49:187;2005.
174. Millen AE, Gruber M, Klein R et al., *Amer J Epidemiol* 158:225;2003.
175. Millen AE, Klein R, Folsom AR et al., *Am J Clin Nutr* 79: 865;73;2004.
176. Mayer-Davis EJ, Bell RA, Reboussin BA et al., *Ophthalmology* 105:2264;1998.
177. Lee C-TC, Gayton EL, Beulens JWJ et al., *Ophthalmology* 117:71;2010.
178. Martinoli L, Di Felice M, Seghieri G et al., *Int J Vit Nutr Res* 63:87;1993.
179. Willems D, Dorchy H, Dufrasne D, *Atherosclerosis* 137:S6;1998.
180. Ward NC, Wu JHY, Clarke MW et al., *J Hypertens* 25:227;2007.
181. Wu JHY, Ward NC, Indrawan AP et al., *Clin Chem* 5:511;2007.
182. Paolisso G, Balbi V, Volpe C, et al. *J Am Coll Nutr* 14:387;1995.
183. Ble-Castillo JL, Carmona-Diaz E, Mendez JD et al., *Biomed Pharmacother* 59:290;2005.
184. Reaven PD, Herold DA, Barnett J, Edelman S., *Diabetes Care* 18:807;1995.
185. Gazis A, White DJ, Page SR, Cockcroft JR, *Diabetic Med* 6:304;1999.
186. Boshtam M, Rafiei M, Golshadi ID et al., *Int J Vit Nutr Res* 75:341;2005.
187. Paolisso G, D'Amore A, Galzerano D et al., *Diabetes Care* 16:1433;1993.
188. Hatwal A, Gujral AS, Bhatia RP et al., *Acta Ophthalmol*, 67:714;1989.
189. Erasmus RT, Olukoga AO, Alanamu RA et al., *Trop Geogr Med* 41:234;1989.
190. Walter RM Jr., Uriu-Hare JY, Olin KL et al., *Diabetes Care* 14:1050;1991.
191. Sharma A, Dabla S, Agrawal RP et al., *J Ind Med Assoc* 105:16;2007.
192. de Valk HW, Hardus PL, van Rijn HJ, Erkelens DW, *Diabetes Care* 22:864;1999.
193. NEI, Vision Problems in the U.S. 2004. www.nei.nih.gov/ eyedata/ (accessed on June 4, 2012).
194. Ritch, R, *J Glaucoma* 10:S33;2001.
195. Kumar DM, Agarwal N, *J Glaucoma* 16:334;2007.
196. Anderson DR, *Am J Ophthalmol* 108:485;1989.
197. Sommer A, Tielsch JM, Katz J et al., *Arch Ophthalmology* 109:1090;1991.
198. Drance SM. *Bowman Lect Eye* 6(Pt 4):337;1992.
199. Coleman AL, Stone KL, Kodjebacheva G et al., *Am J Ophthalmol* 145:1081;2008.
200. Kang JH, Pasquale LR, Willett W et al., *Am J Epidemiol* 58:337;2003.
201. Das UN, *Lipids Health Dis* 7:37;2008.
202. SanGiovanni JP, Chew, EY, *Prog Retina Eye Res* 24:87;2005.
203. Kang JH, Pasquale, LR, Willett WC et al., *Am J Clin Nutr* 79:755;2004.
204. Re, H, Magulike N, Ghebremeskel K, Crawford M. Prostaglandins Leukotrienes Essential Fatty Acids 74:157;2006.
205. Moore P, El-Sherbeny A, Roon P et al., *Exp Eye Res* 73:45;2001.
206. Carroll JF, Tyagi SC, *Am J Hypertens* 8(5 Pt 1):692;2005.
207. Mujumdar VS., Aru GM, Tyag SC, *J Cell Biochem* 82:91;2001.
208. Graham IM, Daly LE, Refsum HM et al., *JAMA* 277:1775;1997.
209. Turacli ME, Tekeli O, Ozdemir F, Akar N, *Clin Exp Ophthalmol* 33:505;2005.
210. Bleich S, Roedl J, Von Ahsen N et al., *Am J Ophthalmol* 138:162;2004.
211. Leibovitch I, Kurtz S, Shemexh G et al., *J Glaucoma* 2:36;2003.
212. Vessani RM, Ritch R, Liebmann JM, Jofe M, *Am J Ophthalmol* 136:41;2003.

213. Clement CI, Goldberg I, Healey PR, Graham SL, *J Glaucoma* 18:73;2009.

214. Cumurcu T, Sahin S, Aydin E. *BMC Ophthalmology* 6:6;2006.

215. Puustjarvi T, Blomster H, Kontkanen M et al., *Graefes Arch Clin Exp Ophthalmol* 242:749;2004.

216. Altintas O, Maral H, Yuksel N et al., *Graefes Arch Clin Exp Ophthalmol* 243:677;2005.

217. Turgut B, Kaya M, Arslan S et al., *Clin Interventions Aging* 5:133;2010.

218. Bleich S, Junemann A, von Ahsen N et al., *J Neural Transm* 109:1499;2002.

219. Micheal S, Qamar R, Akhtar F et al., *Mol Vis* 15:2268;2009.

220. Finkelstein JD, *Eur J Pediatrics* 157(Suppl 2):S40;1998.

221. Rossler CW, Baleanu D, Reulbach U et al., *J Glaucoma* 19:576;2010.

222. Tranchina L, Centofanti M, Oddone F et al., *Graefes Arch Clin Exp Ophthalmol* 249:443;2010.

223. Levin LA, Clark JA, Johns LK, *EIOVS* 37:2744;1996.

224. Gree K, *Ophthalmic Res* 27(Suppl 1):143;1995.

225. Bautista RD, *Int Ophthalmol Clin* 39:57;1999.

226. Zanon-Moreno V, Ciancotti-Olivares L, Asencio J et al., *Mol Vis* 17:2997–3004;2011.

227. Yuki K, *Arch Clin Exp Ophthalmol* 248:243;2010.

228. Asregadoo ER, *Ann Ophthalmol* 11:1095;1979.

229. Engin KN, Yemisci B, Yigit U et al., In: Hatfield DL, Berry MJ, Gladyshev VN, eds. *Selenium: Its Molecular Biology and Role in Human Health.* Springer, New York, p. 99, 2006.

231. Thomson CD, *Analyst* 123:827;1998.

232. Bruhn RL, Stamer WE, Herrygers LA et al., *Br J Ophthalmol* 93:155;2009.

# 69 Nutrition and Brain Health

*Gary W. Small*

## CONTENTS

During the past several decades, physicians and scientists have shown increased interest in the connection between nutrition and brain health. Although the impact of our diet on normal brain development has been appreciated and driven public health recommendations for pregnancy and pediatric care, only recently has attention been focused on brain health and nutrition throughout the life span. Today, research is pointing to the need for a balanced and nutritious diet for maintaining cognitive health as we age. Nutrition also has an impact on other aspects of brain health, helping to maintain normal mood, mental focus, motivation, and attention. This chapter will highlight some of the scientific evidence indicating a relationship between nutrition and brain health and summarize some nutritional recommendations for maintaining cognitive health and mood stability as people age.

## BRAIN HEALTH AND AGING

Brain health is essential to general health since the brain controls all bodily functions.[1] A well-functioning brain has intact neurons and synapses that communicate messages to control basic bodily functions like breathing, heart rate, sensation, and movement, as well as such mental experiences as mood, thinking, reasoning, attention, and visual spatial skills. Age-related alterations in the striatum are accompanied by spatial disorientation, as well as declines in motor function that lead to diminished muscle strength and loss of balance and coordination.

As the brain ages, it atrophies, its synaptic connections become less effective, and its cells do not communicate as well as during youth. A gradual deposition of abnormal protein deposits—amyloid plaques and tau tangles—accumulate in brain regions controlling cognition, and these accumulations

correlate with cognitive decline.[2] Our group[3] performed positron emission tomography (PET) scanning, using a measure of brain plaques and tangles, 2-(1-{6-[(2-[F-18]fluoroethyl)(methyl)amino]-2-naphthyl}ethylidene)malononitrile (FDDNP), on middle-aged and older non-demented adults (median age 64 years) and found that increases in frontal, posterior cingulate, and global FDDNP binding at follow-up correlated with progression of memory decline ($r = -0.32$ to $-0.37$, $P = 0.03$–0.01) after 2 years. Moreover, we found that higher baseline FDDNP binding is associated with future decline in most cognitive domains, including language, attention, executive, and visuospatial abilities ($r = -0.31$ to $-0.56$, $P = 0.05$–0.002). These regional plaque and tangle binding patterns are consistent with known neuropathological patterns of plaque and tangle brain accumulation, spreading from the medial temporal to other neocortical regions as cognitive decline progresses. We also have found these abnormal protein deposits to correlate with late-life major depression and symptoms of anxiety and depression in non-demented volunteers.[4,5]

In addition to plaque and tangle accumulation, numerous neurotransmitter systems decline with aging, particularly cholinergic cells in the basal forebrain that project to brain regions controlling cognitive skills (e.g., frontal, parietal, medial temporal).[6] Neurons in the hippocampus (a brain region critical to forming new memories) show decline,[7] and age-associated general and regional brain atrophy accelerates when people develop mild cognitive impairment and dementia.[8] Loss of such neurotransmitters as dopamine and serotonin leads to decreased sensitivity to stimulation.

Age-related decline in brain health is accompanied by decline in cognitive skills. Although earlier studies suggested that cognitive decline did not begin until age 60, recent research indicates that such decline can be observed as early as age 45. Singh-Manoux et al.[9] observed 5198 men and 2192 women 45–70 years. Their cognitive abilities were assessed three times over a 10-year period. The investigators found that cognitive scores declined in all areas except vocabulary. They reported a 3.6% decline in mental reasoning in those aged 45–49 years and a 9.6% decline in men and 7.4% in women in the age range from 65 to 70 years.

These and other investigators point to the public health implications of such findings for preventing dementia: since these gradual declines in brain health and cognitive abilities precede the onset of dementia symptoms by decades, it might be possible to develop prevention treatments that delay the onset of those symptoms. Moreover, targeting individuals with risk factors for heart disease—obesity, hypertension, or high cholesterol—could not only protect them from future cardiac disease but from cognitive decline and dementia as well.

## LINK BETWEEN LIFESTYLE BEHAVIORS AND BRAIN HEALTH

Considerable scientific evidence points to lifestyle as key to protecting brain health as people age.[10–14] Nutrition, mental and physical exercise, stress reduction, and social engagement can improve cognitive performance and possibly delay the onset of dementia. Our group[15] found that a 6-week healthy lifestyle program including healthy nutrition, physical conditioning, memory training, and stress management improved both encoding and recalling of new verbal information, as well as self-perception of memory ability in older adults residing in continuing care retirement communities. In another study, we found that a 2-week healthy lifestyle program combining mental and physical exercise, stress reduction, and healthy diet was associated with significant effects on cognitive function and brain metabolism.[16] The reduced resting activity in left dorsolateral prefrontal cortex observed following the 2-week program may reflect greater cognitive efficiency of a brain region involved in working memory. Such evidence suggests that the impact of nutrition on brain health could be augmented when combined with several healthy lifestyle behaviors.

## FEEDING THE AGING BRAIN

Numerous nutrients are critical to maintaining brain health and supporting brain structure and function as we age. The ability to perform normal mental activities requires proper maintenance of the structural building blocks that modulate thinking, sensation, and behavior. This connection between nutrition and brain health begins during gestation—protein and energy supplementation of undernourished pregnant mothers and children improves cognitive abilities[17] and continues through the life span and is particularly important to the aging brain.

As the brain ages, inflammation and oxidation appear to contribute to neurodegeneration, just as they do in heart disease, diabetes, cancer, and aging of other body organs.[18,19] In fact, the amyloid plaques that accumulate in the brains of Alzheimer's disease patients show evidence of inflammation, including cytokines (protein molecules that attack foreign material) and activated microglia (cells that clean out cellular waste, ridding the brain of damaged neurons, plaques, and infectious agents). Many scientists theorize that chronic inflammation in the brain destroys neurons, and several investigations have suggested that certain medicines, foods, and healthy behaviors can reduce inflammation. Age-related oxidative stress also damages neurons. Omega-3 (ω-3) fats from nuts and fish and antioxidant fruits and vegetables may diminish age-related inflammatory and oxidative neuronal damage.

Nourishing our brains through a healthy diet appears to protect us from cognitive decline. A recent study[20] of more than 2000 people aged 65 years and older showed that research subjects who ate a greater amount of nuts, fish, tomatoes, poultry, vegetables, and fruits, and a lesser amount of high-fat dairy products, red meat, and butter, had a lower risk for Alzheimer's disease. These kinds of findings point to proper nutrition as a way to bolster brain health as we age.

## OMEGA-3 FATTY ACIDS

Although fat is essential for maintaining brain structure and function, the kinds of fats we ingest are as critical as the amount. Eating too much of any kind of fat can lead to overweight and obesity, so it is important to limit fat intake, but people also need to emphasize ω-3 fatty acids in their diets to protect brain health.

Most American diets are too rich in omega-6 (ω-6) fatty acids from such foods as red meats, margarine, mayonnaise, processed and fried foods, as well as corn and vegetable oils. These polyunsaturated ω-6 fatty acids promote inflammation and contribute to neuronal damage. Minimizing intake of ω-6 fatty acids will protect brain health, so eliminating a meal such as lamb chops and mashed potatoes and substituting grilled wild salmon with a green salad is an example of a brain-healthy alternative that is rich in ω-3 fatty acids and will protect the heart as well. A small amount of dietary ω-6 fatty acid is necessary for optimal brain health. In a typical American diet, the ratio of ingested ω-6 to ω-3 fatty acid is 20–1, whereas a 3 to 1 ω-6 to ω-3 should be the goal.

A diet rich in these anti-inflammatory ω-3 fatty acids is associated with a lower risk for developing Alzheimer's disease.[21] The most abundant ω-3 fatty acid in the brain, docosahexaenoic acid, or DHA, protects brain neurons against the toxic events associated with amyloid plaques and tau tangles. The prevalence of dementia among Nigerians, who eat a diet low in animal fat, is low compared with that of African Americans, who eat a diet with higher intake of ω-6 fatty acids.[22]

Although many Americans seem to prefer animal fat in their diet, at least one study suggested that substituting healthier fats can promote satiety and may help with weight management. This investigation of restaurant goers demonstrated that those who were served olive oil (rich in healthy omega-9 fatty acids) with their bread instead of butter ate 23% less bread compared with those served butter.[23]

Several randomized clinical trials have been performed to follow up on the association observed between ω-3 long-chain polyunsaturated fatty acids and cognitive health in older adults. For example, a 26-week study of cognitively intact subjects aged 65 years or older demonstrated that those subjects with the APOE-4 genetic risk for Alzheimer's disease demonstrated better attention span from ingesting either low daily dose (226 mg EPA, 176 mg DHA) or high dose (1093 mg EPA, 847 mg DHA) of fish oil compared with a placebo group.[24]

Better cognitive health in older adults has been associated with ω-3 polyunsaturated fatty acids (n-3 PUFAs). The n-3 long-chain PUFA eicosapentaenoic acid (EPA) and DHA are necessary for normal brain development and function.[25] Epidemiological studies have demonstrated a clear connection between cognitive performance and ω-3 fatty acids, but clinical trials of DHA supplementation have not been successful in slowing the rate of cognitive and functional decline in patients with mild to moderate Alzheimer's disease compared with placebo.[26] Even though a treatment may not show benefit in patients with dementia, it still may be effective in people with milder forms of cognitive impairment. To this end, an 18-month randomized, double-blind, controlled trial of ω-3 fatty acids in cognitively healthy older adults is currently in progress.[25]

ω-3 fatty acids also may offer a benefit in alleviating symptoms of depression. An 8-week controlled trial of daily 1050 mg of EPA and 150 mg of DHA found improvement in mood in patients with a major depressive episode without comorbid anxiety.[27] EPA appears to be the key ω-3 fatty acid component that is associated with efficacy in major depressive disorder.[28] The American Psychiatric Association recommends that patients with major depression ensure they ingest adequate dietary ω-3 fatty acids.

While ω-3 fatty acids promote brain health, dietary trans-fatty acids inhibit the production of ω-3 fatty acids. Dietary trans-fatty acids may actually result in negative emotions and behaviors. One study of 1018 subjects showed a significant association between dietary trans-fatty acids and aggressive behavior.[29]

## ANTIOXIDANT FOODS

Antioxidant foods protect neurons from oxidative free radicals that damage DNA. Polyphenols are potent antioxidants that can be found in strawberries, blackberries, blueberries, and other colorful berries, as well as grapes, pears, plums, cherries, broccoli, cabbage, celery, onions, and parsley.

Several large-scale studies indicate a link between dietary antioxidants and better brain health, including the Rotterdam Study, which demonstrated an association between higher dietary intake of the antioxidant vitamin E and a lower risk for developing Alzheimer's disease.[30] Another large-scale European study in people aged 65 and older showed an association between daily consumption of fruits and vegetables and a lower risk for all forms of dementia.[31] Although

memory impairment is associated with low antioxidant blood levels, short-term memory has been found to improve in laboratory animals fed with antioxidant-rich berry extracts.[32]

Other research suggests that when study subjects drink fruit or vegetable juice at least three times a week, they have a lower probability of developing Alzheimer's disease compared with those who drink these juices less than once a week.[33] Pomegranate juice is rich in antioxidant polyphenols, and recent studies suggest its brain health benefits for transgenic Alzheimer's mice. After drinking pomegranate juice for 6 months, the transgenic mice demonstrated significantly better memory ability and fewer brain amyloid plaques compared with those drinking placebo.[34] Green tea is another dietary antioxidant source; its phytochemicals have both anti-amyloid and anti-inflammatory properties.[35]

A double-blind, placebo-controlled trial randomized 4447 French participants aged 45–60 years to receive a daily combination of vitamin C (120 mg), β-carotene (6 mg), vitamin E (30 mg), selenium (100 μg), and zinc (20 mg) or a placebo. Subjects receiving the active antioxidant supplementation had better episodic memory scores. Verbal memory also improved by antioxidant supplementation only in subjects who were nonsmokers or who had low serum vitamin C concentrations at baseline.[36]

## OTHER BRAIN–HEALTHY CARBOHYDRATES

The brain uses a considerable amount of energy, and carbohydrates are the main source of that energy. It takes longer to digest whole grains and high-fiber foods than processed foods, and eating whole-grain and high-fiber foods helps control body weight, lower blood pressure, prevent strokes, and reduce the risk for diabetes and heart disease, conditions that can impair cognitive abilities.

Food processing removes some vitamins, minerals, and phytonutrients, as well as fiber from carbohydrates, which increases the glycemic index, the measure of how fast blood sugar rises after eating. Such processed foods as sugared cereals, cookies, and crackers have high-glycemic index ratings, and these foods are digested and absorbed rapidly. By contrast, fresh fruits and vegetables, soybeans, and nuts are digested more slowly, resulting in a slower blood sugar rise. Previous studies suggest that a diet that emphasizes low glycemic index foods may decrease the risk for developing type 2 diabetes.[37] Since diabetes can increase the risk for developing Alzheimer's disease, a low glycemic index diet may protect the brain as well. A low glycemic index diet also may reduce the risk for metabolic syndrome,[38] which increases the risk for heart disease, diabetes, and Alzheimer's disease.

## PROTEINS

Scientists from Columbia University reported that the risk for Alzheimer's disease is lower in people whose diets emphasize proteins from fish and nuts in combination with fruits and vegetables compared with diets that emphasize proteins from red meats and milk products like butter and have fewer fruits and vegetables.[20] Essential amino acids are those that the body cannot synthesize and must be obtained through the diet. Nine of the 20 amino acids are essential and can be obtained through fish, poultry, meat, eggs, milk, yogurt, cheese, and soybeans. The American Heart Association recommends eating fish twice a week; higher amounts could increase the risk for mercury toxicity. Predatory fish like shark and swordfish tend to have higher mercury levels than smaller fish like sole or salmon. Other foods that are sources of brain-healthy proteins include chicken breast, some cheeses (e.g., nonfat or low-fat cottage cheese, goat, mozzarella, ricotta), and nuts (e.g., walnuts, almonds).

## CURCUMIN AND OTHER SPICES

Used for centuries as a treatment for inflammatory diseases, curcumin (diferuloylmethane) is a yellow pigment in the spice turmeric. Considerable research has demonstrated that curcumin mediates its anti-inflammatory effects through the downregulation of inflammatory transcription factors, enzymes and cytokines.[39] A study including more than 1000 volunteers aged 60–93 years[40] showed that volunteers who ate curried foods more frequently had higher scores on the mini–mental state examination. Although evidence suggests that the anti-amyloid and anti-inflammatory effects of curcumin might protect brain health and improve cognitive functioning, a previous study in patients with Alzheimer's dementia did not show cognitive benefits.[41]

It is still possible that the potential anti-inflammatory and anti-amyloid effects of curcumin may only be observed in people at risk for dementia. The mechanism of action for curcumin is not clear, and evidence thus far has not confirmed that it is brain protective when taken as a supplement since the oils used to cook curried dishes may be necessary for it to benefit neuronal health. Moreover, it may not be necessary for curcumin to penetrate the blood–brain barrier for it to exert anti-inflammatory effects, which may be triggered by interactions with immune cells in the gastrointestinal tract. Our research team at UCLA recently initiated a study of curcumin versus placebo in non-demented older adults. Both neuropsychological tests and PET scans of amyloid plaques and tau tangles will be used as outcome measures.

Curcumin is one of many spices and herbs that are antioxidant and have potential to promote brain health. These include cinnamon, oregano, vanilla, parsley, ginger, basil, pepper, and chili. A recent study of the main active antioxidant ingredient in black pepper, piperine, demonstrated that the spice led to improved memory performance in transgenic Alzheimer's mice.[42]

## OVERWEIGHT, OBESITY, AND THE METABOLIC SYNDROME

An estimated 73 million Americans are obese, which increases their risk for heart disease, stroke, and diabetes— all conditions that can impair brain health and memory performance. Approximately 20% of people with obesity also have metabolic syndrome, a symptom cluster of central obesity, and elevated blood sugar, triglycerides, and blood pressure, as well as low levels of HDL cholesterol. This syndrome increases an individual's risk for memory loss. High blood levels of overall cholesterol or low levels of HDL cholesterol, hypertension, and high blood sugar levels have been found to be associated with increased cognitive decline.[43]

People who are overweight or obese in midlife have a higher rate of developing cognitive decline later in life. A recent study from the Swedish Twin Registry of people aged 65 years and older (mean 74 years) showed that both overweight and obesity at midlife independently increased risk for dementia, Alzheimer's disease, and vascular dementia.[44]

Body mass index (BMI) is often used as a measure for overweight and obesity; however, it is not a perfect measure for these conditions. Some individuals have high BMI, yet are at a healthy weight if their lean body mass is greater than that for the average individual. Other people may have BMIs in the normal range, but have large amounts of body fat because of central obesity, which increases their risk for metabolic syndrome.

Despite these caveats, BMI has been used as a measure associated with overweight and obesity. Investigators at Toulouse University in France with 2000 healthy volunteers aged 32–62 years found that a higher BMI at baseline correlated with greater cognitive decline after 5 years. Study volunteers with relatively higher BMIs demonstrated difficulties in list learning information processing.[45]

The fat that is present in central obesity is active in regulating normal and abnormal body function. These fat cells promote insulin resistance, which can lead to diabetes and cardiovascular disease and influence brain health. One study[46] showed that for people with an average age of 60 years, their degree of central obesity was inversely correlated with brain volume and smaller brain size increases dementia risk.

Recent research indicates that losing weight can actually improve memory performance. An investigation that followed obese patients for 12 weeks after weight loss surgery demonstrated significant improvements in memory performance compared with a control group.[47]

## OTHER VITAMIN SUPPLEMENTS

Epidemiological studies have connected dietary vitamin D to brain health and better cognitive abilities. These investigations have led to randomized clinical trials demonstrating cognitive benefits, but these effects may be limited to older adults. For example, a 6-week controlled trial of daily vitamin D (5000 IU cholecalciferol) or placebo included 128 young adult participants (mean age 22 years) and showed no cognitive benefits.[48]

A cross-sectional study of nutrient status and psychometric and imaging indices of brain health was performed in 104 dementia-free older adults, with an average age of 87 years.[49] The investigators reported two nutrient biomarker patterns to be associated with better cognitive performance and MRI measures: one high in plasma vitamins B ($B_1$, $B_2$, $B_6$, folate, and $B_{12}$),

C, D, and E, and another high in plasma marine ω-3 fatty acids. A third pattern that was high in trans fat was associated with less favorable cognitive function and lower total brain volume.

Use of dietary supplements is common among older individuals,[50] but long-term health consequences of many compounds are not known. A recent study[51] assessed the relation of vitamin and mineral supplement use to total mortality in 38,772 older women (mean age 62 years) in the Iowa Women's Health Study. Most of the supplements studied were not associated with a reduced total mortality rate in older women. The use of multivitamins, vitamin B$_6$, folic acid, iron, magnesium, zinc, and copper were associated with increased risk of total mortality compared with non-use. The association was strongest with supplemental iron. By contrast, calcium was associated with decreased risk of mortality.

## ALCOHOL

Clearly, excessive alcohol use is a major health problem worldwide. However, alcohol use in moderation is associated with a lower risk for dementia. A recent study demonstrated that light drinkers had almost a 30% lower risk for developing dementia than did people who either abstain from alcohol or drink in excess.[52] Because this study was not a double-blind placebo-controlled trial, it does not definitely prove a cause and effect relationship. It is possible that drinking in moderation is also associated with some other factor that protects brain health and lowers risk for dementia. For example, moderate drinkers may deal with other aspects of their lives in moderation, which could reflect a personality style associated with lower stress levels.

Precisely what defines light or moderate alcohol use varies among studies, but many experts agree that one glass of wine or spirits for women and two glasses for men per day is a reasonable definition. The male–female differences likely reflect the body weight and size differences between men and women.

Studies of transgenic Alzheimer's mice show that moderate wine consumption leads to fewer brain amyloid plaques.[53] It is possible that antioxidants in alcoholic beverages explain the possible brain protective benefits. Also, resveratrol, which increases life span in animals similar to caloric restriction, is an ingredient in grapes and wine. Clinical trials of resveratrol extracts are in progress to determine their potential benefits in preventing Alzheimer's disease.

## CAFFEINE AND COFFEE

Several epidemiological studies have demonstrated an association between drinking coffee and better brain health. For example, a large-scale Swedish investigation showed that drinking up to three cups of coffee a day was associated with a 65% lower risk for Alzheimer's disease.[54] Coffee consumption is also associated with a lower rate of developing Parkinson's disease and diabetes, both of which increase risk for dementia.[55]

Coffee and other caffeinated beverages also have short-term effects on mental state. Positive effects include an increase in alertness and attention, as well as an elevated mood. Drinking coffee can improve learning and recall; however, excessive caffeine consumption may result in irritability, anxiety, and insomnia. Some people cannot tolerate the acidity of coffee, so they prefer to get caffeine by drinking tea. Chocolate is another source of caffeine: six ounces of brewed coffee contains 100 mg of caffeine, compared with 40 mg from a similar amount of tea, and 10 mg from a chocolate bar.

## BRAIN–HEALTHY NUTRITION MECHANISMS

Clearly our dietary habits have an important effect on our brain health throughout life. Many nutritious foods may protect brain health by reducing inflammation. Other healthy lifestyle strategies, such as exercise, can have a similar effect on inflammation. And chronic inflammation may be an important mechanism for several age-related illnesses, including cancer, heart disease, and Alzheimer's disease.

Pro-inflammatory cytokines present in the adipose tissue of central obesity trigger excess inflammation throughout the body, and a low calorie diet can alter the expression of inflammatory genes in this adipose tissue. A healthy brain diet includes many foods that fight inflammation, including fruits, vegetables, fish, whole grains, legumes, spices, and herbs. Flavonoids, present in cocoa, citrus fruits, and green leafy vegetables, also have anti-inflammatory effects and have been found to benefit cognition in older subjects and laboratory animals.[56]

The interaction between nutrition and brain health is complex. For example, several gastrointestinal hormones or peptides, such as leptin and glucagon-like peptide1 (GLP1), have an influence on emotions and cognitive processes.[57,58] Leptin is synthesized in adipose tissue and sends signals to the brain to reduce appetite (receptors in hypothalamus, cortex, and hippocampus). Leptin also elevates brain-derived neurotrophic factor (BDNF), a protein that stimulates brain cell growth and synaptic connections, leading to a more efficient, sensitive, and adaptive brain. Both leptin and BDNF facilitate synaptic plasticity in the hippocampus. Genetically obese rodents with dysfunctional leptin receptors show impaired spatial learning.[57,58]

Scientists are continuing to tease out the specific components of brain-healthy nutrition in order to develop more evidence-based recommendations for consumers. Adherence to the Mediterranean diet, which includes fruits, vegetables, legumes, cereals, and fish with minimal meat and dairy products, is associated with a lower risk for Alzheimer's disease.[12] Additional studies are elucidating the specificity of mechanisms and effects of the various elements of the Mediterranean as well as other diets, both healthy and unhealthy ones.

In summary, the scientific evidence demonstrates a compelling connection between brain health and nutrition. A diet that emphasizes complex carbohydrates and whole grains;

avoids processed foods and high-glycemic index carbo-hydrates; maintains ideal body weight; includes ω-3 fatty acids, antioxidant fruits and vegetables, and proteins from fish, poultry, or lean beef is likely to support brain health and lower risk for age-related cognitive decline and mood distur-bances throughout life.

## DISCLAIMER

The University of California, Los Angeles, owns a U.S. pat-ent (6, 274, 119) entitled "Methods for Labeling beta-Amyloid Plaques and Neurofibrillary Tangles," and Dr. Small is among the inventors, has received royalties, and may receive royal-ties on future sales. Dr. Small reports having served as an advisor and/or having received lecture fees from Herbalife, Janssen, Lilly, Novartis, and Pfizer. Dr. Small also received a grant from Pom Wonderful.

## REFERENCES

1. Bloom, FE, Beal, F, Kupfer, DJ (Eds). *The Data Guide to Brain Health*. Dana Press, New York, 2011, 733 p.
2. Braak, H, Braak, E. *Acta Neuropathol* 82:239;1991.
3. Small, GW, Siddarth, P, Kepe, V et al. *Arch Neurol* 69:215;2012.
4. Kumar, A, Kepe, V, Barrio, JR et al. *Arch Gen Psychiatry* 68:1143;2011.
5. Lavretsky, H, Siddarth, P, Kepe, V et al. *Am J Geriatr Psychiatry* 17:493;2009.
6. Holmes, C, Ballard, C, Lehmann, D et al. *J Neurol Neurosurg Psychiatry* 76:640;2005.
7. Kepe, V, Barrio, JR, Huang, S-C et al. *Proc Natl Acad Sci U S A* 103:702;2006.
8. Burggren, AC, Renner, B, Jones, M et al. *Int Alzheimers Dis Mar* 15:956053;2011.
9. Singh-Manoux, A, Kivimaki, M, Glymour, MM et al. *Br Med J* 344:7622;2011.
10. Small, GW, Ercoli, LM, Silverman, DHS et al. *Proc Natl Acad Sci U S A* 97:6037;2000.
11. Rolland, Y, AbellanvanKan, G, Vellas, B. *Clin Geriatr Med* 26:75;2010.
12. Sofi, F, Macchi, C, Abbate, R. et al. *J Alzheimers Dis* 20:795;2010s.
13. Lee, Y, Back, JH, Kim, J. *Int Psychogeriatr* 22:174;2010.
14. Merrill, DA, Small, GW. *Psychiatr Clin N Am* 34:249;2011.
15. Miller, KJ, Siddarth, P, Gaines, JM et al. *Am J Geriatr Psychiatry* 20:514;2012.
16. Small, GW, Silverman, DHS, Siddarth, P et al. *Am J Geriatr Psychiatry* 14:538;2006.
17. Freeman, HE, Klein, RE, Kagan, J, Yarbrough, C. *Am J Public Health* 67:233;1977.
18. Akiyama, H, Barger, S, Barnum, S et al. *Neurobiol Aging* 21;383;2000.
19. Serviddio, G, deMatthaeis, A et al. *J Nephrol* 23(Suppl 15):S29;2010.
20. Gu, Y, Nieves, JW, Stern, Y et al. *Arch Neurol* 67:699;2010.
21. Cole, GM et al. *Prostaglandins Leukot Essent Fatty Acids* 81:213;2009.
22. Ogunniyi, A, Baiyewu, O, Gureje, O et al. *Eur J Neurol* 7:485;2000

23. Wansink, B, Linder, LR. *Int J Obes Relat Metab Disord* 27:866;2003.
24. Van de Rest, O, Geleijnse, J, Kok, F et al. *Neurology* 71:430;2008.
25. Danthiir, V, Burns, NR, Nettelbeck, T et al. *Nutr J* 10:117;2011.
26. Quinn, JF, Raman, R, Thomas, RG et al. *JAMA* 304:1903;2010.
27. Lespérance, F, Frasure-Smith, N, St-André, E et al. *J Clin Psychiatry* 72:1054;2011.
28. Martins, JG, Bentsen, H, Puri, BK. *Mol Psychiatry* 17:1144;2012.
29. Golomb, BA, Evans, MA, White, HL, Dimsdale, JE. *PLoS ONE* 332175;2012.
30. Devore, EE, Grodstein, F, vanRooij, FJ et al. *Arch Neurol* 67:819;2010.
31. Raffaitin, C, Letenneur, L. *Neurology* 69:1921;2007.
32. Goyarzu, P, Malin, DH, Lau, FC et al. *Nutr Neurosci* 7:75;2004.
33. Dai, Q, Borenstein, AR, Wu, Y et al. *Am J Med* 119:751;2006.
34. Hartman, RE, Shah, A, Fagan, AM et al. *Neurobiol Dis* 24:506;2006.
35. Kim, J, Lee, HJ, Lee, KW. *J Neurochem* 112:1415;2010.
36. Kesse-Guyot, E, Fezeu, L, Jeandel, C et al. *Am J Clin Nutr* 94:892;2011.
37. Sluijs, I, van der Schouw, YT, van der A, DL et al. *Am J Clin Nutr* 92:905;2010.
38. Finley, CE, Barlow, CE, Halton, TL, Haskell, WL. *J Am Diet Assoc* 110:1820;2010.
39. Aggarwal, BB, Sung, B. *Trends Pharmacol Sci* 30:85;2009.
40. Ringman, JM, Frautschy, SA, Cole, GM et al. *Curr Alzheimer Res* 2:131;2005.
41. Ng, TP, Chiam, PC, Lee, T et al. *Am J Epidemiol* 164:898;2006.
42. Chonpathompikunlert, P, Wattanathorn, J, Muchimapura, S et al. *Food Chem Toxicol* 48:798;2010.
43. Raffaitin, C, Gin, H, Empana, JP et al. *Diabetes Care* 32:169;2009.
44. Xu, WL, Atti, AR, Gatz, M et al. *Neurology* 76:1568;2011.
45. Cournot, M, Marquié, JC, Ansiau, D et al. *Neurology* 67:1208;2006.
46. Debette, S, Beiser, A, Hoffmann, U et al. *Ann Neurol* 68:136;2010.
47. Gunstad, J, Strain, G, Devlin, MJ et al. *Surg Obes Rel Dis* 7:465;2011.
48. Dean, AJ, Bellgrove, MA, Hall, T et al. *PLoS ONE* 6:e25966;2011.
49. Bowman, GL, Silbert, LC, Howieson, D et al. *Neurology* 78:241;2012.
50. Park, K, Harnack, L, Jacobs, DR. *Am J Epidemiol* 169:887;2009.
51. Mursu, J, Robien, K, Harnack, LJ et al. *Arch Intern Med* 171:1625;2011.
52. Anstey, KJ, Mack, HA, Cherbuin, N et al. *Am J Geriatr Psychiatry* 17:542;2009.
53. Wang, J, Ho, L, Zhao, Z et al. *FASEB J* 20:2313;2006.
54. Eskelinen, MH, Kivipelto, M. *J Alzheimers Dis* 20(Suppl 1):S167;2010.
55. Chen, X, Ghribi, O, Geiger, JD et al. *J Alzheimers Dis* 20(Suppl 1):S127;2010.
56. Gomez-Pinilla, F. *Nature Rev* 8:568;2008.
57. Komori, T, Morikawa, Y, Nanjo, K et al. *Neuroscience* 139:1107;2006.
58. Li, XL, Aou, S, Oomura, Y et al. *Neuroscience* 113:607;2002.

# 70 Nutrition and the Skin

*Laura L. Bernet, Christina N. Kim, and Jenny Kim*

## CONTENTS

## INTRODUCTION

Dietary supplements compose a large and lucrative market. One analysis estimated sales of nutritional supplements to exceed $23 billion in 2009.[1] Labels purport an array of benefits, ranging from improved heart health to increased metabolism, to enhanced immunity. Cosmeceuticals, or over-the-counter products proposed to benefit skin appearance, texture, or health, make up a healthy portion of this market, with one 2006 market analysis anticipating sales to exceed $6.4 billion per year by 2010.[2] The question of whether topical nutrients have effects on the skin when taken orally is a good one. Certain vitamin deficiencies and excesses have well-documented effects on skin health. And many nutrients show skin bioavailability when ingested orally and thus warrant study for their cutaneous effects. In this chapter, we aim to review the current literature of certain dietary factors on skin health. We focus mainly on the in vivo human analyses in an attempt to focus the review. Indeed, this work may be limited by studies not included.

## VITAMIN A

Vitamin A derivatives, specifically synthetic retinoids, including isotretinoin, acitretin, and etretinate, are well known to physicians. They are successfully used both topically and systemically to treat numerous skin diseases.[2] A full review of these effects is beyond the scope of this chapter. Here, we will focus on natural sources of vitamin A and its effects on skin.

Vitamin A occurs both as retinol and carotenoids in nature. Retinol or preformed vitamin A, the vitamin's most potent form, is found in animal tissues. It is abundant in milk, liver, and eggs. In addition to other functions, many carotenoids possess vitamin A activity and are thus termed provitamin A.[2,3] They are found in plants and will be discussed subsequently. Retinol is metabolized into all-*trans*-retinoic acid (ATRA) and retinaldehydes. Retinaldehyde palmitate, specifically, is the storage form found in hepatic tissue. Vitamin A is fat soluble and required for epithelial maintenance and differentiation as well as for human reproduction. Humans require 2500–3000 IU/day, and the normal human serum concentration is 0.35–0.75 µg/mL. ATRA acts via a nuclear receptor, the retinoic acid receptor (RAR), which dimerizes with the retinoid X receptor (RXR) to form a transcriptionally active complex. In the epidermis, ATRA has varying action depending on the proliferative state.[3] In normal epidermis, retinoic acid promotes proliferation and thickened skin. In hyperproliferative epidermis, however, retinoic acid has the opposite effect, decreasing and thus normalizing the growth. Additionally, retinoids have anti-inflammatory effects via decreased keratinocyte TNF-alpha and nitric oxide synthesis.[3] Given these effects, vitamin A has been studied for its use in wound healing as well as psoriasis. In addition, thickened epidermis and theoretically better ultraviolet radiation (UVR) absorption as well as the anti-inflammatory properties have led some to study vitamin A's potential anti-skin

cancer effects. Of note, ATRA is photochemically unstable and often converted to both 9-*cis*-retinoic acid and 13-*cis*-retinoic acid or the natural form of isotretinoin. This explains why hypervitaminosis A (occurring at doses >50,000 IU/day in adults) results in a picture similar to the side effect profile of isotretinoin therapy and why vitamin A may have effect in diseases treated by isotretinoin and other derivatives.[3]

### WOUND HEALING

Both topical and dietary supplementation with vitamin A have shown great promise for augmenting impaired wound healing in animals.[4–9] In animals treated with glucocorticoids, inoculated with tumor cells, or with chemically induced diabetes, high-dose vitamin A supplementation speeded wound healing toward the rate of non-impaired controls.[4,6,8,9] It increases collagen production, fibroplasia, and restores the inflammatory response retarded by glucocorticoid treatment.[4,8,10] In humans, dietary studies are lacking. There was an isolated case report that dietary supplementation with vitamin A may increase the rate of wound healing in a prednisone-treated child.[8] Epidemiologic studies have shown decreased levels of vitamin A in people with chronic leg ulcers.[11,12] There have been no randomized controlled trials in this area.

### SKIN CANCER

Vitamin A and its derivatives lead to thickening of the epidermis, which in theory may provide UVR protection and thus skin cancer prevention. Despite the fact that a side effect of isotretinoin is photosensitivity, convincing work has shown that supplementation with retinoids, including high-dose isotretinoin (2 mg/kg) and etretinate, significantly decrease the incidence of non-melanoma skin cancer (NMSC) in patients with xeroderma pigmentosum and renal transplant patients, respectively.[13,14] Lower-dose isotretinoin in normal patients with moderate risk of NMSC has not been effective, however.[15] Unfortunately, dietary supplementation with vitamin A, though better tolerated by patients, has shown mixed results. In 1986, Wald et al. showed lower serum retinol levels in patients who would develop cancer of any form within 1–2 years compared to patients who did not develop skin cancer.[16] Subsequently, in a case-control study, Wei et al. showed an association between basal cell carcinoma (BCC) risk and lower intake of vitamin A.[17] In a randomized controlled trial, Moon et al. showed 25,000 IU of retinol supplementation over 5 years protected against the development of squamous cell carcinoma (SCC) in moderate-risk patients.[18] Another RCT, conducted by Levine et al. in 1997, showed no protective effect of the same dose of retinol over 3 years for either SCC or BCC.[19] Admittedly, these patients were at higher risk for NMSC development than in the Moon et al. study. A case-control study in 1995 actually showed increased levels of serum retinol in cases of BCC compared to controls.[20] Most other studies, however, have shown no relation between dietary vitamin A intake and SCC or BCC incidence.[19,21–25]

## Psoriasis

Although topical and systemic vitamin A derivatives are known to be effective in treating psoriasis, there is little evidence to support a role for dietary supplementation in this disease. There are reports that vitamin A serum levels are low in patients with varying types of psoriasis, although others contradict these findings.[26,27] Vitamin A metabolism may be altered in psoriatic skin, leading to increased retinoic acid synthesis and retinoic acid–binding protein 2 levels.[28] To our knowledge, there are no prospective trials looking at vitamin A dietary supplementation as a therapeutic approach to psoriasis. This is unfortunate, as the use of vitamin A derivatives is often limited by the side effect profile.[26,27]

Despite the wide-ranging effects of synthetic retinoids for skin health, dietary supplementation with vitamin A has less well-defined effects. The work regarding cancer prevention in normal populations is contradictory, and most studies show no association. This is surprising, given the potent effect of synthetic retinoids on patients with xeroderma pigmentosum and immunosuppression. The animal work for wound healing is very provocative. It is noteworthy that the effects are only seen in immunosuppressed animals and points to interesting mechanistic interactions between glucocorticoid and retinoid cell signaling pathways. Further studies in humans are warranted. Psoriasis can be effectively treated with some synthetic retinoids, but dietary evidence for natural vitamin A is sparse and limited to correlation.

## CAROTENOIDS

Carotenoids are found abundantly in plants. They have an extensive networks of double bonds, which make them ideal reactive oxygen species (ROS) scavengers, but also confer their bright colors to many fruits, vegetables, birds, insects, and crustaceons.[28] They also impart color to humans through the well-documented phenomenon of carotenodermia or yellowing of the skin.[29] Humans cannot synthesize carotenoids and thus are reliant upon diet. Carotenoids are bioavailable and concentrate in human skin.[30] Many carotenoids (beta-carotene, alpha-carotene, and beta-cryptoxanthin) have provitamin A activity.[3] It has been estimated that in third-world countries, 70% of dietary vitamin A is actually supplied by carotenoids, although this is likely much less in the developed world.[31] Carotenoids are divided into two groups based on composition. Carotenes, including beta-carotene, alpha-carotene, and lycopene, are composed of only carbon and hydrogen atoms. Xanthophylls, namely, zeaxanthin, lutein, alpha- and beta-cryptoxanthin, canthaxanthin, and astaxanthin, contain an oxygen atom.[31]

In addition to provitamin A activity, carotenoids are biologically active in a number of ways. As antioxidants, they scavenge singlet molecular oxygen and peroxyl radicals, decrease generation of these free radicals, and may prevent lipid peroxidation.[32] Carotenoids also have non-antioxidant effects. They have been shown to induce phase I and phase II metabolism and to have activity on gap junction communication, cell cycle proteins, and intracellular signaling.[31,32] It is through these latter effects that carotenoids, and in particular lycopene, are thought to inhibit cancer cell line growth in vitro.[33–36] Interestingly, under specific conditions, carotenoids may become prooxidant.[37,38] In accordance, animal models have shown differential effects of dietary carotenoids on skin carcinogenesis.[39]

Because of the potent antioxidant activity of carotenoids and their photoprotective action in plants, these nutrients have been studied for their photoprotective, antineoplastic, and immune regulatory properties in humans. While the role for acute photoprotection is promising, unfortunately, the work on cutaneous cancer prevention has been less so. Indeed, certain carotenoids have been recently implicated as procarcinogenic. The initial work regarding skin cell–mediated immunity and carotenoids suggested a supplementary role; however, more recent studies suggest that a well-balanced diet is all one needs. Finally, the most recent work on skin structure and function, while far from conclusive, is suggestive and interesting.

## Photoprotection

Skin carotenoid concentration is known to decrease upon UV irradiation, suggesting a protective role.[40] High doses of beta-carotene supplementation have reportedly improved photosensitivity disorders.[41–43] Accordingly, a number of studies suggest that carotenoids have acute photoprotective effects on human skin. Individual carotenoids, including beta-carotene both alone and with vitamin E, lutein, lycopene, as well as mixture of various carotenoids, increase the minimal erythema dose (MED) and/or decrease UV-induced erythema in human subjects.[43–49] In addition, it has been documented that carotenoids in combination with vitamin E and selenium lead to decreased post-UVR sunburn cell number and p53 expression, suggesting protection at the cellular level.[50] One study showed that tomato paste rich in lycopene reduced UVR-induced MMP-1 expression and mitochondrial DNA damage.[45] Contrary results were shown in a more recent study. No improvement in MED or oxidative stress was seen after 8 weeks of daily 15 mg beta-carotene supplementation.[51] This trial used a lower dose of carotenoids than in the previous studies, and it has been suggested that carotenoids do not exert protective effects until after 10 weeks of supplementation.[52]

## Carcinogenesis

Despite the promising work for photoprotection, carotenoids' roles in cutaneous cancer protection are less encouraging. Older epidemiologic studies associated increased intake of foods high in carotenoids with lower cancer rates.[53] Looking at melanoma, BCC, SCC, and actinic keratoses, several large studies, including multicenter randomized controlled trials with beta-carotene, have shown that carotenoids do not protect against skin cancer. All of these studies were relatively short (4–13 years), therefore not accounting for the slow growing nature of many of these cancers nor the possibility that much of the cellular damage may have been done in childhood, far prior to supplementation.[54–60] Interestingly, one large 5-year study showed an increased risk of melanoma in women supplemented with an antioxidant complex containing vitamin C, vitamin E, beta-carotene, selenium, and zinc.[61] However, in a longer-term follow-up study, this significance was lost, showing no difference from placebo.[62] Surprisingly, it has been found that beta-carotene may in fact be harmful, leading to increased rates of lung cancer and gastric cancer.[63,64] This has led many to recommend against beta-carotene supplementation. A recent study attributed this to a dose effect, showing that 90 mg supplementation led to a nonsignificant increase in thymine-dimer formation while the 30 mg dose led to decreased thymine-dimer formation.[65] Although interesting, even the low dose in this trial was higher than that for previous studies showing increased risk of lung cancer, and therefore this study does not bring order to the mixed results. Some attribute this potential carcinogenic role of beta-carotene to its prooxidant activity or to its ability to alter expression of RAR subtype expression.[31]

## IMMUNE FUNCTION

The evidence for carotenoids contributing to skin cell–mediated immunity is conflicting. In humans, this immunity has been measured by cumulative induration in delayed-type hypersensitivity (DTH) reactions. Bogden et al. showed that 1 year of micronutrient supplementation increased DTH responsiveness in elderly subjects.[66] The studied supplement contained only 0.75 mg of beta-carotene among other nutrients, but this was enough to increase serum beta-carotene concentrations. A second study by Herraiz et al. showed that UVR-induced immunosuppression was significantly decreased in elderly subjects supplemented with 30 mg of daily beta-carotene compared to placebo over 47 days.[67] Contradicting evidence was given in both a short, 3-week, high-dose (90 mg beta-carotene per day) intervention as well as in a larger long-term population-based study by Santos et al.[68] These studies showed no difference in either DTH responses or ex vivo cytokine responses between supplemented and non-supplemented groups. Girodon et al. and Watzl et al. documented similarly negative results with 1 year of daily 6 mg beta-carotene combined with vitamin E and C supplementation and 8 weeks of daily dietary tomato juice containing 47 mg of lycopene, respectively.[69,70] These differences may be explained by the lower baseline plasma levels of beta-carotene seen in the Herraiz et al. study population compared to those in the other trials. In addition, the placebo subjects in Herraiz et al. were subjected to a low-carotenoid diet and subsequently experienced a mean 50% decline in plasma beta-carotene levels. Furthermore, the significant difference between the DTH response in the placebo group compared to the supplement group appears to have resulted from the decline in cell-mediated immunity in the placebo group as opposed to a positive effect in the supplement group. This suggests that dietary deficiency has a negative

effect and says less about supra-physiologic supplementation. Accordingly, it has been shown that a low-carotenoid diet reduces T-lymphocyte function in vivo.[71] The second positive study by Bogden et al. was a trial of numerous combined antioxidants, vitamins, and minerals; thus, the positive effect may be due to substances other than carotenoids.

## SKIN STRUCTURE AND FUNCTION

Many small studies have investigated the in vivo effects of carotenoids on skin structure and function. Heinrich et al. showed that a mixture of carotenoids, selenium, and vitamin E may increase skin density and thickness, while decreasing roughness and scaling.[72] Another study showed lycopene supplementation may increase procollagen expression in UVR-exposed skin.[45] A third study suggested that 12 weeks of lutein and zeaxanthin significantly improves elasticity, increases skin surface lipids, and increases skin hydration.[48] Another showed improved skin hydration after 8 weeks of lutein and zeaxanthin supplementation.[73] Darvin et al. showed that skin lycopene concentrations correlated significantly with objective skin roughness.[74] Although suggestive, these findings are difficult to interpret without clinical correlation.

In summary, carotenoid supplementation, by increasing MED, decreasing UVR-induced erythema, and altering markers of acute photodamage, appears to have an acutely photoprotective effect in humans. Although longer-term studies are needed, carotenoids have no proven anticarcinogenic abilities in humans. Indeed, beta-carotene supplementation may be procarcinogenic, and doses above the daily-recommended value should not be suggested for either long-term photoprotection or cancer prevention. Skin cell–mediated immunity may be affected by beta-carotene, but the current data suggest that baseline deficiency may lead to negative effects, whereas supra-dietary supplementation may not be as important. Studies regarding skin structure and function suggest an effect, but larger studies with clinical correlation are needed.

# VITAMIN E

Vitamin E, also known as alpha- or gamma-tocopherol, was first isolated from wheat germ oil in 1936 by Evans et al. Initially, it was investigated for its fertility-saving properties in mice. Appropriately, the word tocopherol is derived from the Greek word for childbirth. Subsequently, it was discovered that vitamin E was a lipid soluble antioxidant, which quenches singlet oxygen and stabilizes cell membranes.[75] The vitamin is found in numerous fresh vegetables, vegetable oils, cereals, and nuts. The recommended daily intake (RDI) for humans is 30 IU or roughly 15 mg/day. Deficiency leads to hemolysis and neurologic abnormalities, including ataxia. Vitamin E is bioavailable, and its skin concentrations increase after dietary intake. The mechanism for delivery to the skin is not entirely clear, but it has been suggested that sebum excretion plays a role.[76] Vitamin E is the predominant antioxidant found in human epidermis. It is largely located in the stratum corneum. Vitamin E skin levels are decreased by exposure to ozone, benzoyl peroxide, and by almost 50% upon UVR exposure. Interestingly, vitamin E can be regenerated by the presence of other antioxidants, including vitamin C.[77]

In vitro work has shown that vitamin E slows melanoma growth by promoting apoptosis in tumor cells and inhibiting VEGF-signaled angiogenesis. Work in mice has suggested that topical use may improve wound healing, photoprotection, and cutaneous skin cancer.[76] Human topical studies have partially corroborated these findings, showing significantly decreased acute UVR-induced erythema, edema, and sunburn cell formation after topical vitamin application.[2] Mechanistically, topical vitamin E decreases UV-induced lipid peroxidation, immunosuppression, and DNA adduct formation in human skin.[2]

Dietary supplementation has been less well studied in humans. There have been reports of benefit for yellow nail syndrome, vibration disease, and epidermolysis bullosa; however there is little scientific data to confirm these suggestions.[76] Although no definitive therapeutic role has been defined, more recent work has insinuated a place for vitamin E supplementation in photoprotection, skin cancer prevention, atopic dermatitis, and fibrosis.

## PHOTOPROTECTION

In a small 1998 study by Eberlein-Konig et al., 10 subjects were given 1000 IU/day of vitamin E combined with 2000 mg/day of vitamin C for 8 days. Compared to a placebo group and baseline, the supplemented group showed significant increase in MED and significant decrease in cutaneous blood flow.[78] In another 8-day study, Fuchs et al. showed the importance of combining vitamin E with another antioxidant when they observed a significant increase in MED in 10 subjects supplemented with both 2 g of vitamin E per day and 3 g of vitamin C per day, but not in those treated with either vitamin alone or in placebo.[79] A later study showed no change in MED with 8 weeks of 400 IU of vitamin E alone, although there was a small improvement in the UVR-induced skin oxidation as measured by glutathione levels.[51] Vitamin E was combined with carotenoids in a similar study where it led to earlier but not greater improvement in MED than carotenoids alone.[44] Vitamin E, in combination with vitamin C shows promise for photoprotection.

## SKIN CARCINOGENESIS

Given the potential for photoprotection, dietary vitamin E has been investigated for its anticarcinogenic abilities. Despite promising work in animals and epidemiologic efforts, recent human studies have been limited to either mixed prospective interventions or short case-control and cohort studies.[22,76] A prospective trial of vitamin E (30 mg/day) mixed with other antioxidants, including vitamin C, suggested that this combination has no benefit for skin cancer prevention.[61,62] In an Australian population, Heinen et al. showed a small but significantly increased risk (RR 2.6; 95% confidence interval 1.1–6.3) of BCC in patients in the upper tertile of vitamin E

intake (9.7–18.6 mg/day).[25] Non-interventional case-control and cohort studies have shown no relationship between vitamin E serum concentration (not dietary intake) and skin cancer incidence, the longest of which was 17 years.[20,21,54] However, the 17-year study was based on blood draws from a single time point and relied on hospitalization records for diagnosis.[20] This design fails to recognize the incidence of milder skin cancers addressed in private offices as well as the changes in vitamin E serum concentrations that may have occurred over time. The other studies were relatively short (5–8 years), not accounting for the slow growing nature of NMSCs. Indeed, at least one study admitted that many control subjects developed BCCs after the study period.[21] The discrepancy between the apparent photoprotective nature of vitamin E and the disappointing results for skin cancer prevention may be explained in a number of ways. First, the degree of photoprotection achieved with vitamin E supplementation is relatively low compared to that achieved with topical sunscreens. At best, the sun protection factor (SPF) achieved with vitamin E was 1.78.[79] Second, the only prospective study included a dose much lower than that in the photoprotection studies.[61,62] Finally, the retrospective studies showing no benefit for cancer prevention did not account for vitamin C intake, which is important in vitamin E's ability to photoprotect.[79] Thus, it is difficult to determine either a detrimental or beneficial effect of vitamin E for skin cancer prevention from the existing evidence. Longer-term studies including higher-dose vitamin E and vitamin C supplementation may be needed before a conclusion can be drawn.

## IMMUNITY

Interestingly, in a small, 8 day, nine-subject study designed to look at the protective potential for vitamin E and C in polymorphic light eruption (PMLE), the placebo group showed significantly reduced symptoms upon re-exposure to UVR at the end of the trial. The authors postulated that this reduced response in the placebo may represent UV-induced immune suppression and that the negative treatment group results represent protection by vitamin E and C from this immune suppression.[80] Indeed, a number of trials have shown enhanced cell-mediated immunity in subjects supplemented with high-dose vitamin E (100–400 mg/day) compared to baseline or placebo.[81–83] Together, these trials suggest that a serum level of 80% higher than that in average adults leads to improved skin cell–mediated immunity.

## ATOPIC DERMATITIS

Vitamin E's antioxidant nature, as well as its possible immune-modulating abilities, makes it an interesting candidate for study in allergic disease. To our knowledge, prospective treatment trials are limited to 2002 work by Tsoureli-Nikita et al. Here, adult subjects with moderate-to-severe atopic dermatitis showed subjective symptomatic improvement and decreased IgE levels when treated with 400 IU of vitamin E daily for 8 months compared to placebo.[81] This trial was single blind and lacked mention of statistical significance; however, the response to vitamin E (15% remission in treatment group versus 0% in the control, and 8% worsening in the treatment group versus 81% in the control group) was large enough to warrant further more well-controlled studies. Unfortunately, the work since has been limited to associative epidemiologic studies. In 2005, Hoppu et al. showed no correlation between maternal and infant serum vitamin E levels and the presence of atopic dermatitis in the first year of life.[84] When Martindale et al. extended their analysis to 2 years and limited it to children of atopic mothers, however, higher vitamin E intake during pregnancy, as measured by a food frequency questionnaire, was associated with decreased rates of atopic eczema in the second year of life.[85] In this study, similar to the previous, there was no association between maternal or cord blood antioxidant levels and atopic dermatitis. In 2010, Oh et al. and Okuda et al. showed inverse association of atopic dermatitis and vitamin E intake and serum levels, respectively.[86,87] Oh et al. studied preschool age Korean children, while Okuda et al. examined 10–13-year-old Japanese children. Though far from conclusive, together, this work is suggestive of a role for vitamin E intake in atopic dermatitis. It is not yet clear if relative deficiency is predispositional or if supranutritional doses of vitamin E are required for improvement and/or prevention of atopic dermatitis.

## Psoriasis

Vitamin E serum levels were low in patients with active psoriasis in a 2001 case-control study.[26] In a 2009 randomized controlled trial, vitamin E supplementation clinically improved psoriasis in hospitalized patients with erythrodermic and arthropathic psoriasis. PASI scores and oxidative stress decreased more rapidly and to a greater degree in supplemented patients versus placebo. Unfortunately, the intervention included coenzyme Q10 and selenium supplementation as well. It is therefore not clear if vitamin E played an important role.[88] Other than a handful of conflicting studies showing varying levels of vitamin E in the serum of psoriasis patients, there is no evidence to support or refute a role for vitamin E in psoriasis in the absence of other antioxidants.[89–91]

## Fibrosis and Wound Healing

In animal studies, systemic vitamin E retards collagen synthesis and fibroblast proliferation and reduced surgically induced intraperitoneal adhesions.[10] Given this, vitamin E has been endorsed as an effective topical agent to improve the appearance of hypertrophic scars and keloids. The actual scientific evidence for this function in humans is scant and controversial.[92,93] Suggestive work has been done regarding fibrosis and dietary vitamin E, however. In combination with pentoxifylline, 1000 IU of vitamin E per day improved post-breast cancer radiation–induced cutaneous

fibrosis compared to placebo.[94] Neither pentoxifylline nor vitamin E were beneficial on their own. Given this potential, vitamin E has been investigated for a therapeutic role in systemic sclerosis. One small 3-week trial showed no improvement in lipid peroxidation or cutaneous blood flow following cold exposure in patients with systemic sclerosis and Raynaud's phenomenon receiving either 500 or 1000 IU of vitamin E per day compared to placebo or baseline.[95] With a mean decrease of 8.41 points, a longer 24-week trial showed significant improvement in skin thickness, as measured by the Modified Rodnan Skin Score, in patients consuming 800 IU of vitamin E in combination with pentoxifylline compared to baseline.[96] While when compared to a historical control group treated with cyclophosphamide, the significance was lost, there was still a positive trend. The control group did have a higher baseline MRSS, which may have contributed bias. A double-blind, placebo-controlled study is required to assess the efficacy of this treatment in systemic sclerosis.

The role of dietary vitamin E in wound healing, though anecdotally beneficial, is limited to animal studies. Dietary vitamin E may improve the rate of wound healing in diabetic rats.[97,98] However, it decreased the tensile strength of wounds in a nondiabetic rat model.[10] Dietary supplement studies in humans are lacking.

## Safety

There is a growing body of evidence that vitamin E may not be a completely benign supplement. As mentioned, vitamin E supplementation was found to increase BCC incidence in one trial. Vitamin E doses greater than 1000 IU/day may interfere with platelet aggregation. Furthermore, as vitamin E is metabolized by the P450 system, the metabolism of other drugs may be adversely affected.[76] In addition, recent meta-analyses found that vitamin E supplementation at doses greater than 400 IU/day (more than 10 times the RDI) increases all-cause mortality.[99,100] Most of the patients included in these analyses were relatively ill, making their results difficult to extrapolate to a healthy population. However, more studies of the long-term effects on a healthy population would be required before high-dose vitamin E supplementation can be recommended regularly for skin health.

Vitamin E shows promise for photoprotection when combined with another antioxidant, such as vitamin C, but the net effect seems to be small, and the doses studied were many times more the RDI. Vitamin E's role in skin cancer prevention is not supported, but there are limitations to the studies, and their designs are not consistent with those that demonstrated photoprotection. Randomized controlled trials of higher-dose vitamin E in combination with vitamin C or another antioxidant are required before a conclusion can be drawn. The work for vitamin E's effect on the immune system and atopic dermatitis is very suggestive, and further prospective studies are needed to clarify a therapeutic and/or preventative dose. The work combining vitamin E and pentoxifylline potentially warrants further study for this combination and its effect on fibrosis and sclerosis. Importantly, the suggested detrimental effects of vitamin E require a cautious approach for future studies.

## VITAMIN C

Vitamin C or ascorbic acid is found in green leafy vegetables and citrus fruits. It is absorbed in the distal small intestine. Typical intake is 100 mg/day.[2] It plays a number of critical roles in the human body. It is an efficient antioxidant and replenishes stores of vitamin E. It plays a role in folate, tetrahydrofolate, and dihydrofolate reduction. Norepinephrine synthesis, carnitine synthesis, prostaglandin and prostacyclin metabolism all utilize vitamin C. Finally, in a process relevant to skin physiology, vitamin C is critical to collagen synthesis. It acts as a cofactor for prolyl and lysyl hydroxylases, which catalyze the hydroxylation of proline and lysine, respectively. These hydroxylations are critical to the excretion of procollagen from the fibroblast. In addition, these chemical changes may impart increased stability and decreased heat sensitivity to the collagen molecule.[2] Vitamin C's critical effects are demonstrated by at least two different diseases. In Ehlers–Danlos syndrome subtype, there is an absence of the vitamin C catalyzed lysyl hydroxylase, resulting in joint laxity, arterial rupture, scoliosis, and muscle hypotonia.[2] Scurvy results from vitamin C deficiency and is described as early as 1500 BC on papyrus. Skin findings include hyperkeratotic and enlarged follicles, corkscrew and bent hairs, and eventually hemorrhagic follicles. In addition, patients with scurvy may manifest with poor dentition, edematous gingivae, ocular and conjunctival hemorrhage, GI hemorrhage, muscular hemorrhage, and poor bone formation. Anemia is a common finding and is thought to result from hemorrhage and folate and iron deficiencies.[101]

Given the findings of vitamin C deficiency and its known roles as an antioxidant and in collagen synthesis, vitamin C is an attractive study target for a multitude of skin conditions. There is a suggested role for it in atopic dermatitis, bullous disease, wound healing, purpura, and skin cancer prevention. There is no conclusive evidence for dietary supplementation in any of these conditions, but much of the work is provocative.

### ATOPIC DERMATITIS

Given the increased oxidant stress seen in atopic dermatitis, vitamin C has been investigated for a potential protective role.[102] In one 2000 study, women with atopic dermatitis consumed fewer foods rich in vitamin C than healthy controls.[102] In 2003, Leveque et al. showed that the dermis of five patients with atopic dermatitis contained a significantly lower level of ascorbic acid compared to that of five normal controls.[103] This result, although suggestive, is not surprising, as antioxidant levels are known to decrease in the face of inflammation. However, in 2004, Hoppu et al. showed that consumption of breast milk with lower vitamin C levels was associated with

increased risk for atopic dermatitis in the first year of life. This result was confounded by the fact that lower breast milk vitamin C concentration was also associated with mothers who were more likely to have a food allergy.[104] Despite these suggestions of protection, other studies have shown either no relationship or an increased risk of atopy with higher vitamin C and overall fruit intake.[85,86,105] The evidence thus far suggests limited effect of vitamin C intake and the risk of childhood atopic dermatitis; however, there are no randomized controlled trials on this topic.

### BULLOUS DISEASES

Ascorbic acid deficiency has been reported in patients with epidermolysis bullosa. This is likely a consequence of reduced dietary intake secondary to mucous membrane disease. Indeed, nutritional support is recommended to improve outcomes in this entity.[106,107] In other bullous diseases, including porphyria cutanea tarda (PCT), variegate porphyria, and erythropoeitic porphyria, ascorbic acid supplementation may be protective. Porphyria cutanea tarda is a disease characterized by the hepatic deficiency or malfunction of uroporphyrinogen decarboxylase.[107] The excess uroporphyrinogen is oxidized, and the resultant porphyrins deposit and become activated in the skin and other tissues, leading to the characteristic photosensitive blistering phenotype.[108] Patients with symptomatic but not resolved PCT may be deficient in ascorbic acid,[109] and it has been postulated that ascorbic acid may decrease uroporphyrinogen oxidation and thus be protective. Animal studies have shown that this protective role diminishes in the presence of higher serum iron loads.[110] Thus, although maintaining ascorbic acid levels in PCT patients may be beneficial, this likely will not replace the role of phlebotomy and iron depletion.[107] There is limited evidence that vitamin C supplementation may improve photosensitivity and antioxidant status in variegate and erythropoitic porphyrias, respectively.[111–113]

### WOUND HEALING

Vitamin C is a known cofactor in collagen formation, a process important to wound healing.[114,115] Indeed, Balaji et al. suggested that up to 60% of patients with chronic leg ulcers are deficient in vitamin C.[116] In a 2005 meta-analysis, oral nutritional supplementation, which occasionally included vitamin C, suggested benefit in preventing and treating pressure ulcers.[117] The role of isolated vitamin C is far less clear, however. A recent Cochrane review described two studies comparing the effects of twice daily 500 mg vitamin C supplementation to placebo on pressure ulcer healing.[118] One small study of 22 surgical patients showed improved rates of healing in the treatment group. The randomization of this trial was questionable, and the clinical significance of the difference was unclear. A larger trial of 88 mostly nursing home patients showed no difference between supplemented patients and placebo. The control group actually had marginally superior clinical outcomes. Most patients in this trial had nutritional deficiencies at baseline, potentially confounding the effect of sole vitamin C supplementation and making this result difficult to apply to other, non-deficient populations.[118]

## PURPURA

As mentioned, vitamin C plays a critical role in collagen synthesis, and its deficiency results in hemorrhage and potentially arterial rupture. In addition, ascorbic acid improved endothelial cell barrier function in vitro via increased collagen production.[119] Theoretically, then, vitamin C may play an important role in capillary wall stability in vivo, which, in combination with its antioxidant effects, may have implications for capillaritis. Indeed, high-dose vitamin C (500 mg/day) in combination with oral flavonoids has been shown to resolve progressive pigmented purpura in a few case reports.[120,121] Larger studies are required before definitive conclusions can be drawn.

## NON-MELANOMA SKIN CANCER

As a potent antioxidant, vitamin C has been investigated for a protective role in carcinogenesis. In humans, dietary vitamin C may protect against a number of cancers including stomach, cervical, esophageal, stomach, pancreatic, breast, rectal, and lung cancer. In vitro and animal work has suggested that vitamin C is photoprotective. Topical application decreased UV-induced erythema and inflammation in both animals and humans.[2] In addition, dietary vitamin C significantly protected hairless mice from UV-induced SCC development compared to vitamin E.[122] The human work for NMSC is conflicting and limited to retrospective case-control studies and prospective cohort analyses. A 2005 systematic review concluded that the evidence for any relationship between vitamin C and NMSC is at best weak.[123] Although one cohort study[124] showed a decreased risk for SCC in people who consumed more green leafy vegetables, a food high in vitamin C, and a case-control study[17] showed significantly fewer BCCs in those who consumed vitamin C supplements, other studies have shown no relationship[125] or even increased risk for NMSC with increasing vitamin C intake.[23–25,122]

There is no clear role for vitamin C supplementation in any of the aforementioned categories. The evidence for atopic dermatitis and skin cancer prevention is conflicting, and no conclusion can be drawn to date. Theoretically, vitamin C is very important in wound healing given its role in collagen production, but the human studies for dietary supplementation have not been consistent. The role for vitamin C in bullous disease, especially PCT, is quite provocative, but the clinical relevance of supplementation is limited given other more effective therapies. Finally, vitamin C may have therapeutic importance in progressive pigmented purpura, but the data are limited to small case reports. Further study in this area is certainly warranted.

## VITAMIN D

Vitamin D is the most well known for its role in calcium homeostasis and bone health. Humans may derive their vitamin D through two sources. In the diet, vitamin D is found in fatty fish, cod liver oil, as well as fortified dairy products common in the United States. Plant sources provide vitamin D2 (ergocalciferol), while animal sources provide vitamin D3 (cholecalciferol).[126] Recommended dietary intake depends on age and lactation status but is generally 600 IU or 15 µg/day. Humans are also able to synthesize vitamin D with the help of UVB radiation. In the skin, 7-DHC, through photoactivation, is converted to pre-vitamin D3, which can then isomerize to vitamin D3. It is estimated that humans derive 80% of their vitamin D through this cutaneous synthesis. Vitamin D3 is further converted to 25-dihydroxyvitamin D3 then 1,25-dihydroxyvitamin D3 via hydroxylases in the liver and kidney, respectively. This hormonally active form, 1,25-dihydroxyvitamin D3, then binds to the vitamin D receptor located in the nucleus and confers transcriptional changes on the target cell. More immediate, nongenetic effects of vitamin D have also been described. Vitamin D has known effects on keratinocyte proliferation, inflammation, and differentiation, as well as on the immune system.[126,127] It has been studied for a role in a number of cutaneous disorders including skin cancer, atopic dermatitis, and psoriasis. There are no definitive studies to suggest that vitamin D supplementation is helpful or harmful for any of these conditions to date; however, some of the work is very provocative, especially for melanoma.

## ATOPIC DERMATITIS

In addition to its metabolic activities, vitamin D has demonstrated interesting effects on the immune system. The vitamin D receptor is expressed on T lymphocytes, dendritic cells, and peripheral blood mononuclear cells. In vitro studies have supported suppression of Th1 and potentially Th2 responses.[126] In addition, vitamin D supplementation upregulates the expression of antimicrobial peptides in lesional skin from atopic individuals in vivo.[128] Vitamin D deficiency is more common in higher latitudes, as is atopic dermatitis. For these reasons, vitamin D is of increasing interest for a potentially therapeutic role in atopic dermatitis. Three different cohort studies have suggested that higher exposure to vitamin D in utero and in infancy is associated with increased risk of atopic dermatitis.[129–131] A fourth found no association.[132] Conversely, a small trial (n = 11) showed that vitamin D supplementation in childhood may improve the clinical status of seasonal atopic dermatitis.[133] A case-control study from 2008 showed that obese patients with vitamin D deficiency were more likely to report atopic dermatitis compared to replete obese adults.[134] Finally, a more recent 2011 study showed an inverse relationship between vitamin D serum levels and clinical severity of atopic dermatitis in affected children.[135] The mixed results may be secondary to host status at the time of vitamin D exposure.

It is conceivable that the immune system may respond to vitamin D early in life in a fashion that is distinct from that in adulthood or even late childhood. Larger prospective interventional trials will better define a role for vitamin D in atopic dermatitis.

## NON-MELANOMA SKIN CANCER

Vitamin D may have an antiproliferative effect on keratinocytes, depending on their proliferative state. Certain SCCs and BCCs have shown increased expression of the vitamin D receptor. Indeed, in vitro work has suggested that the presence of this vitamin D receptor may impart protection from carcinogenesis.[122] Recent work has shown vitamin D may inhibit the sonic hedgehog pathway, which is known to be involved in BCC development. Together, this suggests a promising role for vitamin D in skin cancer prevention. Unfortunately, in vivo human work is lacking. A few topical studies have shown mixed results.[136,137] Three large, population-based dietary studies have shown no relationship between vitamin D intake and BCC development.[22,23,138] A very recent study showed that increased vitamin D serum levels conferred increased risk for development of NMSC. To try and account for the confounding nature of UV exposure and its impact on both vitamin D synthesis and skin cancer, this study also looked at NMSC incidence on non-sun-exposed skin and found no significant association with vitamin D status.[139] Together, the human data suggest dietary vitamin D intake may not play a role in NMSC development, although conclusive in vivo data are certainly lacking. As a 2008 murine experiment suggested, the discrepancy between the in vivo and in vitro work may be explained by actions of the vitamin D receptor independent to its ligand.[140]

## MELANOMA

In vitro work has suggested that vitamin D has antiproliferative and proapoptotic effects on some melanoma cancer cell lines.[127] Furthermore, certain vitamin D receptor polymorphisms may be associated with increased risk for melanoma.[141] Thus, a therapeutic or preventative role for the vitamin in melanoma is undergoing study. So far, in vivo human data are somewhat mixed. Lower vitamin D levels have been associated with increased risk of melanoma recurrence and increased Breslow thickness at presentation.[142] One study showed decreased vitamin D levels in stage IV melanoma patients compared to stage I.[143] A 2009 meta-analysis by Gandini et al. showed a small protective effect with increased dietary intake.[144] However, smaller case-control studies show no difference between the serum levels of vitamin D in melanoma patients and healthy controls.[145,146] Intermittent, severe sun exposure rather than continuous, low-level sun exposure is thought to lead to increased risk of melanoma.[127] Indeed, a recent study showed that regular weekend exposure may, in fact, be protective. It was suggested that this could be explained by the proposed protective role for vitamin D.[127,147]

It is not clear whether dietary vitamin D would have the same effect, as there are no randomized controlled trials on the subject.

## PSORIASIS

Topical vitamin D has known efficacy in psoriasis. The mechanism is not completely elucidated, but it likely involves its known antiproliferative effects and potentially regulation of the immune system. Oral vitamin D has reported benefits for psoriasis as well. Case reports and small trials have reported skin clearing as well as improvement in psoriatic arthritis.[27] It has been suggested that the use is limited by hypercalcemic side effects.[27] However, the effective doses were within the RDI. In addition, a 1996 study purported its safety for use in psoriasis. The only side effect was a small change in creatinine metabolism, although renal function was not affected.[148] Currently, it is not a recommended systemic treatment for psoriasis,[149] although it should be studied further in this regard.[150]

Vitamin D represents an interesting area of study for multiple skin diseases; however, a clear role is not yet defined for systemic therapy. Work is very suggestive for a protective role in melanoma as well as in psoriasis, and further studies are warranted. The effects of vitamin D on NMSC and atopic dermatitis are less clear, and to date, there is no good evidence suggesting a role either for or against its use in these conditions.

## GREEN TEA

After water, tea is the most commonly consumed beverage in the world. Green tea is made exclusively from the leaves of the evergreen *Camellia sinensis*. It is native to Southeast Asia, though now more than 30 countries cultivate the plant. Unlike black tea production, which involves a lengthy fermentation process, to produce green tea, the leaves of *C. sinesis* are dried rapidly via steaming or pan frying. This rapid process limits the fermentation and oxidation of the active components of the leaves. Thus, like the plant leaves, green tea contains a large amount of biologically active catechins.[151] Catechins compose a class of polyphenols that has demonstrated antioxidant properties in vitro. Indeed, the consumption of green tea has been associated with decreased carcinogenesis in various epidemiologic studies.[152] Mechanistically, catechins act as ROS scavengers and may regulate AP-1 and the MAPK pathway. In addition, epigallocatechin-3-gallate (EGCG), the most abundant catechin in green tea, has been shown to induce apoptosis in skin tumor cells, potentially through NF-kβ regulation.[152]

The antioxidant effects of green tea have produced interest in its potential roles in inflammatory processes in the skin. It has been shown that these catechins are bioavailable to the skin and may increase cutaneous blood flow.[153] Potential roles in photoprotection, photoaging, as well as the overall structure and function of the skin have been purported for green tea.

## PHOTOPROTECTION AND PHOTOAGING

Given the suggested anti-inflammatory effects of green tea, it represents an attractive area of study for dietary photoprotection. Mouse studies have shown that both topical and oral green tea catechin supplementation are photoprotective and anti-carcinogenic.[152] Topical application in humans has also been shown to decrease the sunburn response, reduce UV-induced erythema, and decrease PUVA-induced DNA damage.[152] Dietary human work, however, has been less consistent. In 2003, Chow et al. studied the effect on MED of 800 mg of oral EGCG or Polyphenon E (a proprietary extract of green tea, containing EGCG among other catechins) versus placebo supplementation in 40 volunteers over 4 weeks.[154] At doses equivalent to 16 cups of Japanese-style green tea per day, they saw no improvement in MED in the treatment arms of the study compared to placebo and concluded that EGCG and Polyphenon E may not have photoprotective effects. In an 8-week randomized, controlled, double-blind trial, Chiu et al. showed that combined topical and oral supplementation of green tea extract may lead to histologic improvement in moderately photoaged skin.[155] They found a statistically significant (p = 0.02) increase in elastic tissue content of skin from the treatment group when compared to placebo. This suggests a preventative effect, as the mean loss of tissue in the placebo group was more than twice the gain of tissue in the treatment group. Obviously, this trial is limited in that it combined both topical and oral supplementation. We cannot conclude which administration route may have been beneficial. Furthermore, clinical assessment of photoaging parameters showed no statistically significant difference between groups, suggesting limited clinical importance of these findings. In a 2-year study, Janjua et al. showed no difference between placebo and daily 500 mg green tea extract oral supplementation in terms of clinical photoaging assessment.[156] By 24 months, both treatment and placebo showed statistically significant improvement in clinically assessed erythema, telangiectasia, and overall solar damage. There was no statistically significant difference between groups. By histologic examination, both placebo and green tea–treated subjects showed significant yet similar improvement in overall sun damage, grade of solar elastosis, dermal mucin, and melanin content of skin. As suggested in their discussion, this may be due to improved sun protective activities stimulated by entering a clinical trial. The drop-out rate in the trial was almost 40% but similar in both groups. Finally and conversely, Heinrich et al. showed that 12 weeks of dietary green tea leads to improved photoprotection as measured by erythema response compared to baseline.[153] This trial is interesting in that it contains a much higher dose of catechins (1402 mg/day) than previous trials and purports a positive result, which possibly suggests a dose effect; however, there was no control arm.

## SKIN STRUCTURE AND FUNCTION

A number of studies have assessed green tea's effects on skin structure and function. In 2007, Puch et al. showed improved barrier function measured by TEWL in subjects consuming a mixture containing various catechins.[156] However, the mixture also contained fatty acids, fermented milk, probiotic bacteria, and vitamin E. Therefore, little can be concluded regarding specific nutrient contributions. In a 2-year study by Janjua et al., there was no difference between placebo and daily 500 mg green tea extract oral supplementation in terms of clinical surface evaluation of living skin by Visioscan, self-assessment, and histology.[155] As mentioned, in a limited trial, Chiu et al. showed increased elastic tissue content in skin from patients treated with both oral and topical green tea supplementation compared to placebo.[155] Finally, Heinrich et al. showed that dietary supplementation with 1402 mg of catechins per day over 12 weeks leads to improved elasticity, TEWL, hydration, roughness, scaling, blood flow and oxygen saturation as compared to baseline and placebo.[153]

## SPECIFIC SKIN CONDITIONS

The data for green tea extract in specific skin disorders are limited.[152] There are small amount of data regarding the effects of green tea extract on wound healing, both in vitro and via topical application in mice.[158–160] It has also been suggested that green tea may benefit psoriasis patients given its effects on keratinocyte differentiation. However, the data are limited to topical mouse studies at this point.[161,162]

Overall, our knowledge of green tea's effect on the skin in dietary form on humans is limited. Most studies show no effect of green tea extract on photoprotection, although there is suggestion that the dose may need to be increased to see a benefit. Although there is evidence to suggest an improvement in barrier function and skin structure with green tea supplementation, better clinical correlation is needed. Finally, animal work has suggested a role for green tea in both wound healing and psoriasis, and further studies in humans are warranted.

# OTHER SOURCES OF POLYPHENOLS

Dietary polyphenols are not limited to green tea. A number of other food sources including grape seed, red wine, cocoa, and pine bark extract contain biologically active polyphenols.

Like green tea, cocoa contains epicatechin. Epicatechin from cocoa may improve microcirculation, photoprotection, and skin structure in women.[163,164] As with green tea, it is unclear if these findings are clinically relevant as the studies have not included subjective clinical outcomes.

Proanthocyanidins are found in grape seed extract as well as pine bark. Pine bark extract, which contains procyanidin, has recently been shown in combination with vitamins A, C, and E to improve melasma in Filipino women.[165] Prior studies suggest that procyanidin may be effective for this condition in isolation as well.[166,167] A proprietary supplement containing pine bark extract, among other antioxidants, has been suggested to improve skin elasticity and roughness. However, the observed improvements were small and are not correlated clinically.[168] Furthermore, it is difficult to conclude individual nutrient contributions given the mixed nature of the intervention. A 2006 trial found no significant increase in MED or skin hydration with dietary grape seed extract alone.[169]

Resveratrol, a polyphenol found in red wine, grapes, berries, and peanuts, was initially studied in humans as the explanation for the "French Paradox." It was thought that the resveratrol in red wine may account for why despite the higher fat and alcohol intake of the French, they have better cardiovascular health than Americans. Indeed, resveratrol has been shown to improve cardiovascular health. This is attributed to its potent anti-inflammatory capabilities.[170] Resveratrol also inhibits all three stages of carcinogenesis, that is initiation, promotion, and progression.[171] Accordingly, in vitro and animal work has shown potential for skin anticarcinogenesis.[172] Two recent studies in mice showed potential for modulation of the malignant properties of melanoma.[172,173] Thus far, human studies have shown safety and bioavailability, but efficacy studies are lacking.[172]

The evidence for skin benefits from other sources of dietary polyphenols is even sparser than that for green tea. The most compelling human evidence thus far is that for proanthocyanidins and melasma treatment. Further studies for the role of cocoa in photoprotection and especially resveratrol in carcinogenesis are warranted.

## POLYUNSATURATED FATTY ACIDS

Polyunsaturated fatty acids (PUFAs), especially omega-3 fatty acids, have risen in popularity over the past few decades for their anti-inflammatory abilities. Omega-3 fatty acids studied in human skin disease include the long-chain eicosapentaenoic acid (EPA) and docosahexaenoic acid (DHA), and the short-chain alpha-linolenic acid (ALA). EPA and DHA are primarily found in oily fish and thus fish oil, whereas ALA is typically plant sourced. EPA competes with arachadonic acid (AA) for COX and LOX metabolism, thus altering inflammatory mediator profiles. Omega-3 metabolites include prostaglandins in the three family (PGD3, PGE3, PGF3), hydroxypentanoic acid (HEPE), and leukotrienes in the five family. These mediators are thought to be less potent than the AA metabolites, which include prostaglandin 2s, hydroxyeicosatetraenoic acids (HETE), and leukotriene 4s. Thus, increased availability of the less potent EPA metabolites may dilute the more inflammatory AA metabolites. In addition, omega-3 fatty acids may act at the transcriptional level and modulate intracellular signaling to induce anti-inflammatory actions.[174] Omega-3s, given orally, are bioavailable and alter the skin fatty acid composition significantly. One study showed that skin fatty acid percentage of EPA increased eightfold in supplemented subjects, while controls showed no effect.[175] It is no wonder, then, that omega-3s have been studied for their potential roles in carcinogenesis and immune-mediated inflammatory disease processes of the skin.

### CANCER AND PHOTOPROTECTION

Epidemiologic studies have shown conflicting results regarding the role of dietary omega-3 supplementation with skin cancer. In a 1993 case-control study of 41 women with cutaneous melanoma and 297 age-matched controls, Bain et al. showed that higher intake of PUFA and total fat correlated significantly with lower rates of melanoma.[176] In 2000, van Dam et al. followed >40,000 men over 8 years in a prospective cohort study. They found that higher total fat intake was associated with lower overall risk of BCC and attributed this to mono-unsaturated fat intake, but not PUFA intake.[23] In another case-control study, Hakim et al. showed an increased risk of SCC with higher fat intake, but a decreased risk of SCC with higher EPA and DHA intake. The results of this study, however, were not statistically significant.[177] These epidemiologic studies have many pitfalls and potential confounders, including lack of control for sunlight exposure, family history, and level of health consciousness. However, their findings have led to further interest into the potential mechanism by which omega-3s may be cancer protective.

This mechanism may be through photoprotection. Improvements in hydroa vacciniforme as well as PMLE have been reported after omega-3 supplementation.[178,179] Dietary fish oil has improved MED in healthy subjects as well.[175,180,181] In vivo human experiments have shown that, mechanistically, EPA supplementation may decrease DNA damage in human keratinocytes in vivo as well as affect free radical action.[175,181] Omega-3 supplementation has been associated with decreased cutaneous p53 expression in human populations, and it has been postulated that this may represent "sacrificial oxidation" by PUFAs.[175,181] Overall, the in vitro and mouse results are more promising than the human studies at this point. However, given the difficult nature of these dietary studies, and the modestly positive results, photoprotection and omega-3 supplementation are the areas that warrant further investigation.

### SKIN STRUCTURE AND FUNCTION

In a recent report by Neukam et al., the effect of dietary omega-3 via flaxseed oil on overall skin health was studied. They found significant improvements in skin sensitivity, increased cutaneous blood flow, decreased TEWL, improved hydration, roughness, scaling, and smoothness in 13 subjects supplemented with flaxseed oil compared to 13 controls that were supplemented with safflower seed oil.[182] As opposed to fish oil, flaxseed oil contains the omega-3 ALA, whereas safflower seed oil contains the omega-6 linoleic acid (LA). Interestingly, the flaxseed oil also contained a nonsignificant amount of D-alpha-tocopherol (vitamin E), whereas the control oil did not. This study is limited in the sample size and in that there was no clinical or subjective analysis. In addition, there was no measure of dietary compliance in the study. Despite these limitations, and given previous work that has shown the skin bioavailability of omega-3 fatty acids, this study does suggest that dietary omega-3s may have an acute effect on the structure and function of healthy skin. Additionally, it would be interesting to correlate these parameters with clinical assessment and/or subjective analysis to understand the clinical magnitude of the observed changes in TEWL, hydration, and surface characteristics.

## PSORIASIS

There is some suggestion in the literature that omega-3 supplementation may benefit patients with psoriasis. However, the data from dietary RCTs are conflicting.[183,184] Higher doses of omega-3s given intravenously improved at least short-term outcomes in both stable plaque and acute guttate psoriasis.[185,187] Omega-6 intravenous supplementation, although acting as controls in these studies, led to improvement in short-term outcomes as well, although the results were not as significant as in the omega-3 group.[186,187] Additionally, these higher doses of omega-3s may lead to improved inflammatory mediator profiles in serum of psoriatic patients.[187]

## ATOPIC DERMATITIS

The role of PUFA supplementation in atopic dermatitis has been recently studied in both adults and infants, but the results have been underwhelming. Hempseed oil, which contains both omega-6 and omega-3 fatty acids in the forms of LA and ALA, respectively, showed a nonsignificant trend toward TEWL improvement when given to adults over 4 weeks with atopic dermatitis. It also imparted a statistically significant improvement from baseline in subjective scores of itching, dryness, and frequency of medication usage. However, when compared to olive oil control, this significance is lost.[188] Recently, prenatal, lactational, and infant supplementation with omega-3 fatty acids has been hypothesized to protect children from the development of atopy. A systematic review did show decreased reactivity to skin prick testing in supplemented infants.[189] The CAPS trial, however, has found no association between eczema and fatty acid supplementation in the prenatal and postnatal periods.[188–192] Furuhjelm et al. showed that although IgE-associated eczema may be decreased in supplemented infants, the rate of overall eczema is not significantly different.[193]

## OTHER AREAS

There has been suggestion of a role for omega-3 fatty acids in acne treatment; however, the data are limited to a small case series and an older study looking at fish intake and acne prevalence.[194,195] There may also be a role for dietary PUFAs in wound healing, although it is not clear if this role is helpful or harmful.[196] Omega-3 supplementation has even been looked at as a potential therapy for pruritus in hemodialysis patients.[197] Small, nonsignificant trends suggesting improved pruritus symptoms with omega-3 supplementation have been observed.[196,198]

There is still much work to be done before a definitive role for omega-3 fatty acids is defined for the realm of skin health. There is potential for further work in both psoriasis and photoprotection and subsequent carcinogenesis. We know, at least, that omega-3 supplementation can alter skin fatty acid composition, but more definitive knowledge for their effects on skin health is pending larger and longer trials.

## CONCLUSIONS

The study of the effects of nutrient supplementation is inherently difficult. Almost all studies run into control issues, as it is virtually impossible to control for dietary variability in humans. Thus, it is not surprising that a large amount of the current literature relies on retrospective epidemiologic or prospective cohort studies. Despite these limitations, however, there are certain nutrients that show some promise for skin health. Photoprotection may be provided by many nutrients including polyphenols, PUFAs, vitamin E, and vitamin C, although the results are often mixed. In addition, in all of the positive studies, it should be noted that the degree of photoprotection achieved is far less that of modern day sunscreens. In addition, the measurement used to assess this parameter is usually MED, which does not assess effects that these substances may have on UVA radiation. Indeed, the long-term benefits of photoprotection, that is skin cancer and photoaging, have had mixed results in all nutrients reviewed. NMSC is a slow growing entity, with much of the inciting damage done in younger life. Even the long-term epidemiologic studies are relatively short and do not account for childhood dietary intake or sun exposure. Suggestive work has been done on the potential protective role for vitamin D in melanoma, and a prospective randomized controlled trial is warranted in this area. Regarding photoaging and skin structure and function, although a few studies have purported beneficial results for PUFAs and polyphenols, there have been no clinically relevant correlations made, leaving us with little to conclude.

The data are limited regarding dietary supplementation's impact on psoriasis. The most compelling work thus far has been done with high-dose intravenous omega-3s and improved short-term outcomes in patients hospitalized with severe psoriasis flares. The evidence for long-term benefits for psoriasis and dietary PUFAs is controversial, however. Similarly, vitamins E and A have shown mixed results, and prospective trials for these agents are lacking. Vitamin D has history that suggests dietary benefit for psoriasis, but current studies are lacking. The evidence for green tea is theoretical at this point.

Atopic dermatitis often presents in infancy, and it has thus been postulated that dietary intake in either the prenatal or immediate postnatal period may play a role in the development or prevention of the disease. The evidence to support this theory is mixed, however. Neither PUFAs, vitamins C, D, nor E has shown consistently beneficial or harmful results. The results are similarly confusing for PUFAs and vitamin C in adult populations. Although the work in non-infants has suggested benefit for increased vitamin E intake, the data are limited to one single-blind RCT and two case-control studies. In addition, high-dose vitamin E supplementation may be associated with adverse events, limiting the degree to which this should be recommended.

The data for specific dietary nutrient supplementation for wound healing in humans are lacking. Green tea and vitamins A and E have shown benefit, but the data are limited to animal and retrospective population-based studies.

Vitamin C, given its known role in collagen formation, has been studied in prospective human trials, but to date, the outcomes are conflicting.

Although limited, there are some data to suggest a role for high-dose vitamin E in fibrosis and systemic sclerosis when combined with pentoxifylline. But, again, one should be cautious in recommending high-dose vitamin E given the purported adverse events.

Capillaritis and progressive pigmented purpura may be benefited by high-dose vitamin C. The data are limited to mere case reports, however. Likewise, vitamin C may play a therapeutic role in PCT, though this is probably overshadowed by and not effective in the absence of the current treatment regimen.

Despite the benefits or lack thereof described for nutritional supplements in this review, we would like to emphasize the importance of adequate nutrient intake for skin and overall health. The consequences of nutrient deficiencies are well documented. For example, vitamin A deficiency leads to blindness, phrynoderma, and xerosis. Vitamin D deficiency results in rickets, while lack of vitamin C causes scurvy.[102] In addition, the health benefits derived from a diet rich in fruit and vegetables go beyond those derived from the carotenoids and flavonoids for the skin. Furthermore, we do not want to dissuade any one from using traditional therapies that have proven benefits in favor of dietary remedies. As mentioned, the degree of photoprotection provided by sunscreens and good sun avoidance practices is far greater than that derived from dietary nutrients. Thus, diet cannot be relied upon to prevent sunburn, photoaging, or skin cancer. Although no head-to-head trials have been preformed, this is likely similar for psoriasis, atopic dermatitis, and the other diseases described.

Although beyond the scope of this review, there are numerous studies on the effects of topical vitamins and nutrients on skin health and on skin disease. The authors as well as others have reviewed this elsewhere in depth, but in summary, topical nutrients have shown far greater therapeutic effect on skin, rather than oral supplements, suggesting that for skin health and to improve skin disease, at least for now, evidence suggest that vitamins such as vitamin A, B, C, E and nutrients such as green tea polyphenols should be applied directly to skin rather than via oral ingestion of supplements.

## REFERENCES

1. Hart, A. Annual USA sales of nutritional supplements top $23 billion, but where's the quality control? http://www.examiner.com/article/annual-usa-sales-of-nutritional-supplements-top-23-billion-but-where-s-the-quality-control (Accessed August 1, 2012).
2. Zussman J, Ahdout J, Kim J. *J Amer Acad Dermatol* 63:507;2010.
3. Reichrath J, Lehmann B, Carlberg C et al. *Horm Metab Res* 39:71;2007.
4. Weinzweig J, Levenson SM, Rettura G et al. *Ann Surg* 211:269;1990.
5. Greenwald DP, Sharzer LA, Padawer J et al. *J Surg Res* 49:98;1990.
6. Seifter E, Rettura G, Padawer J et al. *Ann Surg* 194:42;1981.
7. Seifter E, Crowley LV, Rettura G et al. *Ann Surg* 181: 836;1975.
8. Hunt TK, Ehrlich HP, Garcia JA, Dunphy JE. *Ann Surg* 170:633;1969.
9. Ehrlich HP, Hunt, TK. *Ann Surg* 167:324;1968.
10. Ehrlich HP, Tarver H, Hunt TK. *Ann Surg* 175: 235;1972.
11. Rojas AI, Phillips TJ. *Dermatol Surg* 25:601;1999.
12. Ette SI, Ofodile FA, Oluwasanmi JO. *Trop Geograph Med* 34:73;1982.
13. Kraemer KH, DiGiovanna JJ, Moshell AN et al. *NEJM* 318:1633;1988.
14. Kelly JW, Sabto J, Gurr FW, Bruce F. *Lancet* 338:1407;1991.
15. Tangrea JA, Edwards BK, Taylor PR et al. *J Nat Cancer Inst* 84:328;1992.
16. Wald N, Boreham J, Bailey A. *Brit J Cancer* 54:957;1986.
17. Wei Q, Matanoski GM, Farmer ER et al. *J Clin Epidemiol* 47:829;1994.
18. Moon TE, Matanoski GM, Farmer ER et al. 6:949;1997.
19. Levine N, Moon TE, Cartmel B et al. *Cancer Epidemiol Biomarkers Prev* 6:957;1997.
20. Breslow RA, Alberg AJ, Helzlsouer KJ et al. *Cancer Epidemiol Biomarkers Prev* 4:837;1995.
21. Karagas MR, Greenberg ER, Nierenberg D et al. *Cancer Epidemiol Biomarkers Prev* 6:25;1997.
22. Davies TW, Treasure FP, Welch AA, Day NE. *Brit J Dermatol* 146:1017;2002.
23. van Dam RM, Huang Z, Giovannucci E et al. *Am J Clin Nutr* 71:135;2000.
24. Fung TT, Hunter DJ, Spiegelman D et al. *Cancer Causes Control* 13:221;2002.
25. Heinen MM, Hughes MC, Ibiebele TI et al. *Eur J Cancer* 43:2707;2007.
26. Rocha-Pereira P, Santos-Silva A, Rebelo I et al. *Clin Chim Acta* 303:33;2001.
27. Ricketts JR, Rothe MJ, Grant-Kels JM. *Clinics Derm* 28:615;2010.
28. Britton, G. *FASEB J* 9:1551;1995.
29. Micozzi MS, Brown ED, Taylor PR, Wolfe E. *Am J Clin Nutr* 48:1061;1988.
30. Lademann J, Meinke MC, Sterry W, Darvin ME. *Exper Dermatol* 20:377;2011.
31. Stahl W, Sies H. *Biochim Biophys Acta* 1740:101;2005.
32. Stahl W, Ale-Agha N, Polidori MC. *Biol Chem* 383:553;2002.
33. Pastori M, Pfander H, Boscoboinik D et al. *Biochem Biophys Res Commun* 250:582;1998.
34. Amir H, Karas M, Giat J et al. *Nutr Cancer* 33:105;1999.
35. Nahum A, Hirsch K, Danilenko M et al. *Oncogene* 20:3428;2001.
36. Karas M, Amir H, Fishman D et al. *Nutr Cancer* 36:101;2000.
37. Palozza P, Serini S, DiNicuolo F et al. *Carcinogenesis* 25:1315;2004.
38. Palozza P, Serini S, DiNicuolo F et al. *Mol Aspects Med* 24:353;2003.
39. Black HS. *Photochem Photobiol Sci* 3:753;2004.
40. Ribaya-Mercado JD, Garmyn M, Gilchrest BA et al. *J Nutr* 125:1854;1995.
41. Mathews-Roth MM. *Biochimie* 68:875;1986.
42. Alemzadeh R, Feehan T. *Eur J Ped* 163:547;2004.
43. Mathews-Roth MM, Pathak MA, Parrish J et al. *J Invest Dermatol* 59:349;1972.
44. Stahl W, Heinrich U, Jungmann H et al. *Am J Clin Nutr* 71:795;2000.

45. Rizwan M, Rodriguez-Blanco I, Harbottle A et al. *Br J Dermatol* 164:154;2011.
46. Aust O, Stahl W, Sies H et al. *Int J Vitam Nutr Res* 75:54;2005.
47. Stahl W, Heinrich U, Wiseman S et al. *J Nutr* 131:1449;2001.
48. Palombo P, Fabrizi G, Ruocco V et al. *Skin Pharmacol Physiol* 20:199;2007.
49. Heinrich U, Gärtner C, Wiebusch M et al. *J Nutr* 133(1):98–101;January 2003.
50. Césarini JP, Michel L, Maurette JM et al. *Photodermatol Photoimmunol Photomed* 19:182;2003.
51. McArdle F, Rhodes LE, Parslew RA et al. *Am J Clin Nutr* 80:1270;2004.
52. Stahl W, Sies H. *Skin Pharmacol Appl Skin Physiol* 15:291;2002.
53. Block G, Patterson B, Subar A. *Nutr Cancer* 18:1;1992.
54. Greenberg ER, Baron JA, Stukel TA et al. *N Engl J Med* 323:789;1990.
55. Dorgan JF, Boakye NA, Fears TR et al. *Cancer Epidemiol Biomarkers Prev* 13:1276;2004.
56. Green A, Williams G, Neale R et al. *Lancet* 354:723;1999.
57. Darlington S, Williams G, Neale R et al. *Arch Dermatol* 139:451;2003.
58. Frieling UM, Schaumberg DA, Kupper TS et al. *Arch Dermatol* 136:179;2000.
59. Hennekens CH, Buring JE, Manson JE et al. *N Engl J Med* 334:1145;1996.
60. Greenberg ER, Baron JA, Stevens MM et al. *Control Clin Trials* 10:153;1989.
61. Hercberg S, Ezzedine K, Guinot C et al. *J Nutr* 137:2098;2007.
62. Ezzedine K, Latreille J, Kesse-Guyot E et al. *Eur J Cancer* 46:3316;2010.
63. Druesne-Pecollo N, Latino-Martel P, Norat T et al. *Int J Cancer* 127:172;2010.
64. The Alpha-Tocopherol, Beta Carotene Cancer Prevention Study Group, *N Engl J Med* 330:1029;1994.
65. Cho S, Lee DH, Won CH et al. *Dermatology* 221:160;2010.
66. Bogden JD, Bendich A, Kemp FW et al. *Am J Clin Nutr* 60:437;1994.
67. Herraiz LA, Hsieh WC, Parker RS et al. *J Am Coll Nutr* 17:617;1998.
68. Santos MS, Leka LS, Ribaya-Mercado JD et al. *Am J Clin Nutr* 66:917;1997.
69. Girodon F, Galan P, Monget AL et al. *Arch Intern Med* 159:748;1999.
70. Watzl B, Bub A, Blockhaus M et al. *J Nutr* 130:1719;2000.
71. Muller H, Bub A, Watzel B, Rechkemmer G. *Eur J Nutr* 38:35;1999.
72. Heinrich U, Tronnier H, Stahl W et al. *Skin Pharmacol Physiol* 19:224;2006.
73. Morganti P, Fabrizi G, Bruno C. *Skinmed* 3:310;2004.
74. Darvin M, Patzelt A, Gehse S et al. *Eur J Pharm Biopharm* 69:943;2008.
75. Wolf G. *J Nutr* 135:363;2005.
76. Thiele JJ, Ekanayake-Mudiyanselage S. *Mol Aspects Medicine* 28:646;2007.
77. Thiele JJ, Hsieh SN, Ekanayake-Mudiyanselage S. *Dermatol Surg* 31:805;2005.
78. Eberlein-König B, Placzek M, Przybilla B. *J Am Acad Dermatol* 38:45;1998.
79. Fuchs J, Kern H. *Free Radic Biol Med* 25:1006;1998.
80. Eberlein-König B, Fesq H, Abeck D et al. *Photodermatol Photoimmunol Photomed* 16:50;2000.
81. Tsoureli-Nikita E, Hercogova J, Lotti T et al. *Int J Dermatol* 41:146;2002.
82. Wu D, Han SN, Meydani M et al. *J Am Coll Nutr* 25:300;2006.
83. Meydani SN, Meydani M, Blumberg JB et al. *JAMA* 277(17):1380–1386;7 May 1997.
84. Hoppu U, Salo-Väänänen P, Lampi AM, Isolauri E. *Biol Neonate* 88: 24;2005.
85. Martindale S, McNeill G, Devereux G et al. *Amer J Resp Crit Care Med* 171:121;2005.
86. Oh S-Y, Chung J, Kim MK et al. *Eur J Clin Nutr* 64:245;2010.
87. Okuda M, Bando N, Tereo J et al. *Ped Allergy Immunol* 21:e705;2010.
88. Kharaeva Z, Gostova E, DeLuca C et al. *Nutrition* 25:295;2009.
89. Kökçam I, Naziroğlu M. *Clin Chim Acta* 289:23;1999.
90. Severin E, Nave B, Ständer M, Ott R et al. *Dermatol* 198:336;1999.
91. Marrakchi S, Kim I, Delaporte E et al. *Acta Derm Venereol* 74:298;1994.
92. Baumann LS, Spencer J. *Dermatol Surg* 25:311;1999.
93. Zampieri N, Zuin V, Burro R et al. *J Plastic Reconstr Aesthet Surg* 63:1474;2010.
94. Delanian S, Porcher R, Balla-Mekias S et al. *J Clin Oncol* 21:2545;2003.
95. Cracowski JL, Girolet S, Imbert B et al. *Free Rad Biol Med* 38:98;2005.
96. deSouza RB, Macedo AR, Kuruma KA et al. *Clin Rheumatol* 28(10):1207;2009.
97. Musalmah M, Fairuz AH, Gapor MT, Ngah WZ. *Asia Pac J Clin Nutr* 11:S448;2002.
98. Altavilla D, Saitta A, Cucinotta D et al. *Diabetes* 50:667;2001.
99. Bjelakovic G, Nikolova D, Gluud LL et al. *JAMA* 297:842;2007.
100. Miller ER, Pastor-Barriuso R, Dalal D et al. *Ann Int Med* 142:37;2005.
101. Jen M, Yan AC. *Clin Dermatol* 28:669;2010.
102. Finch J, Munhutu MN, Whitaker-Worth DL. *Clinics Dermatol* 28:605;2010.
103. Leveque N, Robin S, Muret P et al. *Dermatology* (Basel, Switzerland) 207:261;2003.
104. Hoppu U, Rinne M, Salo-Väänänen P et al. *Eur J Clin Nutr* 59:123;2005.
105. Laitinen K, Kalliomäki M, Poussa T et al. *Brit J Nutr* 94:565;2005.
106. Gruskay DM. *Arch Dermatol* 124:760;1988.
107. Lechner-Gruskay D, Honig PJ, Pereira G, McKinney S. *Ped Dermatol* 5:22;1988.
108. Anderson KE. *Hepatology* 45:6;2007.
109. Sinclair PR, Gorman N, Shedlofsky SI et al. *J Lab Clinical Med* 130:197;1997.
110. Gorman N, Zaharia A, Trask HS et al. *Hepatology* 45:187;2007.
111. Ferrer MD, Tauler P, Sureda A et al. *Brit J Nutr* 103:69;2010.
112. Boffa MJ, Ead RD, Reed P, Weinkove C. *Photodermatol Photoimmunol Photomed* 12:27;1996.
113. Fedeles F, Murphy M, Roth MJ, Grant-Kels JM. *Clinics Dermatol* 28;627;2010.
114. Brown KL, Phillips TJ. *Clinics Dermatol* 28: 432;2010.
115. Levine M. *NEJM* 314:892;1986.
116. Balaji P, Mosley JG. *Ann Royal CollSurg England* 77:270;1995.
117. Stratton RJ, Ek AC, Engfer M et al. *Ageing Res Rev* 4:422;2005.
118. Langer G, Schloemer G, Knerr A et al. *Cochrane Database Syst Rev* (4):CD003216;2003.
119. Utoguchi N, Ikeda K, Saeki K et al. *J Cell Physiol* 163:393;1995.
120. Laufer F. *J Drugs Dermatol* 5:290;2006.

121. Reinhold U, Seiter S, Ugurel S, Tilgen W. *J Amer Acad Dermatol* 41:207;1999.

122. Payette MJ, Whalen J, Grant-Kels JM. *Clinics Dermatol* 28:650;2010.

123. McNaughton SA, Marks GC, Green AC. *Cancer Epidemiol Biomarkers Prev* 14:1596;2005.

124. Hughes MC, van der Pols JC, Marks GC, Green AC. *Int J Cancer* 119:1953;2006.

125. Fung TT, Spiegelman D, Egan KM et al. *Int J Cancer* 103:110;2003.

126. Searing DA, Leung DYM. *Immunol Allergy Clin N Amer* 30:397;2010.

127. Field S, Newton-Bishop JA. *Molec Oncol* 5:197;2011.

128. Hata TR, Kotol P, Jackson M et al. *J Allergy Clin Immunol* 122:829;2008.

129. Bäck O, Blomquist HK, Hernell O, Stenberg B. *Acta dermato-venereologica* 89:28;2009.

130. Hyppönen E, Sovio U, Wjst M et al. *Ann NY Acad Sci* 1037:84;2004.

131. Gale CR, Robinson SM, Harvey NC et al. *Eur J Clin Nutr* 62:68;2008.

132. Camargo CA, Rifas-Shiman SL, Litonjua AA et al. *Am J Clin Nutr* 85:788;2007.

133. Sidbury R, Sullivan AF, Thadhani RI, Camargo CA Jr. *Brit J Dermatol* 159:245;2008.

134. Oren E, Banerji A, Camargo CA. *J Allergy Clin Immunol* 121:533;2008.

135. Peroni DG, Piacentini GL, Cametti E et al. *Brit J Dermatol* 164:1078;2011.

136. Smit JV, Cox S, Blokx WA et al. *Brit J Dermatol* 147:816;2002.

137. Seckin D, Cerman AA, Yildiz A, Ergun T. *J Drugs Dermatol* 8:451;2009.

138. Hunter DJ, Colditz GA, Stampfer MJ et al. *Annals Epidemiol* 2:231;1992.

139. Eide MJ, Johnson DA, Jacobsen GR. *Arch Dermatol* 147:1379;2011.

140. Ellison TI, Smith MK, Gilliam AC, MacDonald PN. *J Invest Dermatol* 128:2508;2008.

141. Randerson-Moor JA, Taylor JC, Elliott F et al. *Eur J Cancer* 45:3271;2009.

142. Newton-Bishop JA, Beswick S, Randerson-Moor J et al. *J Clin Oncol* 27:5439;2009.

143. Nürnberg B, Gräber S, Gärtner B et al. *Anticancer Res* 29:3669;2009.

144. Gandini S, Raimondi S, Gnagnarella P et al. *Eur J Cancer* 45:634;2009.

145. Cornwell ML, Comstock GW, Holick MF, Bush TL. *Photoderm Photoimmunol Photomed* 9:109;1992.

146. Reichrath J, Querings K. *Cancer Causes Control* 15:97;2004.

147. Newton-Bishop JA, Chang YM, Elliott F et al. *Eur J Cancer* 47:732;2011.

148. Perez A, Raab R, Chen TC et al. *Br J Dermatol* 134:1070;1996.

149. Menter A, Griffiths CE. *Lancet* 370(9583):272;2007.

150. Fu LW, Vender R. *Dermatol Res Pract* 27:6079;2011.

151. Mukhtar H, Ahmad N. *Am J Clin Nutr* 71:1698S;2000.

152. Hsu S. *J Amer Acad Dermatol* 52:1049;2005.

153. Heinrich U, Moore CE, DeSprit S et al. *J Nutr* 141:1202;2011.

154. Chow HH, Cai Y, Hakim IA et al. *Clin Cancer Res* 9:3312;2003.

155. Chiu AE, Chan JL, Kern DG et al. *Dermatol Surg* 31:855;2005.

156. Janjua R, Munoz C, Gorell E et al. *Dermatol Surgery* 35:1057;2009.

157. Puch F, Samson-Villager F et al. *Exper Dermatol* 17:668;2008.

158. Kim H, Kawazoe T, Han DW et al. *Wound Rep Regen* 16:714;2008.

159. Klass BR, Branford OA, Grobbelaar AO, Rolfe KJ. *Wound Rep Regen* 18:80;2010.

160. Park G, Yoon BS, Moon JH et al. *J Invest Dermatol* 128:2429;2008.

161. Hsu S, Dickinson D, Borke J et al. *Exper Dermatol* 16:678;2007.

162. Hsu SD, Dickinson DP, Qin H et al. *Autoimmunity* 40:138;2007.

163. Neukam K, Stahl W, Tronnier H et al. *Eur J Nutr* 46:53;2007.

164. Heinrich U, Neukam K, Tronnier H et al. *J Nutr* 136:1565;2006.

165. Handog EB, Galang DA, deLeon-Godinez MA et al. *Int J Dermatol* 48:896;2009.

166. Yamakoshi J, Sano A, Tokutake S et al. *Phytother Res* 18:895;2004.

167. Ni Z, Mu Y, Gulati O. *Phytother Res* 16:567;2002.

168. Segger D, Schönlau F. *J Dermatolog Treat* 15:222;2004.

169. Hughes-Formella B, Wunderlich O, Williams R. *Skin Pharmacol Physiol* 20:43;2007.

170. Ndiaye M, Philippe C, Mukhtar H et al. *Arch Biochem Biophys* 508:164;2011.

171. Jang M, Cai L, Udeani GO et al. *Science* 275:218;1997.

172. Bhattacharya S, Darjatmoko SR, Polans AS. *Melanoma Res* 21:180;2011.

173. Salado C, Olaso E, Gallot N et al. *J Translational Med* 9:59;2011.

174. Pilkington SM, Watson RE, Nicolaou A, Rhodes LE. *Exper Dermatol* 20:537;2011.

175. Rhodes LE, Shahbakhti H, Azurdia RM et al. *Carcinogenesis* 24(5):919;2003.

176. Bain C, Green A, Siskind V et al. *Annals Epidemiol* 3:235;1993.

177. Hakim IA, Harris RB, Ritenbaugh C. *Nutr Cancer* 36:155;2000.

178. Rhodes LE, Durham BH, Fraser WD et al. *J Invest Dermatol* 105:532;1995.

179. Rhodes LE, White SI. *Br J Dermatol.* 138:173;1998.

180. Orengo IF, Black HS, Wolf JE Jr. *Arch Derm Res* 284:219;1992.

181. Rhodes LE, O'Farrell S, Jackson MJ et al. *J Invest Dermatol* 103:151;1994.

182. van der Pols JC, Xu C, Boyle GM et al. *Cancer Epidemiol Biomarkers Prev* 20:530;2011.

183. Neukam K, De Spirt S, Stahl W et al. *Skin Pharmacol Physiol* 24:67;2011.

184. Søyland E, Funk J, Rajka G et al. *N Engl J Med* 328:1812;1993.

185. Bittiner SB, Tucker WF, Cartwright I et al. *Lancet* 1(8582):378–380; February 1988.

186. Grimminger F, Mayser P, Papavassilis C et al. *Clin Investig* 71:634;1993.

187. Mayser P, Mrowietz U, Arenberger P et al. *J Am Acad Dermatol* 38:539;1998.

188. Callaway J, Schwab U, Harvima I et al. *J Dermatolog Treat* 16:87;2005.

189. Klemens CM, Berman DR, Mozurkewich EL. *BJOG* 118:916;2011.

190. Almqvist C, Garden F, Xuan W et al. *J Allergy Clin Immunol* 119:1438;2007.

191. Marks GB, Mihrshahi S, Kemp AS et al. *J Allergy Clin Immunol* 118:53;2006.

192. Mihrshahi S, Peat JK, Webb K et al. *Control Clin Trials* 22:333;2001.

193. Furuhjelm C, Warstedt K, Fagerås M et al. *Pediatr Allergy Immunol* 22:505;2011.

194. Hitch JM, Greenburg BG, *Arch Dermatol* 84:898;1961.

195. Rubin MG, Kim K, Logan AC. *Lipids Health Dis* 13;36;2008.

196. McDaniel JC, Belury M, Ahijevych K. *Wound Repair Regen* 16:337;2008.

197. Peck LW, Monsen ER, Ahmad S. *Am J Clin Nutr* 64:210;1996.

198. Begum R, Belury MA, Burgess JR, Peck LW. *J Ren Nutr* 14:233;2004.

# 71 Nutrition and Skeletal Health

*Carolyn D. Berdanier*

## CONTENTS

## INTRODUCTION

The skeleton is a complex, metabolically active tissue that serves multiple physiologic functions. It comprises ~8% of the body weight of an adult person's normal weight. It serves as a reservoir for the macrominerals, calcium, phosphorus, and magnesium, yet its most important purpose is to maintain normal posture and locomotion by virtue of its hardness.

## BONE COMPOSITION

Bone consists of both organic and inorganic materials (Table 71.1). Its hardness is due to the deposition of a calcium–phosphorus complex called hydroxyapatite $[Ca_{10}(PO_4)_6(OH)_2]$ in plates that are interspaced within the interstices of a protein matrix composed predominately of type 1 collagen (~90%). This collagen has a unique amino acid composition consisting of large amounts of glycine, proline, and hydroxyproline.[1] A single molecule of type I collagen has a molecular mass of ~285 kD, a width of ~14 Å, and a length of ~300 Å. There are at least 17 different polypeptides found in collagen. The polypeptides used for the collagen protein matrix vary throughout the body and each collagen uses at least three of them.

Collagen is about 30%–33% glycine with another 15%–30% of the amino acid residues as proline and 3, 4, or 5 hydroxyproline. Collagen is a left-handed triple helix stabilized by hydrogen bonding. The hydrogen bonds may involve bridging water molecules between the hydroxyprolines. The collagen fibrils are also held together by covalent cross-linking. These cross-links are between the side chains of lysine and histidine and the linkage is catalyzed by the copper-dependent enzyme lysyl oxidase. Up to four side chains can be covalently bonded to each other. Thus, collagen provides a network of fibers upon which the crystals of hydroxyapatite are deposited. The hydroxyapatite also contains magnesium, iron, sodium, and chloride. These ions are adsorbed onto the surface of the hydroxyapatite crystallites. In addition, strontium, fluoride, and carbonate ions are incorporated into the mineral lattice. The presence of these ions affects the chemical and physical properties of the calcified tissue. Solubility, for example, is decreased when strontium and fluoride ions are present. Hardness is enhanced by the presence of fluoride. Bone also can attract toxic minerals such as cadmium.[2,3]

Collagen synthesis is subject to the influence of ascorbic acid in that three of the key enzymes in the synthetic pathway require ascorbic acid as a coenzyme. Growing children whose diets are deficient in ascorbic acid develop a form of rickets characterized by swellings at the ends of the rib bones. This is called a scorbutic rachitic rosary.

Bone matrix contains, in addition to the hydroxyapatite, a number of noncollagenous proteins, water, lipids, and some incidental compounds such as growth factors and substances such as tetracycline and environmental contaminents.[3] These components are also shown in Table 71.1.

## BONE FORMATION

Bone formation begins in the embryo and continues throughout life. The nature of the process and the cells involved changes as the individual ages. Osteoprogenitor cells in early development synthesize the extracellular matrix described earlier and also regulate the flux of minerals into that matrix. As the

**TABLE 71.1**

**Bone Composition**

| | |
|---|---|
| 35% organic (FFDWᵃ) | Type 1 collagen (90+%) |
| | Noncollagenous proteins: glycosaminoglycans, proteoglycans, glycoproteins, osteocalcin, osteonectin, osteopontin, bone sialoprotein, alkaline phosphatase, etc. |
| | Growth factors and cytokines |
| 65% inorganic (FFDWᵃ) | Hydroxyapatite: $Ca_{10}(PO_4)_6(OH)_2$ |
| | Magnesium, sodium, potassium |
| | Carbonate-containing salts |
| | Fluorine |
| | Deposited "heavy metals" |
| | Trace elements |
| Miscellaneous | Water |
| | Lipids |
| | Deposited molecules: tetracyclines, etc. |

ᵃ Fat-free dry weight.

calcified tissue begins to form, osteoclasts appear on the surface of this tissue and osteoblasts, connected to one another by long processes, are totally surrounded by the mineralizing matrix. Each type of mineralized tissue has some unique properties, but all share several histologic features in the early mineralization process. Hunziker [1] has described this process in the epiphyseal growth plate during the ossification of the endochondral cartilage as it becomes bone. Initial mineral deposition occurs at discrete sites on membrane-bound bodies (matrix vesicles) in the extracellular matrix. These initial deposits are diffuse and lack orientation. The mineral crystals proliferate and mineralization proceeds filling the longitudinal but not the transverse septa. Changes in the activities of enzymes that catalyze the hydrolysis of phosphate esters and those that catalyze certain proteolytic reactions follow or accompany this mineralization. These reactions are prerequisite to vascular invasion. Following vascular invasion, lamellar bone is formed by osteoblasts directly on the surface of the preexisting mineralized cartilage. These osteoblasts secrete type I collagen with very little proteoglycan and few extracellular matrix vesicles. This process is repeated over and over until the bone has finished growing. At this point, the growth plate closes and the mature length and shape of the bone is apparent. This process is called bone modeling. The resultant bone, however, is not metabolically inert. It continues to recycle mineral matter; that is, it is continuously remodeled through the action of the osteoblasts that synthesize the collagen matrix and the osteoclasts that are stimulated by parathyroid hormone (PTH) to reabsorb calcium (and other minerals) in times of need. While the number of osteoblasts declines with age, the number of osteoclasts increases especially in postmenopausal females. This helps to explain some of the age-related loss in bone mineral that occurs in aging females. Osteoclasts act first during bone remodeling by producing cavities on either the cortical or cancellous (trabecular) bone surfaces. When these cavities develop, osteoblasts are

recruited for bone remineralization, thereby filling (or refilling) the cavities. The bone matrix reforms and remineralizes as described earlier with the result of new bone formation. The remodeling process is an ongoing one with rates of resorption equaling the rates of new bone formation as long as the hormones controlling each process are in balance and as long as the nutrients needed to support this ongoing process are provided. Insulin-like growth factor I (IGF-I) and growth hormone play a role in this process.[4–9] If IGF-I is deficient, bone calcium accretion is impaired.[8] Indeed, IGF-I determines the peak bone mineral density that will be achieved at adulthood. IGF-I also serves a role in regulating calcium turnover in bone once full adult stature has been achieved. Some of the IGF-I effect is mediated by its effect on 1, 25-dihydroxyvitamin $D_3$ production.[5,6] This is also true for the growth hormone effect on bone calcium accretion.[5,6] Figure 71.1 illustrates calcium turnover in bone.

Bone mass can remain constant for many decades. However, once the hormone balance changes, this constancy changes.[10–12] In females, bone mass declines by an estimated 1%–2% per year after menopause. In senile men, bone mass loss also occurs. In fact, both senile males and females experience about a 1% loss per year. There is a loss not only in bone mass but also in structural integrity. The bones lose their mineral apatite, become porous (osteoporosis), and as well, lose the architecture upon which the mineral has rested. Some of this loss may be due to a loss in the synthesis of the vitamin K-dependent protein osteocalcin. Subjects prescribed with Coumadin (an antivitamin K substance that delays blood clotting) also synthesize less osteocalcin.[13–15] The very compact cortical portions of the bone disappear, leaving a fragile, largely trabecular bone. The result of these changes is a fragile skeletal system subject to non-trauma-related fracture.

While appropriate hormone balance (PTH, calcitonin, IGF-I, growth hormone, 1, 25-dihydroxyvitamin $D_3$, and estrogen) is important, it should also be recognized that

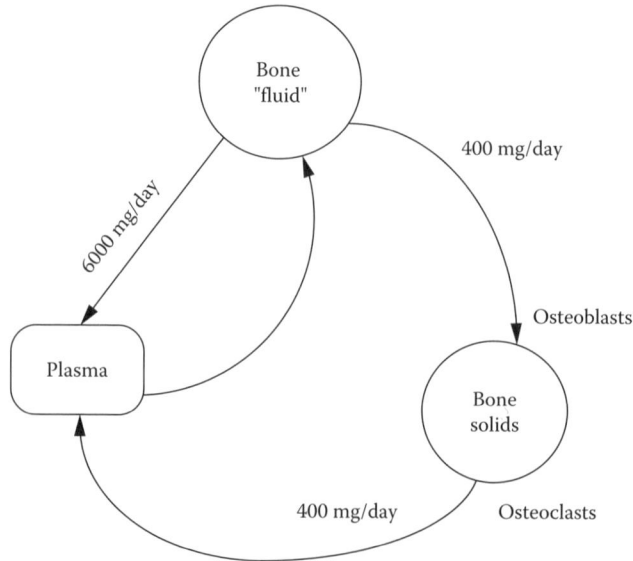

**FIGURE 71.1** Calcium turnover in bone.

## TABLE 71.2
### Nutrients Important to Bone Growth and Density

| Nutrient | Role |
|---|---|
| Calcium | Essential component of the bone apatite |
| Phosphorus | Essential component of the bone apatite |
| 1,25 vitamin $D_3$ | Essential to the synthesis of calbindin |
| Magnesium | Component of bone mineral matrix |
| Ascorbic acid | Essential to normal collagen synthesis |
| Vitamin K | Essential for the synthesis of osteocalcin |
| Protein | Essential for the synthesis of bone protein |
| N-3 fatty acids | Stimulates bone formation |
| Vitamin E | Increases bone formation |
| Boron | Enhances estrogen effect on bone density |
| Zinc | Growth factor for bone |
| Copper | Cofactor in collagen synthesis; stimulates cross-links in bone adding strength |
| Silicon | Enhances skeletal mineralization |
| Vanadium | Enhances skeletal mineralization |
| Manganese | Promotes skeletal growth |
| Selenium | Cofactor for collagen maturation |

## TABLE 71.3
### Food Sources of Calcium in 100 g Portions

| Source | mg | Weight of Average Serving (g) |
|---|---|---|
| Skim milk | 123 | 245 |
| Whole milk | 119 | 244 |
| Ice cream | 129 | 66 |
| Yogurt | 120 | 227 |
| Oysters | 45 | 84 |
| Cheddar cheese | 728 | 28 |
| Spinach | 135 | 90 |
| Mustard greens | 74 | 70 |
| Broccoli | 48 | 44 |
| White bread | 125 | 24 |
| Whole-wheat bread | 72 | 25 |
| Carrots | 26 | 72 |
| Potatoes | 10 | 202 |
| Winter squash | 14 | 102 |
| Egg | 50 | 50 |
| Hamburger | 10 | 100 |
| Hot dog | 19 | 57 |

*Source:* http://www.nal.usda.gov/foodcomposition

a number of nutrients play important roles in the maintenance of bone mass. Listed in Table 71.2 are nutrients deemed important in maintaining normal bone growth and density (see Chapters 11 through 13 for details on these nutrients).

There are some nutrients and food contaminants that have detrimental effects on bone.

Vitamins A in excess can be detrimental to the normal calcium–bone balance. Excess vitamin A can increase bone resorption. Iron in excess decreases bone formation and mineralization and increases bone resorption. Excess molybdenum causes skeletal deformities. Cadmium, tin, and lead, all toxic minerals, decrease bone calcium deposition by replacing this mineral in the mineral matrix.

## CALCIUM AND VITAMIN D

Calcium is the most abundant mineral in bone; the skeleton accounts for greater than 90% of body calcium content. The gastrointestinal (GI) absorption of calcium is affected by a large number of factors such as vitamin D status, transit time, mucosal competence, and calcium binding by phosphates, oxalate, and fiber and the presence of toxic minerals in the gut contents. Vitamin D is the dominant factor influencing calcium absorption. Its active metabolite, 1,25-dihydroxyvitamin D (calcitriol), stimulates production of a specific calcium-binding protein (calbindin) in GI mucosal cells. Calbindin facilitates transcellular transport of calcium through the GI mucosa. In its absence, calcium absorption is minimal with the result of porous, weak bones (osteoporosis).

The average daily calcium intake for adults in the United States ranges from 500 to 1200 mg. The range is quite broad because it depends on the percent of the diet that comes from dairy products. Milk, cheese, ice cream, yogurt, sour cream,

buttermilk, and other fermented and non-fermented milk products can provide as much as 72% of the daily calcium intake. Nuts and whole-grain products are also good sources of calcium, while other foods are relatively poor sources of this mineral. Shown in Table 71.3 are a number of foods and their calcium content. An extensive list of foods and their calcium content can be found on the USDA website: www.ars.usda.gov/nutrientdata. Some foods contain calcium-binding agents that reduce the availability of the calcium to the enterocyte. For example, some plant foods contain calcium in measurable quantities, but these same foods also contain phytate, a six-carbon anomer of glucose having six phosphate groups. Phytate will bind to calcium reducing its availability for absorption. Once the phytate is degraded by the enzyme phytase, the bound calcium is then released and is once again available for absorption. Unfortunately, this release occurs in the lower third of the intestine and in the large intestine, areas which are less active in terms of calcium absorption. Phytate binds other divalent ions (Zn, Fe, Mg) as well and has a similar effect on their absorption. In addition, oxalate and some tannins can have this effect. Foods and food mixtures that provide calcium and phosphorus together in a ratio of 2:1–1:2 optimize calcium absorption. Both minerals are actively transported and yet do not share a single transport mechanism. When the food mixtures are unbalanced with respect to this ratio, then calcium uptake will be impaired.

### Mechanisms of Absorption

Only 20%–50% of ingested calcium is absorbed, yet this mineral is so important to metabolism that two mechanisms exist for its absorption.[16,17] One of these is vitamin D dependent,

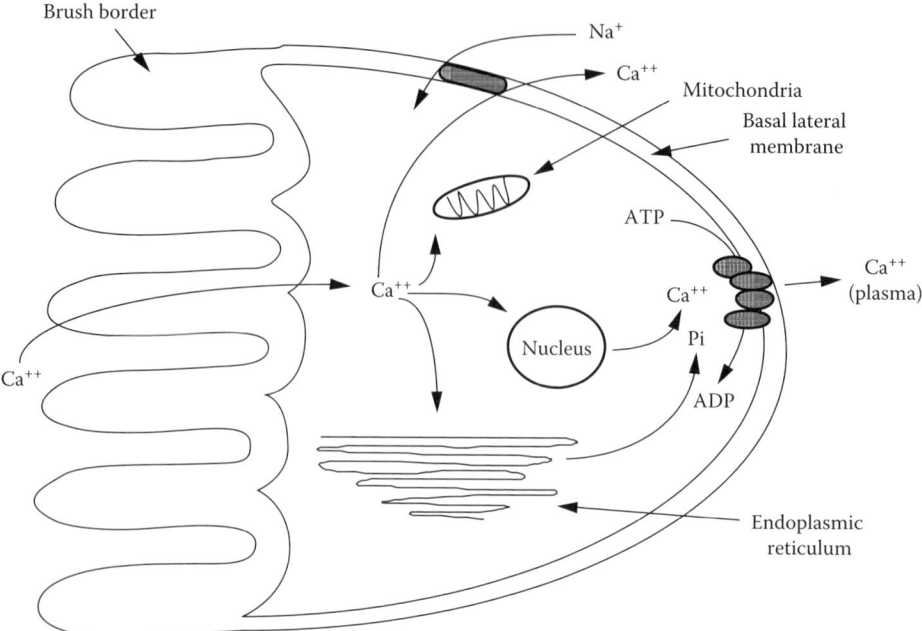

**FIGURE 71.2**    Calcium absorption by the enterocyte. Both the $Ca^{2+}$-$Na^+$ exchange and the energy-dependent systems are shown.

while the other is not. The latter is one that uses passive diffusion. The former is an energy-dependent active transport system and is illustrated in Figure 71.2. This is a saturable system that operates actively when calcium is in short supply in the diet. Thus, when the diet is calcium poor, this system is more active than when a calcium-rich diet is consumed. Thus, a wide range of apparent calcium absorption exists. In the active system, calcium diffuses across the brush border down its thermodynamic gradient into the cell as free unbound $Ca^{++}$. This calcium is then bound by an intracellular protein called calbindin $D_{9k}$ that serves to maintain the level of calcium in the cell at a low, nontoxic level.[18] Calcium released from calbindin enters and leaves the subcell compartments such as the mitochondria[19,20] and endoplasmic reticulum.[21] This occurs in an orderly oscillatory manner.[22] The calcium ion either leaves the enterocyte in exchange for sodium or is extruded from the cell by a calcium-activated ATPase. This ATPase has been found in both the brush border and the basal-lateral membrane. As calcium is extruded, ATP is cleaved to ADP and Pi, hence the energy dependence of this system. Because the sodium that is exchanged for calcium must be actively removed from the intracellular compartment by the $Na^+$-$K^+$ ATPase, this process is also part of this energy-dependent system.

Table 71.4 gives the daily dietary reference intakes of calcium, phosphorus, magnesium, and vitamin D for normal males and females of various ages. Since the average nondairy diet contains only 300–500 mg of calcium, the intentional use of calcium-rich food is necessary to meet recommended intake of this mineral. Examples of calcium-rich foods are shown in Table 71.3. Failing to consume enough calcium-rich foods indicates that a calcium supplement should be added. Similarly, failing to consume enough vitamin D or failing to have sufficient sunlight exposure also indicates the need for

supplementation. There is considerable argument about the need for vitamin D supplementation as well as the need itself for the vitamin. Chapter 57 explores these issues in greater detail.

In individuals with GI, hepatic, or renal deficits, calcium and vitamin D nutrition should be monitored by measurements of calcium, vitamin D metabolite, and PTH levels. Then, should these levels fall outside the normal limits, supplementation should be considered. This is especially important in the anephric patient since the kidney is the major site for the conversion of 25-hydroxyvitamin D to 1,25-dihydroxyvitamin $D_3$.

## OTHER NUTRIENTS

Other nutrients critical to the skeleton include phosphorus (phosphate), magnesium, protein, and lipids. The average American who is not a vegetarian uses meat, dairy products, and phosphoric acid-containing beverages, so the phosphorus intake is usually sufficient, and there is no need for supplementation. In fact, excess phosphorus intake should be avoided since it may increase bone resorption by stimulating excess PTH secretion. Calcium phosphate supplements as a calcium source are not desirable, not only because of a possible stimulatory effect on PTH, but also because the excess phosphate may excessively bind calcium in the GI tract. Excess phosphate may also combine with calcium internally and facilitate its removal from the circulation by deposition within soft tissues and on bone surfaces. The latter does not necessarily contribute to bone integrity, except in undermineralized bone (osteomalacia) in which a high phosphorus intake is often beneficial.

The value of magnesium (Mg) in enhancing or maintaining skeletal vitality is controversial.[23–29]

**TABLE 71.4**

**Daily Dietary Reference Intakes of Various Age/Gender Groups for Calcium, Phosphorus, Magnesium, and Vitamin D**

| Group | Calcium (mg) | Phosphorus (mg) | Magnesium (mg) | Vitamin D (μg) |
|---|---|---|---|---|
| Infants | | | | |
| 0–6 months | 210 | 100 | 30 | 5 |
| 7–12 months | 270 | 275 | 75 | 5 |
| Children | | | | |
| 1–3 years | 500 | 469 | 80 | 5 |
| 4–8 years | 800 | 500 | 130 | 5 |
| Males | | | | |
| 9–13 years | 1300 | 1250 | 240 | 5 |
| 14–18 years | 1300 | 1250 | 410 | 5 |
| 19–30 years | 1000 | 700 | 400 | 5 |
| 31–50 years | 1000 | 700 | 420 | 5 |
| 51–70 years | 1200 | 700 | 420 | 10 |
| 70+ | 1200 | 700 | 420 | 15 |
| Females | | | | |
| 9–13 years | 1300 | 1250 | 240 | 5 |
| 14–18 years | 1300 | 1250 | 360 | 5 |
| 19–30 years | 1000 | 700 | 310 | 5 |
| 31–50 years | 1000 | 700 | 320 | 5 |
| 51–70 years | 1200 | 700 | 320 | 10 |
| 70+ years | 1200 | 700 | 320 | 15 |
| Pregnancy | | | | |
| 14–18 years | 1300 | 1250 | 400 | 5 |
| 19–30 years | 1000 | 700 | 350 | 5 |
| 31–50 years | 1000 | 700 | 360 | 5 |
| Lactation | | | | |
| 14–18 years | 1300 | 1250 | 360 | 5 |
| 19–30 years | 1000 | 700 | 310 | 5 |
| 31–50 years | 1000 | 700 | 320 | 5 |

*Source:* http://www.nal.usda.gov/foodcomposition

Studies conducted in cells and in animal models showed that Mg promotes matrix formation, increases bone mineral content, increases trabecular bone, and increases the mechanical strength of the bone. In excess, magnesium destabilizes the bone crystalline structure. All of these results have been reported to occur in experimental animals; however, in humans, insufficient studies exist to date to verify comparable actions under clinical conditions. Since the U.S. population on the whole has only borderline Mg sufficiency, because of its relatively low concentration in common foodstuffs, there may be some justification in ensuring an adequate Mg intake by the use of supplements (Mg citrate, $MgCl_2$, or Mg–aminoacid salt). However, care must be exercised to avoid an excess intake.

The need for adequate protein of high biologic value to ensure adequate production of bone collagen and noncollagenous bone proteins is obvious. Patients with eating disorders and protein–calorie malnutrition uniformly have deficient skeletons.

Several variable components of the human diet can have important influences on the skeleton by affecting calcium metabolism or affecting the skeleton directly. Excess fiber, caffeine, and acid-containing foods and beverages all have negative effects, whereas the isoflavones and related compounds present in various foods are "weak estrogens" and exert a positive effect. Alcohol, although technically not a nutrient, has multiple adverse actions on bone health.

Aside from vitamin D, four other vitamins have been shown to have an influence on the skeleton. Vitamin A in excess and its more powerful retinoic acid derivatives (used to treat acne, other dermatologic conditions, and certain neoplasms) are powerful stimulators of the osteoclast and can cause bone loss and even hypercalcemia. Vitamin C, on the other hand, is an osteoblast promoter, and severe deficiency is sufficient to cause borderline scurvy accompanied by bony lesions. Vitamin E also increases experimental bone formation, but its clinical significance has not been established. Vitamin K, as a cofactor for gamma-hydroxylation, is responsible for the production of osteocalcin, a noncollagenous matrix protein. Low vitamin K levels have been reported in some osteoporotics, and associations between this vitamin and bone health have been reported.[13–15] A large number of trace elements have either positive or negative effects on the skeleton, but the majority are of interest in experimental systems and have no proven benefits or dangers to patients. Strontium supplementation has been studied in osteoporotics and has been shown to enhance bone density. Lithium, used in the treatment of bipolar disorder, can stimulate the parathyroid glands to excessive activity with increased bone resorption and hypercalcemia. Aluminum overload can occur in chronic renal failure through the use of aluminum-containing antacids and other oral sources or the use of aluminum-contaminated renal dialysis fluid. Aluminum toxicity impairs bone formation and mineralization as well as stimulates bone resorption. Aluminum toxicity in chronic renal failure patients is characterized as a resistant osteomalacia, or so-called aplastic bone disease.

Iron overload, as occurs in hemochromatosis of both primary and secondary etiologies, hemolytic anemias, and some cases of chronic renal failure, uniformly decreases bone formation and mineralization with measurable bone loss. This can be severe enough to cause osteoporosis. In some cases, increased bone resorption has been observed. In chronic renal failure, iron overload can simulate aluminum toxicity. In postmenopausal women on hormone replacement therapy, dietary iron positively influences bone mineral density.[30] Cadmium toxicity, which occurs mainly in individuals with industrial exposure, has similar manifestations to iron overload but tends to present itself as defective mineralization, with predominant osteomalacia. Lead toxicity has similar effects to iron and cadmium but rarely shows skeletal manifestations comparable to its central nervous system (CNS), hematological, and other soft tissue toxicity.

## TABLE 71.5
### Metabolic Bone Diseases

| Disorder | Characteristics |
| --- | --- |
| Rickets | Decreased calcium deposition in bone |
| Osteopetrosis | Decreased resorption |
| Osteogenesis imperfecta | Decreased formation |
| Osteomalacia | Decreased mineralization |
| Skeletal hyperparathyroidism | Increased resorption |
| Paget's disease | Increased resorption, increased formation |
| Enzyme defects | |
| Carbonic anhydrase II | Osteopetrosis |
| 1-Hydroxylase deficiency | Vitamin D-dependent rickets |
| Receptor defects | |
| PTH-related protein receptor | Jansen's metaphyseal chondrodysplasia |
| Fibroblast growth factor 3 receptor | Achondroplasia |
| Calcium sensor receptor | Familial hypocalcemic hypocalciuria (inactivating) |
| Calcium sensor receptor | Autosomal dominant hypoparathyroidism (activating) |
| Vitamin D receptor | Vitamin D-resistant syndromes |
| Signaling mechanism defects | |
| Gs protein excess | McCune–Albright syndrome |
| Gs protein deficiency | Pseudohypoparathyroidism |
| Structural gene defects | |
| Type 1 collagen defects | Osteogenesis imperfect |
| Bone morphogenetic protein 4 | Fibrodysplasia ossificans progressiva (activating) |
| Other genetic defects | |
| Hypophosphatemia | Excessive renal phosphate loss; rickets |

## TABLE 71.6
### Nonpharmacological Approaches to the Prevention and Treatment of Osteoporosis

| Nutrition | Calcium: 1000–1500 mg/Day |
| --- | --- |
| | Permits normal growth and development of the skeleton |
| | Maximizes peak bone mass |
| | Maintains adult bone mass |
| | Minimizes age-related bone loss |
| | Enhances benefits of pharmacological therapy |
| | Vitamin D: 600–1200 IU/day |
| | Intake of calcium/vitamin D should be maintained throughout life, starting before adolescence. Increase awareness in children and adolescents of needed behavioral/nutritional measures |
| | Magnesium: 450–500 mg/day (if tolerated) |
| Exercise fall prevention | |

## METABOLIC BONE DISEASES

The term *metabolic bone disease* refers to an aberration in the modeling and remodeling processes that in turn results in abnormal bone structure/mineralization. Table 71.5 gives examples of the more common disturbances leading to metabolic bone diseases. In addition, there are a number of genetic disorders that also result in abnormal bone formation.

## NUTRITIONAL RECOMMENDATIONS IN METABOLIC BONE DISEASES

### OSTEOPOROSIS

Bone loss sufficient to place patients at immediate risk for fracture should always be treated with a Food and Drug Administration (FDA)-approved drug in addition to a number of nonpharmacological approaches outlined in Table 71.6. The need to achieve an ideal calcium intake cannot be overstated. Opinions vary as to the ideal vitamin D intake, but it

is probable that intakes as high as 25 μg/day would not prove toxic. However, higher vitamin intakes should be avoided. There are also discrepancies in the recommendations for magnesium, but the recommended daily intake of 400–500 mg can be taken, if there is no tendency to frequent or loose bowel movements. In fact, a high magnesium intake may help to relieve the constipating effects of calcium carbonate preparations. During nutrition counseling for osteoporosis, the other nonpharmacological approaches listed in Table 71.6 should be monitored. Falls are particularly serious cofactors in fractures and can be avoided. Adequate protein kilocalorie nutrition promotes muscular strength and agility and therefore helps prevent falls.[31–34]

Although these recommendations are intended for primary types of osteoporosis, they are also applicable, with modifications, in secondary forms of osteoporosis. For example, calcium and vitamin D intakes should be carefully monitored by serum and urine calcium measurements in hyperparathyroidism and idiopathic hypercalciuria, and if urine calcium rises unduly, a thiazide diuretic should be added to reduce urine calcium excretion. In corticosteroid-induced osteoporosis, if the prednisone equivalent dose is 5 mg/day or higher, the vitamin D intake should be drastically increased to the range of 125–175 μg/day. The nonpharmacological approaches in Table 71.6 are equally applicable to patients with lesser degrees of bone loss, or osteopenia. Advanced states of osteopenia may also qualify for a modified drug program.

### OSTEOMALACIA

There are many causes of osteomalacia, and most relate to defects in the vitamin D cascade or an end-organ resistance to active vitamin metabolites, either genetic or acquired. Uncomplicated

**TABLE 71.7**
**Treatment of Osteomalacia**

| Type | Calcium Intake Four Times a Day (q.i.d) | Vitamin D Intake q.i.d | Other Nutrients | Other Agents |
|---|---|---|---|---|
| Nutritional (including post gastrectomy) | Up to 2000 mg | 400–1000 IU | | |
| Malabsorption | Same | Up to 50,000 IU | Other lost nutrients | Gluten-free diet, pancreatic enzymes |
| Dependent rickets | Same | 400–1000 IU plus calcitriol, up to 0.25 mg q.i.d | Same | |
| Familial hypophosphatemic rickets | Same | Up to 150,000 IU and calcitriol, up to 0.25 mg q.i.d | Phosphorus (neutral), up to 3000 mg q.i.d | |
| Oncogenic osteomalacia | Same | Same | | Locate and excise mesenchymal tumor |
| Anticonvulsant-induced osteomalacia | Same | Up to 5000 IU | | |

nutritional deficiencies (of calcium or vitamin D) are rare but do occur in financially and socially stressed individuals and in the institutionalized elderly. A general approach to nutritional therapy of osteomalacia is outlined in Table 71.7, which also indicates modifications to be made in various types of osteomalacia. The reason for advocating a combination of precursor vitamin D and the active metabolite calcitriol is that there is a theoretic possibility that other active metabolites of vitamin D might appear that might have direct stimulatory effects on the mineralization process itself.[35–38]

## RENAL OSTEODYSTROPHY

This term refers to the skeletal complications of chronic renal failure and represents a variable combination of secondary hyperparathyroidism, osteomalacia, osteoporosis, and osteosclerosis.[39–41] Nutritional therapy is an important aspect of treatment, although pharmacologic and surgical approaches may also be necessary in particularly advanced cases. The aim is to suppress the secondary hyperparathyroidism and correct undermineralization by using maximally tolerated doses of the active metabolite of vitamin D, calcitriol (1,25-dihydroxyvitamin D), and calcium. Calcium carbonate is preferred to calcium citrate, although both have the ability to bind phosphorus in the GI tract and thereby reduce the hyperphosphatemia, a major factor in the genesis of the renal osteodystrophy.

## PRIMARY HYPERPARATHYROIDISM

Previously, calcium restriction was advocated to lessen the impact of the hypercalcemia characteristic of the condition. However, the availability of bone density measurements has revealed that this results in greater bone loss and worsens the skeletal complications. Presently, adequate calcium and vitamin D intakes are advocated, preferably as food sources with a minimal use of supplements. The condition is best treated by surgery, although new pharmacologic agents, called calcimimetic agents, are currently under development.

## PAGET'S DISEASE

Although both bone resorption and formation are increased, their quantitative relationship is variable, so that either positive calcium balance (with hypocalciuria) or negative calcium balance (with hypercalciuria) may be present at any given time during the prolonged course of the condition.[42] In any case, the imbalance rarely disturbs the serum calcium level and does not cause serious bone loss in pagetic lesions. Therefore, normal calcium and vitamin D intakes are the best approach, as having Paget's disease does not protect against osteoporosis in nonpagetic areas. Since the bisphosphonates currently in use can occasionally cause transient mild hypocalcemia, some authorities recommend an increased calcium intake during bisphosphonate treatment. On the other hand, calcium should not be supplemented if there is a history of calcium-containing kidney stones. Another type of stone that can occur in Paget's disease is the uric acid stone, as some Paget's disease patients also have a concomitant gouty diathesis.

## REFERENCES

1. Hunziker, E.B., Herrmann, K.W., Schenk, R.K., Mueller, M., Moor, H. *J. Cell Biol.* 98: 267; 1984.
2. Engstrom, A., Hakansson, H., Skerfving, S. et al. *J. Nutr.* 141: 2198; 2011.

3. Surgeon General. http://www.surgeongeneral.gov/library (Accessed January 2, 2012).
4. Gomez, J.M. *Curr. Pharm. Biotech.* 7: 125; 2006.
5. Bianda, T., Hussain, M.A., Glatz, Y. et al. *J. Intern. Med.* 241: 143; 1997.
6. Bianda, T., Glatz, Y., Bouillon, R. et al. *J. Clin. Endocrinol. Metab.* 83: 81; 1998.
7. Mohan, S., Baylink, D.J. *J. Endocrinol.* 185: 415; 2005.
8. Kasukawa, Y., Baylink, D., Wergehal, J.E. et al. *Endocrinol.* 144: 4682; 2003.
9. Breen, M.E., Laing, E.M., Hall, D.B. et al. *J. Clin. Endocrinol. Metab.* 96: 1; 2010.
10. Lewis, R.D., Modlesky, C.M. *Intl. J. Sport Nutr.* 8: 250; 1998.
11. Abrams, S.A. *Horm. Res.* 60: 71S; 2003.
12. Mundy, G.R. *Am. J. Clin. Nutr.* 83: 427S; 2006
13. Bullo, M., Moreno-Navarrete, J.M., Fernandez-Beal, J.M., Salas-Salvado, J. *Am J. Clin. Nutr.* 95: 249; 2012.
14. Cashman, K.D. *Nutr. Rev.* 63: 2284; 2005.
15. Tsugawa, N., Shiraki, M., Suhara, Y. et al. *Am. J. Clin. Nutr.* 83: 380; 2006.
16. Bronner, F. *Am. J. Physiol.* 246: R680; 1984.
17. Bronner, F., Peterlik, M. (Eds.) *Proc. Int. Conf. Prog Bone Min. Res. J. Nutr.* 125: 1963S; 1995.
18. Duflos, C., Bellaton, C., Baghdassarian, N. et al. *J. Nutr.* 126: 834; 1996.
19. Garlid, K.D. *J. Bioenerg. Biomembr.* 26: 537; 1994.
20. Gunter, K.K., Gunter, T.E., *Am. J. Physiol.* 267: C313; 1994.
21. Foletti, D., Guerini, D., Carafoli, E. *FASEB J.* 9: 670; 1995.
22. Sneyd, J., Keizer, J., Sanderson, M.J. *FASEB J.* 9: 1463; 1995.
23. Vormann, J. *Mol. Aspects Med.* 24: 27; 2003.
24. Nieves, J.W. *Am. J. Clin. Nutr.* 81: 1232S; 2005.
25. Nielsen, F.H., Milne, D.B. *Eur. J. Clin. Nutr.* 58: 703; 2004.
26. Miller, K.K. *J. Womens Health* 12: 145; 2003.
27. Panda, D.K., Miao, D., Bolivar, I. et al. *J. Biol. Chem.* 279: 16754; 2004.
28. Wallach, S. *Magnesium and Trace Elements* Vol. 10, p. 281, 1992.
29. Martini, L.A. *Nutr. Rev.* 57: 227; 1999.
30. Maurer, J., Harris, M.M., Stanford, V.A. et al. *J. Nutr.* 135: 863; 2005.
31. Nordin, B.E., Need, A.G., Steurer, T.A., Morris, H.A., Chatterton, B.E., Horowitz, M. *Ann. N. Y. Acad. Sci.* 854: 336; 1998.
32. Lau, E.M., Woo, J. *Nutr. Osteopor. Curr. Opin. Rheumatol.* 10: 368; 1998.
33. Raisz, L.G. *J. Bone Min. Metab.* 17: 79; 1999.
34. Anderson, J.J., Rondano, P., Holmes, A. *Scand. J. Rheumatol.* 103: 65S; 1996.
35. Francis, R.M., Selby, P.L. *Osteomalacia Baillieres. Clin. Endocrinol. Metab.* 11: 145; 1997.
36. Bell, N.H., Key, Jr. L.L. Acquired Osteomalacia. *Curr. Ther. Endocrinol. Metab.* 6: 530; 1997.
37. Klein GL. *Nutrition* 14: 149; 1998.
38. Nightingale, J.M. *Nutrition* 15: 633; 1999.
39. Sakhaee, K., Gonzalez, G.B. *Am. J. Med. Sci.* 317: 251; 1999.
40. Kurokawa, K., Fukagawa, M. *Am. J. Med. Sci.* 317: 355; 1999.
41. Slatopolsky, E. *Nephrol. Dial. Transplant.* 13: 3S; 1998.
42. Delmas, P.D., Meunier, P.J. *N. Eng. J. Med.* 336: 558; 1997.

# 72 Drug Interactions with Nutrients and Natural Products

## Mechanisms and Clinical Importance

*David J. Greenblatt*

## CONTENTS

## INTRODUCTION

The clinical problem of prescription drug interactions with nutrients and natural products is now widely recognized. Initial attention to the problem began with the first report of a pharmacokinetic drug interaction involving grapefruit juice (GFJ) and the calcium channel antagonist agent, felodipine.[1] Since this time, hundreds of publications have appeared in the medical and scientific literature describing the mechanisms and consequences of pharmacokinetic interactions between GFJ and a number of prescription medications.[2–12] There has also been extensive coverage by the lay media, much of which is sensationalized and inaccurate.

Many of the research principles learned in the context of the "grapefruit juice affair" are more broadly applicable to other nutrients and natural substances. This review will focus on the physiological and biochemical mechanisms of such interactions, methodology used to assess these interactions, approaches to evaluating the clinical importance of these events, and potential sources of bias and misinterpretation.

## OVERVIEW OF DRUG–DRUG INTERACTIONS

A pharmacokinetic drug–drug interaction (DDI) is defined as a situation in which one administered drug (the "perpetrator") changes the clearance and plasma concentrations of another (the "substrate" or "victim").[13–16] With a *pharmacokinetic* DDI, the perpetrator may or may not alter the clinical effects of the victim. Whether an actual clinical change accompanies the DDI depends on whether the alteration in plasma concentrations of the substrate victim is sufficient to cause a change in the effects of the drug on the patient. Many statistically significant DDIs are also clinically unimportant, for reasons such as (a) the magnitude of the interaction (that is, the change in plasma levels of the victim drug) is not large enough to be detected clinically or (b) the therapeutic index of the victim drug is large—that is, a wide range of plasma concentrations produce the same clinical effect. DDIs are likely to be of concern in clinical practice if either the size of the interaction is large, or the therapeutic index of the victim is narrow.

**TABLE 72.1**

**Possible Consequences of Drug–Drug Interactions Involving Metabolic Inhibition or Induction**

| | Effect on Substrate Victim | | |
|---|---|---|---|
| Property of Perpetrator | Metabolic Clearance | Plasma Concentration | Possible Clinical Outcome |
| Metabolic inhibition | Decreased | Increased | Increased effectiveness, or toxicity |
| Metabolic induction | Increased | Decreased | Reduced efficacy, or loss of efficacy |

## INDUCTION VERSUS INHIBITION OF DRUG CLEARANCE

DDIs typically occur via the perpetrator's effect on the metabolic mechanisms mediating the clearance of the substrate victim (Table 72.1). With *metabolic inhibition*, the perpetrator inhibits the biotransformation of the victim,[17–21] resulting in higher plasma concentrations of the victim. This raises the possibility that therapeutic effects may be increased, or that toxicity may result. With *metabolic induction*, the perpetrator causes an increase in the clearance of the substrate victim, and plasma concentrations of the victim drug fall to lower levels.[16,20,21] The possible result is that the therapeutic effect of the substrate victim will be reduced, or it may become ineffective altogether.

Inhibition and induction are fundamentally different processes having different mechanisms, and do not simply represent the same biological process going in opposite directions. Inhibition represents a direct effect of an inhibitor on a metabolic enzyme. The inhibitory effect is of rapid onset, and is relatively rapidly reversed when the perpetrator drug is removed. Inhibition can be studied in vitro using mechanical homogenates of liver cells, and the inhibitory potency of a candidate inhibitor can be quantitated using metrics such as an inhibition constant ($K_i$) or a 50% inhibitory concentration ($IC_{50}$).[13–15] In contrast, the process of induction is a more complex phenomenon in which the perpetrator (the inducer) acts as a transcriptional activator via binding to cellular receptors. The result is an increased rate of synthesis of metabolic protein.[22–25] The sequence of transcriptional activation and increased protein synthesis requires several days or more to be complete, and is equally slowly reversed when the inducing agent is discontinued. In vitro study of metabolic induction requires cell cultures of intact hepatocytes such that protein synthetic mechanisms are intact. Unlike inhibition, there is no straightforward quantitative measure analogous to $K_i$ or $IC_{50}$ metric to represent a drug's potency as an inducer.

## DESIGN AND INTERPRETATION OF DRUG–DRUG INTERACTION STUDIES

Clinical DDI studies are now a regular component of the drug development process. The objective of DDI studies is to provide information on the therapeutic benefits and risks of drugs that may be co-administered in clinical practice. There is now reasonable consensus among the regulatory and academic communities as to how DDI studies should be designed and interpreted.[13–15,26–28] The same principles apply to the study of interactions involving drugs and nutrients or natural products.

The area under the plasma concentration curve (AUC) for the substrate victim drug is the principal outcome measure in DDI studies. In single-dose DDI studies, AUC represents the *total* area under the curve from time zero to infinity. If the victim is given in multiple doses such that steady state is attained, AUC is the *segmental* area over a dosing interval at steady state. The customary DDI study has a crossover design, in which AUC for the substrate victim is measured in the same subject on two different occasions: once in the control condition ($AUC_0$); and on a second occasion ($AUC_1$) during coadministration of the candidate perpetrator. For each study participant, an AUC ratio is calculated as follows:

$$AUC\,ratio = \frac{AUC_1}{AUC_0} \qquad (72.1)$$

The individual AUC ratios are then aggregated across the study participants. The most straightforward, transparent, and understandable approach is a calculation of the arithmetic mean and standard deviation of the individual ratios.[29] Statistical significance of the interaction is then easily tested using Student's *t*-test, comparing the arithmetic mean ratio to 1.0. FDA guidance on DDI studies mandates analysis of DDI study data as if it were a bioequivalence study—the geometric mean of individual AUC ratios is calculated, along with the 90% confidence interval (CI).[30] The geometric mean ratio always underestimates the actual arithmetic mean, but the two statistical methods generally yield the same "overall conclusion" about the drug interactions. Either way, an AUC ratio equal to 1.0 indicates no interaction, greater than 1.0 indicates inhibition, and less than 1.0 indicates induction.

## STATISTICAL VERSUS CLINICAL SIGNIFICANCE OF A DDI

A DDI involving metabolic inhibition is more likely to be clinically important if the AUC ratio is large. Regulatory guidelines identify "default" descriptors, consistent with this concept (Table 72.2), but interpretation of the outcome of a

**TABLE 72.2**

**Categorization of Inhibitory DDIs**

| AUC Ratio | Description of Inhibition |
|---|---|
| <1.25 | Negligible |
| ≥1.25 and <2.0 | Weak |
| ≥2.0 and <5.0 | Moderate |
| ≥5.0 | Strong |

DDI study—whether or not the aggregate AUC ratio is significantly different from 1.0—requires supplemental data on the exposure–response relationship for the substrate victim drug.

If a DDI study shows a mean AUC ratio of 1.5, the clinical importance of the interaction depends on the exposure–response properties of the victim. If the victim is administered warfarin, a ratio of 1.5 is very likely to be important, and the DDI would require either avoidance of the drug combination, or reduction in the daily dosage of warfarin. If the victim drug is penicillin, a ratio of 1.5 is unlikely to be important.

## DRUG INTERACTIONS DUE TO METABOLIC INHIBITION: THE GRAPEFRUIT JUICE EXAMPLE

### ROLE OF CYTOCHROME P450-3A (CYP3A)

CYP3A isoforms (referring to CYP3A4 and CYP3A5) are of major quantitative importance in human liver, and are partly or entirely responsible for the metabolic clearance of at least half of the drugs currently used in clinical practice.[18,19,31,32] CYP3A isoforms also are the *only* CYP enzymes present in clinically relevant quantities in enterocyte cells found in the mucosa of the proximal small bowel, which is the site of absorption of the majority of drugs. An orally administered medication that is a substrate for biotransformation by CYP3A is first exposed to CYP3A initially during absorption through small bowel mucosa, and then again during passage through the liver (Figure 72.1). Significant metabolism at either or both of these sites produces incomplete oral bioavailability due to *presystemic extraction* or *first-pass metabolism*.

### MECHANISM OF DRUG INTERACTIONS WITH GRAPEFRUIT JUICE

Interactions of GFJ with prescription medications are caused by inhibition of the activity of CYP3A located in enterocyte cells in the small bowel mucosa. The *furanocoumarins* are among numerous natural substances present in GFJ, and are established as the class of compounds responsible for CYP3A inhibition.[33–41] The most abundant of the furanocoumarins in GFJ is bergamottin, but bergamottin is a weak inhibitor and probably makes only a minor contribution to drug interactions. The most important inhibitor is 6′,7′-dihydroxybergamottin (DHB), which is a strong inhibitor of CYP3A. Also present in GFJ are a series of dimers, termed *spiroesters* or *Paradisins*, formed by linkage of DHB with itself, or DHB with bergamottin. These dimeric compounds are highly potent CYP3A inhibitors, and probably contribute to drug interactions with GFJ.

Usual exposure to GFJ (in the range of 8–12 oz/day of regular-strength GFJ) causes inhibition *only* of enteric CYP3A, without affecting hepatic CYP3A (Figure 72.1). The inhibition process is termed *mechanism-based* or *irreversible*,[41–45] and implies that GFJ does not need to be present in the gastrointestinal tract at the time the substrate victim is given in order to produce an interaction with the victim drug. Prior exposure to GFJ inhibits and inactivates the enzyme, and recovery of function occurs with the normal turnover and regeneration of CYP3A, requiring 48–72 h.[46–51]

### CLINICAL IMPORTANCE OF DRUG INTERACTIONS WITH GFJ

GFJ can be a drug interaction perpetrator only if three conditions are satisfied. First, the substrate drug must be biotransformed by CYP3A. GFJ does not interact with substrates metabolized by other CYP enzymes, such as warfarin[52] (CYP2C9) or theophylline[53] (CYP1A2). Second, the substrate drug must be given orally. Except with unrealistically high doses,[54] GFJ affects only enteric CYP3A enzymes. Hepatic CYP3A is not affected, and clearance of intravenously administered substrates is not impaired by GFJ.[55–59] Finally, the substrate must ordinarily undergo presystemic extraction by enteric CYP3A following oral dosage. Substrates metabolized by CYP3A, but with oral bioavailability close to 100%, are not affected by GFJ. Examples include alprazolam[60] and quinidine.[61] Some substrates (such as midazolam) are subject to first-pass metabolism by a combination of hepatic and enteric CYP3A,[62] in which case GFJ will impair only the enteric CYP3A.

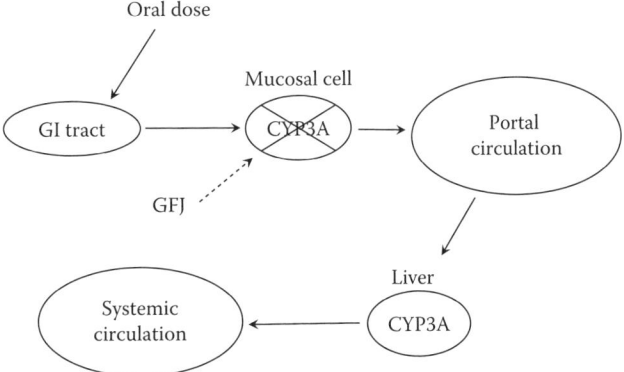

**FIGURE 72.1** Schematic diagram of the fate of an orally administered medication prior to reaching the systemic circulation. The drug undergoes contact with CYP3A enzymes at two different points in the cascade: initially as it passes from the GI tract through small bowel enterocytes to the portal circulation, and again as it passes through the liver. Furanocoumarins in GFJ affect the activity only of enteric CYP3A.

## TABLE 72.3
## Clinical Importance of Drug Interactions with Grapefruit Juice

**Clinically Important Interaction**

| Possible | Probable |
| --- | --- |
| Triazolam | Buspirone |
| Midazolam | Felodipine |
| Diazepam | Simvastatin |
| Nisoldipine | Sirolimus |
| Lovastatin | |
| Carbamazepine | |
| Cyclosporine | |

Given these three necessary conditions, it is not surprising that the number of clinically important drug interactions with GFJ is small (Table 72.3). Only for a few substrates has an interaction been documented such that dosage of the substrate drug may require adjustment in patients taking GFJ, or that GFJ should be avoided. Discussed below are data sources other than controlled pharmacokinetic studies that may be misleading, and yield incorrect conclusions about clinical drug interactions with GFJ.

### INTERACTIONS OF CYP3A SUBSTRATES WITH OTHER NUTRIENTS AND NATURAL SUBSTANCES

Many other juice beverages cause inhibition of CYP3A activity based on in vitro studies (Table 72.4). However, unlike GFJ, those other products do not cause irreversible inhibition of CYP3A, and clinical pharmacokinetic studies show no meaningful interaction with CYP3A substrate drugs in humans. This illustrates an important "disconnection" between in vitro results and clinical implications as applied to these widely consumed food products.[12]

### INHIBITORY INTERACTIONS WITH SUBSTRATES OF OTHER CYPS

Beyond CYP3A, CYP2C9 has received the most attention as a possible target for inhibitory drug interactions with

## TABLE 72.4
## Juice Beverage Products Reported to Produce Inhibition of CYP3A In Vitro

Cranberry
Pomegranate
Blueberry
Raspberry
Black mulberry
Grape
Star fruit
Pumelo
Lime

nutrients and natural products. Unlike CYP3A, CYP2C9 is not present in clinically significant amounts in gastrointestinal mucosal cells.

The anticoagulant agent warfarin is a racemic mixture, of which the S-enantiomer accounts for most of the pharmacologic activity. CYP2C9 is the principal enzyme mediating clearance of S-warfarin.[63] Inhibition of CYP2C9 activity is potentially of major clinical importance, since elevated plasma levels of S-warfarin can produce an excessive anticoagulant effect and a risk of hemorrhage. Many juice beverages—including grapefruit, cranberry, blueberry, grape, and pomegranate—inhibit CYP2C9 activity in vitro, and several isolated, unvalidated case reports suggested potentiation of warfarin anticoagulation by coadministration of cranberry or pomegranate juice.[64,65] However, in no case has a controlled study demonstrated a clinically meaningful inhibition of clearance of warfarin (or any other CYP2C9 substrates) in humans.[65-67] This further exemplifies the in vitro–in vivo "disconnection" as applied to drug interactions with nutrients and natural products.[3,12]

## DRUG INTERACTIONS DUE TO METABOLIC INDUCTION

Induction of drug metabolism by nutrients or natural products is unusual. One clinically important example is St. John's Wort (SJW), an herbal preparation believed to have antidepressant properties.[68] Extended exposure to usual clinical doses of SJW can induce the metabolic activity of CYP3A, CYP2C9, and a number of other metabolic enzymes.[69] As a result, the clearance of substrate drugs metabolized by these CYPs will increase, plasma levels will fall, and therapeutic effectiveness may diminish. The following are examples of clinical events attributed to induction of drug metabolism by SJW: breakthrough bleeding or pregnancy in women taking oral contraceptives; organ rejection in patients taking immunosuppressive agents; recurrence of active HIV infection in patients taking antiretroviral drugs; reduced lipid-lowering efficacy of the statin drug simvastatin.

## LOOKING CRITICALLY AT SOURCES OF DATA

Controlled pharmacokinetic studies in humans represent the only source of biomedical "truth" with respect to prescription drug interactions with nutrients and natural products. However, other data sources are available in the literature. These other sources cannot be assumed to represent biomedical truth, even though such assumptions may be invited or encouraged by the authors, and actually be accepted as truth in some secondary and tertiary sources, and by the lay media.

### SINGLE CASE REPORTS

Case reports describe anecdotal events occurring in individual patients. A typical case report (*hypothetical only*) might go as follows: A patient with atrial fibrillation has been taking warfarin for a period of 6 months, with "stable" anticoagulation (INR in the range of 1.8–3.2). The patient then starts drinking cranberry juice, 8 oz daily with breakfast. Two weeks after starting cranberry juice, the patient develops multiple spontaneous bruises, and the INR is 5.7. The authors of the report speculate that an interaction of cranberry juice with warfarin caused an elevation of plasma S-warfarin concentrations to excessive levels (though the concentrations were not actually measured), thereby explaining the patient's bruising.

The scientific community generally recognizes that anecdotal case reports do not constitute scientific evidence of cause-and-effect.[70–72] Such reports may represent a "signal" of an association that deserves further investigation via controlled studies, but do not by themselves prove causality. This hypothetical report is inconclusive because many warfarin-treated patients who are not drinking cranberry juice spontaneously go "out of control"—with high INR values and evidence of coagulation defects—for no apparent reason. The temporal association with cranberry juice exposure may well have been coincidental. Furthermore, plasma levels of S-warfarin prior to and during cranberry juice exposure were not available.

### Studies in Experimental Animals

The results of DDI studies done in experimental animals are sometimes interpreted as predictive of what will happen with coadministration of the same combination in humans. This kind of extrapolation is not appropriate—there is no known animal model that allows valid prediction of DDIs in humans.

The usual experimental model involves rats or other rodent species. The predictive limitations of the rat model include the following[73–76]: (a) The dosage of the perpetrator in question (on a weight-normalized basis) generally is much higher than the typical human exposure; (b) CYP enzymes in rats are different from the CYP enzymes in humans; (c) the substrate victim drug may or not be metabolized to the same extent by rat CYP isoforms compared to those present in humans; and (d) in the case of CYP3A, the relative distributions of enteric and hepatic CYP3A differs between rats and humans, as does the role of enteric CYP3A in presystemic extraction.

The conclusion is that no assumptions can be made regarding clinical drug interactions involving nutrients and natural products on the basis of experimental animal studies.

### Secondary and Tertiary Sources

All secondary and tertiary sources—including the present review—involve a "filtration" or interpretation of primary research data by the authors or compilers of the document. The tone or "slant" of the interpretation will depend on the training, experience, and biases of the document author(s). Different secondary/tertiary sources may interpret the same primary data differently. Health-care professionals may understandably not have the opportunity to evaluate primary research data themselves, and may come to rely on secondary

or tertiary sources for information on potential drug interactions, but the filtration process should be kept in mind, and a return to the primary data may sometimes be needed to resolve conflicting or uncertain information.

### COMMENTS

Biomedical research on the topic of drug interactions with nutrients and natural products should have the objective of protecting and improving public health. Health-care professionals and patients should be informed of a *realistic* risk of an undesired outcome from combining a prescription drug with a specific natural product so that appropriate modifications and precautions can be taken. However, if there is *not* a realistic risk, warnings do *not* advance public health. Unnecessary alarm may create concern and anxiety, impair compliance with needed pharmacologic treatment plans, and deter consumption of a nutrient that may have health benefits or otherwise enhance quality of life. Health-care professionals should put biases aside and look for the proper balance of caution.

### ACKNOWLEDGMENT

The author is a consultant to the Florida Department of Citrus, Lakeland, FL.

### REFERENCES

1. Bailey DG, Spence JD, Edgar B et al. *Clin. Invest. Med.* 12: 357; 1989.
2. Seden K, Dickinson L, Khoo S, and Back D. *Drugs* 70: 2373; 2010.
3. Hanley MJ, Cancalon P, Widmer WW, and Greenblatt DJ. *Expert Opin. Drug Metab. Toxicol.* 7: 267; 2011.
4. Bailey DG, Arnold JMO, and Spence JD. *Br. J. Clin. Pharmacol.* 46: 101; 1998.
5. Fuhr U. *Drug Saf.* 18: 251; 1998.
6. Greenblatt DJ. *Pharmacy Times* 76: 95; January 2010.
7. Greenblatt DJ, Patki KC, von Moltke LL, and Shader RI. *J. Clin. Psychopharmacol.* 21: 357; 2001.
8. Won CS, Oberlies NH, and Paine ME. *Curr. Drug Metab.* 11: 778; 2010.
9. Bailey DG and Dresser GK. *Am. J. Cardiovasc. Drugs* 4: 281; 2004.
10. Mertens-Talcott SU, Zadezensky I, De Castro WV et al. *J. Clin. Pharmacol.* 46: 1390; 2006.
11. Paine MF and Oberlies NH. *Expert Opin. Drug Metab. Toxicol.* 3: 67; 2007.
12. Farkas D and Greenblatt DJ. *Expert Opin. Drug Metab. Toxicol.* 4: 381; 2008.
13. Greenblatt DJ and von Moltke LL. In: *Enzyme and Transporter-Based Drug-Drug Interaction: Progress and Future Challenges.* K. S. Pang, A. D. Rodrigues, and R. M. Peter (eds.), New York: Springer. p. 625; 2010.
14. Farkas D, Shader RI, von Moltke LL, and Greenblatt DJ. In: *Preclinical Development Handbook: ADME and Biopharmaceutical Properties.* S. C. Gad (ed.), Philadelphia, PA: Wiley-Interscience. p. 879; 2008.
15. Greenblatt DJ. In: *Drug Interactions in Infectious Diseases,* 3rd edn. S. C. Piscitelli, K. A. Rodvold, and M. P. Pai (eds.), New York: Humana Press, p. 1; 2011.

16. Lin JH. *Pharm. Res.* 23: 1089; 2006.
17. Venkatakrishnan K, von Moltke LL, and Greenblatt DJ. *Clin. Pharmacokinet.* 38: 111; 2000.
18. Venkatakrishnan K, von Moltke LL, and Greenblatt DJ. *J. Clin. Pharmacol.* 41: 1149; 2001.
19. Venkatakrishnan K, von Moltke LL, Obach RS, and Greenblatt DJ. *Curr. Drug Metab.* 4: 423; 2003.
20. Pelkonen O, Turpeinen M, Hakkola J et al. *Arch. Toxicol.* 82: 667; 2008.
21. Zhou SF, Xue CC, Yu XQ et al. *Ther. Drug Monit.* 29: 687; 2007.
22. Wang H and LeCluyse EL. *Clin. Pharmacokinet.* 42: 1331; 2003.
23. Willson TM and Kliewer SA. *Nat. Rev. Drug Discov.* 1: 259; 2002.
24. Urquhart BL, Tirana RG, and Kim RB. *J. Clin. Pharmacol.* 47: 566; 2007.
25. Goodwin B, Redinbo MR, and Kliewer SA. *Ann. Rev. Pharmacol. Toxicol.* 42: 1; 2002.
26. Huang SM, Strong JM, Zhang L et al. *J. Clin. Pharmacol.* 48: 662; 2008.
27. Zhang L, Reynolds KS, Zhao P, and Huang SM. *Toxicol. Appl. Pharmacol.* 243: 134; 2010.
28. Huang SM, Temple R, Throckmorton DC, and Lesko LJ. *Clin. Pharmacol. Ther.* 81: 298; 2007.
29. Greenblatt DJ. *J. Clin. Psychopharmacol.* 28: 369; 2008.
30. Steinijans VW, Hartmann M, Huber R, and Radtke HW. *Int. J. Clin. Pharmacol. Ther. Toxicol.* 29: 323; 1991.
31. Greenblatt DJ, He P, von Moltke LL, and Court MH. In: *Cytochrome P450: Role in the Metabolism and Toxicology of Drugs and Other Xenobiotics.* C. Ioannides (ed.), Cambridge, U.K.: Royal Society of Chemistry. p. 354; 2008.
32. Guengerich FP. *Ann. Rev. Pharmacol. Toxicol.* 39: 1; 1999.
33. Kakar SM, Paine MF, Stewart PW, and Watkins PB. *Clin. Pharmacol. Ther.* 75: 569; 2004.
34. Paine MF, Widmer WW, Hart HL et al. *Am. J. Clin. Nutr.* 83: 1097; 2006.
35. Edwards DJ, Bellevue FH, 3rd, and Woster PM. *Drug Metab. Dispos.* 24: 1287; 1996.
36. Fukuda K, Ohta T, Oshima Y et al. *Pharmacogenetics* 7: 391; 1997.
37. Schmiedlin-Ren P, Edwards DJ, Fitzsimmons ME et al. *Drug Metab. Dispos.* 25: 1228; 1997.
38. Guo LQ, Fukuda K, Ohta T, and Yamazoe Y. *Drug Metab. Dispos.* 28: 766; 2000.
39. Cancalon P, Barros SM, Haun C, and Widmer WW. *J. Food Sci.* 76: C543; 2011.
40. Girennavar B, Poulose SM, Jayaprakasha GK et al. *Bioorg. Med. Chem.* 14: 2606; 2006.
41. Greenblatt DJ, Zhao Y, Hanley MJ et al. *Xenobiotica* 42: 1163; 2012.
42. Zhou S, Chan E, Lim LY et al. *Curr. Drug Metab.* 5: 415; 2004.
43. Fontana E, Dansette PM, and Poli SM. *Curr. Drug Metab.* 6: 413; 2005.
44. Zhou S, Yung Chan S, Cher Goh B et al. *Clin. Pharmacokinet.* 44: 279; 2005.
45. Silverman R. *Methods Enzymol.* 249: 240; 1995.
46. Greenblatt DJ, von Moltke LL, Harmatz JS et al. *Clin. Pharmacol. Ther.* 74: 121; 2003.
47. Culm-Merdek KE, von Moltke LL, Gan L et al. *Clin. Pharm. Ther.* 79: 243; 2006.
48. Takanaga H, Ohnishi A, Murakami H et al. *Clin. Pharm. Ther.* 67: 201; 2000.
49. Lundahl J, Regardh CG, Edgar B, and Johnsson G. *Eur. J. Clin. Pharmacol.* 49: 61; 1995.
50. Lilja JJ, Kivistö KT, and Neuvonen PJ. *Clin. Pharmacol. Ther.* 68: 384; 2000.
51. Takanaga H, Ohnishi A, Matsuo H et al. *Br. J. Clin. Pharmacol.* 49: 49; 2000.
52. Sullivan DM, Ford MA, and Boyden TW. *Am. J. Health Syst. Pharm.* 55: 1581; 1998.
53. Fuhr U, Maier A, Keller A et al. *Int. J. Clin. Pharmacol. Ther.* 33: 311; 1995.
54. Lilja JJ, Kivistö KT, Backman JT, and Neuvonen PJ. *Eur. J. Clin. Pharmacol.* 56: 411; 2000.
55. Rashid TJ, Martin U, Clarke H et al. *Br. J. Clin. Pharmacol.* 40: 51; 1995.
56. Uno T, Ohkubo T, Sugawara K et al. *Eur. J. Clin. Pharmacol.* 56: 643; 2000.
57. Ducharme MP, Warbasse LH, and Edwards DJ. *Clin. Pharmacol. Ther.* 57: 485; 1995.
58. Kupferschmidt HHT, Ha HR, Ziegler WH et al. *Clin. Pharmacol. Ther.* 58: 20; 1995.
59. Lundahl J, Regardh CG, Edgar B, and Johnsson G. *Eur. J. Clin. Pharmacol.* 52: 139; 1997.
60. Yasui N, Kondo T, Furukori H et al. *Psychopharmacology* 150: 185; 2000.
61. Min DI, Ku YM, Geraets DR, and Lee H. *J. Clin. Pharmacol.* 36: 469; 1996.
62. Tsunoda SM, Velez RL, von Moltke LL, and Greenblatt DJ. *Clin. Pharmacol. Ther.* 66: 461; 1999.
63. Kaminsky LS and Zhang Z-Y. *Pharmacol. Ther.* 73: 67; 1997.
64. Aston JL, Lodolce AE, and Shapiro NL. *Pharmacotherapy* 26: 1314; 2006.
65. Zikria J, Goldman R, and Ansell J. *Am. J. Med.* 123: 384; 2010.
66. Ngo N, Brantley SJ, Carrizosa DR et al. *J. Exp. Pharmacol.* 2010: 83; 2010.
67. Ansell J, McDonough M, Zhao Y et al. *J. Clin. Pharmacol.* 49: 824; 2009.
68. Linde K, Ramirez G, Mulrow CD et al. *Br. Med. J.* 313: 253; 1996.
69. Zhou S, Chan E, Pan SQ et al. *J. Psychopharmacol.* 18: 262; 2004.
70. Goldman SA. *Clin. Ther.* 20(Suppl C): C40; 1998.
71. Greenblatt DJ and von Moltke LL. *J. Clin. Pharmacol.* 45: 127; 2005.
72. Venning GR. *Br. Med. J.* (*Clin. Res. Ed.*) 284: 249; 1982.
73. Perloff MD, von Moltke LL, and Greenblatt DJ. *Xenobiotica* 34: 133; 2004.
74. Warrington JS, von Moltke LL, Shader RI, and Greenblatt DJ. *Drug Metab. Dispos.* 30: 655; 2002.
75. Warrington JS, Greenblatt DJ, and von Moltke LL. *Xenobiotica* 34: 463; 2004.
76. Kotegawa T, Laurijssens BE, von Moltke LL et al. *J. Pharmacol. Exp. Ther.* 302: 1228; 2002.

# 73 Drugs Used in the Treatment or Management of Human Diseases

*Carolyn D. Berdanier and Theodore Kyle*

## CONTENT

## INTRODUCTION

Chronic and acute diseases are often managed using both drugs and nondrug therapies. Pharmaceutical research has resulted in a wide array of drugs that are useful in helping the body return to its pre-disease state. For some conditions, there is a large selection of drugs to choose from, while for other conditions, the number of drugs available is very small. Some conditions have no pharmaceutical treatments. No drug is without risk. The physician prescribing the drug must weigh the risk of the drug against its possible benefit knowing that there are some diseases that are fatal if left without treatment and also knowing that some drugs have major side effects that can compromise an individual's well-being. The basic function of pharmaceuticals is to help the body repair or normalize itself. If it fails to do this, then the drug has no merit. If it harms the body with no benefit, then the drug not only has no merit but is contraindicated totally and should not be used. There are individual differences in drug tolerances. That is, there can be broad ranges of effectiveness from individual to individual. This can explain why an individual drug may be very effective in one person but not very effective in another. In addition, many drugs may be effective in the individual but may have deleterious effects on the unborn child if the individual taking the drug is pregnant.

Although antiviral drugs are antibiotics in the sense that they interfere with viral activity, the term antibiotic is usually used for that group of drugs that target pathogenic bacteria. A strict definition of the term antibiotic means that the compound in question is the product of one organism against another organism. The actinomycetes, for example, were found to produce streptomycin that attacked gram-negative bacteria. Other bacteria were found to produce penicillin that in turn destroyed gram-positive bacteria. Scientists have learned to modify the original penicillin structure such that new compounds have been made with different characteristics that in turn change the effectiveness of the drug against a wider variety of pathogenic bacteria. Other examples as well can be found and the compounds these organisms produce can be isolated, purified, studied, and, if effective, used to help people harboring their target bacteria. Antibiotics fall into eleven categories based on their structure, composition, and mechanism of action. These are listed in Table 73.1.

Antifungal drugs likewise are not included in the antibiotic drug group. They target pathogenic fungi and are usually man-made compounds that interfere with the metabolism and function of fungi.

Some conditions are not due to pathogenic organisms but are degenerative in nature. That is, they are due to malfunction of organs or metabolic processes that then result in abnormal bodily function. Failure of the $\beta$-cells of the pancreas to produce insulin is an example of this type of disease. When the $\beta$-cells fail, type 1 diabetes results. Type 2 diabetes on the other hand is due to a failure of the target tissues to respond to the hormone insulin. A number of drugs have been developed that assist the body to metabolize glucose and thus "normalize" glucose homeostasis (see Chapter 59). Hypertension and hyperlipemia are two other conditions that are associated with disease, namely, heart disease. Both of these conditions are amenable to pharmacologic management. Tables 73.2 and 73.3 list drugs that are helpful in managing human disease.[1–3] The drugs are grouped by their use. Table 73.2 lists the different drug classes used in nutrition-related disorders, whereas Table 73.3 is organized according to the ATC therapeutic drug class.[3] It provides the generic drug name, the brand name of that drug, and a definition and use for the drug. In this table, drugs are listed alphabetically by generic name within groups of drugs with similar functions. There may be a number of formulations for the same drug and the list may not give all these formulations. Likewise, some drugs have more brand names than there was space to list, so some of these brand names may not be listed. The user should look for the generic name rather than the brand name when seeking information about a given drug.

Hormones, although not strictly drugs, are listed because many have pharmaceutical activity in addition to their use as hormone replacements. For example, there are many formulations of glucocorticoid that are used as anti-inflammatory drugs. Some vitamins and some mineral compounds can be used as drugs, but they are not listed in this table. Similarly, some compounds, although used pharmaceutically, are not included because they are not considered drugs per se. An example of this is charcoal or activated charcoal that is sometimes administered to adsorb ingested noxious compounds or compounds

**TABLE 73.1**

**Categories of Antibiotics**

| Category | Example |
|---|---|
| Carbohydrate-containing compounds | Streptothricin, vancomycin, moenomycin nojirimycin, streptomycin, everninomicin |
| Macrocyclic lactones | Erythromycin, candicidin, rifampin |
| Quinones | Tetracycline, adriamycin, mitomycin |
| Amino acid and peptide analogues | Cycloserine, penicillin, bacitracin, actinomycin, valinomycin, bleomycin |
| Heterocyclic compounds containing nitrogen | Polyoxins |
| Heterocyclic compounds containing oxygen | Monensin |
| Alicyclic derivatives | Cycloheximide, fusidic acid |
| Aromatic compounds | Chloramphenicol, griseofulvin, novobiocin |
| Aliphatic compounds | Fostomycin |
| Quinolone compounds | Nalidixic acid, norfloxacin |
| Oxazolidinone | 2-Oxazolidinone |

produced by the body in the course of the breakdown of food in the gastrointestinal tract. An example of the former is the use of activated charcoal to adsorb a potentially noxious ingested chemical. The charcoal increases the excretion of that chemical before it can be absorbed into the body and harm it. An example of the latter is the use of activated charcoal to reduce the noxious gases produced and released (flatus) following the ingestion of dried beans and pulses. The undigested carbohydrates are acted on by the flora in the intestines and produce short-chain fatty acids as well as a variety of gases. These gases can be noxious.

Some drugs have multiple actions. They may serve as vasodilators and also as antiarrhythmic drugs; both actions are listed. Hormones, as mentioned, fall into this category. They may be hormone replacements and antineoplastic or they may be hormone replacements and anti-inflammatory. Again, both functions are given in the table and the reader will find them under their first listed function.

Although every attempt has been made to include drugs in current use, some drugs may be listed that are no longer in use because the Food and Drug Administration believes they either are not useful or have too many adverse effects. Drug updates can be accessed on eDrugInfo.com. In addition, drugs that have entered the marketplace since this table was constructed may be missing.

## TABLE 73.2
## Drug Classes Used In Nutritionally Impacted Conditions

| Condition | Drug Classes | Examples |
|---|---|---|
| Alcoholism | NO7BB: drugs used in alcohol dependence | Naltrexone, acamprosate |
| | N05C: hypnotics and sedatives | |
| Cancer prevention | G03X: other sex hormones and modulators of the genital system | |
| | G04C: drugs used in benign prostatic hypertrophy | |
| | L02BA: antiestrogens | Tamoxifen |
| | J07BM: papillomavirus vaccines | Gardasil, Cervarix |
| Cancer treatments | L: antineoplastic and immunomodulating agents | |
| | A04: antiemetics and antinauseants | Aprepitant, palonosetron |
| | A07: antidiarrheals, intestinal anti-inflammatory/anti-infective agents | Prednisone |
| | D06: antibiotics and chemotherapeutics for dermatological use | Imiquimod |
| | M05: drugs for treatment of bone diseases | Denosumab, zoledronic acid |
| | V03: all other therapeutic products | Dexrazoxane, leucovorin calcium, rasburicase |
| | V10: therapeutic radiopharmaceuticals | Ibritumomab tiuxetan, tositumomab/iodine I 131 tositumomab |
| Cardiovascular disease | B01: antithrombotic agents | |
| | C01: cardiac therapy | |
| | C03: diuretics | |
| | C07: beta-blocking agents | |
| | C08: calcium channel blockers | |
| | C09: agents acting on the renin–angiotensin system | |
| | C10: lipid-modifying agents | |
| Cataracts | S01A: anti-infectives | Phenylephrine, homatropine |
| | S01F: mydriatics and cycloplegics | |
| Cholesterol control | C10: lipid-modifying agents | |
| Dental disorders | A01AB: anti-infectives and antiseptics for local oral treatment | |
| | J01: antibacterials for systemic use | Amoxicillin, erythromycin, clindamycin |
| | M01A: anti-inflammatory and antirheumatic products, nonsteroidals | Ibuprofen |
| Dermatology | D: dermatologicals | |
| | G01A: anti-infectives and antiseptics, excl. combinations with corticosteroids | |
| | G03A: hormonal contraceptives for systemic use | |
| | J01: antibacterials for systemic use | |
| | J02: antimycotics for systemic use | Diclofenac |
| | J05: antivirals for systemic use | |
| | L01: antineoplastic agents | Methotrexate, fluorouracil, methyl aminolevulinate, aminolevulinic acid |
| | L04A: immunosuppressants | |
| | M03: muscle relaxants | Botulinum toxin |
| | R06: antihistamines for systemic use | |
| Diabetes | A10: drugs used in diabetes | |
| Eating disorders | A04: antiemetics and antinauseants | |
| | N03: antiepileptics | Topiramate |
| | N05: psycholeptics | |
| | N06A: antidepressants | |
| | N06B: psychostimulants, agents used for ADHD and nootropics | |
| | NO7BB: drugs used in alcohol dependence | Naltrexone |
| | R06: antihistamines for systemic use | Cyproheptadine |

(*continued*)

**TABLE 73.2 (continued)**
**Drug Classes Used in Nutritionally Impacted Conditions**

| Condition | Drug Classes | Examples |
|---|---|---|
| Food allergies | A07: antidiarrheals, intestinal anti-inflammatory/anti-infective agents | Cromoglicic acid |
| | A11: vitamins | Vitamin C |
| | C01: cardiac therapy | Epinephrine |
| | H02: corticosteroids for systemic use | |
| | R03: drugs for obstructive airway diseases | Theophylline, zafirlukast, montelukast |
| | R06: antihistamines for systemic use | Diphenhydramine |
| Fatty liver | A05: bile and liver therapy | Ursodiol |
| | A10: drugs used in diabetes | Pioglitazone, rosiglitazone |
| | C10: lipid-modifying agents | Atorvastatin, gemfibrozil, ezetimibe |
| | N06B: psychostimulants, agents used for ADHD and nootropics | Methamphetamine |
| Food addiction and binge eating | A08: antiobesity preparations, excl. diet products | |
| | N03: antiepileptics | Topiramate |
| | N06A: antidepressants | |
| Glaucoma | S01E: antiglaucoma preparations and miotics | |
| Hypertension | C02: antihypertensives | |
| | C03: diuretics | |
| | C07: beta-blocking agents | |
| | C08: calcium channel blockers | |
| | C09: agents acting on the renin–angiotensin system | |
| Macular degeneration | A11: vitamins | Ascorbic acid, beta-carotene, tocopherol |
| | A12: mineral supplements | Cupric oxide, zinc |
| | L01: antineoplastic agents | Bevacizumab |
| | S01L: ocular vascular disorder agents | |
| Metabolic syndrome | Medications for hypertension | |
| | Medications for cardiovascular disease | |
| | Medications for cholesterol control | |
| | Medications for diabetes | |
| Overweight and obesity | A08: antiobesity preparations, excl. diet products | Orlistat, phentermine |
| | A10: drugs used in diabetes | Metformin |
| | N03: antiepileptics | Topiramate, zonisamide |
| | N06A: antidepressants | |
| Renal failure | Medications for hypertension | |
| | A11: vitamins | Calcitriol |
| | B03: antianemic preparations | |
| | V03AE: drugs for treatment of hyperkalemia and hyperphosphatemia | |

*Source:*   ATC/DDD Index 2012 at www.whocc.no/ATC_ddd_index/ (accessed April 27, 2012).

## TABLE 73.3
## Drugs Used to Treat Medical Conditions

| Generic Name | Brand Name(s) | Description or Function |
|---|---|---|
| A: alimentary tract and metabolism | | |
| A01A: stomatological preparations | | |
| A01AB: anti-infectives and antiseptics for local oral treatment | | |
| Amphotericin B | Abelcet, AmBisome, Amphotec, Fungizone | Polyene antifungal |
| Chlorhexidine | Peridex, PerioGard | Antimicrobial |
| Doxycycline | | Tetracycline derivative |
| Miconazole | Oravig | Azole antifungal |
| Natamycin | | Tetraene polyene antifungal |
| Neomycin | | Aminoglycoside |
| Tetracycline | | Streptomyces-derived bacteriostatic agent |
| A04: antiemetics and antinauseants | | |
| Aprepitant | Emend | Substance P/neurokinin 1 receptor antagonist; for nausea and vomiting |
| Palonosetron | Aloxi | 5-HT$_3$ receptor antagonist |
| A05: bile and liver therapy | | |
| Ursodiol | Actigall, Urso | Bile acid |
| A07: antidiarrheals, intestinal anti-inflammatory/anti-infective agents | | |
| Prednisone | | Corticosteroid |
| A08: antiobesity preparations, excl. diet products | | |
| Benzphetamine | Didrex | Anorectic sympathomimetic amine |
| Diethylpropion | | Sympathomimetic amine |
| Phendimetrazine | Bontril, Adipost, Anorex-SR, Appecon, Melfiat, Obezine, Phendiet, Plegine, Prelu-2, Statobex | Anorectic sympathomimetic amine |
| Phentermine | Adipex-P | Anorectic sympathomimetic amine |
| Orlistat | Alli, Xenical | Lipase inhibitor |
| A10: drugs used in diabetes | | |
| Acarbose | Precose | Alpha-glucosidase inhibitor |
| Chlorpropamide | Diabinese | Sulfonylurea (first generation) |
| Exenatide | Byetta | Incretin mimetic |
| Glimepiride | Amaryl | Sulfonylurea (second generation) |
| Glipizide | Glucotrol | Sulfonylurea (second generation) |
| Glyburide | DiaBeta, Glynase, Micronase | Sulfonylurea (second generation) |
| Insulin aspart | NovoLog | Insulin |
| Insulin detemir | Levemir | Insulin |
| Insulin glargine | Lantus | Insulin |
| Insulin glulisine | Apidra | Insulin |
| Insulin human | Humulin, Novolin | Insulin |
| Insulin human NPH | Humulin, Novolin | Insulin |
| Insulin lispro | Humalog | Insulin |
| Metformin | Fortamet, Glucophage, Glumetza, Riomet | Biguanide |
| Miglitol | Glyset | Alpha-glucosidase inhibitor |
| Nateglinide | Starlix | Meglitinide |
| Pioglitazone | Actos | Thiazolidinedione |
| Pramlintide | Symlin | Synthetic amylin analogue |
| Repaglinide | Prandin | Meglitinide |
| Rosiglitazone | Avandia | Thiazolidinedione |
| Sitagliptin | Januvia | Dipeptidyl peptidase-4 inhibitor |
| Tolazamide | | Sulfonylurea (first generation) |
| Tolbutamide | | Sulfonylurea (first generation) |

*(continued)*

**TABLE 73.3 (continued)**
**Drugs Used to Treat Medical Conditions**

| Generic Name | Brand Name(s) | Description or Function |
|---|---|---|
| A11: vitamins | | |
| Ascorbic acid (vitamin C) | Various | Mast cell stabilizer |
| Beta-carotene | | |
| Calcitriol | Calcijex, Rocaltrol, Vectical | Vitamin D analogue |
| Tocopherol (vitamin E) | | |
| A12: mineral supplements | | |
| Cupric oxide | | |
| Zinc | | |
| B: blood and blood-forming organs | | |
| B01: antithrombotic agents | | |
| Abciximab | ReoPro | Glycoprotein IIb/IIIa inhibitor |
| ASA | Aspirin and others | Salicylate |
| Cilostazol | Pletal | Phosphodiesterase III inhibitor |
| Clopidogrel | Plavix | Platelet aggregation inhibitor |
| Dabigatran | Pradaxa | Thrombin inhibitor |
| Dipyridamole | Persantine | Vasodilator |
| Eptifibatide | Integrilin | Glycoprotein IIb/IIIa inhibitor |
| Prasugrel | Effient | Platelet aggregation inhibitor |
| Rivaroxaban | Xarelto | Specific factor Xa inhibitor |
| Tirofiban | Aggrastat | Glycoprotein IIb/IIIa inhibitor |
| Warfarin | Coumadin, Jantoven | Vitamin K-dependent coagulation factor inhibitor |
| B03: antianemic preparations | | |
| Epoetin alfa | Epogen, Procrit | Erythropoiesis stimulator |
| Iron | Bifera, Dexferrum, Elite Iron, Feosol, Fergon, Ferrex 150, Ferrlecit, Hemocyte, INFeD, Venofer | Iron supplement |
| C: cardiovascular system | | |
| C01:cardiac therapy | | |
| Amiodarone | Cordarone, Nexterone, Pacerone | Class III antiarrhythmic |
| Digoxin | Lanoxicaps, Lanoxin | Cardiac glycoside |
| Disopyramide | Norpace | Class I antiarrhythmic |
| Dobutamine | | Inotropic agent |
| Dofetilide | Tikosyn | Class III antiarrhythmic |
| Dopamine | | Inotropic agent |
| Dronedarone | Multaq | Class III antiarrhythmic |
| Epinephrine | Adrenaclick, EpiPen, Twinject | Alpha-adrenergic agonist, sympathomimetic catecholamine |
| Flecainide | Tambocor | Class IC antiarrhythmic |
| Isosorbide dinitrate | Dilatrate-SR, Sorbitrate, Isordil | Nitrate vasodilator |
| Isosorbide mononitrate | Monoket | Nitrate vasodilator |
| Mexiletine | Mexitil | Class IB antiarrhythmic |
| Milrinone | | Bipyridine inotropic/vasodilator |
| Nitroglycerin | | Nitrate vasodilator |
| Norepinephrine | Levophed | Alpha-adrenergic agonist |
| Propafenone | Rythmol | Class IC antiarrhythmic |
| Quinidine | Quinaglute, Quinidex | Class IA antiarrhythmic/schizonticide antimalarial |
| C02: antihypertensives | | |
| Ambrisentan | Letairis | Endothelin receptor antagonist |
| Bosentan | Tracleer | Endothelin receptor antagonist |
| Clonidine | Catapres, Duraclon, Jenloga, Kapvay, Nexiclon | Alpha$_2$-agonist |
| Diazoxide | Proglycem | Nondiuretic benzothiadiazine |
| Doxazosin | Cardura | Alpha$_1$-blocker (quinazoline) |
| Guanfacine | Intuniv | Alpha$_2$-agonist |

**TABLE 73.3 (continued)**
**Drugs Used to Treat Medical Conditions**

| Generic Name | Brand Name(s) | Description or Function |
|---|---|---|
| Hydralazine | | Vasodilator |
| Methyldopa | | Alpha-adrenergic agonist |
| Minoxidil | Rogaine | Peripheral vasodilator |
| Prazosin | Minipress | Alpha$_1$-blocker (quinazoline) |
| Reserpine | | Rauwolfia alkaloid |
| **C03: diuretics** | | |
| Amiloride | Midamor | K$^+$-sparing diuretic |
| Bendroflumethiazide | Corzide | Thiazide diuretic |
| Bumetanide | Bumex | Loop diuretic |
| Chlorothiazide | Diuril | Thiazide diuretic |
| Chlorthalidone | Hygroton, Thalitone | Monosulfamyl diuretic |
| Ethacrynic acid | Edecrin | Aryloxyacetic acid derivative |
| Furosemide | Lasix, Myrosemide | Loop diuretic |
| Hydrochlorothiazide | Microzide, Oretic, Esidrix, Hydro-chlor, Hydro-D, HydroDIURIL | Thiazide diuretic |
| Methyclothiazide | Aquatensen, Enduron | Thiazide diuretic |
| Metolazone | Diulo, Mykrox, Zaroxolyn | Quinazoline diuretic |
| Spironolactone | Aldactone | Aldosterone blocker |
| Torsemide | Demadex | Loop diuretic |
| Triamterene | Dyrenium | K$^+$-sparing diuretic |
| **C07: beta-blocking agents** | | |
| Acebutolol | Sectral | Selective beta$_1$-blocker |
| Atenolol | Tenormin | Selective beta$_1$-blocker |
| Betaxolol | Kerlone | Selective beta$_1$-blocker |
| Bisoprolol | Zebeta | Selective beta$_1$-blocker |
| Carteolol | Cartrol | Nonselective beta-blocker |
| Carvedilol | Coreg | Alpha$_1$-/beta-blocker |
| Esmolol | Brevibloc | Selective beta$_1$-blocker |
| Labetalol | Normodyne, Trandate | Nonselective beta-blocker/alpha$_1$- blocker |
| Metoprolol | Lopressor, Toprol | Selective beta$_1$-blocker |
| Nadolol | Corgard | Nonselective beta-blocker |
| Nebivolol | Bystolic | Selective beta$_1$-blocker |
| Penbutolol | Levatol | Nonselective beta-blocker |
| Pindolol | Visken | Nonselective beta-blocker |
| Propranolol | Inderal, InnoPran | Nonselective beta-blocker |
| Sotalol | Betapace | Beta-blocker (group II/III antiarrhythmic) |
| Timolol | Blocadren | Nonselective beta-blocker |
| **C08: calcium channel blockers** | | |
| Amlodipine | Lotrel, Norvasc | Calcium channel blocker (dihydropyridine) |
| Diltiazem | Cardizem, Tiazac, Tiamate | Calcium channel blocker (nondihydropyridine) |
| Felodipine | Plendil | Calcium channel blocker (dihydropyridine) |
| Isradipine | DynaCirc | Calcium channel blocker (dihydropyridine) |
| Nicardipine | Cardene | Calcium channel blocker (dihydropyridine) |
| Nifedipine | Adalat, Afeditab, Nifedical, Procardia | Calcium channel blocker (dihydropyridine) |
| Nimodipine | Nimotop | Calcium channel blocker |
| Nisoldipine | Sular | Calcium channel blocker (dihydropyridine) |
| Verapamil | Calan, Covera, Isoptin, Verelan | Calcium channel blocker (nondihydropyridine) |
| **C09: agents acting on the renin–angiotensin system** | | |
| Benazepril | Lotensin | ACE inhibitor |
| Candesartan | Atacand | Angiotensin II receptor antagonist |
| Captopril | Captopril | ACE inhibitor |
| Enalapril | Vasotec, Vaseretic | ACE inhibitor |

(continued)

**TABLE 73.3 (continued)**
**Drugs Used to Treat Medical Conditions**

| Generic Name | Brand Name(s) | Description or Function |
|---|---|---|
| Eprosartan | Teveten | Angiotensin II receptor antagonist |
| Fosinopril | Monopril | ACE inhibitor |
| Irbesartan | Avapro | Angiotensin II receptor antagonist |
| Lisinopril | Prinivil, Prinzide, Zestoretic, Zestril | ACE inhibitor |
| Losartan | Cozaar | Angiotensin II receptor antagonist |
| Moexipril | Univasc | ACE inhibitor |
| Olmesartan | Benicar | Angiotensin II receptor antagonist |
| Perindopril | Aceon | ACE inhibitor |
| Quinapril | Accupril | ACE inhibitor |
| Ramipril | Altace | ACE inhibitor |
| Telmisartan | Micardis | Angiotensin II receptor antagonist |
| Trandolapril | Mavik | ACE inhibitor |
| Valsartan | Diovan | Angiotensin II receptor antagonist |
| **C10: lipid-modifying agents** | | |
| Atorvastatin | Lipitor | HMG-CoA reductase inhibitor |
| Colestipol | Colestid | Bile acid sequestrant |
| Cholestyramine | LoCholest, Prevalite, Questran | Bile acid sequestrant |
| Ezetimibe | Zetia | Cholesterol absorption inhibitor |
| Fenofibrate | Antara, Fenoglide, Lipofen, Lofibra, Tricor, Triglide | Fibric acid derivative |
| Fluvastatin | Lescol | HMG-CoA reductase inhibitor |
| Gemfibrozil | Lopid | Fibric acid derivative |
| Lovastatin | Mevacor | HMG-CoA reductase inhibitor |
| Nicotinic acid | Niacor, Nicolar | Nicotinic acid and derivatives |
| Pravastatin | Pravachol | HMG-CoA reductase inhibitor |
| Simvastatin | Zocor | HMG-CoA reductase inhibitor |
| **D: dermatologicals** | | |
| **D01: antifungals for dermatological use** | | |
| Ciclopirox | Loprox, Penlac | Broad-spectrum antifungal |
| Clotrimazole | Gyne-Lotrimin 3, Lotrimin | Azole antifungal |
| Ketoconazole | Extina, Nizoral, Xolegel | Azole antifungal |
| Miconazole | Lotrimin, Monistat, Oravig | Azole antifungal |
| Nystatin | Mycostatin, Nyamyc, Nystop | Polyene antifungal |
| Salicylic acid | Many | Keratolytic agent |
| Selenium sulfide | Various | Antiseborrheic/antifungal |
| Terbinafine | Lamisil | Allylamine antifungal |
| Tolnaftate | | Antifungal |
| Undecylenic acid | Gordochom | Antifungal |
| **D03: preparations for treatment of wounds and ulcers** | | |
| Hyaluronic acid | Restylane | Hyaluronic acid |
| **D04: antipruritics, incl. antihistamines, anesthetics, etc.** | | |
| Diphenhydramine | Benadryl | Antihistamine |
| Promethazine | | Antihistamine |
| **D05: antipsoriatics** | | |
| Acitretin | Soriatane | Retinoid, Oral |
| Acitretin | Soriatane | Retinoid |
| Calcipotriol | Dovonex, Sorilux, Taclonex | Vitamin $D_3$ derivative |
| Calcitriol | Vectical | Vitamin D analogue |
| Methoxsalen | Oxsoralen, 8-Mop | Psoralen |
| Tazarotene | Avage, Tazorac | Retinoid |

## TABLE 73.3 (continued)
## Drugs Used to Treat Medical Conditions

| Generic Name | Brand Name(s) | Description or Function |
|---|---|---|
| D06: antibiotics and chemotherapeutics for dermatological use | | |
| Acyclovir | Xerese, Zovirax | Nucleoside analogue |
| Bacitracin | Baciguent, Neosporin, Polysporin, others | Antibiotic |
| Docosanol | Abreva | Viral entry blocking agent |
| Gentamicin | | Aminoglycoside |
| Idoxuridine | Dendrid | Pyrimidine nucleoside analogue |
| Imiquimod | Aldara, Zyclara | Immune response modifier; used for cancer treatments |
| Metronidazole | Flagyl vaginal cream, MetroCream, MetroGel, MetroLotion, NidaGel, Noritate, Rosasol, Flagystatin | Nitroimidazole |
| Mupirocin | Bactroban | Bacterial protein synthesis inhibitor |
| Neomycin | Various combinations | Aminoglycoside |
| Podofilox | Condylox | Antimitotic |
| Silver sulfadiazine | Flamazine | Topical sulfonamide |
| D07: corticosteroids, dermatological preparations | | |
| Amcinonide | Cyclocort | Corticosteroid |
| Betamethasone | Diprolene, Celestone Soluspan | Corticosteroid |
| Clobetasol | Dermovate, Clobex | Corticosteroid |
| Clobetasone | Spectro eczema care | Corticosteroid |
| Desonide | Desocort, Verdeso | Corticosteroid |
| Desoximetasone | Topicort | Corticosteroid |
| Dexamethasone | Dexasone | Corticosteroid |
| Diflucortolone | Nerisone | Corticosteroid |
| Fluocinolone acetonide | Capex, Derma-smoothe/FS | Corticosteroid |
| Fluocinonide | Lidemol, Lidex | Corticosteroid |
| Halobetasol | Ultravate | Corticosteroid |
| Hydrocortisone | Claritin skin itch relief, Cortate, Cortef, Cortoderm, Emo-Cort, Prevex HC, Sarna HC, Cortef | Corticosteroid |
| Methylprednisolone | Medrol | Corticosteroid |
| Mometasone | Elocom | Corticosteroid |
| Prednicarbate | Dermatop | Corticosteroid |
| Prednisolone | Pediapred | Corticosteroid |
| Triamcinolone | Aristocort, Kenalog | Corticosteroid |
| D09: medicated dressings | | |
| Fusidic acid | Fucidin, Fucidin-H | Bacterial protein synthesis inhibitor |
| D10: antiacne preparations | | |
| Tretinoin | Atralin, Avita, Refissa, Renova, Retin-A | Retinoid |
| Adapalene | Differin | Naphthoic acid derivative (retinoid like), topical |
| Isotretinoin | Amnesteem, Claravis, Sotret | Retinoid |
| Benzoyl peroxide | Many | Antibacterial/keratolytic |
| Clindamycin | Clindasol, Clindets, Dalacin T, Dalacin vaginal cream, Benzaclin, Clindoxyl | Lincomycin derivative |
| Erythromycin | Erysol, Akne-Mycin, Benzamycin, E.E.S., Eryc, EryPed, PCE Dispertab, Stievamycin | Macrolide |
| Azelaic acid | Azelex, Finacea | Dicarboxylic acid antimicrobial |
| Dapsone | Aczone | Sulfone antibiotic |
| D11: other dermatological preparations | | |
| Alitretinoin | Panretin | Retinoid |
| Diclofenac | Cataflam, Cambia, Pennsaid, Solaraze, Voltaren, Zipsor | NSAID |

(continued)

**TABLE 73.3 (continued)**
**Drugs Used to Treat Medical Conditions**

| Generic Name | Brand Name(s) | Description or Function |
|---|---|---|
| Eflornithine | Vaniqa | Ornithine decarboxylase inhibitor |
| Finasteride | Propecia, Proscar | Type II 5 alpha-reductase inhibitor |
| Hydroquinone | Solaquin, Eldoquin, Eldopaque | Depigmentation agent |
| Mequinol | Solage | Depigmentation agent |
| Minoxidil | Rogaine | Peripheral vasodilator |
| Pimecrolimus | Elidel | Macrolactam ascomycin derivative |
| Tacrolimus | Protopic | Macrolide immunosuppressant |
| Zinc pyrithione | | Antifungal/antibacterial |

G: genitourinary system and sex hormones
G01: gynecological anti-infectives and antiseptics
G01A: anti-infectives and antiseptics, excl. combinations with corticosteroids

| | | |
|---|---|---|
| Ascorbic acid | Prevegyne | Vaginal acidifier |
| Butoconazole | Gynazole-1 | Azole antifungal |
| Terconazole | Terazol | Azole antifungal |

G03: sex hormones and modulators of the genital system
G03A: hormonal contraceptives for systemic use

| | | |
|---|---|---|
| Cyproterone and estrogen | Diane-35 | Estrogen/progestogen combination |
| Drospirenone and estrogen | Yasmin, Yaz, Syeda, Ocella | Estrogen/progestogen combination |
| Levonorgestrel and estrogen | Alesse | Estrogen/progestogen combination |
| Norgestimate and estrogen | Tri-Cyclen | Estrogen/progestogen combination |

G03X: other sex hormones and modulators of the genital system

| | | |
|---|---|---|
| Raloxifene | Evista | Breast cancer prevention |

GO4: urologicals
G04C: drugs used in benign prostatic hypertrophy

| | | |
|---|---|---|
| Dutasteride | Avodart | Prostate cancer prevention |
| Finasteride | Proscar | Prostate cancer prevention |

H: systemic hormonal preparations, excl. sex hormones and insulins
H02: corticosteroids for systemic use

| | | |
|---|---|---|
| Cortisone | | Corticosteroid |
| Prednisone | Winpred | Corticosteroid |

J: anti-infectives for systemic use
J01: antibacterials for systemic use

| | | |
|---|---|---|
| Amoxicillin | | |
| Azithromycin | Zithromax, Zmax | Macrolide |
| Cephalexin | Keflex | Cephalosporin |
| Clarithromycin | Biaxin | Macrolide |
| Clindamycin | Dalacin C | Lincomycin derivative |
| Cloxacillin | | Penicillin |
| Daptomycin | Cubicin | Cyclic lipopeptide |
| Demeclocycline | Declomycin | Tetracycline derivative |
| Doxycycline | Atridox, Doryx, Monodox, Oracea, Vibramycin, Vibra-Tabs | Tetracycline derivative |
| Erythromycin | | |
| Linezolid | Zyvox | Oxazolidinone class antibacterial |
| Minocycline | Arestin, Dynacin, Minocin, Solodyn | Tetracycline derivative |
| Moxifloxacin | Avelox, Moxeza, Vigamox | Fluoroquinolone |
| Polymyxin B | Various combinations | Antibiotic |
| Spiramycin | | Experimental macrolide |
| Sulfamethoxazole/trimethoprim | Septra, Bactrim | Sulfonamide/tetrahydrofolic acid inhibitor |
| Tetracycline | Sumycin | *Streptomyces*-derived bacteriostatic agent |
| Tigecycline | Tygacil | Glycylcycline |

**TABLE 73.3 (continued)**
**Drugs Used to Treat Medical Conditions**

| Generic Name | Brand Name(s) | Description or Function |
|---|---|---|
| J02: antimycotics for systemic use | | |
| Fluconazole | Diflucan | Azole antifungal |
| Itraconazole | Sporanox | Azole antifungal |
| Posaconazole | Noxafil | Azole antifungal |
| Voriconazole | Vfend | Azole antifungal |
| J05: antivirals for systemic use | | |
| Acyclovir | Xerese, Zovirax | Nucleoside analogue |
| Famciclovir | Famvir | Nucleoside analogue |
| Valacyclovir | Valtrex | Nucleoside analogue |
| J07: vaccines | | |
| J07B: viral vaccines | | |
| J07BM: papillomavirus vaccines | | |
| Recombinant human papillomavirus (HPV) quadrivalent vaccine | Gardasil | Vaccine |
| HPV bivalent vaccine | Ceravix | Vaccine |
| L: antineoplastic and immunomodulating agents | | |
| L01: antineoplastic agents | | |
| Alemtuzumab | Campath | Monoclonal antibody/CD52 blocker |
| Aminolevulinic acid | Levulan | Protoporphyrin precursor |
| Arsenic trioxide | Trisenox | DNA fragmentation agent |
| Asparaginase *Erwinia chrysanthemi* | Erwinaze, Elspar | Enzyme |
| Axitinib | Inlyta | Tyrosine kinase inhibitor |
| Azacitidine | Vidaza, Mylosar | Pyrimidine nucleoside analogue |
| Bendamustine hydrochloride | Treanda | Alkylating agent |
| Bevacizumab | Avastin | Vascular endothelial growth factor (VEGF) inhibitor |
| Bexarotene | Targretin | Retinoid |
| Bleomycin | Blenoxane | Cytotoxic glycopeptide antibiotic |
| Bortezomib | Velcade | Proteasome inhibitor |
| Brentuximab vedotin | Adcetris | Directed antibody–drug conjugate |
| Cabazitaxel | Jevtana | Antimicrotubule agent |
| Capecitabine | Xeloda | Fluoropyrimidine carbamate |
| Carboplatin | Paraplatin, Paraplat | Platinum coordination compound |
| Cetuximab | Erbitux | Epidermal growth factor receptor (EGFR) antagonist |
| Chlorambucil | Ambochlorin, Amboclorin, Leukeran, Linfolizin | Nitrogen mustard alkylating agent |
| Cisplatin | Platinol | Heavy-metal platinum complex |
| Clofarabine | Clofarex, Clolar | Antimetabolite |
| Crizotinib | Xalkori | Tyrosine kinase inhibitor |
| Cyclophosphamide | Clafen, Cytoxan, Neosar | Nitrogen mustard alkylating agent |
| Cytarabine | Cytosar, Tarabine, Depocyt, Depofoam | Antimetabolite |
| Dacarbazine | Dtic-Dome | Alkylating agent |
| Dasatinib | Sprycel | Kinase inhibitor |
| Daunorubicin | Cerubidine, Rubidomycin | Anthracycline |
| Decitabine | Dacogen | DNA methyltransferase inhibitor |
| Denileukin diftitox | Ontak | Fusion protein |
| Docetaxel | Taxotere | Antimicrotubule agent |
| Doxorubicin | Adriamycin, Doxil, Dox-SL, Evacet | Anthracycline |
| Epirubicin | Ellence | Anthracycline |
| Eribulin mesylate | Halaven | Antimicrotubule agent |
| Erlotinib | Tarceva | EGFR tyrosine kinase inhibitor |
| Etoposide | Etopophos, Toposar, VePesid | Podophyllotoxin derivative |

*(continued)*

**TABLE 73.3 (continued)**
## Drugs Used to Treat Medical Conditions

| Generic Name | Brand Name(s) | Description or Function |
| --- | --- | --- |
| Everolimus | Afinitor | Kinase inhibitor |
| Fludarabine | Fludara, Oforta | Antimetabolite |
| Fluorouracil | Adrucil, Efudex, Fluoroplex | Antimetabolite |
| Gefitinib | Iressa | EGFR inhibitor |
| Gemcitabine | Gemzar | Nucleoside analogue antimetabolite |
| Gemtuzumab ozogamicin | Mylotarg | CD33 monoclonal linked to cytotoxic agent |
| Ifosfamide | Cyfos, Ifex, Ifosfamide | Analogue of the nitrogen mustard cyclophosphamide |
| Imatinib | Gleevec | Protein-tyrosine kinase inhibitor |
| Ipilimumab | Yervoy | Monoclonal antibody |
| Irinotecan | Camptosar | Topoisomerase I inhibitor |
| Ixabepilone | Ixempra | Antimicrotubule agent |
| Lapatinib ditosylate | Tykerb | Kinase inhibitor |
| Lomustine | CeeNU | Nitrosourea alkylating agent |
| Mechlorethamine | Mustargen | Nitrogen mustard alkylating agent |
| Methotrexate | Abitrexate, Folex, Mexate | Dihydrofolic acid reductase inhibitor |
| Mitomycin C | Mitozytrex, Mutamycin | DNA synthesis inhibitor |
| Nelarabine | Arranon | Deoxyguanosine analogue |
| Nilotinib | Tasigna | Kinase inhibitor |
| Ofatumumab | Arzerra | Monoclonal antibody/CD20 blocker |
| Oxaliplatin | Eloxatin | Organoplatinum complex |
| Paclitaxel | Abraxane, Taxol | Antimicrotubule agent |
| Panitumumab | Vectibix | Monoclonal antibody/EGFR blocker |
| Pazopanib | Votrient | Tyrosine kinase inhibitor |
| Pegaspargase | Oncaspar | Protein synthesis inhibitor |
| Pemetrexed | Alimta | Antifolate |
| Pralatrexate | Folotyn | Dihydrofolic acid reductase inhibitor |
| Procarbazine | Matulane | Hydrazine derivative |
| Rituximab | Rituxan | Monoclonal antibody/CD20 blocker |
| Romidepsin | Istodax | Histone deacetylase inhibitor |
| Ruxolitinib | Jakafi | Kinase inhibitor |
| Sorafenib tosylate | Nexavar | Multikinase inhibitor |
| Sunitinib malate | Sutent | Multikinase inhibitor |
| Temozolomide | Methazolastone, Temodar | Alkylating agent (imidazotetrazine derivative) |
| Temsirolimus | Torisel | mTOR inhibitor |
| Topotecan | Hycamtin | Topoisomerase I inhibitor |
| Trastuzumab | Herceptin | Monoclonal antibody/HER2 blocker |
| Vandetanib | Caprelsa | Kinase inhibitor |
| Vemurafenib | Zelboraf | Kinase inhibitor |
| Vinblastine | Velban, Velsar | Vinca alkaloid |
| Vincristine | Vincasar | Vinca alkaloid |
| Vinorelbine tartrate | Navelbine | Vinca alkaloid |
| Vorinostat | Zolinza | Histone deacetylase inhibitor |
| L02: endocrine therapy | | |
| Abiraterone acetate | Zytiga | Nonsteroidal antiandrogen |
| Anastrozole | Arimidex | Nonsteroidal aromatase inhibitor |
| Degarelix | Firmagon | GnRH antagonist |
| Exemestane | Aromasin | Aromatase inactivator |
| Fulvestrant | Faslodex | Estrogen receptor antagonist |
| Letrozole | Femara | Nonsteroidal aromatase inhibitor |
| Leuprolide acetate | Lupron, Viadur | Synthetic gonadotropin-releasing hormone analogue |
| Toremifene | Fareston | Nonsteroidal triphenylethylene derivative |
| Vismodegib | Erivedge | Hedgehog signaling pathway targeting agent |

## TABLE 73.3 (continued)
## Drugs Used to Treat Medical Conditions

| Generic Name | Brand Name(s) | Description or Function |
| --- | --- | --- |
| L02B: hormone antagonists and related agents | | |
| L02BA: antiestrogens | | |
| Tamoxifen | Nolvadex, Istubal, Valodex | Breast cancer prevention; treatment of metastatic breast cancer |
| L03: immunostimulants | | |
| Aldesleukin | Proleukin | Biological response modifier |
| Filgrastim | Neupogen | Granulocyte colony-stimulating factor |
| Plerixafor | Mozobil | Hematopoietic stem cell mobilizer |
| Sipuleucel-T | Provenge | Immunomodulatory agent |
| L04: immunosuppressants | | |
| Lenalidomide | Revlimid | Thalidomide analogue |
| Thalidomide | Synovir, Thalomid | Immunomodulatory agent |
| L04A: immunosuppressants | | |
| Adalimumab | Humira | Monoclonal antibody/TNF-alpha receptor blocker |
| Alefacept | Amevive | Immunosuppressive agent |
| Azathioprine | Azasan, Imuran | Purine antagonist antimetabolite |
| Canakinumab | Ilaris | Monoclonal antibody/IL-1 beta |
| Cyclosporine | Gengraf, Neoral, Restasis, Sandimmune | Cyclic polypeptide immunosuppressant |
| Etanercept | Enbrel | TNF receptor blocker |
| Golimumab | Simponi | Monoclonal antibody/TNF-alpha receptor blocker |
| Infliximab | Remicade | Monoclonal antibody/TNF-alpha receptor blocker |
| Ustekinumab | Stelara | Monoclonal antibody |
| M: musculoskeletal system | | |
| M01A: anti-inflammatory and antirheumatic products, nonsteroidals | | |
| Ibuprofen | Advil, Motrin | NSAID |
| M03: muscle relaxants | | |
| Botulinum toxin | Myobloc, Botox, Dysport, Xeomin | Purified neurotoxin complex |
| M05: drugs for treatment of bone diseases | | |
| Denosumab | Prolia, Xgeva | $IgG_2$ monoclonal antibody; used in osteoporosis and bone mending in cancer |
| Zoledronic acid | Zometa | Bisphosphonate |
| N: nervous system drugs | | |
| N03: antiepileptics | | |
| Topiramate | Topamax | Sulfamate-substituted monosaccharide antiepileptic |
| Zonisamide | Zonegran | Sulfonamide anticonvulsant |
| N05: psycholeptics | | |
| Alprazolam | Niravam, Xanax | Benzodiazepine |
| Lithium carbonate | Lithobid | Antimanic agent |
| Olanzapine | Zyprexa | Thienobenzodiazepine |
| Pimozide | Orap | Diphenylbutylpiperidine |
| N05C: hypnotics and sedatives | | |
| Pentobarbital | Nembutal | Barbiturate; alcoholism |
| N06: psychoanaleptics | | |
| N06A: antidepressants | | |
| Desipramine | Norpramin | Tricyclic antidepressant |
| Imipramine | Tofranil | Tricyclic antidepressant |
| Clomipramine | Anafranil | Tricyclic antidepressant |
| Amitriptyline | | Tricyclic antidepressant |
| Fluoxetine | Prozac | Selective serotonin reuptake inhibitor |
| Citalopram | Celexa | Selective serotonin reuptake inhibitor |

*(continued)*

**TABLE 73.3 (continued)**
**Drugs Used to Treat Medical Conditions**

| Generic Name | Brand Name(s) | Description or Function |
|---|---|---|
| Paroxetine | Paxil, Pexeva | Selective serotonin reuptake inhibitor |
| Sertraline | Zoloft | Selective serotonin reuptake inhibitor |
| Fluvoxamine | Luvox | Selective serotonin reuptake inhibitor |
| Trazodone | Desyrel, Oleptro | Triazolopyridine derivative |
| Mirtazapine | Remeron | Piperazino-azepine |
| Bupropion | Aplenzin, Budeprion, Wellbutrin, Zyban | Aminoketone |
| Venlafaxine | Venlafaxine, Effexor | Serotonin and norepinephrine reuptake inhibitor |
| N06B: psychostimulants, agents used for ADHD and nootropics | | |
| Atomoxetine | Strattera | Selective norepinephrine reuptake inhibitor |
| Methamphetamine | Desoxyn | Sympathomimetic amine |
| N07: other nervous system drugs | | |
| N07B: drugs used in addictive disorders | | |
| N07BB: drugs used in alcohol dependence | | |
| Acamprosate | Campral | GABA analogue |
| Disulfiram | Antabuse | Alcohol oxidation inhibitor |
| Naltrexone | Vivitrol, ReVia | Opioid antagonist |
| P: antiparasitic products, insecticides, and repellents | | |
| P03: ectoparasiticides, incl. scabicides, insecticides, and repellents | | |
| Lindane | | Ectoparasiticide/ovicide |
| Permethrin | Nix, Kwellada-P | Pyrethroid pediculicide |
| R: respiratory system | | |
| R03: drugs for obstructive airway diseases | | |
| Montelukast | Singulair | Leukotriene receptor antagonist |
| Theophylline | Elixophyllin | Xanthine bronchodilator |
| Zafirlukast | Accolate | Leukotriene receptor antagonist |
| R06: antihistamines for systemic use | | |
| Azatadine | Optimine | Antihistamine |
| Cetirizine | Reactine | Antihistamine |
| Cyproheptadine | | Serotonin/histamine antagonist |
| Desloratadine | Aerius | Antihistamine |
| Diphenhydramine | Benadryl | Antihistamine |
| Fexofenadine | Allegra | Antihistamine |
| Loratadine | Claritin | Antihistamine |
| S: sensory organs | | |
| S01: ophthalmologicals | | |
| S01A: anti-infectives | | |
| Azithromycin | Azasite | Macrolide |
| Besifloxacin | Besivance | Fluoroquinolone |
| Ciprofloxacin | Ciloxan | Fluoroquinolone |
| Erythromycin | Ilotycin | Macrolide |
| Gatifloxacin | Zymaxid | Fluoroquinolone |
| Gentamicin | Gentak | Aminoglycoside |
| Levofloxacin | Iquix, Quixin | Fluoroquinolone |
| Moxifloxacin | Moxeza, Vigamox | Fluoroquinolone |
| Ofloxacin | Ocuflox | Fluoroquinolone |
| Sulfacetamide | Bleph-10 | Sulfonamide |
| Tobramycin | Tobrex | Aminoglycoside |
| S01E: antiglaucoma preparations and miotics | | |
| Acetazolamide | Diamox | Carbonic anhydrase inhibitor |
| Apraclonidine | Iopidine | |
| Betaxolol | Betoptic | Selective beta1-blocker |
| Bimatoprost | Lumigan | Prostaglandin analogue |

**TABLE 73.3 (continued)**
**Drugs Used to Treat Medical Conditions**

| Generic Name | Brand Name(s) | Description or Function |
|---|---|---|
| Brimonidine | Alphagan | Selective alpha$_2$-agonist |
| Brinzolamide | Azopt | Carbonic anhydrase inhibitor |
| Carteolol | Ocupress | Nonselective beta-blocker |
| Clonidine | Catapres | Alpha-adrenergic agonist |
| Dorzolamide | Trusopt | Carbonic anhydrase inhibitor |
| Latanoprost | Xalatan | Prostaglandin analogue |
| Levobunolol | Betagan | Nonselective beta-blocker |
| Metipranolol | OptiPranolol | Nonselective beta-blocker |
| Timolol | Betimol, Istalol, Timoptic | Nonselective beta-blocker |
| Travoprost | Travatan Z | Prostaglandin analogue |
| S01F: mydriatics and cycloplegics | | |
| Homatropine | Isopto | Anticholinergic |
| Phenylephrine | Mydfrin, Neo-Synephrine, AK-Dilate | $\alpha$1-adrenergic receptor agonist |
| S01L: ocular vascular disorder agents | | |
| Aflibercept | Eylea | VEGF inhibitor |
| Pegaptanib | Macugen | VEGF inhibitor |
| Ranibizumab | Lucentis | Monoclonal antibody/VEGF-A blocker |
| Verteporfin | Visudyne | Photosensitizing agent |
| V: various | | |
| V03: all other therapeutic products | | |
| Dexrazoxane | Totect, Zinecard | EDTA derivative; treatment for chemotherapy side effects |
| Leucovorin calcium/calcium folinate | Wellcovorin | Cytoprotective agent |
| Rasburicase | Elitek | Recombinant urate-oxidase enzyme; used to prevent high uric acid levels in cancer |
| V03AE: drugs for treatment of hyperkalemia and hyperphosphatemia | | |
| Calcium acetate | PhosLo, Phoslyra | Phosphate binder |
| Lanthanum carbonate | Fosrenol | Phosphate binder |
| Polystyrene sulfonate | Kayexalate, Kionex | Cation-exchange resin |
| Sevelamer | Renagel, Renvela | Phosphate binder |
| V10: therapeutic radiopharmaceuticals | | |
| Ibritumomab tiuxetan | Zevalin | Monoclonal antibody/CD20 blocker |
| Tositumomab/iodine I 131 tositumomab | Bexxar | Monoclonal antibody/CD20 blocker |

*Source:* Physicians Desk Reference 1992, Medical Economics Data, Montvale, NJ, 2563pp; Drugs 2004, Medical Pocket Reference, Lippincott, Williams & Wilkins, Philadelphia, PA, 184pp; ATC/DDD Index 2012 at www.whocc.no/ATC_ddd_index/ (accessed April 27, 2012).

*Note:* This table is organized according to ATC therapeutic drug classes.

## REFERENCES

1. Physicians Desk Reference 1992. Medical Economics Data. Montvale, NJ, 2563pp.

2. Drugs 2004 Medical Pocket Reference, Lippincott, Williams & Wilkins, Philadelphia, PA, 184pp.

3. ATC/DDD Index 2012 at www.whocc.no/ATC_ddd_index/ (accessed April 27, 2012).

# 74 Directory of Clinical Nutrition Websites

*Lynnette A. Berdanier*

The World Wide Web is an excellent resource for information about nutrition and its relation to health and disease. Unfortunately, some of the websites are not scientifically substantiated. Many of the websites are in fact advertisements for products that may or may not be of value in terms of health. There are some sites that promote the use of unproven herbal products. The reader should be aware of the potential for quackery. Listed in Table 74.1 are websites addressing clinical conditions for which nutrition can be useful. Some of these sites are written to address the layman's concerns, while others address the interests of physicians and scientists.

**TABLE 74.1**
**Nutrition-Related Web Resources**

Nutritional effects on chronic alcoholism

    http://www.britannica.com/EBchecked/topic/422916/nutritional-disease/247876/Alcohol—single article with links to related topics such as fetal alcohol syndrome, pancreatitis, and thiamine deficiency

    http://www.niaaa.nih.gov/—links to research and informational papers on many aspects of diet and alcohol consumption

Food allergies and food intolerance

    http://www.fda.gov/Food/—links to papers on allergies and intolerances

    https://www.facebook.com/AmericanAcademyofAllergyAsthmaandImmunology?sk=wall—good site for pubic/professional interaction. Must be on facebook and "like" AAAAI

    http://www.aaaai.org/conditions-and-treatments/allergies/food-allergies.aspx—good overview of food allergies in general with links to specific topics related to food allergies and intolerance

    http://www.nhs.uk/Conditions/food-allergy/—good overview of food allergies and intolerances. UK based

    http://www.niaid.nih.gov/pages/default.aspx?wt.ac=tn

        Home links to

            Bioinformatics        Translational research tools

            Biological materials

    http://www.nutrition.gov/nutrition-and-health-issues/food-allergies-and-intolerances—clearing house site with links to FDA, National Cancer Institute (NIH), and FDA, many connection to specific topics

    http://www.foodallergy.org/—slanted toward nonprofessionals

Nutrition and immune function

    http://www.ajcn.org/—this site is for researchers. Use the search button to look for immune function

Making a nutritional assessment (clinical)

    http://fnic.nal.usda.gov/dietary-guidance/dietary-assessment

        Links to

            Super tracker

            Nutrition analysis tool

            Several calorie trackers

            Fat screener

    http://apps.medsch.ucla.edu/nutrition/dietassess.htm—includes several assessment checklists

Metabolic syndrome (overweight and fatty liver)

    http://www.heart.org/HEARTORG/Conditions/More/MetabolicSyndrome/Metabolic-Syndrome_UCM_002080_SubHomePage.jsp—includes a risk assessment checker, good explanations associated with treatment and symptoms

    http://www.nhlbi.nih.gov/health/health-topics/topics/ms/—national heart lung and blood institute site with links to many areas associated with metabolic syndrome

    http://www.nlm.nih.gov/medlineplus/metabolicsyndrome.html—lots of links to associated topics and diseases; very complete site

Malnourished child

    http://kidshealth.org/

    http://www.bapen.org.uk/—definitions of malnutrition with a malnutrition "calculator" and tracking malnutrition; although based in the United Kingdom, may be of interest to dietetic professionals

Failure to thrive

    http://kidshealth.org/parent/growth/growth/failure_thrive.html#cat162

    http://www.ncbi.nlm.nih.gov/pubmedhealth/—healthcare workers

Definition of failure to thrive and possible causes along with links to assessment and treatment options

Pediatric nutrition

    http://www.eatright.org/—search pediatric nutrition

    http://www.bcm.edu/cnrc/

    http://www.nutritionexplorations.org/

Information about supporting normal growth and development

Childhood obesity

    http://www.cdc.gov/nccdphp/dnpao/index.html

    http://win.niddk.nih.gov/index.htm

    http://www2.aap.org/obesity/

    http://www.med.umich.edu/1libr/yourchild/obesity.htm

    http://www.aafp.org/afp/990215ap/861.html

These sites provide information on childhood obesity, consequences, and treatment options

**TABLE 74.1 (continued)**
**Nutrition-Related Web Resources**

Eating disorders

    http://www.nationaleatingdisorders.org/

    http://www.helpguide.org/—search eating disorders

    http://kidshealth.org/teen/your_mind/mental_health/eat_disorder.html

    http://my.clevelandclinic.org/healthy_living/weight_control/hic_the_psychology_ofeating.aspx

    http://www.recoveryconnection.org/eating-disorders/

    All of these sites list and describe various eating disorders from too little food to ingestion of too much food; there are assessments for evaluating diet distortions

Nutrition and oral health

    http://www.mouthhealthy.org/Home/az-topics/d/diet-and-dental-health—American dental association site. Good review of topic, site deals with nutrition at all life stages

Protein nutrition and muscle mass (appetite)

    http://www.eatright.org/—various topics including suggested means of providing nutrients for building muscles under "nutrition for men" tab

Macro- and micronutrient supplementation

    http://familydoctor.org/familydoctor/prevention-wellness-tab-what-you-need-to-know.html—subtopics include calcium supplementation and antioxidant needs.

    http://fnic.nal.usda.gov/food-composition/individual-macronutrients-phytonutrients-vitamins-min—links for many common vitamins and minerals as well as other related topics in nutrition (see Chapter 1)

Bioactive food components

    http://www.eufic.org/article/en/artid/Nutrient-bioavailability-food/

    http://ec.europa.eu/research/biosociety/food_quality/projects_en.html—contains an A–Z list of project relative to obtain maximum nutrient value from foods

Herbal supplements

    http://nccam.nih.gov/health/supplements/wiseuse.htm—site discusses safety and efficacy factors related to mass-produced herbal supplements

    http://fnic.nal.usda.gov/dietary-supplements/herbal-information—clearing house with links to the American Academy of Physicians and various university research sites

    http://fnic.nal.usda.gov/food-composition/individual-macronutrients-phytonutrients-vitamins-minerals/phytonutrients—clearing house with links to several search engines with information about nutrient supplementation

Nutrition and disease

    http://www.nestlehealthscience.org/—multiple topics including nutrition and cancer, Crohn's disease, dysphagia, malnutrition, pediatrics, weight management, and wound care

    http://fnic.nal.usda.gov/diet-and-disease

Nutrition and renal disease

    http://kidney.niddk.nih.gov/index.aspx—multiple links related to kidney and urologic diseases. In addition, links to chronic kidney disease nutrition management learning modules

Nutrition and cardiovascular disease

    http://fnic.nal.usda.gov/diet-and-disease/heart-health—links to dietary guidelines, childrens' education, cholesterol education program

Nutritional disorders of the GI tract

    http://diabetes.niddk.nih.gov/

    http://digestive.niddk.nih.gov/

    http://fnic.nal.usda.gov/diet-and-disease/digestive-diseases-and-disorders—this is a clearing house site with links to other clearing house pages as well as links for specific section of the GI tract and diseases or structural problems that affect those areas

Nutrition and diabetes

    http://fnic.nal.usda.gov/consumers/eating-health/diabetes-and-prediabetes—clearing house site with links to the American Diabetes Association, NIH, and various university research topics

Nutritional management of the bariatric surgery patient

    http://www.nlm.nih.gov/medlineplus/weightlosssurgery.html—many articles and videos associated with weight-loss surgery

Nutritional management of the frail elderly

    http://www.howtocare.com/diet.htm—links to subjects that most of us don't think about!

Enteral and parenteral nutrition support (hospitalized patient)

    http://guideline.gov/browse/by-organization.aspx?orgid=100—links to subtopic papers; this site is recommended for health professionals

    http://www.fda.gov/Food/GuidanceComplianceRegulatoryInformation/GuidanceDocuments/MedicalFoods/ucm054048.htm—defining and discussion of "medical foods" FDA guidance document

*(continued)*

**TABLE 74.1 (continued)**
**Nutrition-Related Web Resources**

Nutrition and cancer (prevention and treatment)

    http://www.carolinawell.org/healthyliving—use the link for healthy living/healthy behaviors

    http://www.cancer.org/Treatment/SurvivorshipDuringandAfterTreatment/NutritionforPeoplewithCancer/index—there are multiple interrelated
    topics related to food choices and exercise for, during, and after cancer treatment

    http://fnic.nal.usda.gov/diet-and-disease/cancer—this is a clearing house site with multiple links to the NIH, the American Cancer Society and the
    Centers for Disease Control; these sites have specific information about nutrition and physical exercise as a means of preventing cancer and
    suggested guidelines for nourishing the cancer patient

    http://www.cancer.gov/cancertopics/pdq/supportivecare/nutrition/HealthProfessional/page3

Nutrition- and age-related eye disease

    http://www.lighthouse.org/eye-health/—this site covers everything from eye structure to common problems of the eye to diseases affecting the eye to
    nutrition as a preventative for eye problems; click on the prevention tab, then nutrition and eye health

Macular degeneration

    http://www.macular.org/nutrition/index.html—this is a "single article" site but has some good overall information concerning this topic

    http://www.umm.edu/altmed/articles/macular-degeneration-000104.htm—this is a "single article" site but with good information and references for
    further reading

Glaucoma

    http://www.glaucoma.org/treatment/nutrition-and-glaucoma.php—general information focusing on diet as a preventative measure to eye disease

    http://www.umm.edu/altmed/articles/glaucoma-000069.htm—information on complementary medicine associated with glaucoma

Cataracts

    http://www.ars.usda.gov/research/publications/publications.htm?seq_no_115=207417—this is one of a cluster of sites associated with the U.S. DA;
    it specifically links research publications and may not be appropriate for a nonscience reader

Nutrition and CNS health

    http://www.ars.usda.gov/is/ar/archive/aug07/aging0807.htm—single article site on "Food for the Aging Mind"

Nutrition and skin—nothing but commercial sites found

Nutrition and skeletal health

    http://fnic.nal.usda.gov/consumers/eating-health/osteoporosis-and-bone-health—this is a clearing house site with links to the National Osteoporosis
    Foundation, clinical treatment groups, and various university research groups

Drug/nutrient interactions

    http://edis.ifas.ufl.edu/he776—single article site but has chart of common nutrient–drug interactions. Good definitions and guidelines

Quackers

    http://www.fda.gov/

    http://www.quackwatch.com/

    http://fnic.nal.usda.gov/dietary-guidance/fraud-and-nutrition-misinformation

# Index